a **LANGE** medical book

# CURRENT
## Obstetric & Gynecologic
## Diagnosis & Treatment

## Eighth Edition

Edited by

**Alan H. DeCherney, MD**
Louis E. Phaneuf Professor & Chairman
Department of Obstetrics & Gynecology
Tufts University School of Medicine
New England Medical Center
Boston

**Martin L. Pernoll, MD**
Chair
Department of Obstetrics & Gynecology & Maternal Fetal Medicine
MacGregor Association
Houston

**APPLETON & LANGE**
Norwalk, Connecticut

Copyright © 1994 by Appleton & Lange
Paramount Publishing Business and Professional Group
Copyright © 1991, 1987 by Appleton & Lange

97 98 / 10 9 8 7 6

Prentice Hall International (UK) Limited, *London*
Prentice Hall of Australia Pty. Limited, *Sydney*
Prentice Hall Canada, Inc., *Toronto*
Prentice Hall Hispanoamericana, S.A., *Mexico*
Prentice Hall of India Private Limited, *New Delhi*
Prentice Hall of Japan, Inc., *Tokyo*
Simon & Schuster Asia Pte. Ltd., *Singapore*
Editora Prentice Hall do brasil Ltda., *Rio de Janeiro*
Prentice Hall, *Englewood Cliffs, New Jersey*

ISSN: 0197–582x

ISBN 0-8385-1447-2

Acquisitions Editor: Shelley Reinhardt
Production Editor: Christine Langan
Designer: Penny Kindzierski

PRINTED IN THE UNITED STATES OF AMERICA

7/93

# Table of Contents

## SECTION III. PREGNANCY AT RISK

## SECTION IV. GENERAL GYNECOLOGY

## SECTION V. GYNECOLOGIC ONCOLOGY

# The Authors

**D. Ellene Andrew, MD**
Chief Resident, Department of Obstetrics and Gynecology, Tufts University School of Medicine, and New England Medical Center, Boston.

**Michael P. Aronson, MD**
Assistant Professor, Department of Obstetrics and Gynecology, and Chief, Section of Reconstructive Pelvic Surgery and Urogynecology, Tufts University School of Medicine, and New England Medical Center, Boston.

**Emily R. Baker, MD**
Assistant Professor, Department of Obstetrics and Gynecology, Tufts University School of Medicine, and Perinatologist, New England Medical Center, Boston.

**Vicki V. Baker, MD**
Associate Professor, Department of Obstetrics, Gynecology, and Reproductive Sciences and Director, Division of Gynecologic Oncology, The University of Texas Medical School at Houston.

**Harrison G. Ball, MD**
Associate Professor, Department of Obstetrics and Gynecology, and Director, Division of Gynecologic Oncology, Tufts University School of Medicine, and New England Medical Center, Boston.

**David L. Barclay, MD**
Clinical Professor of Obstetrics & Gynecology, University of Arkansas College of Medicine, Little Rock.

**David E. Barnard, MD**
Associate Clinical Professor, Department of Obstetrics and Gynecology, Tulane University School of Medicine, New Orleans.

**Joseph D. Bast, PhD**
Professor, Department of Anatomy and Cell Biology and Department of Obstetrics and Gynecology, University of Kansas School of Medicine, Kansas City.

**Ralph C. Benson, MD**
Professor Emeritus, Department of Obstetrics and Gynecology, Oregon Health Sciences University, Portland.

**Manoj K. Biswas, MD, FACOG, FRCOG**
Associate Professor, Department of Obstetrics and Gynecology, Tulane Medical School, New Orleans.

**Ronald T. Burkman, MD**
C. Paul Hodgkinson Chair of Obstetrics and Gynecology, Henry Ford Hospital, Detroit; Clinical Professor of Obstetrics and Gynecology, University of Michigan Medical School; and Professor of Reproductive Biology, Case Western Reserve University School of Medicine.

**David Chelmow, MD**
Assistant Professor, Department of Obstetrics and Gynecology, Tufts University School of Medicine, Boston, and New England Medical Center.

**Joseph V. Collea, MD**
Professor, Department of Obstetrics and Gynecology, and Director, Antenatal Testing Unit, Georgetown University School of Medicine, Washington, DC.

**David B. Cotton, MD**
Professor, Department of Obstetrics and Gynecology, Hutzel Hospital and Wayne State University School of Medicine, Detroit.

**Sabrina D. Craigo, MD**
Assistant Professor, Department of Obstetrics and Gynecology, Tufts University School of Medicine, and Perinatologist, New England Medical Center, Boston.

**Stephen L. Curry, MD**
Director, Obstetrics and Gynecology, Hartford Hospital, Hartford, and Professor of Obstetrics and Gynecology, University of Connecticut School of Medicine, Farmington.

**Alan H. DeCherney, MD**
Louis E. Phaneuf Professor and Chairman, Department of Obstetrics and Gynecology, Tufts University School of Medicine, and New England Medical Center, Boston.

**Simie Degefu, MD**
Associate Clinical Professor, Department of Obstetrics and Gynecology, Tulane University School of Medicine, New Orleans.

**Clyde H. Dorr, II, MD**
Associate Professor of Obstetrics, Gynecology and Reproductive Sciences, University of Texas Medical School at Houston, and Chief, Gynecology, LBJ General Hospital, Houston.

**Adelina Emmi, MD**
Assistant Professor, Department of Obstetrics and Gynecology, Division of Reproductive Endocrinology, and Director, In Vitro Fertilization, New England Medical Center, Boston.

**Michael D. Fox, MD**
Fellow, Division of Reproductive Endocrinology, Department of Obstetrics and Gynecology, University of Kentucky College of Medicine, Lexington.

**Carol Gagliardi, MD**
Assistant Professor, Department of Obstetrics and Gynecology, University of Medicine and Dentistry of New Jersey, New Jersey Medical School Newark.

**William F. Ganong, MD**
Lange Professor of Physiology Emeritus, University of California, San Francisco.

**Sara H. Garmel, MD**
Fellow, Department of Obstetrics and Gynecology, Division of Maternal Fetal Medicine, Tufts University School of Medicine, and New England Medical Center, Boston.

**Brendan Garry, MB, BCH, FFARCSI**
Assistant Professor, Department of Anesthesia, Tufts University School of Medicine, and New England Medical Center, Boston.

**Melvin V. Gerbie, MD**
Professor of Clinical Obstetrics and Gynecology, Northwestern University Medical School, Chicago.

**Ronald S. Gibbs, MD**
Professor and Chairman, Department of Obstetrics and Gynecology, University of Colorado School of Medicine, Denver.

**William L. Gill, MD**
Professor, Department of Pediatrics, and Head, Section of Neonatology, Tulane University Medical Center, New Orleans.

**Victor Gomel, MD**
Professor of Obstetrics and Gynecology, University of British Columbia School of Medicine, Vancouver, British Columbia.

**Annekathryn Goodman, MD**
Instructor, Department of Obstetrics, Gynecology, and Reproductive Biology, Division of Gynecologic Oncology, Harvard Medical School, and Vincent Memorial Obstetrics & Gynecology Service, Massachusetts General Hospital, Boston.

**Robert A. Graebe, MD**
Head, Reproductive Endocrinology, Monmouth and Riverview Medical Center, Long Branch, New Jersey.

**Ralph W. Hale, MD**
Executive Director, The American College of Obstetricians and Gynecologists, Washington, DC.

**Vivian Halfin, MD**
Assistant Professor of Psychiatry and Obstetrics and Gynecology, Tufts University School of Medicine, and Psychiatric Consultant, Department of Obstetrics and Gynecology, New England Medical Center, Boston.

**Kathleen F. Harney, MD**
Chief Resident, Department of Obstetrics and Gynecology, Tufts University School of Medicine, and New England Medical Center, Boston.

**David B. Hebert, MD**
Clinical Assistant Professor, Department of Obstetrics and Gynecology, Tulane University School of Medicine, New Orleans.

**David L. Hemsell, MD**
Professor, Department of Obstetrics and Gynecology, Director, Division of Gynecology, Southwestern Medical School, The University of Texas Southwestern Medical Center at Dallas.

**Eduardo A. Herrera, MD**
Associate Professor, Department of Obstetrics and Gynecology, Tulane University Medical School and Clinical Director of Operative Gynecology at the Medical Center of Louisiana at New Orleans.

**Darla B. Hess, MD**
Assistant Professor, Departments of Medicine and Obstetrics and Gynecology, and Head, Adult Echocardiography, University of Missouri Medical Center, Columbia.

**L. Wayne Hess, MD**
Associate Professor, Obstetrics and Gynecology, and Head, Obstetrics and Maternal Fetal Medicine, University of Missouri Medical Center, Columbia.

**Edward C. Hill, MD**
Professor Emeritus, Department of Obstetrics, Gynecology & Reproductive Sciences, University of California, San Francisco.

**Howard W. Jones, Jr., MD**
Professor Emeritus, Department of Gynecology & Obstetrics, Johns Hopkins University School of Medicine, Baltimore; Chairman (Hon), Jones Institute, Norfolk, Virginia; and Professor of Obstetrics and Gynecology, Eastern Virginia Medical School, Norfolk.

**Theodore B. Jones, MD**
Assistant Professor, Division of Maternal Fetal Medicine, Department of Obstetrics and Gynecology, Wayne State University School of Medicine and Hutzel Hospital, Detroit.

**Howard L. Judd, MD**
Professor, Department of Obstetrics and Gynecology, and Chief, Division of Reproductive Endocrinology, University of California, Los Angeles School of Medicine, and Executive Director, Division of Reproductive Endocrinology, University of California, Los Angeles and Cedars-Sinai Medical Centers, Los Angeles.

**Peter S. Kapernick, MD**
Clinical Associate Professor of Obstetrics and Gynecology, University of Minnesota Medical School, Minneapolis, and Assistant Chief Obstetrics and Gynecology, Hennepin County Medical Center, Minneapolis.

**Charles Y. Kawada, MD**
Associate Professor, Department of Obstetrics and Gynecology, Tufts University School of Medicine, and New England Medical Center, Boston.

**Robert A. Knuppel, MD, MPH**
Professor and Chairman, Department of Obstetrics and Gynecology, University of Medicine and Dentistry of New Jersey, Robert Wood Johnson Medical School, New Brunswick.

**Kermit E. Krantz, MD, LittD**
University Distinguished Professor, Professor of Gynecology & Obstetrics, and Professor of Anatomy, University of Kansas School of Medicine, Kansas City.

**Wesley Lee, MD, FACOG**
Attending Staff, Department of Obstetrics and Gynecology, William Beaumont Hospital, Royal Oak, Michigan, and Associate Professor, Department of Obstetrics and Gynecology, Wayne State University School of Medicine, Detroit.

**Deborah Lehmann, MD**
Private practice, Fort Worth, Texas.

**William C. Mabie, MD**
Associate Professor, Department of Obstetrics and Gynecology, University of Tennessee College of Medicine, Memphis.

**L. Russell Malinak, MD**
Professor, Department of Obstetrics and Gynecology, Baylor College of Medicine, Houston.

**Mary C. Martin, MD**
Associate Professor, Department of Obstetrics and Gynecology & Reproductive Sciences, and Director, In Vitro Fertilization Program, University of California, San Francisco.

**Rick W. Martin, MD**
Associate Professor, Department of Obstetrics and Gynecology, University of Mississippi School of Medicine, Jackson.

**John S. McDonald, MD**
Professor and Chairman, Department of Anesthesiology, The Ohio State University College of Medicine, Columbus.

**Pamela J. Moore, PhD**
Associate Professor, Department of Obstetrics and Gynecology, and Assistant Dean of Graduate Medical Education, Tulane University School of Medicine, New Orleans.

**John C. Morrison, MD**
Professor of Obstetrics and Gynecology and Pediatrics, Vice Chairman and Director of Research, Department of Obstetrics and Gynecology, University of Mississippi School of Medicine, Jackson.

**David Muram, MD**
Associate Professor and Chief, Section of Pediatric and Adolescent Gynecology, and Director, Division of Gynecology, University of Tennessee College of Medicine, Memphis.

**Kenneth N. Muse, Jr., MD**
Associate Professor, Department of Obstetrics and Gynecology, University of Kentucky College of Medicine, Lexington.

**Stewart E. Niles, Jr., JD**
Senior Partner, Jones, Walker, Waechter, Poitevent, Carrère & Denègre, Attorneys-at-Law, New Orleans.

**Miles J. Novy, MD**
Professor, Department of Obstetrics and Gynecology, Oregon Health Sciences University, Portland.

**April G. O'Quinn, MD**
Professor and Chairman, Department of Obstetrics and Gynecology, Tulane University School of Medicine, New Orleans.

**Sue M. Palmer, MD**
Vice Chair, Department of Obstetrics and Gynecology and Maternal Fetal Medicine, MacGregor Medical Association, Houston.

**Jack W. Pearson, MD**
Professor, Department of Obstetrics and Gynecology, University of Arizona College of Medicine, Tucson.

**Alan S. Penzias, MD**
Assistant Professor, Department of Obstetrics and Gynecology, Division of Reproductive Endocrinology, Tufts University School of Medicine, and New England Medical Center, Boston.

**Dorothee Perloff, MD**
Clinical Professor, Department of Medicine, University of California, San Francisco.

**Martin L. Pernoll, MD**
Chair, Department of Obstetrics and Gynecology and Maternal Fetal Medicine, MacGregor Association, Houston.

**Kenneth G. Perry, Jr., MD**
Assistant Professor, Division of Maternal Fetal Medicine, Department of Obstetrics and Gynecology, University of Mississippi School of Medicine, Jackson.

**Susan M. Ramin, MD**
Assistant Professor, Department of Obstetrics and Gynecology, Southwestern Medical School, University of Texas Southwestern Medical Center at Dallas.

**Jack R. Robertson, MD**
Clinical Professor of Obstetrics and Gynecology, and Chief, Urogynecology, University of Nevada School of Medicine, Las Vegas.

**Miriam B. Rosenthal, MD**
Associate Professor of Psychiatry and Reproductive Biology, Case Western Reserve University School of Medicine, and Division Chief of Behavioral Medicine, Department of Obstetrics and Gynecology, University MacDonald Womens Hospital, Cleveland.

**Timothy C. Rowe, MB BS, FRCOG, FRCSC**
Associate Professor, Department of Obstetrics and Gynecology, Division of Reproductive Endocrinology, University of British Columbia School of Medicine, Vancouver, British Columbia.

**Barbara Shephard, MD**
Assistant Professor, Department of Pediatrics, Tufts University School of Medicine, and Neonatologist, New England Medical Center, Boston.

**Baha M. Sibai, MD**
University Professor, Department of Obstetrics and Gynecology, and Chief, Division of Maternal Fetal Medicine, University of Tennessee College of Medicine, Memphis.

**Donna M. Smith, MD**
Assistant Professor, Department of Obstetrics and Gynecology, Tufts University School of Medicine, and New England Medical Center, Boston.

**Kristen E. Smith, MD**
Fellow, Division of Reproductive Endocrinology, Department of Obstetrics and Gynecology, University of California, Los Angeles School of Medicine.

**Leonard F. Smith, MD**
Associate Professor, Department of Obstetrics and Gynecology, Tufts University School of Medicine, and New England Medical Center, Boston.

**Ramada S. Smith, MD**
Clinical Instructor, Department of Obstetrics and Gynecology, Division of Fetal Imaging, and Division of Maternal Fetal Medicine, Beaumont Hospital, Royal Oak, Michigan.

**Robert J. Sokol, MD**
Dean, Professor of Obstetrics and Gynecology, Wayne State University School of Medicine, Detroit.

**Morton A. Stenchever, MD**
Professor and Chairman, Department of Obstetrics and Gynecology, University of Washington School of Medicine, Seattle.

**Paul Summers, MD**
Associate Professor, Department of Obstetrics and Gynecology, Tulane University School of Medicine, New Orleans.

**Cathy Mih Taylor, MD**
Chief of Obstetrics, Neosho Memorial Regional Medical Center, Chanute, Kansas.

**Ian H. Thorneycroft, MD, PhD**
Professor and Chairman, Department of Obstetrics and Gynecology, University of South Alabama College of Medicine, Mobile.

**Michael W. Varner, MD**
Professor, Department of Obstetrics and Gynecology, University of Utah School of Medicine, Salt Lake City.

**George D. Wendel, Jr., MD**
Associate Professor, Department of Obstetrics and Gynecology, Southwestern Medical School, University of Texas Southwestern Medical Center at Dallas.

**Alvin S. Wexler, MD**
MacGregor Medical Association, Houston.

**Carol A. Wheeler, MD**
Assistant Professor, Department of Obstetrics and Gynecology, Brown University School of Medicine and Women & Infants Hospital, Providence.

**James E. Wheeler, MD**
Professor, Department of Pathology and Laboratory Medicine, Department of Obstetrics and Gynecology, Hospital of University of Pennsylvania, Philadelphia.

**James M. Wheeler, MD**
Assistant Professor, Department of Obstetrics and Gynecology, Baylor College of Medicine, Houston.

**J. Donald Woodruff, MD**
Professor Emeritus of Gynecology and Obstetrics, and Associate Professor of Pathology, Johns Hopkins University School of Medicine, Baltimore.

**Ralph W. Yarnell, MD, FRCPC**
Associate Professor and Director of Obstetric Anesthesia, Department of Anesthesia, Tufts University School of Medicine, New England Medical Center, Boston.

# *Preface*

The 8th edition of *Current Obstetric & Gynecologic Diagnosis & Treatment* offers the health care provider a comprehensive digest of the knowledge necessary for the modern health care of women. In addition to the most up-to-date, clinically relevant information available, *COGDT* provides an incisive look at areas of rapid change in women's health care.

## AUDIENCE

Like all large books, *COGDT* provides a concise, yet comprehensive source of current, clear, and correct information. Medical students will find it an authoritative introduction to the speciality, and an excellent source for reference and review. House officers will welcome the concise, practical information on commonly encountered health problems. Practicing obstetricians and gynecologists, family physicians, internists, and other health care providers whose practice includes women's health care will find *COGDT* a useful reference on all aspects of the subject.

## SCOPE

Sixty-three chapters encompass a wide range of topics, progressing from the basics of health care for women to complicated sub-specialty problems. Information is organized in a logical progression from basic to clinical, simple to complex, and from common to uncommon. Discussions are amplified by detailed anatomic drawings, diagrams, and imaging studies, more than 500 illustrations in all. References at the end of each chapter have been carefully chosen to emphasize current developments in the clinical literature.

## NEW TO THIS EDITION

The 8th edition of *COGDT* reflects greater consumer sensitivity throughout by emphasizing the following themes: **the patient as a person, communication and counseling techniques** and **the patient as participant in decisions about her own health care.**

This edition continues to be **organized into seven sections,** separating fundamental, speciality, and subspecialty information and grouping information likely to be useful to a given level of expertise. This organization results in essentially a series of books within a book.

Section I details the basic material necessary to understand the anatomic and physiologic features unique to the female and to reproduction. Section II is developed to normal obstetrics. Section III, Pregnancy at Risk, describes methods of fetal assessment, reviews early and late pregnancy risks, and details diagnosis and therapy of the maternal or fetal states creating perinatal jeopardy.

Section IV, General Gynecology, comprehensively reviews benign gynecology, continuing the format of basic to increasingly complex issues concerning each topic. Section V is devoted to gynecologic oncology. Section VI discusses reproductive endocrinology and infertility, while Section VII deals with topics not traditionally found in obstetrics and gynecology texts but of obvious importance to the patient and physician—critical care, psychologic aspects of obstetrics and gynecology, sexual assault, the breast, and medicolegal aspects.

Every effort has been made to incorporate the new and exciting changes in obstetrics and gynecology in this edition. It is our continued policy not only to provide basic information but concepts at the cutting edge as well, such as in vitro fertilization and molecular genetics.

New chapters include:

- The Role of Imaging Techniques in Gynecology
- Early Pregnancy Risks
- Pregnancy Complicated by Diabetes Mellitus
- Postpartum Hemorrhage & the Abnormal Puerperium
- Neonatal Resuscitation & Care of the Newborn at Risk
- Gynecologic History, Examination, & Diagnostic Procedures
- Contraception & Family Planning
- Benign Disorders of the Uterine Corpus
- Antimicrobial Chemotherapy
- Premalignant & Malignant Disorders of the Ovaries & Oviducts

Among the extensively revised chapters are the following:

- The Course & Conduct of Normal Labor & Delivery
- The Normal Puerperium
- Methods of Assessment for Pregnancy at Risk
- Late Pregnancy Complications
- Multiple Pregnancy
- Hypertensive States of Pregnancy
- Cardiac, Hematologic, Pulmonary, Renal & Urinary Tract Disorders in Pregnancy
- General Medical Disorders During Pregnancy
- Surgical Diseases & Disorders in Pregnancy
- Pediatric & Adolescent Gynecology
- Complications of Menstruation, Abnormal Uterine Bleeding
- Obstetric Anesthesia & Analgesia
- Benign Disorders of the Vulva & Vagina
- Benign Disorders of the Uterine Cervix
- Benign Disorders of the Ovaries & Oviducts
- Sexually Transmitted Diseases & Pelvic Infections
- Relaxation of Pelvic Supports
- Perioperative Considerations in Gynecology
- Intraoperative & Postoperative Complications of Gynecologic Surgery
- Premalignant & Malignant Disorders of the Vulva & Vagina
- Premalignant & Malignant Disorders of the Uterine Cervix
- Premalignant & Malignant Disorders of the Uterine Corpus
- Radiation Therapy for Gynecologic Cancers
- In Vitro Fertilization & Related Techniques
- Domestic Violence & Sexual Assault

A number of topics have been examined in more detail due to their increasing importance in women's health care. Included in this category are Premenstrual Syndrome (PMS), Abortion, and AIDS.

## ACKNOWLEDGMENTS

*COGDT* continues to represent the collective efforts of leading experts in obstetrics and gynecology. The editors would like to thank these busy and productive individuals for their time and effort in preparing this new edition. Several of our more senior authors have retired, and their expertise will be sorely missed.

A useful clinical text transcends the necessary synthesis of available literature. The well communicated knowledge, experiences, ethics and skills of the authors remains central to being of service to the reader and ultimately of value to their patients. Over the several editions *CODGT* has benefitted from the dedication of many leaders in obstetrics and gynecology. Their contributions have set a standard of excellence as well as providing a framework for future contributions. The 8th edition of *COGDT* continues the evolution begun by previous editions to encompass the many areas of progress in health care for women. As part of that progression this edition adds a new senior editor (Dr. DeCherney) and a host of new authors. The wealth of new material has been assimilated into the strengths of all the previous information to create an ever more comprehensive and useful *COGDT*.

The editors also wish to acknowledge the assistance and support provided by the staff at Appleton & Lange. Space precludes thanking all the deserving, but Martin J. Wonsiewicz, Editor in Chief, Lange Medical Publications and Shelley Reinhardt, Medical Editor, deserve special recognition.

We welcome suggestions and comments concerning *Current Obstetric & Gynecologic Diagnosis & Treatment*. Please address communications to us c/o Appleton & Lange, 25 Van Zant St., E. Norwalk, CT 06855.

A.H. DeCherney, MD
M.L. Pernoll, MD

April 1994

# Section I.
# Reproductive Basics

# Approach to the Patient

**1**

*Mary C. Martin, MD*

An effective relationship between health care provider and patient is based on the knowledge and skill that qualify the provider on effective communication between the individuals, and on the ethical standards that govern the conduct of the participants in the relationship.

## THE KNOWLEDGE BASE

The health care of women encompasses all aspects of medical science and therapeutics. Physicians in the general practice of obstetrics and gynecology are called upon as consultants in specialized areas of medicine pertaining specifically to women; in addition, they frequently act as primary care providers for their patients. Internists in general practice and family practitioners often find that a major component of their clinical activities involves the special needs of women. These special medical needs and concerns vary with the patient's reproductive status, her reproductive potential, and her desire to reproduce, such that no history, examination, interpretation of laboratory data, or therapy can be correctly accomplished without consideration of these aspects of the patient's presentation. Certainly the diagnostic possibilities and the choice of diagnostic or therapeutic intervention will be influenced by the possibility of, or desire for, pregnancy, or in some cases by the patient's hormonal profile. On the other hand, the gynecologic or obstetric assessment must include an evaluation of the patient's general health status and should be placed in the context of the psychologic, social, and emotional status of the patient.

## History

To offer each woman optimal care, the information obtained at each visit should be as complete as possible. Whether the contact is a routine visit or is occasioned by a particular problem or complaint, the woman should be encouraged to view the visit as an opportunity to participate in improving her health. The clinical data base should include general information about the patient and her goals in seeking care. The history of the present problem, past medical history, family history, medications used, allergies, and review of systems should be concise but thorough. Portions of the history provided by questionnaire or by other members of the health care team should be reviewed with the patient, in part to verify the information but also to begin assessing the patient's personality and to determine her attitude toward the health care system. The menstrual history and developmental history may provide a background for presenting complaints in subsequent years. The menstrual history, sexual history, and obstetric history obviously assume central importance for the gynecologic or obstetric visit. In addition, the habit of systematically categorizing the nature of such complaints as pain, abnormal bleeding, or vaginal discharge will usually narrow the differential diagnoses. For example, the categorization of a complaint of pain should include its onset, duration, frequency, and associated behaviors and a description of the nature or type of pain and its location. Such thoroughness will permit assessment of change as well as determination of the appropriate mode of investigation or therapy.

The initial contact with the patient, made while she is fully clothed and comfortable, may be useful in decreasing her anxiety about the physical examination; concerns about the examination may be elicited, and a history of previous unfortunate experiences may alert the examiner to the need for extra attention, time, and gentleness.

## Physical Examination

The second component of the patient assessment, the physical examination, should also be directed toward evaluation of the total patient. The patient should again be encouraged to view the examination as a positive opportunity to gain information about her body, and she should be offered feedback regarding the general physical examination and any significant findings. The examination should always include a breast examination and a discussion of any concerns expressed by the patient. The breast examination provides a good opportunity to reinforce the practice of breast self-examination. The pelvic examination is usually an occasion of heightened anxiety for the patient, and every effort should be made to make the experience a positive one. The physician should give the patient as much control over the process as possible, by asking if she is ready, asking for feedback on whether the examination is painful, and seeking her cooperation in relaxation and muscle control. Information about each step of the examination can be provided so that the patient is involved and appropriately aware of the value of each maneuver.

Inspection of the external genitalia is followed by the gentle insertion of an appropriately sized, warmed speculum to permit inspection of the vagina and the cervix. For patients with pain or increased anxiety, their cooperation must be continually reinforced by slow, gentle placement of the instrument, maintaining downward pressure against the relaxed perineal body and away from the urethral and anterior vaginal areas. Some women may wish to watch, by the use of a mirror, as the genitalia are inspected and may gain confidence from visualizing the cervix and vagina. The Papanicolaou (Pap) smear may be uncomfortable for some women, and they should be alerted when the test is being done. The bimanual examination should also be explained to the patient. When the uterus is anteflexed, the woman may want to appreciate the size and location of her uterus by feeling it with the guidance of the examiner. The rectovaginal and rectal examinations, if performed while the patient relaxes her anal sphincter, provide additional information and can be another source of reassurance for the normal patient or a means of diagnosis for the patient with disease. If an ultrasound is indicated as part of the gynecologic or obstetric examination, additional participation by the patient in the evaluation can be obtained by explanations of the visualized anatomy.

### Implications of Technology

The scientific knowledge base for obstetric and gynecologic care has grown in parallel with general medical advances. Subject areas such as immunologic aspects of reproduction, fertilization in vitro, operative laparoscopy, and infectious diseases in obstetrics and gynecology have only recently been developed or expanded to represent major areas of new information, markedly altering clinical care and challenging the practitioner to remain current. In some cases this proliferation of information and technology has profoundly altered the relationship between health care providers and their patients. For example,

the change from an intuitive management of labor and delivery to active monitoring and subsequent interpretation of data has provided a more rational basis for decision making but has also created a potential for conflict or confusion in the relationship between patient and physician. In seeking to obtain additional information, the physician can be perceived to be intervening unnecessarily. More than ever before, issues of consumerism and participation in decision making require an understanding of the expectations of each individual woman. Whether a woman perceives herself as a "client" or as a "patient," and the degree to which this perception coincides with the views of her physician, may alter her acceptance of recommendations for care. The fact that several options are available in the management of many obstetric or gynecologic situations may further complicate the relationship. However, this situation provides an opportunity to allow the patient to participate actively in choosing the best therapy for her particular circumstance.

## COMMUNICATION

If the first foundation of a strong therapeutic relationship is knowledge, the second is communication. The ability to establish trust, to obtain and deliver complete and accurate information, and to ensure compliance with recommendations depends in large measure on the health care provider's communication skills. In some individuals these skills are innate, but for most the ability to become an effective communicator in a variety of settings requires an active process of learning and a willingness to be evaluated by peers. The information communicated in each encounter, whether by written material, in face-to-face discussion, or by telephone contact, extends beyond the factual content provided to include a demonstration of the provider's willingness to be available for questions and to encourage patient involvement in decision making. For effective resolution of a particular problem or complaint, it may be helpful to encourage the patient to make notes and to elicit her understanding of the assessment and management plan. Compliance with a particular form of therapy may be enhanced if the patient's clear understanding of the diagnosis, the alternative strategies (including anticipated risks and benefits), and the long-term treatment plan is obtained both verbally and in writing. Patients with complicated problems, or those on chronic therapy, may find that keeping a diary of the visits and discussions increases the value of the physician contacts by reinforcing the plan and the outlook.

The counterbalance of a litigious society that may hold the physician responsible for treatment outcome places a high premium on documentation and scientific justification for each intervention or nonintervention and can place the physician in an adversarial position with respect to the patient's desires. The obligation to inform the patient, whether to obtain surgical consent or to advise about choices regarding pregnancy outcome, is becoming in some instances a matter of law rather than established medical practice. These legislative initiatives, while offensive to many, are signals that the public feels it requires protection from manipulation at the hands of those who have the power of knowledge and training not available to all. Regardless of the validity of this perception, it can only be countered by efforts to establish and maintain the trust of each individual with whom the physician has a medical relationship. This trust is founded on the physician's medical knowledge and is maintained by conscientious structured lifetime learning, the frank assessment and acknowledgment of areas of ignorance, and the willingness to discuss with the patient what is known and what is uncertain.

## ETHICS

If the bricks of the foundation of the relationship between physician and patient are knowledge and communication, the mortar that forms the basis for trust is the integrity and ethical behavior of all participants in the relationship. Ethical dilemmas in obstetrics and gynecology are receiving increasing recognition, particularly as they deal with the provocative issues surrounding the beginnings of life, the nature of parenting, and the control of individual patients over their own destiny. Ethical dilemmas only arise when there are conflicting obligations, rights, or claims. Since the delivery of health care involves multiple participants, a consensus of values must often be sought when the patient is cared for by a team, even when significant pluralism of views might be represented. To minimize potential ethical conflicts, to anticipate potential areas of difficulty, and to achieve consistency in behavior, individuals may avail themselves of a number of resources for ethical decision making. In addition to the growing literature in the field, many hospitals and practice settings have formal consultation services for resolution of ethical dilemmas. Before seeking an external framework, however, the practitioner should be aware of his or her own values and understand the basis of these values. The values of the medical profession and of the institutions in which the physician practices, as formulated by codes and standards but also as expressed indirectly through past actions, are usually then helpful in providing a decision making framework. Finally, a familiarity with ethical theories may permit decision-making that achieves an acceptable consensus in the face of conflicting values. Discussions based on consideration of the ethical principles of pa-

tient autonomy (respect for persons), beneficence (doing good), nonmaleficence (refraining from doing harm), and justice (consideration of resources and fairness of opportunity) will prevent capricious and arbitrary decisions.

The principle of autonomy, or respect for each individual person, may form the underlying basis for resolving many ethical questions and will determine appropriate attitudes toward confidentiality, privacy, right to information, and the ultimate primacy of the patient in making treatment decisions. Since caring for women necessarily involves information regarding sensitive and intimate relationships and activities, as well as access to a woman's thoughts, feelings, and emotions, full disclosure of such information by the patient places a burden of trust on the health care provider to protect the rights and privacy of each patient. The relationship established at an initial gynecologic visit between a young adolescent and the physician may potentially extend throughout her adult life and include such major life events as education about reproductive health, assistance in family planning and childbearing, and preservation of physical fitness and well-being through the postmenopausal years. To successfully establish such an enduring clinical relationship requires a sensitivity to the changing goals and needs of the individual patient, as well as the broad fund of knowledge discussed earlier. Offering care to some patients or providing some types of services may not be comfortable for all practitioners. For example, establishing a rapport with an adolescent seeking birth control or providing health care for a lesbian woman may require a nonjudgmental approach when one is interviewing the patient and a balanced consideration of life-style options. The recognition of these special needs has led to a compartmentalization of health care in some regions, so that specialty practices or clinics directed toward adolescent health care, family planning, fertility, oncology, and menopausal care are frequently available. These resources can best be utilized by referral, with guidance provided by a primary provider, so that appropriate use of such resources can be an integral part of the general health care of each woman.

An additional determinant of the relationship that develops between health care provider and patient is economics. It may be either a subtle modifier or a major factor determining the nature of the contact. The rising costs of health care, the increasing degree of government involvement, and the multitude of insurance plans that place restrictions on the delivery of care may significantly affect the choices faced by both provider and patient. Even the continuation of a desired personal relationship between a provider and an individual patient may be determined by the nature of the health plan contracts available to the patient and agreed to by the provider. In some cases, medical decisions—such as treatment for infertility—may be determined in large part not by medical judgment but by economic concerns and what will be supported by third-party payers. Referral patterns may be deter-mined by similar considerations. The patient will be best served in all instances by discussion of the economic consequences of management decisions.

## REFERENCES

Brody DS: The patient's role in clinical decision making. Ann Intern Med 1980;93:718.

Delbarco TL: Enriching the doctor-patient relationship by inviting the patient's perspective. Ann Intern Med 1992; 116(5):414.

Eracher SA, Kirscht JP, Becker MH: Understanding and improving patient's compliance. Ann Intern Med 1984; 100:258.

Quill TE: Recognizing and adjusting to barriers in doctor-patient communication. Ann Intern Med 1989;111:51.

Robbins JA, Bertakis KD, Helms LJ, et al: The influence of physician practice behaviors on patient satisfaction. Family Med 1993;1:17–20.

Roberts DK: Prevention: Patient communication. Clin Obstet Gynecol 1988;31:153.

Stoffelmayr B, Hoppe RB, Weber N: Facilitating patient participation: The doctor-patient encounter. Prim Care 1989;16:265.

# Anatomy of the Female Reproductive System

# 2

*Kermit E. Krantz, MD, LittD*

## ABDOMINAL WALL

### Topographic Anatomy

The anterior abdominal wall is divided into sections for descriptive purposes and to allow the physician to outline relationships of the viscera in the abdominal cavity. The centerpoint of reference is the sternoxiphoid process, which is in the same plane as the tenth thoracic vertebra. The upper 2 sections are formed by the subcostal angle; the lower extend from the lower ribs to the crest of the ilium and forward to the anterior superior iliac spines. The base is formed by the inguinal ligaments and the symphysis pubica.

The viscera are located by dividing the anterolateral abdominal wall into regions. One line is placed from the level of each ninth costal cartilage to the iliac crests. Two other lines are drawn from the middle of the inguinal ligaments to the cartilage of the eighth rib. The 9 regions formed (Fig 2–1) are the epigastric, umbilical, hypogastric, and right and left hypochondriac, lumbar, and ilioinguinal.

Within the right hypochondriac zone are the right lobe of the liver, the gallbladder at the anterior inferior angle, part of the right kidney deep within the region, and, occasionally, the right colic flexure.

The epigastric zone contains the left lobe of the liver and part of the right lobe, the stomach, the proximal duodenum, the pancreas, the suprarenal glands, and the upper poles of both kidneys (Fig 2–2).

The left hypochondriac region marks the situation of the spleen, the fundus of the stomach, the apex of the liver, and the left colic flexure.

Within the right lumbar region are the ascending colon, coils of intestine, and, frequently, the inferior border of the lateral portion of the right kidney.

The central umbilical region contains the transverse colon, the stomach, the greater omentum, the small intestine, the second and third portions of the duodenum, the head of the pancreas, and parts of the medial aspects of the kidneys.

Located in the left lumbar region are the descending colon, the left kidney, and small intestine. Within the limits of the right ilioinguinal region are the cecum and appendix, part of the ascending colon, small intestine, and, occasionally, the right border of the greater omentum.

The hypogastric region includes the greater omentum, loops of small intestine, the pelvic colon, and often part of the transverse colon.

The left ilioinguinal region encloses the sigmoid colon, part of the descending colon, loops of small intestine, and the left border of the greater omentum.

There is considerable variation in the position and size of individual organs due to differences in body size and conformation. Throughout life, variations in the positions of organs are dependent not only on gravity but also on the movements of the hollow viscera, which induce further changes in shape when filling and emptying. The need to recognize the relationships of the viscera to the abdominal regions becomes most apparent when taking into account the distortion that occurs during pregnancy. For example, the appendix lies in the right ilioinguinal region (right lower quadrant) until the 12th week of gestation. At 16 weeks, it is at the level of the right iliac crest. At 20 weeks, it is at the level of the umbilicus, where it will remain until after delivery. Because of this displacement, the symptoms of appendicitis will be different during the 3 trimesters. Similarly, displacement will also affect problems involving the bowel.

### Skin, Subcutaneous Tissue, & Fascia

The abdominal skin is smooth, fine, and very elastic. It is loosely attached to underlying structures except at the umbilicus, where it is firmly adherent. Beneath the skin is the superficial fascia (tela subcutanea) (Fig 2–3). This fatty protective fascia covers the entire abdomen. Below the navel, it consists principally of 2 layers; Camper's fascia, the more superficial layer containing most of the fat; and Scarpa's fascia (deep fascia), the fibroelastic membrane firmly attached to midline aponeuroses and to the fascia lata.

### Arteries

The anterior cutaneous branches of the superficial arteries are grouped with the anterior cutaneous

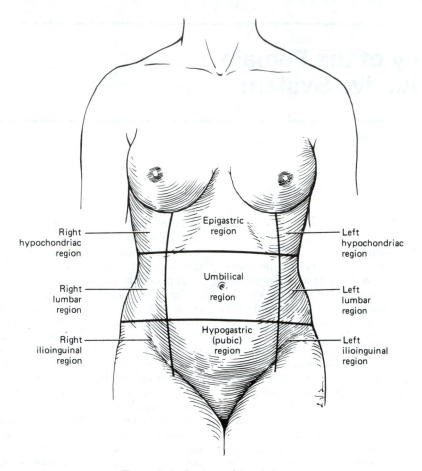

**Figure 2–1.** Regions of the abdomen.

nerves (Fig 2–4). The lateral cutaneous branches stem from the lower aortic intercostal arteries and the subcostal arteries. The femoral artery supplies both the superficial epigastric and the superficial circumflex iliac arteries. From its origin beneath the fascia lata at approximately 1.2 cm beyond the inguinal ligament, the superficial epigastric artery passes immediately through the fascia lata or through the fossa ovalis. From there, it courses upward, primarily within Camper's fascia, in a slightly medial direction anterior to the external oblique muscle almost as far as the umbilicus, giving off small branches to the inguinal lymph nodes and to the skin and superficial fascia. It ends in numerous small twigs that anastomose with the cutaneous branches from the inferior epigastric and internal mammary arteries. Arising either in common with the superficial epigastric artery or as a separate branch from the femoral artery, the superficial circumflex iliac artery passes laterally over the iliacus. Perforating the fascia lata slightly to the lateral aspect of the fossa ovalis, it then runs parallel to the inguinal liga-

ment almost to the crest of the ilium, where it terminates in branches within Scarpa's fascia that anastomose with the deep circumflex iliac artery. In its course, branches supply the iliacus and sartorius muscles, the inguinal lymph nodes, and the superficial fascia and skin.

### Veins

The superficial veins are more numerous than the arteries and form more extensive networks. Above the umbilicus, blood returns through the anterior cutaneous and the paired thoracoepigastric veins, the superficial epigastric veins, and the superficial circumflex iliac veins in the tela subcutanea. A cruciate anastomosis exists, therefore, between the femoral and axillary veins.

### Lymphatics

The lymphatic drainage of the lower abdominal wall (Fig 2–5) is primarily to the superficial inguinal nodes, 10–20 in number, which lie in the area of the inguinal ligament. These nodes may be identified by

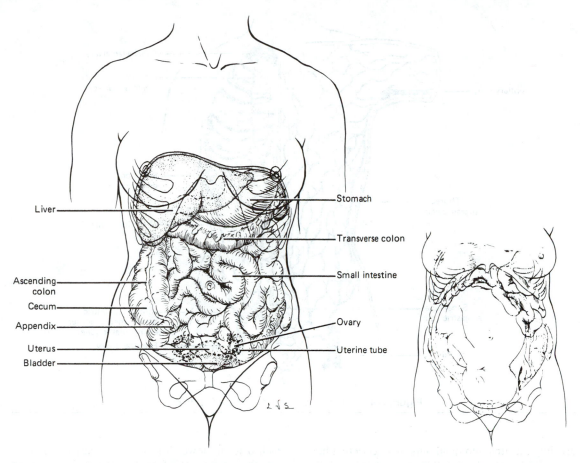

**Figure 2–2.** Abdominal viscera in situ. Inset shows projection of fetus in situ.

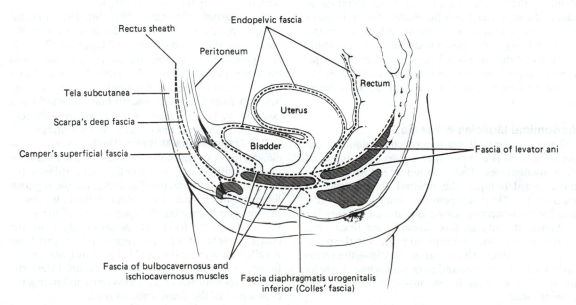

**Figure 2–3.** Fascial planes of the pelvis. (Modified after Netter. Reproduced, with permission, from Benson RC. Handbook of Obstetrics & Gynecology, 8th ed. Lange, 1983.)

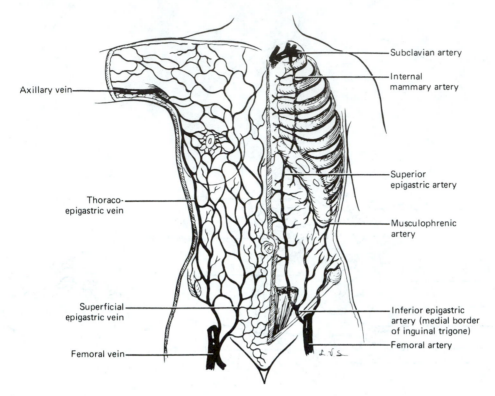

Subclavian artery

Internal
mammary artery

Axillary vein

Superior
epigastric artery

Thoraco-
epigastric vein

Musculophrenic
artery

Superficial
epigastric vein

Inferior epigastric
artery (medial border
of inguinal trigone)

Femoral artery

Femoral vein

**Figure 2–4.** Superficial veins and arteries of abdomen.

dividing the area into quadrants by intersecting horizontal and vertical lines that meet at the saphenofemoral junction. The lateral abdominal wall drainage follows the superficial circumflex iliac vein and drains to the lymph nodes in the upper lateral quadrant of the superficial inguinal nodes. The drainage of the medial aspect follows the superficial epigastric vein primarily to the lymph nodes in the upper medial quadrant of the superficial inguinal nodes. Of major clinical importance are the frequent anastomoses between the lymph vessels of the right and left sides of the abdomen.

### Abdominal Muscles & Fascia

The muscular wall that supports the abdominal viscera (Fig 2–6) is composed of 4 pairs of muscles and their aponeuroses. The 3 paired lateral muscles are the external oblique, the internal oblique, and the transversus. Their aponeuroses interdigitate at the midline to connect opposing lateral muscles, forming a thickened band at this juncture, the linea alba, which extends from the xiphoid process to the pubic symphysis. Anteriorly, a pair of muscles—the rectus abdominis, with the paired pyramidalis muscles at its inferior border with its sheath—constitute the abdominal wall.

**A. External Oblique Muscle:** The external oblique muscle consists of 8 pointed digitations attached to the lower 8 ribs. The lowest fibers insert into the anterior half of the iliac crest and the inguinal ligament. At the linea alba, the muscle aponeurosis interdigitates with that of the opposite side and fuses with the underlying internal oblique.

**B. Internal Oblique Muscle:** The internal oblique muscle arises from thoracolumbar fascia, the crest of the ilium, and the inguinal ligament. Going in the opposite oblique direction, the muscle inserts into the lower 3 costal cartilages and into the linea alba on either side of the rectus abdominis. The aponeurosis helps to form the rectus sheath both anteriorly and posteriorly. The posterior layer extends from the rectus muscle rib insertions to below the umbilicus.

**C. Transversus Muscle:** The transversus muscle, the fibers of which run transversely and arise from the inner surfaces of the lower 6 costal cartilages, the thoracolumbar fascia, the iliac crest, and the inguinal ligament, lies beneath the internal oblique. By inserting into the linea alba, the aponeurosis of the transversus fuses to form the posterior layer of the posterior rectus sheath. The termination of this layer is called the arcuate line, and below it lie transversalis fascia, properitoneal fat, and peritoneum. Inferiorly, the thin aponeurosis of the transversus abdominis becomes part of the anterior rectus sheath.

**D. Rectus Muscles:** The rectus muscles are straplike and extend from the thorax to the pubis.

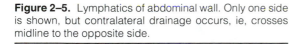

**Figure 2–5.** Lymphatics of abdominal wall. Only one side is shown, but contralateral drainage occurs, ie, crosses midline to the opposite side.

They are divided by the linea alba and outlined laterally by the linea semilunaris. Three tendinous intersections cross the upper part of each rectus muscle, and a fourth may also be present below the umbilicus. The pyramidalis muscle, a vestigial muscle, is situated anterior to the lowermost part of the rectus muscle. It arises from and inserts into the pubic periosteum.

Beneath the superficial fascia and overlying the muscles is the thin, semitransparent deep fascia. Its extensions enter and divide the lateral muscles into coarse bundles.

Abdominal incisions are shown in Fig 2–7. The position of the muscles influences the type of incision to be made. The aim is to adequately expose the operative field, avoiding damage to parietal structures, blood vessels, and nerves. The incision should be so placed as to create minimal tension on the lines of closure.

## Abdominal Nerves

The lower 6 thoracic nerves align with the ribs and give off lateral cutaneous branches (Fig 2–8). The intercostal nerves pass deep to the upturned rib carti-lages and enter the abdominal wall. The main trunks of these nerves run forward between the internal oblique and the transversus. The nerves then enter the rectus sheaths and the rectus muscles, and the terminating branches emerge as anterior cutaneous nerves. The iliohypogastric nerve springs from the first lumbar nerve after the latter has been joined by the communicating branch from the last (12th) thoracic nerve. It pierces the lateral border of the psoas and crosses anterior to the quadratus lumborum muscle but posterior to the kidney and colon. At the lateral border of the quadratus lumborum, it pierces the aponeurosis of origin of the transversus abdominis and enters the areolar tissue between the transversus and the internal oblique muscle. Here, it frequently communicates with the last thoracic and with the ilioinguinal nerve, which also originates from the first lumbar and last thoracic nerves. The iliohypogastric divides into 2 branches. The iliac branch pierces the internal and external oblique muscles, emerging through the latter above the iliac crest and supplying the integument of the upper and lateral part of the thigh. The hypogastric branch, as it passes forward and downward, gives branches to both the transversus abdominis and internal oblique. It communicates with the ilioinguinal nerve and pierces the internal oblique muscle near the anterior superior spine. The hypogastric branch proceeds medially beneath the external oblique aponeurosis and pierces it just above the subcutaneous inguinal ring to supply the skin and symphysis pubica.

## Abdominal Arteries

**A. Arteries of the Upper Abdomen:** The lower 5 intercostal arteries and the subcostal artery accompany the thoracic nerves. Their finer, terminal branches enter the rectus sheath to anastomose with the superior and inferior epigastric arteries. The superior epigastric artery is the direct downward prolongation of the internal mammary artery. This artery descends between the posterior surface of the rectus muscle and its sheath to form an anastomosis with the inferior epigastric artery upon the muscle. The inferior epigastric artery, a branch of the external iliac artery, usually arises just above the inguinal ligament and passes on the medial side of the round ligament to the abdominal inguinal ring. From there, it ascends in a slightly medial direction, passing above and lateral to the subcutaneous inguinal ring, which lies between the fascia transversalis and the peritoneum. Piercing the fascia transversalis, it passes in front of the linea semicircularis, turns upward between the rectus and its sheath, enters the substance of the rectus muscle, and meets the superior epigastric artery. The superior epigastric supplies the upper central abdominal wall, the inferior supplies the lower central part of the anterior abdominal wall, and the deep circumflex supplies the lower lateral part of the abdominal wall.

**B. Arteries of the Lower Abdomen:** The deep

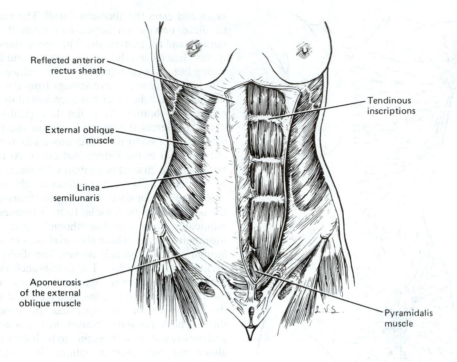

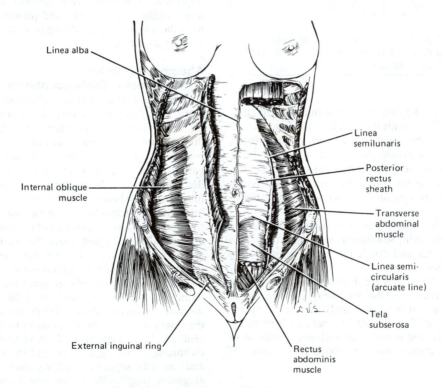

**Figure 2–6.** Musculature of abdominal wall.

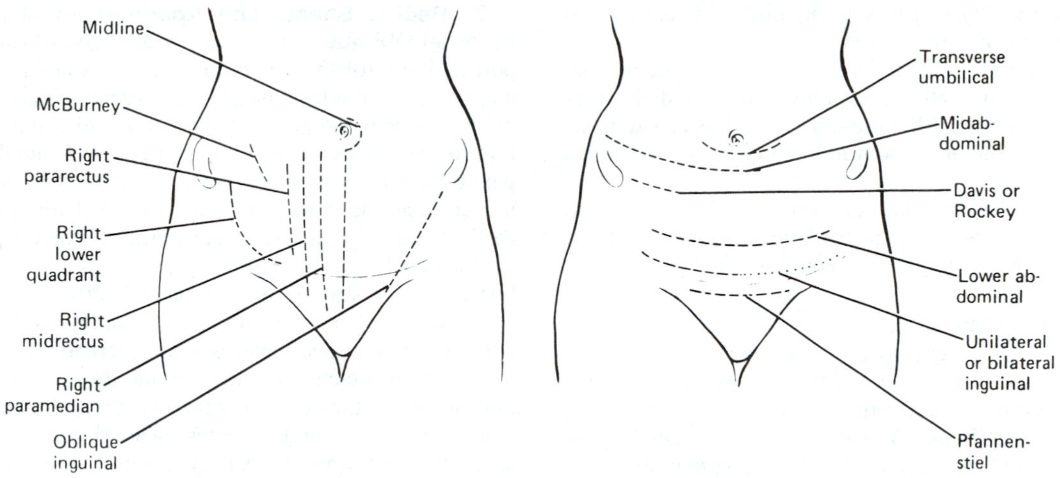

**Figure 2–7.** Abdominal incisions. Transverse incisions are those in which rectus muscles are cut. A Cherney incision is one in which the rectus is taken off the pubic bone and then sewed back; the pyramidalis muscle is left on pubic tubercles.

circumflex iliac artery is also a branch of the external iliac artery, arising from its side either opposite the epigastric artery or slightly below the origin of that vessel. It courses laterally behind the inguinal ligament lying between the fascia transversalis and the peritoneum. The deep circumflex artery perforates the transversus near the anterior superior spine of the ilium and continues between the transversus and in-

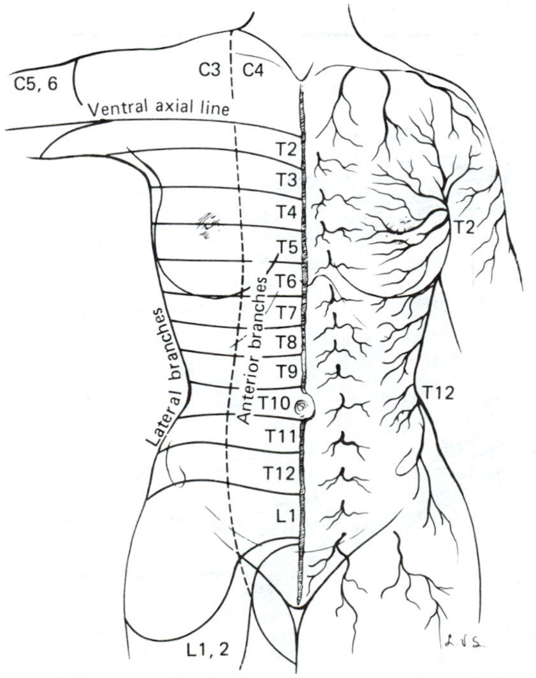

**Figure 2–8.** Cutaneous innervation of the abdominal wall.

ternal oblique along and slightly above the crest of the ilium, finally running posteriorly to anastomose with the ilio lumbar artery. A branch of the deep circumflex iliac artery is important to the surgeon because it forms anastomoses with branches of the inferior epigastric. The deep veins correspond in name with the arteries they accompany. Below the umbilicus, these veins run caudad and medially to the external iliac vein; above that level, they run cephalad and laterally into the intercostal veins. Lymphatic drainage in the deeper regions of the abdominal wall follows the deep veins directly to the superficial inguinal nodes.

The various incisions on the abdomen encounter some muscle planes and vasculature of clinical significance. The McBurney incision requires separation of the external and internal oblique muscles and splitting of the transversus. The deep circumflex artery may be frequently encountered. The paramedian incision is made in the right or left rectus. Below the arcuate line, the fascia of the external and internal oblique, as well as the transversus muscles when present, go over the rectus abdominis; above the arcuate line, the transversus and part of the internal oblique go under the rectus. The vasculature is primarily perforators and frequently the thoracoabdominal vein. Inferiorly, the superficial epigastric may be encountered. In the Pfannenstiel incision, the fascia of the external and internal oblique go over the rectus muscle as well as the transversus muscle when present. After the fascia over the rectus is incised, the muscles can be separated. The superficial epigastric artery and vein are encountered in Camper's fascia. Laterally, the superficial and deep circumflex iliac arteries may be at the margin of the incision. Lying under the transversus muscle and entering the rectus approximately half way to the umbilicus is the inferior epigastric artery.

In the transverse incision, the arcuate line may be encountered. As the rectus muscle is incised, the inferior epigastric within the muscle and its anastomosis with the thoracoabdominal artery must be recognized.

In the Cherny incision, care should be taken to avoid the inferior epigastric artery, which is the primary blood supply to the rectus abdominis.

## Special Structures

There are several special anatomic structures in the abdominal wall, including the umbilicus, linea alba, linea semilunaris, and rectus sheath.

**A. Umbilicus:** The umbilicus is situated opposite the disk between the third and fourth lumbar vertebrae, approximately 2 cm below the mid point of a line drawn from the sternoxiphoid process to the top of the pubic symphysis. The umbilicus is a dense, wrinkled mass of fibrous tissue enclosed by and fused with a ring of circular aponeurotic fibers in the linea alba. Normally, it is the strongest part of the abdominal wall.

**B. Linea Alba:** The linea alba, a fibrous band formed by the fusion of the aponeuroses of the muscles of the anterior abdominal wall, marks the medial side of the rectus abdominis; the linea semilunaris forms the lateral border, which courses from the tip of the ninth costal cartilage to the pubic tubercle. The linea alba extends from the xiphoid process to the pubic symphysis, represented above the umbilicus as a shallow median groove on the surface.

**C. Rectus Sheath and Aponeurosis of the External Oblique:** The rectus sheath serves to support and control the rectus muscles. It contains the rectus and pyramidalis muscles, the terminal branches of the lower 6 thoracic nerves and vessels, and the inferior and superior epigastric vessels. Cranially, where the sheath is widest, its anterior wall extends upward onto the thorax to the level of the fifth costal cartilage and is attached to the sternum. The deeper wall is attached to the xiphoid process and the lower borders of the seventh to ninth costal cartilages and does not extend upward onto the anterior thorax. Caudally, where the sheath narrows considerably, the anterior wall is attached to the crest and the symphysis pubica. Above the costal margin on the anterior chest wall, there is no complete rectus sheath (Fig 2–9). Instead, the rectus muscle is only covered by the aponeurosis of the external oblique. In the region of the abdomen, the upper two-thirds of the internal oblique aponeurosis splits at the lateral border of the rectus muscle into anterior and posterior lamellas. The anterior lamella passes in front of the external oblique and blends with the external oblique aponeurosis. The posterior wall of the sheath is formed by the posterior lamella and the aponeurosis of the transversus muscle. The anterior and posterior sheath join at the midline. The lower third of the internal oblique aponeurosis is undivided. Together with the aponeuroses of the external oblique and transversus muscles, it forms the anterior wall of the sheath. The posterior wall is occupied by transversalis fascia, which is spread over the interior surfaces of both the rectus and the transversus muscles, separating them

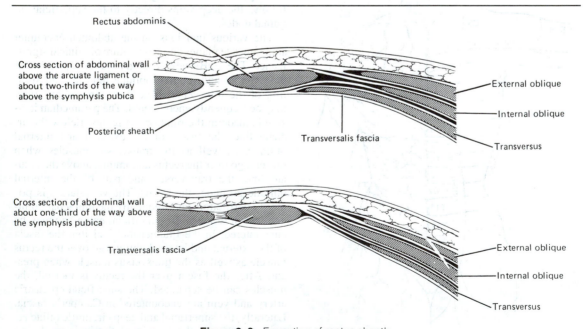

Rectus abdominis

Cross section of abdominal wall above the arcuate ligament or about two-thirds of the way above the symphysis pubica

External oblique

Internal oblique

Posterior sheath

Transversalis fascia

Transversus

Cross section of abdominal wall about one-third of the way above the symphysis pubica

External oblique

Internal oblique

Transversalis fascia

Transversus

**Figure 2–9.** Formation of rectus sheath.

from peritoneum and extending to the inguinal and lacunar ligaments. The transition from aponeurosis to fascia is usually fairly sharp, marked by a curved line called the arcuate line.

**D. Function of Abdominal Muscles:** In general, the functions of the abdominal muscles are 3-fold: (1) support and compression of the abdominal viscera by the external oblique, internal oblique, and transversus muscles; (2) depression of the thorax in conjunction with the diaphragm by the rectus abdominis, external oblique, internal oblique, and transversus muscles, as evident in respiration, coughing, vomiting, defecation, and parturition; and (3) assistance in bending movements of the trunk through flexion of the vertebral column by the rectus abdominis, external oblique, and internal oblique muscles. There is partial assistance in rotation of the thorax and upper abdomen to the same side when the pelvis is fixed by the internal oblique and by the external oblique to the opposite side. In addition, the up per external oblique serves as a fixation muscle in abduction of the upper limb of the same side and adduction of the upper limb of the opposite side. The pyramidalis muscle secures the linea alba in the median line.

### Variations of Abdominal Muscles

Variations have been noted in all of the abdominal muscles.

**A. Rectus Muscle:** The rectus abdominis muscle may differ in the number of its tendinous inscriptions and the extent of its thoracic attachment. Aponeurotic slips or slips of muscle on the upper part of the thorax are remnants of a more primitive state in which the muscle extended to the neck. Absence of part or all of the muscle has been noted. The pyramidalis muscle may be missing, only slightly developed, double, or may extend upward to the umbilicus.

**B. External Oblique Muscle:** The external oblique muscle varies in the extent of its origin from the ribs. Broad fascicles may be separated by loose tissue from the main belly of the muscle, either on its deep or on its superficial surface. The supracostalis anterior is a rare fascicle occasionally found on the upper portion of the thoracic wall. Transverse tendinous inscriptions may also be found.

**C. Internal Oblique Muscle:** The internal oblique deviates at times, both in its attachments and in the extent of development of the fleshy part of the muscle. Occasionally, tendinous inscriptions are present, or the posterior division forms an extra muscle 7–7.5 cm wide and separated from the internal oblique by a branch of the iliohypogastric nerve and a branch of the deep circumflex iliac artery.

**D. Transversus Muscle:** The transversus muscle fluctuates widely in the extent of its development but is rarely absent. Rarely, it extends as far inferiorly as the ligamentum teres uteri (round ligament), and

infrequently it may be situated superior to the anterior superior spine. However, it generally occupies an intermediate position.

**E. Other Variations:** Several small muscles may be present.

1. The pubotransversalis muscle may extend from the superior ramus of the pubis to the transversalis fascia near the abdominal ring.
2. The puboperitonealis muscle may pass from the pubic crest to the transversus near the umbilicus.
3. The posterior rectus abdominis (tensor laminae posterioris vaginae musculi recti abdominis) may spread from the inguinal ligament to the rectus sheath on the deep surface of the rectus muscle near the umbilicus.
4. The tensor transversalis (tensor laminae posterioris vaginae musculi recti et fasciae transversalis abdominis) has appeared from the transversalis fascia near the abdominal inguinal ring to the linea semicircularis.

### Hernias

A hernia (Fig 2–10) is a protrusion of any viscus from its normal enclosure, which may occur with any of the abdominal viscera, especially the jejunum, ileum, and greater omentum. A hernia may be due to increased pressure, such as that resulting from strenuous exercise, lifting heavy weights, tenesmus, or in-

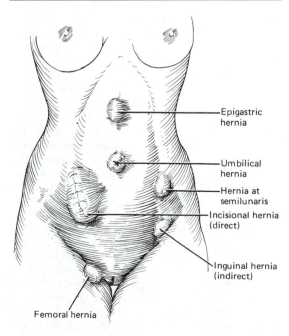

**Figure 2–10.** Hernia sites.

creased expiratory efforts, or may result from decreased resistance of the abdominal wall (congenital or acquired) such as occurs with debilitating illness or old age, prolonged distention from ascites, tumors, pregnancy, corpulence, emaciation, injuries (including surgical incisions), congenital absence, or poor development. Hernias are likely to occur where the abdominal wall is structurally weakened by the passage of large vessels or nerves and developmental peculiarities. Ventral hernias occur through the linea semilunaris or the linea alba. Umbilical hernias occur more frequently and can be one of 3 types. During early fetal development, portions of the mesentery and a loop of the intestine pass through the opening to occupy a part of the body cavity (the umbilical coelom) situated in the umbilical cord. Normally, the mesentery and intestine later return to the abdominal cavity. If they fail to do so, a congenital umbilical hernia results. Infantile umbilical hernias occur if the component parts fail to fuse completely in early postnatal stages. The unyielding nature of the fibrous tissue forming the margin of the ring predisposes to strangulation. Adult umbilical hernias occur frequently in females. When the hernia comes through the ring itself, it is always at the upper part.

## INGUINAL REGION

The inguinal region of the abdominal wall is bounded by the rectus abdominis muscle medially, the line connecting the anterior superior iliac spines superiorly, and the inguinal ligament inferiorly. The region contains 8 layers of abdominal wall. These layers, from the most superficial in ward, are (1) the skin, (2) the tela subcutanea, (3) the aponeurosis of the external oblique muscle, (4) the internal oblique muscle, (5) the transversus abdominis muscle (below the free border, the layer is incomplete), (6) the transversalis fascia, (7) the subperitoneal fat and connective tissue, and (8) the peritoneum. The tela subcutanea consists of the superficial fatty Camper's fascia, which is continuous with the tela subcutanea of the whole body, and the deeper membranous Scarpa's fascia, which covers the lower third of the abdominal wall and the medial side of the groin, both joining below the inguinal ligament to form the fascia lata of the thigh.

### Subcutaneous Inguinal Ring

A triangular evagination of the external oblique aponeurosis, the subcutaneous inguinal ring (external abdominal ring), is bounded by an aponeurosis at its edges and by the inguinal ligament inferiorly. The superior or medial crus is smaller and attaches to the symphysis pubica. The inferior or lateral crus is stronger and blends with the inguinal ligament as it passes to the pubic tubercle. The sharp margins of the ring are attributed to a sudden thinning of the aponeu-

rosis. In the female, the ligamentum teres uteri (round ligament) passes through this ring. The subcutaneous inguinal ring is much smaller in the female than in the male, and the abdominal wall is relatively stronger in this region.

### Ligaments, Aponeuroses, & Fossae

The inguinal ligament itself forms the inferior thickened border of the external oblique aponeurosis, extending from the anterior superior iliac spine to the pubic tubercle. Along its inferior border, it becomes continuous with the fascia lata of the thigh. From the medial portion of the inguinal ligament, a triangular band of fibers attaches separately to the pecten ossis pubis. This band is known as the lacunar (Gimbernat's) ligament. The reflex inguinal ligament (ligament of Colles or triangular fascia) is represented by a small band of fibers, often poorly developed, and derived from the superior crus of the subcutaneous inguinal ring and the lower part of the linea alba. These fibers cross to the opposite side to attach to the pecten ossis pubis. The falx inguinalis or conjoined tendon is formed by the aponeurosis of the transversus abdominis and internal oblique muscles. These fibers arise from the inguinal ligament and arch downward and forward to insert on the pubic crest and pecten ossis pubis, behind the inguinal and lacunar ligaments. The interfoveolar ligament is composed partly of fibrous bands from the aponeurosis of the transversalis muscle of the same and opposite sides. Curving medial to and below the internal abdominal ring, they attach to the lacunar ligament and pectineal fascia.

### Abdominal Inguinal Ring

The abdominal inguinal ring (internal abdominal ring) is the rounded mouth of a funnel-shaped expansion of transversalis fascia that lies approximately 2 cm above the inguinal ligament and midway between the anterior superior iliac spine and the symphysis pubica. Medially, it is bounded by the inferior epigastric vessels; the external iliac artery is situated below. The abdominal inguinal ring represents the area where the round ligament emerges from the abdomen. The triangular area medial to the inferior epigastric artery, bounded by the inguinal ligament below and the lateral border of the rectus sheath, is known as the trigonum inguinale (Hesselbach's triangle), the site of congenital direct hernias.

### Inguinal Canal

The inguinal canal in the female is not well demarcated, but it normally gives passage to the round ligament of the uterus, a vein, an artery from the uterus that forms a cruciate anastomosis with the labial arteries, and extraperitoneal fat. The fetal ovary, like the testis, is an abdominal organ and possesses a gubernaculum that extends from its lower pole downward and forward to a point corresponding to the abdominal inguinal ring, through which it continues into the labia majora. The processus vaginalis is an evagination of peritoneum at the level of the abdominal inguinal ring occurring during the third fetal month. In the male, the processus vaginalis descends with the testis. The processus vaginalis of the female is rudimentary, but occasionally a small diverticulum of peritoneum is found passing partway through the inguinal region; this diverticulum is termed the processus vaginalis peritonei (canal of Nuck). Instead of descending, as does the testis, the ovary moves medially, where it becomes adjacent to the uterus. The intra-abdominal portion of the gubernaculum ovarii becomes attached to the lateral border of the developing uterus, evolving as the ligament of the ovary and the round ligament of the uterus. The extra-abdominal portion of the round ligament of the uterus becomes attenuated in the adult and may appear as a small fibrous band. The inguinal canal is an intermuscular passageway that extends from the abdominal ring downward, medially, and somewhat forward to the subcutaneous inguinal ring (about 3–4 cm). The canal is roughly triangular in shape, and its boundaries are largely artificial. The lacunar and inguinal ligaments form the base of the canal. The anterior or superficial wall is formed by the external oblique aponeurosis, and the lowermost fibers of the internal oblique muscle add additional strength in its lateral part. The posterior or deep wall of the canal is formed by transversalis fascia throughout and is strengthened medially by the falx inguinalis.

## Abdominal Fossae

The abdominal fossae in the inguinal region consist of the foveae inguinalis lateralis and medialis. The fovea inguinalis lateralis lies lateral to a slight fold, the plica epigastrica, formed by the inferior epigastric vessels, and just medial to the abdominal inguinal ring, which slants medially and upward toward the rectus muscle. From the lateral margin of the tendinous insertion of the rectus muscle, upward toward the umbilicus, and over the obliterated artery extends a more accentuated fold, the plica umbilicalis lateralis. The fovea inguinalis medialis lies between the plica epigastrica and the plica umbilicalis lateralis, the bottom of the fossa facing the trigonum inguinale (Hesselbach's triangle). This region is strengthened by the interfoveolar ligament at the medial side of the abdominal inguinal ring and the conjoined tendon lateral to the rectus muscle; however, these bands vary in width and are thus supportive.

## Ligaments & Spaces

The inguinal ligament forms the roof of a large osseoligamentous space leading from the iliac fossa to the thigh. The floor of this space is formed by the superior ramus of the pubis medially and by the body of the ilium laterally. The iliopectineal ligament extends from the inguinal ligament to the iliopectineal emi-

nence, dividing this area into 2 parts. The lateral, larger division is called the muscular lacuna and is almost completely filled by the iliopsoas muscle, along with the femoral nerve medially and the lateral femoral cutaneous nerves laterally. The medial, smaller division is known as the vascular lacuna and is traversed by the external iliac (femoral) artery, vein, and lymphatic vessels, which do not completely fill the space. The anterior border of the vascular lacuna is formed by the inguinal ligament and the transversalis fascia. The posterior boundary is formed by the ligamentum pubicum superius (Cooper's ligament), a thickening of fascia along the public pecten where the pectineal fascia and iliopectineal ligament meet. The transversalis fascia and iliac fascia are extended with the vessels, forming a funnel-shaped fibrous investment, the femoral sheath. The sheath is divided into 3 compartments; (1) the lateral compartment, containing the femoral artery; (2) the intermediate compartment, containing the femoral vein; and (3) the medial compartment or canal, containing a lymph node (nodi lymphatici inguinales profundi [node of Rosenmüller or Cloquet]) and the lymphatic vessels that drain most of the leg, groin, and perineum. The femoral canal also contains areolar tissue, which frequently condenses to form the "femoral septum." Because of the greater spread of the pelvis in the female, the muscular and vascular lacunae are relatively large spaces. The upper or abdominal opening of the femoral canal is known as the femoral ring and is covered by the parietal peritoneum.

## Arteries

In front of the femoral ring, the arterial branches of the external iliac artery are the inferior epigastric and the deep circumflex iliac. The inferior epigastric artery arises from the anterior surface of the external iliac, passing forward and upward on the anterior abdominal wall between peritoneum and transversalis fascia. It pierces the fascia just below the arcuate line, entering the rectus abdominis muscle or coursing along its inferior surface to anastomose with the superior epigastric from the internal thoracic. The inferior epigastric artery forms the lateral boundary of the trigonum inguinale (Hesselbach's triangle). At its origin, it frequently gives off a branch to the inguinal canal, as well as a branch to the pubis (pubic artery), which anastomoses with twigs of the obturator artery. The pubic branch of the inferior epigastric often becomes the obturator artery. The deep circumflex iliac artery arises laterally and traverses the iliopsoas to the anterior superior iliac spine, where it pierces the transversus muscle to course between the transversus and the internal oblique, sending perforators to the surface. It often has anastomoses with penetrating branches of the inferior epigastric via its perforators through the rectus abdominis. The veins follow a similar course.

As the external iliac artery passes through the femoral canal, which underlies the inguinal ligament, it courses medial to the femoral vein and nerve, resting in what is termed the femoral triangle (Scarpa's triangle). The femoral sheath is a downward continuation of the inguinal ligament anterior to the femoral vessel and nerve.

The branches of the femoral artery supplying the groin are (1) the superficial epigastric, (2) the superficial circumflex iliac, (3) the superficial external pudendal, and (4) the deep external pudendal. The superficial epigastric artery passes upward through the femoral sheath over the inguinal ligament, to rest in Camper's fascia on the lower abdomen. The superficial circumflex iliac artery arises adjacent to the superior epigastric, piercing the fascia lata and running parallel to the inguinal ligament as far as the iliac crest. It then divides into branches that supply the integument of the groin, the superficial fascia, and the lymph glands, anastomosing with the deep circumflex iliac, the superior gluteal, and the lateral femoral circumflex arteries. The superficial external pudendal artery arises from the medial side of the femoral artery, close to the preceding vessels. It pierces the femoral sheath and fascia cribrosa, coursing medially across the round ligament to the integument on the lower part of the abdomen and the labium majus, anastomosing with the internal pudendal. The deep external pudendal artery passes medially across the pectineus and adductor longus muscles, supplying the integument of the labium majus and forming, to-

gether with the external pudendal artery, a rete with the labial arteries.

## PUDENDUM

The vulva consists of the mons pubis, the labia majora, the labia minora, the clitoris, and the glandular structures that open into the vestibulum vaginae (Fig 2–11). The size, shape, and coloration of the various structures, as well as the hair distribution, vary between individuals and racial groups. Normal pubic hair in the female is distributed in an inverted triangle, with the base centered over the mons pubis. Nevertheless, in approximately 25% of normal women, hair may extend upward along the linea alba. The type of hair is dependent, in part, on the pigmentation of the individual. It varies from heavy, coarse, crinkly hair in blacks to sparse, fairly fine, lanugo type hair in Oriental women. The length and size of the various structures of the vulva are influenced by the pelvic architecture, as is also the position of the external genitalia in the perineal area. The external genitalia of the female have their exact counterparts in the male.

### Labia Majora

**A. Superficial Anatomy:** The labia majora are comprised of 2 rounded mounds of tissue, originating in the mons pubis and terminating in the perineum.

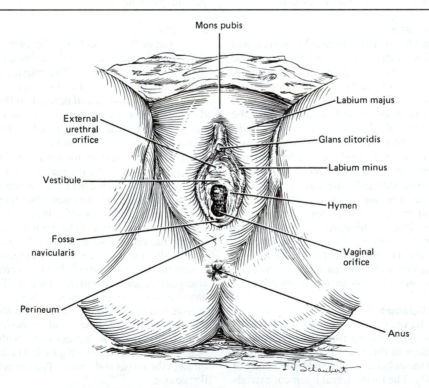

**Figure 2–11.** External genitalia of adult female (parous).

They form the lateral boundaries of the vulva and are approximately 7–9 cm long and 2–4 cm wide, varying in size with height, weight, race, age, parity, and pelvic architecture. Ontogenetically, these permanent folds of skin are homologous to the scrotum of the male. Hair is distributed over their surfaces, extending superiorly in the area of the mons pubis from one side to the other. The lateral surfaces are adjacent to the medial surface of the thigh, forming a deep groove when the legs are together. The medial surfaces of the labia majora may oppose each other directly or may be separated by protrusion of the labia minora. The cleft that is formed by this opposition anteriorly is termed the anterior commissure. Posteriorly, the cleft is less clearly defined and termed the posterior commissure. The middle portion of the cleft between the 2 labia is the rima pudendi.

**B. Deep Structures:** Underlying the skin is a thin, poorly developed muscle layer called the tunica dartos labialis, the fibers of which course, for the most part, at right angles to the wrinkles of the surface, forming a crisscross pattern. Deep to the dartos layer is a thin layer of fascia, most readily recognizable in the old or the young because of the large amount of adipose and areolar tissue. Numerous sweat glands are found in the labia majora, the greater number on the medial aspect. In the deeper substance of the labia majora are longitudinal bands of muscle that are continuous with the ligamentum teres uteri (round ligament) as it emerges from the inguinal canal. Occasionally, a persistent processus vaginalis peritonei (canal of Nuck) may be seen in the upper region of the labia. In most women, it has been impossible to differentiate the presence of the cremaster muscle beyond its area of origin.

**C. Arteries:** The arterial supply into the labia majora comes from the internal and external pudendals, with extensive anastomoses. Within the labia majora is a circular arterial pattern originating inferiorly from a branch of the perineal artery, from the external pudendal artery in the anterior lateral aspect, and from a small artery of the ligamentum teres uteri superiorly. The inferior branch from the perineal artery, which originates from the internal pudendal as it emerges from the canalis pudendalis (Alcock's canal), forms the base of the rete with the external pudendal arteries. These arise from the medial side of the femoral and, occasionally, from the deep arteries just beneath the femoral ring, coursing medially over the pectineus and adductor muscles, to which they supply branches. They terminate in a circular rete within the labium majus, penetrating the fascia lata adjacent to the fossa ovalis and passing over the round ligament to send a branch to the clitoris.

**D. Veins:** The venous drainage is extensive and forms a plexus with numerous anastomoses. In addition, the veins communicate with the dorsal vein of the clitoris, the veins of the labia minora, and the perineal veins, as well as with the inferior hemorrhoidal

plexus. On each side, the posterior labial veins connect with the external pudendal vein, terminating in the great saphenous vein (saphena magna) just prior to its entrance (saphenous opening) in the fossa ovalis. This large plexus is frequently manifested by the presence of large varicosities during pregnancy.

**E. Lymphatics:** The lymphatics of the labia majora are extensive and utilize 2 systems, one lying superficially (under the skin) and the other deeper, within the subcutaneous tissues. From the upper two-thirds of the left and right labia majora, superficial lymphatics pass toward the symphysis and turn laterally to join the medial superficial inguinal nodes. These nodes drain into the superficial inguinal nodes overlying the saphenous fossa. The drainage flows into and through the femoral ring (fossa ovalis) to the nodi lymphatici inguinales profundi (nodes of Rosenmüller or Cloquet; deep subinguinal nodes), connecting with the external iliac chain. The superficial subinguinal nodes, situated over the femoral trigone, also accept superficial drainage from the lower extremity and the gluteal region. This drainage may include afferent lymphatics from the perineum. In the region of the symphysis pubica, the lymphatics anastomose in a plexus between the right and left nodes. Therefore, any lesion involving the labia majora allows direct involvement of the lymphatic structures of the contralateral inguinal area. The lower part of the labium majus has superficial and deep drainage that is shared with the perineal area. The drainage passes, in part, through afferent lymphatics to superficial subinguinal nodes; from the posterior medial aspects of the labia majora, it frequently enters the lymphatic plexus surrounding the rectum.

**F. Nerves:** The innervation of the external genitalia has been studied by many investigators. The iliohypogastric nerve originates from T12 and L1 and traverses laterally to the iliac crest between the transversus and internal oblique muscles, at which point it divides into 2 branches: (1) the anterior hypogastric nerve, which descends anteriorly through the skin over the symphysis, supplying the superior portion of the labia majora and the mons pubis, and (2) the posterior iliac, which passes to the gluteal area.

The ilioinguinal nerve originates from L1 and follows a course slightly inferior to the iliohypogastric nerve, with which it may frequently anastomose, branching into many small fibers that terminate in the upper medial aspect of the labium majus.

The genitofemoral nerve (L1–L2) emerges from the anterior surface of the psoas muscle to run obliquely downward over its surface, branching in the deeper substance of the labium majus to supply the dartos muscle and that vestige of the cremaster present within the labium majus. Its lumboinguinal branch continues downward onto the upper part of the thigh.

From the sacral plexus, the posterior femoral cutaneous nerve, originating from the posterior divisions of S1 and S2 and the anterior divisions of S2 and S3, divides into several rami that, in part, are called the perineal branches. They supply the medial aspect of the thigh and the labia majora. These branches of the posterior femoral cutaneous nerve are derived from the sacral plexus. The pudendal nerve, composed primarily of S2, S3, and S4, often with a fascicle of S1, sends a small number of fibers to the medial aspect of the labia majora. The pattern of nerve endings is illustrated in Table 2–1.

## Labia Minora

**A. Superficial Anatomy:** The labia minora are 2 folds of skin that lie within the rima pudendi and measure approximately 5 cm in length and 0.5–1 cm in thickness. The width varies according to age and parity, measuring 2–3 cm at its narrowest diameter to 5–6 cm at it widest, with multiple corrugations over the surface. The labia minora begin at the base of the clitoris, where fusion of the labia is continuous with the prepuce, extending posteriorly and medially to the labia majora at the posterior commissure. On their medial aspects superiorly beneath the clitoris, they unite to form the frenulum adjacent to the urethra and vagina, terminating along the hymen on the right and left sides of the fossa navicularis and ending posteriorly in the frenulum of the labia pudendi, just superior to the posterior commissure. A deep cleft is formed on the lateral surface between the labium majus and the labium minus. The skin on the labia minora is smooth and pigmented. The color and distention vary, depending on the level of sexual excitement and the pigmentation of the individual. The glands of the labia are homologous to the glandulae preputiales (glands of Littre) of the penile portion of the male urethra.

**B. Arteries:** The main source of arterial supply (Fig 2–12) occurs through anastomoses from the superficial perineal artery, branching from the dorsal artery of the clitoris, and from the medial aspect of the rete of the labia majora. Similarly, the venous pattern and plexus are extensive.

**C. Veins:** The venous drainage is to the medial vessels of the perineal and vaginal veins, directly to the veins of the labia majora, to the inferior hemorrhoidals posteriorly, and to the clitoral veins superiorly.

**D. Lymphatics:** The lymphatics medially may join those of the lower third of the vagina superiorly and the labia majora laterally, passing to the superficial subinguinal nodes and to the deep subinguinal nodes. In the midline, the lymphatic drainage coincides with that of the clitoris, communicating with that of the labia majora to drain to the opposite side.

**E. Nerves:** The innervation of the labia minora originates, in part, from fibers that supply the labia majora and from branches of the pudendal nerve as it emerges from the canalis pudendalis (Alcock's canal) (Fig 2–12). These branches originate from the perineal nerve. The labia minora and the vestibule area are homologous to the skin of the male urethra and penis. The short membranous portion, approximately 0.5 cm of the male urethra, is homologous to the midportion of the vestibule of the female.

## Clitoris

**A. Superficial Anatomy:** The clitoris is the homologue of the dorsal part of the penis and consists of 2 small erectile cavernous bodies, terminating in a rudimentary glans clitoridis. The erectile body, the corpus clitoridis, consists of the 2 crura clitoridis and the glans clitoridis, with overlying skin and prepuce, a miniature homologue of the glans penis. The crura extend outward bilaterally to their position in the anterior portion of the vulva. The cavernous tissue, homologous to the corpus spongiosum penis of the male, appears in the vascular pattern of the labia minora in the female. At the lower border of the pubic arch, a small triangular fibrous band extends onto the clitoris (suspensory ligament) to separate the 2 crura, which turn inward, downward, and laterally at this point, close to the inferior rami of the pubic symphysis. The crura lie inferior to the ischiocavernosus muscles and bodies. The glans is situated superiorly at the fused termination of the crura. It is composed

**Table 2–1.** Quantitative distribution of nerve endings in selected regions of the female genitalia.

| | Touch | | | Pressure | Pain | Other Types | |
|---|---|---|---|---|---|---|---|
| | Meissner Corpuscles[1] | Merkel Tactile Disks[1] | Peritrichous Endings | Vater-Pacini Corpuscles[2] | Free Nerve Endings | Ruffini Corpuscles[2] | Dogiel and Krause Corpuscles[3] |
| Mons pubis | ++++ | ++++ | ++++ | +++ | +++ | ++++ | + |
| Labia majora | +++ | ++++ | ++++ | +++ | +++ | +++ | + |
| Clitoris | + | + | 0 | ++++ | +++ | +++ | +++ |
| Labia minora | + | + | 0 | + | + | + | +++ |
| Hymenal ring | 0 | + | 0 | 0 | +++ | 0 | 0 |
| Vagina | 0 | 0 | 0 | 0 | + Occasionally | 0 | 0 |

[1]Also called corpuscula tactus.
[2]Also called corpuscula lamellosa.
[3]Also called corpuscula bulboidea.

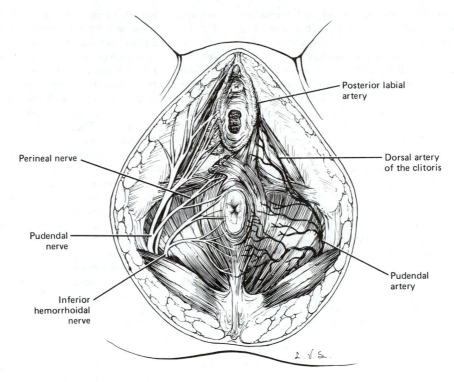

**Figure 2–12.** Arteries and nerves of perineum.

of erectile tissue and contains an integument, hood-like in shape, termed the prepuce. On its ventral surface, there is a frenulum clitoridis, the fused junction of the labia minora.

**B. Arteries:** The blood supply to the clitoris is from its dorsal artery, a terminal branch of the internal pudendal artery, which is the terminal division of the posterior portion of the internal iliac (hypogastric) artery. As it enters the clitoris, it divides into 2 branches, the deep and dorsal arteries. Just before entering the clitoris itself, a small branch passes posteriorly to supply the area of the external urethral meatus.

**C. Veins:** The venous drainage of the clitoris begins in a rich plexus around the corona of the glans, running along the anterior surface to join the deep vein and continuing downward to join the pudendal plexus from the labia minora, labia majora, and perineum, forming the pudendal vein.

**D. Lymphatics:** The lymphatic drainage of the clitoris coincides primarily with that of the labia minora, the right and left sides having access to contralateral nodes in the superficial inguinal chain. In addition, its extensive network provides further access downward and posteriorly to the external urethral meatus toward the anterior portion of the vestibule.

**E. Nerves:** The innervation of the clitoris is through the terminal branch of the pudendal nerve, which originates from the sacral plexus as previously discussed. It lies on the lateral side of the dorsal artery and terminates in branches within the glans, corona, and prepuce. The nerve endings in the clitoris vary from a total absence within the glans to a rich supply primarily located within the prepuce (Table 2–1). A total absence of endings within the clitoris itself takes on clinical significance when one considers the emphasis placed on the clitoris in discussing problems of sexual gratification in women.

### Vestibule

**A. Superficial Anatomy:** The area of the vestibule is bordered by the labia minor laterally, by the frenulum labiorum pudendi (or posterior commissure) posteriorly, and by the urethra and clitoris anteriorly. Inferiorly, it is bordered by the hymenal ring. The opening of the vagina or junction of the vagina with the vestibule is limited by a membrane stretching from the posterior and lateral sides to the inferior surface of the external urethral orifice. This membrane is termed the hymen. Its shape and openings vary and depend on age, parity, and sexual experience. The form of the opening may be infantile, annular, semilunar, cribriform, septate, or vertical; the hymen may even be imperforate. In parous women and in the postcoital state, the tags of the hymenal integument are termed carunculae myrtiformes. The external urethral orifice, which is approximately 2–3 cm posterior to the clitoris, on a slightly elevated and irregular surface with depressed areas on the sides, may appear to be stellate or crescentic in shape. It is characterized by many small mucosal folds around its opening. Bilaterally and on the surface are the orifices of the para- and periurethral glands (ductus paraurethrales [ducts of Skene and Astruc]). At approximately the 5 and 7 o'clock positions, just external to the hymenal rings, are 2 small papular elevations that represent the orifices of the ducts of the glandulae vestibulares majores, or larger vestibular glands (Bartholin) of the female (bulbourethral gland of the male). The fossa navicularis lies between the frenulum labiorum pudendi and the hymenal ring. The skin surrounding the vestibule is stratified squamous in type, with a paucity of rete pegs and papillae.

**B. Arteries:** The blood supply to the vestibule is an extensive capillary plexus that has anastomoses with the superficial transverse perineal artery. A branch comes directly from the pudendal anastomosis with the inferior hemorrhoidal artery in the region of the fossa navicularis; the blood supply of the urethra anteriorly, a branch of the dorsal artery of the clitoris and the azygos artery of the anterior vaginal wall, also contributes.

**C. Veins:** Venous drainage is extensive, involving the same areas described for the arterial network.

**D. Lymphatics:** The lymphatic drainage has a distinct pattern. The anterior portion, including that of the external urethral meatus, drains upward and outward with that of the labia minora and the clitoris. The portion next to the urethral meatus may join that of the anterior urethra, which empties into the vestibular plexus to terminate in the superficial inguinal nodes, the superficial subinguinal nodes, the deep subinguinal nodes, and the external iliac chain. The lymphatics of the fossa navicularis and the hymen may join those of the posterior vaginal wall, intertwining with the intercalated lymph nodes along the rectum, which follow the inferior hemorrhoidal arteries. This pattern becomes significant with cancer. Drainage occurs through the pudendal and the hemorrhoidal chain and through the vestibular plexus onto the inguinal region.

**E. Nerves:** The innervation of the vestibular area is primarily from the sacral plexus through the perineal nerve. The absence of the usual modalities of touch is noteworthy. The vestibular portion of the hymenal ring contains an abundance of free nerve endings (pain).

## Vestibular Glands

The glandulae vestibulares majores (larger vestibular glands or Bartholin glands) have a duct measuring approximately 5 mm in diameter. The gland itself lies just inferior and lateral to the bulbocavernosus muscle. The gland is tubular and alveolar in character, with a thin capsule and connective tissue septa dividing it into lobules in which occasional smooth muscle fibers are found. The epithelium is cuboid to columnar and pale in color, with the cytoplasm containing mucigen droplets and colloid spherules with acidophilic inclusions. The epithelium of the duct is simple in type, and its orifice is stratified squamous like the vestibule. The secretion is a clear, viscid, and stringy mucoid substance with an alkaline pH. Secretion is active during sexual activity. Nonetheless, after about age 30, the glands undergo involution and become atrophic and shrunken.

The arterial supply to the greater vestibular gland comes from a small branch of the artery on the bulbocavernosus muscle, penetrating deep into its substance. Venous drainage coincides with the drainage of the bulbocavernosus body. The lymphatics drain directly into the lymphatics of the vestibular plexus, having access to the posterior vaginal wall along the inferior hemorrhoidal channels. They also drain via the perineum into the inguinal area. Most of this minor drainage is along the pudendal vessels in the canalis pudendalis and explains, in part, the difficulty in dealing with cancer involving the gland.

The greater vestibular gland is homologous to the bulbourethral gland (also known as Cowper's glands, Duverney's glands, Tiedemann's glands, or the Bartholin glands of the male). The innervation of the greater vestibular gland is from a small branch of the perineal nerve, which penetrates directly into its substance.

## Muscles of External Genitalia

The muscles (Fig 2–13) of the external genitalia and cavernous bodies in the female are homologous to those of the male, although they are less well developed.

**A. Bulbocavernosus Muscle:** The bulbocavernosus muscle and deeper bulbus vestibuli or cavernous tissue arise in the midline from the posterior part of the central tendon of the perineum, where each opposes the fibers from the opposite side. Each ascends around the vagina, enveloping the bulbus vestibuli (the corpus cavernosum bodies of the male) to terminate in 3 heads: (1) the fibrous tissue dorsal to the clitoris, (2) the tunica fibrosa of the corpus cavernosa overlying the crura of the clitoris, and (3) decussating fibers that join those of the ischiocavernosus to form the striated sphincter of the urethra at the junction of its mid and lower thirds. The blood supply is derived from the perineal branch of the internal pudendal artery as it arises in the anterior part of the ischiorectal fossa. Deep to the fascia diaphragmatis urogenitalis inferior (Colles' fascia) and crossing between the ischiocavernosus and bulbo

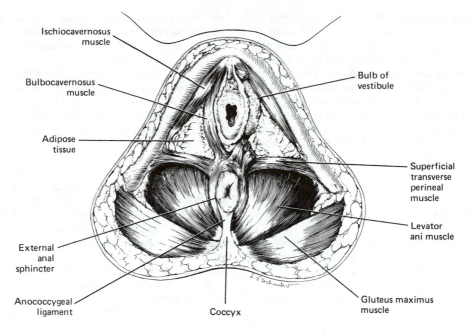

**Figure 2–13.** Pelvic musculature (inferior view).

cavernosus muscles, the pudendal artery sends 1–2 branches directly into the bulbocavernosus muscle and vestibular body, continuing anteriorly to terminate in the dorsal artery of the clitoris. The venous drainage accompanies the pudendal plexus. In addition, it passes posteriorly with the inferior hemorrhoidal veins and laterally with the perineal vein, a branch of the internal pudendal vein. The lymphatics run primarily with those of the vestibular plexus, with drainage inferiorly toward the intercalated nodes of the rectum and anteriorly and laterally with the labia minora and majora to the superficial inguinal nodes. Contralateral drainage in the upper portion of the muscle and body is evident.

**B. Ischiocavernosus Muscle:** The ischiocavernosus muscle and its attendant cavernous tissue arise from the ischial tuberosity and inferior ramus to the ischium. It envelops the crus of its cavernous tissue in a thin layer of muscle ascending toward and over the medial and inferior surfaces of the symphysis pubica to terminate in the anterior surface of the symphysis at the base of the clitoris. It then sends decussating fibers to the region of the upper and middle thirds of the urethra, forming the greater part of the organ's voluntary sphincter. The blood supply is through perforating branches from the perineal artery as it ascends between the bulbocavernosus and ischiocavernosus muscles to terminate as the dorsal artery of the clitoris. The innervation stems from an ischiocavernosus branch of the perineal division of the pudendal nerve.

**C. Transversus Muscle:** The transversus perinei superficialis muscle arises from the inferior ramus of the ischium and from the ischial tuberosity. The fibers of the muscle extend across the perineum and are inserted into its central tendon, meeting those from the opposite side. Frequently, the muscle fibers from the bulbocavernosus, the puborectalis, the superficial transverse perinei, and occasionally the external anal sphincter will interdigitate. The blood supply is from a perforating branch of the perineal division of the internal pudendal artery, and the nerve supply is from the perineal division of the pudendal nerve.

**D. Sensory Corpuscles:** In the cavernous substances of both the bulbocavernosus and ischiocavernosus muscles. Vater-Pacini corpuscles (corpuscula lamellosa) and Dogiel and Krause corpuscles (corpuscula bulboidea) are present.

**E. Inferior Layer of Urogenital Diaphragm:** The inferior layer of urogenital diaphragm is a potential space depending upon the size and development of the musculature, the parity of the female, and the pelvic architecture. It contains loose areolar connective tissue interspersed with fat. The bulbocavernosus muscles, with the support of the superficial transverse perinei muscles and the puborectalis muscles, act as a point of fixation on each side for support of the vulva, the external genitalia, and the vagina.

**F. Surgical Considerations:** A midline perineotomy is most effective to minimize trauma to vital supports of the vulva, bulbocavernosus, and superficial transverse perinei muscles. Overdistention of the vagina caused by the presenting part and body of the infant forms a temporary sacculation. If distention occurs too rapidly or if dilatation is beyond the resilient capacity of the vagina, rupture of the vaginal musculature may occur, often demonstrated by a cuneiform groove on the anterior wall and a tonguelike protrusion on the posterior wall of the vagina. Therefore, return of the vagina and vulva to the nonpregnant state is dependent upon the tonus of the muscle and the degree of distention of the vagina during parturition.

## BONY PELVIS

The pelvis (Fig 2–14) is a basin-shaped ring of bones that marks the distal margin of the trunk. The pelvis rests upon the lower extremities and supports the spinal column. It is composed of 2 innominate bones, one on each side, joined anteriorly and articulated with the sacrum posteriorly. The 2 major pelvic divisions are the pelvis major (upper or false pelvis) and the pelvis minor (lower or true pelvis). The pelvis major consists primarily of the space superior to the iliopectineal line, including the 2 iliac fossae and the region between them. The pelvis minor, located below the iliopectineal line, is bounded anteriorly by the pubic bones, posteriorly by the sacrum and coccyx, and laterally by the ischium and a small segment of the ilium.

### Innominate Bone

The innominate bone is composed of 3 parts: ilium, ischium, and pubis.

**A. Ilium:** The ilium consists of a bladelike upper part or ala (wing) and a thicker, lower part called the body. The body forms the upper portion of the acetabulum and unites with the bodies of the ischium and pubis. The medial surface of the ilium presents as a large concave area: The anterior portion is the iliac fossa; the smaller posterior portion is composed of a rough upper part, the iliac tuberosity; and the lower part contains a large surface for articulation with the sacrum. At the inferior medial margin of the iliac fossa, a rounded ridge, the arcuate line, ends anteriorly in the iliopectineal eminence. Posteriorly, the arcuate line is continuous with the anterior margin of the ala of the sacrum across the anterior aspect of the sacroiliac joint. Anteriorly, it is continuous with the ridge or pecten on the superior ramus of the pubis. The lateral surface or dorsum of the ilium is traversed by 3 ridges: the posterior, anterior, and inferior gluteal lines. The superior border is called the crest, and at its 2 extremities are the anterior and posterior superior iliac spines. The principal feature of the anterior border of the ilium is the heavy anterior inferior iliac spine. Important aspects of the posterior border are the posterior superior and the inferior iliac spines

and, below the the latter, the greater sciatic notch, the inferior part of which is bounded by the ischium. The inferior border of the ilium participates in the formation of the acetabulum.

The main vasculature (Fig 2–15) of the innominate bone appears where the bone is thickest. Blood is supplied to the inner surface of the ilium through twigs of the iliolumbar, deep circumflex iliac, and obturator arteries by foramens on the crest, in the iliac fossa, and below the terminal line near the greater sciatic notch. The outer surface of the ilium is supplied mainly below the inferior gluteal line through nutrient vessels derived from the gluteal arteries. The inferior branch of the deep part of the superior gluteal artery forms the external nutrient artery of the ilium and continues in its course to anastomose with the lateral circumflex artery. Upon leaving the pelvis below the piriform muscle, it divides into a number of branches, a group of which passes to the hip joint.

**B. Ischium:** The ischium is composed of a body, superior and inferior rami, and a tuberosity. The body is the heaviest part of the bone and is joined with the bodies of the ilium and pubis to form the acetabulum. It presents 3 surfaces: (1) The smooth internal surface is continuous above with the body of the ilium and below with the inner surface of the superior ramus of the ischium. Together, these parts form the posterior portion of the lateral wall of the pelvis minor. (2) The external surface of the ischium is the portion that enters into the formation of the acetabulum. (3) The posterior surface is the area between the acetabular rim and the posterior border. It is convex and is separated from the ischial tuberosity by a wide groove. The posterior border, with the ilium, forms the bony margin of the greater sciatic notch. The superior ramus of the ischium descends from the body of the bone to join the inferior ramus at an angle of approximately 90 degrees. The large ischial tuberosity and its inferior portion are situated on the convexity of this angle. The inferior portion of the tuberosity forms the point of support in the sitting position. The posterior surface is divided into 2 areas by an oblique line. The lesser sciatic notch occupies the posterior border of the superior ramus between the spine and the tuberosity. The inferior ramus, as it is traced forward, joins the inferior ramus of the pubis to form the arcus pubis (ischiopubic arch).

The ischium is supplied with blood from the obturator medial and lateral circumflex arteries. The largest vessels are situated between the acetabulum and the sciatic tubercle.

**C. Pubis:** The pubis is composed of a body and 2 rami, superior and inferior. The body contributes to the formation of the acetabulum, joining with the body of the ilium at the iliopectineal eminence and with the body of the ischium in the region of the acetabular notch. The superior ramus passes medially and forward from the body to meet the corresponding

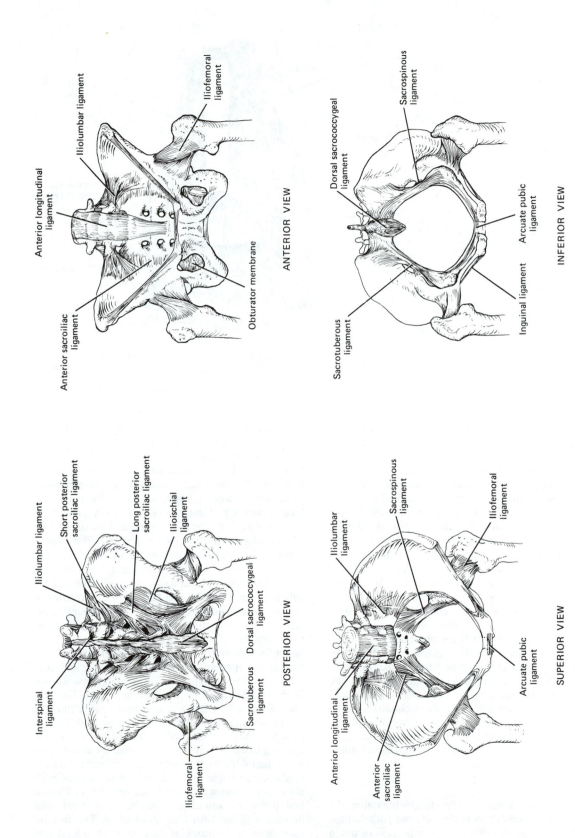

**Figure 2–14.** The bony pelvis. (Reproduced, with permission, from Benson RC: *Handbook of Obstetrics & Gynecology*, 8th ed. Lange, 1983.)

23

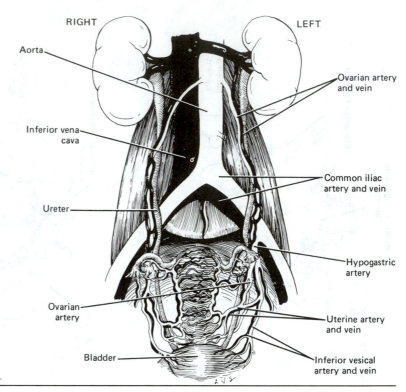

RIGHT                                    LEFT

Aorta

Ovarian artery and vein

Inferior vena cava

Common iliac artery and vein

Ureter

Hypogastric artery

Ovarian artery

Uterine artery and vein

Bladder

Inferior vesical artery and vein

**Figure 2–15.** Blood supply to pelvis.

ramus of the opposite side at the symphysis pubica. The medial or fore portion of the superior ramus is broad and flattened anteroposteriorly. Formerly called "the body," it presents an outer and an inner surface, the symphyseal area, and an upper border or "crest." Approximately 2 cm from the medial edge of the ramus and in line with the upper border is the prominent pubic tubercle, an important landmark. Below the crest is the anterior surface and the posterior or deep surface. The medial portion of the superior ramus is continuous below with the inferior ramus, and the lateral part presents a wide, smooth area anterosuperiorly, behind which is an irregular ridge, the pecten ossispubis. The pecten pubis forms the anterior part of the linea terminalis. In front of and below the pectineal area is the obturator crest, passing from the tubercle to the acetabular notch. On the inferior aspect of the superior ramus is the obturator sulcus. The inferior ramus is continuous with the superior ramus and passes downward and backward to join the inferior ramus of the ischium, forming the "ischiopubic arch." The pubis receives blood from the pubic branches of the obturator artery and from branches of the medial and lateral circumflex arteries.

## Sacrum

The sacrum is formed in the adult by the union of 5 or 6 sacral vertebrae; occasionally, the fifth lumbar vertebra is partly fused with it. The process of union

is known as "sacralization" in the vertebral column. The sacrum constitutes the base of the vertebral column. As a single bone, it is considered to have a base, an apex, 2 surfaces (pelvic and dorsal), and 2 lateral portions. The base faces upward and is composed principally of a central part, formed by the upper surface of the body of the first sacral vertebra, and 2 lateral areas of alae. The body articulates by means of a fibrocartilage disk with the body of the fifth lumbar vertebra. The alae represent the heavy transverse processes of the first sacral vertebra that articulate with the 2 iliac bones. The anterior margin of the body is called the promontory and forms the sacrovertebral angle with the fifth lumbar vertebra. The rounded anterior margin of each ala constitutes the posterior part (pars sacralis) of the linea terminalis. The pelvic surface of the sacrum is rough and convex. In the midline is the median sacral crest (fused spinal processes), and on either side is a flattened area formed by the fused laminae of the sacral vertebrae. The laminae of the fifth vertebra and, in many cases, those of the fourth and occasionally of the third are incomplete (the spines also are absent), thus leaving a wide opening to the dorsal wall of the sacral canal known as the sacral hiatus. Lateral to the laminae are the articular crests (right and left), which are in line with the paired superior articular processes above. The lateral processes articulate with the inferior articular processes of the fifth lumbar vertebra. The inferior extensions of the articular crests form the sacral cornua that bind the sacral hiatus laterally and are attached to the cornua of the coccyx. The cornua can be palpated in life and are important landmarks indicating the inferior opening of the sacral canal (for sacral-caudal anesthesia). The lateral portions of the sacrum are formed by the fusion of the transverse processes of the sacral vertebrae. They form dorsally a line of elevations called the lateral sacral crests. The parts corresponding to the first 3 vertebrae are particularly massive and present a large area facing laterally called the articular surface, which articulates with the sacrum. Posterior to the articular area, the rough bone is called the sacral tuberosity. It faces the tuberosity of the ilium. The apex is the small area formed by the lower surface of the body of the fifth part of the sacrum. The coccyx is formed by 4 (occasionally 3 or 5) caudal or coccygeal vertebrae. The second, third, and fourth parts are frequently fused into a single bone that articulates with the first by means of a fibrocartilage. The entire coccyx may become ossified and fused with the sacrum (the sacrococcygeal joint).

The sacrum receives its blood supply from the middle sacral artery, which extends from the bifurcation of the aorta to the tip of the coccyx, and from the lateral sacral arteries that branch either as a single artery that immediately divides or as 2 distinct vessels from the hypogastric artery. The lowest lumbar branch of the middle sacral artery ramifies over the lateral parts of the sacrum, passing back between the last vertebra and the sacrum to anastomose with the lumbar arteries above and the superior gluteal artery below. The lateral sacral branches (usually 4) anastomose anteriorly to the coccyx with branches of the inferior lateral sacral artery that branch from the hypogastric artery. They give off small spinal branches that pass through the sacral foramens and supply the sacral canal and posterior portion of the sacrum.

## Sacroiliac Joint

The sacroiliac joint is a diarthrodial joint with irregular surfaces. The articular surfaces are covered with a layer of cartilage, and the cavity of the joint is a narrow cleft. The cartilage on the sacrum is hyaline in its deeper parts but much thicker than that on the ilium. A joint capsule is attached to the margins of the articular surfaces, and the bones are held together by the anterior sacroiliac, long and short posterior sacroiliac, and interosseous ligaments. In addition, there are 3 ligaments (Fig 2–16), classed as belonging to the pelvic girdle itself, which also serve as accessory ligaments to the sacroiliac joint: the iliolumbar, sacrotuberous, and sacrospinous ligaments. The anterior sacroiliac ligaments unite the base and the lateral part of the sacrum to the ilium, blending with the periosteum of the pelvic surface and, on the ilium, reaching the arcuate line to attach in the paraglenoid grooves. The posterior sacroiliac ligament is extremely strong and consists essentially of 2 sets of fibers, deep and superficial, forming the short and long

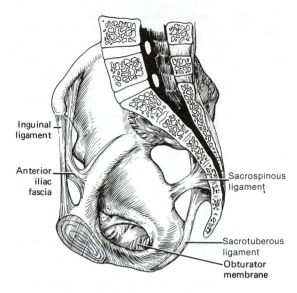

**Figure 2–16.** Ligaments of the pelvis.

posterior sacroiliac ligaments, respectively. The short posterior sacroiliac ligament passes inferiorly and medially from the tuberosity of the ilium, behind the articular surface and posterior interior iliac spine, to the back of the lateral portion of the sacrum and to the upper sacral articular process, including the area between it and the first sacral foramen. The long posterior sacroiliac ligament passes inferiorly from the posterior superior iliac spine to the second, third, and fourth articular tubercles on the back of the sacrum. It partly covers the short ligament and is continuous below with the sacrotuberous ligament. The interosseous ligaments are the strongest of all and consist of fibers of different lengths passing in various directions between the 2 bones. They extend from the rough surface of the sacral tuberosity to the corresponding surface on the lateral aspect of the sacrum, above and behind the articular surface.

## Ligaments

The sacrotuberous ligament, in common with the long posterior sacroiliac ligament, is attached above to the crest of the ilium and posterior iliac spines and to the posterior aspect of the lower 3 sacral vertebrae. Below, it is attached chiefly to the medial border of the ischial tuberosity. Some of the fibers at the other end extend forward along the inner surface of the ischial ramus, forming the falciform process. Other posterior fibers continue into the tendons of the hamstrings.

The sacrospinous ligament is triangular and thin, extending from the lateral border of the sacrum and coccyx to the spine of the ischium. It passes medially (deep) to the sacrotuberous ligament and is partly blended with it along the lateral border of the sacrum.

The iliolumbar ligament connects the fourth and

fifth lumbar vertebrae with the iliac crest. It originates from the transverse process of the fifth lumbar vertebra, where it is closely woven with the sacrolumbar ligament. Some of its fibers spread downward onto the body of the fifth vertebra and others ascend to the disk above. It is attached to the inner lip of the crest of the ilium for approximately 5 cm. The sacrolumbar ligament is generally inseparable from the iliolumbar ligament and is regarded as part of it.

## Pubic Symphysis

The pubic symphysis is a synarthrodial joint of the symphyseal surfaces of the pubic bones. The ligaments associated with it are (1) the interpubic fibrocartilage, (2) the superior pubic ligament, (3) the anterior pubic ligament, and (4) the arcuate ligament. The interpubic fibrocartilage is thicker in front than behind and projects beyond the edges of the bones, especially on the posterior aspect, blending intimately with the ligaments at its margins. Sometimes it is woven throughout, but often the interpubic fibrocartilage presents an elongated, narrow fissure with fluid in the interspace, partially dividing the cartilage into 2 plates. The interpubic cartilage is intimately adherent to the layer of hyaline cartilage that covers the symphyseal surface of each pubic bone. The superior pubic ligament extends laterally along the crest of the pubis on each side to the pubic tubercle, blending in the middle line with the interpubic cartilage. The thick and strong anterior pubic ligament is closely connected with the fascial covering of the muscles arising from the conjoined rami of the pubis. It consists of several strata of thick, decussating fibers of different degrees of obliquity, the superficial being the most oblique and extending lowest over the joint. The arcuate ligament is a thick band of closely connected fibers that fills the angle between the pubic rami to form a smooth, rounded top to the pubic arch. Both on the anterior and posterior aspects of the joint, the ligament gives off decussating fibers that, interlacing with one another, strengthen the joint.

## Hip Joint

The hip joint is a typical example of a ball-and-socket joint, the round head of the femur received by the deep cavity of the acetabulum and glenoid lip. Both articular surfaces are coated with cartilage. The portion covering the head of the femur is thicker above, where it bears the weight of the body, and thins out to a mere edge below. The pit in the femoral head receives the ligamentum teres, the only part uncoated by cartilage. The cartilage is horseshoe-shaped on the acetabulum and, corresponding to the lunate surface, thicker above than below. The ligaments are the articular capsule, transverse acetabular ligament, iliofemoral ligament, ischiocapsular ligament and zona orbicularis, pubocapsular ligament, and ligamentum teres.

**A. Articular Capsule:** The articular capsule is one of the strongest ligaments in the body. It is attached superiorly to the base of the anterior inferior iliac spine at the pelvis, posteriorly to a point a few millimeters from the acetabular rim, and inferiorly to the upper edge of the groove between the acetabulum and tuberosity of the ischium. Anteriorly, it is secured to the pubis near the obturator groove, to the iliopectineal eminence, and posteriorly to the base of the inferior iliac spine. At the femur, the articular capsule is fixed to the anterior portion of the superior border of the greater trochanter and to the cervical tubercle. The capsule runs down the intertrochanteric line as far as the medial aspect of the femur, where it is on a level with the inferior part of the lesser trochanter. It then runs superiorly and posteriorly along an oblique line, just in front of and above the lesser trochanter, and continues along the back of the neck of the femur nearly parallel to and above the intertrochanteric crest. Finally, the capsule passes along the medial side of the trochanteric fossa to reach the anterior superior angle of the greater trochanter. Some of the deeper fibers, the retinacula, are attached nearer the head of the femur. One corresponds to the upper and another to the lower part of the intertrochanteric line; a third is present at the upper and back part of the trochanteric neck.

**B. Transverse Acetabular Ligament:** The transverse ligament of the acetabulum passes across the acetabular notch. It supports the glenoid lip and is connected with the ligamentum teres and the capsule. The transverse ligament is composed of decussating fibers that arise from the margin of the acetabulum on either side of the notch. Those fibers coming from the pubis are more superficial and pass to form the deep part of the ligament at the ischium; those superficial at the ischium are deep at the pubis.

**C. Iliofemoral Ligament:** The iliofemoral ligament is located at the front of the articular capsule and is triangular. Its apex is attached to a curved line on the ilium immediately below and behind the anterior inferior spine; its base is fixed beneath the anterior edge of the greater trochanter and to the intertrochanteric line. The upper fibers are almost straight, while the medial fibers are oblique, giving the appearance of an inverted Y.

**D. Ischiocapsular Ligament:** The ischiocapsular ligament, on the posterior surface of the articular capsule, is attached to the body of the ischium along the upper border of the notch. Above the notch, the ligament is secured to the ischial margin of the acetabulum. The upper fibers incline superiorly and laterally and are fixed to the greater trochanter. The other fibers curve more and more upward as they pass laterally to their insertion at the inner side of the trochanteric fossa. The deeper fibers take a circular course and form a ring at the back and lower parts of the capsule, where the longitudinal fibers are deficient. This ring, the zona orbicularis, embraces the neck of the femur.

**E. Pubocapsular Ligament:** The pubocapsular ligament is fixed proximally to the obturator crest and to the anterior border of the iliopectineal eminence, reaching as far down as the pubic end of the acetabular notch. Below, the fibers reach to the neck of the femur and are fixed above and behind the lowermost fibers of the iliofemoral band, blending with it.

**F. Ligamentum Teres:** The ligamentum teres femoris extends from the acetabular fossa to the head of the femur. It has 2 bony attachments, one on either side of the acetabular notch immediately below the articular cartilage, with intermediate fibers springing from the lower surface of the transverse ligament. At the femur, the ligamentum teres femoris is fixed to the anterior part of the fovea capitis and to the cartilage around the margin of the depression.

### Outlets of the True Pelvis

The true pelvis is said to have an upper "inlet" and a lower "outlet." The pelvic inlet to the pelvis minor is bounded, beginning posteriorly, by (1) the promontory of the sacrum; (2) the linea terminalis, composed of the anterior margin of the alasacralis, the arcuate line of the ilium, and the pecten ossis pubis; and (3) the upper border or crest of the pubis, ending medially at the symphysis. The conjugate or the anteroposterior diameter is drawn from the center of the promontory to the symphysis pubica, with 2 conjugates recognized: (1) the true conjugate, measured from the promontory to the top of the symphysis, and (2) the diagonal conjugate, measured from the promontory to the bottom of the symphysis. The transverse diameter is measured through the greatest width of the pelvic inlet. The oblique diameter runs from the sacroiliac joint of one side to the iliopectineal eminence of the other. The pelvic outlet, which faces downward and slightly backward, is very irregular. Beginning anteriorly, it is bounded by (1) the arcuate ligament of the pubis (in the midline), (2) the ischiopubic arch, (3) the ischial tuberosity, (4) the sacrotuberous ligament, and (5) the coccyx (in midline). Its anteroposterior diameter is drawn from the lower border of the symphysis pubica to the tip of the coccyx. The transverse diameter passes between the medial surfaces of the ischial tuberosities.

### Musculature Attachments

**A. Ilium:** The crest of the ilium gives attachment to the external oblique, internal oblique, transversus (anterior two-thirds), latissimus dorsi and quadratus lumborum (posteriorly), sacrospinalis (internal lip, posteriorly), and tensor fasciae latae and sartorius muscles (anterior superior iliac spine) (Fig 2–17). The posterior superior spine of the ilium gives attachment to the multifidus muscle. The rectus femoris muscle is attached to the anterior inferior iliac spine. The iliacus muscle originates on the iliac fossa. Between the anterior inferior iliac spine and the iliopectineal eminence is a broad groove for the tendon of the iliopsoas muscle. A small portion of the gluteus maximus muscle originates between the pos-

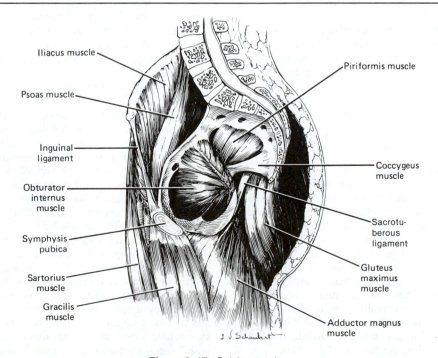

**Figure 2–17.** Pelvic muscles.

terior gluteus line and the crest. The surface of bone between the anterior gluteal line and the crest gives origin to the gluteus medius muscle. The gluteus minimus muscle has its origin between the anterior and inferior gluteal lines.

**B. Ischium:** The body and superior ramus of the ischium give rise to the obturator internus muscle on the internal surface. The ischial spine provides, at its root, attachments for the coccygeus and levator ani muscles on its internal surface and for the gemellus superior muscle externally. The outer surface of the ram is the origin of the adductor magnus and obturator externus muscles. The transversus perinei muscle is attached to the lower border of the ischium. The ischial tuberosity gives rise on its posterior surface to the semimembranosus muscles, the common tendon of the biceps, and semitendinosus muscles and on its inferior surface to the adductor magnus muscle. The superior border is the site of origin of the inferior gemellus and the outer border of the quadratus femoris muscle. The superior ramus of the pubis gives origin to the adductor longus and obturator externus muscles on its anterior surface and to the levator ani and obturator internus muscles. The superior border provides attachment for the rectus abdominis and pyramidalis muscles. The pectineal surface gives origin at its posterior portion to the pectineus muscle. The posterior surface of the superior ramus is the point of attachment of a few fascicles of the obturator internus muscle. The anterior surface of the inferior ramus attaches to the abductor brevis, adductor magnus, and obturator externus muscles, and its posterior surface attaches to the sphincter urogenitalis and the obturator internus.

**C. Sacrum:** The pelvic surface of the sacrum is the origin of the piriform muscle. The lateral part of the fifth sacral vertebra is the point of insertion of the sacrospinalis and gluteus maximus muscles. The ala is attached to fibers of the iliacus muscle.

**D. Coccyx:** The dorsal surface of the coccyx is attached to the gluteus maximus muscle and the sphincter ani externus muscle. The lateral margins receive parts of the coccygeus and of the iliococcygeus muscles.

**E. Greater Trochanter:** The lateral surface of the greater trochanter of the femur receives the insertion of the gluteus medius muscle. The medial surface of the greater trochanter receives the tendon of the obturator externus in the trochanteric fossa, along with the obturator internus and the 2 gemelli. The superior border provides insertion for the piriformis and, with the anterior border, receives the gluteus minimus. The quadratus femoris attaches to the tubercle of the quadratus. The inferior border gives origin to the vastus lateralis muscle. The lesser trochanter attaches to the iliopsoas muscle at its summit. Fascicles of the iliacus extend beyond the trochanter and are inserted into the surface of the shaft.

### Foramens

Several foramens are present in the bony pelvis. The sacrospinous ligament separates the greater from the lesser sciatic foramen. These foramens are subdivisions of a large space intervening between the sacrotuberous ligament and the femur. The piriform muscle passes out of the pelvis into the thigh by way of the greater sciatic foramen, accompanied by the gluteal vessels and nerves. The internal pudendal vessels, the pudendal nerve, and the nerve to the obturator internus muscle also leave the pelvis by this foramen, after which they then enter the perineal region through the lesser sciatic foramen. The obturator internus muscle passes out of the pelvis by way of the lesser sciatic foramen.

The obturator foramen is situated between the ischium and the pubis. The obturator membrane occupies the obturator foramen and is attached continuously to the inner surface of the bony margin except above, where it bridges the obturator sulcus, converting the latter into the obturator canal, which provides passage for the obturator nerve and vessels.

On either side of the central part of the pelvic surface of the sacrum are 4 anterior sacral foramens that transmit the first 4 sacral nerves. Corresponding to these on the dorsal surface are the 4 posterior sacral foramens for transmission of the small posterior rami of the first 4 sacral nerves.

### Types of Pelves

Evaluation of the pelvis is best achieved by using the criteria set by Caldwell and Moloy, which are predicated upon 4 basic types of pelves: (1) the gynecoid type (from Greek gyne woman); (2) the android type (from Greek aner man); (3) the anthropoid type (from Greek anthropos human); and (4) the platypelloid type (from Greek platys broad and pella bowl) (Fig 2–18).

**A. Gynecoid:** In pure form, the gynecoid pelvis provides a rounded, slightly ovoid, or elliptical inlet with a well-rounded forepelvis (anterior segment). This type of pelvis has a well-rounded, spacious posterior segment, an adequate sacrosciatic notch, a hollow sacrum with a somewhat backward sacral inclination, and a Norman-type arch of the pubic rami. The gynecoid pelvis has straight side walls and wide interspinous and intertuberous diameters. The bones are primarily of medium weight and structure.

**B. Android:** The android pelvis has a wedge-shaped inlet, a narrow forepelvis, a flat posterior segment, and a narrow sacrosciatic notch, with the sacrum inclining forward. The side walls converge, and the bones are medium to heavy in structure.

**C. Anthropoid:** The anthropoid pelvis is characterized by a long, narrow, oval inlet, an extended and narrow anterior and posterior segment, a wide sacrosciatic notch, and a long, narrow sacrum, often with 6 sacral segments. The subpubic arch may be an

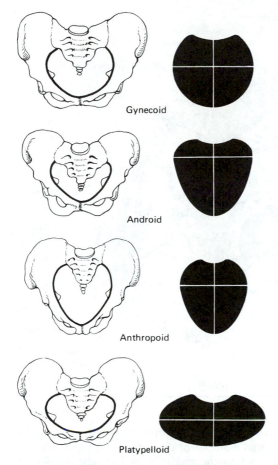

**Figure 2–18.** Types of pelves. White lines in the diagrams at right (after Steele) show the greatest diameters of the pelves at left. (Reproduced, with permission, from Benson RC. *Handbook of Obstetrics & Gynecology*, 8th ed. Lange, 1983.)

angled Gothic type or rounded Norman type. Straight side walls are characteristic of the anthropoid pelvis, whose interspinous and intertuberous diameters are less than those of the average gynecoid pelvis. A medium bone structure is usual.

**D. Platypelloid:** The platypelloid pelvis has a distinct oval inlet with a very wide, rounded retro pubic angle and a wider, flat posterior segment. The sacrosciatic notch is narrow and has a normal sacral inclination, although it is often short. The subpubic arch is very wide and the side walls are straight, with wide interspinous and intertuberous diameters.

The pelvis in any individual case may be one of the 4 "pure" types or a combination of mixed types. When one discusses the intermediate pelvic forms, the posterior segment with its characteristics generally is described first and the anterior segment with its characteristics next, eg, anthropoid-gynecoid, an-droid-anthropoid, or platypelloid-gynecoid. Obviously, it is impossible to have a platypelloid-anthropoid pelvis or a platypelloid-android pelvis.

## Pelvic Relationships

Several important relationships should be remembered, beginning with those at the inlet of the pelvis. The transverse diameter of the inlet is the widest diameter, where bone is present for a circumference of 360 degrees. This diameter stretches from pectineal line to pectineal line and denotes the separation of the posterior and anterior segments of the pelvis. In classic pelves (gynecoid), a vertical plane dropped from the transverse diameter of the inlet passes through the level of the interspinous diameter at the ischial spine. These relationships may not hold true, however, in combination or intermediate (mixed type) pelves. The anterior transverse diameter of the inlet reaches from pectineal prominence to pectineal prominence; a vertical plane dropped from the anterior transverse passes through the ischial tuberosities. For good function of the pelvis, the anterior transverse diameter should never be more than 2 cm longer than the transverse diameter (Fig 2–19).

**A. Obstetric Conjugate:** The obstetric conjugate differs from both the diagonal conjugate and the true conjugate. It is represented by a line drawn from the posterior superior portion of the pubic symphysis (where bone exists for a circumference of 360 degrees) toward intersection with the sacrum. This point need not be at the promontory of the sacrum. The obstetric conjugate is divided into 2 segments: (1) the anterior sagittal, originating at the intersection of the obstetric conjugate with the transverse diameter of the inlet and terminating at the symphysis pubica, and (2) the posterior sagittal, originating at the transverse diameter of the inlet to the point of intersection with the sacrum.

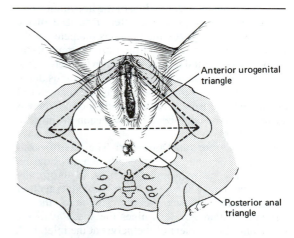

**Figure 2–19.** Urogenital and anal triangles.

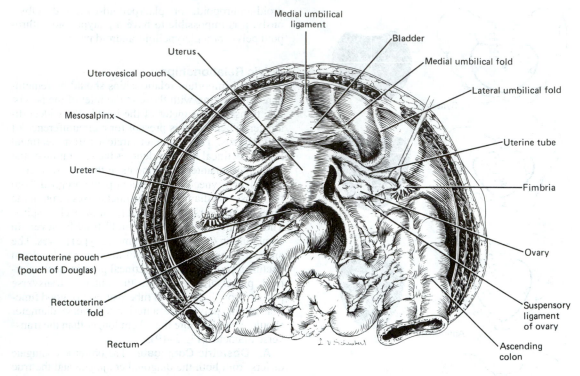

**Figure 2–20.** Female pelvic contents from above.

**B. Interspinous Diameter:** A most significant diameter in the midpelvis is the interspinous diameter. It is represented by a plane passing from ischial spine to ischial spine. The posterior sagittal diameter of the midpelvis is a bisecting line drawn at a right angle from the middle of the interspinous diameter, in the same plane, to a point of intersection with the sacrum. This is the point of greatest importance in the mid pelvis. It is sometimes said that the posterior sagittal diameter should be drawn from the posterior segment of the intersecting line of the interspinous diameter, in a plane from the inferior surface of the symphysis, through the interspinous diameter to the sacrum. However, this configuration often places the posterior sagittal diameter lower in the pelvis than the interspinous diameter. It is the interspinous diameter, together with the posterior sagittal diameter of the mid pelvis, that determines whether or not there is adequate room for descent and extension of the head during labor.

**C. Intertuberous Diameter:** The intertuberous diameter of the outlet will reflect the length of the anterior transverse diameter of the inlet, ie, the former cannot be larger than the latter if convergent or straight side walls are present. Therefore, the intertuberous diameter determines the space available in the anterior segment of the pelvis at the inlet, and, similarly, the degree of convergence influences the length of the biparietal diameter at the outlet.

**D. Posterior Sagittal Diameter:** The posterior sagittal diameter of the outlet is an intersecting line drawn from the middle of the intertuberous diameter to the sacrococcygeal junction and reflects the inclination of the sacrum toward the outlet for accommodation of the head at delivery. It should be noted that intricate measurements of the pelvis are significant only at minimal levels. Evaluation of the pelvis for a given pregnancy, size of the fetus for a given pelvis, and conduct of labor engagement are far more important.

## CONTENTS OF THE PELVIC CAVITY

The organs that occupy the female pelvis (Figs 2–20 to 2–22) are the bladder, the ureters, the urethra, the uterus, the uterine (fallopian) tubes or oviducts, the ovaries, the vagina, and the rectum.* With the exception of the inferior portion of the rectum and most of the vagina, all lie immediately beneath the peritoneum. The uterus, uterine tubes, and ovaries are almost completely covered with peritoneum and are suspended in peritoneal ligaments. The remainder are partially covered. These organs do not completely fill the cavity; the remaining space is occupied by ileum and sigmoid colon.

---

*The rectum is not described in this chapter.

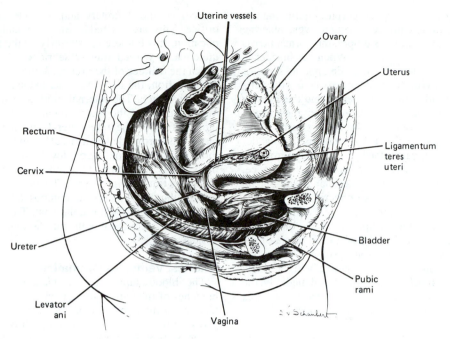

**Figure 2–21.** Pelvic viscera (sagittal view).

## 1. BLADDER

The urinary bladder is a muscular, hollow organ that lies posterior to the pubic bones and anterior to the uterus and broad ligament. Its form, size, and position vary with the amount of urine it contains. When empty, it takes the form of a somewhat rounded pyramid, having a base, a vertex (or apex), a superior sur-

face, and a convex inferior surface that may be divided by a median ridge into 2 inferolateral surfaces.

### Relationships

The superior surface of the bladder is covered with peritoneum that is continuous with the medial umbilical fold, forming the paravesical fossae laterally. Posteriorly, the peritoneum passes onto the uterus at

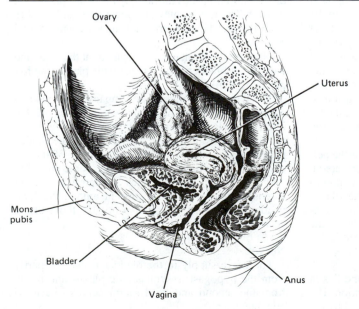

**Figure 2–22.** Pelvic organs (midsagittal view). (Reproduced, with permission, from Benson RC: *Handbook of Obstetrics & Gynecology,* 8th ed. Lange, 1983.)

the junction of the cervix and corpus, continuing upward on the anterior surface to form the vesicouterine pouch. When the bladder is empty, the normal uterus rests upon its superior surface. When the bladder is distended, coils of intestine may lie upon its superior surface. The base of the bladder rests below the peritoneum and is adjacent to the cervix and the anterior fornix of the vagina. It is separated from these structures by areolar tissue containing plexiform veins. The area over the vagina is extended as the bladder fills. The inferolateral surfaces are separated from the wall of the pelvis by the potential prevesical space, containing a small amount of areolar tissue but no large vessels. This surface is nonperitoneal and thus suitable for operative procedures. Posterolateral to the region facing the symphysis, each of the inferolateral surfaces is in relation to the fascia of the obturator internus, the obturator vessels and nerve, the obliterated umbilical artery above, and the fascia of the levator ani below. Posteriorly and medially, the inferior surface is separated from the base by an area called the urethrovesical junction, the most stationary portion of the bladder.

## Fascia, Ligaments, & Muscle

The bladder is enclosed by a thin layer of fascia, the vesical sheath. Two thickenings of the endopelvic fascia, the medial and lateral pubovesical or puboprostatic ligaments, extend at the vesicourethral junction abutting the levator ani muscle from the lower part of the anterior aspect of the bladder to the pubic bones. Similar fascial thickenings, the lateral true ligaments, extend from the sides of the lower part of the bladder to the lateral walls of the pelvis. Posteriorly, the vesicourethral junction of the bladder lies directly against the anterior wall of the vagina.

A fibrous band, the urachus or medial umbilical ligament extends from the apex of the bladder to the umbilicus. This band represents the remains of the embryonic allantois. The lateral umbilical ligaments are formed by the obliterated umbilical arteries and are represented by fibrous cords passing along the sides of the bladder and ascending toward the umbilicus. Frequently, the vessels will be patent, thus forming the superior vesical arteries. The peritoneal covering of the bladder is limited to the upper surface. The reflections of the peritoneum to the anterior abdominal wall and the corresponding walls of the pelvis are sometimes described as the superior, lateral, and posterior false ligaments. The muscle (smooth) of the bladder is represented by an interdigitated pattern continuous with and contiguous to the inner longitudinal and anterior circumferential muscles of the urethra. No distinct muscle layers are apparent.

## Mucous Membrane

The mucous membrane is rose-colored and lies in irregular folds that become effaced by distention. The 3 angles of the vesical trigone are represented by the orifices of the 2 ureters and the internal urethral orifice. This area is redder in color and free from plication. It is bordered posteriorly by the plica interureterica, a curved transverse ridge extending between the orifices of the ureters. A median longitudinal elevation, the uvula vesicae, extends toward the urethral orifice. The internal urethral orifice is normally situated at the lowest point of the bladder, at the junction of the inferolateral and posterior surfaces. It is surrounded by a circular elevation, the urethral annulus, approximately level with the center of the symphysis pubica. The epithelial lining of the bladder is transitional in type. The mucous membrane rests on the submucous coat, composed of areolar tissue superficial to the muscular coat. There is no evidence of a specific smooth muscle sphincter in the vesical neck.

## Arteries, Veins, & Lymphatics

The blood supply to the bladder comes from branches of the hypogastric artery. The umbilical artery, a terminal branch of the hypogastric artery, gives off the superior vesical artery prior to its obliterated portion. It approaches the bladder (along with the middle and inferior vesical arteries) through a condensation of fatty areolar tissue, limiting the prevesical "space" posterosuperiorly, to branch out over the upper surface of the bladder. It anastomoses with the arteries of the opposite side and the middle and inferior vesical arteries below. The middle vesical artery may arise from one of the superior vessels, or it may come from the umbilical artery, supplying the sides and base of the bladder. The inferior vesical artery usually arises directly from the hypogastric artery—in common with or as a branch of the uterine artery—and passes downward and medially, where it divides into branches that supply the lower part of the bladder. The fundus may also receive small branches from the middle hemorrhoidal, uterine, and vaginal arteries.

The veins form an extensive plexus at the sides and base of the bladder from which stems pass to the hypogastric trunk.

The lymphatics, in part, accompany the veins and communicate with the hypogastric nodes (Table 2–2). They also communicate laterally with the external iliac glands, and some of those from the fundus pass to nodes situated at the promontory of the sacrum. The lymphatics of the bladder dome are separate on the right and left sides and rarely cross; but extensive anastomoses are present among the lymphatics of the base, which also involve those of the cervix.

## Nerves

The nerve supply to the bladder is derived partly from the hypogastric sympathetic plexus and partly from the second and third sacral nerves (the nervi erigentes).

**Table 2-2.** Lymphatics of the female pelvis.

Perineum

A. Superficial Lymphatics:

Skin of abdomen (lateral) —————— Superficial nodes

Skin of abdomen (medial) —————— Superficial circumflex vein and nodes

*Frequent anastomoses*

Thigh (medial) and perineal skin ——— Superficial epigastric vein and nodes —————— Frequently cross to contralateral side

Thigh (lateral)

B. Deep Lymphatics:

Clitoral plexus

*Lymphatics through labia majora*

Superior vestibular plexus

Superior network of fourchette

Abdomen ————— To respective superficial inguinal nodes (10—20 along inguinal ligament) (under internal oblique fascia)

Inner rectum ————— Superficial subinguinal nodes (3—4)

Lateral thigh

Saphenous fossa —————— Femoral nodes (3—4); —— External iliac chain nodes in deep inguinal ring (nodi lymphatici inguinales profundi [nodes of Rosenmüller or Cloquet])

**Table 2-2 (cont'd).** Lymphatics of the female pelvis.

**Vagina**

Mucosal plexus
- Inferiorly —— Introitus Superficial vestibular plexus —— Superficial inguinal nodes —— Superficial subinguinal nodes —— Femoral external iliac chain
- Superiorly —— Anastomose with those of cervix (see below)

Muscular plexus
- Posterior wall (intertwine with those of rectum) —— Rectal stalk
- Laterally 4 trunks: 2 posterior trunks, 2 anterior trunks —— Upper part of vagina —— Hypogastrics / External iliac chain / Lateral sacral nodes

**Cervix**

Vaginal plexus —— Cervical plexus —— Uterine plexus: 3 trunks —— Lateral sacral nodes / Broad ligament, uterine pedicle —— Lumbar chain

Lower portion of corpus of uterus —— Isthmus (portio of cervix) —— External iliac chain

# Uterus

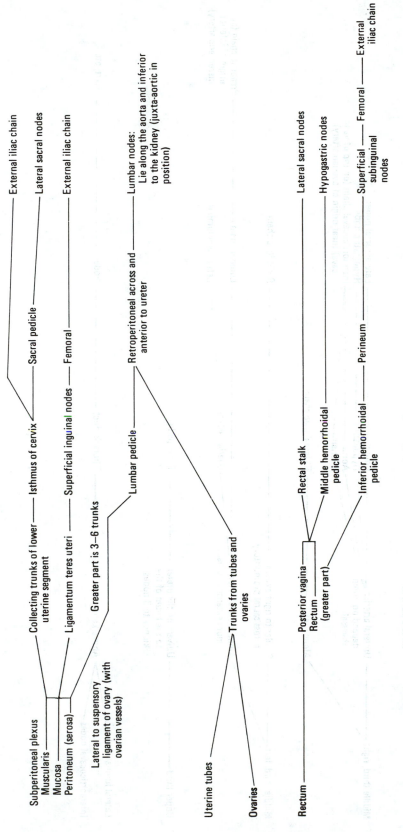

Subperitoneal plexus / Muscularis / Mucosa / Peritoneum (serosa) —— Collecting trunks of lower uterine segment —— Isthmus of cervix —— External iliac chain / Sacral pedicle —— Lateral sacral nodes

Ligamentum teres uteri —— Superficial inguinal nodes —— Femoral —— External iliac chain

Greater part is 3–6 trunks —— Lumbar pedicle —— Retroperitoneal across and anterior to ureter —— Lumbar nodes: Lie along the aorta and inferior to the kidney (juxta-aortic in position)

Lateral to suspensory ligament of ovary (with ovarian vessels)

Uterine tubes —— Trunks from tubes and ovaries

Ovaries

Rectum —— Posterior vagina / Rectum (greater part) —— Rectal stalk —— Lateral sacral nodes / Middle hemorrhoidal pedicle —— Hypogastric nodes / Inferior hemorrhoidal pedicle —— Perineum —— Superficial subinguinal nodes —— Femoral —— External iliac chain

(continued)

**Table 2-2 (cont'd).** Lymphatics of the female pelvis.

Ureters

Lower third
- Along hypogastric vessels —— Large nodes, sacral group on promonotory —— Periaortic chain
- Obliterated hypo-gastrics —— External iliac group (a node is often present on umbilical artery)
- Up the ureters to the middle portion —— Periaortic nodes interaortico-caval nodes

Middle third, right
- Ureteral arteries depend on origin of vessel —— Common iliac / Hypogastric / Aorta / Ovarian —— Lateral sacral nodes / Hypogastric node / Interaorticocaval chain (on top of vena cava) (near origin of ovarian artery)
- Along ureter —— External iliac chain

Middle third, left
- Similar to right except across sacral promontory —— Right iliac chain
- Along ureteral arteries (more extensive spread) —— Ovarian artery —— Lumbar chain / Left lateral lumbar —— Preaortic chain (at origin of inferior mesenteric artery)

Upper third
- Upward on the ureter to the hilum of the kidney to 3 nodes —— Renal pedicle

Lateral lumbar nodes
Interaorticocaval nodes
- Above kidney —— Thoracic duct —— Node —— Heart, etc

36

**Urethra**

Anterior urethra —— Vestibular plexus —— Superficial inguinal nodes —— Superficial subinguinal nodes —— Femoral —— External iliac chain

**Posterior urethra**

1. Anterior superior part —— Trunks —— Interior bladder wall —— Lateral inferior border of umbilical artery —— Middle chain, external iliacs

2. Anterolateral —— Trunks —— Lateral bladder wall —— Internal chain, external iliac group at the obturator nerve (obturator node)

   Posteriorly along internal pudental artery —— Hypogastrics at bifurcation of external and internal iliacs

   Ischiorectal fossa —— Canalis pudendalis (Alcock's canal) —— 3 nodes —— Greater sciatic foramen —— Along inferior gluteal artery —— Onto obturator artery —— Lateral sacral nodes, hypogastric nodes

3. Posterior aspect

   Urethrovaginal septum —— Cervix —— Uterine plexus —— Over ureter —— Along umbilical ligaments —— Lower uterine pedicle —— Middle chain, external iliac nodes, hypogastric nodes

**Bladder**

1. Anterior bladder wall —— (Laterally along umbilical ligaments) —— One trunk near ureter —— Nodes of posterior abdominal group

   Right and left sides remain separate

2. Posterior bladder wall

(Frequent anastomoses between cervix, vagina, and fundus; large vessels upper third, medium middle third, small lower third)

37

## 2. URETERS

### Relationships

The ureter is a slightly flattened tube that extends from the termination of the renal pelvis to the lower outer corner of the base of the bladder, a distance of 26–28 cm. It is partly abdominal and partly pelvic and lies entirely behind the peritoneum. Its diameter varies from 4 to 6 mm, depending on distention, and its size is uniform except for 3 slightly constricted portions. The first of these constrictions is found at the junction of the ureter with the renal pelvis and is known as the upper isthmus. The second constriction—the lower isthmus—is at the point where the ureter crosses the brim of the pelvis minor. The third (intramural) constriction is at the terminal part of the ureter as it passes through the bladder wall. The pelvic portion of the ureter begins as the ureter crosses the pelvic brim beneath the ovarian vessels and near the bifurcation of the common iliac artery. It conforms to the curvature of the lateral pelvic wall, inclining slightly laterally and posteriorly until it reaches the pelvic floor. The ureter then bends anteriorly and medially at about the level of the ischial spine to reach the bladder. In its upper portion, it is related posteriorly to the sacroiliac articulation; then, lying upon the obturator internus muscle and fascia, it crosses the root of the umbilical artery, the obturator vessels, and the obturator nerve. In its anterior relationship, the ureter emerges from behind the ovary and under its vessels to pass behind the uterine and superior and middle vesical arteries. Coursing anteriorly, it comes into close relation with the lateral fornix of the vagina, passing 8–12 mm from the cervix and vaginal wall before reaching the bladder. When the ureters reach the bladder, they are about 5 cm apart. They pass through the bladder wall on an oblique course (about 2 cm long) and in an anteromedial and downward direction. The ureters open into the bladder by 2 slitlike apertures, the urethral orifices, about 2.5 cm apart when the bladder is empty.

### Wall of Ureter

The wall of the ureter is approximately 3 mm thick and is composed of 3 coats: connective tissue, muscle, and mucous membrane. The muscular coat has an external circular and an internal longitudinal layer throughout its course and an external longitudinal layer in its lower third. The mucous membrane is longitudinally plicated and covered by transitional epithelium. The intermittent peristaltic action of the ureteral musculature propels urine into the bladder in jets. The oblique passage of the ureter through the bladder wall tends to constitute a valvular arrangement, but no true valve is present. The circular fibers of the intramural portion of the ureter possess a sphincter like action. Still, under some conditions of overdistention of the bladder, urine may be forced back into the ureter.

### Arteries, Veins, & Lymphatics

The pelvic portion of the ureter receives its blood supply from a direct branch of the hypogastric artery, anastomosing superiorly in its adventitia with branches from the iliolumbar and inferiorly with branches from the inferior vesical and middle hemorrhoidal arteries. Lymphatic drainage passes along the hypogastric vessels to the hypogastric and external iliac nodes, continuing up the ureters to their middle portion where drainage is directed to the periaortic and interaorticocaval nodes (Table 2–2).

### Nerves

The nerve supply is provided by the renal, ovarian, and hypogastric plexuses. The spinal level of the afferents is approximately the same as the kidney (T12, L1, L2). The lower third of the ureter receives sensory fibers and postganglionic parasympathetic fibers from the Frankenhauser plexus and sympathetic fibers through this plexus as it supplies the base of the bladder. These fibers ascend the lower third of the ureter, accompanying the arterial supply. The middle segment appears to receive postganglions of sympathetic and parasympathetic fibers through and from the middle hypogastric plexus. The upper third is supplied by the same innervation as the kidney.

## 3. URETHRA

### Relationships

The female urethra is a canal 2.5–5.25 cm long. It extends downward and forward in a curve from the neck of the bladder (internal urethral orifice), which lies nearly opposite the symphysis pubica. Its termination, the external urethral orifice, is situated inferiorly and posteriorly from the lower border of the symphysis. Posteriorly, it is closely applied to the anterior wall of the vagina, especially in the lower two-thirds, where it is actually integrated with the wall, forming the urethral carina. Anteriorly, the upper end is separated from the prevesical "space" by the pubovesical (pubo prostatic) ligaments, abutting against the levator ani and vagina and extending upward onto the pubic rami.

### Anatomy of Walls

The walls of the urethra are very distensible, composed of spongy fibromuscular tissue containing cavernous veins and lined by submucous and mucous coats. The mucosa contains numerous longitudinal lines when undistended, the most prominent of which is located on the posterior wall and termed the crista urethralis. Also, there are numerous small glands (the homologue of the male prostate, para- and periurethral glands of Astruc, ducts of Skene) that open into the urethra. The largest of these, the paraurethral glands of Skene, may open via a pair of ducts beside the external urethral orifice in the vestibule. The epithelium begins as transitional at the upper end and becomes squamous in the lower part. External to the urethral lumen is a smooth muscle coat composed of an outer circular layer and an inner longitudinal layer in the lower two-thirds. In the upper third, the muscle bundles of the layers interdigitate in a basketlike weave to become continuous with and contiguous to those of the bladder. The entire urethral circular smooth muscle acts as the involuntary sphincter. In the region of the juncture of the mid and lower thirds of the urethra, decussating fibers (striated in type) form the middle heads of the bulbo- and ischiocavernosus muscles and encircle the urethra to form the sphincter urethrae (voluntary sphincter).

### Arteries & Veins

The arterial supply is intimately involved with that of the anterior vaginal wall, with cruciate anastomoses to the bladder. On each side of the vagina are the vaginal arteries, originating in part from the coronary artery of the cervix, the inferior vesical artery, or a direct branch of the uterine artery. In the midline of the anterior vaginal wall is the azygos artery, originating from the coronary or circular artery of the cervix. Approximately 5 branches traverse the anterior vaginal wall from the lateral vaginal arteries to the azygos in the midline, with small sprigs supplying the urethra. A rich anastomosis with the introitus involves the clitoral artery (urethral branches) as the artery divides into the dorsal and superficial arteries of the clitoris, a terminal branch of the internal pudendal artery. The venous drainage follows the arterial pattern, although it is less well defined. In the upper portion of the vagina, it forms an extensive network called the plexus of Santorini (Table 2–3).

### Lymphatics

The lymphatics are richly developed (Fig 2–23). Those of the anterior urethra drain to the vestibular plexus, the superficial inguinal nodes, the superficial subinguinal nodes, and the femoral and external iliac chain. The lymphatic drainage of the posterior urethra can be divided into 3 aspects: the anterior superior, anterolateral, and posterior. The anterior superior portion drains to the anterior bladder wall and up the lateral inferior border of the umbilical artery to the middle chain of the external iliacs. The anterolateral portion drains in several directions. Part extends to the lateral bladder wall and onto the internal chain of the external iliacs at the obturator nerve or to the hypogastrics at the bifurcation of the external and internal iliacs. Another part drains into the ischiorectal fossa and through the canalis pudendalis (Alcock's canal), following the inferior gluteal artery and obturator artery to the lateral sacral and hypogastric nodes. The posterior aspect of the drainage is into the urethrovaginal septum, onto the cervix and the uterine plexus, over the ureter, and along the umbilical ligaments to the middle chain of the external iliacs or to the lower uterine pedicle and the hypogastrics.

### Nerves

The nerve supply is parasympathetic, sympathetic, and spinal. The parasympathetic and sympathetic nerves are derived from the hypogastric plexus; the spinal supply is via the pudendal nerve.

## 4. UTERUS

### Anatomy

The uterus is a pear-shaped, thick-walled, muscular organ, situated between the base of the bladder and the rectum. Covered on each side by the 2 layers of the broad ligament, it communicates above with the uterine tubes and below with the vagina. It is divided into 2 main portions, the larger portion or body above and the smaller cervix below, connected by a transverse constriction, the isthmus. The body is flattened so that the side-to-side dimension is greater than the antero posterior dimension and larger in women who have borne children. The anterior or vesical surface is almost flat; the posterior surface is convex. The uterine tubes join the uterus at the superior (lateral) angles. The round portion that extends above the plane passing through the points of attachment of the 2 tubes is termed the fundus. This portion is the region of greatest breadth. The cavity of the body, when viewed from the front or back, is roughly triangular with the base up. The communication of the cavity below with the cavity of the cervix corresponds in position to the isthmus and forms the internal orifice (internal osuteri). The cervix is somewhat barrel-shaped, its lower end joining the vagina at an angle varying from 45 to 90 degrees. It projects into the vagina and is divided into a supravaginal and a vaginal portion by the line of attachment. About one-fourth of the anterior surface and half of the posterior surface of the cervix belong to the vaginal portion. At the extremity of the vaginal portion is the opening leading to the vagina, the external orifice (external os uteri), which is round or oval before parturition but takes the form of a transverse slit in women who have borne children. It is bounded by anterior and posterior labia. The cavity of the cervix is fusiform in shape, with longitudinal folds or furrows, and extends from the internal to the external orifice.

The size of the uterus varies, under normal conditions, at different ages and in different physiologic states. In the adult who has never borne children, it is approximately 7–8 cm long and 4–5 cm at its widest point. In the prepubertal period, it is considerably smaller. In women who have borne children, it is larger. Its shape, size, and characteristics in the pregnant state become considerably modified depending on the stage of gestation.

**Table 2-3.** Arterial supply to the female pelvis.

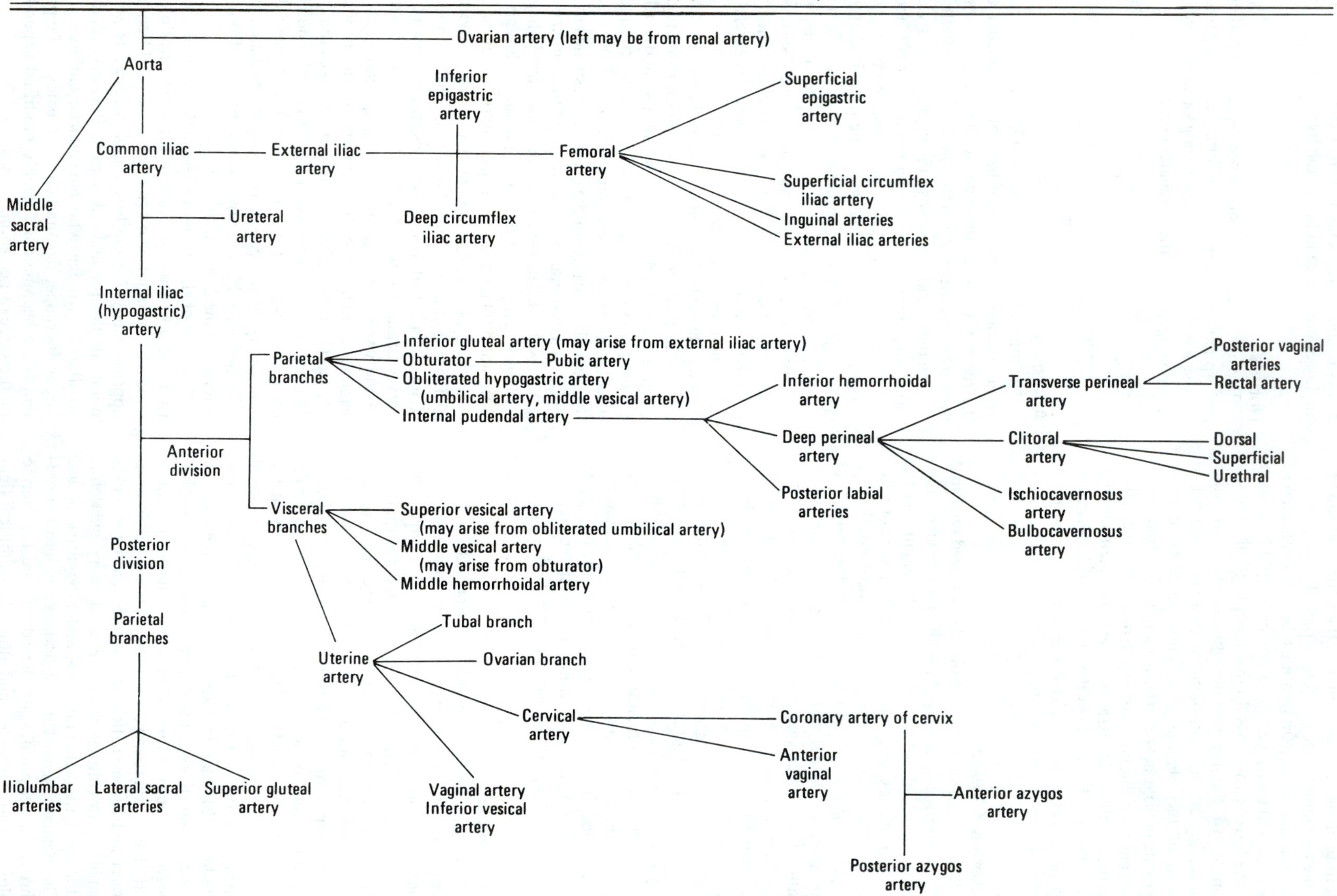

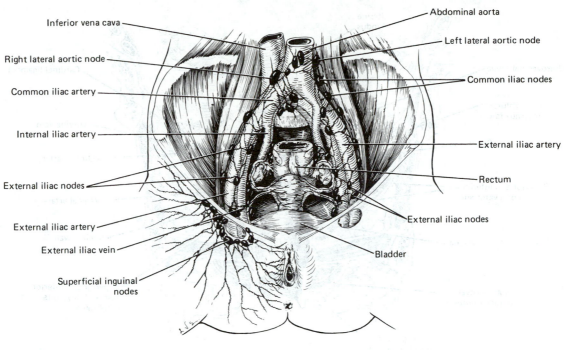

**Figure 2–23.** Lymphatic drainage of pelvis.

## Position & Axis Direction

The direction of the axis of the uterus varies greatly. Normally, the uterus forms a sharp angle with the vagina, so that its anterior surface lies on the upper surface of the bladder and the body is in a horizontal plane when the woman is standing erect. There is a bend in the area of the isthmus, at which the cervix then faces downward. This position is the normal anteversion or angulation of the uterus, although it may be placed backward (retroversion), without angulation (military position), or to one side (lateral version). The forward flexion at the isthmus is referred to as anteflexion, or there may be a corresponding retroflexion or lateral flexion. There is no sharp line between the normal and pathologic state of anterior angulation.

## Relationships

Anteriorly, the body of the uterus rests upon the upper and posterior surfaces of the bladder, separated by the uterovesical pouch of the peritoneum. The whole of the anterior wall of the cervix is below the floor of this pouch, and it is separated from the base of the bladder only by connective tissue. Posteriorly, the peritoneal covering extends down as far as the uppermost portion of the vagina; therefore, the entire posterior surface of the uterus is covered by peritoneum, and the convex posterior wall is separated from the rectum by the rectouterine pouch (cul-de-sac or pouch of Douglas). Coils of intestine may rest upon the posterior surface of the body of the uterus and

may be present in the rectouterine pouch. Laterally, the uterus is related to the various structures contained within the broad ligament: the uterine tubes, the round ligament and the ligament of the ovary, the uterine artery and veins, and the ureter. The relationships of the ureters and the uterine arteries are very important surgically. The ureters, as they pass to the bladder, run parallel with the cervix for a distance of 8–12 mm. The uterine artery crosses the ureter anterosuperiorly near the cervix, about 1.5 cm from the lateral formix of the vagina. In effect, the ureter passes under the uterine artery "as water flows under a bridge."

## Ligaments

Although the cervix of the uterus is fixed, the body is free to rise and fall with the filling and emptying of the bladder. The so-called ligaments supporting the uterus consist of the uterosacral ligaments, the transverse ligaments of the cervix (cardinal ligaments, cardinal supports, ligamentum transversum colli, ligaments of Mackenrodt), the round ligaments, and the broad ligaments (Fig 2–24). The cervix is embedded in tissue called the parametrium, containing various amounts of smooth muscle. There are 2 pairs of structures continuous with the parametrium and with the wall of the cervix: the uterosacral ligaments and the transverse (cardinal) ligament of the neck, the latter of which is the chief means of support and suspends the uterus from the lateral walls of the pelvis minor. The uterosacral ligaments are, in fact, the inferior

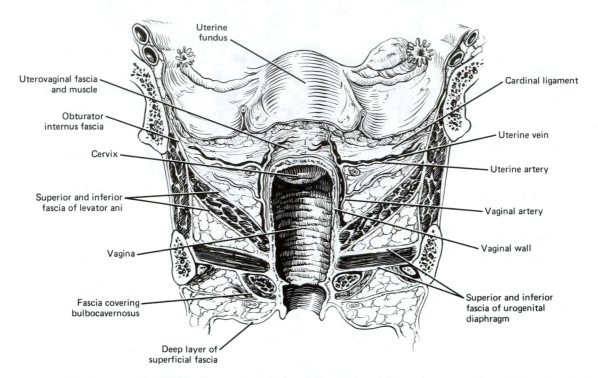

Uterine
fundus

Uterovaginal fascia
and muscle

Obturator
internus fascia

Cervix

Superior and inferior
fascia of levator ani

Vagina

Fascia covering
bulbocavernosus

Deep layer of
superficial fascia

Cardinal ligament

Uterine vein

Uterine artery

Vaginal artery

Vaginal wall

Superior and inferior
fascia of urogenital
diaphragm

**Figure 2–24.** Ligamentous and fascial support of pelvic viscera. (Redrawn from original drawings by Frank H Netter, MD, that first appeared in Ciba *Clinical Symposia*, Copyright © 1950. Ciba Pharmaceutical Co. Reproduced with permission.)

posterior folds of peritoneum from the broad ligament. They consist primarily of nerve bundles from the inferior hypogastric plexus and contain pre- and postganglionic fibers and C fibers of the sympathetic lumbar segments, parasympathetic in part from sacral components and in part from sensory or C fibers of the spinal segments.

The cardinal ligaments are composed of longitudinal smooth muscle fibers originating superiorly from the uterus and inferiorly from the vagina, fanning out toward the fascia visceralis to form, with the internal os of the cervix, the primary support of the uterus. There is a natural defect in the muscle at its sides (hilum of the uterus) and at the cervical isthmus (internal os), where the vasculature and nerve supply enter the uterus. The round ligaments of the uterus, although forming no real support, may assist in maintaining the body of the uterus in its typical position over the bladder. They consist of fibrous cords containing smooth muscle (longitudinal) from the outer layer of the corpus. From a point of attachment to the uterus immediately below that of the ovarian ligament, each round ligament extends downward, laterally, and forward between the 2 layers of the mesometrium, toward the abdominal inguinal ring that it traverses and the inguinal canal, to terminate in a fanlike manner in the labia majora and become continuous with connective tissue. The round ligament is

the gubernaculum (ligamentum teres uteri), vestigial in the female. It is accompanied by a funicular branch of the ovarian artery, by a branch from the ovarian venous plexus, and, in the lower part of its course, by a branch from the inferior epigastric artery, over which it passes as it enters the inguinal ring. Through the inguinal canal, it is accompanied by the ilioinguinal nerve and the external spermatic branch of the genitofemoral nerve.

The broad ligament, consisting of a transverse fold of peritoneum that arises from the floor of the pelvis between the rectum and the bladder, provides minimal support. In addition to the static support of these ligaments, the pelvic diaphragm (levator ani) provides an indirect and dynamic support. These muscles do not actually come in contact with the uterus, but they aid in supporting the vagina and maintain the entire pelvic floor in resisting downward pressure. The effectiveness of these muscles depends on an intact perineum (perineal body, bulbocavernous muscle and body), for if it is lacerated or weakened the ligaments will gradually stretch and the uterus will descend. The uterus and its components and the vagina are, in fact, one continuous unit.

## Layers of Uterine Wall

The wall of the uterus is very thick and consists of 3 layers: serous, muscular, and mucous. The serous layer (perimetrium) is simply the peritoneal covering. It is thin and firmly adherent over the fundus and most of the body, then thickens posteriorly and becomes separated from the muscle by the parametrium. The muscular layer (myometrium) is extremely thick and continuous with that of the tubes and vagina. It also extends into the ovarian and round ligaments, into the cardinal ligaments at the cervix, and minimally into the uterosacral ligaments. Two principal layers of the muscular coat may be distinguished: (1) the outer layer, which is weaker and composed of longitudinal fibers; and (2) a stronger inner layer, the fibers of which are interlaced and run in various directions, having intermingled within them large venous plexuses. The muscle layer hypertrophies with the internal os to form a sphincter. The cervix, from the internal os distally, progressively loses its smooth muscle, finally to be entirely devoid of smooth muscle and elastic in its distal half. It is, in fact, the "dead-end tendon" of the uterus, at which point, during the active component of labor, both the uterus and the vagina direct their efforts. The mucous layer (endometrium) is soft and spongy, composed of tissue resembling embryonic connective tissue. The surface consists of a single layer of ciliated columnar epithelium. The tissue is rather delicate and friable and contains many tubular glands that open into the cavity of the uterus.

## Arteries

The blood supply to the uterus is from the uterine and ovarian arteries. As a terminal branch of the hypogastric artery, the uterine artery runs downward and medially to cross the ureter near the cervix. It then ascends along the lateral border of the uterus in a tortuous course through the parametrium, giving off lateral branches to both uterine surfaces. Above, it anastomoses to join with the ovarian artery in the mesometrium, which creates the main accessory source of blood. The uterine arteries within the uterus form a series of arches over the fundus, creating cruciate anastomoses with the opposite side. Branches of the arcuate arteries (radial) penetrate the myometrium at right angles to terminate in the basilar arterioles for the basilar portion of the endometrium and in the spinal arteries of the endometrium. The spinal arteries are tortuous in structure, not because of endometrial growth but because, ontogenically, an organ carries its arterial supply with it as it changes size and position. Therefore, the spinal arteries are able to maintain adequate arterial flow to the placenta while it is attached within the uterus. On the other hand, the veins of the endometrium are a series of small sinusoids that connect to the larger sinusoids of the myometrium, the latter coalescing into the larger veins of the uterine complex. It is useful here to note the significance of the muscular role of the uterus in helping to control venous bleeding during parturition.

The arterial supply to the cervix is primarily through the cervical branches of the right and left uterine arteries, which form a rete around the cervix (coronary artery), creating the azygos artery in the midlline anteriorly and posteriorly. Anastomoses between this artery and the vaginal artery on both sides afford cruciate flow on the anterior wall, while on the posterior wall of the vagina, anastomoses occur with the right and left middle hemorrhoidal arteries as they supply the wall and the rectum.

## Veins

The veins form a plexus and drain through the uterine vein to the hypogastric vein. There are connections with the ovarian veins and the inferior epigastric by way of the vein accompanying the round ligament.

## Lymphatics

Lymphatic drainage involves several chains of lymph nodes (Table 2–2). From the subperitoneal plexus, the collecting trunks of the lower uterine segment may drain by way of the cervix to the external iliac chain or by way of the isthmus to the lateral sacral nodes. Drainage along the round ligament progresses to the superficial inguinal nodes, then to the femoral, and finally to the external iliac chain. Drainage laterally to the suspensory ligament of the ovary involves the lumbar pedicle and progresses in a retroperitoneal manner across and anteriorly to the ureter, to the lumbar nodes (interaorticocaval) that lie along the aorta, and inferiorly to the kidney.

## Nerves

The pelvic autonomic system can be divided into the superior hypogastric plexus (the presacral plexus and the uterinus magnus), the middle hypogastric plexus, and the inferior hypogastric plexus. The superior hypogastric plexus begins just below the inferior mesenteric artery. It is composed of 1–3 intercommunicating nerve bundles connected with the inferior mesenteric ganglia, but no ganglia are an integral part of the plexus. The intermesenteric nerves receive branches from the lumbar sympathetic ganglia.

**A. Superior Hypogastric Plexus:** The superior hypogastric plexus continues into the mid-hypogastric plexus. The presacral nerves spread out into a lattice-work at the level of the first sacral vertebra, with connecting rami to the last of the lumbar ganglia. The greater part of the superior mid hypogastric plexus may be found to the left of the midline.

**B. Inferior Hypogastric Plexus:** At the first sacral vertebra, this plexus divides into several branches that go to the right and left sides of the pelvis. These branches form the beginning of the right and left inferior hypogastric plexus. The inferior hypogastric plexus, which is the divided continuation of the midhypogastric plexus, the superior hypogastric plexus, the presacral nerve, and the uterinus magnus, is composed of several parallel nerves on each side.

This group of nerves descends within the pelvis in a position posterior to the common iliac artery and anterior to the sacral plexus, curves laterally, and finally enters the sacrouterine fold or ligaments. The medial section of the primary division of the sacral nerves sends fibers (nervi erigentes) that enter the pelvic plexus in the sacrouterine folds. The plexus now appears to contain both sympathetic (inferior hypogastric plexus) and parasympathetic (nervi erigentes) components.

**C. Nervi Erigentes:** The sensory components, which are mostly visceral, are found in the nervi erigentes; however, if one takes into account the amount of spinal anesthetic necessary to eliminate uterine sensation, one must assume that there are a number of sensory fibers in the sympathetic component.

**D. Common Iliac Nerves:** The common iliac nerves originate separately from the superior hypogastric plexus and descend on the surface of the artery and vein, one part going through the femoral ring and the remainder following the internal iliac, finally rejoining the pelvic plexus.

**E. Hypogastric Ganglion:** On either side of the uterus, in the base of the broad ligament, is the large plexus described by Lee and Frankenhauser, the so-called hypogastric ganglion. The plexus actually consists of ganglia and nerve ramifications of various sizes as well as branches of the combined inferior hypogastric plexus and the nervi erigentes. It lies parallel to the lateral pelvic wall, its lateral surface superficial to the internal iliac and its branches; the ureter occupies a position superficial to the plexus. The middle vesical artery perforates and supplies the plexus, its medial branches supplying the rectal stalk. The greater part of the plexus terminates in large branches that enter the uterus in the region of the internal os, while another smaller component of the plexus supplies the vagina and the bladder. The branches of the plexus that supply the uterus enter the isthmus primarily through the sacrouterine fold or ligament. In the isthmus, just outside the entrance to the uterus, ascending rami pass out into the broad ligament to enter the body of the uterus at higher levels—besides supplying the uterine tubes. A part of the inferior hypogastric plexus may pass directly to the uterus without involvement in the pelvic plexus.

Ganglia are in close proximity to the uterine arteries and the ureters, in the adventitia of the bladder and vagina, and in the vesicovaginal septum. The nerve bundles entering the ganglia contain both myelinated and unmyelinated elements. Corpuscula lamellosa (Vater-Pacini corpuscles) may be found within the tissues and are often observed within nerve bundles, especially within those in the lower divisions of the plexus. Both myelinated and unmyelinated nerves are present within the uterus. The nerves enter along the blood vessels, the richest supply lying in the isthmic portion of the uterus. The fibers following the blood vessels gradually diminish in number in the direction of the fundus, where the sparsest distribution occurs. The fibers run parallel to the muscle bundles, and the nerves frequently branch to form a syncytium before terminating on the sarcoplasm as small free nerve endings.

### Sensory Corpuscles

Vater-Pacini corpuscles (corpuscula lamellosa) are present outside the uterus. Dogiel and Krause corpuscles (corpuscula bulboidea) appear in the region of the endocervix. They may also be found in the broad ligament along with Vater-Pacini corpuscles and at the juncture of the uterine arteries with the uterus. These corpuscles may act to modulate the stretch response that reflexly stimulates uterine contractions during labor.

The innervation of the cervix shows occasional free endings entering papillae of the stratified squamous epithelium of the pars vaginalis. The endocervix contains a rich plexus of free endings that is most pronounced in the region of the internal os. The endocervix and the isthmic portion of the uterus in the nonpregnant state both contain the highest number of nerves and blood vessels of any part of the uterus. The presence here of a lamellar type of corpuscle has already been noted.

Nerves pass through the myometrium and enter the endometrium. A plexus with penetrating fibers involving the submucosal region is present in the basal third of the endometrium, with branches terminating in the stroma, in the basilar arterioles, and at the origin of the spiral arterioles. The outer two-thirds of the endometrium is devoid of nerves.

### 5. UTERINE (FALLOPIAN) TUBES (Oviducts)

### Anatomy

The uterine tubes serve to convey the ova to the uterus. They extend from the superior angles of the uterus to the region of the ovaries, running in the superior border of the broad ligament (meso salpinx). The course of each tube is nearly horizontal at first and slightly backward. Upon reaching the lower (uterine) pole of the ovary, the tube turns upward, parallel with the anterior (mesovarian) border, then arches backward over the upper pole and descends posteriorly to terminate in contact with the medial surface. Each tube is 7–14 cm long and may be divided into 3 parts: isthmus, ampulla, and infundibulum. The isthmus is the narrow and nearly straight portion immediately adjoining the uterus. It has a rather long intramural course, and its opening into the uterus, the uterine ostium, is approximately 1 mm in diameter. Following the isthmus is the wider, more tortuous ampulla. It terminates in a funnel-like dilatation, the infundibulum. The margins of the infundibulum are fringed by numerous diverging processes, the fimbriae, the longest of which, the fimbria ovarica, is attached to the ovary. The funnel-shaped mouth of the infundibulum, the abdominal ostium, is about 3 mm in diameter and actually leads into the peritoneal cavity, although it is probably closely applied to the surface of the ovary during ovulation.

## Layers of Wall

The wall of the tube has 4 coats: serous (peritoneal), subserous or adventitial (fibrous and vascular), muscular, and mucous. Each tube is enclosed within a peritoneal covering except along a small strip on its lower surface, where the mesosalpinx is attached. At the margins of the infundibulum and the fimbriae, this peritoneal covering becomes directly continuous with the mucous membrane lining the interior of the tube. The subserous tissue is lax in the immediate vicinity of the tube. The blood and nerve supply is found within this layer. The muscular coat has an outer longitudinal and an inner circular layer of smooth muscle fibers, more prominent and continuous with that of the uterus at the uterine end of the tube. The mucous coat is ciliated columnar epithelium with coarse longitudinal folds, simple in the region of the isthmus but becoming higher and more complex in the ampulla. The epithelial lining extends outward into the fimbriae. The ciliary motion is directed toward the uterus.

## Ligament

The infundibulum is suspended from the pelvic brim by the infundibulopelvic ligament (suspensory ligament of the ovary). This portion of the tube may adjoin the tip of the appendix and fuse with it.

## Arteries & Veins

The blood supply to the tubes is derived from the ovarian and uterine arteries. The tubal branch of the uterine artery courses along the lower surface of the uterine tube as far as the fimbriated extremity and may also send a branch to the ligamentum teres. The ovarian branch of the uterine artery runs along the attached border of the ovary and gives off a tubal branch. Both branches form cruciate anastomoses in the mesosalpinx. The veins accompany the arteries.

## Lymphatics

The lymphatic drainage occurs through trunks running retroperitoneally across and anterior to the ureter, into the lumbar nodes along the aorta, and inferior to the kidney.

## Nerves

The nerve supply is derived from the pelvic plexuses (parasympathetic and sympathetic) and from the ovarian plexus. The nerves of the ampulla are given off from the branches passing to the ovary, while those of the isthmus come from the uterine branches. The nerve fibers enter the muscularis of the tube through the mesosalpinx to form a reticular network of free endings among the smooth muscle cells.

## 6. OVARIES

### Anatomy

The ovaries are paired organs situated close to the wall on either side of the pelvis minor, a little below the brim. Each measures 2.5–5 cm in length, 1.5–3 cm in breadth, and 0.7–1.5 cm in width, weighing about 4–8 g. The ovary has 2 surfaces, medial and lateral; 2 borders, anterior or mesovarian and posterior or free; and 2 poles, upper or tubal and lower or uterine. When the uterus and adnexa are in the normal position, the long axis of the ovary is nearly vertical, but it bends somewhat medially and forward at the lower end so that the lower pole tends to point toward the uterus. The medial surface is rounded and, posteriorly, may have numerous scars or elevations that mark the position of developing follicles and sites of ruptured ones.

### Relationships

The upper portion of this surface is overhung by the fimbriated end of the uterine tube, and the remainder lies in relation to coils of intestine. The lateral surface is similar in shape and faces the pelvic wall, where it forms a distinct depression, the fossa ovarica. This fossa is lined by peritoneum and is bounded above by the external iliac vessels and below by the obturator vessels and nerve; its posterior boundary is formed by the ureter and uterine artery and vein, and the pelvic attachment of the broad ligament is located anteriorly. The mesovarian or anterior border is fairly straight and provides attachment for the mesovarium, a peritoneal fold by which the ovary is attached to the posterosuperior layer of the broad ligament. Since the vessels, nerves, and lymphatics enter the ovary through this border, it is referred to as the hilum of the ovary. Anterior to the hilum are embryonic remnants of the male and female germ cell ducts. The posterior or free border is more convex and broader and is directed freely into the rectouterine pouch. The upper or tubal pole is large and rounded. It is overhung closely by the infundibulum of the uterine tube and is connected with the pelvic brim by the suspensory ligament of the ovary, a peritoneal fold. The lower or uterine pole is smaller and directed toward the uterus. It serves as the attachment of the ligament of the ovary proper.

### Mesovarium

The ovary is suspended by means of the mesovarium, the suspensory ligament of the ovary, and the ovarian ligament. The mesovarium consists of 2 layers of peritoneum, continuous with both the epithelial coat of the ovary and the posterosuperior layer of the broad ligament. It is short and wide and contains branches of the ovarian and uterine arteries, with plexuses of nervers, the pampiniform plexus of veins, and the lateral end of the ovarian ligament. The suspensory ligament of the ovary is a triangular fold of peritoneum and is actually the upper lateral corner of the broad ligament, which becomes confluent with the parietal peritoneum at the pelvic brim. It attaches to the mesovarium as well as to the peritoneal coat of the infundibulum medially, thus suspending both the ovary and the tube. It contains the ovarian artery, veins, and nerves after they pass over the pelvic brim and before they enter the mesovarium. The ovarian ligament is a band of connective tissue, with numerous small muscle fibers, that lies between the 2 layers of the broad ligament on the boundary line between the mesosalpinx and the mesometrium, connecting the lower (uterine) pole of the ovary with the lateral wall of the uterus. It is attached just below the uterine tube and above the attachment of the round ligament of the uterus and is continuous with the latter.

## Structure of Ovary

The ovary is covered by cuboid or low columnar epithelium and consists of a cortex and a medulla. The medulla is made up of connective tissue fibers, smooth muscle cells, and numerous blood vessels, nerves, lymphatic vessels, and supporting tissue. The cortex is composed of a fine areolar stroma, with many vessels and scattered follicles of epithelial cells within which are the definitive ova (oocytes) in various stages of maturity. The more mature follicles enlarge and project onto the free surface of the ovary, where they are visible to the naked eye. They are called graafian follicles. When fully mature, the follicle bursts, releasing the ovum and becoming transformed into a corpus luteum. The corpus luteum, in turn, is later replaced by scar tissue, forming a corpus albicans.

## Arteries

The ovarian artery is the chief source of blood for the ovary. Though both arteries may originate as branches of the abdominal aorta, the left frequently originates from the left renal artery; the right, less frequently. The vessels diverge from each other as they descend. Upon reaching the level of the common iliac artery, they turn medially over that vessel and ureter to descend tortuously into the pelvis on each side between the folds of the suspensory ligament of the ovary into the mesovarium. An additional blood supply is formed from anastomosis with the ovarian branch of the uterine artery, which courses along the attached border of the ovary. Blood vessels that enter the hilum send out capillary branches centrifugally.

## Veins

The veins follow the course of the arteries and, as they emerge from the hilum, form a well-developed plexus (the pampiniform plexus) between the layers of the mesovarium. Smooth muscle fibers occur in the meshes of the plexus, giving the whole structure the appearance of erectile tissue.

## Lymphatics

Lymphatic channels drain retroperitoneally, together with those of the tubes and part of those from the uterus, to the lumbar nodes along the aorta inferior to the kidney. The distribution of lymph channels in the ovary is so extensive that it suggests the system may also provide additional fluid to the ovary during periods of preovulatory follicular swelling.

## Nerves

The nerve supply of the ovaries arises from the lumbosacral sympathetic chain and passes to the gonad along with the ovarian artery.

## 7. VAGINA

The vagina is a strong canal of muscle approximately 7.5 cm long that extends from the uterus to the vestibule of the external genitalia, where it opens to the exterior. Its long axis is almost parallel with that of the lower part of the sacrum, and it meets the cervix of the uterus at an angle of 45–90 degrees. Because the cervix of the uterus projects into the upper portion, the anterior wall of the vagina is 1.5–2 cm shorter than the posterior wall. The circular cul-de-sac formed around the cervix is known as the fornix and is divided into 4 regions; the anterior fornix, the posterior fornix, and 2 lateral fornices. Toward its lower end, the vagina pierces the urogenital diaphragm and is surrounded by the 2 bulbocavernosus muscles and bodies, which act as a sphincter (sphincter vaginae). In the virginal state, an incomplete fold of highly vascular tissue and mucous membrane, the hymen, partially closes the external orifice.

## Relationships

Anteriorly, the vagina is in close relationship to the bladder, ureters, and urethra in succession. The posterior fornix is covered by the peritoneum of the rectovaginal pouch, which may contain coils of intestine. Below the pouch, the vagina rests almost directly on the rectum, separated from it by a thin layer of areolar connective tissue. Toward the lower end of the vagina, the rectum turns back sharply, and the distance between the vagina and rectum greatly increases. This space, filled with muscle fibers, connective tissue, and fat, is known as the perineal body. The lateral fornix lies just under the root of the broad ligament and is approximately 1 cm from the point where the uterine artery crosses the ureter. The remaining lateral vaginal wall is related to the edges of the anterior portion of the levator ani. The vagina is supported at the introitus by the bulbocavernosus muscles and bodies, in the lower third by the levator ani (puborectalis), and superiorly by the transverse (cardinal) ligaments of the uterus. The ductus epoophori longitudinalis (duct of Gartner), the remains of the lower portion of the wolffian duct (mesonephric duct), may often be found on the sides of the vagina as a minute tube or fibrous cord. These vestigial structures often become cystic and appear as translucent areas.

## Wall Structure

The vaginal wall is composed of a mucosal and a muscular layer. The smooth muscle fibers are indistinctly arranged in 3 layers: an outer longitudinal layer, circumferential layer, and a poorly differentiated inner longitudinal layer. In the lower third, the circumferential fibers envelop the urethra. The submucous area is abundantly supplied with a dense plexus of veins and lymphatics. The mucous layer shows many transverse and oblique rugae, which project inward to such an extent that the lumen in transverse section resembles an H-shaped slit. On the anterior and posterior walls, these ridges are more prominent, and the anterior column forms the urethral carina at its lower end, where the urethra slightly invaginates the anterior wall of the vagina. The mucosa of the vagina is lined throughout by stratified squamous epithelium. Even though the vagina has no true glands, there is a secretion present. It consists of cervical mucus, desquamated epithelium, and, with sexual stimulation, a direct transudate.

## Arteries & Veins

The chief blood supply to the vagina is through the vaginal branch of the uterine artery. After forming the coronary or circular artery of the cervix, it passes medially, behind the ureter, to send 5 main branches onto the anterior wall to the midline. These branches anastomose with the azygos artery (originating midline from the coronary artery of the cervix) and continue downward to supply the anterior vaginal wall and the lower two-thirds of the urethra. The uterine artery eventually anastomoses to the urethral branch of the clitoral artery. The posterior vaginal wall is supplied by branches of the middle and inferior hemorrhoidal arteries, traversing toward the midline to join the azygos artery from the coronary artery of the cervix. These branches then anastomose on the perineum to the superficial and deep transverse perineal arteries.

The veins follow the course of the arteries.

## Lymphatics

The lymphatics are numerous mucosal plexuses, anastomosing with the deeper muscular plexuses (Table 2–2). The superior group of lymphatics join those of the cervix and may follow the uterine artery to terminate in the external iliac nodes or form anastomoses with the uterine plexus. The middle group of lymphatics, which drain the greater part of the vagina,

appear to follow the vaginal arteries to the hypogastric channels. In addition, there are lymph nodes in the rectovaginal septum that are primarily responsible for drainage of the rectum and part of the posterior vaginal wall. The inferior group of lymphatics form frequent anastomoses between the right and left sides and either course upward to anastomose with the middle group or enter the vulva and drain to the inguinal nodes.

## Nerves

The innervation of the vagina contains both sympathetic and parasympathetic fibers. Only occasional free nerve endings are seen in the mucosa; no other types of nerve endings are noted.

## STRUCTURES LINING THE PELVIS

The walls of the pelvis minor are made up of the following layers: (1) the peritoneum, (2) the subperitoneal or extraperitoneal fibroareolar layer, (3) the fascial layer, (4) the muscular layer, and (5) the osseoligamentous layer (not further discussed). The anatomy of the floor of the pelvis is comparable to that of the walls except for the absence of an osseoligamentous layer.

## 1. PERITONEUM

The peritoneum presents several distinct transverse folds that form corresponding fossae on each side. The most anterior is a variable fold, the transverse vesical, extending from the bladder laterally to the pelvic wall. It is not the superficial covering of any definitive structure. Behind it lies the broad ligament, which partially covers and aids in the support of the uterus and adnexa.

### Ligaments

The broad ligament extends from the lateral border on either side of the uterus to the floor and side walls of the pelvis. It is composed of 2 layers, anterior and posterior, the anterior facing downward and the posterior facing upward, conforming to the position of the uterus. The inferior or "attached" border of the broad ligament is continuous with the parietal peritoneum on the floor and on the side walls of the pelvis. Along this border, the posterior layer continues laterally and posteriorly in an arc to the region of the sacrum, forming the uterosacral fold. Another fold— the rectouterine fold—frequently passes from the posterior surface of the cervix to the rectum in the midline. The anterior layer of the broad ligament is continuous laterally along the inferior border with the peritoneum of the paravesical fossae and continuous medially with peritoneum on the upper surface of the bladder. Both layers of the attached border continue up the side walls of the pelvis to join with a triangular fold of peritoneum, reaching to the brim of the pelvis to form the suspensory ligament of the ovary or infundibular ligament. This ligament contains the ovarian vessels and nerves. The medial border of the broad ligament on either side is continuous with the peritoneal covering on both uterine surfaces. The 2 layers of the ligament separate to partially contain the uterus, and the superior or "free" border, which is laterally continuous with the suspensory ligament of the ovary, envelops the uterine tube.

The broad ligament can be divided into regions as follows: (1) a larger portion, the mesometrium, which is associated especially with the lateral border of the uterus; (2) the mesovarium, the fold that springs from the posterior layer of the ovary; and (3) the thin portion, the mesosalpinx, which is associated with the uterine tube in the region of the free border. The superior lateral corner of the broad ligament has been referred to as the suspensory ligament of the ovary, or infundibulopelvic ligament, because it suspends the infundibulum as well as the ovary.

### Fossae & Spaces

Corresponding to the peritoneal folds are the peritoneal fossae. The prevesical or retropubic space is a potential space that is crossed by the transverse vesical fold. It is situated in front of the bladder and behind the pubis. When the bladder is displaced posteriorly, it becomes an actual space, anteriorly continuous from side to side and posteriorly limited by a condensation of fatty areolar tissue extending from the base of the bladder to the side wall of the pelvis. The vesicouterine pouch is a narrow cul-de-sac between the anterior surface of the body of the uterus and the upper surface of the bladder when the uterus is in normal anteflexed position. In the bottom of this pouch, the peritoneum is reflected from the bladder onto the uterus at the junction of the cervix and corpus. Therefore, the anterior surface of the cervix is below the level of the peritoneum and is connected with the base of the bladder by condensed areolar tissue. The peritoneum on the posterior surface of the body of the uterus extends downward onto the cervix and onto the posterior fornix of the vagina. It is then reflected onto the anterior surface of the rectum to form a narrow cul-de-sac continuous with the pararectal fossa of either side. The entire space, bounded anteriorly by the cervix and by the fornix in the midline, the uterosacral folds laterally, and the rectum posteriorly, is the rectouterine pouch or cul-de-sac (pouch of Douglas).

### 2. SUBPERITONEAL & FASCIAL LAYERS

The subperitoneal layer consists of loose, fatty areolar tissue underlying the peritoneum. External to the subperitoneal layer, a layer of fascia lines the wall of the pelvis, covering the muscles and, where these are lacking, blending with the periosteum of the pelvic bones. This layer is known as the parietal pelvic fascia and is subdivided into the obturator fascia, the fascia of the urogenital diaphragm, and the fascia of the piriformis. The obturator fascia is of considerable thickness and covers the obturator internus muscle. Traced forward, it partially blends with the periosteum of the pubic bone and assists in the formation of the obturator canal. Traced upward, it is continuous at the arcuate line with the iliac fascia. Inferiorly, it extends nearly to the margin of the ischiopubic arch, where it is attached to the bone. In this lower region, it also becomes continuous with a double-layered triangular sheet of fascia, the fasciae of the urogenital diaphragm, passing across the anterior part of the pelvic outlet. A much thinner portion of the parietal pelvic fascia covers the piriform and coccygeus muscles in the posterior pelvic wall. Medially, the piriformis fascia blends with the periosteum of the sacrum around the margins of the anterior sacral foramens and covers the roots and first branches of the sacral plexus. Visceral pelvic fascia denotes the fascia in the bottom of the pelvic bowl, which invests the pelvic organs and forms a number of supports that suspend the organs from the pelvic walls. These supports arise in common from the obturator part of the parietal fascia, along or near the arcus tendineus. This arc or line extends from a point near the lower part of the symphysis pubica to the root of the spine of the ischium. From this common origin, the fascia spreads inward and backward, dividing into a number of parts classified as either investing (endopelvic) fascia or suspensory and diaphragmatic fascia.

### 3. MUSCULAR LAYER

The muscles of the greater pelvis are the psoas major and iliacus. Those of the lesser pelvis are the piriformis, obturator internus, coccygeus, and levator ani; they do not form a continuous layer.

### Greater Pelvis

**A. Psoas Major:** The fusiform psoas major muscle originates from the 12th thoracic to the fifth lumbar vertebrae. Parallel fiber bundles descend nearly vertically along the side of the vertebral bodies and extend along the border of the minor pelvis, beneath the inguinal ligament, and on toward insertion in the thigh. The medial border inserts into the lesser trochanter, while the lateral border shares its tendon with the iliacus muscle. Together with the iliacus, it is the most powerful flexor of the thigh and acts as a lateral rotator of the femur when the foot is off the ground and free, and a medial rotator when the foot is on the ground and the tibia is fixed. The psoas component flexes the spine and the pelvis and abducts the lumbar region of the spine. The psoas, having longer fibers than the iliacus, gives a quicker but weaker pull.

**B. Iliacus:** The fan-shaped iliacus muscle originates from the iliac crest, the iliolumbar ligament, the greater part of the iliac fossa, the anterior sacroiliac ligaments, and frequently the ala of the sacrum. It also originates from the ventral border of the ilium between the 2 anterior spines. It is inserted in a penniform manner on the lateral surface of the tendon that emerges from the psoas above the inguinal ligament and directly on the femur immediately distal to the lesser trochanter. The lateral portion of the muscle arising from the ventral border of the ilium is adherent to the direct tendon of the rectus femoris and the capsule of the hip joint.

### Lesser Pelvis

**A. Piriformis:** The piriformis has its origin from the lateral part of the ventral surface of the second, third, and fourth sacral vertebrae, from the posterior border of the greater sciatic notch, and from the deep surface of the sacrotuberous ligament near the sacrum. The fiber bundles pass through the greater sciatic foramen to insert upon the anterior and inner portion of the upper border of the greater trochanter. The piriformis acts as an abductor, lateral rotator, and weak extensor of the thigh.

**B. Obturator Internus:** The obturator internus arises from the pelvic surface of the pubic rami near the obturator foramen, the pelvic surface of the ischium between the foramen and the greater sciatic notch, the deep surface of the obturator internus fascia, the fibrous arch that bounds the canal for the obturator vessels and nerves, and the pelvic surface of the obturator membrane. The fiber bundles converge toward the lesser sciatic notch, where they curve laterally to insert into the trochanteric foss of the femur. The obturator internus is a powerful lateral rotator of the thigh. When the thigh is bent at a right angle, the muscle serves as an abductor and extensor.

**C. Coccygeus:** The coccygeus muscle runs from the ischial spine and the neighboring margin of the greater sciatic notch to the fourth and fifth sacral vertebrae and the coccyx. A large part of the muscle is aponeurotic. It supports the pelvic and abdominal viscera and possibly flexes and abducts the coccyx.

**D. Levator Ani:** The levator ani muscle forms the floor of the pelvis and the roof of the perineum. It is divisible into 3 portions: (1) the iliococcygeus, (2) the pubococcygeus, and (3) the puborectalis.

**1. Iliococcygeus—**The iliococcygeus arises from the arcus tendineus, which extends from the ischial spine to the superior ramus of the pubis near the obturator canal and for a variable distance downward below the obturator canal. Its insertion is into the lateral aspect of the coccyx and the raphe that extends from the tip of the coccyx to the rectum. Many fiber bundles cross the median line.

**2. Pubococcygeus—**The pubococcygeus arises from the inner surface of the os pubis, the lower margin of the symphysis pubica to the obturator canal, and the arcus tendineus as far backward as the origin of the iliococcygeus. It passes backward, downward, and medially past the urogenital organs and the rectum, inserting into the anterior sacrococcygeal ligament, the deep part of the anococcygeal raphe, and each side of the rectum. The pubococcygeus lies to some extent on the pelvic surface of the insertion of the iliococcygeus.

**3. Puborectalis—**The puborectalis arises from the body and descending ramus of the pubis beneath the origin of the pubococcygeus, the neighboring part of the obturator fascia, and the fascia covering the pelvic surface of the urogenital diaphragm. Many of the fiber bundles interdigitate with those of the opposite side, and they form a thick band on each side of the rectum behind which those of each side are inserted into the anococcygeal raphe.

The levator ani serves to slightly flex the coccyx, raise the anus, and constrict the rectum and vagina. It resists the downward pressure that the thoracoabdominal diaphragm exerts on the viscera during inspiration.

### Pelvic Diaphragm

The pelvic diaphragm (Fig 2–25) extends from the upper part of the pelvic surface of the pubis and ischium to the rectum, which passes through it. The pelvic diaphragm is formed by the levator ani and coccygeus muscles and covering fasciae. The diaphragmatic fasciae cloaking the levator ani arise from the parietal pelvic fascia (obturator fascia), the muscular layer lying between the fasciae. As viewed from above, the superior fascia is the best developed and is reflected onto the rectum, forming the "rectal sheath." The coccygeus muscle forms the deeper portion of the posterolateral wall of the ischiorectal fossa, helping to bound the pelvic outlet. The diaphragm presents a hiatus anteriorly, occupied by the vagina and urethra. The pelvic diaphragm is the main support of the pelvic floor; it suspends the rectum and indirectly supports the uterus.

### Arteries & Veins

The blood supply to the muscles lining the pelvis is primarily from branches of the hypogastric artery, accompanied by contributions from the external iliac artery. The iliolumbar branch of the hypogastric artery runs upward and laterally beneath the common iliac artery, then beneath the psoas muscle to the superior aperture of the pelvis minor, where it divides into iliac and lumbar branches. The iliac supplies both the iliacus and psoas muscles. It passes laterally beneath the psoas and the femoral nerve and, perforating the iliacus, ramifies in the iliac fossa between the muscle and the bone. It supplies a nutrient artery to the bone and then divides into several branches that can be traced as follows: (1) upward toward the sacroiliac synchondrosis to anastomose with the last lumbar artery, (2) laterally toward the crest of the ilium to anas-

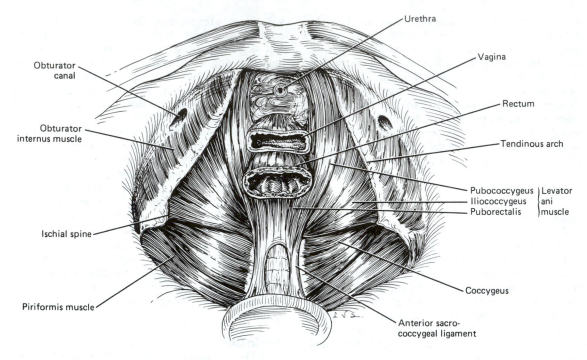

**Figure 2–25.** Pelvic diaphragm from above.

tomose with the lateral circumflex and gluteal arteries, and (3) medially toward the pelvis minor to anastomose with the deep circumflex iliac from the external iliac. The lumbar branch ascends beneath the psoas and supplies that muscle along with the quadratus lumborum. It then anastomoses with the last lumbar artery.

Another branch of the hypogastric artery, the lateral sacral artery, may be represented as 2 distinct vessels. It passes medially in front of the sacrum and turns downward to run parallel with the sympathetic trunk. Crossing the slips of origin of the piriform muscle, it sends branches to that muscle. On reaching the coccyx, it anastomoses in front of the bone with the middle sacral artery and with the inferior lateral sacral artery of the opposite side. The obturator artery usually arises from the hypogastric, but occasionally it may stem from the inferior epigastric or directly from the external iliac artery. It runs forward and downward slightly below the brim of the pelvis, lying between the peritoneum and endopelvic fascia. Passing through the obturator canal, it emerges and divides into anterior and posterior branches that curve around the margin of the obturator foramen beneath the obturator externus muscle.

When the obturator artery arises from the inferior epigastric or external iliac artery, its proximal relationships are profoundly altered, the vessel coursing near the femoral ring where it may be endangered during operative procedures. The anterior branch of the obturator artery runs around the medial margin of

the obturator foramen and anastomoses with both its posterior branch and the medial circumflex artery. It supplies branches to the obturator muscles. The internal pudendal artery is a terminal branch of the hypogastric artery that arises opposite the piriform muscle and accompanies the inferior gluteal artery downward to the lower border of the greater sciatic foramen. It leaves the pelvis between the piriform and coccygeus muscles, passing over the ischial spine to enter the ischiorectal fossa through the small sciatic foramen. Then, running forward through the canalis pudendalis (Alcock's canal) in the obturator fascia, it terminates by dividing into the perineal artery and the artery of the clitoris.

Within the pelvis, the artery lies anterior to the piriform muscle and the sacral plexus of nerves, lateral to the inferior gluteal artery. Among the small branches that it sends to the gluteal region are those that accompany the nerve to the obturator internus. Another of its branches, the inferior hemorrhodial artery, arises at the posterior part of the ischiorectal fossa. Upon perforating the obturator fascia, it immediately breaks up into several branches. Some of those run medially toward the rectum to supply the levator ani muscle. The superior gluteal artery originates as a short trunk from the lateral and back part of the hypogastric artery, associated in origin with the iliolumbar and lateral sacral and sometimes with the inferior gluteal or with the inferior gluteal and the internal pudendal. It leaves the pelvis through the greater sciatic foramen above the piriform muscle, beneath its vein and in front of the superior gluteal nerve. Under cover of the gluteus maximus muscle, it breaks into a superficial and deep division.

The deep portion further divides into superior and inferior branches. The inferior branch passes forward between the gluteus medius and minimus toward the greater trochanter, where it anastomoses with the ascending branch of the lateral circumflex. It supplies branches to the obturator internus, the piriformis, the levator ani, and the coccygeus muscles and to the hip joint. The deep circumflex iliac artery arises from the side of the external iliac artery either opposite the epigastric or a little below the origin of that vessel. It courses laterally behind the inguinal ligament, lying between the fascia transversalis and the peritoneum or in a fibrous canal formed by the union of the fascia transversalis with the iliac fascia. It sends off branches that supply the psoas and iliacus muscles as well as a cutaneous branch that anastomoses with the superior gluteal artery.

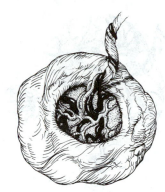

**Figure 2–26.** Marked circumvallate or extrachorial placenta.

## PLACENTA*

At term, the normal placenta is a blue-red, rounded, flattened, meaty discoid organ 15–20 cm in diameter and 2–4 cm thick. It weighs 400–600 g, or about one-sixth the normal weight of the newborn. The umbilical cord arises from almost any point on the fetal surface of the placenta, seemingly at random. The fetal membranes arise from the placenta at its margin. In multiple pregnancy, one or more placentas may be present depending upon the number of ova implanted and the type of segmentation that occurs. The placenta is derived from both maternal and fetal tissue. At term, about four-fifths of the placenta is of fetal origin.

The maternal portion of the placenta amounts to less than one-fifth of the total placenta by weight. It is composed of compressed sheets of decidua basalis, remnants of blood vessels, and, at the margin, spongy decidua. Irregular grooves or clefts divide the placenta into cotyledons. The maternal surface is torn from the uterine wall at birth and as a result is rough, red, and spongy.

The fetal portion of the placenta is composed of numerous functional units called villi. These are branched terminals of the fetal circulation and provide for transfer of metabolic products. The villous surface, which is exposed to maternal blood, may be as much as 12 m² (130 square feet). The fetal capillary system within the villi is almost 50 km (27 miles) long. Most villi are free within the intervillous spaces, but an occasional anchor villus attaches the placenta to the decidua basalis. The fetal surface of the placenta is covered by amniotic membrane and is

smooth and shiny. The umbilical cord vessels course over the fetal surface before entering the placenta.

### Placental Types

**A. Circumvaliate (Circummarginate) Placentas:** In about 1% of cases, the delivered placenta will show a small central chorionic plate surrounded by a thick whitish ring that is composed of a double fold of amnion and chorion with fibrin and degenerated decidua in between. This circumvallate placenta may predispose to premature marginal separation and second-trimester antepartum bleeding (Fig 2–26). This uncommon extrachorial placenta is of uncertain origin. It is associated with increased rates of slight to moderate antepartal bleeding, early delivery, and perinatal death. Older multiparas are more prone to its development. Low-birthweight infants and extrachorial placentas seem related.

**B. Succenturiate Lobe:** Occasionally there may be an accessory cotyledon, or succenturiate lobe, with vascular connections to the main body of the placenta. A succenturiate lobe may not always deliver with the parent placenta during the third stage of labor. This leads to postpartal hemorrhage. If a careful examination of the delivered membranes reveals torn vessels, immediate manual exploration of the uterus is indicated for removal of an accessory lobe (Fig 2–27).

*This section is contributed by Robert C. Goodlin, MD.

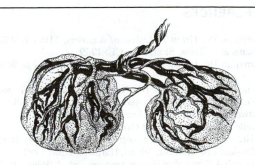

**Figure 2–27.** Succenturiate placenta.

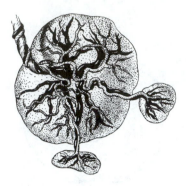

**Figure 2–28.** Bipartite placenta.

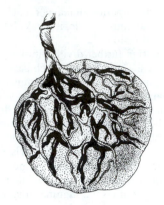

**Figure 2–29.** Marginal insertion of battledore placenta.

**C. Bipartite Placenta:** A bipartite placenta is an uncommon variety. The placenta is divided into 2 separate lobes but united by primary vessels and membranes. Retention of one lobe after birth will cause hemorrhagic and septic complications. Examine the vasculature and note the completeness of membranes of a small placenta for evidence of a missing lobe, and recover the adherent portion without delay (Fig 2–28).

**D. Marginal Insertion of Cord (Battledore Placenta):** The umbilical cord may be found inserted into the chorionic plate at almost any point, but when it inserts at the margin it is sometimes called a battledore placenta (Fig 2–29).

**E. Placenta Membranacea:** This type of placenta is one in which the decidua capsularis is so well vascularized that the chorion laeve does not atrophy and villi are maintained. Hence, the entire fetal envelope is functioning placenta.

**F. Placenta Accreta:** In rare cases, the placenta is abnormally adherent to the myometrium, presumably because it developed where there was a deficiency of decidua. Predisposing factors include placenta previa (one-third of cases), previous cesarean (one-fourth), a prior D&C (one-fourth), and grand multiparity. The adherence may be partial or total. Rarely, the placenta may invade the myometrium deeply (placenta increta) or even perforate the uterus (placenta percreta). When attempts are made to remove a placenta accreta manually, hemorrhage may be severe. The treatment is hysterectomy.

**G. Placenta Previa:** This abnormality is discussed in Chapter 23.

**H. Multiple Pregnancy Placenta:** In fraternal twins, the placentas may be 2 distinct entities or fused. There are 2 distinct chorions and amnions. In the case of identical twins, the picture may be more confusing. Depending upon the time of division of the fertilized ovum, the position of the placentas and number of membranes will vary. If the division occurs soon after fertilization, 2 distinct placentas and sets of membranes are the result. From that point on, many variations, eg monochorionic monoamniotic fused placentas and, possibly, interchange of blood supply, may occur. Further variations may be noted when triplets or more are derived from one ovum. When the presence of identical twins is suspected, it is always wise to clamp the cord on the placental side at the time it is clamped on the infant to minimize the chance of exsanguination of the uterine twin.

## REFERENCES

Basmajian JV: *Grant's Method of Anatomy,* 11th ed. Williams & Wilkins, Slonecker, CE: 1989.

Basmajian JV: *Primary Anatomy,* 8th ed. Williams & Wilkins, 1982.

Brooks SM, Brooks NP: *The Human Body: Structure and Function in Health and Disease,* 2nd ed. Mosby, 1980.

Caldwell WE, Moloy HC: Anatomical variations in the female pelvis. *Am J Obstet Gynecol* 1933:26:479.

Christensen JB, Telford I: *Synopsis of Gross Anatomy With Clinical Correlations,* 4th ed. Harper & Row, 1982.

Crafts RC: *A Textbook of Human Anatomy,* 3rd ed. Wiley, 1985.

Dienhart CM: *Basic Human Anatomy and Physiology,* 3rd ed. Saunders, 1979.

Donnelly JE: *Living Anatomy.* Human Kinetics, 1982.

Goss CM: *Gray's Anatomy of the Human Body,* 30th ed. Lea & Febiger, 1985.

Harrison RJ, Navarainam V (editors): *Progress in Anatomy.* Vol. 2. Cambridge Univ Press, 1982.

Hollinshead WH: *Anatoma Humana,* 3rd ed. Harper & Row, 1982.

Junqueira LC, Carneiro J, Kelley, RO: *Basic Histology,* 7th ed. Appleton & Lange, 1992.

Jones HW III, Wentz AC, and Burnett LS: *Novak's Textbook of Gynecology,* 11th ed. Williams & Wilkins, 1988.

Lane A: *Functional Human Anatomy: The Regional Approach,* 3rd ed. Kendall-Hunt, 1981.

Lockart RD et al: *Anatomy of the Human Body.* Faber & Faber, 1981.

Moore KL: *Clinically Oriented Anatomy.* 3rd ed. Williams & Wilkins, 1992.

Netter FH et al: *The Ciba Collection of Medical Illustrations.* Vol. 2: Reproductive System, Ciba, 1970.

Schlossberg L, Zuidema GD (editors): *The Johns Hopkins Atlas of Human Functional Anatomy,* 2nd ed. Johns Hopkins Univ Press, 1980.

Scicka D, Murawski E: Tendinous intersections of the rectus abdominis muscle in human fetuses. *Folia Morpho* 1980; 39:427.

Wilson DB, Wilson WJ: *Human Anatomy,* 2nd ed. Oxford Univ Press, 1983.

# 3

# The Role of Imaging Techniques in Gynecology

*Robert A. Graebe, MD*

## Case Report

C.O. is a 29-year-old white female, who presented with a history of infertility for several years, followed by a history of recurrent pregnancy losses.

Her past medical and surgical histories were negative. Gynecologically, she was remarkable in that she reported severe dysmenorrhea for the previous several years relieved by NSAIDs (nonsteroidal anti-inflammatory drugs). Her gynecologist found a low luteal phase progesterone and treated her with 50 mg of clomiphene citrate (CC) days 5–9 of the cycle.

She responded very well to the medication with a conception. The pregnancy resulted in a spontaneous abortion 5 weeks later. No D&C was required and she recovered well. She was still unable to conceive on her own and was again placed on CC. Again, she conceived and again had a spontaneous abortion—this time at 7 weeks' gestation. No D&C was performed.

The patient was then evaluated for recurrent pregnancy losses. Karyotype was normal for both partners. Hormonal evaluation was normal with the exception of a low mid-luteal phase progesterone. Immunologic and infectious screening also failed to reveal a cause for the recurrent losses. The hystero-salpingogram (HSG) demonstrated a midline filling defect similar to the one seen in Figure 3–1.

The patient was informed of the results and the potential for future miscarriages. The need for further evaluation and possible repair hysteroscopically or abdominally was carefully explained to the patient together with its risks and benefits. She elected to try CC one more time and hoped to avoid surgery.

At 8 weeks' gestation, vaginal ultrasonography revealed positive fetal cardiac activity in a CC-induced ovulation. While still on micronized progesterone, 100 mg 3 times daily, she was referred to her gynecologist for routine obstetric care.

At 12 weeks' gestation, the patient had an incomplete abortion that required a D&C. She recovered uneventfully and later returned to the office for further evaluation and treatment.

Several months were allowed to lapse before a hysteroscopy/laparoscopy revealed a broad-based intrauterine septum and stage I endometriosis. To evaluate the depth and width of the septum, a LaparoScan™ (EndoMedix, Irvine, CA) laparoscopic 7.5 Hz probe was used during the procedure. The septum was removed with the Storz™ (Storz K, Irvine CA) hysteroscopic resectoscope loop on a 40-watt setting. After the resection had been carried out, the ultrasonic probe was again used to measure the thickness of the myometrium and to verify the resection of the septum. A 30-mL 18F Foley catheter with the distal tip resected was placed in the fundus and inflated. The patient was discharged and placed on a broad-spectrum antibiotic and conjugated estrogen, 2.5 mg daily.

## Discussion

Recently, a proliferation of imaging techniques used in medical practice has occurred. Nowhere is this more apparent than in gynecology.

The HSG has been considered the "gold standard" in the imaging of the uterine corpus for benign disorders (submucous myomas, submucous polyps, localization of tubal occlusion, and evaluation of müllerian fusion defects) and malignant disease (endometrial carcinoma).

In the case reported, the standard scout film was obtained and the cervix was prepared after the following were assured: the position of the uterus, absence of pelvic tenderness, and a negative pregnancy test. The water-soluble contrast medium was injected into the uterine cavity and oblique and anteroposterior films were obtained. These showed a midline uterine filling defect of the type usually seen with septate or bicornuate uteri.

Ultrasonography performed on this patient during her pregnancies failed to show the filling defect. If suspected, the septum may have been encountered by more careful scanning. The scans of the last pregnancy revealed only an eccentrically placed pregnancy that might have been seen ultrasonographically even in normally structured uteri. Although not helpful at this point, ultrasonographic examination of the uterus between conceptions might have been helpful if used with a distending medium. (This is especially useful in patients allergic to iodine contrast medium.)

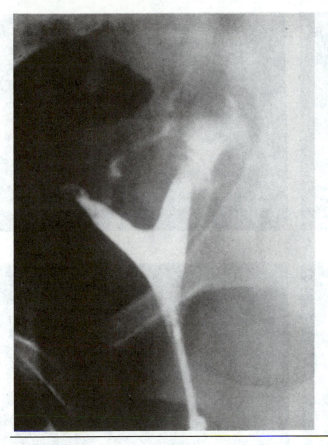

**Figure 3–1.** Müllerian anomaly as demonstrated by hysterosalpingogram. (Reproduced, with permission, from Doyle MB: Magnetic resonance imaging in müllerian fusion defects. J Reprod Med 1992;37:33.)

This technique of ultrasonic HSG has been described by Richman et al (1984) and is performed by occluding the cervix with a uterine injector and distending the uterus. This method can demonstrate the separate cavities as well as the possible difference between the septate and the bicornuate uterus while demonstrating tubal patency. This technique was adopted for this patient during her uterine septum resection to add ultrasonic contrast between the endometrial cavity and septum and the myometrium.

Using 2 video cameras (one for the resectoscope and the other for the laparoscope and the Laparo-Scan™ laparoscopic ultrasound probe), all aspects of the surgery were evaluated. This setup allowed the operating surgeon adequate visualization of the uterine cavity during the resection and enabled other personnel in the operating room to follow the progress of the surgery. The laparoscopic video allowed the careful monitoring of the uterine surface and provided the surgeon with the security that there would be less likelihood of a uterine perforation. This complication could have resulted in possible bowel injury.

The usefulness of the laparoscopic ultrasound probe with a picture within a picture was that it allowed the visualization of the 2 separate cavities and measurement of the length and width of the septum. It also enabled the operator to demonstrate the complete removal of the septum (Fig 3–2).

## Imaging of the Uterus

Pelvic ultrasonography has demonstrated itself to have a significant role in the diagnosis of uterine leiomyomas (submucous, intramural, and subserosal). The laparoscopic probe may be very useful in evaluating myomas, their position, and their vascular supply. Ultrasonography may also be useful in evaluating the feasibility of continuing the procedure pelviscopically.

Occasionally, the detection and localization of myomas, assessment of size, and their differential diagnosis are difficult. In these circumstances it is sometimes useful to perform magnetic resonance imaging (MRI) of the pelvis. MRI can accurately measure the volume of the myoma (Andreyko et al, 1988). This is an aid in determining whether medical management of myomas has resulted in shrinkage or if conservatively treated myomas are growing. Malignant degeneration of myomas visualized by MRI as described by some authors would allow for early and appropriate intervention (Pellerito et al, 1992).

MRI also may be useful in the differential diagnosis of myomas and adenomyosis, benign and malig-

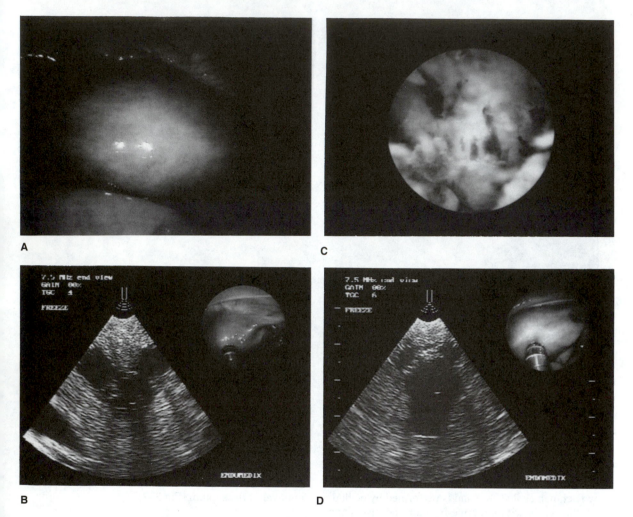

**Figure 3–2.** Uterine septum. **A:** Laparoscopic view shows a broad uterine fundus. **B:** Laparoscopic probe on the fundus of the uterus demonstrates the depth and width of the septum. **C:** Hysteroscopic view showing the resection of the uterine septum. **D:** Laparoscopic probe on the fundus of the uterus demonstrates the resected septum. (Note the echogenicity of the debris in the fundus.)

nant ovarian pathology, pelvic kidney, and pelvic abscess.

Pellerito et al (1992) have described MRI of müllerian defects to be an effective method of evaluation between the septate and the bicornuate uterus thus avoiding the more costly laparoscopy. In patients with very complicated müllerian fusion defects (didelphys with transverse vaginal septum or noncommunicating uterine segment), MRI may give a clear anatomic picture of the condition and allow for a properly planned surgical repair. If pelvic MRI had been performed on the patient in the case report, it would probably have had the same appearance as that of the MRI in Figure 3–3. (Readers are referred to the review of MRI in müllerian fusion defects in Table 3–1.)

## Imaging of the Ovaries

About 12,000 women in the USA die annually as a result of ovarian cancer. Unfortunately, the ability of the pelvic examination to detect small ovarian malignancy is low. The same can be said of CA-125 monoclonal marker for ovarian cancer, which has been found to be a poor predictor of early cases (Di-Xia et al, 1988).

The flat plate of the abdomen may still be useful in the diagnosis of dermoid cysts of the ovary. However, cystic and solid structures of the ovary are now better evaluated by transabdominal ultrasonography (TAUS) and transvaginal ultrasonography (TVUS), computerized tomography (CT), and MRI.

Morphologic criteria have been assigned to give additional caution concerning the ultrasound finding when ovarian cancer is suspected. Cysts > 4 cm, solid

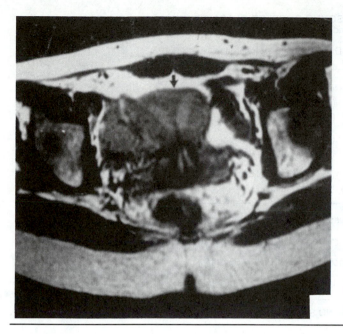

**Figure 3–3.** Complete uterine septum extending to the cervix. (Reprinted, with permission, from Doyle MB: Magnetic resonance imaging in müllerian fusion defects. J Reprod Med 1992; 37:33.)

and cystic components, septa and papillary nodules have all been described (Meire et al, 1978).

Recently, transvaginal ultrasonography combined with color flow and Doppler waveform was shown by Kurjak et al (1992) to be sensitive and specific enough for application in an ovarian cancer screening program. Color flow allows for the identification of vessels not previously identified with gray scale. With the use of the Doppler waveform, high- and low-resistance vessels in the ovaries can be separated. The resistance index (RI) is the systolic flow velocity peak minus the diastolic trough divided by the sys-

**Table 3–1.** Types of müllerian anomalies and associated MRI findings (Reprinted with permission from Doyle.)

| Class and Type | No. | Finding |
|---|---|---|
| I: Segmental agenesis/hypoplasia | 7 (24%) | Agenesis: no identifiable organ or small amorphous tissue |
| A. Vaginal | 0 | remnant. Hypoplasia: uterus small for patient's age, main- |
| B. Cervical | 0 | tains adult body/cervix ratio of 2:1, reduced intercornual |
| C. Fundal | 0 | distance (< 2 cm), low signal intensity on $T_2$-weighted im- |
| D. Tubal | 0 | ages with poor zonal differentiation, endometrial/myome- |
| E. Combined | 7 | trial width reduced. |
| II: Unicornuate uterus | 5 (17%) | Banana-shaped uterus, normal width of endometrium and |
| A1. Rudimentary horn with endometrium | | myometrium, endometrial/myometrial ratio preserved |
|   (A) Communicating with main uterine cavity | 0 | |
|   (B) Not communicating with main uterine cavity | 1 | |
| A2. Rudimentary horn without endometrium | 1 | |
| B. No rudimentary horn | 3 | |
| III: Didelphys (Figure 7) | 5 (17%) | Double, separate uterus, cervix and upper vagina; each uter- |
| | | ine cavity of normal volume; endometrium and myome- |
| | | trium of normal width; endometrial/myometrial ratio normal |
| IV: Bicornuate uterus (Figure 6) | 10 (34%) | Uterine fundus concave or flattened outward, two horns visi- |
| A. Complete | 3 | ble with increased intercornual distance (> 4 cm), septum- |
| B. Partial | 3 | high-signal-intensity myometrium on $T_2$-weighted images |
| C. Arcuate | 4 | at level of fundus; high-signal-intensity myometrium (7 pa- |
| | | tients) or low-signal-intensity fibrous tissue at level of |
| | | lower uterine segment (3 patients) |
| V: Septate (Figure 5) | 2 (7%) | Uterine fundus convex outward, normal intercornual dis- |
| A. Complete (Figure 5B, C) | 1 | tance (2–4 cm), each uterine cavity reduced in volume, |
| B. Incomplete (Figure 5A) | 1 | endometrial/myometrial width and ratio normal, septum— |
| | | low signal intensity on $T_1$- and $T_2$-weighted images |

Because of rounding, the percentages do not add up to 100.

## OVARIAN TUMOR ULTRASOUND-DOPPLER CLASSIFICATION
Circle all characteristics seen and add numbers in parentheses for a score.

Patient name _____ Date _____ Institution _____

|  | FLUID |  | INTERNAL BORDERS |  | SIZE |
|---|---|---|---|---|---|
| **UNILOCULAR** | Clear | (0) | Smooth | (0) |  |
|  | Internal echoes | (1) | Irregular | (2) |  |
| **MULTILOCULAR** | Clear | (1) | Smooth | (1) |  |
|  | Internal echoes | (1) | Irregular | (2) |  |
| **CYSTIC-SOLID** | Clear | (1) | Smooth | (1) |  |
|  | Internal echoes | (2) | Irregular | (2) |  |

| | | | | | |
|---|---|---|---|---|---|
| **PAPILLARY PROJECTIONS** | Suspicious | (1) | Definite | (2) |
| **SOLID** | Homogenous | (1) | Echogenic | (2) |
| **PERITONEAL FLUID** | Absent | (0) | Present | (1) |
| **LATERALITY** | Unilateral | (0) | Bilateral | (1) |

### ULTRASOUND SCORE
≤ 2    Benign
3–4    Questionable
> 4    Suspicious

| **COLOR DOPPLER** | | **RI (resistance index)** | |
|---|---|---|---|
| No vessels seen | (0) | | (0) |
| Regular separate vessels | (1) | > 0.40 | (1) |
| Randomly dispersed vessels | (2) | < 0.41 | (2) |

If suspected corpus luteum, repeat in next menstrual cycle in proliferative phase.

### COLOR DOPPLER SCORE
≤ 2    Benign
3–4    Questionable

**Figure 3–4.** Scoring system used to evaluate the morphology of adnexal tumor. RI = resistance index. (Reprinted, with permission, from Kurjak A, Shulman H, Sosic A, et al: Transvaginal ultrasound, color flow, and Doppler waveform of the postmenopausal adnexal mass. Obstet Gynecol 1992;80:917.

tolic peak. Using these techniques in 1000 women, Kurjak et al (1992) were able to identify 83 women with the signs ultrasonographically or symptoms that led to surgery (Fig 3–4). Twenty-nine tumors were malignant, 4 from the asymptomatic group (Table 3–2). Color flow was not seen in only 2 of the malignant tumors. This demonstrates a sensitivity of 93% (Table 3–3). With a specificity of 65% for color flow alone, Doppler measurements are needed (Table 3–4). On the basis of distribution of RI values in benign and malignant tumors, a statistical cutoff value for the RI is 0.41 (Fig 3–5). Ability to identify malignant ovarian tumors with a combination of the above-mentioned techniques may allow for timely referral to gynecologic oncologists rather than the simpler laparoscopic approaches to benign adnexal disease.

Not all studies are in agreement. Hata et al (1992), in an evaluation of 63 patients with ovarian tumors (36 benign, 27 malignant), found that transvaginal Doppler ultrasonography does not provide any more useful diagnostic information than transvaginal sonography, MRI, or CA-125 for the differentiation of malignant from benign ovarian tumors. Clearly, additional clinical studies are needed to realize the full diagnostic potential of these imaging techniques.

CT may be useful for staging ovarian cancer preoperatively or for planning second-look procedures. In patients with benign-appearing adnexal masses (ovarian cysts or tubo-ovarian abscesses), CT may be very useful for biopsy and drainage. The contraindications to needle biopsy and drainage include lack of a safe unobstructed path for the needle, bleeding disorders, and lack of a motivated patient.

**Table 3–2.** Histology and blood flow characteristics. (Reprinted with permission from Kurjak et al.)

| Histology | N | Flow Detected | RI |
|---|---|---|---|
| **Malignant** | | | |
| Papillary adenocarci-noma | 13 | 12 | 0.39 ± 0.04 |
| Serous cystadeno-carcinoma | 3 | 3 | 0.30 ± 0.04 |
| Endometrioid adenocar-cinoma | 4 | 4 | 0.38 ± 0.02 |
| Metastatic carcinoma | 7 | 7 | 0.37 ± 0.07 |
| Theca-granulosa cell | 2 | 1 | 0.37 |
| Total | 29 | 27 | 0.37 ± 0.08 |
| **Benign** | | | |
| Simple cyst | 25 | 5 | 0.75 ± 0.17 |
| Papillary serous cyst | 4 | 1 | 0.6 |
| Mucinous cyst | 5 | 3 | 0.62 ± 0.09 |
| Inflammatory mass | 2 | 1 | 0.62 |
| Parasitic cyst | 1 | 0 | 0 |
| Fibroma | 4 | 3 | 0.56 ± 0.03 |
| Thecoma | 2 | 2 | 0.60 |
| Cystadenofibroma | 1 | 1 | 0.56 |
| Endometrioma | 4 | 1 | 0.56 |
| Cystic teratoma | 1 | 1 | 0.36 |
| Pseudo- and parovar-ian cyst | 4 | 0 | 0 |
| Brenner tumor | 1 | 1 | 0.50 |
| Total | 54 | 19 | 0.62 ± 0.11* |

RI = resistance index.
Data are presented as N or mean ± SD.
*P < .001.

## Imaging of the Fallopian Tubes

The best direct evaluation of the patency and architecture of the fallopian tubes is by means of endoscopic techniques. The best evaluation of tubal function indirectly is with HSG. This method allows demonstration of tubal patency and visualization of tubal rugations while avoiding the more costly laparoscopic surgery. Some disadvantages of HSG are pelvic infection, dye allergies, failure to detect adnexal adhesions, and false-positives for tubal occlusion. For patients with dye allergies, the procedure described by Richman et al (1984) could be useful in demonstrating tubal patency.

## Imaging in Ectopic Pregnancy

Romero et al (1985) found that when the serial human chorionic gonadotropin (hCG) levels reach

**Table 3–3.** Color flow in ovarian masses. (Reprinted with permission from Kurjak et al.)

| | Present | Absent |
|---|---|---|
| Benign | 19 | 35 |
| Malignant | 27 | 2 |

Fisher exact two-tailed test: < 1 × 10^-7. Sensitivity = 93%; specificity = 65%; positive predictive value = 59%; negative predictive value = 95%.

**Table 3–4.** Flow pattern in benign and malignant ovaries. (Reprinted with permission from Kurjak et al.)

| Vessel Type | RI Benign | RI Malignant |
|---|---|---|
| Peripheral | 0.56 (0.48–1.0) | 0.40 (0.31–0.61)* |
| Central | 0.54 (0.46–0.62) | 0.38 (0.27–0.41)* |
| Septal | 0.48 (0.47–0.50) | 0.37 (0.32–0.42)* |

RI = resistance index.
Data are presented as mean (range).
*P < .01.

6500 mU/mL, most normal intrauterine pregnancies can be detected by TAUS as a gestational sac. The value of adnexal sonography in the management of ectopic pregnancies was demonstrated by Batzer et al. They showed that if no gestational sac was seen on TAUS by 28 days and a HCG level was greater then 7500 mU/mL, an ectopic gestation should be suspected (Batzer et al 1983). In a second related report, Romero et al (1988) stated that the presence of fluid in cul-de-sac and a noncystic adnexal mass has a predictive value of 94% in the diagnosis of ectopic pregnancy. However, the sonographic appearance of a pseudogestational sac should not be confused with the gestational sac. In the latter, a double-ring sign caused by the decidua parietalis is seen abutting against the decidua capsularis (Bradley et al, 1983).

TVUS, on the other hand, has the advantage of earlier and improved localization of the pregnancy in the diagnosis of ectopic and intrauterine pregnancy with less pelvic discomfort since the bladder is not painfully distended (Thorsen et al, 1990). Shapiro et al (1988) noted that when using TVUS, they were able to identify correctly 92% of the time the presence of an ectopic when the HCG titer was less than 3600 mU/mL.

CT and MRI studies in the evaluation of ectopic pregnancies are limited at the present time, but clinical application of the newer color flow and Doppler flow in the diagnosis of ectopic pregnancies holds great promise when combined with pelvic ultrasound and serial hCG determinations (Taylor et al, 1990).

## Conclusion

The rapidly developing imaging techniques prevalent today have proved to be a valuable aid in the diagnosis and early treatment of benign and malignant gynecologic disorders. To provide the patient with the highest level of medical care, the contemporary practicing gynecologist must keep constantly abreast of the new developments and applications of diagnostic imaging.

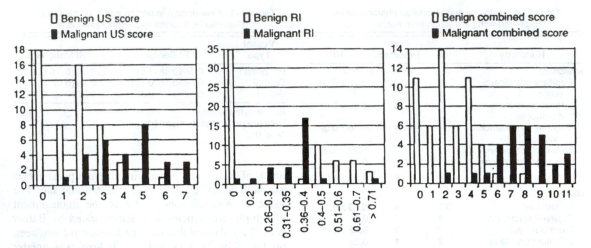

**Figure 3–5.** Distribution of data results in this study. **A:** The ultrasound (US) score; **B:** resistance index (RI); and **C:** combination of the two. In (**B**), an RI of zero means that no flow was seen. (Reprinted, with permission from Kurjak A, Shulman H, Sosic A, et al: Transvaginal ultrasound, color flow, and Doppler waveform of the postmenopausal adnexal mass. Obstet Gynecol 1992;80:917.)

## REFERENCES

Andreyko JL, Blumenfeld Z, Marshall LA, et al: Use of an agonistic analog of gonadotropin-releasing hormone (nafarelin) to treat leiomyomas: Assessment by magnetic resonance imaging. Am J Obstet Gynecol 1988;158:903.

Batzer FR, Weiner SW, Corson SL, et al: Landmarks during the first forty-two days of gestation demonstrated by the β subunit of human chorionic gonadotropin and ultrasound. Am J Obstet Gynecol 1983;146:973.

Bradley WG, Fiske CE, Filly RA: The double sac sign of early intrauterine pregnancy: Use in exclusion of ectopic pregnancy. Radiology 1983;143:223.

Di-Xia C, Schwartz PE, Xinguo ZI, et al: Evaluation of Ca 125 levels in differentiating malignant from benign tumor in patients with pelvic masses. Obstet Gynecol 1988;72:23.

Doyle MB: Magnetic resonance imaging in müllerian fusion defects. J Reprod Med 1992;37:33.

Hata K, Hata T, Manabe A, et al: A critical evaluation of transvaginal Doppler studies, transvaginal sonography, magnetic resonance imaging, and CA 125 in detecting ovarian cancer. Obstet Gynecol 1992;80:922.

Janus C, White M, Dottino P, et al: Uterine leiomyosarcoma magnetic resonance imaging. Gynecol Oncol 1989; 32: 79.

Kurjak A, Shulman H, Sosic A, et al: Transvaginal ultrasound, color flow, and Doppler waveform of the postmenopausal adnexal mass. Obstet Gynecol 1992;80:917.

Meire HB, Farrant P, Guha T: Distinction of benign from malignant ovarian cysts by ultrasound. Br J Obstet Gynaecol 1978;85:893.

Pellerito JS, McCarthy SM, Doyle MB, et al: Diagnosis of uterine anomalies: Relative accuracy of MR imaging, endovaginal sonography, and hysterosalpingography. Radiology 1992;183:795.

Richman TS, Viscomi GN, DeCherney Ah, et al: Fallopian tubal patency assessed by ultrasound following fluid injection. Radiology 1984;152:507.

Romero R, Kadar N, Castro D, et al: The value of adnexal sonographic findings in the diagnosis of ectopic pregnancy. Am J Obstet Gynecol 1988;158:52.

Romero R, Kadar N, Jeanty P, et al: Diagnosis in ectopic pregnancy: Value of the discriminatory human chorionic gonadotropin zone. Obstet Gynecol 1985;66:357.

Shapiro BS, Cullen M, Taylor KJW, et al: Transvaginal ultrasonography for the diagnosis of ectopic pregnancy. Fertil Steril 1988;50:425.

Taylor K, Ramos I, Feyock A, et al: Ectopic pregnancy: Duplex Doppler evaluation. Radiology 1990;176:359.

Thorsen MK, Lawson TL, Aiman EJ, et al: Diagnosis of ectopic pregnancy: Endovaginal vs. transabdominal sonography. Radiology 1990;155:307.

# Embryology of the Urogenital System & Congenital Anomalies of the Female Genital Tract

# 4

*Joseph D. Bast, PhD*

The adult genital and urinary systems are distinct both in function and in anatomy, except for the male urethra. During development, however, the 2 systems are closely associated. Primordial elements in the urinary system participate in the formation of genital structures; this requisite initial developmental overlap of the 2 systems covers approximately 4–12 weeks after fertilization. The complexity of developmental events in these systems is evident by the incomplete separation of the 2 systems found in some congenital anomalies (eg, female pseudohermaphroditism with persistent urogenital sinus). For the sake of clarity, this chapter describes the embryology of each system separately, rather than following a strict developmental chronology.

This chapter also presents descriptive overviews of some congenital malformations of the female genital tract and, when possible, an explanation of their embryonic origins. In view of the complexity and duration of differentiation and development of the genital and urinary systems, it is not surprising that the incidence of malformations involving these systems is one of the highest (10%) of all body systems. Etiologies of congenital malformations are sometimes categorized on the basis of genetic, environmental, or genetic-plus-environmental (so-called polyfactorial inheritance) factors. Known genetic and inheritance factors reputedly account for about 20% of anomalies detected at birth, aberration of chromosomes for nearly 5%, and environmental factors for nearly 10%. The significance of these statistics must be viewed against reports that (1) an estimated one-third to one-half of human zygotes are lost during the first week of gestation and (2) the cause of possibly 70% of human anomalies is unknown. Even so, congenital malformations remain a matter of concern because they are detected in nearly 6% of infants, and 20% of perinatal deaths are purportedly due to congenital anomalies.

The inherent pattern of normal development of the genital system can be viewed as one directed toward somatic "femaleness," unless development is directed by factors for "maleness." The presence and expression of a Y chromosome (and its testis-determining genes) in a normal 46,XY karyotype of somatic cells directs differentiation toward a testis, and normal development of the testis makes available its steroidal and proteinaceous hormones for the selection and differentiation of the genital ducts. In the normal absence of these testicular products, the "female" paramesonephric (müllerian) ducts persist. Normal feminization or masculinization of the external genitalia is also a result of the respective timely absence or presence of androgen.

An infant usually is reared as female or male according to the appearance of the external genitalia. However, genital sex is not always immediately discernible, and the choice of sex of rearing can be an anxiety-provoking consideration. Unfortunately, even when genital sex is apparent, later clinical presentation may unmask disorders of sexual differentiation that can lead to problems in psychologic adjustment. Whether a somatic disorder is detected at birth or later, investigative backtracking through the developmental process is necessary for proper diagnosis and treatment.

## OVERVIEW OF THE FIRST FOUR WEEKS OF DEVELOPMENT*

The transformation of the bilaminar embryonic disk into a trilaminar disk composed of **ectoderm, mesoderm,** and **endoderm** (the 3 embryonic germ layers) occurs during the third week by a process called **gastrulation** (Fig 4–1). All 3 layers are derived from epiblast. During this process, a specialized longitudinal thickening of epiblast, the **primitive streak,** forms near the margin (future caudal region) of the bilaminar disk and eventually elongates cephalad through the midline of the disk and extends to the

---

*Embryonic or fetal ages given in this chapter are relative to the time of fertilization and should be considered estimates rather than absolutes.

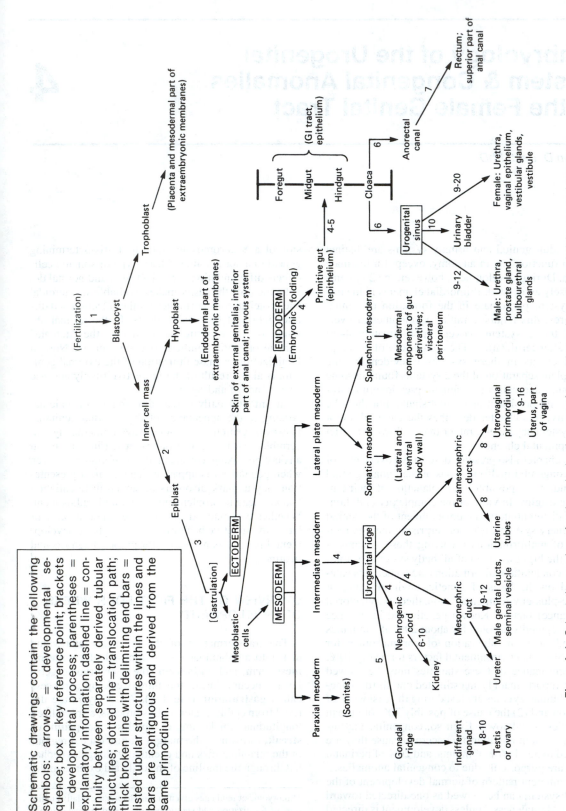

**Figure 4–1.** Schematic overview of embryonic development of progenitory urinary and genital tissues and structures considered to be derivatives of embryonic ectoderm, mesoderm, or endoderm. Numbers indicate the weeks after fertilization when the indicated developmental change occurs.

Schematic drawings contain the following symbols: arrows = developmental sequence; box = key reference point; brackets = developmental process; parentheses = explanatory information; dashed line = continuity between separately derived tubular structures; dotted line = translocation path; thick broken line with delimiting end bars = listed tubular structures within the lines and bars are contiguous and derived from the same primordium.

central region. Some epiblastic cells migrate medially through a midline depression of the streak to the ventral aspect of the streak, whereafter they become **mesoblastic cells.** The mesoblastic cells migrate peripherally between most of the epiblast and the hypoblast, forming the middle layer (**embryonic mesoderm**) of the now trilaminar disk. Other mesoblastic cells migrate into the hypoblastic layer, causing lateral displacement of most, if not all, of the hypoblastic cells. This new ventral layer of the disk becomes the **embryonic endoderm.** With formation of the new mesodermal layer, the overlying epiblast becomes the **embryonic ectoderm,** of which the medial part gives rise to **neuroectoderm,** the forerunner of the neural tube and neural crest (ie, the nervous system). By the end of the third week, 3 clusters of embryonic mesoderm are organized on both sides of the midline-developing notochord and neural tube.

The medial cluster is a thickened longitudinal column of mesoderm called **paraxial mesoderm,** from which **somites,** and in turn much of the axial skeleton, will form. The lateralmost cluster is called **lateral plate mesoderm,** in which a space (or coelom) develops, creating dorsal and ventral mesodermal layers (Fig 4–2). The **intermediate mesoderm** is located between the paraxial and lateral plate mesoderm and is the origin of the urogenital ridge and, hence, much of the reproductive and excretory systems (Fig 4–1). The primitive streak regresses after the fourth week. Rarely, degeneration of the streak is incomplete and presumptive remnants form a teratoma in the sacrococcygeal region of the fetus (more common in females than in males).

Weeks 4 through 8 of development are called the **embryonic period** (the **fetal period** is from week 9 to term) because formation of all major internal and external structures, including the 2 primary forerunners of the urogenital system (urogenital ridge and urogenital sinus), begins during this time. During this period the embryo is most likely to develop major congenital or acquired morphologic anomalies in response to the effects of various agents. During the fourth week, the shape of the embryo changes from that of a trilaminar disk to that of a crescentic cylinder. The change results from "folding," or flexion, of the embryonic disk in a ventral direction through both its transverse and longitudinal planes. Flexion occurs as midline structures (neural tube and somites) develop and grow at a faster pace than more lateral tissues (ectoderm, 2 layers of lateral plate mesoderm enclosing the coelom between them, and endoderm). Thus, during transverse folding, the lateral tissues on each side of the embryo curl ventromedially and join the respective tissues from the other side, creating a midline ventral tube (the endoderm-lined **primitive gut**), a mesoderm-lined coelomic cavity (the **primitive abdominopelvic cavity**), and the incomplete ventral and lateral body wall. Concurrent longitudinal flexion ventrally of the caudal region of the disk establishes the pouch-like distal end, or **cloaca,** of the primitive gut as well as the distal attachment of the cloaca to the yolk sac through the allantois of the sac (Fig 4–4).

A noteworthy point (see Gonads, in text that follows) is that the primordial germ cells of the later-developing gonad initially are found close to the allantois and later migrate to the gonadal primordia. Subsequent partitioning of the cloaca during the sixth week results in formation of the anorectal canal and the **urogenital sinus,** the progenitor of the urinary bladder, urethra, vagina, and other genital structures (Fig 4–1 and Table 4–1; see Subdivision of the Cloaca & Formation of the Urogenital Sinus in following text).

Another consequence of the folding process is the repositioning of the intermediate mesoderm, the forerunner of the urogenital ridge. Laterally adjacent to developing somites (from paraxial mesoderm) before flexion, the intermediate mesoderm is located after flexion just lateral to the dorsal mesentery of the gut and in the dorsal wall of the new body cavity. Thickening of this intermediate mesoderm with subsequent bulging into the cavity will form the longitudinal **urogenital ridge** (Figs 4–1 and 4–4). Thus, by the end of the fourth week of development, the principal structures (urogenital ridge and cloaca) and tissues that give rise to the urogenital system are present.

Tables 4–1 and 4–2 provide a general overview of urogenital development.

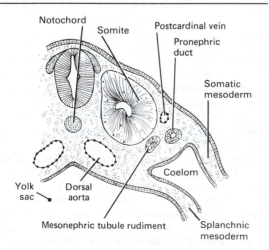

Notochord
Somite
Postcardinal vein
Pronephric duct
Somatic mesoderm
Coelom
Yolk sac
Dorsal aorta
Mesonephric tubule rudiment
Splanchnic mesoderm

**Figure 4–2.** Cross section of embryo at the level of the rudimentary mesonephros. The tubule will form a lumen, grow, and connect with the duct. About 4 weeks' gestation, during embryonic flexion.

## THE URINARY SYSTEM

Three excretory "systems" form successively, with temporal overlap, during the embryonic period. Each

**Table 4–1.** Adult derivatives and vestigial remains of embryonic urogenital structures.[1,2]

| Embryonic Structure | Male | Female |
|---|---|---|
| Indifferent gonad | *Testis* | *Ovary* |
| Cortex | *Seminiferous tubules* | *Ovarian follicles* |
| Medulla | *Rete testis* | *Medulla* |
| | | Rete ovarii |
| Gubernaculum | Gubernaculum testis | *Ovarian ligament* |
| | | *Round ligament of uterus* |
| Mesonephric tubules | *Ductus efferentes* | Epoophoron |
| | Paradidymis | Paroophoron |
| Mesonephric duct | Appendix of epididymis | Appendix vesiculosa |
| | *Ductus epididymidis* | Duct of epoophoron |
| | *Ductus deferens* | Duct of Gartner |
| | *Ureter, pelvis, calices,* and *collecting tubules* | *Ureter, pelvis, calices,* and *collecting tubules* |
| | *Ejaculatory duct and seminal vesicle* | |
| Paramesonephric duct | Appendix of testis | Hydatid (of Morgagni) |
| | | *Uterine tube* |
| | | *Uterus* |
| | | *Vagina (fibromuscular wall)* |
| Urogenital sinus | *Urinary bladder* | *Urinary bladder* |
| | *Urethra* (except glandular portion) | *Urethra* |
| | | *Vagina* |
| | Prostatic utricle | *Urethral* and *paraurethral glands* |
| | *Prostate gland* | |
| | *Bulbourethral glands* | *Greater vestibular glands* |
| Müllerian tubercle | Seminal colliculus | Hymen |
| Genital tubercle | *Penis* | *Clitoris* |
| | *Glans penis* | *Glans clitoridis* |
| | *Corpora cavernosa penis* | *Corpora cavernosa clitoridis* |
| | *Corpus spongiosum* | *Bulb of the vestibule* |
| Urogenital folds | *Ventral aspect of penis* | *Labia minora* |
| Labioscrotal swellings | *Scrotum* | *Labia majora* |

[1]Modified and reproduced, with permission, from Moore KL, Persaud TVN: *The Developing Human: Clinically Oriented Embryology,* 5th ed. Saunders, 1993.
[2]Functional derivatives are in italics.

system has a different excretory "organ," but the 3 systems share anatomic continuity through development of their excretory ducts. The 3 systems are mesodermal derivatives of the urogenital ridge (Figs 4–3 and 4–4), part of which becomes a longitudinal mass, the **nephrogenic cord.** The **pronephros,** or organ of the first system, exists rudimentarily, is nonfunc-

tional, and regresses during the fourth week. However, the developing pronephric ducts continue to grow and become the mesonephric ducts of the subsequent kidney, the **mesonephros.** The paired mesonephroi exist during 4–8 weeks as simplified morphologic versions of the third, or permanent, set of kidneys, and they may have transient excretory function. The permanent kidney, the **metanephros,** begins to form in response to an inductive influence of a diverticulum of the mesonephric ducts during the fifth week and becomes functional at 10–13 weeks. During nephric differentiation, the urogenital mass becomes suspended from the dorsal wall by a double-layered urogenital mesentery.

## Pronephros

Segmented clusters of cells form in each urogenital ridge opposite the cervical somitic region and give rise to **pronephric tubules.** The lateral end of a tubule in one segment of the ridge grows caudally to fuse with the end of the pronephric tubule in the next segment, thus initiating the cephalic portion of each of the bilateral **pronephric ducts** (Fig 4–3). The pronephroi degenerate by the end of the fourth week, but, by initiating formation of pronephric ducts, they set in motion the developmental sequence for the formation of the permanent excretory ducts and kidneys. The pronephric ducts continue to grow caudally until week 5, when they contact and open into the lateral posterior wall of the cloaca.

## Mesonephros

Development of the mesonephric glomerulotubular units begins while the pronephric tubules are regressing. Cells in each nephrogenic cord condense to form cell clusters just caudal to the pronephros and adjacent to the caudally growing pronephric duct (now called the **mesonephric duct**). Each cluster differentiates into a hollow **mesonephric vesicle** and then a **mesonephric tubule.** Subsequently, the lateral end of a tubule joins the mesonephric duct (Figs 4–4 and 4–5), while the medial end of the tubule expands into a double-layered, cup-shaped primitive glomerular capsule (**Bowman's capsule**; Fig 4–6). The capsule is vascularized by a capillary tuft, the **glomerulus,** derived from the aorta. Proliferation of the tubule's midportion produces a primitive version of a convoluted tubule.

While differentiation of the mesonephros is taking place in the caudal region, regression of mature tubules in the cranial region is also occurring (Fig 4–7). This craniocaudal gradient of differentiation followed by regression can give the impression that the relatively large, ovoid mesonephric kidney "descends" along the posterior wall of the body cavity during the embryonic period. By the end of this period, most remaining mesonephric tubules and glomeruli have begun to degenerate. Some of these tu-

**Table 4–2.** Developmental chronology of the human urogenital system.[1]

| Age in Weeks[2] | Size (C-R)[3] in mm | Urogenital System |
|---|---|---|
| 2.5 | 1.5 | Allantois present. |
| 3.5 | 2.5 | All pronephric tubules formed.<br>Pronephric duct growing caudad as a blind tube.<br>Cloaca and cloacal membrane present. |
| 4 | 5 | Primordial germ cells near allantois.<br>Pronephros degenerated.<br>Pronephric (mesonephric) duct reaches cloaca.<br>Mesonephric tubules differentiating rapidly.<br>Metanephric bud pushes into secretory primodrium. |
| 5 | 8 | Mesonephros reaches its caudal limit.<br>Ureteric and pelvic primordia distinct. |
| 6 | 12 | Cloaca subdividing into urogenital sinus and anorectal canal.<br>Sexless gonad and genital tubercle prominent.<br>Paramesonephric duct appearing.<br>Metanephric collecting tubules begin branching. |
| 7 | 17 | Mesonephros at peak of differentiation.<br>Urogenital sinus separated from anorectal canal (cloaca subdivided).<br>Urogenital and anal membranes rupturing. |
| 8 | 23 | Earliest metanephric secretory tubules differentiating.<br>Testis (8 weeks) and ovary (9–10 weeks) identifiable as such.<br>Paramesonephric ducts, nearing urogenital sinus, are ready to unite as uterovaginal<br>    primordium.<br>Genital ligaments indicated. |
| 10 | 40 | Kidney able to excrete urine.<br>Bladder expands as sac.<br>Genital duct of opposite sex degenerating.<br>Bulbourethral and vestibular glands appearing.<br> Vaginal bulbs forming. |
| 12 | 56 | Kidney in lumbar location.<br>Early ovarian folliculogenesis begins.<br>Uterine horns absorbed.<br>External genitalia attain distinctive features.<br>Mesonephros and rete tubules complete male duct.<br>Prostate and seminal vesicle appearing.<br>Hollow viscera gaining muscular walls. |
| 16 | 112 | Testis at deep inguinal ring.<br>Uterus and vagina recognizable as such.<br>Mesonephros involuted. |
| 20–38<br>(5–9 months) | 160–350 | Female urogenital sinus becoming a shallow vestibule (5 months).<br>Vagina regains lumen (5 months).<br>Uterine glands begin to appear (5 months).<br>Scrotum solid until sacs and testes descend (7–8 months).<br>Kidney tubules cease forming at birth. |

[1]Modified and reproduced, with permission, from Arey LB: *Developmental Anatomy,* 7th ed. Saunders, 1965.
[2]After fertilization.
[3]C–R, crown-rump length.

bules (descriptively called **epigenital mesonephric tubules**) persist in the mesonephric region laterally adjacent to the developing gonad and will participate in formation of the gonad and the male ductuli efferentes (Fig 4–8). A few tubules at other levels may persist as vestigial remnants near the gonad and sometimes become cystic (see Figs 4–14 and 4–15).

Differentiation of the caudal segment of the mesonephric ducts results in (1) incorporation of part of the ducts into the wall of the urogenital sinus (early vesicular trigone, see following text), and (2) formation of a ductal diverticulum, which plays an essential role in formation of the definitive kidney. If male sex differentiation occurs, the major portion of each duct becomes the epididymis, ductus deferens, and ejaculatory duct. Only small vestigial remnants of the duct sometimes persist in the female (**Gartner's duct; duct of the epoophoron**).

## Metanephros (Definitive Kidney)

**A. Collecting Ducts:** By the end of the fifth week, a **ureteric bud,** or metanephric diverticulum, forms on the caudal part of the mesonephric duct

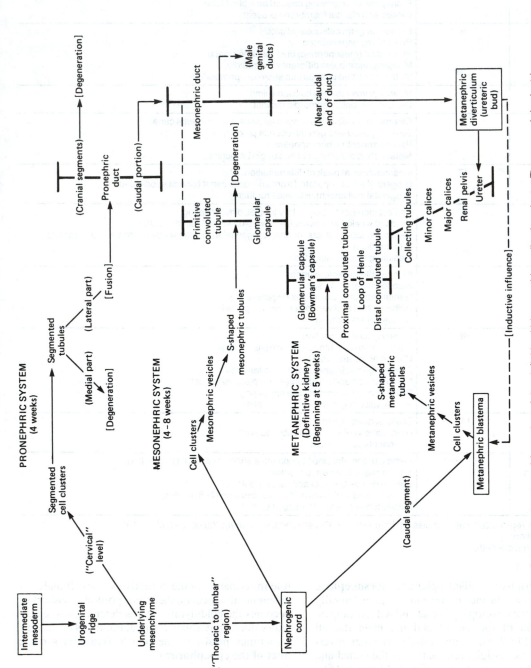

**Figure 4–3.** Schematic drawing of formation of the definitive kidney and its collecting ducts. The pronephric duct is probably the only structure that participates in all 3 urinary systems, as its caudal portion continues to grow and is called the mesonephric duct when the mesonephric system develops. (Explanatory symbols are given in Fig 4–1.)

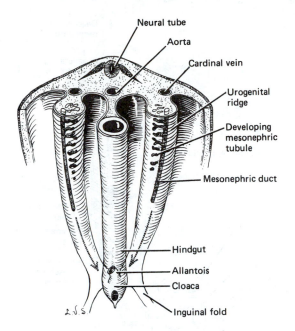

**Figure 4–4.** Early stage in the formation of the meso-nephric kidneys and their collecting ducts in the urogeni-tal ridge. The central tissue of the ridge is the nephrogenic cord, in which the mesonephric tubules are forming. The mesonephric ducts grow toward (*arrows*) and will open into the cloaca. About 5 weeks' gestation.

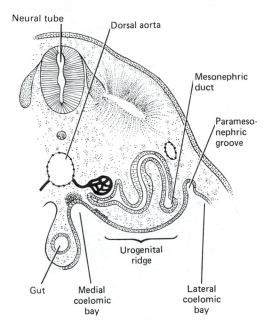

**Figure 4–5.** Cross section of embryo during early differ-entiation of the S-shaped mesonephric tubule. A primitive glomerular unit is forming, and the tubule has opened into the duct. Note the invagination of coelomic epithelium, a very early stage of formation of the paramesonephric duct. Between 5 and 6 weeks' gestation.

close to the cloaca (Fig 4–7). The bud gives rise to the collecting tubules, calices, renal pelvis, and ureter (Fig 4–3). The stalk of the elongating bud will be-come the **ureter** when the ductal segment between the stalk and the cloaca becomes incorporated into the wall of the urinary bladder (which is a derivative of the partitioned cloaca, see text that follows; Figs 4–9 through 4–12). The expanded tip, or **ampulla,** of the bud grows into the adjacent metanephric mesoderm (**blastema**), and continued growth of the bud eventu-ally relocates the ampulla and associated blastema dorsal to the mesonephros (ie, "retroperitoneal").

Between week 6 and weeks 20–24, the ampulla subdivides, and successive divisions yield approxi-mately 12–15 generations of buds, or eventual **col-lecting tubules.** From weeks 10–14, dilatation of the early generations of tubular branches successively produces the **renal pelvis,** the **major calices,** and the **minor calices,** while the middle generations form the medullary collecting tubules. The last several genera-tions of collecting tubules grow centrifugally into the cortical region of the kidney between weeks 24 and 36.

**B. Nephrons:** Dorsocranial growth of the ure-teric bud into the caudal end of the nephrogenic cord brings the bud into contact with the metanephric me-soderm, or **metanephric blastema** (Fig 4–7). The blastema becomes a cap-like structure over the

ampullated end of the bud, and continued mainte-nance of this intimate relationship is necessary for normal metanephric organogenesis. Formation of the definitive excretory units starts at about the eighth week. Blastemic cells are influenced by the ampulla to form clusters. Subsequent early stages of differen-tiation of the blastema are similar to those in the de-velopment of the mesonephric tubule.

The cell clusters form **metanephric vesicles, which elongate and differentiate into metanephric tubules.** Differential proliferation of segments of the midportion of the tubule produces the **proximal** and **distal convoluted tubules,** whereas the central mid-portion forms the **loop of Henle** (Fig 4–3). The loops eventually grow centripetally toward the developing medullary zone. The end of the nephric tubule nearest the ampulla of the subdividing bud joins the newly formed collecting duct of that bud. The other end of the metanephric tubule expands, infolds somewhat, and becomes the cup-shaped **Bowman's capsule.** The capsule is invaginated by a tuft of capillaries, the **glomerulus.** Formation of urine purportedly begins at about weeks 10–13, when an estimated 20% of the nephrons are morphologically mature.

The last month of gestation is marked by interstitial growth, hypertrophy of existing components of uri-niferous tubules, and the disappearance of bud pri-mordia for collecting tubules. Opinions differ about

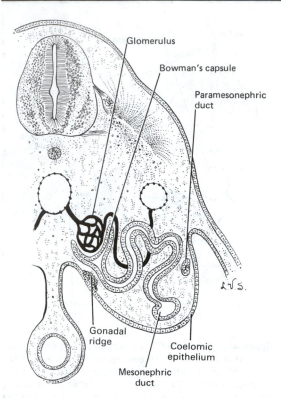

**Figure 4–6.** Cross section of embryo after formation of the mesonephric excretory unit (a simplified depiction of the primitive convoluted tubule is presented). The collection of cells beneath the epithelium of the urogenital ridge facing the medial coelomic bay is part of the developing gonadal ridge, from which the gonad will differentiate. About 6 weeks' gestation.

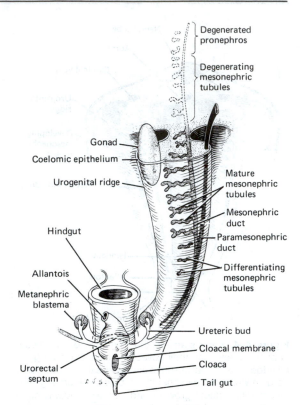

**Figure 4–7.** Metanephric diverticulum (ureteric bud) and blastema and the relationships between the mesonephric and genital structures in the urogenital ridge. The paramesonephric duct crosses ventral to the mesonephric duct and grows toward the cloaca. The urorectal septum begins to subdivide the cloaca. About 6 weeks' gestation.

whether formation of nephrons ceases prenatally at about 28 or 32 weeks or, postnatally, during the first several months. If the ureteric bud fails to form, undergoes early degeneration, or fails to grow into the nephrogenic mesoderm, aberrations of nephrogenesis result. These may be nonthreatening (**unilateral renal agenesis**), severe, or even fatal (**bilateral renal agenesis, polycystic kidney**).

**C. Positional Changes:** Figure 4–13 illustrates relocation of the kidney to a deeper position within the posterior body wall, as well as the approximately 90-degree medial rotation of the organ on its longitudinal axis. Rotation and lateral positioning are probably facilitated by the growth of midline structures (axial skeleton and muscles). The "ascent" of the kidney between weeks 5 and 8 can be attributed largely to differential longitudinal growth of the rest of the lumbosacral area and to the reduction of the rather sharp curvature of the caudal region of the embryo. Some migration of the kidney may also occur. Straightening of the curvature is perhaps attributable also to relative changes in growth, especially the development of the infraumbilical abdominal wall. As

the kidney moves into its final position (lumbar 1–3 by the 12th week), its arterial supply shifts to successively higher aortic levels. Ectopic kidneys can result from abnormal "ascent." During the seventh week, the "ascending" metanephroi closely approach each other near the aortic bifurcation. The close approximation of the 2 developing kidneys can lead to fusion of the lower poles of the kidneys, resulting in formation of a single **horseshoe kidney,** the ascent of which would be arrested by the stem of the interior mesenteric artery. Infrequently, a **pelvic kidney** results from trapping of the organ beneath the umbilical artery, which restricts passage out of the pelvis.

## THE GENITAL SYSTEM

Sexual differentiation of the genital system occurs in a basically sequential order: genetic, gonadal, ductal, and genital. **Genetic sex** is determined at fertilization by the complement of sex chromosomes (ie, XY specifies a genotypic male and XX a female). How-

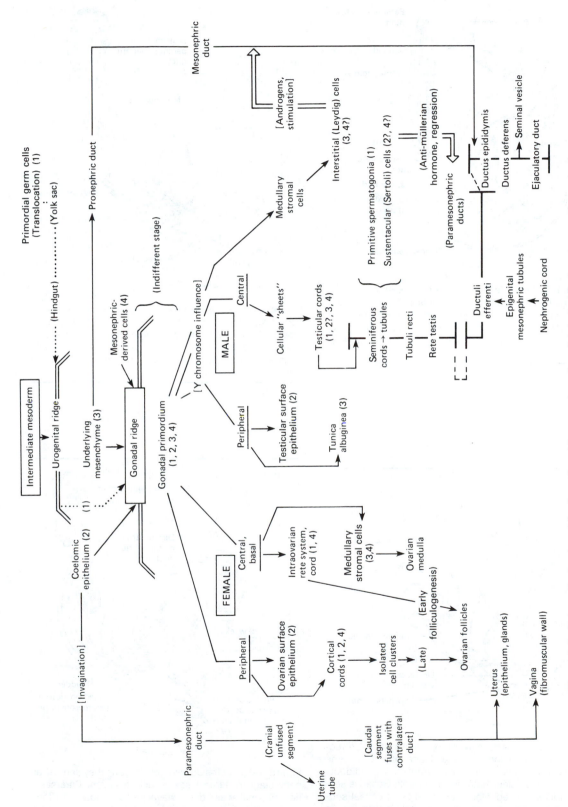

**Figure 4–8.** Schematic drawing of the formation of the gonads and genital ducts. Numbers in parentheses by tissues after the indifferent stage indicate the presumed cellular origin from the urogenital ridge (see text for details; explanatory symbols are given in Fig 4–1).

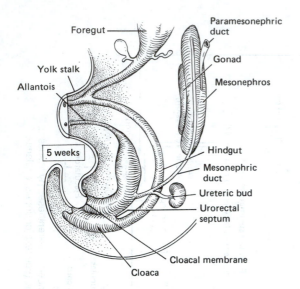

**Figure 4–9.** Left-side view of urogenital system and cloacal region prior to subdivision of cloaca by urorectal septum (Tourneux and Rathke folds). Position of future paramesonephric duct is shown (begins in the sixth week). Gonad is in the indifferent stage (sexually undifferentiated).

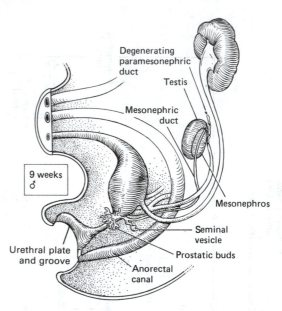

**Figure 4–11.** Left-side view of urogenital system at an early stage of male sexual differentiation. Phallic part of urogenital sinus is proliferating anteriorly to form the urethral plate and groove. Seminal vesicles and prostatic buds are shown at a more advanced stage (about 12 weeks) for emphasis.

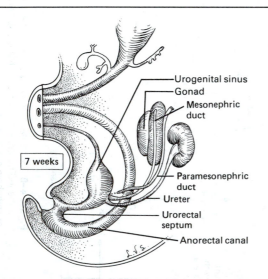

**Figure 4–10.** Left-side view of urogenital system. Urorectal septum nearly subdivides the cloaca into the urogenital sinus and the anorectal canal. Paramesonephric ducts do not reach the sinus until the ninth week. Gonad is sexually undifferentiated. Note incorporation of caudal segment of mesonephric duct into urogenital sinus (compare with Fig 4–9).

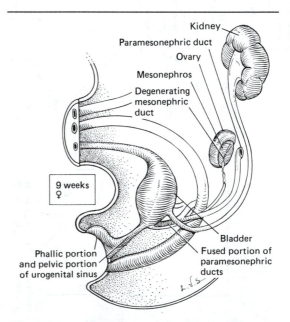

**Figure 4–12.** Left-side view of urogenital system at an early stage of female sexual differentiation. Paramesonephric (müllerian) ducts have fused caudally (to form uterovaginal primordium) and contacted the pelvic part of the urogenital sinus.

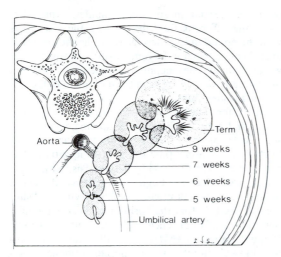

**Figure 4–13.** Positional changes of the definitive kidney at 5 different stages but projected on one cross-sectional plane. (Redrawn and modified, with permission, from Kelly HA, Burnam CF: *Diseases of Kidneys, Ureters and Bladder.* Appleton-Century-Crofts, 1972.)

ever, early morphologic indications of the sex of the developing embryo do not appear until about the eighth or ninth week after conception. Thus, there is a so-called **indifferent stage,** when morphologic identity of sex is not clear or when preferential differentiation for one sex has not been imposed on the sexless primordia. This is characteristic of early developmental stages for the gonads, genital ducts, and external genitalia. When the influence of genetic sex has been expressed on the indifferent gonad, **gonadal sex** is established. The **SRY** (**sex-determining region of the Y chromosome**) gene in the short arm of the Y chromosome of normal genetic males is considered the best candidate for the gene encoding for the **testis-determining factor** (**TDF**). TDF initiates a chain of events that results in differentiation of the gonad into a testis with its subsequent production of anti-müllerian hormone and testosterone, which influences development of somatic "maleness" (see Testis, in following text). Normal genetic females do not have the SRY gene, and the early undifferentiated medullary region of their presumptive gonad does not produce the TDF (see Ovary).

The testis and ovary are derived from the same primordial tissue but histologically visible differentiation toward a testis occurs sooner than that toward an ovary. An "ovary" is first recognized by the absence of testicular histogenesis (eg, thick tunica albuginea) or by the presence of germ cells entering meiotic prophase between the eighth and about the 11th week. The different primordia for male and female genital ducts exist in each embryo during overlapping periods, but establishment of male or female **ductal sex** depends on the presence or absence, respectively, of

testicular products and the sensitivity of tissues to these products. The 2 primary testicular products are androgenic steroids (**testosterone** and nonsteroidal **anti-müllerian hormone** (see Testis). Stimulation by testosterone influences the persistence and differentiation of the "male" mesonephric ducts (**wolffian ducts**), whereas anti-müllerian hormone influences regression of the "female" paramesonephric ducts (**müllerian ducts**). Absence of these hormones in a nonaberrant condition specifies persistence of müllerian ducts and regression of wolffian ducts, ie, initiation of development of the uterus and uterine tubes. **Genital sex** (external genitalia) subsequently develops according to the absence or presence of androgen. Thus, *the inherent pattern of differentiation of the genital system can be viewed as one directed toward somatic "femaleness" unless the system is dominated by certain factors for "maleness" (eg, gene expression of the Y chromosome, androgenic steroids, and anti-müllerian hormone).*

## THE GONADS

### Indifferent (Sexless) Stage

Gonadogenesis temporally overlaps metanephrogenesis and interacts with tissues of the mesonephric system. Formation of the gonad is summarized schematically in Fig 4–8.

About the fifth week, the midportion of each urogenital ridge ventromedially adjacent to the mesonephros thickens as cellular condensation forms the **gonadal ridge** (Fig 4–6). For the next 2 weeks, this ridge is an undifferentiated cell mass, lacking either testicular or ovarian morphology. As shown in Fig 4–8, the cell mass consists of (1) **primordial germ cells,** which translocate into the ridge, and a mixture of **somatic cells** derived by (2) proliferation of the **coelomic epithelial cells,** (3) condensation of the **underlying mesenchyme** of part of the urogenital ridge, and (4) in-growth of **mesonephric-derived cells.** The epithelial cells are not confined to the coelomic surface because the basal lamina of the coelomic epithelium is discontinuous in the area of the gonadal ridge.

The **mesonephric-derived cells** enter the basal aspect of the undifferentiated gonad, and some of these cells move peripherally, while some epithelial cells penetrate the mesenchyme and move centrally. During the indifferent stage, the germ cells and different somatic cells "intermingle" in the compact mass of the primordium. Later differentiation of the gonadal primordium results from interaction of the germ cells and the 3 types of somatic cells listed above. The end of the gonadal indifferent stage in the male is near the middle of the seventh week, when a basal lamina delineates the coelomic epithelium and the developing tunica albuginea separates the coelomic epithelium from the developing testicular cords. The indifferent stage in the female ends around the ninth week, when the first oogonia enter meiotic prophase.

**Primordial germ cells,** presumptive progenitors of the gametes, become evident in the late third to early fourth weeks in the dorsocaudal wall of the yolk sac and the mesenchyme around the allantois. The **allantois** is a caudal diverticulum of the yolk sac that extends distally into the primitive umbilical stalk and, after embryonic flexion, is adjacent proximally to the cloacal hindgut. The primordial germ cells are translocated from the allantoic region (about the middle of the fourth week) to the urogenital ridge (between the middle of the fifth week and late in the sixth week). The mechanism of translocation is uncertain (perhaps partially by ameboid movement and also passively owing to positional change of tissues). It is not known whether primordial germ cells must be present in the gonadal ridge for full differentiation of the gonad to occur. The initial stages of somatic development appear to occur independently of the germ cells. Later endocrine activity in the testis, but not in the ovary, is known to occur in the absence of germ cells. The germ cells appear to have some influence on gonadal differentiation at certain stages of development.

## Testis

During early differentiation of the testis, there are condensations of germ cells and somatic cells (see previous text), which have been described as platelike groups, or sheets. These groups are at first distributed throughout the gonad and then become more organized as primitive **testicular cords.** The cords begin to form centrally and are somewhat arranged perpendicular to the long axis of the gonad. In response to testis-determining factor (TDF), these cords will differentiate into Sertoli cells (see following text). The first characteristic feature of male gonadal sex differentiation is evident around week 8, when the **tunica albuginea** begins to form in the mesenchymal tissue underlying the coelomic epithelium. Eventually, this thickened layer of tissue causes the developing testicular cords to be separated from the surface epithelium and placed deeper in the central region of the gonad. The surface epithelium reforms a basal lamina and later thins to a mesothelial covering of the gonad. The testicular cords coil peripherally and thicken as their cellular organization becomes more distinct. A basal lamina eventually develops in the testicular cords, although it is not known if the somatic cells, germ cells, or both are primary contributors to the lamina.

Throughout gonadal differentiation, the developing testicular cords appear to maintain a close relationship to the basal area of the mesonephric-derived cell mass. An interconnected network of cords, **rete cords,** develops in this cell mass and gives rise to the **rete testis.** The rete testis joins centrally with neigh-

boring epigenital mesonephric tubules, which become the **efferent ductules** linking the rete testis with the epididymis, a derivative of the mesonephric duct. With gradual enlargement of the testis and regression of the mesonephros, a cleft forms between the 2 organs, slowly creating the mesentery of the testis, the **mesorchium.**

The differentiating testicular cords are made up of primordial germ cells (primitive spermatogonia) and somatic "supporting" cells (**sustentacular cells,** or **Sertoli cells**). Some precocious meiotic activity has been observed in the fetal testis. Meiosis in the germ cells usually does not begin until puberty; the cause of this delay is unknown. Besides serving as "supporting cells" for the primitive spermatogonia, Sertoli cells also produce a glycoprotein, **anti-müllerian hormone** (AMH; also called **müllerian-inhibiting substance**). Anti-müllerian hormone causes regression of the paramesonephric (müllerian) ducts, apparently during a very discrete period of ductal sensitivity in male fetuses. At puberty, the seminiferous cords mature to become the seminiferous tubules, and the Sertoli cells and spermatogonia mature.

Shortly after the testicular cords form, the steroid-producing **interstitial (Leydig) cells** of the extracordal compartment of the testis differentiate from stromal mesenchymal cells, probably due to anti-müllerian hormone. Mesonephric-derived cells may also be a primordial source of Leydig cells. Steroidogenic activity of Leydig cells begins near the tenth week. High levels of testosterone are produced during the period of differentiation of external genitalia (weeks 11–12) and maintained through weeks 16–18. Steroid levels then rise or fall somewhat in accordance with changes in the concentration of Leydig cells. Both the number of cells and the levels of testosterone decrease around the fifth month.

## Ovary

**A. Development:** In the normal absence of the Y chromosome or the sex-determining region of the Y chromosome (SRY gene; see The Genital System, above), the somatic sex cords of the indifferent gonad do not produce testis-determining factor (TDF). In the absence of TDF, differentiation of the gonad into a testis and its subsequent production of anti-müllerian hormone and testosterone do not occur (see Testis, above). The indifferent gonad becomes an ovary. Complete ovarian differentiation seems to require 2 X chromosomes (XO females exhibit ovarian dysgenesis, in which ovaries have precociously degenerated germ cells and no follicles and are present as gonadal "streaks"). The first recognition of a developing ovary around weeks 9–10 is based on the temporal absence of testicular-associated features (most prominently, the tunica albuginea) and on the presence of early meiotic activity in the germ cells.

Early differentiation toward an ovary involves mesonephric-derived cells "invading" the basal region (adjacent to mesonephros) and central region of the gonad (central and basal regions represent the primitive "medullary" region of the gonad). At the same time, clusters of germ cells are displaced somewhat peripherally into the "cortical" region of the gonad. Some of the central mesonephric cells give rise to the rete system that subsequently forms a network of cords (**intraovarian rete cords** extending to the primitive cortical area. As these cords extend peripherally between germ clusters, some epithelial cell proliferations extend centrally, and some mixing of these somatic cells apparently takes place around the germ cell clusters. These early cord-like structures are more irregularly distributed than early cords in the testis and not distinctly outlined. The cords open into clusters of germ cells, but all germ cells are not confined to cords. The first oogonia that begin meiosis are located in the innermost part of the cortex and are the first germ cells to contact the intraovarian rete cords.

**Folliculogenesis** begins in the innermost part of the cortex when the central somatic cells of the cord contact and surround the germ cells and an intact basal lamina is laid down. These somatic cells are morphologically similar to the mesonephric cells that form the intraovarian rete cords associated with the oocytes and apparently differentiate into the presumptive granulosa cells of the early follicle. Folliculogenesis continues peripherally. Between weeks 12 and 20 of gestation, proliferative activity causes the surface epithelium to become a thickened, irregular multilayer of cells, and in the absence of a basal lamina, the cells and apparent epithelial cell cords mix with underlying tissues. These latter cortical cords often retain a connection to and appear similar to the surface epithelium. The epithelial cells of these cords probably differentiate into granulosa cells and contribute to folliculogenesis, although this is after the process is well under way in the central region of the gonad. Follicles fail to form in the absence of oocytes or with precocious loss of germ cells, and oocytes not encompassed by follicular cells degenerate.

Stromal mesenchymal cells, connective tissue, somatic cells of cords not participating in folliculogenesis, and a vascular complex form the **ovarian medulla** in the late fetal ovary. Individual **primordial follicles** containing diplotene oocytes populate the inner and outer cortex of this ovary. The rete ovarii may persist, along with a few vestiges of mesonephric tubules, as the vestigial epoophoron near the adult ovary. Finally, similar to the testicular mesorchium, the **mesovarium,** eventually forms as a gonadal mesentery between the ovary and old urogenital ridge. Postnatally, the epithelial surface of the ovary consists of a single layer of cells continuous with peritoneal mesothelium at the ovarian hilum. A thin, fibrous connective tissue, the tunica albuginea, forms beneath the surface epithelium and separates it from the cortical follicles.

**B. Anomalies of the Ovaries:** Anomalies of the ovaries encompass a broad range of developmental errors from complete absence of the ovaries to supernumerary ovaries. The many variations of gonadal disorders usually are subcategorized within classifications of disorders of sex determination. Unfortunately, there is little consensus for a major classification, although most include pathogenetic consideration. Extensive, excellent summaries of the different classifications are offered in the references to this chapter.

Congenital absence of the ovary (no gonadal remnants found) is very rare. Two types have been considered, agenesis and agonadism. By definition, **agenesis** implies that the primordial gonad did not form in the urogenital ridge, whereas **agonadism** indicates the absence of gonads that may have formed initially and subsequently degenerated. It can be difficult to distinguish one type from the other on a practical basis. For example, a patient with female genital ducts and external genitalia and a 46,XY karyotype could represent either gonadal agenesis or agonadism. In the latter condition, the gonad may form but undergo early degeneration and resorption before any virilizing expression is made. *Whenever congenital absence of the ovaries is suspected, careful examination of the karyotype, the external genitalia, and the genital ducts must be performed.*

Descriptions of agonadism have usually indicated that the external genitalia are abnormal (variable degree of fusion of labioscrotal swellings) and that either very rudimentary ductal derivatives are present or there are no genital ducts. The cause of agonadism is unknown, although several explanations have been suggested, such as (1) failure of the primordial gonad to form, along with abnormal formation of ductal anlagen, and (2) partial differentiation and then regression and absorption of testes (accounting for suppression of müllerian ducts but lack of stimulation of mesonephric, or wolffian, ducts). Explanations that include teratogenic effects or genetic defects are more likely candidates in view of the associated incidence of nonsexual somatic anomalies with the disorder. The **streak gonad** is a product of primordial gonadal formation and subsequent failure of differentiation, which can occur at various stages. The gonad usually appears as a fibrous-like cord of mixed elements (lacking germ cells) located parallel to a uterine tube. Streak gonads are characteristic of **gonadal dysgenesis** and a 45,XO karyotype (**Turner's syndrome**; distinctions are drawn between Turner's syndrome and **Turner's stigmata** when consideration is given to the various associated somatic anomalies of gonadal dysgenesis). However, streak gonads may be consequent to genetic mutation or hereditary disease other than the anomalous karyotype.

Ectopic ovarian tissue occasionally can be found as **accessory ovarian tissue** or as **supernumerary ovaries.** The former may be a product of disaggregation of the embryonic ovary, and the latter may arise from the urogenital ridge as independent primordia.

## SUBDIVISION OF THE CLOACA & FORMATION OF THE UROGENITAL SINUS

The endodermally lined urogenital sinus is derived by partitioning of the endodermal cloaca; it is the precursor of the urinary bladder in both sexes and the urinary and genital structures specific to each sex (see Fig 4–1). The cloaca is a pouch-like enlargement of the caudal end of the hindgut and is formed by the process of "folding" of the caudal region of the embryonic disk between 4 and 5 weeks' gestation (see Overview of Development, above; Figs 4–1 and 4–4). During the "tail-fold" process, the posteriorly placed allantois, or allantoic diverticulum of the yolk sac, becomes an anterior extension of the cloaca (Figs 4–4 and 4–9). Soon after the cloaca forms, it receives posterolaterally the caudal ends of the paired mesonephric ducts and hence becomes a junctional cistern for the allantois, the hindgut, and the ducts (Fig 4–7). A **cloacal membrane,** composed of ectoderm and endoderm, is the caudal limit of the primitive gut and temporarily separates the cloacal cavity from the extraembryonic confines of the amniotic cavity (Figs 4–7 and 4–9).

Between weeks 5 and 7, 3 wedges of splanchnic mesoderm, collectively called the **urorectal septum,** proliferate in the coronal plane in the caudal region of the embryo to eventually subdivide the cloaca (Figs 4–9 through 4–12). The superior wedge, called the **Tourneux fold,** is in the angle between the allantois and the primitive hindgut, and it proliferates caudally into the superior end of the cloaca (Fig 4–9). The other 2 mesodermal wedges, called the **Rathke folds,** proliferate in the right and left walls of the cloaca. Beginning adjacent to the cloacal membrane, these laterally placed folds grow toward each other and the Tourneux fold. With fusion of the 3 folds creating a urorectal septum, the once single chamber is subdivided into the primitive **urogenital sinus** (ventrally) and the **anorectal canal** of the hindgut (dorsally; see Figs 4–10 through 4–12). The mesonephric ducts and allantois then open into the sinus. The uterovaginal primordium of the fused paramesonephric ducts will contact the sinusal wall between the mesonephric ducts early in the ninth week of development. Formation of the external genitalia is discussed below. However, it can be noted that the junctional point of fusion of the cloacal membrane and urorectal septum forms the **primitive perineum** (later differentiation creates the so-called perineal body of tissue) and subdivides the cloacal membrane into the **urogenital membrane** (anteriorly) and the **anal membrane** (posteriorly; Figs 4–9, 4–12, 4–14 and 4–24).

## THE GENITAL DUCTS

### Indifferent (Sexless) Stage

Two pairs of genital ducts are initially present in both sexes: (1) the **mesonephric (wolffian) ducts,** which give rise to the male ducts and a derivative, the seminal vesicles; and (2) the **paramesonephric (müllerian) ducts,** which form the oviducts, uterus, and part of the vagina. When the adult structures are described as derivatives of embryonic ducts, this refers to the epithelial lining of the structures. Muscle and connective tissues of the differentiating structures originate from splanchnic mesoderm and mesenchyme adjacent to ducts. Mesonephric ducts are originally the excretory ducts of the mesonephric "kidneys" (see previous text), and they develop early in the embryonic period, about 2 weeks before development of paramesonephric ducts (weeks 6–10). The 2 pairs of genital ducts share a close anatomic relationship in their bilateral course through the urogenital ridge. At their caudal limit, both sets contact the part of the cloaca that is later separated as the urogenital sinus (Figs 4–9, 4–10, and 4–14). Determination of the ductal sex of the embryo (ie, which pair of ducts will continue differentiation rather than undergo regression) is established initially by the gonadal sex and later by the continuing influence of hormones.

Formation of each paramesonephric duct begins early in the sixth week as an invagination of coelomic epithelium in the lateral wall of the cranial end of the urogenital ridge, and adjacent to each mesonephric duct (Fig 4–5). The free edges of the invaginated epithelium join to form the duct except at the site of origin, which persists as a funnel-shaped opening, the future **ostium of the oviduct.** At first, each paramesonephric duct grows caudally through the mesenchyme of the urogenital ridge and laterally parallel to a mesonephric duct. More inferiorly, the paramesonephric duct has a caudomedial course, passing ventral to the mesonephric duct (Fig 4–7). As it follows the ventromedial bend of the caudal portion of the urogenital ridge, the paramesonephric duct then lies medial to the mesonephric duct, and its caudal tip lies in close apposition to its counterpart from the opposite side (Fig 4–14). At approximately the eighth week, the caudal segments of the right and left ducts fuse medially and their lumens coalesce to form a single cavity. This conjoined portion of the Y-shaped paramesonephric ducts becomes the uterovaginal primordium, or canal.

### Male: Genital Ducts

**A. Mesonephric Ducts:** The mesonephric ducts persist in the male and, under the stimulatory influence of testosterone, differentiate into the internal

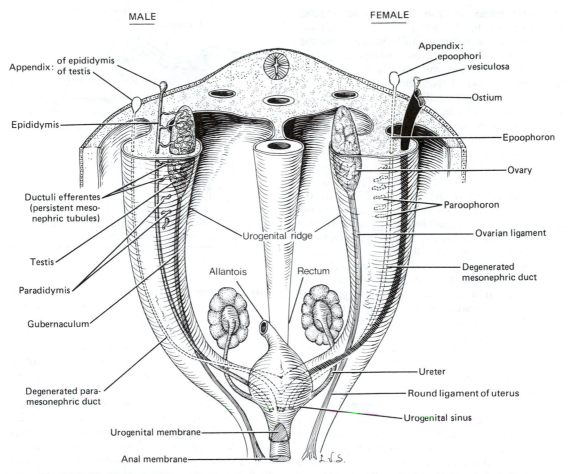

**Figure 4–14.** Diagrammatic comparison between male and female differentiation of internal genitalia.

genital ducts (epididymis, ductus deferens, and ejaculatory ducts). Near the cranial end of the duct, some of the mesonephric tubules (epigenital mesonephric tubules) of the mesonephric kidney persist lateral to the developing testis. These tubules form a connecting link, the **ductuli efferentes,** between the duct and the rete testis (Fig 4–14). The cranial portion of each duct becomes the convoluted **ductus epididymis.** The **ductus deferens** forms when smooth muscle from adjacent splanchnic mesoderm is added to the central segment of the mesonephric duct. The seminal vesicle develops as a lateral bud from each mesonephric duct just distal to the junction of the duct and the urogenital sinus (Fig 4–11). The terminal segment of duct between the sinus and seminal vesicle forms the **ejaculatory duct,** which becomes encased by the developing prostate gland early in the 12th week (see Differentiation of the Urogenital Sinus later in chapter). A vestigial remnant of the duct may persist cranially near the head of the epididymis as the **appendix epididymis,** whereas remnants of mesonephric tubules near the inferior pole of the testis and

tail of the epididymis may persist as the **paradidymis** (Fig 4–14).

**B. Paramesonephric Ducts:** The paramesonephric ducts begin to undergo morphologic regression centrally (and progress cranially and caudally) about the time they meet the urogenital sinus caudally (approximately the start of the ninth week). Regression is effected by nonsteroidal anti-müllerian hormone produced by the differentiating Sertoli cells slightly before androgen is produced by the Leydig cells (see Testis). Anti-müllerian hormone is produced from the time of early testicular differentiation until birth (ie, not only during the period of regression of the paramesonephric duct). However, ductal sensitivity to anti-müllerian hormone in the male seems to exist for only a short "critical" time preceding the first signs of ductal regression. Vestigial remnants of the cranial end of the ducts may persist as the **appendix testis** on the superior pole of the testis (Fig 4–14). Caudally, a ductal remnant is considered to be part of the prostatic utricle of the seminal colliculus in the prostatic urethra.

## C. Relocation of the Testes and Ducts:

Around weeks 5–6, a band-like condensation of mesenchymal tissue in the urogenital ridge forms near the caudal end of the mesonephros. Distally, this gubernacular precursor tissue grows into the area of the undifferentiated tissue of the anterior abdominal wall and toward the genital swellings. Proximally, the **gubernaculum** contacts the mesonephric duct when the mesonephros regresses and the gonad begins to form. By the start of the fetal period, the mesonephric duct begins differentiation and the gubernaculum adheres indirectly to the testis via the duct, which lies in the mesorchium of the testis. The external genitalia differentiate over the seventh to about the 19th week. By the 12th week, the testis is near the deep inguinal ring, and the gubernaculum is virtually at the inferior pole of the testis, proximally, and in the mesenchyme of the scrotal swellings, distally.

Although the testis in early development is near the last thoracic segment, it is still close to the area of the developing deep inguinal ring. With rapid growth of the lumbar region and "ascent" of the metanephric kidney, the testis remains relatively immobilized by the gubernaculum, although there is the appearance of a lengthy transabdominal "descent" from an upper abdominal position. The testis descends through the inguinal canal around the 28th week and into the scrotum about the 32nd week. Testicular blood vessels form when the testis is located on the dorsal body wall and retain their origin during the transabdominal and pelvic descent of the testis. The mesonephric duct follows the descent of the testis and hence passes anterior to the ureter, which follows the retroperitoneal ascent of the kidney (Fig 4–14).

## Female: Uterus and Uterine Tubes

**A. Mesonephric Ducts:** Virtually all portions of these paired ducts degenerate in the female embryo, with the exception of the most caudal segment between the ureteric bud and the cloaca, which is later incorporated into the posterior wall of the urogenital sinus (Figs 4–9 and 4–10) as the **trigone of the urinary bladder.** Regression begins just after gonadal sex differentiation and is finished near the onset of the third trimester. Cyst-like or tubular vestiges of mesonephric duct (Fig 4–15) may persist to variable degrees parallel with the vagina and uterus (**Gartner's cysts**). Other mesonephric remnants of the duct or tubules may persist in the broad ligament (**epoophoron**).

**B. Paramesonephric Ducts:** Differentiation of müllerian ducts in female embryos produces the uterine tubes, uterus, and probably the fibromuscular wall of the vagina. In contrast to the ductal/gonadal relationship in the male, ductal differentiation in the female does not require the presence of ovaries. Formation of the bilateral paramesonephric ducts during the second half of the embryonic period has been described (see Indifferent Stage, in previous

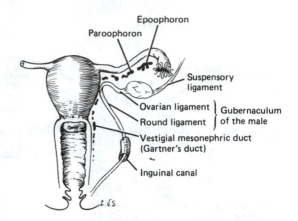

**Figure 4–15.** Female genital tract. Gubernacular derivatives and mesonephric vestiges are shown.

text). By the onset of the fetal period, the 2 ducts are joined caudally in the midline, and the fused segment of the new Y-shaped ductal structure is the **uterovaginal primordium** (Fig 4–12). The nonfused cranial part of each paramesonephric duct gives rise to the **uterine tubes** (oviducts), and the distal end of this segment remains open and will form the **ostium of the oviduct.**

Early in the ninth week, the uterovaginal primordium contacts medially the dorsal wall of the urogenital sinus. This places the primordium at a median position between the bilateral openings of the mesonephric ducts, which joined the dorsal wall during the fifth week before subdivision of the urogenital sinus from the cloaca occurred (Figs 4–12 and 4–13). A ventral protrusion of the dorsal wall of the urogenital sinus forms at the area of contact of the uterovaginal primordium with the wall and between the openings of the mesonephric ducts. In reference to its location, this protrusion is called the **sinusal tubercle (sinus tubercle, paramesonephric tubercle, müllerian tubercle).** This tubercle may consist of several types of epithelia derived from the different ducts as well as from the wall of the sinus.

Shortly after the sinusal tubercle forms, midline fusion of the middle and caudal portions of the paramesonephric ducts is complete, and the vertical septum (apposed walls of the fused ducts) within the newly established uterovaginal primordium degenerates, creating a single cavity or canal (Fig 4–19). The solid tip of this primordium continues to grow caudally, while a mesenchymal thickening gradually surrounds the cervical region of the uterovaginal primordium. The primordium gives rise to the fundus, body, and isthmus of the uterus, specifically the endometrial epithelium and glands of the uterus. The endometrial stroma and smooth muscle of the myometrium are derived from adjacent splanchnic mesenchyme. The epithelium of the cervix forms from the lower aspect of the primordium. Development of the various components of the uterus covers the 3 trimesters of gestation. The basic structure is generated during the latter part of the first trimester. The initial formation of glands and muscular layer occurs near midgestation, whereas mucinous cells in the cervix appear during the third trimester.

The formation of the vagina is discussed below with differentiation of the urogenital sinus, even though it has not been resolved whether the vaginal epithelium is a sinusal or paramesonephric derivative (or both). The fibromuscular wall of the vagina is generally considered to be derived from the uterovaginal primordium (Fig 4–18).

**C. Relocation of the Ovaries and Formation of Ligaments:** Transabdominal "descent" of the ovary, unlike that of the testis, is restricted to a relatively short distance, presumably (at least partly) because of attachment of the gubernaculum to the paramesonephric duct. Hence, relocation of the ovary appears to involve both (1) a passive rotatory movement of the ovary as its mesentery is drawn by the twist of the developing ductal mesenteries and (2) extensive growth of the lumbosacral region of the fetus. The ovarian vessels (like the testicular vessels) originate or drain near the point of development of the gonad, the arteries from the aorta just inferior to the renal arteries and the veins to the left renal vein or to the vena cava from the right gonad.

Initial positioning of the ovary on the anteromedial aspect of the urogenital ridge is depicted in Fig 4–14, as is the relationship of the paramesonephric duct lateral to the degenerating mesonephros, the ovary, and the urogenital mesentery. The urogenital mesentery between the ridge and the dorsal body wall represents the first mesenteric support for structures developing in the ridge.

Alterations within the urogenital ridge eventually result in formation of contiguous double-layered mesenteries supporting the ovary and segments of the paramesonephric ducts. Enlargement of the ovary and degeneration of the adjacent mesonephric tissue bring previously separated layers of coelomic mesothelium into near apposition, establishing the mesentery of the ovary, the **mesovarium.** Likewise, mesonephric degeneration along the region of differentiation of the unfused cranial segment of the paramesonephric ducts establishes the **mesosalpinx.** Caudally, growth and fusion ventromedially of these bilateral ducts "sweeps" the once medially attached mesenteries of the ducts toward the midline. These bilateral mesenteries merge over the fused uterovaginal primordium and extend laterally to the pelvic wall to form a continuous double-layered "drape," the **mesometrium of the broad ligament,** between the upper portion of the primordium and the posterolateral body wall. This central expanse of mesentery creates the rectouterine and vesicouterine pouches. The midline caudal fusion of the ducts also alters the previous longitudinal ori-

entation of the upper free segments of the ducts (the oviducts) to a near transverse orientation. During this alteration, the attached mesovarium is drawn from a medial relationship into a posterior relationship with the paramesonephric mesentery of the mesosalpinx and the mesometrium.

The **suspensory ligament of the ovary,** through which the ovarian vessels, nerves, and lymphatics traverse, forms when cranial degeneration of the mesonephric tissue and regression of the urogenital ridge adjacent to the ovary reduces these tissues to a peritoneal fold.

The **round ligament of the uterus** and the **proper ovarian ligament** are both derivatives of the **gubernaculum,** which originates as a mesenchymal condensation at the caudal end of the mesonephros and extends over the initially short distance to the anterior abdominal wall (see Relocation of the Testes and Ducts in previous text). As the gonad enlarges and the mesonephric tissue degenerates, the cranial attachment of the gubernaculum appears to "shift" to the inferior aspect of the ovary. Distally, growth of the fibrous gubernaculum continues into the inguinal region. However, the midportion of the gubernaculum becomes attached, inexplicably, to the paramesonephric duct at the uterotubal junction. Formation of the uterovaginal primordium by caudal fusion of the paramesonephric ducts apparently carries the attached gubernaculum medially within the cover of the encompassing mesentery of the structures (ie, the parts of the developing broad ligament). This fibrous band of connective tissue eventually becomes 2 ligaments.

Cranially, the band is the proper ligament of the ovary, extending between the inferior pole of the ovary and the lateral wall of the uterus just inferior to the oviduct. Caudally, it continues as the uterine round ligament from a point just inferior to the proper ovarian ligament and extending through the inguinal canal to the labium majus.

**D. Anomalies of the Uterine Tubes (Oviducts, Fallopian Tubes):** The uterine tubes are derivatives of the cranial segments of the paramesonephric (müllerian) ducts, which differentiate in the urogenital ridge between the sixth and ninth weeks (Figs 4–7 and 3–14). Ductal formation begins with invagination of the coelomic epithelium in the lateral coelomic bay (Fig 4–5). The initial depression remains open to proliferate and differentiate into the ostium (Fig 4–14). Variable degrees of **duplication of the ostium** sometimes occur; in such cases, the leading edges of the initial ductal groove presumably did not fuse completely or anomalous proliferation of epithelium around the opening occurred.

**Absence of a uterine tube** is very rare when otherwise normal ductal and genital derivatives are present. This anomaly has been associated with (1) ipsilateral absence of an ovary and (2) ipsilateral unicornuate uterus (and probable anomalous broad ligament). Bilateral absence of the uterine tubes is most frequently associated with lack of formation of the uterus and anomalies of the external genitalia. Interestingly, absence of the derivatives of the lower part of the müllerian ducts with persistence of the uterine tubes occurs more frequently than the reverse condition. This might be expected, as the müllerian ducts form in a craniocaudal direction.

**Partial absence** of a uterine tube (middle or caudal segment) also has been reported. The cause of partial absence is unknown, although several theories have been advanced. One theory holds that when the unilateral anomaly coincides with ipsilateral ovarian absence, a "vascular accident" might occur following differentiation of the ducts and ovaries. Obviously, various factors resulting in somewhat localized atresia could be proposed. From a different perspective, bilateral absence of the uterine tubes as an associated disorder in a female external phenotype is characteristic of **testicular feminization syndrome** (nonpersistence of the rest of the paramesonephric ducts, anomalous external genitalia, hypoplastic male genital ducts, and testicular differentiation with usual ectopic location).

**E. Anomalies of the Uterus:** The epithelium of the uterus and cervix and the fibromuscular wall of the vagina are derived from the paramesonephric (müllerian) ducts, the caudal ends of which fuse medially to form the uterovaginal primordium. Most of the primordium gives rise to the uterus (Fig 4–18). Subsequently, the caudal tip of the primordium contacts the pelvic part of the urogenital sinus, and the interaction of the sinus (sinovaginal bulbs) and primordium leads to differentiation of the vagina. Various steps in this sequential process can go awry, such as (1) complete or partial failure of one or both ducts to form (agenesis), (2) lack of or incomplete fusion of the caudal segments of the paired ducts (abnormal uterovaginal primordium), or (3) failure of development *after* successful formation (aplasia or hypoplasia). Many types of anomalies may occur because of the number of sites for potential error, the complex interactions necessary for the development of the müllerian derivatives, and the duration of the complete process.

Complete **agenesis of the uterus** is very rare, and associated vaginal anomalies are usually expected. Also, a high incidence of associated structural or positional abnormalities of the kidney has been reported; there has been speculation that the initial error in severe cases may be in the development of the urinary system and then in the formation of the paramesonephric ducts.

Aplasia of the paramesonephric ducts **(müllerian aplasia)** is more common than agenesis and could occur after formation and interaction of the primordium with the urogenital sinus. A rudimentary uterus or a vestigial uterus (ie, varying degrees of fibromuscular tissue present) is most frequently accompanied by partial or complete absence of the vagina (see text that follows). As in uterine agenesis, ectopic kidney or absence of a kidney is frequently associated with uterine aplasia (in about 40% of cases). **Uterine hypoplasia** variably yields a rudimentary or infantile uterus and is associated with normal or abnormal uterine tubes and ovaries. Unilateral agenesis or aplasia of the ducts gives rise to **uterus unicornis**, whereas unilateral hypoplasia may result in a rudimentary horn that may or may not be contiguous with the lumen of the "normal" horn (**uterus bicornis unicollis** with one unconnected rudimentary horn; Fig 4–16). The status of the rudimentary horn must be considered for potential hematometra at puberty.

Anomalous **unification** caudally of the paramesonephric ducts results in many uterine malformations (Fig 4–16). The incidence of defective fusion is estimated to be 0.1–3% of females. Furthermore, faulty unification of the ducts has been cited as the primary error responsible for most anomalies of the female genital tract. Partial or complete retention of the apposed walls of the paired ducts can produce slight **(uterus subseptus unicollis)** to complete **(uterus bicornis septus)** septal defects in the uterus. Complete failure of unification of the paramesonephric ducts can result in a double uterus **(uterus didelphys)** with either a single or double vagina.

**F. Anomalies of the Cervix:** Because the cervix forms as an integral part of the uterus, cervical anomalies are often the same as uterine anomalies. Thus, absence or hypoplasia of the cervix is rarely found with a normal uterovaginal tract. The cervix appears as a fibrous juncture between the uterine corpus and the vagina.

## DIFFERENTIATION OF THE UROGENITAL SINUS

Until differentiation of the genital ducts begins, the urogenital sinus appears similar in both sexes during the middle and late embryonic period. For purposes of describing the origin of sinusal derivatives, the sinus can be divided into 3 parts: (1) the **vesical part,** or the large dilated segment superior to the entrance of the mesonephric ducts; (2) the **pelvic part,** or the narrowed tubular segment between the level of the mesonephric ducts and the inferior segment; and (3) the **phallic part,** often referred to as the definitive urogenital sinus (the anteroposteriorly elongated, transversely flattened inferiormost segment) (Fig 4–12). The **urogenital membrane** temporarily closes the inferior limit of the phallic part. The superior limit of the vesical part becomes delimited by conversion of the once tubular allantois to a thick fibrous cord, the **urachus,** by about 12 weeks. After differentiation of the vesical part of the sinus to form the epithelium of the **urinary bladder,** the urachus maintains its continuity between the apex of the bladder and the

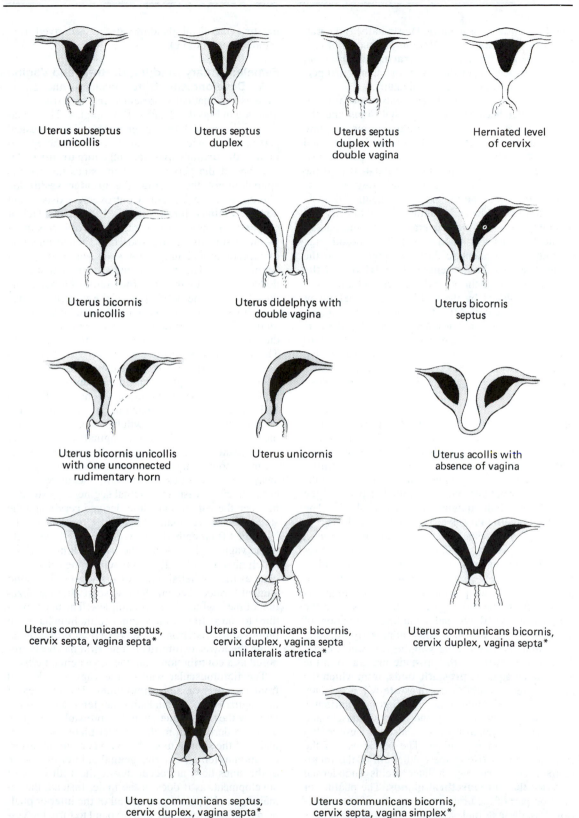

**Figure 4–16.** Uterine anomalies. (*Redrawn and reproduced, with permission, from Toaff R: A major genital malformation: Communicating uteri. Obstet Gynecol 1974;43:221.)

umbilical cord and is identified postnatally as the **median umbilical ligament.** Various anomalies of urachal formation can present as **urachal fistula, cyst,** or **sinus,** depending on the degree of patency that persists during obliteration of the allantois.

In both sexes, the caudal segments of each mesonephric duct between the urogenital sinus and the level of the ureter of the differentiating metanephric diverticulum (or ureteric bud) become incorporated into the posterocaudal wall of the vesical part (ie, urinary bladder) of the sinus (Figs 4–9 and 4–10). As the dorsal wall of the bladder grows and "absorbs" these caudal segments, the ureters are gradually "drawn" closer to the bladder and eventually open directly and separately into it, dorsolateral to the mesonephric ducts (Figs 4–10 and 4–11). The mesodermal segment of mesonephric duct incorporated into the bladder defines the epithelium of the **trigone of the bladder,** although this mesodermal epithelium is secondarily replaced by the endodermal epithelium of the sinusal bladder. After formation of the trigone, the remainder of each mesonephric duct (ie, the portion that was cranial to the metanephric diverticulum) is joined to the superior end of the pelvic part of the urogenital sinus. Thereafter, the ducts either degenerate (in females) or undergo differentiation (in males), as already discussed.

## Male: Urinary Bladder and Urethra (Fig 4–17)

The urogenital sinus gives rise to the endodermal epithelium of the **urinary bladder,** the prostatic and membranous urethra, and most of the spongy (penile) urethra (except the glandular urethra). Outgrowths from its derivatives produce epithelial parts of the prostate and bulbourethral glands (Fig 4–17). The **prostatic urethra** receives the ejaculatory ducts (derived from the mesonephric ducts) and arises from 2 parts of the urogenital sinus. The portion of this urethral segment superior to the ejaculatory ducts originates from the inferiormost area of the vesical part of the sinus. The lower portion of the prostatic urethra is derived from the pelvic part of the sinus near the entrance of the ducts and including the region of the sinusal tubercle–the latter apparently forming the seminal colliculus. Early in the 12th week, endodermal outgrowths of the prostatic urethra form the prostatic anlage, the **prostatic buds,** from which the glandular epithelium of the **prostate** will arise. Differentiation of splanchnic mesoderm contributes other components to the gland (smooth muscle and connective tissue), as is the case also for mesodermal parts of the urinary bladder. The pelvic part of the sinus also gives rise to the epithelium of the **membranous urethra,** which later yields endodermal buds for the **bulbourethral glands.** The phallic, or inferior, part of the urogenital sinus proliferates anteriorly as the external genitalia form (during weeks 9–12) and results in incorporation of this phallic part as the endodermal epithelium of the **spongy (penile) urethra** (the distal glandular urethra is derived from ectoderm; see below).

## Female: Urinary Bladder, Urethra, and Vagina

**A. Development:** Differentiation of the female sinus is schematically presented in Fig 4–18 and illustrated in Figs 4–12 and 4–19 through 4–21. In contrast to sinusal differentiation in the male, the vesical part of the female urogenital sinus forms the epithelium of the **urinary bladder** and entire **urethra.** Derivatives of the pelvic part of the sinus include the epithelium of the **vagina,** the **greater vestibular glands,** and the **hymen.** Controversy exists about how the vagina is formed, mainly because of a lack of consensus about the origin and degree of inclusion of its precursory tissues (mesodermal paramesonephric duct, endodermal urogenital sinus, or even mesonephric duct). The most common theory is that 2 endodermal outgrowths, the **sinovaginal bulbs,** of the dorsal wall of the pelvic part of the urogenital sinus form bilateral to and join with the caudal tip of the uterovaginal primordium (fused paramesonephric ducts) in the area of the sinusal tubercle (Fig 4–19). This cellular mass at the end of the primordium occludes the inferior aspect of the canal, creating an endodermal **vaginal plate** within the mesodermal wall of the uterovaginal primordium. Eventually, the vaginal segment grows, approaching the vestibule of the vagina. The process of growth has been described either as "down-growth" of the vaginal segment away from the uterine canal and along the urogenital sinus or, more commonly, as "up-growth" of the segment away from the sinus and toward the uterovaginal canal. In either case, the vaginal segment is extended between the paramesonephric-derived cervix and the sinus-derived vestibule (Figs 4–19 through 4–21). Near the fifth month, the breakdown of cells centrally in the vaginal plate creates the vaginal lumen, which is delimited peripherally by the remaining cells of the plate as the epithelial lining of the vagina. The solid vaginal fornices become hollow soon after canalization of the vaginal lumen is complete. The upper one-third to four-fifths of the vaginal epithelium has been proposed to arise from the uterovaginal primordium, while the lower two-thirds to one-fifth has been proposed as a contribution from the sinovaginal bulbs.

The fibromuscular wall of the vagina is derived from the uterovaginal primordium. The cavities of the vagina and urogenital sinus are temporarily separated by the thin **hymen,** which is probably a mixture of tissue derived from the vaginal plate and the remains of the sinusal tubercle. With concurrent differentiation of female external genitalia, inferior closure of the sinus does not occur during the 12th week of development, as it does in the male. Instead, the remainder of the pelvic part and all of the inferior phallic part of the urogenital sinus expand to form the **vestibule of the vagina.** Presumably, the junctional zone of pigmentation on the labia minora represents the

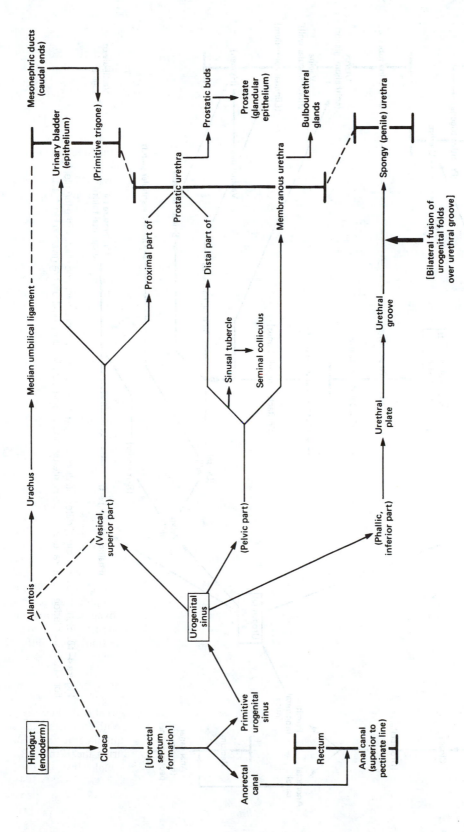

**Figure 4–17.** Schematic drawing of male differentiation of the urogenital sinus; formation of urinary bladder and urethra. (Explanatory symbols are given in Fig 4–1.)

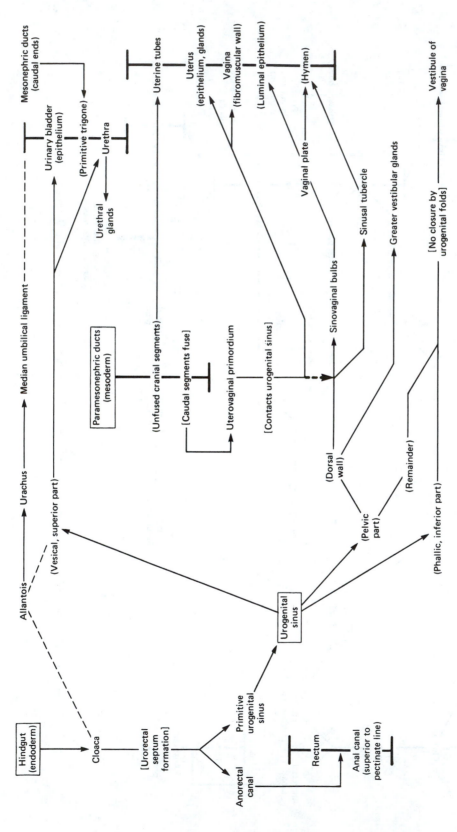

**Figure 4–18.** Schematic drawing of differentiation of urogenital sinus and paramesonephric ducts in the female; formation of urinary bladder, urethra, uterine tubes, uterus, and vagina. (Explanatory symbols are given in Fig 4–1.)

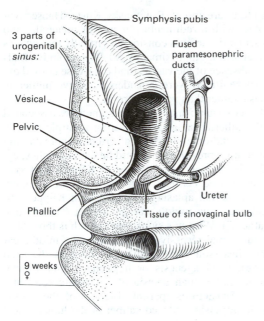

**Figure 4–19.** Sagittal cutaway view of female urogenital sinus and uterovaginal primordium (fused paramesonephric ducts). Sinovaginal bulbs form in the tenth week.

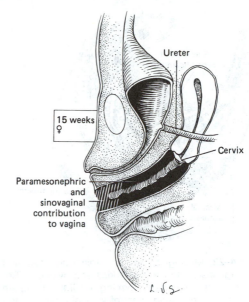

**Figure 4–21.** Sagittal cutaway view of differentiated urogenital sinus and precanalization stage of vaginal development. The drawing depicts one of several theories about the relative contributions of paramesonephric ducts and sinovaginal bulbs to the vagina (there is little consensus of opinion [see text]).

distinction between endodermal derivation from the urogenital sinus (medially) and ectodermal skin (laterally).

**B. Anomalies of the Vagina:** The vagina is derived from interaction between the uterovaginal primordium and the pelvic part of the urogenital sinus (Fig 4–18; see previous section, 'A. Development').

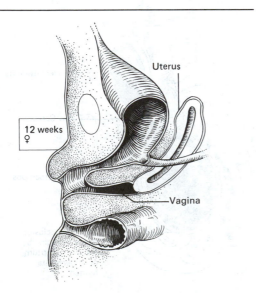

**Figure 4–20.** Sagittal cutaway view of developing vagina and urethra.

above). The causes of vaginal anomalies are difficult to assess because integration of the uterovaginal primordium and the urogenital sinus in the *normal* differentiation of the vagina remains a controversial subject. Furthermore, an accurate breakdown of causes of certain anomalous vaginal presentations, as with many anomalies of the external genitalia, would have to include potential moderating factors of endocrine and genetic origin as well.

The incidence of absence of the vagina due to suspected **vaginal agenesis** is about 0.025%. Agenesis may be due to failure of the uterovaginal primordium to contact the urogenital sinus. The uterus is usually absent (Fig 4–22). Ovarian agenesis is not usually associated with vaginal agenesis. The presence of greater vestibular glands has been reported with presumed vaginal agenesis; their presence emphasizes the complexity of differentiation of the urogenital sinus.

Simpson (1976) has presented a useful classification and perhaps clarification of the clinical presentation of absence of the vagina, in which a distinction is made between müllerian aplasia and vaginal atresia. According to this classification, **vaginal atresia** is considered when the lower portion of the vagina consists merely of fibrous tissue while the contiguous superior structures (the uterus, in particular) are well differentiated (perhaps because the primary defect is in the sinusal contribution to the vagina). In **müllerian aplasia,** almost all of the vagina and most of

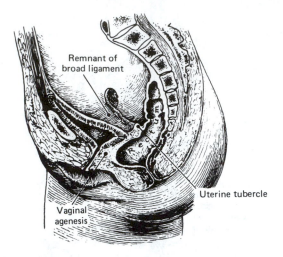

**Figure 4–22.** Midsagittal view of vaginal agenesis and uterine agenesis with normal ovaries and oviducts. (Reproduced, with permission, from Ingram JM: The Ingram technique for the management of vaginal agenesis and stenosis. The Pelvic Surgeon 1981;2:1.)

the uterus are absent (Rokitansky-Küster-Hauser syndrome, with a rudimentary uterus of bilateral, solid muscular tissue, was considered virtually the same as this aplasia). Approximately 80–90% of individuals with absence of the vagina (and otherwise normal external genitalia) were considered to have müllerian aplasia rather than vaginal atresia.

Other somatic anomalies are sometimes associated with müllerian aplasia, suggesting multiple malformation syndrome. Associated vertebral anomalies are much more prevalent than middle ear anomalies, eg, müllerian aplasia associated with **Klippel-Feil syndrome** (fused cervical vertebrae) is more common than müllerian aplasia associated with Klippel-Feil syndrome plus middle ear anomalies ("conductive deafness"). **Winter's syndrome,** which is thought to be autosomal recessive, is evidenced by middle ear anomalies (somewhat similar to those in the triad above), renal agenesis or hypoplasia, and vaginal atresia (rather than aplasia of the paramesonephric ducts). **Dysgenesis** (partial absence) of the vagina and **hypoplasia** (reduced caliber of the lumen) have also been described.

**Transverse vaginal septa** (Fig 4–23) are probably

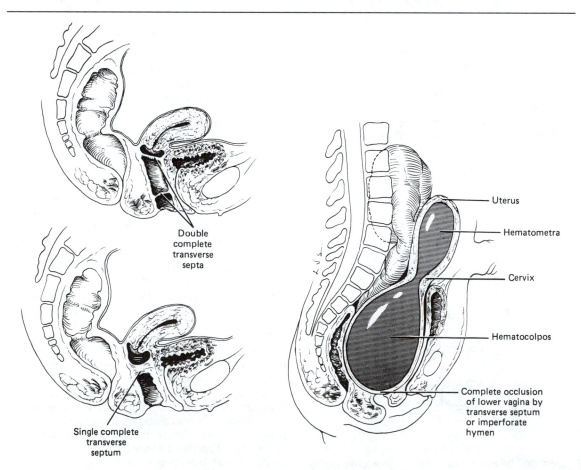

**Figure 4–23.** Transverse vaginal septa.

not the result of vaginal atresia but rather of incomplete canalization of the vaginal plate or discrete fusion of sinusal and primordial (ductal) derivatives. Alternative explanations are likely, as the histologic composition of septa is not consistent. A rare genetic linkage has been demonstrated. A single septum or multiple septa can be present, and the location may vary in upper or lower segments of the lumen. **Longitudinal vaginal septa** can also occur. A variety of explanations have been advanced, including true duplication of vaginal primordial tissue, anomalous differentiation of the uterovaginal primordium, abnormal variation of the caudal fusion of the müllerian ducts, persistence of vaginal plate epithelium, and anomalous mesodermal proliferation. Septa may be imperforate or perforated. A transverse septum creates the potential for various occlusive manifestations (eg, hydrometrocolpos, hematometra, or hematocolpos, depending on the composition of the trapped fluid). (See Chapter 31.)

Abnormalities of the vagina are often associated with anomalies of the urinary system and the rectum, because differentiation of the urogenital sinus is involved in formation of the bladder and urethra as well as the vagina and vestibule. Furthermore, if partitioning of the cloaca into the sinus and anorectal canal is faulty, then associated rectal defects can occur. Compound anomalies may affect the urinary tract or rectum. The urethra may open into the vaginal wall; even a single vesicovaginal cavity has been described. On the other hand, the vagina can open into a persistent urogenital sinus, as in certain forms of female pseudohermaphroditism. Associated rectal abnormalities include vaginorectal fistula, vulvovaginal anus, rectosigmoidal fistula, and vaginosigmoidal cloaca in the absence of the rectum (see also Cloacal Dysgenesis, below).

**C. Anomalies of the Hymen:** The hymen is probably a mixture of tissue derived from remains of the sinusal tubercle and the vaginal plate. Usually, the hymen is patent, or perforate, by puberty, although an **imperforate hymen** is not rare. The imperforate condition can be a congenital error of lack of central degeneration or a result of inflammatory occlusion after perforation. Obstruction of menstrual flow at puberty may be the first sign (Fig 4–23).

**D. Cloacal Dysgenesis (Including Persistence of the Urogenital Sinus):** Anomalous partitioning of the cloaca by the abnormal development of the urorectal septum is rare, at least based on reported cases in the literature. As anticipated from a developmental standpoint, the incidence of associated genitourinary anomalies is high. Five types of cloacal or anorectal malformations are summarized in Table 4–3.

**Rectocloacal fistula with a persistent cloaca** provides a common canal or outlet for the urinary, genital, and intestinal tracts. The distinction between a canal and an outlet is one of depth (deep versus very

**Table 4–3.** Cloacal malformations.[1]

| | |
|---|---|
| **Rectocloacal Fistula** | |
| Vestibule | Deformed; flanked by labia; clitoris in front, fourchette behind; anterior vestibule short, shallow, and moist; single external orifice in posterior half of vestibule (common conduit for urine, cervical mucus, and feces). |
| Bladder/urethra | Anterior; directed cranially and ventrally. |
| Vagina | Opens into the vault of cloaca. |
| Anus/rectum | Enters at highest and most posterior point; orifice is in midline and stenotic. |
| Disposition | Lengths of urethra and vagina are inversely proportionate to length of cloacal canal. |
| **Rectovaginal Fistula** | |
| Vestibule | Normal anatomy (2 orifices: urethral & vaginal). |
| Bladder/urethra | Normal. |
| Vagina | May be septate or normal. |
| Anus/rectum | Internal in the midposterior vaginal wall. |
| Disposition | Anus absent from perineum. |
| **Rectovestibular Fistula** | |
| Vestibule | Contains rectum, otherwise normal. |
| Urethra | Normal. |
| Vagina | Normal. |
| Anus/rectum | Small, sited at the fossa navicularis. |
| Disposition | Rectum is parallel with both vagina and urethra. |
| **Covered Anus** | |
| Vestibule | Normal. |
| Urethra | Normal. |
| Vagina | (Probably normal.) |
| Anus | At any point between the normal site and the fourchette; anocutaneous; anovulvar. |
| Disposition | Genital folds are abnormally fused anterior and posterior to common orifice and give rise to hypertrophied perineal raphe. |
| **Ectopic Anus** | |
| Vestibule | Normal. |
| Urethra | Normal. |
| Vagina | Normal. |
| Anus | Anterior to the normal site; normal function. |
| Disposition | Fault lies in the development of the perineum. |

[1]Modified and reproduced, with permission, from Okonkwo JEN, Crocker KM: Cloacal dysgenesis. Obstet Gynecol 1977; 50:97.

shallow, respectively) of the persistent lower portion of the cloaca and, thus, the length of the individual urethral and vaginal canals emptying into the cloaca. The inverse relationship between depth (or length) of the cloaca and length of the vaginal and urethral canals is probably a reflection of the time when arrest of formation of the urorectal septum occurs. Although the bladder, the vagina, and the rectum can empty into a common cloaca as just described, other unusual variations of persistent cloaca can also occur.

For example, the vagina and rectum develop, but the urinary bladder does not develop as a separate entity from the cloaca. Instead, the vagina and rectum open separately into a "urinary bladder," which has ureters entering posterolaterally to the vagina (vaginal orifice is in the "anatomic trigone" of the bladder-like structure). The external orifice from the base of this cloacal "bladder" is a single narrow canal. One explanation for this variant might be that arrest of formation of the urorectal septum occurs much earlier than does the separate development of distal portions of the 3 tracts (urethra, vagina, and anorectum) to a more advanced (but still incomplete) stage before urorectal septal formation ceases. The anomaly is probably rare.

With a **rectovaginal fistula,** the vestibule may appear anatomically normal but the anus does not appear in the perineum. The defect probably results from anorectal agenesis due to incomplete subdivision of the cloaca (similar agenesis in the male could result in a rectourethral fistula). The development of the anterior aspect of the vagina completes the separation of the urethra from the vagina, so there is not a persistent urogenital sinus. **Anorectal agenesis** is reputedly the most common type of anorectal malformation, and usually a fistula occurs. Rectovaginal, anovestibular (or rectovestibular; Table 4–2), and anoperineal fistulas account for most anorectal malformations.

In the absence of the anorectal defect (normal anal presentation) but presence of a **persistent urogenital sinus** with a single external orifice, various irregularities of the urethra and genitalia can appear. The relative positions of urethral and vaginal orifices in the sinus can even change as the child grows. In the discussion of anomalies of the labia majora (see following text), note is made of the association of a persistent urogenital sinus in female pseudohermaphroditism due to congenital adrenal hyperplasia. The vagina opens into the persisting pelvic part of the sinus, which extends with the phallic part of the sinus to the external surface at the urogenital opening. The sinus can be deep and narrow in the neonate, approximating the size of a urethra, or it can be relatively shallow.

Urinary tract disorders associated with persistent urogenital sinus include duplication of the ureters, unilateral ureteral and renal agenesis or atresia, and lack of or abnormal ascent of the kidneys. Variations in the anomalies of derivatives of the urogenital sinus appear to be related in part to the time of arrest of normal differentiation and development of the urogenital sinus, as well as to the impact of other factors associated with abnormal sexual differentiation, such as the variable degrees of response to adrenal androgen in congenital adrenal hyperplasia.

## THE EXTERNAL GENITALIA

### Undifferentiated Stage

The external genitalia begin to form early in the embryonic period, shortly after development of the cloaca. The progenitory tissues of the genitalia are common to both sexes, and the early stage of development is virtually the same in females and males. Although differentiation of the genitalia can begin around the onset of the fetal period if testicular differentiation is initiated, definitive genital sex is usually not clearly apparent until the 12th week. Formation of external genitalia in the male involves the influence of androgen on the interaction of subepidermal mesoderm with the inferior parts of the endodermal urogenital sinus. In the female, this androgenic influence is absent.

The external genitalia form within the initially compact area bounded by the umbilical cord (anteriorly), the developing limb buds (laterally), the embryonic tail (posteriorly), and the cloacal membrane (centrally). Two of the primordia for the genitalia first appear bilaterally adjacent to the cloacal membrane (a medial pair of cloacal folds and a lateral pair of genital [labioscrotal] swellings). The **cloacal folds** are longitudinal proliferations of caudal mesenchyme located between the ectodermal epidermis and the underlying endoderm of the phallic part of the urogenital sinus. Proliferation and bilateral anterior fusion of these folds create the **genital tubercle,** which protrudes near the anterior edge of the cloacal membrane by the sixth week (Figs 4–24 to 4–26). Extension of the tubercle forms the phallus, which at this stage is the same size in both sexes.

By the seventh week, the urorectal septum subdivides the bilayered (ectoderm and endoderm) cloacal membrane, into the **urogenital membrane** (anteriorly) and the **anal membrane** (posteriorly). The area of fusion of the urorectal septum and the cloacal membrane becomes the **primitive perineum,** or **perineal body.** With formation of the perineum, the cloacal folds are divided transversely as **urogenital folds** adjacent to the urogenital membrane and **anal folds** around the anal membrane. As the mesoderm within the urogenital folds thickens and elongates between the perineum and the phallus, the urogenital membrane sinks deeper into the fissure between the folds. Within a week, this membrane ruptures, forming the **urogenital orifice** and, thus, opening the urogenital sinus to the exterior. Similar thickening of the anal folds creates a deep anal pit, in which the anal membrane breaks down to establish the **anal orifice** of the anal canal (Figs 4–24 and 4–25).

Subsequent masculinization or feminization of the external genitalia is a consequence of the respective

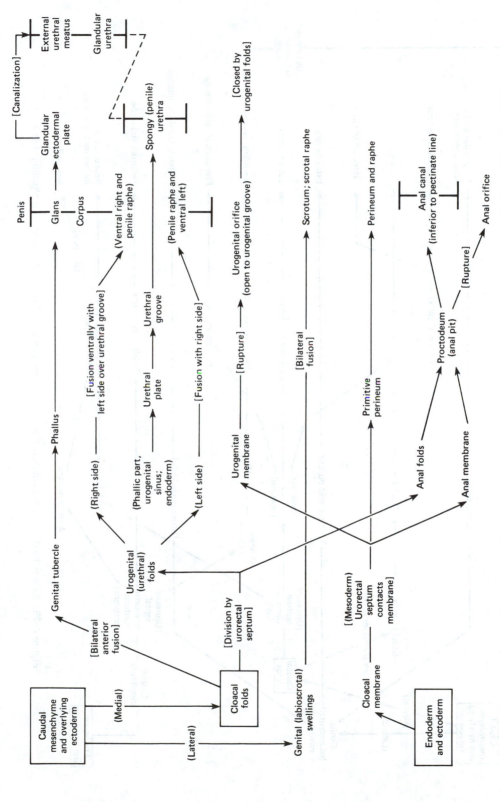

**Figure 4–24.** Schematic drawing of formation of male external genitalia. (Explanatory symbols are given in Fig 4–1.)

87

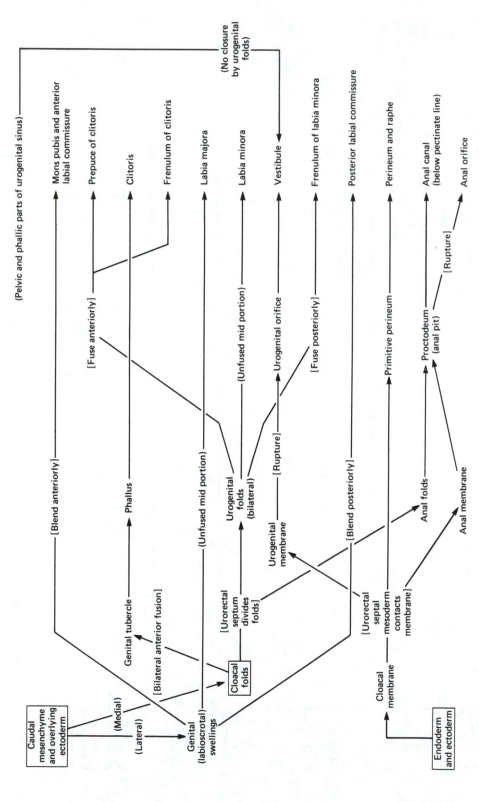

**Figure 4–25.** Schematic drawing of formation of female external genitalia. (Explanatory symbols are given in Fig 4–1.)

88

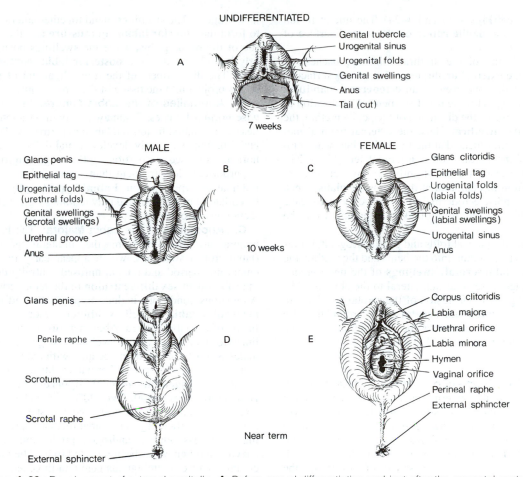

**Figure 4–26.** Development of external genitalia. **A:** Before sexual differentiation and just after the urorectal septum divides the cloacal membrane. **B** and **D:** Male differentiation at about 10 weeks and near term, respectively. The urogenital folds fuse ventrally over the urethral groove to form the spongy urethra and close the inferior phallic part of the urogenital sinus. The glandular urethra forms by canalization of invaginated ectoderm from the tip of the glans. **C** and **E:** Female differentiation at about 10 weeks and near term, respectively. Until about 12 weeks, there is little difference in the appearance of female and male external genitalia. The urogenital folds fuse only at their anterior and posterior extremes, while the unfused remainder differentiates into the labia minor. (See also Figs 4–24 and 4–25.)

presence or absence of androgen and the androgenic sensitivity or insensitivity of the tissues. The significance of both of these factors (availability of hormone and sensitivity of target tissue) is exemplified by the rare condition (about 1 in 50,000 "females") of **testicular feminization,** wherein testes are present (usually ectopic) and produce testosterone and anti-müllerian hormone. The anti-müllerian hormone suppresses formation of the uterus and uterine tubes (from the paramesonephric ducts), whereas testosterone supports male differentiation of the mesonephric ducts to form the epididymis and ductus deferens. The anomalous feminization of the external genitalia is considered to be due to androgenic insensitivity of the precursor tissues consequent to an abnormal androgen receptor or postreceptor mechanism set by genetic inheritance.

## Male

Early masculinization of the undifferentiated or indifferent genitalia takes place during the first 3 weeks of the fetal period (weeks 9–12) and is caused by androgenic stimulation. The phallus and urogenital folds gradually elongate to initiate development of the **penis.** The subjacent endodermal lining of the inferior part (phallic) of the urogenital sinus extends anteriorly along with the urogenital folds, creating an endodermal plate, the **urethral plate.** The plate deepens into a groove, the **urethral groove,** as the urogenital folds (now called **urethral folds**) thicken on each side of the plate. The urethral groove extends into the ventral aspect of the developing penis, and the bilateral urethral folds slowly fuse in a posterior to anterior direction over the urethral groove to form the **spongy (penile) urethra,** thereby closing the urogenital orifice (Figs 4–17 and 4–24). The line of fusion becomes the **penile raphe** on the ventral surface of the penis.

As closure of the urethral folds approaches the glans, the external urethral opening on this surface is eliminated. Concurrently, an **ectodermal glandular plate** invaginates the tip of the penis. Canalization of the plate forms the distal end of the penile urethra, the **glandular urethra.** Thus, the external urethral meatus becomes located at the tip of the glans when closure of the urethral folds is completed (Fig 4–24). The **prepuce** is formed slightly later by a circular invagination of ectoderm at the tip of the **glans penis.** This cylindric ectodermal plate then cleaves to leave a double-layered fold of skin extending over the glans.

While the cloacal folds and phallic urogenital sinus were differentiating into the penis and the urethra, the **genital (labioscrotal) swellings** of the undifferentiated stage were enlarging lateral to the cloacal folds. Medial growth and fusion of the scrotal swellings to form the **scrotum** and **scrotal raphe** around the 12th week virtually complete the differentiation of the male external genitalia (Fig 4–24 and 4–26).

### Female

**A. Development of External Genitalia:** Feminization of the external genitalia proceeds in the absence of androgenic stimulation (or nonresponsiveness of the tissue). The 2 primary distinctions in the general process of feminization versus masculinization are (1) the lack of continued growth of the phallus and (2) the near absence of fusion of the urogenital folds and the labioscrotal swellings. Female derivatives of the indifferent sexual primordia for the external genitalia are virtual homologous counterparts of the male derivatives. Formation of the female genitalia is schematically presented in Fig 4–25.

The growth of the phallus slows relative to that of the urogenital folds and labioscrotal swellings and becomes the diminutive **clitoris.** The anterior extreme of the urogenital folds fuses superior and inferior to the clitoris, forming the **prepuce** and **frenulum of the clitoris,** respectively. The midportions of these folds do not fuse but give rise to the **labia minora.** Lack of closure of the folds leaves the urogenital orifice patent and results in formation of the **vestibule of the vagina** from the inferior portion of the pelvic part and the phallic part of the urogenital sinus at about the fifth month (Fig 4–25). Derivatives of the vesical part of the sinus (the **urethra**) and the superior portion of the pelvic part of the sinus (**vagina and greater vestibular glands**) then open separately into the vestibule. The **frenulum of the labia minora** is formed by fusion of the posterior ends of the urogenital folds. The mesoderm of the labioscrotal swellings proliferates beneath the ectoderm and remains virtually unfused to create the **labia majora** lateral to the

labia minora. The swellings blend together anteriorly to form the **anterior labial commissure** and the tissue of the **mons pubis,** while the swellings posteriorly less clearly define a **posterior labial commissure.** The distal fibers of the round ligament of the uterus project into the tissue of the labia majora.

**B. Anomalies of the Labia Minora:** In otherwise normal females, 2 somewhat common anomalies occur—labial fusion and labial hypertrophy. True labial fusion as an early developmental defect in the normally unfused midportions of the urogenital folds is purportedly less frequent than "fusion" due to inflammatory-type reaction. **Labial hypertrophy** can be unilateral or bilateral and may require surgical correction in extreme cases.

**C. Anomalies of the Labia Majora:** The labia majora are derived from the bilateral genital (labioscrotal) swellings, which appear early in the embryonic period and remain unfused centrally during subsequent sex differentiation in the fetal period. Anomalous conditions include **hypoplastic** and **hypertrophic labia** as well as different gradations of fusion of the labia majora. Abnormal fusion (masculinization) of labioscrotal swellings in genetic females is most commonly associated with ambiguous genitalia of female pseudohermaphroditism consequent to **congenital adrenal hyperplasia (adrenogenital syndrome).** Over 90% of females with congenital adrenal hyperplasia have a steroid 21-hydroxylase deficiency (autosomal recessive), resulting in excess adrenal androgen production. This enzyme deficiency has been reported to be "the most common cause of ambiguous genitalia in genetic females" (Oshima and Troen, 1981). Associated anomalies include clitoral hypertrophy and persistent urogenital sinus. Formation of a penile urethra is extremely rare.

**D. Anomalies of the Clitoris:** Clitoral agenesis is extremely rare and is due to lack of formation of the genital tubercle during the sixth week. Absence of the clitoris could also result from **atresia** of the genital tubercle. The tubercle forms by fusion of the anterior segments of the cloacal folds. Very rarely, these anterior segments fail to fuse, and a **bifid clitoris** forms. This anomaly also occurs when unification of the anterior parts of the folds is restricted by exstrophy of the cloaca or bladder. Duplication of the genital tubercle with consequent formation of a **double clitoris** is equally rare. **Clitoral hypertrophy** alone is not common but may be associated with various intersex disorders.

**E. Anomalies of the Perineum:** The primitive perineum originates at the area of contact of the mesodermal urorectal septum and the endodermal dorsal surface of the cloacal membrane (at 7 weeks). During normal differentiation of the external genitalia in the fetal period, the primitive perineum maintains the separation of the urogenital folds and ruptured urogenital membrane from the anal folds and ruptured anal membrane, and later develops the perineal body. Malformations of the perineum are rare and usually associated with malformations of cloacal or anorectal development consequent to abnormal development of the urorectal septum. **Imperforate anus** has an incidence of about 0.02%. The simplest form (rare) is a thin membrane over the anal canal (the anal membrane failed to rupture at the end of the embryonic period). **Anal stenosis** can arise by posterior deviation of the urorectal septum as the septum approaches the cloacal membrane, causing the anal membrane to be smaller (with a relatively increased anogenital distance through the perineum). **Anal agenesis** with a fistula detected as an ectopic anus is considered to be a urorectal septal defect. The incidence of agenesis with a fistula is only slightly less than that without a fistula. In females, the fistula commonly may be located in the perineum (**perineal fistula**) or open into the posterior aspect of the vestibule of the vagina (**anovestibular fistula**; see Cloacal Dysgenesis).

## REFERENCES

Beekhuis JR, Hage JC: The double uterus associated with an obstructed hemivagina and ipsilateral renal agenesis. Eur J Obstet Gynecol Reprod Biol 1983;16:47.

Berta P, Hawkins JR, Sinclair AH et al: Genetic evidence equating SRY and the testis-determining factor. Nature 1990;348:448.

Blyth B, Duckett JW Jr: Gonadal differentiation: A review of the physiological process and influencing factors based on recent experimental evidence. J Urol 1991; 145:689.

Brumsted JR, Riddick DH: Hysteroscopic evaluation and therapy of müllerian anomalies, pp 64–65. In: *Current Therapy in Obstetrics and Gynecology*, vol 3. Quilligan EJ, Zuspan FP (editors). Saunders, 1990.

Buttram VC Jr, Gibbons WE: Müllerian anomalies: A proposed classification (an analysis of 144 cases). Fertil Steril 1979;32:40.

Byskov AG: Differentiation of mammalian embryonic gonad. Physiol Rev 1986;66:71.

Byskov AG, Hoyer PE: Embryology of mammalian gonads and ducts pp 265–302. In: *The Physiology of Reproduction*, vol 1. Knobil E, Neill JD (editors). Raven Press, 1988.

Carr BR, Casey ML: Growth of the adrenal gland of the normal human fetus during early gestation. Early Hum Dev 1982;6:121.

Casey ML, Carr BR: Growth of the kidney in the normal human fetus during early gestation. Early Hum Dev 1982;6:11.

Cruikshank SH, Van Drie DM: Supernumerary ovaries: Update and review. Obstet Gynecol 1982;60:126.

Elias S et al: Genetics studies in incomplete müllerian fusion. Obstet Gynecol 1984;63:276.

George FW, Wilson JD: Sex determination and differentiation, pp 1–26. In: *The Physiology of Reproduction*, vol 1. Knobil E, Neill JD (editors). Raven Press, 1988.

Gondos B: Diagnosis of abnormalities in gonadal development. Ann Clin Lab Sci 1982;12:276.

Gray SW, Skandalakis JE: *Embryology for Surgeons*, 2nd ed. Williams & Wilkins, 1993.

Grumbach MM, Conte FA: Disorders of sexual differentiation, pp 853–952. In: *Williams' Textbook of Endocrinology*, 8th ed. Wilson JD, Foster DW (editors). Saunders, 1992.

Hansen N, Coury DL: Congenital anomalies of the neonate, pp 305–312. In: *Current Therapy in Obstetrics and Gynecology*, vol 3. Quilligan EJ, Zuspan FP (editors). Saunders, 1990.

Heinonen PK, Pystynen PP: Primary infertility and uterine anomalies. Fertil Steril 1982;40:311.

Jirasek JE: *Morphogenesis of the genital system in the human*. Birth Defects: Original Article Series. 1977; 13(2):13.

Jones HW Jr: Reconstruction of congenital uterovaginal anomalies, pp 246–286; Surgical procedures for disorders of sexual development, pp 287–378. In: *Female Reproductive Surgery*. Rock JA, Murphy AA, Jones HW Jr (editors). Williams & Wilkins, 1992.

Josso N, Picard J-Y: Anti-müllerian hormone. Physiol Rev 1986;66:1038.

Jost A: Sexual organogenesis, pp 3–19. In: *Reproduction*, vol 7. *Handbook of Behavioral Neurobiology*. Adler N, Pfaff D, Goy RW (editors). Plenum Press, 1985.

Larsen WJ: Development of the urogenital system, pp 235–279. In: *Human Embryology*. Churchill Livingstone, 1993.

McCrory WW: Normal organogenesis of the human kidney, pp 259–280. In: *Abnormal Functional Development of the Heart, Lungs, and Kidney: Approaches to Functional Teratology*. Kavlock RJ, Grabowski CT (editors). Liss, 1983.

McDonough PG: Gonadal dysgenesis, pp 56–60. In: *Current Therapy in Obstetrics and Gynecology*, vol 3. Quilligan EJ, Zuspan FP (editors). Saunders, 1990.

McLaren A: What makes a man a man? Nature 1990; 346:216.

Mittwoch U: Sex determination and sex reversal: Genotype, phenotype, dogma and semantics. Hum Genet 1992; 89:467.

Moore KL, Persaud TVN: *The Developing Human: Clinically Oriented Embryology*, 5th ed. Saunders, 1993.

Nhan VQ, Huisjes HJ: Double uterus with a pregnancy in each half. Obstet Gynecol 1983;61:115.

Okonkwo JEN, Crocker KM: Cloacal dysgenesis. Obstet Gynecol 1977;50:97.

O'Rahilly R: The timing and sequence of events in the development of the human reproductive system during the embryonic period proper. Anat Embryol 1983;166:247.

Oshima H, Troen P: Disorders of sexual differentiation and development, pp 725–758. In: *Endocrinology and Metabolism*. Felig P et al (editors). McGraw-Hill, 1981.

Page DC, Fisher EMC, McGillivray B, Brown LG: Additional deletion in sex-determining region of human Y chromosome resolves paradox of X,t(Y;22) female. Nature 1990; 346:279.

Peters H, McNatty KP: *The Ovary: A Correlation of Structure and Function in Mammals*. University of California Press, 1980.

Porter IH, Hook EB (editors): *Human Embryonic and Fetal Death*. Birth Defects Institute Symposium, Series X. Academic Press, 1980.

Ross GT: Disorders of the ovary and female reproductive tract, pp 733–798. In: *Williams' Textbook of Endocrinology*, 8th ed. Wilson JD, Foster DW (editors). Saunders, 1992.

Saenger P: Abnormal sex differentiation. J Pediatr 1984; 104:1.

Serio M et al (editors): *Sexual Differentiation: Basic and Clinical Aspects* (Serono Symposium 11). Raven Press, 1984.

Shepard TH: *Catalog of Teratogenic Agents*, 7th ed. The Johns Hopkins University Press, 1992.

Simpson JL: Anomalies of internal ducts, pp 341–359. In: *Disorders of Sexual Differentiation: Etiology and Clinical Delineation*. Academic Press, 1976.

Sinclair AH, Berta P, Palmer MS et al: A gene from the human sex-determining region encodes a protein with homology to a conserved DNA-binding motif. Nature 1990;346:240.

Singh J, Devi YL: Pregnancy following surgical correction of nonfused müllerian bulbs and absent vagina. Fertil Steril 1983;61:267.

Smith ED: *Incidence, frequency of types, and etiology of anorectal malformations*. Birth Defects Original Article Series 1988;24:231.

Stephens FD: *Embryology of the cloaca and embryogenesis of anorectal malformations*. Birth Defects Original Article Series 1988;24:177.

Suidan FG, Azoury RS: The transverse vaginal septum: A clinicopathologic evaluation. Obstet Gynecol 1979; 54:278.

Thomas DFM: Cloacal malformations: embryology, anatomy and principles of management. Prog Pediatr Surg 1989;23:135.

Verkauf BS (editor): *Congenital Malformations of the Female Reproductive Tract and Their Treatment*. Appleton & Lange, 1993.

Warkany J: Prevention of congenital malformations. Teratology 1981;23:175.

Wartenberg H: Development of the early human ovary and role of the mesonephros in the differentiation of the cortex. Anat Embryol 1982;165:253.

# Genetic Disorders & Sex Chromosome Abnormalities

# 5

*Morton A. Stenchever, MD, & Howard W. Jones, Jr., MD*

## GENETIC DISORDERS

## MENDELIAN LAWS OF INHERITANCE

### 1. TYPES OF INHERITANCE

#### Autosomal Dominant

In autosomal dominant inheritance, it is assumed that a mutation has occurred in one gene of an allelic pair and that the presence of this new gene produces enough of the changed protein to give a different phenotypic effect. Environment must also be considered because the effect may vary under different environmental conditions. The following are characteristic of autosomal dominant inheritance:

(1) The trait appears with equal frequency in both sexes.

(2) For inheritance to take place, at least one parent must have the trait unless a new mutation has just occurred.

(3) When a homozygous individual is mated to a normal individual, all offspring will carry the trait. When a heterozygous individual is mated to a normal individual, 50% of the offspring will show the trait.

(4) If the trait is rare, most persons demonstrating it will be heterozygous (see Table 5–1).

#### Autosomal Recessive

The mutant gene will not be capable of producing a new characteristic in the heterozygous state in this circumstance under customary environmental conditions—ie, with 50% of the genetic material producing the new protein, the phenotypic effect will not be different from that of the normal trait. When the environment is manipulated, the recessive trait occasionally becomes dominant. The characteristics of this form of inheritance are as follows:

(1) The characteristic will occur with equal frequency in both sexes.

(2) For the characteristic to be present, both parents must be carriers of the recessive trait.

(3) If both parents are homozygous for the recessive trait, all offspring will have it.

(4) If both parents are heterozygous for the recessive trait, 25% of the offspring will have it.

(5) In pedigrees showing frequent occurrence of individuals with rare recessive characteristics, consanguinity is often present (see Table 5–2).

#### X-Linked Recessive

This condition occurs when a gene on the X chromosome undergoes mutation and the new protein formed as a result of this mutation is incapable of producing a change in phenotype characteristic in the heterozygous state. Because the male has only one X chromosome, the presence of this mutant will allow for expression should it occur in the male. The following are characteristic of this form of inheritance:

(1) The condition occurs more commonly in males than in females.

(2) If both parents are normal and an affected male is produced, it must be assumed that the mother is a carrier of the trait.

(3) If the father is affected and an affected male is produced, the mother must be at least heterozygous for the trait.

(4) A female with the trait may be produced in one of 2 ways: (1) She may inherit a recessive gene from both her mother and her father; this suggests that the father is affected and the mother is heterozygous. (2) She may inherit a recessive gene from one of her parents and may express the recessive characteristic as a function of the Lyon hypothesis; this assumes that all females are mosaics for their functioning X chromosome. It is theorized that this occurs because at about the time of implantation each cell in the developing female embryo selects one X chromosome as its functioning X and that all progeny cells thereafter use this X chromosome as their functioning X chromosome. The other X chromosome becomes inactive. Since this selection is done on a random basis, it is conceivable that some females will be produced who will be using primarily the X chromosome bearing the reces-

| Table 5–1. Examples of autosomal dominant conditions and traits. |
| :--- |
| Achondroplasia |
| Acoustic neuroma |
| Aniridia |
| Cataracts, cortical and nuclear |
| Chin fissure |
| Color blindness, yellow-blue |
| Craniofacial dysostosis |
| Deafness (several forms) |
| Dupuytren's contracture |
| Ehlers-Danlos syndrome |
| Facial palsy, congenital |
| Huntington's chorea |
| Hyperchondroplasia |
| Intestinal polyposis |
| Keloid formation |
| Lipomas, familial |
| Marfan's syndrome |
| Mitral valve prolapse |
| Muscular dystrophy |
| Neurofibromatosis (Recklinghausen's disease) |
| Night blindness |
| Pectus excavatum |
| Adult polycystic renal disease |
| Tuberous sclerosis |
| Von Willebrand's disease |
| Wolff-Parkinson-White syndrome (some cases) |

| Table 5–2. Examples of autosomal recessive conditions and traits. |
| :--- |
| Acid maltase deficiency |
| Albinism |
| Alkaptonuria |
| Argininemia |
| Ataxia-telangiectasia |
| Bloom's syndrome |
| Cerebrohepatorenal syndrome |
| Chloride diarrhea, congenital |
| Chondrodystrophia myotonia |
| Color blindness, total |
| Coronary artery calcinosis |
| Cystic fibrosis |
| Cystinosis |
| Cystinuria |
| Deafness (several types) |
| Dubowitz's syndrome |
| Laron's dwarfism |
| Dysautonomia |
| Fructose-1,6-diphosphatase deficiency |
| Galactosemia |
| Gaucher's disease |
| Glaucoma, congenital |
| Histidinemia |
| Homocystinuria |
| Maple syrup urine disease |
| Mucolipidosis I, II, III |
| Mucopolysaccharidosis I-H, I-S, III, IV, VI, VII |
| Muscular dystrophy, autosomal recessive type |
| Niemann Pick disease |
| Phenylketonuria |
| Sickle cell anemia |
| 17α-Hydroxylase deficiency |
| 18-Hydroxylase deficiency |
| 21-Hydroxylase deficiency |
| Tay-Sachs disease |
| Wilson's disease |
| Xeroderma pigmentosum |

sive gene. Thus, a genotypically heterozygous individual may demonstrate a recessive characteristic phenotypically on this basis (see Table 5–3).

## X-Linked Dominant

In this situation, the mutation will produce a protein that, when present in the heterozygous state, is sufficient to cause a change in characteristic. The following are characteristic of this type of inheritance:

(1) The characteristic occurs with the same frequency in males and females.

(2) An affected male mated to a normal female will produce the characteristic in 50% of the offspring.

(3) An affected homozygous female mated to a normal male will produce the affected characteristic in all offspring.

(4) A heterozygous female mated to a normal male will produce the characteristic in 50% of the offspring.

(5) Occasional heterozygous females may not show the dominant trait on the basis of the Lyon hypothesis (see Table 5–4).

## 2. APPLICATIONS OF MENDELIAN LAWS

### Identification of Carriers

When a recessive characteristic is present in a population, carriers may be identified in a variety of ways. If the gene is responsible for the production of a protein (eg, an enzyme), the carrier often possesses 50% of the amount of the substance present in homozygous normal persons. Such a circumstance is found in galactosemia, where the carriers will have approximately half as much galactose-1-phosphate uridyl transferase activity in red cells as do noncarrier normal individuals.

At times, the level of the affected enzyme may be only slightly below normal, and a challenge with the substance to be acted upon may be required before the carrier can be identified. An example is seen in carriers of phenylketonuria, in whom the deficiency in phenylalanine hydroxylase is in the liver cells and serum levels may not be much lower than normal. Nonetheless, when the individual is given an oral loading dose of phenylalanine, plasma phenylalanine levels may remain high because the enzyme is not present in sufficient quantities to act upon this substance properly.

In still other situations where the 2 alleles produce different proteins that can be measured, a carrier state will have 50% of the normal protein and 50% of the other protein. Such a situation is seen in sickle cell trait, where one gene is producing hemoglobin A and

**Table 5–3.** Examples of X-linked recessive conditions and traits.

Androgen insensitivity syndrome (complete and incomplete)
Color blindness, red-green
Diabetes insipidus (most cases)
Fabry's disease
Glucose-6-phosphate dehydrogenase deficiency
Gonadal dysgenesis (XY type)
Gout (certain types)
Hemophilia A (factor VIII deficiency)
Hemophilia B (factor IX deficiency)
Hypothyroidism, X-linked infantile
Hypophosphatemia
Immunodeficiency, X-linked
Lesch-Nyhan syndrome
Mucopolysaccharidosis II
Muscular dystrophy, adult and childhood types
Otopalatodigital syndrome
Reifenstein's syndrome

the other hemoglobin S. Thus, the individual has half the amount of hemoglobin A as a normal person and half the hemoglobin S of a person with sickle cell anemia. An interesting but important problem involves the detection of carriers of cystic fibrosis. This is the most common autosomal recessive disease in Caucasian populations of European background occurring in 1 in 2500 births in such populations, but being found in the carrier state in 1 in 25 Americans. By 1990, over 230 alleles of the single gene responsible have been discovered. The gene is known as the cystic fibrosis transmembrane conductance regulator (CFTR) and the commonest mutation, delta F508, accounts for about 70% of all mutations, with 5 specific point mutations accounting for over 85% of cases. Because so many alleles are present, population screening poses logistic problems that have yet to be worked out. Most programs screen for the commonest mutations using DNA replication and amplification studies.

## Expressivity & Penetrance

Expressivity and penetrance are examples of how an autosomal characteristic may not be expressed in quite the form that it ordinarily would be. With regard to expressivity, while the gene is present, the entire genome of the individual must be taken into consideration. Other genetic influences may be operating— even environmental ones—that may modify the manner in which the gene expresses itself. Penetrance, on the other hand, involves the expression of a dominant gene and takes into consideration the fact that while

**Table 5–4.** Examples of X-linked dominant conditions and traits.

Acro-osteolysis, dominant type
Cervico-oculo-acoustic syndrome
Hyperammonemia
Orofaciodigital syndrome I

the gene may express itself in most individuals in a similar fashion, there may be some circumstance of environment or other gene activity during the development of the individual that may modify its action so that the phenotypic factor is not seen. Thus, one could state that during embryonic development, there is a requirement of some environmental factor to allow the gene to express itself, and, in an occasional rare case, this may not take place. Hence, the gene is not allowed to operate at its specific time.

## Incidence of Diseases With Known Inheritance Patterns

If the incidence of a particular condition known to be autosomal recessive is known in a given population, then, applying mendelian law, it is possible to calculate the number of carriers in that population. The key to this circumstance, which will prevent error, is the testing of a large number of individuals within a population to calculate the true incidence of the autosomal recessive state.

## Prenatal Diagnosis as an Aid

It is now possible to detect carrier and affected individuals of a large number of metabolic diseases prenatally. By using cells obtained from chorionic villus sampling, amniocentesis, or funiocentesis (umbilical vein puncture), genetic testing for specific proteins, linkage studies or DNA studies may be carried out. These tests may be offered to couples where carrier state is present or where one parent is affected.

## 3. POLYGENIC INHERITANCE

Polygenic inheritance is defined as the inheritance of a single phenotypic feature as a result of the effects of many genes. Most physical features in humans are determined by polygenic inheritance. Many common malformations are determined in this way also. For example, cleft palate with or without cleft lip, clubfoot, anencephaly, meningomyelocele, dislocation of the hip, and pyloric stenosis each occur with a frequency of 0.5–2 per 1000 in white populations. Altogether, these anomalies account for slightly less than half of single primary defects noted in early infancy. They are present in siblings of affected infants— when both parents are normal—at a rate of 2–5%. They are also found more commonly among relatives than in the general population. The increase in incidence is not environmentally induced because the frequency of such abnormalities inmonozygotic twins is 4–8 times that of dizygotic twins and other siblings. The higher incidence inmonozygotic twins is called concordance.

Sex also plays a role. Certain conditions appear to be transmitted by polygenic inheritance and are passed on more frequently by the mother who is affected than by the father who is affected. Cleft lip occurs in 6% of the offspring of women with cleft lip, as opposed to 2.8% of offspring of men with cleft lip.

There are many racial variations in diseases believed to be transmitted by polygenic inheritance, making racial background a determinant of how prone an individual will be to a particular defect. In addition, as a general rule, the more severe a defect, the more likely it is to occur in subsequent siblings. Thus, siblings of children with bilateral cleft lip are more likely to have the defect than are those of children with unilateral cleft lip.

Environment undoubtedly plays a role in polygenic inheritance, because seasonal variations alter some defects and their occurrence rate from country to country in similar populations.

## CYTOGENETICS

### 1. IDENTIFICATION OF CHROMOSOMES

In 1960, 1963, 1965, and 1971, international meetings were held in Denver, London, Chicago, and Paris, respectively, for the purpose of standardizing the nomenclature of human chromosomes. These meetings resulted in a decision that all autosomal pairs should be numbered in order of decreasing size from 1 to 22. Autosomes are divided into groups on the basis of their morphology, and these groups are labeled by the letters A–G. Thus, the A group is comprised of pairs 1–3; the B group, pairs 4 and 5; the C group, pairs 6–12; the D group, pairs 13–15; the E group, pairs 16–18; the F group, pairs 19 and 20; and the G group, pairs 21 and 22. The sex chromosomes are labeled X and Y, the X chromosome being similar in size and morphology to the No. 7 pair and thus frequently included in the C group (C-X) and the Y chromosome being similar in morphology and size to the G group (G-Y) (Fig 5–1).

The short arm of a chromosome is labeled p and the long arm q. If a translocation occurs in which the short arm of a chromosome is added to another chromosome, it is written p+. If the short arm is lost, it is p−. The same can be said for the long arm (q+ and q−).

It has been impossible to separate several chromosome pairs from one another on a strictly morphologic basis because the morphologic variations have been too slight. However, there are other means of identifying each chromosome pair in the karyotype. The first of these is the incorporation of $^3$H-thymidine, known as the autoradiographic technique. This

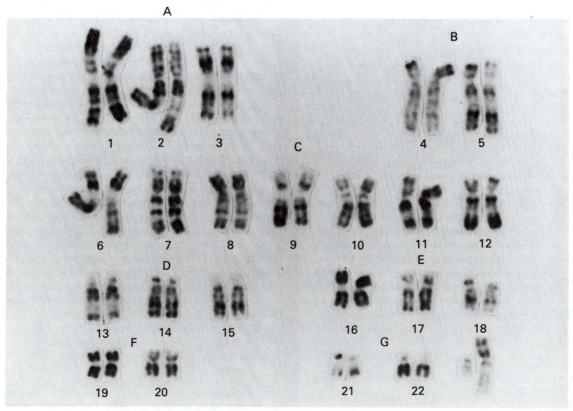

**Figure 5–1.** A karyotype of a normal male demonstrating R banding.

procedure involves the incorporation of radioactive thymidine into growing cells in tissue culture just before they are harvested. Cells that are actively undergoing DNA replication will pick up the radioactive thymidine, and the chromosomes will demonstrate areas of activity. Each chromosome will incorporate thymidine in a different pattern, and several chromosomes can therefore be identified by their labeling pattern. Nonetheless, with this method it is not possible to identify each chromosome, although it is possible to identify chromosomes involved in pathologic conditions, eg, $D_1$ trisomy and Down's syndrome.

Innovative staining techniques have made it possible to identify individual chromosomes in the karyotype and to identify small anomalies that might have evaded the observer using older methods. These involve identification of chromosome banding by a variety of staining techniques, at times with predigestion with proteolytic agents. Some of the more commonly used techniques are the following:

**(1) Q banding:** Fixed chromosome spreads are stained without any pretreatment using quinacrine mustard, quinacrine, or other fluorescent dyes and observed with a fluorescence microscope.

**(2) G banding:** Preparations are incubated in a variety of saline solutions using any one of several pretreatments and stained with Giemsa's stain.

**(3) R banding:** Preparations are incubated in buffer solutions at high temperatures or at special pH

and stained with Giemsa's stain. This process yields the reverse bands of G banding (see Fig 5–1).

**(4) C banding:** Preparations are either heated in saline to temperatures just below boiling or treated with certain alkali solutions and then stained with Giemsa's stain. This process causes prominent bands to develop in the region of the centromeres.

## 2. CELL DIVISION

Each body cell goes through successive stages in its life cycle. As a landmark, cell division may be considered as the beginning of a cycle. Following this, the first phase, which is quite long but depends on how rapidly the particular cell is multiplying, is called the $G_1$ stage. During this stage, the cell is primarily concerned with carrying out its function. Following this, the S stage, or period of DNA synthesis, takes place. Next there is a somewhat shorter stage, the $G_2$ stage, during which time DNA synthesis is completed and chromosome replication begins. Following this comes the M stage, when cell division occurs.

Somatic cells undergo division by a process known as **mitosis** (Fig 5–2). This is divided into 4 periods. The first is the **prophase,** during which the chromosome filaments shorten, thicken, and become visible. At this time they can be seen to be composed of 2 long parallel spiral strands lying adjacent to one an-

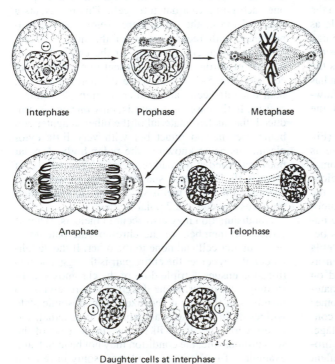

Interphase    Prophase    Metaphase

Anaphase    Telophase

Daughter cells at interphase

**Figure 5–2.** Mitosis of a somatic cell. (Reproduced, with permission, from Stenchever MA: *Human Cytogenetics: A Workbook in Reproductive Biology.* The press at Case Western Reserve University, 1972.)

other and containing a small clear structure known as the **centromere.** As prophase continues, the strands continue to unwind and may be recognized as chromatids. At the end of the prophase, the nuclear membrane disappears and **metaphase** begins. This stage is heralded by the formation of a spindle and the lining up of the chromosomes in pairs on the spindle. Following this, **anaphase** occurs, at which time the centromere divides and each daughter chromatid goes to one of the poles of the spindle. **Telophase** then ensues, at which time the spindle breaks and cell cytoplasm divides. A nuclear membrane now forms, and mitosis is complete: Each daughter cell has received chromosome material equal in amount and identical to that of the parent cell. Because each cell contains 2 chromosomes of each pair and a total of 46 chromosomes, a cell is considered to be **diploid.** Occasionally, an error takes place on the spindle, and instead of chromosomes dividing, with identical chromatids going to each daughter cell, an extra chromatid goes to one daughter cell and the other lacks that particular member. After the completion of cell division, this leads to a trisomic state (an extra dose of that chromosome) in one daughter cell and a monosomic state (a missing dose of the chromosome) in the other daughter cell. Any chromosome in the karyotype may be involved in such a process, which is known as mitotic nondisjunction. If these cells thrive and produce their own progeny, a new cell line is established within the individual. The individual then has more than one cell line and is known as a **mosaic.** A variety of combinations and permutations have occurred in humans.

Germ cells undergo division for the production of eggs and sperm by a process known as **meiosis.** In the female it is known as oogenesis and in the male as spermatogenesis. The process that produces the egg and the sperm for fertilization essentially reduces the chromosome number from 46 to 23 and changes the normal diploid cells to anaploid cell, ie, a cell that has only one member of each chromosome pair. Following fertilization and the fusion of the 2 pronuclei, the diploid status is reestablished.

Meiosis can be divided into several stages (Fig 5–3). The first is **prophase I.** Early prophase is known as the **leptotene stage,** during which chromatin condenses and becomes visible as a single elongated threadlike structure. This is followed by the **zygotene stage,** when the single threadlike chromosomes migrate toward the equatorial plate of the nucleus. At this stage, homologous chromosomes become arranged close to one another to form **bivalents** that exchange materials at several points known as **synapses.** In this way, genetic material located on one member of a pair is exchanged with similar material located on the other member of a pair. Next comes the **pachytene stage** in which the chromosomes contract to become shorter and thicker. During this stage, each chromosome splits longitudinally into 2 chromatids united at the centromere. Thus, the bivalent

becomes a structure composed of 4 closely opposed chromatids known as a **tetrad.** The human cell in the pachytene stage demonstrates 23 tetrads. This stage is followed by the **diplotene stage,** in which the chromosomes of the bivalent are held together only at certain points called bridges or chiasms. It is at these points that crossover takes place. The sister chromatids are joined at the centromere so that crossing-over can only take place between chromatids of homologous chromosomes and not between identical sister chromatids. In the case of males, the X and Y chromosomes are not involved in crossing-over. This stage is followed by the last stage of prophase, known as **diakinesis.** Here the bivalents contract, and the chiasms move toward the end of the chromosome. The homologs pull apart, and the nuclear membrane disappears. This is the end of prophase I.

**Metaphase I** follows. At this time, the bivalents are now highly contracted and align themselves along the equatorial plate of the cell. Paternal and maternal chromosomes line up at random. This stage is then followed by **anaphase I** and **telophase I,** which are quite similar to the corresponding events in mitosis. Nevertheless, the difference is that in meiosis the homologous chromosome of the bivalent pair separates and not the sister chromatids. The homologous bivalents pull apart, one going to each pole of the spindle, following which 2 daughter cells are formed at telophase I.

Metaphase, anaphase, and telophase of meiosis II take place next. A new spindle forms in metaphase, the chromosomes align along the equatorial plate, and, as anaphase occurs, the chromatids pull apart, one each going to a daughter cell. This represents a true division of the centromere. Telophase then supervenes, with reconstitution of the nuclear membrane and final cell division. At the end, a haploid number of chromosomes is present in each daughter cell (see Fig 5–3). In the case of spermatogenesis, both daughter cells are similar, forming 2 separate sperms. In the case of oogenesis, only one egg is produced, the nuclear material of the other daughter cell being present and intact but with very little cytoplasm, this being known as the **polar body.** A polar body is formed at the end of meiosis I and the end of meiosis II. Thus, each spermatogonium produces 4 sperms at the end of meiosis, whereas each oogonium produces one egg and 2 polar bodies.

Nondisjunction may also occur in meiosis. When it does, both members of the chromosome pair go to one daughter cell and none to the other. If the daughter cell that receives the entire pair is the egg, and fertilization ensues, a triple dose of the chromosome, or trisomy, will occur. If the daughter cell receiving no members of the pair is fertilized, a monosomic state will result. In the case of autosomes, this is lethal, and a very early abortion will follow. In the case of the sex chromosome, the condition may not be lethal, and examples of both trisomy and monosomy have been

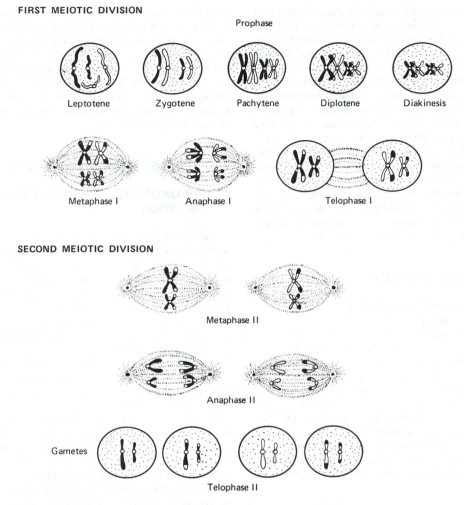

**FIRST MEIOTIC DIVISION**

Prophase

Leptotene Zygotene Pachytene Diplotene Diakinesis

Metaphase I Anaphase I Telophase I

**SECOND MEIOTIC DIVISION**

Metaphase II

Anaphase II

Gametes

Telophase II

**Figure 5–3.** Meiosis in the human. (Reproduced, with permission, from Stenchever MA: Human Cytogenetics: *A Workbook in Reproductive Biology.* The press at Case Western Reserve University, 1972.)

seen in humans. Any chromosome pair may be involved in trisomic or monosomic conditions.

## 3. ABNORMALITIES IN CHROMOSOME MORPHOLOGY & NUMBER

As has been stated, nondisjunction may give rise to conditions of trisomy. In these cases, the morphology of the chromosome is not affected, but the chromosome number is. Be this as it may, breaks and rearrangements in chromosomes may have a variety of results. If 2 chromosomes undergo breaks and exchange chromatin material between them, the outcome is 2 morphologically new chromosomes known as **translocations.** If a break in a chromosome takes place, and the fragment is lost, **deletion** has occurred. If the deletion is such that the cell cannot survive, the condition may be lethal. Nonetheless, several examples

of deleted chromosomes in individuals who have survived have been identified. If a break takes place at either end of a chromosome, and the chromosome heals by having the 2 ends fuse together, a ring chromosome is formed. Examples of these have been seen clinically in all of the chromosomes of the karyotype, and generally they exhibit a variety of phenotypic abnormalities.

At times a chromosome will divide by a horizontal rather than longitudinal split of the centromere. This leaves each daughter cell with a double dose of one of the arms of the chromosome. Thus, one daughter cell receives both long arms and the other both short arms of the chromosome. Such a chromosome is referred to as an **isochromosome,** the individual being essentially trisomic for one arm and monosomic for the other arm of the chromosome. Examples of this abnormality have been seen in humans.

Another anomaly that has been recognized is the

occurrence of 2 breaks within the chromosome and rotation of the center fragment 180 degrees. Thus, the realignment allows for a change in morphology of the chromosome although the original number of genes is preserved. This is called an **inversion**. At meiosis, however, the chromosome has difficulty in undergoing chiasm formation, and abnormal rearrangements of this chromosome, leading to partial duplications and partial losses of chromatin material, do take place. This situation may lead to several bizarre anomalies. If the centromere is involved in the inversion, the condition is called a **pericentric inversion**.

Breaks occasionally occur in 2 chromosomes, and a portion of one broken chromosome is inserted into the body of another, leading to a grossly abnormal chromosome. This is known as an **insertion** and generally leads to gross anomalies at meiosis.

## 4. METHODS OF STUDY

### Sex Chromatin (X-Chromatin) Body (Barr Body)

The X-chromatin body was first seen in the nucleus of the nerve cell of a female cat in 1949 by Barr and Bertram. It has been found to be the constricted, nonfunctioning X chromosome. As a general rule, only one X chromosome functions in a cell at a given time. All other X chromosomes present in a cell may be seen as X-chromatin bodies in a resting nucleus. Thus, if one knows the number of X chromosomes, one can anticipate that the number of Barr bodies will be one less. If one counts the number of Barr bodies, the number of X chromosomes may be determined by adding one.

### Drumsticks on Polymorphonuclear Leukocytes

Small outpouchings of the lobes of nuclei in polymorphonuclear leukocytes of females have been demonstrated to be the X-chromatin body in this particular cell. Hence, leukocyte preparations may be used to detect X-chromatin bodies in much the same way as buccal cells are used.

### Chromosome Count

In the karyotypic analysis of a patient, it is the usual practice to count 20–50 chromosome spreads for chromosome number. The purpose of this is to determine whether mosaicism exists because if a mosaic pattern does exist, there will be at least 2 cell lines of different counts. Photographs are made of representative spreads, and karyotypes are constructed so that the morphology of each chromosome may be studied.

### Banding Techniques

As previously described, it is possible after appropriate pretreatment to stain metaphase spreads with special stains and construct a karyotype that demonstrates the banding patterns of each chromosome. In this way, it is now possible to identify with certainty every chromosome in the karyotype. This is of value in such problems as translocations and trisomic conditions. Another use depends on the fact that most of the long arm of the Y chromosome is heterochromic and stains deeply with fluorescent stains. The Y chromosome may be identified at a glance, therefore, even in the resting nucleus.

## APPLIED GENETICS & TERATOLOGY

### 1. CHROMOSOMES & SPONTANEOUS ABORTION

An entirely new approach to reproductive biology problems became available with the advent of tissue culture and cytologic techniques that made it possible to culture cells from any tissue of the body and produce karyotypes that could be analyzed. In the early 1960s, investigators in a number of laboratories began to study chromosomes of spontaneous abortions and demonstrated that the earlier the spontaneous abortion occurred, the more likely it was to be due to a chromosomal abnormality. It is now known that in spontaneous abortions occurring in the first 8 weeks, the fetuses have about a 50% incidence of chromosome anomalies.

Of abortuses that are abnormal, approximately one-half are trisomic, suggesting an error of meiotic nondisjunction. One-third of abortuses with trisomy have trisomy 16. While this abnormality does not occur in live-born infants, it apparently is a frequent problem in abortuses. The karyotype 45,X occurs in nearly one-fourth of chromosomally abnormal abortuses. This karyotype occurs about 24 times more frequently in abortuses than in live-born infants, a fact that emphasizes its lethal nature. Over 15% of chromosomally abnormal abortuses have polyploidy (triploidy or tetraploidy). These lethal conditions are seen only in abortuses except in extremely rare circumstances and are due to a variety of accidents, including double fertilization and a number of meiotic errors. Finally, a small number of chromosomally abnormal abortuses have unbalanced translocations and other anomalies.

### Habitual Abortion

Couples who experience habitual abortion make up about 0.5% of the population. The condition is defined as 3 or more spontaneous abortions. Several investigators have studied groups of these couples using banding techniques and have found that 10–25% of them will have a chromosome anomaly in either the male or female partner. Those seen are 47,XXX, 47,XYY, and a variety of balanced translocation carriers. Those with sex chromosome abnormalities will frequently demonstrate other nondisjunctional events. Chromosome anomalies are thus a major cause of habitual abortion, and the incorporation of genetic evaluation into such a workup is potentially fruitful.

Lippman-Hand and Bekemans recently reviewed the world literature and studied the incidence of balanced translocation carriers among 177 couples who had 2 or more spontaneous abortions. These studies suggest that in 2–3% of couples experiencing early fetal loss, one partner will have balanced translocations. This percentage is not markedly increased when more than 2 abortions occur. Females had a somewhat higher incidence of balanced translocations than did males.

## 2. CHROMOSOMAL DISORDERS

This section will be devoted to a brief discussion of various autosomal abnormalities. Table 5–5 summarizes some of the autosomal abnormalities that have been diagnosed. These are represented as syndromes,

together with some of the signs typical of these conditions. In general, autosomal monosomy is so lethal that total loss of a chromosome is rarely seen in an individual born alive. Only a few cases of monosomy 21–22 have been reported to date, which attests to the rarity of this disorder. Trisomy may occur with any chromosome. The 3 most common trisomic conditions seen in living individuals are trisomies 13, 18, and 21. Trisomy of various C group chromosomes has been reported sporadically. The most frequently reported is trisomy 8. Generally, trisomy of other chromosomes must be assumed to be lethal, because they occur only in abortuses, not in living individuals. To date, trisomy of every autosome except chromosome 1 has been seen in abortuses.

Translocations can occur between any 2 chromosomes of the karyotype, and a variety of phenotypic expressions may be seen after mediocre arrangements. Three different translocation patterns have been identified in Down's syndrome: 15/21, 21/21, and 21/22.

Deletions may also occur with respect to any chromosome in the karyotype and may be brought about

**Table 5–5.** Autosomal disorders.

| Type | Synonym | Signs |
|------|---------|-------|
| Monosomy<br>  Monosomy 21–22 | | Moderate mental retardation, antimongoloid slant of eyes, flared nostrils, small mouth, low-set ears, spade hands. |
| Trisomy<br>  Trisomy 13 | Trisomy D: The "$D_1$" syndrome | Severe mental retardation, congenital heart disease (77%), polydactyly, cerebral malformations (especially aplasia of olfactory bulbs), eye defects, low-set ears, cleft lip and palate, low birth weight. Characteristic dermatoglyphic pattern. |
| Trisomy 18 | Trisomy E: The "E" syndrome, Edward's syndrome | Severe mental retardation, long narrow skull with prominent occiput, congenital heart disease, flexion deformities of fingers, narrow palpebral fissures, low-set ears, harelip and cleft palate. Characteristic dermatoglyphics, low birth weight. |
| Trisomy 21 | Down's syndrome | Mental retardation, brachycephaly, prominent epicanthal folds. Brushfield spots, poor nasal bridge development, congenital heart disease, hypotonia, hypermobility of joints, characteristic dermatoglyphics. |
| Translocations<br>  15/21 | Down's syndrome | Same as trisomy 21. |
| 21/21 | Down's syndrome | Same as trisomy 21. |
| 21/22 | Down's syndrome | Same as trisomy 21. |
| Deletions<br>  Short arm chromosome 4(4p-) | Wolf's syndrome | Severe growth and mental retardation, midline scalp defects, seizures, deformed iris, beak nose, hypospadias. |
| Short arm chromosome 5(5p-) | Cri du chat syndrome | Microcephaly, catlike cry, hypertelorism with epicanthus, low-set ears, microganthism, abnormal dermatoglyphics, low birth weight. |
| Long arm chromosome 13(13q-) | . . . | Microcephaly, psychomotor retardation, eye and ear defects, hypoplastic or absent thumbs. |
| Short arm chromosome 18(18p-) | . . . | Severe mental retardation, hypertelorism, low-set ears, flexion deformities of hands. |
| Long arm chromosome 18(18q-) | . . . | Severe mental retardation, microcephaly, hypotonia, congenital heart disease; marked dimples at elbows, shoulders, and knees. |
| Long arm chromosome 21(21q-) | . . . | Associated with chronic myelogenous leukemia. |

by a translocation followed by a rearrangement in meiosis, which leads to the loss of chromatin material, or by a simple loss of the chromatin material following a chromosome break. Some of the more commonly seen deletion patterns are listed in Table 5–5.

The most frequent abnormality related to a chromosome abnormality is Down's syndrome. Down's syndrome serves as an interesting model for the discussion of autosomal diseases. The 21 trisomy type is the most common form and is responsible for approximately 95% of Down's syndrome patients. There is a positive correlation between the frequency of Down's syndrome and maternal age. Babies with Down's syndrome are more often born to teenage mothers and, even more frequently, to mothers over 35. Al-

though it is not entirely clear why this is so, it may be that in older women, at least, the egg has been present in prophase of the first meiotic division from the time of fetal life and that, as it ages, there is a greater tendency for nondisjunction to occur, leading to trisomy. A second theory is that coital habits are more erratic in both the very young and the older mothers, and this may lead to an increased incidence in fertilization of older eggs. This theory maintains that these eggs may be more likely to suffer nondisjunction or to accept abnormal sperm. Be this as it may, the incidence of Down's syndrome in the general population is approximately 1 in 600 deliveries and at age 40 approximately 1 in 100 deliveries. At age 45, the incidence is approximately 1 in 40 deliveries (Table 5–6). The

**Table 5–6.** Estimates of rates per thousand of chromosome abnormalities in live births by single-year interval.[1]

| Maternal Age | Down's Syndrome | Edward's Syndrome (Trisomy 18) | Patau's Syndrome (Trisomy 13) | XXY | XYY | Turner's Syndrome Genotype | Other Clinically Significant Abnormality[2] | Total[3] |
|---|---|---|---|---|---|---|---|---|
| < 15 | 1.0[4] | < 0.1[4] | < 0.1–0.1 | 0.4 | 0.5 | < 0.1 | 0.2 | 2.2 |
| 15 | 1.0[4] | <0.1[4] | < 0.1–0.1 | 0.4 | 0.5 | < 0.1 | 0.2 | 2.2 |
| 16 | 0.9[4] | < 0.1[4] | < 0.1–0.1 | 0.4 | 0.5 | < 0.1 | 0.2 | 2.1 |
| 17 | 0.8[4] | <0.1[4] | < 0.1–0.1 | 0.4 | 0.5 | < 0.1 | 0.2 | 2.0 |
| 18 | 0.7[4] | <0.1[4] | < 0.1–0.1 | 0.4 | 0.5 | < 0.1 | 0.2 | 1.9 |
| 19 | 0.6[4] | < 0.1[4] | < 0.1–0.1 | 0.4 | 0.5 | < 0.1 | 0.2 | 1.8 |
| 20 | 0.5–0.7 | < 0.1–0.1 | < 0.1–0.1 | 0.4 | 0.5 | < 0.1 | 0.2 | 1.9 |
| 21 | 0.5–0.7 | < 0.1–0.1 | < 0.1–0.1 | 0.4 | 0.5 | < 0.1 | 0.2 | 1.9 |
| 22 | 0.6–0.8 | < 0.1–0.1 | < 0.1–0.1 | 0.4 | 0.5 | < 0.1 | 0.2 | 2.0 |
| 23 | 0.6–0.8 | < 0.1–0.1 | < 0.1–0.1 | 0.4 | 0.5 | <0.1 | 0.2 | 2.0 |
| 24 | 0.7–0.9 | 0.1–0.1 | < 0.1–0.1 | 0.4 | 0.5 | < 0.1 | 0.2 | 2.1 |
| 25 | 0.7–0.9 | 0.1–0.1 | < 0.1–0.1 | 0.4 | 0.5 | < 0.1 | 0.2 | 2.1 |
| 26 | 0.7–1.0 | 0.1–0.1 | < 0.1–0.1 | 0.4 | 0.5 | < 0.1 | 0.2 | 2.1 |
| 27 | 0.8–1.0 | 0.1–0.2 | < 0.1–0.1 | 0.4 | 0.5 | < 0.1 | 0.2 | 2.2 |
| 28 | 0.8–1.1 | 0.1–0.2 | < 0.1–0.2 | 0.4 | 0.5 | < 0.1 | 0.2 | 2.3 |
| 29 | 0.8–1.2 | 0.1–0.2 | < 0.1–0.2 | 0.5 | 0.5 | < 0.1 | 0.2 | 2.4 |
| 30 | 0.9–1.2 | 0.1–0.2 | < 0.1–0.2 | 0.5 | 0.5 | < 0.1 | 0.2 | 2.6 |
| 31 | 0.9–1.3 | 0.1–0.2 | < 0.1–0.2 | 0.5 | 0.5 | < 0.1 | 0.2 | 2.6 |
| 32 | 1.1–1.5 | 0.1–0.2 | 0.1–0.2 | 0.6 | 0.5 | < 0.1 | 0.2 | 3.1 |
| 33 | 1.4–1.9 | 0.1–0.3 | 0.1–0.2 | 0.7 | 0.5 | < 0.1 | 0.2 | 3.5 |
| 34 | 1.9–2.4 | 0.2–0.4 | 0.1–0.3 | 0.7 | 0.5 | < 0.1 | 0.2 | 4.1 |
| 35 | 2.5–3.9 | 0.3–0.5 | 0.2–0.3 | 0.9 | 0.5 | < 0.1 | 0.3 | 5.6 |
| 36 | 3.2–5.0 | 0.3–0.6 | 0.2–0.4 | 1.0 | 0.5 | < 0.1 | 0.3 | 6.7 |
| 37 | 4.1–6.4 | 0.4–0.7 | 0.2–0.5 | 1.1 | 0.5 | < 0.1 | 0.3 | 8.1 |
| 38 | 5.2–8.1 | 0.5–0.9 | 0.3–0.7 | 1.3 | 0.5 | < 0.1 | 0.3 | 9.5 |
| 39 | 6.6–10.5 | 0.7–1.2 | 0.4–0.8 | 1.5 | 0.5 | < 0.1 | 0.3 | 12.4 |
| 40 | 8.5–13.7 | 0.9–1.6 | 0.5–1.1 | 1.8 | 0.5 | < 0.1 | 0.3 | 15.8 |
| 41 | 10.8–17.9 | 1.1–2.1 | 0.6–1.4 | 2.2 | 0.5 | < 0.1 | 0.3 | 20.5 |
| 42 | 13.8–23.4 | 1.4–2.7 | 0.7–1.8 | 2.7 | 0.5 | < 0.1 | 0.3 | 25.5 |
| 43 | 17.6–30.6 | 1.8–3.5 | 0.9–2.4 | 3.3 | 0.5 | < 0.1 | 0.3 | 32.6 |
| 44 | 22.5–40.0 | 2.3–4.6 | 1.2–3.1 | 4.1 | 0.5 | < 0.1 | 0.3 | 41.8 |
| 45 | 28.7–52.3 | 2.9–6.0 | 1.5–4.1 | 5.1 | 0.5 | < 0.1 | 0.3 | 53.7 |
| 46 | 36.6–68.3 | 3.7–7.9 | 1.9–5.3 | 6.4 | 0.5 | < 0.1 | 0.3 | 68.9 |
| 47 | 46.6–89.3 | 4.7–10.3 | 2.4–6.9 | 8.2 | 0.5 | < 0.1 | 0.3 | 89.1 |
| 48 | 59.5–116.8 | 6.0–13.5 | 3.0–9.0 | 10.6 | 0.5 | < 0.1 | 0.3 | 115.0 |
| 49 | 75.8–152.7 | 7.6–17.6 | 3.8–11.8 | 13.8 | 0.5 | < 0.1 | 0.3 | 149.3 |

[1]Reproduced, with permission, from Hook EB: Rates of chromosome abnormalities at different maternal ages. *Obstet Gynecol* 1981;**58**:282.
[2]XXX is excluded.
[3]Calculation of the total at each age assumes rate for autosomal aneuploidies is at the mid points of the ranges given.
[4]No range may be constructed for those under 20 years by the same methods as for those 20 and over.

other 5% of Down's syndrome patients are the result of translocations, the most common being the 15/21 translocation. Nevertheless, 21/21 and 21/22 examples have been noted. In the case of 15/21, the chance of recurrence in a later pregnancy is theoretically 25%. In practice, a rate of 10% is observed if the mother is the carrier. When the father is the carrier, the odds are less, because there may be a selection not favoring the sperm carrying both the 15/21 translocation and the normal 21 chromosome. In the case of 21/21 translocation, there is no chance for a normal child to be formed, because the carrier will contribute either both 21s or no 21 and, following fertilization, will produce either a monosomic 21 or trisomic 21. With regard to 21/22 translocation, the chance of producing a baby with Down's syndrome is 1 in 2.

In general, other trisomic states occur with greater frequency in older women, and the larger the chromosome involved, the more severe the syndrome. Since trisomy 21 involves the smallest of the chromosomes, the phenotypic problems of Down's syndrome are the least severe, and a moderate life expectancy may be anticipated. Even these individuals will be grossly abnormal, however, because of mental retardation and defects in other organ systems. The average life expectancy of patients with Down's syndrome is much lower than for the general population.

## 3. GENETICS & CANCER

Certain families have a greater tendency to develop cancer. It is also recognized that certain cancers occur more frequently in families with notable cancer histories. Cancer of the endometrium, ovary, colon, and breast are good examples of these. On the other hand, cancer of the cervix is a tumor that does not occur with increased frequency in women with a family history of cancer. A patient with a strong family history of cancer should be checked frequently for cancer.

A number of families with hereditary diseases associated with chromosome breakage have also been noted to have a high incidence of cancer. Examples of these are families with high incidences of Bloom's syndrome, Fanconi's anemia, or ataxia-telangiectasia. In addition, chromosome-breaking agents, eg, x-rays and certain viruses, seem to predispose exposed individuals to higher tumor incidences.

Studies of **oncogenes** provide some insight into the mechanisms by which normal cells are transformed into cancer cells. It was first believed that retroviruses (RNA viruses) entered cells and encoded their message onto the DNA by reverse transcription, thereby introducing an oncogenic tendency into that cell. These viruses are found in both humans and animals; the first described was the Rous sarcoma virus. Careful study has now shown that retroviruses are attracted to DNA already present within the cell (oncogenes). In their natural state, oncogenes, which are present in all cells, are responsible for orderly cell division. They direct the synthesis of a variety of protein products acting on the plasma membrane, in the cytoplasm, and in the nucleus of the cell. They seem to be responsible for the production of small peptides, and a number of other cell functions are attributed to them, including production of protein kinase, guanosine, growth factor, and growth factor receptors and effects on triphosphate and DNA binding. Conversion of normal cell function to cancerous cell activity seems to occur when the oncogene function is changed. Oncogenes may be adversely influenced by point mutation, by translocation from their position on their usual chromosome, by amplification of their function due to some other agent such as a virus, or by a variety of other mechanisms. As we learn more about oncogenes, we will learn more about cell division and the development of cancer and, most likely, about embryonic development as well.

An example of an oncogene that is probably involved in the initial phase of some neoplastic diseases and its progression is the breast-ovarian gene (BRCA1). Seen in families with a strong tendency to these diseases, the gene has several mutant alleles and is located on the short arm of chromosome 17.

## 4. AMNIOCENTESIS

Amniocentesis for prenatal diagnosis of genetic diseases is an extremely useful tool in the following circumstances or classes of patients:

(1) Maternal age 35 years or above.

(2) Previous chromosomally abnormal child.

(3) Three or more spontaneous abortions.

(4) Patient or husband with chromosome anomaly.

(5) Family history of chromosome anomaly.

(6) Possible female carrier of X-linked disease.

(7) Metabolic disease risk (because of previous experience or family history).

(8) Neural tube defect risk (because of previous experience or family history).

Currently, so many metabolic diseases may be diagnosed prenatally by amniocentesis that when the history elicits the possibility of one being present, it is prudent to check with a major center to ascertain the availability of a diagnostic method. In addition, it is possible to diagnose the sex of the infant, using the X-chromatin body or fluorescent method for the Y chromosome or tissue culture and karyotypic analysis of the amniotic cells. It is also possible to diagnose a chromosome abnormality by this latter method. Before attempting amniocentesis, the patient and her husband should be told that no therapy is currently available for most of the affected infants but that, when the risk of a serious disease is present, induced abortion may be a solution. Amniocentesis generally is carried out at the 15th to 17th weeks of gestation but can be offered earlier (12–14 weeks) and is best done transabdominally. The fluid must be sent directly to the laboratory. It should not be frozen, because freezing kills the cells. Table 5–7 lists some of the conditions that now can be diagnosed prenatally by biochemical means.

## 5. CHORIONIC VILLUS SAMPLING

Recent techniques allow sampling of chorionic villi for genetic analysis. Sampling may be carried out either transcervically or transabdominally under direct ultrasound visualization. The risk of spontaneous abortion with this technique is 2–5%, and septic abortion may occur occasionally. The risk of abortion becomes less in more experienced hands. Cells obtained may be analyzed for karyotype and biochemical markers, and DNA probes may be used to detect specific genes. This technique may be performed between 9 and 11 weeks' gestation, providing earlier diagnosis than amniotic fluid studies, but the risk of complications is somewhat greater than with amniocentesis.

## 6. OTHER TOOLS FOR PRENATAL DIAGNOSIS

Other tools useful in prenatal diagnosis of genetic problems are the following:

**(1) X-ray:** X-ray study can be useful in diagnosing structural defects as well as other selected conditions associated with defects discernible by radiologic examination.

**(2) Ultrasonography:** This is useful in diagnosing structural defects including those involving the cardiovascular, genitourinary, gastrointestinal,neuromuscular, and skeletal systems.

**(3) Direct fetal blood sampling:** In the past few years the technique of sampling fetal blood from the umbilical vein transabdominally, by using ultrasound guidance, has become more widely practiced and with minimal risk to mother and fetus. Fetal blood sampling offers access both to fetal cells and serum, making a wide variety of fetal evaluations both genetically and physiologically possible.

**Table 5–7.** Examples of hereditary diseases diagnosable prenatally.

---

Lipidoses (at least 7): Gaucher's, Tay-Sachs, Fabry's, etc.
Mucopolysaccharidoses (at least 6): Hurler's, Hunter's, etc.
Aminoacidurias (at least 11): Cystinosis, homocystinuria, maple syrup urine disease, etc.
Diseases of carbohydrate metabolism (at least 8): Glucose-6-phosphate dehydrogenase deficiency, glycogen storage disease, etc.
Miscellaneous (at least 11): Adrenogenital syndrome, Lesch-Nyhan syndrome, etc.

---

**(4) Linkage studies:** This technique utilizes the fact that 2 genes may be closely aligned on the same chromosome. Therefore, if both genes exist in a given individual, it is possible to detect the presence of one by testing for the other. Thus, indirect evidence for a defect can be ascertained even though no specific test is available for that defect. This technique is still quite experimental and has only limited potential at present.

Kan and Dozy (1978) described one of the early uses of linkage studies when they observed polymorphism of DNA sequences adjacent to the human beta-globin structural gene and its relationship to the sickle cell anemia mutation. Recombinant DNA technology, however, permits the isolation of DNA sequences from several genetic complexes comprised of either an entire genome or a short sequence. Gene-specific probes will identify specific DNA sequences necessary for normal gene function; results of these probes can be used for study of mutation and rearrangement. DNA sequence polymorphism can be used to construct genetic linkage maps of entire genomes; this permits antenatal diagnosis of genetic diseases caused by a single gene mutation, even in the absence of an understanding of the biochemical defect. An excellent review by Davies (1981) discusses this procedure in detail.

**(5) DNA analysis:** By using a variety of techniques, including DNA amplification and cloning, the human genome is now open to detailed investigation. There are currently many clinical applications including prenatal diagnosis, disease identification, and forensic, and disease therapy.

## GENETIC COUNSELING

While genetic counseling should generally be carried out by persons with experience in both genetics and clinical medicine, an individual physician can play a significant role in this aspect of patient care. This role begins with the careful taking of a medical and family history. A family tree can be constructed (Fig 5–4). In doing so, it is important to account for each individual in each generation in both the husband's and wife's families. Abortions should be included, as should persons who have died. When a specific diagnosis is known in the proband and the relatives are dead or otherwise not available, the physician may ask to see photographs, which may show characteristics of the suspected condition. In many cases, when the pedigree is constructed, the inheritance pattern can be determined. If this can be done, the relative risks that future progeny will be affected can be estimated. This pedigree information is also useful in discussing the case with a genetic counselor.

### Single Gene Defects

If one parent is affected and the condition is caused

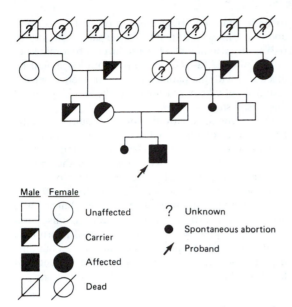

Male Female

☐ ○ Unaffected     **?** Unknown

◨ ◖ Carrier     ● Spontaneous abortion

■ ● Affected     ↗ Proband

⊘ ⊘ Dead

**Figure 5–4.** Pedigree showing unaffected offspring, carrier offspring, and affected offspring in a family with an autosomal recessive trait (sickle cell anemia).

by an autosomal dominant disorder, the chances are 1 in 2 that a child will be affected. If both parents are carriers of an autosomal recessive condition, the chances are 1 in 4 that the child would be affected and 1 in 2 that the child would be a carrier. Carrier status of both parents can be assumed if an affected child has been produced or if a carrier testing program was available and both parents were discovered to be carriers by this means. Tay-Sachs disease and sickle cell disease detection programs are examples of the latter possibility.

When carrier testing is available and the couple is at risk, as with Tay-Sachs disease in Jewish couples and sickle cell disease in blacks, the physician should order these tests before pregnancy is undertaken, or immediately if the patient is already pregnant. When parents are carriers and pregnancy has been diagnosed, prenatal diagnostic testing is indicated if there is a test. If a physician does not know whether or not a text exists or how to obtain one, the local genetic counseling program, local chapter of the National Foundation/March of Dimes, or state health department should be called for consultation. These sources may be able to inform the physician about new research that may have produced a prenatal test. A new test may be likely, because this area of research is very dynamic. If genetic counseling services are readily available, patients with specific problems should be referred to those agencies for consultation. It is impossible for a physician to keep track of all of the current developments in the myriad of conditions caused by single gene defects.

X-linked traits are frequently amenable to prenatal diagnostic testing. When such tests are not available, the couple has the option of testing for the sex of the fetus. If a fetus is noted to be a female, the odds are overwhelming that it will not be affected, although a carrier state may be present. If the fetus is a male, the chances are 1 in 2 that it will be affected. With this information, the couple can decide whether or not to continue the pregnancy in the case of a male fetus. Again, checking with genetic counseling agencies may reveal a prenatal diagnostic test that has only recently been described, or information such as gene linkage studies that may apply in the individual case.

## Neural Tube Disease

Most neural tube diseases, eg, anencephaly, spina bifida, and meningomyelocele, are associated with a multifactorial inheritance pattern. The frequency of their occurrence varies in different populations—eg, as high as 10 per 1000 births in Ireland and as low as 0.8 per 1000 births in the western USA. Ninety percent are index cases, ie, they occur spontaneously without previous occurrence in a family. The remaining 10%, however, are proper subjects for genetic counseling. In general, if a couple has a child with such an anomaly, the chance of producing another affected child is 2–5%. If they have had 2 such children, the risk can be as high as 10%. However, other diagnostic possibilities involving different modes of inheritance should be considered. Siblings also run greater risks of having affected children, with the highest risk being to female offspring of sisters and the lowest to male offspring of brothers. For the couple at high risk—Irish descent, previous affected child, or sibling of an individual with an affected child—a maternal serum alpha-fetoprotein test between 16 and 18 weeks' gestation is indicated. If an elevation of 2.5 or more standard deviations above the mean is noted, amniocentesis for alpha-fetoprotein should be done along with a careful ultrasound study of the fetus for structural anomalies. In questionable cases, fetal x-ray may be helpful also. Evidence for a neural tube defect noted on ultrasound or x-ray and suspected by amniotic fluid alpha-fetoprotein elevation of 3.0 or more standard deviations above the mean makes termination of pregnancy a reasonable course to follow if this is the desire of the couple.

Radioimmunoassay kits for maternal screening are now commercially available. It has not been determined whether the cost is outweighed by the benefits in a low-risk population. However, the American College of Obstetricians and Gynecologists recently recommended that all mothers be informed that maternal serum alpha-fetoprotein (AFP) screening is available. This is best conducted at 16-18 weeks' gestation. A number of states have set up screening programs or will have them soon.

Approximately 5–5.5% of women screened will

have abnormally elevated values ($\geq$ 2.5 times the mean). Most of these will be false-positive results (a repeat test should determine this) or due to inaccurate dating of gestational age, multiple gestation, fetal demise or dying fetus, or a host of other structural abnormalities. In most cases, repeat AFP testing and ultrasound examination will identify the problem. If serum AFP remains elevated and ultrasound examination does not yield a specific diagnosis, amniotic fluid AFP levels should be measured as well as amniotic fluid acetylcholinesterase levels. Further testing and counseling may be necessary before a final diagnosis can be made.

Recently, low maternal AFP levels (<0.5 times the mean) have been implicated in fetuses with chromosome abnormalities. Such cases should be referred for amniocentesis with chromosome analysis.

## Chromosome Abnormalities

In most parts of the USA where prenatal diagnostic screening facilities are available, it is standard policy to offer prenatal diagnostic testing to all women over age 35, because they are at greater risk than the general population for the occurrence of trisomic offspring. The risk increases with age, from roughly 1 in 200 for all chromosomal trisomies at age 35 to 1 in 20 at age 45 (see Table 5–6). It is the physician's responsibility to recommend prenatal diagnostic studies in such cases and to point out the possible consequences if the studies are refused.

The benefits of designating a specific age after which prenatal diagnostic testing should be performed are debatable. Most infants with chromosome abnormalities are born to mothers under age 35 years, simply because more women have children in this younger age group. The incidence of infants born with chromosome abnormalities increases with each year of maternal age, and age 35 is only an arbitrary cutoff point. Costs of testing are high (about $1000 per patient), and facilities would be overtaxed and costs even higher if all women underwent testing. It is probably reasonable to provide information about the procedure to all pregnant women and allow each one to decide whether or not the procedure would be worth it to her.

In the section on prenatal diagnosis, other indications for prenatal diagnostic testing have been mentioned. Individuals who are known carriers of chromosome abnormalities should certainly be offered prenatal diagnosis, since their offspring are at very high risk for an anomaly. The indication for prenatal diagnosis in the case of habitual aborters is less compelling than the others listed. This assumes that roughly half of fetuses aborted in the first trimester will have a chromosome abnormality, and that in about half of these the anomaly will consist of autosomal trisomy. If this is actually the case, one would expect that after 3 spontaneous miscarriages the mother would probably already have produced one trisomic abortion. If she has produced a trisomic abortion, she would then be in the same category of risk as any woman who has produced a trisomic live-born child—ie, 2–5%. These possibilities should be discussed with the patient and may influence her decision about whether or not to go ahead with prenatal diagnostic studies.

Physicians have an obligation to counsel patients known to be at high risk who for that reason are reluctant to become pregnant. The patient should be informed about resources available so that she and her husband can realistically decide whether or not to conceive a child. If she is at high risk for an affected child and a prenatal diagnostic test exists but she will not consider abortion, she may be less anxious to undertake a pregnancy than if the option of abortion is available to her. All possibilities must be set out during the counseling process so that the patient will know what her options are.

## Conclusions

Genetic counseling involves interaction between the physician, the family, and the genetic counselor. It is the physician's responsibility to utilize the services of the genetic consultant in the best interest of the patient. All options should be presented in a nonjudgmental fashion and with no attempt to persuade, based on the best information available at the time. The couple should then be encouraged to decide on a course of action that suits their particular needs. If the decision is appropriate, it should be supported by the physician and the genetic counselor. Very rarely, the patient will make a decision the physician regards as unwise or unrealistic. Such a decision may be based on superstition, religious or mystical beliefs, simple naiveté, or even personality disorder. The physician should make every attempt to clarify the issues for the patient. Rarely, other resources such as family members or spiritual leaders may be consulted in strict confidence. The physician and the genetic counselor must clearly set forth the circumstances of the problem in the record, in case the patient undertakes a course of action that ends in tragedy and perhaps attempts to blame the professional counselors for not preventing it. Fortunately, these problems occur infrequently. In most instances, the physician, genetic counselor, and couple working together can arrive at a solution in keeping with the family's best interests.

# GYNECOLOGIC CORRELATES

## THE CHROMOSOMAL BASIS OF SEX DETERMINATION

### Syngamy

The sex of the fetus is normally determined at fertilization. The cells of normal females contain two X chromosomes; those of normal males contain one X and one Y. During meiotic reduction, half of the male gametes receive a Y chromosome and the other half an X chromosome. In as much as the female has two X chromosomes, all female gametes contain an X chromosome. If a Y-bearing gamete fertilizes an ovum, the fetus is male; conversely, if an X-bearing gamete fertilizes an ovum, the fetus is female.

Arithmetically, the situation described previously should yield a male:female sex ratio of 100—the sex ratio being defined as 100 times the number of males divided by the number of females. However, for many years, the male:female sex ratio of the newborns in the white population has been approximately 105. Apparently the sex ratio at fertilization is even higher than at birth: most data on the sex of abortuses indicate a preponderance of males.

### Abnormalities of Meiosis-Mitosis

The discussion in this section will be limited to anomalies of meiosis and mitosis that result in some abnormality in the sex chromosome complement of the embryo.

Chromosome studies in connection with various clinical conditions suggest that errors in meiosis and mitosis do indeed occur. These errors result in any of the following principal effects: (1) an extra sex chromosome, (2) an absent sex chromosome, (3) 2 cell lines having different sex chromosomes and arising by mosaicism, (4) 2 cell line shaving different sex chromosomes and arising by chimerism, (5) a structurally abnormal sex chromosome, and (6) a sex chromosome complement inconsistent with the phenotype.

By and large, an extra or a missing sex chromosome arises as the result of an error of disjunction in meiosis I or II in either the male or the female. In meiosis I, this means that instead of each of the paired homologous sex chromosomes going to the appropriate daughter cell, both go to one cell, leaving that cell with an extra sex chromosome and the daughter cell with none. Failure of disjunction in meiosis II simply means that the centromere fails to divide normally.

A variation of this process, known as anaphase lag, occurs when one of the chromosomes is delayed in arriving at the daughter cell and thus is lost. Theoretically, chromosomes may be lost by failure of associ-

ation in prophase and by failure of replication, but these possibilities have not been demonstrated.

Persons who have been found to have 2 cell lines apparently have had problems in mitosis in the very early stage of embryogenesis. Thus, if there is nondisjunction or anaphase lag in an early (first, second, or immediately subsequent) cell division in the embryo, mosaicism may be said to exist. In this condition, there are 2 cell lines; one has a normal number of sex chromosomes, and the other is deficient in a sex chromosome or has an extra number of sex chromosomes. A similar situation exists in chimerism, except that there may be a difference in the sex chromosome: one may be an X and one may be a Y. This apparently arises by dispermy, by the fertilization of a double oocyte, or by the fusion, very early in embryogenesis, of 2 separately fertilized oocytes. Each of these conditions has been produced experimentally in animals.

Structural abnormalities of the sex chromosomes—deletion of the long or short arm or the formation of an isochromosome (2 short arms or 2 long arms)—result from injury to the chromosomes during meiosis. How such injuries occur is not known, but the results are noted more commonly in sex chromosomes than in autosomes—perhaps because serious injury to an autosome is much more likely to be lethal than injury to an X chromosome, and surviving injured X chromosomes would therefore be more common.

The situation in which there is a sex chromosome complement with an inappropriate genotype arises in special circumstances of true hermaphroditism and XX males (see later sections).

### The X Chromosome in Humans

At about day 16 of embryonic life, there appears on the undersurface of the nuclear membrane of the somatic cells of human females a structure 1 μm in diameter known as the X-chromatin body. There is genetic as well as cytogenetic evidence that this is one of the X chromosomes (the only chromosome visible by ordinary light microscopy during interphase). In a sense, therefore, all females are hemizygous with respect to the X chromosome. However, there are genetic reasons for believing that the X chromosome is not entirely inactivated during the process of formation of the X-chromatin body. In normal females, inactivation of the X chromosome during interphase and its representation as the X-chromatin body are known as the Lyon phenomenon (for Mary Lyon, a British geneticist). This phenomenon may involve, at random, either the maternal or the paternal X chromosome. Furthermore, once the particular chromosome has been selected early in embryogenesis, it is always the same X chromosome that is inactivated in the progeny of that particular cell. Geneticists have found that the ratio of maternal to paternal X chromosomes inactivated is approximately 1:1.

The germ cells of an ovary are somewhat of an exception to the X inactivation concept in that X inactivation does not characterize the meiotic process. Apparently, meiosis is impossible without 2 genetically active X chromosomes. While random structural damage to one of the X chromosomes seems to cause meiotic arrest, oocyte loss, and therefore failure of ovarian development, an especially critical area necessary for oocyte development has been identified on the long arm of the X. This essential area involves almost all of the long arm and has been specifically located from Xq13 to Xq26. If this area is broken in one of the X chromosomes as in a deletion or translocation, oocyte development does not occur. However, a few exceptions to this rule have been described.

It is a curious biologic phenomenon that if one of the X chromosomes is abnormal, it is always this chromosome that is genetically inactivated and becomes the X-chromatin body, irrespective of whether it is maternal or paternal in origin. While this general rule seems to be an exception to the randomness of X inactivation, this is more apparent than real. Presumably, random inactivation does occur, but the disadvantaged cells—ie, those left with a damaged active X—do not survive. Consequently, the embryo develops only with cells with a normal active X chromosome (X-chromatin body) (Fig 5–5).

If there are more than two X chromosomes, all X chromosomes except one are genetically inactivated and become X-chromatin bodies; thus, in this case, the number of X-chromatin bodies will be equal to the number of X chromosomes minus one. This type of inactivation applies to X chromosomes even when

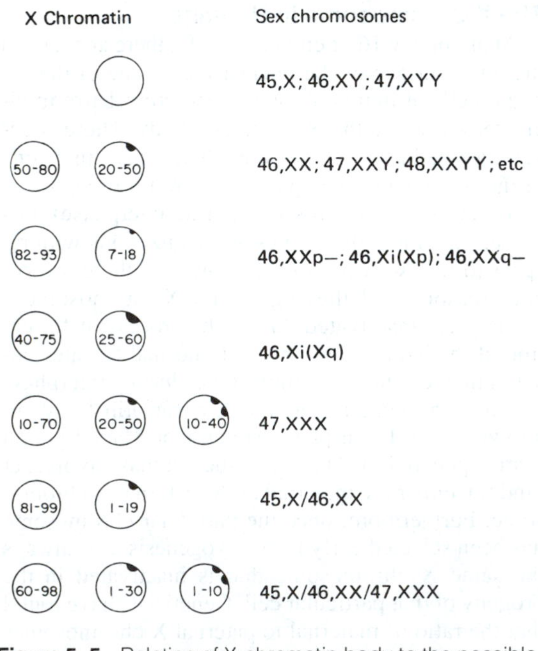

a Y chromosome is present, eg, in Klinefelter's syndrome.

Although the X chromosomes are primarily concerned with the determination of femininity, there is abundant genetic evidence that loci having to do with traits other than sex determination are present on the X chromosome. Thus, in the catalog of genetic disorders given in the 10th edition of *Mendelian Inheritance in Man* (McKusick, 1992), 320 traits are listed as more or less definitely X-linked. Substantial evidence for X linkage has been found for about 160 of these traits; the rest are only suspected of having this relationship. Hemophilia, color blindness, childhood muscular dystrophy (Duchenne's dystrophy), Lesch-Nyhan syndrome, and glucose-6-phosphate dehydrogenase deficiency are among the better known conditions controlled by loci on the X chromosome. These entities probably arise from the expression of a recessive gene due to its hemizygous situation in males.

X-linked dominant traits are infrequent in the human. Vitamin D-resistant rickets is an example.

There is at least one disorder that can be classified somewhere between a structural anomaly of the X chromosome and a single gene mutation. X-linked mental retardation in males is associated with a fragile site at q26, but a special culture medium is required for its demonstration. Furthermore, it has been shown that heterozygote female carriers for this fragile site have low IQ test scores.

## The Y Chromosome in Humans

Just as the X chromosome represents the only chromosome visible by ordinary light microscopy in interphase, the Y chromosome is the only chromosome visible in interphase, after exposure to quinacrine compounds, by the use of fluorescence microscopy. This is a very useful diagnostic method.

In contrast to the X chromosome, few traits have been traced to the Y chromosome except those having to do with testicular formation and those at the very tip of the short arm, homologous with those at the tip of the short arm of the X. Possession of the Y chromosome alone, ie, without an X chromosome, apparently is lethal, because such a case has never been described.

From the study of chromosome phenotype correlations of persons with abnormal sex chromosomes at the gene level, there is considerable evidence that there is a factor that determines testicular differentiation. This is located on the Y short arm and has been referred to as the testis determining factor (TDF). In 1966, Ferguson-Smith proposed that XY chromosomal interchange during male meiosis might result in the transfer of Y material to the paternal X chromosomes. It was thought that such an abnormal interchange could explain the presence of testicular development in patients who could not be demonstrated to have a Y chromosome. In that same publication, Ferguson-Smith proposed that variations in the extent of

| X Chromatin | Sex chromosomes |
|---|---|
| ◯ | 45,X; 46,XY; 47,XYY |
| (50-80) (20-50) | 46,XX; 47,XXY; 48,XXYY; etc |
| (82-93) (7-18) | 46,XXp−; 46,Xi(Xp); 46,XXq− |
| (40-75) (25-60) | 46,Xi(Xq) |
| (10-70) (20-50) (10-40) | 47,XXX |
| (81-99) (1-19) | 45,X/46,XX |
| (60-98) (1-30) (1-10) | 45,X/46,XX/47,XXX |

**Figure 5–5.** Relation of X-chromatin body to the possible sex chromosome components.

inactivation of the Y-bearing X chromosome could result either in subjects with complete testicular determination or with incomplete determination.

The availability of Y chromosome probes has made it possible to attempt to locate more precisely why specific sequences seem to be associated with testicular development. At one time, the gene for the zinc finger protein on Y (ZFY), a 160 kilobase segment, seemed to be a candidate to be the TDF.

Palmer, in 1989, identified individuals with testicular development where ZFY seemed to be eliminated, but where a 35-kilobase region adjacent to the pseudoautosomal boundary called the sex-determining region of the Y chromosome (SRY) was a more promising sequence.

While SRY is a prime suspect to be the TDF, there are a few cases with testicular development that do not seem to have the SRY sequence. It cannot be excluded that SRY is a regulatory sequence and that the real TDF has not yet been identified with certainty.

At one time, it was thought that the HY antigen was the determining factor for testicular development, ie, was the TDF. However, it has been shown that the locus for HY is near but quite distinct from ZFY and SRY. The exact function of HY remains undetermined, but there is circumstantial evidence that deletion of HY in men with testes is associated with azoospermia. This has been referred to as the AZF. It may indeed be identical with HY, because it maps to a very close region.

## ABNORMAL DEVELOPMENT

### 1. OVARIAN AGENESIS-DYSGENESIS

In 1938, Turner described 7 girls 15–23 years of age with sexual infantilism, webbing of the neck, cubitus valgus, and retardation of growth. A survey of the literature indicates that "Turner's syndrome" means different things to different writers. After the later discovery that ovarian streaks are characteristically associated with the clinical entity described by Turner, "ovarian agenesis" became a synonym for Turner's syndrome. After discovery of the absence of the X-chromatin body in such patients, the term ovarian agenesis gave way to "gonadal dysgenesis," "gonadalagenesis," or "gonadal aplasia."

Meanwhile, some patients with the genital characteristics mentioned previously were shown to have a normally positive X-chromatin count. Furthermore, a variety of sex chromosome complements have been found in connection with streak gonads. As if these contradictions were not perplexing enough, it has been noted that streaks are by no means confined to patients with Turner's original tetrad of infantilism, webbing of the neck, cubitus valgus, and retardation of growth but may be present in girls with sexual infantilism only. Since Turner's original description, a

host of additional somatic anomalies (varying in frequency) have been associated with his original clinical picture; these include shield chest, overweight, high palate, micrognathia, epicanthal folds, low-setears, hypoplasia of nails, osteoporosis, pigmented moles, hypertension, lymphedema, cutix laxa, keloids, coarctation of the aorta, mental retardation, intestinal telangiectasia, and deafness.

For our purpose, the eponym Turner's syndrome will be used to indicate sexual infantilism with ovarian streaks, short stature, and 2 or more of the somatic anomalies mentioned earlier. In this context, such terms as ovarian agenesis, gonadalagenesis, and gonadal dysgenesis lose their clinical significance and become merely descriptions of the gonadal development of the person. At least 21 sex chromosome complements have been associated with streak gonads (Fig 5–6), but only about 9 sex chromosome complements have been associated with Turner's syndrome. However, approximately two-thirds of patients with Turner's syndrome have a 45,X chromosome complement, whereas only one-fourth of patients without Turner's syndrome but with streak ovaries have a 45,X chromosome complement.

Karyotype/phenotype correlations in the syndromes associated with ovarian agenesis are not completely satisfactory. Nonetheless, if gonadal development is considered as one problem and if the somatic difficulties associated with these syndromes are considered as a separate problem, one can make certain correlations.

With respect to failure of gonadal development, it

45,X
46,XX
46,XY
46,XXp−
46,XXq−
46,Xi(Xp)
46,Xi(Xq)
46,XXq−?
45,X/46,XX
45,X/46,XY
45,X/46,Xi(Xq)
45,X/46,XXp−
45,X/46,XXq−
45,X/46,XXq−?
45,X/46,XX       ⎫
45,X/46,Xi(Xq)  ⎭
45,X/46,XX/47,XXX ⎫
45,X/47,XXX         ⎭
45,X/46,XX/47,XXX       ⎫
45,X/46,Xi(Xq)/47,XXX ⎭
45,X/46,XXr(X)
45,X/46,XX/46,XXr(X)
45,X/46,XXr(X)/47,XXr(X)r(X)
45,X/46,XX/47,XXX ⎫
45,X/46,XXq−        ⎭

**Figure 5–6.** The 21 sex chromosome complements that have been found in patients with streak gonads.

is important to recall that diploid germ cells require 2 normal active X chromosomes. This is in contrast to the somatic cells, where only one sex chromosome is thought to be genetically active, at least after day 16 of embryonic life in the human, when the X-chromatin body first appears in the somatic cells. It is also important to recall that in 45,X persons, no oocytes persist, and streak gonads are the rule. From these facts, it may be inferred that failure of gonadal development is not the result of a specific sex chromosome defect but rather of the absence of two X chromosomes with the necessary critical zones.

Karyotype/phenotype correlations with respect to the somatic abnormalities are even sketchier than the correlations with regard to gonadal development. However, there is good evidence to show that monosomy for the short arm of the X chromosome is related to somatic difficulties, although some patients with long-arm deletions have somatic abnormalities.

### History of Gonadal Agenesis

The histologic findings in these abnormal ovaries in patients with gonadal streaks are essentially the same regardless of the patient's cytogenetic background (Fig 5–7).

Fibrous tissue is the major component of the streak. It is indistinguishable microscopically from that of the normal ovarian stroma. The so-called germinal epithelium, on the surface of the structure, is a layer of low cuboid cells; this layer appears to be completely inactive.

Tubules of the ovarian rete are invariably found in sections taken from about the midportion of the streak.

In all patients who have reached the age of normal puberty, hilar cells are also demonstrated. The number of hilar cells varies among patients. In those with some enlargement of the clitoris, hilar cells are present in large numbers. It may be that these developments are causally related. Nevertheless, hilar cells are also found in many normal ovaries. The origin of hilar cells is not precisely known, but they are associated with development of the medullary portion of the gonad. Their presence lends further support to the concept that in ovarian agenesis the gonad develops along normal lines until just before the expected appearance of early oocytes. In all cases in which sections of the broad ligament have been available for study, it has been possible to identify the mesonephric duct and tubules—broad ligament structures found in normal females.

### Clinical Findings

#### A. Symptoms and Signs:

**1. In newborn infants–**The newborn with streak ovaries often shows edema of the hands and feet. Histologically, this edema is associated with large dilated vascular spaces. With such findings, it is obviously desirable to obtain a karyotype. However, some children with streak ovaries—particularly those who have few or no somatic abnormalities—cannot be recognized at birth.

**2. In adolescents–**The arresting and characteristic clinical finding in many of these patients is their short stature. Typical patients seldom attain a height of 1.5 m (5 ft) (Fig 5–8). In addition, sexual infantilism is a striking finding. As was mentioned earlier, a variety of somatic abnormalities may be present; by definition, if 2 or more of these are noted, the patient may be considered to have Turner's syndrome. Most

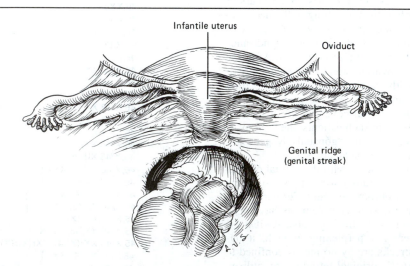

**Figure 5–7.** Gonadal streaks in a patient with the phenotype of Turner's syndrome. (Redrawn and reproduced, with permission, from Jones HW Jr, Scott WW: *Hermaphroditism, Genital Anomalies and Related Endocrine Disorders,* 2nd ed. Williams & Wilkins, 1971.)

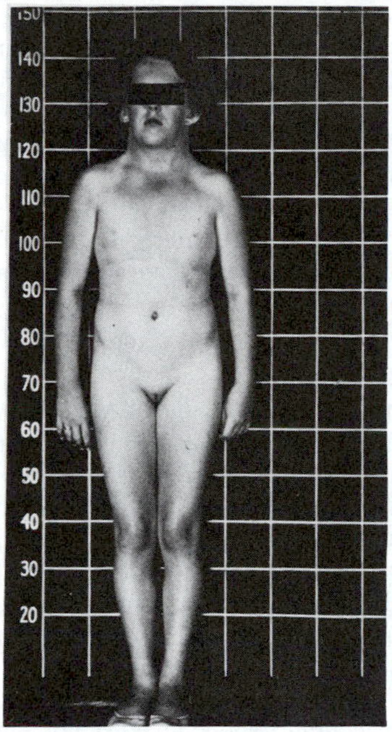

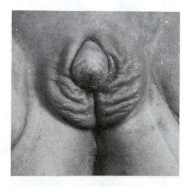

**Figure 5–8.** Patient with Turner's syndrome. (Reproduced, with permission, from Jones HW Jr, Scott WW: Hermaphroditism, *Genital Anomalies and Related Endocrine Disorders,* 2nd ed. Williams & Wilkins, 1971.)

of these patients have only one normal X chromosome, and two-thirds of them have no other sex chromosome. Patients of normal height without somatic abnormalities may also have gonadal streaks. Under these circumstances, there is likely to be a cell line with 2 normal sex chromosomes but often a second line with a single X. The internal findings are exactly the same as in patients with classic Turner's syndrome, however.

**B. Laboratory Findings:** An important finding in patients of any age–but especially after that of expected puberty, ie, about 12 years—is elevation of total gonadotropin production. From a practical point of view, ovarian failure in patients over age 15 cannot be considered as a diagnostic possibility unless the serum FSH is more than 50 mIU/mL and LH is more than 90 mIU/mL.

Nongonadal endocrine functions are normal. Urinary excretion of estrogens is low, and the maturation index and other vaginal smear indices are shifted well to the left.

### Treatment

Substitution therapy with estrogen is necessary for development of secondary characteristics.

Therapy with growth hormone will increase height. There remain some uncertainties over whether ultimate height will be greater than it otherwise would be. Current evidence suggests that it will be.

The incidence of malignant degeneration is increased in the gonadal streaks of patients with a Y chromosome, as compared with normal males. Surgical removal of streaks from all patients with a Y chromosome is recommended.

## 2. TRUE HERMAPHRODITISM

By classic definition, true hermaphroditism exists when both ovarian and testicular tissue can be demonstrated in one patient. In humans, the Y chromosome carries genetic material that is normally responsible for testicular development; this material is active even when multiple X chromosomes are present. Thus, in Klinefelter's syndrome, a testis develops with up to four Xs and only one Y. Conversely (with rare exceptions), a testis has not been observed to develop in the absence of the Y chromosome. The exceptions are found in true hermaphrodites and XX males, in whom testicular tissue has developed in association with an XX sex chromosome complement.

### Clinical Findings

**A. Symptoms and Signs:** No exclusive features clinically distinguish true hermaphroditism from other forms of intersexuality. Hence, the diagnosis must be entertained in an infant with any form of intersexuality, except only those with a continuing virilizing influence, eg, congenital adrenal hyperplasia. Firm diagnosis is possible after the onset of puberty, when certain clinical features become evident, but the diagnosis can and should be made in infancy.

In the past, most true hermaphrodites have been reared as males because they have rather masculine-appearing external genitalia (Fig 5–9). Nevertheless, with early diagnosis, most should be reared as females.

Almost all true hermaphrodites develop female-

**Figure 5–9.** External genitalia of a patient with true hermaphroditism. (Reproduced, with permission, from Jones HW Jr, Scott WW: *Hermaphroditism, Genital Anomalies and Related Endocrine Disorders,* 2nd ed. Williams & Wilkins, 1971.)

type breasts. This helps to distinguish male hermaphroditism from true hermaphroditism, because few male hermaphrodites other than those with familial feminizing hermaphroditism develop large breasts.

Many true hermaphrodites menstruate. The presence or absence of menstruation is partially determined by the development of the uterus; many true hermaphrodites have rudimentary or no development of the müllerian ducts (Fig 5–10).

A few patients who had a uterus and menstruated after removal of testicular tissue have become pregnant and delivered normal children.

**B. Sex Chromosome Complements:** Most true hermaphrodites have X-chromatin bodies and karyotypes that are indistinguishable from those of normal females. In contrast to these, a few patients who cannot be distinguished clinically from other true hermaphrodites have been reported to have a variety of other karyotypes—eg, several chimeric persons with karyotypes of 46,XX/46,XY have been identified.

In true hermaphrodites, the testis is competent in its müllerian-suppressive functions, but an ovotestis may behave as an ovary insofar as its müllerian-suppressive function is concerned. The true hermaphroditic testis or ovotestis is as competent to masculinize the external genitalia as is the testis of a patient with the virilizing type of male hermaphroditism. This is unrelated to karyotype.

Deletion mapping by DNA hybridization has shown that most (but not all) XX true hermaphrodites have Y-specific sequences. Abnormal crossing-over of a portion of the Y chromosome to the X, in meiosis, may explain some cases. This latter is further supported by the finding of a positive H-Y antigen assay in some patients with 46,XX true hermaphroditism.

In general, the clinical picture of true hermaphroditism is not compatible with the clinical picture in other kinds of gross chromosomal anomalies. For example, very few true hermaphrodites have associated somatic anomalies, and mental retardation almost never occurs.

### Treatment

The principles of treatment of true hermaphroditism do not differ from those of the treatment of hermaphroditism in general. Therapy can be summarized by stating that surgical removal of contradictory organs is indicated, and the external genitalia should be reconstructed in keeping with the sex of rearing. The special problem in this group is how to establish with certainty the character of the gonad. This is particularly difficult in the presence of an ovotestis, because its recognition by gross characteristics is notoriously inaccurate, and one must not remove too much of the gonad for study. In some instances, the gonadal tissue of one sex is completely embedded within a gonadal structure primarily of the opposite sex.

### 3. KLINEFELTER'S SYNDROME

This condition, first described in 1942 by Klinefelter, Reifenstein, and Albright, occurs only in apparent males. As originally described, it is characterized by small testes, azoospermia, gynecomastia, relatively normal external genitalia, and otherwise average somatic development. High levels of gonadotropin in urine or serum are characteristic.

### Clinical Findings

**A. Symptoms and Signs:** By definition, this syndrome applies only to persons reared as males. The disease is not recognizable before puberty except by routine screening of newborn infants (see below). Most patients come under observation at 16–40 years of age.

Somatic development during infancy and childhood may be normal. Growth and muscular development may also be within normal limits. Most patients have a normal general appearance and no complaints referable to this abnormality, which is often discovered in the course of a routine physical examination or an infertility study.

In the original publication by Klinefelter and others, gynecomastia was considered an essential part of the syndrome. Since then, however, cases without gynecomastia have been reported.

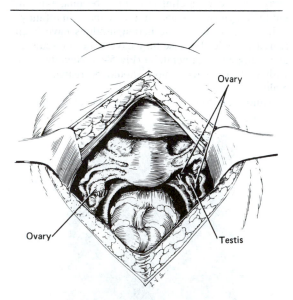

**Figure 5–10.** Internal genitalia of a patient with true hermaphroditism. (Reproduced, with permission, from Jones HW Jr, Scott WW: *Hermaphroditism, Genital Anomalies and Related Endocrine Disorders,* 2nd ed. Williams & Wilkins, 1971.)

Labels on figure: Ovary, Ovary, Testis

The external genitalia are perfectly formed and in most patients are quite well developed. Erection and intercourse usually are satisfactory.

There is no history of delayed descent of the testes in typical cases, and the testes are in the scrotum. Neither is there any history of testicular trauma or disease. Although a history of mumps orchitis is occasionally elicited, this disease has not been correlated with the syndrome. The testes, however, in contrast to the rest of the genitalia, are often very small (about $1.5 \times 1.5$ cm).

Psychologic symptoms are often present. Most studies of this syndrome have been done in psychiatric institutions. The seriousness of the psychological disturbance seems to be partly related to the number of extra X chromosomes—eg, it is estimated that about one-fourth of XXY patients have some degree of mental retardation.

**B. Laboratory Findings:** One of the extremely important clinical features of Klinefelter's syndrome is the excessive amount of pituitary gonadotropin found in either urine or serum assay.

The urinary excretion of neutral 17-ketosteroids varies from relatively normal to definitely subnormal levels. There is a rough correlation between the degree of hypoleydigism as judged clinically and a low 17-ketosteroid excretion rate.

**C. Histologic and Cytogenetic Findings:** Klinefelter's syndrome may be regarded as a form of primary testicular failure.

Several authors have classified a variety of forms of testicular atrophy as subtypes of Klinefelter's syndrome. Be this as it may, Klinefelter believed that only those patients who have a chromosomal abnormality could be said to have this syndrome. Microscopic examination of the adult testis shows that the seminiferous tubules lack epithelium and are shrunken and hyalinized. They contain large amounts of elastic fibers. Leydig cells are present in large numbers.

Males with positive X-chromatin bodies are likely to have Klinefelter's syndrome. The nuclear sex anomaly reflects a basic genetic abnormality in sex chromosome constitution. All cases studied have had at least two X chromosomes and one Y chromosome. The commonest abnormality in the sex chromosome constitution is XXY, but the literature also records XXXY, XXYY, XXXXY, and XXXYY and mosaics of XX/XXY, XY/XXY,XY/XXXY, and XXXY/XXXXY. In all examples except the XX/XXY mosaic, a Y chromosome is present in all cells. From these patterns, it is obvious that the Y chromosome has a very strong testis-forming impulse, which can operate in spite of the presence of as many as four X chromosomes.

Thus, patients with Klinefelter's syndrome will have not only a positive X-chromatin body but also a positive Y-chromatin body.

The abnormal sex chromosome constitution causes differentiation of an abnormal testis, leading to testicular failure in adulthood. At birth or before puberty, such testes show a marked deficiency or absence of germinal cells.

By means of nursery screening, the frequency of males with positive X-chromatin bodies has been estimated to be 2.65 per 1000 live male births.

### Treatment

There is no treatment for the 2 principal complaints of these patients: infertility and gynecomastia. No pituitary preparation has been effective in the regeneration of the hyalinized tubular epithelium or the stimulation of gametogenesis. Furthermore, no hormone regimen is effective in treating the breast hypertrophy. When the breasts are a formidable psychologic problem, surgical removal may be a satisfactory procedure. In patients who have clinical symptoms of hypoleydigism, substitution therapy with testosterone is an important physiologic and psychologic aid. Donor sperm may be offered for the treatment of the infertility.

### 4. DOUBLE-X MALES

A few cases have been reported of adult males with a slightly hypoplastic penis and very small testes but no other indication of abnormal sexual development. These males are sterile. Unlike those with Klinefelter's syndrome, they do not have abnormal breast development. They are clinically very similar to patients with Del Castillo's syndrome (testicular dysgenesis). Nevertheless, the XX males have a positive sex chromatin and a normal female karyotype. These may be extreme examples of the sex reversal that is usually partial in true hermaphroditism.

### 5. MULTIPLE-X SYNDROMES

The finding of more than one X-chromatin body in a cell indicates the presence of more than two X chromosomes in that particular cell. In many patients, such a finding is associated with mosaicism, and the clinical picture is controlled by this fact—eg, if one of the strains of the mosaicism is 45,X, gonadal agenesis is likely to occur. There also are persons who do not seem to have mosaicism but do have an abnormal number of X chromosomes in all cells. In such persons, the most common complement is XXX (triplo-X syndrome), but XXXX (tetra-X syndrome), and XXXXX (penta-X syndrome) have been reported.

An additional X chromosome does not seem to have a consistent effect on sexual differentiation. The body proportions of these persons are normal, and the external genitalia are normally female. A number of such persons have been examined at laparotomy, and no consistent abnormality of the ovary has been found. In a few cases, the number of follicles appeared to be reduced, and in at least one case the ovaries were very small and the ovarian stroma poorly differentiated. About 20% of postpubertal patients with the triplo-X syndrome report various degrees of amenorrhea or some irregularity in menstruation. For the most part, however, these patients have a normal menstrual history and are of proved fertility.

Almost all patients known to have multiple-X syndromes have some degree of mental retardation. A few have mongoloid features. (The mothers of these patients tended to be older than the mothers of normal children—as is true also in Down's syndrome.) Perhaps these findings are in part circumstantial, since most of these patients have been discovered during surveys in mental institutions. The important clinical point is that mentally retarded infants should have chromosomal study.

Uniformly, the offspring of triplo-X mothers have been normal. This is surprising, because theoretically in such cases meiosis should produce equal numbers of ova containing one or two X chromosomes, and fertilization of the abnormal XX ova should give rise to XXX and XXY individuals. Nevertheless, the triplo-X condition seems selective for normal ova and zygotes.

The diagnosis of this syndrome is made by identifying a high percentage of cells in the buccal smear with double X-chromatin bodies and by finding 47 chromosomes with a karyotype showing an extra X chromosome in all cells cultured from the peripheral blood. It should be noted that in the examination of the buccal smear, some cells have a single X-chromatin body. Hence, on the basis of the chromatin examination, one might suspect XX/XXX mosaicism. Actually, in triplo-X patients, only a single type of cell can be demonstrated in cultures of cells from the peripheral blood. The absence of the second X-chromatin body in some of the somatic cells may result from the time of examination of the cell (during interphase) and from the spatial orientation, which could have prevented the two X-chromatin bodies (adjacent to the nuclear membrane) from being seen. In this syndrome, the number of cells containing either one or 2 X-chromatin bodies is very high—at least 60–80%, as compared with an upper limit of about 40% in normal females.

## 6. FEMALE HERMAPHRODITISM DUE TO CONGENITAL ADRENAL HYPERPLASIA

### Essentials of Diagnosis

- Female pseudohermaphroditism, ambiguous genitalia with clitoral hypertrophy, and, occasionally, persistent urogenital sinus.

- Early appearance of sexual hair; hirsutism, dwarfism.
- Urinary 17-ketosteroids elevated; pregnanetriol may be increased.
- Elevated serum 17-hydroxyprogesterone.
- Occasionally associated with water and electrolyte imbalance—particularly in the neonatal period.

### General Considerations

Female hermaphroditism due to congenital adrenal hyperplasia is a clearly delineated clinical syndrome. The syndrome has been better understood since the discovery that cortisone may successfully arrest virilization. The problem is usually due to a deficiency of a gene required for 21 hydroxylation in the biosynthesis of cortisol.

If the diagnosis is not made in infancy, an unfortunate series of events ensues. Because the adrenals secrete an abnormally large amount of virilizing steroid even during embryonic life, these infants are born with abnormal genitalia (Fig 5–11). In extreme cases, there is fusion of the scrotolabial folds and, in rare instances, even the formation of a penile urethra. The clitoris is greatly enlarged, so that it may be mistaken for a penis (Fig 5–12). No gonads are palpable within the fused scrotolabial folds, and their absence has sometimes given rise to the mistaken impression of male cryptorchidism. Usually, there is a single urinary meatus at the base of the phallus and the vagina

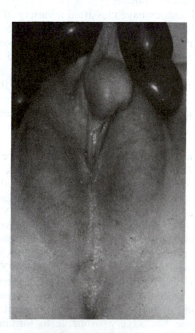

**Figure 5–11.** External genitalia of a female patient with congenital virilizing adrenal hyperplasia. Compare with Fig 5–12. (Reproduced, with permission, from Jones HW Jr, Scott WW: *Hermaphroditism, Genital Anomalies and Related Endocrine Disorders,* 2nd ed. Williams & Wilkins, 1971.)

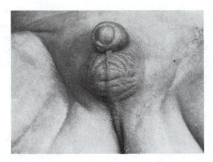

**Figure 5–12.** External genitalia of a female patient with congenital virilizing adrenal hyperplasia. This is a more severe deformity than that shown in Fig 5–11.

enters the persistent urogenital sinus as noted in Figure 5–13.

During infancy, provided there are no serious electrolyte disturbances, these children grow more rapidly than normal. For a time, they greatly exceed the average in both height and weight. Unfortunately, epiphyseal closure occurs by about age 10, with the result that as adults these people are much shorter than normal (Fig 5–14).

The process of virilization begins at an early age. Pubic hair may appear as early as age 2 years but usually somewhat later. This is followed by growth of axillary hair and finally by the appearance of body hair and a beard, which may be so thick as to require daily shaving. Acne may develop early. Puberty never ensues. There is no breast development. Menstruation does not occur. During the entire process, serum adrenal androgens and 17-hydroxyprogesterone are abnormally high.

Although our principal concern here is with this abnormality in females, it must be mentioned that adrenal hyperplasia of the adrenogenital type may also occur in males, in whom it is called macrogenitosomia precox. Sexual development progresses rapidly, and the sex organs attain adult size at an early age. Just as in the female, sexual hair and acne develop unusually early, and the voice becomes deep. The testes are usually in the scrotum; however, in early childhood they remain small and immature, although the genitalia are of adult dimensions. In adulthood, the testes usually enlarge and spermatogenesis occurs, allowing impregnation rates similar to those of a control population. Somatic development in the male corresponds to that of the female; as a child, the male exceeds the average in height and strength, but (if untreated) as an adult he is stocky, muscular, and well below average height.

Both the male and the female with this disorder—but especially the male—may have the complicating problem of electrolyte imbalance. In infancy, it is manifested by vomiting, progressive weight loss, and dehydration and may be fatal unless recognized promptly. The characteristic findings are an exceed-

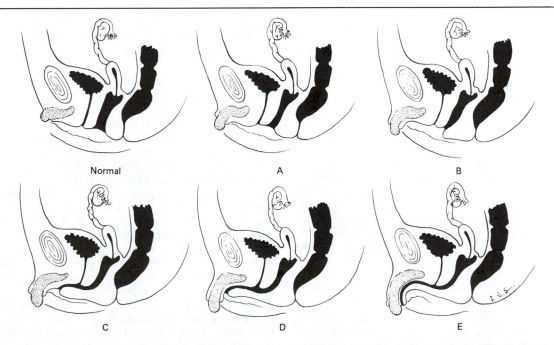

**Figure 5–13.** Sagittal view of genital deformities of increasing severity (A–E) in congenital virilizing adrenal hyperplasia. (Redrawn and reproduced, with permission, from Verkauf BS, Jones HW Jr: Masculinization of the female genitalia in congenital adrenal hyperplasia. South Med J 1970;63:634.)

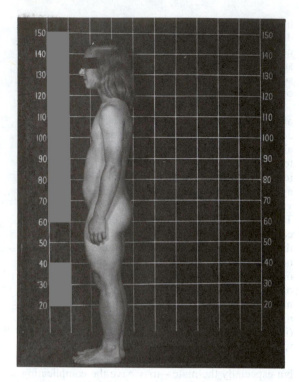

**Figure 5–14.** An untreated adult with virilizing adrenal hyperplasia. Note the short stature and the relative shortness of the limbs. (Reproduced, with permission, from Jones HW Jr, Scott WW: *Hermaphroditism, Genital Anomalies and Related Endocrine Disorders,* 2nd ed. Williams & Wilkins, 1971.)

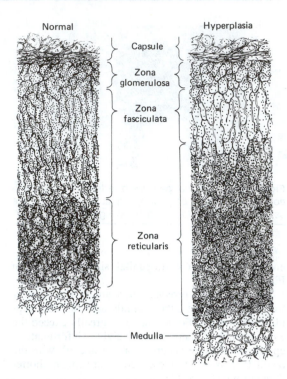

**Figure 5–15.** Normal adrenal architecture and adrenal histology in congenital virilizing adrenal hyperplasia. Note the great relative increase in the zona reticularis.

ingly low serum sodium level and low $CO_2$ combining power level and a high potassium level. The condition is sometimes misdiagnosed as congenital pyloric stenosis.

A few of these patients have a deficiency in 11-hydroxylation which is associated with hypertension in addition to virilization.

### Adrenal Histology

The adrenal changes center on a reticular hyperplasia, which becomes more marked as the patient grows older. In some instances, the glomerulosa may participate in the hyperplasia, but the fasiculata is greatly diminished in amount or entirely absent. Lipid studies show absence of fascicular and glomerular lipid but an abnormally strong lipid reaction in the reticularis (Fig 5–15).

### Ovarian Histology

The ovarian changes may be summarized by stating that in infants, children, and teenagers, there is normal follicular development to the antrum stage but no evidence of ovulation. With increasing age, less and less follicular activity occurs, and primordial follicles disappear. This disappearance must not be complete, however, because cortisone therapy, even in adults, usually results in ovulatory menstruation after 4–6 months of treatment.

### Developmental Anomalies of the Genital Tubercle & Urogenital Sinus Derivatives

The phallus is composed of 2 lateral corpora cavernosa, but the corpus spongiosum is normally absent. The external urinary meatus is most often located at the base of the phallus (Fig 5–11). An occasional case may be seen in which the urethra does extend to the end of the clitoris (Fig 5–12). The glans penis and the prepuce are present and indistinguishable from these structures in the male. The scrotolabial folds are characteristically fused in the midline, giving a scrotumlike appearance with a median perineal raphe; however, they seldom enlarge to normal scrotal size. No gonads are palpable within the scrotolabial folds. When the anomaly is not severe (eg, in patients with postnatal virilization), fusion of the scrotolabial folds is not complete, and by gentle retraction it is often possible to locate not only the normally located external urinary meatus but also the orifice of the vagina.

An occasional patient has no communication between the urogenital sinus and the vagina. In no case does the vagina communicate with that portion of the urogenital sinus that gives rise to the female urethra or the prostatic urethra. Instead, the vaginal communication is via caudal urogenital sinus derivatives; thus, fortunately, the sphincter mechanism is not involved, and the anomalous communication is with that portion of the sinus that develops as the vaginal vestibule in the female and the membranous urethra in the male. From the gynecologist's point of view, it is much more meaningful to say that the vagina and (female) urethra enter a persistent urogenital sinus than to say that the vagina enters the (membranous [male]) urethra. This conclusion casts some doubt on the embryologic significance of the prostatic utricle, which is commonly said to represent the homologue of the vagina in the normal male.

## Hormone Changes

Important and specific endocrine changes occur in congenital adrenal hyperplasia of the adrenogenital type. The ultimate diagnosis depends on demonstration of these abnormalities.

**A. Urinary Estrogens:** The progressive virilization of female hermaphrodites caused by adrenal hyperplasia would suggest that estrogen secretion in these patients is low, and this hypothesis is further supported by the atrophic condition of both the ovarian follicular apparatus and the estrogen target organs. Actually, the determination of urinary estrogens, both fluorometrically and biologically, indicates that they are elevated.

**B. Serum Steroids:** The development of satisfactory radioimmunoassay techniques for measuring steroids in blood serum has resulted in an increased tendency to measure serum steroids rather than urinary metabolites in diagnosing the condition and monitoring therapy. Serum steroid profiles of many patients with this disorder show that numerous defects in the biosynthesis of cortisol may occur. The most common defect is at the 21-hydroxylase step. Less frequent defects are at the 11-hydroxylase step and the 3β-ol-dehydrogenase step. Rarely, the defect is at the 17-hydroxylase step. In the most common form of the disorder—21-hydroxylase deficiency—the serum 17-hydroxyprogesterone level and, to a lesser extent, the serum progesterone level are elevated. This is easily understandable when it is recalled that 17-hydroxyprogesterone is the substrate for the 21-hydroxylation step (Fig 5–16). Likewise, in the other enzyme defects, the serum steroid substrates are greatly elevated.

## Pathogenesis of Virilizing Adrenal Hyperplasia

The basic defects in congenital virilizing adrenal hyperplasia are one or more enzyme deficiencies in the biosynthesis of cortisol (Fig 5–16). With the reduced production of cortisol, normal feedback to the hypothalamus fails, with the result that increased amounts of ACTH are produced. This excess production of ACTH stimulates the deficient adrenal gland to produce relatively normal amounts of cortisol—but also stimulates production of abnormally large amounts of estrogen and androgens by the zona reticularis. In this overproduction, a biologic preponderance of androgens causes virilization. These abnormal sex steroids suppress the gonadotropins, so that untreated patients never reach puberty and do not menstruate.

The treatment of this disorder, therefore, consists in part of the administration of sufficient exogenous cortisol to suppress ACTH production to normal levels. This in turn should reduce the overstimulation of the adrenal, so that the adrenal will cease to produce abnormally large amounts of estrogen and androgen. The gonadotropins generally return to normal levels,

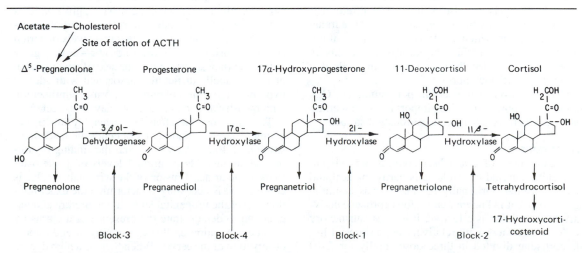

**Figure 5–16.** Enzymatic steps in cortisol synthesis. Localization of defects in congenital adrenal hyperplasia.

with consequent feminization of the patient and achievement of menstruation.

The pathogenesis of the salt-losing type of adrenal hyperplasia involves a deficiency in aldosterone production.

## Diagnosis

Hermaphroditism due to congenital adrenal hyperplasia must be suspected in any infant born with ambiguous or abnormal external genitalia. It is exceedingly important that the diagnosis be made at a very early age if undesirable disturbances of metabolism are to be prevented.

All patients with ambiguous external genitalia should have an appraisal of their chromosomal characteristics. In all instances of female pseudohermaphroditism due to congenital hyperplasia, the chromosomal composition is that of a normal female. A pelvic ultrasound in the newborn to determine the presence of a uterus is very helpful and, if positive, strongly suggests a female infant.

The critical determinations are those of the urinary 17-ketosteroid and serum 17-hydroxyprogesterone levels. If these are elevated, the diagnosis must be either congenital adrenal hyperplasia or tumor. In the newborn, the latter is very rare, but in older children and adults with elevated 17-ketosteroids the possibility of tumor must be considered. One of the most satisfactory methods of making this different diagnosis is to attempt to suppress the excess androgens by the administration of dexamethasone. In an adult or an older child, a suitable test dose of dexamethasone is 1.25 mg/45 kg (100 lb) body weight, given orally for 7 consecutive days. In congenital adrenal hyperplasia, there should be suppression of the urinary 17-ketosteroids on the seventh day of the test to less than 1 mg/24 h; in the presence of tumor, either there will be no effect or the 17-ketosteroid levels will rise.

Determination of urinary dehydroepiandrosterone (DHEA) or serum dehydroepiandrosterone sulfate (DHEA=S) levels can also be helpful in differentiating congenital adrenal hyperplasia from an adrenal tumor. Levels in patients with congenital adrenal hyperplasia may be double normal levels, whereas an adrenal tumor is usually associated with levels that are much higher than normal.

Determination of the serum, potassium, and $CO_2$ combining power is also important to ascertain whether electrolyte balance is seriously disturbed.

## Treatment

The treatment of female hermaphroditism owing to congenital adrenal hyperplasia is partly medical and partly surgical. Originally, cortisone was administered; today, it is known that various cortisone derivatives are at least as effective. It is most satisfactory to begin treatment with relatively large doses of hydrocortisone divided in three doses orally for 7–10 days to obtain rapid suppression of adrenal activity.

In young infants, the initial dose is about 25 mg/d; in older patients, 100 mg/d. After the output of 17-ketosteroids has decreased to a lower level, the dose should be reduced to the minimum amount required to maintain adequate suppression. This requires repeated measurements of plasma 17$\alpha$-hydroxyprogesterone in order to individualize the dose.

It has been found that even with suppression of the urinary 17-ketosteroids to normal levels, the more sensitive serum 17-hydroxyprogesterone may still be elevated. It seems difficult and perhaps undesirable to suppress the serum 17-hydroxyprogesterone values to normal, because to do so may require doses of hydrocortisone which tend to cause cushingoid symptoms.

In the treatment of newborns with congenital adrenal hyperplasia who have a defect of electrolyte regulation, it is usually necessary to administer sodium chloride in amounts of 4–6 g/d, either orally or parenterally, in addition to cortisone. Furthermore, fludrocortisone acetate (Florinef) usually is required initially. The dose is entirely dependent on the levels of the serum electrolytes, which must be followed serially but is generally 0.05–0.1 mg/d.

In addition to the hormone treatment of this disorder, surgical correction of the external genitalia is usually necessary.

During acute illness or other stress, as well as during and after an operation, additional hydrocortisone is indicated to avoid the adrenal insufficiency of stress. Doubling the maintenance dose is usually adequate in such circumstances.

## 7. FEMALE HERMAPHRODITISM WITHOUT PROGRESSIVE MASCULINIZATION

Females with no adrenal abnormality may have fetal masculinization of the external genitalia with the same anatomic findings as in patients with congenital virilizing adrenal hyperplasia. Unlike patients with adrenogenital syndrome, patients without adrenal abnormality do not have elevated levels of serum steroids or urinary 17-ketosteroids nor—as they grow older—do they show precocious sexual development or the metabolic difficulties associated with adrenal hyperplasia. At onset of puberty, normal feminization with menstruation and ovulation may be expected.

The diagnosis of female hermaphroditism not owing to adrenal abnormality depends on the demonstration of 46,XX karyotype and the finding of normal serum steroids or normal levels of 17-ketosteroids in the urine. If fusion of the scrotolabial folds is complete, it is necessary to determine the exact relationship of the urogenital sinus to the urethra and vagina and to demonstrate the presence of a uterus by rectal examination or ultrasonography or endoscopic observation of the cervix. When there is a high degree of masculinization, the differential diagnosis between this condition and true hermaphroditism may be very difficult; an exploratory laparotomy may be required in some cases.

## Classification

Patients with this problem may be seen because of a variety of conditions.

1. Exogenous androgen:
   a. Maternal ingestion of androgen.
   b. Maternal androgenic tumor.
   c. Luteoma of pregnancy.
   d. Adrenal androgenic tumor.
2. Idiopathic: No identifiable cause.
3. Special or nonspecific: The same as (2) except that it is associated with various somatic anomalies and with mental retardation.
4. Familial: A very rare anomaly.

## 8. MALE HERMAPHRODITISM

Persons with abnormal or ectopic testes may have external genitalia so ambiguous at birth that the true sex is not identifiable (Fig 5–17). At puberty, these persons tend to become masculinized or feminized depending on factors to be discussed below. Thus, the adult habitus of these persons may be typically male, ie, without breasts, or typically female, with good breast development. In some instances, the external genitalia may be indistinguishable from those of a normal female; in others, the clitoris may be enlarged; and in still other instances there may be fusion

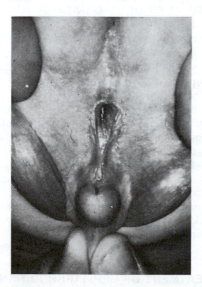

**Figure 5–17.** External genitalia in male hermaphroditism. (Reproduced, with permission, from Jones HW Jr, Scott WW: *Hermaphroditism, Genital Anomalies and Related Endocrine Disorders*, 2nd ed. Williams & Wilkins, 1971.)

of the labia in the midline, resulting in what seems to be a hypospadiac male. A deep or shallow vagina may be present. A cervix, a uterus, and uterine tubes may be developed to varying degrees; however, müllerian structures are often absent. Mesonephric structures may be grossly or microscopically visible. Body hair may be either typically feminine in its distribution and quantity or masculine in distribution and of sufficient quantity as to require plucking or shaving if the person is reared as a female. In a special group, axillary and pubic hair is congenitally absent. Although there is a well-developed uterus in some instances, all patients so far reported have been amenorrheic—in spite of the interesting theoretic possibility of uterine bleeding from endometrium stimulated by estrogen of testicular origin. There is no evidence of adrenal malfunction. In the feminized group and, less frequently, in the nonfeminized group, there is a strong familial history of the disorder. Male hermaphrodites reared as females may marry and be well adjusted to their sex role. Others, especially when there has been equivocation regarding sex of rearing in infancy, may be less than attractive as women because of indecisive therapy. Psychiatric studies indicate that the best emotional adjustment comes from directing endocrine, surgical, and psychiatric measures toward improving the person's basic characteristics. Fortunately, this is consonant with the surgical and endocrine possibilities for those reared as females, because current operative techniques can produce more satisfactory feminine than masculine external genitalia. Furthermore, the testes of male hermaphrodites are nonfunctional as far as spermatogenesis is concerned. Only about one-third of male hermaphrodites are suitable for rearing as males.

## Classification

Since about 1970, considerable progress has been made in identifying specific metabolic defects that are etiologically important for the various forms of male hermaphroditism. Details are beyond the scope of this text. Nevertheless, it is important to point out that all cases of male hermaphroditism have a defect in either the biologic action of testosterone or the müllerian inhibiting factor of the testis. Furthermore, it now seems apparent that nearly all—if not all—of these defects have a genetic or cytogenetic background. The causes and pathogenetic mechanisms of these defects may vary, but the final common pathway is one of the 2 problems just mentioned; in the adult a study of the serum gonadotropins and serum steroids, including the intermediate metabolites of testosterone, can often pinpoint a defect in the biosynthesis of testosterone. In other cases, the end organ action of testosterone may be defective. In children, the defect is sometimes more difficult to determine before gonadotropin levels rise at puberty, but one may suspect a problem by observing abnormally high levels of steroids that act as substrates in the metabolism of testosterone. A working classification of male hermaphroditism is as follows:

I. Male hermaphroditism due to a central nervous system defect.
   A. Abnormal pituitary gonadotropin secretion.
   B. No gonadotropin secretion.
II. Male hermaphroditism due to a primary gonadal defect.
   A. Identifiable defect in biosynthesis of testosterone.
      1. Pregnenolone synthesis defect (lipoid adrenal hyperplasia).
      2. 3β-Hydroxysteroid dehydrogenase deficiency.
      3. 17α-Hydroxylase deficiency.
      4. 17,20-Desmolase deficiency.
      5. 17β-Ketosteroid reductase deficiency.
   B. Unidentified defect in androgen effect.
   C. Defect in duct regression (Figs 5–18 and 5–19).
   D. Familial gonadal destruction.
   E. Leydig cell agenesis.
   F. Bilateral testicular dysgenesis.
III. Male hermaphroditism due to peripheral end organ defect.
   A. Androgen insensitivity syndrome (Fig 5–20).
      1. Androgen binding protein deficiency.
      2. Unknown deficiency.
   B. 5α-Reductase deficiency.
   C. Unidentified abnormality of peripheral androgen effect.
IV. Male hermaphroditism due to Y chromosome defect.

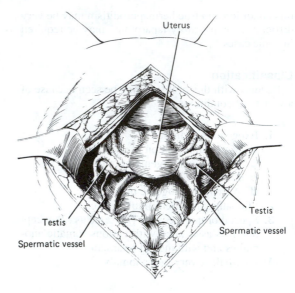

**Figure 5–19.** Internal genitalia of the patient whose external genitalia are shown in Fig 5–18. (Reproduced, with permission, from Jones HW Jr, Scott WW: *Hermaphroditism, Genital Anomalies and Related Endocrine Disorders,* 2nd ed. Williams & Wilkins, 1971.)

   A. Y chromosome mosaicism (asymmetric gonadal differentiation) (Fig 5–21).
   B. Structurally abnormal Y chromosome.
   C. No identifiable Y chromosome.

## 9. DIFFERENTIAL DIAGNOSIS IN INFANTS WITH AMBIGUOUS GENITALIA

Accurate differential diagnosis is possible in most patients with ambiguous genitalia (Table 5–8). This requires a complex history of the mother's medication, a complex sex chromosome study, rectal examination for the presence or absence of a uterus, measurement of serum steroid levels, pelvic ultrasonography, and information about other congenital anomalies. The following disorders, however, do not yield to differentiation by the parameters given in Table 5–8: (1) idiopathic masculinization, (2) the "special" forms of female hermaphroditism, (3) 46,XX true hermaphroditism; and, occasionally, (4) the precise type of male hermaphroditism. For these differentiations, laparotomy may be necessary for diagnosis and also for therapy.

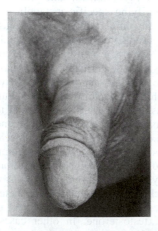

**Figure 5–18.** External genitalia in male hermaphroditism. (Reproduced, with permission, from Jones HW Jr, Scott WW: *Hermaphroditism, Genital Anomalies and Related Endocrine Disorders,* 2nd ed. Williams & Wilkins, 1971.)

## 10. TREATMENT OF HERMAPHRODITISM

The sex of rearing is much more important than the obvious morphologic signs (external genitalia, hor-

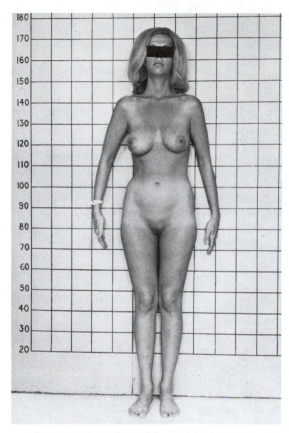

**Figure 5–20.** Androgen insensitivity syndrome.

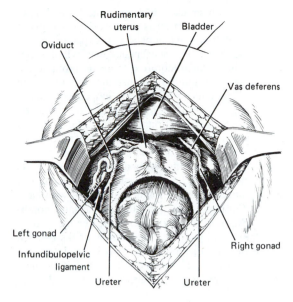

**Figure 5–21.** Internal genitalia in asymmetric gonadal differentiation. (Reproduced, with permission, from Jones HW Jr, Scott WW: *Hermaphroditism, Genital Anomalies and Related Endocrine Disorders,* 2nd ed. Williams & Wilkins, 1971.)

mone dominance, gonadal structure) in forming the gender role. Furthermore, serious psychologic consequences may result from changing the sex of rearing after infancy. Therefore, it is seldom proper to advise a change of sex after infancy to conform to the gonadal structure of the external genitalia. Instead, the physician should exert efforts to complete the adjustment of the person to the sex role already assigned. Fortunately, most aberrations of sexual development are discovered in the newborn period or in infancy, when reassignment of sex causes few problems.

Regardless of the time of treatment (and the earlier the better), the surgeon should reconstruct the exter-

nal genitalia to correspond to the sex of rearing. Any contradictory sex structures that may function to the patient's disadvantage in the future should be eradicated. Specifically, testes should always be removed from male hermaphrodites reared as females, regardless of hormone production. In cases of testicular feminization, orchiectomy is warranted because a variety of tumors may develop in these abnormal testes if they are retained, but the orchiectomy may be delayed until after puberty in this variety of hermaphroditism.

In virilized female hermaphroditism due to adrenal hyperplasia, the suppression of adrenal androgen production by the use of cortisone from an early age will result in completely female development. It is no longer necessary to explore the abdomen and the internal genitalia in this well-delineated syndrome. The surgical effort should be confined to reconstruction of the external genitalia along female lines.

**Table 5–8.** Differential diagnosis of ambiguous external genitalia.[1]

| Diagnosis | Karyotype | History | Uterus | Anomalies | 17-KS | Sex Chromosomes |
|---|---|---|---|---|---|---|
| Adrenal hyperplasia | 46,XX | + | + | − | E | XX |
| Maternal androgen | 46,XX | + | + | − | N | XX |
| Idiopathic masculinization | 46,XX | − | + | − | N | XX |
| Special or nonspecific | 46,XX | − | + | − | N | XX |
| Female familial | 46,XX | + | + | + | N | XX |
| True hermaphroditism | 46,XX; 46,XY; etc | − | + or − | − | N | XX or other |
| Male hermaphroditism | 46,XY | + | + or − | − | N | XY or other |
| Streak gonad | 45,X; 46,XX; 46,XY; etc | − | + | + or − | N | XO or other |

[1]+ = positive, − = negative, N = normal, E = elevated.

Patients with streak gonads or Turner's syndrome, who are invariably reared as females, should be given exogenous estrogen when puberty is expected. Those hermaphrodites reared as females who will not become feminized also require estrogen to promote the development of the female habitus, including the breasts. In patients with a well-developed system, cyclic uterine withdrawal bleeding can be produced even though reproduction is impossible. Estrogen should be started at about age 12 and may be given as conjugated estrogens, 1.5 mg/d orally (or its equivalent). In some patients, after a period of time, this dosage may have to be increased for additional breast development. In patients without ovaries who have uteri and in male hermaphrodites in the same condition, cyclic uterine bleeding can often be induced by the administration of estrogen for 3 weeks of each month. In other instances, this may be inadequate to produce a convincing "menstrual" period; if so, the 3 weeks of estrogen may be followed by 3–4 days of progestin (eg, medroxyprogesterone acetate) orally or a single injection of progesterone. Prolonged estrogen therapy increases the risk of subsequent development of adenocarcinoma of the corpus, so that periodic endometrial sampling is mandatory in such patients.

### Reconstruction of Female External Genitalia

The details of the operative reconstruction of abnormal external genitalia are beyond the scope of this chapter. However, it should be emphasized that the procedure should be carried out at the earliest age possible so as to enhance the desired psychologic, social, and sexual orientation of the patient and also to obtain an easier adjustment by the parents. Sometimes the reconstruction can be done during the neonatal period. In any case, operation should not be delayed beyond the first several months of life. From a technical point of view, early operation is possible in all but the most exceptional circumstances.

## REFERENCES

Anderson A: Some clinical implications of recombinant DNA technology with emphasis on prenatal diagnosis of hemoglobinopathies. Clin Biochem 1984;17:112.

Antonarakis SE et al: Prenatal diagnosis of haemophilia A by factor VIII gene analysis. Lancet 1985;1:1407.

Bardoni B et al: A deletion map of the human Yq11 region: implications for the evolution of the Y chromosome and tentative mapping of a locus involved in spermatogenesis. Genomics 1991;11:443.

Barnabei VM, Wyandt HE, Kelly TE: A possible exception to the critical region hypothesis. Am J Hum Genet 1981;33:61.

Bercu BB, Schulman JD: Genetics of abnormalities of sexual differentiation and of female reproductive failure. Obstet Gynecol Surv 1980;35:1.

Berkovitz GD et al: The role of the sex-determining region of the Y chromosome (SRY in the etiology of 46,XX true hermaphroditism). Hum Genet 1992;88:411.

Berthezenage F et al: Leydig-cell agenesis: A cause of male pseudohermaphroditism. N Engl J Med 1976;295:969.

Bostock CJ, Summer AT: *The Eukaryotic Chromosome.* North Holland Publishing Co, 1978.

Bowcock AM et al: THRA1 and D17S183 flank an interval of <cM for the breast-ovarian gene (BRCA1) on chromosome 17q21. Am J Hum Genet 1993;52:718.

Ferguson-Smith MA: Karyotype-phenotype correlations in gonadal dysgenesis and their bearing on the pathogenesis of malformations, J Med Genet 1965;2:142.

Ferguson-Smith MA: Progress in the molecular cytogenetics of man. Phil Trans R Soc Lond 1988;319:239.

Feunteun J et al: A breast-ovarian cancer susceptibility gene maps to chromosome 17q21. Am J Hum Genet 1993; 52:736.

Golbus MS et al: Prenatal genetic diagnosis in 3000 amniocenteses. N Engl J Med 1979;300:157.

Gordon H: Oncogenes. Mayo Clin Proc 1985;60:697.

Gyorki S et al: Defective nuclear accumulation of androgen receptors in disorders of sexual differentiation. J Clin Invest 1983;72:819.

Haseltine F, Ohno S: Mechanisms of gonadal differentiation. Science 1981;211:1272.

Hsia DY-Y: The detection of heterozygote carriers. Med Clin North Am 1969;53:857.

Hook EB: Rates of chromosome abnormalities at different maternal ages. Obstet Gynecol 1981;58:282.

Jones HW Jr: A long look at the adrenogenital syndrome. Johns Hopkins Med J 1979;145:143.

Jones HW Jr, Ferguson-Smith MA, Heller RH: Pathologic and cytogenetic findings in true hermaphroditism: Report of six cases and review of 23 cases from the literature. Obstet Gynecol 1965;25:435.

Kajii T et al: Anatomic and chromosomal anomalies in 639 spontaneous abortuses. Hum Genet 1980;55:87.

Kan YW, Dozy AM: Polymorphism of DNA sequence adjacent to human beta-globin structural gene: Relationship to sickle mutation. Proc Natl Acad Sci USA 1978; 75:5631.

Klinefelter HF Jr, Reifenstein EC Jr, Albright F: Syndrome characterized by gynecomastia, aspermatogenesis without aleydigism and increased excretion of follicle-stimulating hormone. J Clin Endocrinol 1942;2:615.

Kosanovic M et al: Infrequent structural chromosomal aberrations in women with primary amenorrhea. Int J Fertil 1979;24:68.

Lidsky AS, Guttler F, Woo SLC: Prenatal diagnosis of classic phenylketonuria by DNA analysis. Lancet 1985; 1:549.

Lippman-Hand A, Bekemans M: Balanced translocations among couples with two or more spontaneous abortions: Are males and females equally likely to be carriers? Hum Genet 1983;68:252.

Main DM, Mennuti MT: Neural tube defects: Issues in prenatal diagnosis and counseling. Obstet Gynecol 1986; 67:1.

McKusick VA: *Mendelian Inheritance in Man,* 10th ed. Johns Hopkins Univ Press, 1992.

Meizner I, Glezerman M: Cordocentesis in the evaluation of the growth-retarded fetus. Clin Obstet Gynecol 1992; 35:126.

Menutti MT et al: An evaluation of cytogenetic analysis as a primary tool in the assessment of recurrent pregnancy wastage. Obstet Gynecol 1978;52:308.

National Institutes of Health: *Antenatal Diagnosis. Publication No. 79–1973.* National Institutes of Health, 1979.

Nihoul-Faaekaaetaae C et al: Preservation on gonadal function in true hermaphroditism. J Pediatr Surg 1984;19:50.

Page DC et al: The sex determining region of the human Y chromosome encodes a finger protein. Cell 1987; 51: 1091.

Pao CC, Kao S-M, Hor JJ, Chang SY: Lack of mutational alteration in the conserved regions of ZFY and SRY genes of 46,XY females with gonadal dysgenesis. Hum Reprod 1993;8:224.

Park IJ, Aimakhu VE, Jones HW Jr: An etiologic and pathogenetic classification of male hermaphroditism. Am J Obstet Gynecol 1975;123:505.

Park IJ, Jones HW Jr: Familial male hermaphroditism with ambiguous external genitalia. Am J Obstet Gynecol 1970; 108:1197.

Raskin S et al: Cystic fibrosis genotyping by direct PCR analysis of Guthrie blood spots. PCR Methods Appl 1992;2:154.

Rosenfeld R et al: Six-year results of a randomized prospective trial of human growth hormone and oxandrolone in Turner syndrome. J Pediatr 1992;121:49.

Sant-Cassia LJ, Cooke P: Chromosomal analysis of couples with repeated spontaneous abortions. Br J Obstet Gynaecol 1981;88:52.

Simpson E et al: Separation of the genetic loci for the H-Y antigen and for testis determination on human Y chromosome. Nature 1987;326:876.

Speiser PW, New MI, White PC: Molecular genetic analysis of nonclassic steroid 21-hydroxylase deficiency associated with HLA-B14, DR1. Obstet Gynecol Surv 1988; 43:693.

Stenchever MA: Chromosome evaluation: Clinical applications. Chapter 2 In: *Progress in Gynecology.* Vol 6. Taymor ML, Green TH (editors). Grune & Stratton, 1975.

Stenchever MA et al: Cytogenetics of habitual abortion and other reproductive wastage. Am J Obstet Gynecol 1977;127:143.

Stoll CG et al: Interchromosomal effect in balanced translocation. Birth Defects 1978;14:393.

Tiepalo L, Zuffardi O: Location of factors controlling spermatogenesis in the nonfluorescent portion of the human Y chromosome long arm. Hum Genet 1976;34:119.

Tsuji K, Nakano R: Chromosome studies of embryos from induced abortions in pregnant women age 35 and over. Obstet Gynecol 1978;52:542.

Turner G et al: Heterozygous expression of X-linked mental retardation and X-chromosome marker fra(X)(q27). N Engl J Med 1980;303:662.

Turner HH: A syndrome of infantilism, congenital webbed neck, and cubitus valgus. Endocrinology 1938;23:566.

# Physiology of Reproduction in Women*

*William F. Ganong, MD*

This chapter is concerned with the function of the female reproductive system from birth through puberty and adulthood to the menopause.

## PUBERTY

After birth, the gonads are quiescent until they are activated by gonadotropins from the pituitary to bring about the final maturation of the reproductive system. This period of final maturation is known as **adolescence.** It is often called **puberty,** although strictly defined, puberty is the period when the endocrine and gametogenic functions of the gonads first develop to the point where reproduction is possible. In girls, the first event is **thelarche,** the development of breasts, followed by **pubarche,** the development of axillary and pubic hair, and then **menarche,** the first menstrual period. The initial periods are generally anovulatory, and regular ovulation begins about one year later. In contrast to the situation in adulthood, removal of the gonads during the period from soon after birth to puberty causes little or no increase in gonadotropin secretion, so gonadotropin secretion is not being held in check by the gonadal hormones. In children between the ages of 7 and 10, a slow increase in estrogen and androgen secretion precedes the more rapid rise in the early teens (Fig 6–1).

The age at the time of puberty is variable; in Europe and the USA, it has been declining at the rate of 1–3 months per decade for more than 175 years. In the USA in recent years, puberty has generally been occurring between the ages of 8 and 13 in girls and 9 and 14 in boys.

Another event that occurs in humans at the time of puberty is an increase in the secretion of adrenal androgens (Fig 6–2). The onset of this increase is called **adrenarche,** which occurs at age 8–10 years. There are no changes in the secretion of cortisol or ACTH.

Adrenarche may be due to a change in the enzyme systems in the adrenal, so that more pregnenolone is diverted to the androgen pathway, but there is some evidence that it is due to increased secretion of an as yet unisolated **adrenal androgen-stimulating hormone (AASH)** from the pituitary gland.

The adrenal androgens contribute significantly to the growth of axillary and pubic hair. The breasts develop under the influence of the ovarian hormones estradiol and progesterone, with estradiol primarily responsible for the growth of ducts and progesterone primarily responsible for the growth of lobules and alveoli. The sequence of the changes that occur at puberty in girls are summarized in Fig 6–3.

### Control of the Onset of Puberty

A neural mechanism is responsible for the onset of puberty. In children, the gonads can be stimulated by gonadotropins, the pituitary contains gonadotropins, and the hypothalamus contains gonadotropin-releasing hormone(GnRH). However, the gonadotropins are not secreted. In addition, estrogens do not produce a surge of luteinizing hormone (LH) secretion in girls via the positive feedback mechanism that is operative once puberty has occurred (see below). In immature monkeys, normal menstrual cycles can be brought on by pulsatile injection of GnRH, and the cycles persist as long as the pulsatile injection is continued. In addition, GnRH is secreted in a pulsatile fashion in adults. Thus, it seems clear that during the period from birth to puberty, a neural mechanism is operating to prevent the normal pulsatile release of GnRH. The nature of the mechanism inhibiting the GnRH pulse generator is unknown.

### Sexual Precocity

The major causes of precocious sexual development in human are listed in Table 6–1. Early development of secondary sexual characteristics without gametogenesis is caused by abnormal exposure of immature males to androgen or females to estrogen. This syndrome should be called **precocious pseudopuberty** to distinguish it from true precocious puberty due to an early but otherwise normal pubertal

---

*This chapter is based in large part on Chapter 23 in: Ganong WF: *Review of Medical Physiology,* 16th ed. Appleton & Lange, 1993.

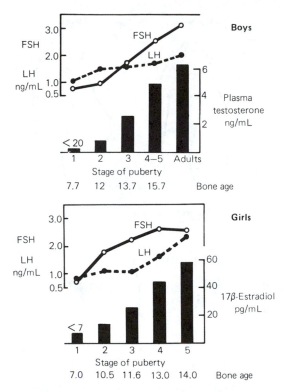

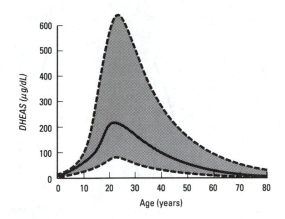

**Figure 6–2.** Change in serum dehydroepiandrosterone sulfate (DHEAS) with age. There are no significant differences between males and females. The middle line is the mean, and the dashed lines identify -1.96 standard deviations. (Modified and reproduced, with permission, from Smith MR et al: A radioimmunoassay for the estimation of serum dehydroepiandrosterone sulfate in normal and pathological sera. Clin Chim Acta 1975;65:5).

**Figure 6–1.** Changes in plasma hormone concentrations during puberty in boys (top) and girls (bottom). Stage 1 of puberty is preadolescence in both sexes. In boys, stage 2 is characterized by beginning enlargement of the testes, stage 3 by penile enlargement, stage 4 by growth of the glans penis, and stage 5 by adult genitalia. The stages of puberty in girls are summarized in Fig 6–3. (Reproduced, with permission, from Grumbach MM: Onset of puberty. In: *Puberty: Biologic and Psychosocial Components.* Berenberg SR [editor]. HE Stenfoert Kroese BV, 1975.)

pattern of gonadotropin secretion from the pituitary (Fig 6–4).

In one large series of cases, precocious puberty was the most frequent endocrine symptom of hypothalamic disease. It is interesting that in experimental animals and humans, lesions of the ventral hypothalamus near the infundibulum cause precocious puberty. The effect of the lesions may be due to interruption of neural pathways that produce inhibition of the GnRH pulse generator, or to chronic stimulation of GnRH secretion originating in irritative foci around the lesion. Pineal tumors are sometimes associated with precocious puberty, but there is evidence that these tumors are associated with precocious puberty only when there is secondary damage to the hypothalamus. Precocity due to this and other forms of hypothalamic damage probably occurs with equal frequency in both sexes, although the constitutional form of precocious puberty is more common in girls. In addition, it has now been proved that precocious gametogenesis and steroidogenesis can occur without the pubertal pattern of gonadotropin secretion (gonadotropin-independent precocity).

### Delayed or Absent Puberty

The normal variation in the age at which adolescent changes occur is so wide that puberty cannot be considered to be pathologically delayed until menarche has failed to occur by the age of 17. Failure of maturation due to panhypopituitarism is associated with dwarfing and evidence of other endocrine abnormalities. Patients with the XO chromosomal pattern and gonadal dysgenesis are also dwarfed. In some individuals, puberty is delayed and menarche does not occur (primary amenorrhea), even though the gonads are present and other endocrine functions are normal.

### REPRODUCTIVE FUNCTION AFTER SEXUAL MATURITY

### Menstrual Cycle

The anatomy of the reproductive system of adult women is described in Chapter 2. Unlike the reproductive system of men, this system shows regular cyclic changes that teleologically may be regarded as periodic preparation for fertilization and pregnancy. In primates, the cycle is a **menstrual cycle,** and its most conspicuous feature is the periodic vaginal bleeding that occurs with the shedding of the uterine mucosa (**menstruation**). The length of the cycle is notoriously variable, but an average figure is 28 days from the start of one menstrual period to the start of

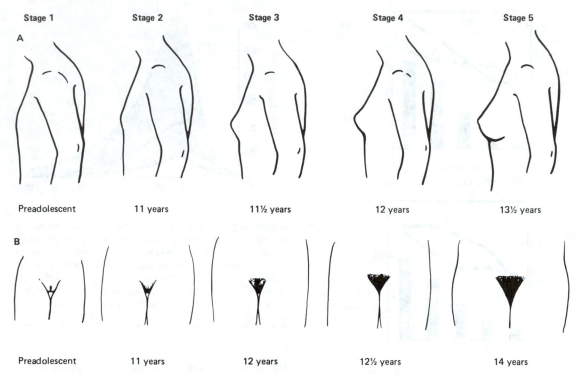

**Figure 6–3.** Sequence of events at adolescence in girls. *A:* Stage 1: Preadolescent; elevation of papillae only. Stage 2: Breast bud stage (may occur between ages 8 and 13); elevation of breasts and papillae as small mounds, with enlargement of areolar diameter. Stage 3: enlargement and elevation of breasts and areolas with no separation of contours. Stage 4: Areolas and papillae project from breast to form a secondary mound. Stage 5: Mature; projection of papillae only, with recession of areolas into general contour of breast. *B:* Stage 1: Preadolescent; no pubic hair. Stage 2: Sparse growth along labia of long, slightly pigmented, downy hair that is straight or slightly curled (may occur between ages 8 and 14). Stage 3: Darker, coarser, more curled hair growing sparsely over pubic area. Stage 4: Resembles adult in type but covers smaller area. Stage 5: Adult in quantity and type. (Redrawn, with permission, from Tanner JM: *Growth at Adolescence,* 2nd ed. Blackwell, 1962.)

**Table 6–1.** Classification of the causes of precocious sexual development in humans.

**True precocious puberty**
  Constitutional
  Cerebral: Disorders involving posterior hypothalamus
  Tumors
  Infections
**Precocious pseudopuberty** (no spermatogenesis or ovarian development)
  Adrenal
    Congenital virilizing adrenal hyperplasia (without treatment in males; following cortisone treatment in females)
    Androgen-secreting tumors (in males)
    Estrogen-secreting tumors (in females)
  Gonadal
    Interstitial cell tumors of testis
    Granulosa cell tumors of ovary
  Miscellaneous

the next. By common usage, the days of the cycle are identified by number, starting with the first day of menstruation.

## Ovarian Cycle

From the time of birth, there are many **primordial follicles** under the ovarian capsule. Each contains an immature ovum (Fig 6–5). At the start of each cycle, several of these follicles enlarge and a cavity forms around the ovum (antrum formation). This cavity is filled with follicular fluid. In humans, one of the follicles in one ovary starts to grow rapidly on about the sixth day and becomes the **dominant follicle.** The others regress, forming **atretic follicles.** It is not known how one follicle is singled out for development during this **follicular phase** of the menstrual cycle, but it seems to be related to the ability of the follicle to secrete the estrogen inside it that is needed for final maturation. However, when women are given highly purified human pituitary gonadotropin preparations by injection, many follicles develop simultaneously.

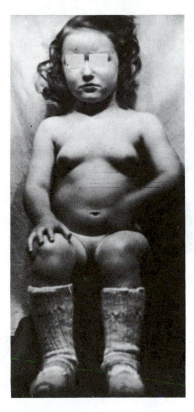

**Figure 6–4.** Constitutional precocious puberty in a 3 ½-year-old girl. The patient developed pubic hair and started to menstruate at the age of 17 months. (Reproduced, with permission, from Jolly H: *Sexual Precocity.* Thomas, 1955.)

The structure of a maturing ovarian follicle (**graafian follicle**) is shown in Fig 6–5. The cells of the **theca interna** of the follicle are the primary source of circulating estrogens. However, the follicular fluid has a high estrogen content, and much of this estrogen appears to come from the granulosa cells.

At about the 14th day of the cycle, the distended follicle ruptures, and the ovum is extruded into the abdominal cavity. This is the process of **ovulation.** The ovum is picked up by the fimbriated ends of the uterine tubes (oviducts) and transported to the uterus. Unless fertilization occurs, the ovum degenerates or is passed on through the uterus and out the vagina.

The follicle that ruptures at the time of ovulation promptly fills with blood, forming what is sometimes called a **corpus hemorrhagicum.** Minor bleeding from the follicle into the abdominal cavity may cause peritoneal irritation and fleeting lower abdominal pain ("mittelschmerz"). The granulosa and theca cells of the follicle lining promptly begin to proliferate, and the clotted blood is rapidly replaced with yellowish, lipid-rich **luteal cells,** forming the **corpus luteum.** This is the **luteal phase** of the menstrual cycle, during which the luteal cells secrete estrogens

and progesterone. If pregnancy occurs, the corpus luteum persists, and there are usually no more menstrual periods until after delivery. If there is no pregnancy, the corpus luteum begins to degenerate about 4 days before the next menses (day 24 of the cycle) and is eventually replaced by fibrous tissue, forming a **corpus albicans.**

In humans, no new ova are formed after birth. During fetal development, the ovaries contain over 7 million germ cells; however, many undergo involution before birth, and others are lost after birth. At the time of birth, there are approximately 2 million primordial follicles containing ova, but approximately 50% of these are atretic. The million or so ova that are normal undergo the first part of the first meiotic division at about this time and enter a stage of arrest in prophase in which those that survive persist until adulthood. Atresia continues during development, and the number of ova in both the ovaries at the time of puberty is less than 300,000 (Fig 6–6). Normally, only one of these ova per cycle (or about 500 in the course of a normal reproductive life) is stimulated to mature; the remainder degenerate. Just before ovulation, the first meiotic division is completed. One of the daughter cells, the **secondary oocyte,** receives most of the cytoplasm, while the other, the **first polar body,** fragments and disappears. The secondary oocyte immediately begins the second meiotic division, but this division stops at metaphase and is completed only when a sperm penetrates the oocyte. At that time, the **second polar body** is cast off and the fertilized ovum proceeds to form a new individual. The arrest in metaphase is due, at least in some species, to formation in the ovum of the protein **pp39**$^{mos}$, which is encoded by the **c-mos** proto-oncogene. When fertilization occurs, the pp39$^{mos}$ is destroyed within 30 minutes by **calpain,** a calcium-dependent cysteine protease.

## Uterine Cycle & Menstruation

The events that occur in the uterus during the menstrual cycle terminate in the menstrual flow. By the end of each menstrual period, all but the deep layers of the endometrium has sloughed. Under the influence of estrogens from the developing follicles, the endometrium regenerates from the deep layer and increases rapidly in thickness during the period from the 5th to 16th days of the menstrual cycle. As the thickness increases, the uterine glands are drawn out so that they lengthen (Fig 6–7), but they do not become convoluted or secrete to any degree. These endometrial changes are called proliferative, and this part of the menstrual cycle is sometimes called the **proliferative phase.** It is also called the preovulatory or follicular phase of the cycle. After ovulation, the endometrium becomes more highly vascularized and slightly edematous under the influence of estrogen and progesterone from the corpus luteum. The glands become coiled and tortuous (Fig 6–7), and they begin to secrete a clear fluid. Consequently, this

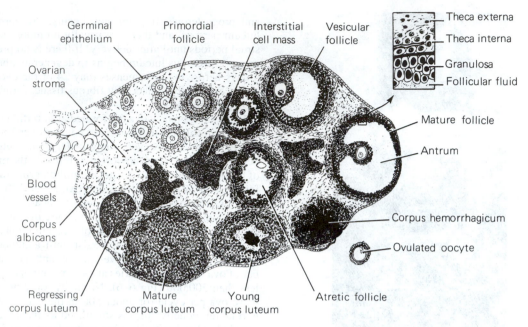

**Figure 6–5.** Diagram of a mammalian ovary, showing the sequential development of a follicle, formation of a corpus luteum, and, in the center, follicular atresia. A section of the wall of a mature follicle is enlarged at the upper right. The interstitial cell mass is not prominent in primates. (After Patten B, Eakin RM. Reproduced, with permission, from Gorbman A, Bern H: *Textbook of Comparative Endocrinology.* Wiley, 1962.)

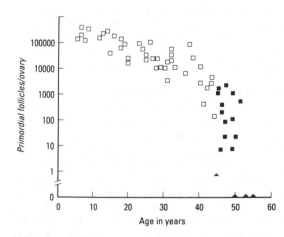

**Figure 6–6.** Number of primordial follicles per ovary in women at various ages. □, premenopausal women (regular menses); ■, perimenopausal women (irregular menses for at least 1 year); ▲, postmenopausal women (no menses for at least 1 year). Note that the vertical scale is a log scale and that the values are from one rather than 2 ovaries. (Redrawn by PM Wise and reproduced, with permission, from Richardson SJ, Senikas V, Nelson JF: Follicular depletion during the menopausal transition: evidence for accelerated loss and ultimate exhaustion. J Clin Endocrinol Metab 1987;65:1231.)

phase of the cycle is called the **secretory** or **luteal phase.**

The endometrium is supplied by 2 types of arteries. The superficial two-thirds of the endometrium that is shed during menstruation, the **stratum functionale,** is supplied by long, coiled **spiral arteries** (Fig 6–8), whereas the deep layer that is not shed is supplied by short, straight **basilar arteries.**

When the corpus luteum regresses, hormonal support for the endometrium is withdrawn. The endometrium becomes thinner, which adds to the coiling of the spiral arteries. Foci of necrosis appear in the endometrium, and these coalesce. There is, in addition, necrosis of the walls of the spiral arteries, leading to spotty hemorrhages that become confluent and produce the menstrual flow.

The cause of the vascular necrosis is unknown, but it is associated with spasm of the blood vessel walls, which may be reproduced by locally released prostaglandins. There are large quantities of protaglandins in the secretory endometrium and in menstrual blood, and infusions of $PGF_{2a}$ produce endometrial necrosis and bleeding. One theory of the onset of menstruation holds that in necrotic endometrial cells, lysosomal membranes break down with the release of enzymes that foster the formation of prostaglandins from cellular phospholipids, and the prostaglandins produce vasospasm, vascular necrosis, and menstrual flow. After menstruation, a new endometrium regenerates from cells that remain in the stratum basalis.

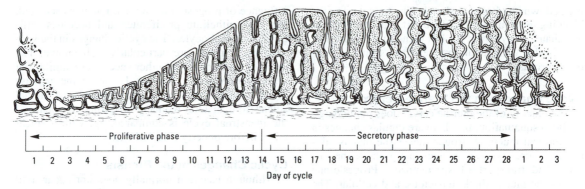

Proliferative phase

Day of cycle

**Figure 6–7.** Changes in the endometrium during the menstrual cycle. (Reproduced, with permission, from Ganong WF: *Review of Medical Physiology,* 16th ed. Appleton & Lange, 1993.)

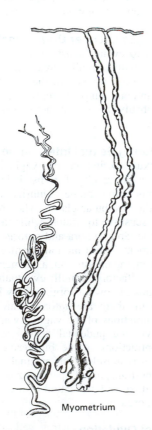

Myometrium

**Figure 6–8.** Spiral artery of endometrium. Drawing of a spiral artery (left) and 2 uterine glands (right) from the endometrium of a rhesus monkey; early progestational phase. The uterine cavity is at the top. (Reproduced, with permission, from Daron GH: The arterial pattern of the tunica mucosa of the uterus in the macacus rhesus. Am J Anat 1936;58:349.)

From the point of view of endometrial function, the proliferative phase of the menstrual cycle represents the restoration of the epithelium from the preceding menstruation, and the secretory phase represents the preparation of the uterus for implantation of the fertilized ovum. The length of the secretory phase is remarkably constant, at about 14 days, and the variations seen in the length of the menstrual cycle are due for the most part to variations in the length of the proliferative phase. When fertilization fails to occur during the secretory phase, the endometrium is shed, and a new cycle starts.

## Normal Menstruation

Menstrual blood is predominantly arterial, with only 25% of the blood being of venous origin. It contains tissue debris, prostaglandins, and relatively large amounts of fibrinolysin from the endometrial tissue. The fibrinolysin lyses clots, and so menstrual blood does not normally contain clots unless the flow is excessive.

The usual duration of the menstrual cycle is 3–5 days, but flows as short as 1 day and as long as 8 days can occur in normal women. The average amount of blood lost is 30 mL but may range normally from slight spotting to 80 mL. Loss of more than 80 mL is abnormal. Obviously, the amount of flow can be affected by various factors, including thickness of the endometrium and medications and diseases that affect the clotting mechanism.

## Anovulatory Cycles

In some instances, ovulation fails to occur during the menstrual cycle. Such anovulatory cycles are common for 17–18 months after menarche and again before the onset of menopause. When ovulation does not occur, no corpus luteum is formed, and the effects of progesterone on the endometrium are absent. Estrogens continue to cause growth, however, and the proliferative endometrium becomes thick enough to break down and begin to slough. The time it takes for bleeding to occur is variable, but it usually occurs in less than 28 days from the last menstrual period. The flow is also variable and ranges from scanty to relatively profuse.

## Cyclic Changes in the Uterine Cervix

The mucosa of the uterine cervix does not undergo cyclic desquamation, but there are regular changes in the cervical mucus. Estrogen makes the mucus thinner and more alkaline, changes that promote the survival and transport of spermatozoa. Progesterone makes the mucus thick, tenacious, and cellular. The mucus is thinnest at the time of ovulation, and its elasticity, or **spinnbarkeit,** increases so that by midcycle, a drop can be stretched into a long, thin thread that may be 8–12 cm or more in length. In addition, it dries in an arborizing, fernlike pattern when a thin layer is spread on a slide (Fig 6–9). After ovulation and during pregnancy, the mucus becomes thick and fails to form the fern pattern.

## Vaginal Cycle

Under the influence of estrogens, the vaginal epithelium becomes cornified, and cornified epithelial cells can be identified in the vaginal smear. Under the

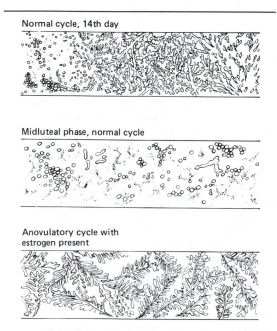

**Figure 6–9.** Patterns formed when cervical mucus is smeared on a slide, permitted to dry, and examined under the microscope. Progesterone makes the mucus thick and cellular. In the smear from a patient who failed to ovulate (*bottom*), there is no progesterone to inhibit the estrogen-induced fern pattern. (Reproduced, with permission, from Ganong WF: *Review of Medical Physiology,* 16th ed. Appleton & Lange, 1993.)

influence of progesterone, a thick mucus is secreted, and the epithelium proliferates and becomes infiltrated with leukocytes. The cyclic changes in the vaginal smear in rats are particularly well known. The changes in humans and other species are similar but unfortunately not so clear-cut. However, the increase in cornified epithelial cells is apparent when a vaginal smear from an adult woman in the follicular phase of the menstrual cycle is compared, eg, with a smear taken before puberty (Fig 6–10).

## Cyclic Changes in the Breasts

Although lactation normally does not occur until the end of pregnancy, there are cyclic changes in the breasts during the menstrual cycle. Estrogens cause proliferation of mammary ducts, whereas progesterone causes growth of lobules and alveoli (see below). The breast-swelling, tenderness, and pain experienced by many women during the 10 days preceding menstruation are probably due to distention of the ducts, hyperemia, and edema of the interstitial tissue of the breasts. All of these changes regress, along with the symptoms, during menstruation.

## Cyclic Changes in Other Body Functions

In addition to cyclic breast swelling and tenderness, there is usually a small increase in body temperature during the luteal phase of the menstrual cycle. This change in body temperature, which is discussed below, is probably due to the thermogenic effect of progesterone.

## Changes During Sexual Intercourse

During sexual excitation, the vaginal walls become moist as a result of transudation of fluid through the mucus membrane. A lubricating mucus is secreted by the vestibular glands. The upper part of the vagina is sensitive to stretch, while tactile stimulation from the labia minora and clitoris adds to the sexual excitement. The stimuli are reinforced by tactile stimuli from the breasts and, as in men, by visual, auditory, and olfactory stimuli; eventually, the crescendo or climax known as orgasm may be reached. During orgasm, there are autonomically mediated rhythmic contractions of the vaginal wall. Impulses also travel via the pudendal nerves and produce rhythmic contractions of the bulbocavernosus and ischiocavernosus muscles. The vaginal contractions may aid in the transport of spermatozoa but are not essential for it, since fertilization of the ovum is not dependent on orgasm.

## Indicators of Ovulation

It is often important in clinical practice to know that ovulation has occurred and to know when during the cycle it has occurred. It is also important to be able to predict when ovulation will occur. The finding of a secretory pattern in a biopsy of the endometrium (Fig 6–7) indicates that a functioning corpus

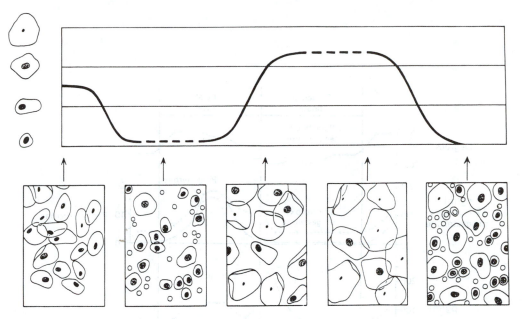

**Figure 6–10.** Vaginal cytologic picture in various stages of life. *Top:* Graphic representation of the maturation of vaginal epithelium. *Bottom:* Left to right: Epithelial maturation at birth; atrophic cell picture in childhood; beginning of estrogenic influence in puberty; complete maturation in the reproduction period; regression in old age. (Reproduced, with permission, from Beller FK et al: *Gynecology: A Textbook for Students.* Springer-Verlag, 1974.)

luteum is present. A less reliable indicator of a functioning corpus luteum in a woman who has regular menses and does not have an infection or bleeding is the finding of thick, cellular cervical mucus that does not form a fern pattern. A convenient and more reliable indicator of the time of ovulation is a rise in the basal body temperature (Fig 6–11). Accurate temperatures can be obtained by use of a thermometer with wide gradations. The woman should take her temperature orally, vaginally, or rectally in the morning before getting out of bed. The cause of the temperature change at the time of ovulation is unknown but is probably due to the increase in progesterone secretion, since progesterone is thermogenic. A rise in urinary LH occurs during the rise in circulating LH that causes ovulation, and this increase can be measured as another indicator of ovulation. Kits employing dipsticks or simple color tests for detection of urinary LH are available for home use; although they are expensive, they are beginning to be used in place of basal body temperature by women interested in defining their fertile period.

The ovum lives approximately 72 hours after it is extruded from the follicle but is probably fertilizable for less than half this time. Sperms apparently survive in the female genital tract for no more than 48 hours. Consequently, the "fertile period" during a 28-day cycle is no longer than 120 hours and is probably much shorter. Unfortunately for those interested in the "rhythm method" of contraception, the time of ovulation varies even from one menstrual cycle to an-

other in the same woman. Before day 9 and after day 20, there is little chance of conception, but there are documented cases of pregnancy resulting from isolated coitus on every day of the cycle.

## ESTROGENS

### Chemistry, Biosynthesis, & Metabolism

The naturally occurring estrogens are $17\beta$-estradiol, estrone, and estriol (Fig 6–12). They are $C_{18}$ steroids, ie, they do not have an angular methyl group attached to the 10 position or a $\Delta^4$-3 keto configuration in the A ring (Fig 6–12). They are secreted by the theca interna and granulosa cells of the ovarian follicles, by the corpus luteum, and by the placenta. The biosynthetic pathway involves their formation from androgens. They are also formed by aromatization of androstenedione in the circulation. Aromatase is the enzyme that catalyzes the conversion of $\Delta^4$-androstenedione to estrone (Fig 6–12). It also catalyzes the conversion of testosterone to estradiol.

Theca interna cells have many LH receptors, and LH acts on them via cyclic AMP (cyclic adenosine 3′, 5′-monophosphate) to increase conversion of cholesterol to androstenedione. Some androstenedione is converted to estradiol, which enters the circulation. The theca interna cells also supply androstenedione to the granulosa cells. The granulosa cells only make estradiol when provided with androgens (Fig 6–13), and they secrete the estradiol that they produce into

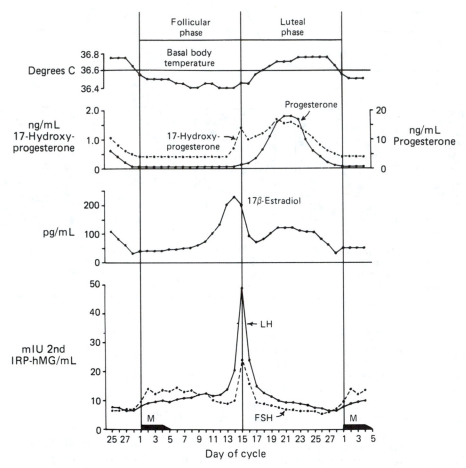

**Figure 6–11.** Typical basal body temperature and plasma hormone concentrations during a normal 28–day human menstrual cycle. M, menstruation; IRP-hMG, international reference standard for gonadotropins. (Reproduced, with permission, from Midgley AR. In: *Human Reproduction,* Hafez ESE, Evans TN [editors]. Harper & Row, 1973.)

the follicular fluid. They have many FSH receptors, and FSH facilitates the secretion of estradiol by acting via cyclic AMP to increase the aromatase activity in these cells. Mature granulosa cells also acquire LH receptors, and LH stimulates estradiol production.

The stromal tissue of the ovary also has the potential to produce androgens and estrogens. However, it probably does so in insignificant amounts in normal premenopausal women. **17β-estradiol,** the major secreted estrogen, is in equilibrium in the circulation with **estrone.** Estrone is further metabolized to **estriol** (Fig 6–12), probably mainly in the liver. Estradiol is the most potent estrogen of the 3 and estriol the least.

Two percent of the circulating estradiol is free. The remainder is bound to protein: 60% to albumin, 38%

to the same gonadal steroid-binding globulin (GBG) that binds testosterone Table 6–2.

In the liver, estrogens are oxidized or converted to glucuronide and sulfate conjugates. Appreciable amounts are secreted in the bile and reabsorbed in the bloodstream (enterohepatic circulation). There are at least 10 different metabolites of estradiol in human urine.

## Secretion of Estrogens

The concentration of estradiol in plasma during the menstrual cycle is shown in Fig 6–11. Almost all of the estrogen comes from the ovary. There are 2 peaks of secretion: one just before ovulation and one during the midluteal phase. The estradiol secretion rate is 36

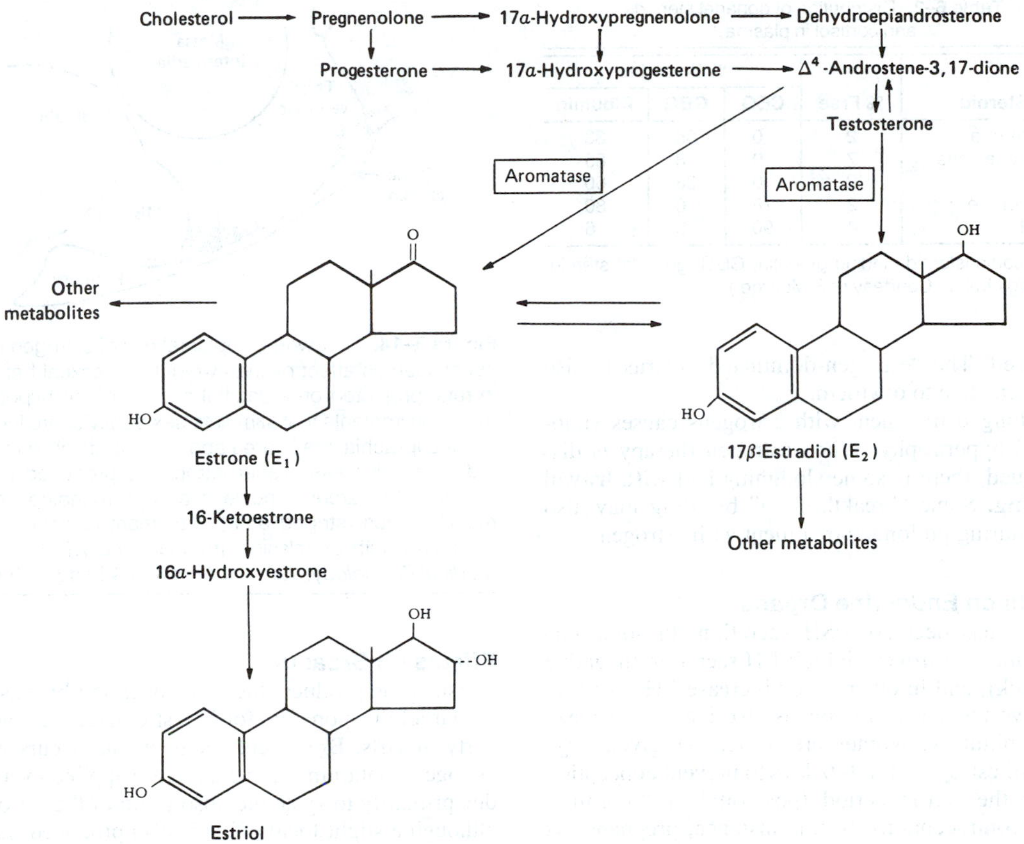

Cholesterol
Pregnenolone
17α-Hydroxypregnenolone
Dehydroepiandrosterone
Progesterone
17α-Hydroxyprogesterone
Δ4-Androstene-3,17-dione
Testosterone
Aromatase
Aromatase
Other metabolites
Estrone (E1)
17β-Estradiol (E2)
16-Ketoestrone
16α-Hydroxyestrone
Other metabolites
Estriol

**Figure 6–12.** Biosynthesis and metabolism estrogens. (Reproduced, with permission, from Ganong WF: *Review of Medical Physiology,* 16th ed. Appleton & Lange, 1993.)

μg/d (133 μmol/d) in the early follicular phase, 380 μg/d just before ovulation, and 250 μg/d during the midluteal phase (Table 6–3). After menopause, estrogen secretion declines to low levels. For comparison, the estradiol production rate in men is about 50 μg/d (180 μmol/d).

## Effects on Female Genitalia

Estrogens facilitate the growth of the ovarian follicles and increase the motility of the uterine tubes. Their role in the cyclic changes in the endometrium, cervix, and vagina is discussed above. They increase uterine blood flow and have important effects on the smooth muscle of the uterus. In immature and ovariectomized females, the uterus is small and the myometrium atrophic and inactive. Estrogens increase the amount of uterine muscle and its content of contractile proteins. Under the influence of estrogens, the myometrium becomes more active and excitable, and action potentials in the individual muscle fibers are

CIRCULATION
THECA INTERNA CELLS
GRANULOSA CELLS
ANTRUM
Cholesterol
Cholesterol
Androstenedione
Androstenedione
Estradiol
Estradiol
Estradiol
Estradiol

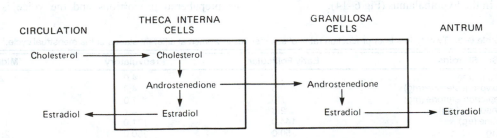

**Figure 6–13.** Interactions between theca and granulosa cells in estradiol synthesis and secretion. (Reproduced, with permission, from Ganong WF: *Review of Medical Physiology,* 16th ed. Appleton & Lange, 1993.)

**Table 6–2.** Distribution of gonadal steroids and cortisol in plasma.[1]

| Steroid | % Free | % Bound to | | |
| --- | --- | --- | --- | --- |
| | | CBG | GBG | Albumin |
| Testosterone | 2 | 0 | 65 | 33 |
| Androstenedione | 7 | 0 | 8 | 85 |
| Estradiol | 2 | 0 | 38 | 60 |
| Progesterone | 2 | 18 | 0 | 80 |
| Cortisol | 4 | 90 | 0 | 6 |

[1]CBG, corticosteroid-binding globulin; GBG, gonadal steroid-binding globulin. (Courtesy of S Munroe.)

increased. The "estrogen-dominated" uterus is also more sensitive to oxytocin.

Prolonged treatment with estrogens causes endometrial hypertrophy. When estrogen therapy is discontinued, there is some sloughing and **withdrawal bleeding.** Some "breakthrough" bleeding may also occur during prolonged treatment with estrogens.

### Effects on Endocrine Organs

Estrogens decrease FSH secretion. In some circumstances, estrogens inhibit LH secretion (negative feedback), and in others, they increase LH secretion (positive feedback). Estrogens also increase the size of the pituitary. Women are sometimes given large doses of estrogens for 4–6 days to prevent conception during the fertile period (postcoital or "morning-after" contraception). In this instance, pregnancy is probably prevented by interference with implantation of the fertilized ovum rather than by changes in gonadotropin secretion.

Estrogens cause increased secretion of angiotensinogen and thyroid-binding globulin. They exert an important protein anabolic effect in chickens and cattle, possibly by stimulating the secretion of androgens from the adrenal; estrogens have been used commercially to increase the weight of domestic animals. Estrogens have been reported to exert anabolic effects, and they cause epiphyseal closure.

### Behavioral Effects

Estrogens are responsible for estrus behavior in animals, and they increase libido in humans. They apparently exert this action by a direct effect on certain neurons in the hypothalamus (Fig 6–14).

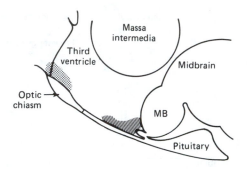

**Figure 6–14.** Loci where implantations of estrogen in the hypothalamus affect ovarian weight and sexual behavior in rats, projected on a sagittal section of the hypothalamus. The implants that stimulate sex behavior are located in the suprachiasmatic area above the optic chiasm (dotted area), whereas ovarian atrophy is produced by implants in the arcuate nucleus and surrounding ventral hypothalamus (striped area). MB, mamillary body. (Reproduced, with permission, from Ganong WF: *Review of Medical Physiology,* 16th ed. Appleton & Lange, 1993.)

### Effects on Breasts

Estrogens produce duct growth in the breasts and are largely responsible for breast enlargement at puberty in girls. Breast enlargement that occurs when estrogen-containing skin creams are applied locally is due primarily to systemic absorption of the estrogen, although a slight local effect is also produced. Estrogens are responsible for the pigmentation of the areolas; pigmentation usually becomes more intense during the first pregnancy than it does at puberty.

### Effects on Female Secondary Sex Characteristics

The body changes that develop in girls at puberty—in addition to enlargement of the breasts, uterus, and vagina—are due in part to estrogens, which are the "feminizing hormones," and in part simply to the absence of testicular androgens. Women have narrow shoulders and broad hips, thighs that converge, and arms that diverge (wide **carrying angle**). This body configuration, plus the female distribution of fat in the breasts and buttocks, is also seen in castrated males. In women, the larynx retains its prepubertal proportions and the voice is high-

**Table 6–3.** Twenty-four hour production rates of sex steroids in women at different stages of the menstrual cycle.[1]

| Sex Steroids | Early Follicular | Preovulatory | Midluteal |
| --- | --- | --- | --- |
| Progesterone (mg) | 1.0 | 4.0 | 25.0 |
| 17-Hydroxyprogesterone (mg) | 0.5 | 4.0 | 4.0 |
| Dehydroepiandrosterone (mg) | 7.0 | 7.0 | 7.0 |
| Androstenedione (mg) | 2.6 | 4.7 | 3.4 |
| Testosterone (µg) | 144.0 | 171.0 | 126.0 |
| Estrone (µg) | 50.0 | 350.0 | 250.0 |
| Estradiol (µg) | 36.0 | 380.0 | 250.0 |

[1]Modified and reproduced, with permission, from Yen SSC, Jaffe RB: *Reproductive Endocrinology,* 3rd ed. Saunders, 1991.

pitched. There is less body hair and more scalp hair, and the pubic hair generally has a characteristic flat-top pattern (**female escutcheon**). Growth of pubic and axillary hair in the female is due primarily to androgens rather than estrogens, although estrogen treatment may cause some hair growth. The androgens are produced by the adrenal cortex and, to a lesser extent, by the ovaries.

## Other Actions of Estrogens

Estrogens are said to make sebaceous gland secretions more fluid and thus to counter the effects of testosterone and inhibit formation of comedones (blackheads) and acne. The liver palms, spider angiomas, and slight breast enlargement seen in advanced hepatic disease are due to increased circulating estrogens. The increase appears to be due to decreased hepatic metabolism of androstenedione, making more of this androgen available for conversion to estrogen.

Estrogens have a significant plasma cholesterol-lowering effect, and they inhibit atherogenesis. They contribute to the low incidence of myocardial infarction and other complications of atherosclerotic vascular disease in premenopausal women. However, large doses of orally active estrogens appear to promote thrombosis because they reach the liver in high concentrations in the portal blood and alter hepatic production of clotting factors.

## Mechanism of Action of Estrogens

Most actions of estrogens on their target cells, like those of other steroid hormones (Fig 6–15), involve entry of the steroid into the cell; binding to a receptor, which in the case of estrogen is in the nucleus; transformation of the receptor to expose a DNA-binding domain; and binding of the steroid-receptor complex to enhancer-like elements in DNA. This in turn increases the transcription of certain genes with the production of mRNAs. The mRNAs code for proteins that bring about the changes in cell function. Almost all estrogen actions are produced in this fashion, although there also appear to be poorly understood rapid actions on cell membranes in some situations.

## Synthetic Estrogen

The ethinyl derivative of estradiol (Fig 6-16) is a potent estrogen. Unlike naturally occurring estrogens it is relatively active when given orally, because it has an ethinyl group in position 17, which makes it resistant to hepatic metabolism. Naturally occurring hormones have low activity when given orally, because the portal venous drainage of the intestine carries them to the liver, where they are largely inactivated before they can reach the general circulation. Some nonsteroidal substances and a few compounds found in plants have estrogenic activity. Plant estrogens rarely affect humans but may cause undesirable effects in farm animals. Diethylstilbestrol (Fig 6–16) and a number of related compounds are strongly es-

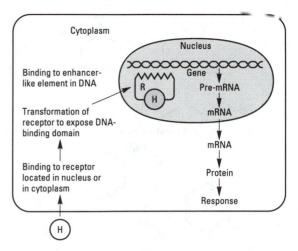

**Figure 6–15.** Mechanism of action of steroid and thyroid hormones. H, receptor; R, receptor. The estrogen, progestin, androgen, glucocorticoid, mineralocorticoid, 1,25-dihydroxycholecalciferol, and thyroid hormone receptors have different molecular weights, but all have a ligand-binding domain and a DNA-binding domain that is exposed when the ligand binds. The receptor-hormone complex then binds to DNA, producing increased transcription. (Reproduced, with permission, from Ganong, WF: *Review of Medical Physiology*, 16th ed. Appleton & Lange, 1993.)

trogenic, possibly because they are converted to steroidlike ring structures in the body.

## PROGESTERONE

### Chemistry, Biosynthesis, & Metabolism

Progesterone (Fig 6–17) is a $C_{21}$ steroid secreted in large amounts by the corpus luteum and the placenta. It is an important intermediate in steroid biosynthesis in all tissues that secrete steroid hormones, and small amounts enter the circulation from the testes and adrenal cortex. 17α-hydroxyprogesterone is secreted along with estrogens from the ovarian follicle, and its secretion parallels that of 17β-estradiol (Fig 6–11). The 20α- and 20β- hydroxy derivatives of progesterone are formed in the corpus luteum. About 2% of the progesterone in the circulation is free (Table 6–2), whereas 80% is bound to albumin and 18% is bound to corticosteroid-binding globulin. Progesterone has a short half-life and is converted in the liver to pregnanediol, which is conjugated to glucuronic acid and excreted in the urine (Fig 6–17).

### Secretion of Progesterone

In women, the plasma progesterone level is approximately 0.9 ng/mL (3 nmol/L) during the follicular phase of the menstrual cycle, whereas in men, the level is approximately 0.3 ng/mL (1 nmol/L). The dif-

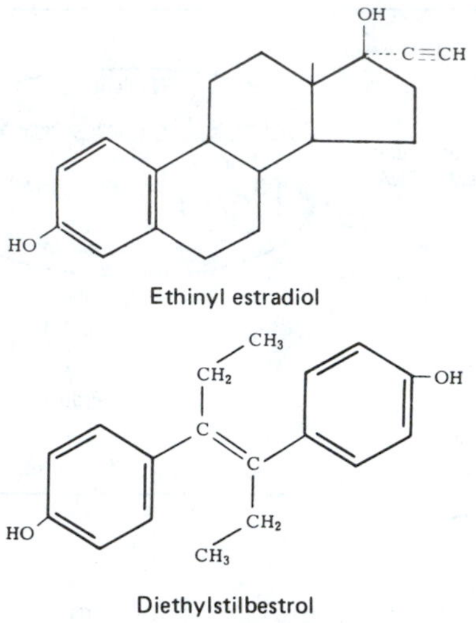

**Figure 6–16.** Synthetic estrogens (Reproduced, with permission, from Ganong WF: *Review of Medical Physiology*, 16th ed. Appleton & Lange, 1993.)

ference is due to secretion of small amounts of progesterone by cells in the ovarian follicle. During the luteal phase, the large amounts secreted by the corpus luteum cause ovarian secretion to increase about 20-fold (Fig 6–3). The result is an increase in plasma progesterone to a peak value of approximately 18 ng/mL (60 nmol/L) (Fig 6–11).

The stimulating effect of LH on progesterone secretion by the corpus luteum is due activation of adenylyl cyclase and involves a subsequent step that is dependent on protein synthesis.

## Actions of Progesterone

The principal target organs of progesterone are the uterus, the breasts, and the brain. Progesterone is responsible for the progestational changes in the endometrium and the cyclic changes in the cervix and vagina described above. It has anti-estrogenic effects on the myometrial cells, decreasing their excitability, their sensitivity to oxytocin, and their spontaneous electrical activity, while increasing their membrane potential. It decreases the number of estrogen receptors in the endometrium and increases the rate of conversion of 17β-estradiol to less active estrogens.

In the breast, progesterone stimulates the development of lobules and alveoli. It induces differentiation of estrogen-prepared ductal tissue and supports the secretory function of the breast during lactation.

The feedback effects of progesterone are complex and are exerted at both the hypothalamic and the pituitary level. Large doses of progesterone inhibit LH secretion and potentiate the inhibitory effects of estrogens, preventing ovulation.

Progesterone is thermogenic and is probably responsible for the rise in basal body temperature at the

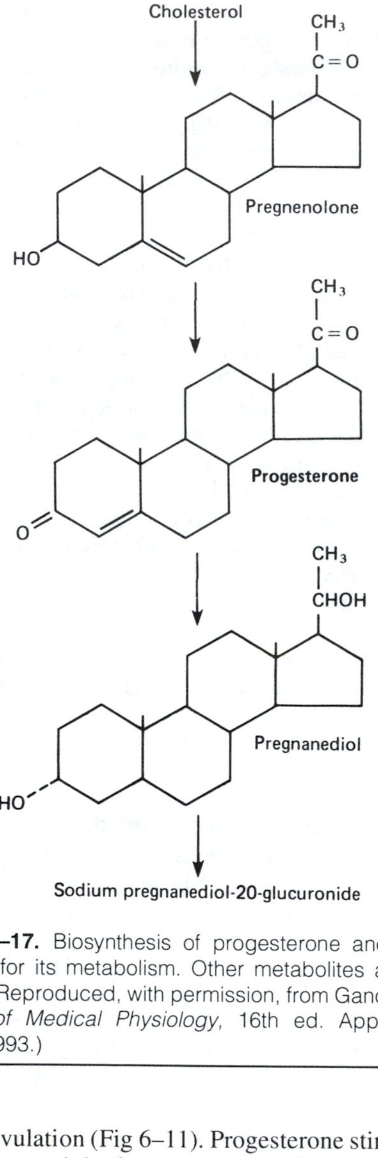

**Figure 6–17.** Biosynthesis of progesterone and major pathway for its metabolism. Other metabolites are also formed. (Reproduced, with permission, from Ganong WF: *Review of Medical Physiology*, 16th ed. Appleton & Lange, 1993.)

time of ovulation (Fig 6–11). Progesterone stimulates respiration, and the fact that alveolar $PCO_2$ in women during the luteal phase of the menstrual cycle is lower than that in men is attributed to the action of secreted progesterone. In pregnancy, alveolar $PCO_2$ falls as progesterone secretion rises.

Large doses of progesterone produce natriuresis, probably by blocking the action of aldosterone on the kidney. The hormone does not have a significant anabolic effect. The effects of progesterone, like those of other steroids, are brought about by an action on DNA to initiate synthesis of new mRNA. The progesterone receptor is bound to a heat shock protein in the absence of the steroid, and progesterone binding releases the heat shock protein, exposing the DNA-binding domain of the receptor. The synthetic steroid **mifepristone (RU-486)** binds to the receptor but does not release the heat shock protein, and it blocks the binding of progesterone. Since the maintenance of early pregnancy depends on the stimulatory effect of progesterone on endometrial growth and its inhibition of uterine contractility, mifepristone causes abortion. In some countries, mifepristone combined with a prostaglandin is used to produce elective abortions.

Substances that mimic the action of progesterone are sometimes called **progestational agents, gestagens,** or **progestins.** They are used along with synthetic estrogens as oral contraceptive agents.

## PREMENSTRUAL SYNDROME

Some women develop symptoms such as irritability, bloating, edema, emotional lability, decreased ability to concentrate, depression, headache, and constipation during the last 7–10 days of their menstrual cycles. These symptoms of the **premenstrual syndrome (PMS)** have been attributed to salt and water retention. However, it seems unlikely that this or any of the other hormonal alterations that occur in the late luteal phase are responsible because the time course and severity of the symptoms are not modified if the luteal phase is terminated early and menstruation produced by administration of mifepristone. Therefore, at present the cause of the premenstrual syndrome must be listed as unknown.

## RELAXIN

Relaxin is a polypeptide hormone that is secreted by the corpus luteum in women and the prostate in men. During pregnancy, it relaxes the pubic symphysis and other pelvic joints and softens and dilates the uterine cervix during pregnancy. Thus, it facilitates delivery. It also inhibits uterine contractions and may play a role in the development of the mammary glands. In nonpregnant women, relaxin is found in the corpus luteum and the endometrium during the secretory but not the proliferative phase of the menstrual cycle. Its function in nonpregnant women is unknown.

In most species, there is only one relaxin gene, but in humans there are 2 genes on chromosome 9 that code for 2 structurally different polypeptides that both have relaxin activity. However, only one of these genes is active in the ovary and the prostate. The structure of the polypeptide produced in these 2 tissues is shown in Fig 6–18.

## INHIBINS AND ACTIVINS

Polypeptides called **inhibins** that inhibit FSH secretion were first isolated from testes, but it was soon discovered that they were also produced by the ovaries. There are 2 inhibins, and they are formed from 3 polypeptide subunits: a glycosylated α subunit with a molecular weight of 18,000, and 2 nonglycosylated β subunits, $\beta_A$ and $\beta_B$, each with a molecular weight of 14,000. The subunits are formed from precursor proteins (Fig 6–19). The α subunit combines with $\beta_A$ to form a heterodimer and with $\beta_B$ to form another heterodimer, with the subunits linked by disulfide bonds. Both $\alpha\beta_A$ (inhibin A) and $\alpha\beta_B$ (inhibin B) inhibit FSH secretion by a direct action on the pituitary. Inhibins are produced by Sertoli cells in males and granulosa cells in females.

The heterodimer $\beta_A\beta_B$ and the $\beta_A\beta_A$ and $\beta_B\beta_B$ stimulate rather than inhibit FSH secretion and consequently are called **activins.** Their function in reproduction is unsettled. However, the inhibins and activins are members of the TGFβ superfamily of dimeric growth factors that also includes the Müllerian inhibitory substance (MIS) that is important in embryonic development of the gonads. Two **activin receptors** have been cloned, and both appear to be serine kinases. Inhibins and activins are found not only in the gonads but also in the brain and many other tissues. In the bone marrow, activins are involved in the development of white blood cells. In embryonic life, activins are involved in the formation of mesoderm. All mice in which a targeted deletion of the α-inhibin gene was produced initially grew in a normal fashion but then developed gonadal stromal tumors, so the α-inhibin gene is a tumor-suppressor gene.

In plasma, $\alpha_{-2}$ macroglobulin binds activins and inhibins. In tissues, activins bind to a family of 4 glycoproteins called **follistatins.** Binding of the activins inactivates their biologic activity, but the relation of

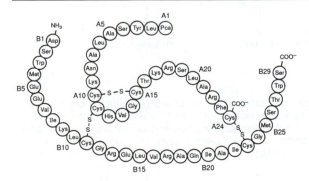

**Figure 6–18.** Structure of human luteal and prostatic relaxin. Note the A and B chains connected by disulfide bridges. Pca, pyroglutamic acid residue at N terminal of A chain. (Modified and reproduced, with permission, from Winslow, JW et al: Human seminal relaxin is a product of the same gene as human luteal relaxin. Endocrinology 1992;130:2660.)

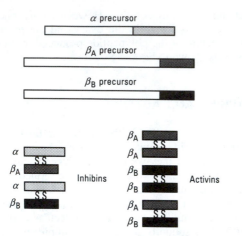

**Figure 6–19.** Inhibins and activins. The heterodimers formed by the combination of the α subunit with the $\beta_a$ subunit or the $\beta_b$ subunit are inhibins that suppress FSH secretion. The $\beta_a\beta_b$ heterodimer and the $\beta_a\beta_a$ and $\beta_b\beta_b$ homodimers are artivins that stimulate FSH secretion. SS, disulfide bonds. (Modified from Ganong WF: *Review of Medical Physiology*, 16th ed. Appleton & Lange, 1993).

follistatins to inhibin and their physiologic function are unsettled.

## PITUITARY HORMONES

Ovarian secretion depends on the action of hormones secreted by the anterior pituitary gland. The anterior pituitary gland secretes 6 established hormones: adrenocorticotropic hormone (ACTH) growth hormone, thyrotropic hormone (TSH) follicle-stimulating hormone (FSH) luteinizing hormone (LH) and prolactin (Fig 6–20). It also secretes one putative hormone β-lipotropic hormone (β-LPH).

## GONADOTROPINS

The gonadotropins FSH and LH act in concert to regulate the cyclic secretion of the ovarian hormones. They are glycoproteins made up of α and β subunits. The α subunits have the same amino acid composition as the α subunits in the glycoproteins TSH and human chorionic gonadotropin (hCG); the specificity of these 4 glycoprotein hormones is imparted by the different structures of their β subunits. The carbohydrates in the gonadotropin molecules increase the potency of the hormones by markedly slowing their metabolism. The half-life of human FSH is about 170 minutes; the half-life of LH is about 60 minutes.

The receptors for FSH and LH are serpentine receptors coupled to adenylyl cyclase through $G_S$. In addition, each has an extended, glycosylated extracellular domain.

### Hypothalamic Hormones

The secretion of the anterior pituitary hormones is regulated by the hypothalamic hypophysiotropic hormones. These substances are produced by neurons and enter the protal hypophysial vessels (Fig 6–21), a special group of blood vessels that transmit substances directly from the hypothalamus to the anterior

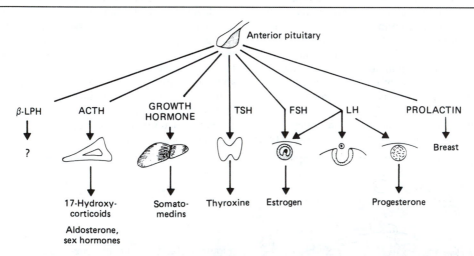

**Figure 6–20.** Anterior pituitary hormones. gb-LPH, gb-lipotropic hormone; ACTH, adenocorticotropic hormone; TSH, thyrotropic hormone; FSH, follicle-stimulating hormone; LH, luteinizing hormone. In women, FSH and LH act in sequence on the ovary to produce growth of the ovarian follicle, which secretes estrogen; ovulation; and formation and maintenance of the corpus luteum, which secretes estrogen and progesterone. In men, FSH and LH control the functions of the testes. Polactin stimulates lactation. (Reproduced, with permission, from Ganong WF: *Review of Medical Physiology,* 16th ed. Appleton & Lange, 1993.)

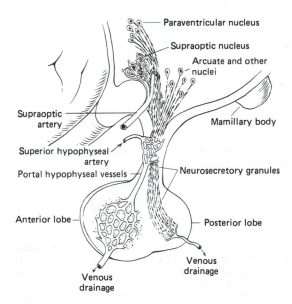

**Figure 6–21.** Simplified schematic reconstruction of the hypothalamus and the pituitary. (After Hansel; courtesy International Journal of Fertility. Redrawn and reproduced, with permission, from Schally et al: Hypothalamic regulatory hormones. Science 1973;179:341. Copyright 1973 by the American Association for the Advancement of Science.)

pituitary gland. The actions of these hormones are summarized in Fig 6–22. The structure of 6 established hypophysiotropic hormones is known (Fig 6–23). No single prolactin-releasing hormone has been isolated and identified. However, several polypeptides that are found in the hypothalamus can increase prolactin secretion, and one or more of these may stimulate prolactin secretion under physiologic conditions.

The posterior pituitary differs from the anterior in that its hormones, oxytocin and arginine vasopressin, are secreted by neurons directly in the systemic circulation. These hormones are produced in the cell bodies of neurons located in the supraoptic and paraventricular nuclei of the hypothalamus and transported down the axons of these neurons to their endings in the posterior lobe of the pituitary. The hormones are released from the endings into the circulation when action potentials pass down the axons and reach the endings. The structures of the hormones are shown in Fig 6–24.

## CONTROL OF OVARIAN FUNCTION

FSH from the pituitary is responsible for early maturation of the ovarian follicles, and FSH and LH together are responsible for final follicle maturation. A burst of LH secretion (Fig 6–11) triggers ovulation and the initial formation of the corpus luteum. There is also a smaller midcycle burst of FSH secretion the significance of which is uncertain. LH stimulates the secretion of estrogen and progesterone from the corpus luteum.

### Hypothalamic Components

The hypothalamus occupies a key role in the control of gonadotropin secretion. Hypothalamic control is exerted by GnRH secreted into the portal hypophyseal vessels. GnRH stimulates the secretion of FSH as well as LH and it is unlikely that there is an additional separate follicle-stimulating hormone-releasing hormone (FRH).

GnRH is normally secreted in episodic bursts (**circhoral secretion**). These bursts are essential for normal secretion of gonadotropins, which are also exerted in an episodic fashion (Fig 6–25). If GnRH is administered by constant infusion, the number of GnRH receptors in the anterior pituitary decreases (**down regulation**), and LH secretion falls to low levels. However, if GnRH is administered episodically at a rate of 1 pulse per hour, LH secretion is stimulated. This is true even when endogenous GnRH secretion has been prevented by a lesion of the ventral hypothalamus.

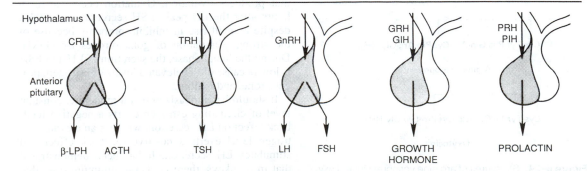

**Figure 6–22.** Effects of hypophysiotropic hormones on the secretion of anterior pituitary hormones. (Reproduced, with permission, from Ganong WF: *Review of Medical Physiology,* 14th ed. Appleton & Lange, 1989.)

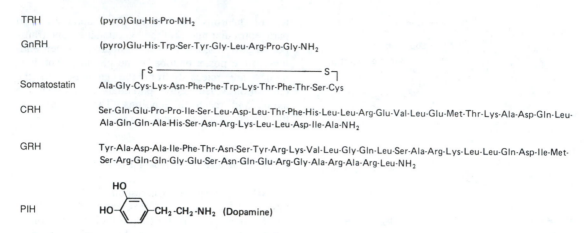

**Figure 6–23.** Structure of hypophyseotropic hormones in humans. The structure of somatostatin that is shown is the tetradecapeptide (somatostatin 14). In addition, presomotostatin is the source of an N-terminal extended polypeptide containing 28 amino acid residues (somatostatin 28) and a polypeptide containing 12 amino acid residues from the extended portion (somatostatin 28 [1–12]. These residues are found in many tissues.

It is now clear not only that episodic secretion of GnRH is a general phenomenon, but that fluctuations in the frequency and amplitude of the GnRH bursts are important in generating the other hormonal changes that are responsible for the menstrual cycle. Frequency is increased by estrogens and decreased by progesterone and testosterone. The frequency increases late in the follicular phase of the cycle, culminating in the LH surge. During the secretory phase, the frequency decreases as a result of the action of progesterone, but when estrogen and progesterone secretion decrease at the end of the cycle, frequency once again increases.

At the time of the midcycle LH surge, the sensitivity of the gonadotropins to GnRH is greatly increased because of their exposure to GnRH pulses of the frequency that exist at this time. This self-priming effect of GnRH is important in producing a maximum LH response.

The nature and the exact location of the GnRH pulse generator in the hypothalamus are still unsettled. However, it is known in a general way that norepinephrine and possibly epinephrine in the hypothalamus increase GnRH pulse frequencies. Conversely, opioid peptides such as the enkephalins and β-endorphin reduce the frequency of GnRH pulses.

The down regulation of pituitary receptors and the consequent decrease in LH secretion produced by constantly elevated levels of GnRH has led to the use of long-acting GnRH agonists to inhibit LH secretion in precocious puberty and cancer of the prostate.

**Feedback Effects**

Changes in plasma LH, FSH, sex steroids, and inhibin during the menstrual cycle are shown in Fig 6–11, and their feedback relations are diagrammed in Fig 6–26. During the early part of the follicular phase, inhibin is low and FSH is modestly elevated, fostering follicular growth. LH secretion is held in check by the negative feedback effect of the rising plasma estrogen level. At 36–48 hours before ovulation, the estrogen feedback effect becomes positive, and this initiates the burst of LH secretion (LH surge) that produces ovulation. Ovulation occurs about 9 hours after the LH peak. FSH secretion also peaks, despite a small rise in inhibin, probably because of the strong stimulation of gonadotropes by GnRH. During the luteal phase, the secretion of LH and FSH is low because of the elevated levels of estrogen, progesterone, and inhibin.

It should be emphasized that a moderate, constant level of circulating estrogen exerts a negative feedback effect on LH secretion, whereas an elevated estrogen level exerts a positive feedback effect and stimulates LH secretion. It has been demonstrated that in monkeys, there is also a minimum time that estrogens must be elevated to produce positive feed-

Cys-Tyr-Phe-Gln-Asn-Cys-Pro-Arg-Gly-NH₂

Arginine vasopressin

Cys-Tyr-Ile-Gln-Asn-Cys-Pro-Leu-Gly-NH₂

Oxytocin

**Figure 6–24.** Structures of arginine vasopressin and oxytocin. (Reproduced, with permission, from Ganong WF: *Reivew of Medical Physiology*, 16th ed. Appleton & Lange, 1993.)

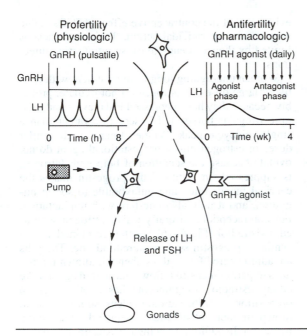

**Figure 6–25.** Profertility and antifertility actions of GnRH and its agonists. The normal secretion of GnRH is pulsatile, occurring at 30–60 minute intervals. This mode, which can be mimicked by timed injections, produces circhoral peaks of LH and FSH secretion and promotes fertility. If GnRH is administered by continuous infusion, or if one of its long-acting synthetic agonists is injected, there is initial stimulation of the pituitary receptors. However, this lasts for only a few days, and is followed by receptor down-regulation with inhibition of gonadotropin secretion (antifertility effect). (Reproduced, with permission, from Conn PM, Crowley WF Jr,: Gonadotropin-releasing hormone and its analogues. New Engl J Med 1991;324:93).

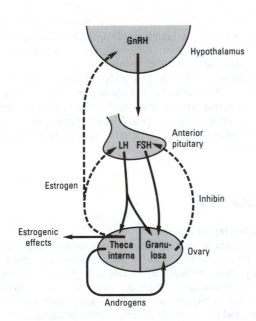

**Figure 6–26.** Feedback regulation of ovarian function. The cells of the theca interna provide androgens to the granulosa cells, and the thecal cells produce the circulating estrogens, which inhibit the secretion of LH, GnRH, and FSH. Inhibins from the granulosa cells also inhibit FSH secretion. LH regulates thecal cells, whereas the granulosa cells are regulated by both LH and FSH. The dashed arrows indicate inhibition, and the solid arrows indicate stimulation. (Reproduced, with permission, from Ganong WF: *Review of Medical Physiology*, 16th ed. Appleton & Lange, 1993.)

back. When circulating estrogen was increased about 300% for 24 hours, only negative feedback was seen; but when it was increased about 300% for 36 hours or more, a brief decline in secretion was followed by a burst of LH secretion that resembled the midcycle surge. When circulating levels of progesterone were high, the positive feedback effect of estrogen was inhibited. There is evidence that in primates, both the negative and the positive feedback effects of estrogen are exerted in the mediobasal hypothalamus, but exactly how negative feedback is switched to positive feedback and then back to negative feedback in the luteal phase remains unknown.

## Control of Menstrual Cycle

In an important sense, regression of the corpus luteum (**luteolysis**) is the key to the menstrual cycle. There is some evidence that prostaglandins may play a role in this process, possibly by inhibiting the effect of LH on cyclic AMP. In some domestic animals, oxytocin secreted by the corpus luteum appears to exert a local luteolytic effect, possibly via release of prostaglandins. Once luteolysis begins, the estrogen and progesterone levels fall and the secretion of FSH and LH increases. A new crop of follicles develops and then a single dominant follicle matures as the result of the action of FSH and LH. Near midcycle, there is a rise in estrogen secretion from the follicle. This rise augments the responsiveness of the pituitary to GnRH and triggers a burst of LH secretion. The resulting ovulation is followed by formation of a corpus luteum. There is a drop in estrogen secretion, but progesterone and estrogen levels then rise together.

The elevated estrogen and progesterone levels inhibit FSH and LH secretion for a while, but luteolysis again occurs, and a new cycle starts.

## Reflex Ovulation

Female cats, rabbits, mink, and certain other animals have long periods of **estrus,** or heat, during which they ovulate only after copulation. Such **reflex ovulation** is brought about by afferent impulses from the genitalia and the eyes, ears, and nose that converge on the ventral hypothalamus and provoke an ovulation-inducing release of LH from the pituitary. In species such as rats, monkeys, and humans, ovulation is a spontaneous periodic phenomenon, but afferent impulses converging on the hypothalamus can also exert effects. Ovulation can be delayed for 24 hours in rats by administering pentobarbital or other neurally active drugs 12 hours before the expected time of follicle rupture. In women, menstrual cycles may be markedly influenced by emotional stimuli.

## Contraception

Methods commonly used to prevent conception are listed in Table 6–4, along with their failure rates. Once conception has occurred, abortion can be produced by progesterone antagonists such as mifepristone.

Implantation of foreign bodies in the uterus causes changes in the duration of the sexual cycle in a number of mammalian species. In humans, such foreign bodies do not alter the menstrual cycle, but they act as effective contraceptive devices. Intrauterine implantation of pieces of metal or plastic **intrauterine devices, IUDs)** has been used in programs aimed at controlling population growth. Although their mechanism of action is still unsettled, there is

evidence that the contraceptive effect of IUDs is due in part, to a spermicidal action. Their usefulness is limited by their tendency to cause intrauterine infections.

Women undergoing long-term treatment with relatively large doses of estrogen do not ovulate, probably because they have depressed FSH levels and multiple irregular bursts of LH secretion rather than a single midcycle peak. Women treated with similar doses of estrogen plus a progestational agent do not ovulate because the secretion of both gonadotropins is suppressed. In addition, the progestin makes the cervical mucus thick and unfavorable to sperm migration, and it may also interfere with implantation. For contraception, an orally active estrogen such as ethinylstradiol (Fig 6–16) is often combined with a synthetic progestin such as norethindrone. The pills are administered for 21 days, then withdrawn for 5–7 days to permit menstrual flow, and started again. Like ethinyl estradiol, norethindrone has an ethinyl group on position 17 of the steroid nucleus, so it is resistant to hepatic metabolism and consequently is effective by mouth. In addition to being a progestin, it is partly metabolized to ethinyl estradiol, and for this reason it also has estrogenic activity. It is now clear that small as well as large doses of estrogen are effective (Table 6–4); the use of small dose reduces the risk of thromboses or other complications. Progestins alone can be used for contraception, although they are more effective when combined with estrogens.

Implants made up primarily of progestins are now seeing increased use in some parts of the world. The implants are inserted under the skin and can prevent pregnancy for up to 5 years. They often produce amenorrhea but otherwise appear to be well tolerated.

**Table 6–4.** Relative effectiveness of frequently used contraceptive methods.[1]

| Method | Failures per 100 Woman-Years |
|---|---|
| Vasectomy | 0.02 |
| Tubal ligation and similar procedures | 0.13 |
| Oral contraceptive | |
| > 50 μg estrogen and progestin | 0.32 |
| < 50 μg estrogen and progestin | 0.27 |
| Progestin only | 1.2 |
| IUD | |
| Copper 7 | 1.5 |
| Loop D | 1.3 |
| Diaphragm | 1.9 |
| Condom | 3.6 |
| Withdrawal | 6.7 |
| Spermicide | 11.9 |
| Rhythm | 15.5 |

[1]Data from Vessey M, Lawless M, Yeates D: Efficacy of different contraceptive methods. Lancet 1982;1:841. Reproduced with permission.

# PROLACTIN

## Chemistry of Prolactin

Prolactin is another anterior pituitary hormone that has important functions in reproduction and pregnancy. It is difficult to distinguish prolactin from growth hormone in humans, because growth hormone has lactogenic activity and, except during pregnancy and lactation, there is very little prolactin in the human pituitary. The prolactin molecule contains 199 amino acid residues and 3 disulfide bridges (Fig 6–27) and has considerable structural similarity to human growth hormone and human chorionic somatomammotropin (hCS). The half-life of prolactin, like that of growth hormone, is about 20 minutes. Structurally similar prolactins are secreted by the endometrium and by the placenta.

The human prolactin receptor resembles the growth hormone receptor and is one of the super-

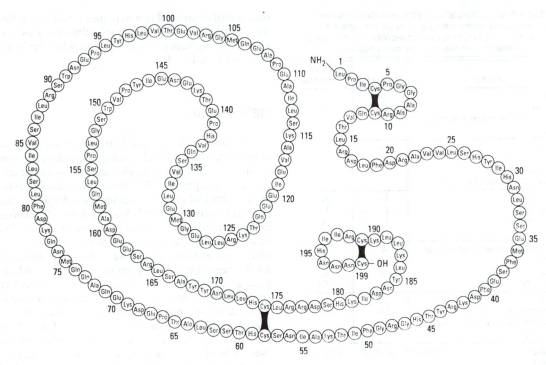

**Figure 6–27.** Structure of human prolactin. (Reproduced, with permission, from Bondy PK, Rosenberg LE: *Metabolic Control and Disease,* 8th ed. Saunders, 1980.)

family of receptors that includes the growth hormone receptor and receptors for many cytokines and hematopoietic growth factors. When activated, its cytoplasmic domain may have tyrosine kinase activity, but the exact mechanism of signal transduction is unknown.

## Actions

Prolactin causes milk secretion from the breast after estrogen and progesterone priming. Its effect on the breast involves increased action of mRNA and increased production of casein and lactalbumin. However, the action of the hormone is not exerted on the cell nucleus and is prevented by inhibitors of microtubules. Prolactin also inhibits the effects of gonadotropins, possibly by an action at the level of the ovary.

## Regulation of Prolactin Secretion

In laboratory animals and in humans, the secretion of prolactin is clearly independent of that of growth hormone. The normal plasma prolactin concentration is approximately 8 ng/mL in women and 5 ng/mL in men. Secretion is tonically inhibited by the hypothalamus, and section of the pituitary stalk leads to an increase in circulating prolactin. Thus, the effect of hypothalamic **prolactin-inhibiting hormone (PIH)** usually overbalances the effect of the putative **pro-**

**lactin-releasing hormone (PRH).** As noted above, PIH is dopamine secreted by the tuberoinfundibular dopaminergic neurons into the portal hypophyseal vessels, and there are several hypothalamic polypeptides with PRH activity. These include thyrotropin-releasing hormone (TRH), vasoactive intestinal polypeptide (VIP), and oxytocin. In humans, prolactin secretion is increased by exercise, surgical and psychologic stresses, and stimulation of the nipples (Table 6–5). Plasma prolactin rises during sleep, the rise starting after the onset of sleep and persisting throughout sleep. Secretion is increased during pregnancy, reaching a peak at the time of parturition. After delivery, plasma concentration falls to nonpregnant levels in about 8 days. Suckling produces a prompt increase in secretion, but the magnitude of this rise gradually declines after a woman has been nursing for longer than 3 months. With prolonged lactation, milk secretion occurs with prolactin levels that are in the normal range.

L-dopa decreases prolactin secretion by increasing the formation of dopamine. Drugs such as apomorphine and bromocriptine inhibit prolactin secretion because they stimulate dopamine receptors. Chlorpromazine and related drugs that block dopamine receptors increase prolactin secretion. Estrogens produce a slowly developing increase in prolactin secretion.

**Table 6–5.** Factors affecting the secretion of human prolactin and growth hormone. I, moderate increase; I+, marked increase; I++, very marked increase; N, no change; D, moderate decrease; D+, marked decrease.[1]

| Factor | Prolactin | Growth Hormone |
|---|---|---|
| Sleep | I+ | I+ |
| Nursing | I++ | N |
| Breast stimulation in nonlactating women | I | N |
| Stress | I+ | I+ |
| Hypoglycemia | I | I+ |
| Strenuous exercise | I | I |
| Sexual intercourse in women | I | N |
| Pregnancy | I++ | N |
| Estrogens | I | I |
| Hypothyroidism | I | N |
| TRH | I+ | N |
| Phenothiazines, butyrophenones | I+ | N |
| Opiates | I | I |
| Glucose | N | D |
| Somatostatin | N | D+ |
| L-Dopa | D+ | I+ |
| Apomorphine | D+ | I+ |
| Bromocriptine and related ergot derivatives | D+ | I |

[1]Modified from Frantz A: Prolactin. N Eng J Med 1978; 298:201.

It is now established that prolactin facilitates the secretion of dopamine in the median eminence. Thus, prolactin acts in the hypothalamus in a negative feedback fashion to inhibit its own secretion.

## Hyperprolactinemia

Up to 70% of patients with chromophobe adenomas of the anterior pituitary have elevated plasma prolactin levels. In some instances, the elevation may be due to damage to the pituitary stalk, but in most cases, the tumor cells actually secrete the hormone. The hyperprolactinemia may cause galactorrhea, but in many individuals, there are no demonstrable abnormalities. Indeed, most women with galactorrhea have normal prolactin levels; definite elevations are found in less than one-third of patients with this condition.

It is also interesting to note that 15–20% of women with secondary amenorrhea have elevated prolactin levels and that when prolactin secretion is reduced, normal menstrual cycles and fertility return. It appears that prolactin may produce amenorrhea by blocking the action of gonadotropins on the ovaries,

but definitive proof of this hypothesis must await further research. In men, hyperprolactinemia is associated with impotence that disappears when prolactin secretion is reduced.

## MENOPAUSE

The human ovary gradually becomes unresponsive to gonadotropins with advancing age, and its function declines, so that sexual cycles and menstruation disappear (menopause). This unresponsiveness is associated with and probably caused by a decline in the number of primordial follicles (Fig 6–6). The ovaries no longer secrete progesterone and 17β-estradiol in appreciable quantities. Estrogen is formed by aromatization of androstenedione in the circulation, but the amounts are normally small. The uterus and vagina gradually become atrophic. As the negative feedback effect of the estrogens and progesterone is reduced, secretion of FSH and LH is increased, and plasma FSH and LH rise to high levels. Old female mice and rats have long periods of diestrus and increased levels of gonadotropin secretion, but a clearcut "menopause" has apparently not been described in animals.

In women, the menses usually become irregular and cease between the ages of 45 and 55. The average age at onset of the menopause has increased since the turn of the century and is currently about 52 years.

Sensations of warmth spreading from the trunk to the face ("hot flushes," also called hot flashes) and various psychic symptoms are common after ovarian function has ceased. The hot flushes are prevented by administration of estrogen. They are not peculiar to the menopause; they also occur in premenopausal women and men whose gonads are removed surgically or destroyed by disease. Their cause is unknown. However, it has been demonstrated that they coincide with surges of LH secretion. LH is secreted in episodic bursts at intervals of 30–60 minutes or more (circhoral secretion), and in the absence of gonadal hormones, these bursts are large. Each hot flush begins with the start of a burst. However, LH itself is not responsible for the symptoms, because they can continue after removal of the pituitary. Instead, it appears that some event in the hypothalamus initiates both the release of LH and the episode of flushing. The menopause and the clinical management of patients with menopausal symptoms are discussed in more detail in Chapter 57.

# REFERENCES

Baird DT, Glasier AF: Hormonal contraception. N Engl J Med 1993;328:1543.

Baulieu EE: Contragestion and other clinical applications of RU 486, an antiprogesterone at the receptor. Science 1989;245:1351.

Bulleti C, Gurpide F (editors): The primate endometrium. Ann NY Acad Sci 1991;622:1.

Conn PM, Crowley WJ Jr: Gonadotropin-releasing hormone and its analogs. N Engl J Med 1991;324:93.

Falkner F, Tanner JM (editors): *Human Growth,* 2nd ed, 2 vols. Plenum, 1986.

Ganong WF: *Review of Medical Physiology,* 16th ed. Appleton & Lange, 1993.

Knobil E, Neill JD (editors): *The Physiology of Reproduction.* 2 vols. Raven Press, 1987.

Weiss G: The physiology of human relaxin. Contrib Gynecol Obstet 1991;18:130.

Wilson JB, Foster DW: *Williams' Textbook of Endocrinology,* 7th ed. Saunders, 1985.

Winston RML, Handyside AH: New challenges in human in vitro fertilization. Science 1993;260:932.

Yen SSC, Jaffe RB (editors): *Reproductive Endocrinology,* 3rd ed. Saunders, 1991.

# 7

# Maternal Physiology During Pregnancy

*Pamela J. Moore, PhD*

The physiologic, biochemical, and anatomic changes that occur during pregnancy are extensive and may be systemic or local. However, most systems return to prepregnancy status between the time of delivery and 6 weeks postpartum.

Teleologic alterations during pregnancy maintain a healthy environment for the fetus without compromising the mother's health. Thus, in most instances, physiologic activity is increased in pregnant women, but smooth muscle (eg, urinary and gastrointestinal tracts) demonstrates decreased activity. Many laboratory values are dramatically altered from nonpregnant values. An understanding of the normal physiologic changes induced by pregnancy is essential in understanding coincidental disease processes.

## GASTROINTESTINAL TRACT

During pregnancy, nutritional requirements, including those for vitamins and minerals, are increased, and several maternal alterations occur to meet this demand. Pregnant women tend to rest more often, conserving their energy and thereby enhancing fetal nutrition. Although the mother's appetite usually increases, so that food intake is greater, some women have a decreased appetite or experience nausea and vomiting (see Chapter 9). These symptoms may be related to relative levels of human chorionic gonadotropin (hCG). In rare instances, women may crave bizarre substances such as clay, cornstarch, soap, or even coal.

### Oral Cavity

During pregnancy, several changes may occur in the oral cavity. Salivation may seem to increase due to swallowing difficulty associated with nausea, and, if pH of the oral cavity decreases, tooth decay may occur. Tooth decay during pregnancy, however, is not due to lack of calcium in the teeth. Indeed, dental calcium is stable and not mobilized during pregnancy as is bone calcium.

The gums may become hypertrophic and hyperemic; often, they are so spongy and friable that they bleed easily. This may be due to increased systemic estrogen; similar problems sometimes occur with the use of oral contraceptives. Vitamin C deficiency also can cause tenderness and bleeding of the gums. The gums should return to normal in the early puerperium.

### Gastrointestinal Motility

Gastrointestinal motility may be reduced during pregancy due to increased levels of progesterone, which in turn decrease the production of motilin, a hormonal peptide that is known to stimulate smooth muscle in the gut. Gastric emptying has generally been considered to be slowed during pregnancy; however, recent work by Macfie et al (1991) via indirect methods have shown no changes in gastric emptying rates of women in the first or second trimesters or at term. Transit time of food through the gastrointestinal tract may be so much slower that more water than normal is reabsorbed, leading to constipation.

### Stomach and Esophagus

Gastric production of hydrochloric acid is variable and sometimes exaggerated, especially during the first trimester. More commonly, gastric acidity is reduced. Production of the hormone gastrin (which may be manufactured by the placenta) increases significantly, resulting in increased stomach volume and decreased stomach pH. Gastric production of mucus may be increased. Esophageal peristalsis is decreased, accompanied by gastric reflux because of the slower emptying time and dilatation or relaxation of the cardiac sphincter. Gastric reflux is more prevalent in later pregnancy owing to elevation of the stomach by the enlarged uterus. These conditions may simulate hiatal hernia. Besides leading to heartburn, all of these alterations (increased stomach acidity, slower emptying time, and increased intragastric pressure caused by the enlarged uterus), as well as lying in the supine lithotomy position, make the use of anesthesia more hazardous because of the increased possibility of regurgitation and aspiration.

### Small and Large Bowel and Appendix

As the uterus grows and the stomach is pushed upward, most areas of the large and small bowel move upward and laterally. The appendix is displaced superiorly in the right flank area (see Fig 24–1). These organs return to their normal positions in the early puerperium. As noted previously, motility is generally decreased and gastrointestinal tone is decreased.

## Gallbladder

Gallbladder function is also altered during pregnancy because of hypotonia of the smooth muscle wall. Emptying time is slowed and often incomplete. Thus, at the time of cesarean section, the gallbladder often appears dilated and atonic. Bile can become thick, and bile stasis may lead to gallstone formation. The chemical composition of bile is not appreciably altered. Plasma cholinesterase activity is decreased during normal pregnancy.

## Liver

There are no apparent morphologic changes in the liver during normal pregnancy, but there are functional alterations. Serum alkaline phosphatase activity can double, probably because of increased placental alkaline phosphatase isozymes. There is also a decrease in plasma albumin and a slight decrease in plasma globulins. Thus, a decrease in the albumin/globulin ratio occurs normally in pregnancy. In nonpregnant patients, such a decrease could be an indication of liver disease.

## KIDNEYS & URINARY TRACT

### Renal Dilatation

During pregnancy, each kidney increases in length by 1–1.5 cm, with a concomitant increase in weight. The renal pelvis is dilated up to 60 mL (10 mL is the normal volume in nonpregnant women). The ureters are dilated above the brim of the bony pelvis, more so on the right side than on the left. The ureters also elongate, widen, and become more curved, although kinking is rare. Thus, there is an increase in urinary stasis. As much as 200 mL of residual urine may be present in the dilated collecting system.

Although the absolute cause of hydronephrosis and hydroureter in pregnancy is unknown, there may be several contributing factors: (1) Elevated progesterone levels may contribute to hypotonia of smooth muscle in the ureter. However, high progesterone levels do not cause hydroureter in nonpregnant women. (2) The ovarian vein complex in the suspensory (infundibulopelvic) ligament of the ovary may enlarge enough to compress the ureter at the brim of the bony pelvis, thus causing dilatation above that level. (3) Dextrorotation of the uterus during pregnancy may explain why the right ureter is usually dilated more than the left. (4) Hyperplasia of smooth muscle in the distal one-third of the ureter may cause reduction in luminal size, leading to dilatation in the upper two-thirds. Whatever the cause of dilatation, the effect is stasis of urine. This may lead to infection and may make tests of renal function difficult to interpret.

### Renal Function

The changes in renal function that occur during pregnancy are probably due to increased maternal and placental hormones, including adrenocorticotropic hormone (ACTH), antidiuretic hormone (ADH), aldosterone, cortisol, human chorionic somatomammotropin (hCS), and thyroid hormone. An additional factor is the increase in plasma volume. The glomerular filtration rate (GFR) increases during pregnancy by about 50%; the increase begins early in pregnancy, and levels remain relatively high until term, with value returning to normal by 20 weeks postpartum. The renal plasma flow (RPF) rate increases by as much as 25–50% throughout early and mid pregnancy (Table 7–1). Differences exist in observations of RPF in late pregnancy. Lind (1985) suggests that the maximum rate of RPF occurs by the end of the second trimester, with the rate remaining constant until term. Posture has little effect on the rate. Urinary flow and sodium excretion rates in late pregnancy can be altered by posture, being twice as great in the lateral recumbent position as in the supine position. Thus, posture must be taken into account whenever measurements of urinary function are taken. Collection periods should be at least 12–24 hours to allow for errors caused by the greatly dilated areas of the urinary tract.

At rest, 20% of the cardiac output is delivered to the kidneys. As much as 80% of the filtrate is resorbed by the proximal tubules independent of hormonal control. If this were not so, urine volume would be approximately 150 L/d. The sodium resorbed in the distal tubules is responsive to aldosterone. The concentration of the urine is ultimately determined by ADH activity. Even though the GFR increases dramatically during pregnancy, the volume

**Table 7–1.** Changes in kidney function during pregnancy.[1]

| Time | Renal Plasma Flow (mL/min) | Glomerular Filtration Rate (mL/min) |
|---|---|---|
| **Pregnancy** | | |
| 13 weeks | 804.67 | 161.33 |
| 20.8 weeks | 749.13 | 157.11 |
| 38 weeks | 589 | 146 |
| **Postpartum** | | |
| 20 weeks | 491 | 100 |
| 80 weeks | 549 | 97 |

[1]Reproduced, with permission, from Sims EAH, Krantz KE: Serial studies of renal function during pregnancy and the puerperium in normal women. *J Clin Invest* 1958;**37:**1764. Copyright permission from the American Society for Clinical Investigation. Tabulation from Danforth DN (editor): Page 334 in: *Obstetrics and Gynecology,* 4th ed. Harper & Row, 1982.

of urine passed each day is not increased. Thus, the urinary system appears to be even more efficient during pregnancy.

With the increase in GFR, there is an increase in endogenous clearance of creatinine; the peak increase at 50% above nonpregnancy levels occurs at about 32 weeks' gestation, after which time creatinine clearance decreases as term approaches. The concentration of creatinine in serum is reduced in proportion to the increase in GFR, and the concentration of blood urea nitrogen is similarly reduced. A nonpregnant woman excretes an average of 0.7–1 g/24 h of creatinine. In pregnant women, serum creatinine is 0.46 ± 0.13 mg/100 mL (nonpregnant values = 0.67 ± 0.14 mg/100 mL). Blood urea nitrogen is reduced in pregnancy (8.17 ± 1.5 mg/100 mL; nonpregnant values = 13 ± 3 mg/100 mL).

Glucosuria during pregnancy is not necessarily abnormal; glucose is excreted in the urine at sometime during pregnancy in more than 50% of women. Glucosuria may be explained by the increase in GFR with impairment of tubular resorption capacity for filtered glucose. Glucose is excreted in varying amounts and in a random pattern not related to blood glucose levels. Glucosuria during pregnancy, though common, should be monitored closely because it may also be a sign of diabetes mellitus. Increased levels of urinary glucose also contribute to increased susceptibility of pregnant women to urinary tract infection. For unknown reasons, normal pregnant women demonstrate increased loss of nutrients in the urine (eg, amino acids, water–soluble vitamins).

Proteinuria changes little during pregnancy; 200–300 mg/24 h of protein is lost normally. If more than 500 mg/24 h is lost (except during vigorous labor), a disease process should be suspected.

Levels of the enzyme renin, which is produced in the kidney, increase early in the first trimester, and continue to rise until term. This enzyme acts on its substrate angiotensinogen, which is formed in the liver, to first form angiotensin I and then angiotensin II, which acts as a vasoconstrictor. Levels of angiotensin I and angiotensin II also increase, but the vasoconstriction that might be expected does not occur, and there is no subsequent rise in blood pressure. Normal pregnant women are resistant to the pressor effect of elevated levels of angiotensin II (Fig 7–1), but those suffering from preeclampsia are not resistant (see Chapter 19). Angiotensin II is also a major stimulus for adrenocortical secretion of aldosterone, which in conjunction with ADH encourages salt and water retention in pregnancy.

### Bladder

As the uterus enlarges, the urinary bladder is displaced upward and flattened in the anterior-posterior or diameter. Pressure from the uterus leads to increased urinary frequency. Bladder vascularity in-

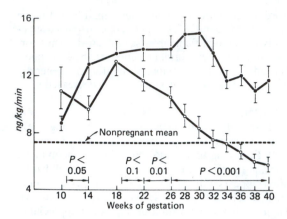

**Figure 7–1.** Comparison of mean angiotensin II doses required to evoke a pressor response in 120 primigravidas who remained normotensive (●) and 72 primigravidas who ultimately developed preeclampsia (○). (Reproduced, with permission, from Gant NF et al: A prospective study of angiotensin II pressor response throughout primigravid pregnancy. J Clin Invest 1973;52: 2682. Copyright permission from the American Society for Clinical Investigation.)

creases and muscle tone decreases, increasing capacity up to 1500 mL.

## HEMATOLOGIC SYSTEM

### Blood Volume

Perhaps the most striking maternal physiologic alteration occurring during pregnancy is the increase in blood volume. The magnitude of the increase varies according to the size of the woman, the number of pregnancies she has had, the number of infants she has delivered, and whether there is one or multiple fetuses. A small woman may have an increase in blood volume of only 20%, whereas a large woman may have an increase of 100%. The increase progresses until term (Fig 7–2); the average increase in volume at term is 45–50%. Hypervolemia begins in the first trimester,increases rapidly in the second trimester, and plateaus at about the 30th week; some studies have demonstrated a slight decline in the last 10 weeks of gestation.

The mechanisms responsible for increased blood volume are not totally understood. Aldosterone, which is elevated during pregnancy, may contribute to this effect, as may elevated levels of estrogen and progesterone. The increase is needed for extra blood flow to the uterus, extra metabolic needs of the fetus, and increased perfusion of other organs, especially the kidneys. There is also extra blood flow to the skin, allowing dissipation of heat caused by the increased metabolic rate. Extra volume also compensates for

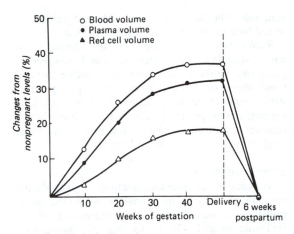

**Figure 7–2.** Changes in total blood volume, plasma volume, and red blood cell volume during pregnancy and the postpartum period. Graph constructed from several reports in the literature. (Reproduced, with permission, from Peck TM, Arias F: Hematologic changes associated with pregnancy. Clin Obstet Gynecol 1979;22:785.)

maternal blood loss at delivery. The average blood loss with vaginal delivery is 500–600 mL, and with cesarean section, 1000 mL.

**A. Red Blood Cells:** The increase in red blood cell mass is about 33%, or approximately 450 mL of erythrocytes. Erythrocyte volume increases steadily whether or not iron supplementation is given, but the increase is greater with supplementation. Since plasma volume increases earlier in pregnancy and faster than red blood cell volume, the hematocrit falls until the end of the second trimester, when the increase in red blood cells is synchronized with the plasma volume increase. The hematocrit then stabilizes or may increase slightly near term.

**B. Iron:** With the increase in red blood cells, the need for iron for the production of hemoglobin naturally increases. If supplemental iron is not added to the diet, **iron deficiency anemia** will result (see Chapter 22). Maternal requirements can reach 6–7 mg/d in the latter half of pregnancy. If iron is not readily available, the fetus uses iron from maternal stores. Thus, the production of fetal hemoglobin is usually adequate even if the mother is severely iron-deficient. Therefore, anemia in the newborn is rarely a problem; instead, maternal iron deficiency more commonly may cause preterm labor and late spontaneous abortion, increasing the incidence of infant wastage and morbidity.

**C. White Blood Cells:** The total blood leukocyte count increases during normal pregnancy from a prepregnancy level of 4300–4500/μL to 5000–12,000/μL in the last trimester, although counts as high as 16,000/μL have been observed in the last trimester. Counts as high as 25,000–30,000/μL have

been noted in normal patients during labor. Lymphocyte and monocyte numbers stay essentially the same throughout pregnancy; polymorphonuclear leukocytes are the primary contributors to the increase. Studies by Krause et al (1987) indicate an impairment in polymorphonuclear leukocyte chemotaxis that appears to be a cell-associated defect. Pregnant women in the third trimester demonstrated a decrease in polymorphonuclear leukocyte adherence. These results may explain an increased incidence of infection in pregnant women, which has been reported by other investigators. Basophils decrease slightly. There is controversy about whether eosinophil numbers increase, decrease, or remain the same as pregnancy advances. There is no apparent explanation for these discrepancies. Levels are only plus or minus 2–3% from normal prepregnancy levels.

**D. Platelets:** Recent studies (Tygart, 1986) have reported an apparent increase in the manufacture of platelets (thrombocytopoiesis) during pregnancy that is accompanied by progressive platelet consumption. Levels of prostacyclin ($PGI_2$), a platelet aggregation inhibitor, and thromboxane $A_2$, an inducer of platelet aggregation and a vasoconstrictor, both increase during pregnancy.

**E. Clotting Factors:** During pregnancy, levels of several essential coagulation factors increase. There are marked increases in fibrinogen (factor I) and factor VIII. Factors VII, IX, X, and XII also increase but to a lesser extent.

Plasma fibrinogen concentrations begin to increase from normal, nonpregnant levels (1.5–4.5 g/L) during the third month of pregnancy and progressively rise until late pregnancy (4–6.5 g/L). Indeed, with the increase in plasma volume, circulating fibrinogen levels toward the end of pregnancy approach double that of the nonpregnant state. Fibrinogen synthesis may be increased because of its utilization in the uteroplacental circulation, or it may be the result of hormonal changes, particularly high levels of estrogen.

Prothrombin (factor II) is only slightly affected by pregnancy, if at all. Some investigators have noted small increases; others have reported normal values. Recent studies have also noted mild increases in factor V, and suggest a "thrombin like" influence on the activity of factor V. Factor XI decreases slightly toward the end of pregnancy, and factor XIII (fibrin-stabilizing factor) is appreciably reduced, up to 50% at term.

Fibrinolytic activity is depressed during pregnancy and labor, although the precise mechanism is unknown. The placenta may be partially responsible for this alteration in fibrinolytic status. Plasminogen levels increase concomitantly with fibrinogen levels, causing an equilibration of clotting and lysing activity.

Clearly, coagulation and fibrinolytic systems undergo major alterations during pregnancy. Understanding these physiologic changes is necessary to manage 2 of the more serious problems of pregnancy—hemorrhage and thromboembolic disease—both caused by disorders in the mechanism of hemostasis (see Chapter 58).

## CARDIOVASCULAR SYSTEM

### Position & Size of Heart

As the uterus enlarges and the diaphragm becomes elevated, the heart is displaced upward and somewhat to the left with rotation on its long axis, so that the apex beat is moved laterally. Cardiac capacity increases by 70—80 mL; this may be due to increased volume or to hypertrophy of cardiac muscle. The size of the heart appears to increase by about 12%.

### Heart Rhythms & Murmurs

With the anatomic changes in the heart, there may also be alterations in heart rhythm and electrocardiographic findings, and nonpathologic murmurs may occur. Electrocardiographic changes are probably due to the change in position of the heart and may include a 15–20-degree shift to the left in the electrical axis. There may be reversible ST, T, and Q wave changes. The first heart sound may be split, with increased loudness of both portions, and the third heart sound may also be louder. As many as 90% of pregnant women may have a late systolic or ejection murmur attributable to the increase in stroke volume. This murmur disappears soon after delivery. There also may be a soft diastolic murmur, which is transient and sometimes coincident with the third heart sound. Continuous murmurs or bruits may be heard at the left sternal edge, arising from the internal thoracic (mammary) artery. Caution is needed in interpreting murmurs during pregnancy, particularly systolic murmurs, because such physiologic alterations do not necessarily indicate heart disease and must be differentiated from pathologic changes.

### Cardiac Output

Cardiac output increases approximately 40% during pregnancy, reaching its maximum at 20–24 weeks' gestation and continuing at this level until term. The increase in output can be as much as 1.5 L/min over the nonpregnant level. Cardiac output is very sensitive to changes in body position. This sensitivity increases with lengthening gestation, presumably because the uterus impinges upon the inferior vena cava, thereby decreasing blood return to the heart.

Cardiac output is the product of **stroke volume** and **heart rate**. In early pregnancy, stroke volume accounts for nearly all of the increase in cardiac output. The heart rate increases with lengthening gestation and by term is 15 beats/min higher than the nonpregnant rate. The heart rate is variable and can be affected by exercise, emotional stress, or heat.

Stroke volume increases 25–30% during pregnancy, reaching its maximum level at 12–24 weeks' gestation. Stroke volume is very sensitive to positional alteration. For example, in the supine position stroke volume decreases after 20 weeks, reaching normal, nonpregnancy levels by term; in the lateral recumbent position, stroke volume remains the same from 19 weeks' gestation until term.

### Blood Pressure

Systemic blood pressure declines slightly during pregnancy. There is little change in systolic blood pressure, but diastolic pressure is reduced (5–10 mm Hg) from about 12–26 weeks. Diastolic pressure increases thereafter to prepregnancy levels by about 36 weeks.

Venous pressure in the upper body is basically unchanged during pregnancy, but pressure increases significantly in the lower extremities as pregnancy progresses, particularly when the patient is supine, sitting, or standing. The obstruction posed by the uterus on the inferior vena cava and the pressure of the fetal presenting part on the common iliac veins can result in decreased blood return to the heart. This decreases cardiac output, leads to a fall in blood pressure, and causes edema in the lower extremities. The elevated venous pressure returns toward normal if the woman lies in the lateral recumbent position. Venous pressure also falls immediately following cesarean section.

### Peripheral Resistance

Peripheral resistance equals blood pressure divided by cardiac output. Because blood pressure either decreases or remains the same during pregnancy and cardiac output increases appreciably, there is good evidence that peripheral resistance declines markedly.

### Blood Flow

As in the kidneys, blood flow to the uterus and breasts increases during gestation, but the amount of increase depends on the stage of gestation (Fig 7–3). The increase in uterine blood flow is probably about 500 mL/min but may be as high as 700–800 mL/min. The uterus and placenta have increased blood flow because their vascular resistance is lower than that of the systemic circulation.

Renal blood flow increases approximately 400 mL/min above nonpregnant levels, and blood flow to the breasts increases approximately 200 mL. Blood flow to the skin also increases, particularly in the feet and hands. Heat due to increased maternal metabolism and heat produced by the fetus are dissipated via increased blood flow to the skin.

Diversion of blood flow to large muscles during

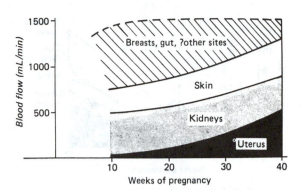

**Figure 7–3.** The distribution of cardiac output during pregnancy. (Reproduced, with permission, from Hytten FE, Leitch I: The Physiology of Human Pregnancy. Blackwell, 1964.)

physical exercise may decrease uteroplacental blood flow. The extent to which this may compromise the fetus is unknown. An additional load may be placed on uteroplacental oxygen transfer mechanism, and this may cause an abnormal fetal heart rate pattern. Interpretation of these heart rate changes must take into account the stage of gestation. A normal fetus in a normal mother can probably tolerate mild to moderate exercise without difficulty. The effects of vigorous exercise on a normal infant are unknown.

## Effects of Labor on the Cardiovascular System

When a patient is in the supine position, uterine contractions can cause a 25% increase in maternal cardiac output, a 15% decrease in heart rate, and a resultant 33% increase in stroke volume. However, when the laboring patient is in the later recumbent position, the hemodynamic parameters stabilize, with only a 7.6% increase in cardiac output, a 0.7% decrease in heart rate, and a 7.7% increase in stroke volume. These significant differences are attributable to inferior vena caval occlusion caused by the gravid uterus. During contractions, pulse pressure increases 26% in the supine position but only 6% in the lateral recumbent position. Central venous pressure increases in direct relationship to the intensity of uterine contraction and increased intra-abdominal pressure. Additionally, cardiopulmonary blood volume increases 300–500 mL during contractions. At the time of delivery, hemodynamic alterations vary with the method of anesthesia used (see Chapter 26).

## PULMONARY SYSTEM

### Anatomic & Physiologic Changes

Pregnancy produces anatomic and physiologic changes that affect respiratory performance. Early in pregnancy, capillary dilatation occurs throughout the respiratory tract, leading to engorgement of the nasopharynx, larynx, trachea, and bronchi. This causes the voice to change and makes breathing through the nose difficult. Respiratory infections and preeclampsia aggravate these symptoms. Chest x-rays reveal increased vascular markings in the lungs.

As the uterus enlarges, the diaphragm is elevated as much as 4 cm, and the rib cage is displaced upward and widens, increasing the lower thoracic diameter by 2 cm and the thoracic circumference by up to 6 cm. Elevation of the diaphragm does not impede its movement. Abdominal muscles have less tone and are less active during pregnancy, causing respiration to be more rather than less diaphragmatic.

### Lung Volumes & Capacities

In respiration physiology, there are 4 defined lung "volumes" and 4 "capacities." The 4 volumes do not overlap. They are defined as follows: **Tidal volume** is the volume of gas inspired or expired during each respiration. It varies with body requirements, but the term usually refers to quiet respiration at rest. The position of the chest at the end of quiet expiration is known as the end-expiratory position. **Inspiratory reserve volume** is the maximum amount of air that can be inspired beyond normal tidal inspiration. **Expiratory reserve volume** is the maximum amount of air that can be expired from the resting end-expiratory position. **Residual volume** is the volume of gas remaining in the lungs at the end of maximal expiration.

The 4 "capacities" each include 2 or more of the "volumes" defined above. **Total lung capacity** includes them all; it is the total amount of gas in the lung at the end of maximum inspiration. **Vital capacity** includes all but residual volume; it is the maximum volume of gas that can be expired after a maximum inspiration. **Inspiratory capacity** is tidal volume plus inspiratory reserve volume; it is the maximum volume of gas that can be inspired from the resting end-expiratory position. **Functional residual capacity** is expiratory reserve volume plus residual volume; it is the amount of gas remaining in the lungs at the resting end-expiratory position and the volume of gas with which the tidal air must mix.

Alterations occurring in lung volumes and capacities during pregnancy include the following (Fig 7–4). Dead space volume increases owing to relaxation of the musculature of conducting airways. Tidal volume increases gradually (35–50%) as pregnancy progresses. Total lung capacity is reduced (4–5%) by the elevation of the diaphragm. Functional residual capacity, residual volume, and expiratory reserve volume all decrease by about 20%. Larger tidal volume and smaller residual volume cause increased alveolar

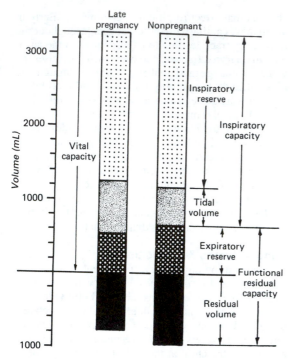

**Figure 7–4.** The components of lung volume in late pregnancy compared with those in nonpregnant women. (Reproduced, with permission, from Hytten FE, Leitch I: The Physiology of Human Pregnancy. Blackwell, 1964.)

ventilation (about 65%) during pregnancy. Inspiratory capacity increases 5–10%, reaching a maximum at 22–24 weeks' gestation.

Functional respiratory changes include a slight increase in respiratory rate, a 50% increase in minute ventilation, a 40% increase in tidal volume, and a progressive increase in oxygen consumption of up to 15–20% above nonpregnant levels by term. The in-

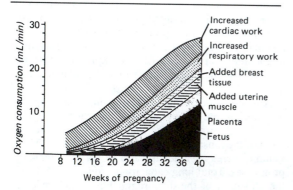

**Figure 7–5.** Components of increased oxygen consumption during pregnancy. (Reproduced, with permission, from Hytten FE, Leitch I: The Physiology of Human Pregnancy. Blackwell, 1964.)

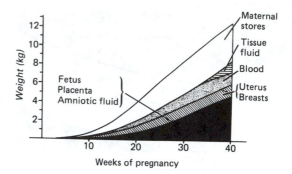

**Figure 7–6.** Components of weight gain during pregnancy. (Reproduced, with permission, from Hytten FE, Leitch I: The Physiology of Human Pregnancy. Blackwell, 1964.)

crease in oxygen consumption is caused by the increased metabolic needs of the mother (cardiac and respiratory muscles) and fetus (Fig 7–5).

With the increase in respiratory tidal volume associated with a normal respiratory rate, there is an increase in respiratory minute volume of approximately 26%. As the respiratory minute volume increases, **"hyperventilation of pregnancy"** occurs, causing a decrease in alveolar $CO_2$. This decrease lowers the maternal blood $CO_2$ tension; however, alveolar oxygen tension is maintained within normal limits. Maternal hyperventilation is probably due to the action of progesterone on the respiratory center, although it has been suggested that changes may occur in the sensitivity of peripheral chemoreceptors in the carotid body. Maternal hyperventilation is considered a protective measure that prevents the fetus from exposure to excessive levels of $CO_2$.

## Effects of Labor on the Pulmonary System*

During labor, anxiety, fear, and other emotional reactions may affect the rate and depth of respiration and, consequently, the $CO_2$ content of the blood. Frequently, patients become dyspneic, hyperventilate, and develop respiratory alkalosis, which may lead to carpopedal spasm and acid-base imbalance.

There is a further decrease in functional residual capacity (FRC) during the early phase of each uterine contraction, resulting from redistribution of blood from the uterus to the central venous pool. Because this decrease in FRC occurs without a concomitant change in dead space, there is little residual dilution and, therefore, presumably more efficient gas exchange. Administration of anesthesia must be adjusted accordingly, because of the more rapid changes in the concentration of gas in the lungs. Oxygen saturation decreases with each contraction and

*This section is contributed by Martin L. Pernoll, MD.

**Table 7–2.** Estimate of extracellular and intracellular water added during pregnancy.[1]

| | Total Water (mL) | Extracellular (mL) | Intracellular (mL) |
|---|---|---|---|
| Fetus | 2343 | 1360 | 983 |
| Placenta | 540 | 260 | 280 |
| Amniotic fluid | 792 | 792 | ... |
| Uterus | 743 | 490 | 253 |
| Mammary glands | 304 | 148 | 156 |
| Plasma | 920 | 920 | ... |
| Red cells | 163 | ... | 163 |
| Extracellular, extravascular water | 1195 | 1195 | ... |
| Total | 7000 | 5165 | 1835 |

[1]Reproduced, with permission, from Hytten FE, Leitch I: *The Physiology of Human Pregnancy.* Blackwell, 1964.

then returns to precontraction levels. During labor, the increase in ventilation, decrease in FRC, and increase in cardiac output significantly influence the induction of and emergence from inhalation anesthesia. The increase in cardiac output increases the uptake of soluble anesthetics by the blood and retards the rate at which alveolar concentration approaches inspired concentration, in turn retarding the induction of anesthesia.

## METABOLISM

As the fetus and placenta grow and place increasing demands on the mother, phenomenal alterations in metabolism occur. The most obvious physical changes are weight gain and altered body shape. **Weight gain** is due not only to the uterus and its contents but also to increased breast tissue, blood volume, and water volume (about 6.8 L) in the form of extravascular and extracellular fluid. Deposition of fat and protein and increased cellular water are added to maternal stores. The average weight gain during pregnancy is 12.5 kg (27.5 lb). Distribution of weight gain is shown in Fig 7–6 and distribution of extracellular and intracellular water in Table 7–2.

During normal pregnancy, approximately 1000 g of the weight gain is attributable to protein. Half of this is found in the fetus and the placenta, with the rest being distributed as uterine contractile protein, breast glandular tissue, plasma protein, and hemoglobin. Plasma albumin levels are decreased and fibrinogen levels increased.

Total body fat increases during pregnancy, but the amount varies with the total weight gain. During the second half of pregnancy, plasma lipids increase (plasma cholesterol increases 50%, plasma triglyceride concentration may triple), but triglycerides, cholesterol, and lipoproteins decrease soon after delivery. The ratio of low-density lipoproteins (LDLs) to high-density proteins (HDLs) increases during pregnancy. It has been suggested that most fat is stored centrally during mid pregnancy and that as the fetus demands more nutrition in the latter months, fat storage decreases.

The metabolism of carbohydrates and insulin during pregnancy is discussed in Chapter 18. A "diabetic-type" condition can appear during pregnancy in a nondiabetic woman and then totally disappear after delivery.

## REFERENCES

Borell U et al: Influence of uterine contractions on uteroplacental blood flow at term. Am J Obstet Gynecol 1965;93:44.

Chesley LC: Plasma and red cell volumes during pregnancy. Am J Obstet Gynecol 1972;112:440.

Fainstat T: Ureteral dilation in pregnancy: A review. Obstet Gynecol Surv 1963;18:845.

Ganong WF: *Review of Medical Physiology,* 12th ed. Lange, 1985.

Gant NF et al: A prospective study of angiotensin II pressor response throughout primigravid pregnancy. J Clin Invest 1973;52:2682.

Gibbs CP: Maternal physiology. Clin Obstet Gynecol 1981;24:525.

Hathaway WE, Bonnar J: *Perinatal Coagulation, Monographs in Neonatology.* Grune and Stratton, 1978.

Hytten FE, Chamberlain G: *Clinical Physiology of Obstetrics,* 3rd ed. Blackwell, 1981.

Lind T: *Maternal Physiology: Basic Science Monograph in Obstetrics and Gynecology.* Council on Resident Education in Obstetrics and Gynecology (CREOG), 1985.

Metcalfe J, McAnulty JH, Ueland K: Cardiovascular physiology. Clin Obstet Gynecol 1981;24:693.

Milsom I, Forssman L: Factors influencing aortocaval com-

pression in late pregnancy. Am J Obstet Gynecol 1984;
148:764.

Peck TM, Arias F: Hematologic changes associated with
pregnancy. Clin Obstet Gynecol 1979;22:785.

Pernoll ML et al: Oxygen consumption at rest and during
exercise in pregnancy. Respir Physiol 1975;25:285.

Pernoll ML et al: Ventilation during rest and exercise in
pregnancy and postpartum. Respir Physiol 1975;25:295.

Pritchard JA: Changes in blood volume during pregnancy
and delivery. Anesthesiology 1965;26:393.

Sims EAH, Krantz KE: Serial studies of renal function during pregnancy and the puerperium in normal women. J
Clin Invest 1985;37:1764.

Tygart SG et al: Longitudinal study of platelet indices during pregnancy. Am J Obstet Gynecol 1986;154:883.

# Maternal-Placental-Fetal Unit; Fetal & Early Neonatal Physiology

Robert A. Knuppel, MD, MPH

Fetal genetics, physiology, anatomy, and biochemistry can now be studied with the use of ultrasonography, fetoscopy, chorionic villus sampling, amniocentesis, and fetal cord and scalp blood sampling. Embryology and fetoplacental physiology must now be considered when providing direct patient care.

---

## THE PLACENTA

---

A **placenta** may be defined as any intimate apposition or fusion of fetal organs to maternal tissues for the purpose of physiologic exchange. The basic parenchyma of all placentas is the **trophoblast;** when this becomes a membrane penetrated by fetal **mesoderm,** it is called the chorion.

In the evolution of viviparous species, the yolk sac presumably is the most archaic type of placentation, having developed from the egg-laying ancestors of mammals. In higher mammals, the **allantoic sac** fuses with the chorion, forming the chorioallantoic placenta, which has mesodermal vascular villi. When the trophoblast actually invades the maternal endometrium (which in pregnancy is largely composed of decidua), a deciduate placenta results. In humans, maternal blood comes into direct contact with the fetal trophoblast. Thus, the human placenta may be described as a discoid, deciduate, hemochorial chorioallantoic placenta.

### DEVELOPMENT OF THE PLACENTA

Soon after ovulation, the endometrium develops its typical secretory pattern under the influence of progesterone from the corpus luteum. The peak of development occurs at about 1 week after ovulation, coinciding with the expected time for implantation of a fertilized ovum.

Pregnancy occurs when healthy spermatozoa in ad-

equate numbers penetrate receptive cervical mucus, ascend through a patent uterotubal tract, and fertilize a healthy ovum without about 24 hours following ovulation. The spermatozoa that penetrate favorable mucus travel through the uterine cavity and the uterine tubes at a rate of about 6 mm/min. During this transit, an enzymatic change occurs that renders the spermatozoa capable of fertilizing the ovum. This process is called **capacitation.** The cellular union between the sperm and the egg is referred to as **syngamy.** The tip of the sperm head (**acrosome**) loses its cell membrane and probably releases a lytic enzyme that facilitates penetration of the zona pellucida surrounding the ovum.

Once the sperm head containing all of the paternal genetic material enters the cytoplasm of the ovum, a **"zona reaction"** occurs that prevents the entrance of a second sperm. The first cleavage occurs during the next 36 hours. As the conceptus continues to divide and grow, the peristaltic activity of the uterine tube slowly transports it to the uterus, a journey that requires 6–7 days. Concomitantly, a series of divisions creates a hollow ball, the **blastocyst,** which then implants within the endometrium. Most cells in the wall of the blastocyst are trophoblastic; only a few are destined to become the embryo.

Within a few hours after implantation, the trophoblast invades the endometrium and begins to produce **human chorionic gonadotropin (hCG)** which is thought to be important in converting the normal corpus luteum into the corpus luteum of pregnancy. As the cytotrophoblasts (**Langhans' cells**) divide and proliferate, they form transitional cells that are ultrastructurally more mature and a likely source of hCG. Next, these transitional cells fuse, lose their individual membranes, and form the multinucleated **syncytiotrophoblast.** Mitotic division then ceases. Thus, the syncytial layer becomes the front line of the invading fetal tissue. Maternal capillaries and venules are tapped by the invading fetal tissue to cause extravasation of maternal blood and the formation of small lakes (lacunae), the forerunners of the intervillous space. These lacunae fill with maternal blood by reflux from previously tapped veins. An occasional maternal artery then opens, and a sluggish circulation is established (hematotropic phase of the embryo).

The lacunar system is separated by trabeculae, many of which develop buds or extensions. Within these branching projections, the cytotrophoblast forms a mesenchymal core.

The proliferating trophoblast cells then branch to form secondary and tertiary villi. The **mesoblast,** or central stromal core, also formed from the original trophoblast, invades these columns to form a supportive structure within which capillaries are formed. The **embryonic body stalk** (later to become the umbilical cord) invades this stromal core to establish the fetoplacental circulation. If this last step does not occur, the embryo will die. Sensitive tests for hCG suggest that at this stage, more embryos die than live.

Where the placenta is attached, the branching villi resemble a leafy tree (the **chorion frondosum**), whereas that portion of the placenta covering the expanding conceptus is smoother (**chorion laeve**). When the latter is finally pushed against the opposite wall of the uterus, the villi atrophy, leaving the amnion and chorion to form the 2-layered sac of fetal membranes (Fig 8–1).

About 40 days after conception, the trophoblast has invaded approximately 40–60 spiral arterioles, of which 12–15 may be called major arteries. The pulsatile arterial pressure of blood that spurts from each of these major vessels pushes the chorionic plate away from the decidua to form 12–15 "tents," or maternal **cotyledons.** The remaining 24–45 tapped arterioles form minor vascular units that become crowded between the larger units. As the chorionic plate is pushed away from the basal plate, the anchoring villi pull the maternal basal plate up into septa (columns of fibrous tissue that virtually surround the major cotyledons). Thus, at the center of each maternal vascular unit there is one artery that terminates in a thin-walled sac, but there are numerous maternal veins that open through the basal plate at random. The human placenta has no peripheral venous collecting system. Within each maternal vascular unit is the fetal vascular "tree," with the tertiary free-floating villi (the major area for physiologic exchange) acting as thousands of baffles that disperse the maternal bloodstream in many directions. A cross-sectional diagram of the mature placenta is shown in Fig 8–2.

Table 8–1 summarizes the major morphologic-functional correlations that take place during placental development.

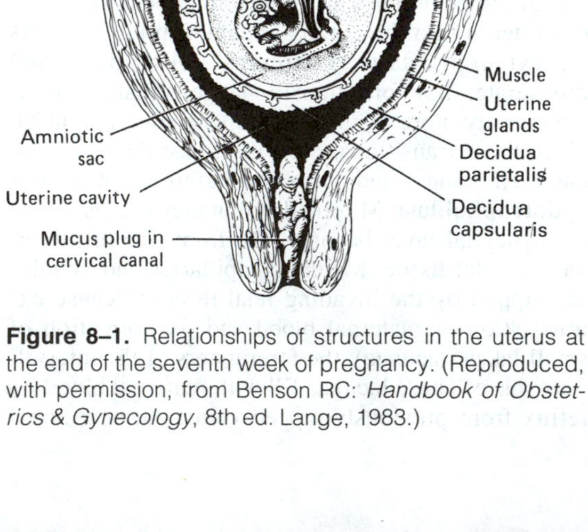

## FUNCTIONS OF THE MATERNAL-PLACENTAL-FETAL UNIT

The placenta is a complex organ of internal secretion, releasing numerous hormones and enzymes into

**Figure 8–1.** Relationships of structures in the uterus at the end of the seventh week of pregnancy. (Reproduced, with permission, from Benson RC: *Handbook of Obstetrics & Gynecology*, 8th ed. Lange, 1983.)

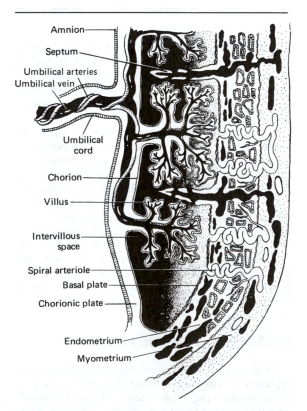

**Figure 8–2.** Schematic cross section of the circulation of the mature placenta. (Reproduced, with permission, from Benson RC: *Handbook of Obstetrics & Gynecology*, 8th ed. Lange, 1983.)

**Table 8–1.** Development of the human placenta.[1]

| Days After Ovulation | Important Morphologic-Functional Correlations |
|---|---|
| 6–7 | Implantation of blastocyst. |
| 7–8 | Trophoblast proliferation and invasion. Cytotrophoblast gives rise to syncytium. |
| 9–11 | Lacunar period. Endometrial venules and capillaries tapped. Sluggish circulation of maternal blood. |
| 13–18 | Primary and secondary villi form; body stalk and amnion form. |
| 18–21 | Tertiary villi, 2–3 mm long, 0.4 mm thick. Mesoblast invades villi, forming a core. Capillaries form in situ and tap umbilical vessels, which spread through blastoderm. Fetoplacental circulation established. Sluggish lacunar circulation. |
| 21–40 | Chorion frondosum; multiple anchored villi, which form free villi shaped like "inverted trees." Chorionic plate forms. |
| 40–50 | Cotyledon formation: <br><br>(1) Cavitation. Trophoblast invasion opens 40–60 spiral arterioles. Further invasion stops. Spurts of arterial blood form localized hollows in chorion frondosum. Maternal circulation established. <br><br>(2) Crowning and extension. Cavitation causes concentric orientation of anchoring villi around each arterial spurt, separating chorionic plate from basal plate. <br><br>(3) Completion. Main supplying fetal vessels for groups of second-order vessels are pulled from the chorioallantoic mesenchyme to form first-order vessels of fetal cotyledons. <br><br>(4) About 150 rudimentary cotyledons with anchoring villi remain, but without cavitation and crowning ("tent formation"). Sluggish, low-pressure (5–8 mm Hg) flow of maternal blood around them. |
| 80–225 | Continued growth of definitive placenta. Ten to 12 large cotyledons form, with high maternal blood pressures (40–60 mm Hg) in the central intervillous spaces; 40–50 small to medium-sized cotyledons and about 150 rudimentary ones are delineated. Basal plate pulled up between major cotyledons by anchoring villi to form septa. |
| 225–267 (term) | Cellular proliferation ceases, but cellular hypertrophy continues. |

[1]Adapted from Reynolds SRM: Formation of fetal cotyledons in the hemichorial placenta. Am J Obstet Gynecol 1966;94:425. (Reproduced, with permission, from Page EW, Villee CA, Villee DB: *Human Reproduction*. Saunders, 1976.)

the maternal bloodstream. In addition, it serves as the organ of transport for all fetal nutrients and metabolic products as well as for the exchange of oxygen and $CO_2$. Although fetal in origin, the placenta depends almost entirely on maternal blood for its nourishment.

The arterial pressure of maternal blood (60–70 mm Hg) causes it to pulsate toward the chorionic plate into the low-pressure (20 mm Hg) intervillous space. Venous blood in the placenta tends to flow along the basal plate and out through the venules directly into maternal veins. The pressure gradient within the fetal circulation changes slowly with the mother's posture, fetal movements, and physical stress. The pressure within the placental intervillous space is about 10 mm Hg when the pregnant woman is lying down. After a few minutes of standing, this pressure exceeds 30 mm Hg. In comparison, the fetal capillary pressure is 20–40 mm Hg.

Clinically, placental perfusion can be altered by many physiologic changes in the mother or fetus. When a precipitous fall in maternal blood pressure occurs, increased plasma volume improves placental perfusion. An increased rate of rhythmic uterine contractions benefits placental perfusion, but tetanic labor contractions are detrimental to placental and fetal circulation. An increased fetal heart rate tends to expand the villi during systole, but this is a minor aid in circulatory transfer.

### Circulatory Function

**A. Uteroplacental Circulation:** The magnitude of the uteroplacental circulation is difficult to measure in humans. The consensus is that total uterine blood flow near term is 500–700 mL/min. Not all of this blood traverses the intervillous space. It is generally assumed that about 85% of the uterine blood flow goes to the cotyledons and the rest to the myometrium and endometrium. One may assume that blood flow in the placenta is 400–500 mL/min in a patient near term who is lying quietly on her side and is not in labor.

As the placenta matures, thrombosis decreases the number of arterial openings into the basal plate. At term, the ratio of veins to arteries is 2:1 (approximately the ratio found in other mature organs).

Near their entry into the intervillous spaces, the terminal maternal arterioles lose their elastic reticulum. Since the distal portions of these vessels are lost with the placenta, bleeding from their source can be controlled only by uterine contraction. Thus, uterine atony causes postpartum hemorrhage.

**B. Plasma Volume Expansion and Spiral Artery Changes:** Structural alterations occur in the human uterine spiral arteries found in the decidual part of the placental bed. As a consequence of the action of cytotrophoblast on the spiral artery vessel wall, the normal musculoelastic tissue is replaced by a mixture of fibrinoid and fibrous tissue. The small spiral arteries are converted to large tortuous channels, creating low-resistance channels or arteriovenous shunts.

In dogs, when a surgically created arteriovenous shunt is opened, there soon appears a marked increase in plasma volume, cardiac output, and retention of sodium. An apparent anemia occurs, as the red blood cell mass is slower to expand. The reverse happens when the shunt is closed. This situation is similar to that of early normal pregnancy, when there is an early increase in plasma volume and resulting physiologic anemia as the red blood cell mass slowly expands. Immediately after delivery, with closure of the placental shunt, diuresis and natriuresis occur. When the spiral arteries fail to undergo these physiologic changes, fetal growth retardation often occurs with preeclampsia. Campbell (1983) and more recently Voigt et al (1992) used gated, pulsed Doppler ultrasound to study the uterine arcuate arteries serving the spiral arteries and placenta in pregnant women. Among the patients who showed evidence of failure of the spiral arteries to dilate and increased vascular resistance, there was subsequently a high frequency of proteinuric hypertension, poor fetal growth, and fetal hypoxia. Voigt et al (1992) also noted that Doppler ultrasound profiles correlated well with the histologic findings on subsequent biopsy of the placental bed.

Fleischer et al (1986) reported that normal pregnancy is associated with a uterine artery Doppler velocimetry systolic/diastolic ratio of less than 2:6. With a higher ratio and a notch in the wave form, the pregnancy is usually complicated by stillbirth, premature birth, intrauterine growth retardation, or preeclampsia.

Wells et al (1984) demonstrated that the decidual spiral arteries that have been attacked by the cytotrophoblast have a fibrinoid matrix that develops amniotic antigens, apparently to maintain the structural integrity of the vessel wall. Thus, there are histologic and immunologic explanations for the presence or absence of the marked increase in uterine blood flow and plasma volume expansion seen in human pregnancies.

Goodlin et al (1984) believed that failure of the spiral arteries to dilate and adequately expand plasma volume evokes increased maternal venous reactivity and multiple organ dysfunction. This disorder probably cannot be corrected by medical therapy, but therapy may modify secondary effects.

**C. Fetoplacental Circulation:** At term, a normal fetus has a total umbilical blood flow of 350–400 mL/min. Thus, the maternoplacental and fetoplacental flows are of a similar order of magnitude.

The villous system is best compared with an inverted tree. The branches pass obliquely downward and outward within the intervillous spaces. This arrangement probably permits preferential currents or gradients of flow and undoubtedly encourages inter-

villous fibrin deposition, commonly seen in the mature placenta.

**Cotyledons** (subdivisions of the placenta) can be identified early in placentation. Although they are separated by the placental septa, some communication occurs via the subchorionic lake in the roof of the intervillous spaces.

Prior to labor, placental filling occurs whenever the uterus contracts (*Braxton Hicks contractions*). At these times, the maternal venous exits are closed but the thicker-walled arteries are only slightly narrowed. When the uterus relaxes, blood drains out through the maternal veins. Hence, blood is not squeezed out of the placental lake with each contraction, nor does it enter the placental lake in appreciably greater amounts during relaxation.

During the height of an average first-stage contraction, most of the cotyledons are devoid of any flow and the remainder are only partially filled. Thus, intermittently—for periods of up to a minute—maternoplacental flow virtually ceases. Therefore, it should be evident that any extended prolongation of the contractile phase, as in uterine tetany, could lead to fetal hypoxia.

### Maternal Circulation

Aortocaval compression is a common cause of abnormal fetal heart rate during labor. In the third trimester, the contracting uterus obstructs its own blood supply to the level of L3–4 (**Poseiro effect**) when the mother is supine. This obstruction is completely relieved by turning the patient on her side. Although only about 30% of pregnant women will demonstrate aortocaval compression when supine, women in labor (particularly after epidural anesthesia) should not be maintained in a supine position.

In all supine pregnant women at term, obstruction of the inferior vena cava by uterine pressure is relatively complete. However, only about 10% have inadequate collateral circulation (intervertebral venous plexus, lumbar venous plexus, abdominal wall superficial and deep veins, hemorrhoidal plates, vertebral azygous and portal system), and develop **maternal supine hypotension syndrome.** This syndrome is characterized by decreased cardiac output, bradycardia, and hypotension. Relief is obtained when the woman is placed in the lateral position. Most pregnant women near term sleep on their sides instinctively to avoid such problems.

Uterine blood flow and placental perfusion values are directly correlated with the pregnancy-related increase in maternal plasma volume. Relative maternal hypovolemia is found in association with most complications of pregnancy, including preeclampsia, SGA fetus, premature labor, and various fetal anomalies.

### Endocrine Function
**A. Secretions of the Maternal-Placental-**

**Fetal Unit:** The placenta and the maternal-placental-fetal unit produce increasing amounts of steroids late in the first trimester. Of greatest importance are the steroids required in fetal development from 7 weeks' gestation through parturition. Immediately following conception and until 12–13 weeks' gestation, the principal source of circulating gestational steroids (progesterone is the major one) is the corpus luteum of pregnancy. However, after 42 days, the placenta assumes an increasingly important role in the production of several steroid hormones. Steroid production by the embryo occurs even before implantation is detectable in utero. Prior to implantation, production of progesterone by the embryo may be of importance in ovum transport.

Once implantation occurs, there is secretion of trophoblastic hCG and other pregnancy-related peptides. A more sophisticated array of fetoplacental steroids is produced during organogenesis and with the development of a functioning hypothalamic-pituitary-adrenal axis. Adrenohypophyseal basophilic cells first appear at about 8 weeks in the fetus and indicate the presence of significant quantities of adrenocorticotropic hormone (ACTH). The first adrenal primordial structures are identified at approximately 4 weeks, and the fetal adrenal cortex develops in concert with the adenohypophysis.

The fetus and the placenta acting in concert are the principal steroid regulators controlling intrauterine growth, maturation of vital organs, and parturition.

The fetal adrenal cortex is much larger than its adult counterpart. From mid trimester until term, the large inner mass of the fetal adrenal gland (80% of the adrenal tissue) is known as the **fetal zone**. This tissue is supported by factors unique to the fetal status and regresses rapidly after birth. The outer zone ultimately becomes the bulk of the postnatal and adult cortex.

Trophoblastic mass increases exponentially through the seventh week, after which time the growth velocity gradually increases to an asymptote close to term. The fetal zone and placenta share and exchange steroid precursors to make possible the full complement of fetoplacental steroids. Formation and regulation of steroid hormones also take place within the fetus itself.

In addition to the steroids, another group of placental hormones unique to pregnancy are the polypeptide hormones, each of which has an analogue in the pituitary. These placental protein hormones include hCG and human chorionic somatomammotropin. The existence of placental human chorionic corticotropin also has been suggested.

A summary of the hormones produced by the maternal-placental-fetal unit is shown in Table 8–2.

**B. Placental Secretions:**

**1. Human chorionic gonadotropin**–Human chorionic gonadotropin (hCG) was the first of the placental protein hormones to be described. Its molecu-

**Table 8–2.** Summary of maternal-placental-fetal endocrine-paracrine functions.

**Peptides of exclusively placental origin**
Human chorionic gonadotropin (hCG)
Human chorionic somatomammotropin (hCS)
Human chorionic corticotropin (hCC)
SP1—pregnancy specific $\beta$-1 glycoprotein
SP4—pregnancy specific $\beta$-1 glycoprotein
Pregnancy-associated plasma proteins (PAPP)
  PAPP-A
  PAPP-B
  PAPP-C
  PAPP-D [hCS]
Pregnancy-associated $\beta_1$ macroglobulin ($\beta_1$, PAM)
Pregnancy-associated $\alpha_2$ Macroglobulin ($\alpha_2$ PAM)
Pregnancy-associated major basic protein (pMBP)
Placental Proteins (PP) 1 through 21
Placental Membrane Proteins (MP) 1 through 7.
  MP1 also known as placental alkaline phosphatase (PLAP)
Hypothalamic like hormone ($\beta$ endorphin, ACTH-like)
**Steroid of mainly placental origin**
Progesterone
**Hormones of maternal-placental-fetal origin**
Estrone
Estradiol 50% from maternal androgens
**Hormone of placental-fetal origin**
Estriol
**Hormone of corpus luteum of pregnancy**
Relaxin
**Fetal hormones**
Thyroid hormone
Fetal adrenal zone hormones
$\alpha$-Melanocyte-stimulating hormone
Corticotropin intermediate lobe peptide (CLIP)
Anterior pituitary hormone
Adrenocorticotropic hormone (ACTH)
Tropic hormones for fetal zone of placenta
$\beta$-Endorphin
$\beta$-Lipotropin
Intermediate pituitary hormones

lar weight is 36,000–40,000. It is a glycoprotein that has biologic and immunologic similarities to luteinizing hormone from the pituitary. Recent evidence suggests that hCG is produced by the syncytiotrophoblast of the placenta. hCG is elaborated by all types of trophoblastic tissue, including that of hydatidiform moles, chorioadenoma destruens, and choriocarcinoma. As with all glycoprotein hormones (LH, FSH, TSH), hCG is composed of 2 subunits, alpha and beta. The alpha subunit is common to all glycoproteins, and the beta subunit confers unique specificity to the hormone. Typically, neither subunit is active by itself; only the intact molecule exerts hormonal effects.

Antibodies have been developed to the betasubunit of hCG. This specific reaction allows for differentiation of hCG from pituitary LH. hCG is detectable 9 days after the midcycle LH peak, which occurs 8 days after ovulation and only 1 day after implantation. This measurement is useful because it can detect pregnancy in all patients on day 11 after fertilization.

Concentrations of hCG rise exponentially until 9–10 weeks' gestation, with a doubling time of 1.3–2 days. Knowledge of hCG doubling times has important practical applications. Normally, doubling values during early pregnancy augur well for a successful outcome. Conversely, abnormally slow doubling times are considered a bad prognostic sign indicating an imminent miscarriage or, far worse, an ectopic pregnancy. Concentrations peak at 60–90 days' gestation. Afterwards, hCG levels decrease to a plateau that is maintained until delivery. The half-life of hCG is approximately 32–37 hours, in contrast to that of most protein and steroid hormones, which have half-lives measured in minutes. Structural characteristics of the hCG molecule allow it to interact with the human TSH receptor in activation of the membrane adenylate cyclase that regulates thyroid cell function. The finding of hCG-specific adenylate stimulation in the placenta may mean that hCG provides "order regulation" within the cell of the trophoblast.

**2. Human chorionic somatomammotropin**– Human chorionic somatomammotropin (hCS) is a protein hormone with immunologic and biologic similarities to pituitary growth hormone. It has also been designated **human placental lactogen (hPL)** and is synthesized in the syncytiotrophoblastic layer of the placenta. It can be found in maternal serum and urine in both normal and molar pregnancies. However, it disappears so rapidly from serum and urine after delivery of the placenta or evacuation of the uterus that it cannot be detected in the serum after the first postpartum day. The somatotropic activity of hCS is 3% or less than that of human growth hormone (hGH). In vitro, hCS stimulates thymidine incorporation into DNA and enhances the action of hGH and insulin. It is present in microgram per milliliter quantities in early pregnancy, but its concentration increases as pregnancy progresses, with peak levels reached during the last 4 weeks. Prolonged fasting at mid gestation and insulin-induced hypoglycemia are reported to raise hCS concentrations. Amniotic instillation of prostaglandin $PGF_2$ causes a marked reduction in hCS levels. hCS may exert its major metabolic effect on the mother to ensure that the nutritional demands of the fetus are met.

It has been suggested that hCS is the "growth hormone" of pregnancy. The in vivo effects of hCS owing to its growth hormonelike and anti-insulin characteristics result in impaired glucose uptake and stimulation of free fatty acid release, with resultant decrease in insulin effect. The maternal metabolism appears to be directed toward mobilization of maternal sources to furnish substrate for the fetus.

**3. Human chorionic corticotropin**–Human chorionic corticotropin (hCC) is another pituitarylike hormone. The physiologic role of hCC and its regulation are unknown.

**4. Placental proteins**–A number of proteins thought to be specific to the pregnant state have been isolated. The most commonly known are the 4 pregnancy-associated plasma proteins (PAPP) designated as PAPP-A, PAPP-B, PAPP-C, and PAPP-D. PAPP-D is the hormone hCS (described earlier). All these proteins are produced by the placenta and/or decidua. The physiologic role of these proteins except for PAPP-D are at present unclear. Numerous investigators have postulated various functions ranging from facilitating fetal "allograft" survival and the regulation of coagulation and complement cascades to the maintenance of the placenta and the regulation of carbohydrate metabolism in pregnancy. A host of other pregnancy specific/associated proteins have since been isolated. The greatest challenge, however, lies in the divination of their function. Such knowledge will provide important insights into placental function and hopefully allow us to understand more completely the pregnant state.

**C. Fetoplacental Secretions:** The placenta may be an incomplete steroid-producing organ that must rely on precursors reaching it from the fetal and maternal circulations (an integrated maternal-placental-fetal unit). The adult steroid-producing glands can form progestins, androgens, and estrogens, but this is not true of the placenta. Estrogen production by the placenta is dependent upon precursors reaching it from both the fetal and maternal compartments. Placental progesterone formation is accomplished in large part from circulating maternal cholesterol.

In the placenta, cholesterol is converted to pregnenolone and then rapidly and efficiently to progesterone. Production of progesterone approximates 250 mg/d by the end of pregnancy, at which time circulating levels are on the order of 130 mg/mL. To form estrogens, the placenta, which has anactive aromatizing capacity, utilizes circulating androgens obtained primarily from the fetus but also from the mother. The major androgenic precursor is **dehydroepiandrosterone sulfate (DHEA-S)**.

This compound comes from the fetal adrenal gland. Because the placenta has an abundance of sulfatase (sulfate-cleaving) enzyme, DHEA-S is converted to free unconjugated DHEA when it reaches the placenta, then to androstenedione, testosterone, and finally estrone and 17β-estradiol.

The major estrogen formed in pregnancy is estriol. Ninety percent of the estrogen in the urine of pregnant women is estriol. It is excreted into the urine as sulfate and glucuronide conjugates. Concentrations increase with advancing gestation, ranging from approximately 2 mg/24 h at 16 weeks to 35–40 mg/24 h at term. Estriol is formed during pregnancy by a unique biosynthetic process that demonstrates the interdependence of the fetus, placenta, and mother. DHEA-S is quantitatively the major steroid produced by the fetal adrenal gland, with most of it being produced in the fetal zone. When DHEA-S of the fetus or mother reaches the placenta, estrone and estradiol are formed. However, little of either is converted to estriol by the placenta; instead, some of the DHEA-S undergoes 16ga-hydroxylation, primarily in the fetal liver. When the 16-hydroxydehydroepiandrosterone sulfate (16-OHDHEA-S) reaches the placenta, the placental sulfatase enzyme acts to cleave the sulfate side chain, and the unconjugated 16-OHDHEA-S is aromatized to form estriol. The estriol is then secreted into the maternal circulation. When it reaches the maternal liver, it is conjugated to estriol sulfate and estriol glucosiduronate in a mixed conjugate. These forms are excreted into the maternal urine.

Circulating progesterone and estriol are thought to be important during pregnancy because they are present in such large amounts. Progesterone may play a role in maintaining the myometrium in a state of relative quiescence during much of pregnancy. A high local (intrauterine) concentration of progesterone may block cellular immune responses to foreign antigens. Progesterone appears to be essential for the maintenance of pregnancy in almost all mammals examined. This suggests that progesterone may be instrumental in conferring immunologic privilege to the uterus.

The functional role of estriol in pregnancy is the subject of wide speculation. It appears to be effective in increasing uteroplacental blood flow, as it has a relatively weak estrogenic effect on other organ systems. Indeed, estrogens may exert their effect on blood flow via prostaglandin stimulation.

## Placental Transport

The placenta has a high rate of metabolism, with consumption of oxygen and glucose occurring at a faster rate than in the fetus. Presumably, this high requirement is due to multiple transport and biosynthesis activities.

The primary function of the placenta is the transport of oxygen and nutrients to the fetus and the reverse transfer of $CO_2$, urea, and other catabolites back to the mother. In general, those compounds that are essential for the minute-by-minute homeostasis of the fetus (eg, oxygen, $CO_2$, water, sodium) are transported very rapidly by diffusion. Compounds required for the synthesis of new tissues (eg, amino acids, enzyme cofactors such as vitamins) are transported by an active process. Substances such as certain maternal hormones, which may modify fetal growth and are at the upper limits of admissible molecular size, may diffuse very slowly, whereas proteins such as IgG immunoglobulins probably reach the fetus by the process of pinocytosis.

This transfer takes place by at least 5 mechanisms: simple diffusion, facilitated diffusion, active transport, pinocytosis, and leakage.

**A. Mechanisms of Transport:**

**1. Simple diffusion**–Simple diffusion is the method by which gases and other simple molecules cross the placenta. The rate of transport depends on the chemical gradient, the diffusion constant of the compound in question, and the total area of the placenta available for transfer (Fick's law). The chemical gradient—ie, the differences in concentration in fetal and maternal plasma—is in turn affected by the rates of flow of uteroplacental and umbilical blood. Simple diffusion is also the method of transfer for exogenous compounds such as drugs.

**2. Facilitated diffusion**–The prime example of a substance transported by facilitated diffusion is glucose, the major source of energy for the fetus. The transfer of glucose from mother to fetus occurs more rapidly than can be accounted for by the Fick equation. Presumably, a carrier system operates with the chemical gradient (as opposed to active transport, which operates against the gradient) and may become saturated at high glucose concentrations. In the steady state, the glucose concentration in fetal plasma is about two-thirds that of the maternal concentration, reflecting the rapid rate of fetal utilization. Substances of low molecular weight, minimal electric charge, and high lipid solubility diffuse across the placenta with ease.

**3. Active transport**–When compounds such as the essential amino acids and water-soluble vitamins are found in higher concentration in fetal blood than in maternal blood, and when this difference cannot be accounted for by differential protein-binding effects, the presumption is that the placenta concentrates the materials during passage by an active transport system. This has been proved in the case of selected amino acids in human subjects by observing that the natural L forms are transferred with greater rapidity than the unnatural D forms, which are simply optical isomers of identical molecular size. Thus, the selective transport of specific essential nutrients is accomplished by enzymatic mechanisms.

**4. Pinocytosis**–Electron microscopy has shown pseudopodial projections of the syncytiotrophoblastic layer that reach out to surround minute amounts of maternal plasma. These particles are carried across the cell virtually intact to be released on the other side, whereupon they promptly gain access to the fetal circulation. Certain other proteins (eg, foreign antigens) may be immunologically rejected. This process may work both to and from the fetus, but the selectivity of the process has not been determined. Complex proteins, small amounts of fat, and immune bodies and even viruses may traverse the placenta in this way. For the passage of complex proteins, highly selective processes involving special receptors are involved. For example, maternal antibodies of the IgG class are freely transferred, whereas other antibodies are not.

**5. Leakage**–Gross breaks in the placental membrane may occur, allowing the passage of intact cells. Despite the fact that the hydrostatic pressure gradient is normally from fetus to mother, tagged red cells and white cells have been found to travel in either direction. Such breaks probably occur most often during labor or with placental disruption (abruptio placentae, placenta previa, or trauma), cesarean section, or intrauterine fetal death. It is at these times that fetal red cells can most often be demonstrated in the maternal circulation. This is the mechanism by which the mother may become sensitized to fetal red cell antigens such as Rh factor.

**B. Placental Transport of Drugs:** The placental membranes are often referred to as a "barrier" to fetal transfer, but there are few substances (eg, drugs) that will not cross the membranes at all. A few compounds, such as heparin and insulin, are of sufficiently large molecular size or charge that minimal transfer occurs. This lack of transfer is almost unique among drugs. Most medications are transferred from the maternal to the fetal circulation by simple diffusion, the rate of which is determined by the respective gradients of the drugs.

These diffusion gradients are influenced in turn by a number of serum factors, including the degree of drug-protein binding. Since serum albumin concentration is considerably less during pregnancy, drugs that bind almost exclusively to plasma albumin (eg, warfarin, salicylates) may have relatively higher unbound concentrations and, therefore, an effectively higher placental gradient. By contrast, a compound such as carbon monoxide may attach itself so strongly to the increased total hemoglobin that there will be little left in the plasma for transport.

The placenta also acts as a lipoidal resistance factor to the transfer of water-soluble foreign organic chemicals; as a result, chemicals and drugs that are readily soluble in lipids are transferred much more easily across the placental barrier than are water-soluble drugs or molecules. Ionized drug molecules are highly water soluble and are therefore poorly transmitted across the placenta. Because ionization of chemicals depends in part on their pH-pK relationships, there are multiple factors that determine this "simple diffusion" of drugs across the placenta. *Obviously, drug transfer is not simple, and one must assume that some amount of almost any drug will cross the placenta.*

**C. Placental Transfer of Heat:** The core temperature of the human fetus is only about 0.5° C above that of the maternal colon (core temperature) and about 0.2° C above that of the amniotic fluid. There is a further temperature gradient of approximately 0.1° C between the amniotic fluid and the uterine wall. Given these low fetal-maternal temperature gradients, it appears that virtually all fetal heat loss is from the umbilical flow through the placenta, as the thermal diffusion capacity of the placental villous surface is considerably greater than that of the fetal body surface.

## ANATOMIC DISORDERS OF THE PLACENTA

Observation of structural alterations within the placenta may indicate fetal and maternal disease that otherwise might go undetected.

### Twin-Twin Transfusion Syndrome

Nearly all monochorionic twin placentas show an anastomosis between the vessels of the 2 umbilical circulations. These usually involve the major branches of the arteries and veins in the placental surface. Artery-to-artery communications are by far the most common, but the less frequent venovenous anastomosis may also occur. Of great pathologic significance are deep arteriovenous communications between the 2 circulations. This occurs when there are shared lobules supplied by an umbilical arterial branch from one fetus and drained by an umbilical vein branch of the other fetus. Fortunately, one-way flow to the shared lobule may be compensated for by reverse flow through a superficial arterioarterial or venovenous anastomosis, if they coexist.

Twin-twin transfusion syndrome is believed to arise when shared lobules causing blood flow from one twin to the other are not compensated for by the presence of superficial anastomosis or by shared lobules causing flow in the opposite direction. This syndrome occurs in 15–30% of cases of monochorial placentation and is defined in terms of a difference in cord hemoglobin between the pair of greater than 5 dL. The twin receiving the transfusion is plethoric and polycythemic and may show cardiomegaly. The donor twin is pale and anemic and may have organ weights similar to those seen in the intrauterine malnutrition form of SGA.

### Placental Infarction

A placental infarct is an area of ischemic necrosis of placental villi resulting from obstruction of blood flow through the spiral arteries as a result of thrombosis. The lesions have a lobular distribution. However, the spiral arteries are not true end arteries, and if there is adequate flow through the arteries supplying adjacent lobules, sufficient circulation will be maintained to prevent necrosis. Thus, ischemic necrosis of one placental lobule probably indicates not only that the spiral artery supplying the infarcted lobule is thrombosed but that flow through adjacent spiral arteries is severely impaired. Placental infarction may serve as a mechanism allowing the fetus to redistribute blood flow to those placental lobules that are adequately supplied by the maternal circulation. The infarct is usually extensive before the fetus is physiologically impaired.

### Chorioangioma of the Placenta

A benign neoplasm composed of fetoplacental capillaries may occur within the placenta. It is grossly visible as a purple-red, apparently encapsulated mass, variable in size, and occasionally multicentered. Placental hemangioma, or "chorioangioma," may be linked with maternal, fetal, and neonatal complications. Many placental tumors are accompanied by hydramnios, and some have been associated with preeclampsia-eclampsia. The developing fetus may be subjected to hypoxia, resulting in low birth weight, because blood within the tumor fails to reach the placental villi (and become oxygenated). The tumor may act as an arteriovenous shunt requiring increased fetal cardiac output, with resulting cardiomegaly. Fetal hydrops may occur, as may hypoalbuminemia and a microangiopathic type of hemolytic anemia. Neonatal thrombocytopenia has been associated with disseminated intravascular coagulation secondary to the liberation of thromboplastic substances.

### Amniotic Bands

Close inspection of the fetal membranes, particularly near the umbilical cord insertion, may reveal band or stringlike membrane segments that are easily lifted above the placental surface. Such amniotic bands appear to be the result of a tear in the amnion early in pregnancy. They may cause constriction of the developing limbs or other fetal parts. Amputation has been known to result. Syndactyly, clubfoot, and fusion deformities of the cranium and face may also be explained in certain instances on the basis of amniotic bands. Myometrial bands also have been found within the intrauterine cavity but do not appear to place the same amount of tension on fetal anatomy as do amniotic bands.

### Amnion Nodosum

Examination of the fetal surface of the placental peripheral membranes after delivery may disclose small elevated nodules several millimeters in diameter. Microscopic examination of these nodules may reveal areas of ulceration of amniotic epithelium covered with deposits of celluloid debris probably representing vernix caseosa. These nodules reflect oligohydramnios regardless of cause. They frequently occur in association with underlying congenital anomalies of the fetal genitourinary system. With this information, one is alerted to the possibility that Potter's syndrome or a variant with pulmonary hypoplasia may affect the infant.

### Chronic Intrauterine Infection

Chronic intrauterine infection may have a deleterious effect on organogenesis and interfere with organ development. Infections such as toxoplasmosis, rubella, cytomegalovirus, herpes, and syphilis are seen most frequently. It has been only in the past 2 decades that chronic inflammation within placental villi has been recognized and linked with intrauterine infection. Such inflammatory foci have an incidence of approximately 20% in referral institutions. Usually, no

causative organism is found, and the term **chronic villitis of unknown etiology** is used. This is an inflammatory lesion that focuses on placental villi. It has a significant correlation with unexplained stillbirth and a considerable association with fetal morbidity and SGA newborns. An increased risk of recurrence with associated adverse pregnancy outcome is suggested.

The placenta should be sent to the pathology laboratory for examination in the following cases: (1) perinatal death; (2) malformation, edema, or anemia; (3) extremes of amniotic fluid volume; (4) extreme SGA; (5) unexpected severe birth asphyxia; (6) preterm birth; (7) multiple gestation; (8) abnormal placenta; and (9) perinatal infection.

## THE UMBILICAL CORD

### Development

In the early stages, the embryo has a thick embryonic stalk containing 2 umbilical arteries, one large umbilical vein, the allantois, and primary mesoderm. The arteries carry blood from the embryo to the chorionic villi, and the umbilical vein returns blood to the embryo. The umbilical vein and 2 arteries twist around one another.

In the fifth week of gestation, the amnion expands to fill the entire extraembryonic coelom. This process forces the yolk sac against the embryonic stalk and covers the entire contents with a tube of amniotic ectoderm, forming the umbilical cord. The cord is narrower in diameter than the embryonic stalk and rapidly increases in length. The connective tissue of the umbilical cord is called **Wharton's jelly** and is derived from the primary mesoderm. The umbilical cord can be found in loops around the baby's neck in approximately 23% of normal spontaneous vertex deliveries.

At birth, the mature cord is about 50–60 cm in length and 12 mm in diameter. A long cord is defined as more than 100 cm and a short cord as less than 30 cm. There may be as many as 40 spiral twists in the cord, as well as false knots and true knots. When umbilical blood flow is interrupted at birth, the intra-abdominal sections of the umbilical arteries and vein gradually become fibrous cords. The course of the left umbilical vein is discernible in the adult as a fibrous cord from the umbilicus to the liver (ligamentum teres) contained within the falciform ligament. The umbilical arteries are retained proximally as the internal iliac arteries and give off the superior vesicle arteries and the medial umbilical ligaments within the medial umbilical folds to the umbilicus. When the umbilical cord is cut and the end examined at the time of delivery, the vessels ordinarily are collapsed (Fig 8–3A), but if a segment of cord is fixed while the vessels are distended, the characteristic appearance is as shown in Fig 8–3B.

## Analysis of the Umbilical Cord in Fetal Abnormalities

A segment of umbilical cord should be kept available as a source of umbilical cord blood for blood gas measurements at the time of delivery. Cord blood gases are a more objective measure of oxygenation than Apgar scores, especially in dark-skinned babies.

The umbilical cord has recently become a means of evaluating the fetus in utero. Umbilical cord sampling under ultrasonographic guidance has opened new vistas in perinatal physiology, teratology, genetics, and therapeutic endeavors to correct Rh isoimmunization.

## ABNORMALITIES OF THE UMBILICAL CORD

### Velamentous Insertion

In velamentous insertion, the umbilical vessels divide to course through the membranes before reaching the chorionic plate. When these vessels present themselves ahead of the fetus (vasa praevia), they may rupture during labor to cause fetal exsanguination. Velamentous insertion occurs in about 1% of placentas, and 25–50% of these infants will have structural defects. Testing of all episodes of painless vaginal bleeding for fetal hemoglobin (Apt test or hemoglobin electrophoresis) will allow detection of this cause of fetal distress or death.

### Short Umbilical Cord

It appears from indirect evidence in the human fetus that the length of the umbilical cord at term is determined by the amount of amniotic fluid present during the first and second trimesters and by the mobility of the fetus. If oligohydramnios, amniotic bands, or limitation of fetal motion occur for any reason, the umbilical cord will not develop to an average length. Amniocentesis performed to produce oligohydramnios in pregnant rats at 14-16 days results in significant reduction of umbilical cord length. The length of the umbilical cord does not vary with fetal weight, presentation, or placental size. Simple mechanical factors may determine the eventual length of the cord.

### Knots in the Umbilical Cord

True knots occur in the cord in 1% of deliveries, leading to a perinatal loss of 6.1% in such cases. False knots are developmental variations with no clinical importance.

### Loops of the Umbilical Cord

Twisting of the cord about the fetus may be the reason for excessive cord length. One loop of cord is present about the neck in 21% of deliveries, 2 loops in 2.5%, and 3 loops in 0.2%. When 3 loops are present, the cord is usually longer than 70 cm. One study of 1000 consecutive deliveries found one or more loops of cord around the neck in approximately 24% of cases. Single or multiple loops of umbilical cord around the neck caused no fetal morbidity or mortality in that series, but Naeye's recent report (1987) illustrates that cord entanglement may be an important cause of still birth.

### Torsion of the Umbilical Cord

Torsion of the cord occurs counterclockwise in most cases. If twisting is extreme, fetal asphyxia may result.

### Single Artery

A 2-vessel cord (absence of one umbilical artery) occurs about once in 500 deliveries (6% of twins). The cause may be aplasia or atrophy of the missing vessel. The anomaly is more common in blacks than whites but equally frequent in primiparas and multiparas. About 30% of these infants will have structural defects. There is also a strong association between fetal structural anomalies and placental vascular occlusion or thrombosis. Perinatal examination for such vascular defects should be routine.

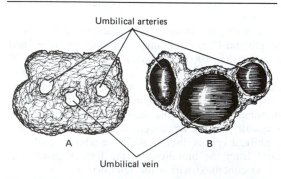

**Figure 8–3.** Drawings of cross sections of umbilical cord (A) after blood vessels are empty and (B) while they are filled, as in utero. The central vein and 2 arteries occupy most of the space. (Based on photography by SRM Reynolds.)

## THE FETUS

The human fetus is born about 40 weeks after the first day of the last menstrual period (LMP). The gestational age is measured from the first day of the LMP, although obviously conception can not occur until 2 weeks after the beginning of this calculation. The 9.5 calendar months are divided into trimesters for convenient classification of certain obstetric events. The term fetus is born 9.5 lunar cycles (29.53 days each) after conception, and the postconceptional age in weeks is used to denote the stage of development of the embryo.

An estimate of **conceptional age** can be made by measuring the embryo or fetus. Various methods of measurement have been developed, each with its own limitations and inaccuracies. Crown-rump and crown-heel lengths are the most common measurements. Crown-heel lengths are difficult to measure because the legs are often flexed in different positions. Most methods based on measurement are inaccurate because the fetus may move about or stretch while it is being measured. Embryologists most often use the term *conceptual age*, which begins with the date of conception or fertilization. Unfortunately, the confusion in terminology is often transmitted to the patient. It is appropriate to utilize weeks in discussing the length of gestation with the patient, so that communication and understanding is enhanced.

## GROWTH & DEVELOPMENT

During the first 8 weeks, the term embryo is used to denote the developing organism because it is during this time that all the major organs are formed (Table 8–3). After the eighth week, the word fetus is proper; this is a period when further growth and organ maturation occur. The loss of a fetus weighing less than 500 g (about 22 weeks' gestational age) is called a **spontaneous abortion**. A fetus weighing 500–1000 g (22-28 weeks) is called **immature**. From 28–36 weeks, it is referred to as premature. A **term fetus** is arbitrarily defined as one that has attained 37 weeks' gestational age.

The growth of the fetus may be conveniently described in units of 4 weeks' gestational age, beginning with the first day of the LMP:

**8 weeks:** The embryo is 2.1–2.5 cm long and weighs 1 g, and the head makes up almost half the bulk. The hepatic lobes may be recognized. Red blood cells are forming in the yolk sac and liver and contain hemoglobin. The kidneys are beginning to form.

**12 weeks:** The fetus is 7–9 cm long and weighs 12–15 g. The fingers and toes have nails, and the external genitalia may be recognizable as male or female. The volume of amniotic fluid is about 30 mL. The intestines undergo peristalsis and are capable of absorbing glucose.

**16 weeks:** The length is 14–17 cm and the weight about 100 g. The sex is discernible. Hemoglobin F is present, and formation of hemoglobin A begins.

**20 weeks:** The weight is about 300 g. Heart tones may often be detected by stethoscope. Movements have been perceived by the mother for 2–3 weeks. The uterine fundus is near the level of the umbilicus.

**24 weeks:** The weight is 600 g. Some fat is beginning to be deposited beneath the wrinkled skin. Viability is reached by the 24th week, but survival at this stage is still relatively rare.

**28 weeks:** The weight is about 1050 g and the length about 37 cm. The lungs are now capable of breathing, but the surfactant content is low; survival is possible in level II or level III neonatal centers.

**32 weeks:** The weight is about 1700 g and the length 42 cm. If born at this stage, about 5 of 6 infants survive.

**36 weeks:** The weight is about 2500 g and the length about 47 cm. The skin has lost its wrinkled appearance. The chances for survival are good.

**40 weeks:** The term fetus averages 50 cm in length and 3200–3500 g in weight. The head has a maximal transverse (biparietal) diameter of 9.5 cm, and when the neck is well flexed, the diameter from the brow to a point beneath the occiput (suboccipitobregmatic) is also 9.5 cm. The average fetus, therefore, requires cervical dilatation of almost 10 cm before it can descend into the vagina.

## FETAL & EARLY NEONATAL PHYSIOLOGY

During the past 2 decades, improved neonatal care has led to increased survival rates for very low birth weight infants, even those as young as 24 weeks. Obviously, an understanding of fetal and early neonatal physiology is critical in the appropriate management of these babies. The recent introduction of fetoscopy, pulsed Doppler evaluation, and umbilical cord blood sampling allows detection and treatment of fetal disorders in utero. A greater understanding of fetal physiology is needed to perform therapeutic techniques via the umbilical cord or within the intrauterine environment.

### Hematology

The fetal circulation is established at about 25 postconceptional days. At that time, the major sources of red blood cells are blood islands in the body stalk. By 10 weeks, the liver assumes the major role in erythropoiesis, but the spleen and bone marrow gradually take over this function. At term, the bone marrow is the source of at least 90% of the red cells. The hormone erythropoietin is produced in considerable quantities by 32 weeks, but levels fall almost to zero during the first week after birth, unless the infant is anemic, in which case the values are higher.

**Erythrocytes** are the first blood cells produced by the fetus and have a life span of 120 days. The earliest erythrocytes are megaloblastic and circulate as nucle-

**Table 8–3.** Embryonic and fetal growth and development.

| Fertilization Age (weeks) | Crown-Rump Length | Crown-Heel Length | Weight | Gross Appearance | Internal Development |
|---|---|---|---|---|---|
| **Embryonic stage** | | | | | |
| 1 | 0.5 mm | 0.5 mm | ? | Minute clone free in uterus. | Early morula. No organ differentiation. |
| 2 | 2 mm | 2 mm | ? | Ovoid vesicle superficially buried in endometrium. | External trophoblast. Flat embryonic disk forming 2 inner vesicles (amnioectomesodermal and endodermal). |
| 3 | 3 mm | 3 mm | ? | Early dorsal concavity changes to convexity; head, tail folds form; neural grooves close partially. | Optic vesicles appear. Double heart recognized. Fourteen mesodermal somites present. |
| 4 | 4 mm | 4 mm | 0.4 g | Head is at right angle to body; limb rudiments obvious, tail prominent. | Vitelline duct only communication between umbilical vesicle and intestines. Initial stage of most organs has begun. |
| 8 | 3 cm | 3.5 cm | 2 g | Eyes, ears, nose, mouth recognizable; digits formed, tail almost gone. | Sensory organ development well along. Ossification beginning in occiput, mandible, and humerus (diaphysis). Small intestines coil within umbilical cord. Pleural pericardial cavities forming. Gonadal development advanced without differentiation. |
| **Fetal stage** | | | | | |
| 12 | 8 cm | 11.5 cm | 19 g | Skin pink, delicate; resembles a human being, but head is disproportionately large. | Brain configuration roughly complete. Internal sex organs now specific. Uterus no longer bicornuate. Blood forming in marrow. Upper cervical to lower sacral arches and bodies ossify. |
| 16 | 13.5 cm | 19 cm | 100 g | Scalp hair appears. Fetus active. Arm-leg ratio now proportionate. Sex determination possible. | External sex organs grossly formed. Myelination. Heart muscle well developed. Lobulated kidneys in final situation. Meconium in bowel. Vagina and anus open. Ischium ossified. |
| 20 | 18.5 cm | 22 cm | 300 g | Legs lengthen appreciably. Distance from umbilicus to pubis increases. | Sternum ossifies. |
| 24 | 23 cm | 32 cm | 600 g | Skin reddish and wrinkled. Slight subcuticular fat. Vernix. Primitive respiratorylike movements. | Os pubis (horizontal ramus) ossifies. |
| 28 | 27 cm | 36 cm | 1100 g | Skin less wrinkled; more fat. Nails appear. If delivered may survive with optimal care. | Testes at internal inguinal ring or below. Talus ossifies. |
| 32 | 31 cm | 41 cm | 1800 g | Fetal weight increased proportionately more than length. | Middle fourth phalanges ossify. |
| 36 | 34 cm | 46 cm | 2200 g | Skin pale, body rounded. Lanugo disappearing. Hair fuzzy or wooly. Ear lobes soft with little cartilage. Umbilicus in center of body. Testes in inguinal canals; scrotum small with few rugae. Few sole creases. | Distal femoral ossification centers present. |
| 40 | 40 cm | 52 cm | 3200+ g | Skin smooth and pink. Copious vernix. Moderate to profuse silky hair. Lanugo hair on shoulders and upper back. Ear lobes stiffened by thick cartilage. Nasal and alar cartilages distinguishable. Nails extend over tips of digits. Testes in full, pendulous, rugous scrotum (or labia majora) well developed. Creases cover sole. | Proximal tibial ossification centers present. Cuboid, tibia (proximal epiphysis) ossify. |

ated cells. Mean red cell values change as the fetus grows (Table 8–4).

After the first week of life, erythrocyte concentrations begin to decline gradually, reaching zero by 6–12 weeks after birth. The hemoglobin concentration decreases to about 10 g/dL and by term, to as low as 7–8 g/dL (**physiologic anemia of the newborn**).

The synthesis of **hemoglobin** occurs in the proerythroblast, normoblast, and reticulocyte but not in the mature red blood cell. Types of fetal hemoglobin present prior to 12 weeks are Gower I and II and Portland I. There are at least 7 types of hemoglobin chains. The synthesis of each chain is under the genetic control of a separate structural gene locus. The complete amino acid sequences of the 7 normal globin chains have been determined. A functional hemoglobin molecule is a tetramer composed of 4 globin chains and 4 hemo groups. From the eighth week of gestation to term, **hemoglobin F** is the major hemoglobin in the fetus, but a small amount of hemoglobin A can also be detected. The ratio of beta to gamma synthesis remains approximately 1:10 during this period and until term. The beta to gamma ratio in the fetus is a criterion used for prenatal diagnosis by fetal blood analysis (Fig 8–4). Around the time of birth, the ratio changes because of the gradually decreased synthesis of gamma chains and increased synthesis of beta chains (Table 8–5).

Fortuitously, blood in the fetus has a 50% higher hemoglobin concentration than in the adult and a greater oxygen affinity than maternal blood. Even though fetal oxygen tension is less, fetal blood carries an amount of oxygen comparable to that in maternal blood. The alkali resistance of hemoglobin F makes it possible to demonstrate hemoglobin F-containing cells in the maternal circulation (**Apt test**).

The higher affinity of hemoglobin F for oxygen is accentuated by **2,3-diphosphoglycerate (2,3-DPG),** which is present in adult red cells. Fetal and maternal blood have differing oxygen saturation curves, mostly because 2,3-DPG competes with oxygen for binding sites on adult cells.

## Immunology

There are 3 basic types of leukocytes found in the blood: **granulocytes, monocytes,** and **lymphocytes.** The granular acidic leukocytes are subdivided into 3 types, based on the sustaining characteristics of the acidic plasma granules and their function—eosinophilic, basophilic, and neutrophilic granulocytes. A functional difference also exists among the lymphocytes, which are divided into 2 broad groups designated as **T cells** and **B cells.** The functions of monocytes vary greatly during maturation or with environmental influences; thus, it is not currently possible to divide them into distinct subgroups. Although all these cells are generally regarded as white blood cells, they should be viewed as cell types that merely use the blood as a means of transportation from sites of production to sites of function. Both the sites of production and (for the most part) sites of function are extravascular. The fetus presents with relative leukocytosis, the white count being 15,000–20,000/gmLxxx at term.

Circulating white cells constitute the first line of defense against pathogenic bacteria, as outlined in Table 8–6. Leukocytes appear in the fetal circulation after 2 months' gestation. The prothymocytes migrate from the fetal liver or bone marrow to enter the embryonic thymus at approximately 8 weeks' gestation. Soon after, the splenic anlage begins to mature. Both produce lymphocytes, a major source of the antibodies that constitute the second line of defense against harmful foreign antigens. Both antibody-mediated immunity and cell-mediated immunity depend on the activity of small lymphocytes derived from bone marrow precursors. The stem cells, which during the early embryonic stage originate in the yolk sac, in later stages of development in the liver, and in adults in the bone marrow, differentiate to form 2 distinct lymphocyte populations. One group is **thymus-derived (T lymphocytes)** and the other is **bone marrow-derived (B lymphocytes).** T lymphocytes can be detected in the thymus after 11 weeks' gestation, they appear in the peripheral blood, spleen, and lymph nodes by 16–18 weeks, and by 30–32 weeks the fetus has a near adult number of circulating T lymphocytes.

The life span of lymphocytes is not uniform. Recent studies suggest that B and T cell populations contain similar proportions of long- and short-lived lymphocytes. The T lymphocytes constitute 65-85% of the lymphocytes present in the thoracic duct, blood, and lymph nodes. The long-lived lymphocytes represent the major portion (90%) of the thoracic duct cells, whereas the short-lived lymphocytes are located mainly in the thymus, spleen, and bone marrow. The T cells are effector cells in delayed sensitivity reactions and elimination of foreign tissues. They also play an important role in the expression of some humoral immune responses. The T cells can release a variety of nonspecific chemical mediators called **lymphokines,** eg, **interferon, transfer factor, mitogenic factor, migration** and **inhibition factors,** and **cytotoxic** and **growth inhibitory factors.**

B lymphocytes originate in the bone marrow of most mammals. B cells seem to be more sessile than T cells. B cells are found primarily in the perilymphoid organs, lymph nodes, and the thymic-independent areas around germinal centers. They are also present in very small amounts in the peripheral blood. They seem to be short-lived. B cells differentiate into **plasma cells,** which are ultimately repsonsible for the synthesis and secretion of all forms of antibody and all circulating immunoglobulins. The average life span of plasma cells is 0.5–2 days.

**Table 8–4.** Mean red cell values during gestation.[1]

| Age (weeks) | Hemoglobin (g/dL) | Hematocrit (%) | Red Blood Cells ($10^6/\mu$L) | Mean Corpuscle Volume ($\mu m^3$/L) | Mean Corpuscle Hemoglobin (pg) | Mean Corpuscle Hemoglobin Concentration (g/dL) | Nucleated Red Blood Cells (% or red blood cells) | Reticulocytes (%) | Diameter ($\mu$m) |
|---|---|---|---|---|---|---|---|---|---|
| 12 | 8–10 | 33 | 1.5 | 180 | 60 | 34 | 5–8 | 40 | 10.5 |
| 16 | 10 | 35 | 2 | 140 | 45 | 33 | 2–4 | 10–25 | 9.5 |
| 20 | 11 | 37 | 2.5 | 135 | 44 | 33 | 1 | 10–20 | 9 |
| 24 | 14 | 40 | 3.5 | 123 | 38 | 31 | 1 | 5–10 | 8.8 |
| 28 | 14.5 | 45 | 4 | 120 | 40 | 31 | 0.5 | 5–10 | 8.7 |
| 34 | 15 | 47 | 4.4 | 118 | 38 | 32 | 0.2 | 3–10 | 8.5 |

[1]Reproduced, with permission, from Oskl FA, Naiman JL: *Hematologic Problems in the Newborn*, 3rd ed Saunders, 1982.

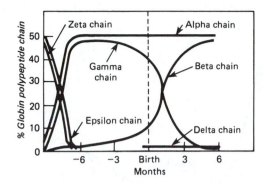

**Figure 8–4.** Hemoglobin chains.

**Table 8–6.** Defense mechanisms against infectious pathogens.

| | Humoral Defense | Cellular Defense |
|---|---|---|
| General | Complement system Properdin system | Granulocytes Monocytes Reticuloendothelial system |
| Immune | Immunoglobulins | Lymphocytes |

**Immunoglobulins (Ig)** are serum globulins with antibody activity as their primary property. The 5 classes of Ig have been designated IgG, IgM, IgA, IgD, and IgE. In the human newborn, plasma cells are absent from the bone marrow and the lamina propria of the ileum and appendix. They appear only 4–6 weeks after birth. However, beginning at 20 weeks' gestation, the fetal spleen synthesizes IgG and IgM but not IgA or IgD (Fig 8–5).

**IgG** is normally produced only in trace amounts prenatally, its full synthesis beginning 3–4 weeks after birth. **IgM** globulins are also found in small amounts in the fetus, primarily in the circulation but not diffused into extravascular spaces. They are synthesized in lymphocytoid plasma cells and reticular cells of the spleen and lymph nodes. Fetal production of IgG and IgM is low, however, in comparison with adult production. The fetal spleen synthesizes relatively more IgM than IgG. IgM is the first class to appear in the circulation after initial immunization and is the predominant class produced by infants in the neonatal period. At birth, the plasma level of IgM is about 5% of the normal adult level, with most, if not all, of this antibody being of fetal origin. Within 2–5 days after birth, the rate of IgM synthesis in-

creases rapidly. IgM, unlike IgG, does not cross the human placenta, and the half-life of IgM is 5 days.

This comparison between IgG and IgM is important in determining possible intrauterine infection. The fetal IgG serum concentration at term equals the maternal concentration because IgG crosses the placenta. IgG constitutes 90% of all serum antibodies in the fetus because of the maternal contribution. IgM is predominantly of fetal origin and, therefore, is used to determine whether fetal infection is present, but there are many false-positive and false-negative results. After birth, the IgG half-life in the newborn circulation is 3–4 weeks. IgE does not cross the placenta, and cord levels are only 10% of maternal levels.

The fetus and newborn are not as well equipped immunologically as the adult to combat infection. The primary deficiency is both cellular and humoral. T lymphocytes do not respond to specific antigens, and B lymphocytes do not develop into plasma cells. This results in IgG levels that are below maternal levels until late in the third trimester, and complement and properdin proteins, which are necessary for opsonization of bacteria, are consistently reduced.

IgA production does not begin until several weeks after birth. Because IgA is produced in response to the antigens of enteric organisms, the newborn is particularly susceptible to intestinal infections.

The response of the fetus to antigens of maternal origin depends on the level of immunologic competence achieved by the fetus. During the first trimester, for example, rubella virus elicits no response from the embryo, whose tissues are therefore subject to damage. Fetal and maternal tissues are no more tolerant of each other than are the tissues of any 2 first-degree relatives (as contrasted to identical twins).

## Endocrinology

The thyroid is the first endocrine gland to develop in the fetus. As early as the fourth postconceptional week, the thyroid can synthesize thyroxine. The **pancreas** develops early as an outgrowth of the duodenal endoderm, and as early as 12 weeks' gestation, **insulin** may be extracted from the B cells of the pancreas. Maternal insulin is not transferred to the fetus in physiologic quantities, and the fetus must supply whatever is needed for the metabolism of glucose. Insulin is thus the primary hormone regulating the rate of fetal growth. The B cells of the normal fetus respond poorly to hyperglycemia unless the stimulus is repeated many times, eg, diabetes in the mother may

**Table 8–5.** Embryonic, fetal, and adult hemoglobin concentrations.

| Hemoglobin | Globin Polypeptides | Percent in Cord Blood |
|---|---|---|
| **Embryo** | | |
| Gower I | Zeta-2, epsilon-2 | — |
| Gower II | Alpha-2, epsilon-2 | — |
| Portland I | Zeta-2, gamma-2 | — |
| Portland II | Zeta-4 | — |
| **Fetus** | | |
| Bart's | Gamma-4 | < 1 |
| Hemoglobin F | Alpha-2f, gamma-2 | 60–85 |
| **Adult** | | |
| Hemoglobin A | Alpha-2, beta-2 | 15–40 |
| Hemoglobin $A_2$ | Alpha-2, delta-2 | < 1 |

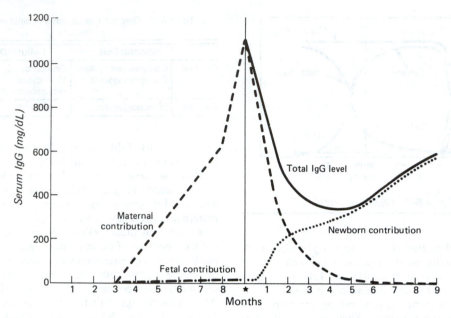

**Figure 8–5.** Development of IgG levels with age. Relationship of development of normal serum levels of IgG during fetal and newborn stages, and maternal contribution. (Modified from Allansmith M et al: The development of immunoglobulin levels in man. J Pediatr 1968;72:289.)

cause hyperplasia of fetal B cells so that larger quantities of insulin will be produced. This may be why some infants of diabetic mothers grow to an excessive size or show evidence of hyperinsulinism immediately after birth.

All the tropic hormones synthesized by the **anterior pituitary gland** are present in the fetus, although the precise role of these protein hormones in fetal growth and metabolism is not well understood. **ACTH** plays a vital role, however, in stimulating growth of the adrenal cortex, because the tropic hormones are too large for placental transfer from the mother in significant quantities.

The fetal **adrenal cortex** consists mainly of a fetal zone that disappears about 6 months after birth. The cortex is an active endocrine organ that produces large quantities of steroid hormones. There is evidence that the steadily increasing activity of the fetal zone triggers the sequence of events that leads to the initiation of labor. Atrophy of the fetal adrenal gland (as in anencephalic fetuses) may result in marked prolongation of pregnancy. The fetal adrenal cortex is larger in premature infants when the cause of labor is unknown than when the pregnancy is terminated by placental abruption or by elective induction of labor. The fetal adrenal gland is an important source of catecholamines, which will respond to stress placed on the fetal myocardium. There is a preferential blood flow to the fetal adrenal in acidosis, unlike the adult response to acidosis.

## CIRCULATORY FUNCTION IN THE FETUS & NEWBORN

The abrupt transition from intrauterine life to independent existence necessitates circulatory adaptations in the newborn. These include diversion of blood flow through the lungs, closure of the ductus arteriosus and foramen ovale, and obliteration of the ductus venosus and umbilical vessels.

Infant circulation has 3 phases: (1) the predelivery phase, in which the fetus depends on the placenta; (2) the intermediate phase, which begins immediately after delivery with the infant's first breath; and (3) the adult phase, which is normally completed during the first few months of life.

### Predelivery Phase

The umbilical vein carries oxygenated blood from the placenta to the fetus (Figs 8–6, 8–7). In the abdomen, the vein branches and enters the liver; a small branch bypasses the liver as the ductus venosus to enter the inferior vena cava directly.

Almost all the blood from the superior vena cava is directed through the tricuspid valve into the right ventricle, which ejects into the pulmonary trunk. Most of this relatively deoxygenated blood then passes directly through the ductus arteriosus to the descending aorta and on to the placenta. Blood from the inferior vena cava, which includes the oxygenated umbilical venous blood, largely passes directly

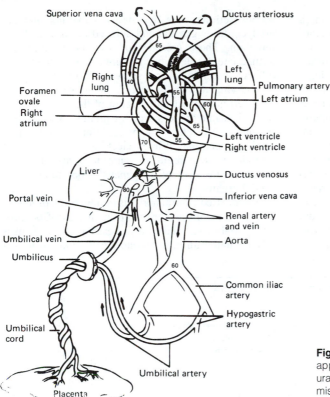

**Figure 8–6.** The fetal circulation. Numbers represent approximate values of the percentage of oxygen saturation of the blood in utero. (Reproduced, with permission, from Parer JT: *Handbook of Fetal Heart Rate Monitoring.* WB Saunders, 1983.)

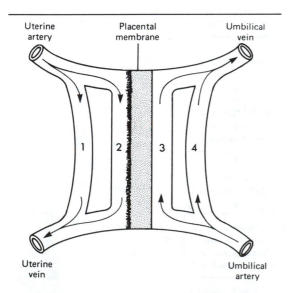

**Figure 8–7.** Schematic diagram of the placental circulation. (1) Shunting of maternal blood away from exchange surfaces. (2) Intervillous space. (3) Fetal capillaries of chorionic villi. (4) Shunting of fetal blood away from capillary exchange surfaces. (Modified and reproduced, with permission, from Parer JT: *Handbook of Fetal Heart Rate Monitoring.* WB Saunders, 1983.)

through the foramen ovale into the left atrium and left ventricle to be ejected into the ascending aorta. The left ventricle ejects about one-third of the combined ventricular output of the fetus. Most of the left ventricular output passes to the fetal head, while the right ventricle, with blood of lower oxygen content, ejects mainly into the descending aorta. The aortic oxygen saturation difference is related not only to superior and inferior vena caval flow patterns but also to flow of the umbilical venous blood as it enters the inferior vena cava. This well-oxygenated blood preferentially passes to the cerebral and coronary circulations. Both ventricles pump in parallel, unlike the situation in adults.

The fetal cardiovascular responses to stress represent a complex interplay between state of arousal, changes in blood gases, hydrogen ion concentration, reflex effects initiated by chemoreceptor or baroreceptor stimulation, and hormonal levels.

Superficially, the fetal hypoxemic-asphyxial response is much like the adult diving response in that they both involve selective vasoconstriction and the baroreceptor reflex, a primitive reflex involving changes in heart rate, arterial and venous dilatation, and cardiac performance. This reflex is evoked by changes in mean blood pressure and is modified by blood gas levels. The ability of some mammals to remain submerged for long periods of time remained a mystery until it was recognized that they become a "heart-brain" preparation through selective vasoconstriction. Likewise, during the fetal hypoxemic response, selective vasoconstriction diverts cardiac output to the brain, heart, placenta, and adrenal gland. With widespread vasoconstriction, hypertension occurs, inducing bradycardia through the baroreceptor reflex mechanism and vagal stimulation. The bradycardia is acute, meaning that it begins with the event and ends with the event. Bradycardia behaves like other vagal stimuli, such as head or uterine compression, umbilical cord compression, or even fetal grunting. A healthy fetus is usually able to tolerate bradycardia, providing it is neither severe nor constant. In contrast, the fetal asphyxial response represents depressed myocardial or central nervous system performance. Under these circumstances, even though va-

soconstriction occurs, hypertension does not, and any bradycardia is gradual and delayed in onset and termination. These episodes of fetal bradycardia are termed late decelerations and are often ominous. The different mechanisms are shown in Fig 8–8.

In diving mammals, lactic acid is washed out of hypoperfused tissues after relief of the vasoconstriction. The same process occurs with the hypoxic fetus, producing a brief period of acidemia after birth or after oxygenation. While selective vasoconstriction provides a "heart-brain" preparation, at the same time it disturbs the flow of oxygenated blood to other essential organs.

A depressed central nervous system often produces a relatively constant heart rate with lack of beat-to-beat variability. Fetal beat-to-beat variability is usually mediated through autonomic stimulation result-

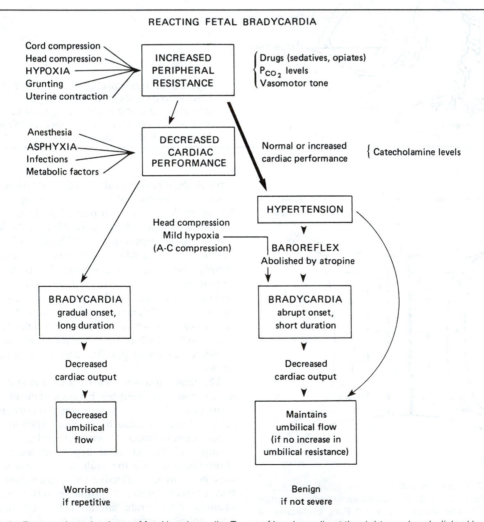

**REACTING FETAL BRADYCARDIA**

**Figure 8–8.** Proposed mechanisms of fetal bradycardia. Types of bradycardia at the right may be abolished by atropine, those at the left by inotropic agents. Fetal head compression, mild hypoxia, and maternal aorta caval compression may all produce direct vagal bradycardia without baroreceptor reflex. (Reproduced, with permission, from Goodlin RC, Haesslein HG: Fetal reacting bradycardia. Am J Obstet Gynecol 1977;129:845.)

ing from activity of both higher and lower brain centers. Such central nervous system activity reflects general fetal arousal levels and is decreased when the fetus is immature, asleep, drugged, or asphyxiated. Lack of fetal heart rate variability plus other signs of fetal stress can be an ominous sign. The central nervous system and cardiovascular system respond differently to hypoxia according to gestational age.

The umbilical vessels are relatively nonreactive, but the systemic and pulmonary circulations respond, when stressed, with vasoconstriction. The fetal pulmonary circulation receives a small portion (8–10%) of the fetal cardiac output, and therefore it does not play a central role in the fetal cardiovascular hypoxia response. Changes in fetal arterial pressure tend to be buffered by the fetal umbilical-placental circulation. Likewise, the decrease in fetal cardiac output seen during bradycardia is modified by the redistribution of cardiac output to vital organs such as the brain, heart, placenta, and adrenal gland, so that the baroreceptor reflex may not be as effective during fetal life. The response of the fetus to hypoxia is even more complex with chemoreceptor reflex stimulation from the aortic receptors, baroreceptor reflexes, and direct myocardial depression. Fetal tachycardia may result from sympathetic nervous stimulation and circulating catecholamines. Since the capacity to respond to any one of these different stimuli varies with gestational age, arousal levels, general health, and the presence of drugs and hormones, there are no universal, precise fetal heart rate responses to distress.

When placental transfer of oxygen is inadequate, anaerobic glycolysis leads to the accumulation of excessive amounts of lactic acid in the fetus. There is then an associated accumulation of $CO_2$ and hydrogen ion ($H^+$), which results in decreased fetal pH. Although the maternal and fetal $H^+$ values maintain a relatively constant gradient, differences in the bicarbonate levels allow for variation in fetal pH. Thus, determination of fetal scalp or cord blood gases is useful in the assessment of fetal well-being. During

fetal distress (seriously altered homeostasis), fetal blood levels of prostaglandins, catecholamines, steroids, endorphins, and pituitary hormones are often elevated (Table 8–7).

When the fetus shows signs of distress during labor, placental transfer can be improved by use of several maneuvers. First, a vaginal examination should be performed, and if prolapse of the umbilical cord has occurred, compression of the cord should be relieved immediately by lifting the presenting fetal part off the cord. The second maneuver is to roll the mother from one side to the other to check for maternal aortocaval compression. Third, it may be helpful to administer oxygen to the mother; however, this only slightly increases the oxygen content of the uterine arterial blood, because the arterial hemoglobin is already nearly saturated. Fourth, discontinue oxytocin and consider administration of a tocolytic agent to inhibit uterine activity. Fifth, rapidly administer 1 L of intravenous fluids to acutely expand the maternal plasma volume; a colloid solution such as 5% albumin is preferred, but a balanced salt solution is acceptable.

## Intermediate Phase

At birth, 2 events occur that alter the fetal hemodynamics: (1) ligation of the umbilical cord causes an abrupt though transient rise in arterial pressure, and (2) a rise in plasma $CO_2$ and fall in blood $PO_2$ help to initiate regular breathing.

With the first few breaths, the intrathoracic pressure of the newborn remains low (–40 to –50 mm Hg); after distention of the airways, however, the pressure rises to the normal adult level (–7 to –8 mm Hg). The initially high vascular resistance of the pulmonary bed is probably reduced by 75–80%. Pressure in the pulmonary artery falls by at least 50%, whereas pressure in the left atrium doubles.

In the fetus, the high resistance of the pulmonary bed causes most of the deoxygenated blood in the pulmonary artery to enter the descending aorta via the

**Table 8–7.** Average "normal" fetal scalp[1] and cord acid-base values.[2]

|  | Before Labor | Second Stage of Labor |
|---|---|---|
| **Scalp** | | |
| pH | 7.37 | 7.3 |
| $CO_2$ pressure (mm Hg) | 38 | 43 |
| Bicarbonate (mmol/L) | 21 | 21 |
| Base excess (mmol/L) | –3 | –5 |
|  | **Umbilical Vein** | **Umbilical Artery** |
| **Cord** | | |
| pH | 7.32 | 7.26 |
| $PO_2$ | 38.9 | 17.7 |
| $PCO_2$ | 37.1 | 40 |
| Base deficit | 6.8 | 6.7 |

[1]Population unrelated to cord sample population.
[2]Related to babies 28–43 weeks with Apgar scores greater than 7 at 1.5 minutes.

ductus arteriosus. At birth, expansion of the lungs occurs in the newborn, and most of the blood from the right ventricle then enters the lungs via the pulmonary artery. Furthermore, increased systemic arterial pressure reverses the flow of blood through the ductus arteriosus. Neonatal blood flows from the high-pressure aorta to the low-pressure pulmonary artery.

The increased pressure in the left atrium would normally result in backflow into the right heart through a patent foramen ovale. However, the anatomic configuration of the foramen is such that the increased pressure causes closure of the foramen by a valvelike fold situated in the wall of the left atrium.

The neonatal circulation is complete with closure of the ductus arteriosus and foramen ovale, but adjustments continue for 1–2 months, until the adult phase begins.

### Adult Phase

The ductus arteriosus usually is obliterated in the early postnatal period, probably by reflex action secondary to elevated oxygen tension and the interaction of prostaglandins. If the ductus remains open, a systolic crescendo murmur that diminishes during diastole (**"machinery murmur"**) is often heard over the second left interspace.

Obliteration of the foramen ovale is usually complete in 6–8 weeks, with fusion of its valve to the left interatrial septum. The foramen may remain patent in some individuals, however, with few or no symptoms. The obliterated ductus venosus from the liver to the vena cava becomes the ligamentum venosum. The occluded umbilical vein becomes the ligamentum teres of the liver.

The hemodynamics of the normal adult differ from those of the fetus in the following respects: (1) venous and arterial blood no longer mix in the atria; (2) the vena cava carries only deoxygenated blood into the right atrium, where it goes to the right ventricle and then is pumped into the pulmonary arteries and finally to the pulmonary capillary bed; and (3) the aorta carries only oxygenated blood from the left heart via the pulmonary veins for distribution to the rest of the body.

## RESPIRATORY FUNCTION IN THE FETUS & NEWBORN

Gas exchange in the fetus occurs in the placenta. Transfer of gases is proportionate to the difference in partial pressure of each gas and surface area and inversely proportionate to membrane thickness. Thus, the placenta can be viewed as the fetal "lungs in utero."

Until about 12 weeks, placental permeability is low because of the small surface area of the placental "lake" and the early relative thickness of the tropho-blastic membrane. From 12–32 weeks, the membrane thins and the surface area steadily increases. However, placental oxygen utilization makes accurate quantitation of oxygen transfer difficult.

The partial pressure of oxygen ($PO_2$) of fetal blood is less than that of maternal blood. Although not compatible with extrauterine life, the $PO_2$ is adequate for the fetus, as there is a higher concentration of hemoglobin in fetal blood, much of which is hemoglobin F. Hemoglobin F has a much greater affinity for oxygen than adult hemoglobin A, resulting in greater fetal oxygen saturation. However, the enhanced ability of the fetus to deliver oxygen to the peripheral tissues seems primarily dependent upon a cardiac output that is 2.5–3 times greater than in the adult.

Both the $PCO_2$ and the $CO_2$ content of fetal blood are slightly greater than levels in the mother's blood. As a result, $CO_2$ diffuses from fetus to mother for elimination.

The central and motor pathways of the fetal respiratory system are active, and respiration at birth is the culmination of in utero processes. Two main types of fetal breathing movements are recognized. One is a paradoxic irregular sequence, in which the abdominal wall moves outward as the chest wall moves inward. The other is a regular gentle movement, in which the chest and abdominal wall move outward and inward together. Fetal respiratory activity permits neuromuscular and skeletal maturation as well as development of the respiratory epithelium. As term approaches, the fetal diaphragm is usually active only during fetal REM sleep. Without such activity, the lungs would be hypoplastic and inadequate for gas exchange. Curiously, the alveolar membrane does excrete chloride into tracheal fluid and perhaps absorbs nutrients from amniotic fluid. Consequently, it has been proposed that, like the fish gill, the fetal alveolar membrane functions as an organ of osmoregulation. In sheep, prolactin has been shown to act on both the fetal lung and amniotic membrane in facilitating sodium transport, and this may be a mechanism of control of fetal blood volume.

Hypoxia or maternal cigarette smoking reduces fetal breathing movements, while hyperglycemia increases fetal breathing movements. In general, these movements are governed by the same central nervous system patterns that control changes in fetal heart rate and body movements. The greatest clinical accuracy in the biophysical identification of the abnormal fetus is achieved when multiple variables are considered, eg, fetal breathing, general movements, heart rate patterns, and response to stimuli. In both sheep and humans, fetal breathing movements diminish or cease 24–36 hours before the onset of true labor. In preterm labor with intact membranes, the presence of fetal breathing movements may indicate that pregnancy will continue, while fetal apnea may indicate early delivery.

The first breath of the newborn normally occurs within the first 10 seconds after delivery. The first breath usually is a gasp, the result of central nervous system reaction to sudden pressure, temperature change, and other external stimuli. With the first breath, the slight increase in $PO_2$ may activate chemoreceptors to send impulses to the central nervous system respiratory center and then to the respiratory musculature. As a result, a rhythmic but rapid breathing sequence occurs, which persists into the neonatal period. The amniotic fluid usually drains from the respiratory tract or is absorbed. If meconium is present, it may be aspirated, and if not cleared shortly after birth, it will migrate peripherally as continued respiration is established. Complete or partial obstruction of the respiratory tract or chemical pneumonitis may result.

Contrary to popular belief, the fetal lungs are not highly plastic. As development progresses, tissue elastin probably falls as the density of tissue to potential air space decreases. At the same time, liquid and future air space is enriched with phospholipid surfactants secreted by maturing type 2 saccular alveolar cells. When air breathing begins at birth, dispersion of air into the surfactant-rich liquid of the mature lungs results in formation of stable alveoli. Overall, a mature volume-pressure diagram is developed, characterized by relatively low opening pressures, high maximal volume, wide hysteresis, and retention of large volumes at end deflation or expiration.

With the onset of breathing, pulmonary vascular resistance is reduced and the capillaries fill with blood. Normally, the foramen ovale closes and pulmonary circulation is established.

Surfactant-poor lungs do not have the capacity to produce alveolar stability. As a consequence, initial aeration requires greater opening pressure, achieves a smaller maximal volume, and results in little hysteresis and gas retention during deflation. This is the underlying pathophysiologic mechanism of neonatal respiratory distress syndrome. One may anticipate inadequate phospholipid surfactant when the lecithin/sphingomyelin (L/S) ratio is less than 2. Conversely, one can anticipate mature fetal lungs and a 1–2% chance of respiratory distress syndrome if the L/S ratio is greater than 2.

## GASTROINTESTINAL FUNCTION IN THE FETUS & NEWBORN

The gastrointestinal tract is not truly functional until after birth, because the placenta is the organ of alimentation during fetal life. Nevertheless, when contrast medium is injected into the amniotic fluid as early as the fourth month of gestation, it may be promptly observed within the stomach and small intestine.

The full development of proteolytic activity does not develop until after birth, but the fetal gastrointestinal tract is quite capable of absorbing amino acids, glucose, and other soluble nutrients.

Meconium is produced during late pregnancy, but the amount is small. Passage of meconium in utero probably occurs with asphyxia, which increases intestinal peristalsis and relaxation of the anal sphincter.

Intrahepatic erythropoiesis begins during the eighth week in the embryo, and the liver is well developed histologically by mid pregnancy. During fetal life, the liver acts as a storage depot for glycogen and iron. Reasonably complete liver function is not achieved until well after the neonatal period has passed. Liver deficiencies at birth are many, including reduced hepatic production of fibrinogen and coagulation factors II, VII, IX,XI, and XII.

Vitamin K stored in the liver is deficient at birth because its formation is dependent upon bacteria in the intestine. These deficiencies predispose the newborn to hemorrhage during the first few days of life.

The formation of glucose from amino acids (gluconeogenesis) in the liver and adequate storage of glucose are not well established in the newborn. Moreover, levels of carbohydrate-regulating hormones such as cortisol, epinephrine, and glucagon may be initially insufficient. As a consequence, neonatal hypoglycemia is common after stressful stimuli such as exposure to cold or malnutrition.

Glucuronidation is limited during the early neonatal period, with the result that bilirubin is not readily conjugated for excretion as bile. After physiologic hemolysis of excess red blood cells in the first week of life or with pathologic hemolysis in isoimmunized newborns, jaundice occurs. If marked hyperbilirubinemia develops, kernicterus may ensue.

Metabolism of drugs by the liver is poor in the newborn period (eg, sulfonamides and chloramphenicol). Moreover, numerous inborn errors of metabolism (eg, galactosemia) may be diagnosed soon after birth. Neonatal liver function gradually improves, assuming proper food, freedom from infection, and a favorable environment.

Secretory and absorptive functions are accelerated after delivery. Most digestive enzymes are present, but the gastric contents are neutral at birth, although acidity soon develops. The initial neutrality may briefly delay the growth in the bowel of bacteria necessary for the formation of vitamin K in the intestine. The newborn can assimilate simple solutions and breast milk immediately after birth but cannot digest cow's milk as well until the second or third day after elimination of excessive gastric mucus. Slow progress of milk through the stomach and upper intestine is usual during the early neonatal period.

Normally, some air enters the stomach during feedings. Pocketing of air in the upper curvature of the stomach occurs when the newborn is lying flat.

Hence, turning of the infant and "burping" with the infant upright are necessary.

Large bowel peristalsis promptly increases after delivery, and 1–6 stools per day are passed. Absence of stool within 48 hours after birth is indicative of intestinal obstruction or imperforate anus.

## RENAL FUNCTION IN THE FETUS & NEWBORN

During uterine growth and development, the placenta serves as the major regulator of fluid and electrolyte balance. The kidneys are unnecessary for fetal growth and development, as demonstrated by the rare neonate born with renal agenesis. Hence, the placenta and maternal lungs and kidneys normally maintain fetal fluid and electrolyte balance. When the connection between fetal circulation and the placenta is interrupted during delivery, the kidneys are called upon to assume the homeostatic functional demands of extrauterine life.

The placenta (the major homeostatic organ) receives 40–65% of the fetal cardiac output. Renal blood flow in fetal lambs has been shown to be constant when expressed per gram of renal tissue, and renal vascular resistance is maintained at a constant value. Following birth, renal blood flow increases significantly and renal vascular resistance decreases by about 25%. However, renal blood flow is low and vascular resistance high when compared with adult levels.

The high neonatal vascular resistance may be attributable to increased renal adrenergic activity in the newborn. The neonatal renal vasculature has been shown to be sensitive to catecholamines, and the kidneys have been shown to have a high density of high-affinity alpha-adrenoceptors. At birth, a greater percentage of blood perfuses the deeper cortical nephrons. With maturation, the rise in blood flow to the outer cortical region increases faster than the rise to the inner cortex.

The **glomerular filtration rate (GFR)** in fetal animals, particularly lambs, increases proportionately with growth of the kidney (GFR expressed per gram of kidney weight) and rises significantly after birth. Renal blood flow has a similar pattern. During the first 24 hours of life, measurements of the GFR reflect the status of renal function during intrauterine life; at least 24 hours are needed for the GFR to adapt to the extrauterine environment. The GFR and renal blood flow follow a similar postnatal pattern, with values more than doubling during the first 2 weeks of life. This is also true in preterm neonates, although values start at lower levels.

Preterm infants have a negative sodium balance during the first 1–3 weeks of life. The mechanism for sodium wasting in premature infants probably involves proximal and distal tubule function. Preterm infants have a lower rate of sodium resorption in the proximal tubule than term infants. Newborns also have a limited ability to excrete a salt load when compared with adults. The functional tubular immaturity of the kidney in newborns is also demonstrated by increased renal excretion of glucose and amino acids and by decreased ability to concentrate, dilute, and acidify the urine. A normal serum bicarbonate level for a preterm infant may be as low as 14–16 mmol/L, but this level increases to 21 mmol/L during the first week of life (the value is similar in term newborns). Thus, newborn infants have a limited ability to excrete an acid load as well as a lower renal threshold for bicarbonate. Preterm infants do not concentrate urine as well as term infants. Most infants do not concentrate urine as well as adults until 6–12 months of age. Maximal urine osmolality in preterm newborns is 500–600 mosm/kg water; in term infants, maximum osmolality is 500–700 mosm/kg water.

Formation of urine is thought to begin at 9–12 weeks' gestation. By 32 weeks, fetal production of urine approaches 12 mL/h, and by term, 28 mL/h. At that point, urine is the major component of amniotic fluid. As mentioned before, the relative amounts of amniotic fluid can provide information on the status of fetal renal function. Oligohydramnios may be associated with renal hypoplasia, dysplasia, or obstructive uropathy. A normal amount of amniotic fluid indicates that there is some function in at least one kidney.

Ninety-three percent of all infants, either term or preterm, will void within the first 24 hours of life; 99% will void within 48 hours. Inadequate urine formation by the neonate can be associated with intravascular volume depletion, hypoxia, congenital nephrotic syndrome, tubular necrosis, renal agenesis, bilateral renal arterial or venous thrombosis, or obstructve uropathy. Normal infants may have transient glycosuria or proteinuria and a urine pH of 6.0–7.0.

Ultrasonography allows diagnosis of hydronephrosis prenatally and has stimulated research into therapeutic use of antenatal urinary aspiration or diversion techniques. A registry has been formed that has compiled data regarding fetal surgery. These attempts continue to be experimental, but the hope is that early "decompression" may prevent renal dysplasia. Prospective studies are warranted to determine whether early neonatal corrective surgery for congenital obstruction (pyeloplasty or ureteral reimplant) is truly worthwhile.

## CENTRAL NERVOUS SYSTEM FUNCTION IN THE FETUS & NEWBORN

It has been known for at least a century that the fetus is capable of sustained motor activity well before quickening. Through the eighth week of gestation, nearly 95% of responses are contralateral. Ipsilateral responses (torso stimulus) begin to appear with much greater frequency during the ninth week. By 12–13 weeks, local reflexes have almost completely replaced the total pattern of response. Recent ultrasonographic evaluations have followed motor activity in utero and all confirm a transition from simple whole body movements to complex motor responses. Thus, the sensation of fetal movement is an increasing part of the sensory input to the brain stem.

The cortex begins to develop during the eighth week. The neural maturational events that have been evaluated have emphasized 2 transitional periods: (1) a possible consolidation of brain stem influence over motor activity and sensory input near the end of the first trimester, and (2) establishment of the sensory input channel to the neothalamocortical connection around mid gestation. However, it is apparent that the brain stem is only partially developed and functional at term.

The functional development of the human central nervous system is too complex to summarize. Nevertheless, a few clinical correlates must be mentioned. An individual's development neither begins nor ends at birth. Abnormal neuronal migrations in the developing human brain are generally early gestational events induced by genetic factors, teratogens, or infections. Although the major neuronal migrations have formed the cortical plate by 16 weeks' gestation, late migrations from the germinal matrix into the cerebral cortex continue until 5 months postnatally. The external granular layer of the cerebellar cortex continues to migrate until age 1 year. Thus, ample opportunity exists for disturbances of these migratory processes in the postnatal period. Moreover, myelination is only rudimentary in the cerebral cortex of term infants. Axons of the large pyramidal cells of the motor cortex are myelinated only as far cortically as the cerebral peduncles of the midbrain, as demonstrated by light microscopy, and pyramidal tract axons in the medulla oblongata have only 1 or 2 turns of myelin, as seen on electron microscopy.

Neurologic development not only implies acquisition of perceptual, motor, linguistic, and intellectual skills but also signifies progressive organization of the anatomic and physiologic substrates of those achievements. Formation of the nervous system begins with the embryonic neural plate and terminates with completion of the final myelination cycle in the brain, ie, the frontal temporal association bundle at age 32–34 years. It is obvious that there are many things that can interrupt the normal migration, eg, a premature infant who suffers a subependymal hemorrhage affecting the radial glial process that is guiding a neuron to the surface. The neuron may retract from the cortical surface after its cell origin is destroyed. The maturation is in situ, but the migrating neuron unable to establish the intended synaptic relations

with the cortex. Perhaps the faulty synaptic circuitry of this "incidental finding" at autopsy contributes to the development of an epileptic focus. Another mechanism of prenatal or postnatal cerebral dysgenesis involves toxins that destroy the cytoskeletal elements of glial and nerve cells, eg, methyl-mercury poisoning. Methyl-mercury chloride abruptly arrests the active movement of migrating neurons in vitro, causing damage to the neural membrane of the growth zone, interferes with DNA synthesis, and ultimately compromises cytoskeletal proteins.

Psychiatrists and psychologists have long recognized in utero modifying influences, and Freud stated that "each individual ego is endowed from the beginning with its own peculiar disposition and tendencies." For example, maternal anxiety levels do affect fetal development, and intrauterine stimuli determine, to a degree, the maturation of nerve cells and structural patterns of the developing brain. Maternal emotional stress can have immediate and long-term effects on fetal development, but it is unclear whether effects are predictable.

Between 10 and 20 weeks' gestational age, the fetus displays several basic motor patterns that are later integrated into specific actions. The first jerky patterns of the second trimester become the functional movement patterns that allow the fetus to move about in utero. After mid pregnancy, these motor patterns mature in a manner similar to the mature repertoire of the newborn. Clues to future central nervous system development may be found in the study of these various fetal motor patterns, and failure to progress at various stages seems to indicate subsequent cerebral dysfunction. Real-time ultrasonic examination of such fetal motor patterns may lead to improved care in high-risk situations.

The fetus demonstrates various sleep-wake patterns throughout its development in utero. During most of its antenatal life, fetal electrocortical activity is of low voltage, associated with rapid eye movements, slow heart rate, and fetal breathing activity. In the third trimester, high-voltage activity is associated with the more lively activity. Finally, near term, the fetus appears to be awake at least 30% of the time. These fetal states may be discerned by ultrasonic study of eye movements, which may be altered by drugs or maternal anxiety levels. These, in turn, affect fetal heart rate responses to stress.

The term fetus has high **endorphin** levels that may modify the behavioral state, including heart rate responses. Endorphin levels may be responsible for the primary apnea of the newborn and for the lack of heart rate reactivity in otherwise normal intrapartum fetuses. The fetus probably suffers pain, as does any other individual, and high endorphin levels may limit pain and other effects of stress. The near-term fetus, then, has nearly all the neurologic attributes of the newborn infant.

# INTRAUTERINE NUTRITION

Maternal diet among mammals is incredibly varied. For instance, the female black bear hibernates during her pregnancy, but she supplies metabolites to her fetus while neither eating nor drinking. In contrast, the pregnant guinea pig eats continuously. Obviously, forced fasting may have different effects on these different species during pregnancy. As shown in Fig 8–9, many maternal and placental modifications of nutrients occur before the nutrients reach the fetus. The mother and the placenta have first priority in use of these nutrients. Although vitamin B accumulates in greater concentrations in fetal blood than in maternal blood, the placental release of most vitamins to the fetus seems to depend on the degree of saturation of the vitamin reserve in the placenta. Because these nutrient-modifying factors differ markedly in different species, it is hazardous to interpolate data from laboratory animals to humans. The human newborn is 16% fat. Normally, the human fetus has a large accumulation of high-calorie fat, which during the last few weeks of gestation represents over 80% of the fetal caloric accretion. There are 2 components of fetal caloric intake: the building-block, or accretion, component and the growth, or heat production, component. Starvation and protein-turnover studies suggest that the fetus uses calories primarily for maintenance rather than growth.

In pregnant sheep at term (pregnancy in sheep and humans is comparable in terms of relative fetal/maternal weights), one-third of the maternal glucose is used by the uterus; of this amount, two-thirds is consumed by the uteroplacental tissue and only one-third by the fetus. In sheep, the placenta rather than the fetus is clearly the primary intrauterine glucose consumer. This large glucose uptake by the placenta is partially explained by its high rate of lactate production. Laboratory studies have shown that when the human fetus is well oxygenated, the umbilical arterial lactate concentration, and the umbilical arteriovenous difference is positive, indicating that lactate is also an important nutrient for the human fetus.

Ammonia is another compound produced in large quantities by the placenta and, like lactate, is released into the umbilical circulation. In humans, ketones and free fatty acids play a large role in fetal nutrition. The fetus actively synthesizes fatty acids in the liver, brain, and lung, which have special requirements for myelin and surfactant. Although fatty acids can be transported across the placenta, their oxidation does not seem to add much to the total energy economy of the fetus. The fetus regularly uses protein for oxidative metabolism. The metabolism of the human brain is very active during the perinatal period, and the brain is an obligatory consumer of glucose. Ketone bodies may partially replace glucose during periods of hypoglycemia and may also be a source of carbon for central nervous system lipids and proteins.

The placenta transports more water than any other substance. Since maternal hydrostatic and serum colloid osmotic pressures vary significantly during a normal day, unknown placental mechanisms protect the fetus against rapid shifts of water, which could cause either hydrops or dehydration. It may be that placental water transport is a passive process resulting from active solute transfer, as in the intestine.

The most widely recognized fetal hormone known to modify the rate of fetal growth is insulin. Fetuses with anomalies that preclude the availability of fetal growth hormone, thyroxine, adrenocortical steroids, or sex steroids achieve normal birth weights. Inasmuch as maternal insulin is not transferred to the fetus in physiologic quantities, the fetal pancreas must supply sufficient insulin for the oxidation of glucose. Under the stimulus of recurring hyperglyce-

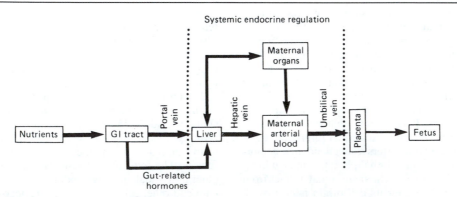

**Figure 8–9.** Schematic diagram showing the pathway of nutrients in the mother as they are broken down into different concentrations in the maternal portal vein and, finally, the umbilical vein. (Modified and reproduced, with permission, from Battaglia FC: The comparative physiology of fetal nutrition. Am J Obstet Gynecol 1984;148:850.)

mia—as with maternal diabetes mellitus—the B cells of the fetal pancreas may become hyperplastic and secrete larger quantities of insulin.

## THE AMNIOTIC FLUID

There is a vital need for a nonrestricting intrauterine environment, which develops before the fetus. This environment can only be ensured if it is part of the development of the fetus. Every fetus is surrounded by a protective cushion of amniotic fluid, whether the fetus develops inside the mother as a viviparous species or in an egg. In the first half of pregnancy, amniotic fluid volume appears to increase in association with growth of the fetus, and the correlation between fetal weight and amniotic fluid is very close. The serum osmolality and sodium, urea, and creatinine content of maternal serum and amniotic fluid are not significantly different. This suggests that amniotic fluid is an ultrafiltrate of maternal serum. Ultrasonographic evaluation during the first half of pregnancy reveals that the fetus does empty its bladder during the first half of gestation.

The average volume of amniotic fluid at term is 800 ml, and the sodium concentration is fairly constant. The volume and sodium concentration remain the same in spite of the fact that a normal fetus will swallow some of the fluid and will also contribute urine, which concentrates sodium. Analysis of amniotic fluid provides unique information about the fetus. In the first half of pregnancy, amniotic fluid appears to maintain the extracellular fluid chemistry of the fetus. In the second half, amniotic fluid reflects the development of renal function and, by virtue of the cells it sheds, the morphologic development of skin and mucous membranes. Amniotic fluid has a low specific gravity (1.008) and a pH of 7.2. Pathways of solute and water exchange in amniotic fluid are shown in Fig 8–10.

Diagnostic amniocentesis has provided a means of determining amniotic fluid content. Much of the work initially emanated from amniograms followed by spectrophotometric analysis of amniotic fluid in Rh factor isoimmunization. When an Rh-positive fetus is developing erythroblastosis, the severity of the anemia is closely correlated with the bilirubin concentration. The usual technique is to obtain a spectrophotometric tracing between the wavelengths of 550 nm and 350 nm and then determine the deviation of the optical density (OD) at 450 nm. An illustration of such a determination is shown in Fig 14–9. In this example, the OD 450-nm peak has an OD difference of 0.069, which, if found at 37 weeks' gestation, would be an indication for immediate cesarean delivery. Further details about the management of the affected fetus are given in Chapter 14.

In the past decade, morphologic chromosomal ab-

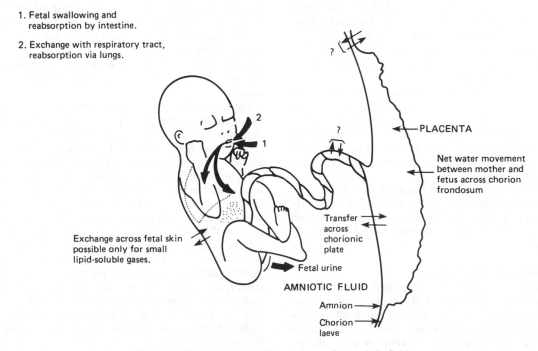

1. Fetal swallowing and reabsorption by intestine.

2. Exchange with respiratory tract, reabsorption via lungs.

PLACENTA

Net water movement between mother and fetus across chorion frondosum

Transfer across chorionic plate

Exchange across fetal skin possible only for small lipid-soluble gases.

Fetal urine

AMNIOTIC FLUID

Amnion

Chorion laeve

**Figure 8–10.** Solute and water exchange in amniotic fluid.

normalities and more than 100 inborn errors of metabolism have been identified. The amniotic fluid collects cells shed from the skin, amnion, and gastrointestinal and genitourinary tracts. In amniotic fluid obtained by amniocentesis at about 16 weeks, 30–80% of these cells are usually alive. Recent cytotechnologic advances may allow karyotyping from amniotic fluid as early as 11 weeks of gestation. The total number of cells increases with the length of gestation, but the proportion of viable cells does not increase, and at about 24 weeks, only 10–15% of the total number of cells are viable. The live cells are induced to adhere to the bottom of a tissue culture vessel after 3–4 days in culture, and they develop either an epithelial or fibroplastic morphology. The cells eventually form a monolayer, and when introduced into a suitable culture medium (containing nutrients and supplied with serum) are induced to divide. The dividing cells are arrested at metaphase with demecolcine or colchicine to prevent formation of the mitotic spindle. The advantage of this method is that a number of slides can be prepared, so that specific stain methods can be used and the chromosome preparation can be banded satisfactorily.

There is no simple or accurate method currently available to measure amniotic fluid volume. **Oligohydramnios** almost always indicates the presence of some abnormality. Polyhydramnios may occur in normal pregnancy but is associated with some abnormality of mother or fetus in approximately 50% of cases. Quantitation of amniotic fluid volume by ultrasound is subjective. The term **polyhydramnios (hydramnios)** has been classically associated with amniotic fluid volume of 2000 mL or more. Oligohydramnios may be more objectively determined by identification of the largest pocket of fluid measuring less than 2 cm × 2 cm. However, this definition is associated with many false-positive and false-negative readings.

Oligohydramnios is associated with SGA fetus, renal tract abnormalities such as renal agenesis, and urinary tract dysplasia. The clinical manifestation of oligohydramnios is a direct result of the impairment of urine flow to the amniotic fluid in the late part of the first half of pregnancy or during the second and third trimesters.

Amniotic fluid inhibits bacterial growth; the phosphate to zinc ratio is a predictor of inhibitory activity. In cases of intraamniotic fluid infection, "inorganic phosphorus" levels in amniotic fluid are often elevated.

## Amniotic Fluid Markers

Alpha-fetoprotein (AFP) is of fetal origin, and concentrations in amniotic fluid and maternal serum are of value in prenatal diagnosis of neural tube defects and other fetal malformations. Fetal serum contains AFP in a concentration 150 times that of maternal serum. High levels of maternal serum AFP are associated with an elevated level of amniotic fluid protein and subsequent findings of open neural tube defects.

In neural tube defects where there is an open lesion (even when covered with a membrane) in the spinal canal, fetal cerebrospinal fluid passes into the amniotic fluid. A suitable neural marker to determine whether cerebrospinal fluid is leaking into the amniotic fluid would be a protein of molecular size so large that it would not normally be excreted in the urine. The enzyme **acetylcholinesterase** has a molecular weight on the order of 300,000. Acetylcholinesterase levels in amniotic fluid appear to be more specific than the AFP test in predicting neural tube defects.

The clinical importance of low levels of AFP in maternal serum has also been recognized. Low levels of AFP in conjunction with estriol and comparatively high levels of hCG (roughly twice normal for given gestational age) have been shown to be predictive for Down's syndrome. As an illustration, if one assumes a base rate of diagnostic amniocentesis of 5% (the approximate proportion of pregnancies occurring beyond age 35), the likelihood of detecting Down's syndrome using only maternal age as a risk factor would be only 30%. However, if amniocenteses were to be performed on the basis of age, AFP, estriol, and hCG levels, the yield would rise to almost 60%. Down's syndrome is the most common congenital cause of severe mental retardation, occurring with an incidence of about 1.3 per 1000 live births. Advanced maternal age is the most common consideration in selecting women for diagnostic amniocentesis. This policy derives from the fact that the risk of Down's syndrome rises with advancing maternal age. The greatly improved detection rate (Table 8–8) afforded by combining serum screening and age as screening criteria is fast establishing this method as the screening test of choice in many centers throughout the world.

Other proteins may enter the amniotic fluid from the maternal plasma. Some proteins enter the fluid by transudation of placental components, but they also enter from other sources, including maternal uterine decidua, fetal skin, amnion, chorion, the umbilical cord, amniotic fluid cells, fetal urine, meconium, and fetal nasopharyngeal, oral, and lacrimal secretions. It is assumed that the relative contribution of these tissues will change during pregnancy. The major proportion of soluble proteins in amniotic fluid between 10 weeks' gestation and term is thought to be (1) of serum type and (2) of maternal origin entering the fluid by diffusing through the amniotic chorion. The observed concentration gradient for AFP between fetal serum and amniotic fluid should not be taken to imply that AFP's presence in amniotic fluid is explained largely by permeation. Indeed, the concentration of AFP in fetal urine during the second trimester

**Table 8–8.** Detection rate of Down's syndrome and open neural defects when different markers are considered alone and in combination.

| Parameter | Detection Rate (%) | False Positive Rate (%) |
|---|---|---|
| **Down's syndrome** | | |
| Maternal Age | 30 | 7.5 |
| AFP + Age | 35 | |
| Estriol + Age | 43 | Based on a |
| hCG + Age | 47 | false positive |
| AFP + Estriol + Age | 45 | rate of 5% and |
| AFP + hCG + Age | 54 | risk cut off of |
| Estriol + hCG + Age | 54 | 1/250 |
| AFP + Estriol + hCG + Age | 58 | |
| **Spina bifida/open neural tube defects** | | |
| Acetylcholinesterase | 99 | 0.34 |
| AFP | 85 | 0.36 |
| Acetylcholinesterase if maternal AFP is | | |
| ≥ 1.0 MOM | 98 | 0.29 |
| ≥ 2.0 MOM | 96 | 0.14 |
| ≤ 3.0 MOM | 91 | 0.11 |

AFP = Alpha Feto Protein, MOM = Multiples of Median.
(Adapted from Wald NJ et al: Prenatal biochemical screening for Downs Syndrome and neural tube defects. Curr Opin Obstet Gynecol 1992;4:302.)

is comparable with levels of AFP in amniotic fluid at this time.

The amniotic fluid serves a number of important functions besides being a valuable source for analysis of fetal tissues and fluids. It cushions the fetus against severe injury; provides a medium in which the fetus can move easily; may be a source of fetal nutrients; and, in early pregnancy, is essential for fetal lung development. The amniotic fluid is continuously exchanged at a rapid rate. Indeed, it is possible, at least on a temporary basis, to increase amniotic fluid volume by rapid expansion of maternal plasma volume with an intravenous infusion of colloid fluid such as 5% albumin. After 34–36 weeks, determination of amniotic fluid volume becomes even more complicated because the larger fetus swallows more fluid, upsetting the relationship between fetal size and fluid volume. After 38 weeks, both amniotic fluid and maternal plasma volume decrease. These relative decreases are even more apparent in postmature pregnancy.

Studies have shown that the fetus near term drinks 400–500 mL of amniotic fluid per day; this is about the same as the amount of milk consumed by a newborn infant. To maintain a reasonable stability of volume, the fetus must excrete about the same volume of urine into the amniotic fluid each day.

During late pregnancy, the amniotic fluid contains increasing quantities of particulate material, including desquamated cells of fetal origin; lanugo and scalp hairs; vernix caseosa; a few leukocytes; and small quantities of albumin, urates, and other organic and inorganic salts. The calcium content of amniotic fluid is low (5.5 mg/dL), but the electrolyte concentration is otherwise equivalent to that of maternal plasma. As mentioned previously, meconium is ordinarily absent but is excreted by the fetus in response to vagal activity.

## REFERENCES

Battaglia FC: The comparative physiology of fetal nutrition. Am J Obstet Gynecol 1984;148:850.

Bonds DR et al: Fetal weight/placental weight ratio and perinatal outcome. Am J Obstet Gynecol 1984;149:195.

Bonds DR et al: Human fetal weight and placental weight growth curves: A mathematical analysis from a population at sea level. Biol Neonate 1984;45:261.

Campbell S et al: New Doppler technique for assessing uteroplacental blood flow. Lancet 1983;1:675.

Castle BM, Turnbull AC: The presence or absence of fetal breathing movements predicts the outcome of preterm labour. Lancet 1983;2:471.

Dawes GS: The central control of fetal breathing and skeletal muscle movements. J Physiol 1984;346:1.

Farmakides G et al: Prenatal surveillance using non stress testing and Doppler velocimetry. Obstet Gynecol 1988; 71:184.

Fisher DJ: Oxygenation and metabolism in the developing heart. Semin Perinatol 1984;8:217.

Fleischer A et al: Uterine artery Doppler velocimetry in pregnant women with hypertension. Am J Obstet Gynecol 1986;154:806.

Fritz MA, Guo SM: Doubling time of human chorionic gonadotrophin (hCG) in normal early pregnancy: relationship to hCG concentration and gestational age. Fertil Steril 1987;47:584.

Goldenberg RL, Huddleston JF, Nelson KG: Apgar scores and umbilical arterial pH in preterm newborn infants. Am J Obstet Gynecol 1984;149:651.

Goodlin RC: Expanded toxemia syndrome or gestosis. Am J Obstet Gynecol 1986;154:1227.

Goodlin RC, Anderson JC, Gallagher TF: Relationship between amniotic fluid volume and maternal plasma volume expansion. Am J Obstet Gynecol 1984;146:505.

Harris R, Andrews T : Prenatal screening for Down's syndrome. Arch Dis Child 1988;63:705.

Hustin J, Foidart JM, Lambote R: Maternal vascular lesions in preeclampsia and intrauterine growth retardation. Placenta 1983;4:489.

Jaffe RB: Fetoplacental endocrine and metabolic physiology. Clin Perinatol 1983;10:669.

Juchau MR, Faustman-Watts E: Pharmacokinetic considerations in the maternal-placental-fetal unit. Clin Obstet Gynecol 1983;26:379.

Kauaauapaua P: Prostanoids in neonatology. Ann Clin Res 1984;16:330.

Longo LD: Maternal blood volume and cardiac output during pregnancy: A hypothesis of endocrinologic control. Am J Physiol 1983;245(5-Part 1):R720.

Naeye RL: Functionally important disorders of the placenta, umbilical cord, and fetal membranes. Hum Pathol 1987;18:680.

Rosenfeld CR: Consideration of the uteroplacental circulation in intrauterine growth. Semin Perinatol 1984;8:42.

Reed KL: Fetal pulmonary artery and aorta: Two-dimensional Doppler echocardiography. Obstet Gynecol 1987;69:175.

Sarnat HB: Disturbances of late neuronal migrations in the perinatal period. Am J Dis Child 1987;141:969.

Scarpelli EM: Perinatal lung mechanics and the first breath. Lung 1984;162:61.

Silverman F et al: The Apgar score: Is it enough? Obstet Gynecol 1985;66:331.

Suidan JS, Wasserman JF, Young BK: Placental contribution to lactate production by the human fetoplacental unit. Am J Perinatol 1984;1:306.

Voigt HJ, Becker V. Doppler flow measurements and histomorphology of the placental bed in uteroplacental insufficiency. J Perinat Med 1992;20(2): 139.

Wald NJ, Cuckle HS, Nanchahal K: Amniotic fluid acetylcholinesterase measurement in the prenatal diagnosis of open neural tube defects: Second report of the Collaborative Acetylcholinesterase study. Prenat Diagn 1989;9:813.

Wasmoen TL: Placental Proteins. In *Fetal and Neonatal Physiology*, Polin RA, Fox WW (editors). WB Saunders, 1992.

Wells M et al: Spiral (uteroplacental) arteries of the human placental bed show the presence of amniotic basement membrane antigens. Am J Obstet Gynecol 1984; 150:973.

# Normal Pregnancy & Prenatal Care

# 9

*Martin L. Pernoll, MD & Cathy Mih Taylor, MD*

## NORMAL PREGNANCY

Pregnancy (gestation) is the maternal condition of having a developing fetus in the body. The human conceptus from fertilization through the eighth week of pregnancy is termed an **embryo;** from the eighth week until delivery, it is a **fetus.** For obstetric purposes, the duration of pregnancy is based on **gestational age**: the estimated age of the fetus calculated from the first day of the last (normal) menstrual period (LMP), assuming a 28-day cycle. Gestational age is expressed in completed weeks. This is in contrast to **developmental age (fetal age),** which is the age of the offspring calculated from the time of implantation.

The term **gravid** is a general one meaning pregnant, and **gravidity** is the total number of pregnancies (normal or abnormal). Parity is the state of having given birth to an infant or infants weighing 500 g or more, alive or dead. In the absence of known weight, an estimated duration of gestation of 20 completed weeks or more (calculated from the first day of the LMP) may be used. From the practical clinical viewpoint, a fetus is considered viable when it has reached a gestational age of 23–24 weeks and a weight of 600 g or more. However, only very rarely will a fetus of 20–23 weeks weighing 500–600 g or less survive, even with optimal care. With regard to parity, a multiple birth is a single parous experience.

### Live Birth

Live birth is the complete expulsion or extraction of a product of conception from the mother, regardless of the duration of pregnancy, which, after such separation, breathes or shows other evidence of life (eg, beating of the heart, pulsation of the umbilical cord, or definite movements of the involuntary muscles) whether or not the cord has been cut or the placenta detached. An **infant** is a live-born individual from the moment of birth until the completion of 1 year of life.

In the most recent nomenclature, a **preterm infant** is defined as one born at any time through the 37th completed week of gestation (259 days). Unfortunately, for purposes of evaluating statistical data, this definition does not specify that there are great differences among fetuses in this group. Therefore, it is useful to preserve the classification by weight or duration of gestation still used by many (Fig 9–1). Using the latter system, an **abortion** is the expulsion or extraction of all (complete) or any part (incomplete) of the placenta or membranes, without an identifiable fetus or with a fetus (alive or dead) weighing less than 500 g. In the absence of known weight, an estimated duration of gestation of under 20 completed weeks (139 days) calculated from the first day of the LMP may be used.

An **immature infant** weighs 500–1000 g and has completed 20 to less than 28 weeks of gestation. A **premature infant** is one with a birth weight of 1000–2500 g and a duration of gestation of 28 to less than 38 weeks. A **low-birth-weight infant** is any live-born infant weighing 2500 g or less at birth. An **undergrown** or **small-for-date infant** is one who is significantly undersized (< 2 SD) for the period of gestation. A **mature infant** is a live-born infant who has completed 38 weeks of gestation (and usually weighs over 2500 g). A **postmature infant** is one who has completed 42 weeks or more of gestation. The **postmature syndrome** is characterized by prolonged gestation, sometimes an excessive-size fetus (see Large-For-Gestational-Age Pregnancy in Disproportionate Fetal Growth Chapter), and diminished placental capacity for sufficient exchange, associated with cutaneous and nutritional changes in the newborn infant.

A fetus or infant of **excessive size** is one who is larger than the gestation would indicate or who at the time of birth weighs over 4500 g. Significantly increased morbidity and mortality rates may be associated with the relative dystocia created by the large fetus. About 10% of newborn infants are **oversized** (over 4000 g), and 2% are of "excessive" size (over 4500 g). With better nutrition and heavier infants, there has not been a commensurate increase in maternal pelvic dimensions. Excessive fetal size should be

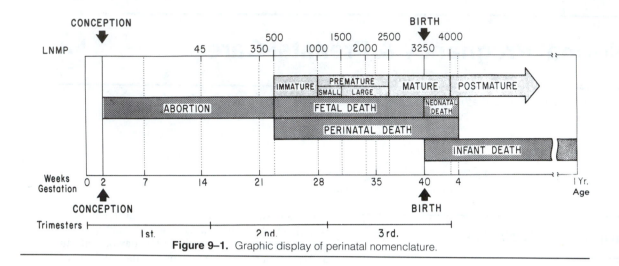

**Figure 9–1.** Graphic display of perinatal nomenclature.

suspected in large multiparous or obese mothers, those with diabetes mellitus, or those whose weight gain during pregnancy has been greater than anticipated.

The untimely termination of pregnancy constitutes one of the major problems of perinatal care. The factors that lead to the initiation of labor and the subsequent termination of pregnancy remain unknown. This is the case for both late termination and premature termination. A prolonged pregnancy is a gestation that has advanced beyond 2 SD from the mean and with a duration of 42½ weeks or longer (297 days). The perinatal mortality rate at 43 weeks is twice that at 39–42 weeks. The fetus probably develops a relatively restricted placental exchange capability, leading to an increased intrauterine death rate.

Each of the above terms is numerically expressed by a rate per 1000 births over a given interval.

## Birth Rate & Fertility Rate

**Birth rate** is commonly expressed in terms of the number of live births per 1000 population. The fertility rate is expressed as the number of live births per 1000 women aged 15–44 years and is thus a more sensitive measure of the reproductive activity of a given population. There were an estimated 4,084,000 live births in the USA during the year ending December 1992. This number is slightly lower than the 4,111,000 reported for the similar 1991 interval. Likewise, during the same interval, the 1992 fertility rate (69.3) was less than that of 1991 (69.6).* Indeed,

the fertility rate appears to have peaked in 1990 at 71.1, after having been 67.1 in 1988.

## Neonatal Interval

The neonatal interval is from birth until 28 days of life. During this interval, the infant is referred to as a newborn infant. The interval may be divided into 3 periods:

Neonatal period I: birth through 23 hours, 59 minutes.

Neonatal period II: 24 hours of life through 6 days, 23 hours, 59 minutes.

Neonatal period III: seventh day of life through 27 days, 23 hours, 59 minutes.

## Perinatal Interval

The perinatal interval is the span of fetal and neonatal life. It is an important concept because many of the stresses and hazards that affect the fetus have either a direct or an indirect effect in the neonatal period. An arbitrary division of authority (between obstetrician and pediatrician) and attention only to the product of conception at birth may be hazardous and unwarranted. The perinatal interval of life may be divided into 2 periods:

Perinatal period I: 28 weeks of completed gestation to the first 7 days of life.

Perinatal period II: 20 weeks of gestation through 27 days of life.

## Perinatal Mortality Rates

Jeopardy to life is greater during the perinatal interval than at any subsequent time. Current data indicates that the number of lives lost during the 5-month period from the 20th week of gestation to the seventh day after birth is almost equal to the number lost during the next 40 years of life. Table 9–1 illustrates death rates by age, race, and sex in the USA. Of those

---

*These data are provisional and are from the *Monthly Vital Statistic Report* 1993;41:1, the preeminent source of data concerning births, marriages, divorces, and deaths. It is available on a monthly basis from the National Center for Health Statistics (Centers for Disease Control, Public Health Service), US Department of Health and Human Services.

**Table 9–1.** USA estimated death rates by age, race, and sex for the 12 months ending December 1992 (per 100,000 specified population).

| Age | All Races, Both Sexes | Black Female | White Female | Black Male | White Male |
|---|---|---|---|---|---|
| < 1 | 834.3 | 1497.1 | 629.8 | 1701.7 | 729.2 |
| 1–4 | 44.2 | 66.1 | 33.8 | 70.8 | 43.9 |
| 5–14 | 22.2 | 24.6 | 15.8 | 39.0 | 25.2 |
| 15–24 | 99.5 | 72.8 | 44.1 | 269.6 | 127.7 |
| 25–34 | 134.1 | 154.3 | 56.6 | 405.6 | 170.0 |
| 35–44 | 233.4 | 326.3 | 117.5 | 712.2 | 282.1 |
| 45–54 | 448.6 | 603.8 | 288.4 | 1,184.6 | 526.1 |
| 55–64 | 1,144.3 | 1,399.7 | 806.0 | 2,242.7 | 1,385.5 |
| 65–74 | 2,528.2 | 2,602.5 | 1,910.2 | 4,200.3 | 3,176.6 |
| 75–84 | 5,867.3 | 5,782.5 | 4,809.0 | 8,750.0 | 7,508.1 |
| ≥ 85 | 14,052.1 | 12,068.4 | 13,264.2 | 14,900.0 | 16,927.2 |

These data are provisional and are from the Monthly Vital Statistics Report 1993;41:1.

deaths occurring in the first year of life, approximately 70% will occur in the first 28 days. If one adds this to the fetal loss, then it is the period of greatest threat to life for a given interval. Additionally, Table 9–1 demonstrates the marked sexual and racial differences in the mortality rates for each age group.

There are many causes of death during the perinatal period. The relative importance of each can only be assessed in the context of overall mortality rates and appraisal of those factors that present the greatest hazard to the fetus and infant. Fetal deaths after 20 weeks account for about 50% of all perinatal deaths.

## DIAGNOSIS

The diagnosis of pregnancy is usually made on the basis of a history of amenorrhea, an enlarging uterus, and a positive pregnancy test. Nausea and breast tenderness are also often present. It may be crucial to diagnose pregnancy before the first missed menstrual period to prevent exposure of the fetus to hazardous substances (eg, x-ray, teratogenic drugs), to manage ectopic or nonviable pregnancies, or to provide better health care for the mother.

The manifestations of pregnancy are classified into 3 groups: presumptive, probable, and positive.

### Presumptive Manifestations
**A. Symptoms:**
**1. Amenorrhea–**Cessation of menses is caused by increasing estrogen and progesterone levels produced by the corpus luteum. Thus, amenorrhea is a fairly reliable sign of conception in women with regular menstrual cycles. In women with irregular cycles, amenorrhea is not a reliable sign. Delayed menses may also be caused by other factors such as emotional tension, chronic disease, opioid and dopaminergic medications, endocrine disorders, and certain genitourinary tumors. Spotting due to bleed-

ing at the implantation site may occur from the time of implantation (about 6 days after fertilization) until 29–35 days after the LMP in many women. Some women have unexplained cyclic bleeding throughout pregnancy.

**2. Nausea and vomiting–**This common symptom occurs in approximately 50% of pregnancies and is most marked at 2–12 weeks' gestation. It is usually most severe in the morning but may occur at any time and may be precipitated by cooking odors and pungent smells. Emotional tension may play a role in the severity of nausea and vomiting. Extreme nausea and vomiting may be a sign of multiple gestation or molar pregnancy. Protracted vomiting associated with dehydration and ketonuria (**hyperemesis gravidarum**) may require hospitalization.

Treatment for uncomplicated nausea consists of light dry foods, small frequent meals, and emotional support. Some improvement can be seen with the addition of high-dose $B_6$ therapy and the preconceptional use of prenatal vitamins. Antinauseant drugs are used only as a final measure. The nausea probably results from rapidly rising serum levels of human chorionic gonadotropin (hCG). During the first trimester, serum hCG levels may be as high as 100,000 mU/mL.

**3. Breasts–**
**a. Mastodynia–**Mastodynia, or **breast tenderness,** may range from tingling to frank pain caused by hormonal responses of the mammary ducts and alveolar system. Circulatory increases result in breast engorgement and venous prominence. Similar tenderness may occur just before menses.

**b. Enlargement of circumlacteal sebaceous glands of the areola (Montgomery's tubercles)–**Enlargement of these glands occurs at 6–8 weeks' gestation and is due to hormonal stimulation.

**c. Colostrum secretion–**Colostrum secretion may begin after 16 weeks' gestation.

**d. Secondary breasts–**Secondary breasts may become more prominent both in size and in coloration. These occur along the nipple line. Hypertrophy of axillary breast tissue often causes a symptomatic lump in the axilla.

**4. Quickening–**The first perception of fetal movement occurs at 18–20 weeks in primigravidas and at 14–16 weeks in multigravidas. Fetal movement may be mistaken for peristalsis; therefore, it is not a reliable symptom of pregnancy by itself but may be useful in determining the duration of pregnancy.

**5. Urinary tract–**

**a. Bladder irritability, frequency, and nocturia–**These conditions occur because of increased bladder circulation and pressure from the enlarging uterus.

**b. Urinary tract infection–**Urinary tract infection must always be ruled out because pregnant women are more likely than nonpregnant women to have significant bacteriuria (7% versus 3%).

**B. Signs:**

**1. Increased basal body temperature–**Persistent elevation of basal body temperature over a 3-week period usually indicates pregnancy if temperatures have been carefully charted.

**2. Skin–**

**a. Chloasma–**Chloasma, or the **mask of pregnancy,** is darkening of the skin over the forehead, bridge of the nose, or cheekbones and is most marked in those with dark complexions. It usually occurs after 16 weeks' gestation and is intensified by exposure to sunlight.

**b. Linea nigra–**Linea nigra is darkening of the skin in the areola, nipples, and lower midline of the abdomen from the umbilicus to the pubis (darkening of the linea alba). The basis of these changes is stimulation of the melanophores by an increase in melanocyte-stimulating hormone.

**c. Stretch marks–**Stretch marks, or striae of the breast and abdomen, are caused by separation of the underlying collagen tissue and appear as irregular scars. This is probably an adrenocorticosteroid response. These marks generally appear later in pregnancy when the skin is under greater tension.

**d. Spider telangiectases–**Spider telangiectases are common skin lesions that result from high levels of circulating estrogen. These vascular stellate marks blanch when compressed. Palmar erythema is often an associated sign. Both of these signs are also seen in patients with liver failure.

## Probable Manifestations

**A. Symptoms:** Symptoms are the same as those discussed under Presumptive Manifestations, above.

**B. Signs:**

**1. Pelvic organs–**Many changes in the pelvic organs are perceivable to the experienced physician, including the following:

**a. Chadwick's sign–**Congestion of the pelvic vasculature causes bluish or purplish discoloration of the vagina and cervix.

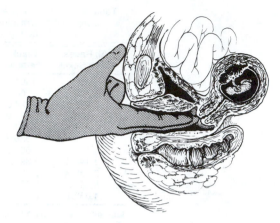

**Figure 9–2.** Softening of the cervix (Goodell's sign).

**b. Leukorrhea–**An increase in vaginal discharge consisting of epithelial cells and cervical mucus is due to hormone stimulation. Cervical mucus that has been spread on a glass slide and allowed to dry no longer forms a fern-like pattern but has a granular appearance.

**c. Goodell's sign–**Cyanosis and softening of the cervix (Fig 9–2) is due to increased vascularity of the cervical tissue. This change may occur as early as 4 weeks.

**d. Ladin's sign–**At 6 weeks, the uterus softens in the anterior midline along the uterocervical junction (Fig 9–3).

**e. Hegar's sign–**This is widening of the softened area of the isthmus, resulting in compressibility of the isthmus on bimanual examination. This occurs by 6–8 weeks (Fig 9–4).

**f. McDonald's sign–**The uterus becomes flexible at the uterocervical junction at 7–8 weeks.

**g. Von Fernwald's sign–**An irregular softening of the fundus develops over the site of implantation at

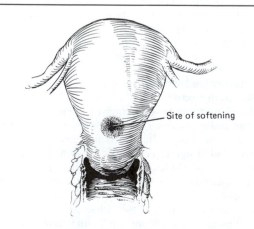

Site of softening

**Figure 9–3.** Ladin's sign.

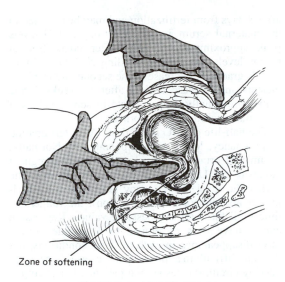

Zone of softening

**Figure 9–4.** Hegar's sign.

during pregnancy. There is slight but definite relaxation of the joints. Relaxation is most pronounced at the pubic symphysis, which may separate to an astonishing degree.

**2. Abdominal enlargement–**There is progressive abdominal enlargement from 7 to 28 weeks. At 16–22 weeks, growth may appear more rapid as the uterus rises out of the pelvis and into the abdomen (Fig 9–6).

**3. Uterine contractions–**As the uterus enlarges, it becomes globular and often rotates to the right. Painless uterine contractions (**Braxton Hicks contractions**) are felt as tightening or pressure. They usually begin at about 28 weeks' gestation and increase in regularity. These contractions usually disappear with walking or exercise, whereas true labor contractions become more intense.

4–5 weeks (Fig 9–5). If this occurs in the cornual area (Piskacek's sign), it may be confused with a uterine leiomyoma or abnormal uterine development. By 10 weeks, the uterus becomes symmetric and enlarges to double its nonpregnant size.

**h. Bones and ligaments of pelvis–**The bony and ligamentous structures of the pelvis also change

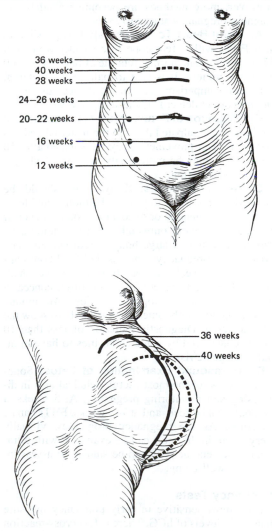

36 weeks
40 weeks
28 weeks
24–26 weeks
20–22 weeks
16 weeks
12 weeks

36 weeks
40 weeks

**Figure 9–6.** Height of fundus at various times during pregnancy.

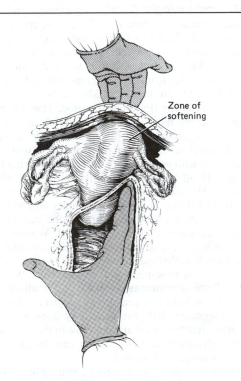

Zone of softening

**Figure 9–5.** Von Fernwald's sign.

**4. Ballottement of the uterus—**At 16–20 weeks, ballottement of the uterus on bimanual examination may give the impression that a floating object occupies the uterus. This is a valuable sign but is not diagnostic. A similar sign may also be elicited with uterine leiomyomas, ascites, or ovarian cysts.

**5. Uterine souffle—**Auscultation of the abdomen after 16 weeks often elicits a rushing sound synchronous with the pulse (caused by the movement of maternal blood filling the placental vessels and sinuses). The intensity may vary from a whisper to a loud rush. With anterior implantation, this sound may mask the fetal heart sounds for several months.

## Positive Manifestations

The various signs and symptoms of pregnancy are often reliable, but none is diagnostic. A positive diagnosis must be made upon objective findings, many of which are not produced until after the first trimester. However, more methods are becoming available to diagnose pregnancy at an early stage.

**A. Fetal Heart Tones (FHTs):** It is possible to hear FHTs with a fetoscope in a slender woman at 17–18 weeks. The normal fetal heart rate is 120–160 beats per minute. It is best to palpate the maternal pulse for comparison. Electronic devices using the Doppler effect detect FHTs as early as 8 weeks.

**B. Palpation of Fetus:** After 22 weeks, the fetal outline can be palpated through the maternal abdominal wall. Fetal movements may be palpated after 18 weeks. This may be more easily accomplished by a vaginal examination.

**C. X-Ray of Fetus:** X-ray films should be avoided in pregnancy to protect the mother and fetus from possible genetic or oncogenic risk. However, if the potential benefit outweighs the risk, radiographs may be of value. A large body of radiographic data exists about pregnancy. The ossified fetal bones appear at 12–14 weeks. Before 16 weeks, bowel shadows and pelvic bone configuration often conceal a pregnancy in the anteroposterior view. An oblique view of the lower abdomen is most likely to show the fetal skeleton. Diagnostic radiation of less than 10 rads is considered by some authorities to have minimal teratogenic risk.

**D. Ultrasound Examination of Fetus:** Sonography is one of the most useful technical aids in diagnosing and monitoring pregnancy. At 5 weeks, a fetal pole can be seen, and at 7–8 weeks, FHTs can be discerned. As the pregnancy progresses, virtually every organ in the fetus can be examined with ultrasound, and fetal activity can be studied to assess intrauterine well-being.

## Pregnancy Tests

Tests most sensitive in early pregnancy measure changes in levels of hCG. There is less cross-reaction and testing is more accurate with the beta subunit of hCG. hCG is produced by the syncytiotrophoblast after 8 days from fertilization and may be detected in the maternal serum as early as 9 days. hCG levels peak approximately 65 days after conception at serum levels generally exceeding 50,000 mU/mL. Levels gradually decrease in the second and third trimesters and increase slightly after 34 weeks. Urine values are usually proportionate to serum values if maternal renal function is normal.

The half-life of hCG is 1.5 days. After termination of pregnancy, levels drop exponentially. Normally, serum and urine hCG levels return to nonpregnant values (< 5 mU/mL) 21–24 days after delivery. The higher the level at pregnancy termination (first-trimester abortion or molar gestation), the longer the time until the return to baseline values. Regression curves have been developed to determine normal hCG disappearance in each of these conditions, but they are difficult to apply to specific cases because of varying circumstances among patients. For example, minimal residual trophoblast in the uterus after a D&C may delay the fall in hCG levels. In such cases, it may be important to at least establish that levels are falling and eventually reach nonpregnant values (Fig 9–7).

**A. Biologic Tests:** Biologic tests have been replaced by more sensitive and economical methods. In 1928, urine from pregnant women was injected into immature mice. If sufficient hCG was present, the mice ovulated and, on sacrifice, corpora lutea could be observed. Testing in rabbits was begun in 1931. Rats and frogs have also been used.

**B. Immunologic Tests:** Immunologic tests are based on antigenic properties of the polypeptide protein hCG. The tests available all use direct or indirect agglutination of sensitized red blood cells or latex particles. Testing time is 2 minutes to 2 hours, and sensitivity varies from 250–3500 mU/mL of hCG, depending on the product used. Most tests are positive 4–7 days after the first missed period. Test accuracy may be altered by (1) proteinuria, which inactivates anti-hCG agglutination; (2) immunologic disease, which causes false-positive reactions because of IgM interaction with test reagents; and (3) luteinizing hormone (LH; all immunologic tests cross-react with elevated LH levels). Any condition that stimulates release of LH from the anterior pituitary may result in a false-positive reaction. Antipsychotic agents and tranquilizers may cause release of LH. Women who have undergone ovariectomy, who are menopausal, who have hypothyroidism, or who are in renal failure may also have false-positive tests (see Table 9–2).

**C. Radioimmunoassay for hCG:** Radioimmunoassay for hCG is a sensitive and specific test for early pregnancy. LH cross-reactivity does not occur when the reagents used are sensitive to the β-subunit of the glycoprotein. Laboratories can detect serum levels as low as 2–4 mU/mL.

This test requires scintillation counting and 24–48 hours of incubation time. A quantitative analysis of

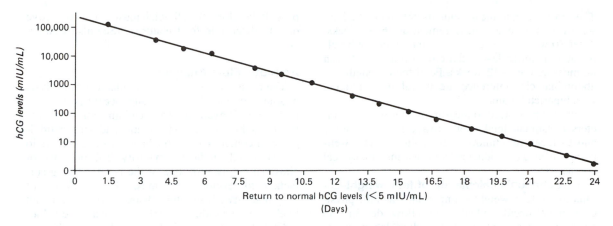

**Figure 9–7.** Regression of hCG following delivery, assuming a 1.5-day half-life.

hCG can be obtained and used to determine the normalcy and viability of early pregnancy.

**D. Radioreceptor Assay:** Radioreceptor assay measures receptor sites by a competitive binding mechanism and is capable of measuring levels as low as 200 mU. This test may be completed in 2–4 hours. Unfortunately, this test also cross-reacts with LH.

**E. Home Pregnancy Tests:** Home pregnancy tests are immunologic tests and have the same problems mentioned above in addition to the possibility of misinterpretation. hCG is detected in a first-voided morning urine sample. A positive test is indicated by a color change or confirmation mark in the test well. If negative, the test may be repeated in 2 weeks or a radioimmunoassay could be performed. If still negative, amenorrhea due to another condition should be considered.

## CALCULATION OF GESTATIONAL AGE & ESTIMATED DATE OF CONFINEMENT

After the diagnosis of pregnancy is made, it is imperative to determine the duration of pregnancy and the estimated date of confinement (EDC).

**Table 9–2.** Immunologic tests for pregnancy.

| Method | Materials | Results |
|---|---|---|
| Direct coagulation | Latex particles coated with anti-hCG + serum or urine. | Coagulation if hCG is present (pregnant). |
| Inhibition of coagulation | Anti-hCG + serum or urine **plus** Sensitized red cells **or** Latex particles coated with hCG. | Coagulation if hCG is absent (not pregnant); inhibition if hCG is present (pregnant). |

### Calculation of Gestational Age

**A. Pregnancy Calendar or Calculator:** Normally, human pregnancy lasts 280 days or 40 weeks (9 calendar months or 10 lunar months) from the last normal menstrual period (LMNP). This may also be calculated as 266 days or 38 weeks from the last ovulation in a normal 28-day cycle. The easiest method of determining gestational age is with the pregnancy calendar or calculator.

**B. Clinical Parameters of Gestational Age:**

**1. Uterine size–**An early first-trimester examination usually correlates well with the estimated gestational age. The uterus is palpable just at the pubic symphysis at 8 weeks. At 12 weeks, the uterus becomes an abdominal organ and at 15 weeks is usually at the midpoint between the pubic symphysis and the umbilicus. The uterus is palpable at 20 weeks at the umbilicus. Fundal size correlates roughly with the estimated gestational age at 26–34 weeks. After 36 weeks, the fundal height may decrease as the fetal head descends into the pelvis. Fundal height is determined by measuring the distance in centimeters from the pubic symphysis to the fundus (Fig 9–6).

**2. Quickening–**The first fetal movement is usually appreciated at 17 weeks in the average multipara and at 18 weeks in the average primipara.

**3. Fetal heart tones–**FHTs may be heard by fetoscope at 20 weeks, whereas Doppler ultrasound usually detects heart rates by 10 weeks.

**4. X-ray examination–**Fetal age can only be approximated by x-ray evaluation of bony calcification. Fortunately, this method has been largely replaced by the use of ultrasound.

**5. Ultrasonography–**Ultrasonography is now the most widely used technique for determination of gestational age; there is now little or no justification for the use of x-ray for this purpose.

Measurement of fetal biparietal diameter is an accurate method of determining fetal age at 20–30 weeks. Fetal growth at this time is linear and rapid.

The most accurate measurements are taken at 20–24 weeks, with a repeat measurement at 26–30 weeks. After 30 weeks, the accuracy of measurement by ultrasound is much less. Fetal crown-rump length can be measured at 5–12 weeks. Fetal femur length and abdominal circumference are useful in correlation with biparietal diameter.

Ultrasound is used to measure fetal growth parameters, to estimate fetal weight, to access fetal anatomy and to measure amniotic fluid volume. Fetal well-being can also be evaluated by measuring biophysical characteristics.

**6. Johnson's calculation of fetal weight–**Estimation of fetal weight is important when the physician must decide whether to allow delivery to proceed as a natural event, to induce labor, to use tocolytic agents, or to perform cesarean section. Johnson's formula for estimation of fetal weight in vertex presentations is as follows:

**Fetal weight (in grams) =**
**fh (in centimeters) – n × 155**
**n = 12 if vertex is above ischial spines**
**n = 11 if vertex is below ischial spines**
**fh = fundal height (measured from the pubic symphysis)**

If the patient weighs more than 91 kg (200 lb), 1 cm is subtracted from the fundal height, as in the following example:

**fh = 30 cm, station = – 2**
**therefore, (29 – 12) × 155 = 2635 g**

This calculation is accurate within 375 g in 75% of newborns.

### Estimated Date of Confinement (Nägele's Rule)

The EDC can be determined mathematically using Nägele's rule: Subtract 3 from the month of the LNMP, and add 7 to the first day of the LNMP. Example: With an LNMP of July 14, the EDC is April 21. This rule is based on a normal 28-day cycle. In women with a longer proliferative phase, add to the first day of the LNMP the usual 7 days plus the number of days that the cycle extends beyond 28 days.

## DIAGNOSIS OF PREGNANCY AT TERM

A **term fetus** has reached a stage of development that will allow the best chance for extrauterine survival (37–42 weeks). Whether a fetus has reached this stage can be determined by the methods outlined above for ascertaining fetal age and EDC.

At term, a fetus usually weighs over 2500 g. Depending on maternal factors such as obesity and diabetes, amniotic fluid volume, and genetic and racial factors, the baby may be larger or smaller than expected; therefore, the clinician must rely on objective data to determine fetal maturity. (See also Chapter 16.)

### Amniotic Fluid Analysis

The most accurate test of fetal maturity is analysis of amniotic fluid obtained by amniocentesis. The amniotic fluid is evaluated for creatinine concentration, lecithin/sphingomyelin (L/S) ratio, and phosphatidylglycerol content (see also Chapter 13). An L/S ratio of 2:1 usually indicates maturity. The presence of phosphatidylglycerol, one of the last fetal lung surfactants to develop, is the most reliable indicator of lung maturity. Respiratory distress syndrome is not likely to occur following delivery when these values indicate fetal maturity. Values may be less reliable if the mother is diabetic or if amniotic fluid is contaminated by blood, meconium, or other body fluids (eg, urine or vaginal contents).

The **shake test** may be used if biochemical assays are not available. A vial containing 1 mL amniotic fluid mixed with 1 mL 95% ethanol is compared with a second vial containing 1 mL amniotic fluid, 0.5 mL ethanol, and 0.5 mL normal saline solution. If a ring of bubbles appears in the second vial after 30 seconds of vigorous shaking, an L/S ratio of 2 or greater can be assumed. Bubbles in the 1:1 mixture but not in the second vial mean that the fetus is in a borderline stage of development and that the pregnancy should be allowed to continue if possible.

### Ultrasonography

Multiple early prenatal ultrasound examination are most accurate in diagnosing fetal maturity. A late biparietal diameter of 9.8 cm or more, however, is usually indicative of fetal maturity.

## DIAGNOSIS OF POSTDATES PREGNANCY

The diagnosis and management of prolonged pregnancy are discussed in Chapter 13.

## DIAGNOSIS OF FETAL DEATH

Early in pregnancy, the first sign of fetal death is absence of uterine growth. In such cases, when pregnancy testing is initially positive but then negative on 2 subsequent occasions, fetal death is likely. Descending serial blood hCG values are usually predictive of spontaneous abortion.

In later pregnancy, the first sign of fetal death is usually absence of fetal movement noted by the mother. This is followed by absence of FHTs. Signs and symptoms of pregnancy may subside. A roentgenogram of the fetus may show evidence of fetal death, including overlapping skull bones (**Spalding's sign**), gas in the great vessels (**Robert's sign**), and exaggeration of the fetal spinal curvature or angulation of the spine. These signs are due to postmortem changes in the degenerating fetus.

Real-time ultrasonography is nearly 100% accurate in determining the absence of fetal heart motion. Clot formation in the fetal heart chambers is an early diagnostic sign of fetal death.

**Hypofibrinogenemia** develops 4–5 weeks after fetal death as thromboplastic substances are released from the degenerating products of conception. Coagulation studies should be started 2 weeks after intrauterine death, and delivery should be attempted by 4 weeks or if serum fibrinogen falls below 200 mg/mL.

## DETECTION OF PREVIOUS PREGNANCY

Occasionally, the physician is called on to determine whether a patient has had a previous pregnancy. This diagnosis can rarely be made with certainty, but a reasonably accurate opinion can often be formulated. The appraisal is based on the status of the reproductive organs and the changes that pregnancy usually causes. The breasts of the multiparous patient are in most cases less firm and more pendulous and have increased pigmentation of the areolar areas. A lax abdominal wall may be noted, with separation of the rectus muscles. The scar of a cesarean section may be present. Striae over the abdomen or breasts, although not diagnostic, are suggestive of prior pregnancy. The perineum may reveal the scars of a previous episiotomy or laceration. The vaginal canal may show extreme relaxation. Following delivery, the external cervical os usually appears as a transverse slit or stellate gap, as contrasted with the small circular cervical opening in the nulliparous woman.

## PRENATAL CARE

Prenatal care as we know it today is a relatively new development in medicine. It originated in Boston in the first decade of this century. Before that time, the patient who thought she was pregnant may have visited a physician for confirmation but did not visit again until delivery was imminent. The nurses of the Instructive Nursing Association in Boston, thinking they might contribute to the health of pregnant mothers, began making house calls on all mothers registered for delivery at the Boston Lying-In Hospital. These visits were so successful that the principle behind them was gradually accepted by physicians, and our present system of prenatal care, which stresses prevention, evolved.

Pregnancy is a normal physiologic event that is complicated by pathologic processes dangerous to the health of the mother and fetus in only 5–20% of cases. The physician who undertakes care of pregnant patients must be familiar with the normal changes that occur during pregnancy, so that significant abnormalities can be recognized and their effects minimized.

Prenatal care should have as a principal aim the identification and special treatment of the high-risk patient—the one whose pregnancy, because of some factor in her medical history or significant development during pregnancy, is likely to have a poor outcome.

The purpose of prenatal care is to ensure, as far as possible, an uncomplicated pregnancy and the delivery of a live healthy infant. There is evidence that mothers and offspring who receive prenatal care have a lower risk of complications. There is also evidence that the mother's emotional state during pregnancy may have a direct effect on fetal outcome. Lederman et al (1981) reported that anxiety in labor is positively correlated with plasma epinephrine levels, which in turn seem to result in abnormal fetal heart rate patterns and low Apgar scores. Similarly, Crandon (1979) measured anxiety in women in the third trimester and noted that in newborns of anxious women, the 5-minute Apgar score was distinctly lower.

Ideally, a woman planning to have a child should have a medical evaluation before she becomes pregnant. This allows the physician to establish by history, physical examination, and laboratory studies the patient's overall fitness for undertaking pregnancy. This is the ideal time to stress the dangers of cigarette smoking, alcohol and drug use, and exposure to teratogens. Instruction on proper diet and exercise habits can be given. Vitamins, especially folic acid, taken 3 months before conception may be beneficial (decreased incidence of open neural tube defects). Unfortunately, most patients do not seek preconceptional care, and the initial prenatal visit is scheduled well after pregnancy is under way.

Common reasons why pregnant women may not receive adequate prenatal care are inability to pay for health care; fear of or lack of confidence in health care professionals, lack of self-esteem, delays in suspecting pregnancy or in reporting pregnancy to others, different individual or cultural perceptions of the importance of prenatal care, adverse initial feelings about being pregnant, and religious or cultural prohibitions. These factors should be screened for and addressed.

### INITIAL OFFICE VISIT

The purpose of the first visit to the physician is to identify all risk factors involving the mother and fetus. Once identified, high-risk pregnancies require individualized specialized care. The diagnosis of pregnancy is made on the basis of physical signs and symptoms and the results of laboratory tests discussed earlier in this chapter.

## History

**A. Present Pregnancy:** The interview should begin with a full discussion of the symptoms. The patient should have time to express her ideas on childbearing and parenting and to discuss the effect of pregnancy on her life situation.

The patient with regular menses may be able to accurately calculate the EDC using the first day of the LMP and Nägele's rule (LMP – 3 months + 7 days = EDC). Determination of the EDC may be difficult if menses have been irregular or if conception has occurred during use of oral contraceptives. The date of the LNMP may be helpful if there has been some recent irregular bleeding. The EDC may also be determined if the patient knows the probable date of conception.

The common symptoms of pregnancy may be helpful in diagnosing and dating the pregnancy (see previous text).

**B. Previous Pregnancy:** Events of prior pregnancies (regardless of outcome) provide important clues to potential problems in the current one. The following information is necessary: length of gestation, birth weight, fetal outcome, length of labor, fetal presentation, type of delivery, and complications (prenatal, during labor, postpartum).

**C. Medical History:** Many medical disorders are exacerbated by pregnancy (see Chapter 23). Many cardiovascular, gastrointestinal, and endocrine disorders require careful evaluation and counseling concerning possible deleterious effects on the mother. A history of previous blood transfusion may suggest the rare possibility of associated hemolytic disease of the newborn because of maternal antibodies from a minor blood group mismatch. Knowledge of drug sensitivities is also important.

A history of maternal infections during pregnancy should be obtained. Precautions should be taken to avoid reinfection. If possible, current infections should be treated to prevent hazardous fetal effects. Review of the patient's knowledge about avoiding mutagenic and teratogenic risks (see Chapter 14) is prudent.

The prenatal history should include important social aspects such as the number of sexual partners, the history of sexually transmitted diseases, and possible contact with intravenous drug users. HIV testing has become mandatory in some clinics and should be considered in high-risk individuals.

**D. Surgical History:** Of special importance is a history of previous gynecologic surgery. Prior uterine surgery may necessitate cesarean delivery. A history of multiple induced abortions or midtrimester losses may suggest an incompetent cervix. Patients with previous cesarean deliveries may be candidates for vaginal delivery if they are adequately counseled and meet established guidelines.

**E. Family History:** A family history of diabetes mellitus should alert the physician to this disorder, especially if the patient has a history of large or anomalous babies or previous stillbirths. Glucose tolerance testing must be done to determine current endocrine function.

Awareness of familial disorders is also important in pregnancy management. Thus, a brief 3-generation pedigree is most useful. Antenatal screening tests are available for many hereditary diseases (see Chapter 30).

A history of twinning is important, since dizygotic twinning (polyovulation) may be a maternally inherited trait.

## Physical Examination

**A. General Examination:** A complete physical examination must be performed on every new patient. In a young healthy woman, this may be the first complete examination she has ever had.

**B. Pelvic Examination:** The pelvic examination is of special importance to the obstetrician.

**1. Pelvic soft tissue**–Any pelvic mass should be described accurately and examined by ultrasonography.

**2. Bony pelvis**–The pelvic configuration should be appraised to determine which patients are more likely to develop cephalopelvic disproportion in labor. X-ray pelvimetry is the most accurate method of assessing the diameters of the vault, midpelvis, and outlet. However, x-ray pelvimetry should be postponed until near term and then used only if the potential benefit exceeds the risk. This technique allows assessment of the fetal head and position as well as the pelvic diameters.

**a. Pelvic inlet**–Although the transverse diameter of the inlet cannot be measured clinically, the anteroposterior diameter or diagonal conjugate usually can be estimated. For this measurement, the middle finger of the examining hand reaches for the promontory of the sacrum, and the tissue between the examiner's index finger and thumb is pushed against the pubic symphysis while the point of pressure is noted (Fig 9–8). The distance between the tip of the examining finger and this point of pressure measures the diagonal conjugate of the inlet. Subtracting 1.5 cm from the diagonal conjugate gives a satisfactory estimate of the true conjugate (conjugata vera), or the true anterior diameter of the pelvic inlet.

**b. Midpelvis**–Precise clinical measurement of the diameter of the midpelvic space is not feasible. With some experience, however, the physician can estimate this distance by noting the prominence and relative closeness of the ischial spines. If the walls of

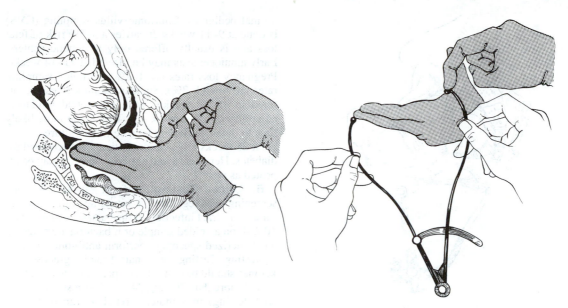

**Figure 9–8.** Measurement of the diagonal conjugate (DC) (conjugata diagonalis, CD). (Reproduced, with permission, from Benson RC: *Handbook of Obstetrics & Gynecology*, 8th ed. Lange, 1983.)

the pelvis seem to converge; if the curve of the sacrum is straightened or shallow; or if the sacrosciatic notches are unusually narrow, doubt about the adequacy of the mid pelvis is justified.

   **c. Pelvic outlet**–For clinical purposes, the outlet can be adequately estimated by physical examination. The shape of the outlet can be determined by palpating the pubic rami from the symphysis to the ischial tuberosities and noting the angle of the rami. A subpubic angle of more than 90 degrees suggests inadequacy of the outlet. The intertuberous (biischial) diameter can be accurately measured with Thoms's pelvimeter (Fig 9–9). A diameter of more than 8.5 cm usually is adequate for delivery of a term infant. The posterior sagittal diameter can also be measured with Thoms' pelvimeter (Fig 9–10). If the sum of the tuberischial diameter and the posterior sagittal diameter is more than 15 cm, the pelvic outlet is usually adequate. A prominent or angulated coccyx diminishes the anteroposterior diameter of the pelvic outlet.

   Martin's pelvimeter or Breisky's pelvimeter may be used to measure the distance from the inferior border of the pubic symphysis to the posterior aspect of the tip of the sacrum (ie, the anteroposterior diameter; normal = 11.9 cm).

   On rare occasions, extreme abnormality of the pelvis precludes vaginal delivery. In most cases, below average clinical measurements alert the obstetrician to the possibility of fetopelvic disproportion and, therefore, dystocia. However, an adequate trial of labor is usually the final determinant of true adequacy of the bony pelvis.

## Laboratory Tests

   The following laboratory assessments should be performed as early as possible in pregnancy and repeated at least once (ideally twice) between 24 and 36 weeks' gestation.

   **A. Blood Screening:** At the first visit, measure hematocrit, hemoglobin, white blood cell count, and differential. Determine blood group type, Rh factor, and antibodies to blood group antigens. Additionally,

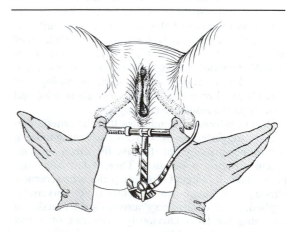

**Figure 9–9.** Measurement of the biischial (BI) or intertuberous (tuberischial [TI]) diameter with Thoms's pelvimeter. (Reproduced, with permission, from Benson RC: *Handbook of Obstetrics & Gynecology*, 8th ed. Lange, 1983.)

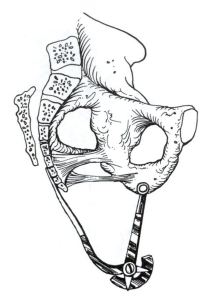

**Figure 9–10.** Posterior sagittal (PS) measurements with Thoms's pelvimeter. (Reproduced, with permission, from Benson RC: *Handbook of Obstetrics & Gynecology,* 8th ed. Lange, 1983.)

a serologic test for syphilis (VDRL) and rubella antibody titer should be obtained. Patients with risk factors may need initial screening for hepatitis B, toxoplasmosis, and HIV. Indeed, some authorities indicate the desirability to screen all patients for glucose intolerance, e.g., by a 1-hour blood sugar after ingestion of 50 g glucose. Patients with risk factors may need initial screening for toxoplasmosis.

Maternal serum alpha-fetoprotein (AFP) testing is now recommended for all pregnancies at 16–18 weeks as a means of screening for open neural tube defects or chromosomal abnormalities (primarily trisomy 21). Unfortunately, the test has a high level of false-positive results. Multiple marker studies measure AFP, estriol, and hCG to screen for Down's syndrome. These marker assays seem promising, but Down's syndrome detection is only about 60% and false-negative results remain high.

Recent information indicates that the criteria previously suggested by the CDC for screening those at risk for hepatitis are not effective for screening an indigent obstetric population. Thus, it has been suggested that all indigent obstetric patients be screened, although this suggestion currently is not universally applied. More controversy surrounds the practice of screening for HIV. Obviously, screening of at-risk populations (drug addicts, partners of bisexual men, prostitutes, partners of those with the virus, and those with known exposure) is warranted.

**C. Genetics testing:** Genetic studies should be offered to women over age 35 and to those with ab-

normal pedigrees. Chorionic villus sampling (CVS) is done at 9–11 weeks. It carries a 3–5% risk of fetal loss and is usually offered only at genetic centers. Early amniocentesis may be offered at 11–14 weeks. Pregnancy loss rates are 1–2% and failed sampling rates are low (1–2%). Standard amniocentesis is offered at 16–18 weeks. With ultrasound guidance, complication rates are < 1%. This is the most likely time to obtain sufficient fetal cells for culture.

At 28 weeks of gestation, patients are screened for diabetes. Hematocrit and antibody screens may be repeated as well.

**B. Urine Testing:** Perform urinalysis and screening tests (eg, dipstick nitrite testing) or culture for urinary tract infection. If the bacteria count is over $10^5$/mL on a voided sample or if bacteria are noted on a catheterized specimen, perform antibiotic sensitivity testing. Testing for urinary protein, glucose, and ketones should be done at each prenatal visit. Proteinuria of more than 300 mg/24 h ($\geq$ 2+ on standard dipstick testing) may indicate renal dysfunction or, if associated with relative hypertension, the onset or progression of preeclampsia-eclampsia. The presence of glucosuria signifies that the delivery of glucose to the kidneys exceeds renal resorptive capacity. This is not important if blood levels are normal, but elevated blood levels indicate carbohydrate intolerance. During pregnancy, the presence of ketones in the urine usually indicates inadequate intake of carbohydrates but not fetal jeopardy or maternal diabetes. The diet should be evaluated in this case to make certain that carbohydrate intake is adequate.

**C. Papanicolaou Smear:** Papanicolaou smears are performed unless recent results are available. Some obstetricians routinely screen for gonorrhea and chlamydia; others reserve this for high-risk patients. Microscopic examination of vaginal secretions is performed if indicated.

**D. Group B streptococcus:** Some authorities currently recommend culture in late pregnancy (at or beyond the 36th week) of the lower vaginal tract for group B streptococcus. The rationale being that if the mother is positive, she may be treated (usually with ampicillin) at the time of admission in labor, thus decreasing the risk of group B streptococcal sepsis in the newborn.

**E. Stool Culture:** A stool culture for ova and parasites may be indicated in some cases, particularly in recent immigrants from endemic areas such as southeast Asia.

**F. Tuberculin Skin Test:** A tuberculin skin test is appropriate for high-risk patients.

## SUBSEQUENT VISITS

The standard schedule for prenatal office visits is 0–32 weeks, once every 4 weeks; 32–36 weeks, once every 2 weeks; and 36 weeks to delivery, once each week. At each visit, weight gain, blood pressure, fundal height, and findings on abdominal examination by Leopold's maneuvers should be recorded. Additionally, FHTs heart tones should be documented and urine should be checked for glucose and protein. These findings should be reviewed and compared with those of previous examinations.

## MATERNAL WELL-BEING AS A SIGN OF FETAL WELL-BEING

In modern obstetric practice, fetal well-being has been determined mainly by direct monitoring and testing. It is important not to overlook the status of the mother when determining fetal well-being. Maternal health is obviously crucial to fetal development and must be continuously assessed during pregnancy.

### Maternal Height & Weight

Maternal height and weight and the rate and amount of weight gain during pregnancy are important in fetal development. Women who are underweight or of short stature tend to have smaller babies, and are at risk for low birth weight and preterm delivery. A teenage mother is compromised if her diet is not adequate to meet her own growth requirements as well as those of her fetus. In such circumstances, women less than 157 cm (5 ft) tall and especially those weighing less than 45 kg (100 lb) should be encouraged to gain at least the minimum of 11–12 kg (25 lb), if not more.

Inadequate progressive weight gain may reflect nutritional deficit, maternal illness, or a hormonal milieu that does not promote proper volume expansion and anabolic state. Often, this is associated with poor fundal growth and a small fetus and placenta, suggesting fetal growth retardation. Weight gain and fundal height should be closely monitored during pregnancy.

### Blood Pressure

Blood pressure levels may provide a clue to subtle circulatory compromise. Normally, the mean arterial pressure drops somewhat from prepregnancy or early pregnancy values during the midtrimester. It is important to note this decline so that it does not mask a subsequent rise in blood pressure that may signal the onset of hypertension. In the third trimester, blood pressure recordings taken in the supine position may be higher than those taken in the recumbent position; this may also indicate the onset of hypertension. Normal patients may have a significant drop in blood pressure in the supine position (supine hypotensive syndrome).

### Fundal Height

Fundal height should be measured and recorded at each visit. Measurements should be made with a centimeter tape (**McDonald technique**) from the pubic symphysis to the top of the uterine mass over the curvilinear abdominal surface. Caliper measurements are not recommended, because they are linear and therefore not progressive. Progress is especially important in the third trimester, when fetal growth retardation is most easily determined.

### Fetal Heart Tones

FHTs can usually be heard by 10–12 postmenstrual weeks using a hand-held Doppler device. This may be helpful when gestational age is in doubt or in the presence of threatened abortion or other abnormal observations in the late first trimester. Routine exposure of the fetus to ultrasound has not been shown to be harmful but is still controversial. As soon as possible (18–22 weeks), it is probably best to record heart tones by standard obstetric stethoscopic means. Attention should be paid both to rate and rhythm and to any accelerations, decelerations, or irregularities. Significant abnormalities may be further assessed by ultrasonography, fetal echocardiography, or electronic fetal heart rate monitoring, depending on gestational age. Term gestation can be assumed 18–20 weeks after FHTs have first been heard with the standard unamplified obstetric stethoscope. However, prudence demands use of other clinical landmarks in determining gestational age.

### Edema

At each prenatal visit, abnormal or potentially abnormal findings should be noted, and a careful record should be made of any unusual events that have occurred since the last visit. Transient episodes of general edema or swelling should be noted. Lower extremity edema in late pregnancy is a natural consequence of hydrostatic compromise of lower body circulation.

Edema of the upper body (eg, face and hands), especially in association with relative or absolute increases in blood pressure, may be the first sign of preeclampsia. Subtle changes may precede the more obvious picture (eg, finger rings may become too tight; this is a convenient index of early difficulties). A moderate rise in blood pressure without excessive fluid retention may suggest a predisposition to chronic hypertension.

### Fetal Size & Position

Manual assessment of fetal size and position is always indicated after about 26 weeks. The fetus may assume a number of positions before late gestation, but persistence of an abnormal lie into late pregnancy suggests abnormal placentation, uterine anomalies, or other problems that should certainly be investigated further. If an abnormal lie persists, consider external version after 37 weeks. Suspected abnormal fetal size should also be investigated, and failure to palpate fetal parts easily (confirmed by uterine measurements departing from expectations) suggests polyhydramnios.

## PREPARATION FOR LABOR

As term approaches, the patient must be instructed on the physiologic changes associated with labor. She is usually admitted to the hospital when contractions are occurring at 5- to 10-minute intervals. She should be told to seek medical advice for any of the following danger signals: (1) rupture of membranes, (2) vaginal bleeding, (3) evidence of preeclampsia (eg, marked swelling of the hands and face, blurring of vision, headache, epigastric pain, convulsions), (4) chills or fever, (5) severe or unusual abdominal or back pain, or (6) any other severe medical problems.

## NUTRITION IN PREGNANCY

The mother's nutrition from the moment of conception is an important factor in the development of the infant's metabolic pathways and future well-being. The pregnant woman should be encouraged to eat a balanced diet and should be made aware of special needs for iron, folic acid, calcium, and zinc.

The average woman weighing 58 kg (127 lb) has a

normal dietary intake of 2300 kcal/d. An additional 300 kcal/d is needed during pregnancy and an additional 500 kcal/d during breast-feeding (Table 9–3). Consumption of fewer calories could result in inadequate intake of essential nutrients.

## WEIGHT GAIN

The American College of Obstetricians and Gynecologists recommends a weight gain of 10–12 kg (22–27 lb) during pregnancy. Underweight women may need to gain more, while obese women should gain only 6–9 kg (15–20 lb). Heavier women or those with excessive weight gain during pregnancy are likely to have macrosomic infants. Inadequate weight gain is associated with small-for-gestational age (SGA) infants (Fig 9–11).

The fetus accounts for about one-third of the normal weight gain (3500 g); the placenta, amniotic fluid, and uterus for 650–900 g; interstitial fluid and blood volume for 1200–1800 g each; and breast enlargement for 400 g. The remaining 1640 g or more is largely maternal fat.

## NUTRITIONAL REQUIREMENTS

**A. Protein:** Protein needs in the second half of pregnancy are 1 g/kg plus 20 g per day (approxi-

**Table 9–3.** Recommended daily dietary allowances for nonpregnant, pregnant, and lactating women.

| | Nonpregnant Women (Years) | | | | | Pregnant Women | Lactating Women |
|---|---|---|---|---|---|---|---|
| | 11–14 | 15–18 | 19–22 | 23–50 | 51+ | | |
| **Energy (kcal)** | 2400 | 2100 | 2100 | 2000 | 1800 | +300 | +500 |
| **Protein (g)** | 44 | 48 | 46 | 46 | 46 | +30 | +20 |
| **Fat-soluble vitamins** | | | | | | | |
| Vitamin A activity (RE) | 800 | 800 | 800 | 800 | 800 | 1000 | 1200 |
| (IU) | 4000 | 4000 | 4000 | 4000 | 4000 | 5000 | 6000 |
| Vitamin D (IU) | 400 | 400 | 400 | . . . | . . . | 400 | 400 |
| Vitamin E activity (IU) | 12 | 12 | 12 | 12 | 12 | 15 | 15 |
| **Water-soluble vitamins** | | | | | | | |
| Ascorbic acid (mg) | 45 | 45 | 45 | 45 | 45 | 60 | 80 |
| Folacin (μg) | 400 | 400 | 400 | 400 | 400 | 800 | 600 |
| Niacin (mg) | 16 | 14 | 14 | 13 | 12 | +2 | +4 |
| Riboflavin (mg) | 1.3 | 1.4 | 1.4 | 1.2 | 1.1 | +0.3 | +0.5 |
| Thiamin (mg) | 1.2 | 1.1 | 1.1 | 1 | 1 | +0.3 | +0.3 |
| Vitamin $B_6$ (mg) | 1.6 | 2 | 2 | 2 | 2 | 2.5 | 2.5 |
| Vitamin $B_{12}$ (μg) | 3 | 3 | 3 | 3 | 3 | 4 | 4 |
| **Minerals** | | | | | | | |
| Calcium (mg) | 1200 | 1200 | 800 | 800 | 800 | 1200 | 1200 |
| Iodine (μg) | 115 | 115 | 100 | 100 | 80 | 125 | 150 |
| Iron (mg) | 18 | 18 | 18 | 18 | 10 | +18 | 18 |
| Magnesium (mg) | 300 | 300 | 300 | 300 | 300 | 450 | 450 |
| Phosphorus (mg) | 1200 | 1200 | 800 | 800 | 800 | 1200 | 1200 |
| Zinc (mg) | 15 | 15 | 15 | 15 | 15 | 20 | 25 |

Reproduced, with permission, from Babson SG, Pernoll ML, Benda GI: *Diagnosis and Management of the Fetus and Neonate at Risk.* Mosby, 1980. Modified from Committee on Dietary Allowances, Food and Nutrition Board: *Recommended Dietary Allowances,* 9th ed. National Academy of Sciences, 1980.

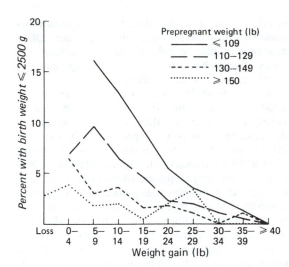

**Figure 9–11.** Risk of low birth weight among infants of white patients in relation to gravida's prepregnancy weight and weight gain. (Reproduced, with permission, from Niswander KR et al: Weight gain during pregnancy and prepregnancy weight: Association with birth weight of term gestation. Obstet Gynecol 1969;33:482.)

**Table 9–4.** Recommended daily dietary allowances for women 18–35 years old, 162 cm (64 inches) tall, and weighing 57.5 kg (128 lb) when not pregnant. (Food and Nutrition Board, National Research Council. Revised, 1973.)

| Nutrient | Nonpregnant | Increase | |
| | | Pregnant | Lactating |
| --- | --- | --- | --- |
| Kilocalories | 2000 | 300 | 500 |
| Protein (g) | 55 | 10 | 20 |
| Vitamin A (IU) | 5000 | 2000 | 3000 |
| Vitamin D (IU) | 400 | None | None |
| Vitamin E (IU) | 12 | 3 | 3 |
| Ascorbic acid (mg) | 45 | 15 | 15 |
| Folacin* (mg) | 0.4 | 0.4 | 0.2 |
| Niacin[†] (mg) | 14 | 2 | 4 |
| Thiamine (mg) | 1.4 | 0.3 | 0.3 |
| Riboflavin (mg) | 1.4 | 0.3 | 0.5 |
| Vitamin $B_6$ (mg) | 2 | 0.5 | 0.5 |
| Vitamin $B_{12}$ (µg) | 3 | 1 | 1 |
| Calcium (g) | 0.8 | 0.4 | 0.4 |
| Phosphorus (g) | 0.8 | 0.4 | 0.4 |
| Iodine (µg) | 100 | 25 | 50 |
| Iron (mg) | 18 | 30–60 | 30–60 |
| Magnesium (mg) | 300 | 150 | 150 |

*Refers to dietary sources ascertained by *Lactobacillus casei* assay; pteroylglutamic acid may be effective in smaller doses.
[†]Includes dietary sources of the vitamin plus 1 mg equivalent for each 60 mg of dietary tryptophan.

mately 80 g/d for the average woman). Protein intake is essential for embryonic development.

**B. Calcium:** Calcium intake should be increased to 1.5 g/d in the later months and during lactation. If calcium intake is inadequate, fetal needs will be met through demineralization of the maternal skeleton. Maternal calcium stores may be further drained during lactation.

**C. Iron:** Iron supplements (30–60 mg/d) are currently recommended for pregnant and lactating women. It is estimated that 300–500 mg of iron is transported to the fetus during pregnancy.

**D. Vitamins and Minerals:** Vitamin and mineral preparations are commonly given but should not be substituted for adequate food intake. Folic acid has been shown to effectively reduce the risk of neural tube defects (NTD) in high risk patients. A daily 4-mg dose is recommended for patients who have had a previous pregnancy affected by NTD. It should be begun more than 1 month prior to pregnancy (preferably 3 months) and continued through the first trimester. Patients with insulin-dependent diabetes mellitus and those with seizure disorders treated by valproic acid and carbamazapine are also at greater risk. Vitamin $B_{12}$ supplements are also desirable for vegetarian patients and those with known megaloblastic anemia (Table 9–4).

### Salt Restriction

Moderate amounts of foods containing sodium are not harmful during normal pregnancy. In fact, sodium restriction may be potentially dangerous. There is no evidence that rapid weight gain in preeclampsia can be controlled with sodium restriction.

## COMMON COMPLAINTS DURING PREGNANCY

Most of the minor complaints during pregnancy can be minimized with patient education and prompt treatment. It is best to refrain from using all medications during pregnancy unless they are absolutely essential.

### Ptyalism

Excessive salivation (sialism, ptyalism) is an infrequent but troublesome complaint of pregnant women. Belladonna extract, 8–15 mg orally 4 times a day, may be tried.

### Pica

Pica (cissa) is the ingestion of substances that have no value as food or are unwholesome. Common examples are clay and laundry starch. This practice probably does not derive from physiologic craving; rather, it seems to be a curious folk way and is still widespread, especially in the southeastern USA. Pica is harmful because it interferes with good nutrition by substituting nonnutritious bulk for nutritionally important foods. The necessity for good nutrition must be explained to these patients.

### Abnormal Frequency of Urination

Urinary frequency is a common complaint

throughout pregnancy. Vascular engorgement of the pelvis and hormonal changes are responsible for altered bladder function. Late in pregnancy, when pressure on the bladder by the enlarging uterus and the fetal presenting part decreases bladder capacity, urination becomes even more frequent.

Dysuria or hematuria may be signs that infection has developed and diagnostic and therapeutic measures are called for.

## Sexually Transmitted Diseases (STD)

**A. Syphilis:** Syphilis screening tests such as the Venereal Disease Research Laboratory (VDRL) slide test or the rapid plasma reagent (RPR) test are not specific and will remain positive even after disease treatment. Treponemal antibody tests are used to confirm positive cases. Penicillin remains the treatment of choice with treatment protocols correlating with disease severity. Erythromycin or ceftriaxone are treatment alternatives for the pregnant patient. Monthly serologic tests are followed to assess treatment response.

**B. Chlamydia:** The most effective screening consists of DNA probe analysis for this infection. Treatment usually consists of 7 days of erythromycin in the pregnant woman. Amoxicillin is used for patients with intolerance to erythromycin base or ethylsuccinate.

**C. Gonorrhea:** Gonorrhea is best detected by cervical culture. Since many strains are penicillin-resistant, ceftriaxone has become the drug of choice. Amoxicillin is used for nonresistant strains and spectinomycin is recommended for the penicillin-allergic patient.

**D. Herpes Simplex Virus:** Tissue culture is the best confirmation of herpes infection. Topical acyclovir may improve symptoms, but oral and parenteral therapy is reserved only for the immunocompromised patient or those with life-threatening disease. Cultures are recommended when a lesion is suspected. If no lesions are noted, vaginal delivery is recommended. Cesarean delivery is the route of choice for patients with active lesions at the time of delivery or with prodromal symptoms at the time of delivery or rupture of membranes.

## Other Infections

**A. Trichomoniasis:** *Trichomonas vaginalis* can be found in 20–30% of pregnant patients, but only 5–10% complain of leukorrhea or irritation. This flagellated, pear-shaped, motile organism can be seen under magnification when the vaginal discharge is diluted with warm normal saline solution and examined microscopically. Suspect trichomoniasis when the discharge is fetid, foamy, or greenish or when there are reddish (" strawberry") petechiae on the mucous membranes of the cervix or vagina.

Treatment is discussed in Chapter 34. Metronidazole (Flagyl), a good trichomonacide, is not recommended during the first trimester of pregnancy because its safety has not been fully established. Other medications may be helpful and safe during pregnancy. Acceptable antitrichomonas therapy can also be afforded by vaginal clindamycin.

**B. Candidiasis:** *Candida albicans* can be cultured from the vagina in many pregnant women, symptoms occur in less than 50%. When symptoms do occur, they consist of severe vaginal burning and itching and a profuse caseous white discharge. Marked inflammation of the vagina and introitus may be noted. The symptoms are likely to be aggravated by intercourse, and the male partner not infrequently develops mild irritation of the penis. Topical application of miconazole nitrate in a cream base (Monistat) or nystatin (Mycostatin) by suppository usually relieves the symptoms. The infection often flares up during pregnancy, in which case retreatment is necessary.

**C. Nonspecific Infections:** If irritation is obviously present but a pathogen cannot be identified, symptomatic therapy may be of value. This may include application of a cortisone cream to the vulva to alleviate itching or burning.

## Varicose Veins

Varicosities may develop in the legs or in the vulva. A family history of varicosities is often present. Pressure by the enlarging uterus on the venous return from the legs is a major factor in the development of varicosities. The physician should warn the patient, early in pregnancy, of the need for elastic stockings and elevation of the legs if varices develop. Specific therapy (injection or surgical correction) usually is contraindicated during pregnancy. Superficial varicosities may signal deeper venous disease. These patients should be examined carefully for signs of deep vein thrombosis.

## Edema

Dependent edema due to impedance of venous return is a common but rarely serious complaint late in pregnancy. Generalized edema is seen in the hands and face and may be an ominous sign of preeclampsia-eclampsia. Edema in pregnancy is due to fluid retention under the influence of ovarian, placental, and steroid hormones. Preeclampsia-eclampsia of pregnancy must be excluded. Dependent edema should be treated only if the patient is uncomfortable. Elevation of the legs (especially in the lateral decubitus) will improve the circulation. Diuretics (eg, thiazides, ethacrynic acid) are contraindicated and may be hazardous.

## Joint Pain, Backache, & Pelvic Pressure

Although the main bony components of the pelvis consist of 3 separate bones, the symphysial and sacroiliac articulations permit practically no motion in the nonpregnant state. In pregnancy, however, endocrine relaxation of these joints permits some movement. The pregnant patient may develop an unstable pelvis, which produces pain. A tight girdle or a belt worn about the hips, together with frequent bed rest, may relieve the pain; however, hospitalization is sometimes necessary.

Improvement in posture often relieves backache. The increasingly protuberant abdomen causes the patient to throw her shoulders back to maintain her balance; this causes her to thrust her head forward to remain erect. Thus, she increases the curvature of both the lumbar spine and the cervicothoracic spine. A maternity girdle to support the abdominal protuberance and shoes with 2-inch heels, which tend to keep the shoulders forward, may reduce the lumbar lordosis and thus relieve backache. Local heat and back rubs may relax the muscles and ease discomfort. Exercises to strengthen the back are most rewarding.

### Leg Cramps

Leg cramps in pregnancy may be due to a reduced level of diffusible serum calcium or elevation of serum phosphorus. Treatment should include curtailment of phosphate intake (less milk and nutritional supplements containing calcium phosphate) and increase of calcium intake (without phosphorus) in the form of calcium carbonate or calcium lactate tablets. Aluminum hydroxide gel, 8 mL orally 3 times a day before meals, adsorbs phosphate and may increase calcium absorption. Symptomatic treatment consists of leg massage, gentle flexing of the feet, and local heat. Tell the patient to avoid pointing toes when she stretches her legs (eg, on awakening in the morning): this triggers a gastrocnemius cramp. She should also practice "leading with the heel" in walking.

### Breast Soreness

Physiologic breast engorgement may cause discomfort, especially during early and late pregnancy. A well-fitting brassiere worn 24 hours a day affords relief. Ice bags are temporarily effective. Hormone therapy is of no value.

### Discomfort in the Hands

Acrodysesthesia of the hands consists of periodic numbness and tingling of the fingers. (The feet are never involved.) It affects at least 5% of pregnant women. It is a brachial plexus traction syndrome due to drooping of the shoulders during pregnancy. The discomfort is most common at night and early in the morning. It may progress to partial anesthesia and impairment of manual proprioception. The condition is apparently not a serious one, but it may persist after delivery as a consequence of lifting and carrying the baby.

### Other Common Complaints

See Chapters 23 and 24 for discussions of other common complaints during pregnancy, including ab-

dominal pain, nausea and vomiting, syncope and faintness, heartburn, constipation, hemorrhoids, genital tract complications, headache, and carpal tunnel syndrome.

## DRUGS, CIGARETTE SMOKING, & ALCOHOL DURING PREGNANCY

### Drugs

Teratogenicity has been established for only a few drugs, but many more are still not proved to be safe for use during pregnancy. The physician should have a good reason for prescribing any drug early in pregnancy or, indeed, during the last half of the menstrual cycle, when any fertile, sexually active woman might be pregnant.

Little is known about the effects of marijuana on the fetus, but major deleterious consequences have not been reported. Heroin, cocaine, and methadone, on the other hand, are associated with major problems in the neonate, especially potentially fatal withdrawal symptoms.

### Cigarette Smoking

An increased incidence of low-birth-weight infants have been ascribed to heavy cigarette smoking by pregnant women. This effect seems to be dose-related. Smoking also increases the risk of fetal death or damage in utero. Smoking similarly increases the risk of abruptio placentae and placenta previa, each of which increases the fetal risk as well as the maternal risk of death or damage. Since there are many potentially hazardous substances in tobacco smoke, the particular one responsible for these adverse effects has not been identified. Pregnant women should be encouraged not to smoke. If quitting is too stressful, the patient should at least cut down on the number of cigarettes smoked per day.

### Alcoholic Beverages

Moderate ingestion of alcohol has been thought in the past to cause no ill effects on the uterus or fetus despite the easy passage of alcohol across the placenta. Instances of newborns showing alcoholic withdrawal symptoms have been reported, but only in infants born to chronic alcoholics who drank heavily during pregnancy. Moreover, the chronic alcoholic may suffer from malnutrition, to the extent that the craving for alcohol exceeds the desire for food.

A **fetal alcohol syndrome** following maternal ethanol ingestion has recently been described, with an incidence varying from 1 in 1500 to 1 in 600 live births, depending apparently on variations in drinking practices. The major features include growth retardation, characteristic facial dysmorphology (including microcephaly and microphthalmia), central nervous system deficiencies, and other abnormalities. Rosett et al (1981) have reported a dose-effect relationship, with full-blown fetal alcohol syndrome occurring in those who reported heavy drinking. They further noted an improved neonatal outcome when the mothers were able to reduce maternal alcohol consumption before the third trimester. These researchers believe that counseling to reduce alcohol intake during pregnancy need not be performed by a special professional but can be integrated into routine prenatal care. Pregnant women should be encouraged to avoid alcohol intake completely during pregnancy. If this is not possible, the intake should be reduced to a minimum.

## OTHER MATTERS OF CONCERN DURING PREGNANCY

### Intercourse

There has always been a suspicion that intercourse may be responsible for early abortion. Certainly, if cramps or spotting has followed coitus, it should be proscribed. There is also evidence that coitus late in pregnancy may initiate labor, perhaps because of an orgasm—uterine contraction reflex. All in all, it may be best to proscribe intercourse for patients who have had a previous premature delivery or are currently experiencing uterine bleeding.

### Bathing

Bath water does not enter the vagina. Even swimming is not contraindicated during normal pregnancy. Diving should be avoided because of possible trauma.

A woman in the last trimester of pregnancy is clumsy and has poor balance. For this reason, she should be cautioned about slipping and falling in the tub or shower.

### Douching

Douching, seldom necessary, may be harmful.

### Dental Care

There may be generalized gum hypertrophy and bleeding during pregnancy. Interdental papillae (epulis) may also form in the upper gingivae. This rarely resorbs and must be excised. Normal dental procedures under local anesthesia (ie, drilling and filling) may be carried out at any time during gestation. Long procedures should be postponed until the second trimester. Antibiotics are given for dental abscesses and in cases of rheumatic heart disease and mitral valve prolapse.

### Immunization

All pregnant women should be vaccinated against poliomyelitis if not already immune. Poliovaccine may be administered safely during pregnancy. Live virus vaccines should be avoided during pregnancy because of possible deleterious effects on the fetus.

The American College of Obstetricians and Gynecologists recommends that diphtheria and tetanus toxoid be administered in pregnancy if exposure to pathogens is likely. The hepatitis B vaccine series may be given in pregnancy to women at risk. Measles, mumps, and rubella vaccine should be given 3 months prior to pregnancy or immediately postpartum. Viral shedding occurs in children receiving vaccination but they do not transmit the virus; thus vaccination may be safely given to the children of pregnant women. Immune globulin is recommended for pregnant women exposed to measles, hepatitis A, hepatitis B, tetanus, chickenpox, or rabies.

### Clothing

Loose-fitting conventional clothing often suffices until late in pregnancy, although maternity garments may be used as desired. A well-fitted brassiere is essential. A maternity girdle is rarely prescribed except for the relief of back pain or for abdominal weakness. Panty girdles and garters should be avoided because they interfere with circulation in the legs. Well-fitted shoes with heels of medium height are best in pregnancy.

### Exercise

Exercise in moderation is acceptable during pregnancy, but the patient should also rest an hour or 2 during the day. Dangerous sports (eg, horseback riding) and undue physical stress should be avoided. Aerobic and exercise classes have to be designed for pregnancy. Target heart rates are adjusted for age and weight, and routines are aimed to protect joints and promote flexibility.

### Employment

Women who have sedentary jobs may continue to work throughout the pregnancy. Employment that requires physical exertion calls for a careful evaluation by the obstetrician and an occupational medical practitioner. It is unwise to adopt rigid policies regarding work during pregnancy—each patient has a different level of capability, a different level of prepregnancy conditioning, a different exercise tolerance, and a different physique.

Substantial physical effort increases maternal oxygen consumption and places an increased demand on cardiac reserve that may result in decreased uterine blood flow. There are no studies as yet that prove this theory beyond doubt, but a conservative approach to the problem is recommended.

### Travel

Travel (by automobile, train, or plane) does not adversely affect a pregnancy, but separation from the physician may be hazardous. For this reason, instruct patients with a history of spontaneous abortion and those who have experienced vaginal bleeding in the course of the present pregnancy to avoid travel to distant places.

# REFERENCES

Abrams BF, Laros RK Jr: Prepregnancy weight, weight gain, and birth weight. Am J Obstet Gynecol 1986; 154:503.

Ahmed AG, Klopper A: Estimation of gestational age by last menstrual period, by ultrasound scan and by SP1 concentration: Comparisons with date of delivery. Br J Obstet Gynaecol 1986;93:122.

American College of Obstetricians and Gynecologists: Immunization During Pregnancy. ACOG Technical Bulletin 160. Washington, DC, ACOG 1991.

American College of Obstetricians and Gynecologists: Folic Acid and the Prevention of Recurrent Neural Tube Defects. ACOG Committee Opinion 120. Washington, DC, ACOG 1993.

Crandon AJ: Maternal anxiety and neonatal well-being. J Psychosom Res 1979;23:113.

Czeizel AE et al: The effect of preconceptional multivitamin-mineral supplementation on vertigo, nausea and vomiting in the first trimester of pregnancy. Arch Gynecol Obstet 1992;251:181.

Edozien JC, Switzer BR, Bryan RB: Medical evaluation of the special supplemental food program for women, infants and children. Am J Clin Nutr 1979;32:677.

Golbus M: Teratology for the obstetrician: Current status. Obstet Gynecol 1980;55:269.

Howard F, Hill J: Drugs in pregnancy. Obstet Gynecol Surv 1979;34:643.

Ingram DD, Makuc D, Kleinman JC: National and state trends in use of prenatal care, 1970-83. Am J Public Health 1986;76:415.

Isikoff SK, Civantos F, Deforge MJ: Evaluation of a new pregnancy test claiming beta-subunit specificity. Am J Clin Pathol 1980;74:98.

Kosasa TS et al: Early detection of implantation using a radioimmunoassay specific for human chorionic gonadotropin. J Clin Endocrinol 1978;36:622.

Lederman E et al: Maternal psychological and physiologic correlates of fetal-newborn health status. Am J Obstet Gynecol 1981;139:956.

McCalum WD, Brinkley JF: Estimation of fetal weight from ultrasonic measurements. Am J Obstet Gynecol 1979; 133:195.

Morrison JC, Whybrew WJ, Bucovaz ET: The L/S ratio and "shake" test in normal and abnormal pregnancies. Obstet Gynecol 1978;52:410.

Nasrat HA, Al-Hachim GM, Mahmood FA: Perinatal effects of nicotine. Biol Neonate 1986;49:8.

Poland ML et al: Barriers to receiving adequate prenatal care. Am J Obstet Gynecol 1987;157:297.

Rayburn WF: Drugs during pregnancy: Are any really safe? Nebr Med J 1986;71:45.

Robinson ET, Barber JH: Early diagnosis of pregnancy in general practice. J R Coll Gen Pract 1977;27:335.

Rosett HL, Weiner L, Edelin KC: Strategies for prevention of fetal alcohol effects. Obstet Gynecol 1981;57:1.

Selbing A: Conceptual dating using ultrasonically measured fetal femur length and abdominal diameters in early pregnancy. Br J Obstet Gynaecol 1986;93:116.

Sullivan TF, Barg WF Jr, Stiles GE: Evaluation of a new rapid slide test for pregnancy. Am J Obstet Gynecol 1979;133:411.

Sutter CB: Maternal and infant nutrition recommendations: A review. J Am Diet Assoc 1984;84:572.

# 10

# The Course & Conduct of Normal Labor & Delivery

*Manoj K. Biswas, MD, FACOG, FRCOG, & Sabrina D. Craigo, MD*

**Labor** may be defined as a coordinated effective sequence of involuntary uterine contractions that result in effacement and dilatation of the cervix and voluntary bearing-down efforts leading to the expulsion per vagina of the products of conception. **Delivery** is the mode of actual expulsion of the fetus and placenta. A delivery that occurs before 20 weeks of gestation is called an **abortion.**

**Parturition** is the birth process; a **parturient** is a patient in labor. **Parity** is the state of having given birth to an infant or infants weighing 500 g or more, alive or dead. If the weight is not known, an estimated length of gestation of 24 weeks or more may be used. A **nullipara** is a woman who has not delivered an offspring weighing 500 g or more or of 24 weeks' gestation or more. A **primipara** has given birth to such a fetus once, and a **multipara** has done so more than once.

**Gravidity** refers to the total number of pregnancies, including abortions, hydatidiform moles, ectopic pregnancies, and normal intrauterine pregnancies. A **nulligravida** has never been pregnant, a **primigravida** has been pregnant only once, and a **multigravida** has been pregnant more than once.

**True labor** is characterized by regular uterine contractions ("pains") that become more frequent and forceful and of longer duration with the passage of time, accompanied by effacement and dilatation of the cervix. **False labor,** which is quite common in late pregnancy, is characterized by irregular brief uterine contractions evoking back or abdominal pain. The contractions of false labor are inconsistent in interval, duration, and strength, and cause no change in the cervix. False labor has no significance except as a frequent cause of anxiety and premature hospital admission.

During the course of several days to several weeks before the onset of true labor, the cervix begins to soften and dilate. In many cases, when labor starts, the cervix is already dilated 1–3 cm in diameter. This is usually more marked in the multiparous patient, the cervix being relatively more firm and closed in nulliparous women.

In true labor, the woman is usually aware of her contractions during the first stage. The intensity of pain depends on the fetopelvic relationships, the quality and strength of uterine contractions, and the emotional and physical status of the patient. Very few women experience no discomfort during the first stage of labor. With the beginning of true normal labor, some women describe slight low back pain that radiates around to the lower abdomen. Each contraction starts with a gradual buildup of intensity, and dissipation of discomfort promptly follows the climax. Normally, the contraction will be at its height well before discomfort is reported. Dilatation of the lower birth canal and distention of the perineum during the second stage of labor will almost always cause discomfort.

The average duration of the first stage of labor in primipara patients is 8–12 hours; in subsequent pregnancies, 6–8 hours. If the first stage of labor lasts longer than 12 hours or if cervical dilatation fails to advance over a period of 2 hours, the labor is considered abnormal. The second stage of labor varies from a few minutes to 1–2 hours. Formerly, the upper limit of the duration of the second stage of labor was considered to be 2 hours. Currently, greater individualization is allowed in the duration of the second stage.

The fetal membranes—a protective barrier against infection—rupture before the onset of labor in about 10% of cases (premature rupture of the membranes). At full term, 9 women out of 10 will be in labor within 24 hours after rupture of the membranes. If labor does not begin within 24 hours after rupture, the case must be considered to be complicated by prolonged premature rupture of the membranes.

In rare instances, actual leakage of fluid ceases in premature rupture or premature prolonged rupture of the membranes, presumably as a result of sealing off of a small "high leak" in the membranes. More often, however, drainage ceases because the presenting part descends to obstruct the free egress of amniotic fluid.

Just before the beginning of labor, a small amount of red-tinged mucus called "show" may be passed. This is a plug of cervical mucus mixed with blood and is possible evidence of cervical dilatation and effacement.

## FETAL PRESENTATION, POSITION, & LIE

**Fetal presentation** designates that fetal part that is the most dependent structure in the birth canal. Under normal circumstances, about 95% of parturients have a cephalic (vertex) presentation. Breech presentation occurs in 4–5% of pregnancies at term; face, brow, or shoulder presentations are rare. **Fetal lie** refers to the relationship of the long axis of the fetus to the long axis of the uterus. Fetal lie may be either longitudinal—the normal situation—or transverse, which is uncommon and usually presents serious problems of delivery. Oblique lie technically is a variant of transverse lie.

**Fetal position** of a particular presentation refers to the relationship of an arbitrary reference point on the fetus to a specific point in the right or left side of the maternal pelvis. In cephalic presentation with fully flexed head, the reference point is the occiput. The occiput, when it lies in contact with left or right iliopubic eminence, is called left occipito or right occipito anterior; similarly when occiput lies in contact with left or right sacroiliac joints, it is called left or right occipito posterior position of the vortex presentation. Reference point for face presentation in mentum (chin), and for breech it is sacrum. If in any specific presentation, the point of direction is in the transverse diameter, it is called left or right transverse, like left or right occipito transverse position of the vertex presentation.

The various positions, presentations, and lies are affected by a number of factors, both maternal and fetal. Maternal factors include tumors of the uterus, congenital anomalies of the uterus, ovarian tumors, abnormalities of the maternal pelvis and lumbar spine, and extragenital factors such as pelvic kidney. Fetal factors include size of the baby, size of the fetal head—eg, hydrocephalus or anencephaly—and congenital fetal abnormalities of the bony or soft parts, eg, fetal abdominal tumors. The location of the placenta may also affect fetal lie and presentation: a partial or total placenta previa alter fetal lie and presentation. Moreover, the amount of amniotic fluid has an indirect effect on fetal position and presentation, eg, with excessive fluid present, transverse lie is more common. Most commonly, the fetus tends to assume a position facing the placenta.

Generally, fetal presentation and position can be determined by abdominal examination. One abdominal examination consists of 4 maneuvers of Leopold (Fig 10–1). In markedly obese patients or in primigravid patients with good abdominal muscles, it may be difficult to effectively perform the Leopold maneuvers. In such cases, vaginal examination or ultrasound will help to define the presenting part.

Sonography can delineate placental location, fetal head flexion, fetal anatomic abnormalities, and amniotic fluid volume. Abdominal x-ray may provide more information regarding fetal station and bony fetal abnormalities.

It is very important in the conduct of labor and delivery to ascertain as carefully as possible the presentation, position, and lie of the fetus. Variations from normal can lead to dystocia or difficult delivery.

## ESSENTIAL FACTORS OF LABOR

The progress and final outcome of labor are influenced by 4 factors (1) the passage (the bony and soft tissues of the maternal pelvis), (2) the powers (the contractions or forces of the uterus), (3) the passenger (the fetus), and (4) the psyche. Abnormalities of any of these components, singly or in combination, may result in dystocia. The first is not subject to change by therapeutic manipulation during delivery; the second and third can be influenced by medications or by manual or forceps intervention. The psyche is profoundly influenced by preparation for labor, familial support, trust in the care providers, previous life experiences, and by behavior of those in her environment during labor. In turn the psyche can materially influence the powers and the passenger.

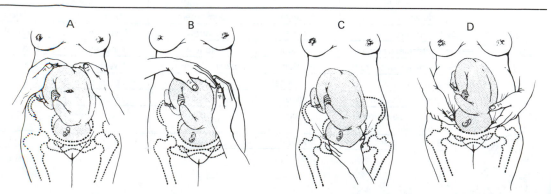

**Figure 10–1.** Determining fetal presentation (A, B), position (C), and engagement (D). (The 4 maneuvers of Leopold (Reproduced, with permission, from Benson RC: Handbook of Obstetrics & Gynecology, 8th ed. Lange, 1983.)

## 1. THE PASSAGE

### Bony Pelvis

The physician must carefully evaluate variations in pelvic architecture because the progress of delivery is directly determined by the sequence of attitudes and positions the fetus must assume in its passage through the birth canal. For this reason, a reasonably accurate assessment of the pelvic architecture and the pelvic diameters is an important part of obstetric care.

The obstetrician is concerned essentially with the true (rather than the false) pelvis, which includes the inlet, the midpelvis, and the outlet. Modern concepts of obstetric pelvic types and their influence on the conduct of labor are based for the most part on the classic work of Caldwell and Moloy in the 1930s. The 4 basic pelvic types identified by these workers and generally adopted throughout the world are the gynecoid, android, anthropoid, and platypelloid pelvic configurations.

These designations are based essentially on the inlet configurations, but certain features of the lower true pelvis are also characteristic of each type. Most pelves are "mixed" types, the anterior segment resembling one type and the posterior segment another. The characteristics of the 4 basic pelvic types are shown in Table 10–1.

The capacity of the bony pelvis can be estimated accurately enough for practical purposes by careful clinical examination. Long experience in the examination of human pelves is necessary, since x-ray films and mechanical models are no substitute for the careful assessment of the characteristics of the bones of the pelvic girdle. Clinical examination may have to be repeated during the course of pregnancy and even during labor if progress is unsatisfactory. It may be best to delay definitive typing and mensuration of the pelvis until shortly before term because by then the fetus has achieved maximal size, against which the pelvic capacity can be more effectively assessed.

**A. Pelvic Landmarks:** In evaluating the course and conduct of labor, a thorough knowledge of the following pelvic landmarks and their spatial relationships is mandatory.

**1. Pelvic inlet–**The pelvic inlet is bounded anteriorly by the superior rami of the symphysis pubis, laterally by the iliopectineal lines, and posteriorly by the superior portion of the sacrum. Technically, the superior portion of the symphysis and the uppermost point of the sacral promontory lie just above the inlet (Fig 10–2). Thus, the anteroposterior diameter of the superior strait (**true conjugate** or **conjugata vera**) does not represent the shortest diameter. This actually lies just below the upper margin of the symphysis. The slightly shorter diameter, the **obstetric conjugate,** is the critical one through which the head must pass at this level.

The plane of the inlet, when considered as a flat surface, is inclined at an angle of about 55 degrees from the horizontal when the patient is standing. This angle is referred to as the **pelvic inclination** (Fig 10–2). When this angle is wide, the prognosis for sat-

**Table 10–1.** Characteristics of 4 types of pelves.

| | Gynecoid | Android | Anthropoid | Platypelloid |
|---|---|---|---|---|
| Widest transverse diameter of inlet | 12 cm | 12 cm | <12 cm | 12 cm |
| Anteroposterior diameter of inlet | 11 cm | 11 cm | >12 cm | 10 cm |
| Side walls | Straight | Convergent | Narrow | Wide |
| Forepelvis | Wide | Narrow | Divergent | Straight |
| Sacrosciatic notch | Medium | Narrow | Backward | Forward |
| Inclination of sacrum | Medium | Forward (lower 1/3) | Wide | Narrow |
| Ischial spines | Not prominent | Prominent | Not prominent | Not prominent |
| Suprapubic arch | Wide | Narrow | Medium | Wide |
| Transverse diameter of outlet | 10 cm | <10 cm | 10 cm | 10 cm |
| Bone structure | Medium | Heavy | Medium | Medium |

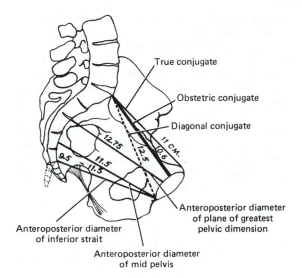

**Figure 10–2.** Pelvic measurements. (Reproduced, with permission, from Benson RC: Handbook of Obstetrics & Gynecology, 8th ed. Lange, 1983.)

isfactory labor is better than when a narrow inclination is noted.

In actual practice, the true conjugate cannot be measured directly. For clinical purposes, however, its length is estimated indirectly by measuring the distance from the lower margin of the symphysis to the promontory of the sacrum. From this measurement—the **diagonal conjugate**—the true conjugate is determined by subtracting 1.5–2 cm (depending on the height and inclination of symphysis). Normally, the true conjugate measures 11 cm or more.

The transverse diameter of the inlet is at right angles to the true conjugate and represents the greatest distance between the iliopectineal lines on either side. Unfortunately, it cannot be measured manually. The transverse diameter usually intersects the true conjugate at a point about 5 cm anterior to the sacral promontory, somewhat posterior to the true center of the inlet.

**2. Midpelvis**—The midpelvis is bounded anteriorly by the lower margin of the symphysis, laterally by the ischial spines, and posteriorly by the sacrum at the level of S3–S4. The midpelvis usually is the plane of narrowest pelvic dimensions. Its normal anteroposterior diameter is about 11.5 cm, and its transverse (interspinous) diameter is approximately 10 cm.

**3. Pelvic outlet**—The pelvic outlet is bounded anteriorly by the subpubic arch, laterally by the ischial tuberosities, and posteriorly by the tip of the sacrum (not the coccyx). The outlet actually consists of 2 triangular planes with a common base, the latter being a line between the two ischial tuberosities. The latter measurement (intertuberous) averages 11 cm. The anteroposterior diameter of the outlet is 9.5–11.5

cm, while the posterior sagittal is about 7.5 cm in the average pelvis.

The side walls of the pelvis extend from the inlet at the point of the transverse diameter inferiorly and anteriorly to the lower levels of the ischial tuberosities. The side walls generally are straight; if they converge, they may limit the capacity of the midpelvis or outlet.

The axis of the pelvis refers to the curve of the birth canal (curve of Carus) as described by a line drawn through the center of each of the above planes. This line curves anteriorly as the outlet is approached (Fig 10–2).

**B. Pelvic Contractures:** The inlet is considered to be contracted if the anteroposterior diameter is less than 10 cm or if the transverse diameter of the inlet is less than 12 cm. One cause of inlet contraction is rickets, which affects about 5% of black women in the USA. Debilitating diseases in childhood also may lead to poor pelvic development, with a generally contracted pelvis.

Midpelvic contraction generally is considered to exist when the diameter between the ischial spines is less than 9.5 cm or the sum of the interischial spinous and posterior sagittal diameters of the midpelvis falls to 13.5 cm or less. Based on the sum of the transverse and anteroposterior diameters of the pelvic inlet and that of the midpelvis, an adequate pelvic size is defined as values greater than 22 cm for the inlet and greater than 20 cm for the midpelvis. In addition, the capacity of the midpelvis is directly related to the posterior sagittal diameter of this plane, which normally is 5 cm. Midpelvic contracture is suggested by prominent ischial spines, converging pelvic side walls, and narrowed sacrosciatic notches.

Outlet contraction is considered to exist when the intertuberous (ischial) diameter is 8 cm or less. Contracture here, as in the midpelvis, is directly related to the posterior sagittal diameter and the subpubic arch configuration. It should be noted that the relationship between the interspinous diameter and the intertuberous diameter of a given pelvis is quite constant; outlet contraction of measurable degree is seldom seen without concomitant midpelvic contraction.

**C. Prognosis for Vaginal Delivery:** Pelvic (bony) dystocia may be due to the abnormalities and variations of any of the planes of the pelvis discussed earlier as well as to the various factors involved in fetal size, position, and presentation, and moldability of the fetal head. In addition to clinical evaluation of the pelvis, other details are helpful in predicting vaginal delivery in a given patient. These include data from the past obstetric history, ie, the duration and description of previous labors, the types of deliveries, and the sizes of infants born previously. A history of difficult forceps delivery, of neonatal death or morbidity, or of previous cesarean section after prolonged labor may suggest the possibility of pelvic contracture or relative cephalopelvic disproportion. In the primigravid patient, such factors as previous debilitating illnesses or pelvic girdle injury, nonengagement of the fetal head at term, or failure to progress in labor, with primary or secondary inertia, all must be considered in the pelvic assessment.

**D. Trial of Labor:** In cases of borderline pelvic contraction, a trial of labor may be indicated. Such a trial should not be considered safe in cases of malpresentation, or outlet contraction, and should be considered with caution in cases of preeclampsia or significant medical complications.

No specific time limit can be imposed on the definition of trial of labor. All that is necessary is an adequate period of time in labor to provide reasonable evidence that vaginal delivery may be accomplished with safety to both mother and child. A trial of labor is often interpreted to mean 4–6 hours of good labor. If definite cervical dilatation occurs, continuing and satisfactory progress in labor should be anticipated. A definite timetable should be set up, with periodic reevaluation of all factors that might contribute to dystocia or failure of labor to progress. In addition to pelvic size and configuration, fetal size and position and the character and effectiveness of uterine contractions must be assessed. The station of the fetal head, the presence or absence of molding, and the development of a fetal caput are helpful in evaluating the success of labor and the degree of disproportion.

**E. X-Ray Pelvimetry:** X-ray pelvimetry is not needed in most patients. Moreover, the information obtained by x-ray pelvimetry rarely alters the clinical management of the case. Collectively, the data compiled from various studies indicate the incidence of leukemia in children exposed to radiation in utero show a relative risk for childhood leukemia of 1.5.

Ultrasound technology has been tried for pelvic mensuration but noted to be complicated, tedious, incomplete, and without clinical utility. X-ray pelvimetry has been replaced currently by computed tomographic pelvimetry by digital radiography in many centers. This technique has been noted to be accurate and simple with films that are easier to interpret than conventional films. Recently, MRI pelvimetry has been noted to be very accurate with errors that are less than 1%, and the technique is not influenced by uterine or fetal motion. Despite advanced imaging technology, fetopelvic disproportion and delivery outcome have been predicted with limited accuracy.

There are several factors singularly or in combination that can determine the outcome of labor. Among these factors are the force and effectiveness of the uterine contractions, the size and malleability of the fetal head, and the presentation and position of the fetus. Other considerations involve the axis of the pelvis, the status of the fetal membranes, and the flexion of the fetal head.

The type of maternal pelvis might influence the course of labor. The gynecoid pelvis is most condu-

cive to normal labor. In anthropoid pelves the fetal head is often engaged in an occipitoposterior position, and the patient often must deliver the fetus in that position. In android pelves the fetal head tends to engage in the transverse or posterior position. The android pelvis predisposes to a persistent occipitoposterior position of the vertex presentation, deep transverse arrest, and deflexion on the fetal head. Perineal tears are common because the undue posterior pressure is occasioned by fetal passage below the narrow subpubic arch. In a platypelloid pelvis, the fetal head might not engage because of the short anteroposterior diameter of the pelvic inlet.

### Pelvic Soft Tissues

The maternal pelvic soft tissues have an effect on the type and progress of labor. The muscles and fascia of the pelvis have been previously described in Chapter 2. The levator ani muscles, which are the main soft tissue components of the pelvic cavity in the midportion, consist of three parts, pubococcygeus, iliococcygeus, and ischiococcygeus. The disposition of the levator ani muscles helps in the forward rotation of the presenting part during labor. Also, the anatomy of the uterus and the vagina may vary the progress of labor. Occasionally, congenital malformations of these organs, eg, vaginal septa or constrictions, will obstruct labor. These and other vaginal abnormalities should be noted prior to the onset of labor.

### 2. THE POWERS

The uterus remains relatively quiescent during the first half of pregnancy. Studies indicate, however, that recurrent myometrial contractions occur throughout pregnancy. Small uterine contractions with an intensity of 2–4 mm Hg often occur 1–3 times a minute recorded as early as around 10 weeks of gestation. Contractions of the intensity of 10–15 mm Hg lasting 30 seconds or more called Braxton-Hicks contractions occur once per hour or so between 12 and 30 weeks of gestation with increasing frequency to about every 10 minutes during the last 2 weeks preceding labor. About 48 hours prior to onset of labor, contractions with an amplitude of 20–30 mm Hg occur at intervals of 5–10 minutes. During the latest phase of labor, 2–4 contractions with an amplitude of 20–30 mm Hg occur during each 10 minute period. In active phase, the intensity of the contractions increase and cervical dilations progresses, mean intensity remains about 35mm Hg increasing to 48 mm Hg as the cervix approaches full dilatation. With the maternal pushing effort, the intraamniotic pressure reaches to about 100–150 mm Hg. The frequency of uterine contractions increases with the progress in labor from 2 to 4 contractions per 10 minutes in early labor to 5–4 contractions per 10 minutes at the end of labor. During the early labor, the baseline pressure generally is less than 10 mm Hg to about 12–15 mm Hg with the established active phase of labor with intact membranes. Transcervical intrauterine catheters can be used to measure the force of uterine contractions following rupture of the membranes. The intensity and duration of contractions are recorded on a tocograph, which may be useful in evaluating the effectiveness of labor. The internal pressure catheter is especially helpful in determining responses to oxytocin augmentation, thereby preventing hyperstimulation of the myometrium.

Since the upper part of the uterus contains many more myometrial elements than the lower portion, the usual contraction progresses through the uterus from top to bottom. In addition, each individual myometrial cell as it contracts does not quite regain its normal length on relaxation. This process is known as brachystasis of the uterine muscle fibers. As this mechanism progresses, an upper and a lower uterine segment are developed. Before the onset of labor, the lower uterine segment usually is thinner than the upper segment. The transition area between the 2 segments is designated the physiologic retraction ring. The lower uterine segment becomes progressively thinner as labor advances and the upper segment becomes progressively thicker. With these changes, the junction becomes more and more distinct.

## 3. THE PASSENGER

The diameters of the fetal head at term usually are greater than those of the body, and the head is thus the most difficult part to deliver. (In certain fetal abnormalities such as massive ascites, the abdomen may be larger, but this is rare.) The fetal skull is composed of 3 major parts: the face, the vault or roof, and the base. The face and the base of the skull are composed of bones that are heavy and more or less fused. The bones of the vault are not joined. Thus, changes in shape are possible as the head passes through the pelvis and is subjected to constriction by external forces. This mechanism leads to temporary changes, known as **molding,** in the general shape of the fetal head.

The vault is composed of 2 frontal bones, 2 parietal bones, and one occipital bone. They are slightly separated from one another at the sutures or margins of abutment and by wider spaces, the anterior and posterior fontanelles. The sutures and fontanelles can usually be identified by direct palpation. However, excessive molding of the head or scalp edema may obscure these landmarks. The widest lateral diameter of the head, the biparietal diameter, averages 8.5–9.5 cm. In most cases, the head enters the pelvis with the sagittal suture line in the transverse plane of the mother's pelvis. When this suture is midway between the pubis and the sacrum, the relationship is referred to as **synclitism.** When the sagittal suture line deviates from the midline toward the symphysis or the sacrum, it is termed **asynclitism.** Asynclitism often is an indication that the pelvis is too small for descent of the fetal head, although asynclitism may be present in normal labor, particularly when the head is small. Flexion of the fetal head on the body is important in normal labor because flexion determines which diameter of the head will pass through the narrowest portion of the pelvis. In most cases, full flexion of the head is due to the pressures of the bony and soft tissues of the passage upon the fetal head as fetal descent occurs. When the head is fully flexed, the suboccipitobregmatic diameter is presented to the pelvis. This measures 9.5 cm in the average term infant. The common flexions are shown in Fig 10–3.

## 4. THE PSYCHE

There is ample evidence in the literature to assume the influence of psychologic factors on the course of labor and delivery. A high level of anxiety during pregnancy has been associated with decreased uterine activity and with longer and dysfunctional labor. Therefore, it is important for the prospective first-time mother to attend prenatal education classes to alleviate her fears, to make labor and delivery more understandable, and to learn that she will be supported psychologically as well as physically. She should also be encouraged to participate in prenatal exercise classes and to learn various psychoprophylactic techniques to alleviate pain during labor.

## MECHANISM OF INITIATION OF LABOR

Many theories have been proposed over the years to explain the sequence of events that culminate in labor and delivery, but the exact metabolic and endocrine pathways are not yet known. A consideration of several of the more plausible theories suggests that the mother, the fetus, and the placenta all contribute to the maintenance of pregnancy, and that the removal of certain restraints finally triggers progressively more rhythmic and forceful uterine contractions.

The common occurrence of prolonged gestation in gravidas with anencephalic fetuses and those with fetal adrenal hypoplasia lends support to the concept of a role for the fetal adrenal glands in human parturition. Moreover, in the human fetus there is extensive hypertrophy of the adrenals, caused principally by the enlargement of the fetal zone. There is extensive secretion of $C_{19}$-steroids (specifically dehydroepiandrosterone [DHEA] sulfate) by the fetal adrenals, and these compounds function as precursors in the production by the placenta of estrogens (primarily estradiol and indirectly estriol). Estrogen is known to stimulate phospholipid synthesis, phospholipid turn-

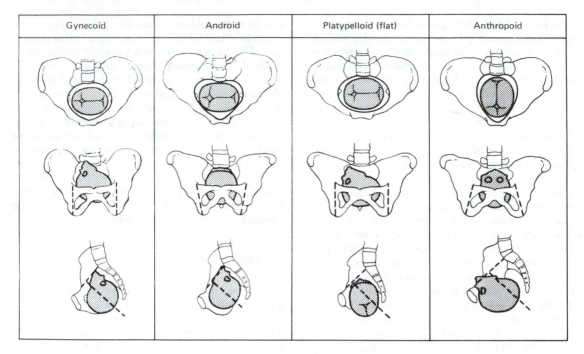

|  Gynecoid | Android | Platypelloid (flat) | Anthropoid  |

**Figure 10–3.** Flexions of the fetal head in the 4 major pelvic types. (Reproduced, with permission, from Danforth DN, Ellis AH: Midforceps delivery: A vanishing art? Am J Obstet Gynecol 1963;86:29.)

over, rates of incorporation of arachidonic acid into phospholipids, prostaglandin biosynthesis, and the formation of lysosomes in the uterine endometrium. These metabolic consequences of estrogen may be critical to the preparatory events requisite to the process of normal human parturition.

The key role of prostaglandin production as the initiator of labor in human beings has not been established; however, it is interesting to note that the administration of large doses of aspirin (a prostaglandin inhibitor) to pregnant women results in prolonged gestation. Indomethacin inhibits prostaglandin synthetase and has also been shown to prolong gestation in the subhuman primate. These observations are consistent with prostaglandin formation as the initiator of myometrial contractions. Additionally, arachidonic acid is the precursor of prostaglandin and is stored in esterified form in the amnion and chorion. Uterine decidua is also a site for prostaglandin synthetase activity. Phospholipase $A_2$ is the enzymatic liberator of arachidonic acid from its esterified form.

From observations made years ago in pregnant rabbits, theories have been proposed in which progesterone withdrawal is the initiating event in human labor. Although the results of most human studies have not confirmed this theory, it is possible that progesterone suppresses the activity of phospholipase $A_2$ except near the end of normal gestation. The withdrawal of progesterone could result in augmented expression of phospholipase $A_2$ activity. Arachidonic acid is con-

verted by the incorporation of 2 molecules of oxygen into a highly unstable endoperoxide, prostaglandin $G_2$ ($PGG_2$), which then lose an oxygen radical to become PGH2, from which are formed all the prostaglandins of the 2 series, as well as thromboxane A2 (Fig 10–4).

Both $PGE_2$ and $PGF_2$ stimulate contractility in the gravid human uterus. The action of prostaglandin on the contractile proteins of smooth muscle cells is thought to depend on enhancement of calcium transport through the plasma membranes of the intracellular organelles. Uterine muscle requires calcium, and it has been suggested that calcium also is involved in adrenergic stimulation and prostaglandin action. The sarcoplasmic reticulum is a system of channels surrounding the myofibrils. The intracellular free calcium binds to one of the contractile proteins and removes the inhibition to actin-myosin interaction, so that the actin and myosin filaments slide past each other and combine temporarily, resulting in a contraction.

Oxytocin released by the neurohypophysis may have a physiologic role in the onset of labor. However, there is little evidence that increased maternal levels of oxytocin are responsible for initiating parturition, but a low fixed level may be an essential permissive factor. Once labor has begun, oxytocin levels do rise, especially during the second stage. Thus, oxytocin may be important for developing more intense uterine contractions. Extremely high concentra-

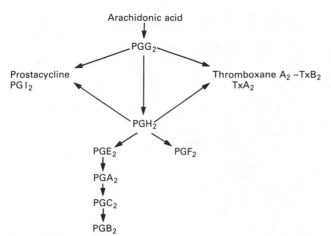

**Figure 10–4.** Production of prostaglandins during human parturition.

tions of oxytocin are found in the cord blood at delivery; thus, release of oxytocin from the fetal pituitary may also play a role in labor. It may be that the prostaglandins are essential mediators of oxytocin's effect on the uterus, although prostaglandins could function in a more permissive role. In addition, prostaglandins and oxytocin may work together to inhibit calcium binding within myometrial cells, thereby raising intracellular calcium levels and activating contractions.

The uterine smooth muscle cells are dispersed throughout extracellular material composed mainly of collagen fibers, which act as intramuscular tendons. The connective tissue integrates the myometrial contractile force generated within the individual muscle cells. The cells communicate with one another through connections called gap junctions. Gap junctions are composed of aggregates of proteins lodged in the plasma membranes. These cell-to-cell contacts may synchronize and coordinate myometrial function by conducting electrophysiologic stimuli during labor. The absence of gap junctions may maintain the muscle in an inactive state, thus maintaining pregnancy. The mechanism responsible for stimulating the formation of gap junctions at term during pregnancy has not been established.

# THE COURSE OF NORMAL LABOR

Labor commonly is divided into 3 stages:

(1) The first stage begins with the onset of labor and ends when dilatation of the cervix (10 cm) is complete. This is usually the longest stage of labor. The average duration of the first stage of labor in a primigravida is 8–12 hours; in a multipara 6–8 hours.

(2) The second stage of labor extends from full dilatation of the cervix to the birth of the baby and varies from a few minutes to about two hours depending on both fetal and maternal factors.

(3) The third stage of labor is the period from the birth of the infant to delivery of the placenta. The hour immediately after delivery of the placenta, during which time the danger of postpartal hemorrhage is greatest, is often referred to as the fourth stage of labor; it will be considered here as part of the third stage.

During the first stage, effacement accompanies dilatation. It is often difficult to determine exactly when labor begins, but as a rule contractions that occur every 2–3 minutes and last 30–45 seconds result in significant dilatation or effacement of the cervix and descent of the presenting part.

The average duration of the first stage of labor in primigravida is about 8 hours; however, there are individual variations depending on (1) the parity of the patient; (2) the frequency, intensity, and duration of uterine contractions; (3) the ability of the cervix to dilate and efface; (4) the fetopelvic diameters; and (5) the presentation and position of the fetus.

The median duration of the second stage of labor is 50 minutes in primigravida and 20 minutes in multigravida women. However, it could be highly variable depending on (1) fetal presentation and position; (2) fetopelvic relationships; (3) resistance of maternal pelvic soft tissue; (4) frequency, intensity, duration, and regularity of uterine contractions; and (5) efficiency of maternal voluntary expulsive efforts.

The rapidity of separation and means of delivery of the placenta determine the duration of the third stage.

### MECHANISM OF LABOR

(Tables 10–2 and 10–3, Figs 10–4 to 10–13)

**Table 10–2.** Mechanisms of labor: vertex presentation.

| Engagement | Flexion | Descent | Internal Rotation | Extension | External Rotation (Restitution) |
|---|---|---|---|---|---|
| Generally occurs in late pregnancy or at onset of labor. Mode of entry into superior strait depends on pelvic configuration; posterior occiput is most common position. | Good flexion is noted in most cases. Flexion aids engagement and descent. (Extension occurs in brow and face presentations.) | Depends on pelvic architecture and cephalopelvic relationships. Descent is usually slowly progressive. | Takes place during descent. After engagement, vertex usually rotates to the transverse. It must next rotate to the anterior or posterior to pass the ischial spines, whereupon, when the vertex reaches the perineum, rotation from a posterior to an anterior position generally follows. | Follows distention of the perineum by the vertex. Head concomitantly stems beneath the symphysis. Extension is complete with delivery of the head. | Following delivery, head normally rotates to the position it originally occupied at engagement. Next, the shoulders descend (in a path similar to that traced by the head). They rotate anteroposteriorly for delivery. Then the head swings back to its position at birth. The body of the baby is then delivered. |

## Vertex Presentation

The mechanism of labor in the vertex as well as the breech presentation (see later) consists of engagement of the presenting part, flexion, descent, internal rotation, extension, external rotation, and expulsion. The mechanism of labor is dictated by the pelvic dimensions and configuration, the size of the passenger, and the strength of the contractions. In essence, delivery proceeds along the "line of least resistance," ie, by adaptation of the smallest achievable diameters of the presenting part to the most favorable dimensions and contours of the birth canal. Particularly in the case of vertex presentations, delivery is somewhat like the passage of a rounded object through a short bent stove pipe equipped with several dampers (baffles).

The sequence of events in vertex presentation is as follows:

**A. Engagement:** This usually occurs late in pregnancy–in the primigravida, commonly in the last

**Table 10–3.** Mechanisms of labor: frank breech presentation.

| Flexion | Descent | Internal Rotation | Lateral Flexion | External Rotation (Restitution) |
|---|---|---|---|---|
| Hips: Engagement usually occurs in one of oblique diameters of pelvic tent. | | | | |
| | Anterior hip generally descends more rapidly than posterior, both at inlet and outlet. | Ordinarily takes place when breech reaches levator musculature. Fetal bitrochanteric rotates to anteroposterior diameter. | Occurs when anterior hip stems beneath symphysis; posterior hip is born first. | After birth of breech and legs, infant's body turns toward mother's side to which its back was directed at engagement of breech. This accommodates engagement of the shoulders. |
| Shoulders: Bisacromial diameter engages in same diameter as breech. | | | | |
| | Gradual descent is the rule | Anterior shoulder rotates so as to bring shoulders into anteroposterior diameter of outlet. | Anterior shoulder at symphysis and posterior shoulder is delivered first (when body is supported). | |
| Head: Engages in the same diameter as shoulders. | | | | |
| Flexes on entry into superior strait. Biparietal occupies oblique used by shoulders. At outlet, neck or chin arrests beneath symphysis and head is delivered by gradual flexion. | Follows the shoulders. | Occiput (if a posterior) or face (if an occiput anterior) rotates to hollow of sacrum. This brings presenting part to anteroposterior diameter of outlet. | | |

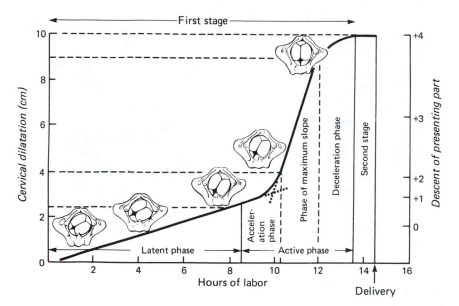

**Figure 10–5.** Schematic illustration of progress of rotation of occipitoanterior presentation in the successive stages of labor.

2 weeks. In the multiparous patient, engagement usually occurs with the onset of labor. The head usually enters the superior strait in the occiput transverse position in 70% of women with a gynecoid pelvis.

**B. Flexion:** In most cases, flexion is essential for both engagement and descent. This will vary, of course, if the head is small in relation to the pelvis or if the pelvis is unusually large. When the head is improperly fixed—or if there is significant narrowing of the pelvic strait (as in the platypelloid type of pelvis)—there may be some degree of deflexion if not actual extension. Such is the case with a brow (deflexion) or face (extension) presentation.

**C. Descent:** Descent is gradually progressive and is affected by the forces of labor and thinning of the lower uterine segment. Other factors also play a part, eg, pelvic configuration and the size and position of the presenting part. The greater the pelvic resistance or the poorer the contractions, the slower the descent.

**D. Internal Rotation:** With the descent of the head into the midpelvis, rotation occurs so that the sagittal suture occupies the anteroposterior diameter of the pelvis. Internal rotation normally begins with the presenting part at the level of the ischial spines. The levator ani muscles form a V-shaped sling that tends to rotate the vertex anteriorly. In cases of occipitoanterior vertex, the head has to rotate 45 degrees, and in occipitoposterior vertex, 135 degrees, to pass beneath the pubic arch.

**E. Extension:** Extension follows extrusion of

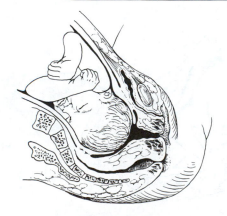

**Figure 10–6.** Engagement of LOA.

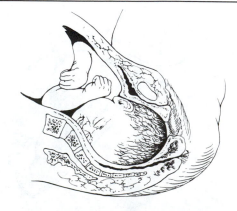

**Figure 10–7.** Descent in LOA position.

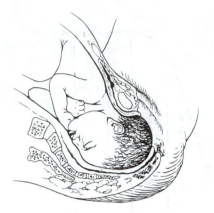

**Figure 10–8.** Anterior rotation of head.

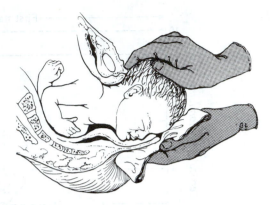

**Figure 10–9.** Modified Ritgen maneuver.

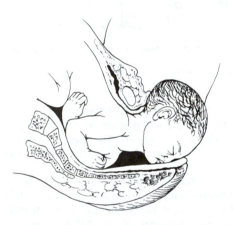

**Figure 10–10.** Extension of the head.

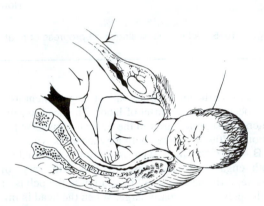

**Figure 10–11.** External rotation of the head.

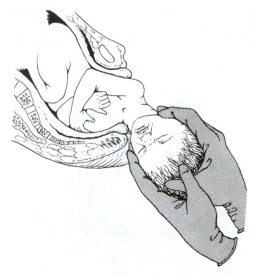

**Figure 10–12.** Delivery of anterior shoulder.

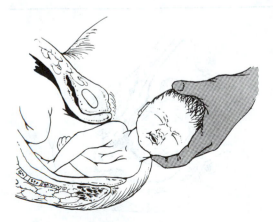

**Figure 10–13.** Delivery of posterior shoulder.

the head beyond the introitus, with the occiput beneath the symphysis pubis.

**F. External Rotation:** External rotation (restitution) follows delivery of the head when it rotates to the position it occupied at engagement. Following this, the shoulders descend in a path similar to that traced by the head. The anterior shoulder rotates internally about 45 degrees to come under the pubic arch for delivery. As this occurs, the head swings back to its position at birth. Following these maneuvers, the body, legs, and feet are delivered.

## Breech Presentation

The mechanism of labor varies for breech presentations. The bitrochanteric diameter usually engages in one of the oblique diameters of the pelvic inlet. As descent occurs, the anterior hip generally descends more rapidly than the posterior hip both at the inlet and the outlet. Internal rotation occurs when the breech reaches the levator muscles and the fetal bitrochanteric diameter rotates to the anteroposterior diameter. Lateral flexion occurs when the anterior hip stems beneath the symphysis; this allows the posterior hip to be born first. The infant's body turns toward the mother's side to which its back was directed at engagement. This allows accommodation for engagement of the shoulders. Hence, the bisacromial diameter engages in the same diameter as the breech. There is gradual descent. The anterior shoulder rotates to bring the shoulders into the anteroposterior diameter of the outlet just as did the fetal trochanteric diameter. The anterior shoulder then follows lateral flexion to appear beneath the symphysis, and the posterior shoulder is delivered first as the body is supported. The head in breech presentation tends to engage in the same diameter as the shoulders. It flexes on entry into the superior strait, and the biparietal diameter occupies the oblique used by the shoulders. Descent follows the path of the shoulders, and internal rotation occurs to the hollow of the sacrum.

## MANAGEMENT OF EARLY LABOR

When a patient believes that she is in labor, she should be carefully examined to confirm labor and to identify significant abnormalities (eg, fetopelvic disproportion, ineffectual uterine contractions). The history of the onset of contractions, the presence or absence of bleeding, the possible loss of amniotic fluid, and the fetal heart tones (FHTs) and activity of the fetus should be recorded. A record of the prenatal care visits, examinations, laboratory reports, and any treatment given should be reviewed if it is available. The review of recent events should include not only data regarding intercurrent infections or other illnesses but also the time of the patient's last meal.

## Initial Examination & Procedures

Examination of a woman in early or suspected early labor should consist of a basic evaluation of her current clinical condition. How the patient reacts to labor (eg, anxiety, tension) is also an important part of the total evaluation.

On admission to the labor unit (or initial home visit if home delivery is anticipated), the following procedures should be performed.

(1) Obtain a history of relevant medical details since the last examination.

(2) Record the vital signs: temperature, pulse, respiratory rate, and blood pressure. Make an appraisal of the patient's general condition together with any grossly abnormal physical findings.

(3) Obtain a clean-catch urine specimen and test for protein and glucose to establish a baseline for subsequent management of the patient.

(4) Do a brief general physical examination.

(5) Examine the abdomen, noting such things as scars or evidence of old trauma. Palpate the uterus to determine the fetal presentation, engagement, position, and level of the most dependent part (see Fig 10–1). Count the FHTs for 1 minute with a stethoscope or electronic instrument (eg, Doptone). (It is helpful to indicate the location of the FHTs with suitable markings on the skin for the benefit of other examiners and to note rotation and descent of the fetus.)

(6) Note the frequency, regularity, intensity, and duration of the uterine contractions.

(7) If there is evidence of vaginal bleeding or loss of amniotic fluid, record the type and amount. (It is particularly important to note the color and character of the amniotic fluid, eg, the presence or absence of meconium or staining. Nitrazine indicator paper will turn from yellow [acid] to deep blue-green [alkaline] when moistened with amniotic fluid.)

(8) Vaginal examination: Aseptic vaginal examination should be done to determine the degree of dilatation and effacement of the cervix as well as any abnormalities of the soft tissues of the birth canal. This evaluation should identify the presenting fetal part and the station of the presenting part in relation to the level of the ischial spines (Fig 10–14). The long axis of the birth canal between the ischial spines and the pelvic inlet, also between the ischial spines and the outlet of the pelvis, have been arbitrarily divided into thirds. Thus, if the presenting part is at the level of the inlet, it is at −3 station; if it has descended one-third the distance from the pelvic inlet to the ischial spines, it is at −2 station, similarly, two-thirds the distance indicates −1; at the level of the spin 0 station, +1 indicates the presenting part to be one-third the distance below the spine. Similarly, +2, two-thirds below, and +l3 indicates fetal part to be at the level of the perineum.

(a) Dilatation of the cervical os is expressed in centimeters, indicating the diameter of the cervical opening. Ten centimeters constitutes full dilatation. A di-

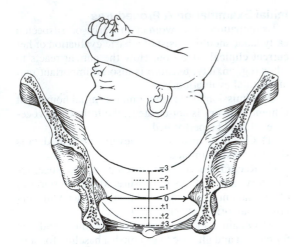

**Figure 10–14.** Stations of the fetal head. (Reproduced, with permission, from Benson RC: Handbook of Obstetrics & Gynecology, 8th ed. Lange, 1983.)

ameter of 6 cm or less can be measured directly; when the distance is more than 6 cm, however, it is often easier to subtract twice the width of the remaining "rim" from 10 cm. For example, if a 1-cm rim is felt anteriorly, posteriorly, and laterally, this indicates 8 cm dilatation.

(b) Effacement of the cervix is a process of thinning out that is accomplished before and (especially) during the first stage of labor. The cervix thins by retraction. In this manner, it "gets out of the way" of the presenting part, allowing more room for the birth process.

Effacement is expressed in percentage from 0% (uneffaced) to 100% (cervix less than about 0.25 cm thick).

(c) The position of the presenting part can usually be confirmed by vaginal examination:

(i) Vertex presentations. In fully flexed vertex presentation, posterior fontanelle, part of sagittal suture, and lambdoidal sutures are palpable. The position is determined by the relation of the fetal occiput to the mother's right or left side. This is expressed as OA (occiput precisely anterior), LOA (left occiput anterior), LOP (left occiput posterior), etc.

(ii) Breech presentations are determined by palpating both ischial tuberosities, the feet may be felt alongside the buttocks in complete breech, and in footling breech one or both feet are inferior to the buttocks. Breech could be left or right sacroanterior (LSA, RSA) or left or right sacroposterior (LSP, RSP).

(iii) Face presentations. Extension of the fetal head on the neck causes the face to be the presenting part. The chin, a prominent and identifiable facial landmark, is used as a point of reference. As with vertex presentations, the position of the fetal chin is related

to the mother's pelvis, left or right side, and the anterior or posterior portion. This is expressed as left mentum posterior (LMP), right mentum anterior (RMA), and right mentum posterior. Face could be diagnosed by vaginal examination by palpating the landmarks of face like chin, mouth, nose, orbital ridges, and the malar bones.

(iv) Brow occurs as a result of partial extension of cephalic presentation. It usually is a temporary presentation, which converts during labor to face or vertex presentation. The frontal sutures, large anterior fontanel, supraorbital ridges, and the root of the nose can be palpated vaginally.

(v) In transverse lie, the long axis of the body of the fetus is perpendicular to that of the mother. In transverse lie, the shoulder is usually over the pelvic inlet, with the head lying in one iliac fossa and the buttocks in the other. This condition is also referred to as a shoulder presentation. The side of the mother toward which the acromion is directed determines the designation of the lie as right or left acromial. In either position, the back may be directed anteriorly, posteriorly, superiorly, or inferiorly; it is known as dorsoanterior or dorsoposterior.

(vi) Compound presentations represent an extremity lying alongside or below the presenting part, with both trying to enter the pelvis simultaneously.

(9) Other examinations: If there are questions about the presentation of the fetus, ultrasonograms may be helpful in determining the presence of fetal abnormalities as well as the differentiation of abnormal presentations from normal ones, eg, breech, face, compound, or transverse lie. It may be particularly difficult to determine these findings clinically in the markedly obese patient, in the gravida who is in extremely active labor with a contraction or tight uterus, or when there may be partial placental separation or abnormal uterine function. At times, although the initial physical examination may be confusing, further examination as labor progresses may help clarify the situation.

### Preparation of the Patient for Labor

If the patient definitely is in early labor and therefore is to remain in the home or hospital for anticipated delivery, further preparation should be carried out.

(1) Cleansing of the perineum should be performed with a soap solution or nonirritating detergent preparation. Shaving labial and pubic hair was once routine. Shaving does not decrease infection or improve wound healing, and women experience discomfort and irritation with regrowth of the hair, so perineal shaving is no longer part of routine "preparation" in most hospitals. If better exposure is needed (eg, for laceration repair) long labial hair can be cut with scissors.

(2) Enemas were routinely given to patients in early labor until the 1980s. Attitudes have changed,

however, since enemas are uncomfortable for the patient and do not prevent fecal contamination of the perineum. An enema or laxative suppository can be used to empty the rectum if necessary, but should not be given routinely.

(3) The patient in mild labor should be advised to remain in bed if the membranes have been ruptured, if she is bleeding, or if a sedative has been administered. Otherwise, if the fetal heart rate pattern is reassuring ambulation can be encouraged. Ambulation may be effective in augmenting the efficacy of labor and decreasing the need for analgesia.

(4) Analgesics are helpful for the patient with significant discomfort. The preferred analgesic in most institutions is meperidine (pethidine, Demerol), 50–75 mg intramuscularly or intravenously. Butorphanol (Stadol) and nalbuphine (Nubain) can also be used safely for analgesia during labor. These drugs are not known to cause neonatal depression. Naloxone hydrochloride (Narcan) is a narcotic antagonist capable of reversing respiratory depression induced by opioid narcotics by displacing the narcotic from specific receptors in the central nervous systems. It is usually administered in a dose of 0.1 mg per kg of fetal body weight injected into the umbilical vein.

Analgesics should be coordinated with anesthesia (see Chapter 26). Small doses of analgesics are not injurious to the fetus and may be beneficial to the mother.

If analgesic preparations are used, they should not be administered too frequently. An interval of 2–4 hours between doses is advisable. Sedatives or analgesic drugs should not be given immediately before anticipated delivery because of possible depressive effects on the infant. Analgesia should not be given too early in labor because it may slow the progress of labor. This is true also if analgesia is given in excessive amounts. Drug therapy must be individualized for each patient. The progress of labor, the intensity of contractions, the patient's pain threshold, and the presence or absence of complications—all are features in the decision whether to administer sedative or analgesic medications.

Conduction anesthesia (epidural) may be used late in the first stage of labor for analgesia and carried through delivery as anesthesia. These methods are usually reserved for the second stage of labor and delivery.

(6) Diet and fluids: Controversy exists surrounding the issue of oral intake during labor. Small amounts of clear liquids are permissible, but the patient should not be given solid food during labor. Gastric motility is greatly inhibited by uterine contractions, and gastroesophageal reflux is common in pregnancy. Aspiration of gastric contents has been a significant cause of maternal mortality in the past. The risk of aspiration pneumonitis is related to the risk of general anesthesia, since the patient's ability to protect her airway is compromised while under general anesthesia. Although any pregnant patient has a risk of emergent delivery for an intrapartum complication, this risk is small for a patient with an otherwise uncomplicated pregnancy. For these patients, oral intake of liquids during early labor may be reasonable. Any patient with a known risk for operative delivery should have oral intake restricted to small amounts of water or ice chips. Small amounts of nonparticulate antacids may be given to prevent possible tracheal irritation in case of vomiting and increase the pH of gastric contents. Similarly, low risk patients do not routinely require intravenous catheters. IV access is indicated when regional anesthetics are used, for prolonged labor, for access for medications, and if a risk factor for postpartum hemorrhage is identified. The intravenous route has an additional advantage in that the actual amount of fluid being administered can be recorded. A continuous slow intravenous drip (5% dextrose in lactated Ringer's solution or balanced electrolyte solution at a rate of 125 mL/h) is recommended in most patients when fluids are infused during labor and delivery. Large boluses of glucose should be avoided because of a risk of causing neonatal hyperglycemia, hyperinsulinemia, and subsequent hypoglycemia.

## Supervision of the First Stage of Labor

(1) The fetal heart tones should be recorded every 10–15 minutes. If it is suspected that problems may arise in labor or delivery or if the patient has been categorized as "high-risk" on the basis of her obstetric history or prior examination, electronic fetal monitoring should be utilized. If the presence of complications is established or anticipated, continuous fetal heart tone monitoring will be necessary. With or without external or internal uterine contraction monitoring, the tracing should be evaluated at least every 15 minutes during the first stage and every 5 minutes during the second stage of labor. (Fig 10–15.)

Despite widespread use of electronic monitoring, there has been no demonstrated impact or incident of longterm neurologic handicap. (See Chapter 13).

(2) The patient should be examined abdominally and vaginally as necessary to follow the progress of labor.

Vaginal examinations are facilitated by offering thorough explanation and allowing the patient to indicate when she is prepared for the examination. Additionally, perineal relaxation may be evoked by placing slight pressure on the posterior fourchette and requesting relaxation of "this muscle." Sterile lubrication, gentleness, conducting the examination between contractions, discussion during, and explanation after the procedure all assist in enhancing the patient's comfort.

Early in the uncomplicated case, such examinations may be done hourly. As labor progresses, more frequent examinations are usually required. However,

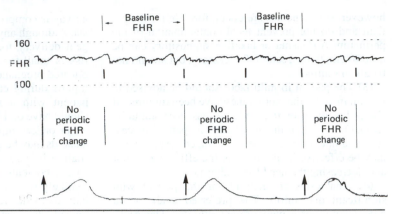

**Figure 10–15.** Normal fetal heart rate (FHR) with average variability. Periodic FHR changes are, by definition, changes in FHR associated with uterine contractions (UC). Baseline FHR is the FHR between periodic FHR changes. (Reproduced, with permission, from Hon EH: An Atlas of Fetal Heart Rate Patterns. Harty Press, 1968.)

too frequent vaginal examinations are uncomfortable for the patient and increase the incidence of intrauterine infection, particularly after rupture of the membranes. Descent of the fetus and internal rotation can often be determined by external palpation alone. Shift of the point of maximal impulse of the fetal heartbeat is a useful indication of fetal descent.

On vaginal examination, dilatation and effacement of the cervix, the station and position of the presenting part, or the presence of an abnormality should be noted; in the case of vertex presentation, one should note the size of caput and degree of molding of fetal head, particularly if the presenting part is high. The passage of blood, or meconium stained amniotic fluid should be recorded.

(3) The frequency and character of the uterine contractions, the tone of the uterus, and the general reaction of the patient in labor should be recorded periodically. Graphic display of cervical dilatation and the

time elapsed provides a visual concept of the progress of labor (compare Figs 10–16 to 10–19).

(4) The patient should be encouraged to void as labor progresses. This usually can be accomplished with a commode at the bedside or with a bedpan in bed. If the patient cannot void, however, she should be catheterized to prevent overdistention of the bladder. If the latter occurs, the patient may suffer from bladder atony postpartum.

(5) The normal laboring woman should have the liberty to move around during early labor prior to the use of analgesic drugs. Subsequently, the patient can sit in a comfortable chair, or she can use the bed if she prefers. She should not be restricted to the supine position.

### Preparation for Delivery

Adequate delivery room facilities include anesthesia and resuscitation equipment and drugs as well as

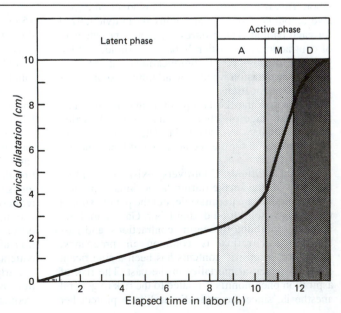

**Figure 10–16.** Dilatation of the cervix at various phases of labor (primiparous labor). A, acceleration phase. M, phase of maximum slope. D, deceleration phase.

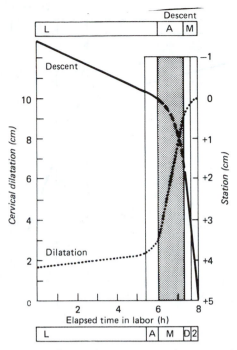

**Figure 10–17.** Composite mean curves for descent (solid line) and dilatation (broken line) for 389 multiparas. Intervals: L, latent; A, acceleration; M, maximum slope; D, deceleration; 2, second stage. Relationship is shown between acceleration period of descent and maximum slope of dilatation (shaded area), between latent period of descent and latent plus acceleration phases of dilatation, and between maximum slope of descent and deceleration phase plus second stage. (Redrawn and reproduced, with permission, from Friedman EA, Sachtleben MR: Station of the fetal presenting part. 1. Pattern of descent. Am J Obstet Gynecol 1965;93:522.)

the sterile surgical instruments that may be needed. Drapes, sponges, and sutures should be on the delivery table. (Most delivery rooms have a standard setup, but variations are permissible if they are in conformity with sound surgical principles.)

The patient should be transported from the labor to the delivery room on a wheeled litter with side rails. Many obstetric units now have LDR (labor, delivery, and recovery) rooms where the patient can labor and deliver without changing rooms. For delivery, knee crutches should be available so that the legs can be supported when the patient is in the lithotomy position. Some women may choose to support their own legs during the second stage or even deliver in a lateral recumbent or sitting position. The patient's body should not be allowed to extend beyond the end of the delivery table because of the possibility of back injury.

The use of birthing chairs or tables allows the patient to be placed in a more upright position for the second stage of labor as maternal comfort is noted to

be an advantage attributed to such posture. There is no clear difference between upright position and conventional recumbent position in the length of the second stage, the mode of delivery, or the rise of potential trauma. Increased postpartum hemorrhage has been noted with the upright position in the second stage of labor.

After the patient is properly positioned on the delivery table, surgical preparation of the vulvar area should be carried out with detergent and antiseptic solution such as povidone-iodine (Betadine). Surgical drapes can be applied so that the legs and abdomen are covered. The physician and assistants must scrub their hands and wear masks and sterile gowns and gloves for their own protection.

## MANAGEMENT OF THE SECOND STAGE OF LABOR (Vertex Delivery)

Spontaneous delivery of the fetus presenting by the vertex is divided into 3 phases: (1) delivery of the head, (2) delivery of the shoulders, and (3) delivery of the body and legs. The second stage of labor begins when the cervix is fully dilated. The obstetrician should be alert to the imminence of delivery following complete dilatation of the cervix. However, this stage may last as long as 1–2 hours.

Delivery should be anticipated when the presenting part reaches the pelvic floor. This may be sooner if the patient is a multipara or if labor is progressing rapidly.

Preparations for delivery should be made as noted earlier. When the presenting part distends the perineum, anesthesia may be administered. Pudendal block may be performed at this time. If conduction anesthesia is being used, it is usually administered in the late first stage or in the second stage as previously noted. Local anesthesia can be injected in the posterior area of the perineum if episiotomy is planned, and the patient does not have perineal anesthesia from regional or pudendal block.

Episiotomy, when indicated, is carried out when delivery is imminent. Median episiotomy is preferred in most cases. If the perineum is short or if there are contraindications to a median episiotomy, mediolateral episiotomy may be performed. Bleeding should be controlled by hemostats. In the case of a breech presentation, the episiotomy should be generous so as not to impede delivery of the aftercoming head.

Between uterine contractions the presenting part tends to recede slightly, but "crowning" occurs when the head is visible at the vaginal introitus surrounded by the labial margin and not receding in between contractions.

In all cases, delivery should be controlled so as to prevent forceful, sudden expulsion or extraction of the baby. A controlled delivery should prevent fetal

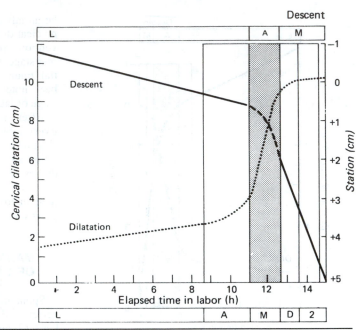

**Figure 10–18.** Relationship between cervical dilatation and descent of the presenting part in a primipara. L, latent phase. A, acceleration phase. M, phase of maximum slope. D, deceleration phase. 2, second stage.

and maternal injury. Thus, as the head advances, flexion of the head should be maintained, when necessary, by pressure over the perineum.

Gentle, gradual delivery is desirable. Pressure applied from the coccygeal region upward (modified Ritgen maneuver [see Fig 10–9]) will extend the head at the proper time and thereby protect the perineal musculature.

### Delivery of the Head (Figs 10–6 to 10–11)

In vertex presentations, the forehead appears first (after the vertex) and then the face and chin. The neck appears next. The umbilical cord is around the baby's neck in about 15–20% of deliveries. Fortunately, the cord is rarely tight enough to cause fetal hypoxia. It should be loosened cautiously and pulsations checked. If the cord is pulsating well, there is no need

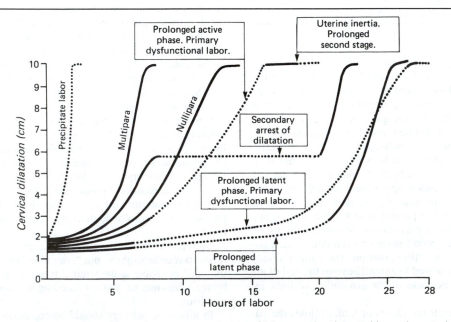

**Figure 10–19.** Major types of deviation from normal progress of labor may be detected by noting cervical dilatation at various intervals after labor begins.

to hasten delivery. Gently slip the cord over the infant's head. If this cannot be done easily, double clamp the cord with forceps, cut between the forceps, and proceed with the delivery. Once the head has been delivered, the infant's airway should be cleared by pressure on the trachea and nose. Wipe fluid from the nose and mouth and then aspirate the nasal and oral passages with a soft rubber suction bulb or with a small catheter attached to a DeLee suction trap.

Before external rotation (restitution), which occurs next, the head is usually drawn back toward the perineum. This movement precedes engagement of the shoulders, which are now entering the pelvic inlet. From this time on, support the infant manually and facilitate the mechanism of labor.

Following delivery of the head, gentle traction should be exerted on it downward or posteriorly; this aids progression of the anterior shoulder beneath the symphysis. The forward shoulder will gradually appear. Next, the head should be lifted upward to aid delivery of the posterior shoulder. If it becomes necessary to expedite delivery of the shoulders, the posterior arm of the fetus may be delivered by inserting the fingers into the vagina to bring the arm down across the baby's chest and out the introitus. Traction on the head should be gentle to avoid excessive stretching so as to avoid bracheal plexus palsey.

### Delivery of the Shoulders (Figs 10–12 and 10–13)

Delivery of the shoulders should be slow and gradual; the shoulders should be rotated if necessary to the anteroposterior diameter of the outlet.

In vertex presentations, a hand may present after the head. This need not obstruct delivery of the shoulders. Merely sweep the baby's hand and arm over its face, draw the arm out, and deliver the other shoulder as outlined above.

### Delivery of the Body & Extremities

The body and legs should be delivered gradually by easy traction after the shoulders have been freed.

### Immediate Care of the Infant

As soon as the infant is delivered, it should be held with the head lower than the body (no more than 15 degrees) to facilitate drainage by gravity of accumulated mucus and bronchial secretions in the airways. Record the Apgar rating at 1 minute and at 5 minutes (see Chapter 11). The air passages should be cleared by means of a soft rubber bulb syringe. Resuscitation measures must be instituted immediately if there is evidence of cardiopulmonary distress. The baby should be placed under radiant heat or in a heated newborn care cart to preserve body heat. Cooling of the infant should be avoided at all times.

Some physicians place the child on the mother's abdomen. This is a safe alternative if the infant is near

term and vigorous at birth, but should be avoided if the newborn is premature, has meconium, or needs any resuscitation. The infant should be dried while on the mother's abdomen, to avoid heat loss.

The body temperature of the newborn must be maintained by radiant heat from above to avoid chilling. The cord must be clamped and cut. The umbilical cord should be examined to identify the number of vessels. Two arteries and one vein are normal.

Apply a sterile cord clamp, cord tie of umbilical tape, or a rubber band just distal to the skin edge at the cord insertion at the umbilicus. Cover the cord stump with a dry gauze dressing held by a belly band, preferably of elastic material. It is best to clamp the umbilical cord approximately 1 cm from the skin reflection. Wipe the eyelids with moist cotton. Next, 1 drop of 1% aqueous silver nitrate must be instilled into each eye. The medication must be freshly prepared or expressed from commercial wax "pearls," which maintain the safe concentration. (Tetracycline or erythromycin ophthalmic ointment is as effective as silver nitrate against gonococci and pneumococci and costs about the same, but the law in some jurisdictions calls for silver nitrate.) Excessive silver nitrate should be washed out with sterile saline after about 30–60 seconds.

A general physical examination is next in order, and any gross abnormalities or congenital malformations are noted in the record. Record also the weight, total length, shoulder circumference, and head circumference.

It is imperative that proper identification be affixed in the form of a necklace or bracelet before the newborn is transferred from the labor room to the nursery, and this must be verified by checking with the mother's identification.

When feasible, the mother should be given the infant to hold or even to nurse. The infant is then transferred to the nursery for further observation and care. Loss of body heat by the newborn must be avoided.

### Immediate Care of the Mother Postpartum

Following delivery of the placenta (described below), the perineum, vagina, and cervix must be inspected thoroughly for lacerations, hematomas, or extension of episiotomy incisions. The cervix may be examined by manual retraction of the vaginal walls for visualization or by placement of a self-retaining retractor. The cervix should be examined circumferentially and any significant lacerations noted. Lacerations longer than 1 cm should be repaired at this time with interrupted absorbable sutures. The mattress-type suture, tied not too tightly because of cervical edema, should ensure hemostasis and healing. Lacerations of the vaginal vault must be sought and repaired also. Enlarging hematomas should be excised and drained and deep mattress sutures placed for control of bleeding. Following inspection of the cervix and the vaginal vault, a temporary pack may be placed in the vagina to maintain a clear field of visualization during the episiotomy repair.

The extent of laceration of the birth canal may be designated roughly in degrees (Fig 10–20). In first-degree lacerations, only mucosa or skin (or both) is damaged. Bleeding is usually minimal. Second-degree lacerations include tears of the mucosa or skin (or both) plus disruption of the superficial fascia and the transverse perineal muscle. (The sphincter ani muscle is spared.) Bleeding is often brisk. Third-degree lacerations involve the previous structures plus the anal sphincter. Moderate blood loss is to be expected. Fourth-degree lacerations include entry into the rectal lumen. Bleeding may be profuse, and fecal soiling is inevitable.

Sulcus lacerations, urethral and cervical damage, etc, are documented specifically.

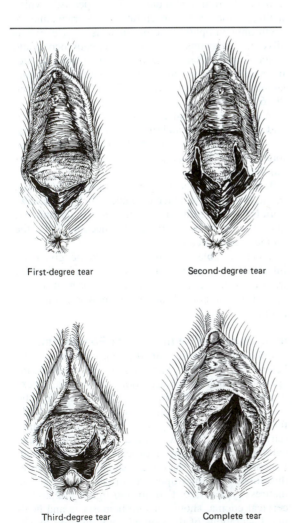

First-degree tear     Second-degree tear

Third-degree tear     Complete tear

**Figure 10–20.** Perineal tears. (Reproduced, with permission, from Benson RC: Handbook of Obstetrics & Gynecology, 8th ed. Lange, 1983.)

## MANAGEMENT OF THE THIRD STAGE OF LABOR

The third stage of labor extends from the delivery of the infant's body to delivery of the placenta. Because the hour immediately following delivery of the placenta may be a critical one, it is often called the fourth stage of labor.

Management of the third stage of labor can usually be facilitated by the use of oxytocic drugs (oxytocin), 10 IU added to the infusion bottle; or methylergonovine maleate (Methergine), 0.2 mg intramuscularly. After delivery of the infant, the uterus will continue to contract. This causes considerable reduction of the placental site and aids in separation of the placenta. The placenta is attached to the uterine wall only by anchor villi and thin-walled blood vessels, all of which eventually tear. In some instances the placental margin separates first; in others, when the central portion of the placenta is freed initially, there may be retroplacental bleeding that helps to shear the placenta from the uterine wall. Placental separation usually occurs within 5 minutes following delivery of the infant. There may be incomplete or gradual separation of the placenta, however, due to uterine relaxation, minimal retroplacental bleeding, or placental or uterine abnormalities that lead to fibrosis and firm attachment of the placenta to the uterine wall. When the placenta is morbidly adherent with the uterine wall, it is called **placenta accreta**. The condition may be partial or total. When the placenta separates incompletely, it may allow retroplacental blood sinuses to remain open, so that severe blood loss may result. Moreover, the presence of the placenta in the uterus may prevent contraction of the uterus, thus allowing considerable blood loss during the third stage. Normal placental separation is indicated by a firmly contracting and rising uterine fundus.

As the uterus contracts and becomes smaller, it changes in shape from discoid to globular. The umbilical cord, which is still attached to the placenta, becomes longer as the placenta descends. When the placenta is ready for expulsion or extraction, it will present at the cervical os and may even dilate the cervix slightly. Do not attempt to pull on the cord until the placenta is completely detached, or uterine inversion may occur. Do not knead the fundus and use the uterus as a piston to expel the placenta. This "Credé" maneuver may be traumatic, leading to hemorrhage or to inversion of the uterus, which is further compounded by shock and infection. As the placenta passes from the uterus into the vagina, it may present by either the fetal surface or the maternal surface of the placenta. These have been termed the Schultze and Duncan mechanisms, respectively, but such designations are archaic and without significance. The mechanism preferred for the recovery of the placenta is the Brandt-Andrews maneuver (Fig 10–21), in which pressure is placed abdominally just above the

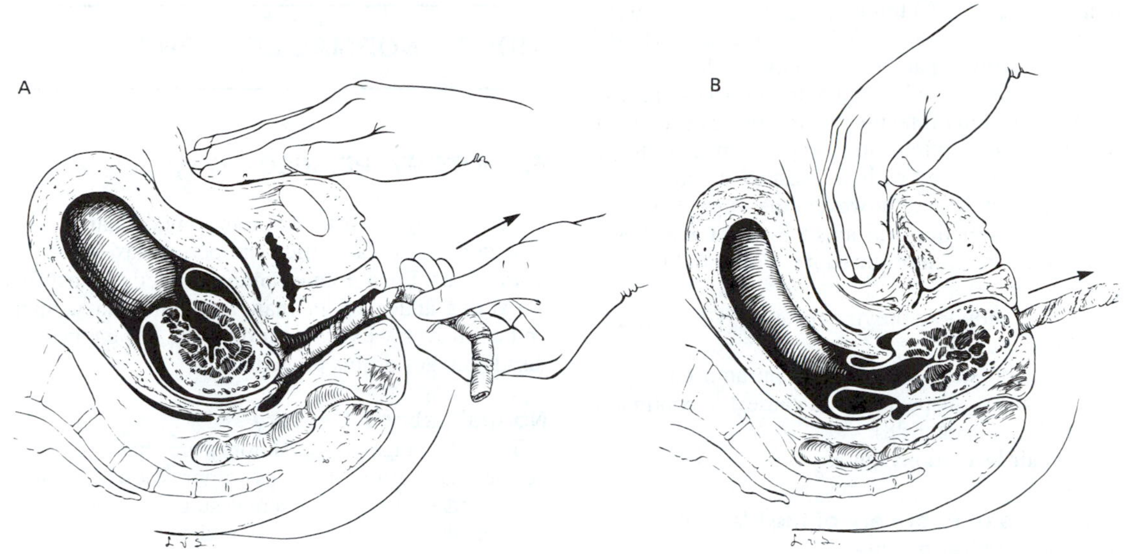

**Figure 10–21.** Brandt-Andrews maneuver. (A) Traction is exerted on the cord as the uterus is gently elevated. (B) Pressure is exerted between the symphysis and the uterine fundus, forcing the uterus upward and the placenta outward, as traction on the cord is continued.

symphysis to elevate the uterus into the abdomen and at the same time express the placenta into the vagina. Gentle cord traction will then help to guide the placenta out of the birth canal.

The placenta must be carefully inspected to make certain that there are no missing cotyledons and that the membranes have been totally recovered.

The uterus should be palpated and elevated at completion of the third stage of labor. Firm compression of the uterus may express clots and stimulate the corpus to contract. This reduces total blood loss. If there is persistent bleeding from a flaccid uterus, gentle massage and oxytocics may be employed as necessary during repair of the episiotomy and in the immediate postpartum period. When there is excessive bleeding, it is always important to have an intravenous route available for administration of blood, fluids, and such drugs as may be required. For this purpose, a large-bore needle (16 or 18 gauge) should be in-dwelling for emergency therapy.

## Obstetric Procedures That Minimize Complications During the Third Stage

See Chapter 28 for a complete discussion of the complications of the third stage of labor.

The following procedures will usually prevent entrapment of the placenta and conserve blood:

(1) Give oxytocin (Pitocin, Syntocinon), 10 IU (1.0 mL) intramuscularly, or 20 IU in a liter of fluid, given at a rate of about 125cc/hour. Bolus intravenous administration of undiluted oxytocin must never be used, as there is a potential risk of profound hypotension.

(2) Another method utilizes the intravenous injection of 0.2 mg of methylergonovine maleate (Methergine) or its equivalent with delivery of the anterior shoulder. This is not recommended because some ergot products may cause sudden dangerous hypertension plus entrapment of the placenta as a result of marked cervicouterine contraction.

Methylergonovine maleate (Methergine), 0.2 mg, is best given intramuscularly after the placenta is separated and is in the vagina. This is complementary to the Brandt-Andrews maneuver. Intravenous methylergonoric should be avoided secondary to a risk of severe hypotension, cardiac arrythmia, or cardiac arrest.

(3) Recover the placenta by the Pastore or Brandt-Andrews technique (see later).

(4) The uterus should be elevated and compressed manually to express all clots. (Clots may form when brisk bleeding occurs, especially from vaginal and cervical lacerations. Slight bleeding from the uterus ordinarily clots and liquefies to pass finally as fluid blood.)

(5) Another procedure is to give the synthetic oxytocin intravenously. Not more than 2–3 units as a direct infusion should be administered in this manner. If oxytocin is added to a continuous intravenous drip, it may be given in a concentration of 10 IU/500 mL of fluid. However, this is more commonly used for extended intravenous administration to ensure continued contraction of an atonic uterus. The total amount of fluids administered should always be monitored to avoid overhydration.

(6) If bleeding continues and intravenous fluids have not been started, insert a No. 16 or No. 18 needle

into a large vein and administer 20 IU (1 mL) of oxytocin in 1 L of 5% glucose in balanced electrolyte solution. Have cross-matched blood available.

(a) Examine the lower genital tract for lacerations.

(b) Exploration of the uterus for rupture or retained products of conception must be performed. Usually this can be conducted without anesthesia and the additional risk it poses; however, the importance of complete examination warrants the use of anesthesia if examination cannot be done comfortably and quickly.

(7) Give methylergonovine maleate, 0.2 mg intramuscularly.

(8) Give prostaglandin $F_2\alpha$mg intramuscularly if uterine atony is suspected as a cause for continued bleeding (see Chapter 28).

(9) Repair lacerations quickly.

### Techniques of Recovery of the Placenta
**A. Pastore Technique:**

1. Stand to the patient's left and elevate the fundus with the fingers of the right hand.

2. If the placenta separates, massage the fundus gently; otherwise, leave it alone until contractions occur.

3. Place the left hand flat over the abdomen with the fingers superior to the symphysis.

4. When contractions occur and the placenta separates, squeeze the fundus gently and push it downward slightly with the right hand.

5. Prevent the fundus from entering the pelvis by holding the left hand above and behind the symphysis. The placenta can be felt to slide beneath the hand through the lower uterine segment into the cervix or vagina.

6. Lift the fundus upward to leave the placenta free in the vagina.

7. Extract the placenta from the vagina by gentle cord traction.

**B. Brandt-Andrews Technique (Modified):**

1. Immediately after delivery of the infant, clamp the umbilical cord close to the vulva. Palpate the uterus gently without massage to determine whether firm contractions are occurring (Fig 10–21).

2. After several uterine contractions and a change in size and shape, indicate separation of the placenta, hold the clamp at the vulva firmly with one hand, place the fingertips of the other hand on the abdomen, and press between the fundus and symphysis to elevate the fundus. If the placenta has separated, the cord will extrude into the vagina.

3. Further elevate the fundus, apply gentle traction on the cord, and deliver the placenta.

**C. Manual Separation and Removal of the Placenta:** See Chapter 28.

## AIDS TO NORMAL DELIVERY

### EPISIOTOMY (PERINEOTOMY)

Episiotomy consists of making a pudendal incision to widen the vulvar orifice and permit easier passage of the fetus. Episiotomies are performed in most first deliveries and even in many multigravida women, and controversy exists regarding the advantages and disadvantages of this procedure.

#### Normal Labor & Delivery

The advantages of episiotomy are that it prevents perineal lacerations, relieves compression of the fetal head, and shortens the second stage of labor by removing the resistance of the pudendal musculature. Furthermore, a surgical incision can be repaired more successfully than a jagged tear. The disadvantages of episiotomy are that the incidence of 3rd and 4th degree extensions is increased, blood loss is higher, more pain experienced in the postpartum period, and the incidence of subsequent dyspareunia may be higher.

Episiotomy is indicated (1) when a tear is imminent, (2) in most forceps and breech deliveries, and (3) to facilitate delivery.

#### Types of Episiotomy (Fig 10–22)

The tissues incised by an episiotomy are (1) posterior vaginal wall mucous membrane, (2) perineal skin

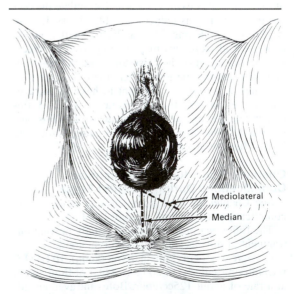

**Figure 10–22.** Types of episiotomy. (Reproduced, with permission, from Benson RC: Handbook of Obstetrics & Gynecology, 8th ed. Lange, 1983.)

and subcutaneous tissue, and (3) perineal body, which is the median raphe of the levator ani located between the anus and the vagina reinforced by the central tendon of the perineum, which consists of the bulbocavernosus muscles, superficial and deep transverse perineal muscles, and sphincter ani externus and internus muscles.

**A. Median:** This is the easiest episiotomy to accomplish and to repair. It is almost bloodless and is less painful than other episiotomies. The median raphe of the perineum is incised. Extension to fourth-degree laceration is common with this type, noted in the literature to be as high as 23.9%.

**B. Mediolateral:** The mediolateral incision may not result in a third- or fourth-degree laceration but there may be more bleeding or pain than with a median incision. Incise downward and outward in the direction of the lateral margin of the anal sphincter. Postpartum dyspareunia is common with this type. Third-degree extension is described in up to 9% of the cases.

### Timing of the Episiotomy

Episiotomy should be done when the presenting part begins to distend the perineum, and prior to application of forceps.

### Repair of Episiotomy & Lacerations (Fig 10–23)

The repair of a midline episiotomy must be done under local infiltration anesthesia or under conduction anesthesia if that has been used for delivery. Chromic catgut or polyglycolic suture is usually used in a running locking fashion, starting about 0.5 cm above the apex of the incision in the posterior vaginal wall, to close both underlying tissue and the vaginal mucosa up to the hymenal ring. The suture is then tied. Three or 4 interrupted sutures are then placed in the muscle and fascia of the perineum. The superficial fascia of the perineum is repaired with continuous suture, and the same suture is then carried upward as subcuticular stitch in the perineum to be tied at the level of the hymenal ring.

In fourth-degree laceration repairs, close the rectal wall with fine interrupted polyglycolic sutures, and close the overlying fascia. Reapproximate the ends of the rectal sphincter with interrupted cat gut sutures, preferably in the perimuscular fascia rather than the friable muscle itself. Then suture lacerations in the more superficial structures.

## INDUCTION OF LABOR

Induction of labor by medical or surgical means usually should be performed only upon specific indications. Induction of labor indicates initiations of labor with oxytocin with or without artificial rupture of membranes. Elective inductions, meaning initia-

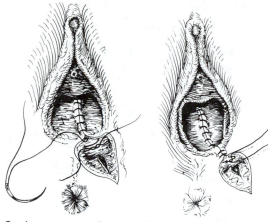

Continuous suture of mucosa with inverted suture of perineal musculature

Mucosal suture continued in skin and tied with inverted suture

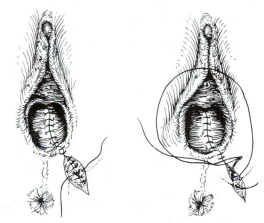

Closure of fascia

Skin closed subcutaneously

**Figure 10–23.** Episiotomy repair. (Reproduced, with permission, from Benson RC: Handbook of Obstetrics & Gynecology, 8th ed. Lange, 1983.)

tion of labor solely for convenience, is not recommended. Generally speaking, induction of labor should be considered when further prolongation of pregnancy might expose the mother or fetus or both to certain risk and when vaginal delivery is not contraindicated. Careful evaluation of the cervix is predictive of the potential success of induction (Table 10–4) and is highly recommended before induction. To avoid iatrogenic prematurity, the gestational criteria for the fetus should be evaluated carefully before elective induction, ie, early ultrasound, lecithin/sphingomyelin ratio, and amniotic fluid phosphatidyl glycerol levels.

### Indications

The following are common indications for induction of labor:

(1) Prolonged pregnancy.

Table 10–4. Bishop method of pelvic scoring for elective induction of labor.[1,2]

| Examination | Points | | |
|---|---|---|---|
| | 1 | 2 | 3 |
| Cervical dilatation (cm) | 1–2 | 3–4 | 5–6 |
| Cervical effacement (%) | 40–50 | 60–70 | 80 |
| Station of presenting part | – 1, – 2 | 0 | + 1, + 2 |
| Consistency of cervix | Medium | Soft | . . . |
| Position of cervix | Middle | Anterior | . . . |

[1]Modified and reproduced, with permission, from Bishop EH: Pelvic scoring for elective induction. *Obstet Gynecol* 1964; 24:66.
[2]Elective induction of labor may be performed safely when pelvic score is 9 or more.

(2) Diabetes mellitus.
(3) Rh isoimmunization.
(4) Preeclampsia.
(5) Premature rupture of membranes.
(6) Chronic hypertension.
(7) Placental insufficiency.
(8) Suspected intrauterine growth retardation.

## Contraindications

Absolute contraindications to induction of labor include the following:

(1) Cephalopelvic disproportion.
(2) Placenta previa.
(3) Uterine scar due to previous classical cesarean section, myomectomy, entering the endometrium, hysterotomy, or unification surgery.
(4) Transverse lie.

Relative contraindications to induction of labor include the following:

(1) Breech presentation.
(2) Polyhydramnios.
(3) Multiple gestation.
(4) Grand multiparity.
(5) Prematurity.

## Complications of Induction of Labor

**A. For the Mother:** In many cases, induction of labor exposes the mother to more distress and discomfort than judicious delay and subsequent vaginal or cesarean delivery. The following hazards must be borne in mind: (1) failure of induction; (2) uterine inertia and prolonged labor; (3) tumultuous labor and tetanic contractions of the uterus, causing premature separation of the placenta, rupture of the uterus, and laceration of the cervix; (4) intrauterine infection; (5) postpartum hemorrhage.

**B. For the Fetus:** An induced delivery exposes the infant to the risk of prematurity if the EDC has been inaccurately calculated. Precipitous delivery may result in physical injury. Prolapse of the cord may follow amniotomy. Injudicious administration of oxytocin or inadequate observation during induc-

tion could lead to fetal demise in utero or delivery of a baby with poor apgars score.

**Methods of Cervical Ripening:** Cervical ripening prior to induction of labor could significantly facilitate the labor onset and progression of labor and increase the chance of vaginal delivery particularly in primigravid patients.

(1) Prostaglandin: Small doses of $PGE_2$ applied locally intravaginally can provide significant improvement in the Bishop's score. Currently, commercially available prostaglandin gel (Prepidil) comes prepackaged in a single-dose syringe containing 0.5 mg of $PGE_2$ in 2.5 mL of a viscous gel compound of colloidal silicon dioxide in triacetin. The syringe is attached to a soft plastic catheter for intracervical administration, and the catheter is shielded to help prevent application above the internal cervical os. Patients with the history of asthma, glaucoma, vaginal bleeding, chorioammonitis, ruptured membranes, or previous cesarean section must be excluded for prostagladin gel ripening of the cervix.

With the Prepidil, usually 12 hours should be given for cervical ripening, following which oxytocin induction should be started. Although stated in the literature, with prostaglandin cervical ripening method, side effects like fetal heart rate deceleration, fetal distress, emergency cesarean section, uterine hypertonicity, nausea, vomiting, fever, peripartum infection, uterine atony, and excess blood loss, current literature review does not indicate any significant differences between the control and the treatment group with intracervical protein $E_2$ gel.

(2) Relaxin: It is a polypeptide hormone that is produced in the human corpus luteum, decidua, and chorion. Purified porein relaxin in the dose of 2 mg in tylose gel vaginally or intracervically is noted to induce cervical ripening in 80% of the cases and labor in about one-third of patients over a 12-hour period.

(3) Balloon catheter: Generally a Foley catheter with a 25–50 mL balloon is passed into the endocervix above the internal os using tissue forceps. The balloon is passed into the endocervix above the internal os using tissue forceps. The balloon is then inflated with sterile saline, and the catheter is withdrawn gently to the level of internal cervical os. This method should induce cervical ripening over 8–12 hours. The cervix will be 2–3 cm dilated when the balloon falls out, which will make amniotomy possible, but effacement may be unchanged.

(4) Hygroscopic dilators: Laminaria tents are made from desiccated stems of cold water seaweed–*Laminaria digitata* or *L. japonica*. Laminaria, when placed in the endocervix for 6–12 hours, increase in diameter 3 to 4 fold, by extracting water from cervical tissues, gradually swelling and applying expansive radial force to the cervical canal. Currently, synthetic dilators like Lamicel, a polyvinyl alcohol polymer sponge impregnated with 450 mg magnesium sulfate,

and Dilapan made from a stable nontoxic hydrophilic polymer of polyacrylonitrile, are noted to be highly effective in cervical ripening.

## Methods of Induction of Labor
### A. Pharmacologic Methods:
**1. Oxytocin–**Parenteral administration of a very dilute solution of oxytocin is the most effective medical means of inducing labor. (Note: Ergot preparations cause sustained contractions and must not be used before delivery for any reason. Oxytocin exaggerates the inherent rhythmic pattern of uterine motility, which often becomes clinically evident during the last trimester and increases as term is approached.

The dosage must be individualized. The administration of oxytocin is really a biologic assay: the smallest possible effective dose must be determined for each patient and then utilized to initiate labor.

Note: Constant observation by qualified attendants (preferably the physician) is required if this method is used.

The intravenous route is preferred. (Intramuscular administration of oxytocics may be dangerous.)

It is the physician's responsibility (not the nurse's) to determine that the correct amount of oxytocin has been added to the infusion bottle and that a specific dose in milliunits (mU) per minute is delivered.

In most cases, it is sufficient to add 0.1 mL of oxytocin (1 unit, Pitocin, Syntocinon) to 1 L of 5% dextrose in water (1 mU/mL). Thus, each 1 mL of solution will contain 1 mU of oxytocin.

One acceptable oxytocin infusion regimen is to begin induction or augmentation at 1 mU/min, preferably with an infusion pump or other accurate delivery system.

Increase oxytocin arithmetically in 2-mU increments—1, 3, 5, etc, mU/min—at 15-minute intervals.

When contractions of 50–60 mm Hg (internal monitor pressure) or 40–60 seconds (on the external monitor) occur at 2.5- to 4-minute intervals, the oxytocin dose should not be increased further.

**2. Prostaglandins–**Prostaglandins in the form of vaginal suppositories have been used to induce labor for midtrimester pregnancy termination. The $F_{2\alpha}$ fraction of prostaglandins ($PGF_{2\alpha}$) has been used intravenously to initiate labor; however, it has not received approval by the Food and Drug Administration for use for this purpose at term. A more standard approach for midtrimester pregnancy termination involves intra-amniotic injection of $PGF_{2\alpha}$ or vaginal $PGE_2$ suppositories. Side effects include nausea, vomiting, hyperthermia, and uterine hypertonicity. The E2 fraction of prostaglandins ($PGE_2$) has been applied as a local extra-amniotic cervical vaginal gel to prime or ripen the cervix prior to induction. $PGE_2$ gel is currently approved for use in the USA for cervical ripening doses of 0.5 mg. Use of $PGE_2$ gel does not reduce the incidence of cesarian delivery and or

failed induction, but does shorten the time interval from induction to delivery.
### B. Surgical Methods:
(1) Amniotomy is an effective way to induce labor in certain cases with high Bishop's score. Release of amniotic fluid shortens the muscle bundles of the myometrium; the strength and duration of the contractions are thereby increased and a more rapid contraction sequence follows.

The membranes should be ruptured with an amnihook. Make no effort to strip the membranes, and do not displace the head upward to drain off amniotic fluid. Amniotomy has not been proven effective in augmenting labor uniformly; it is probably wise to await the onset of active phase of labor to do this procedure. Early and variable deceleration of fetal heart rate is noted to be relatively common with amniotomy. Amniotomy in selected cases could shorten the course of labor without reducing the incidence of operative delivery.

(2) Stripping of the membranes may be a safe method of attempting to induce labor, but it should not be performed if there is a possibility of placenta previa.

(3) When performed in women at term there is a higher rate of spontaneous labor and lower incidence of post"xxx" pregnancies than in women who did not have sweeping of membranes performed.


## NATURAL CHILDBIRTH

In modern obstetrics, numerous procedures and drugs are used for the purpose of reducing discomfort and shortening labor. These techniques range from elective induction of labor to continuous conduction analgesia-anesthesia and prophylactic forceps delivery. Admittedly, overenthusiastic or ill-advised use of such methods may complicate parturition and perhaps "cheat" the mother of the satisfaction to be gained from a significant natural experience. For these reasons, Grantly Dick-Read postulated that fear results in tension, which in turn causes pain, and that this can retard the progress and intensify the discomforts of labor and delivery.

Natural childbirth programs are popular in current obstetric practice. Properly utilized, these require the adequate preparation of the patient and her partner so that both will understand the nature and progress of labor and delivery. In addition, they must be apprised of the actual delivery procedure and the physical appearance and reactions of the infant. Properly performed, natural childbirth usually calls for the father to be an active participant and aide during parturition rather than simply an observer. This in turn requires his full understanding and assistance in timing contractions, aiding in breathing mechanisms and relaxation techniques used by the patient, and giving emotional support.

Natural childbirth has come to mean different things to different people, and there are some erroneous concepts that should be explained. One widespread notion that must be corrected is that "natural" childbirth means "painless" delivery. Even the most enthusiastic adherents of natural childbirth do not make this claim. Nor does natural childbirth necessarily mean drugless labor—although lower doses of medications usually are employed. Natural childbirth is an attempt to make labor easier through the elimination of fear and tension. It is based on the perfectly valid premise that labor is easier for women who are self-assured, relaxed, and cooperative. This can be accomplished in 3 ways. First, the main prerequisite is complete confidence in the obstetric team; the presence of able, dedicated attendants is an effective obstetric anodyne. Second, knowledge of the natural physiologic changes that take place as pregnancy advances will enable the patient to know what to expect; an understanding of what will transpire in labor, including what the doctors in attendance must do, will alleviate anxiety. And third, the patient should learn how to relax, to avoid apprehension, and to cooperate confidently during labor.

If these objectives can be achieved, the advantages of natural childbirth or related methods will be apparent.

## PSYCHOPROPHYLAXIS: THE LAMAZE TECHNIQUE FOR PREPARED CHILDBIRTH

The Lamaze method calls for the individual instruction of both partners, viewing of films of actual deliveries, visits to labor and delivery rooms, and prenatal explanation by the attending physician. When properly performed, these methods generally are successful and reduce or even eliminate the need for analgesia and anesthesia in many patients. The program must be individualized, however, because many patients are not suitable candidates or do not wish this type of delivery. Also, on large obstetric services that serve many unwed mothers, the fathers often are not available to function as assistants at the time of labor and delivery.

The psychoprophylaxis program of preparation for childbirth emphasizes bodybuilding exercises, relaxation, breathing techniques, and comfort aids. It has been successful in alleviating tension and pain during labor. A trained "teacher" (often a nurse or midwife) assists the patient in physical education and relaxation procedures. Exercises such as sitting in "tailor" fashion, squatting, and abdominal and pelvic floor muscle contractions are employed. Relaxation concentrates on muscle groups and includes contraction and relaxation on command. Breathing techniques involve chest (not abdominal) breathing. The patient uses her intercostal muscles, but the diaphragm is relaxed. In abdominal breathing, the diaphragm tenses with uterine contractions, so that it may actually press down on the uterus and interfere with relaxation.

During the first stage of labor, the patient uses slow, deep, chest breathing. Rapid, shallow breathing and panting are recommended just before full dilatation of the cervix ("transition phase"), immediately prior to the phase of voluntary expulsive efforts.

During the second stage of labor, pushing alternates with panting. The patient sits in the tailor position, holding her flexed knees. This allows her to brace during bearing-down efforts. Panting between the contractions helps in the relaxation phase.

Comfort aids include light massage of the back, pressure on the sacrum, and lying "on the side of the occiput."

This preparation for childbirth generally requires 6–8 weeks of practice sessions. The patient's self-confidence and her ability to cope with the labor process are improved by such a program, which is especially popular in western Europe and in Russia as "psychoprophylaxis."

The Leboyer method of "natural childbirth," a modification of the Lamaze concept, calls for birth of the infant in a darkened room free of bright lights and immediate immersion of the infant in a tepid tub to simulate the fetal state, followed by stroking or gently massaging the infant as it adjusts to its extrauterine environment. There is emphasis on immediate bonding with the mother by means of cuddling and stroking of the newborn by the mother, plus putting the infant to breast while the mother is still on the delivery table.

Both the methods discussed earlier call for partner participation in the antenatal training and in the delivery process. The mate participates as an active member of the supporting team—a participant in the birth process rather than simply an observer. He is educated in the process of labor and delivery and assists the patient in her breathing and relaxation exercises. He is present in the delivery room during the actual birth and is encouraged to hold and caress the newborn.

Fears that partner participation would lead to increased puerperal and neonatal infections have been largely eliminated by requiring aseptic conditions for the partner, including proper gowning and handwashing techniques. Similarly, concerns over the possibility of the partner fainting or interfering and presenting an obstacle when emergencies arise have been eliminated by providing him with proper prelabor and predelivery instruction and education, including viewing films of childbirth. Thus, "childbirth education" is an important component of family-centered maternity care. The concept of family-centered maternity care is a logical extension of the natural childbirth principles exemplified by the Lamaze and Leboyer methods. This concept extends the father's participation throughout the postpartum and nursing periods in the hospital and includes rooming-in of the infant with the mother. It calls again for teaching and education in aseptic techniques and contagious dis-ease prevention measures, including proper gowning and handwashing procedures. The ultimate goal is a strongly bonded family unit as well as a healthy one, with all the advantages of modern obstetric care.

## REFERENCES

Coats PM et al: A comparison between midline and mediolateral episiotomies. Br J Obstet Gynaecol 1980;87:408.

Costs of normal births: Regional variations, 1986. Stat Bull Metrop Insur Co 1988;69(4):24.

DeJong RN Jr, Shy KK, Carr KC: An out-of-hospital birth center using university referral. Obstet Gynecol 1981; 58:703.

Devoe LD, Ruedrich DA, Searle N: Does the onset of spontaneous labor at term influence fetal biophysical test parameters? Obstet Gynecol 1988;72:838.

Earn AA: The partographic labor board: An alternative for earlier decisions regarding management during labor. Am J Obstet Gynecol 1982;144:858.

Fraser WD, Sokol R: Amniotomy and Maternal Position in Labor. Clinical Obstet Gynecol 1992;

El-Turkey M, Grant JM: Sweeping of the membrane is an effective method of induction of labour in prolonged pregnancy: A report of a randomized trial. Br J Obstet Gynecol 1992:99:455.

Flynn AM et al: Ambulation in labour. Br Med J 1978; 2:591.

Fraser WD, Sokol R: Amniotomy and Maternal position in labor. Clin Obstet Gynecol 1992;35:535.

Forman A et al: Evidence for a local effect of intracervical prostaglandin E2. Am J Obstet Gynecol 1982;143:756.

Hadlock FP, Harrist RB, et al: Sonographic estimation of fetal wieght. Radiology 1984;150:535.

Harbort GM Jr: Assessment of uterine contractility and activity. Clinical Obstet Gynecol 1992;35:546.

Hill LM: Abnormal labor. Primary Care 1983;10:285.

Ingemarsson E et al: Influence of occiput posterior position on the fetal heart rate pattern. Obstet Gynecol 1980; 55:301.

Jagani N et al: The predictability of labor outcome from a comparison of birth weight and x-ray pelvimetry. Am J Obstet Gynecol 1981;139:507.

Kazzi GM, Bottoms SF, Rosen MG: Efficacy and safety of Laminaria digitata for preinduction ripening of the cervix. Obstet Gynecol 1982;60:440.

Laifer SA: Oral intake during labor. Clin Consultations Obstet Gynecol 1992;4:206.

Lange AP et al: Prelabor evaluation of inducibility. Obstet Gynecol 1982;60:137.

Liggins GC: Initiation of parturition. Br Med Bull 1979; 35:145.

Martin JN Jr, Morrison JC, Wiser WL: Vaginal birth after cesarean section: The demise of routine repeat abdominal delivery. Obstet Gynecol Clin North Am 1988;15:719.

McColgin SW et al: Stripping membranes at term: Can it safely reduce the incidence of posterm pregnancy? Obstet Gynecol 1990;76:678.

Modanlow HD et al: Macrosomia: Maternal, fetal and neonatal implications. Obstet Gynecol 1980;56:35.

Morgan MA, Thurnau GR.: Efficacy of fetal-pelvic index for delivery of neonats weighing 4000 grams or greater. Am J Obstet Gynecol 1988;158:1133.

Nelson NM et al: A randomized clinical trial of the Leboyer approach to childbirth. N Engl J Med 1980;302:655.

Owen J, Hauth JC: Oxytocin for the induction or augmentation of labor. Clinical Obstet Gyncol 1992;35:464

Patterson RM: Estimation of fetal weight during labor. Obstet Gynecol 1985;65:330.

Pello LC et al: Screening of the fetal heart rate in early labour. Br J Obstet Gynaecol 1988;95:1128.

Prendiville WJ et al: The Bristol third stage trial: Active versus physiological management of third stage of labour. Br Med J 1988;297:1295.

Read JA, Miller FC, Paul RH: Randomized trial of ambulation versus oxytocin for labor enhancement: A preliminary report. Am J Obstet Gynecol 1981;139:669.

Read JA et al: Urinary bladder distention: Effect on labor and uterine activity. Obstet Gynecol 1980;56:565.

Roberts J, Malasanos L, Mendez-Bauer C: Maternal positions in labor: Analysis in relation to comfort and efficiency. Birth Defects 1981;17:97.

Russell JGB: The rationale of primitive delivery positions. Br J Obstet Gynaecol 1982;89:712.

St. James-Roberts I et al: Biofeedback as an aid to childbirth. Br J Obstet Gynaecol 1983;90:56.

Thaler I, Timor IE, Goldberg I: Interpretation of the fetal ECG during labor: The effect of uterine contractions. J Perinat Med 1988;16:373.

X-ray pelvimetry. (Policy statement.) American College of Obstetricians and Gynecologists (Sept), 1979.

Yoshida Y, Manabe Y: Stretch-induced delivery is independent of the functional fetal role and dysfunction of the amnion and decidua: A morphologic and enzyme cytochemical study. Am J Obstet Gynecol 1988;159:1293.

Zimmer EZ, Divon MY, Vadasz A: Fetal heart rate beat-to-beat variability in uncomplicated labor. Gynecol Obstet Invest 1988;25:80.

# 11 Essentials of Normal Newborn Assessment & Care

*William L. Gill, MD*

## Essentials of Diagnosis

- Apgar score at 1 and 5 minutes.
- Airway patency and adequacy of ventilation.
- Maintenance of infant temperature.
- Screening physical examination for life threatening conditions.
- Determination of appropriateness for gestational age.
- Complete physical examination after infant is stabilized.
- Laboratory screening for disease.
- Discharge examination.

## General Considerations

**Term newborns** are defined as those born at 36 weeks' gestation or more. The initial physical examination done in the delivery room is a rapid screening for life-threatening anomalies that require immediate attention. The most important assessments are airway patency and adequacy of ventilation.

A more complete physical examination is appropriate after a transition period of 1–6 hours during which the infant is observed for stability of temperature and vital signs. The weight, length, and head circumference are carefully recorded and used to classify the neonate as large-for-gestational age (LGA), appropriate-for-gestational age (AGA), or small-for-gestational age (SGA).

Brief examinations should also be performed daily and at the time of discharge. The discharge examination should be performed in the presence of the mother to discuss the findings and review infant care and feeding.

## THE INFANT IMMEDIATELY AFTER BIRTH

### Apgar Score

Apgar scoring is used to evaluate the neonate at 1 and 5 minutes after birth (Table 11–1). A score of 0, 1, or 2 is given for each of 5 objective signs. A total score of 10 indicates that the infant is in the best possible condition.

A term infant with an Apgar score of 8–10 is con-sidered to be making an excellent transition to extrauterine life and needs no intervention. A moderately depressed infant (score of 5–7) will need tactile stimulation, blow-by oxygen to the face, or assisted ventilation with a resuscitation bag and face mask. A severely depressed infant (score of 0–4) is considered to be asphyxiated, and immediate intubation is indicated if rapid positioning, suction, stimulation, and bag and mask ventilation do not effect immediate improvement in heart rate and color. The 1-minute Apgar score is used to evaluate cardiorespiratory function—spontaneous or during resuscitation. The 5-minute Apgar score is more useful in predicting long-term outcome. Term newborns with 5-minute scores of less than 6 have a higher risk of neurologic sequelae or death. Premature newborns often have lower Apgar scores, but the correlation is not as direct.

### Caring for the Infant Immediately After Delivery

The immediate needs of the infant at delivery are several.

**A. Drying the Skin:** The skin should be dried with warmed blankets or towels to remove amniotic fluid, preventing evaporative heat loss and cold stress. This procedure also provides tactile stimulation to the skin, which encourages increased movement.

**B. Warming the Infant:** Place the infant under a radiant warmer heat source. This is currently the only practical way to guarantee enough heat gain for the infant to avoid cold stress. Cold stress evokes a dangerous combination of responses, including increased oxygen consumption, vasoconstriction, and decreased peripheral perfusion.

**C. Clearing the Airway:** Clearance of the airway and bulb suctioning of the nares and oropharynx are recommended in the first 5 minutes after birth for infants with Apgar scores of 5 or greater. Suctioning by catheter of the posterior pharynx and stomach should be delayed until after the assignment of the 5-minute Apgar score to avoid vasovagal bradycardia or asystole. In infants with Apgar scores of 4 or less

**Table 11–1.** Apgar scoring.

| Signs | Points Scored | | |
|---|---|---|---|
| | **0** | **1** | **2** |
| Heartbeats per minute | Absent | Slow (<100) | Over 100 |
| Respiratory effort | Absent | Slow, irregular | Good, crying |
| Muscle tone | Limp | Some flexion of extremities | Active motion |
| Reflex irritability | No response | Grimace | Cry or cough |
| Color | Blue or pale | Body pink, extremities blue | Completely pink |

requiring immediate intubation and resuscitation, suctioning of the airway by catheter will improve visualization of the airway. If meconium staining is present, endotracheal intubation and suctioning should be done prior to initiation of any ventilation if the particulate meconium is "pea-soup" thick or thicker.

## Physical Examination

The goal of physical examination in the delivery room is exclusion of life-threatening problems.

**A. Airway:** Since most neonates are obligate nose breathers, it is essential that patency of the nasal passages be confirmed (ie, choanal atresia excluded). If the passages are not patent, insertion and maintenance of an oral airway are essential. Infants with a large protruding tongue may also require insertion of an oral airway.

**B. Chest:** Since the tracheobronchial tree is filled with fluid before birth, auscultation of the lungs usually reveals rales with the first few breaths. These should clear within 1 hour. Respiratory rates are 30–60/min for the first 2 hours and are usually irregular. The heart rate is also usually irregular, averaging more than 100 beats/ min but sometimes dropping to as low as 80 beats/min in term infants. The maximum systolic blood pressure in a term newborn should not exceed 80 mm Hg, and the diastolic pressure should not exceed 50 mm Hg. A mean arterial blood pressure of less than 30 mm Hg is associated with poor peripheral perfusion and shock.

**C. Abdomen:** The abdomen is usually soft and appears flat at birth. As the bowel fills with gas, abdominal fullness increases. The liver is usually palpable 1.5–2 cm below the right costal margin. The kidneys can be palpated immediately after birth. A scaphoid abdomen associated with increasing respiratory distress suggests diaphragmatic hernia with bowel in the thorax. Marked abdominal distention may indicate abdominal masses, ascites, or bowel obstruction.

**D. Skin:** Acrocyanosis of the peripheral extremities is common after birth. Petechiae are usually present over the presenting part and are common over the shoulders and thorax.

Pallor may be indicative of anemia, hypotension, or hypercapnia. Expansion of blood volume with plasmanate or a 5% albumin solution should be done slowly, with careful observation of blood pressure. Anemia should be corrected to a minimum hematocrit of 40% in any infant requiring oxygen supplementation or having a hematocrit less than 35% at term. This is accomplished with 10–15 mL/kg of packed red blood cells.

Pronounced plethora of the skin suggests the possibility of polycythemia. This occurs frequently in infants of diabetic mothers, SGA infants, and the recipient twin in twin-twin transfusion syndrome. Infants with hematocrits of 70% or more should receive a partial exchange transfusion of plasmanate or fresh-frozen plasma. Jaundice at birth requires immediate evaluation for hemolytic or infectious causes.

**E. General:** Malformations and deformations of the extremities, face, and neural tube should be noted. Palsies, asymmetric movements, or other evidences of birth injury should be observed. The infant should be identified by arm and leg bands identical to those placed on the mother.

## THE INFANT DURING THE FIRST FEW HOURS AFTER BIRTH

The initial 6 hours after birth are the **transitional period,** during which the infant is observed closely for signs of distress or abnormality. Excessive handling is avoided, since it is not well tolerated during this period. Those providing initial care should observe the infant closely for pallor, cyanosis, respiratory distress, plethora, jaundice, seizures, tremors, abdominal distention, and extreme lethargy or hyperactivity.

The initial assessment by the nursing staff should include vital signs; hematocrit; and peripheral blood sugar in infants of diabetic mothers, LGA and SGA infants, and any infant appearing jittery or having seizures. During this period, routine care should include use of a radiant warmer to stabilize the temperature and prophylaxis for ocular infection with either silver nitrate drops or drops of an antibiotic such as erythromycin. Vitamin K (AquaMEPHYTON), 1 mg intramuscularly, should be given to prevent hemorrhagic disease of the newborn.

As vital signs stabilize, a feeding tube should be gently passed through each of the orifices to check for patency and rule out problems such as choanal atresia, esophageal atresia, imperforate hymen, and imperforate anus.

Once the temperature has stabilized, the infant can be bathed to remove vernix, blood, and debris from the skin and scalp.

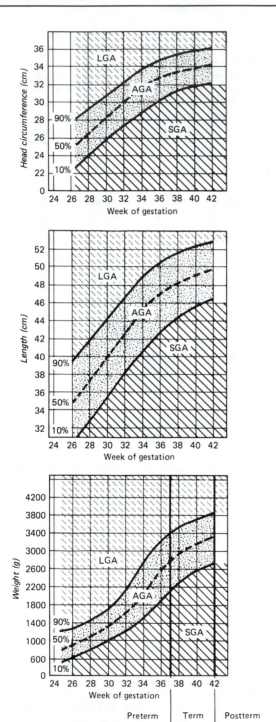

**Figure 11–1.** Classification of newborns based on gestational age plotted against head circumference, length, and weight. AGA, appropriate-for-gestational age; LGA, large-for-gestational age; SGA, small-for-gestational age. (Adapted and reproduced, with permission, from Lubchenco LO, Hansman C, Boyd E: Intrauterine growth in length and head circumference as estimated from live births at gestational ages from 26 to 42 weeks. Pediatrics 1966;37:403 and Battaglia FC, Lubchenco LO: A practi-

An initial feeding can also be given during this time.

## CLINICAL ESTIMATION OF GESTATIONAL AGE

Estimation of fetal gestational age is based on the date of the last menstrual period, serial fundal height measurements, onset of fetal movement, and detection of fetal heartbeat. Ultrasound measurements of biparietal diameter of the fetal skull, femur length, and abdominal girth may be particularly helpful, especially serial measurements. (See Table 13–3.) The L/S ratio and phospholipid profile are useful measures of fetal pulmonary maturity. (See also Chapter 9.)

Gestational age can be determined by examination after birth, since physical characteristics and neurologic development progress in a predictable fashion with increasing gestational age.

Table 11–2 shows the clinical criteria used to rate neuromuscular and physical maturity in a shortened version of the Dubowitz estimate of gestational age. These scoring sheets are available in the USA from major infant formula companies. Each aspect of neuromuscular and physical development is scored on a scale from 0 to 5. The total score gives the maturity rating. If levels of maturity differ for physical and neuromuscular characteristics, problems of intrauterine growth are often present.

Fig 11–1 shows the normal growth curves for fetal length, weight, and head circumference. These measurements are plotted for the gestational age determined in the maturity rating (Fig 11–1). SGA, LGA, or AGA can then be plotted.

## COMPLETE PHYSICAL EXAMINATION OF THE NEWBORN

A complete physical examination of the newborn should be performed within 24 hours of delivery but after the 6-hour transition period, when the infant has stabilized. Observation for abnormal findings during the transition period will identify those infants who require earlier evaluation.

### General Appearance & Vital Signs

The vital signs, physical measurements, and maturity ratings noted during the transition period should be reviewed. Patterns of heart rates and respiratory

cal classification of newborn infants by weight and gestational age. J Pediatr 1967;71:159. This form is available from the Mead Johnson Nutritional Group, Evansville, IN 47721.)

**Table 11–2.** Newborn maturity rating and classification.

| | 0 | 1 | 2 | 3 | 4 | 5 |
|---|---|---|---|---|---|---|
| **Neuromuscular maturity** | | | | | | |
| Posture | | | | | | |
| Square window (wrist) | 90° | 60° | 45° | 30° | 0° | |
| Arm recoil | 180° | | 100°–180° | 90°–100° | <90° | |
| Popliteal angle | 180° | 160° | 130° | 110° | 90° | <90° |
| Scarf sign | | | | | | |
| Heel to ear | | | | | | |
| **Physical maturity** | | | | | | |
| Skin | Gelatinous, red, transparent | Smooth, pink; visible veins | Superficial peeling and/or rash; few veins | Cracking, pale area; rare veins | Parchment, deep cracking; no vessels | Leathery, cracked, wrinkled |
| Lanugo | None | Abundant | Thinning | Bald areas | Mostly bald | |
| Plantar creases | No crease | Faint red marks | Anterior transverse crease only | Creases anterior two-thirds | Creases cover entire sole | |
| Breast | Barely perceptible | Flat areola; no bud | Stippled areola; bud, 1–2 mm | Raised areola; bud, 3–4 mm | Full areola; bud, 5–10 mm | |
| Ear | Pinna flat; stays folded | Slightly curved pinna; soft; slow recoil | Well-curved pinna; soft; ready recoil | Formed and firm; instant recoil | Thick cartilage; ear stiff | |
| Genitalia (male) | Scrotum empty; no rugae | | Testes descending; few rugae | Testes down; good rugae | Testes pendulous; deep rugae | |
| Genitalia (female) | Prominent clitoris and labia minora | | Majora and minora equally prominent | Majora large; minora small | Clitoris and minora completely covered | |

The following information should be recorded: Birth date and Apgar score at 1 and 5 minutes. Two separate examinations should be made within the first 24 hours to determine the estimated gestational age according to maturity rating. Each examination and the age of the infant at each examination should be noted.

Maturity rating:

| Score | 5 | 10 | 15 | 20 | 25 | 30 | 35 | 40 | 45 | 50 |
|---|---|---|---|---|---|---|---|---|---|---|
| Weeks | 26 | 28 | 30 | 32 | 34 | 36 | 38 | 40 | 42 | 44 |

Reproduced, with permission, from Ballard JL et al: A simplified assessment of gestational age. Pediatr Res 1977;11:374. Figures adapted from Sweet AY: Classification of the low-birth-weight infant. In: Care of the High-Risk Infant, 3rd ed. Klaus MH, Fanaroff AA (editors). Saunders, 1986. This form is available from the Mead Johnson Nutritional Group, Evansville, IN 47721.

rates should be evaluated. Normal blood pressures are related to the size and postnatal age of the infant, but in most cases, the mean should be greater than 30 mm Hg. Blood pressures should be determined in both the upper and lower extremities using the Doppler method and a cuff that covers two-thirds of the extremity.

## Skin

**Vernix caseosa,** a whitish cheesy material, normally covers the body of the fetus, increasing in amount as term approaches. The amount may decrease once term is reached, and the substance may be completely absent in postterm infants. Dry skin with cracking and peeling of superficial layers is common in postterm infants and SGA infants. Edema may be generalized, as in renal, cardiac, hematologic, or other systemic disease, or localized, as in Turner's syndrome (dorsum of hands and feet). Meconium staining of the umbilical cord, nails, and skin suggests prior fetal intrauterine stress. The skin of preterm infants is more translucent and may be covered with fine lanugo hair.

**Mongolian spots** are bluish-black areas of increased pigmentation over the back and buttocks, most frequently seen in blacks. **Neonatal pustular melanosis** is also seen in black infants as a small vesicle that leaves a pigmented freckle when the vesicle ruptures. **Erythema toxicum neonatorum** is a benign rash presenting like flea bites, with a raised center on an erythematous base that may progress to vesicles. Wright's stain of the vesicle exudate shows numerous eosinophils. **Milia** are small white papules over the nose and face. **Capillary hemangiomas** are common over the eyelids, forehead, nares, lips, occiput, and neck.

Staphylococcal or streptococcal infection of the skin may present as vesicles similar to those of erythema toxicum, but Gram's stain shows polymorphonuclear cells with bacteria often visible. Herpesvirus can also present as vesicular lesions, usually in clusters. Tzanck preparation of a scraping from the base of the vesicles shows multinucleated giant cells, which also show fluorescent antibodies to herpesvirus.

## Head

The size, shape, and symmetry of the head should be noted. The head circumference should be plotted on the growth curves (Fig 11–1). Molding of the skull in vertex deliveries is due to passage through the birth canal, which causes transient elongation. **Caput succedaneum** is an area of edema over the presenting scalp that extends across suture lines. It is also seen at the application site of vacuum extractors. **Cephalohematomas** represent bleeding in the subperiosteal space of the skull bones; the margins of the hematoma are limited by the edges of the bone involved.

The **anterior fontanelle** varies greatly in size from 1 to 4 cm, and the suture lines vary from palpably open to overriding. The fontanelle is usually concave, pulsates with the infant's heartbeat, may flatten with crying, and becomes slightly depressed when the infant is upright and quiet. The **posterior fontanelle** is usually less than 1 cm in diameter and may not be palpable. A third fontanelle representing a widening of the sagittal suture in the parietal bones may also be palpable, especially in infants with Down's syndrome. **Craniosynostosis** presents as an immobile ridge along one or more sutures and is associated with increasing cranial deformity.

## Face, Nose, & Mouth

Symmetry and general appearance of the facial structures should be observed. Unusual facial features may suggest specific syndromes, eg, bushy connected eyebrows in Cornelia de Lange syndrome or widened upper lip frenulum in fetal alcohol syndrome. Detection of one anomaly indicates that others may also be present.

Contusions and localized swelling and asymmetry of facial movement may result from passage through the birth canal or from the use of forceps during delivery. Facial nerve palsy is observed when the infant cries; the unaffected side of the mouth droops downward, giving a distorted facial grimace. With extensive nerve injury, the eyelid will remain partially open on the affected side.

The shape of the nose may be suggestive of specific chromosomal anomalies (eg, the broad beaked nose of trisomy 18). Nose deformity due to intrauterine pressure is common, but nasal fracture is rare. Nasal obstruction not related to structural narrowing or choanal atresia may be caused by congenital infections such as syphilis or cytomegalovirus infection.

Cleft lip and palate may occur as an isolated anomaly or as part of a syndrome such as trisomy 13. A high arched palate may be present as an isolated finding or may be associated with abnormal facies. Most newborns have relatively small mandibles, but micrognathia is seen with Pierre Robin anomaly and may be associated with blockage of the airway by the tongue.

## Eyes

The eyes should be examined at least once during the nursery stay. The overall size and shape of the eyes and orbits may suggest chromosomal anomalies. Examination should include the periorbital structures and anterior orbital structures (ie, cornea, iris, and lens). Nerve function and the red light reflex of the retina should be observed. Absence of the red light reflex or detection of a yellowish-white mass in the eye suggests congenital retinoblastoma. Mydriatic and cycloplegic ophthalmic drops, in concentrations not to exceed 0.2% cyclopentolate and 1% phenylephrine, may be instilled to dilate the pupils for a thorough examination. Corneal and lens opacities, pupil size, and iris abnormalities (eg, Brushfield spots and colobomas) should be noted. Congenital glaucoma presents with an enlarged "ox eye" cornea (> 11 mm), which is often cloudy due to edema. Chorioretinitis may result from congenital infection with *Toxoplasma gondii,* cytomegalovirus, rubella virus, or herpesvirus hominis.

## Ears

Malformed ears may suggest specific syndromes (eg, Treacher Collins syndrome), and low-set malpositioned ears may be associated with other congenital anomalies, especially of the urinary tract. The tympanic membranes are difficult to visualize before removal of vernix and debris. Fluid may be present in the middle ear for the first few hours. Otitis media may occur in infants with cleft palate and in those intubated with nasotracheal tubes for long periods.

Congenital deafness may be detected by standardized neonatal screening tests involving infant movement in response to measured levels of sound or by use of scalp electrodes to monitor brain-stem-evoked response to sound. If potentially ototoxic drugs were used during pregnancy, screening for hearing deficit is especially important. Brain-stem-evoked auditory response (BEAR) screening is also advised in infants < 1500 g birth weight, infants suspected of having congenital infections, those with central nervous system infections, or those with a family history of a syndrome associated with deafness.

## Neck

The symmetry, position, range of motion, and muscle tone of the neck should be observed. Webbing or excessive skin folds on the nape of the neck suggest chromosomal abnormalities (eg, Turner's syndrome, Down's syndrome). Torticollis due to shortening or spasm of the sternocleidomastoid may occur if hemorrhage into the body of the muscle occurs at birth. Enlargement of the thyroid may occur, and sinus tracts may be seen as remnants of branchial clefts.

## Thorax

The shape and symmetry of the thorax and nipples are noted. Absent clavicles permit unusual anterior movement of the shoulders. Fracture of the clavicle is common in shoulder dystocia and is detected by tenderness and crepitus at the fracture site and decreased movement of the arm. Asymmetry of the chest wall may indicate pulmonary distress, airway obstruction, or air leaks (eg, pneumothorax).

## Lungs

Auscultation of the lungs will determine equality of bronchial breath sounds, equal air entry, and the presence of fine rales. In the first few hours of life, rales indicate normal lung expansion. If pneumothorax is present, breath sounds and heart sounds may be distant, percussion may be hyperresonant, and the area lighted on chest transillumination will be larger than the normal 2-cm diameter. Decreased air entry and expiratory grunting are signs of respiratory distress. A chest x-ray must be obtained when abnormal lung findings are suspected. The presence of bowel sounds over the thorax and gas-filled intestinal loops in the chest on x-ray suggest the presence of diaphragmatic hernia.

## Heart & Vascular System

Clamping of the umbilical cord and expansion of the lungs initiate the change from fetal circulation to neonatal pulmonary circulation. Fetal shunts at the ductus arteriosus, foramen ovale, and ductus venosus close, and pulmonary blood flow increases as the lungs expand and pulmonary vascular resistance decreases. Because the pressures in the right side of the heart are essentially equal to those in the left in the normal newborn, flow across septal defects does not occur in the immediate newborn period. Cardiac murmurs are heard with valvular narrowing, and abnormal flow patterns cause inequality of pressures in the heart. Clicks are always abnormal in the neonate. General signs of heart disease include tachypnea, cyanosis, and shock or sudden decompensation associated with hypoxemia and metabolic acidosis. The heart size, location and intensity of the cardiac impulse, heart rate and rhythm, peripheral pulse intensity, and blood pressures in the arms and legs should be determined in the cardiovascular evaluation. Further evaluation may require chest x-ray, ECG, M-mode or 2-dimensional echocardiography, and, possibly, cardiac catheterization.

Sudden decompensation of oxygenation accompanied by metabolic acidosis in an infant who had previously been stable is suggestive of a ductal-dependent cardiac anomaly in which closure of the ductus arteriosus leads to a critical decrease in pulmonary or systemic blood flow. 2-D Echocardiography should be done immediately to confirm the presence or absence of a ductal-dependent cardiac lesion.

## Abdomen

The abdomen appears flat at birth and becomes more protuberant as the bowel fills with air. A markedly scaphoid abdomen associated with respiratory distress suggests diaphragmatic hernia (more common on the left side).

**Omphalocele** is a midline abdominal wall defect that involves the umbilicus and is covered by the yolk sac membrane. **Gastroschisis** is an abdominal wall defect that is distinctly separate from the umbilicus, and the exposed bowel is not covered by a membrane. Complete absence of abdominal musculature (**prune-belly syndrome**) may occur in association with severe urinary tract anomalies or bladder obstruction. The liver, spleen, and kidneys are easily palpated in the first 24 hours after birth.

## Genitalia

**A. Male Genitalia:** In the term male infant, the testes have descended into the pendulous scrotum, and rugae completely cover the scrotal sac. The size of the scrotum varies, depending on the presence of hydroceles. Inguinal hernias may be present at birth; they are usually reducible and can be distinguished from hydroceles by scrotal transillumination. The foreskin is adherent to the glans and cannot be retracted. The complete formation of the penile shaft and the urethral orifice should be noted. With hypospadias, the urethra may open at any point from the base of the shaft to the corona of the glans.

**B. Female Genitalia:** In the term female, the labia majora completely cover the labia minora and clitoris. A fully developed hymenal ring is usually visible, often with excess tissue tags. The hymen should be perforate, with a white mucous discharge from the vagina. An imperforate hymen presents as a solid septum sealing the vaginal opening. Persistence of imperforate hymen can lead to the development of hydrometrocolpos. The imperforate hymen is usually easily disrupted with a blunt probe. Within the first 14 days after birth, vaginal bleeding may occur as a result of withdrawal from maternal estrogen. The mother should be reassured that this is normal and will stop within 3 days.

**C. Ambiguous Genitalia:** If the genitalia appear ambiguous, gender assignment should not be made until a complete evaluation (sometimes including karyotyping) determines the true sex of the infant.

## Anus & Rectum

The patency of the rectum and location of the anal opening should be determined, rectal muscle tone should be observed, and passage of meconium should be noted. If an imperforate anus is present, ultrasonography or x-ray will determine the distance between the rectal atresia and the anal surface. Fistulas may open into the vagina or bladder in females or into the bladder or onto the perineum in males.

Hard meconium producing total rectosigmoid blockage is referred to as **meconium plug syndrome.** Abdominal distention is relieved by passage of the plug; a saline enema, 3–5 mL, may be required. Rectal fissures with bleeding can occur in the newborn period.

## Extremities

The extremities should be symmetric and equal in size. Hemihypertrophy may be indicative of severe anomalies. Other major abnormalities of the extremities include absence of a bone, clubfoot, syndactyly of digits, extra digits, or absent parts of extremities. Congenital hip dislocation is suspected with limitation of hip abduction or when a "click" can be felt when the femurs are pressed downward and then abducted. Nerve palsies and fractures present as decreased movement of the extremities. Hand and foot deformities are frequent with chromosomal abnormalities.

## Central Nervous System

General observations of tone and movement are important in the neonate. Activity may range from complete absence of movement to tremors, jerks, or convulsions as well as opisthotonos and hyperactivity in infants with central nervous system damage. Hypoxic-ischemic central nervous system injury in a term infant is frequently associated with seizures and abnormal tone and reflexes. Intracerebral hemorrhage may be seen in the area of injury, leading to infarction of central nervous system tissue.

Neurologic screening should include the following assessments:

**A. Muscle Tone:** A good test is recoil of the extremities after stretching. The hypertonic baby is frequently jittery, startles easily, and exhibits "tight fisting." The hypotonic infant is "floppy." The extremities fall to the bed loosely when picked up and released.

**B. Rooting Reflex:** The rooting reflex is elicited by stroking the infant at the corners of the mouth and at the midline of the upper and lower lips. The mouth opens, the head turns toward the stimulus, and there is an oral search. Absence of such behavior warrants further investigation.

**C. Sucking Reflex:** This reflex may be observed by placing a finger in the infant's mouth and noting the vigor of movement and suction produced. Hypertonic infants making biting rather than sucking movements.

**D. Traction Response:** To initiate the traction response, pull the infant to a sitting position by traction on the arms at the wrists. After an initial head lag, active neck muscle flexion normally moves the head and chest into line as the infant reaches the vertical position.

**E. Grasp Reflex:** Stroking the palm or sole normally causes active grasping by the involved extremity.

**F. Biceps, Triceps, Knee, and Ankle Tendon Reflexes:** Percussion with a finger or thin rubber hammer should elicit the jerk characteristic of deep tendon reflexes. Reflexes should be symmetric.

**G. Trunk Incurvation:** The infant is draped prone over the supporting examiner's hand. Stroking the back parallel with the spine causes the normal infant to twist the pelvis toward the stimulated side.

**H. Righting Response:** When the infant is lifted vertically, the legs normally will step. When the soles of the feet are placed on the table, the infant will normally attempt to exhibit upright posture by extension of the leg followed by the trunk and head.

**I. Placing:** When the infant is held vertically and the dorsum of the foot is stroked against the edge of the table, the normal infant will flex the knee and attempt to place the foot as though trying to step onto the table.

**J. Moro Reflex (Startle Reflex):** Quick release of traction on the arms or allowing the head to drop suddenly a few centimeters will normally cause a startle reaction. Shoulder abduction and elbow extension will be followed by adduction of the arms associated with spreading and extension of the fingers.

Any abnormal neurologic reactions should be noted and a repeat examination done when the infant is quiet. A Brazelton examination may be indicated to determine a more comprehensive neurologic behavioral status.

## CARE OF THE NORMAL NEWBORN

Every effort must be made to allow the mother to see, touch, and examine her infant in the delivery room to begin the bonding process. Some mothers wish to initiate breastfeeding in the delivery room as a means of reinforcing the bonding experience. Although this usually can be easily accomplished, care must be taken to avoid cold stress, since the infant's only source of heat in most air-conditioned delivery rooms will be conduction from the mother's skin.

In order to facilitate observation during the transition period (6 hours after birth), infants are usually moved from the delivery room to an observation-transition nursery. Most mothers will accept the 6 hours of separation if bonding needs are satisfied by initial contact. For care of the infant during this period, see p. 229. At the end of this period, the infant can be returned to the mother for feedings or rooming-in.

### Duration of Hospitalization Following Delivery

The trend during the past few years has been toward shortened hospital stays after delivery. Most normal newborns who have been delivered vaginally are now discharged with the mother 36–48 hours after delivery. Mothers who have undergone cesarean delivery usually remain in the hospital for an average of 4 days. Discharge prior to 36 hours after delivery carries a definite risk of delay in detecting problems such as jaundice, poor feeding patterns, and infection. Another recent trend has been delivery in a birthing room using natural childbirth methods; the infant remains with the mother, and both are discharged within 6–12 hours. Although this is safer than home birth, serious problems may escape detection because of the short period of observation. If such a program is to be as safe as possible, parents should attend prenatal classes that include infant care sessions, and a nurse should visit the home within 1–2 days. Medical follow-up should be made 3–5 days after birth for physical examination, screening for phenylketonuria and thyroid function, and evaluation of feeding and weight gain.

### Screening for Disease

Laboratory testing to screen for potential medical problems is part of routine newborn care. Some tests are required by law. Tests should include the following:

(1) Blood types of mother and infant and direct Coombs' test for the infant (to detect antibody-mediated blood group incompatibilities).

(2) Serologic test for syphilis.

(3) Whole blood screen for phenylalanine (standard requirement in the USA). The Guthrie method on filter paper is usually used. Aminoacidurias, including valine, leucine, isoleucine, and homocystine, can be tested in some states.

(4) Thyroid function tests ($T_4$ and TSH).

(5) Sickle cell and other hemoglobinopathies.

(6) Hematocrit screening.

(7) Galactosemia in any infant with jaundice (urine test with Clinitest tablets for reducing substances).

Maternal hepatitis B surface antigen status should also be known. If positive, hepatitis B immune globulin as well as hepatitis B vaccine should be given to the infant within 18–24 hours of birth.

### Circumcision

Although the American Academy of Pediatrics has stated that there is no longer any medical reason for neonatal circumcision, a high percentage of males in the USA are circumcised. Parents must be advised of the risks and benefits of the procedure and be allowed to make an individual choice.

### Infant Feeding

**A. Infant Formulas:** Table 11–3 shows the composition of the major formulas available in the USA. No conclusive data show that any one formula is superior. Selection is often made according to the preference of the mother, the physician, or the current nursery "house formula." All standard formulas contain 20 kcal/oz. Formulas prepared for use in newborn nurseries are ready to feed in 4-oz bottles with disposable nipples. No preparation or sterilization is required, and the formula can be stored and fed at room temperature. Formula preparation after discharge is simplified by the use of formula concentrates that are mixed with equal parts of water. The American Academy of Pediatrics recommends use of a formula containing iron for the first year of life.

**B. Breastfeeding:** Over the past several years, enthusiasm for breastfeeding has grown. Breast milk not only supplies optimal caloric needs in the most digestible form but also offers added protection against infection because of its antibodies (princi-

Table 11–3. Normal and special infant formulas.

| Formula | Protein | Fat | Carbohydrate | Osmolality (mosm/L) | Sodium (meq/L) | Calcium (mg/L) | Phosphorus (mg/L) |
|---|---|---|---|---|---|---|---|
| **Standard** | | | | | | | |
| Similac (plain, low iron) (Ross) | 18% whey, 82% casein | 40% coconut oils, 60% soy oils | Lactose | 290 | 11 | 510 | 390 |
| Similac with iron (Ross) | 18% whey, 82% casein | 40% coconut oils, 60% soy oils | Lactose | 290 | 11 | 510 | 390 |
| Enfamil (plain, low iron) (Mead Johnson) | 60% whey, 40% casein | ?45% palm oil, 20% soy oil, 20% coconut oil & 15% high oleic sunflower | Lactose | 290 | 9 | 440 | 300 |
| Enfamil with iron (Mead, Johnson) | 60% whey, 40% casein | ?45% palm oil, 20% soy oil, 20% coconut oil & 15% high oleic sunflower | Lactose | 290 | 9 | 440 | 300 |
| Lacto-free (Mead Johnson) | 18% whey, 82% casein | 45% palm oil, 20% soy oil, 20% coconut oil, 15% high oleic sunflower oil | 100% glucose polymers | 20 | 20 | 550 | 370 |
| SMA, SMA lo-iron (Wyeth) | 60% whey, 40% casein | 33% oleo, 27% coconut, 15% soy, 25% safflower oils | Lactose | 300 | 6.5 | 440 | 330 |
| **Soy** | | | | | | | |
| Isomil (Ross) | Soy protein isolate | 60% coconut oils, 40% soy oils | 50% corn syrup solids, 50% sucrose | 250 | 13 | 700 | 500 |
| Isomil SF (Ross) | Soy protein isolate | 60% coconut oils, 40% soy oils | 100% corn syrup solid | 150 | 13 | 700 | 500 |
| Prosobee (Mead Johnson) | Soy protein isolate | ?same % ages as written in | Glucose polymers, corn syrup solids | 160 | 13 | 630 | 500 |
| Nursoy (Wyeth) | Soy protein isolate | Oleo, coconut, soy, oleic (safflower) oils | Sucrose | 145 | 13 | 630 | 500 |
| **Premature** | | | | | | | |
| Special Care 24 calorie (Ross) | 60% whey, 40% casein | 50% MCT, 30% corn oils, 20% coconut oils | 50% lactose, 50% polycose | 300 | 15 | 1440 | 720 |
| **Standard** | | | | | | | |
| Similac (plain, low iron) (Ross) | 18% whey, 82% casein | 40% coconut oils, 60% soy oils | Lactose | 290 | 11 | 510 | 390 |
| Similac with iron (Ross) | 18% whey, 82% casein | 40% coconut oils, 60% soy oils | Lactose | 290 | 11 | 510 | 390 |
| Enfamil (plain, low iron) (Mead Johnson) | 60% whey, 40% casein | 45% palm olein, 20% soy oil, 20% coconut oil, 15% high oleic sunflower | 100 glucose polymers | 290 | 9 | 440 | 300 |
| Enfamil (with iron) (Mead Johnson) | 60% whey, 40% casein | 45% palm olein, 20% soy oil, 20% coconut oil, 15% high oleic sunflower | 100 glucose polymers | 290 | 9 | 440 | 300 |

| | Protein | Fat | Carbohydrate | | | | |
|---|---|---|---|---|---|---|---|
| Lacto free (Mead Johnson) | 18% whey, 82% casein | 45% palm olein, 20% soy oil, 20% coconut oil, 15% high oleic sunflower | 100 glucose polymers | 20 | 20 | 550 | 370 |
| SMA, SMA lo-iron (Wyeth) | 60% whey, 40% casein | 33% oleo, 27% coconut, 15% soy, 25% safflower oils | Lactose | 300 | 6.5 | 440 | 330 |
| **Soy** | | | | | | | |
| Isomil (Ross) | Soy protein isolate | 60% coconut oils, 40% soy oils | 50% corn syrup solids, 50% sucrose | 250 | 13 | 700 | 500 |
| Isomil SF (Ross) | Soy protein isolate | 60% coconut oils, 40% soy oils | 100% corn syrup solids | 150 | 13 | 700 | 500 |
| Prosobee (Mead Johnson) | Soy protein isolate | 45% palm olein, 20% soy oil, 20% coconut oil, 15% high oleic sunflower | Glucose polymers, corn syrup solids | 160 | 13 | 630 | 500 |
| Nursoy (Wyeth) | Soy protein isolate | Oleo, coconut, soy, oleic (safflower) oils | Sucrose | 145 | 13 | 630 | 500 |
| **Premature** | | | | | | | |
| Special Care 24 calorie (Ross) | 60% whey, 40% casein | 50% MCT, 30% corn oils, 20% coconut oils | 50% lactose, 50% polycose | 300 | 15 | 1440 | 720 |
| Special Care 20 calorie (Ross) | 60% whey, 40% casein | 50% MCT, 30% corn oils, 20% coconut oils | 50% lactose, 50% polycose | 220 | 13 | 1200 | 600 |
| Low Birth Weight 24 calorie (Ross) | 18% whey, 82% casein | 50% MCT, 20% soy oils, 30% coconut oils | 50% lactose, 50% polycose | 300 | 16 | 730 | 560 |
| Enfamil Premature 24 calorie (Mead Johnson) | 60% whey, 40% casein | 40% MCT, 40% corn oils, 20% coconut oils | 60% polycose, 40% lactose | 264 | 14 | 940 | 470 |
| Enfamil Premature 20 calorie (Mead Johnson) | 60% whey, 40% casein | 40% MCT, 40% corn oils, 20% coconut oils | 70% polycose, 30% lactose | 300 | 14 | 1000 | 470 |
| SMA "Premie" 24 calorie (Wyeth) | 60% whey, 40% casein | Oleo, coconut, soy, and safflower oils, 13% MCT | 50% lactose, 50% maltodextrans | 235 | 15 | 950 | 400 |
| **Low Mineral** | | | | | | | |
| Similac PM 60/40 (Ross) | 60% whey, 40% casein | 60% coconut oils | Lactose | 260 | 7 | 400 | 200 |
| **Carbohydrate Free** | | | | | | | |
| RCF (Ross) | Soy protein isolate | 60% coconut oils, 40% soy oils | . . . | . . . | 13 | 700 | 500 |

Table 11–3 (cont'd). Normal and special infant formulas.

| | Protein | Fat | Carbohydrate | Osmolality (mosm/L) | Sodium (meq/L) | Calcium (mg/L) | Phosphorus (mg/L) |
|---|---|---|---|---|---|---|---|
| **Specialty** | | | | | | | |
| Pregestimil (Mead Johnson) | Casein hydrolysates | 40% MCT, 60% corn oils | Corn syrup, glucose polymers | 348 | 15 | 600 | 400 |
| Alimentum (Ross) | Casein hydrolysates | 40% MCT, 60% corn oils | Sucrose, Glucose polymers | 346 | 15 | 600 | 400 |
| Breast milk | 60% whey, 40% casein | Human milk fat | Lactose | 300 | 6.5–10 | 330 | 150 |
| Whole cow's milk | 18% whey, 82% casein | Butterfat | Lactose | 290 | 22 | 1230 | 960 |
| Special Care 20 calorie (Ross) | 60% whey, 40% casein | 50% MCT, 30% corn oils, 20% coconut oils | 50% lactose, 50% polycose | 220 | 13 | 1200 | 600 |
| Low Birth Weight 24 calorie (Ross) | 18% whey, 82% casein | 50% MCT, 20% soy oils, 30% coconut oils | 50% lactose, 50% polycose | 300 | 16 | 730 | 560 |
| Enfamil Premature 24 calorie (Mead Johnson) | 60% whey, 40% casein | 40% MCT, 40% corn oils, 20% coconut oils | 60% polycose, 40% lactose | 264 | 14 | 940 | 470 |
| Enfamil Premature 20 calorie (Mead Johnson) | 60% whey 40% casein | 40% MCT, 40% corn oils, 20% coconut oils | 70% polymers, 30% lactose | 300 | 14 | 1000 | 470 |
| SMA "Premie" 24 calorie (Wyeth) | 60% whey, 40% casein | Oleo, coconut, soy, and safflower oils, 13% MCT | 50% lactose, 50% maltodextrans | 235 | 15 | 950 | 400 |
| **Low Mineral** | | | | | | | |
| Similac PM 60/40 (Ross) | 60% whey, 40% casein | 60% coconut oils | Lactose | 260 | 7 | 400 | 200 |
| **Carbohydrate Free** | | | | | | | |
| RCF (Ross) | Soy protein isolate | 60% coconut oils, 40% soy oils | ... | ... | 13 | 700 | 500 |
| **Specialty** | | | | | | | |
| Pregestimil (Mead Johnson) | Casein hydrolysates | 40% MCT, 60% corn oils | Corn syrup, glucose polymers | 348 | 15 | 600 | 400 |
| Alimentum (Ross) | Casein hydrolysates | 40% MCT 60% corn oils | Sucrose glucose polymers | 346 | 15 | 600 | 400 |
| **Breast milk** | 60% whey, 40% casein | Human milk fat | Lactose | 300 | 6.5–10 | 330 | 150 |
| **Whole cow's milk** | 18% whey, 82% casein | Butterfat | Lactose | 290 | 22 | 1230 | 960 |

pally secretory IgA) and active macrophages and lymphocytes. These offer protection against gastrointestinal pathogens that cause diarrhea.

Preparation for breastfeeding should begin in the prenatal period. Rolling and stretching the nipple will increase elasticity and "toughen" the nipple to minimize soreness and cracking. Following delivery, production of colostrum begins and continues until the milk "comes in" on approximately the third day. The nursing staff must be supportive of the nursing mother and reassure her that she will be able to supply the baby's needs. They should teach her techniques to minimize nipple trauma and instruct her on infant position and nasal airway maintenance. Supplemental water feedings after breast feedings should be discouraged in the neonatal period unless the infant demonstrates signs of dehydration with urine specific gravity of 1.020 or more and the loss of over 10% of birth weight. Use of artificial nipples for any type of supplementation can lead to "nipple confusion" by the infant, who will begin showing preference for the nipple from which it is easiest to obtain milk. This may lead to decreased interest and difficulty in nursing.

There are relatively few contraindications to breastfeeding. Those that must be considered include active tuberculosis and hepatitis B in the mother and maternal use of certain drugs including tetracyclines, antithyroid medication, and certain antimetabolites.

## Discharge Examination

Since a complete physical examination is performed within the first 24 hours after birth, only supplemental rechecking of heart sounds, vital signs, and weight need be performed at discharge. The discharge examination should ideally be performed in the presence of the mother to discuss any findings, answer any questions, and give instructions about routine care and feeding. Plans for medical follow-up are made at this time.

## Car Seats

Safe transportation of infants should begin with the first ride home from the hospital. Most states in the USA require safety-approved car seats for children up to 4 years of age. Car seat instructions and literature should be distributed well in advance of discharge and should be discussed in prenatal classes. Many hospitals have a rental or purchase program for infant car seats.

## Immunization

The American Academy of Pediatrics now recommends immunization of all newborns with hepatitis B vaccine in the nursery at discharge or in the physician's office within 2 weeks.

## REFERENCES

American Academy of Pediatrics Committee on Fetus and Newborn: Criteria for early infant discharge and follow-up evaluation. Pediatrics 1980;65:651.

Avery GB (editor): *Neonatology: Pathophysiology and Management of the Newborn,* 3rd ed. Lippincott, 1987.

Barness LA: Nutritional requirements of the full-term neonate, pp. 21–28. In: *Textbook of Pediatric Nutrition.* Suskind RM (editor). Raven Press, 1981.

Bloom RS: *Textbook of Neonatal Resuscitation.* American Heart Association, 1987.

Christophersen ER, Sullivan MA: Increasing the protection of newborn infants in cars. Pediatrics 1982;70:21.

Dubowitz LMS, Dubowitz V: *Gestational Age of the Newborn: A Clinical Manual.* Addison-Wesley, 1977.

Graham TP, Bender HW: Preoperative diagnosis and management of infants with critical congenital heart disease. Ann Thorac Surg 1980;29:272.

*Guidelines for Perinatal Care.* American Academy of Pediatrics/American College of Obstetricians and Gynecologists, 1983.

Lawrence RA: *Breast Feeding: A Guide for the Medical Profession,* 2nd ed. Mosby, 1984.

Odell GB: *Neonatal Hyperbilirubinemia.* Grune & Stratton, 1980.

Patel DA, Flaherty EG, Dunn J: Factors affecting the practice of circumcision. Am J Dis Child 1982;136:634.

Remington JR, Klein JO: *Infectious Diseases of the Fetus and Newborn Infant,* 2nd ed. Saunders, 1983.

Smith DW: Recognizable Patterns of Human Malformations, 3rd ed. Saunders, 1982.

Thibeault DW, Gregory GA: *Neonatal Pulmonary Care.* Addison-Wesley, 1979.

Volpe JJ: *Neurology of the Newborn.* Saunders, 1981.

# The Normal Puerperium

*Miles J. Novy, MD*

The puerperium is the period of adjustment after pregnancy and delivery when the anatomic and physiologic changes of pregnancy are reversed and the body returns to the normal nonpregnant state. The postpartum period has been arbitrarily divided into the **immediate puerperium**—the first 24 hours after parturition—when acute postanesthetic or postdelivery complications may occur; the **early puerperium,** which extends until the first week postpartum; and the **remote puerperium,** which includes the period of time required for involution of the genital organs. Traditionally, the latter period has extended through the sixth week postpartum, a practice that may have originated in biblical times.*

The reproductive organs return to virtually the normal state by 6 weeks after delivery, and a majority of nonlactating women resume menstrual cycles at this time or soon thereafter.

## ANATOMIC & PHYSIOLOGIC CHANGES DURING THE PUERPERIUM

### Uterine Involution

The uterus increases markedly in size and weight during pregnancy (about 11 times the nonpregnant weight) but involutes rapidly after delivery. Estrogens, progesterone, and the chronic stretching of muscle induced by the enlarging fetus exert synergistic effects on the synthesis of actomyosin and collagen. Progesterone alone is not a prominent cause of myometrial hyperplasia, but estrogen stimulates both uterine hyperplasia and hypertrophy. Withdrawal of the steroid sex hormones of pregnancy increases the activity of uterine collagenase and the release of proteolytic enzymes. At the same time, macrophages migrate into the endometrium and myometrium. Involution of the uterus after delivery occurs chiefly as a result of a decrease in myometrial cell size.

Immediately following delivery, the uterus weighs

about 1 kg and its size approximates that of a 20-week pregnancy (at the level of the umbilicus). At the end of the first postpartum week, it normally will have decreased to the size of a 12-week gestation to be just palpable at the symphysis pubis (Fig 12–1). Ultrasonography can be used to measure length and width of the uterine cavity. During the first week, there is a 31% decrease in uterine area; during the second and third weeks, a 48% decrease; and subsequently, an 18% decrease. The observed changes in uterine area are mainly due to changes in uterine length, since the transverse diameter remains relatively constant during the puerperium. Uterine involution is nearly complete by 6 weeks, at which time the organ weighs less than 100 g.

The increase in the amount of connective tissue and elastin in the myometrium and blood vessels and the increase in numbers of cells are permanent to some degree, so that the uterus is slightly larger following pregnancy.

Because of the decreased volume of the uterus following expulsion of the fetus and placenta, myometrial force and intrauterine pressures are higher in the early puerperium than they are before delivery. Myometrial contractions can develop pressures of 150 mm Hg or more. These contractions (referred to as **afterpains**) are less disturbing than the contractions of labor, however, because no cervical dilatation or stretching of the perineal floor occurs. Afterpains occur during the first 2–3 days of the puerperium and are more common in multiparas than in primiparas. Such pains are accentuated during nursing as a result of oxytocin release from the posterior pituitary. During the first 12 hours postpartum, uterine contractions are regular, strong, and coordinated (Fig 12–2). The intensity, frequency, and regularity of contractions decrease after the first postpartum day as involutional changes proceed.

### Changes in the Placental Implantation Site

Following delivery of the placenta, there is immediate contraction of the placental site to a size less than half the diameter of the original placenta. This contraction causes constriction and permits occlusion

---

*For medicolegal purposes, some states classify a maternal death as one related to obstetric causes occurring within 90 days of delivery.

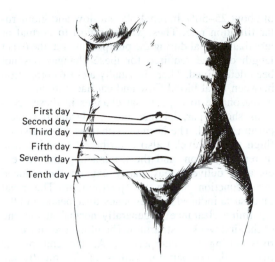

**Figure 12–1.** Involutional changes in the height of the fundus and the size of the uterus during the first 10 days postpartum.

end of the third postpartum week except at the placental site, where regeneration is usually not complete until 6 weeks postpartum. In the disorder termed **subinvolution of the placental site,** complete obliteration of the vessels in the placental site fails to occur. Patients with this condition have persistent lochia and are subject to brisk hemorrhagic episodes. Curettage reveals partly obliterated hyalinized blood vessels.

**Lochia rubra** is blood-tinged uterine discharge that includes shreds of tissue and decidua. It is termed **lochia serosa** after a few days when it becomes serous and paler. During the second or third postpartum week, the lochia becomes thicker, mucoid, and yellowish-white (**lochia alba**), coincident with a predominance of leukocytes and degenerated decidual cells. During the fifth week postpartum, the lochial secretions cease as healing nears completion. Although the lochia provides a good culture medium for the growth of microorganisms, the bactericidal properties of the uterine granulation tissue ensure a virtually sterile uterine cavity if adequate drainage is available. A mild chronic cellular infiltrate of leukocytes persists in the myometrium for as long as 4 months postpartum. These findings must be taken into account if pelvic surgery during the puerperium is contemplated.

of underlying blood vessels. It also accomplishes hemostasis and presumably leads to endometrial necrosis. Initially, the placental site is elevated and somewhat ragged and friable in appearance. Involution occurs by means of the extension and downgrowth of marginal endometrium and by endometrial regeneration from the glands and stroma in the decidua basalis. Endometrial regeneration is completed by the

## Changes in the Cervix, Vagina, & Muscular Walls of the Pelvic Organs

The cervix gradually closes during the puerperium; at the end of the first week, it is little more than 1 cm

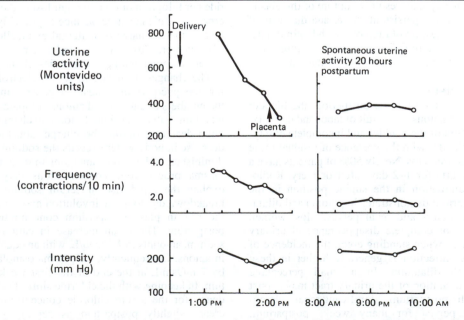

**Figure 12–2.** Uterine activity during the immediate puerperium (*left*) and at 20 hours postpartum (*right*). (Adapted from Hendricks CH et al: Am J Obstet Gynecol 1962;83:890.)

dilated. The external os is converted into a transverse slit, thus distinguishing the parous woman who delivered vaginally from the nulliparous woman or from one who delivered by cesarean section. Colposcopic examination soon after delivery may reveal ulceration, ecchymosis, and laceration. Complete healing and reepithelialization occur 6–12 weeks later. Stromal edema and round cell infiltration and the endocervical glandular hyperplasia of pregnancy may persist for up to 3 months. Cervical lacerations heal in most uncomplicated cases, but the continuity of the cervix may not be restored, so that the site of the tear may remain as a scarred notch.

After vaginal delivery, the overdistended and smooth-walled vagina gradually returns to its antepartum condition by about the third week. Thickening of the mucosa, cervical mucus production, and other estrogenic changes may be delayed in a lactating woman. The torn hymen heals in the form of fibrosed nodules of mucosa, the **carunculae myrtiformes.** Two weeks after delivery, the uterine tube reflects a hypoestrogenic state marked by atrophy and partial deciliation of the epithelium. Normal changes in the pelvis after uncomplicated term vaginal delivery include widening of the symphysis and sacroiliac joints and occasionally gas in these joints. Gas is often seen by ultrasonography in the endometrial cavity after uncomplicated vaginal delivery and does not necessarily indicate the presence of endometritis.

The voluntary muscles of the pelvic floor and the pelvic supports gradually regain their tone during the puerperium. Tearing or overstretching of the musculature or fascia at the time of delivery predisposes to genital hernias. Overdistention of the abdominal wall during pregnancy may result in rupture of the elastic fibers of the cutis, persistent striae, and diastasis of the rectus muscles. Involution of the abdominal musculature may require 6–7 weeks, and vigorous exercises are not recommended until after that time.

## Urinary System

In the immediate postpartum period, the bladder mucosa is edematous as a result of labor and delivery. Overdistention of the bladder and incomplete emptying of the bladder with the presence of residual urine are common problems. Nearly 50% of patients have a mild proteinuria for 1–2 days after delivery. Radiographic examination in the supine position in the early puerperium demonstrates hypotonia and dilatation of the ureters and renal pelves. Most women show partial or complete disappearance of urinary tract dilatation when standing erect; the incidence of urinary tract infection is generally higher in these women with dilatation. In a small percentage of women, dilatation of the urinary tract may persist for 3 months postpartum. Significant renal enlargement may persist for many weeks postpartum. Pregnancy is accompanied by an estimated increase

of about 25–50% in renal plasma flow and glomerular filtration rate. These values return to normal or less than normal during the puerperium, but the exact length of time required for these changes has not been determined. There is usually a close correlation between renal blood flow and cardiac output, and it is reasonable to expect that changes in these functions should parallel one another during the puerperium as well. The hormonal changes of pregnancy (high steroid levels) also contribute to the increase in renal function, and the diminishing steroid levels after delivery may partly explain the reduced renal function during the puerperium. The renal glycosuria induced by pregnancy disappears, and the creatinine clearance is generally normal at the end of the first week postpartum. The blood urea nitrogen rises during the puerperium: At the end of the first week postpartum, values of 20 mg/dL are reached, compared with 15 mg/dL in the late third trimester.

## Fluid Balance & Electrolytes

An average decrease in maternal weight of 5.5 kg (12 lb) occurs during labor and after delivery of the infant and placenta and the loss of amniotic fluid. The average patient may lose an additional 4 kg (9 lb) during the puerperium as a result of excretion of the fluids and electrolytes accumulated during pregnancy.

There is an average net fluid loss of at least 2 L during the first week postpartum and an additional loss of approximately 1.5 L during the next 5 weeks. The water loss in the first week postpartum represents a loss of extracellular fluid. A negative balance must be expected of slightly more than 100 meq of chloride per kilogram of body weight lost in the early puerperium. This negative balance is probably attributable to the discharge of maternal extracellular fluid. The puerperal losses of salt and water are generally larger in women with preeclampsia-eclampsia.

The changes occurring in serum electrolytes during the puerperium indicate a general increase in the numbers of cations and anions compared with antepartum values. Although total exchangeable sodium decreases during the puerperium, the relative decrease in body water exceeds the sodium loss. The diminished aldosterone antagonism due to falling plasma progesterone concentrations may partially explain the rapid rise in serum sodium. Cellular breakdown due to tissue involution may contribute to the rise in plasma potassium concentration noted postpartum. The mean increase in cations, chiefly sodium, amounts to 4.7 meq/L, with an equal increase in anions. Consequently, the plasma osmolality rises by 7 mOsm/L at the end of the first week postpartum. In keeping with the chloride shift, there is a tendency for the serum chloride concentration to decrease slightly postpartum as serum bicarbonate increases.

## Metabolic & Chemical Changes

Total fatty acids and nonesterified fatty acids return to nonpregnant levels on about the second day of the puerperium. Both cholesterol and triglyceride concentrations decrease significantly within 24 hours after delivery, and this change is reflected in all lipoprotein fractions. Plasma triglycerides continue to fall and approach nonpregnant values 6–7 weeks postpartum. By comparison, the decrease in plasma cholesterol levels is slower; LDL cholesterol remains above nonpregnant levels for at least 7 weeks postpartum. Lactation does not influence lipid levels, but, in contrast to pregnancy, the postpartum hyperlipidemia is sensitive to dietary manipulation.

During the early puerperium blood glucose concentrations (both fasting and postprandial) tend to fall below the values seen during pregnancy and delivery. This fall is most marked on the second and third postpartum days. Accordingly, the insulin requirements of diabetic patients are lower. Reliable indications of the insulin sensitivity and the blood glucose concentrations characteristic of the nonpregnant state can be demonstrated only after the first week postpartum. Thus, a glucose tolerance test performed in the early puerperium may be interpreted erroneously if nonpuerperal standards are applied to the results.

The concentration of free plasma amino acids increases postpartum. Normal nonpregnant values are regained rapidly on the second or third postpartum day and are presumably a result of reduced utilization and an elevation in the renal threshold.

## Enzyme Changes
## (See also Chapter 6.)

Hepatic sulfobromophthalein (Bromsulphalein; BSP) storage capacity is increased 2-fold in late pregnancy, whereas the maximal tubular excretory rate is decreased. However, BSP retention in serum may remain in the normal range because hepatic clearance is increased as a result of the relative hypoalbuminemia of pregnancy. These changes in BSP metabolism are probably estrogen-related and revert to normal soon after delivery. Serum alkaline phosphatase of hepatic origin returns to nonpregnant levels by the third week postpartum. Serum glutamic-oxaloacetic transaminase (SGOT) and serum glutamic-pyruvic transaminase (SGPT) are unchanged in normal pregnancy and the puerperium unless there is hepatocellular injury. As a result of the muscular activity of labor, creatine phosphokinase and lactic dehydrogenase activities may be elevated in maternal blood for several days after delivery. Lipoprotein lipase activity is increased during pregnancy and returns to nonpregnant levels by 10 days postpartum. Pregnancy-associated proteins believed to be of placental origin disappear from blood within a few days after delivery. Alpha-fetoproteins and oxytocinase can be detected in plasma for many weeks postpartum, suggesting that they are not solely of placental origin.

## Cardiovascular Changes

**A. Blood Coagulation:** The production of both prostacyclin ($PGI_2$), an inhibitor of platelet aggregation, and thromboxane $A_2$, an inducer of platelet aggregation and a vasoconstrictor, is increased during pregnancy and the puerperium. Possibly, the balance between thromboxane $A_2$ and $PGI_2$ is shifted to the side of thromboxane $A_2$ dominance during the puerperium, since platelet reactivity is increased at this time. Rapid and dramatic changes in the coagulation and fibrinolytic systems occur after delivery (Table 12–1). A decrease in the platelet count occurs immediately after separation of the placenta, but a secondary elevation occurs in the next few days together with an increase in platelet adhesiveness. The plasma fibrinogen concentration begins to decrease during labor and reaches its lowest point during the first day postpartum. Thereafter, rising plasma fibrinogen levels reach prelabor values by the third or fifth day of the puerperium. This secondary peak in fibrinogen activity is maintained until the second postpartum week, after which the level of activity slowly returns to normal nonpregnant levels during the following 7–10 days. A similar pattern occurs with respect to factor VIII and plasminogen. Circulating levels of antithrombin III are decreased in the third trimester of

**Table 12–1.** Changes in blood coagulation and fibrinolysis during the puerperium.

| | Time Postpartum | | | | |
|---|---|---|---|---|---|
| | 1 Hour | 1 Day | 3–5 Days | 1st Week | 2nd Week |
| Platelet count | ↓ | ↑ | ↑↑ | ↑↑ | ↑ |
| Platelet adhesiveness | ↑ | ↑↑ | ↑↑↑ | ↑ | 0 |
| Fibrinogen | ↓ | ↓ | ↑ | 0 | ↓ |
| Factor V | | ↑ | ↑↑ | ↑ | 0 |
| Factor VIII | ↓ | ↓ | ↑ | ↑ | ↓ |
| Factors II, VII, X | | ↓ | ↓ | ↓↓ | ↓↓ |
| Plasminogen | ↓ | ↓↓ | 0 | ↓ | ↓ |
| Plasminogen activator | ↑↑↑ | ↑↑ | 0 | | |
| Fibrinolytic activity | ↑ | ↑↑ | ↑↑ | ↑ | |
| Fibrin split products | ↑ | ↑↑ | ↑↑ | | |

The arrows indicate the direction and relative magnitude of change compared with the late third trimester or antepartum values. Zero indicates a return to antepartum but not necessarily nonpregnant values. (Prepared from the data of Manning FA et al: Am J Obstet Gynecol 1971;110:900, Bonnar J et al: Br Med J 1970;2:200; Ygge J: Am J Obstet Gynecol 1969;104:2; and Shaper AG et al: J Obstet Gynaecol Br Commonw 1968;75:433.)

pregnancy and in women taking estrogens for post-partum lactation suppression. Patients with a congenital deficiency of antithrombin III (an endogenous inhibitor of factor X) have recurrent venous thromboembolic disease, and a low level of this factor has been associated with a "hypercoagulable state."

The fibrinolytic activity of maternal plasma is greatly reduced during the last months of pregnancy but increases rapidly after delivery. In the first few hours postpartum, an increase in tissue plasminogen activator (t-PA) develops, together with a slight prolongation of the thrombin time, a decrease in plasminogen activator inhibitors, and a significant increase in fibrin split products. Protein C is an important coagulation inhibitor that requires the non-enzymatic cofactor protein S (which exists as a free protein and as a complex) for its activity. The level of protein S, both total and free, increases on the first day after delivery and gradually returns to normal levels after the first week postpartum.

According to current concepts, the fibrinolytic system is in dynamic equilibrium with the factors that promote coagulation. Thus, after delivery, the increased plasma fibrinolytic activity coupled with the consumption of several clotting factors suggests a large deposition of fibrin in the placental bed. Because of the continued release of fibrin breakdown products from the placental site, the concentration of fibrin split products continues to rise even after spontaneous plasma fibrinolytic activity decreases. Increased levels of soluble fibrin monomer complexes are observed during the early puerperium compared with levels at 3 months postpartum.

The increased concentration of clotting factors normally seen during pregnancy can be viewed as teleologically important in providing a reserve to compensate for the rapid consumption of these factors during delivery and in promoting hemostasis after parturition. Nonetheless, extensive activation of clotting factors together with immobility, sepsis, or trauma during delivery may set the stage for later thromboembolic complications (see Chapter 43). The secondary increase in fibrinogen, factor VIII, or platelets (which remain well above nonpregnant values in the first week postpartum) also predisposes to thrombosis during the puerperium. The abrupt return of normal fibrinolytic activity after delivery may be a protective mechanism to combat this hazard. A small percentage of puerperal women who show a diminished ability to activate the fibrinolytic system appear to be at high risk for the development of postpartum thromboembolic complications.

**B. Blood Volume Changes:** The total blood volume normally decreases from the antepartum value of 5–6 L to the nonpregnant value of 4 L by the third week after delivery. One third of this reduction occurs during delivery and soon afterward, and a similar amount is lost by the end of the first postpartum week. Additional variation occurs with lactation. The hypervolemia of pregnancy may be viewed as a protective mechanism that allows most women to tolerate considerable loss of blood during parturition. The quantity of blood lost during delivery generally determines the blood volume and hematocrit during the puerperium. Normal vaginal delivery of a single fetus entails an average blood loss of about 400 mL, whereas cesarean section leads to a blood loss of nearly 1 L. If total hysterectomy is performed in addition to cesarean section delivery, the mean blood loss increases to approximately 1500 mL. Delivery of twins and triplets entails blood losses similar to those of operative delivery, but a compensatory increase in maternal plasma volume and red blood cell mass is observed during multiple pregnancy.

Dramatic and rapid readjustments occur in the maternal vasculature after delivery, so that the response to blood loss during the early puerperium is different from that occurring in the nonpregnant woman. Delivery leads to obliteration of the low-resistance uteroplacental circulation and results in a 10–15% reduction in the size of the maternal vascular bed. Loss of placental endocrine function also removes a stimulus to vasodilatation.

A declining blood volume with a rise in hematocrit is usually seen 3–7 days after vaginal delivery (Fig 12–3). In contrast, serial studies of patients after cesarean section indicate a more rapid decline in blood volume and hematocrit and a tendency for the hematocrit to stabilize or even decline in the early puerperium. Hemoconcentration occurs if the loss of red cells is less than the reduction in vascular capacity. Hemodilution takes place in patients who lose 20% or

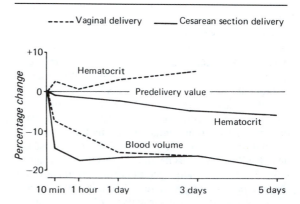

**Figure 12–3.** Postpartum changes in hematocrit and blood volume in patients delivered vaginally and by cesarean section. Values are expressed as the percentage change from the predelivery hematocrit or blood volume. (From the data of Ueland K et al: Maternal cardiovascular dynamics. 1. Cesarean section under subarachnoid block anesthesia. Am J Obstet Gynecol 1968;100:42; and Ueland K, Hansen J: Maternal cardiovascular dynamics. 3. Labor and delivery under local and caudal analgesia. Am J Obstet Gynecol 1969;103:8.)

more of their circulating blood volume at delivery. In patients with preeclampsia-eclampsia, resolution of peripheral vasoconstriction and mobilization of excess extracellular fluid may lead to a significant expansion of the vascular volume by the third postpartum day. Plasma atrial natriuretic peptide levels nearly double during the first days postpartum in response to atrial stretch caused by blood volume expansion and may have relevance for postpartum natriuresis and diuresis. Occasionally, a patient sustains minimal blood loss at delivery. In such a patient, marked hemoconcentration may occur in the puerperium, especially if there has been a preexisting polycythemia or a considerable increase in the red cell mass during pregnancy.

**C. Hematopoiesis:** The red cell mass increases by about 30% during pregnancy, whereas the average red cell loss at delivery is approximately 14%. Thus, the mean postpartum red cell mass level should be about 15% above nonpregnant values. The sudden loss of blood at delivery, however, leads to a rapid and short-lived reticulocytosis (with a peak on the fourth postpartum day) and moderately elevated erythropoietin levels during the first week postpartum.

The bone marrow in pregnancy and in the early puerperium is hyperactive and capable of delivering a large number of young cells to the peripheral blood. Prolactin may play a minor role in bone marrow stimulation.

A striking leukocytosis occurs during labor and extends into the early puerperium. In the immediate puerperium the white blood cell count may be as high as 25,000/μL, with an increased percentage of granulocytes. The stimulus for this leukocytosis is not known, but it probably represents a release of sequestered cells in response to the stress of labor.

The serum iron level is decreased and the plasma iron turnover is increased between the third and fifth days of the puerperium. Normal values are regained by the second week postpartum. The shorter duration of ferrokinetic changes in puerperal women compared with the duration of changes in nonpregnant women who have had phlebotomy is due to the increased erythroid marrow activity and the circulatory changes described above.

Most women who sustain an average blood loss at delivery and who have had iron supplementation during pregnancy show a relative erythrocytosis during the second week postpartum. Since there is no evidence of increased red cell destruction during the puerperium, any red cells gained during pregnancy will disappear gradually according to their normal life span. A moderate excess of red blood cells after delivery, therefore, may lead to an increase in iron stores. Iron supplementation is not necessary for normal postpartum women if the hematocrit or hemoglobin concentration 5–7 days after delivery is equal to or greater than a normal predelivery value. In the late

puerperium, there is a gradual decrease in the red cell mass to nonpregnant levels as the rate of erythropoiesis returns to normal.

**D. Hemodynamic Changes:** The hemodynamic adjustments in the puerperium depend largely on the conduct of labor and delivery, eg, maternal position, method of delivery, mode of anesthesia or analgesia, and blood loss. Cardiac output increases progressively during labor in patients who have received only local anesthesia. The increase in cardiac output peaks immediately after delivery, at which time it is approximately 80% above the prelabor value. During a uterine contraction there is a rise in central venous pressure, arterial pressure, and stroke volume—and, in the absence of pain and anxiety, a reflex decrease in the pulse rate. These changes are magnified in the supine position. Only minimal changes occur in the lateral recumbent position because of unimpaired venous return and absence of aortoiliac compression by the contracting uterus (Poseiro effect). Epidural anesthesia modifies the progressive rise in cardiac output during labor and reduces the absolute increase observed immediately after delivery, probably by limiting pain and anxiety.

The hemodynamic effects of uterine contractions are avoided when cesarean section delivery is performed prior to the onset of labor. Nonetheless, the rise in cardiac output noted in the immediate puerperium still occurs. Major fluctuations in blood pressure, cardiac output, heart rate, and stroke volume occur during cesarean section delivery under subarachnoid block or balanced general anesthesia. Extradural anesthesia without epinephrine provides hemodynamic stability during cesarean section and only a small rise in cardiac output after delivery, suggesting that this would be the preferred mode of analgesia in patients with heart disease.

Although major hemodynamic readjustments occur during the period immediately following delivery, there is a return to nonpregnant conditions in the early puerperium. A trend for normal women to increase their blood pressure slightly in the first 5 days postpartum reflects an increased uterine vascular resistance and a temporary surplus in plasma volume. Cardiac output (measured by Doppler and cross-sectional echocardiography) declines 28% within 2 weeks postpartum from peak values observed at 38 weeks' gestation. This change is associated with a 20% reduction in stroke volume and a smaller decrease in myocardial contractility indices. Postpartum resolution of the pregnancy-induced ventricular hypertrophy takes longer than the functional postpartum changes (Fig 12–4). There are no hemodynamic differences between lactating and nonlactating mothers.

## Respiratory Changes

The pulmonary functions that change most rapidly are those influenced by alterations in abdominal contents and thoracic cage capacity. Lung volume

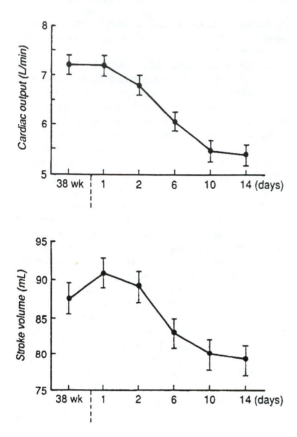

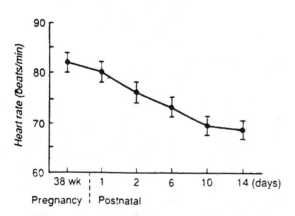

**Figure 12–4.** Changes in cardiac output, stroke volume, and heart rate during the puerperium after normal delivery. From Hunter S, Robson SC: Adaptation of the maternal heart in pregnancy. Br Heart J 1992;68:540.

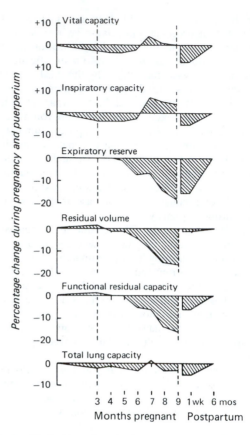

**Figure 12–5.** Alterations in lung volumes during pregnancy and 1 week and 6 months postpartum. (Modified from Cugell DW et al: Pulmonary function in pregnancy. Am Rev Tuberc 1953;67:568.)

changes in the puerperium are compared with those occurring during pregnancy in Figure 12–5. The residual volume increases, but the vital capacity and inspiratory capacities decrease. The maximum breathing capacity is also reduced after delivery. An increase in resting ventilation and in oxygen consumption and a less efficient response to exercise

may persist during the early postpartum weeks. Comparisons of aerobic capacity prior to pregnancy and again postpartum indicate that lack of activity and weight gain contribute to a generalized detraining effect 4–8 weeks postpartum. It is possible that an exercise program throughout pregnancy would prevent or ameliorate the decline in aerobic capacity that is observed postpartum.

Changes in acid-base status generally parallel changes in respiratory function. The state of pregnancy is characterized by respiratory alkalosis and compensated metabolic acidosis, whereas labor represents a transitional period. A significant hypocapnia ($< 30$ mm Hg), a rise in blood lactate, and a fall in pH are first noted at the end of the first stage of labor and extend into the puerperium. Within a few days, a rise toward the normal nonpregnant values of $P_{CO_2}$(35–40 mm Hg) occurs. Progesterone influences the rate of ventilation by means of a central effect, and rapidly decreasing levels of this hormone are largely responsible for the increased $P_{CO_2}$ seen in the first week postpartum. An increase in base excess and plasma bicarbonate accompanies the relative postpartum hypercapnia. A gradual increase in pH and base excess occurs until normal levels are reached at about 3 weeks postpartum.

The resting arterial $PO_2$ and oxygen saturation during pregnancy are higher than those in nonpregnant women. During labor, the oxygen saturation may be depressed, especially in the supine position, probably as a result of a decrease in cardiac output and a relative increase in the amount of intrapulmonary shunting. However, a rise in the arterial oxygen saturation to 95% is noted during the first postpartum day. An apparent oxygen debt incurred during labor extends into the immediate puerperium and appears to depend on the length and severity of the second stage of labor. Many investigators have commented on the continued elevation of the basal metabolic rate for a period of 7–14 days following delivery. The increased resting oxygen consumption in the early puerperium has been attributed to mild anemia, lactation, and psychologic factors.

## Pituitary-Ovarian Relationships

The plasma levels of placental hormones decline rapidly following delivery. Human placental lactogen has a half-life of 20 minutes and reaches undetectable levels in maternal plasma during the first day after delivery. Human chorionic gonadotropin (hCG) has a mean half-life of about 9 hours. The concentration of hCG in maternal plasma falls below 1000 mU/mL within 48–96 hours postpartum and falls below 100 mU/mL by the seventh day. Follicular phase levels of immunoreactive luteinizing hormone (LH)-hCG are reached during the second postpartum week. Highly specific and sensitive radioimmunoassays for the beta subunit of hCG indicate virtual disappearance of hCG from maternal plasma between the 11th and 16th days following normal delivery. The regressive pattern of hCG activity is slower after first-trimester abortion than it is after term delivery and even more prolonged in patients who have had a suction curettage for molar pregnancy.

Within 3 hours after removal of the placenta, the plasma concentration of estradiol-17β falls to 10% of the antepartum value. The lowest levels are reached by the seventh postpartum day (Fig 12–6). Plasma estrogens do not reach follicular phase levels (> 50 pg/mL) until 19–21 days postpartum in nonlactating women. The return to normal plasma levels of estrogens is delayed in lactating women. Lactating women who resume spontaneous menses achieve follicular phase estradiol levels (> 50 pg/mL) during the first 60–80 days postpartum. Lactating amenorrheic persons are markedly hypoestrogenic (plasma estradiol < 10 pg/mL) during the first 180 days postpartum. The onset of breast engorgement on days 3–4 of the puerperium coincides with a significant fall in estrogens and supports the view that high estrogen levels suppress lactation.

The metabolic clearance rate of progesterone is high, and, as with estradiol, the half-life is calculated in minutes. By the third day of the puerperium, the plasma progesterone concentrations are below luteal phase levels (< 1 ng/mL).

Prolactin levels in maternal blood rise throughout pregnancy to reach concentrations of 200 ng/mL or more. After delivery, prolactin declines in erratic fashion over a period of 2 weeks to the nongravid range in nonlactating women (Fig 12–6). In women who are breastfeeding, basal concentrations of prolactin remain above the nongravid range and increase dramatically in response to suckling. As lactation progresses, the amount of prolactin released with each suckling episode declines. If breastfeeding occurs only 1–3 times each day, serum prolactin levels return to normal basal values within 6 months postpartum; if suckling takes place more than 6 times each day, high basal concentrations of prolactin will persist for more than 1 year. The diurnal rhythm of peripheral prolactin concentrations (a daytime nadir followed by a nighttime apogee) is abolished during late pregnancy but is reestablished within 1 week postpartum in nonnursing women.

Serum follicle-stimulating hormone (FSH) and LH concentrations are very low in all women during the first 10–12 days postpartum whether or not they lactate. The levels increase over the following days and reach follicular phase concentrations during the third week postpartum (Fig 12–6). At this time, a marked LH pulse amplification occurs during sleep, but it disappears as normal ovulatory cycles are established. In this respect, the transition from postpartum amenorrhea to cyclic ovulation is reminiscent of puberty, when gonadotropin secretion increases during sleep. There is a preferential release of FSH over LH postpartum during spontaneous recovery or after stimulation by exogenous gonadotropin-releasing hormone (GnRH). In the early puerperium, the pituitary is relatively refractory to GnRH, but 4–8 weeks postpartum the response to GnRH is exaggerated. The low levels of FSH and LH postpartum are most likely related to an insufficiency of endogenous GnRH secretion during pregnancy and the early puerperium, resulting in the depletion of pituitary gonadotropin stores. The high estrogen and progesterone milieu of late pregnancy is associated with increased endogenous opioid activity, which may be responsible for suppression of GnRH activity in the puerperium. Resumption of FSH and LH secretion can be accelerated by administering a long-acting GnRH agonist during the first 10 days postpartum.

The frequency with which menstruation is reestablished in the puerperium in lactating and nonlactating women is shown in Figure 12–7. The first menses after delivery usually follows an anovulatory cycle or one associated with inadequate corpus luteum function. The ovary may be somewhat refractory to exogenous gonadotropin stimulation during the puerperium in both lactating and nonlactating women. When

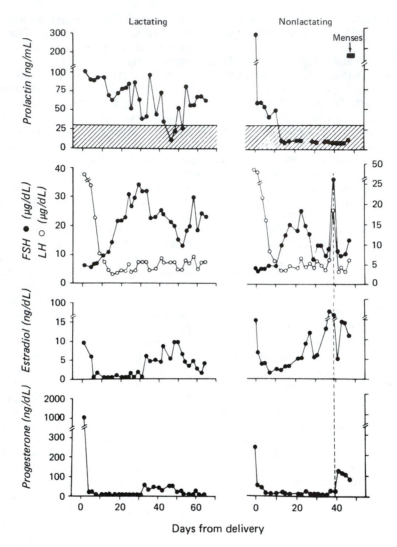

**Figure 12–6.** Serum concentrations of prolactin, FSH, LH, estradiol, and progesterone in a lactating and nonlactating woman during the puerperium. The hatched bars for the prolactin data represent the normal nongravid range. To convert the FSH and LH to milli-International units per milliliter, divide the FSH values by 2 and multiply the LH values by 4.5 FSH, follicle-stimulating hormone; LH, luteinizing hormone. (From Reyes FI, Winter JS, Faiman C: Pituitary-ovarian interrelationships during the puerperium. Am J Obstet Gynecol 1972;114:589.)

prolactin is suppressed with bromocriptine, postpartum ovarian refractoriness to gonadotropin stimulation persists, suggesting that hyperprolactinemia plays only a small role in the diminished gonadal response. Lactation is characterized by an increased sensitivity to the negative feedback effects and a decreased sensitivity to the positive feedback effects of estrogens on gonadotropin secretion.

Because ovarian activity normally resumes upon weaning, either the suckling stimulus itself or the raised level of prolactin is responsible for the suppression of pulsatile gonadotropin secretion. Hyperprolactinemia may not account entirely for the inhibition of gonadotropin secretion during lactation, since

bromocriptine treatment abolishes the hyperprolactinemia of suckling but not the inhibition of gonadotropin secretion. Sensory inputs associated with suckling (if sufficiently intense), as well as oxytocin and endogenous opioids that are released during suckling may affect the hypothalamic control of gonadotropin secretion, may affect the hypothalamic control of gonadotropin secretion, possibly by inhibiting the pulsatile secretion of GnRH. It appears that by 8 weeks after delivery, while ovarian activity still remains suppressed in fully breastfeeding women, pulsatile secretion of LH has resumed at a low and variable frequency in most women. However, the presence or absence of GnRH or LH pulses at 8

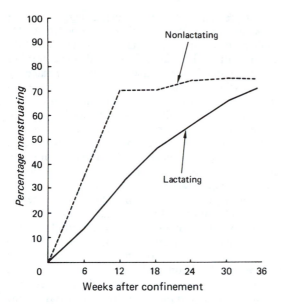

**Figure 12–7.** Frequency at which menstruation is reestablished in the puerperium in lactating and nonlactating multiparous women. (Adapted from Sherman A: *Reproductive Physiology of the Post-partum Period.* Livingstone, 1966.)

weeks does not predict the time of resumption of ovarian activity.

The time of appearance of the first ovulation is variable, but it is delayed by breastfeeding. Approximately 10–15% of nonnursing mothers ovulate by the time of the 6-week postpartum examination, and approximately 30% ovulate within 90 days postpartum. An abnormally short luteal phase is noted in 35% of first ovulatory cycles. The earliest reported time of ovulation as determined by endometrial biopsy is 33 days postpartum. Patients who have had a first-trimester abortion or ectopic pregnancy generally ovulate sooner after termination of pregnancy (as early as 14 days) than do women who deliver at term. Moreover, the majority of these women do ovulate before the first episode of postabortal bleeding—in contrast to women who have had a term pregnancy.

Endometrial biopsies in lactating women do not show a secretory pattern before the seventh postpartum week. Provided that nursing is in progress and that menstruation has not returned, ovulation before the tenth week postpartum is rare. In well-nourished women who breastfeed for an extended period of time, less than 20% had ovulated by 6 months postpartum. Much of the variability in the resumption of menstruation and ovulation observed in lactating women may be due to individual differences in the strength of the suckling stimulus and to partial weaning (formula supplementation). This emphasizes the fact that suckling is not a reliable form of birth control. Since the period of lactational infertility is rela-

tively short in Western societies, some form of contraception must be used if pregnancy is to be avoided. Among women who have unprotected intercourse only during lactational amenorrhea but adopt other contraceptive measures when they resume menstruation, only 2% will become pregnant during the first 6 months of amenorrhea. In underdeveloped countries, lactational amenorrhea and infertility may persist for 1–2 years owing to frequent suckling and poor maternal nutrition. When maternal dietary intake is improved, menstruation resumes at least 6 months earlier.

## Other Endocrine Changes

A progressive enlargement of the pituitary gland occurs during pregnancy with a 30–100% increase in weight achieved at term. Magnetic resonance imaging indicates a linear gain in pituitary gland height of about 0.08 mm/wk during pregnancy. An additional increase in size occurs during the first week postpartum. Beyond the first week postpartum, however, the pituitary gland returns rapidly to its normal size in both lactating and nonlactating women.

The physiologic hypertrophy of the pituitary gland is associated with an increase in the number of pituitary lactotroph cells at the expense of the somatotropic cell types. Thus, growth hormone secretion is depressed during the second half of pregnancy and the early puerperium. Because levels of circulating insulin-like growth factor (IGF-1) increase throughout pregnancy, a placental growth hormone has been postulated and recently identified. Maternal levels of IGF-1 correlate highly with this distinct placental growth hormone variant but not placental lactogen during pregnancy and in the immediate puerperium.

Late pregnancy and the early puerperium are also characterized by pituitary somatotroph hyporesponsiveness to growth hormone-releasing hormone and to insulin stimulation. Whatever the inhibitory mechanism may be (possibly increased somatostatin secretion), it persists during the early postpartum period.

The rapid disappearance of placental lactogen and the low levels of growth hormone after delivery lead to a relative deficiency of anti-insulin factors in the early puerperium. It is not surprising, therefore, that low fasting plasma glucose levels are noted at this time and that the insulin requirements of diabetic patients usually drop after delivery. Glucose tolerance tests performed in women with gestational diabetes demonstrate that only 30% have abnormal tests 3–5 days after delivery and 20% have abnormal glucose tolerance at 6 weeks postpartum. When the relative hyperinsulinism and hypoglycemia of pregnancy return to the nonpregnant range at 6–8 weeks postpartum, a paradoxic decline in fasting glucagon levels is found. Since the early puerperium represents a transitional period in carbohydrate metabolism, the results of glucose tolerance tests may be difficult to interpret.

The evaluation of thyroid function is also difficult

in the period immediately after birth because of rapid fluctuations in many indices. Characteristically, the plasma thyroxine and other indices of thyroid function are highest at delivery and in the first 12 hours thereafter. A decrease to antepartum values is seen on the third or fourth day after delivery. Reduced available estrogens postpartum lead to a subsequent decrease in circulating thyroxine-binding globulin and a gradual diminution in bound thyroid hormones in serum. Serum concentrations of thyroid-stimulating hormone (TSH) are not significantly different postpartum from those of the pregnant or nonpregnant state. Administration of thyroid-releasing hormone (TRH) in the puerperium results in a normal increase in both TSH and prolactin, and the response is similar in lactating and nonlactating patients. Because pregnancy is associated with some immunosuppressive effects, hyperthyroidism or hypothyroidism may recur postpartum in autoimmune thyroid disease. Failure of lactation and prolonged disability may be the result of hypothyroidism postpartum. In Sheehan's syndrome of pituitary infarction, postpartum cachexia and myxedema are seen secondary to anterior hypophyseal insufficiency.

Maternal concentrations of total and unbound (free) plasma cortisol, adrenocorticotropic hormone (ACTH) and immunoreactive corticotropin-releasing hormone (CRH) and β-endorphin rise progressively during pregnancy and increase further during labor. Plasma 17-hydroxycorticosteroids increase from a concentration of 4–14 μg/dL at 40 weeks' gestation. A 2- to 3-fold increase is seen during labor. ACTH, CRH, and β-endorphin decrease rapidly after delivery and return to nonpregnant levels within 24 hours. Prelabor cortisol values are regained on the first day postpartum but a return to normal, nonpregnant cortisol and 17-hydroxycorticosteroid levels is not reached until the end of the first week postpartum.

Much of the rise in total cortisol (but not in the unbound fraction) can be explained by the parallel increase in corticosteroid-binding globulin (CBG) during pregnancy. Displacement of cortisol from CBG by high concentrations of progesterone cannot account for the increased free cortisol levels because saliva progesterone levels (a measure of the unbound hormone) do not fluctuate, whereas a normal diurnal rhythm of saliva cortisol is maintained during pregnancy and postpartum. An extrapituitary source of ACTH, a progesterone-modulated decrease in the hypothalamic-pituitary sensitivity to glucocorticoid feedback inhibition, and an extrahypothalamic (eg, placental) source of CRH have been suggested as explanations for elevated plasma ACTH levels and the inability of dexamethasone to completely suppress ACTH in pregnant women.

The placenta produces large amounts of CRH in the third trimester, which is released into the maternal circulation and may contribute to the hypercotisole-mia of pregnancy. Present evidence suggests that it stimulates the maternal pituitary to produce ACTH while desensitizing the pituitary to further acute stimulation with CRH. Maternal hypothalamic control of ACTH production is retained (perhaps mediated by vasopressin secretion); this permits a normal response to stress and a persistent diurnal rhythm.

Overall, it is most likely that under the influence of rising estrogens and progesterone, there is a resetting of the hypothalamic-pituitary sensitivity to cortisol feedback during pregnancy, which persists for several days postpartum. Several studies have suggested a relationship between peripartum alterations in maternal levels of cortisol and β-endorphin and the development of postnatal mood disturbances.

The excretion of urinary 17-ketosteroids is elevated in late pregnancy as a result of an increase in androgenic precursors from the fetoplacental unit and the ovary. An additional increase of 50% in the amount of excretion occurs during labor. Excretion of 17-ketosteroids returns to antepartum levels on the first day after delivery and to the nonpregnant range by the end of the first week. The mean levels of testosterone during the third trimester of pregnancy range from 3 to 7 times the mean values for nonpregnant women. The elevated levels of testosterone decrease after parturition parallel with the gradual fall in sex hormone-binding globulin (SHBG). Androstenedione, which is poorly bound to SHBG, falls rapidly to nonpregnant values by the third day postpartum. Conversely, the postpartum plasma concentration of dehydroepiandrosterone sulfate (DHEA-S) remains lower than that of nonpregnant women, because its metabolic clearance rate continues to be elevated in the early puerperium. Persistently elevated 17-ketosteroids or androgens during the puerperium are an indication for investigation of ovarian abnormalities. Plasma renin and angiotensin II levels fall during the first 2 hours postpartum to levels within the normal nonpregnant range. This suggests that an extrarenal source of renin has been lost with the expulsion of the fetus and placenta.

There is little direct information about the puerperal changes in numerous other hormones, including, aldosterone, parathyroid hormone, calcitonin, and others. More research should be done on these important endocrine relationships in the puerperium.

## COMPLICATIONS DURING THE PUERPERIUM

### Postpartum Complications

**A. Postanesthetic Problems:** Serious and acute obstetric and postanesthetic complications often occur during the first few hours immediately following delivery. The patient should therefore be transferred to a recovery room where she can be constantly attended and where observation of bleeding, blood pressure, pulse, and respiratory change can be made every 15 minutes for at least 1–2 hours after delivery or until the effects of general or major regional anesthesia have disappeared. Upon return to the patient's room or ward, the patient's blood pressure should be taken and the measurement repeated every 12 hours for the first 24 hours and daily thereafter for several days. Preeclampsia-eclampsia, infection, or other medical or surgical complications of pregnancy may require more prolonged and intensive postpartum care.

The most common respiratory complications that follow general anesthesia and delivery are airway obstruction or laryngospasm and vomiting with aspiration of vomitus. Bronchoscopy, tracheostomy, and other related procedures must be done promptly as indicated. Hypoventilation and hypotension may follow an abnormally high subarachnoid block. Because serum cholinesterase activity is lower during labor and the postpartum period, hypoventilation during the early puerperium may also follow the use of large amounts of succinylcholine during anesthesia for cesarean section. Brief postpartum shivering is commonly seen after completion of the third stage of labor and is no cause for alarm. The cause is unknown, but it may be related to loss of heat or it may be a sympathetic response. Subcutaneous emphysema may make its appearance postpartum after vigorous bearing-down efforts. Most cases resolve spontaneously.

Hypertension in the immediate puerperium is most often due to excessive use of vasopressor or oxytocic drugs. It must be treated promptly with a vasodilator. Hydralazine, 5 mg slowly intravenously, usually reduces the blood pressure.

Postanesthetic complications that manifest themselves later in the puerperium include postsubarachnoid puncture headache, atelectasis, renal or hepatic dysfunction, and neurologic sequelae.

Postpuncture headache is usually located in the forehead, deep behind the eyes; occasionally, the pain radiates to both temples and to the occipital region. It usually begins on the first or second postpartum day and lasts 1–3 days. Because new mothers frequently develop various types of headache, the correct diagnosis is essential. An important characteristic of postspinal puncture headache is increased pain in the sitting or standing position and significant improvement when the patient is supine. The mild form is relieved by aspirin or other analgesics. Headache is due to leakage of cerebrospinal fluid through the site of dural puncture into the extradural space. It is advisable to supplement the daily oral intake of fluids with at least 1 L of 5% glucose in saline intravenously. Administration of 7–10 mL of the patient's own blood into the thecal space at the point of previous needle insertion will "patch" the leaking point and relieve

the patient in most cases. Subdural hematoma is a rare complication of chronic leakage of cerebrospinal fluid and resultant loss of support to intracranial structures.

A small percentage of women who develop headaches during this time also show symptoms of meningeal irritation. Headache due to aseptic chemical meningitis is not relieved by lying down. Lumbar puncture reveals a slightly elevated pressure and an increase in spinal fluid protein and white blood cells but no bacteria. Symptoms usually disappear 1–3 days later, and the spinal fluid returns to normal within 4 days with no sequelae. Treatment is conservative and includes supportive measures, analgesics, and fluids.

Neurologic problems in the puerperium sometimes follow traumatic childbirth, eg, injury to the femoral nerve caused by forceps when the patient was in the lithotomy position. Such complications are rarely bilateral, which aids in the differential diagnosis of a spinal cord lesion. Evidence of more serious neurologic sequelae following regional or general anesthesia for delivery requires consultation with the anesthesiologist and a neurologist.

**B. Postpartum Hemorrhage:** After the third stage of labor, the uterus must be palpated frequently to make certain that the fundus remains firmly contracted and that no excessive vaginal bleeding occurs. Estimates of blood loss are imprecise, especially when clots are passed, but the loss of more than 300 mL of blood constitutes excessive loss and, traditionally, if more than 500 mL is lost, postpartum hemorrhage is said to have occurred. Lack of clotting or clot formation indicates a coagulation defect. Puerperal inversion of the uterus is an obstetric emergency associated with hemorrhage and shock. Immediate recognition and prompt manual replacement will ensure a normal postpartum course.

If uterine atony develops, the fundus should be elevated and massaged to stimulate uterine contractions. Compression of the uterus with the hand placed on the abdomen and a fist in the vagina with anteflexion of the uterus may be necessary to control the bleeding. Methylergonovine (Methergine), 0.2 mg intramuscularly (or its equivalent), should be administered unless contraindicated (as in cardiac or hypertensive patients). Start an oxytocin (Pitocin, Syntocinon) intravenous drip of 10–20 U in 1 L of 5% dextrose in water, using a large-bore needle. If needed, blood transfusion should be given early before shock occurs. Prostaglandin $F_{2\alpha}$ ($PGF_{2\alpha}$), 0.25–1 mg injected directly into the myometrium, or 15-methyl prostaglandin $F_{2\alpha}$, 0.25 mg injected intramuscularly every 2 hours, is highly effective as a hemostatic agent in controlling postpartum hemorrhage. A 20-mg $PGE_2$ suppository placed in the posterior vaginal fornix can be used to treat persistent postpartum uterine atony. When the degree of postpartum bleeding is significant but not serious enough to warrant immediate exploration of the uterine cavity, ultrasonic evaluation may differentiate retained placental tissue and blood clots from an empty uterus. When bleeding cannot be controlled, the patient should be returned to the delivery room for inspection of the birth canal. It may be necessary to suture lacerations, remove placental fragments, pack the uterus, or perform bilateral internal iliac artery ligation or even hysterectomy to control hemorrhage.

An effective alternative approach to the control of pelvic hemorrhage consists of angiographic localization of the specific bleeding vessel and transcatheter embolization with Gelfoam fragments. The complications of labor and delivery that lead to postpartum hemorrhage and the specific management of these problems are discussed in Chapter 28.

**C. Postpartum Infections:** Febrile morbidity in the puerperium is defined as a temperature elevation of 38°C (100.4°F) or more occurring after the first 24 hours postpartum on 2 or more occasions that are not within the same 24 hours. The most frequent causes of fever in the postpartum period are infections of the genital tract, urinary tract, and breasts. Cesarean section delivery presents a much higher risk of postpartum infection and subsequent death or morbidity. The risk of death from cesarean section delivery is estimated to be 4 times greater than that from vaginal delivery. Prolonged labor, rupture of the membranes, and chorioamnionitis increase the risk of postpartum uterine infection.

Fever during the puerperium must be regarded as resulting from genital tract infection unless evidence to the contrary is found. The most common pathogens in puerperal infection are anaerobic nonhemolytic streptococci, coliform bacteria, *Bacteroides,* and staphylococci. Because of improved obstetric care, there has been a reduced incidence of beta-hemolytic streptococcal infection. Genital tract colonization with *Mycoplasma hominis* is detected in almost 40% of lower socioeconomic group patients and in about 20% of higher income patients. Peripartum tissue invasion by *M hominis* (as determined by antibody titer rise) is commonly associated with moderate fever and minimal or no physical findings in colonized women who lack protective antibody. Chlamydiae are associated with approximately 25% of the uterine infections that occur from 48 hours to 6 weeks postpartum among patients who deliver vaginally. Mycoplasmas are sensitive to tetracycline or lincomycin; chlamydiae are sensitive to tetracycline or erythromycin. A low-grade fever on the second or third postpartum day commonly results from retention of the lochia or a saprophytic infection of retained fragments of fetal membranes. There may be a delay in uterine involution, but the pulse rate generally remains normal. Resolution of the fever follows improved uterine drainage after the administration of oxytocic agents or removal of free placental fragments from the cervical os. Postpartum toxic shock syndrome should be considered in the presence of a macular rash and hypotension. Infection in uterine fibroids is unusual, but when it occurs it tends to be in the early puerperium. After delivery, the blood supply to fibroids is greatly diminished, and they tend to undergo ischemic degeneration.

**1. Endometritis–**The majority of patients with puerperal infection have endometritis. On the third postpartum day, the temperature often rises to 38.8–39.4°C (102–103°F) and remains elevated. Associated signs and symptoms are tachycardia, uterine tenderness, and malaise. The lochia is often profuse and has a foul odor. The infection may spread to the parametrium and pelvic peritoneum. Paralytic ileus may be an associated problem. In puerperal sepsis caused by group A or B beta-hemolytic *Streptococcus,* the lochia may be scanty and free of odor, but rapid lymphatic spread of the infection, bacteremia, and toxicity constitute a classic sequence. The most striking clinical signs include the onset of uterine tenderness and an abrupt temperature elevation to 38.8°C (102°F) or higher within the first 24 hours after delivery. Serious late complications of pelvic peritonitis include abscess formation, pelvic thrombophlebitis, disseminated intravascular coagulation, septic shock, and subsequent infertility.

Aseptic technique during labor and the early puerperium and the avoidance of trauma during delivery will reduce the incidence of puerperal infection. Multivariant analysis has identified cesarean delivery as the dominant overall predictor of puerperal endometritis (relative risk, 12.8) with bacterial vaginosis and high virulence organisms as the other significant predictors. Isolation precautions are appropriate. Intrauterine cultures and blood cultures should be obtained and treatment with broad-spectrum antibiotics instituted until more specific therapy can be selected on the basis of bacteriologic studies. Patients who do not respond to an initial antibiotic regimen of ampicillin and an aminoglycoside (kanamycin, gentamicin) or a cephalosporin should be reexamined for the presence of anaerobic organisms, eg, *Bacteroides.* Therapy with a broad-spectrum, single agent (cefoxitin, cefotaxime, cefoperazone, moxalactam, or piperacillin) has been demonstrated to be safe and effective for postcesarean endometritis. The most common combinations of drugs for treating anaerobes are an aminoglycoside and clindamycin, penicillin and chloramphenicol, and an aminoglycoside and metronidazole.

Treatment for postpartum endometritis or parametritis includes bed rest in the semi-Fowler position, hydration and intravenous fluids, decompression of the bowel, and maintenance of electrolyte balance.

**2. Urinary tract infections–**Urinary tract infections occur during the puerperium in about 5% of patients. Most are caused by coliform bacteria. Symptoms of acute cystitis usually develop on the first or second postpartum day, often following urinary retention, instrumentation, or trauma to the bladder. Operative delivery and vaginal or vulvar lacerations may interfere with normal micturition. Predisposing factors include prolonged labor, administration of a large volume of intravenous fluid, and conduction anesthesia. On the first postpartum day, 17% of patients have asymptomatic bacteriuria (> 100,000 colonies/mL). Spontaneous resolution of bacteriuria occurs in 75% of these women by the third postpartum day, the most appropriate time to obtain a clinically meaningful urine culture. A patient with bacteriuria during pregnancy is at higher risk of developing this complication than patients with negative urine cultures.

Upper urinary tract infection characteristically develops on the third or fourth postpartum day and is manifested by chills, spiking fever, costovertebral angle tenderness, and frequently nausea and vomiting. Diagnosis must be confirmed by urinalysis and a culture, colony count, and bacterial sensitivity study of an uncontaminated urine specimen. Treatment consists of a high fluid intake, good drainage of urine, and appropriate antibiotic therapy. If the patient does not improve, urinary tract obstruction should be suspected. All patients who have had a puerperal urinary tract infection should have urine cultures repeated at the 4- or 6-week postpartum visit.

## Other Medical Complications in the Puerperium

The patient with a preexisting medical or surgical illness that complicates pregnancy requires special attention during the puerperium. Women with pulmonary disease, especially those with an obstructive component, are at increased risk of developing atelectasis and pneumonia, partly as a result of impaired diaphragmatic motion after delivery. Careful attention to pulmonary toilet and avoidance of both heavy sedation and dehydration will reduce the incidence of pulmonary complications.

Before optimal management of pregnant cardiac patients became available, most maternal cardiac deaths occurred postpartum. After the stress of labor and delivery, patients with severe mitral stenosis may develop pulmonary edema in the immediate or early puerperium, when there are significant shifts in extracellular and intravascular fluid volumes. In patients with rheumatic heart disease, cardiac and extracardiac factors such as ectopic beats, tachycardia, upper respiratory infection, emotional upset, and anemia can so affect the patient's condition in the span of 24 hours as to precipitate congestive heart failure. Factors predisposing to the development of thrombophlebitis or pulmonary embolism pose additional hazards to the cardiac patient during the puerperium.

Routine antibiotic prophylaxis against endocarditis is not necessary at normal delivery but is probably indicated after abortion, cesarean section, or manual removal of the placenta.

The immediate and early puerperium are especially hazardous for the patient with cyanotic congenital heart disease and pulmonary hypertension (eg, Eisenmenger's syndrome). Systemic hypotension and metabolic and respiratory acidosis may lead to exaggeration of a right-to-left shunt or to reversal of a left-to-right shunt. Death characteristically occurs during labor or within the first 10 days postpartum. Deterioration is characterized by increasing cyanosis and decreasing cardiovascular function. Treatment must concentrate on the prevention of contributing factors such as blood loss, hypoxemia, pulmonary irritants, venous pooling, spinal anesthesia, and sepsis.

It is pertinent to emphasize here that the interaction of other medical illnesses with pregnancy and the puerperium is not entirely predictable. Papular and herpetiform eruptions and idiopathic jaundice precipitated by pregnancy characteristically improve after the first week postpartum. On the other hand, aggravation of the following conditions may occur during the puerperium: myasthenia gravis, sarcoidosis, ulcerative colitis, rheumatoid arthritis, and the collagen diseases. In asthma and allergic manifestations, the pattern observed during pregnancy tends to reverse itself during the puerperium. These observations provide the basis for the clinical impression that a state of relative hypoadrenocorticism exists in the early puerperium. Corticosteroid therapy initiated during pregnancy for the management of collagen disorders should be continued and the dosage probably increased during the puerperium to reduce the hazards of exacerbations. Treated hypoparathyroid patients should be carefully followed during the immediate puerperium because hypercalcemia may occur.

A relatively high incidence of thyroid dysfunction occurs in the postpartum interval. Approximately 6% of women have transient thyrotoxicosis or hypothyroidism after delivery. Most of these women have thyroid microsomal autoantibodies; this supports the hypothesis that postpartum thyroid dysfunction is induced by aggravation of preexisting subclinical autoimmune thyroiditis. Immunologic regulation may be altered after delivery, causing proliferation of immunocompetent cell clones directed against thyroid antigens. The thyrotoxic phase is probably caused by cytotoxic destruction of thyroid cells and leakage of thyroid hormones into the circulation. The hypothyroidism is considered transient, but nearly 50% of women with silent postpartum hypothyroidism have laboratory evidence of chronic thyroid hypofunction at follow-up. Postpartum thyroiditis should be suspected in any woman who presents with fatigue, palpitations, emotional lability, or thyroid enlargement during the first year after delivery. The diagnosis is usually not made at the time of the postpartum visit because most cases have their onset later.

**A. Postpartum Cardiomyopathy:** Postpartum cardiomyopathy, a disorder of the heart muscle, presents clinically with the onset of cardiac failure. The cause is unknown. This serious, even critical, complication is seen most commonly in older multiparous women without evidence of prior heart disease and in women who have had preeclampsia-eclampsia or a multiple pregnancy, but the syndrome can follow stillbirths and even early abortions. Pathologic findings include focal degeneration and fibrosis of muscle fibers, with mural thrombi but without coronary artery disease. Catheter studies have demonstrated low-output cardiac failure with dilated, poorly contracting ventricles, pulmonary and systemic hypertension, and absence of significant pericardial effusions. Most patients with postpartum cardiomyopathy develop this disorder in the first month postpartum, but it may occur as late as 3–5 months postpartum. In about 7% of reported cases, onset of the disorder has been noted in the last month of pregnancy. Postpartum cardiomyopathy should be considered in the differential diagnosis of a patient without preexisting evidence of heart disease who develops moderate respiratory distress and chest pain with signs of left heart failure postpartum. A holosystolic murmur indicating mitral insufficiency and evidence of cardiomegaly on chest x-ray should aid in excluding other causes of these symptoms.

Patients with postpartum cardiomyopathy respond to digitalis and the conventional management of pulmonary edema. Anticoagulation is recommended to minimize pulmonary and systemic emboli. Extended bed rest accelerates the rate of recovery. Patients whose heart size returns to normal within 6 months have a good prognosis and may resume their normal activity. Historically, repeat pregnancy has been discouraged, but recent prospective echocardiography studies indicate that patients whose left ventricular function has returned to normal may undertake subsequent pregnancy with a low risk of recurrent left ventricular dysfunction.

**B. Postpartum Hemolytic Uremia:** The syndrome of postpartum hemolytic uremia has been recently described. Renal failure due to intrarenal intravascular coagulation is associated with a microangiopathic hemolytic anemia. Most of the patients have an uncomplicated pregnancy and delivery, but in a few instances there has been a mild preexisting preeclampsia. A brief influenza-like illness has also been described. Cases of postpartum hemolytic uremia differ from other cases of this disorder in that the patient is reasonably well for a period of 1–10 weeks following childbirth before renal failure becomes apparent. The pathogenesis is obscure, but the condition may be similar to thrombotic thrombocytopenic purpura. It is hypothesized that an antecedent infection triggers either the generalized Shwartzman reaction or the formation of an antigen-antibody complex that circulates and produces immune complex glomerulonephritis and subsequent intravascular coagulation.

The patient may present with nausea, vomiting, dyspnea, cyanosis, a bleeding tendency, oliguria or anuria, convulsions, and abdominal and back pain. Prompt diagnosis is essential if treatment is to be successful. Helpful laboratory studies include tests for intravascular coagulation and fibrinogen degradation products. Intravenous heparin (approximately 20,000 U/day with appropriate controls) should be instituted, although heparin therapy is not uniformly successful. Although the cause of hemolytic-uremic syndrome remains undetermined, some cases are associated with a marked decrease in plasma antithrombin III levels. Since heparin increases the turnover rate of antithrombin, the administration of heparin to antithrombin III-deficient patients may therefore paradoxically increase the risk of thrombosis.

Common supportive measures include digitalis, transfusion, and drug therapy for hypertension, hyperkalemia, and hyperuricemia. Immunosuppressive therapy is ineffective and potentially harmful. Dipyridamole is advocated in combination with aspirin or prostacyclin infusion as in other disorders involving rapid platelet destruction. Plasma exchange (plasmapheresis with plasma infusions) may be dramatically beneficial. Renal biopsy should be postponed because of the danger of hemorrhage at the biopsy site. Despite treatment of this disorder with hemodialysis, the prognosis is poor.

**C. Postpartum Eclampsia:** Eclampsia occurs before labor in about 25% of reported cases, during labor in approximately 50%, and postpartum in the remaining 25%. The onset of postpartum convulsions usually occurs near delivery; the risk declines progressively with each 12-hour postpartum period. After 48 hours, the disorder is rare but can occur up to 14 days postpartum (late postpartum eclampsia). It has been postulated that retained placental fragments play a role in some patients with late postpartum convulsions and that these patients require curettage for management. Eclamptic patients must be differentiated from those with any of the following conditions: epilepsy; metabolic, infectious, or hypertensive diseases; space-occupying central nervous system lesions; and cerebrovascular accidents. Some patients with late postpartum eclampsia do not manifest any signs or symptoms of preeclampsia in the antenatal or intrapartum periods and thus are not treated prophylactically. Other patients develop late postpartum seizures in spite of intrapartum and early postpartum magnesium sulfate therapy (see Chapter 19). At present, it is difficult to identify those patients who need prolonged therapy.

**D. Postpartum Psychosis:** Controversy exists as to whether or not postpartum psychosis is a specific entity distinct from other major diagnostic categories of mental illness (see also Chapter 60). The onset of psychiatric symptoms soon after delivery may be acute and dramatic. The postpartum reaction syndrome includes a spectrum of psychiatric disorders (schizophrenia, manic-depressive psychosis, psychoneuroses, and depression). Affective disorders are by far the most common. Early symptoms include withdrawal, paranoia, and refusal to eat. Depression may soon alternate with manic behavior. During these mood swings, patients may harm themselves or their infants. Nonetheless, mothers should be kept in contact with their babies whenever possible. Childbirth with its attendant stress is seen as the precipitating event that leads to the exacerbation of an underlying or latent disorder. The woman who feels unloved, is involved in a discordant marital relationship, or did not want the baby is at a higher risk for postpartum depression. Emotional support and physical assistance from family, friends, and medical personnel during pregnancy, delivery, and the puerperium are important preventive measures. Psychotherapy holds a prominent place in management.

The usual drugs and supportive treatment appropriate to the patient's disorder should be given—phenothiazines for schizophrenia, mood-elevating drugs and other appropriate therapy for depression, and sedatives for manic states. Vitamin $B_6$ supplementation has no place in the prevention or treatment of postpartum depression. Rarely, patients with puerperal psychosis associated with folic acid deficiency will respond to appropriate therapy. The prospect of recovery from postpartum mental illness is good, although in some studies, recurrence after subsequent pregnancy and delivery has been 10–20%.

### Surgical Complications

Surgical problems during the puerperium mainly concern complications of labor and delivery such as hemorrhage, wound infections and dehiscence, uterine rupture and inversion, urinary tract injuries, and thrombophlebitis (see Chapter 28). Surgical complications are more common with cesarean section or operative delivery. Postpartum surgical problems may also follow adjunctive surgery such as sterilization procedures performed at delivery or soon thereafter. Certainly, the increased vascularity and edema of pelvic tissues predispose to a higher incidence of postoperative bleeding from ligated vascular pedicles.

The mild adynamic ileus commonly seen after labor and delivery predisposes to gastrointestinal complications in the puerperium. Dramatic distention of the cecum and colon may follow cesarean section. Mechanical obstruction must be ruled out if bowel problems do not respond to nasogastric tube decompression.

Appendicitis may occur less frequently postpartum than during pregnancy. Torsion of the spleen or rupture of a splenic aneurysm, or ovarian artery aneurysm, although rare, do occur in the puerperium. Cholecystectomy, not usually recommended during pregnancy, may be required in the puerperium for serious gallbladder disease. The acute surgical abdomen is particularly dangerous in the early puerperium because there is a tendency to attribute symptoms such as pain and vomiting to the recent delivery and the stretched abdominal muscles do not respond normally to peritoneal irritation.

Management of venous thrombosis and thrombophlebitis is discussed in Chapters 22 and 59. Pregnancy and the puerperium may predispose to ovarian and cerebral venous thrombosis and Budd-Chiari syndrome (hepatic vein thrombosis), but this is rare.

## CONDUCT OF THE PUERPERIUM

All patients will benefit from 3–5 days of hospitalization after delivery. Increasing hospital costs and a trend toward earlier discharge have reduced the duration of the traditional lying-in period. Most women can now return home safely 3 days after normal vaginal delivery if proper instructions are given. Earlier discharge may be unwise, especially for the unselected primiparous patient. Selected mothers and infants who have had uncomplicated labors and deliveries may be discharged safely 24 hours postpartum if discharge criteria are met and follow-up care is provided. Optimal care includes daily visits by a perinatal nurse practitioner through the fourth postpartum day.

### Emotional Reactions

Several basic emotional responses occur in almost every woman who has given birth to a normal baby. A woman's first emotion is usually one of extreme relief followed by a sense of happiness and gratitude that the new baby has arrived safely. A regular pattern of behavior occurs in the human mother immediately after birth of the infant. Touching, holding, and grooming of the infant under normal conditions rapidly strengthen maternal ties of affection. However, not all mothers react in this way, and some may even feel detached from the new baby. Such feelings are usually temporary and should not give rise to anxiety. In the first few days after delivery, the mother may experience feelings of inadequacy and depression, commonly referred to as postpartum blues. The "blues" occur most frequently between the third and tenth postpartum days. The symptoms vary in their intensity but include feelings of anxiety, tearfulness, mood swings, forgetfulness, and difficulty in concentration. The blues are self-limiting, but the distress can be diminished by physical comfort and reassurance. Evidence suggests that rooming-in during the hospital stay reduces maternal anxiety and results in more successful breastfeeding.

Prematurity or illness of the newborn delays early

intimate maternal-infant contact and may have an adverse effect on the rapid and complete development of normal mothering responses. Stressful factors during the puerperium (eg, marital infidelity or loss of friends as a result of the necessary confinement and preoccupation with the new baby) may leave the mother feeling unsupported and may interfere with the formation of a maternal bond with the infant.

When a baby dies or is born with a congenital defect, the obstetrician should tell the mother and father about the problem together, if possible. The baby's normal healthy features and potential for improvement should be emphasized, and positive statements should be made about the present availability of corrective treatment and the promises of ongoing research. In the event of a perinatal loss, parents should be assisted in the grieving process. They should be encouraged to see and touch the baby at birth or later, even if maceration or anomalies are present. Mementos such as footprints, locks of hair, or a photograph can be a solace to the parents after the infant has been buried. During the puerperium, the obstetrician has an important opportunity to help the mother whose infant has died work through her period of mourning or discouragement and to assess abnormal reactions of grief that suggest a need for psychiatric assistance. Pathologic grief is characterized by the inability to work through the sense of loss within 3–4 months, with subsequent feelings of low self-esteem.

## Ambulation & Rest

The policy of early ambulation after delivery benefits the patient. Early ambulation provides a sense of well-being, hastens involution of the uterus, improves uterine drainage, and lessens the incidence of postpartum thrombophlebitis. After the second postpartum day, the patient may be out of bed as desired, but early ambulation does not mean return to normal activity or work. Rest is essential after delivery, and the demands on the mother should be limited to allow for adequate relaxation and adjustment to her new responsibilities. It is helpful to set aside a few hours each day for rest periods. Many mothers do not sleep well for several nights after delivery, and it is surprising how the day is occupied with the care of the newborn. Sedatives such as secobarbital, 100 mg orally, or flurazepam (Dalmane), 30 mg orally, at bedtime as necessary, generally ensure a good night's rest.

## Diet

A regular diet is permissible as soon as the patient regains her appetite and is free from the effects of analgesics and anesthetics. Protein foods, fruits, vegetables, milk products, and a high fluid intake are recommended, especially for nursing mothers. However, even lactating women probably require no more than 2600–2800 kcal/day. It may be advisable to continue the daily vitamin-mineral supplement during the early puerperium.

## Care of the Bladder

Most women empty the bladder during labor or have been catheterized at delivery. Even so, serious bladder distention may develop within 12 hours. A long and difficult labor or a forceps delivery may traumatize the base of the bladder and interfere with normal voiding. In some cases, overdistention of the bladder may be related to pain or spinal anesthesia. The marked polyuria noted for the first few days postpartum causes the bladder to fill in a relatively short time. Hence, obstetric patients require catheterization more frequently than most surgical patients. The patient should be catheterized every 6 hours after delivery if she is unable to void or empty her bladder completely. Intermittent catheterization is preferable to an indwelling catheter because the incidence of urinary tract infection is lower. However, if the bladder fills to more than 1000 mL, at least 2 days of decompression by a retention catheter is usually required to establish voiding without significant residual urine. If the catheter is left in the bladder for more than 12 hours, bacteriuria is likely. Prophylaxis may include urinary acidifying agents, but urine cultures are necessary to ascertain the nature of the invading organism.

Therapy should be instituted with ampicillin, amoxicillin, cephalexin, nitrofurantoin, or another appropriate antibiotic. The incidence of true asymptomatic bacteriuria is approximately 5% in the early puerperium. Postpartum patients with a history of previous urinary tract infection, conduction anesthesia, and catheterization during delivery and operative delivery, should have a bacterial culture of a midstream urine specimen. In cases of confirmed bacteriuria, antibiotic treatment should be given; otherwise bacteriuria will persist in nearly 30% of patients. Three days of therapy are sufficient and this therapy avoids prolonged antibiotic exposure to the lactating mother.

## Bowel Function

Pregnancy itself is associated with increased gastric emptying but gastrointestinal motility is commonly delayed after labor and delivery. The mild ileus that follows delivery, together with perineal discomfort and postpartum fluid loss by other routes, predisposes to constipation during the puerperium. Obstruction of the colon by a retroverted uterus is a rare complication during the puerperium. If an enema was given before delivery, the patient is unlikely to have a bowel movement for 1–2 days after childbirth. Milk of magnesia, 15–20 mL orally on the evening of the second postpartum day, usually stimulates a bowel movement by the next morning. If not, a rectal suppository such as bisacodyl or a small tap water or oil retention enema may be given. Less bowel stimulation will be needed if the diet contains sufficient roughage. Stool softeners such as dioctyl sodium sulfosuccinate may ease the discomfort of early bowel movements. Hemorrhoidal discomfort is a common complaint postpartum and usually responds to conservative treatment with suppositories and sitz baths. It is rarely necessary to treat hemorrhoids surgically postpartum unless thrombosis is extensive.

Laxatives, enemas, and a diet with ample roughage are contraindicated in the early puerperium in the patient who has had suture repair of severe childbirth lacerations. Phenolphthalein, senna, and jalap laxatives should not be used if the patient is nursing, because slight contamination of breast milk may occur.

### Bathing

As soon as the patient is ambulatory, she may take a shower. Sitz or tub baths after the second postpartum day are probably safe if the tub is clean, because bath water will not gain access to the vagina unless it is directly introduced. Most patients prefer showers to tub baths because of the profuse flow of lochia immediately postpartum. Vaginal douching is contraindicated in the early puerperium.

### Care of the Episiotomy

Postpartum perineal pain symptoms are related to the duration of the second stage of labor even when an episiotomy is not used.

Immediately after delivery, cold compresses (usually ice) applied to the perineum decrease traumatic edema and discomfort. The perineal area should be gently cleansed with plain soap at least once or twice a day and after voiding or defecation. If the pudendum is kept clean, healing should occur rapidly. Dry heat applied to the perineum with an infrared lamp for 20 minutes 3 times daily should relieve local discomfort and promote healing. Some obstetricians recommend cool sitz baths for relief of perineal pain. Episiotomy pain is easily controlled by simple analgesics. The use of sanitary napkins should be avoided during the first day after delivery. Ointments and anesthetic solutions have little value.

The episiotomy or repaired pudendal lacerations should be inspected daily. A vaginal or rectal examination should be performed only if a hematoma or infection seems likely and, if so, aseptic technique should be used. Episiotomy wounds rarely become infected, which is remarkable when one considers the difficulty of avoiding contamination of the perineal area. In the event of sepsis, local heat and irrigation should cause the infection to subside. Appropriate antibiotics may be indicated if an immediate response to these measures is not observed. In rare instances, the wound should be opened widely and sutures removed for adequate drainage.

Necrotizing fasciitis is a rare but serious complication of episiotomy incision extension caused by anaerobic bacteria. When the wound has been cleaned, secondary closure may be attempted, even though only a minority of such closures heal well. Perineorrhaphy may be required several weeks later if there has been considerable distortion of the normal tissue relationships.

### Oxytocic Agents

Administration of oxytocic agents beyond the immediate puerperium should be limited to patients who have specific indications such as postpartum hemorrhage or endometritis. The routine use of ergot preparations such as methylergonovine maleate (Methergine), 0.2 mg orally every 6 hours for extended periods of time, is of questionable value in hastening uterine involution. Potential disadvantages include interference with normal lactation as a result of inhibition of prolactin release and the possibility of ergot poisoning if prolonged therapy is permitted.

### Postpartum Immunization

**A. Prevention of Rh Isoimmunization:** The postpartum injection of $Rh_o$ (D) immunoglobulin* will prevent sensitization in the Rh-negative woman who has had a fetal-to-maternal transfusion of Rh-positive fetal red cells. The risk of maternal sensitization rises with the volume of fetal transplacental hemorrhage. The usual amount of fetal blood that enters the maternal circulation is less than 0.5 mL. The usual dose of 300 $\mu$g of $Rh_o$ (D) immunoglobulin is in excess of the dose generally required, because 25 $\mu$g of RhoGAM per milliliter of fetal red cells is sufficient to prevent maternal immunization. If neonatal anemia or other clinical symptoms suggest that a large transplacental hemorrhage has occurred, the amount of fetal blood in the maternal circulation can be estimated by the Kleihauer-Betke smear, and the amounts of RhoGAM to be administered can be adjusted accordingly. An alternative to the acid-elution smear is the Du test, which will detect 20 mL or more of Rh-positive fetal blood in the maternal circulation.

$Rh_o$ (D) immunoglobulin is administered after abortion without qualifications or after delivery to women who meet all of the following criteria: (1) The mother must be $Rh_o$ (D)-negative without Rh antibodies; (2) the baby must be $Rh_o$ (D) or Du-positive; and (3) the cord blood must be Coombs-negative. If these criteria are met, a 1:1000 dilution of $Rh_o$ (D) immunoglobulin is cross-matched to the mother's red cells to ensure compatibility, and 1 mL (300 $\mu$g) is given intramuscularly to the mother within 72 hours after delivery. If the 72-hour interval has been exceeded, it is advisable to give the globulin rather than withhold it, for it may still protect against sensitization. $Rh_o$ (D) immunoglobulin should also be given after delivery or abortion when serologic tests of maternal sensitization to the Rh factor are questionable. ***Caution:*** Do not inject the infant. Do not give intravenously.

The average risk of maternal sensitization after

---

*Trade names include Gamulin Rh, $HypRh_o$-D, and $Rh_o$GAM.

abortion is approximately half the risk incurred by full-term pregnancy and delivery; the latter has been estimated at 11%. Even though mothers have received $Rh_o$ (D) immunoglobulin, they should be screened with each subsequent pregnancy, since occasional failures are related to inadequate $Rh_o$ (D) immunoglobulin administration postpartum or an undetected very low titer in the previous pregnancy.

**B. Rubella Vaccination:** A significant number of women of childbearing age have never had rubella. When tested by the hemagglutination inhibition method, 10–20% of women are seronegative (titer of 1:8 or less). Women who are susceptible to rubella can be vaccinated safely and effectively with a live attenuated rubella virus vaccine (RA 27/3 strain) during the immediate puerperium. Seroconversion occurs in approximately 90% of women vaccinated postpartum. The puerperium is an ideal time for vaccination because there is no risk of inadvertently vaccinating a pregnant woman. Although there have been no reports of human fetal malformations due to vaccine virus, the theoretic possibility of teratogenicity exists. Nursing mothers need not be excluded from immunization. There is concern, however, about recent evidence that 75% of such women shed rubella virus in the breast milk, and persistent rubella carrier state with periodic viral reactivation may rarely occur in the child. The neonate's exposure to the virus in breast milk is not associated with an alteration of responses to subsequent immunization.

Vaccinated patients should be informed that transient side effects (arthralgia or rash) are common and that contraception for 2 months postpartum is mandatory. Among adult women there is a 10–15% incidence of acute polyarthritis following immunization. Since $Rh_o$ (D) immunoglobulin may contain rubella antibodies, there has been some concern that these may prevent successful vaccination against rubella. However, it has been shown that the serologic response to rubella vaccination in the puerperium was satisfactory even when anti-D immunoglobulin was given shortly before vaccination. On the other hand, it has been shown that a blood transfusion can prevent successful rubella vaccination if it is performed soon after the transfusion.

## Discharge Examination & Instructions

Before the patient's hospital discharge, the breasts and abdomen should be examined. The degree of uterine involution and tenderness should be noted. The calves and thighs should be palpated to rule out thrombophlebitis. The characteristics of the lochia are important and should be observed. The episiotomy wound should be inspected to see whether the sutures are healing satisfactorily. A blood sample should be obtained for hematocrit or hemoglobin determination. Unless the patient has an unusual pelvic complaint, there is little need to perform a vaginal ex-

amination. Occasionally, a sponge may be left in the vagina at delivery, but with proper technique this should not occur. The obstetrician should be certain that the patient has had a bowel movement, is voiding normally, and is physically able to assume her new responsibilities at home.

The patient will require some advice on what she is allowed to do when she arrives home. Hygiene is essentially the same as practiced in the hospital, with a premium on cleanliness. Upon discharge from the hospital, the patient should be instructed to rest for at least 2 hours during the day, and her usual household activities should be curtailed. She should not take over her full household duties for at least 3 weeks; thereafter, most normal activities can be resumed. She may climb up and down stairs, but walking or riding outdoors should be minimized during the first 2 weeks. She should avoid carrying heavy packages or doing taxing household chores for about 3–4 weeks after delivery. It is inadvisable for the patient to return to work until 5–6 weeks after delivery. Generally, sports and athletic activities may be resumed after the postpartum evaluation (see next section).

Various forms of social support are critical for mothers, especially those employed outside the home: available, high-quality day care; parental leave for both mothers and fathers; and support provided by the workplace such as flexible hours, opportunity to breastfeed, on-site day care, and care for sick children. The patient who has had frequent prenatal visits to her obstetrician may feel cut off from the doctor during the interval between discharge and the first postpartum visit. She will feel reassured in this period of time if she receives thoughtful advice on what she is allowed to do and what she can expect when she arrives home. She should be instructed to take her temperature at home twice daily and to notify the physician or nurse in the event of fever, vaginal bleeding, or back pain. At the time of discharge, the patient should be informed that she will note persistent but decreasing amounts of vaginal lochia for about 3 weeks and possibly a small period during the fourth or fifth week after delivery. A consultation with the pediatrician before the first postpartum visit with the obstetrician will be helpful.

## Postpartum Exercises

Exercises to strengthen the muscles of the back, pelvic floor, and abdomen are advocated, but strenuous exercises should be postponed until approximately 3 weeks after delivery. This allows the abdominal muscles to partially regain their original length and tone and prevents undue patient fatigue. The recommended forms of postpartum exercises are illustrated in Figure 12–8. The patient should begin with a single exercise performed 5 times and repeated several times daily. On subsequent days, additional exercises are added sequentially. Strengthening of the

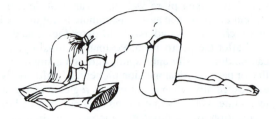

Rest on the elbows and knees, keeping the upper arms and legs perpendicular to the body. Hump the back upward. Contract the buttocks and draw the abdomen in vigorously. Relax, breathe deeply.

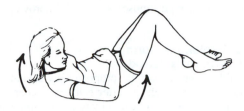

Lie flat on the back with the knees and hips flexed. Tilt the pelvis inward and contract the buttocks tightly. Lift the head while contracting the abdominal muscles.

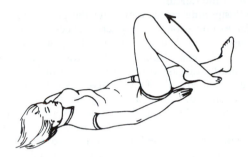

Slowly flex the knee and then the thigh on the abdomen. Lower the foot to the buttock. Straighten and lower the leg to the floor.

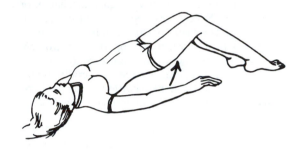

Lie flat on the back with the arms at the sides. Draw the knees up slightly. Arch the back.

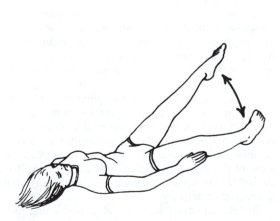

Raise first the right and then the left leg as high as possible. Keep the toes pointed and the knee straight. Lower the leg gradually, using the abdominal muscles but not the hands.

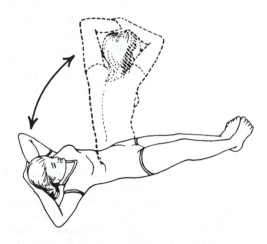

Lie flat on the back with the arms clasped behind the head. Then sit up slowly. (If necessary, hook feet under furniture.) Slowly lie back.

**Figure 12–8.** Recommended postpartum exercises. Exercises to strengthen the muscles of the back, pelvic floor, and abdomen are advocated but should be postponed for approximately 3 weeks after delivery. This allows the abdominal muscles to partially regain their original length and tone and prevents undue patient fatigue. The patient should begin with a single exercise that is performed 5 times and repeated twice daily. On subsequent days, additional exercises are added sequentially. Strengthening of the back and abdominal muscles will correct lordosis and the diastasis of the rectus muscles and will improve posture.

back and abdominal muscles will correct lordosis and diastasis of the rectus muscles and will improve posture.

## Sexual Relations During the Postpartum Period

Establishment of normal prepregnancy sexual response patterns is delayed after delivery. According to Masters and Johnson, genital vasocongestion, vaginal lubrication and distention, and orgasmic intensity are reduced for 6–8 weeks postpartum. At 12 weeks, sexual response patterns return to the prepregnant state. There is considerable variation in sexual interest during the puerperium. Most women report low or absent sexual desire during the early puerperium and ascribe this to fatigue, weakness, pain on intromission, irritative vaginal discharge, or fear of injury. Nearly 50% report a return of sexual desire within 2–3 weeks postpartum. In spite of minimal desire in a substantial proportion of women, nearly all resume sexual intercourse by 6–8 weeks after delivery. Lactating women generally report higher sexual interest than do bottle-feeding mothers. Postpartum vaginal atrophy may interfere with satisfactory coitus.

Sexual counseling is indicated before the mother is discharged from the hospital. A discussion of the normal fluctuations of sexual interest during the puerperium is appropriate, as are suggestions for noncoital sexual options that enhance the expression of mutual pleasure and affection. The importance of sleep and rest and of the husband's emotional and physical support is emphasized. If milk ejection during sexual relations is a concern, nursing the baby prior to sexual intimacy can help. Sexual relations can generally be resumed by the third week postpartum, if desired. A water-soluble lubricant or vaginal estrogen cream is especially helpful in lactating amenorrheic mothers in whom vaginal atrophy occurs, usually because of low circulating estrogen levels.

## Contraception & Sterilization

The immediate puerperium has long been recognized as a convenient time for the performance of tubal ligation. If the sterilization procedure is not performed within 3 days postpartum, the risk of infection may be increased and the advantage of easy access to the tubes via minilaparotomy is diminished. Parous women should be informed of the availability of postpartum sterilization during their prenatal visits. Despite the increasing success rate of microsurgical tubal reanastomosis, the permanence of tubal ligation should be emphasized. Sterilization is not recommended in young women of low parity, at emergency cesarean section or when the outcome of the pregnancy is in doubt and survival of the infant is not assured. Appropriate counseling regarding risks of failure, permanency of the procedure, medical risks, and potential psychosocial reactions to the procedure shall have taken place well in advance of delivery. Patient ambivalence at the last minute is not unusual, in which case it is advisable to defer the procedure until after the puerperium. Postpartum tubal ligation can be done easily and rapidly through a small midline or periumbilical incision immediately after delivery (especially when a continuous regional analgesic technique is already in use) and does not prolong hospitalization or significantly increase morbidity. A major anesthetic should be initiated only after careful evaluation by the anesthesia service, since the parturient may have an increased risk of regurgitation and aspiration of gastric contents. Laparoscopic sterilization is not advisable in the immediate puerperium, because of increased pelvic vascularity and the large size of the fundus.

Postponing coitus until after the postpartum visit and examination is considered excessive by most couples, but abstinence should be practiced for at least 2–3 weeks. Nonetheless, contraceptive methods should be discussed prior to hospital discharge and the patient advised of the relative risks of conception, depending on whether she is nursing or not (see Chapter 33). During lactational amenorrhea, the pregnancy rate is approximately 8%; however, once menstruation has resumed, the rate rises to 36% despite continued lactation. The earliest reported time of ovulation as determined by endometrial biopsy is 33 days postpartum in nonlactating women and 49 days in lactating women. Contraceptive advice should take into account the possibility that conception may occur as early as the second or third week after abortion or ectopic pregnancy.

The use of vaginal foam, a condom, or both may be prescribed until the postpartum examination. Fitting of a diaphragm is not practical until involution of the reproductive organs has taken place. Many obstetricians avoid the use of oral contraceptives in the immediate puerperium in the nonlactating woman to allow time for the hypothalamic-pituitary axis to recover from the prolonged suppression of pregnancy. However, no firm data exist showing that immediate postpartum institution of oral contraceptives leads to an increased incidence of postpill amenorrhea. In view of the hypercoagulable state postpartum, it is advisable to postpone oral contraceptive therapy until 2 weeks after delivery.

The intramuscular injection of a long-acting progestin such as medroxyprogesterone acetate (Depo-Provera), 50–200 mg, provides effective contraception for the lactating woman for a 3- to 6-month period without provoking maternal thromboembolism or decreasing milk yield. However, questions relating to prolonged amenorrhea or the inconvenience of irregular bleeding limit the usefulness of this method. Even low-dose combined oral contraceptives (containing 30 μg of estrogen) have small but definite negative effects on milk yield and infant growth during the first few postpartum months. The extent of mammary transfer of ethinyl estradiol is small. After the daily administration of 50 μg of ethinyl estradiol to the mother, the concentration in milk is below the practical detection limit of the radioimmunoassay (15 pg/mL). It has been estimated that the baby ingesting about 600 mL of milk per day would receive about 0.02% of the estrogen dose to the mother. A combination pill containing 20 μg of ethinyl estradiol and 1 mg of norethindrone acetate (Loestrin) or one with 0.35 mg of norethindrone (Micronor) may be useful in this instance.

Insertion of an intrauterine device immediately after placental delivery has been advocated in some clinics as a means of providing birth control to a large number of women in lower socioeconomic groups who may not return to the hospital postpartum. Although this practice appears to be safe, the cumulative rates for pregnancy, expulsion (10–20%), and removal because of side effects are higher than after interval insertion. The immediate puerperium is not the optimal time for insertion of an intrauterine device if the patient will return for a postpartum visit. The risk of uterine perforation during IUD insertion is higher in lactating women, probably because of the accelerated rate of uterine involution.

## Postpartum Examination

At the postpartum visit—4–6 weeks after discharge from hospital—the patient's weight and blood pressure should be recorded. Most patients retain about 60% of any weight in excess of 11 kg (24 lb) that was gained during pregnancy. A suitable diet may be prescribed if the patient has not returned to her approximate prepregnant weight. If the patient was anemic upon discharge from the hospital or has been bleeding during the puerperium, a complete blood count should be determined. Persistence of uterine bleeding demands investigation and definitive treatment.

The breasts should be examined, and the adequacy of support, abnormalities of the nipples or lactation, and the presence of any masses should be noted. The patient should be instructed concerning self-examination of the breasts. A complete rectovaginal evaluation is required.

Profuse vaginal discharge is usually not present at 4–6 weeks postpartum unless there is an associated vaginitis, which will generally respond to specific treatment. Nursing mothers may show a hypoestrogenic condition of the vaginal epithelium. Prescription of a vaginal estrogen cream to be applied at bedtime should relieve local dryness and coital discomfort without the side effects of systemic estrogen therapy. The cervix should be inspected and a Papanicolaou (Pap) smear obtained. Women whose prenatal smears are normal are still at risk for an abnormal Pap smear at their postpartum visit. When minimal cervicitis or eversion is present, mild acetic acid douches or application of an antibiotic vaginal cream (eg, 2% cleocin gel) may be all that is necessary. If there is persistent eversion of the squamocolumnar junction, the patient should return for treatment by cervical cauterization or cryotherapy.

The episiotomy incision and repaired lacerations must be examined and the adequacy of pelvic and perineal support noted. Bimanual examination of the uterus and adnexa is indicated. At the time of the postpartum examination, most patients have some degree of retrodisplacement of the uterus, but this may soon correct itself.

Asymptomatic retroposition of the uterus is not regarded as an abnormal condition. If pain, abnormal bleeding, or other symptoms are present, a vaginal pessary may be inserted as a trial procedure to encourage anteversion of the fundus. However, pessary support for long periods of time is not recommended. In the absence of pelvic disease, uterine retrodisplacement rarely if ever requires surgical correction. If marked uterine descensus is noted or if the patient develops stress incontinence, symptomatic cystocele, or rectocele, surgical correction should be considered. Hysterectomy or vaginal repair is best postponed for at least 3 months after delivery to allow maximal restoration of the pelvic supporting structures.

The patient may resume full activity or employment if her course to this point has been uneventful. Once again, the patient should be advised regarding family planning and contraceptive practices. The postnatal visit is an important opportunity to consider general disorders such as backache and depression and to discuss infant feeding and immunization. A further gynecologic and cytologic examination is desirable about 6 months after delivery. The rapport established between the obstetrician and the patient during the prenatal and postpartum periods provides a unique opportunity to establish a preventive health program in subsequent years.

# LACTATION PHYSIOLOGY

## PHYSIOLOGY

The mammary glands are modified exocrine glands that undergo dramatic anatomic and physiologic changes during pregnancy and in the immediate puerperium. Their role is to provide nourishment for the newborn and to transfer antibodies from mother to infant.

During the first half of pregnancy, proliferation of alveolar epithelial cells, formation of new ducts, and development of lobular architecture occur. Later in pregnancy, proliferation declines, and the epithelium differentiates for secretory activity. At the end of gestation, each breast will have gained approximately 400 g. Factors contributing to increase in mammary size include hypertrophy of blood vessels, myoepithelial cells, and connective tissue; deposition of fat; and retention of water and electrolytes. Blood flow is almost double that of the nonpregnant state.

The mammary gland has been called the mirror of the endocrine system, because lactation depends on a delicate balance of several hormones. An intact hypothalamic-pituitary axis is essential to the initiation and maintenance of lactation. Lactation can be divided into 3 stages: (1) mammogenesis, or mammary growth and development; (2) lactogenesis, or initiation of milk secretion; and (3) galactopoiesis, or maintenance of established milk secretion (Table 12–2). Estrogen is responsible for the growth of ductular tissue and alveolar budding, whereas progesterone is required for optimal maturation of the alveolar glands. Glandular stem cells undergo differentiation into secretory and myoepithelial cells under the influence of prolactin, growth hormone, insulin, cortisol, and an epithelial growth factor. Although alveolar secretory cells actively synthesize milk fat and proteins from midpregnancy onward, only small amounts are released into the lumen. However, lactation is possible if pregnancy is interrupted during the second trimester.

Prolactin is an obligatory hormone for milk production, but lactogenesis also requires a low estrogen environment. Although prolactin levels continue to rise as pregnancy advances, placental sex steroids block prolactin-induced secretory activity of the glandular epithelium. It appears that sex steroids and prolactin are synergistic in mammogenesis but antagonistic in galactopoiesis. Therefore, lactation is not initiated until plasma estrogens, progesterone, and human placental lactogen (hPL) fall after delivery. Progesterone inhibits the biosynthesis of lactose and α-lactalbumin; estrogens directly antagonize the lactogenic effect of prolactin on the mammary gland by inhibiting α-lactalbumin production. hPL may also

exert a prolactin-antagonist effect through competitive binding to alveolar prolactin receptors.

The maintenance of established milk secretion requires periodic suckling and the actual emptying of ducts and alveoli. Growth hormone, cortisol, thyroxine, and insulin exert a permissive effect. Prolactin is required for galactopoiesis, but high basal levels are not mandatory, because prolactin concentrations in the nursing mother decline gradually during the late puerperium and approach that of the nonpregnant state. However, if a woman does not suckle her baby, her serum prolactin concentration will return to nonpregnant values within 2–3 weeks. If the mother suckles twins simultaneously, the prolactin response is about double that when one baby is fed at a time, illustrating an apparent synergism between the number of nipples stimulated and the frequency of suckling. The mechanism by which suckling stimulates prolactin release probably involves the inhibition of dopamine, which is thought to be the hypothalamic prolactin-inhibiting factor.

Stimulation of the nipples by suckling or other physical stimuli evokes a reflex release of oxytocin from the neurohypophysis. Because retrograde blood flow can be demonstrated within the pituitary stalk, oxytocin may reach the adenohypophysis in very high concentrations and affect pituitary release of prolactin independently of any effect on dopamine. The release of oxytocin is mediated by afferent fibers of the fourth to sixth intercostal nerves via the dorsal roots of the spinal cord to the midbrain.

The paraventricular and supraoptic neurons of the hypothalamus make up the final afferent pathway of the milk ejection reflex. The central nervous system modulates the release of oxytocin; stress or fear may inhibit the letdown reflex, whereas the cry of an infant may provoke it. Oxytocin levels may rise during orgasm, and sexual stimuli may trigger milk ejection. Psychic factors associated with the expectation of nursing are sufficient to release oxytocin prior to milk letdown but are not effective in releasing prolactin in the absence of suckling.

## SYNTHESIS OF HUMAN MILK

Milk is secreted by apocrine (with pinching-off of the cellular apex) and porous merocrine (with no change in cellular morphology) processes. The principal carbohydrate in human milk is lactose. Glucose metabolism is a key function in human milk production, because lactose is derived from glucose and galactose; the latter originates from glucose-6-phosphate. A specific protein, α-lactalbumin, catalyzes lactose synthesis. This rate-limiting enzyme is inhibited by gonadal hormones during pregnancy. Prolactin and insulin, which enhance the uptake of glucose by mammary cells, also stimulate the formation of triglycerides. Fat synthesis takes place in the endoplas-

**Table 12–2.** Multihormonal interaction in mammary growth and lactation.

| Mammogenesis | Lactogenesis | Galactopoiesis |
|---|---|---|
| Estrogens | Prolactin | ↓Gonadal hormones |
| Progesterone | ↓Estrogens | Suckling (oxytocin, prolactin) |
| Prolactin | ↓Progesterone | Growth hormone |
| Growth hormone | ↓hPL(?) | Glucocorticoids |
| Glucocorticoids | Glucocorticoids | Insulin |
| Epithelial growth factor | Insulin | Thyroxine and parathyroid hormone |

Arrows signify that lower than normal levels of the hormone are necessary for the effect to occur.

mic reticulum. Most proteins are synthesized de novo in the secretory cells from essential and nonessential plasma amino acids. The formation of milk protein and mammary enzymes is induced by prolactin and enhanced by cortisol and insulin.

Mature human milk contains 7% carbohydrate as lactose, 3–5% fat, 0.9% protein, and 0.2% mineral constituents expressed as ash. Its energy content is 60–75% kcal/dL. About 25% of the total nitrogen of human milk represents nonprotein compounds, eg, urea, uric acid, creatinine, and free amino acids. The principal proteins of human milk are casein, $\alpha$-lactalbumin, lactoferrin, IgA, lysozyme, and albumin. Milk also contains a variety of enzymes that may contribute to the infant's digestion of breast milk, eg, amylase, catalase, peroxidase, lipase, xanthine oxidase, and alkaline and acid phosphatase. The fatty acid composition of human milk is rich in palmitic and oleic acids and varies somewhat with the diet. The major ions and mineral constituents of human milk are $Na^+$, $K^+$, $Ca^{2+}$, $Mg^{2+}$, $Cl^-$, phosphorus, sulfate, and citrate. Calcium concentrations vary from 25 to 35 mg/dL and phosphorus concentrations from 13 to 16 mg/dL. Iron, copper, zinc, and trace metal contents vary considerably. All the vitamins except vitamin K are found in human milk in nutritionally adequate amounts. The composition of breast milk is not greatly affected by race, age, or parity and does not differ between the 2 breasts unless 1 breast is infected.

**Colostrum,** the premilk secretion, is a yellowish alkaline secretion that may be present in the last months of pregnancy and for the first 2–3 days after delivery. It has a higher specific gravity (1.040–1.060); a higher protein, vitamin A, immunoglobulin, and sodium and chloride content; and a lower carbohydrate, potassium, and fat content than mature breast milk. Colostrum has a normal laxative action and is an ideal natural starter food.

Ions and water pass the membrane of the alveolar cell in both directions. Human milk differs from the milk of many other species by having a lower concentration of monovalent ions and a higher concentration of lactose. The aqueous phase of milk is isosmotic with plasma; thus, the higher the lactose, the lower the ion concentration. The ratio of potassium to sodium is 3:1 in both milk and mammary intracellular fluid. Because milk contains about 87% water and lactose is the major osmotically active solute, it follows that milk yield is largely determined by lactose production.

## IMMUNOLOGIC SIGNIFICANCE OF HUMAN MILK

The neonate is immunologically immature, and maternal antibody will bolster the infant's defenses against infection. The transfer of IgG is accomplished during fetal life chiefly by active transport across the placenta. All classes of immunoglobulins are found in milk, but IgA constitutes 90% of immunoglobulins in human colostrum and milk. The output of immunoglobulins by the breast is maximal in the first week of life and declines thereafter as the production of milk-specific proteins increases. Lacteal antibodies against enteric bacteria and their antigenic products are largely of the IgA class. IgG and IgA lacteal antibodies provide short-term systemic and long-term enteric humoral immunity to the breastfed neonate. IgA anti-poliomyelitis virus activity present in breastfed infants indicates that at least some transfer of milk antibodies into serum does occur. However, maternal lacteal antibodies are absorbed systemically by human infants for only a very short time after birth. Long-term protection against pathogenic enteric bacteria is provided by the adsorption of lacteal IgA to the intestinal mucosa. In addition to providing passive immunity, there is evidence that lacteal immunoglobulins can modulate the immunocompetence of the neonate, but the exact mechanisms have not been described. For instance, the secretion of IgA into the saliva of breastfed infants is enhanced in comparison with bottle-fed controls.

Breast milk also contains more than 100,000 blood cells per milliliter, most of which are leukocytes. The total cell count is even higher in colostrum. In human milk, the leukocytes are predominantly mononuclear cells and macrophages. Both T and B lymphocytes are present. The immunologic value of the lymphoid and reticuloendothelial cells in human milk is yet to be clarified, but data from animal experiments indicate that maternal lymphocytes can be incorporated into the suckling's tissues and function in a variety of immunologic contexts. In humans, the evidence is circumstantial and is based on the transfer of tuberculin sensitivity to infants from their tuberculin-positive mothers and on the greater histocompatibility between mother and infant compared with that between father and infant. Finally, sensitized T lymphocytes and other immunocompetent cells in mammary secretions may protect the breast itself against bacterial colonization.

Elements in breast milk other than immunoglobulins and cells have prophylactic value against infections. The marked difference between the intestinal flora of breastfed and bottle-fed infants is due to a dialyzable nitrogen-containing carbohydrate (bifidus factor) that supports the growth of *Lactobacillus bifidus* in breastfed infants. The stool of bottle-fed infants is more alkaline and contains predominantly coliform organisms and *Bacteroides* sp. *L bifidus* inhibits the growth of *Shigella* sp, *Escherichia coli,* and yeast. Human milk also contains a nonspecific antimicrobial factor, lysozyme (a thermostable and acid-stable enzyme that cleaves the peptidoglycans of bacteria), and a "resistance factor," which protect the infant against staphylococcal infection. Lactoferrin, an iron chelator, exerts a strong bacteriostatic effect on staphylococci and *E coli* by depriving the organisms of iron. Both C3 and C4 components of complement and antitoxins for neutralizing *Vibrio cholerae* are found in human milk. Unsaturated vitamin $B_{12}$-binding protein in milk renders the vitamin unavailable for utilization by *E coli* and *Bacteroides*. Finally, interferon in milk may provide yet another nonspecific anti-infection factor.

Human milk may also have prophylactic value in childhood food allergies. During the neonatal period, permeability of the small intestine to macromolecules is increased. Secretory IgA in colostrum and breast milk reduces the absorption of foreign macromolecules until the endogenous IgA secretory capacity of the newborn intestinal lamina propria and lymph nodes develops at 2–3 months of age. Protein of cow's milk can be highly allergenic in the infant predisposed by heredity. The introduction of cow's milk-free formulas (see Table 11–3) has considerably reduced the incidence of milk allergy. Thus, comparative studies on the incidence of allergy, bacterial and viral infections, severe diarrhea, necrotizing enterocolitis, tuberculosis, and neonatal meningitis in breastfed and bottle-fed infants support the concept that breast milk fulfills a protective function.

## ADVANTAGES & DISADVANTAGES OF BREASTFEEDING

### For the Mother

**A. Advantages:** Breastfeeding is economical, and it is emotionally satisfying to most women. It helps to contract the uterus and accelerates the process of uterine involution in the postpartum period. It promotes mother-infant bonding. According to epidemiologic studies, breastfeeding may help to protect the suckled breast against cancer. Over a 6-month period postpartum, weight loss is greater in lactating than in nonlactating women, although body fat is not significantly affected.

**B. Disadvantages and Contraindications:** Regular nursing restricts activities and may be perceived by the mother as an inconvenience. In cultures in which nursing in public is commonplace, nursing is less inconvenient. Twins can be nursed successfully, but few women are prepared for the first weeks of almost continual feeding. Cesarean section may necessitate modifications of early breastfeeding routines. Difficulties such as nipple tenderness and mastitis may develop. Compared with nonlactating women, breastfeeding women have a significant decrease (mean, 6.5%) in bone mineral content of the lumbar spine at 6 months postpartum.

Breastfeeding by a hypoparathyroid mother is undesirable, because adequate calcium supplementation to replace losses in breast milk is difficult in these patients. Furthermore, large amounts of 25-hydroxy-

vitamin $D_3$ appear in the milk of mothers receiving therapy for hypoparathyroidism. There are few absolute contraindications other than breast cancer. Augmentation mammoplasty with silicone implants should not affect breastfeeding, but reduction mammoplasty involving nipple autotransplantation severs the lactiferous ducts and precludes nursing.

### For the Infant

**A. Advantages:** Breast milk is digestible, available at the right temperature, and free of bacterial contamination. Its composition is ideal, it has anti-infectious properties, and there are fewer allergy problems in breastfed infants. Breastfed infants are not so likely to become obese as are formula-fed babies. Suckling promotes infant-mother bonding.

**B. Disadvantages and Contraindications:** Absolute contraindications to breastfeeding are breast cancer; active pulmonary tuberculosis in the mother; severe mastitis; or maternal intake of cancer chemotherapeutic agents or certain other drugs (Table 12–3). Breastfeeding does not protect against the deleterious effects of congenital hypothyroidism. The milk of a nursing mother with cystic fibrosis is high in sodium and places the infant at risk for hypernatremia. Hepatitis B antigen has been found in breast milk, but transmission by this route is unlikely to occur. A small number of otherwise healthy breastfed infants develop unconjugated hyperbilirubinemia (sometimes exceeding 20 mg/dL) during the first few weeks of life owing to higher than normal glucuronyl transferase inhibitory activity of the breast milk. The inhibitor may be a pregnanediol, although increased milk lipase activity and free fatty acids are likely the critical factors.

Breastfeeding is not usually possible for weak, ill, or very premature infants or for infants with cleft palate, choanal atresia, or phenylketonuria. It is common practice in many nurseries to feed premature infants human milk collected fresh from their mothers or processed from donors. The effects of processing and storage on the persistence of viral agents are not well studied. Cytomegalovirus transmission through breast milk has been documented and may pose a significant hazard for preterm infants. It is recommended that seronegative preterm infants receive milk from seronegative donors only.

## ANTENATAL PREPARATION FOR BREASTFEEDING

Patient education and the decision to breastfeed should ideally be accomplished in the prenatal period. The first step in patient education is to explain to the mother the advantages and disadvantages of nursing the infant. The next step is instruction in preparation techniques.

The attitudes of the mother and those about her are

**Table 12–3.** Transmission of drugs and toxins in breast milk.

| | Drug Transfer to Milk | Drug-Induced Neonatal Problem | Use In Nursing Women |
|---|---|---|---|
| **Anticoagulants** | | | |
| Dicumarol | Very slight | — | Acceptable |
| Warfarin (Coumadin) | Traces | — | Acceptable |
| Heparin | None | — | Safe |
| **Antihypertensive diuretics** | | | |
| Guanethidine (Ismelin) | Minimal | — | Acceptable |
| Propranolol (Inderal) | Minimal | — | Acceptable |
| Chlorthalidone (Hygroton) | Significant | Diuresis | Contraindicated |
| Chlorothiazide (Diuril) | Significant | Thrombocytopenia | Contraindicated |
| Methyldopa | Slight | Hypotension | Acceptable |
| Labetalol | Significant | Bradycardia, hypotension | Use cautiously |
| Atenolol | Significant | Bradycardia | Acceptable |
| Digitalis | Slight | — | Safe |
| Dipyridamole | Insignificant | — | Safe |
| Hydralazine | Moderate | — | Acceptable |
| Amiodarone | Significant | Potential goiter | Contraindicated |
| **Antimicrobials** | | | |
| Chloramphenicol (Chloromycetin) | Significant | Induction of "gray disease" in neonate Bone marrow suppression | Contraindicated |
| Metronidazole (Flagyl) | Significant | Blood dyscrasias: Neurologic disorders | Contraindicated |
| Penicillins, aminoglycosides, cephalosporins | Moderate | Modification of bowel flora | Safe |
| Clindamycin | Significant | — | Acceptable |
| Erythromycin | Significant | — | Safe |
| Nitrofurantoin | Slight | G6PD anemia | Use with caution |
| Trimethoprim | Slight | — | Use with caution |
| Tetracycline | ?Significant | Permanent discoloration of teeth | Contraindicated |
| Sulfonamides | Varies with product | G6PD anemia or kernicterus with Rh or ABO incompatibility | Use with caution |
| Nalidixic acid (NegGram) | Significant | G6PD anemia | Contraindicated |
| Pyrimethamine | Significant | Vomiting, marrow suppression, Thrombocytopenia | Contraindicated |
| Quinolones | | | Use with caution |
| Amantadine | Low | Potential vomiting and skin rash | Use with caution |
| Quinine | Significant | Thrombocytopenia occasionally | Use with caution |
| Chloroquine | None | — | Safe |
| Isoniazid (INH) | Significant | Hepatic toxicity | Contraindicated |
| **Antithyroid Drugs** | | | |
| [131]I and other radioactive products | Very significant | Permanent athyrosis | Contraindicated |
| Thiouracils | Slight | Hypothyroidism potentially | Acceptable in usual doses |
| Methimazole | Significant | Thyroid dysfunction | Contraindicated |
| **Drugs Affecting Central Nervous System** | | | |
| Alcohol | Slight | Sedative, pseudo-Cushing's disease | May use in small amounts occasionally |
| Chloral hydrate | Minimal | — | Safe |
| Meprobamate | 4 × plasma level | Sedation | Contraindicated |
| Diazepam (Valium) | Moderate | Sedation | Use judiciously |
| Lithium | 1/3–1/2 plasma level | Hypotonia, hypothermia, cyanosis ECG changes | Contraindicated |

(continued)

**Table 12–3 (cont'd).** Transmission of drugs and toxins in breast milk.

| | Drug Transfer to Milk | Drug-Induced Neonatal Problem | Use in Nursing Women |
|---|---|---|---|
| Phenothiazines | ?Significant | Drowsiness | Use cautiously |
| Amitryptiline | Minimal | — | Safe |
| Tricyclic antidepressants | Slight | — | Acceptable |
| Fluoxetine (Prozac) | Slight | — | Use with caution |
| Phenobarbital | ?Significant | Hepatic microsomal enzymes produced | Minimal dosage safe |
| Phenytoin (Dilantin) | Minimal | — | Safe |
| Carbamazepine | Slight | — | Safe |
| MgSO$_4$ | Significant | Hypotonia | Acceptable |
| Clonazepam | Significant | Potential apnea | Use cautiously |
| Propoxyphene (Darvon) | Minimal | — | Safe |
| Naproxen | Slight | Altered platelet function | Acceptable |
| Ibuprofen | Minimal | Altered platelet function | Safe |
| Indomethacin | Moderate | Altered platelet function | Safe in small doses |
| Aspirin | ?Significant | Altered platelet function | Safe in small doses |
| Acetaminophen | Slight | — | Safe |
| Morphine | Trace | — | Acceptable |
| Methadone | Significant | Narcotic addiction | Acceptable |
| Meperidine (Demerol) | Significant | Narcotic addiction | Short-term use |
| Heroin | Significant | Narcotic addiction | Contraindicated |
| Cocaine | Data not available | Tremulousness | Contraindicated |
| Codeine | Minimal | — | Safe |
| Caffeine | Moderate | Irritability | Avoid excessive doses |
| Nicotine (tobacco smoking) | ?Significant | — | ?Safe |
| **Hormones and Metabolic Agents** | | | |
| Insulin | None | — | Safe |
| Corticotropin | None | — | Safe |
| Prednisone | Slight | — | Acceptable |
| Medroxyprogesterone (Provera) | Slight | — | Safe |
| Chlorpropamide | Moderate | Unknown | Use cautiously |
| Tolbutamide | Moderate | Unknown | Use cautiously |
| Thyroxine | Slight to moderate | — | Probably safe |
| Oral contraceptives | ?Significant | Gynecomastia in males ?Carcinogenic | Contraindicated |
| **Bronchodilators, Antihistamines** | | | |
| Ephedrine | Moderate | Irritability | Use cautiously |
| Diphenlydramine | Moderate | Drowsiness | Avoid excessive doses |
| Ranitidine | Moderate | Decreased gastric acidity | Contraindicated |
| Dimetidine | Significant | CNS stimulation | Contraindicated |
| Meclizine, cyclizine | Variable | Irritability, sleep disturbance | Use with caution |
| **Antineoplastics, Immunosuppressants** | Variable | Potential leukopenia, thrombocytopenia | Contraindicated |
| **Laxatives** | | | |
| Phenolphthalein | Significant | Loose stools | Safe in small doses |
| Cascara sagrada | Significant | Loose stools | Safe in small doses |

For additional information, see Briggs GG, Freeman RK, Yaffee JS: *Drugs in Pregnancy and Lactation* (pp 1–503). Williams & Wilkins, 1986, and publications such as the *Physicans Desk Reference*.

especially important. If she regards breastfeeding as abnormal, unclean, or embarrassing, no amount of persuasion or antenatal preparation will influence the outcome, particularly if she is compelled to nurse. In contrast, a woman who has a very strong desire to breastfeed her baby may succeed even if her breasts are small and the nipples poorly protractile. Antenatal discussion of the patient's desire is most important. In some cases, the maternal instinct does not become strong until after the baby is born. A woman may have no inclination toward breastfeeding during pregnancy, but she may change her mind after delivery. The patient who is antagonistic to the idea of breastfeeding—especially if she has been unsuccessful in the past—should be assured that she will not be obliged to breastfeed after her present delivery. This may eliminate a major source of anxiety and guilt.

Although many methods of preventing breast and nipple problems have been advocated, the majority of women have never used any type of antenatal breast preparation. No convincing evidence exists that successful lactation depends on the application of this cream or that lotion. Moreover, it is doubtful whether a woman can "toughen" the skin of the nipples successfully, although tenderness may be reduced by washing and by the application of hydrous lanolin or similar unguents. Alcohol, benzoin tincture, and other drying agents should not be used on the nipples, because they remove natural skin oils and may do more harm than good by causing irritation and fissures. Support of the enlarged breast is important to prevent "sagging" following pregnancy.

Flat or inverted nipples that the baby cannot grasp may cause failure of nursing. Gentle traction by the patient may elevate the nipples during the latter part of pregnancy, but some nipple protraction during gestation should be expected even without special manipulation. Nipple shields worn under a brassiere during the last trimester have been recommended for retracted nipples.

Regular gentle manual expression of colostrum during the final weeks of pregnancy may be of value in the initiation of lactation. Emptying the breasts during the puerperium is beneficial, and the patient may learn the technique before painful engorgement occurs.

A popular method of manual expression consists of 2 movements. The first is compression of the whole breast between the hands, starting at the margins and continuing inward as far as the areola. Firm pressure is maintained throughout this movement, which is repeated 10 times. Its object is to move colostrum from the finer into the larger ducts and the lacteal sinuses. The second movement is designed to empty the sinuses. The latter are pinched sharply and repeatedly between the thumb and forefinger of one hand while the breast is held firmly in the other hand. Success in expelling colostrum depends on the direction in which the force of the pinch is applied. The force must be directed somewhat backward, toward the center of the breast, rather than toward the base of the nipple.

## PRINCIPLES & TECHNIQUES OF BREASTFEEDING

The interrelationships of mother, father, baby, and environment (including the medical personnel who care for mother and baby in the prenatal and postnatal periods) influence the nursing experience. Consideration must be given to (1) the mother's attitude toward nursing and her emotional status, breast anatomy, and general health; (2) the father's interest; (3) conditions in the home; and (4) the baby's maturity, normality, weight, vigor, and appetite. Each case must be managed individually, using the guidelines outlined below.

In the absence of anatomic or medical complications, the timing of the first feeding and the frequency and duration of subsequent feedings largely determine the outcome of breastfeeding. Infants and mothers who are able to initiate breastfeeding within 1–2 hours of delivery are more successful than those whose initial interactions are delayed for several hours. Suckling has a propitious oxytocic effect, and colostrum is good for the newborn. Unfortunately, feeding may be delayed by hospital routine or custom. Lactation is established most successfully if the baby remains with the mother and she can feed on demand for adequate intervals throughout the first 24-hour period. The initial feeding should last 5 minutes at each breast in order to condition the letdown reflex. At first, the frequency of feedings may be very irregular (8–10 times a day), but after 1–2 weeks a fairly regular 4- to 6-hour pattern will emerge.

When the milk "comes in" abruptly on the third or fourth postpartum day, there is an initial period of discomfort caused by vascular engorgement and edema of the breasts. The baby does not nurse so much by developing intermittent negative pressure as by a rhythmic grasping of the areola; the infant "works" the milk into its mouth. Little force is required in nursing, because the breast reservoirs can be emptied and refilled without suction. Nursing mothers notice a sensation of drawing and tightening within the breast at the beginning of suckling after the initial breast engorgement disappears. They are thus conscious of the milk ejection reflex, which may even cause milk to spurt or run out.

Some women expend a great deal of emotion on the subject of breastfeeding, and a few are almost overwhelmed by fear of being unable to care for their babies in this way. If attendants are sympathetic and patient, however, a woman who wants to nurse usually can do so. Attendants must be certain that the baby "fixes" on (actually over) the nipple and the areola so as to feed properly without pain to the mother (Fig 12–9).

The baby should nurse at both breasts at each feeding, because overfilling of the breasts is the main deterrent to the maintenance of milk secretion. Nursing at only one breast at each feeding inhibits the reflex that is provoked simultaneously in both breasts. Thus, nursing at alternate breasts from one feeding to the next may increase discomfort due to engorgement and reduce milk output. It is helpful for the mother to be taught to empty the breasts after each feeding; a sleepy baby may not have accomplished this. The use of supplementary formula or other food during the first 6–8 weeks of breastfeeding can interfere with lactation and should be avoided except when absolutely necessary. The introduction of an artificial nipple, which requires a different sucking mechanism, will weaken the sucking reflex required for breastfeeding. Some groups such as the La Leche League recommend that other fluids be given by spoon or dropper rather than by bottle.

In preparing to nurse, the mother should (1) wash her hands with soap and water, (2) clean her nipples and breasts with water, and (3) assume a comfortable position in, preferably, a rocking or upright chair. If the mother is unable to sit up to nurse her baby because of painful perineal sutures, she may feel more comfortable lying on her side. A woman with large pendulous breasts may find it difficult to manage both the breasts and the baby. If the baby lies on a pillow, the mother will have both hands free to guide the nipple.

Each baby nurses differently; however, the following procedure is generally successful:

(1) Allow the normal newborn to nurse at each breast on demand or approximately every 3–4 hours, for 5 minutes per breast per feeding the first day. Over the next few days, gradually increase feeding time to initiate the letdown reflex, but do not exceed 10–15 minutes per breast. Suckling for longer than 15 minutes may cause maceration and cracking of the nipples and thus lead to mastitis.

(2) Compressing the periareolar area and expressing a small amount of colostrum or milk for the baby to taste may stimulate the baby to nurse.

(3) Try to keep the baby awake by moving or patting, but do not snap its feet, work its jaw, push its head, or press its cheeks.

(4) Place the nipple well back in the baby's mouth so that it rests against the palate and the baby can compress the periareolar area with its jaws. Hold the breast away from the baby's nostrils.

(5) Before removing the infant from the breast, gently open its mouth by lifting the outer border of the upper lip to break the suction.

After nursing, gently wipe the nipples with water and dry them.

## MILK YIELD

The prodigious energy requirements for lactation are met by mobilization of elements from maternal tissues and from dietary intake. Physiologic fat stores laid down during pregnancy are mobilized during lactation, and the return to prepregnant weight and figure is promoted. A variety of studies suggest that a lactating woman should increase her normal daily food intake by 600 kcal/day but intakes of 2000–2300 calories are sufficient for lactating women. The recommended daily dietary increases for lactation are 20 g of protein; a 20% increase in all vitamins and minerals except folic acid, which should be increased by 50%; and a 33% increase in calcium, phosphorus, and magnesium. There is no evidence that increasing fluid intake will increase milk volume. Fluid restric-

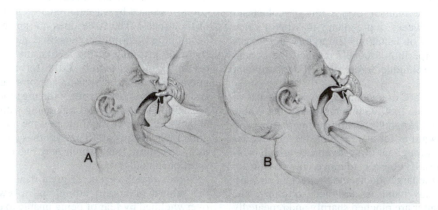

**Figure 12–9.** Mechanism of suckling in the neonate. **A:** Tongue moves forward to draw nipple in as glottis still permits breathing. **B:** Tongue moves along nipple, pressing it against palate with glottis closed. Ductules under the areola are compressed, and milk flow begins. The cheeks fill the mouth and provide negative pressure.

tion also has little effect, because urine output will diminish in preference to milk output.

With nursing, average milk production on the second postpartum day is about 120 mL. The amount increases to about 180 mL on the third postpartum day and to as much as 240 mL on the fourth day. In time, milk production reaches about 300 mL/d.

A good rule of thumb for the calculation of milk production for a given day in the week after delivery is to multiply the number of the postpartum day by 60. This gives the approximate number of milliliters of milk secreted in that 24-hour period.

If all goes well, sustained production of milk will be achieved by most patients after 10–14 days. A yield of 120–180 mL per feeding is common by the end of the second week. When free secretion has been established, marked increases are possible; a wet nurse can often suckle 3 babies successfully for weeks.

Early diminution of milk production often is due to failure to empty the breasts because of weak efforts by the baby or ineffectual nursing procedures; emotional problems, such as aversion to nursing; or medical complications, such as mastitis, debilitating systemic disease, Sheehan's syndrome. Late diminution of milk production results from too generous complementary feedings of formula, emotional or other illness, and pregnancy.

Adequate rest is essential for successful lactation. Sometimes it is difficult to ensure an adequate milk yield if the mother is working outside the home. If it is not possible to rearrange the nursing schedule to fit the work schedule or vice versa, it may be necessary to empty the breasts manually or by pump. The Loyd-B-Pump is a simple hand-triggered pump easy to carry in a large handbag. The Egnell Breast Pump is a larger, more sophisticated, and costlier piece of equipment for use on the maternity floor. Milk output can be estimated by weighing the infant before and after feeding. If there has been a bowel movement during feeding, the baby should be weighed before the diaper is changed.

The baby's behavior and sleep periods and the character of its stools are the best measures of success of feeding. The baby who is still hungry at the end of a session of nursing should be given water and should be patted to expel gas. This baby should also be fed earlier the next time. Supplementary feeding of formula should be reserved for the baby who does not gain weight because of not getting enough food. Measures that are popularly supposed to improve the milk supply (eg, drinking beer, eating rich foods) probably do little more than relax or reassure the mother. Further study is needed to evaluate the safety of galactagogues such as domperidone, metoclopramide, and sulpiride, which may have side effects such as dyskinesias. Domperidone is secreted in considerably smaller amounts in breast milk relative to the thera-

peutic dosage than is either metoclopramide or sulpiride. These drugs act as dopamine antagonists and stimulate the release of prolactin and milk in puerperal women without stimulating the secretion of TRH and thyroid hormones. Milk yield is favorably increased by sulpiride during the early puerperium in primiparous mothers not accustomed to nursing.

It may be necessary to substitute bottle-feeding for breastfeeding if the mother's supply continues to be inadequate (less than 50% of the infant's needs) after 3 weeks of effort; if nipple or breast lesions are severe enough to prevent pumping; or if the mother is either pregnant or severely (physically or mentally) ill. Nourishment from the inadequately lactating breast can be augmented with the Lact-Aide Nursing Trainer, a device that provides a supplemental source of milk via a plastic capillary tube placed beside the breast and suckled simultaneously with the nipple. Disposable plastic bags serve as reservoirs, and the supplemental milk is warmed by hanging the bag next to the mother. The Lact-Aide supplementer has also been used to help nurse premature infants and to reestablish lactation after untimely weaning due to illness. The long-term success of breastfeeding is increased by a structured home support system of postnatal visiting by allied health personnel or experienced volunteers.

## DISORDERS OF LACTATION

### Painful Nipples

Tenderness of the nipples, a common symptom during the first days of breastfeeding, generally begins when the baby starts to suck. As soon as milk begins to flow, nipple sensitivity usually subsides. If maternal tissues are unusually tender, dry heat may help between feedings. Nipple shields should be used only as a last resort, since they interfere with normal sucking. Glass or plastic shields with rubber nursing nipples are preferable to shields made entirely of rubber.

Nipple fissures cause severe pain and prevent normal letdown of milk. Local infection around the fissure can lead to mastitis. Unless the fissures heal, lactation will fail. The application of vitamin A and D ointment or hydrous lanolin, which do not have to be removed, is often effective. Benzoin tincture is a traditional remedy for cracked nipples, but this gummy substance may occlude the nipple ducts and should not be used. Dilute silver nitrate is much too irritating to be recommended. To speed healing, the following steps are recommended. Apply dry heat for 20 minutes 4 times a day with a 60-watt bulb held 18 inches away from the nipple. Conduct prefeeding manual expression. Begin nursing on the side opposite the fissure with the other breast exposed to air to allow the initial letdown to occur atraumatically. Apply expressed breast milk to nipples and let it dry in between feedings. If necessary, use a nipple shield while nursing, and take aspirin with or without codeine just after nursing. On rare occasions, it may be necessary to stop nursing temporarily on the affected side and to empty the breast either manually or by gentle pumping. If a painful fissure persists or recurs despite therapy, the success of breastfeeding is remote, and suppression of lactation is indicated.

A cause of chronic severe sore nipples without remarkable physical findings is candidal infection. Prompt relief is provided by topical nystatin cream. Thrush or candidal diaper rash or maternal candidal vaginitis must be treated as well.

## Engorgement

Engorgement of the breasts occurs in the first week postpartum and is due to vascular congestion and accumulation of milk. The primiparous patient and the patient with inelastic breasts are more prone to engorgement. Vascularity and swelling increase on the second day after delivery; the areola or breast may become engorged. Prepartum breast massage and around-the-clock demand feedings help to prevent engorgement in these patients. When the areola is engorged, the nipple is occluded and proper grasping of the areola by the infant is not possible. With moderately severe engorgement, the breasts become firm and warm, and the lobules may be palpable as tender, irregular masses. Considerable discomfort and, often, a slight fever can be expected, and the patient may become frustrated and tearful. All this is a threat to milk production.

Mild cases may be relieved by aspirin or other analgesics, cool compresses, and partial expression of the milk before nursing. In severe cases, administer hypnotics, and have the patient empty the breasts manually. The patient should support the breast with her fingers and with her thumbs distally and massage gently toward the areola. When the peripheral lobules have been softened, areolar expression is carried out. Hand pumps exert negative pressure only on the areola and must be accompanied by massage of the distal lobules. The Egnell mechanical pump simulates the stroking action of the infant's tongue. Oxytocin—by injection or intranasally—to augment the milk letdown reflex may help certain patients with engorged breasts. Nevertheless, persistent engorgement carries a poor prognosis, and suppression of lactation may be necessary.

## Mastitis

Mastitis occurs most frequently in primiparous nursing patients and is usually caused by coagulase-positive *Staphylococcus aureus*. High fever should never be ascribed to simple breast engorgement alone. Inflammation of the breast seldom begins before the fifth day postpartum. Most frequently, symptoms of a painful erythematous lobule in an outer quadrant of the breast are noted during the second or third week of the puerperium. Inflammation may occur with weaning when the flow of milk is disrupted, or the nursing mother may acquire the infection during her hospital stay and then transmit it to the infant. The demonstration of antibody-coated bacteria in the milk indicates the presence of infectious mastitis. Many infants harbor an infection and, in turn, infect the mother's breast during nursing. Neonatal streptococcal infection should be suspected if mastitis is recurrent or bilateral. Indeed, if the infants of mothers with breast abscesses are scrutinized, the majority will be found to have furunculosis.

Prevention of breast infection requires meticulous breast hygiene. If a fissure of the nipple develops, a nipple shield should be tried in order to allow nursing to continue. Infection may be limited to the subareolar region but more frequently involves an obstructed lactiferous duct and the surrounding breast parenchyma. If cellulitis is not properly treated, a breast abscess may develop. When only mastitis is present, it is best to prevent milk stasis by continuing breastfeeding (unless fissures are present) or by using a breast pump. Apply local heat, provide a well-fitted brassiere, and institute appropriate antibiotic treatment. Cephalosporins, methicillin sodium, and cloxacillin sodium are the antibiotics of choice to combat penicillinase-producing bacteria. The dosage of cloxacillin is 500 mg every 6 hours for 1–3 days until symptoms subside and then 250 mg every 6 hours for a total of 10 days.

Pitting edema over the inflamed area and some degree of fluctuation are evidence of abscess formation. It is necessary to incise and open loculated areas and provide wide drainage. Unlike with mastitis, continuing breastfeeding is not recommended in the presence of a breast abscess.

## Miscellaneous Complications

A galactocele, or milk-retention cyst, is caused by the blockage of a milk duct. Diagnosis may be made by mammography. The cyst may be aspirated but will fill up again. It can be removed surgically under local anesthesia without discontinuing nursing. Sometimes the infant will reject one or both breasts. Strong foods such as beans, cabbage, turnips, broccoli, onions, garlic, or rhubarb may cause aversion to milk or neonatal colic. A common cause of nursing problems is maternal fatigue.

## Transmission of Drugs in Breast Milk

The benefits of prescribing drugs for the breastfeeding mother must be weighed against the potential hazards of the drug to the infant. As a general rule, administration of a drug immediately after the infant suckles will result in a lower concentration of the substance in the milk at the next feeding. Drugs that can be given in a single daily dose should be taken just prior to the infant's longest sleep period. Since milk is continuously produced, milk levels reflect simultaneous plasma drug levels. The quantity of a drug that will be ingested by a neonate can be estimated if one knows the concentration of the drug in the breast milk. An infant's average intake of milk is 165 mL/kg/day. The maximal daily drug dose ingested can be calculated as peak milk level 165 mL/kg/day.

The physicochemical determinants of the rate of passage of a drug into milk are pKa and lipid solubility (oil/water partition coefficient). Compounds that exist primarily in the ionized form at physiologic pH diffuse slowly into milk, as do compounds that are extensively protein-bound. Highly lipid-soluble drugs pass more rapidly into milk than do more water-soluble ones. For the most part, drugs are transported more efficiently across the placenta than into breast milk.

Drugs that may have an adverse effect on lactation include oral contraceptive steroids, ergot derivatives, and pyridoxine (vitamin $B_6$) in large doses. Drugs that may have an adverse effect on the breast-fed infant when taken by the mother include anticancer agents; certain antimicrobials such as chloramphenicol, isoniazid, metronidazole, nitrofurantoin, and sulfonamides; and diazepam and other tranquilizers in protracted use. Since the levels of propylthiouracil (PTU) are only about 10% of the maximum maternal serum levels, the calculated daily dosage received by a nursing infant is very small; therefore, it is reasonable to permit a patient taking PTU to nurse her infant providing the infant's thyroid status is periodically evaluated. Heparin does not appear in milk and is safe to use during lactation. The safety of thiazide diuretics is controversial. The excretion characteristics and compatibility with breastfeeding of various pharmacologic compounds are given in Table 12–3.

Exposure to environmental agents is of special concern to lactating women. Moderate alcohol or nicotine intake poses little if any risk to the infant. Marihuana and organic pesticides raise serious concerns because they are lipid soluble and undergo prolonged storage in body fat. Plasma fluoride is poorly transferred to breast milk; infants thus receive almost no fluoride during breastfeeding, and consideration should be given to fluoride supplementation.

Breast feeding has been recognized as a mode of human immunodeficiency virus (HIV) transmission. Breast feeding might pose an additional risk (about 15%) for an infant above that already present at birth because the mother had HIV. The risk of HIV transmission through breast milk is substantially higher among women who become infected during the postpartum lactation period. Most mothers in developed countries who know of their seropositivity choose not to breast feed; in underdeveloped countries where lactation is critical to infant survival, HIV-infected mothers may choose to breast feed their infants.

## INHIBITION & SUPPRESSION OF LACTATION

Despite a recent upsurge in breastfeeding in Western countries, there are many women who will not or cannot breastfeed and others who fail in the attempt. Supervised lactation inhibition is desirable in the event of fetal or neonatal death as well. Approximately 50% of parturients are candidates for postpartum lactation suppression.

The oldest and simplest method of suppressing lactation is to stop nursing, to avoid nipple stimulation, to refrain from expressing or pumping the milk, and to bind the breasts snugly for 48–72 hours. Ice bags and analgesics are helpful. Patients who receive no medication will complain of breast engorgement (45%), pain (45%), and leaking breasts (55%). Although the breasts will become considerably engorged and the patient may experience discomfort, the collection of milk in the duct system will suppress its production, and resorption will occur. After approximately 2–3 days, engorgement will begin to recede, and the patient will be comfortable again.

A variety of naturally occurring and synthetic estrogens used alone or in combination with an androgenic hormone are effective in suppressing lactation. Antiestrogenic compounds, eg, clomiphene (100 mg orally daily for 5 days), also inhibit lactation postpartum, probably by reducing prolactin secretion. Estrogens probably suppress galactopoiesis at the level of breast tissue, since estrogens stimulate rather than inhibit prolactin release. Estrogenic compounds have been shown to be superior to placebo in relieving breast engorgement and milk leakage. However, rebound lactation has been noted in some patients 8–10 days after cessation of estrogen therapy.

The possibility that estrogen therapy during the puerperium may increase the incidence of venous thromboembolism is supported by certain retrospective studies, but not all groups of patients are equally affected. Specifically, the risk of thromboembolic disease is not increased in women under 25 years of age who have had a normal delivery, but it is increased 10-fold in women over 35 years who have had a cesarean section and received estrogens. Although estrogens probably are not contraindicated in most normal patients, their use for lactation suppression should be discouraged, because other pharmacologic methods are safer and more effective.

Combinations of estrogen and androgen have been used to improve the effect of estrogens alone. The most successful regimen is to inject intramuscularly the following after the first stage of labor: 3 mL of a solution containing (in oil, per milliliter) 90 mg of testosterone enanthate and 4 mg of estradiol valerate. This procedure prevents symptoms of breast engorgement in 90% of patients. Although virilization is not seen with the usual doses, elevated serum androgens may persist for 6–8 weeks, and some women report increase in facial hair and oiliness of skin. This medication is not associated with significant thromboembolic risk in the young patient who has delivered vaginally.

Lactation suppression by inhibiting prolactin secretion with synthetic ergot alkaloids such as bromocriptine (Parlodel) is safe and highly effective both immediately postpartum and after lactation has been established. Bromocriptine is a specific dopamine receptor agonist that has a direct action on the anterior pituitary lactotrophs to inhibit prolactin secretion. Because it accelerates the natural postpartum fall in prolactin, it suppresses both lactogenesis and galactopoiesis. Bromocriptine is, on physiologic

grounds, the most logical medication to use, but it requires prolonged therapy and is not without unpleasant side affects. The recommended dosage is 2.5 mg orally twice daily for 3 weeks after vital signs have stabilized, beginning no sooner than 4 hours after delivery. Some patients complain of nasal congestion, mild constipation, nausea, headache, dizziness, and postural hypotension. In the event of side effects, the daily dose can be halved. A single dose of cabergoline (0.5 mg, 2 tablets) is as effective as the standard bromocriptine regimen, but rebound and other adverse symptoms are less common.

Recent reports suggest that oral prostaglandin $E_2$ (2 mg every 6 hours on the fourth and fifth days postpartum) is an effective inhibitor of milk secretion and breast engorgement. The mechanism of action is not known, but a $PGE_2$-induced decrease in prolactin may be mediated by hypothalamic dopaminergic neurons.

## REFERENCES

### ANATOMY & PHYSIOLOGY OF THE PUERPERIUM

Allolio B, Hoffmann J, Linton EA et al: Diurnal salivary cortisol patterns during pregnancy and after delivery: Relationship to plasma corticotrophin-releasing-hormone. Clin Endocrinol 1990;33:279.

Bacigalupo G, Riese S, Rosendahl H, Saling E: Quantitative relationships between pain intensities during labor and beta-endorphin and cortisol concentrations in plasma: Decline of the hormone concentrations in the early postpartum period. J Perinat Med 1990;18:289.

Battin DA et al: Effect of suckling on serum prolactin, luteinizing hormone, follicle-stimulating hormone, and estradiol during prolonged lactation. Obstet Gynecol 1985;65:785.

Bremme K, Ostlund E, Almqvist I et al: Enhanced thrombin generation and fibrinolytic activity in normal pregnancy and the puerperium. Obstet Gynecol 1992;80:132.

Brewer MM, Bates RM, Vannoy LP: Postpartum changes in maternal weight and body fat deposits in lactating versus nonlactating women. Am J Clin Nutr 1989;49:259.

Dawood MY et al: Oxytocin release and plasma anterior pituitary and gonadal hormones in women during lactation. J Clin Endocrinol Metab 1981;52:678.

De Leo V, Lanzetta D, D'Antona D et al: Control of growth hormone secretion during the postpartum period. Gynecol Obstet Invest 1992;33:31.

Elster AD, Sanders TG, Vines FS, Chen MYM: Size and shape of the pituitary gland during pregnancy and postpartum: Measurement with MR imaging. Radiology 1991;181:531.

Garagiola DM, Tarver RD, Gibson L et al: Anatomic changes in the pelvis after uncomplicated vaginal de-

livery: A CT study on 14 women. AJR 1989;153:1239.

Gerbasi FR, Bottoms S, Farag A, Mammen EF: Changes in hemostasis activity during delivery and the immediate postpartum period. Am J Obstet Gynecol 1990;162:1158.

Hatjis CG, Kofinas AD, Greelish JP et al: Atrial natriuretic factor concentrations during pregnancy and in the postpartum period. Am J Perinatol 1992;9:275.

Hornnes PJ, Kuhl C: Plasma insulin and glucagon responses to isoglycemic stimulation in normal pregnancy and postpartum. Obstet Gynecol 1980;55:425.

Howie PW et al: The relationship between suckling-induced prolactin response and lactogenesis. J Clin Endocrinol Metab 1980;50:670.

Kremer JAM, Borm G, Schellekens LA et al: Pulsatile secretion of luteinizing hormone and prolactin in lactating and nonlactating women and the response to naltrexone. J Clin Endocrinol Metab 1991;72:294.

Lewis PR, Brown JB, Renfree MB, Short RV: The resumption of ovulation and menstruation in a well-nourished population of women breastfeeding for an extended period of time. Fertil Steril 1991;55:529.

Liu JH, Park KH: Gonadotropin and prolactin secretion increases during sleep during the puerperium in nonlactating women. J Clin Endocrinol Metab 1988;66:839.

Liu J, Rebar RW, Yen SSC: Neuroendocrine control of the postpartum period. Clin Perinatol 1983;10:723.

McNeilly AS: Prolactin and the control of gonadotrophin secretion in the female. J Reprod Fertil 1980;58:537.

Moore P et al: Insulin binding in human pregnancy: Comparisons to the postpartum, luteal and follicular states. J Clin Endocrinol Metab 1981;52:937.

Oats JN, Beisher NA: The persistence of abnormal glucose tolerance after delivery. Obstet Gynecol 1990; 75:397.

Oppenheimer LW et al: The duration of lochia. Br J Obstet Gynecol 1986;93:754.

Potter JM, Nestel PJ: The hyperlipidemia of pregnancy in normal and complicated pregnancies. Am J Obstet Gynecol 1979;133:165.

Robson SC et al: Hemodynamic changes during the puerperium: A Doppler and M-mode echocardiographic study. Br J Obstet Gynecol 1987;94:1028.

Sheehan KL, Yen SSC: Activation of pituitary gonadotropic function by an agonist of luteinizing hormone-releasing factor in the puerperium. Am J Obstet Gynecol 1979;135:755.

Smith R, Thomson M: Neuroendocrinology of the hypothalamo-pituitary-adrenal axis in pregnancy and the puerperium. Ballieres Clin Endocrinol Metab 1991;5:167.

South-Paul JE, Rajagopal KR, Tenholder MF: Exercise responses prior to pregnancy and in the postpartum state. Med Sci Sports Exerc 1992;24:410.

Tay CCK, Glasier AF, McNeilly AS: The 24 h pattern of pulsatile luteinizing hormone, follicle stimulating hormone and prolactin release during the first 8 weeks of lactational amenorrhoea in breastfeeding women. Hum Reprod 1992;7:951.

Van Rees D, Bernstine RL, Crawford W: Involution of the postpartum uterus: An ultrasonic study. J Clin Ultrasound 1981;9:55.

Walters BNJ et al: Blood pressure in the puerperium. Clin Sci 1986;71:589.

Ylikorkala O, Viinikka L: Thromboxane $A_2$ in pregnancy and puerperium. Br Med J 1980;281:1601.

## COMPLICATIONS DURING THE PUERPERIUM

Bigrigg A, Chissel S, Read MD: Use of intramyometrial 15-methyl prostaglandin $F_{2\alpha}$ to control atonic postpartum hemorrhage following vaginal delivery and failure of conventional therapy. Br J Obstet Gynaecol 1991;98:734.

Bowes W: The puerperium and its complications. Curr Opin Obstet Gynecol 1990;20:780.

Cox SM, Gilstrap LC III: Postpartum endometritis. Obstet Gynecol Clin North Am 1989;16:363.

Gilbert WM, Moore TR, Resnik R et al: Angiographic embolization in the management of hemorrhagic complications of pregnancy. Am J Obstet Gynecol 1992;166:493.

Lev-Toaff AS, Baka JJ, Toaff ME et al: Diagnostic imaging in puerperal febrile morbidity. Obstet Gynecol 1990;75:402.

Roti E, Emerson CH: Clinical Review 29: Postpartum thyroiditis. J Clin Endocrinol Metab 1992;74:3.

Sutton MSJ, Cole P, Plappert M et al: Effect of subsequent pregnancy on left ventricular function in peripartum cardiomyopathy. Am Heart J 1991;121:1776.

Watson AB Jr: The puerperium and its complications. Curr Opin Obstet Gynecol 1990;2:780.

## CONDUCT OF THE PUERPERIUM

Black NA et al: Postpartum rubella immunization: A controlled trial of two vaccines. Lancet 1983;2:990.

Chi IC, Gates D, Thapa S: Performing tubal sterilizations during women's postpartum hospitalization: A review of the United States and international experiences. Obstet Gynecol Surv 1992;47:71.

Freda VJ et al: Prevention of Rh hemolytic disease: Ten years' clinical experience with Rh-immunoglobulin. N Engl J Med 1975;292:1014.

Fuller WE: Family planning in the postpartum period. Clin Obstet Gynecol 1980;23:1081.

Hume AL, Hijab JC: Oral contraceptives in the immediate postpartum period. J Fam Pract 1991;32:423.

Kennedy K, Visness C: Contraceptive efficacy of lactational amenorrhea. Lancet 1992;339:227.

Kowalski K: Managing perinatal loss. Clin Obstet Gynecol 1980;23:1113.

Mabray CR: Postpartum examination: A reevaluation. South Med J 1979;72:1433.

O'Hanley K, Huber DH: Postpartum IUDs: Keys for success. Contraception 1992;45:351.

Perez A, Labbok M, Queenan J: Clinical study of the lactational amenorrhea method for family planning. Lancet 1992;339:968.

Reamy K, White SE: Sexuality in pregnancy and the puerperium: A review. Obstet Gynecol Surv 1985;40:1.

## LACTATION

Aono T et al: Effect of sulpiride on poor puerperal lactation. Am J Obstet Gynecol 1982;143:927.

Anderson PO: Drug use during breast-feeding. Clin Pharm 1991;10:595.

Berlin CM Jr: Pharmacologic considerations of drug use in the lactating mother. Obstet Gynecol 1981;58(5 Suppl):17S.

Cunningham A, Jelliffe D, Jelliffe P: Breast-feeding and health in the 1980s: A global epidemiologic review. J Pediatr 1991;118:659.

Dusdieker LB et al: Effect of supplemental fluids on human milk production. J Pediatr 1985;106:207.

European Multicenter Study Group for Cabergoline in Lactation Inhibition: Single dose cabergoline versus bromocriptine in inhibition of puerperal lactation: Randomized, double blind, multicentre study. Br Med J 1991;302:1367.

Glass RI et al: Protection against cholera in breast-fed children by antibodies in breast milk. N Engl J Med 1983;308:1389.

Hayslip CC, Klein TA, Wary L, Duncan WE: The effects of lactation on bone mineral content in healthy postpartum women. Obstet Gynecol 1989;73:588.

Kleinberg DL et al: Estradiol inhibits prolactin induced $\alpha$-lactalbumin production in normal primate mammary tissue in vitro. Endocrinology 1982;110:279.

Kochenour NK: Lactation suppression. Clin Obstet Gynecol 1980;23:1045.

Kramer MS: Does breast feeding help protect against atopic disease? Biology, methodology and a golden jubilee of controversy. J Pediatr 1988;112:2.

Lawrence R: The puerperium, breastfeeding, and breast milk. Curr Opin Obstet Gynecol 1990;2:23.

Lawrence RA: *Breast-Feeding: A Guide for the Medical Profession.* Mosby, 1980.

McNeilly AS: Effects of lactation on fertility. Br Med Bull 1979;35:151.

Specker B, Tsang R, Ho M: Changes in calcium homeostasis over the first year postpartum: Effect of lactation and weaning. Obstet Gynecol 1991;78:56.

Van de Perre P, Simonon A, Msellati P et al: Postnatal transmission of HIV type 1 from mother to infant. N Engl J Med 1991;325:593.

West CP: The acceptability of a progestin-only contraceptive during breast-feeding. Contraception 1983; 27:563.

Whitehead RG: Nutritional aspects of human lactation. Lancet 1983;1:167.

Ziegler JB: Breast feeding and HIV. Lancet 1993; 342:1437.

Zinaman M, Highes V, Queenan J et al: Acute prolactin and oxytocin response and milk yield to infant suckling and artificial methods of expression in lactating women. Pediatrics 1992;89:437.

# Section III.
# The Pregnancy at Risk

# Methods of Pregnancy Assessment for Pregnancy at Risk

# 13

*Robert J. Sokol, MD, Theodore B. Jones, MD, & Martin L. Pernoll, MD*

## Essentials of Diagnosis

- A careful history to reveal specific risk factors.
- A maternal physical examination organized to identify or exclude risk factors.
- Routine maternal laboratory screening for common disorders.
- Special maternal laboratory evaluations for disorders suggested by any evaluative process.
- Comprehensive fetal assessment over the course of pregnancy.
- Recognition of the method most likely to effect an atraumatic delivery.
- Careful neonatal examination and assessment.

## General Considerations

Human reproduction is neither as physiologic nor as successful as was once thought. Probably more than 50% of conceptions are lost before pregnancy is even recognized; another 15–40% are lost in the first trimester. Of the latter group, over 60% have abnormal karyotypes, defying current methodologies for prevention of loss. However, many other causes of reproductive jeopardy are amenable to diagnosis and treatment. Thus,one of the major purposes of antenatal care is to detect disorders that place either mother or fetus at risk. Proper identification of those at risk may allow timely intervention with prevention of morbidity and mortality. Indeed, unanticipated maternal, fetal, or neonatal losses are less frequent if sustained care has been provided throughout pregnancy. Moreover, although the higher maternal and perinatal morbidity and mortality rates of some nations or populations may be related to a less advanced state of economic and industrial development, differences in groups at similar levels are more directly related to variations in the availability and quality of maternal and neonatal care.

## HIGH-RISK PREGNANCY

High-risk pregnancy is broadly defined as one in which the mother, fetus, or newborn is or will be at increased risk for morbidity or mortality before or after delivery. Many factors may be involved, including poor nutrition, inadequate prenatal care, unintended pregnancy, genetic abnormalities, and preexisting maternal or fetal disease. Obstetric disorders that commonly impose higher risks on the mother and fetus include preeclampsia-eclampsia, abruptio placentae, prematurity, and small size for gestational age (SGA) infant, among many others (Table 13–1). The purpose of this chapter is to detail essential aspects of the diagnostic modalities available for determination of pregnancies at risk.

## Maternal & Infant Morbidity & Mortality Related to High-Risk Pregnancy

The incidence of high-risk pregnancy varies according to the criteria used to define it. A great many factors are involved, and the outcome of any given factor may be quite different in different patients. Risk factors are often identified only in retrospect.

In the USA in 1980, the incidence of maternal deaths directly related to obstetric causes was 1.2 per 100,000 births. Leading causes of maternal death are pulmonary thromboembolic disease and pregnancy-induced hypertension, followed by uterine hemorrhage and sepsis.

Statistics on perinatal infant deaths in the USA usually count stillbirths as well as deaths of preterm infants weighing 500 g or more and infants up to 28 days of age. Neonatal mortality (ie, excluding stillbirths) in the USA has fallen steadily in recent years to the present level of 10 deaths per 1000.

Most perinatal deaths not directly due to congenital anomalies are associated with breech presentation, abruptio placentae, preeclampsia-eclampsia, twinning, pyelonephritis, placenta previa, or polyhydramnios. Stillbirth has been associated with advanced maternal age, massive obesity, and a high antepartum risk score.

**Table 13–1.** Risk factors related to specific pregnancy problems.

**Preterm labor**
  Age below 16 or over 35 years
  Low socioeconomic status
  Maternal weight below 50 kg (110 lb)
  Poor nutrition
  Previous preterm birth
  Incompetent cervix
  Uterine anomalies
  Smoking
  Drug addiction and alcohol abuse
  Pyelonephritis, pneumonia
  Multiple gestation
  Anemia
  Abnormal fetal presentation
  Preterm rupture of membranes
  Placental abnormalities
  Infection
**Polyhydramnios**
  Diabetes mellitus
  Multiple gestation
  Fetal congenital anomalies
  Isoimmunization (Rh or ABO)
  Nonimmune hydrops
  Abnormal fetal presentation
**Intrauterine growth retardation (IUGR)**
  Multiple gestation
  Poor nutrition
  Maternal cyanotic heart disease
  Chronic hypertension
  Pregnancy-induced hypertension
  Recurrent antepartum hemorrhage
  Smoking
  Maternal diabetes with vasculopathy
  Fetal infections
  Fetal cardiovascular anomalies
  Drug addiction and alcohol abuse
  Fetal congenital anomalies
  Hemoglobinopathies
**Oligohydramnios**
  Renal agenesis (Potter's syndrome)
  Prolonged rupture of membranes
  Intrauterine growth retardation
  Intrauterine fetal demise
**Postterm pregnancy**
  Anencephaly
  Placental sulfatase deficiency
  Perinatal hypoxia, acidosis
  Placental insufficiency
**Chromosomal abnormalities**
  Maternal age 35 years or more at delivery
  Balanced translocation (maternal and paternal)

# PRECONCEPTIONAL EVALUATION

The concept of preconceptional evaluation and counseling of women of reproductive age has gained increasing acceptance as an important component of women's health. Care given in the family planning and gynecology office should be based on the premise that the patient is a reproductive-capable woman. Issues of potential consequence to a pregnancy (ie, medical problems, harmful lifestyle habits, genetic issues) should be investigated and interventions devised.

# MATERNAL ASSESSMENT FOR POTENTIAL FETAL OR PERINATAL RISK

## UNIFORM PERINATAL RECORD

A number of forms have been developed to assist the physician in evaluating risk factors in pregnancy. Some forms are simple lists; others rate factors numerically according to their importance. Records such as the HOLLISTER and POPRAS forms, which provide uniform data for each patient, are helpful both in diagnosis and in management decision-making.

## INITIAL SCREENING

### History

**A. Maternal Age:** Women ages 20–29 years have the lowest rates of maternal, perinatal, and infant morbidity and mortality; younger and older women have higher rates.

**1. Adolescent pregnancy**–Pregnancy in adolescents is often associated with emotional stress and poor nutrition. Patients age 16 years or younger have an increased risk of preeclampsia-eclampsia. Low birth weight in infants of adolescents is increased and is probably due to organic causes such as placental abnormalities, poor nutrition, smoking, and drug use. Programs for pregnant adolescents that provide emotional support and nutritional supplements reduce the risks in this age group.

**2. Pregnancy in older women**–Advanced maternal age (age 35 or older at delivery) is more likely to be associated with pregnancy-induced hypertension. Obesity, diabetes, and uterine myomas are also more common in older women.

Chromosomal abnormalities (especially trisomy syndromes) are more common in infants born to older women. The age-specific risk of chromosomal trisomy rises from 0.9% at age 35–36 years to 7.8% at age 43–44 years. Since 50% of abnormal pregnancies end in spontaneous abortion, the actual rate of trisomy in newborns is about 50% of the fetal rate. Even if there is no family history of genetic abnormality, genetic counseling (see Chapter 5) should be provided for pregnant women age 35 years and older; some authorities recommend it for women age 33 and older. Amniocentesis in the early midtrimester or chorionic villus sampling in the first trimester should be offered. An increased risk of trisomy has been noted in association with low levels of maternal serum alpha-fetoprotein (AFP; % of the gestational age-related median). Testing followed by an appropriate genetic workup may detect up to 70% of all trisomies prenatally. Women 35 and older are often delivered by cesarean section in current clinical practice. This may reflect the patient's and the physician's attitudes toward the "premium pregnancy"—eg, making sure nothing goes wrong with what may be perceived as a "last chance" to have a child—rather than the presence of obstetric indications for cesarean delivery. Age alone is not an acceptable indication for delivery by cesarean section.

**B. History of Previous Pregnancies:** The outcome of previous pregnancies is relevant to the current pregnancy. The more term deliveries in the obstetric history (up to 5), the better the chance of a successful outcome, and vice versa. Second pregnancies have the lowest perinatal mortality rates.

The following historical events should be considered high-risk factors.

**1. Habitual abortion**–Habitual abortion is defined as 3 or more consecutive spontaneous losses of a nonviable fetus. In some series, an association with preterm delivery has been noted; this may be related to difficulty in differentiating between spontaneous abortion early in the second trimester, spontaneous abortion due to incompetent cervical os, and very early preterm birth. Habitual abortion is best investigated before another pregnancy occurs. Parental balanced chromosomal translocations, uterine and cervical anomalies, infections, connective tissue diseases, and hormonal abnormalities should be ruled out. (See also Chapters 5 and 14.)

**2. Previous stillbirth or neonatal death**–A history of stillbirth or neonatal death may suggest fetal or parental cytogenetic abnormality, but the first task is to investigate and rule out systemic maternal diseases such as diabetes, chronic renovascular disease, and chronic hypertension. Exclusion of connective tissue disease is important, since stillbirth and repeated early pregnancy loss may be associated with the presence of circulating antibodies, most notably the lupus anticoagulant or anticardiolipin antibody. Autopsy, radiographs, and skin biopsy of the stillborn infant to identify cytogenetic disorders may be of help in counseling about future pregnancies.

**3. Previous preterm or SGA infant**–It is important to distinguish between previous preterm and previous SGA infants. The mother may remember the birth weight and the estimated gestational age but may not realize that the infant was SGA rather than premature. The greater the number of previous preterm deliveries, the greater the risk at present and the more closely the patient should be watched for early onset of contractions. A woman who has had a previous SGA infant should be evaluated for associated risks such as hypertension, renal disease, inadequate weight gain, infection, cigarette smoking, or alcohol abuse. (See also Chapter 16.)

**4. Previous large infant**–A previous macrosomic infant (> 4000 g) suggests maternal diabetes mellitus. It is now recommended that all women be screened between the 24th and 28th gestational weeks with a 50-g 1-hour oral glucose challenge test. Women with a previous macrosomic infant, poor obstetric history, or family history of diabetes should be screened at their initial visit and, if normal, tested again as outlined. (See Chapters 16 and 18.)

**5. Grand multiparity**–Many clinicians believe that women who have had 6 or more previous deliveries are at increased risk of uterine inertia during labor and of postpartum hemorrhage due to uterine atony. Precipitous labor and delivery may occur in multiparas, with resulting soft tissue trauma and hemorrhage. Blood products for rapid transfusion should be readily available. Placenta previa is more common in the multiparous patient. (See also Chapter 17.)

**6. Previous infant with Rh isoimmunization or ABO incompatibility**–Blood typing of both parents and blood group antibody screening of the mother should be done at the first prenatal visit. Women at risk for Rh(D) isoimmunization should be screened for anti-Rh(D) antibody at varying intervals during pregnancy.

**7. Previous preeclampsia-eclampsia**–Previous preeclampsia-eclampsia increases the risk for hypertension in the current pregnancy, especially if there is underlying chronic hypertension or renal disease. (See Chapter 18.)

**8. Previous infant with known or suspected genetic disorder or congenital anomaly**–A woman who has had an infant with a genetic disorder or congenital anomaly should be offered genetic counseling. Testing is available for some defects with ultrasonography, amniocentesis, chorionic villus sampling, DNA linkage studies, and DNA analysis. Elevated maternal serum alpha-fetoprotein levels in the second midtrimester can assist in identification of fetuses with neural tube defects. (See Chapter 5 for discussions of genetic defects, counseling, and testing.)

**9. Previous birth-damaged infant or infant requiring special neonatal care**–A history of shoulder dystocia or other mechanical problems during delivery should be sought. Preterm delivery is the most common situation requiring admission of the neonate to the intensive care unit.

**10. Previous pregnancy terminated upon medical indication (rare)**–Termination of pregnancy due to maternal disease is usually limited to those with Marfan's syndrome, severe cardiovascular disease, advanced diabetes mellitus, or severe renal disease with high serum creatinine levels. (See also Chapters 23 and 24.)

**11. Other risk factors from the history of previous pregnancies**–These include rapidly succeeding pregnancies (< 3 months between delivery and conception); operative deliveries (cesarean, midforceps, breech extraction; see Chapter 27); prolonged labor or dystocia (see Chapter 25); and severe psychologic disturbances associated with labor and delivery (see Chapter 60).

**C. History of Reproductive Tract Disorders:**

**1. Genital tract abnormalities**–Incompetent cervical os is the most common example. Uterine anomalies such as septate uterus or bicornuate uterus are difficult to detect during pregnancy and are best evaluated by hysteroscopy or hysterosal pingography between pregnancies. (See Chapters 4, 35, 36, 47, and 48.)

**2. Uterine leiomyomas**–Uterine leiomyomas occur more frequently in older women and may be associated with an increased risk of recurrent pregnancy loss, hemorrhagic degeneration during pregnancy or in the postpartum period, dystocia or malpresentation (if the myoma is large), and adherent placenta. Submucous myomas present the greatest problem. (See Chapter 36.)

**3. Cervical lesions**–Appropriate management of cervical disorders varies with their nature (cell type) and severity. Cervical colposcopy is usually done early. Biopsy examination of a lightly atypical lesion may be deferred until after delivery to avoid the increased risk of bleeding from the site during pregnancy. Because of the risk of malignant spread, a patient with invasive cervical carcinoma should be delivered by cesarean section, sometimes followed by radical hysterectomy. The clinician should be aware of the association between papillomavirus and herpes simplex virus infections. (See Chapters 35 and 47.)

**4. Ovarian mass**–Malignant ovarian tumors are relatively rare during the reproductive years. Rupture of an ovarian dermoid cyst with resulting peritonitis may occur during labor or delivery. Symptomatic or enlarging ovarian masses may require operative removal. The optimal time for laparotomy is during the second trimester, when the risks of abortion and preterm delivery are thought to be minimal. Luteomas of pregnancy identified at cesarean section should not be removed. (See Chapter 37.)

**5. Other historical risk factors**–History of infertility (see Chapter 53) or of operative procedures involving the uterus or cervix.

**D. Medical Complications of Pregnancy:** Specific disease states may adversely affect the outcome of pregnancy for the mother or infant. Pregnancy itself may aggravate certain medical disorders and ameliorate others. Table 13–2 lists the most important disorders that may complicate pregnancy. (See also Chapters 23 and 24.)

**E. Exposure to Teratogens:** A teratogen is any substance, agent, or environmental factor that can adversely affect the development of the fetus. Less than 1% of all malformations are related to chemicals, radiation, or drug exposure. Drugs known to have teratogenic effects include alcohol, phenytoin, folic acid antagonists, lithium, mercury, valproic

**Table 13–2.** Some diseases and disorders complicating pregnancy.

Chronic hypertension
Renal disease
Diabetes mellitus
Heart disease
Previous endocrine ablation (eg, thyroidectomy)
Maternal cancer
Sickle cell trait and disease
Substance use or abuse
Pulmonary disease (eg, tuberculosis, sarcoidosis, asthma)
Thyroid disorders
Gastrointestinal and liver disease
Epilepsy
Blood disorders (eg, anemia, coagulopathy)
Others, including previous pelvic injury or disease producing pelvic deformity, connective tissue disorders, mental retardation, psychiatric disease

acid, streptomycin, tetracycline, thalidomide, trimethadione, androgens, diethylstilbestrol, chemotherapeutic compounds, antithyroid agents, and warfarin. Infections that have been proved to be teratogenic include coxsackievirus infection, cytomegalovirus, herpes simplex, viral hepatitis, influenza, mumps, poliomyelitis, rubella, varicella, syphilis, listeriosis, mycoplasmosis, and toxoplasmosis. *Listeria monocytogenes* may cause fetal death in utero. Other infections such as herpes simplex, hepatitis B, and human immunodeficiency virus are significant risk factors for perinatal infection. Certain chemicals and x-radiation may be detrimental, and some nutrients needed for normal development may cause fetal anomalies if taken in excessive amounts (eg, vitamin A). Indeed, it currently may be worthwhile to query the patient concerning possible use of isotretrinoin (Acutane). The patient should be asked about possible exposures and advised what to avoid. Information on nutritional needs during pregnancy should be provided. (See Chapter 9.)

**F. Family History:** A detailed family history is important to determine whether mental retardation, twinning, or heritable diseases have occurred. The risk assessment of the current pregnancy is facilitated by a 3-generation pedigree. (See Chapter 5.)

## Physical Examination

At the initial prenatal visit, a complete physical examination should be performed. The obstetrician-gynecologist may be the patient's only physician, and the examination done as part of antenatal care may occasionally uncover a previously unsuspected medical problem. Particular attention should be paid to the thyroid, breasts, lungs, heart, and abdomen. Findings on physical examination that bear on pregnancy risk are discussed briefly here.

**A. Stature:** The mother's height correlates with pelvic capacity. Women under 150 cm (5 ft) tall have an increased likelihood of fetopelvic disproportion.

Short stature is an indication for careful assessment of the bony pelvis. (See Chapter 16.)

**B. Weight:** Women who weigh less than 45 kg (100 lb) when not pregnant have an increased likelihood of delivering an SGA infant. Weight gain should be encouraged for these women. Maternal obesity is a risk factor for fetal macrosomia, probably both as a direct cause and because diabetes mellitus may be associated with obesity. Few clinicians use weight-for-height charts, so obesity is often defined as weight of more than 90 kg (200 lb) regardless of height. Morbid obesity is often defined as weight of more than 115 kg (250 lb). Such patients also have increased risk of dysfunctional labor and shoulder dystocia, according to some studies. Some clinicians feel that restricted (rather than normal) weight gain during pregnancy is beneficial for obese women, but this view is controversial. (See Chapter 16.)

**C. Blood Pressure:** The normal tendency of both systolic and diastolic blood pressures to decrease in the midtrimester may complicate the diagnosis of chronic hypertension in patients first evaluated at this time. A rapid increase in blood pressure, often in association with proteinuria and central edema, is characteristic of preeclampsia.

**D. Eyes:** Retinal changes associated with chronic hypertension are sometimes seen, but diabetic retinopathy is of greater concern. Careful evaluation of the ocular fundi for evidence of neovascularization is indicated in patients with diabetes. Ophthalmologic referral is usually indicated. A detached retina in a pregnant diabetic woman is an emergency, since permanent blindness may result unless the detachment is treated promptly, usually by laser.

**E. Thyroid:** Some clinicians believe that the thyroid feels somewhat "fuller" during pregnancy, although objective evidence is lacking. If the thyroid is palpably enlarged, further workup, including serum total thyroxine (T4), resin uptake of triiodothyronine (RT3U), and free thyroxine index (FT4I), is indicated. Hyperthyroidism, particularly with thyroid storm, poses a major maternal risk during pregnancy.

**F. Breasts:** Breast engorgement during pregnancy makes detection of masses more difficult, so that breast cancer is often detected at a later stage. If a mass is palpable, the usual breast cancer workup should be performed without delay. (See Chapter 62.)

**G. Heart:** Abnormalities noted by cardiac auscultation call for electrocardiography and perhaps cardiologic referral for diagnosis. Diastolic murmurs always require further workup. Systolic ejection murmurs are extremely common.

**H. Vascular System:** Severe varicosities may cause major discomfort during pregnancy. If associated with incompetent perforating veins, varicosities probably increase the risk of development of thrombophlebitis.

## Pelvic Examination

The pelvic examination may reveal abnormalities that will affect the outcome of pregnancy:

**A. Uterus:**

**1. Uterine prolapse–**Prolapse of the uterus, particularly if the cervix extends beyond the introitus, usually requires temporary artificial support with a pessary until normal uterine growth lifts the pregnancy out of the pelvis. Chronic cervicitis may require treatment with antibiotics.

**2. Uterine retroflexion–**Incarcerated retroflexed uterus may be associated with pelvic pain and possibly lead to abortion near the end of the first trimester. There may be associated maternal urinary retention. Timely manipulation of the incarcerated uterus while the patient is in the knee-chest position usually is successful in moving the uterus out of the pelvis.

**3. Uterine anomalies–**Uterine anomalies may lead to preterm labor and increased perinatal losses and are often difficult to detect during pregnancy. (See Chapter 4.)

**B. Cervix:** Cervical tumors or dilatation or prior deep lacerations may predispose to cervical incompetency.

**C. Vagina and Vulva:** Some abnormalities of the vagina and vulva may distort the birth canal (eg, large Gartner duct cysts, surgical scarring, septation, or massive condylomata acuminata. Condylomas may be associated with severe hemorrhage in relation to laceration or episiotomy. (See Chapters 4, 34, and 46.)

**D. Ovaries and Uterine Tubes:** Adnexal tumors over 5 cm in diameter may require intervention during pregnancy. (See Chapters 37 and 49.)

**E. Pelvic Architecture:** Severe orthopedic deformity is now rare because of improved nutrition. Scoliosis may cause slight deformity of the pelvis, which should be carefully evaluated. Restricted range of motion of the hips is sometimes seen in patients with rheumatoid arthritis and may be severe enough to prevent delivery in the lithotomy position. Such patients often are delivered in the Sims position.

**F. Pelvic Capacity:** Methods of measuring pelvic capacity are outlined in Chapter 9. Vaginal delivery may be difficult if there is a palpable promontory of the inlet (diagonal conjugate of < 11.5 cm); if the midpelvis has prominent ischial spines, convergent side walls, a flat sacrum, or a sacrospinous ligament of less than 5 cm; or if the outlet has an intertuberous diameter of less than 8.5 cm or a narrow suprapubic angle (< 90 degrees).

## Estimation of Gestational Age

Methods of estimating gestational age are outlined in Chapter 9. Inappropriate uterine size for dates presents a major management problem. Many decisions that must be made later in pregnancy (eg, when or whether to do a cesarean section) depend on accurate assessment of the duration of the pregnancy. Thus, size-for-dates discrepancy is a clear indication for both sonographic evaluation and serial height measurements throughout pregnancy. Possible reasons for size-for-dates discrepancies are inaccurate dating of conception, multiple pregnancy, polyhydramnios, SGA fetus, the presence of uterine leiomyomas, and fetal death in utero. The SGA fetus is perhaps the most commonly missed problem, often misinterpreted as an error in dating of the conception. Since the SGA fetus is at risk for intractable neurobehavioral abnormalities, every effort should be made to avoid overlooking that diagnosis.

### Estimation of Fundal Height and Fetal Presenting Position and Lie

See Chapters 9 and 10.

## COURSE OF PREGNANCY

Every antenatal visit should be regarded as an opportunity to anticipate problems that may beset the mother and fetus. At these visits, special attention should be paid to the following problems.

**A. Weight Gain:** Inadequate progressive weight gain may reflect nutritional deficit, maternal illness, or a hormonal milieu that does not promote proper volume expansion and anabolic state. Often, this is associated with poor fundal growth and a small fetus and placenta, suggesting fetal growth retardation. Weight gain and fundal height should be closely monitored during pregnancy.

**B. Hypertension:** Repeated blood pressure readings of 140/90 mm Hg, of a rise in systolic pressure of 30 mm Hg, or of a diastolic pressure 15 mm Hg higher than in early pregnancy should be considered evidence of preeclampsia. The need for hospitalization is controversial, but increased bed rest is certainly indicated. Diuretics are controversial and generally contraindicated. (See Chapter 19.)

**C. Pyelonephritis:** At the first antenatal visit, urinalysis should be done and a clean voided specimen collected for culture and sensitivity testing. Patients with bacteriuria of more than 100,000 organisms per milliliter should be given antibiotics to minimize the risk of pyelonephritis. If pyelonephritis develops, hospitalization and treatment with intravenous hydration and antibiotics may be necessary. After completing initial antibiotic therapy, the patient should be monitored for recurrent bacteriuria, which may require retreatment. Several authors have suggested using oral antibiotics prophylactically for the remainder of pregnancy after an episode of pyelonephritis, whereas others suggest its use after any recurrence.

**D. Fever:** High maternal fever (> 39.5°C [103°F]) is thought to trigger preterm labor. It may also injure the fetal central nervous system. The cause of fever should be determined, appropriate treatment given, and uterine activity carefully monitored. Antipyretics or a cooling blanket may be necessary to lower the temperature. If chorioamnionitis is suspected, amniocentesis for microscopy and culture should be considered; delivery may be necessary.

**E. Isoimmunization:** Blood typing and screening for Rh isoimmunization and abnormal antibodies should be done at the initial visit. If antibodies are detected, they are usually quantitated as a titer. The most common type of sensitization is to Rh(D) antigen, for others see Table 13–3. If the patient is Rh-negative and screening reveals no Rh antibodies at the initial visit, the screening test should be repeated at 24 weeks of gestation. If the screening test gives positive results, follow-up with amniocentesis may be appropriate depending on the antibody titer. All Rh-negative women carrying a pregnancy fathered by an Rh-positive man and who have a negative indirect Coombs' test (no free circulating antibodies) should be given 300 µg of Rh-immune globulin at the beginning of the third trimester (about 28 weeks) to prevent sensitization by the fetus during the last trimester.

**F. Diabetes Mellitus:** Routine screening consists of determining blood sugar 1 hour after a 50-g oral glucose load. If the plasma blood sugar level is over 135–140 mg/dL, a 3-hour glucose tolerance test should be performed. If 2 out of the 4 values on the glucose tolerance test are in the abnormal range, the patient is considered to have gestational diabetes and needs to be treated. Oral hypoglycemic agents are contraindicated in pregnancy.

**G. Third-Trimester Uterine Bleeding:** Any uterine bleeding late in the second trimester or at any time during the third trimester is a serious matter calling for prompt investigation and management. The most common causes of third-trimester bleeding are placenta previa, abruptio placentae, and lower genital tract trauma. "Bloody show"—discharge of blood-tinged mucus—usually means that the cervix has dilated somewhat and that the onset of labor is imminent. Bleeding related to placenta previa is usually not accompanied by pain, and the uterus is soft and relaxed. Sonography is a fairly reliable means of

**Table 13–3.** The most common blood antigens with the potential for severe isoimmunization.

| Blood Group | Antigen |
| --- | --- |
| Kell | K |
| Duffy | Fy$^a$ |
| Kidd | Jk$^a$ |
| | Jk$^b$ |
| MNSs | M |
| | S |
| | s |
| | U |
| Diego | Di$^a$ |

diagnosing low-lying placenta. In abruptio placentae, the patient typically complains of abdominal pain with associated uterine tenderness and uterine contractions.

**H. Uterine Size-for-Dates Discrepancy:** Sonography is helpful in establishing gestational age. In general, the earlier that sonography is done in the second trimester, the more precise is the estimate. Repeated ultrasound examinations at least 3 weeks apart improve the accuracy of the data obtained.

**I. Polyhydramnios and Oligohydramnios:** Polyhydramnios (hydramnios) is the excessive accumulation of amniotic fluid. The diagnosis is usually made sonographically. In severe cases, it can cause severe maternal dyspnea and premature labor. Polyhydramnios may be caused by maternal diabetes, fetal anomalies (esophageal atresia, trisomy 18, anencephaly, and spina bifida), placental abnormalities, multiple gestation, or isoimmunization; in about one-third of cases, the cause is unknown.

Oligohydramnios is severe deficiency of amniotic fluid (sometimes defined as maximum vertical pocket of < 1 cm determined by sonography). It may be caused by premature rupture of membranes, obstruction of the fetal urinary tract, severe intrauterine growth retardation, or fetal demise. Some congenital fetal anomalies (eg, Potter's syndrome) are also associated with oligohydramnios. When oligohydramnios occurs early in pregnancy, it is often associated with a poor fetal outcome and can lead to fetal pulmonary hypoplasia, amniotic band syndrome, and fetal compression. (See also Chapter 15.)

**J. Preterm Labor:** Onset of labor prior to 37 weeks of pregnancy is considered preterm labor. Incompetent cervix, previous uterine surgery, uterine anomalies, excessive cigarette smoking or maternal stress, multiple gestation, polyhydramnios, and antepartum bleeding can be associated with preterm labor. Maternal infections (eg, bacterial pneumonia, cystitis and pyelonephritis and appendicitis) can cause preterm labor. Intrauterine infection with intact membranes can also cause preterm labor. A patient with a history of premature labor is at increased risk for recurrence and should be followed closely. Once detected, idiopathic premature labor should be vigorously treated with intravenous hydration and tocolytic agents (ritodrine, terbutaline, and magnesium sulfate). An important consideration is an evaluation of the pregnancy for evidence of intraamniotic infection.

**K. Multiple Gestation:** The most common type of multiple gestation is twins. Twins may be "identical" (monozygotic) or "fraternal" (dizygotic). The incidence of multiple gestation is increased by induction of ovulation, particularly if gonadotropin therapy has been used. Multiple gestation is associated with an increased incidence of fetal malformations, premature labor, and complications of labor and delivery. Early detection of multiple gestation by sonography may help in management. Some authors have advocated early selective abortion if more than 3 fetuses are detected.

**L. Postterm Pregnancy:** Pregnancy that continues beyond 42 weeks (or beyond 294 days from the last menstrual period) is considered prolonged or postterm. There is general agreement that without proper management, the neonatal mortality rate in such cases is increased considerably, perhaps 3- to 5-fold. Some clinicians believe that all—or almost all—such pregnancies should be delivered promptly. This approach may decrease the risks of perinatal morbidity and mortality, but in some cases it has been associated with high rates of cesarean birth. Careful evaluation of the postterm pregnancy must be done to ensure that the fetus is not asphyxiated, as can occur in postmaturity syndrome, a diagnosis that can only be made after delivery. Postmature babies have meconium staining of the skin and membranes, decreased subcutaneous fat, and peeling skin. Oligohydramnios is also present. Antepartum surveillance, usually starting at 41 weeks, includes biweekly nonstress tests (NSTs) or contraction stress tests (CSTs) combined with sonographic evaluation of amniotic fluid volume. An abnormal NST or CST, the presence of oligohydramnios, or meconium-stained amniotic fluid may identify the postmature fetus. These are generally considered indications for delivery.

**M. Acute Surgical Problems:** Any problem that occurs in nonpregnant women may also occur in pregnant patients (eg, appendicitis, cholecystitis, peptic ulcer disease). Appendicitis during pregnancy often presents in an atypical manner and may be difficult to diagnose. This can lead to delay in operative intervention with increased maternal morbidity rates and risk of preterm labor. (See also Chapter 24.)

## COURSE OF LABOR

When a patient has been admitted to the labor and delivery area, risk assessment must not only be continued but intensified. The prenatal history should be reviewed for any factors that may predispose to intrapartum risk. Any problems that have developed since the last antepartum visit must be recorded and evaluated by physical examination. Attention is then turned to risks that may develop during labor. A review of risks listed in the preceding section on perinatal morbidity will indicate the importance of the intrapartum period and its complications as determinants of infant outcome. In this section, the focus will be on labor complications and fetal factors associated with increased risk.

### Abnormal Progress of Labor

Major dysfunctional labor patterns include a prolonged latent phase, protraction patterns (eg, protracted active phase, dilatation and protracted descent, and arrest abnormalities), secondary arrest of dilatation, and arrest of descent. For management of these abnormalities, see Chapter 26. Prior to the use of fetal monitoring, arrest disorders were associated with increased risk of fetal distress and lowered IQ in children 3–4 years of age. More recent studies suggest that with appropriate conservative management, including a judicious trial of labor with oxytocin augmentation, fetal monitoring, and cesarean delivery in appropriate cases, risks to the fetus can be eliminated. A key component of management is appropriate diagnosis, which may be facilitated by charting the progress of labor.

## Fetal Distress

**A. Fetal Monitoring:** Monitoring of the fetal heart rate and uterine contractions during labor allows early detection of abnormalities that may endanger the fetus. The tracing must be assessed continuously to detect problems as soon as they develop. Interpretation of the tracing is an art.

Risk factors detected by monitoring are abnormal uterine contraction patterns (including uterine tachysystole and tetanic contractions) and fetal heart rate abnormalities (including tachycardia, bradycardia, flattened heart rate baseline, late decelerations, and extreme variable decelerations). A useful rule of thumb is that the later, deeper, and longer the deceleration, the more threatening it is. In addition, the combination of meconium in the amniotic fluid and fetal heart rate decelerations indicate increased risk. The presence of more than one sign of fetal distress on the monitor tracing should be more worrisome than intermittent isolated findings.

**B. Fetal Scalp Blood Sampling:** Fetal scalp blood sampling for determination of pH can be helpful in arriving at a diagnosis of true fetal distress. A pH of more than 7.25 is usually considered to be in the normal range. A pH of 7.0–7.25 should be interpreted as preacidosis, and testing should be repeated immediately. A pH of less than 7.0 indicates acidosis and the need for prompt intervention.

## Other Abnormalities of Labor

**A. Meconium Staining:** The presence of meconium in the amniotic fluid should be considered an indicator of fetal risk and is an indication for fetal monitoring. Meconium staining is much more common in term and postterm pregnancies than in preterm pregnancies and may be a marker of full fetal

**Table 13–4.** Mean ultrasound measurements at given gestational ages.

| Menstrual Age (weeks) | Biparietal Diameter (cm) | Head circumference (cm) | Abdominal Circumference (cm) | Femur Length (cm) |
|---|---|---|---|---|
| 12 | 2.0 | 7.1 | 5.6 | 0.8 |
| 13 | 2.3 | 8.4 | 6.9 | 1.1 |
| 14 | 2.7 | 9.8 | 8.1 | 1.5 |
| 15 | 3.0 | 11.1 | 9.3 | 1.8 |
| 16 | 3.3 | 12.4 | 10.5 | 2.1 |
| 17 | 3.7 | 13.7 | 11.7 | 2.4 |
| 18 | 4.0 | 15.0 | 12.9 | 2.7 |
| 19 | 4.3 | 16.3 | 14.1 | 3.0 |
| 20 | 4.6 | 17.5 | 15.2 | 3.3 |
| 21 | 5.0 | 18.7 | 16.4 | 3.6 |
| 22 | 5.3 | 19.9 | 17.5 | 3.9 |
| 23 | 5.6 | 21.0 | 18.6 | 4.2 |
| 24 | 5.8 | 22.1 | 19.7 | 4.4 |
| 25 | 6.1 | 23.2 | 20.8 | 4.7 |
| 26 | 6.4 | 24.2 | 21.9 | 4.9 |
| 27 | 6.7 | 25.2 | 22.9 | 5.2 |
| 28 | 7.0 | 26.2 | 24.0 | 5.4 |
| 29 | 7.2 | 27.1 | 25.0 | 5.6 |
| 30 | 7.5 | 28 | 26.0 | 5.8 |
| 31 | 7.7 | 28.9 | 27.0 | 6.1 |
| 32 | 7.9 | 29.7 | 28.0 | 6.3 |
| 33 | 8.2 | 30.4 | 29.0 | 6.5 |
| 34 | 8.4 | 31.2 | 30.0 | 6.6 |
| 35 | 8.6 | 31.8 | 30.9 | 6.8 |
| 36 | 8.8 | 32.5 | 31.8 | 7.0 |
| 37 | 9.0 | 33.1 | 32.7 | 7.2 |
| 38 | 9.1 | 33.6 | 33.6 | 7.3 |
| 39 | 9.3 | 34.1 | 34.5 | 7.5 |
| 40 | 9.5 | 34.5 | 35.4 | 7.6 |

Reproduced, with permission, from Hadlock FP et al: Computer assisted analysis of fetal age in the third trimester using multiple fetal growth parameters. J Clin Ultrasound 1983;11:313. Copyright © 1983 by John Wiley & Sons, Inc. Reprinted by permission of John Wiley & Sons, Inc.

maturation. Its presence during labor should be noted and taken seriously, so that internal electrical fetal monitoring can be instituted, through DeLee nasopharyngeal suctioning performed at delivery and postdelivery. Recent evidence indicates that the potential morbidity of meconium in the amniotic fluid may be largely eliminated by amnioinfusion of normal saline during labor. In those with fetal distress, in the depressed neonate, in those with respiratory distress, and in those with thick meconium, the suctioning must be carried below the level of the vocal cords to avoid meconium aspiration.

**B. Uterine Atony:** When oxytocin augmentation of labor is necessary, the possibility of uterine atony in the immediate postdelivery period with associated hemorrhage is materially enhanced. Uterine atony may also be seen after delivery of multiple fetuses and in grand multiparas.

## DELIVERY

Risks to the mother and fetus during delivery include the following.

### Analgesia and Anesthesia

The major maternal risk of anesthesia (and one of the major causes of maternal death today) is aspiration pneumonia. The risk is considerably increased during labor because of slowed gastric emptying.

Another hazard is inadequate placental perfusion secondary to hypotension. This may be a direct result of supine hypotension syndrome, which may occur when the pregnant woman is placed in the supine position and the enlarged uterus compresses the venous system, producing decreased venous return, lowered cardiac output, and hypotension. The syndrome may be more severe when regional anesthesia has been given (eg, spinal or epidural anesthesia), causing general systemic hypotension. The syndrome can be avoided by adequate hydration and by placing the patient on her left side, thereby displacing the uterus to the left so that venous return is not obstructed.

Injection of local anesthetic directly into the fetus (eg, during paracervical or pudendal block) can lead to rapid fetal demise.

Other risks include overdosage of general anesthesia, inadequate pulmonary ventilation, and inadequate oxygenation. Pregnant patients tend to become hypoxic more rapidly than nonpregnant ones because of reduced residual lung volume. Therefore, 100% oxygen should be administered prior to induction of general anesthesia for operative delivery.

### Trauma

Direct trauma may affect the mother or fetus during vaginal or cesarean delivery.

**A. Maternal Trauma:** The theory that episiotomy prevents pelvic relaxation in later years is diffi-

cult to prove; however, an appropriately sized and placed episiotomy is more easily repaired than a jagged laceration. Postpartum pain may be minimized by the use of polyglycolic suture rather than chromic catgut. With either laceration or episiotomy, placement of the first stitch above the highest point is a key in reducing the risk of dangerous continued postpartum hemorrhage. Development of vesicovaginal fistula is now extremely rare, probably because of fewer neglected labors. With cesarean delivery, the clinician must assess the risk of tearing the uterine artery with a low transverse cervical incision. The lower uterine segment may be poorly developed in early preterm labor, particularly if the fetus is in preterm breech presentation or transverse lie. Tears of the uterine artery may be avoided by the use of a low vertical incision, although there may be more bleeding from the vertical incision.

**B. Fetal Trauma:** Trauma to the fetus may also occur during delivery. Difficult breech extraction, especially in association with internal podalic version, may result in fetal trauma. This procedure is now used only for the delivery of the second twin in transverse lie, although many physicians consider external version and cesarean section to be safer alternatives. Skull fractures in the parietal area may occur spontaneously during delivery. Basilar skull fractures are more frequently related to difficult midforceps procedures. Fetal trauma is generally considered iatrogenic and constitutes not only a significant medical risk for the fetus but a legal risk for the physician. Difficult midforceps procedures should surely be avoided, although the easier low midforceps operations are still acceptable. With suspected macrosomia, midforceps procedures should be avoided because of the association with shoulder dystocia and the risk of brachial plexus damage. Although unusual, fetal injuries to the scalp or underlying tissue may also occur in association with the use of fetal spiral electrodes used for direct fetal heart rate monitoring, fetal scalp sampling for assessment of blood pH, or vacuum extraction cups used to facilitate delivery.

## POSTPARTUM PERIOD

The mother is still at risk for complications during the immediate and late postpartum periods. To minimize the risk of immediate postpartum hemorrhage, the obstetrician must have a clear plan of action. The placenta must be carefully examined and the uterus carefully explored to rule out cervical or vaginal laceration or retained products of conception. If uterine atony occurs, direct uterine compression is the first step, followed by use of oxytocic agents. Use of prostaglandin preparations produces effective uterine contractions and decreased bleeding associated with uterine atony. Thus, in some cases, the risks associated with ligation of the uterine or hypogastric artery or with postpartum hysterectomy have been avoided. Oxytocin should not be given to prevent bleeding upon delivery of the anterior shoulder because there may be an oncoming undiagnosed second twin. (Twinning is undiagnosed in about 5% of cases, even when prenatal ultrasound is used.)

Appropriate management of the third stage of labor can minimize the risk of uterine inversion (rare). Other postpartum risks include infection (endometritis; wound infection in cesarean delivery), thrombophlebitis and thromboembolism, urinary retention, late postpartum hemorrhage, and postpartum psychosis.

## NEONATAL PERIOD

The obstetrician should perform a rapid and immediate assessment of the neonate in the delivery room. Apgar scores at 1, 5, and sometimes 10 minutes after birth are assigned by the obstetric or neonatal nurse or by the pediatrician. The obstetrician should look for signs of prematurity and intrauterine growth retardation. Low-birth-weight infants should be immediately dried to minimize heat loss, since hypothermia may lead to respiratory distress and acidosis. The obstetrician should carefully examine the genitalia and look for any major congenital anomalies as well as signs of respiratory difficulty (eg, chest wall retraction with respiration, nasal flaring, "grunting").

The rate of neonatal risk depends on the patient population served by the clinician; 5–10% of infants commonly require special or intensive neonatal care. The most common significant problems are associated with low birth weight related to preterm delivery or SGA. Macrosomic infants may also develop significant problems. Term infants who are appropriate for gestational age (AGA)—approximately 85% of births—seldom develop significant neonatal problems in the absence of severe asphyxia or birth trauma. Some of the more common neonatal problems are discussed below. (See also Chapter 29.)

### General Problems

Preterm and postterm infants and those who are growth-retarded or macrosomic are at increased risk. Blood glucose measurements for infants of diabetic mothers must be followed closely to avoid severe hypoglycemia. Hypoglycemia, particularly when associated with neonatal seizures, probably constitutes a risk for long-term neurobehavioral abnormality. Infants of drug-dependent mothers are at risk for withdrawal symptoms.

### Skin

A rash may signify viral infection (eg, herpes simplex, varicella, cytomegalovirus infection). Neonatal disseminated herpesvirus infection remains a life-threatening complication, even with the use of antiviral agents. This risk can be minimized by appropriate prenatal diagnosis of maternal herpesvirus infection and cesarean delivery if the mother has recent positive cultures or active disease.

### Head and Neck

Craniofacial abnormalities may be markers for fetal alcohol syndrome or fetal hydantoin syndrome. Cataracts may suggest in utero rubella infection. Bulging fontanelles may reflect intracerebral bleeding.

### Respiratory System

Transient tachypnea of the newborn tends to be associated with preterm delivery and is generally self-limited, but respiratory distress syndrome continues to be a problem, particularly in very low-birth-weight infants (< 1500 g) or asphyxiated infants. Other serious neonatal risks include meconium aspiration, persistent apnea, and bronchopulmonary dysplasia related to high oxygen concentrations and prolonged use of the respirator. Recurrent apnea and bradycardia, particularly in low-birth-weight infants, are considered by some to be risk factors for later development of sudden infant death syndrome (SIDS). Finally, intrauterine stress may enhance the possibility of perinatal pulmonary hypertension.

### Cardiovascular System

Cardiac abnormalities sometimes require extensive workup and surgical correction in the neonatal period. Patent ductus arteriosus may require surgical closure. Persistent fetal circulation may be associated with perinatal asphyxia.

### Gastrointestinal System

A major risk is necrotizing enterocolitis, which sometimes occurs in nursery epidemics and may be associated with retrovirus infection. It tends to be a problem among low-birth-weight infants but often develops late, after they have been advanced to the progressive care nursery.

### Neurologic System

Withdrawal symptoms may occur in infants of drug-addicted mothers. A major problem is neonatal seizures, which are possibly the most reliable predictor of later neurobehavioral abnormality. The inciting factors and risks related to intracerebral bleeding are receiving intensive attention in the literature as a result of their serious medical and legal implications.

### Other Risks

Renal failure may be associated with perinatal asphyxia. Sepsis is a frequent concern in the neonatal intensive care unit.

## SUMMARY & CONCLUSIONS

It is often said that pregnancy and labor and delivery are normal physiologic processes. This is an obvious truth, but the many problems discussed here emphasize the necessity for close observation and the importance of early detection of abnormalities.

Abnormalities tend to occur in clusters or in association with one another. Awareness of these relationships and the patterns in which they occur is the mark of a seasoned clinician. Ideal obstetric care in high-risk pregnancy might be described as "intensive observation and minimal but appropriate and timely intervention." No pregnancy should be considered routine.

## ANTEPARTUM TESTING IN PREGNANCIES AT RISK

### ULTRASONOGRAPHY

Ultrasonography has been applied clinically in several forms. B-scan ultrasound provides a static 2-dimensional representation of fetal structures; real-time scans show movement of these structures. Both rely on the same principle. As a pulsed ultrasonic beam strikes a tissue interface, an echo is obtained where densities differ. In the interval between pulses, the transducer acts as a receiver for the reflected sound. The sound is then converted into electrical energy, amplified, and recorded. Real-time ultrasonography uses a linear array of sequentially pulsating transducers, and a sector scanner uses an oscillating transducer. Integrative hardware and software allow for viewing of soft tissue structures. Ultrasound scans have no adverse fetal effects as far as is known.

Until the advent of sonography, it was not possible to measure fetal growth accurately. Because the normal fetus and placenta constitute an ever-enlarging entity, various methods of evaluation have been devised in an attempt to measure growth as a function of fetal gestational age and health. Serial sonographic measurements of the fetal parts now provide a more precise means of determining pregnancy dating and fetal growth and obtaining other useful information.

Diagnostic ultrasonography may be used to measure fetal biparietal diameter, abdominal circumference, and femur length, which may be used in estimation of gestational age, assessment of fetal growth, and estimation of fetal weight (see Table 13–4 on p 282). Transvaginal ultrasonography has aided the clinician by allowing reliable imaging at early gestational ages( beginning at 5–6 weeks). Such imaging allows for the clinician to: clarify the location of a pregnancy where in doubt, establish early gestational criteria, and, in expert hands, provide early diagnosis of fetal anomalies. It is also useful in assessing placental location, molar or multiple gestation, fetal location and attitude, fetal abnormalities (anencephaly, hydrocephaly), and fetal death. Other uses include early identification of intrauterine or extrauterine pregnancy, assessment of amniotic fluid volume, identification of uterine or ovarian tumors, detection of foreign bodies, assistance with therapeutic procedures, and assessment of fetal well-being by viewing fetal heart rate and activity.

Newly developed ultrasonic Doppler techniques have been recently applied to obstetrics. Assessment of umbilical blood flow using Doppler waveform analyses may help to identify a fetus at risk for intrauterine growth retardation.

The application of real-time ultrasonic evaluation to the evaluation of fetal well-being is discussed in the section on Biophysical Profile, which follows. Because radiography may be hazardous, and because of the greater accuracy and detail provided by ultrasonography, radiography is rarely done, except in rare instances in which fetal bony abnormalities must be precisely defined.

### PRENATAL DIAGNOSIS

Prenatal diagnosis can be offered for a number of disorders (Table 13–5). The techniques (amniocentesis, chorionic villus sampling, and fetal blood sampling) involve obtaining fetal cells for analysis.

#### Amniocentesis

Amniocentesis is performed under the guidance of ultrasonography. A needle is inserted through the mother's abdominal wall—directly into the amniotic sac—and amniotic fluid is obtained. The most common use of this procedure is to collect fetal cells from the amniotic fluid to use in performing cytogenetic analysis. Amniocentesis is usually done between 16 and 18 weeks of gestation, but it can be performed as early as 12 weeks. Early samples may have fewer cells available for study. Risks associated with the procedure are considered very low; the risk of abortion as a result of amniocentesis is generally considered to be 1 in 200 or less at most centers. Because many other disorders are now or soon will be detectable, when a specific case is encountered, a tertiary care center doing antenatal genetic diagnosis should be consulted. Only experienced personnel should undertake this procedure, which must be accomplished

**Table 13–5.** Disorders that may be detected by antenatal diagnosis.

**Chromosome disorders**
  Abnormalities of chromosome number, eg, trisomy 21, trisomy 18, Turner's syndrome.
  Aberrations of chromosome structure, eg, cri du chat syndrome.
**Fetal sex in X-linked disorders,** eg, Duchenne muscular dystrophy, factor VIII hemophilia.
**Neural tube defects,** eg, anencephaly, myelomeningocele.
**Inborn errors of metabolism**
  Lipidoses, eg, Fabry's disease, Gaucher's disease, generalized gangliosidosis, juvenile GM gangliosidosis, Tay-Sachs disease, Sandhoff's disease, Krabbe's disease, metachromatic leukodystrophy, Niemann-Pick disease type A.
  Mucopolysaccharidoses, eg, type I (Hurler), type II (Hunter), type III (Sanfilippo A).
  Amino acid and related disorders, eg, argininosuccinicaciduria, citrullinemia, cystinuria, severe infantile maple sugar urine disease, methylmalonic aciduria responsive to vitamin $B_{12}$.
  Carbohydrate metabolism disorders, eg, galactosemia, glycogen storage disease types II and IV.
**Miscellaneous,** eg, adenosine deaminase deficiency, congenital nephrosis, cystinosis, hypophosphatasia, I cell disease, Lesch-Nyhan syndrome, lysosomal acid phosphatase deficiency, xeroderma pigmentosum, sickle cell anemia, cystic fibrosis, beta-thalassemia.

by a team (an obstetrician experienced in early amniocentesis, a medical genetic group with biochemical and cytogenetic expertise, a genetic counseling service, and the full range of professional referral services).

## Chorionic Villus Sampling

An alternative to amniocentesis is chorionic villus sampling. It is performed transcervically or transabdominally, at between 9 and 11 weeks of gestation. Under sonographic guidance, a sterile catheter is placed into the uterine cavity and directed toward the placental site. Chorionic villi are aspirated and later analyzed. Worldwide studies are still in progress regarding the safety and efficacy of this procedure, but it appears to have risks similar to or slightly greater than those associated with amniocentesis. Reports of limb reduction deformities of distal extremities appear to be rare and time-critical (performed before the 66th day.) The benefit of chorionic villus sampling is that since it can be performed earlier in gestation, termination of pregnancy can still be performed in the first trimester if a result that shows fetal abnormalities is obtained. The procedure should be performed only by carefully trained personnel.

## Fetal Blood Sampling

Fetal blood sampling, also referred to as cordocentesis or percutaneous umbilical blood sampling, is a very recent addition to the techniques of prenatal diagnosis. It is performed only in very selected cases and by a limited number of carefully trained personnel. The umbilical cord is identified using sonography, and a sterile needle is placed within the umbilical vessels to obtain fetal blood. The procedure is done in the second and third trimesters, and the blood can be analyzed for chromosomal or metabolic abnormalities. The benefit of this procedure is the rapidity with which results can be obtained; however, it may be associated with a 1–2% risk of fetal death in certain situations.

## Clinical Application

Fetal cells can be analyzed for chromosomal or metabolic disorders. This is especially important if the mother is 35 years of age or older at the time of delivery, has had a previously affected child, or has a significant family history of such disorders. For evaluation of chromosomes, the fetal cells are grown and a karyotype analysis is performed. Results can be completed within several days (on fetal blood cells) or several weeks, depending on the rate of cell growth. Specific enzymes can be assayed in certain metabolic diseases (eg, Tay-Sachs disease or Gaucher's disease). New techniques in molecular genetics are becoming available for the detection of other diseases. Using restriction endonucleases, DNA sequences can be evaluated. These capabilities have aided in the prenatal diagnosis of sickle cell anemia and other disorders in which the molecular defect is known. In disorders such as cystic fibrosis or polycystic kidney disease, in which the molecular defect has not yet been determined, however, DNA linkage analysis may be available in certain situations.

Maternal serum **alpha-fetoprotein (AFP) testing** is now done often for neural tube defects and other rarer abnormalities. AFP levels are raised in any situation with increased exposure of fetal blood to the maternal circulation, including threatened abortion, twin gestation, and abruptio placentae, as well as in more advanced gestations that have been misdated. Elevated levels in accurately dated pregnancies are followed up by amniocentesis for determination of amniotic fluid AFP levels. Elevated levels suggest the presence of neural tube, abdominal wall, and other fetal anomalies, including fetal death, many of which are detectable by ultrasonography; a moderate amount of elevated AFP values may represent false-positive results. It has been shown that of 25 women with one elevated serum AFP level, in only one instance will it eventually prove to be associated with a fetal neural tube defect. Low values of AFP have been reported to be associated with fetuses with chromosome abnormalities, esp. Down's syndrome. Women with such testing results have a risk level greater than that accorded a 35-year-old woman. Low values of AFP and maternal age increased the incidence of detection from 20% detectable by age alone to nearly 50%. Recently, the addition of either human chorionic gonadotropin alone or with unconjugated estriol (UE3) to MSAFP and maternal age has been reported to increase the detection rate to between 60–65%. However, the majority of the trisomies diagnosed are trisomy 21, and such testing has not yet been acknowledged as standard of care. In cases of known or suspected Rh isoimmunization, amniocentesis may be done from the midpoint of gestation to evaluate fetal bilirubin levels (see Chapter 13).

Amniocentesis has also been performed to detect amniotic fluid infection following premature spontaneous rupture of the membranes. The amount of amniotic fluid available will be reduced, however, and risks must be carefully weighed against benefits. Some authorities feel that bacteria in the amniotic fluid in these cases does not present a significant fetal risk and recommend against amniocentesis. This opinion presumes that cervical cultures have ruled out group A or B streptococcus, gonococcus, *Listeria monocytogenes*, and *Staphylococcus aureus*.

## PULMONARY MATURITY TESTING

Analysis of the phospholipids present in the amniotic fluid has aided in the timing of delivery in certain circumstances. The major problem faced by premature infants is respiratory distress syndrome (RDS). When phospholipids have been synthesized by the fetus at a certain point in gestation, the risk of RDS is minimized.

Pulmonary surfactant is an anti-atelectasis factor that normally prevents the collapse of alveoli. Surfactant is synthesized by the type II alveolar cells. The major phospholipids that are analyzed in amniotic fluid to assess fetal pulmonary maturity are lecithin (L), sphingomyelin (S), and phosphatidylglycerol (PG).

The amniotic fluid concentration of lecithin increases dramatically at approximately 35 weeks of gestation, whereas the level of sphingomyelin remains stable (Fig 13–1). These facts have led to the use of the L/S ratio, which has proved to be the most valuable assay of fetal pulmonary maturity. In general, an L/S ratio of 2 or greater has been associated with pulmonary maturity in repeated studies. With an L/S ratio of 1.5–1.9, approximately 50% of infants will have RDS. The risk of RDS increases to 73% if the L/S ratio is below 1.5.

More recently, the presence or absence of PG has become important as a marker for completed pulmonary maturation. PG does not appear until 35 weeks of gestation and then increases in amount over the next few weeks. However, most infants who lack PG in the presence of a mature L/S ratio will not develop RDS. Research continues on other phospholipids

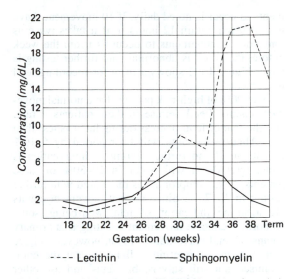

**Figure 13–1.** Measurement of the relationship of amniotic fluid lecithin to that of sphingomyelin has provided a practical means of evaluating maturity of the fetal lung. As shown, mean concentrations of surface-active lecithin and sphingomyelin normally do not differ significantly until about the 30th week of pregnancy; the sharp increase in lecithin at 35 weeks reflects activation of the choline incorporation pathway of lecithin synthesis and signifies that pulmonary maturity is sufficient to prevent respiratory distress syndrome from occurring.

present in the amniotic fluid and their potential applicability in determining fetal lung maturity.

## BIOMETRIC EVALUATION OF FETAL WELL-BEING

Antepartum surveillance is used to identify potential fetal compromise. Although typically the nonstress test (NST), contraction stress test (CST), and biophysical profile (BPP) are used in office or hospital settings, opinion differs as to which test is preferable. In general, each has a different end point, and the tests can be used together in assessing fetal status. Some disorders that may be detected by antenatal diagnosis are listed in Table 13–5.

## 1. FETAL MOVEMENT COUNTING

Fetal movements are noted subjectively by most pregnant women. After the fetus has reached viability, the mother is asked to report any diminution in activity as a possible sign of fetal compromise. Several formal methods of counting in high-risk pregnancies have been studied. The time required for 10 movements to occur is noted daily. If 10 movements have not occurred within 12 hours or if it takes twice as long for 10 movements to occur as it did the week before, the count is abnormal, and further testing is done. Figure 13–2 shows a form for recording fetal movements.

Over 90% of high-risk patients have normal movement counts. Fetal demise in these patients is rare, and the rate of fetal distress during labor is less than 5%. Abnormal counts will be reported by 5–10% of patients. If no further testing or intervention is done, fetal death will occur in 10–30% of these patients. Fetal compromise is diagnosed with further testing in 40–70%. Since normal movement counts are a strong indication of fetal well-being, some authorities endorse movement counting as a primary means of fetal surveillance. Most, however, believe that movement counting will not reveal the compromised but still salvageable fetus and use other tests as well (eg, NST, CST, BPP). At the very least, fetal movement counting remains a helpful adjuvant in the surveillance of the fetus for evidence of well-being.

## 2. NONSTRESS TEST

The normal fetus has sleep-wake cycles of 20–45 minutes, with cycle length gradually increasing with advancing gestational age. During rapid eye movement (REM) sleep and during awake periods, movements of the limbs and trunk and breathing movements occur. Body movements are usually associated with accelerations in fetal heart rate. The presence of normal movements and accompanying fetal heart rate accelerations strongly suggests that the uteroplacental unit is functioning normally. Movements are absent during non-REM sleep, when there are certain anomalies of the fetal central nervous system,

after administration of sedative-hypnotic drugs or ingestion of alcohol, and when the fetus is hypoxic-acidotic.

### Indications

The NST is usually the primary means of fetal surveillance for most conditions that place the fetus at high risk for placental insufficiency.

### Protocol

The external fetal monitor is used. The mother should be in the lateral or supine position with a lateral tilt to prevent supine hypotensive syndrome. Fetal movements are recorded, and fetal heart rate changes are monitored. The test is classified as reactive if, during a 20-minute period, at least 2 accelerations of the fetal heart rate are present, each at least 15 beats above the baseline rate and lasting at least 15 seconds. The test is nonreactive if fewer than 2 such accelerations are present in a 45-minute period. The baseline fetal heart rate, apparent beat-to-beat and long-term variability, and the presence of contractions or fetal heart rate decelerations are also noted.

Typical reactive and nonreactive tracings are shown in Figures 13–3 and 13–4.

The NST is performed weekly or twice weekly, depending on the reason for testing (Table 13–6). If the test is reactive (negative for evidence of fetal compromise), the pregnancy is allowed to continue and the test is repeated at the appropriate interval. If the test is nonreactive (positive for evidence of fetal compromise), additional testing is performed.

The fetus is more active 1–2 hours after meals; thus, the NST is ideally performed in the postprandial interval.

### Clinical Usefulness

A reactive NST with an otherwise normal tracing is an excellent indicator of fetal well-being. When the NST is used as the primary means of antepartum sur-

## Fetal Movement Record

|  | M | Tu | W | Th | F | Sat. | Sun. |
|---|---|---|---|---|---|---|---|
| 8 AM |  |  |  |  |  |  |  |
| 10 AM |  |  |  |  |  |  |  |
| 12 PM |  |  |  |  |  |  |  |
| 2 PM |  |  |  |  |  |  |  |
| 4 PM |  |  |  |  |  | Name: |  |
| 6 PM |  |  |  |  |  | Date: |  |
| 8 PM |  |  |  |  |  | EGA: |  |

**Figure 13–2.** Fetal movement record. The patient begins to count movements at 8:00 AM daily and marks the time at which the 10th movement is felt. If 10 movements are not felt by 8:00 PM or if it takes twice as long to feel 10 movements as on prior days, the physician is contacted.

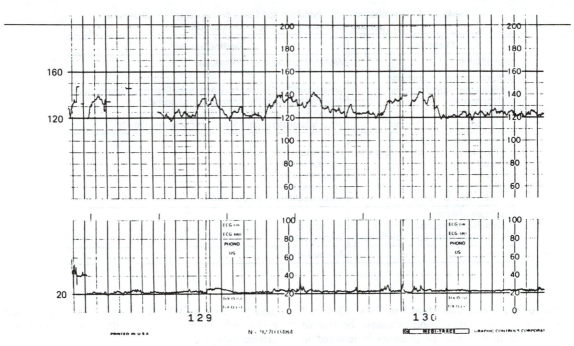

**Figure 13–3.** Reactive tracing in nonstress test. Two accelerations of 15-beat amplitude lasting more than 15 seconds are seen in this 7-minute segment of recording.

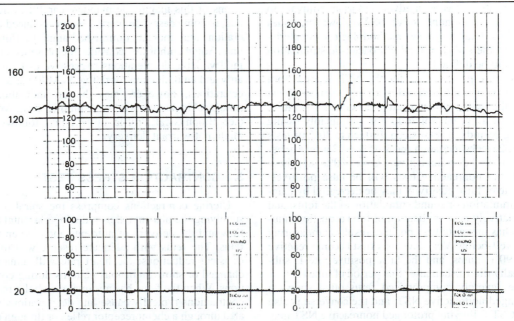

**Figure 13–4.** Nonreactive tracing in nonstress test. No accelerations are seen in this segment of recording. No accelerations were seen subsequently for 25 minutes, but the test showed reactive accelerations after 45 minutes.

**Table 13–6.** Nonstress testing schedule in conditions predisposing to fetal demise (presuming fetal viability has been reached).

| Diagnosis | Testing Interval |
|---|---|
| Prior stillbirth | Weekly (starting at 32–35 weeks) |
| Maternal medical conditions | |
|   Insulin-dependent diabetes | Weekly at 32–35 weeks (earlier if indicated), then twice weekly |
|   Hypertension | Weekly (starting at 32–35 weeks or when indicated) |
|   Renal disease | Weekly (starting at 32–35 weeks or when indicated) |
|   Collagen vascular disease | Weekly (starting at 28–35 weeks or when indicated) |
| Obstetric complications | |
|   Premature rupture of membranes | At admission to hospital |
|   Preeclampsia | Twice weekly if stable |
|   Discordant twins | Twice weekly |
|   Intrauterine growth retardation | Twice weekly |
|   Postdates pregnancy | Twice weekly from 41.5 weeks |
| Fetal abnormalities | |
|   Diminished movement | As needed |
|   Decreased amniotic fluid volume | Twice weekly |
| Labor | As needed |

veillance at the intervals shown in Table 13–6 and when appropriate intervention is made, the rate of fetal demise in high-risk pregnancies is reduced to 1–3 per 1000; this is below the rate for unmonitored low-risk pregnancies.

The NST may be nonreactive even when the fetus is healthy. Use of drugs or alcohol by the mother or testing during a period of non-REM sleep may result in absence of movement or accelerations. In cases of drug or alcohol use, the CST will still be valid.

Vibroacoustic stimulation has been demonstrated to elicit a response in fetuses, the most common of which are FHR accelerations and fetal gross body movements. It has been advocated as an adjuvant to aid in clarifying nonreactive NSTs. However, issues regarding fetal response, methodologic characteristics, and the safety of fetal vibroacoustic stimulation remain to be defined.

The false-positive rate for the NST depends to a great extent on the duration of observation. Most NSTs that will become reactive do so within 45 minutes of testing, but some do not, presumably owing to long periods of fetal sleep. Fifteen to 30% of tests at 28–32 weeks' gestation and 3–15% at 33 weeks or beyond will be nonreactive. Over 80% of these 45-minute nonreactive tests will be false positives. The rate of false positivity may be decreased by manual stimulation or sound stimulation of the fetus, and the relatively new application of fetal acoustic stimulation has met with very positive results in measuring fetal well-being. Very few tests first become reactive after 90 minutes, and the false-positive rate is substantially diminished after this period of time.

The severely compromised fetus often shows a prolonged nonreactive NST, and the converse is also true. CST following prolonged nonreactive NST may result in profound decelerations of fetal heart rate in up to one-third of cases. Despite appropriate neonatal management, 5–30% of infants with unexplained prolonged nonreactive NSTs will die of chronic intrauterine asphyxia.

### Antepartum Fetal Heart Rate Decelerations

When decelerations are associated with contractions, interpretation and management are as the same as for CSTs. However, spontaneous decelerations may occur during nonstress testing. Decelerations of more than 40 beats/min or to rates of less than 90 beats/min with a duration of longer than 60 seconds are associated with extremely high rates of fetal demise (25%) and fetal distress in labor (50%). Decelerations of this magnitude mandate careful evaluation and, in some cases, delivery. Less pronounced decelerations may indicate diminished amniotic fluid volume. Some authorities consider the presence of even mild variable decelerations suggestive of fetal jeopardy and an indication for delivery. Mild variable decelerations, however, may be an indication for sonographic assessment of amniotic fluid volume (see Biophysical Profile in text that follows) and might not warrant delivery.

### 3. CONTRACTION STRESS TEST

Uterine contractions compress the spiral arteries supplying the placenta, thus reducing placental blood flow and the delivery of nutrients and oxygen to the fetus. The fetus with adequate reserve will tolerate transient reductions; the heart rate will remain unchanged or show innocuous patterns during contractions. When the fetus has minimal metabolic reserve, contractions typically cause late decelerations mediated through a chemoreceptor reflex or through direct myocardial depression. Thus, the presence of late decelerations is suggestive of fetal compromise, and the absence of late decelerations correlates with fetal well-being. However, late decelerations may occur whenever placental blood flow or oxygen supply is reduced (eg, with supine hypotensive syndrome, maternal hypoxia, or severe anemia) or may merely reflect transient reductions in fetal $PO_2$.

## Protocol

With the mother in the semi-Fowler position or with a lateral tilt to prevent supine hypotensive syndrome, external fetal monitors are applied. The fetal heart rate and any contractions are observed for a period of 20 minutes. Contractions are then induced by means of intermittent nipple stimulation or dilute oxytocin infusion. When oxytocin is used, the procedure is often referred to as an oxytocin challenge test (OCT). The fetal heart rate pattern is observed as the frequency of contractions increases to at least 3 but not more than 5 in 10 minutes. Uterine stimulation is then discontinued, and the fetal heart rate is observed until induced contractions have subsided.

The test was originally performed by infusing oxytocin at a rate of 0.5 mU/min, with the rate increased every 20–30 minutes until adequate contractions were observed. However, experience has shown that intermittent nipple stimulation may obviate the need for oxytocin infusion in most patients. The patient stimulates the nipple of one breast through her clothing for 2 minutes and then ceases stimulation for 5 minutes. Coupled contractions—series of multiple contractions without uterine relaxation between—are sometimes seen with nipple stimulation, but the test can be successfully performed in over 80% of patients. With either oxytocin or nipple stimulation, the test often requires 1–2 hours to complete.

The test is judged reactive or nonreactive according to the same criteria as for the NST (see previous text). It is further categorized as follows: negative (no late decelerations); equivocal (nonrepetitive late decelerations); hyperstimulated (late decelerations following coupled contractions, contractions at a rate of more than 5 every 10 minutes, or contractions individually lasting more than 90 seconds); or positive (late decelerations occurring with each of 3 contractions in a 10-minute period).

## Contraindications

Unlike the NST, the CST involves uterine stimulation and thus may involve risk in some situations (Table 13–7). The CST does not ordinarily provoke labor but may do so in predisposed patients. In patients with prior uterine incisions, uterine rupture is a theoretic hazard. In most instances, when the test is performed in a facility fully prepared to respond to fetal or maternal emergencies, evaluation of fetal well-being is sufficiently important to justify the risk.

## Clinical Application

Negative CSTs are repeated at weekly (or more fre-

**Table 13–7.** Relative contraindications to contraction stress testing.

Predisposition to uterine rupture
    Previous classic cesarean section
    Previous full-thickness hysterectomy incision
Predisposition to premature delivery
    Premature rupture of membranes
    Premature labor
    Twins
    Hydramnios
    Incompetent cervix
Predisposition to bleeding
    Placenta previa
    Unexplained vaginal bleeding

quent) intervals; equivocal or "hyperstimulated" tests are repeated within 24 hours; and positive CSTs require further evaluation or immediate delivery.

Negative CSTs are excellent predictors of fetal health. The rate of false-negative tests (fetal demise within 1 week of a negative test) is approximately 1 per 1000.

Equivocal CSTs may be indicative of early fetal compromise or of a healthy fetus. When an equivocal CST is seen in conjunction with a reactive NST, the fetus is likely to be in good health. Fetal demise within the recommended 24-hour retesting interval is exceedingly rare and unrelated to predictable causes. Positive CSTs may occur because of supine hypotensive syndrome, fetal anomalies, diminished maternal blood oxygen-carrying capacity, or true uteroplacental insufficiency.

Twenty-five to 75% of positive CSTs occur in the absence of fetal compromise. It is possible to reduce the rate of unnecessary interventions by considering the presence or absence of fetal heart rate accelerations as well as the presence of late decelerations. These reactive-positive CSTs are frequently false-positive tests. Some authorities argue that the false-positive test represents the transition between the healthy and the severely compromised fetus, whereas others believe the fetus is unlikely to be suffering from uteroplacental insufficiency if fetal heart rate accelerations are still present. Management of the reactive-positive CST requires careful assessment and sound clinical judgment. For the mature fetus, delivery may be considered. Otherwise, the test may be repeated within 24 hours or an alternative means of fetal assessment, the BPP, may be considered (see following text). Doppler waveform analysis of umbilical blood flow may aid in the diagnosis of the compromised fetus.

The nonreactive-positive CST is more frequently indicative of fetal compromise but still can occur when the fetus will tolerate labor. In the near-term pregnancy, unless a correctable cause such as severe maternal anemia or hypotension can be found, delivery is mandated. If the fetus is very premature, a BPP may be done; if the score is 8 or more, it is likely that the fetus is in good health, and delivery may be delayed.

When the decision has been reached to deliver the fetus based on a positive CST, induction of labor with extremely close fetal monitoring may be appropriate if the cervix is favorable (see Chapter 10). Following nonreactive-positive CSTs, 25–50% of fetuses may tolerate labor. When the cervix is not favorable, cesarean delivery is appropriate. Even with expeditious delivery, a significant proportion of infants showing nonreactive-positive CSTs will succumb to sequelae of chronic intrauterine compromise or prematurity. However, if left in utero, a much larger proportion will die.

## 4. BIOPHYSICAL PROFILE

The fetal BPP is based on assessment of fetal heart rate, breathing movements, limb movements, and trunk attitude and movements and on measurement of amniotic fluid volume. The total score is obtained by addition of the numerical rating (2–0) for each parameter. Although some investigators have advocated adding the sonographic assessment of placental maturation known as "grading" to the BPP, this practice has not been widely accepted at this time. It is believed that hypoxia due to chronic uteroplacental insufficiency has varying effects on the central nervous system centers responsible for fetal tone, movement, breathing, and heart rate. Heart rate is thought to be the most affected, ie, the most sensitive to intrauterine stress and the earliest detectable factor, and tone is thought to be least affected. However, the fetal breathing is also very sensitive to stress and its absence may be the earliest sign of fetal compromise. Amniotic fluid volume is not acutely influenced by central nervous system alterations. The assessment of amniotic fluid volume in the BPP reflects the high correlation between low amniotic fluid amount and abnormal pregnancy outcome. The mechanism by which chronic fetal stress causes oligohydramnios is not well understood.

### Protocol

An NST is performed in association with the BPP. Depending on the results, this may take 45–90 minutes. Continuous real-time ultrasonography is then performed to obtain the remaining information included in the BPP. This may take only 15–20 minutes if the fetus is found to be normal or as long as 30 minutes if abnormalities are discovered. Scoring of the test is shown in Table 13–8. Fetal movement is reduced if the mother has ingested drugs or alcohol and reduced or absent during non-REM sleep. Oligohydramnios (reduced amniotic fluid volume) occurring in the presence of intact membranes and a normal fetal urinary system may be due to redistribution of fetal blood away from the kidneys to preserve the heart and brain.

Fetal activity is greatest 1–2 hours after the mother has had a meal; the same is true for breathing movements. Thus, the period of observation may be minimized by arranging testing inappropriate relation to meals or by offering the mother caloric liquids prior to testing. A score of 0 or 2 (positive test) indicates fetal jeopardy. Delivery should take place immediately. With a score of 4 or 6, delivery may be indicated or testing may be repeated within 24 hours, depending on the clinical situation. A score of 8 or 10 (negative test) indicates fetal well-being.

### Clinical Application

Advocates of the BPP point out that the ultrasound scan may detect lethal congenital anomalies; that the false-negative rate is about the same as that of the CST; and that the false-positive rate is substantially lower than that of either the NST or the CST.

Clinical experience with the BPP as a primary means of surveillance is not so extensive as with the other tests, but the rate of fetal demise is lower than 1 per 1000 patients tested.

The false-positive rate for the BPP appears to be quite low. In a blind trial conducted prior to general use of the test, test results were not used in planning management. Fetal distress during labor occurred in 100% of fetuses with a score of 0 and in 75% with a score of 2. Corresponding 5-minute Apgar scores below 7 were 80% and 50%, respectively. The false-positive rate of the BPP is reported to be less than 30%.

The BPP may not be accurate if sedative-hypnotic drugs have been given prior to testing or if alcohol has been ingested; that is, if a low BPP score is obtained under these circumstances, its accuracy must be questioned and the test either repeated when the

**Table 13–8.** Scoring of the biophysical profile.

|  | Normal (2) | Abnormal (1) |
|---|---|---|
| Amniotic fluid volume | Fluid pocket of 1 cm$^2$ or more | Oligohydramnios |
| Nonstress test | Reactive | Nonreactive |
| Breathing | At least one episode of breathing lasting at least 30 seconds | No episode of breathing |
| Limb movement | Three discrete movements | Two or fewer movements |
| Fetal tone | At least one episode of limb or trunk extension followed by return to flexion | No episode of movement |

offending agents have been metabolized or a CST performed. Furthermore, unlike the NST and CST, at least one component of the BPP may be affected by labor. Fetal breathing movements are thought to stop at the onset of true but not false labor; thus, the test may be invalid in the patient with productive uterine activity, although this, by definition, will lead to delivery. The test must be interpreted with caution when amniotic fluid volume is reduced because of rupture of the membranes. It is interesting that although it may no longer serve as a test of fetal compromise, the BPP may be a predictor of fetal infection during conservative management of premature rupture of the membranes. Indeed, over 90% of those with marginal or low scores proved to have infection. Absent or diminished fetal breathing movement is the most common abnormality. In less than 2% of infected fetuses, a normal BPP is recorded.

The BPP has a high rate of detection of anomalies among pregnancies showing intrauterine compromise. In one study, 1.5% of the fetuses tested were found to have serious anomalies. Based on this experience, even if the BPP is not the first line of antepartum fetal surveillance, an ultrasound scan to evaluate the possibility of a fetal anomaly is indicated when the result of any test of compromise is positive.

The BPP involves no fetal risk and relatively little time. Ultrasonographic examination requires some expertise and may involve physician time. If the amniotic fluid volume is normal and the NST is reactive, observation of the other factors usually adds little information (scores for these infants are almost always 8 or 10). Some institutions perform the NST and fluid assessment first; if these are normal, the testing is terminated, but in abnormal cases, ultrasonography or the CST is performed.

## ACCURACY OF ANTEPARTUM FETAL SURVEILLANCE

### False-Negative Tests

Although the introduction of fetal surveillance programs has regularly resulted in dramatic lowering of stillbirth rates, the tests are by no means perfect. The rate of fetal demise in unmonitored high-risk pregnancies is 10–30 per 1000; with antepartum surveillance, this rate is reduced to 1–3 per 1000, which is lower than the rate for unmonitored low-risk pregnancies (2–4 per 1000).

For each of the tests now in use (NST, CST, and BPP), any negative test for fetal compromise is repeated at weekly to twice-weekly intervals as long as the patient is clinically stable. If an underlying medical or obstetric condition deteriorates; if diminished fetal movement is reported; or when regular contractions begin, more intensive monitoring is indicated.

Apart from labor itself, 2 conditions place pregnancies at particularly high risk for intrauterine demise: insulin-dependent diabetes and postdates pregnancy. The mechanism by which diabetes mellitus predisposes to stillbirth is incompletely understood. It is thought that most fetal deaths among monitored patients (which may occur within 1 day of completely reassuring testing) may be related to erratic blood glucose control.

For postdates pregnancy, the CST is a good predictor of fetal well-being, but the NST alone may not be. In one series of 4000 patients, 8 potentially preventable stillbirths occurred in patients monitored by NSTs. Six of these were in postdates pregnancies; this was out of proportion to the percentage of postdates pregnancies in the monitored patients. In a smaller series of 125 postdates pregnancies in which the presence of fetal heart rate accelerations alone was taken to be a negative test for fetal compromise, 4 fetal deaths occurred. Induction of labor is commonly recommended in postdates pregnancies, particularly after 42.5 weeks, when the physician is confident that the duration of pregnancy has been measured correctly.

### True-Positive Tests

Anomalous infants commonly have "positive" tests for fetal compromise, nonreactive NSTs, positive CSTs, and low BPP scores. Many anomalies are not detectable by ultrasonography; however, others, such as anencephaly, are readily seen. A significant rate of detectable anomalies does occur among ultrasonically examined pregnancies and may be of great importance in planning obstetric intervention. The cost-benefit ratio of ultrasonographic screening of all pregnancies can be argued, but examination of the fetus showing signs of compromise is indicated.

Some fetuses may have suffered such extreme asphyxia that, despite prompt delivery, irreversible damage will have occurred and death may result. This is not an insignificant problem (Table 13–9). For infants with BPP scores of 0 or 2 and for those with

**Table 13–9.** Perinatal mortality rates following various test results.

| Test Outcome | Perinatal Mortality Rate (per 1000 deliveries) |
|---|---|
| Biophysical profile 8–10 | <10 |
| Contraction stress test negative | <10 |
| Nonstress test reactive | <10 |
| Biophysical profile 6 | ? |
| Contraction stress test reactive positive | 51 |
| Biophysical profile 4 | 90 |
| Biophysical profile 2 | 120 |
| Contraction stress test nonreactive positive | 211 |
| Biophysical profile 0 | 600 |

Data adapted from Freeman (1982) and Manning (1982).

nonreactive positive CSTs, intervention may come too late in 10–60% of cases.

When surveillance is positive for fetal compromise, a decision must be made regarding the timing of delivery. This may be particularly difficult if the infant must be delivered prematurely. The possibility of false-positivity must be considered, and the level of neonatal care available is also important. Most centers now have neonatal survival rates above 75%, even in the 26- to 28-week group. If test results are considered to be reliable and fetal compromise is strongly suspected, there is no choice but to deliver.

## SUMMARY

Each test of fetal compromise has significant shortcomings as well as advantages. Fetal movement counting is inexpensive and simple but is too subjective for use as a primary means of surveillance in most settings. The NST is inexpensive and entails no fetal risk but is affected by alcohol and drugs and has a higher false-positive and possibly false-negative rate than the BPP or CST. The CST is more expensive and inconvenient to perform than the NST, may provoke premature labor in predisposed patients, and may cause frank distress in the compromised fetus. The false-negative rate is low, but the false-positive rate may be as high as 25%, even when reactive-positive tests are eliminated. The BPP, when implemented on a large scale, is somewhat more expensive as a primary means of surveillance than the NST. Like the NST, it entails no fetal risk but may be affected by drugs and alcohol. The false-negative rate is comparable to that for the CST, but the false-positive rate appears to be substantially lower than for any of the other tests (Table 13–10).

The question of which means of primary antepartum fetal surveillance is the "best" is unsettled. Each practitioner and institution must choose, on the basis of published and personal experiences, how to assess high-risk obstetric conditions in a cost-effective and risk-beneficial fashion. Some perinatologists use the CST or BPP as a primary means of surveillance. At most institutions, facilities and finances do not permit this approach, and the NST is used as the primary test. Except in the postdates pregnancy, the NST may be supportable based on outcomes.

# INTRAPARTUM ASSESSMENT OF FETAL WELL-BEING

## COURSE OF LABOR

When a patient has been admitted to the labor and delivery area, risk assessment must not only be continued but intensified. The prenatal history should be reviewed for any factors that may predispose to intrapartum risk. Any problems that have developed since the last antepartum visit must be recorded and evaluated by physical examination. Attention is then turned to risks that may develop during labor. A review of risks listed in the previous section on perinatal morbidity will indicate the importance of the intrapartum period and its complications as determinants of infant outcome. In this section, the focus will be on the detection of labor complications and fetal factors associated with increased risk.

### Abnormal Progress of Labor

Major dysfunctional labor patterns include a prolonged latent phase, protraction patterns (protracted active phase, dilatation, and protracted descent) and arrest abnormalities (secondary arrest of dilatation, and arrest of descent). For management of these abnormalities, see Chapter 25. Prior to the use of fetal monitoring, arrest disorders were associated with increased risk of fetal distress and lowered IQ in children 3–4 years of age. More recent studies suggest that with appropriate conservative management, including a judicious trial of labor with oxytocin augmentation, fetal monitoring, and cesarean delivery in appropriate cases, risks to the fetus can be eliminated. A key component of management is appropriate diagnosis, which may be facilitated by charting the progress of labor.

### Meconium Staining

The presence of meconium in the amniotic fluid should be considered an indicator of fetal risk and is an indication for fetal monitoring. Meconium staining is much more common in term and postterm pregnancies than in preterm pregnancies and may be a marker of full fetal maturation. Its presence during

**Table 13–10.** Comparison of some tests of fetal well-being.

| Test | Cost | Risk | Time | False-Positive Rate | False-Negative Rate |
|---|---|---|---|---|---|
| Fetal movement counting | 0 | 0 | (0) | 30–60% | ?<5%) |
| Nonstress test | + | 0 | 30 minutes–2 hours | Depends on duration | 0.2–0.3% |
| Contraction stress test | +++ | + | 1–2 hours | 25–50% | 0.1% |
| Biophysical profile | +++ | 0 | 1–2 hours | <30% | 0.1% |

labor should be noted and taken seriously, so that internal electrical fetal monitoring can be instituted and DeLee suction prepared for at delivery to avoid meconium aspiration. Thorough nasopharyngeal suctioning of the fetus must be performed during delivery.

## Uterine Atony

When oxytocin augmentation of labor is necessary, the possibility of uterine atony in the immediate postdelivery period is materially enhanced.

## FETAL HEART RATE MONITORING

Fetal heart rate (FHR) monitoring as a means of assessing well-being has been the subject of some controversy. There is agreement that heart rate monitoring is based on clinical and laboratory studies demonstrating that fetal hypoxia reliably produces changes in FHR patterns. However, these abnormal patterns may also occur in the absence of fetal distress. There is general agreement concerning the desirability of detection of the compromised fetus, because current estimates indicate that about 20% of stillbirths, 20–40% of cases of cerebral palsy, and approximately 10% of cases of severe mental retardation arise from intrapartum events leading to asphyxia. Therefore, guidelines for clinical application are necessary.

The following discussion of electronic fetal monitoring conforms to the recommendations for current clinical practice set forth in the Report of the National Institute of Child Health and Human Development Consensus Development Task Force: *Predictors of Intrapartum Fetal Distress: The Role of Electronic Fetal Monitoring.*

Risk factors detected by monitoring include abnormal uterine contraction patterns (including uterine tachysystole and tetanic contractions) and FHR abnormalities (including tachycardia, severe bradycardia, flattened heart rate baseline, late decelerations, and extreme variable decelerations). A useful rule of thumb is that the later, deeper, and longer the deceleration, the more threatening it is. The presence of more than one sign of fetal distress on the monitor tracing should be more worrisome than intermittent isolated findings.

### Auscultatory Monitoring

The most widely used means (worldwide) of fetal assessment during labor is the head stethoscope. Even the most meticulous auscultatory monitoring is subject to considerable human error, so it must be undertaken with considerable care. The fetal heart tones should be recorded for 30 seconds immediately after a uterine contraction at least every 30 minutes during the first stage of labor, every 15 minutes during the second stage, and every 10 minutes in the delivery room. These methods require adequate numbers of fully trained personnel at the bedside.

Some evidence exists that auscultatory monitoring suffices for determining the effect of labor on the fetus in situations in which no risk factors have been identified. However, intrapartum hypoxic events may occur in any pregnancy, and subtle changes in FHR reflecting these may not be diagnosed by auscultation.

### Electronic Monitoring

Even when appropriately obtained and interpreted, electronic fetal monitoring screens only for intrapartum fetal distress. It is not specifically diagnostic. Furthermore, the diagnosis of fetal distress during labor cannot be assessed by any single clinical or laboratory measurement. One must appreciate this limitation to avoid basing inappropriate clinical decisions on data derived from monitoring. To date, however, fetal distress is a diagnosis largely based on monitoring criteria, with or without supplemental testing.

A normal FHR pattern on continuous monitoring indicates a greater than 95% probability of fetal well-being. Moreover, there is a suggestion of beneficial effect (as measured by perinatal morbidity and mortality) of electronic fetal monitoring in high-risk pregnancy. Although the specific risk factors most amenable to assessment by electronic fetal monitoring have not been detailed, the situations listed in Table 13–11 certainly warrant fetal monitoring. Currently, electronic FHR monitoring may be accomplished externally (from the maternal abdominal wall) or internally (directly from the fetus).

**A. External Monitoring:** The most common external method demonstrates FHR by pulsed ultrasonography (Doppler ultrasound); direct fetal electrocardiography and phonocardiography are others. The latter 2 are more difficult technically than the former, especially for routine use. Therefore, the focused Doppler technique has enjoyed wide popularity. All 3 methods may be combined with an external strain gauge secured over the abdomen for recording the motion of the uterus during contractions (Fig 13–5). Doppler ultrasound external monitors have a limited capability for accurately reflecting short-term variability unless it is seriously depressed. Also, with external monitoring, the strength of uterine contractions cannot be quantitated. However, as a screening method, these disadvantages are outweighed by the ease of application and the acceptance by patients and attending personnel. If an abnormal FHR pattern is detected, direct FHR monitoring should be instituted promptly.

**B. Internal Monitoring:** The fetal electrocardiographic impulse, obtained directly, potentially provides the greatest amount of accurate information about FHR patterns. To accomplish this, a spiral electrode is attached directly to the fetal presenting part, either through an endoscope or by palpation. The

**Table 13–11.** Risk problems warranting electronic fetal monitoring.

**Maternal disease predisposing to fetal problems**
Hypertensive states of pregnancy
Diabetes mellitus
Isoimmunization
Premature labor
Amniocentesis
Maternal fever of any origin
Cyanotic maternal heart disease
Maternal respiratory insufficiency
Collagen diseases
History of previous stillbirth
Anemia

**Uterine problems predisposing to fetal problems**
Failure to progress
Uterine hypertonia or polysystole
Use of uterine relaxants
Oxytocin administration
Previous cesarean section in labor

**Placenta and cord problems**
Abruptio placentae
Placenta previa (external only)
Unexplained third-trimester bleeding
Prolapsed cord (while awaiting cesarean or rapid vaginal delivery)
Vasa previa (while awaiting cesarean, external only)

**Fetal problems**
Meconium staining of amniotic fluid
Abnormal FHR by auscultation
Intrauterine growth retardation
Postterm pregnancy
Abnormalities on antepartum testing prior to labor
Premature pregnancy
Multiple gestation

Modified after Freeman RK, Parer JT, Puttler OL: Page 70 in: *A Clinical Approach to Fetal Monitoring.* Berkeley Bio-engineering, Inc., 1974.

electrocardiographic impulses are amplified and then transmitted to a cardiotachometer (Fig 13–6). The cardiotachometer uses a filter to convert the fetal electrocardiographic pattern into relatively discrete electronic impulses. Detection and counting devices then measure the interval between successive impulses. A potential that is inversely proportional to the time between the successive impulses is computed, and this is displayed as the heart rate series.

To determine the changes in FHR evoked by the stress of uterine contractions (a period of decreased placental blood flow), it is necessary to measure each contraction concomitantly. This is done directly by inserting a pliable plastic catheter attached to a strain gauge through the dilated cervix into the amniotic sac to a point behind the fetal presenting part. This is accomplished by using a guide that is insinuated just beyond the lip of the cervix.

Maternal and fetal complications associated with direct electronic monitoring may occur, but the risks are low. The most frequent fetal complication is scalp abscess at the site of electrode application. This complication is not related to the type of electrode used and is usually noted at 1–14 days after birth in up to 3% of directly monitored deliveries. Local therapy is

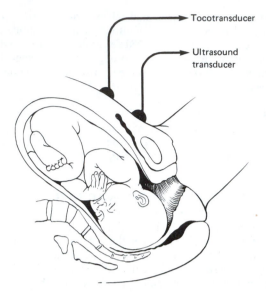

**Figure 13–5.** External fetal heart rate monitoring. (Redrawn, with permission, from Hon EH: Hosp Pract [Sept] 1970;5:91.)

usually sufficient. Maternal complications, eg, infection, are unusual. The fetal scalp electrode has also been associated with introduction of herpesvirus into the fetal scalp in mothers who shed the virus from the cervix and should be used in women with a history of genital herpes infection only if indicated.

**1. Basal fetal heart rate**—The normal FHR is 120–160 beats/min. This rate is defined as the average between the peaks and the depressions. Tracings of FHRs obtained from normal mature fetuses not

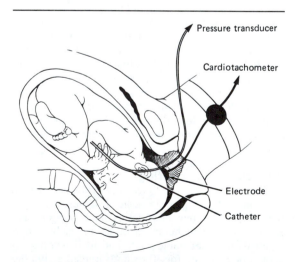

**Figure 13–6.** Internal fetal heart rate monitoring. (Redrawn, with permission, from Hon EH: Hosp Pract [Sept] 1970;5:91.)

under the influence of medications (such as narcotics, barbiturates) show small, rapid, rhythmic fluctuations, with an amplitude of 5–15 beats/min. These fluctuations are superimposed on the basal FHR and are often referred to as "beat-to-beat variability." They are a sign of good autonomic interplay in the fetal heart regulatory mechanism and are a paramount sign of fetal well-being. Some flattening of these fluctuations is seen during sleep; on occasion, with anomalies; following ingestion of certain drugs; and, most important and most seriously, with fetal hypoxia-acidosis (Figs 13–7 to 13–12).

**2. Transitory changes–**

**a. Decelerations–**A deceleration is a transient fall in FHR in relation to a uterine contraction. The amplitude of the deceleration, in beats/min, is the difference between the basal FHR recorded preceding the dip and the minimum FHR recorded at the bottom of the dip. The lag time (in seconds) is the interval between the peak of the contraction and the bottom of the corresponding deceleration (Fig 13–13A). These decelerations are of 3 types; early, late, and variable.

**(1) Early deceleration–**(Fig 13–13B.) This occurs during normal labor, particularly in the later stages. Presumably, uterine contractions apply pressure to the fetal skull, and reflex bradycardia occurs at the beginning of the contraction phase. The FHR promptly returns to normal when the contraction ends. The patterns of these decelerations are of uniform shape, and they reflect the uterine pressure curve. Rupture of the membranes is associated with an 8-fold increase in the incidence of this deceleration pattern because the fetal head is exposed to much stronger compression than when the membranes are intact. These FHR patterns are not worrisome. Babies with deviations of this type usually are born healthy. In most cases, the FHR does not fall below 100 beats/min, and these patterns are less than 90 seconds in duration.

**(2) Late deceleration–**(Fig 13–13C.) This is a transitory decrease in FHR that occurs after the contraction begins. The lag time is considerably greater than that of early deceleration. Like the pattern of early deceleration, late deceleration is of uniform shape, but the FHR does not return to baseline levels until well after the uterine contraction, and the nadir occurs beyond the apex of the associated contraction. These changes are presumed to be caused by any of the factors that reduce uteroplacental gas exchange. Babies with such deviations may be born depressed. In general, late decelerations last less than 90 seconds and are associated with a baseline FHR in the normal range. Late-deceleration FHR patterns may be associated with persistent hypoxia or fetal acidosis resulting from decreased maternal-fetal exchange. The pattern is frequently associated with high-risk pregnancies, uterine hyperactivity, or maternal hypotension. If beat-to-beat variability persists in the normal range despite late decelerations and if the normal baseline rate is present, acidosis will rarely be found. This can be confirmed by fetal scalp stimulation resulting in

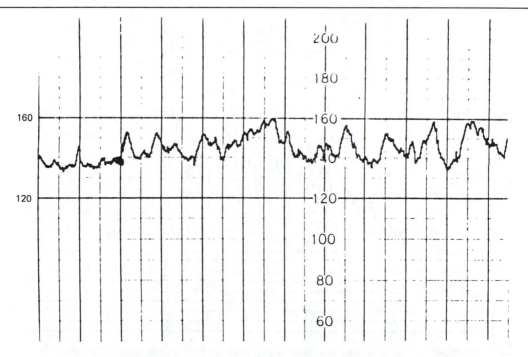

**Figure 13–7.** Normal short-term and long-term beat-to-beat variability.

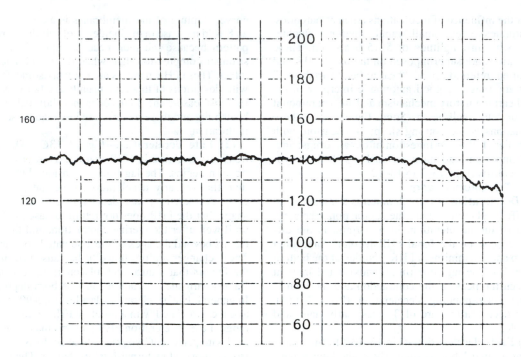

**Figure 13–8.** Reduced variability. This may occur during fetal sleep, following maternal intake of drugs, or with reduced fetal central nervous system function, as in asphyxia.

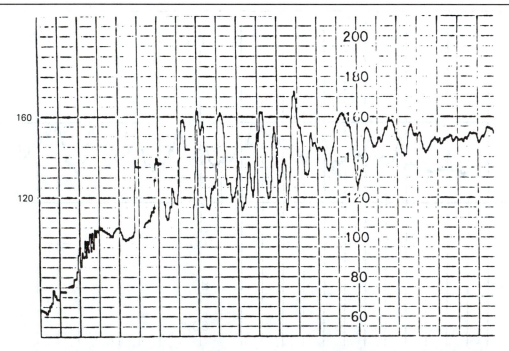

**Figure 13–9.** Increased variability, as frequently seen during recovery from a prolonged deceleration. This has been correlated with reduced and subsequently recovering transcutaneous $Po_2$ measurements.

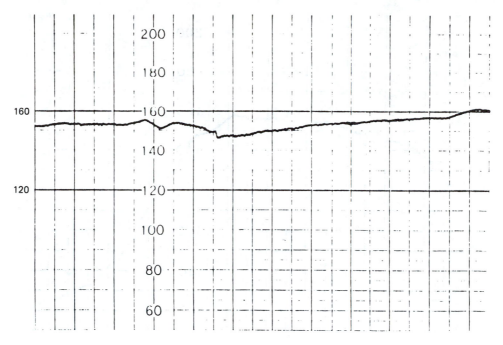

**Figure 13–10.** Markedly reduced variability. This is evidence of fetal acidosis and distress unless proved otherwise.

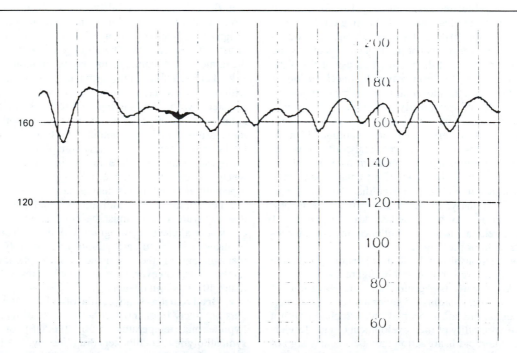

**Figure 13–11.** Markedly reduced variability with apparent preservation of long-term variability. Although preservation of long-term variability may be reassuring, the complete absence of short-term variability is worrisome. This pattern appeared in late labor in a baby with gastroschisis and extruded bowel. Blood gases were normal.

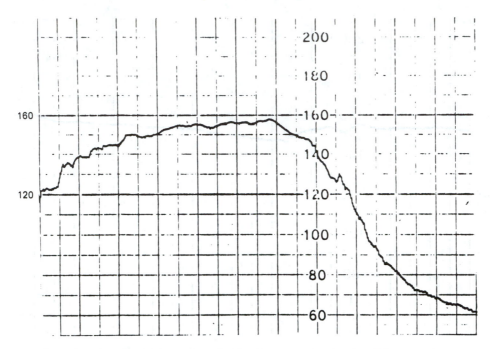

**Figure 13–12.** Severely reduced variability and terminal fetal heart rate deceleration. This pattern is never normal but is most worrisome in a postmature fetus with heavy meconium staining.

acceleration of the heart rate or by scalp blood pH determination.

**(3) Variable deceleration–**(Fig 13–13*D*.) When the umbilical cord is compressed during contractions, changes in the FHR pattern include variable waveforms. These forms also occur at odd times during the contraction phase of the uterus. Because of this variable behavior, the term **variable deceleration** is used. These are the most common FHR patterns associated with stethoscopically diagnosed fetal distress. The deceleration patterns are not always of uniform shape, and they vary widely in amplitude. In most cases, compression of the umbilical cord can be relieved by turning the mother from back to side or from one side to the other. Cord compression may cause transient FHRs of fewer than 100 beats/min and, occasionally, of fewer than 10–60 beats/min. The duration may be a few seconds or more than 1 minute. Fetal acidosis does not occur unless episodes are frequent or prolonged.

The relationship of FHR decelerations to uterine contractions are summarized in Figure 13–14.

**b. Accelerations–**Accelerations are elevations of the FHR. Accelerations are generally very reassuring; if accelerations are sustained and associated with a lack of variability or the development of late decelerations, the rapid heart action may be an early sign of fetal distress. However, accelerations usually may be interpreted as a solidly reliable sign of fetal well-being.

**3. Sustained changes–**Sustained changes fall into 3 categories:

**a. Beat-to-beat variability–**Beat-to-beat or short-term variability observed in normal mature fetuses is a sign of well-being, although it may be altered by a variety of medications. The absence of variability in the unmedicated mature fetus may be ominous.

**b. Tachycardia–**Tachycardia may be associated with maternal fever, maternal hyperthyroidism (if associated with long-acting thyroid stimulator), amnionitis, use of parasympatholytic or sympathomimetic drugs, fetal hypovolemia, fetal heart failure, or fetal hypoxia. It may be an early sign of fetal distress. Tachycardia may indicate recovering fetal distress when it occurs following a prolonged deceleration, especially if variability is decreased.

If none of the above conditions is found, a fetal cardiac tachyarrhythmia must be considered. In such cases, a fetal electrocardiogram will aid in diagnosis of the exact type of arrhythmia and possibly alter management of the pregnancy. Such phenomena rarely occur, however, with recordable rates of fewer than 240 beats/min or more.

**c. Bradycardia–**Bradycardia of mild degree occurs relatively frequently, either because of maternal hypothermia (temperature < 36°C[96.8°F]) or beta-sympatholytic (beta blocker) drug therapy. Bradycardia regularly follows anesthesia with paracervical block, which is now rarely used when the fetus is alive. Persistent bradycardia may reflect congenital

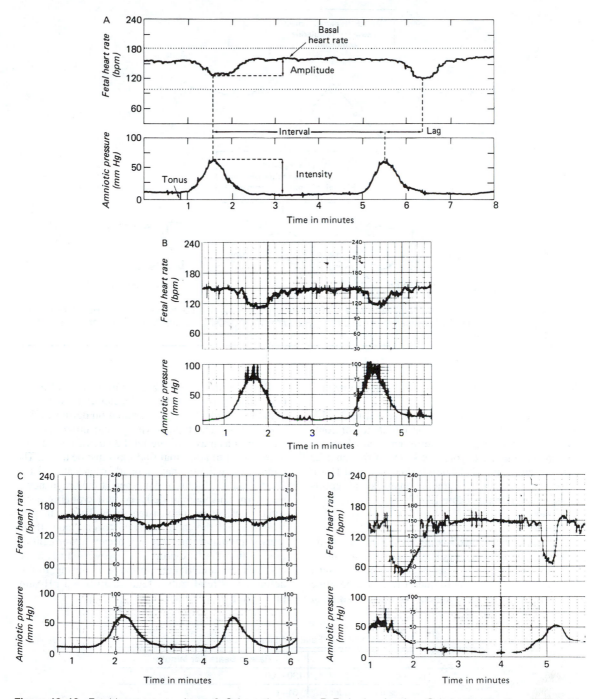

**Figure 13–13.** Fetal heart rate tracings. **A:** Schematic tracing. **B:** Early deceleration. **C:** Late deceleration. **D:** Variable deceleration. (Reproduced, with permission, from Babson SG et al: *Management of High-Risk Pregnancy and Intensive Care of the Neonate,* 3rd ed. Mosby, 1975.)

cardiac conduction defects, particularly in mothers with systemic lupus erythematosus.

**d. Sinusoidal pattern–**Sinusoidal FHR patterns have been reported with extreme fetal jeopardy (in association with Rh isoimmunization and fetal anemia resulting from fetomaternal transfusion). However, this pattern has also been encountered following administration of narcotics to the mother. The sinusoidal pattern should be viewed as a probable sign of fetal compromise, unless it is observed in the pre-

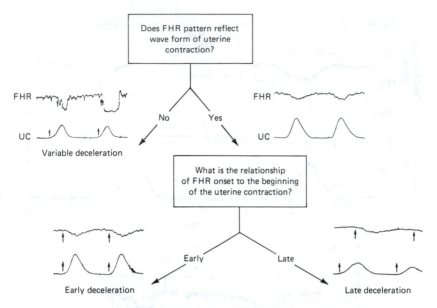

**Figure 13–14.** The relationship of fetal heart rate (FHR) decelerations to uterine contractions (UC). (Reproduced, with permission, from Hon EH: *An Introduction to Fetal Heart Rate Monitoring.* Postgraduate Division, University of Southern California School of Medicine, 1973.)

viously reassuring fetal tracing following administration of narcotic medication.

FHR patterns are summarized in Table 13–12. More detailed discussions of the intricacies of combined FHR deceleration patterns and fetal beat-to-beat arrhythmia are beyond the scope of this chapter (see references for Catanzarite, Freeman, and Hon). A useful format for FHR tracing analysis and reporting is summarized in Table 13–13.

## Summary

Diagnosis of fetal well-being by use of electronic fetal monitoring alone requires awareness of a number of factors. Any maternal or fetal risk factors must be considered. The baseline heart rate and baseline variability must be determined. Reassuring signs of fetal well-being include accelerations not following or intimately associated with decelerations and accelerations provoked by fetal stimulation during vaginal examination. The type, severity, and progression of decelerations may indicate fetal distress. The success of treatment of abnormal findings must be noted. The method of delivery may depend on gestational age and the status of fetus and mother. If the pregnancy is near term and vaginal delivery will probably occur soon, transient or inconsistent irregularities may be tolerated and the labor allowed to continue. If the fetus is premature but has significant abnormalities, especially if they are progressively worsening, delivery must be undertaken. In cases requiring further definition of fetal status, fetal scalp blood pH sampling can be carried out.

**Table 13–12.** Fetal heart rate patterns.

| | | | Rate in Beats Per Minute |
|---|---|---|---|
| Basal FHR | Normal | | 120–160 |
| | Tachycardia | Moderate | 161–180 |
| | | Marked | 181 or more |
| | Bradycardia | Moderate | 100–119 |
| | | Marked | 90 or less |
| Transitory FHR changes | Variability | | 5–15 beats/min amplitude |
| | Accelerations | | Increased by 15 or more |
| | Decelerations Early Late Variable | | Decreased by 10–40 Decreased by 5–60 Decreased by 10–60, occasionally more |

**Table 13–13.** Fetal heart rate monitoring.

---

**Monitoring uterine activity**
  Baseline tonus
  Contractions: amplitude, frequency, duration
**Monitor fetal heart rate**
  Baseline: rate, variability
  Periodic changes
    Accelerations
    Decelerations: early, late, variable
    Combined accelerations/decelerations
Assessment and comment

---

## FETAL SCALP BLOOD SAMPLING

Ascertaining the fetal scalp blood pH may assist in assessing fetal distress during the course of labor. However, the cervix must be dilated more than 2 cm and the fetal vertex well applied to the cervix. Fetal scalp sampling is facilitated when the vertex is low in the pelvis.

To obtain the specimen, one must insert an amnioscope and wipe the scalp clean. A thin layer of silicone gel is applied to allow a drop of blood to form at the site of the incision. The incision is made with a special narrow blade that can penetrate no more than 2 mm. Blood is aspirated into a heparinized capillary tube and the pH promptly determined. It is necessary to observe the incision carefully to be certain that bleeding stops.

If the pH is over 7.25, the fetus probably is normal; if the pH is between 7.2 and 7.24, the fetus may be somewhat compromised; and if the pH is less than 7.2, the fetus may not be expected to tolerate this indefinitely. Simultaneous maternal sampling can be used to make certain that fetal acidosis is not secondary to maternal acidosis. When the mother is found to be acidotic, the fetus should be considered acidotic also if the scalp pH is more than 0.2 pH units below that of the maternal arterial pH. Causes of maternal acidosis include muscular activity, starvation, dehydration, long first or second stage of labor, and metabolic disease. In practice, maternal pH is seldom measured unless there is some reason to suspect maternal acidosis as a possible cause of the apparent fetal distress.

In interpreting fetal pH values, bear in mind that respiratory acidosis is merely an accumulation of $CO_2$, whereas metabolic acidosis also includes the accumulation of lactic acid from anaerobic metabolism. The diagnosis of fetal asphyxia requires evidence of multisystem organ damage in the newborn as well as hypercapnia, hypoxia, and acidosis. Metabolic acidosis is marked by a base deficit (negative base excess) of greater than 10. In the case of asphyxia, $PO_2$ is likely to be under 16 mm Hg and $PCO_2$ over 60 mm Hg.

Physiologic responses by the fetus to compensate for low $PO_2$ ideally include high hemoglobin concentration, high oxygen-carrying capability, an oxyhemoglobin curve shifted to the left, high oxygen saturation, increased cardiac output, and selective shunting of oxygenated blood. However, if oxygen supplies are inadequate, the fetus will revert to anaerobic metabolism.

The most common causes of the development of acidosis are supine hypotension, amniotomy, maternal narcosis, and fetal bradycardia. Because of the variability of the other components of asphyxia, the scalp blood pH, which is reflective of fetal arterial pH, may be less well correlated with the Apgar score. In both term and preterm infants, a relationship has been demonstrated between pH and electronic fetal monitoring patterns, but not all fetuses with abnormal FHR patterns have acidotic pH values on sampling.

The confidence limit of fetal scalp blood sampling is 0.05 pH units. (Cord blood = 0.02 pH units.) However, fetal scalp blood sampling may produce both false abnormals and false normals. The most common causes of false abnormals (low pH with a vigorous newborn) are maternal acidosis and the variable central nervous system response of the neonate to acidosis in a basically healthy baby. Other possible causes of false low pH are sampling from an area of local stasis, contamination of the sample with other substances or the operator's expired air if mouth suction on the capillary tube is used, and prolonged storage of blood samples at room temperature before analysis. The usual causes of false normals (normal pH with a depressed newborn) are narcosis, infection, prematurity, asphyxia occurring after the sample was taken, neonatal airway obstruction, trauma during delivery, congenital anomalies, and incomplete recovery from asphyxia. Carbon dioxide may be lost from the sample following undue exposure of the drop of blood to air before collection into the capillary tube.

Indications for fetal blood sampling include the presence of meconium, FHR over 160 or less than 100, late decelerations, severe variable decelerations, complex patterns, and other clinical indications of fetal distress that cannot be explained or judged on monitoring alone. Obvious contraindications include a fetus with possible clotting abnormalities, an inaccessible fetal presenting part, and maternal infection with herpesvirus.

The most common fetal complication of scalp blood sampling is persistent bleeding from the sample site. Hemostasis is imperative. Other risks include sampling from improper areas, deep incisions, and infection.

## UMBILICAL CORD BLOOD SAMPLING AT DELIVERY

Apgar scoring has been the conventional means of evaluating the status of the infant at birth. It is usually assumed that this score reflects the degree of neonatal asphyxia. Neonatal asphyxia and neonatal depression are often considered to be synonymous terms. However, recent studies using cord blood analysis have cast serious doubts on the reliability of Apgar scoring for asphyxia, especially in preterm infants. One large study demonstrated only a 15–20% correlation between low Apgar scores and abnormal cord blood pH in term infants. Of those with a pH of 7.11 or less, only 14% had 5-minute Apgar scores of less than 7; of those with an Apgar score of less than 7 at 5 minutes, only 19% had pH values in this abnormal range.

Studies of correlations between gestational age, Apgar scores, and cord blood pH have shown even poorer correlations between Apgar scores and the degree of acidosis in very premature babies. There is, in fact, a rather linear correlation between gestational age and Apgar scores, unrelated to pH. Although most studies do show a relationship between Apgar scores and survival rates, even when corrected for gestational age, gestational age is by far the more influential factor in determining outcome.

Asphyxia should be diagnosed only following cord blood determinations and evidence of multisystem

**Table 13–14.** Umbilical cord blood gas measurements in term nulliparous pregnancies.

|  | Artery | Vein |
|---|---|---|
| pH | $7.24 \pm 0.07$ | $7.32 \pm 0.06$ |
| $P_{CO_2}$ (mm Hg) | $56.3 \pm 8.6$ | $43.8 \pm 6.7$ |
| $P_{O_2}$ (mm Hg) | $17.9 \pm 6.9$ | $28.7 \pm 7.3$ |
| Bicarbonate (mEq/L) | $24.1 \pm 2.2$ | $22.6 \pm 2.1$ |
| Base deficit (mEq/L) | $3.6 \pm 2.7$ | $2.9 \pm 2.4$* |

*All values listed as mean ± SD.
Modified from Thorp JA et al: Routine umbilical cord blood gas determinations? Am J Obstet Gynecol 1989;161:601.

organ damage in the newborn. The more general term "depression" should be used for babies with low Apgar scores. The range of normal umbilical cord pH and blood gases in mature infants is noted in Table 13–14. Most normal newborns become more acidotic during the first 10–20 minutes of life before recovering. An infant should not be considered seriously asphyxiated unless both cord blood values and neonatal blood values indicate the requisite abnormalities.

# REFERENCES

American College of Obstetricians and Gynecologists: Antepartum Fetal Surveillance. ACOG Technical Bulletin No. 107, 1987.

American College of Obstetricians and Gynecologists: Antenatal Diagnosis of Genetic Disorders. ACOG Technical Bulletin No. 108, 1987.

American College of Obstetricians and Gynecologists: Teratology. ACOG Technical Bulletin No. 84, 1985.

American College of Obstetricians and Gynecologists: Prevention of D Isoimmunization. ACOG Technical Bulletin No. 147, 1990.

American College of Obstetricians and Gynecologists: Operative Vaginal Delivery. ACOG Technical Bulletin No. 152, 1991.

American College of Obstetricians and Gynecologists: Alpha-Fetoprotein. ACOG Technical Bulletin No. 154, 1991.

Arduini D, Rizzo G, Romanini C: The development of abnormal heart rate patterns after absent end-diastolic in umbilical artery: Analysis of risk factors. Am J Obstet Gynecol 1993;168:43.

Bourgeois FJ et al: The significance of fetal heart rate decelerations during nonstress testing. Am J Obstet Gynecol 1984;150:213.

Bowes WA Jr et al: Fetal heart rate monitoring in premature infants weighing 1,500 grams or less. Am J Obstet Gynecol 1980;137:791.

Bowman JM, Pollock JM: Antenatal prophylaxis of Rh isoimmunization: 28-weeks'-gestation program. Can Med Assoc J 1978;118:627.

Brendt RL, Beckman DA: Teratology. In: Eden RD, Boehm FH (editors): Assessment and care of the fetus. Appleton & Lange, 1990.

Clark SL, Paul RH: Intrapartum fetal surveillance: The role of fetal scalp blood sampling. Am J Obstet Gynecol 1985;153:717.

Cohen W (editor): Management of Labor. University Park Press, 1983.

Cunningham FG, MacDonald PC, Gant NF (editors): Williams Obstetrics, 19th ed. Appleton & Lange, 1993.

Devoe LD et al: Clinical sequelae of the extended nonreactive NST. Am J Obstet Gynecol 1985;151:1074.

Druzin ML et al: Antepartum fetal heart rate testing. 7. The significant of fetal bradycardia. Am J Obstet Gynecol 1981;139:194.

D'Alton ME, DeCherney AH: Prenatal diagnosis. N Engl J Med 1993;328:114.

Elkington KW: At the waters edge: Where obstetrics and anesthesia meet. Obstet Gynecol 1991;77:304.

Freeman RK, Garite T: Fetal Heart Rate Monitoring. Williams & Wilkins, 2nd ed. 1991.

Gabbe SG, Niebyl JR, Simpson JL (editors): Obstetrics: Normal and Problem Pregnancies. Churchill Livingstone, 2nd ed, 1991.

Gelbons MJ: Chromosomes, aberrations, and mammalian reproduction. In: Fertilization and Embryonic Development in Vitro. Mastroigmil L et al (editors). Plenum Press, 1981.

Gibbs RS et al: A review of premature birth and subclinical infection. Am J Obstet Gynecol 1992;166:1515.

Gratacos JA, Paul RH: Antepartum fetal heart rate monitoring: Nonstress test versus contraction stress test. Clin Perinatol 1980;7:387.

Grix A et al: Patterns of multiple malformations in infants of diabetic mothers. In: Prenatal Diagnosis and Mechanisms of Teratogenesis. Alan R. Liss, 1981.

Gross TL et al: Amniotic fluid phosphatidylglycerol: A potentially useful predictor of intrauterine growth retardation. Am J Obstet Gynecol 1981;140:277.

Hon EH: *An Atlas of Fetal Heart Rate Patterns*. Harty, 1968.0000

Hoskins IA, Frieden FJ, Young BK: Variable decelerations in reactive nonstress tests with decreased amniotic fluid index predict fetal compromise. Am J Obstet Gynecol 1991;165:1094.

Huddleston JF et al: Oxytocin challenge test for antepartum fetal assessment. Am J Obstet Gynecol 1979;135:609.

Johnson TRB et al: Significance of the sinusoidal fetal heart rate pattern. Am J Obstet Gynecol 1981;139:446.

Jones TB et al: Preconceptional planning. Clin Obstet Gynecol 1990;17,4:801.

Keegan KA Jr, Paul RH: Antepartum fetal heart rate testing. 4. The nonstress test as a primary approach. Am J Obstet Gynecol 1980;136:75.

Keegan KA Jr et al: Antepartum fetal heart rate testing. 5. The nonstress test: An outpatient approach. Am J Obstet Gynecol 1980;136:81.

Knox GE et al: Management of prolonged pregnancy: Results of a prospective randomized trial. Am J Obstet Gynecol 1979;134:376.

Landy HJ et al: Genetic implications of idiopathic hydramnios. Am J Obstet Gynecol 1987;157:114.

Low JA: The current status of maternal and fetal blood flow velocimetry. Am J Obstet Gynecol 1991;164:1049.

MacDonald ML, Wagner RM, Slotnich RN: Sensitivity and specificity of screening for Down's syndrome with alphafetoprotein, hCG, unconjugated estriol, and maternal age. Obstet Gynecol 1991;77:63.

Manning FA et al: Fetal biophysical profile scoring: A prospective study in 1,184 high-risk patients. Am J Obstet Gynecol 1981;140:289.

Mendenhall HW et al: The nonstress test: The value of a single acceleration in evaluating the fetus at risk. Am J Obstet Gynecol 1980;136:87.

Merkatz IR, et al: An association between low maternal serum alpha-fetoprotein and fetal chromosomal abnormalities. Am J Obstet Gynecol 1984;148:886.

Milunsky A: *Genetic Disorders and the Fetus,* 2nd ed. Plenum Press, 1986.

Molsted-Pedersen L: Pregnancy and diabetes: A survey. Acta Endocrinol 1980;238(Suppl):13.

Moore TR, Piacquadio K: A prospective evaluation of fetal movement screening to reduce the incidence of antepartum fetal death. Am J Obstet Gynecol 1989;160:1075.

Muneshige A et al: A rapid and specific enzymatic method for the quantification of phosphatidylcholine, disaturated phosphatidylcholine, and phosphatidylglycerol in amniotic fluid. Am J Obstet Gynecol 1983;145:474.

Naeye RI: Causes of perinatal mortality excess in prolonged gestations. Am J Epidemiol 1978;108:429.

O'Sullivan JB: Establishing criteria for gestational diabetes. Diabetes Care 1980;3:437.

Perkins RP: Perinatal observations in a high-risk population managed without intrapartum fetal pH studies. Am J Obstet Gynecol 1984;149:327.

Phelan JP: The nonstress test: A review of 3,000 tests. Am J Obstet Gynecol 1981;139:7.

Redman CWG, Roberts JM: Management of pre-eclampsia. Lancet 1993;341:1451.

Reece EA et al: The safety of obstetric ultrasonography: Concern for the fetus. Obstet Gynecol 1990;76:139.

Romero R, et al: Amniotic fluid white blood cell count: A rapid and simple test to diagnose microbial invasion of the amniotic cavity and predict preterm delivery. Am J Obstet Gynecol 1991;165:821-30.

Rosen MG, Dickinson JC: The paradox of electronic fetal monitoring: More data may not enable us to predict or prevent infant neurologic morbidity. Am J Obstet Gynecol 1993;745-51.

Sever JL et al: *Handbook of Perinatal Infections*, 2nd ed. Little, Brown, 1988.

Shepard TH: *Catalog of Teratogenic Agents*, 5th ed. John Hopkins Univ Press, 1986.

Simpson JL et al: *Genetics in Obstetrics and Gynecology*. Grune & Stratton, 1982.

Slomka C, Phelan JP: Pregnancy outcome in the patient with a nonreactive nonstress test and a positive contraction stress test. Am J Obstet Gynecol 1981;139:11.

Sokol RJ et al: Clinical application of high-risk scoring on an obstetric service. Am J Obstet Gynecol 1977;128:652.

Sokol RJ, Brindley BA, Dombrowski MP: Practical diagnosis and management of abnormal labor. In: *Danforth's Obstetrics and Gynecology*. Scott JR et al (editors). Lippincott, 1990.

Van Dortsen JP, Leuke RR, Schifrin BS: Pyelonephritis in pregnancy: The role of in-hospital management and introfarautoin suppression. J Reprod Med 1987;32:895.

Vintzileos AM et al: The use and misuse of the fetal biophysical profile. Am J Obstet Gynecol 1987;156:527.

Weinberger SE et al: Pregnancy and the lung. Am Rev Respir Dis 1980;121:559.

Weingold AB et al: Nonstress testing. Am J Obstet Gynecol 1980;138:195.

Zanini B, Paul RH, Huey JR: Intrapartum fetal heart rate: Correlation with scalp pH in the preterm fetus. Am J Obstet Gynecol 1980;136:43.

Zimmer EZ, Divon MY: Fetal vibroacoustic stimulation. Obstet Gynecol 1993;81:451-7.

Zuspan FP et al: NICHD Consensus Development Task Force Report. Predictors of intrapartum fetal distress: The role of electronic fetal monitoring. J Reprod Med 1979;23:207.

# 14

# Early Pregnancy Risks

*Martin L. Pernoll, MD, & Sara H. Garmel, MD*

More than 25% of all gestations will present to a health care provider in early pregnancy with vaginal bleeding and/or pelvic pain. The acuity of these symptoms may vary from a casual comment or phone message to presentation in profound shock. However, after the symptoms are encountered several pressing issues must be confronted:

1. Is there a life-threatening emergency?
2. Is there a pregnancy?
3. If there is a pregnancy, is it an intrauterine pregnancy?
4. Is the pregnancy progressing normally?

Successful management of any early pregnancy emergency rests on timely diagnosis. Every patient should receive a complete history (eg, previous reproductive history, last menstrual period, last normal menstrual period, precipitating events, extent and duration of pain, duration and amount of bleeding). Determination of the vital signs and ruling out shock are the next steps in assessment. A brief general physical may be conducted, but much of the attention will be focused on the abdominal examination and a careful pelvic examination.

The abdominal examination is conducted to establish the presence of any localizing tenderness (peritoneal irritation) and to assist in ascertaining the presence or absence of blood in the peritoneal cavity. The pelvic examination assists in establishing the amount of vaginal bleeding, the type of vaginal bleeding, the status of cervical dilatation, any pain on cervical motion, uterine configuration and size, and adnexal masses or tenderness. Significant bleeding or peritoneal bleeding signal a life-threatening condition.

If there is a life-threatening emergency, the patient must be evaluated in an appropriate facility with full capability for blood transfusion, surgical intervention, and more intensive care. If the situation is less critical, the evaluation may proceed in a less acute setting.

Laboratory studies generally include a complete blood count, blood type and Rh (if not already known), a quantitative β-hCG (human chorionic gonadotropin) and pelvic ultrasonography (either vaginal or transabdominal). The latter two tests quickly and efficiently assist in determining whether a pregnancy exists and whether it is in the uterus. On a single determination these studies may not be able to give full details of whether the pregnancy is progressing normally. However, strong evidence to the contrary may be provided by ultrasonographic findings of an empty gestational sac, a molar gestation, or a fetal disorganization. Likewise, a β-HCG that is very low or has not risen appropriately from a preceding study is strong presumptive evidence of a compromised pregnancy. Additional studies that may be useful are serum progesterone, cultures of the cervix (with antibiotic sensitivity testing) or cervical contents to determine pathogens in case of infection, and blood cross-matching.

More complicated circumstances may require serial ultrasound and quantitative β-HCG evaluations as well as the addition of other studies, the most useful of which is serum progesterone.

## SPONTANEOUS ABORTION

### Essentials of Diagnosis
- Suprapubic pain and uterine cramping.
- Vaginal bleeding.
- Cervical dilatation.
- Extrusion of products of conception.
- Disappearance of symptoms and signs of pregnancy.
- Negative pregnancy test or quantitative β-hCG that is not properly increasing.
- Adverse ultrasonic findings (eg, empty gestational sac, fetal disorganization, lack of fetal growth).

### Definitions
**Spontaneous abortion** is defined as a pregnancy terminating before the 20th completed week (139 days) of gestation. It implies the expulsion of any or all of the placenta or membranes. Although the definition includes cases with a live-born or stillborn infant weighing less than 500 g, there may not be an identifiable fetus. **Complete abortion** is the expulsion of all of the products of conception before the

20th completed week of gestation, whereas **incomplete abortion** is the expulsion of some, but not all, of the products of conception in the same interval. **Early abortion** occurs before 12 weeks and **late abortion** between 12 and 20 weeks. **Threatened abortion** is intrauterine bleeding occurring before the 20th completed week, with or without uterine contractions, without expulsion of the products of conception, and without dilatation of the cervix. **Inevitable abortion** refers to the state in which bleeding of intrauterine origin occurs before the 20th completed week with continuous and progressive dilatation of the cervix, but without expulsion of the products of conception. Although spontaneous abortion generally occurs 1–3 weeks after the death of the embryo or fetus, in **missed abortion,** the embryo or fetus dies in utero before the 20th completed week of gestation, but the products of conception are retained. **Infected abortion** is abortion associated with infection of the genital organs and is contrasted to **septic abortion**, in which there is infected abortion with systemic dissemination of infection. In **undiagnosed (subclinical) spontaneous abortion**, the pregnancy is reabsorbed or aborted before it has been recognized. **Induced abortion** is accomplished for therapeutic or elective termination of pregnancy (see Chapter 33).

## Incidence

In the spectrum of reproductive wastage, spontaneous abortion is probably the largest single contributor, with an incidence of 15–40%. Other causes are infertility (15%), prematurity (10%), fetal death (1%), ectopic pregnancy (1%), and neonatal death (1%).

Approximately 75% of spontaneous abortions occur before 16 weeks and 62% before 12 weeks. The incidence of subclinical spontaneous abortion has been estimated at 8% but is probably much higher, based on observations made during in vitro fertilization.

The incidence of abortion is influenced by the age of the couple and by a number of pregnancy-related factors, including whether a previous full-term normal pregnancy has occurred, the number of previous spontaneous abortions, whether there has been a previous stillbirth, and whether a previous infant was born with malformations or known genetic defects. In addition, parental influences, including balanced translocation carriers and medical complications (eg, diabetes mellitus) may influence the rate of spontaneous abortion.

## Etiology

Most spontaneous abortions are associated with abnormal products of conception and occur prior to clinical evidence of pregnancy. Over 15% of fertilized ova do not divide. Fifteen percent are lost before implantation (first week of gestation), approximately 25% are lost during implantation (second week of gestation), and 10% are lost following the first missed menses. In about 60% of spontaneous abortions occurring during the first trimester, there is an abnormal karyotype (about 50% are aneuploid and 50% are euploid). Overall, at least 10% of human conceptions are thought to have chromosomal abnormalities.

Other causes of spontaneous abortion account for a smaller percentage of losses, with the next largest category after genetic abnormalities being "unknown." Other known factors include infection, anatomic defects (eg, maternal müllerian defects), endocrine factors (probably related to failure of the corpus luteum), immunologic factors (currently under active investigation), and maternal systemic disease (eg, diabetes mellitus, hyperthyroidism). Please see the section on Recurrent Abortion that follows for further discussion of potential etiologies and recurrences.

The major causes of second-trimester abortion are anatomic defects of the uterus or cervix, fetal demise, and circumvallate placentation (with subsequent bleeding and labor). In the past syphilis and erythroblastosis were causes of second-trimester loss, but fortunately both are rare today.

Occasionally trauma is related to abortion. This may occur either directly—eg, local injury to the pregnant uterus, especially penetrating wounds or steering wheel or seat belt injury in midtrimester pregnancy—or indirectly. Examples of the latter include surgical trauma (eg, removal of an ovary containing the corpus luteum of pregnancy; appendectomy), total-body irradiation greater than 3000 rads, and electric shock (lightning or power line contact).

## Pathology

In spontaneous early abortion, hemorrhage into the decidua basalis often occurs. Necrosis and inflammation appear in the region of implantation. The pregnancy becomes partially or entirely detached and is, in effect, a foreign body in the uterus. Uterine contractions and dilatation of the cervix result in expulsion of most or all of the products of conception.

There are distinct patterns of spontaneous abortion. The amniotic sac and contents may be evacuated with the chorion and decidua; the embryo may be expelled, with rupture of the amniotic sac and passage of the fetus alone; or the entire pregnancy and the decidua may be passed intact.

In cases of missed abortion, there may be partial organization of the blood clot surrounding the conceptus. This results in the formation of a fleshy, nodular, dark red mass called a **carneous mole**, or **blood (Breus) mole**.

Hydropic villous degeneration, a common finding in abortions caused by chromosomal defects, may be due to an abnormal germ cell or accidental injury to the developing embryo.

**Laboratory Findings:**

**1. Pregnancy tests–**Since chorionic gonadotropin is produced by the syncytiotrophoblast, falling or abnormally low plasma levels of β-HCG are predictive of spontaneous abortion.

**2. Complete blood count**–If significant bleeding has occurred, blood studies will indicate anemia. If infection is present, the white blood cell count will be elevated (12,000–20,000/μL). The sedimentation rate, already elevated by pregnancy, increases with infection and anemia.

**3. Blood type and Rh**–Knowing the blood type and Rh in patients with threatened or actual abortion is mandatory. Not only does it assist in rapidly accomplishing cross-match if blood loss becomes excessive, it also delineates those that are Rh-negative. Knowing whether a patient is Rh-negative facilitates administration of Rh immune globulin for prevention of Rh isoimmunization. In early gestation with threatened abortion, 50 μg may be sufficient to prevent isoimmunization, but in more advanced gestations or other forms of abortion the full dose (300 μg) should be administered within 72 hours of the event.

**4. Progesterone**–During the first trimester, the principal source of progesterone is the corpus luteum. Thereafter, the principal source is the chorioplacental system. Pregnanediol (the major catabolite of progesterone) and serum progesterone drop precipitously in abortion. Moreover, some abortions are due to a luteal defect and inadequate progesterone production. Thus, progestogen therapy may benefit those patients with a demonstrated deficiency, but will not be useful in those with adequate progesterone.

**5. Ultrasonography**–Ultrasonography is highly accurate in diagnosing impending spontaneous abortion and is being used increasingly, especially transvaginally. X-rays are of no value in diagnosis of early abortion. In advanced missed abortion, x-rays may reveal a distorted fetal skeleton and intravascular gas in the fetus.

## Clinical Presentations and Therapy

**A. Threatened Abortion:** The previable pregnancy may be in jeopardy, but pregnancy continues. The cervix remains closed, although slight bleeding or cramping may be noted.

Place the patient at bed rest, interdict intercourse, and observe the patient's progress. Mild sedatives may be helpful, but drug therapy is generally ineffective in preventing abortion because so many of these uncertain pregnancies are abnormal. Although progesterone has been widely used in treatment for threatened abortion, its use is controversial because no clear data support its benefits, except for a few patients with documented luteal defects or progesterone deficiency. Advocates of progesterone's use note one other potential benefit–smooth muscle relaxation. However, even this action may increase the incidence of missed abortion, and an abnormal pregnancy, even a hydatidiform mole, may be retained.

The prognosis in the case of threatened abortion is good when all abnormal signs and symptoms disappear and when resumption of the progress of pregnancy is apparent. Ultrasonography is helpful in the management of threatened abortion by detecting fetal movement or heart beat. This prognostic sign is most reliable after 7 weeks' gestation.

**B. Inevitable Abortion:** Pain (uterine cramping) and bleeding with an open cervix indicate impending abortion; the expulsion of the uterine contents is imminent. Abortion is inevitable when 2 or more of the following are noted:

(a) Moderate effacement of the cervix.
(b) Cervical dilatation greater than 3 cm.
(c) Rupture of the membranes.
(d) Bleeding for more than 7 days.
(e) Persistence of cramps despite narcotic analgesics.
(f) Other signs of termination of pregnancy (eg, partial extrusion of products of conception).

Inevitable and incomplete abortion both require similar therapy.

**C. Incomplete Abortion:** Although some products of conception have passed from the uterine cavity, retained tissue is evidenced by continued bleeding, a patulous cervix, and an enlarged, boggy uterus (Fig 14–1). Cramps are usually present but may not be severe. Bleeding generally is persistent and is often severe enough to constitute frank hemorrhage. Examination should be both manual and by speculum. Tissue at the external os should be removed with sponge forceps and examined by a pathologist. If abortion is complicated or has occurred after the first trimester, the patient may require hospitalization.

Type and cross-match for possible blood transfusion if bleeding is brisk or if the initial hemoglobin is less than 10 g/dL. Administer 5% dextrose in lactated Ringer's solution intravenously with 10 units of oxy-

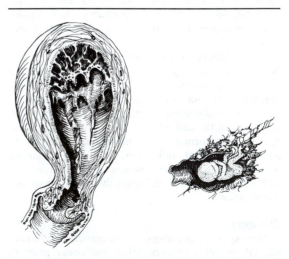

**Figure 14–1.** Incomplete abortion. **Right:** Product of incomplete abortion. (Reproduced, with permission, from Benson RC: *Handbook of Obstetrics & Gynecology,* 8th ed. Lange, 1983.)

tocin per 500 mL. The oxytocin contracts the uterus, aids in the expulsion of tissue or clots, and limits blood loss. Ergot preparations, which contract the cervix as well as the uterus, should be given acutely only when the diagnosis of complete abortion is certain, chronic hypertension has been ruled out, and blood loss is not controlled by oxytocin. Prostaglandins are an alternative. Blood replacement is dictated by the extent of hemorrhage and shock.

D&C should be performed for possible retained tissue. Evacuate the uterus promptly. Suction D&C is most effective. Intravenous oxytocin prior to uterine instrumentation decreases the possibility of uterine perforation. A sharp curet may be used to ensure complete removal of all tissue after suction curettage, but a vigorous "total curettage" should not be performed because uterine synechia (Asherman's syndrome) may result. When completeness of abortion is in doubt, D&C should always be accomplished.

The prognosis for the mother is good if the retained tissue is promptly and completely evacuated. Rh-negative mothers who are candidates for Rh immune globulin should receive it as soon after the abortion as possible.

**D. Complete Abortion:** Although slight bleeding may continue for a short time after passing the entire conceptus, complete abortion is marked by cessation of pain as well as termination of brisk bleeding (Fig 14–2). The fetus and the placenta may be expelled separately. It is important that the conceptus be very carefully examined for completeness and for trophoblastic disease.

The patient should be observed for further bleeding. All products of conception must be thoroughly examined for completeness and characteristics. The prognosis is excellent when all products of conception have been removed and when molar gestation and choriocarcinoma can be ruled out.

**E. Missed Abortion:** Missed abortion implies that despite fetal death the pregnancy has been retained. Any of the causes of abortion may be responsible. Why the pregnancy is maintained remains unknown, but viable placental function may be one cause and exogenous long-acting progestogens may be another. In both cases it is possible that progestogen production reduces uterine contractility.

Missed abortion is often manifested by loss of symptoms of pregnancy and a decrease in uterine size. The embryo or fetus has succumbed, but no tissue is passed. Pain or tenderness is unusual. There may be a brownish vaginal discharge. The cervix remains firm and closed, and no adnexal abnormality can be identified.

Ultrasonography is effective for following a pregnancy suspected of being a missed abortion. The quantitative β-HCG may decline, and urine pregnancy tests may become negative. In markedly prolonged (> 4 weeks) midtrimester missed abortion, absorption of the products of conception may result in a coagulopathy most notable for a low plasma fibrinogen.

The differential diagnosis of missed abortion includes continued pregnancy, inaccurate dating of a continuing pregnancy, and pelvic tumor without pregnancy.

In the past it was common to simply await the onset of an abortion when missed abortion was detected. Currently, a more interventional route is usually undertaken, with the uterus being evacuated soon after diagnosis. In the first trimester this is usually accomplished by suction curettage, whereas in the second trimester evacuation is most frequently accomplished using prostaglandin E suppositories. If evidence of a seriously reduced fibrinogen level, infection, or anemia exists, appropriate therapy must also be instituted. When coagulopathy or infection is not present, the maternal prognosis is good, since serious sequelae with uncomplicated missed abortion are uncommon.

**F. Septic Abortion:** Infected and septic abortion constitute a continuum of the extent to which infection has spread. Fever and generalized pelvic discomfort may indicate infected abortion, whereas septic abortion is often manifested by a malodorous discharge from the vagina and cervix, pelvic and abdominal pain, marked suprapubic tenderness, signs of peritonitis, tenderness with movement of the uterus or cervix, fever of 37.8–40.6°C (100–105°F)—although hypothermia often heralds or accompanies endotoxic shock (see below), jaundice due to hemolysis or oliguria (or both) secondary to septicemia. Trauma to the cervix or upper vagina may be recognized if there has been a clumsy attempt to induce an abortion.

The extent of the infection is usually confirmed by

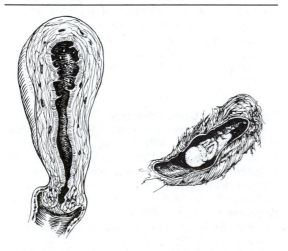

**Figure 14–2.** Complete abortion. (**Right:** Product of complete abortion. (Reproduced, with permission, from Benson RC: Handbook of Obstetrics & Gynecology, 8th ed. Lange, 1983.)

an elevated white blood count and other systemic signs of infection. The appropriate studies include a complete blood count, a urinalysis, culture of the discharge from the uterus, and blood cultures. In addition, electrolytes, liver function tests, blood urea nitrogen, creatinine, coagulation studies, and arterial blood gases may be useful in the seriously compromised patient. Imaging studies may include a chest x-ray and abdominal x-rays to exclude free air in the peritoneal cavity, the presence of gas-forming bacteria or the presence of a foreign body.

Although a minor endometritis may be managed with outpatient care (antibiotics, oxytocics, and fluid replacement), always hospitalize the seriously ill or anyone in whom there is a question of sepsis. Invasive monitoring is often necessary to adequately treat the critically ill patient (see Chapter 57–treatment of septic shock). Intravenous antibiotic coverage for anaerobic and aerobic bacteria is begun (eg, ampicillin, gentamicin, Cleocin) and the patient is observed carefully for signs of worsening sepsis.

Individualize antibiotic therapy if a specific organism is suspected or if the patient has a known antibiotic sensitivity. Give blood transfusion as required and intravenous 5% glucose lactated Ringer's solution with 20 units of oxytocin/1000 mL through a large-bore intravenous line. Monitor urinary output.

A D&C should be performed to make certain all of the products of conception have been removed. Abdominal hysterectomy should be considered when *Clostridia* is the causative organism, when uterine perforation has occurred, when the sepsis fails to respond adequately to treatment, or when the patient responds incompletely after being in septic shock. Vena caval clipping and ovarian vein ligation may be indicated when repeated septic pulmonary embolization occurs.

### Differential Diagnosis

**Ectopic pregnancy** is the probable cause of menstrual abnormality, unilateral pelvic pain, uterine bleeding, and a tender adnexal mass. **Membranous dysmenorrhea** is characterized by cramps, bleeding, and passage of an endometrial cast. Decidua and villi are absent; amenorrhea does not occur. **Prolonged hyperestrogenism** in the nonpregnant woman may also lead to abnormal uterine bleeding that must be differentiated from abortion.

**Hydatidiform mole** usually ends in abortion before the 5th month. Theca lutein cysts, when present, cause bilateral ovarian enlargement; the uterus may be unusually large. Bloody discharge may contain hydropic villi.

Other entities that may be confused with abortion are extruding **pedunculated myoma** and **cervical neoplasia** (such as polyps, carcinoma). The entire range of septic pelvic conditions, including **ruptured tubo-ovarian abscess** must be considered in septic abortion.

### Complications

Severe or persistent hemorrhage during or following abortion may be life-threatening. Obviously, the more advanced the gestation, the greater the likelihood of excessive blood loss.

Sepsis develops most frequently after criminal or self-induced abortion but may also occur in women who are sexually active immediately following abortion. The sequelae of infection, eg, salpingitis and intrauterine synechia or infertility, are other complications of abortion.

Perforation of the uterine wall may occur during D&C because of the soft and vaguely outlined uterine wall; it may be accompanied by injury to the bowel and bladder, hemorrhage, infection, and fistula formation. Death may result from salpingitis, peritonitis, septicemia, intravascular coagulation, or septic shock. Thrombophlebitis and septic embolization may also occur.

Choriocarcinoma is a rare complication of abortion.

Multiple pregnancy with the loss of one fetus and retention of another is not only possible but has been well-documented early in pregnancies closely monitored by ultrasonography. Usually, the fetus is simply reabsorbed, but the loss of one fetus in multiple gestation may be accompanied by cramping or vaginal bleeding.

### Prevention

Most abortions cannot be prevented, nor is there adequate evidence that it would be reasonable to do so, since many are the result of chromosomal abnormality. Some abortions can be prevented by study and treatment of maternal disorders before pregnancy; by early obstetric care, with adequate treatment of maternal disorders such as diabetes and hypertension; and by protection of pregnant women from environmental hazards to health and from exposure to rubella or other infectious diseases.

Cerclage closure of an incompetent cervix is effective in prevention of midtrimester abortion (Fig 14–3).

### Treatment of Complications

Coitus and douches are contraindicated after abortion, and pelvic rest will decrease the incidence of postabortal infections. Uterine perforation is manifested by signs of intraperitoneal bleeding, rupture of the bowel or bladder, or peritonitis. When uterine perforation is suspected, laparoscopy is indicated to determine the extent of laceration or bowel injury. The need for laparotomy is primarily based on these findings.

Pelvic thrombophlebitis and septic emboli are critical sequelae. Consider antibiotics, anticoagulants, ligation of the internal iliac and ovarian veins, and clipping or ligation of the vena cava.

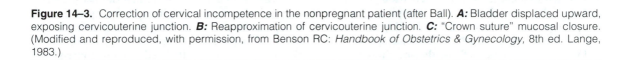

**Figure 14–3.** Correction of cervical incompetence in the nonpregnant patient (after Ball). **A:** Bladder displaced upward, exposing cervicouterine junction. **B:** Reapproximation of cervicouterine junction. **C:** "Crown suture" mucosal closure. (Modified and reproduced, with permission, from Benson RC: *Handbook of Obstetrics & Gynecology,* 8th ed. Lange, 1983.)

## RECURRENT ABORTION

### Definitions

**Habitual abortion** is defined as 3 consecutive spontaneous pregnancy wastages before 20 weeks' gestation with a fetus weighing less than 500 g. **Recidive abortion** is 2 consecutive spontaneous pregnancy wastages before 20 weeks' gestation with a fetus weighing less than 500 g. Distinct identification of the number of consecutive spontaneous abortions is very desirable.

### Incidence

The risk of one spontaneous abortion is 15–40%; 2 consecutive losses occur in 2–3% of all women, and it is only when 3 consecutive losses are reached that the incidence (< 1%) exceeds that which could be experienced simply as a result of random chance. Most important, the monitoring of subsequent pregnancy is crucial and should be initiated as early as it is ascertained that the patient has conceived.

### Etiology and Therapy

**A. Genetic:** No etiologic factor is identified in approximately 50% of recurrent abortion cases. Of the known causative factors, there are both similarities and differences between the first and second trimester. The similarities are infection (~15% for both trimesters) and uterine defects (~12% for both trimesters); whereas the dissimilarities include cervical incompetence (~3% for the first trimester compared with ~30% for the second trimester), endocrine causes (~7% for the first trimester compared with ~1.5% for the second trimester), chromosomal aberration (4–10% for the first trimester, but few in the

second trimester) and systemic disorders (almost none in the first trimester and ~ 3% in the second trimester.

Knowing the karyotype of aborted material is important in counseling the couple with recurrent abortion. There is a 50–60% incidence of abnormal karyotype in any spontaneous first-trimester abortion (compared with a 7.3% incidence in planned abortions). The most common abnormalities are trisomy (52%), polyploidy (26%), and X monosomy (15%). The remainder include double trisomies, mosaicism, and translocations. If the first pregnancy has a normal karyotype but ends in first-trimester abortion, a subsequent pregnancy will be chromosomally abnormal in 50% of cases. However, if the first abortus is chromosomally abnormal, the next pregnancy has an 80% chance of karyotypic abnormality.

Possible causes of genetic errors include translocation of parental chromosomes (an important cause of fetal abnormalities as well as abortions), chromosomal variation (recombination defects), various other genetic factors (including biochemical disorders and homozygous dominant inheritance), environmental agents (including radiation, chemicals, medications), viral agents (TORCH infections are the primary ones), and delay in fertilization of the ovulated egg.

Trisomy, the most common nondisjunction, occurs at the first meiotic division. Autosomal trisomy appears to be a nonrandom event. Approximately two-thirds of trisomy 21 anomalies are of maternal origin. Triploidy may be either maternal or paternal in origin. Parents who are carriers of a balanced translocation have an increased risk of spontaneous abortion (as well as a 50% chance of karyotypic or phenotypic abnormality in the offspring). Parental chromosomal variance has also been suggested as a cause of cytogenetic error.

The incidence of abnormal karyotypes appears to be between 4% and 10% in couples who have habitual spontaneous abortion. The abnormalities most frequently noted are translocation (44%), mosaicism (48%), and deletions or inversions (8%). When a couple has had one spontaneous abortion and malformed children, there is an abnormal chromosomal pattern in one of the parents in as up to 20% of couples. In additional, over 10% of couples with habitual abortion demonstrate multifactorial problems in previous offspring or close family members. Examples reported include neural tube defects, Potter's syndrome, diaphragmatic hernia, omphalocele, and cleft lip or palate. Most recently, hypermodality has been implicated as a cause of habitual abortion. The incidence of habitual abortion and aneuploidy in offspring appears to be more than 10-fold higher in parents who have hypermodal chromosomal spreads.

For serious genetic defects, therapy must be tailored to which of the parents is affected. If the defect is paternal, the only option now available is artificial insemination. For a maternal defect, a donor egg may be fertilized by the husband's semen. Table 14–1 details possible therapies for habitual abortion.

**B. Anatomic Abnormalities of the Reproductive Tract:** Anatomic abnormalities were the first described causes of habitual abortion and account for up to 15% of first-trimester and ~33% of second-trimester recurrent pregnancy losses. Defects include congenital uterine anomalies, cervical incompetence, submucous leiomyomas, abnormalities due to diethylstilbestrol exposure in utero, or Asherman's syndrome (see also Chapter 4).

A major difficulty in counseling couples with anatomic abnormalities of the reproductive tract is that ~50% of women with uterine defects have no reproductive problem. Bicornuate uterus and single uterine horn each account for approximately one-third of spontaneous abortions due to anatomic abnormalities and septate uterus for another 20–25%.

Generally, losses from anatomic abnormalities occur either very early (as a result of inadequate blood flow to the implantation site) or in the second trimester (presumably due to structural defects, although blood supply may also be an important factor).

Diagnosis of anatomic abnormalities is usually accomplished by hysterosalpingography, hysteroscopy, or laparoscopy. Treatment is primarily surgical. The Jones, Tompkins, or Strassman procedures or myomectomy are usually used to correct uterine abnormalities. Cervical abnormalities are usually corrected by means of cerclage (McDonald or Shirodkar procedure, Fig 14–4) or isthmic reconstruction. Surgical treatment is successful in ~70% of cases.

**C. Hormonal Abnormalities:** Hormonal causes of habitual abortion (25%) include thyroid dysfunction, progesterone insufficiency, and diabetes mellitus. For potential hypothyroidism, the usual hormonal tests performed are T3, T4, and TSH. Although the association between thyroid dysfunction

**Table 14–1.** Diagnosis and treatment of habitual abortion.

| Cause | Diagnosis | Treatment |
|---|---|---|
| Genetic error | Obtain a 3-generation pedigree and karyotyping of both parents and any previous aborted material. | Artificial insemination by donor, possible embryo transfer. |
| Anatomic abnormalities of reproductive tract | Perform hysterosalpingogram, hysteroscopy, laparoscopy. | Uterine operation: Jones, Tompkins, Strassman procedure, myomectomy. Cervical cerclage (abdominal or vaginal), reconstruction of cervical isthmus. |
| Hormonal abnormalities | Perform laboratory studies for $T_3$, $T_4$, and TSH and serum progesterone; biopsy of endometrium during luteal phase; and glucose screening (1 or 2 hours postprandial and Hgb $A_{lc}$). | Thyroid replacement, progesterone, clomiphene citrate, pergonal. |
| Infection | Obtain cervical or endometrial tissue for culture of *L monocytogenes, Chlamydia, Mycoplasma, U urealyticum, N gonorrhoeae,* cytomegalovirus, herpes simplex. Obtain serum titers for *T pallidium, B abortus, T gondii.* | Appropriate antibiotics. |
| Immunologic factors | HLA-A and -B typing of both parents, transferrin C typing of both parents. | Purified paternal lymphocytes (possibly). |
| Systemic disease | Antinuclear antibodies or antibodies to double-stranded DNA, SMA. | Variable according to specific disease. |

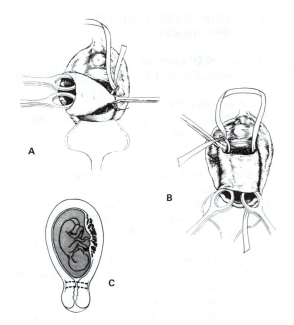

A

B

C

**Figure 14–4.** Cerclage of the cervix (Shirodkar) with incompetent os in pregnant patient. (Reproduced, with permission, from Benson RC: *Handbook of Obstetrics & Gynecology,* 8th ed. Lange, 1983.)

and habitual abortion has been challenged, occasional cases appear to respond favorably to thyroid therapy.

Progesterone deficiency may account for most cases of habitual abortion due to hormonal causes. Unfortunately, the diagnosis is usually retrospective or empiric because there is a poor correlation between pregnancy loss and serum or urine progesterone levels (or their metabolites). However, diagnosis is usually made by serum progesterone levels or luteal phase endometrial biopsies.

Most studies supporting hormonal abnormalities are based on the response to exogenous progesterone treatment. The risk:benefit ratio of exposing the fetus to exogenous progesterone must be considered. Vaginal suppositories (100 mg once or twice daily) are usually given, or attempts are made to increase corpus luteum progesterone production by use of clomiphene or other ovulatory agents. (See Chapter 5 for discussion of inadequate luteal phase.)

**D. Infections:** Infections that may lead to recurrent abortion include those due to *Mycoplasma, Ureaplasma urealyticum, Toxoplasma gondii, Neisseria gonorrhoeae, Chlamydia,* Listeria monocytogenes, herpes simplex, Treponema pallidum, *Brucella,* and cytomegalovirus. The incidence of spontaneous abortion due to these agents is not known because of a lack of controlled prospective trials. In women who have had habitual abortion, cervical or endometrial tissue should be obtained for culture of *L monocytogenes, Chlamydia, Mycoplasma, N gonor-*

*rhoeae,* cytomegalovirus, and herpes simplex. Serum titers may be obtained for *T pallidum, B abortus,* or *T gondii.*

Antibiotics should be given if infection is confirmed, and appropriate follow-up should be done to monitor therapy.

**E. Immunologic Factors:** Compared with women who carry a pregnancy to term, women who are habitual aborters have the following characteristics:

(1) They share more HLA-A and -B antigens with their partners.

(2) They have fewer inhibitors of cell-mediated immunity.

(3) They are more likely to have an absence of transplantation antigen.

(4) They have more fetuses that are transplantation-antigen compatible (in such cases, maternal protecting or blocking factors may not be stimulated, and the blastocyst may be rejected).

(5) They have increased sharing of transferrin type G with their partner.

(6) They have a low prevalence of serum anticytomegalovirus response.

(7) They have a lower lymphocytotoxic antibody titer than would be expected.

(8) They have a lower antisperm antibody titer than would be expected.

Despite this information, the diagnosis of immunologic abnormalities currently remains unclear and is largely retrospective; thus, diagnostic modalities should be considered on a case-by-case basis. Experimental treatment has been attempted with administration of purified paternal lymphocytes to the mother.

Women with blood group P or PK produce anti-P antibody, which may be a factor in recurrent abortion. Plasmapheresis has been successful in the treatment of these women.

**F. Systemic Disease:** Systemic causes of recurrent abortion are easily diagnosed (eg, chronic hypertensive or chronic renal disease). Collagen vascular disease may be more subtle and is associated with a marked increase in the rate of spontaneous abortion (eg, 40% with systemic lupus erythematosus [SLE]). Screening for collagen vascular disease and any other suspected diseases should be performed. The incidence of systemic disease as a cause of habitual abortion is unknown. Therapy involves treatment of the specific disease. A discussion of SLE can be found in Chapter 22.

Overt diabetes mellitus is associated with at least a 3-fold increase in the rate of spontaneous abortion. Screening for glucose intolerance should be performed in women with habitual abortion (either routine screening techniques or testing for hemoglobin $A_{1c}$). Indeed, a clear correlation has been demonstrated between elevated levels of hemoglobin $A_{1c}$ and spontaneous abortion.

## Diagnosis

A careful reproductive history and a 3-generation pedigree should be taken for both partners. Ascertain whether congenital anomalies, early pregnancy losses or chromosomal problems have been experienced by other family members. The physical examination is keyed to exclude uterine or cervical anomalies. Any medical illness must be appropriately worked up (eg, diabetes, SLE, rheumatoid arthritis). It may be useful to determine T3, T4, TSH and to perform glucose screening, if symptomatology or family history is positive. Luteal phase defects may be ruled out with luteal phase progesterone levels and late luteal phase endometrial biopsy. Obtain cervical cultures for *Chlamydia*, *N gonorrhoeae*, *Mycoplasma*, and *U urealyticum*.

Antinuclear antibodies, ACA (anticardiolipin antibodies) and activated PTT are the most commonly suggested methods to rule out immune disorders. Hysterosalpingograms or hysteroscopy may be of use to rule out uterine defects and laparoscopy used to clarify types of müellerian defects. Indeed because second-trimester losses account for <10% of all recurrent abortions and there is a high incidence of anatomic factors, investigation for a uterine defect may be warranted in certain circumstances after a single second-trimester loss. A karyotype may be performed on both partners. As noted previously, it is also useful to know the karyotype of aborted material. The best chance for cellular growth will be from the amniotic fluid, amnion, or residual fetal tissue. The placenta is more difficult to culture and in all cases care must be taken to keep the tissue aseptic. Table 14–1 summarizes a diagnostic workup for habitual abortion.

## Prognosis

Repeated abortion is very difficult psychologically for patients and their families. However, even without therapy, it is not a hopeless situation. The incidence of first-trimester abortion following one loss is 24%; after 2 losses, 26%; and after 3 losses, 32%.

Current recommendations for early pregnancy monitoring in a patient who has recurrent abortions includes prenatal vitamins with folic acid for 3 months before conception and 3-month spacing between pregnancies. The pregnancy should be confirmed by quantitative β-hCG as soon as the patient is late for menses and weekly β-HCG titers repeated to confirm an appropriate rise. A single serum progesterone at 6–8 weeks confirms adequate progesterone production in early pregnancy. A vaginal probe ultrasonography at 6–8 weeks substantiates fetal development and heart beat. Subsequent ultrasonographic examinations (interval based on physician judgment) monitor growth and continued viability. The patient should be instructed to come in early if abortion threatens and to save any tissue for karyotype. Obviously cervical checks are imperative if cervical incompetence is likely.

## EXTRAUTERINE PREGNANCY (Ectopic Pregnancy)

### Essentials of Diagnosis

- Amenorrhea followed by irregular vaginal bleeding.
- Adnexal tenderness or mass.
- Ultrasonographic evidence of adnexal mass and no intrauterine gestation.
- Positive β-hCG.

**Abdominal Pain and Tenderness:** An extrauterine pregnancy (ectopic pregnancy) is one in which a fertilized ovum implants in an area other than the uterine cavity (Fig 14–5). At least 99% of extrauterine pregnancies occur in the uterine tube.

The incidence is about 1 in 100 pregnancies (1 in 80–200 pregnancies); over 75% are diagnosed before the 12th week of gestation. The rate increased from 4.8 in 1000 term births in 1970 to 14.5 in 1000 in 1980 and is expected to be even higher today. Ectopic pregnancy may occur at any time from menarche to menopause, but 40% of these pregnancies occur in women between ages 20 and 29 years. More ectopic pregnancies occur in "infertile" women, in lower socioeconomic groups, and in women who have had a previous ectopic pregnancy. Ten to 20% will have a second ectopic pregnancy, and 4–5% of these will occur in the opposite tube. Women who have been treated for salpingitis or have had tuboplasty are more prone to tubal ectopic pregnancy.

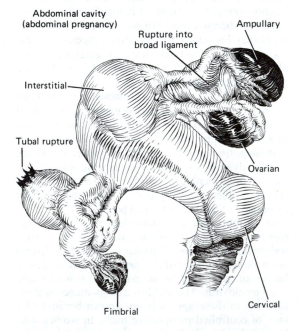

**Figure 14–5.** Sites of ectopic pregnancies. (Reproduced, with permission, from Benson RC: *Handbook of Obstetrics & Gynecology*, 8th ed. Lange, 1983.)

## Classification & Specific Incidence

Tubal pregnancies account for more than 99% of total ectopic pregnancies. The locations within the tube are as follows: ampullary (55%), isthmic (25%), fimbrial (17%), interstitial (2%), bilateral, and distal with segmental absence of the tube.

Ovarian pregnancy (<0.5%) may be classified as ovarian, tubo-ovarian, abdomino-ovarian (secondary abdominal pregnancy).

Abdominal pregnancies (<0.1%) are classified as primary, secondary, abdomino-ovarian, or tubo-abdominal.

Compound or heterotrophic (combined with intrauterine pregnancy, are seen 1 in 17,000–30,000 pregnancies).

Cervical are very rare extrauterine pregnancies and may be intraligamentous, in the vesicovaginal space, and may occur following hysterectomy (in a cervical stump, in a uterine tube, in a prolapsed uterine tube [fimbria], or abdominal).

Although it occurs rarely, it is also possible to have abnormal placements of pregnancy in the uterus including (in descending order of occurrence): cornual, angular, within a uterine diverticulum, in a uterine sacculation, in a rudimentary horn, or intramural.

## Etiology

The primary causes of ectopic pregnancy include conditions that either prevent or impede passage of a fertilized ovum through the uterine tube.

**A. Tubal Factors:** Up to 50% of women with ectopic pregnancies have had salpingitis previously. Chronic salpingitis will be identified histologically in about 50% of excised tubal pregnancy specimens. Other tubal factors that interfere with the progress of the fertilized ovum are adherent folds of tubal lumen due to salpingitis isthmica nodosa, developmental abnormalities of the tube (congenital diverticula, accessory ostia, or atresia), abnormal tubal anatomy due to diethylstilbestrol (DES) exposure in utero, previous tubal or pelvic organ microsurgery, tubal ligation, conservative treatment of unruptured tubal pregnancy, extrinsic adhesions (after peritonitis, kidney transplants, diverticulitis), pelvic tumors, endometriosis, excessive length or tortuosity, physiologic failure such as tubal spasm or inadequate peristalsis, and problems associated with intrauterine devices.

**B. Zygote Abnormalities:** A variety of zygote abnormalities have been reported in ectopic pregnancy, including chromosomal abnormalities, gross malformation, and neural tube defects. An increased incidence of ectopic pregnancy has been reported in partners of males with abnormal sperm counts or a high incidence of abnormal spermatozoa.

**C. Ovarian Factors:** Ovarian factors possibly resulting in the development of an ectopic pregnancy are fertilization of an unextruded ovum, transmigration of the ovum, post-midcycle ovulation and fertilization, and ovarian enlargement due to use of clomiphene (Clomid) or menotropins (Pergonal).

**D. Exogenous Hormones:** Evidence is mounting that the administration of exogenous hormones may play a role in ectopic gestation. For example, of pregnancies occurring in women taking progestin-only oral contraceptives, 4–6% have been ectopic pregnancies. If a "morning-after pill" (which contains a large amount of estrogen) has been given but fails to prevent a pregnancy, there is a 10-fold increase in the incidence of ectopic gestation. Up to 16% of pregnancies occurring in women who have a progesterone-bearing IUD are ectopic pregnancies.

**E. Other Factors:** Other factors associated with ectopic pregnancy are tubal abortion and subsequent implantation, the proclivity of a fertilized ovum to implant in an unusual area, endometriosis, the presence of an IUD (4–9% rate of ectopic pregnancy [2 in 1000 IUD users], with 1 in 8 being primary ovarian pregnancies), in vitro fertilization and embryo transfer, abnormal early implantation, and any form of intraperitoneal bleeding.

## Pathology

One important aspect of ectopic pregnancy is the lack of resistance of the endosalpinx to invasion by the trophoblast; thus, implantation occurs beneath the endosalpinx in the muscle and connective tissue next to the tubal serosa. There may be little or no decidual reaction and minimal defense against the penetrating trophoblast. Therefore, the trophoblast invades the blood vessels to cause local hemorrhage. A hematoma in the subserosal space enlarges as pregnancy progresses, with possible bleeding out of the distal end of the tube but not out of the tubal lumen. Distention, thinness of the tube, and invading trophoblast all predispose to rupture.

Rupture may be intracapsular or extracapsular. Extracapsular rupture occurs when the villous ovum erodes through the tubal wall and the tubal serosa ruptures when stretched to the breaking point. In intracapsular rupture, the embryo, fluid, and blood are expelled from the fimbriated ostium of the tube after rupture of the amniotic and chorionic membranes.

Bleeding may cease temporarily after either extracapsular or intracapsular rupture, but the embryo rarely survives. However, occasionally, pregnancy may continue if an adequate portion of the placental attachment is retained or if secondary implantation occurs elsewhere.

Generally, an abdominal pregnancy is primary; very rarely, it may be secondary to a tubal rupture or abortion with the trophoblast maintaining its tubal attachment or the entire ovum implanting again at another site. There may be serious effects from invasion of vital organs in cases of abdominal pregnancy. The invasive characteristics of trophoblast resemble those of carcinoma. In any event, the embryo rarely survives the initial hemorrhage. The incidence of abdominal pregnancy is one per 15,000 pregnancies; the fetal mortality rate is about 90%.

The corpus luteum of pregnancy continues only as long as there is viable trophoblastic tissue. The uterus enlarges slightly and is softened because of the added circulation and the decidual reaction in the endometrium. There may be endometrial separation and uterine bleeding when the ectopic pregnancy terminates and separates; only in interstitial ectopic nidation is there drainage of blood from the tube through the uterus, cervix, and vagina.

### Endometrial Changes & Vaginal Bleeding

In tubal ectopic pregnancy, bleeding is of uterine origin and is caused by endometrial involution and slough of the superficial tissues—largely decidua. Atypical changes in the endometrium occasionally are suggestive but not diagnostic of ectopic pregnancy. The **Arias-Stella** reaction consists of great variation in nuclear size, numerous mitoses in atypical areas, nuclear hypertrophy, focal enlargement of glandular cells, loss of cell boundaries and "stacking" of gland cells, increase in quantity of cytoplasm, disappearance of lumina of glands owing to cellular hypertrophy, vacuolization, loss of cellular polarity, nuclear lobulation, and frothy appearance of the cytoplasm. Arias-Stella reaction, probably due to hormonal overstimulation, may resemble endometriosis.

Occasionally, endometrial tissue may be passed as a so-called decidual cast. Superficial secretory endometrium usually is present, but there are no trophoblastic cells.

### Termination of the Pregnancy

This occurs in various ways depending on the site of implantation.

**A. Tubal:** A tubal pregnancy may terminate by abortion or missed abortion, extratubal rupture into the broad ligament, or intratubal rupture leading to tubal abortion or formation of hematosalpinx or pelvic hematocele. Pregnancy may proceed to an advanced stage with or without rupture but rarely to viability. Approximately 50% of all ectopic pregnancies abort, are reabsorbed, or become "chronic."

Isthmic rupture often occurs at 6–8 weeks' gestation, ampullary rupture at 8–12 weeks, and interstitial rupture at about 4 months depending on such factors as the size of the uterus and whether or not trauma occurs.

**B. Interstitial, Angular, Cornual:** Since the pregnancy begins in the portion of the tube that crosses the myometrium, the fate of the gestation resembles that of intrauterine pregnancies that implant in the cornu or near to it. In these 3 types, the pregnancy may rupture into the uterine cavity; the uterine wall may divide, causing severe local destruction to the myometrium; or the rupture may be directed into

the broad ligament or directly into the peritoneal cavity. An angular ectopic pregnancy may carry to term, since the nidation point is just inside the uterine cavity. This is a serious, potentially lethal form of ectopic pregnancy that often requires hysterectomy as an emergency procedure. Occasionally, these pregnancies may abort into the uterine cavity.

**C. Cervical:** A cervical pregnancy may rupture into the cervical canal, may go directly into the vagina, and rarely may rupture into the base of the broad ligament, with an intra-abdominal complication of hematoma formation.

**D. Abdominal:** Abdominal pregnancy may rupture into the peritoneal cavity, into the retroperitoneal space, or into a vital organ. The pregnancy may form an unrecognizable mass (adipocere), or an intraperitoneal abscess may be formed from infected fetal parts, or a lithopedion may be the end result. The pregnancy may continue to an advanced stage.

**E. Ovarian:** Ovarian pregnancy usually ruptures into the peritoneal cavity but may dissect into the folds of the ovarian ligament or form a lithopedion. An ovarian pregnancy almost never reaches viability.

**F. Combined:** The tubal pregnancy may abort or rupture, and the uterine pregnancy may abort, terminate prematurely, or continue to term. A bilateral tubal pregnancy may abort or rupture on both sides— not always simultaneously. Neither pregnancy continues to viability.

### Clinical Findings

No specific symptoms or signs are pathognomonic of ectopic pregnancy, but a combination of findings may be suggestive. Ectopic pregnancy should be suspected when symptoms of early pregnancy (amenorrhea, breast tenderness, and nausea) are followed by bleeding (usually spotting) and diffuse lower abdominal pain within the first 1–8 weeks after the missed period. The patient may experience a progressive course of faintness, exacerbation of pain (rupture or impending rupture), syncope, and shoulder pain. The symptoms and signs of blood loss must be carefully evaluated (see Chapters 19 and 57). Over 16% of ectopic gestations present as surgical emergencies.

**A. Symptoms:** The following symptoms may assist in the diagnosis of ectopic pregnancy:

- Pelvic or lower abdominal pain is present in over 99% of cases. Approximately 44% of women experience generalized pain, and roughly 33% have unilateral lower abdominal pain. Subdiaphragmatic pain or sharp shoulder pain (caused by extensive intra-abdominal bleeding irritating the diaphragm) occurs in approximately 22% of cases.
- Abnormal uterine bleeding occurs in roughly 75% of cases regardless of the site.
- Secondary amenorrhea of less than 2 weeks' duration occurs in about 68% of cases.

- Syncope is present in 37% of cases.
- In only about 7% of ectopic pregnancies is a uterine cast passed vaginally.

**B. Signs:** On examination, the following signs are important in the diagnosis of ectopic gestation:

**1. Abdominal tenderness**–Diffuse or localized abdominal tenderness is present in over 80% of ectopic pregnancies. The presence of "fixed abdominal tenderness" on turning the patient (positive Adler sign) may be useful but is highly inconsistent.

**2. Adnexal tenderness**–Adnexal tenderness is present in over 75% of cases. The pain may be exquisitely severe on palpation or slight movement of the cervix and uterus.

**3. Adnexal mass**–A unilateral adnexal mass is palpated in more than 53% of patients. The mass is usually boggy and poorly delineated. Occasionally, a cul-de-sac mass is present.

**4. Uterine changes**–The typical changes of pregnancy in the uterus are not correlated with the duration of an advanced ectopic pregnancy. In nearly 71%, the uterus is perceived to be of normal size, while in 26%, it is 6–8 weeks' size and in slightly more than 3%, it is 9–12 weeks' size.

**6. Fever**–Fever is unusual, occurring in only about 2% of patients.

**Laboratory Findings:**

**1. Pregnancy tests**–($\beta$-hCG, 700 mU/mL in urine) are positive in 82.5% of ectopic pregnancies and negative in only 17.5%. Of course, a positive test only confirms pregnancy and does not indicate whether it is intrauterine or extrauterine. Moreover, because diagnosis is often needed early in pregnancy when hCG levels are low, a negative test does not rule out an ectopic gestation. A serum $\beta$-hCG test with a sensitivity of 35 mU/mL will be negative in only 2% of ectopic gestations.

Recently, it was observed (Stovall, 1989) that over 80% of patients with ectopic pregnancy have a serum progesterone of less than 15 ng/mL, whereas nearly 90% of comparable intrauterine gestations exceed that value. This finding led to the suggestion that a single serum progesterone may be useful in screening for ectopic pregnancy.

**2. Hematocrit**–The hematocrit will be more than 39% in over 72% of cases and 21–30% in 23% of cases with ectopic pregnancies. In 4.7%, the hematocrit will be less than 21%.

**3. White blood cell count**–The white blood count is variable, but nearly 50% of patients have a count of less than 10,000/$\mu$L, whereas nearly 36% have 10,000–15,000/$\mu$L, over 10% have 15,000–21,000/$\mu$L, and nearly 5% have more than 20,000/$\mu$L.

**4. Reticulocytes**–The reticulocytes may be increased to more than 2%. Hematin is detected by spectroscopy in peripheral blood 2 days after 100 mL or more of blood accumulates intraperitoneally. The

icterus index may be elevated in chronic cases. Serum amylase may be as high as 1600 Somogyi units per deciliter (normal = 80–100 units/dL) if narcotics have not been given. Urine urobilinogen is elevated, indicating decomposition of blood. Slight porphyrinuria is present with hemoperitoneum or hematocele, but this finding may also be noted with torsion of an ovarian cyst.

**Special Examinations:**

Ultrasonically the diagnosis of ectopic gestation depends on finding an empty uterine cavity and products of conception outside the uterus (in the adnexa or cul-de-sac as clearly defined products of conception or as a cystic or complex mass).

**1. Culdocentesis**–Culdocentesis is the transvaginal passage of a needle (posterior to the cervix) into the cul-de-sac (pouch of Douglas) for the purpose of determining whether free blood is present in the abdomen (Fig 14–6). The procedure is simple and safe and may be useful in the diagnosis of intraperitoneal bleeding. It is generally accomplished with the unanesthetized patient in the dorsal lithotomy position. A speculum is placed in the vagina and the posterior lip of the cervix grasped with an Allis clamp or a tenaculum. The vagina is cleansed (eg, with povidone iodine), and local anesthetic may or may not be injected into the area posterior to the cervix between the uterosacral ligaments. An 18-gauge spinal needle is attached to a 10-mL syringe, and with gentle traction on the cervix, the needle is passed the short distance into the cul-de-sac.

Culdocentesis reveals nonclotting blood in approximately 95% of cases with ectopic gestation. In 97.5% of those cases, the hematocrit will exceed 15%, and in 2.5% it will be less than 15%. The blood obtained is generally nonclotting owing to intraperitoneal bleeding from ectopic gestation (the blood first undergoes clotting and, subsequently, fibrinolysis). If the blood clots it is probably from a vessel punctured in the wall of the vagina. Obviously, no blood is obtained if the cul-de-sac is not entered or if a tubal pregnancy is not bleeding intraperitoneally. Usually, the cul-de-sac contains some straw-colored fluid, and this may be used to determine whether the needle has been properly placed when there is no bleeding. If culdocentesis yields a negative result, further diagnostic tests should be performed (ie, pregnancy test, ultrasonography, and, possibly, laparoscopy). If culdocentesis is positive, laparoscopy or laparotomy should be performed immediately.

**2. Laparoscopy**–Laparoscopy has been very useful in the diagnosis of early and unruptured ectopic pregnancy. Moreover, it will rule out ectopic pregnancy in the difficult differential diagnosis of acute abdominal pain. Laparoscopy has largely replaced the very hazardous practice of attempting to diagnose ectopic gestation by examination under an-

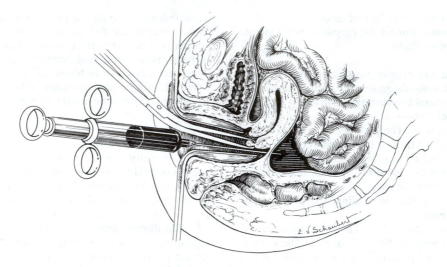

**Figure 14–6.** Culdocentesis.

esthesia. (At one time, examination under anesthesia was advocated as a means of avoiding the need for laparotomy. However, all too frequently even gentle pressure would rupture the ectopic site; thus, no mass was palpated and the anesthetized patient simply slipped into shock.) Finally, laparoscopy is increasingly being used for definitive surgical management in unruptured or early ectopic gestation (see Chapter 43).

**3. Dilatation and curettage**–D&C may exclude intrauterine pregnancy. In contrast to either incomplete abortion or dysfunctional uterine bleeding, the amount of tissue obtained is scant. Pathologic analysis of the tissue should reveal the Arias-Stella reaction, further reinforcing the presumptive diagnosis of ectopic pregnancy. When trophoblastic tissue is recovered (usually chorionic villi), the diagnosis of intrauterine pregnancy is confirmed. In such cases, ectopic gestation is unlikely simply because of the extraordinary rarity of combined ectopic and intrauterine pregnancies. Unfortunately, D&C may interrupt an intrauterine gestation, and after 4–5 days of continued bleeding it is unlikely to be diagnostic (in such cases, degenerating tissue inadequate for analysis may be all that is obtained).

**4. Exploratory laparoscopy**–This is the final diagnostic procedure. It establishes the presence or absence of ectopic (but not cervical) pregnancy. Laparotomy is indicated when the presumptive diagnosis of ectopic pregnancy with profound hemorrhage necessitates immediate control of the bleeding or when definitive therapy is not possible by laparoscopy.

## Differential Diagnosis (Table 14–2)

About 50 pathologic conditions may be confused with extrauterine pregnancy. The most common of these are appendicitis, salpingitis, ruptured corpus luteum cyst or ovarian follicle, uterine abortion, twisted ovarian cyst, and urinary tract disease. Less commonly, degenerating leiomyomas and normal intrauterine pregnancy with other abdominal or pelvic problems must be included in the differential diagnosis.

## Complications

About 1 in 1000 ectopic pregnancies result in maternal death. Hemorrhage is the major cause of maternal death in untreated ruptured ectopic pregnancy. Untreated or mistreated ruptured ectopic tubal pregnancy is responsible for 8–12% of all maternal deaths and about 16% of deaths from hemorrhage during pregnancy. The majority of these deaths are preventable.

Chronic salpingitis often follows neglected ruptured tubal ectopic pregnancy. Infertility or sterility develops in many patients who have undergone surgery for extrauterine pregnancy. Intestinal obstruction and fistulas may develop after hemoperitoneum and peritonitis.

## Prevention

Treat salpingitis early and vigorously; perform D&C promptly for incomplete abortion, avoiding adhesions. Early diagnosis of unruptured tubal pregnancy will obviate later extensive surgery. Most forms of ectopic pregnancy other than tubal are not preventable.

## Treatment

**A. Emergency Treatment:** Immediate surgery is indicated when the diagnosis of ectopic pregnancy with hemorrhage is made. Transfusion with whole blood or appropriate blood component therapy as soon as possible is indicated when the patient is in

**Table 14–2.** Differential diagnosis of ectopic pregnancy.

| | Ectopic Pregnancy | Appendicitis | Salpingitis | Ruptured Corpus Luteum Cyst | Uterine Abortion |
|---|---|---|---|---|---|
| Pain | Unilateral cramps and tenderness before rupture. | Epigastric, periumbilical, then right lower quadrant pain; tenderness localizing at McBurney's point. Rebound tenderness. | Usually in both lower quadrants, with or without rebound. Dysuria sometimes present. | Unilateral, becoming general with progressive bleeding. | Midline cramps. |
| Nausea and vomiting | Occasionally before, frequently after rupture. | Usual. Precedes shift of pain to right lower quadrant. | Infrequent. | Rare. No symptoms or signs of pregnancy. | Almost never. |
| Menstruation | Some aberration; missed period, spotting. | Unrelated to menses. | Hypermenorrhea or metrorrhagia, or both. | Period delayed, then bleeding, often with pain. | Longer amenorrhea, then spotting, then brisk bleeding. |
| Temperature and pulse | 37.2–37.8°C (99–100°F). Pulse variable: normal before, rapid after rupture. | 37.2–37.8°C (99–100°F). Pulse rapid: 99–100 | 37.2–40°C (99–104°F). Pulse elevated in proportion to fever. | Not over 37.2°C (99°F). Pulse normal unless blood loss marked, then rapid. | To 37.2°C (99°F) if spontaneous; to 40°C (104°F) if induced (infected). |
| Pelvic examination | Unilateral tenderness, especially on movement of cervix. Crepitant mass on one side or in cul-de-sac. | No masses. Rectal tenderness high on right side. | Bilateral tenderness on movement of cervix. Mass only when pyosalpinx or hydrosalpinx is present. | Tenderness over affected ovary. No masses. Uterus firm and not enlarged. | Cervix slightly patulous. Uterus slightly enlarged, irregularly softened. Tender only with infection. |
| Laboratory findings | White cell count of 15.000/μL. Red cell count strikingly low if blood loss large. Sedimentation rate slightly elevated. | Negative β-hCG. White cell count 10,000–18,000/μL (rarely normal). Red cell count normal. Sedimentation rate slightly elevated. | Negative β-hCG. White cell count 15,000–30,000/μL. Red cell count normal. Sedimentation rate markedly elevated. | Negative β-hCG. White cell count normal to 10,000/μL. Red cell count normal. Sedimentation rate normal. | White cell count 15,000/μL if spontaneous; to 30,000 μL if induced (infection). Red cell count normal. Sedimentation rate slightly to moderately elevated. |

shock. Blood should be warmed, if possible, to prevent chilling. Also administer antishock measures as indicated; that is, keep the patient comfortably warm, give oxygen, and apply moderately snug tourniquets around the upper legs.

Rapid entry into the abdomen should be accomplished in cases of extensive bleeding, since control of hemorrhage can be lifesaving. Careful, fast exploration of the abdominal cavity should be done at once, because the bleeding may be from a site other than the adnexa. Remove products of conception, clots, and free blood, exposing the area of nidation. If the pregnancy is advanced, do not disturb an adherent placenta but leave it in situ. Do not insert drains. If necessary, give an autotransfusion, using the patient's own citrated and filtered blood; this may be lifesaving if no other blood is available. Stimulant general anesthesia should be used; avoid depressants such as regional block or thiopental.

**B. Surgical Treatment:** As noted above, many unruptured ectopic gestations as well as some ruptured ectopic gestations may be managed by laparoscopic techniques. Many of these nonemergency cases can be managed in outpatient surgeries or surgicenters, eliminating the necessity for hospitalization. More severe cases require more intensive care situations as well as laparotomy.

**C. Medical Treatment:** Very early unruptured ectopic pregnancies as well as some chronic ectopic pregnancies have been treated with systemic methotrexate. Therapy response is then monitored carefully with every 48-hour quantitative hCG determinations. Preliminarily, this technique appears very promising.

**D. Supportive Treatment:** If symptoms and signs of infection are present, give broad-spectrum antibiotics, prescribe oral or intravenous iron therapy (or both), and order a high-protein diet with vitamin and mineral supplements as soon as the patient is on oral intake.

**Prognosis**

Another tubal pregnancy will occur in 10–20% of patients treated. Infertility develops in approximately 50% of patients who have undergone surgery for the treatment of an ectopic pregnancy, and of these, about 30% become sterile. Normal pregnancies are achieved in about 50% of patients who have one ectopic pregnancy. The maternal mortality rate due to ectopic pregnancy in the USA is 1–2%; the perinatal mortality rate is virtually 100%.

## TUBAL ECTOPIC PREGNANCY
## (Not Including Interstitial Type)

Tubal pregnancy is the most common form of ectopic pregnancy, and for this reason the terms "tubal pregnancy" and "ectopic pregnancy" are frequently taken to be synonymous (Fig 14–7). At least 50% of tubal ectopic pregnancies resolve spontaneously before diagnosis and without rupture. In the past 5 years, the incidence of tubal ectopic pregnancy has increased more than 50% owing to the following factors: epidemic salpingitis; microscopic tubal surgery of all kinds; conservative management of the tube with preservation of an organ that still retains the causative factor; the timing of artificial insemination and natural methods of contraception, which lead to fertilization of a late ovum; an increased number of tubal ligations with increased failures; and DES syndrome. The incidence of tubal ectopic pregnancy is higher in black women than in white women.

### Etiology

Conditions and contributing factors that may lead to tubal pregnancy include acute or chronic salpingitis, peritubular adhesions or tumor with fixation of the tube, congenital anomalies such as accessory tubes, infantile tubal development or abnormal length, functional failure with poor peristalsis or tubal spasm, endosalpingosis, endometriosis, postperitonitis inflammatory reaction, inhibition of ciliary action, microsurgery of the tube (eg, anastomosis, fimbrioplasty, salpingostomy, reimplantation), tubal sterilization procedures (eg, electrocoagulation, fimbriectomy, Pomeroy method).

### Clinical Findings

**A. Acute Tubal Rupture:** (Almost 40% of tubal ectopic pregnancies.) A history of abnormal menstruation and infertility is present in about 60% of cases, with scanty persistent vaginal bleeding in 80%. Findings may include sharp abdominal or pelvic pain; adnexal mass; peritoneal irritation; shoulder pain and backache; falling blood pressure, hemoglobin, and hematocrit; and classic symptoms of hemorrhagic shock with weakness, thirst, profuse perspiration, "air hunger," and oliguria. Coma and narrowing pulse pressure are ominous signs. Complications of acute tubal rupture may be life-threatening.

**B. Chronic Tubal Rupture:** (Almost 60% of tubal ectopic pregnancies.) When the point of rupture is small and bleeding slow, the symptoms generally are vague and inconclusive.

**C. Unruptured Tubal Pregnancy:** (Currently 2% of tubal ectopic pregnancies, but rapidly increasing as diagnostic methods are more widely applied.) This may be suspected if there is a history of amenorrhea, with symptoms and signs of early pregnancy, scanty dark vaginal bleeding, and discomfort in the affected adnexal area, especially when the uterus is moved. The diagnosis should be more clear when a definite tender, slightly fixed mass is felt, particularly when the ovary can be felt separately on the same side.

### Treatment

See general treatment discussion earlier in this chapter.

Selection of a conservative surgical procedure depends on the status of the patient and the location of the pregnancy. If the woman is not a candidate for conservative operation, total tubal excision is advised. Ampullary pregnancy may be treated with salpingostomy and isthmic pregnancy with segmental resection (never salpingostomy). Details of conservative surgery may be found in Chapter 58.

When the tube must be removed, clamp the tube from the fimbrial end inward and then on the uterine side. Excision of the tube against the uterine cornu at the level of the uterine body prevents uterine cornual rupture, which may lead to intrauterine abortion, repeat ectopic pregnancy, or endosalpingitis of the tubal remnant.

Correction of tubal disease and lysis of adhesions in the opposite adnexa are indicated in cases with minimal or no bleeding and in those without rupture.

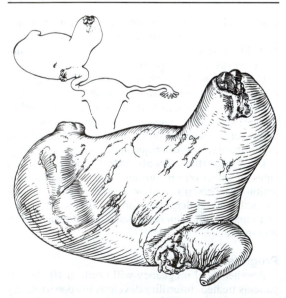

**Figure 14–7.** Tubal pregnancy. (Modified from a drawing by Ashworth.)

Fimbrioplasty and salpingostomy can be performed, and occasional uterine or ovarian suspension is indicated. However, tubal uterine implantation is not indicated at this time. Intraoperative patency tests may be obscured by pregnancy changes and hyperemia.

## INTERSTITIAL ECTOPIC PREGNANCY

In interstitial pregnancy, the fertilized ovum implants in the portion of the uterine tube that traverses the uterine wall. This type of ectopic pregnancy occurs in 2–4% of all pregnancies, most frequently in multiparas 25–35 years of age. It may occur following previous salpingectomy. The nidation site may be in the uterointerstitial (inner) portion, the true interstitial (middle) portion, or the tubointerstitial (outer) portion.

### Etiology

Descent of the fertilized ovum through the tube proceeds at a reduced rate through the interstitial portion, and the ovum may be arrested here. This is often due to obstruction of the tubal lumen or failure of the transport mechanism. The question of increased incidence of interstitial pregnancy associated with the use of IUDs is not settled. The following factors influence the formation of obstruction or interfere with passage of the gamete:

(1) Developmental anomalies, eg, partial atresia, accessory tube, or diverticula.

(2) Intra-abdominal fertilization, with a developing morula too large for the tubal lumen.

(3) Pelvic infections, eg, salpingitis, ciliary destruction, and interference with tubal peristalsis and perisalpingitis and parametritis, which causes adhesions, edema, and fibrosis.

(4) Peritubal adhesions, with kinking or angulation of the tube from pelvic surgery, endometriosis, previous ectopic pregnancy, and ovarian or other pelvic tumors.

(5) Adjacent uterine tumor such as intramural or subserous myomas, which often occlude or impair the tubal lumen in the interstitial area.

(6) An endometrium-like transformation of the tubal epithelium, which may encourage implantation.

(7) Interstitial pregnancy in the stump of a tube previously removed either for a previous tubal ectopic pregnancy or other adnexal disease.

### Course of the Disease

The tubal epithelium becomes eroded by the trophoblast, and the myometrium is invaded. The muscle is destroyed by infiltration in the area of least resistance. The gestational sac is composed of serosa, a small amount of connective tissue, and thinned uterine muscle lying in the posterior-superior part of the involved cornu. The pregnancy has thus become intramural and extracanalicular.

The embryo or fetus may die at any stage of development as a result of periovular hemorrhage. If the fetus dies early, the tissues generally are absorbed.

Rupture of the uterine wall is the most common outcome until the 10th—14th weeks. The duration of pregnancy seems to depend on the nidation site. Implantation in either the utero- or tubointerstitial area favors early rupture. No living children have been reported with interstitial pregnancy. Implantation in the middle third or true interstitial portion somewhat prolongs the gestation. Occasionally, the pregnancy will abort into the uterine cavity if the implantation is in the uterointerstitial area. A lithopedion may be formed with rupture.

### Clinical Findings

**A. Symptoms and Signs:** The manifestations are generally nonspecific, with the usual signs of early normal intrauterine pregnancy. Intermittent, recurrent, sharp abdominal pain occurs at 4–6 weeks. Sudden abdominal pain is followed by collapse. Localized tenderness occurs over the affected cornu. Vaginal bleeding occurs in only about 25% of cases.

Pelvic examination may reveal uterine findings compatible with early uterine pregnancy and a palpable mass in the area of pregnancy with a broad base extending outward (Baart de la Faille's sign). This mass will be softer than the uterus and may be very sensitive.

Unruptured interstitial pregnancy may be diagnosed by ultrasonography. Laparoscopy allows visualization of the pathologic process.

Diagnostic findings at surgery (Ruge-Simon syndrome) are displacement of the uterine fundus to the opposite side, elevation of the involved cornu, and rotation of the uterus on its long axis. In addition to the tube, the round and ovarian ligaments will be lateral to the sac. Manipulation of the uterus may make the cornual mass more apparent, or the administration of oxytocin may cause uterine contraction and better visualization of the gestation.

**B. Laboratory Findings:** There are no characteristic laboratory findings except those that occur following rupture with massive intraperitoneal hemorrhage. Pregnancy tests usually are positive.

### Differential Diagnosis

Interstitial pregnancy must be differentiated from tubal ectopic pregnancy near the uterus, cornual pregnancy, angular pregnancy, cornual myoma, cornual abscess, pregnancy in one horn of a bicornuate uterus, large endometrioma at the uterotubal junction, and endosalpingosis. Angular pregnancy should be differentiated from interstitial pregnancy by laparoscopy, because such a pregnancy can carry to term. Angular pregnancy forces the round ligament to lie lateral to the mass, which is not the case with interstitial pregnancy.

A benign tumor may occasionally be confused with interstitial pregnancy.

## Complications

Rupture is a catastrophic event because massive hemorrhage, shock, and early maternal death may follow, especially if the uterine artery is lacerated. The uterine wall below the tubal insertion is the most common site of rupture, and this may extend downward into the uterine vasculature and cause extensive uterine damage. The ovarian circulation may be involved also, and the pregnancy may be extruded intra- or extraperitoneally.

## Prevention

Interstitial pregnancy may recur in cases of previous salpingectomy with cornual resection; hence, this procedure does not ensure against recanalization. Excision of the cornual area with careful—preferably double—peritonization is the procedure of choice. The round ligament may be brought over and sutured for reinforcement.

## Treatment

**A. Emergency Measures:** Management of shock due to hemorrhage, as in any other case, requires rapid massive blood replacement, perhaps intra-arterial administration.

**B. Surgical Measures:** Once the diagnosis of interstitial ectopic pregnancy is made—either before or after rupture—immediate laparotomy is required. Simple wedge resection, reconstruction of the uterine wall, and salpingectomy may be the best procedure. Preservation of the ovary should be attempted if feasible. The extent of surgery depends on the degree of damage to the uterus and adnexa. Total abdominal hysterectomy and unilateral salpingo-oophorectomy on the affected side may be necessary. In the patient with severe shock, a supracervical hysterectomy may be lifesaving. A conservative, extensive, prolonged uterine reconstruction is ill-advised in a patient with massive hemorrhage.

## Prognosis

The prognosis for viability of the fetus in interstitial pregnancy is nil. The reconstructed uterus may rupture during a subsequent pregnancy, and delivery after uterine repair or reconstruction should be by elective cesarean section. Careful exploration of the area following placental removal must be performed because of the possibility of placenta accreta in the region of repair.

The prognosis is good for the mother if adequate blood transfusion and early surgery are accomplished, but poor if shock is deep and occurs early after rupture or if treatment is delayed. The mortality

rate in interstitial pregnancy is 2–3%; following a previous salpingectomy, it is about 7%.

## ABDOMINAL ECTOPIC PREGNANCY

Abdominal pregnancy has an incidence of 1 in 8000 term births. Diagnosis of primary abdominal pregnancy depends on the presence of normal tubes and ovaries without evidence of trauma; the absence of a uteroplacental fistula; and attachment of the conceptus exclusively to the peritoneal surface. Secondary abdominal pregnancies (more common) occur when the fetus escapes from the tube through a rupture or through the fimbriated end. Abdominal pregnancy seems to occur in older women of low parity, but endometriosis is rarely reported.

There have been 6 primary abdominal pregnancies reported in the spleen and 4 in the liver. The predominant presenting symptom is hemorrhage. If a pregnancy is not found in the pelvis when abdominal gestation is suspected, exploration of the upper abdomen may reveal omental, splenic, or hepatic sites. Treatment frequently requires splenectomy and omentectomy. Excision with local hemostasis using exact suture placement is the procedure of choice in hepatic pregnancy. A retained placenta may be managed with methotrexate. In cases of intractable hemorrhage, use of a MAST suit (military antishock trousers) will control bleeding for 48 hours or until the patient becomes stable. If bleeding persists with the first release of pressure from the suit, pressure can be restored for another 24 hours.

In secondary abdominal pregnancy, the primary site of the gestation may have been tubal, ovarian, or even uterine.

The pregnancy usually develops normally if the implantation sites provide sufficient blood supply to the placenta. Discomfort, genitourinary symptoms, and actual pain are the rule as the pregnancy progresses. If undiagnosed and untreated, the fetus will die and suppurate, with abscess formation; form a true lithopedion or calcified fetus; develop into an adipocere; or result in undetermined retention of bony fetal parts with absorption of soft tissues. Massive intra-abdominal hemorrhage may ensue; fetal parts may extrude through the rectum, bladder, or vagina; or an abdominal fistula may form.

## Clinical Findings

**A. Symptoms and Signs:** Abdominal pregnancy may be suspected in relation to bizarre pregnancy symptoms, ie, a history suggestive of tubal rupture or abortion; a pregnancy complicated by unusual gastrointestinal symptoms; fetal movements that are very marked or painful; easy palpation of the fetal parts and movement; pregnancy described by a multipara as "different"; false labor near term (a small uterus may be felt in the pelvis by examination early in the pregnancy); high-lying fetus in abnormal presentation—often transverse; displacement of a firm, long cervix; palpation of fetal parts through the vaginal fornix; or a palpable placental mass and an unusually loud vascular souffle.

**B. X-Ray Findings:** The fetus rides high in the abdomen over the maternal spine in the lateral view. The fetal skeleton is unusually clear in relation to maternal organs.

Ultrasonography is useful in making a diagnosis of abdominal pregnancy and also in following regression in the size of a retained placenta associated with abdominal pregnancy.

### Differential Diagnosis

Differential diagnosis of abdominal ectopic pregnancy concerns intrauterine or abdominal pregnancy. Usually the diagnosis may be made by ultrasound examination. In the rare case in which ultrasound is not diagnostic, it may be useful to give oxytocin; if uterine contractions can be felt, abdominal pregnancy is ruled out. The same is true if the fetus can be felt through the cervical canal.

### Complications

Most complications are related to preoperative intra-abdominal hemorrhage or the postoperative course after removal of the fetus. Reoperation may be necessary because of obstruction, abscess, fistula, or bleeding.

### Treatment

Treatment for abdominal ectopic pregnancy consists of immediate surgical removal of the fetus and membranes and ligation of the cord near the placenta. The placenta should be removed only when the operator is absolutely certain that total hemostasis can be accomplished (very rare). The abdomen should be closed without drainage except in the presence of infection. If the placenta is allowed to remain, methotrexate or dactinomycin in full antitumor dosage may be given to destroy the trophoblast and speed resorption of the placenta.

### Prognosis

The maternal mortality rate for patients with abdominal ectopic pregnancy is approximately 10%. About 50% of fetuses are alive at surgery, but only about 20% survive.

## COMBINED & COMPOUND EXTRA- & INTRAUTERINE ECTOPIC PREGNANCY

Combined intrauterine and extrauterine pregnancy means the existence of simultaneous pregnancies. Compound intrauterine and extrauterine pregnancy is superposition of the intrauterine pregnancy on the extrauterine one. It may be classified according to the duration of gestation. Along with the general increase in incidence of tubal ectopic pregnancies there has been an increase in heterotopic pregnancies. A history of spontaneous or elective abortion with subsequent persistent pain should be examined by means of ultrasonography or laparoscopy for concomitant tubal pregnancy. Multiparas are more commonly affected. A compound pregnancy of the extra- and intrauterine type is one in which a normal intrauterine pregnancy occurs when an ectopic pregnancy has died, ruptured, or resolved.

### Clinical Findings

If the patients gives a history compatible with ectopic pregnancy but presents with a large, soft uterus and accentuated symptoms and signs of pregnancy, she may have a combined pregnancy. Unusual abdominal pain in the presence of spontaneous abortion or profuse uterine bleeding with signs of peritoneal irritation should suggest combined pregnancy.

Ultrasonographic evaluation usually reveals an intrauterine gestation as well as an adnexal mass and more than one corpus luteum. It is occasionally necessary to resort to laparoscopy for diagnosis.

### Differential Diagnosis

Consider retained products of conception, salpingitis, myoma, twisted ovarian cyst, or acute appendicitis. Rarely is the correct diagnosis made prior to surgery.

### Complications

Massive intra-abdominal hemorrhage with shock often occurs in combined ectopic pregnancy. There may also be excessive bleeding from the uterus, with simultaneous spontaneous uterine abortion. A normal intrauterine pregnancy may be removed by an ill-timed diagnostic D&C.

### Treatment

The treatment for combined ectopic pregnancy is the same as that for ruptured or unruptured ectopic pregnancy with an intrauterine pregnancy. If possible, the intrauterine pregnancy should be preserved, but if abortion is inevitable or incomplete, a D&C must be done as soon as possible to avoid blood loss.

If 2 living premature fetuses are diagnosed, immediate hospitalization and treatment should be arranged. Delivery by abdominal laparotomy and cesarean section may be indicated. If the placenta remains in situ, the mother may be given methotrexate following the surgery.

### Prognosis

The maternal mortality rate is about 1%; most fetuses of a uterine pregnancy survive following removal of a concomitant ectopic pregnancy.

# OTHER UNCOMMON
# ECTOPIC PREGNANCIES

## Cervical Pregnancy

A large, dark, highly vascularized cervix with bleeding or extrusion of dark tissue through the external os will be noted in a cervical pregnancy. There may be backache or dysuria, and abdominal pain is described. Distention of the cervix and dilatation of the external os are thought to cause the low abdominal pain.

The diagnosis is suggested clinically by continuous bleeding after amenorrhea; a soft and disproportionately enlarged cervix equal to or greater than the uterine corpus (an hourglass effect); a tight internal cervical os and a patulous external cervical os; and a dilated, thin-walled cervical canal with histologic evidence of the products of conception. Diagnosis may be made by ultrasonographic demonstration of a characteristic cervical enlargement. The differential diagnosis includes cervical phase uterine abortion, cervical abortion, placenta previa, and uterine or cervical cancer.

Immediate surgery is indicated as soon as the diagnosis is suspected. Hemorrhage may be massive and sometimes fatal. Ligation of the hypogastric arteries or the cervical branches of the uterine arteries may be effective in controlling excessive bleeding. Curettage of the endocervix and endometrium may stop the heavy bleeding. Sutures and Gelfoam or gauze packing may be necessary. Packing of the endometrial cavity, dilated cervical canal, and vagina with gauze for counterpressure may control bleeding. If tissue damage or necrosis is great, hysterectomy is necessary. Amputation of the cervix is not recommended.

The prognosis for continued reproductive capability is grave and if adequate hemostasis cannot be achieved, maternal life is jeopardized.

## Ovarian Pregnancy

Ovarian pregnancy cannot be diagnosed on the basis of clinical signs. Pain and cramps, a pelvic mass, vaginal bleeding after a period of amenorrhea, and clinical shock are the most common findings. A positive pregnancy test is also common. A preoperative diagnosis of ectopic pregnancy is made in 63% of cases. Ovarian twin pregnancy is a rarity.

The incidence of ovarian pregnancy is 1 in 7000 term births. In women who use IUDs, the ratio of ovarian to tubal ectopic pregnancies is 1 to 9, with the former representing 3% of all ectopic pregnancies.

A diagnosis of primary ovarian pregnancy is made when trophoblastic tissue is found by microscopic examination exclusively in either intra- or extrafollicular ovarian tissue. Fertilization always takes place outside the ovary. Involvement may be bilateral; the ovaries are ruptured in 90% of cases. The ovarian gestation is discovered during the first trimester in 90% of cases. The differential diagnosis includes

ectopic pregnancy, postsurgical pelvic hematoma, and rapidly growing ovarian cyst.

Treatment for cervical pregnancy is surgical removal. Sacrifice of the ovary and occasionally the tube is usually necessary, although some cases lend themselves to ovarian wedge resection. Preservation of the ovary is especially indicated when the other ovary and uterine tube are diseased or have been removed. Hysterectomy is rarely indicated, especially if hemorrhage has occurred. Excessive blood loss requires all of the usual supportive measures.

## Multiple Tubal Ectopic Pregnancy

Multiple tubal ectopic pregnancy presents essentially the same as single ectopic pregnancy, with the possible exception of bilateral palpable, tender adnexal masses. Treatment should be as conservative as possible, and the tube should be preserved when feasible. However, successive coexistent tubal pregnancies have been recorded that required bilateral salpingectomy with or without abdominal hysterectomy.

## Intraligamentous Pregnancy

Intraligamentous pregnancies are rare (1 in 50,000 pregnancies). The conceptus is contained within the anatomic confines of the broad ligament. Clinical findings are similar to those of an abdominal pregnancy. The patient may be hospitalized several times before the diagnosis is made. The uterus is usually displaced to the opposite side. If the pregnancy persists, the mass may become palpable abdominally and occasionally may be detected by pelvic or rectovaginal examination.

Diagnosis is made when labor induction fails or when the uterus can be palpated or is seen on ultrasound. Ultrasonography may improve diagnostic accuracy in this rare condition.

Treatment must be individualized, but inevitably involves laparotomy. The condition is often discovered late and cases in which pregnancy is followed to fetal viability have been reported. The placenta should be removed when possible, and bleeding is usually well controlled.

## Pregnancy in a Uterine Diverticulum
## or Sacculation

Uterine diverticula are rare, and a pregnancy within one is exceptional. It resembles abdominal pregnancy or a uterine saccular pregnancy. Delivery by abdominal laparotomy and hysterotomy are necessary. Saccular pregnancy, because of the thin wall, suggests an abdominal pregnancy, except that the pregnancy is not high in the abdomen and there are no gastrointestinal symptoms. Removal of the pregnancy must be by incision through the saccular wall.

## Angular Pregnancy

In this case, the conception becomes implanted in the angle of the uterus just inside the uterotubal attachment on the side of the uterine cavity. This is often over the tubal ostium. The symptoms may differ from normal uterine pregnancy either at the time of spontaneous abortion or labor and delivery. Diagnosis usually is made following delivery, with manual removal of the placenta, or at cesarean section. Angular pregnancy may present as a painful, tender sacculation of the uterus; vaginal bleeding may be present. Manual removal of the placenta during the third stage of labor may be required. Curettage for bleeding after incomplete abortion may identify the placental site.

## Pregnancy in a Rudimentary Horn

It is very difficult to make this diagnosis before surgery. However, the condition is most hazardous to maternal life because pregnancy frequently progresses into the midtrimester or later and delivery is possible only by abdominal surgery. Rupture of such a pregnancy usually occurs and is accompanied by serious intraperitoneal hemorrhage. Surgical exploration in cases of rupture and hemorrhage should be immediate. A viable infant may be delivered by cesarean section. Total excision of the abnormal horn is advised, although total hysterectomy is occasionally necessary.

## Intramural Pregnancy

Intramural pregnancy is defined as a gestation separate from the uterine tubes or uterine cavity that is surrounded by the myometrium. This diagnosis is almost never made prior to termination of the pregnancy; however, unruptured intramural pregnancies have been described. Irregular development of the uterine mass and abnormal or persistent pain and tenderness may point to an abnormal gestation. The definitive diagnosis may be made on pathologic examination during which an incomplete or absent decidua basalis is found. The placenta may be percreta or accreta. Uterine wall rupture often occurs in the area of the pregnancy and in most cases the rupture also extends into the uterine cavity.

Treatment consists of surgical removal of the pregnancy with reconstruction of the area of rupture. It may be possible to detach the tissue mass without entering the uterine cavity. If damage is severe, total hysterectomy may be necessary; but subtotal hysterectomy has been performed in the presence of massive hemorrhage with extensive tissue damage and a patient in severe shock.

## Vaginal Pregnancy

A suburethral cyst containing chorionic villi and trophoblastic cells indicating a vaginal pregnancy has been described. Possible causes include fertilization of an ovum in the vagina and passage of an early conceptus from the cervix. Treatment is simple excision and pathologic identification.

## Pregnancy Subsequent to Hysterectomy

The pregnancy follows the course of a tubal ectopic gestation if nidation takes place in the tube and may develop as an abdominal pregnancy if implantation is in the abdomen. Posthysterectomy ovarian pregnancy has been reported in 31 patients. Clinical findings are those of a postoperative and rapidly growing intra-abdominal tumor and ectopic pregnancy. Laparotomy is the treatment of choice. Surgical excision of the ectopic pregnancy is required.

## EXPOSURE TO FETOTOXIC AGENTS

Many variations occur in the complex biologic process of human development. Although population heterogeneity and even the evolutionary process are based on such events, some deviations from the usual developmental process result in aberrations of normal structure and function that may lead to impairment. These adverse structural and functional alterations have been closely scrutinized since antiquity in a considerable effort to detail their causation. The clinician investigating the effects of exposure to fetotoxic agents usually must consider 3 important factors: whether the patient is known to have reproductive defects or potential reproductive risks (discussed throughout this text; see also Chapter 13); whether there has been actual or potential hazardous exposure to fetotoxic agents during pregnancy; and whether it can be determined that structural or functional abnormalities are likely to develop in the fetus of a patient exposed to fetotoxic agents. Assessment of these factors requires a thorough understanding of genetics (see Chapter 4) and early fetal development and growth (see Chapter 2). Assessment of developmental defects in newborn offspring is briefly discussed in Chapter 29.

Many harmful agents are responsible for altering the complex biologic process of human development (eg, irradiation, viruses, gases, and drugs). However, even the most careful investigation will fail to reveal the cause in 60–70% of developmental handicaps. At least 20% of all abnormalities are due to known parental genetic influences and another 3–5% to mutations. Thus, only a small minority of abnormalities can be ascribed to fetal exposure to harmful agents. Infections (Table 14–3) account for 2–3%; drugs and hostile environmental agents (eg, irradiation) account for only 4–5%. Aberrations that result from fetal exposure to harmful agents is tragic because such exposure is often preventable.

Approximately 3–7% of newborns in the USA have abnormalities at birth that are serious enough to require some form of treatment. Moreover, full recognition of malformations, anomalies, or defects may take years. Thus, estimates that as high as 10% of the total population suffer from some structural or functional developmental disability do not appear unrea-

**Table 14–3.** Infections affecting the fetus or newborn.

| Maternal Infection | Effects on Fetus or Newborn |
|---|---|
| **Specific viral infections** | |
| Rubella | Malformations, bleeding, hepatosplenomegaly, pneumonitis, hepatitis, encephalitis |
| Cytomegalovirus | Microcephaly, chorioretinitis, deafness, mental retardation |
| Herpes simplex | Generalized herpes, encephalitis, death |
| Mumps | Fetal death, endocardial fibroelastosis (?), malformations (?) |
| Rubeola | Increased abortions and stillbirths |
| Western equine encephalitis | Encephalitis |
| Chickenpox, shingles | Chickenpox or shingles, increased abortions and stillbirths |
| Smallpox | Smallpox, increased abortions and stillbirths |
| Vaccinia | Generalized vaccinia, increased abortions |
| Influenza | Malformations (?) |
| Poliomyelitis | Spinal or bulbar poliomyelitis |
| Hepatitis | Hepatitis |
| Coxsckie B viruses | Myocarditis |
| **Nonspecific viral infections** | |
| Upper respiratory infections | None |
| Severe viral infections | |
| **Syphilis** | Congenital syphilis |
| **Baceterial infections** | |
| Gonorrhea | Ophthalmitis |
| Acute bacterial infections | Prematurity |
| Tuberculosis | Congenital tuberculosis |
| Listeriosis | Abortions, stillbirths, septicemia, meningoencephalitis, habitual abortion (?) |
| Pyelonephritis | Premature labor |
| **Protozoan infections** | |
| Toxoplasmosis | Microcephaly, chorioretinitis, jaundice |
| Malaria | Low birth weight, perinatal mortality (?) |

Modified from Sever JL: Perinatal infections affecting the developing fetus and newborn. In: *The Prevention of Mental Retardation Through Control of Infectious Diseases.* Public Health Service Publication No. 1692, 1968.

**Table 14–4.** Potential adverse effects of fetotoxic exposure at selected stages of development.

| Week Since Ovulation | Potential Adverse Effect |
|---|---|
| 1 | Abortion |
| 2–7 | Fetal wastage<br>Structural malformations (see specific defects below)<br>Carcinogenesis<br>Severe intrauterine growth retardation |
| 3 | Ectopia cordis<br>Omphalocele<br>Ectomelia<br>Sympodia |
| 4 | Omphalocele<br>Ectomelia<br>Tracheoesophageal fistula<br>Hemivertebra |
| 5 | Tracheoesophageal fistula<br>Hemivertebra<br>Nuclear cataract<br>Microphthalmia<br>Facial clefts<br>Carpal of pedal ablation |
| 6 | Microphthalmia<br>Carpal or pedal ablation<br>Cleft lip<br>Agnathia<br>Lenticular cataract<br>Congenital heart disease<br>Gross cardiac septal and/or aortic anomalies |
| 7 | Congenital heart disease<br>Interventricular septal defects<br>Pulmonary stenosis<br>Digital ablation<br>Cleft palate<br>Micrognathia<br>Epicanthus<br>Brachycephaly |
| 8 | Congenital heart disease<br>Epicanthus<br>Brachycephaly<br>Persistent ostium primum<br>Nasal bone ablation<br>Digital stunting |
| 9–40 | Central nervous system anomalies<br>Behavioral disorders<br>Functional abnormalities<br>Reproductive effects<br>Intrauterine growth retardation |

Modified and reproduced, with permission, from Pernoll ML: Abortion induced by chemicals encountered in the environment. Clin Obstet Gynecol 1986;29:955.

sonable. Such a figure is probably very conservative given the current epidemic of substance abuse, eg, of tobacco, alcohol, methamphetamine, cocaine, during pregnancy.

## Evaluation

The highly individualized diagnosis and counseling of patients with actual or potential exposure to fetotoxic agents is facilitated by an organized plan for evaluation.

**A. Diagnosis:**

**1. Timing of exposure**—Obtain complete information about gestational stage at the time of exposure. Usually, fetal organs or structures are most vulnerable to adverse influences during the periods of most rapid development. Table 14–4 lists some of the potential adverse effects related to the timing of fetotoxic exposure. Such information may be useful

**Table 14–5.** Factors influencing the ability of a chemical to induce alteration in the normal process of fetal development.[1]

**Gross host factors influencing the amount of agent to which the DNA is exposed**
  Absorption
  Penetration
  Transport
  Activation
  Inactivation
  Excretion
**Local host factors influencing outcome**
  Removal of mutated cells
  pH
  Temperature
**Genetic mechanisms potentially influencing outcome**
  Condensation of nuclear membrane
  Condensation of chromosomes
  Specific nucleotide kinases and DNA replicase (avoids incorporation of wrong nucleotides into DNA)
  Excision of wrong bases and repair
  Repair of single-stranded lesions
  Repair of double-stranded lesions
  Recombination

Reproduced, with permission, from Pernoll ML: Abortion induced by chemicals encountered in the environment. Clin Obstet Gynecol 1986;29:956.

to target fetal areas for investigation and to provide a general picture, but it must not be too rigidly interpreted because the interaction of any given agent with the fetal genome is not always fully known.

**2. Characteristics of exposure**–Obtain complete information about the characteristics of the exposure, eg, the route of exposure, the length of time that the exposure occurred, the total dose received during exposure, and any simultaneous or other exposures that might influence the pregnancy. The manifestations of abnormal development range from no effect to lethal effects as a function of fetal tissue dose, in which the access of the adverse agent to developing tissue is evaluated and its ability to alter the normal process is estimated. Factors that may influence the fetal tissue dose are summarized in Table 14–5.

**3. Risks associated with exposure**–Review the scientific data concerning the risks associated with exposure, keeping in mind the overall validity of various studies as well as their applicability to the

**Table 14–6.** Criteria used to recognize teratogens in humans.

Abrupt increase in the incidence of a particular defect or association of defects.
Known environmental change coincident with this increase.
Known exposure to the environmental change early in pregnancy, yielding characteristically defected infants.
Absence of other factors common to all pregnancies, yielding infants with the characteristic defects.

Modified and reproduced, with permission, from Wilson JG: Embryotoxicity of drugs in man. In: *Handbook of Teratology.* Vol 1. Wilson JG, Fraser FC (editors). Plenum Press, 1977.

**Table 14–7.** General principles of teratology.

| | |
|---|---|
| **Mechanisms** (initiating changes associated with teratogenic influence) | Mutation. Chromosome disruption. Mitotic interference. Altered nucleic acid integrity or function. Precursor or substrate deprivation. Altered energy sources. Changed membrane characteristics. Altered osmolar balance. Enzyme inhibition. |
| **Pathogenesis** (manifestation of abnormal development created by above mechanisms) | Excessive or reduced cell interactions. Failed cell interactions. Reduced biosynthesis. Impeded morphogenetic movement. Mechanical disruption of tissues. |
| **Common pathways** | Too few cells or cell products to affect localized morphogenesis or functional maturation. Other imbalances in growth and differentiation. |
| **Final defects** (final manifestations of abnormal development) | Death. Malformation. Growth retardation. Functional disorder. |

Modified and reproduced, with permission, from Wilson JG: Current status of teratology: General principles and mechanisms derived from animal studies. In: *Handbook of Teratology.* Vol 1. Wilson JG, Fraser FC (editors): Plenum Press, 1977.

**Table 14–8.** Teratogenicity drug labeling now required by FDA.*

**Category A:** Well-controlled human studies have not disclosed any fetal risk.
**Category B:** Animal studies have not disclosed any fetal risk; or have suggested some risk not confirmed in controlled studies in women; or there are not adequate studies in women.
**Category C:** Animal studies have revealed adverse fetal effects; there are no adequate controlled studies in women.
**Category D:** Some fetal risk, but benefits may outweigh risk (eg, life-threatening illness, no safer effective drug). Patient should be warned.
**Category X:** Fetal abnormalities in animal and human studies; risk not outweighed by benefit. *Contraindicated in pregnancy.*

*The FDA has established 5 categories of drugs based on their potential for causing birth defects in infants born to women who use the drugs during pregnancy. By law, the label must set forth all available information on teratogenicity.

**Table 14–9.** Risk/benefit assessment of drugs administered to pregnant women in first trimester.

| Drug | Effects Reported | Drug | Effects Reported |
|------|------------------|------|------------------|
| **I. Risk outweighs benefit in first trimester** | | | |
| Acetazolamide | Limb defects | Phenmetrazine | Skeletal and visceral malformations |
| Amphetamines | Transposition of great vessels, cleft palate | Phenytoin | Multiple anomalies |
| Chlorquine | Retinal damage, eighth nerve damage | Podophyllin (in laxatives) | Multiple anomalies |
| Chlorpropamide | Increase of anomalies | Serotonin | Increase of anomalies |
| Dicumarol | Skeletal and facial anomalies, mental retardation | Sex steroids | VACTERL syndrome |
| | | Streptomycin | Eighth nerve damage, micromelia, multiple skeletal anomalies |
| Diethylstilbestrol | Clear cell adenocarcinoma of vagina and cervix, genital tract anomalies | Tetracycline | Inhibition of bone growth, micromelia, syndactyly, discoloration of teeth |
| Ethanol | Fetal alcohol syndrome | Thalidomide | Limb, auricle, eye, and visceral malformations |
| Iodide | Congenital goiter, hypothyroidism, mental retardation | | |
| LSD | Chromosomal abnormalities, increase of anomalies | Tolbutamide | Increase of anomalies |
| | | Trimethadione | Multiple anomalies |
| Meclizine | Multiple anomalies | Warfarin sodium | Skeletal and facial anomalies, mental retardation |
| Methotrexate (for psoriasis) | Multiple anomalies | | |
| Paramethadione | Multiple anomalies | | |
| **II. Risk versus benefits uncertain in first trimester** | | | |
| Barbiturates | Increase of anomalies | Metronidazole | None |
| Benzodiazepines | Cardiac defects | Propylthiouracil | Goiter, hypothyroidism, mental retardation |
| Cannabis | Increase of anomalies | | |
| Clofibrate | None | Pyrimethamine | Increase of anomalies |
| Cytotoxic drugs | Increase of anomalies | Quinine | Increase of anomalies |
| Diazoxide | Increase of anomalies | Thiouracil | Goiter, hypothyroidism, mental retardation |
| EDTA | Increase of anomalies | | |
| Gentamicin | Eighth nerve damage | Trimethoprim/ sulfamethoxazole | Cleft palate |
| Kanamycin | Eighth nerve damage | | |
| Lithium | Goiter, eye anomalies, cleft palate | | |
| **III. Benefit outweighs risk in first trimester** | | | |
| Acetaminophen | None | Isoniazid | Increase of anomalies |
| Antacids | Increase of anomalies | Isoproterenol | None |
| Antihistamines | None | Monoamine oxidase inhibitors | None |
| Chloramphenicol | None | | |
| Clomiphene | Increase of anomalies, neural tube defects, Down's syndrome | Pencillamine | Connective tissue defects |
| | | Penicillins | None |
| General anesthesia | Increase of anomalies | Phenothiazines | None |
| Glucocorticoids | Cleft palate, cardiac defects | Rifampin | Spina bifida, cleft palate |
| Haloperidol | Limb malformations | Salicylates | CNS, visceral, and skeletal malformations |
| Heprain | None | | |
| Hydralazine | Increase of anomalies | Sulfonamides | Cleft palate, facial, and skeletal defects |
| Idoxuridine | Increase of anomalies | Terbutaline | None |
| Imipramine | CNS and limb anomalies | Theophylline | None |
| Insulin | Skeletal malformations | Tricyclic antidepressants | CNS and limb malformations |

Modified and reproduced, with permission, from Howard F, Hill J: Drugs in pregnancy. Obstet Gynecol Surv 1979:34:643.

case. Determine the properties of the agent that create risk.

Evaluation of the studies of fetal exposure to harmful agents is difficult owing to the large number of potential fetotoxic influences and possible combined or interactive effects of certain agents; the retrospective nature of most studies; the incomplete knowledge of the types of defects created; the difficulty evaluating damage, even if target areas can be identified; the presence or absence of influences that may alter the potential biologic effects of a particular agent; and the presence or absence of potential genotype or group variations that might alter an individual's susceptibility. Therefore, certain criteria that may be used to recognize teratogens in humans have been defined (Table 14–6). The known mechanisms of abnormal development are summarized in Table 14–7, which also outlines a working hypothesis of the pathogenesis, common pathways, and final manifestations of abnormal development.

**4. Susceptibility to exposure**—Obtain complete medical, reproductive, and genetic histories to the existence of host factors that may mitigate or amplify the effects of the exposure.

**5. Extent of exposure**—Use available diagnostic modalities to ascertain exposure status as soon as possible. Acute and convalescent sera should be obtained for viral infections; it is also possible to obtain heavy metal levels. Other diagnostic technologies may also be helpful, including ultrasound for direct evaluation of potential target tissues (see Chapter 13).

**6. Counseling:** Counseling of the parents should compare what is known about the exposure of their fetus to harmful agents and what is known about the "normal, usual, or natural" rate of abortion or alteration of the normal course of pregnancy. If available information is inadequate, the parents should be so advised. In some cases, intervention (eg, hydrocephalic decompression) may be possible. To be effectively performed, most such interventions require a highly sophisticated team. In other cases, the parents

may elect to abort an affected fetus. Effective counseling should provide the best information available to assist the parents in what is always a very difficult decision.

Often the clinician is faced with the possibility of maternal or fetal harm unless therapeutic measures are instituted. The risks versus the benefits of such measures should always be carefully assessed. It is helpful to note the FDA standards for drug labeling with regard to teratogenicity (Table 14–8) when referring to drug package inserts for such information. Publications such as the *Physician's Desk Reference* are also useful. Table 14–9 summarizes risks versus benefits for some compounds.

# REFERENCES

A.C.O.G. Technical Bulletin: Management of Isoimmunization in Pregnancy. No. 90. American College of Obstetrics and Gynecology, 1986.

Anderson SG: Management of threatened abortion with real-time sonography. Obstet Gynecol 1980;55:259.

Bernard B et al: Maternal fetal hemorrhage: Incidence and sensitization. (Abstract.) Pediatr Res1977;11:467.

Bowman JM: Controversies in Rh prophylaxis: Who needs Rh immune globulin and where should it be given? Am J Obstet Gynecol 1985;151:289.

Brenner PF et al: Ectopic pregnancy: A study of 300 consecutive surgically treated cases. JAMA 1980;243:673.

Carapella-de Luca E et al: Maternofetal transfusion during delivery and sensitization of the newborn against the rhesus D-antigen. Vox Sang 1978;34:241.

Cartwright PS, DiPietro DL: Ectopic pregnancy: Changes in serum human chorionic gonadotropin concentration. Obstet Gynecol 1984;63:76.

Cohen F, Zuelzer WW: The transplacental passage of maternal erythrocytes into the fetus. Am J Obstet Gynecol 1965;93:566.

Coupet E: Ectopic pregnancy: The surgical epidemic. J Natl Med Assoc 1989;81:567.

DeCherney A, Polan ML: Evaluation and management of habitual abortion. Br J Hosp Med 1984;31:261.

Delke I, Veridiano NP, Tancer ML: Abdominal pregnancy: Review of current management and addition of 10 cases. Obstet Gynecol 1982;60:200.

DeStefano F et al: Risk of ectopic pregnancy following tubal sterilization. Obstet Gynecol 1982;60:326.

Dorfman SF: Deaths from ectopic pregnancy, United States, 1979 to 1980. Obstet Gynecol 1983;62:334.

Duckman S, Suarez J, Spitaleri J: Vaginal pregnancy presenting as a suburethral cyst. Am J Obstet Gynecol 1984;149:572.

Edmonds DK et al: Early embryonic mortality in women. Obstet Gynecol Surv 1983;38:433.

Freda VJ: The Rh problem in obstetrics and a new concept of its management using amniocentesis and spectrophotometric scanning of amniotic fluid. Am J Obstet Gynecol 1965;92:341.

Gitstein S et al: Early cervical pregnancy: Ultrasonic diagnosis and conservative treatment. Obstet Gynecol 1979;54:758.

Graber CD et al: T Mycoplasma in human reproductive failure. Obstet Gynecol 1979;54:558.

Grimes HG, Nosal RA, Gallgher JC: Ovarian pregnancy: A series of 24 cases. Obstet Gynecol 1983;61:174.

Gustavii B: Missed abortion and uterine contractility. Am J Obstet Gynecol 1978;130:18.

Holzgreve W et al: X-chromosome hyperploidy in couples with multiple spontaneous abortions. Obstet Gynecol 1984;63:237.

Huber J, Hosmann J, Vytiska Binstorfer E: Laparoscopic surgery for tubal pregnancies utilizing laser. Int J Gynaecol Obstet 1989;29:153.

Husslein P et al: Chromosome abnormalities in 150 couples with multiple spontaneous abortions. Fertil Steril 1982;37:379.

Jansen RPS, Elliott PM: Angular intrauterine pregnancy. Obstet Gynecol 1981;58:167.

Juberg RC, Knops J, Mowrey PN: Increased frequency of lymphocytic mitotic nondisjunction in recurrent spontaneous aborters. J Med Genet 1985;22:32.

Kadar N, DeCherney AH, Romero R: Receiver operating characteristic (ROC) curve analysis of the relative efficacy of single and serial chorionic gonadotropin determinations in the early diagnosis of ectopic pregnancy. Fertil Steril 1982;37:542.

Khoury MJ, Flanders WD, James LM, Erickson JD: Human teratogens, prenatal mortality, and selection bias. Am J Epidemiol 1989;130:361.

Kleihauer E, Braun H, Betke K: Demonstration von Fetalen Haemoglobin in den Erythrozyten eines Blutaus striches. Klin Wochenschr 1957;35:637.

Langer A, Iffy L (editors): *Extrauterine Pregnancy*. PSG Publishing Company, 1986.

Leach RE, Ory SJ: Modern management of ectopic pregnancy. J Reprod Med 1989;34:324.

Liley AW: Liquor amnii analysis in the management of pregnancy complicated by rhesus immunization. Am J Obstet Gynecol 1961;82:1359.

Loffer FD et al: Current concepts in the management of ectopic pregnancies: A symposium. J Reprod Med 1986; 31:73.

Mashiach S et al: Nonoperative management of ectopic pregnancy. J Reprod Med 1982;27:133.

McArdle CR: Failed abortion in a septate uterus. Am J Obstet Gynecol 1978;131:910.

McCausland A: High rate of ectopic pregnancy following laparoscopic coagulation failures. Am J Obstet Gynecol 1980;136:97.

McIntyre JA et al: Clinical, immunologic, and genetic definitions of impary and secondary recurrent spontaneous abortions. Fertil Steril 1984;42:849.

Menge AC, Beer AE: The significance of human leukocyte antigen profiles in human infertility, recurrent abortion, and pregnancy disorders. Fertil Steril 1985;43:693.

Michels VV et al: Chromosome translocations in couples with multiple spontaneous abortions. Am J Hum Genet 1982;34:507.

Morton NE et al: Cytogenetic surveillance of spontaneous abortions. Obstet Gynecol Surv 1983;38:425.

Narod SA, Khazen R: Spontaneous abortions in Ontario, 1979 to 1984. Can J Public Health 1989;80:209.

Nelson DM: Bilateral internal iliac artery ligation in cervical pregnancy: Conservation of reproductive function. Am J Obstet Gynecol 1979;134:145.

Sachs ES et al: Chromosome studies of 500 couples with two or more abortions. Obstet Gynecol 1985;65:375.

Schenker JG, Evron S: New concepts in the surgical management of tubal pregnancy and the consequent postoperative results. Fertil Steril 1983;40:709.

Schinfeld JS, Reedy G: Mesosalpingeal vessel ligation for conservative treatment of ectopic pregnancy. J Reprod Med 1983;28:823.

Scott JR; Immunologic aspects of recurrent spontaneous abortion. Fertil Steril 1982;38:301.

Siegler AM, Wang CF, Westoff C: Management of unruptured tubal pregnancy. Obstet Gynecol Surv 1981; 36:599.

Simpson JL et al: Parental chromosomal rearrangements associated with repetitive spontaneous abortions. Fertil Steril 1981;36:584.

Stabile I, Campbell S, Grudzinskas JG: Threatened miscarriage and intrauterine hematomas: Sonographic and biochemical studies. J Ultrasound Med 1989;8:289.

Stabile I, Grudzinskas G, Chord T (editors): *Spontaneous Abortion, Diagnosis and Treatment*. Springer-Verlag, 1992.

Stenchever MA: Habitual abortion. Contemp Obstet Gynecol (Jan)1983;1:162.

Stovall TG et al: Preventing ruptured ectopic pregnancy with a single serum progesterone. Am J Obstet Gynecol 1989;160:1425.

Taylor P, Cumming D: Combined laparoscopy and minilaparotomy in the management of unruptured tubal pregnancy. Fertil Steril 1979;32:521.

Tharapel AT, Tharapel SA, Bannerman RM: Recurrent pregnancy losses and parental chromosome abnormalities: A review. Br J Obstet Gynaecol 1985;92:899.

Timor Tritsch IE et al: The use of transvaginal ultrasonography in the diagnosis of ectopic pregnancy. Am J Obstet Gynecol 1989;161:157.

Valle RF, Sabbagha RE: Management of first trimester pregnancy termination failures. Obstet Gynecol 1980; 55:625.

Watson WJ: Management of unruptured ectopic gestation by linear salpingostomy: A prospective, randomized clinical trial of laparoscopy versus laparotomy. [Letter.] Obstet Gynecol 1989;74:282.

Weathersbee PS: Early reproductive loss and the factors that may influence its occurrence. J Reprod Med 1982; 25:315.

Weckstein LN: Current perspective on ectopic pregnancy. Obstet Gynecol Surv 1985;40:259.

Weckstein LN et al: Accurate diagnosis of early ectopic pregnancy. Obstet Gynecol 1985;65:393.

Weitkamp LR, Schacter BZ: Transferrin and HLA: Spontaneous abortion, neural tube defects, and natural selection. N Engl J Med 1985;313:925.

Wentz AC, Martens P, Wilroy RS Jr: Luteal phase inadequacy and a chromosomal anomaly in recurrent abortion. Fertil Steril 1984;41:142.

Wolf GC, Thompson NJ: Female sterilization and subsequent ectopic pregnancy. Obstet Gynecol 1980;55:17.

# Late Pregnancy Complications

# 15

*Martin L. Pernoll, MD*

## PREMATURE LABOR

### Essentials of Diagnosis
- Gestation less than 36 weeks.
- Two 30-second contractions within 10 minutes over a 30-minute observation period.
- Progressive cervical effacement or dilatation.
- Intact membranes.
- No abruptio placentae or placenta previa.

### General Considerations

Labor is the process of coordinated uterine contractions leading to progressive cervical effacement and dilatation by which the fetus and placenta are expelled. Premature labor is defined as labor occurring after 20 weeks' but before 36 weeks' gestation. Regular, painful uterine contractions must be present, occurring at least twice every 10 minutes for at least 30 minutes. There must be demonstrated cervical effacement or dilatation and intact membranes. Cases of premature labor with ruptured membranes are categorized as premature rupture of the membranes. Depending on socioeconomic status and a number of other factors, premature labor will complicate 5–15% of all pregnancies.

Rates of morbidity and mortality in premature infants are high (80% of all perinatal deaths in some institutions). Thirteen percent of infants are classified as having low birth weight (< 2500 g). Three percent of these are mature low-birth-weight infants, and about 10% are truly premature. The latter group accounts for nearly two-thirds of infant deaths (approximately 25,000 in the USA annually). One to 3% of premature births are due to miscalculation of gestational age or to medical intervention needed by the mother or fetus.

The care of premature (birth weight 1000–2500 g) and immature (birth weight < 1000 g) infants is costly. Compared with term infants, those born prematurely suffer greatly increased morbidity and mortality (eg, functional disorders, abnormalities of growth and development). Thus, every effort is made to prevent or inhibit premature labor. If preterm labor cannot be inhibited or is best allowed to continue, it should be conducted with the least possible trauma to the mother and infant.

### Pathogenesis

Many obstetric, medical, and anatomic disorders are associated with premature labor. Some of these are shown in Table 15–1. Detailed discussions of these conditions are given in other chapters. Causes of prematurity and low birth weight may be similar. Although several prospective risk-scoring tools are in use, they have not been convincingly demonstrated to be of value.

### Clinical Findings

**A. Symptoms:**

**1. Uterine contractions**–Regular uterine contractions occurring at least twice during a 10-minute period with a duration of at least 30 seconds are diagnostic if they occur for 30 minutes.

**2. Dilatation and effacement of cervix**–Cervical dilatation or effacement that is progressive over a 30- to 60-minute interval or a cervix that is well effaced and dilated (at least 2 cm) on admission is considered diagnostic.

**3. Premature rupture of membranes (PROM)**–Premature onset of labor often occurs with premature rupture of membranes (20-25% of all premature deliveries).

**4. Vaginal bleeding**–In most pregnancies complicated by abruptio placentae or placenta previa, the birth weight of infants is less than 2500 g.

**5. Increased vaginal discharge and vaginal pressure**–Incompetent cervix usually presents with increased vaginal discharge and vaginal pressure.

**B. Signs:**

**1. Gestational age**–Gestational age must be between 20 and 30 weeks.

**2. Fetal size**–Care must be taken to determine fetal size by ultrasonography (and well-being by electronic fetal monitoring).

**3. Presenting part**–The presenting part must be noted because abnormal presentation is more common in earlier stages of gestation.

**Table 15–1.** Diseases and disorders associated with premature labor.

**Obstetric complications**
In previous or current pregnancy
  Severe hypertensive state of pregnancy
  Anatomic disorders of the placenta (eg, abruptio placentae, placenta previa, circumvallate placenta)
  Placental insufficiency
  Premature rupture of membranes
  Polyhydramnios or oligohydramnios
Previous premature or low-birth-weight infant
Complications due to poor prenatal care (often due to low socioeconomic or educational status)
Multiple pregnancy
Short interval between pregnancies (<3 months)
Inadequate or excessive weight gain during pregnancy
Previous abortion
Previous laceration of cervix or uterus
**Medical complications**
Pulmonary or systemic hypertension
Renal disease
Heart disease
Infection: pyelonephritis, acute systemic infection, urinary tract infection, genital tract infection, (eg, gonorrhea, herpes simplex, mycoplasmosis), feto-toxic infection (eg, cytomegalovirus infection, toxoplasmosis, listeriosis), maternal systemic infection (eg, pneumonia, influenza, malaria), maternal intra-abdominal sepsis (eg, appendicitis, cholecystitis, diverticulitis)
Heavy cigarette smoking
Alcoholism or drug addiction
Severe anemia
Malnutrition or obesity
Leaking benign cystic teratoma
Perforated gastric or duodenal ulcer
Adnexal torsion
Maternal trauma or burns
**Surgical complications**
Any intra-abdominal procedure
Conization of cervix
Previous incision in uterus or cervix (eg, cesarean delivery)
**Genital tract anomalies**
Bicornuate, subseptate, or unicornuate uterus
Congenital cervical incompetency

**C. Laboratory Studies:** 1. Complete blood count with differential.

2. Urine obtained by catheter for urinalysis, culture, and sensitivity testing.

3. Ultrasound examination for fetal size, position, and placental location.

4. Amniocentesis for equivocal diagnosis of fetal maturity (L/S ratio, phosphatidylglycerol levels, or rapid surfactant test). Bacteriologic studies may also be done in some cases (microscopic observation of bacteria and white blood cells on culture and sensitivity testing).

5. Electrolytes and serum glucose testing in cases requiring tocolysis.

6. Hematologic workup in cases associated with hemorrhage (see Chapter 20).

**Treatment**

The patient should be observed for 30–60 minutes to determine appropriate management. Decisions regarding management are made depending on the presence of uterine contractions and the degree of cervical dilatation and effacement as well as the absence of contraindications to continued pregnancy (Table 15–2). A longer period of observation is not desirable, because the effectiveness of therapy diminishes as labor advances. Suppression of labor (tocolysis) should be necessary in only about 25% of cases of premature labor. In the remaining 75%, attempts are either contraindicated or unlikely to be successful.

**A. Cases in Which Premature Labor Should Be Allowed to Continue:** Table 15–3 shows cases in which premature labor should be allowed to continue.

**B. Sedation and Hydration:** A regimen of hydration and sedation is being used increasingly as "pretherapy" before tocolysis is attempted. In Group II patients (see Table 15–2), this regimen alone is successful in suppressing premature labor. Pregnancy lasts 2 more weeks without further therapy in up to 80% of patients who respond to this regimen. The protocol is shown in Table 15–4. If this fails, tocolysis is initiated or other therapy undertaken as noted in Table 15–3.

**C. Tocolysis:** In Group IV patients and failed Group II patients, tocolytic therapy is initiated if the following criteria are met: (1) the fetus is apparently healthy; (2) gestational age is 20–34 weeks (up to 37 weeks if intensive neonatal care is not available); (3) cervical dilatation is less than 4 cm and effacement is less than 80%; and (4) the membranes are intact. In some cases in which membranes are not intact, tocolysis may be initiated anyway to allow the necessary 24–48 hours for administration of corticosteroids to accelerate maturation of fetal lungs.

The decision to use a tocolytic and the choice of agent must be carefully considered. The beta-mimetics, particularly ritodrine, and magnesium sulfate are the most commonly used. There are contraindications to each agent. Newer agents under investigation are the prostaglandin inhibitors and calcium channel blockers.

**1. Beta-mimetic adrenergic agents**–Beta-mimetic adrenergic agents act directly on beta receptors ($\beta_2$) to relax the uterus and uterine vessels. Their use is limited by dose-related major cardiovascular side effects, including pulmonary edema, adult respiratory distress syndrome, elevated systolic and reduced diastolic blood pressure, and both maternal and fetal tachycardia. Other dose-related effects are decreased serum potassium and increased blood glucose, plasma insulin, and lactic acidosis. Maternal medical contraindications to the use of beta- adrenergic agents include cardiac disease, hyperthyroidism, uncontrolled hypertension, or pulmonary hypertension; asthma requiring sympathomimetic drugs or corticosteroids for relief; uncontrolled diabetes; and chronic hepatic or renal disease. Commonly observed effects

**Table 15–2.** Management of premature labor based on the presence of uterine contractions and the degree of cervical dilatation and effacement.

| Group | Uterine Contractions[1] | Cervical Effacement and Dilatation | Diagnosis | Management |
|---|---|---|---|---|
| I | No | No | No labor | None |
| II | Yes | No[2] | Premature labor | Hydration and sedation |
| III | No | Yes[3] | Incompetent cervix | Bed rest; consider cerclage |
| IV | Yes | Yes[3] | Premature labor | Tocolytic protocol |

[1]Two or more contractions every 10 minutes for 30 minutes.
[2]Dilatation less than 4 cm and effacement less than 80%.
[3]Effacement of 80% with dilatation of more than fingertip width, or change with observation.

during intravenous administration are palpitations, tremors, nervousness, and restlessness.

**a. Ritodrine**–Ritodrine is the standard by which other agents are judged. Table 15–5 shows a detailed protocol for ritodrine.

**b. Terbutaline**–Although not FDA-approved in the USA, terbutaline has been studied in the USA and used elsewhere as a tocolytic agent. The mode of action is similar to that of ritodrine, and the precautions and contraindications are the same. A bolus of 250 µg followed by 10–80 µg/min until labor stops may be effective. The drug is then administered subcutaneously, 0.25–0.5 mg every 2–4 hours for 12 hours. A maintenance dose of 2.5–5 mg may be given orally 2–4 times a day. Intravenous terbutaline may not be as easily controlled as ritodrine and is more costly, but intramuscular terbutaline is effective (ritodrine is not available in an intramuscular form).

**c. Isoxsuprine**–Isoxsuprine also is not FDA-approved in the USA for tocolysis and is not recommended, because of its narrow therapeutic range.

**Table 15–3.** Some cases in which premature labor should not be suppressed.

**Maternal diseases and disorders**
  Severe hypertensive disease (eg, acute exacerbation of chronic hypertension, eclampsia, severe preeclampsia)
  Pulmonary or cardiac disease (eg, pulmonary edema, adult respiratory distress syndrome, valvular disease, tachyarrhythmias)
  Maternal hemorrhage (eg, abruptio placentae, placenta previa, disseminated intravascular coagulation)
**Fetal diseases and disorders**
  Fetal death
  Fetal distress
  Intrauterine infection (chorioamnionitis)
  Polyhydramnios
  Therapy adversely affecting the fetus (eg, fetal distress due to attempted suppression of labor)
  Erythroblastosis fetalis
  Severe intrauterine growth retardation
**Conditions in which labor cannot be arrested**
  Ruptured membranes
  Bulging membranes
  Cervical dilatation of more than 4 cm and effacement of more than 80%
  Inaccurate dating of gestational age (ie, fetus is mature)

**2. Magnesium sulfate**–Although magnesium sulfate has not been FDA-approved for use as a tocolytic, it is widely used. Apparently less effective than ritodrine or terbutaline, magnesium sulfate is the best alternative if beta-mimetic drugs are contraindicated or cause toxicity. A protocol for use of magnesium sulfate is shown in Table 15–6. Magnesium sulfate may appear less likely to cause serious side effects than the beta-mimetics, but its therapeutic range is close to the range in which it will cause respiratory and cardiac depression. These symptoms may

**Table 15–4.** Sedation and hydration protocol for premature labor.

**Criteria for admission to protocol**
  Observe the patient for 30 minutes with fetal monitoring (Table 15–3).
  Confirm that gestational age is more than 20 weeks (variable in different institutions).
  Perform necessary examinations and tests to rule out any contraindications to sedation-hydration therapy.
**Protocol**
  Give sedation and hydration for 1 hour. Observation of the patient and fetal monitoring must be continuous during this time.
    Sedation: Give morphine sulfate, 8–12 mg intramuscularly (provided no allergy exists, delivery is not imminent, and naloxone hydrochloride [Narcan] is available should delivery occur and fetal respiration be depressed).
    Hydration: Give 0.5% normal saline in 5% dextrose, 500 mL intravenously for 30 minutes. An alternative solution is lactated Ringer's solution in 5% dextrose.
  At the end of one hour, patients are divided into 3 groups as follows:
    Group 1: Cervical dilatation and effacement are progressing. Proceed to tocolytics or other appropriate therapy (eg, delivery; administration of magnesium sulfate). This group is usually only a small percentage of patients.
    Group 2: There is no cervical change, but uterine contractions continue. Proceed to tocolytics. This group is usually less than half of patients. Even if suppression of labor is successful at this time, there is still a risk of subsequent premature labor and delivery.
    Group 3: There is no cervical change, and uterine contractions cease. Observation of the patient should continue. Over half of patients will be in this group. There is a continued risk of premature labor and delivery.

**Table 15–5.** Protocol for use of ritodrine in suppression of premature labor.[1]

**Criteria for admission to protocol**

Premature labor has been confirmed.

Gestational age of 20–34 weeks has been confirmed by physiologic maturity studies. Therapy may be initiated before physiologic maturity studies are obtained if prematurity is strongly suspected or if the case is judged an emergency.

Examinations and tests have ruled out any cases of maternal or fetal diseases or disorders in which it would be best to allow labor to continue.

Any specific contraindications to ritodrine therapy have been ruled out (eg, antepartum hemorrhage requiring immediate delivery, severe preeclampsia or eclampsia, intrauterine fetal death, chorioamnionitis, maternal cardiac disease, maternal pulmonary hypertension, maternal hyperthyroidism, uncontrolled maternal diabetes mellitus, preexisting maternal medical conditions that would be seriously affected by the known pharmacologic properties of beta-mimetic drugs [eg, hypovolemia, cardiac arrhythmias associated with tachycardia or digitalis intoxication, uncontrolled hypertension, pheochromocytoma, bronchial asthma already treated by beta-mimetics or steroids], known hypersensitivity to any component of the solution or tablets).

**Protocol**

The initial intravenous administration should usually be followed by oral administration. The dosage is determined by uterine response and avoidance of side effects. *Note the precautions and side effects listed below.*

**Intravenous therapy:** Do not use any ritodrine solution that is discolored or contains precipitate or particulate matter. *Use the solution promptly after preparation. Do not use after 48 hours.*

Place the patient in the left lateral position.

Monitor the amount and rate of administration carefully to avoid circulatory overload (overhydration).

Use of a controlled infusion device is recommended to adjust the rate of flow in drops per minute (eg, intravenous microdrip chamber).

The recommended dilution is 150 mg ritodrine hydrochloride (three 5-mL ampules **or** one 10-mL vial **or** one 10-mL syringe) in 500 mL fluid, yielding a final concentration of 0.3 mg/mL. In those cases where fluid restriction is medically desirable, a more concentrated solution may be prepared. Ritodrine for intravenous infusion should be diluted with 5% weight per volume dextrose solution. Because of the increased probability of pulmonary edema, saline diluents such as 0.9% weight per volume sodium chloride solution; compound sodium chloride solution (Ringer's solution); and Hartmann's solution should be reserved for cases where dextrose solution is medically undesirable (eg, diabetes mellitus).

Start intravenous therapy as soon as possible after the diagnosis is made. The usual initial dose is 0.1 mg/min (0.33 mL/min, or 20 drops/min). The dosage is gradually increased (according to uterine response) by 0.05 mg/min, (0.17 mL/min, or 10 drops/min) every 10 minutes until the desired result is attained. The effective dosage is usually 0.15–0.35 mg/min (0.5–1.17 mL/min, or 30–70 drops/min).

Frequent monitoring of uterine contractions, maternal heart rate and blood pressure, and fetal heart rate is required, with dosage individually titrated according to response. If other drugs must also be given intravenously, piggyback tubing or use of a second intravenous site will permit independent control of ritodrine.

The infusion should usually be continued for at least 12 hours after uterine contractions cease. With the recommended dilution, the maximum volume of fluid administered after 12 hours at the highest dose (0.35 mg/min) will be approximately 840 mL.

**Oral therapy:** Initial oral therapy is 1 tablet (10 mg) given approximately 30 minutes before the termination of intravenous therapy. The usual dosage schedule for the first 24 hours of oral administration is 1 tablet every 2 hours. Then, give 1–2 tablets (10–20 mg) every 4–6 hours, depending on uterine activity and occurrence of side effects. The total daily dose should not exceed 120 mg. Treatment may be continued as long as is desirable to prolong pregnancy.

**Protocol for recurrent premature labor**

Repeated intravenous infusion may be given.

**Precautions to be observed with intravenous ritodrine therapy**

The patient must be hospitalized.

Administration must be closely monitored. Those in attendance must have knowledge of the pharmacology of the drug and must be qualified to identify and manage complications of drug administration and pregnancy.

Cardiovascular responses (including maternal pulse and blood pressure and fetal heart rate) must be closely monitored. Danger signs (because of the propensity for cardiovascular response or the unmasking of occult cardiac disease) include persistent high tachycardia (> 140/min), tachypnea (either or both of the above may be signs of impending pulmonary edema), and chest pain or tightness of the chest (temporarily discontinue medication and obtain an ECG as soon as possible).

Maternal pulmonary edema (even up to the point of death) has been reported both antepartum and postpartum. This appears to be more frequent with concomitant corticosteroid usage. Fluid overload must be avoided, and the state of hydration must be carefully monitored. Discontinue the drug immediately if signs of pulmonary edema develop.

Plasma glucose and serum electrolytes must be carefully monitored (particularly important with prolonged administration). Intravenous administration of ritodrine elevates the plasma insulin and glucose and decreases plasma potassium concentrations. The heomogram may be helpful in assessing hydration.

**Side effects of ritodrine**

Adverse effects of ritodrine are related to beta-mimetic activity. The effects noted below are for intravenous therapy. The only adverse effects of oral therapy are small increases in maternal heart rate (maternal blood pressure and fetal heart rate are unaffected), palpitations, tremor, nausea, jitteriness, rash, and cardiac arrhythmias (about 1%). Impaired liver function (ie, increased transaminase levels and hepatitis) has also been reported infrequently (< 1% of cases) with use of ritodrine and other beta sympathomimetics.

**Common effects (80–100%):** Increased maternal heart rate (average = 130/min). Increased systolic blood pressure (average increase = 12 mm Hg). Decreased diastolic blood pressure (average decrease = 23 mm Hg). Increased fetal heart rate (average = 164/min).

**Frequent effects (10–50%):** Tremor, nausea, vomiting, headache, erythema.

**Occasional effects (5–10%):** Nervousness, jitteriness, restlessness, emotional upset or anxiety, malaise.

**Infrequent effects (1–3%):** Chest pain or tightness (rarely associated with ECG abnormalities) and arrhythmia.

**Table 15–5 (cont'd).** Protocol for use of ritodrine in suppression of premature labor.

**Other reported adverse effects:** Anaphylactic shock, heart murmur, ileus, constipation, dyspnea, hemolytic icterus, lactic acidosis, rash, epigastric distress, bloating, diarrhea, hyperventilation, glycosuria, sweating, drowsiness, weakness.
**Neonatal side effects (infrequent):** Hypoglycemia, ileus. In addition, hypocalcemia and hypotension have been reported in neonates whose mothers were treated with beta-mimetic agents other than ritodrine.
**Side effects due to overdosage:** The amount of ritodrine required to produce symptoms of overdosage in humans is individually variable. No reports of death due to overdose have been received. Symptoms of overdosage are those of excessive beta-adrenergic stimulation, eg, tachycardia, (maternal or fetal), palpitation, cardiac arrhythmia, hypotension, dyspnea, nervousness, tremor, nausea, vomiting.

Revised and reproduced with permission, from *YUTOPAR® Sterile Solution and Tablets (Ritodrine Hydrochloride)* (package insert). Astra Pharmaceutical Products, Inc.

be reversed by calcium gluconate (10 mL of a 10% solution given intravenously), and this antidote should be kept at the bedside when magnesium sulfate is used. The reflexes must be tested periodically for magnesium overdosage. Several recent protocols have used both magnesium sulfate and ritodrine, suggesting that the 2 agents have an additive effect.

**3. Ethyl alcohol**–Ethyl alcohol was used extensively in the past to inhibit labor. It is thought to inhibit release of oxytocin. However, its side effects (eg, nausea, drunkenness) occur to such an extent that most patients are intolerant of its use.

**4. Other tocolytics**–Two exciting new classes of tocolytics are now being tested but have not been released for clinical use and are therefore not recommended. The prostaglandin inhibitors appear to be effective but may cause premature closure of the fetal ductus arteriosus. The calcium blockers (calcium channel blockers) may have fewer side effects and appear to be effective in preliminary trials.

**5. Results of tocolytic therapy**–With all tocolytics, a point may be reached where further therapy is not indicated. This may be due to adverse maternal or fetal response to the progress of labor.

**Table 15–6.** Protocol for use of magnesium sulfate in suppression of premature labor.

**Criteria for admission to protocol**
Premature labor has been confirmed.
Gestational age of 20–34 weeks has been confirmed.
Examinations and tests have ruled out any cases of maternal or fetal diseases or disorders in which it would be best to allow labor to continue.
Any specific contraindications to magnesium sulfate therapy have been ruled out.
**Protocol**
Begin intravenous infusion of magnesium sulfate, 4 g (40 ml of 10% solution). The rate of infusion should be slow enough to prevent flushing or vomiting. Give continuous infusion of magnesium sulfate 10%, 200 mL, in 5% dextrose, 800 mL, at a rate of 100 mL/h until labor subsides or progresses to an irreversible stage (spontaneous rupture of membranes or cervical dilatation of 5 cm).
Reduce the rate of infusion if magnesium toxicity is observed.
**Protocol for recurrent premature labor**
If contractions recur after discontinuation of the infusion, the procedure may be repeated.

Thus, if cervical dilatation reaches 5 cm, the treatment should be considered a failure and abandoned. If labor resumes after a period of quiescence, treatment may be reinstituted using the same or a different drug.

The results of tocolytic therapy are difficult to judge because of the lack of well-controlled studies. However, it is estimated that labor was halted for 72 hours or more in 90% of patients who received ritodrine.

Ritodrine is credited in one series with reducing the neonatal death rate from 13% to 5% and the incidence of respiratory distress from 20% to 11%. Fifty-eight percent of the infants had a birth weight in excess of 2500 g, and no adverse long-term effects have been observed over a 2-year period.

**D. Glucocorticoids:** Glucocorticoid therapy has significantly reduced the incidence of neonatal respiratory distress in noncaucasian and female infants in a multicenter study. Some other studies (but not all) have indicated a beneficial effect in all infants due to increased production of pulmonary surfactant. The agent most commonly used is beta-methasone, 12 mg intramuscularly, repeated once in 12–24 hours. If therapy is successful and pregnancy is prolonged, the dose is sometimes given weekly; whether this is truly efficacious remains to be determined.

## Conduct of Labor & Delivery

Small premature infants should be delivered in a hospital equipped for intensive neonatal care whenever possible, because transfer following birth is more hazardous. Premature breech infants weighing less than 1500–2000 g are generally delivered by cesarean section. If the presentation is cephalic, vaginal birth is preferred in the absence of fetal distress.

Every effort should be made to avoid fetal hypoxia and intraventricular hemorrhage. Adequate hydration should assist in preventing maternal acidosis. Internal fetal monitoring or scalp sampling, or both, for blood pH should be done if hypoxia is suspected. Sedative and analgesic drugs in reduced dosages should be used sparingly. Paracervical block should be avoided because of potential adverse fetal effects.

Conduction anesthesia (particularly epidural) may be the best choice because it provides maximum relaxation of the birth canal and reduces transplacental transfer of agents potentially capable of depressing the fetus. Pudendal block anesthesia is also satisfactory if the pelvic floor and perineum are pliable or relaxed. A generous episiotomy should be made to further reduce the risk of injury. Delivery can be aided by forceps with a short cephalic curve (eg, Tucker-McLean forceps) serving as a sort of helmet to protect and guide the fetal head over the perineum. Before clamping the cord, wait 45–60 seconds—while holding the neonate below placental level—to ensure that adequate blood is received from the placental circulation.

If a cesarean section is indicated, the decision to operate is based on maturity of the fetus and prognosis for survival. In borderline cases, good criteria on which to base a decision are lacking. When performing a cesarean section, it is important to ascertain that the uterine incision is adequate for extraction of the fetus without delay or unnecessary trauma. This often requires a vertical incision when the lower uterine segment is incompletely developed.

In managing the premature newborn infant, the avoidance of heat loss is of critical importance. When birth follows the unsuccessful use of parenteral tocolytic agents, keep in mind the potential residual adverse effects of these drugs. Beta-adrenergic agents may cause neonatal hypotension, hypoglycemia, hypocalcemia, and ileus. Magnesium sulfate may be responsible for respiratory and cardiac depression. In addition, oral maintenance doses of a beta-adrenergic agent can produce hypoglycemia in the newborn.

## Cord pH & Blood Gases

Apgar scores are often low in low-birth-weight babies. This does not indicate asphyxiation or compromised status but merely reflects the immaturity of the physiologic systems. Therefore, it is crucial to obtain cord pH and blood gas measurements for premature (and other high-risk) infants in order to document the status at birth. These measurements can also be correlated with intrapartum fetal heart rate monitoring, scalp sampling, and Apgar scores. Cord pH and blood gas measurements may also be helpful in reconstructing intrapartum events; auditing fetal acidemia; evaluating the efficacy of the clinical diagnosis, detection, and therapy; clarifying resuscitative measures; and determining the need for more intensive neonatal care.

## Prognosis

Excellent neonatal care in the delivery room and nursery will do much to ensure a good prognosis for the preterm infant (see Chapter 29). Lower-birth-weight babies have a lesser chance of survival and a greater chance of permanent sequelae in direct relationship to size. It is difficult to make generalizations regarding survival rates and sequelae because of the many causes of premature delivery, the different levels of perinatal care, and the institutional differences

in reported series. However, infants weighing 2000–2500 g usually have survival rates of more than 97%; those weighing 1500–2000 g, more than 90%; and those weighing 1000–1500 g, 65–80%. Two-thirds of infants weighing 800–1350 g survive, and handicaps occur in fewer than 20%. Mortality and morbidity rates are much higher in smaller fetuses.

## PREMATURE RUPTURE OF MEMBRANES

### Essentials of Diagnosis

- History of a gush of fluid from the vagina.
- Continued leakage of fluid from the vagina.
- Demonstration of amniotic fluid leakage from the cervix.
- Demonstration of oligohydramnios by ultrasound examination.

### General Considerations

Rupture of the membranes may happen at any time during pregnancy. It becomes a problem if the fetus is premature (preterm rupture of membranes) or, in the case of a mature fetus, if the period of time between rupture of the membranes and the onset of labor is prolonged (prelabor rupture of the membranes). If 24 hours elapse between rupture of the membranes and the onset of labor, the problem is one of prolonged premature rupture of the membranes.

The exact cause of rupture is not known, although there are many associated conditions (Table 15–7). Premature rupture of the membranes occurs in approximately 10.7% of all pregnancies. In approximately 94% of cases, the fetus is mature (approximately 20% of these are cases of prolonged rupture). Premature fetuses (1000–2500 g) account for about 5% of the total number (about 50% of cases are prolonged), while immature fetuses (< 1000 g) account for less than 0.5% (about 75% of cases are prolonged).

### Pathology & Pathophysiology

Premature rupture of the membranes is an important cause of premature labor, prolapse of the cord, and intrauterine infection. Amnionitis is an important cause of endomyometritis and puerperal sepsis.

**Table 15–7.** Diseases and disorders associated with premature rupture of the membranes.

Maternal infection (eg, urinary tract infection, lower genital tract infection, sexually transmitted diseases)
Intrauterine infection
Cervical incompetency
Multiple previous pregnancies
Hydramnios
Nutritional deficit
Decreased tensile strength of membranes
Familial history of premature rupture of membranes

In extremely prolonged rupture of the membranes, the fetus may have an appearance similar to that of Potter's syndrome (eg, extraordinary flexion, wrinkling of the skin). It has been reported, but not confirmed, that various anomalies may result from chronically decreased amniotic fluid volume.

## Clinical Findings

**A. Symptoms:** The diagnostic evaluation must be efficient and impeccably conducted to minimize the number of vaginal examinations and the risk of chorioamnionitis. Symptoms are the key to diagnosis; the patient usually reports a sudden gush of fluid or continued leakage. Continued leakage has a worse prognosis. Occasionally, patients will report a persistent trickle, suggesting a small tear or perforation of the membranes. Additional symptoms that may be useful include the color and consistency of the fluid and the presence of flecks of vernix, reduced size of the uterus, and increased prominence of the fetus to palpation.

**B. Sterile Speculum Examination:** A most important step in accurate diagnosis is examination with a sterile speculum. This is conducted only after careful abdominal examination reveals no contraindications to vaginal examination. The posterior vaginal fornix is exposed by means of the speculum, and the pH of the pool fluid is tested with nitrazine paper (amniotic fluid has a pH of 7.0–7.25). Additional studies and procedures of importance should be done as follows: (1) Cervical secretions should be collected for culture. (2) Fluid should be collected from the vaginal pool for potassium hydroxide and wet mount examinations, nitrazine test, and fern test (air-dry a drop of the fluid on a slide and examine for arborization). (3) Observe leakage of fluid from the cervical os with the Valsalva maneuver, cough, or fundal pressure. (4) If fluid flows cleanly into the posterior lip of the speculum (uncontaminated), it may be collected for determination of the L:S ratio, phosphatidylglycerol, or rapid surfactant test.(5) Determine the degree of cervical dilatation and effacement. (6) Check for cord prolapse. (7) If no free fluid is found, place a dry pad under the patient's hips and observe for subsequent leakage.

Occasionally, there will be such concern about whether or not membranes are ruptured that it will be necessary to perform amniocentesis and inject a dilute solution of Evans blue or indigo carmine dye. This is done following removal of amniotic fluid for physiologic maturity testing, analysis for white blood cells or bacteria, and possible culture and sensitivity testing. After 15–20 minutes, insertion of a vaginal speculum should reveal blue dye in the vagina if the membranes are ruptured.

**C. Physical Examination:** A careful physical examination should be done to search for other signs of infection.

**D. Laboratory Studies:** Initial laboratory studies should include a complete blood count with differential; urine collected by catheterization for urinalysis, culture, and sensitivity testing; ultrasound examination for fetal size; and amniocentesis in some cases for studies detailed above.

**E. Amnionitis:** In all cases of amnionitis, it is safer for the fetus to be delivered than to be retained in utero. The most common organisms causing amnionitis are those that would ascend from the vagina (eg, streptococci B and D and anaerobes). The most reliable signs of infection include the following: (1) Fever (the temperature should be checked every 4 hours and a morning value of more than 37.2 °C [99 °F] viewed with alarm). (2) Maternal leukocytosis. A daily leukocyte count and differential should be obtained. If any abnormalities are encountered, this may be repeated more frequently. In most laboratories, a white blood cell count of more than 16,000/μL is considered alarming. (3) Uterine tenderness (check every 4 hours). (5) Tachycardia (either maternal pulse > 100/min or fetal heart rate of > 160/min is worrisome). (5) Amniotic fluid C-reactive protein measurements and gas-liquid chromatography have both been suggested as useful in detecting amnionitis.

A number of confounding factors may complicate the diagnosis of amnionitis. For example, frequent fundal examinations may cause uterine tenderness. Corticosteroid administration may cause mild leukocytosis (increase of 20–25%), and labor is associated with leukocytosis. If the diagnosis of amnionitis is equivocal, amniocentesis may be performed to search for bona fide evidence (eg, amniotic fluid containing numerous leukocytes or bacteria on Gram's stain or anaerobic or aerobic culture).

The differential diagnosis of ruptured membranes includes hydrorrhea gravidarum, vaginitis, increased vaginal fluid, and urinary incontinence.

## Treatment

Differences of opinion bordering on controversy exist regarding details of management of premature or prolonged rupture of the membranes. One group believes that nonintervention (no vaginal manipulations or attempts at delivery) may be more beneficial for both preterm and term fetuses than attempts to deliver. A second group holds that delivery should be induced within a reasonable interval (usually no more than 8–12 hours) if gestational age is greater than 33 weeks or if the fetus is mature according to physiologic maturity tests. Both groups agree on the desirability of delivery when there is premature rupture of membranes and amnionitis. Differences in populations studied may account for the disparate findings and differences of opinion. Thus, it has been suggested that for maternity services where rates of infection are low, nonintervention may be appropriate. For institutions with high rates of morbidity due to infection, the mother and infant may benefit from delivery within 24 hours.

**A. Intervention:** If intervention is selected, the following recommendations have been helpful.

**1. Estimated gestational age over 36 weeks; fetal weight over 2500 g**–Although there is a 90% expectation of spontaneous labor within 24 hours, whenever the latent period exceeds 8–12 hours, induction by means of oxytocin infusion is indicated to minimize the risk of infection.

**2. Estimated gestational age 34–36 weeks; fetal weight 2000–3000 g**—Induction as above is probably indicated. Some may prefer to wait 24–48 hours in the expectation of accelerated lung surfactant production.

**3. Estimated gestational age 26–34 weeks; fetal weight 500–2000 g**—Management should be based on diagnostic amniocentesis. If there is evidence of lung maturation (mature lecithin: sphingomyelin ratio or presence of phosphatidylglycerol) or amnionitis (bacteria in amniotic fluid), labor should be induced. If the lecithin:sphingomyelin ratio is in the immature range and there is no evidence of amnionitis, the patient should be maintained at bed rest, with vital signs taken every 4 hours and white blood count daily. Adrenocorticosteroid drugs for lung maturation may be beneficial.

If leakage of fluid stops and the patient remains afebrile, without evidence of increasing uterine irritability, she may initially be allowed to walk and may subsequently be dismissed from the hospital, but monitored very closely as an outpatient. She should be advised to avoid vaginal douches and coitus and instructed to monitor her temperature at least four times a day. If amnionitis develops, delivery should be performed. If subsequent leakage of amniotic fluid occurs, the patient will need additional evaluation.

**4. Estimated gestational age under 26 weeks; fetal weight under 500 g**–Once the diagnosis is established, the outcome of the pregnancy must be discussed with medical personnel and the family. There is very little chance of fetal salvage and considerable maternal risk.

**B. Nonintervention:** In cases where nonintervention is selected, care must be taken to rule out amnionitis. The guidelines noted above may be helpful. Most protocols for nonintervention recommend bed rest with bathroom privileges, no intercourse, no use of douches or tampons, and recording of temperatures 3–6 times a day and white blood cell counts every other day. It has been demonstrated that a daily biophysical profile (see Chapter 13) is as accurate as amniocentesis in detecting chorioamnionitis. The patient must know how to immediately reach the physician and is instructed to call should any of the following occur: fever, chills, pain, symptoms suggesting "flu" or viral syndrome, change in vaginal discharge, onset of labor, vaginal bleeding, or abdominal or back pain.

For management of retardation of labor, use of corticosteroids, progression of labor and delivery, and use of cord blood sampling for determination of infant status at birth, see Premature Labor, above.

## PROLONGED PREGNANCY

### Essentials of Diagnosis

- Confirmation of gestational age greater than 42 completed weeks.
- Biophysical evaluations 2-3 times weekly.
- Exclusion of risk factors, including oligohydramnios, placental insufficiency, dysmaturity, malposition, fetopelvic disproportion, and meconium staining of amniotic fluid.

### General Considerations

Prolonged pregnancy is defined as pregnancy that has reached 42 weeks of completed gestation from the first day of the LMP or 40 weeks' gestation from the time of conception. Most fetuses will show effects of impairment of the nutritional supply (weight loss, reduced subcutaneous tissue, scaling, parchmentlike skin). This condition is referred to as dysmaturity. The cause of most cases of dysmaturity remains unknown, but anencephalic fetuses and those with placental sulfatase deficiency are often associated with prolonged pregnancy.

At least 3% of infants are born after 42 completed weeks' gestation (in some series, as many as 12%). Because of the potential risks of dysmaturity, these infants deserve particular attention.

The maternal risks usually relate to extraordinary fetal size (ie, dysfunctional labor, arrested progress of labor, fetopelvic disproportion). Extraordinary fetal size may result in birth injury (eg, shoulder girdle dystocia). Placental insufficiency is thought to be associated with aging of the placenta; this is the basis for another group of fetal problems. Oligohydramnios, which is more common in postterm gestation, may lead to cord compromise.

Complications resulting from prolonged pregnancy result in a sharp rise in perinatal morbidity rates (2–3 times those of infants born at 37-42 weeks). Complications in the survivors increase the chance of mental retardation and neurologic sequelae.

### Diagnosis

Diagnosis of this condition is usually made by ultrasound. A frequent finding is decreased amniotic fluid volume.

To adequately evaluate the risk of fetal compromise, the following is a useful protocol for pregnancies beyond 41 weeks' gestation:

A. Confirm gestational age by referring to records of early pregnancy tests and ultrasound examinations, the exact time of conception (if known), and clinical parameters (eg, LMP, LNMP, quickening, early examination, sequential fundal measurements).

B. Perform nonstress testing 2–3 times weekly. (Some authorities believe that contraction stress testing, a biophysical profile, or both are necessary to detect the jeopardized fetus and recommend weekly or biweekly testing.)

C. Perform ultrasonic monitoring at least twice weekly to assess amniotic fluid volume (biophysical profiles may be obtained at the same time).

D. Have the mother count fetal movements each day.

## Treatment

Many authorities will not allow a gestation to progress beyond 41 completed weeks and nearly all agree with delivery by 42 ½ weeks, believing that risks to the infant exceed the risks associated with induced labor. If the choice is to continue the pregnancy, it may be advisable to have the patient monitor fetal activity. The following precautions should be taken:

A. Decreased fetal movement warrants an immediate biophysical profile evaluation. Despite the concerns of some authorities, many continue to use the nonstress test as their primary screening device.

B. Abnormalities in the nonstress test mandate an immediate contraction stress test.

C. An abnormal contraction stress test, decreased amniotic fluid volume, abnormal biophysical profile, or detection of meconium or other signs of fetal compromise warrants serious consideration of delivery.

D. A large or compromised fetus may require cesarean delivery.

E. In the absence of fetopelvic disproportion or fetal distress, labor may be induced. Fetal monitoring should be continuous.

## Rh ISOIMMUNIZATION & OTHER BLOOD GROUP INCOMPATIBILITIES

### Essentials of Diagnosis

- Maternal Rh-negativity and presence of antibody on indirect Coombs' test.

- Rh or other antibody titer posing fetal risk.
- Previous infant with hemolytic disease of the newborn.
- Postnatal fetal cord blood findings of Rh-positivity and anemia (hemoglobin < 10 g).

### General Considerations

A fetus receives half of its genetic components from its mother and half from its father and may therefore have different blood groups than those of its mother. Some blood groups may act as antigens in individuals not possessing those blood groups. The antigens reside on red blood cells. If enough fetal cells leak into the maternal blood, a maternal antibody response may be provoked. Some blood types specifically produce antibodies capable of crossing the placenta. They then enter the fetal circulation and react with the fetal erythrocytes, causing hemolytic anemia. This leads to responses in the fetus to meet the jeopardy of enhanced blood cell breakdown. These changes in the fetus and newborn are called erythroblastosis fetalis. As noted below, several blood groups are capable of producing fetal risk, but those in the Rh group have caused the overwhelming majority of cases of erythroblastosis fetalis, so that the Rh group will be used as the example.

The Rh blood group is the most complex human blood group. The Rh antigens are grouped in 3 pairs: Dd, Cc, and Ee. The major antigen in this group, $Rh_o$, (D), or Rh factor, is of particular concern. A woman who is lacking the Rh factor (Rh-negative) may carry an Rh-positive fetus. If fetal red blood cells pass into the mother's circulation in sufficient numbers, maternal antibodies to the Rh-positive antigen may develop and cross the placenta, causing hemolysis of fetal blood cells (Fig 15–1). Hemolytic disease of the newborn may occur, and severe disease may cause fetal death.

In standard testing when the father is Rh-positive, 2 possibilities exist, ie, he may be homozygous or heterozygous. Forty-five percent of Rh-positive persons are homozygous for D, and 55% are heterozygous. If the father is homozygous, all of his children will be Rh-positive; if he is heterozygous, half of his

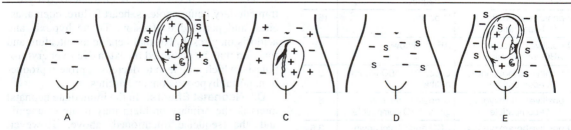

**Figure 15–1.** A: Rh-negative woman before pregnancy. B: Pregnancy occurs. The fetus is Rh-positive. C: Separation of the placenta. D: Following delivery, Rh isoimmunization occurs in the mother, and she develops antibodies (S) to the Rh-positive antigen. E: The next pregnancy with an Rh-positive fetus. Maternal antibodies cross the placenta, enter the fetal bloodstream, and attach to Rh-positive red cells, causing hemolysis.

children will be Rh-positive and half will be Rh-negative. By way of contrast, the Rh-negative individual is always homozygous.

## Incidence

Basque populations have the highest incidence of Rh-negativity (30–35%). Caucasian populations in general have a higher incidence (15–16%; Finland, 10–12%). Blacks in the USA have a rate of 8%; African blacks, 4%; Indoeurasians, 2%; and North American Indians, 1%. The incidence among mongoloid races is nil.

The overall risk of isoimmunization for an Rh-positive ABO-compatible infant with an Rh-negative mother is about 16%. Of these, 1.5–2% of reactions will occur antepartum, 7% within 6 months of delivery, and the remainder (7%) early in the second pregnancy, most likely as the result of an amnestic response. ABO incompatibility between an Rh-positive fetus and an Rh-negative mother provides some protection against Rh isoimmunization; the overall incidence is 1.5–2% in these cases. Some risks for other potential paternal and fetal blood groups are demonstrated in Table 15–8.

## Pathogenesis

**A. Maternal Rh Isoimmunization:** Rh antigens are lipoproteins that are confined to the red cell membrane. Isoimmunization may occur by 2 mechanisms: (1) following incompatible blood transfusion or (2) following fetomaternal hemorrhage between a mother and an incompatible fetus. Fetomaternal hemorrhage may occur during pregnancy or at delivery. With no apparent predisposing factors, fetal red cells have been detected in maternal blood in 6.7% of women during the first trimester, 15.9% during the second trimester, and 28.9% during the third trimester. There are a number of predispositions to fetomaternal hemorrhage, including spontaneous or

induced abortion, amniocentesis, abdominal trauma (eg, due to motor vehicle accidents or external version), placenta previa, abruptio placentae, fetal death, multiple pregnancy, manual removal of the placenta, and cesarean section.

Although the exact number of Rh-positive cells necessary to cause isoimmunization of the Rh-negative pregnant women is unknown, as little as 0.1 mL of Rh-positive cells will cause sensitization. Even with delivery, this amount occurs in less than half of cases.

Fortunately, there are other mitigating factors to Rh isoimmunization. A very important one is that about 30% of Rh-negative persons never become sensitized (nonresponders) when given Rh-positive blood. As noted above, ABO incompatibility also confers a protective effect.

The initial maternal immune response to Rh sensitization is low levels of IgM. Within 6 weeks to 6 months, IgG antibodies become detectable. In contrast to IgM, IgG (7S immunoglobulins) is capable of crossing the placenta and destroying fetal Rh-positive cells.

**B. Other Blood Group Isoimmunization:** Of the other blood groups that may evoke immunoglobulins capable of crossing the placenta (often called atypical or irregular immunizing antibodies), those that may cause severe fetal hemolysis (listed in descending order of occurrence) are Kell, Duffy, Kidd, MNSs, Diego, and P. Lutheran and Xg groups may cause fetal hemolysis, but it is usually less severe (also see Table 12–2).

**C. Fetal Effects:** Hemolytic disease of the newborn occurs when the maternal antibodies destroy the Rh-positive fetal red blood cells. Fetal anemia results, stimulating extramedullary erythropoietic sites to produce high levels of nucleated red cell elements. Immature erythrocytes are present in the fetal blood owing to poor maturation control. Hemolysis produces heme, which is converted to bilirubin; both of these substances are neurotoxic. However, while the fetus is in utero, heme and bilirubin are effectively removed by the placenta and the mother metabolizes them.

When fetal red blood cell destruction far exceeds production and severe anemia occurs, erythroblastosis fetalis may occur. This is characterized by extramedullary hematopoiesis, heart failure, edema, ascites, and pericardial effusion. Tissue hypoxia and acidosis may result. Normal hepatic architecture and function may be disturbed by extensive liver erythropoiesis, which may lead to decreased protein production, portal hypertension, and ascites.

**D. Neonatal Effects:** In the immediate neonatal interval, the primary problem may relate to anemia and the sequelae mentioned above. However, hyperbilirubinemia may also pose an immediate risk and certainly poses a risk as further red cell breakdown occurs. The immature (and often compromised) liver, with its low levels of glucuronyl-

**Table 15–8.** Risk of Rh isoimmunization in infants of fathers with various blood groups.[1]

| Father | Baby | Risk (%) |
|---|---|---|
| D-negative | D-negative | 0 |
| D-positive homozygous, ABO-compatible | D-positive | 16 |
| D-positive homozygous, ABO-incompatible | ABO unknown | 7 |
| D-positive homozygous, ABO-compatible | D-positive, ABO-incompatible | 2 |
| D-positive heterozygous, ABO-compatible | D-positive heterozygous, ABO-compatible | 8 |
| D-positive heterozygous, ABO-incompatible | ABO and Rh unknown | 3.5 |

[1]Modified and reproduced, with permission, from Bowman JM: Hemolytic disease of the newborn. In: Conn HF, Conn RB Jr (editors): *Current Diagnosis 6*. Saunders, 1980.

transferase, is unable to conjugate the large amounts of bilirubin. This results in high serum bilirubin, with resultant kernicterus (bilirubin deposition in the basal ganglia).

## Management of the Unsensitized Rh-Negative Pregnancy

**A. Prepregnancy or First Prenatal Visit:** On the first prenatal visit, all pregnant women should be screened for the ABO blood group and the Rh group, including Du. They should also undergo antibody screening (indirect Coombs' test). If the woman is Rh-negative, testing for paternal ABO and Rh blood groups may be useful.

**B. Visit at 28 Weeks:** Antibody screening is performed. If negative, 300 µg of Rh immuneglobulin (RhIgG) is given.

**C. Visit at 35 Weeks:** Antibody screening is repeated. If it is negative, the patient is merely observed. If screening is positive, the patient is managed as Rh-sensitized.

**D. Postpartum Visit:** If the infant is Rh-positive or Du-positive, 300 µg of RhIgG is administered to the mother (provided maternal antibody screening is negative). If antibody is positive, the patient is managed as if she will be Rh-sensitized during the next pregnancy.

**E. Special Fetomaternal Risk States:** Several circumstances may occur during pregnancy that mandate giving RhIgG to the unsensitized patient. Problems in the prevention of Rh isoimmunization are summarized in Table 15–9.

**1. Abortion**–Sensitization will occur in 2% of spontaneous abortions and 4–5% of induced abortions. In the first trimester, due to the small amount of fetal blood, 50 µg of RhIgG is apparently enough to prevent sensitization.

**2. Amniocentesis**–If the placenta is traversed by the needle, there is up to an 11% chance of sensitization. It is recommended that 300 µg of RhIgG be administered when amniocentesis is performed in the unsensitized patient.

**3. Antepartum hemorrhage**–In cases of placenta previa or abruptio placentae, it is recommended

**Table 15–9.** Problems in prevention of Rh isoimmunization.[1]

Allergic reactions to Rh IgG.
Failure to give treatment after delivery of Rh-positive baby.
Failure to give treatment after abortion or amniocentesis.
Failure of RhIgG to confer protection (because of massive transplacental hemorrhage or inadvertent Rh-positive transfusion).
Occurrence of Rh immunization late in pregnancy or soon after delivery, before prophylaxis is given.
Occurrence of Rh immunization during infancy.
Very weak Rh antibody in an Rh-negative woman.

[1]Reproduced, with permission, from Creasy RK, Resnick R: *Maternal-Fetal Medicine: Principles and Practice.* Saunders, 1984.

that 300 µg of RhIgG be given. If the pregnancy is carried more than 12 weeks from the time of RhIgG administration, it is recommended that the prophylactic dose be repeated.

**F. Delivery With Fetomaternal Hemorrhage:** In only about 0.4% of patients will fetomaternal hemorrhage be so great that it cannot be managed with 300 µg of RhIgG. There are a number of studies to determine if this has occurred (eg, Kleihauer-Betke test); however, these are not commonly employed as screening tests because of the rarity of the circumstance and because fetomaternal hemorrhage rarely occurs without antecedent clinical evidence (eg, precipitous delivery, anemicneonate, abruptio placentae, placenta previa, tetanic labor, manual removal of the placenta).

## Management of the Pregnancy With Isoimmunization

Once the maternal antibody titers indicate isoimmunization (> 1 in 8 pregnancies) with one of the blood groups likely to cause fetal hemolysis, the fetus must be closely monitored. Generally, ultrasound is performed at 14–16 weeks to search for signs of fetal ascites or edema and to confirm gestational age. It will also be necessary to perform amniocentesis, usually first at 18–22 weeks. Because of the risk of transplacental hemorrhage and other side effects, ultrasound should be used to guide the needle.

The amniotic fluid is analyzed by spectrophotometry and by the amount of light absorbed by the blood breakdown products plotted on a semilogarithmic scale versus gestational age. It is known that the concentration of these pigments in the unsensitized case gradually decreases as pregnancy progresses. Thus, the severity of fetal affliction may be approximated (Fig 15–2) and this information used as a guide for further studies and treatment.

**A. Mildly Affected Fetus:** The unaffected or mildly affected fetus will fall into zone 1. Amniocentesis should be repeated every 2–3 weeks, and delivery should be near term and certainly after the fetus has achieved pulmonary maturity.

**B. Moderately Affected Fetus:** The moderately affected fetus will fall into zone 2. It will be necessary to repeat amniocentesis every 1–2 weeks. Delivery generally is required prior to term, and the fetus is delivered as soon as pulmonary maturity is reached. In some cases, it may be necessary to enhance pulmonary maturity by the use of betamethasone.

**C. Severely Affected Fetus:** The severely affected fetus falls into zone 3. Intervention is usually needed to allow the fetus to reach a gestational age at which delivery and neonatal risks are fewer than the risks of in utero therapy. Amniocentesis will generally have to be repeated weekly. Ultrasound is used to search for fetal ascites or edema.

Intrauterine transfusion may be necessary to pre-

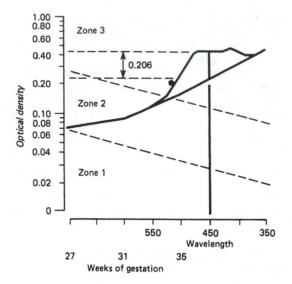

**Figure 15–2.** Amniotic fluid spectrophotometric reading (Liley method) is 0.206 in this example. The value falls into zone 3, indicating impending fetal death. This first affected infant was delivered at 35 weeks' gestation with a cord hemoglobin level of 4.7 g/l00 mL and a cord bilirubin level of 8 mg/100 mL and required 5 exchange transfusions to survive. (Reproduced, with permission, from Creasy RK, Resnick R: Page 575 in: Maternal-Fetal Medicine: Principles and Practice. Saunders, 1984.

vent the fetus from dying. This is performed using O-negative, low-titer, glycerolized or irrigated packed red cells. The volume to be transfused is roughly approximated by the following formula: (Weeks of gestation – 20) × 10 mL.

The fetal heart rate is closely monitored during the procedure, and if tachycardia occurs, the transfusion is stopped. Although most transfusions have been introduced into the fetal abdominal cavity, recent use of ultrasonically directed fetal vascular injections at one of 3 sites (in the placenta, near the cord insertion into the fetus, or near the placental cord insertion) appears

to be so promising that this is the current method of choice. After the procedure, the fetal heart tones are monitored carefully for at least 4 hours.

After transfusion, repeat transfusions or delivery will be necessary as production of fetal blood markedly decreases or ceases. Timing of these transfusions may be assisted by ultrasonic determination of increasing or decreasing fetal peritoneal fluid. When the fetus has sufficient pulmonary maturity for survival, delivery should take place.

## ABO HEMOLYTIC DISEASE

ABO hemolytic disease is much milder than the isoimmunization evoked by $Rh_0$ and the other antigens noted above. The reason for this difference is poorly understood, because both IgG and IgM are produced antenatally. Although 20–25% of pregnancies have potential maternal-infant ABO incompatibility, a recognizable process in the neonate occurs in only 10% of those cases. Those affected are almost always group A (especially A1) or B infants of group O mothers. The neonatal direct Coombs' test may be positive or negative, and maternal antibodies are also variable.

In Rh isoimmunization, only 1–2% of cases occur in the first-born infant, whereas 40–50% of ABO incompatibilities occur in the first-born infant. Serious fetal sequelae (eg, stillbirth, hydrops) almost never occur, and severe fetal anemia is also rare.

ABO hemolytic disease is primarily manifest following birth, with early neonatal onset of jaundice (at < 24 hours) with variable elevation of the indirect bilirubin. The management of ABO incompatibility relates to bilirubin surveillance and phototherapy (required in 10% of cases). The infants may have hepatosplenomegaly. Exchange transfusion is necessary in only 1% of cases, and the incidence of late anemia is rare. Sequelae such as kernicterus almost never occur.

## REFERENCES

A.C.O.G. Technical Bulletin: *Management of Isoimmunization in Pregnancy.* No. 90. American College of Obstetrics and Gynecology, 1986.

Andreyko JL et al: Results of conservative management of premature rupture of the membranes. Am J Obstet Gynecol 1984;148:600.

Arias: Predictability of complications associated with prolongation of pregnancy. Obstet Gynecol 1987;70:101.

Barford DAG, Rosen MG: Cervical incompetence: Diagnosis and outcome. Obstet Gynecol 1984;64:159.

Bartolucci L et al: Ultrasonography in preterm labor. Am J Obstet Gynecol 1984;149:52.

Bochner CJ et al: Antepartum predictors of fetal distress in postterm pregnancy. Am J Obstet Gynecol 1987;157:353.

Bottoms SF et al: Clinical Interpretation of ultrasound measurements in preterm pregnancies with premature rupture of the membranes. Obstet Gynecol 1987;69:358.

Cotton DB et al: Use of amniocentesis in preterm gestation with ruptured membranes. Obstet Gynecol 1984;63:38.

Curet LB et al: Association between ruptured membranes, tocolytic therapy, and respiratory distress syndrome. Am J Obstet Gynecol 1984;148:263.

Dyson DC: Management of prolonged pregnancy: Induction of labor versus antepartum fetal testing. Am J Obstet Gynecol 1987;156:928.

Eden RD et al: Perinatal characteristics of uncomplicated postdate pregnancies. Obstet Gynecol 1987;69:296.

Fuchs AR, Fuchs F, Stubblefield PG: Preterm Birth, Second Edition. McGraw-Hill, New York, 1993.

Goldenberg RL, Huddleston JF, Nelson KG: Apgar scores and umbilical arterial pH in preterm newborn infants. Am J Obstet Gynecol 1984;149:651.

Hameed C et al: Silent chorioamnionitis as a cause of preterm labor refractory to tocolytic therapy. Am J Obstet Gynecol 1984;149:726.

Hatjis CG et al: Addition of magnesium sulfate improves effectiveness of ritodrine in preventing premature delivery. Am J Obstet Gynecol 1984;150:142.

Hatjis CL et al: Efficiency of combined administration of magnesium sulfate and ritodrine in the treatment of premature labor. Obstet Gynecol 1987;69:317.

Iams JD et al: Management of preterm prematurely ruptured membranes. Am J Obstet Gynecol 1985;151:32.

Minkoff H et al: Risk factors for prematurity and premature rupture of membranes. Am J Obstet Gynecol 1984; 150:965.

Moberg LJ, Garite TJ, Freeman RK: Fetal heart rate patterns and fetal distress in patients with preterm premature rupture of membranes. Obstet Gynecol 1984;64:60.

Morrison JC et al: Prevention of preterm birth by ambulatory assessment of uterine activity: A randomized study. Am J Obstet Gynecol 1987;156:536.

Nicolaides KH, Sadovsky G, Cetin E: Fetal heart rate patterns in red blood cell isoimmunized pregnancies. Am J Obstet Gynecol 1989;161:351.

Pitkin RM, Scott JR (editors): *Clinical Obstetrics and Gynecology.* (Crenshaw C, Coulam CB, guest editors.) Lipincott, 1986.

Sampson MB et al: Tocolysis with terbutaline sulfate in patients with placenta previa complicated by premature labor. J Reprod Med 1984;29:248.

Reece EA et al: Ultrasound versus amniotic fluid spectral analysis: Are they sensitive enough to predict neonatal complications associated with isoimmunization? Obstet Gynecol 1989;74:357.

Ronkin S, et al: Intravascular exchange and bolus transfusion in the severely isoimmunized fetus. Am J Obstet Gynecol 1989;160:429.

Socol ML et al: Perinatal outcome following prior delivery in the late second or early third trimester. Obstet Gynecol 1984;150:228.

Tamura RK et al: Diminished growth in fetuses born preterm after spontaneous labor or rupture of membranes. Am J Obstet Gynecol 1984;148:1105.

Taylor J, Garite TJ: Premature rupture of membranes before fetal viability. Obstet Gynecol 1984;64:615.

Vintzileos AM et al: Preterm premature rupture of the membranes: A risk factor for the development of abruptio placenta. Am J Obstet Gyncol 1987;156:1235.

# Disproportionate Fetal Growth

*Michael W. Varner, MD*

Weight at delivery was once considered evidence of prematurity (birth weight < 2500 g) or postmaturity (macrosomia; birth weight > 4500 g). These criteria were later revised when it was realized that abnormal growth was reflected in factors other than birth weight. Normative standards were developed that include birth weight, length, and head circumference according to gestational age. Abnormal fetal growth is now defined according to percentiles: Infants classified as small for gestational age (SGA) are in the 10th percentile or below, and those classified as large for gestational age (LGA) are in the 90th percentile or above. Standards now also vary among different populations.

Improved ultrasound technology has provided more information regarding gestational age. For example, fetal weights determined by ultrasonography at 20–32 weeks' gestation (accurate within 100 g) suggest that many infants born prematurely are smaller than infants of the same gestational age who are later delivered at term.

Both SGA and LGA fetuses have an increased risk of perinatal morbidity and mortality (Tables 16–1 and 16–2). The pathogenesis, differential diagnosis, and treatment are different for the 2 extremes of growth. The term intrauterine growth retardation, often used in association with SGA fetuses, is not used here because of the negative connotation of the word "retardation."

Some fetuses may show effects of genetic disorders, infectious disease, or toxic factors but may not be so extensively affected as to be included in the SGA category. These infants have been called non-SGA SGA. They are at some increased risk for adverse perinatal and long-term sequelae but probably not to the same extent as SGA infants.

## SMALL-FOR-GESTATIONAL-AGE PREGNANCY

### Pathophysiology

When compared with average-for-gestational-age (AGA) fetuses, the SGA fetus has altered body com-

position (including decreased body fat, total protein, whole body DNA and RNA, glycogen, and free fatty acids), altered distribution of weight among organs, and altered body proportions. About 20% of SGA infants are symmetrically small, with a relatively proportionate decrease in many organ weights. Eighty percent are asymmetrically small, with relative sparing of brain weight, especially when compared with that of the liver or thymus.

Diminished placental function is the most common causative factor in SGA pregnancy. Although this finding sometimes reflects abnormal placental anatomy (eg, battledore placenta, velamentous insertion of the cord, single umbilical artery, circumvallate placenta, placenta previa), it more frequently reflects abnormal function of a normal placenta (eg, due to cigarette smoking, diminished perfusion, infection, infarction, premature placental aging, chronic idiopathic villitis). In some cases abnormal placental function may be due to abnormal platelet-vessel or platelet-platelet interactions caused by insufficient production of prostacyclin, resulting in a relative dominance of thromboxane $A_2$, a powerful vasoconstrictor.

In asymmetric SGA infants, brain weight is decreased only slightly compared with that of AGA controls, primarily owing to decreased brain cell size and not to decreased brain cell numbers. Cerebral abnormalities include decreased myelination, decreased utilization of metabolic substrates other than glucose, and altered protein synthesis. At least in experimental animals, these changes are more likely to produce adverse effects in the brain stem and cerebellum. This differential sparing is particularly prominent when deprivation occurs in the latter half of pregnancy. Deprivation early in pregnancy is associated with less cerebral sparing and diffusely slowed brain growth.

Symmetric SGA infants have proportionately small brains, usually because of a decreased number of brain cells. Although this may be the result of early, severe nutritional deprivation, the cause is more often a genetic disorder, infection, or other problem. The thymus is usually small, being decreased by an average of 25%. This may in part ex-

**Table 16–1.** Some complications of SGA pregnancy.

**Maternal Complications**
Complications due to underlying disease, preeclampsia, premature labor, cesarean delivery
**Fetal Complications**
Stillbirth, hypoxia and acidosis, malformations
**Neonatal Complications**
Hypoglycemia, hypocalcemia, hypoxia and acidosis, hypothermia, meconium aspiration syndrome, polycythemia, congenital malformations, sudden infant death syndrome
**Long-Term Complications**
Lower IQ, learning and behavior problems, major neurologic handicaps (seizure disorders, cerebral palsy, severe mental retardation, hypertension)

plain the decreased cellular immunity seen in SGA infants.

The liver is also frequently affected, at least partly because of diminished glycogen deposition. The liver may also have functional (metabolic) abnormalities, as manifested by abnormal cord blood and neonatal serum chemistries. Such abnormalities often reflect the underlying cause of decreased size.

Blood flow to the lungs may be decreased, lessening the pulmonary contribution to amniotic fluid volume; this may be partly responsible for the often-encountered oligohydramnios. Decreased pulmonary blood flow may also be associated with accelerated functional pulmonary maturity.

Renal blood flow is frequently reduced in asymmetric SGA pregnancies. The resultant diminished glomerular filtration rate may further contribute to oligohydramnios.

The SGA fetus is at risk for in utero complications, including hypoxia and metabolic acidosis, which may occur at any time but are likely to occur during labor. Hypoxia is the result of increasing fetal oxygen requirements during pregnancy (both total requirement and requirement per kilogram of ideal fetal body weight), with a rapid increase during the third trimester. If, for whatever reason, the fetus receives inadequate oxygen, hypoxia and subsequent metabolic acidosis will ensue. If undetected or untreated, this will lead to decreased glycogen and fat stores, ischemic end organ damage, meconium-stained amniotic fluid, and oligohydramnios, with eventual vital organ damage and intrauterine death.

**Table 16–2.** Some complications of LGA pregnancy.

**Maternal Complications**
Cesarean section, postpartum hemorrhage, shoulder dystocia, perineal trauma, operative vaginal delivery
**Fetal Complications**
Stillbirth, anomalies, shoulder dystocia
**Neonatal Complications**
Low Apgar score, hypoglycemia, birth injury, hypocalcemia, polycythemia, jaundice, feeding difficulties
**Long-Term Complications**
Obesity, type II diabetes, neurologic or behavioral problems, childhood onset of cancer

## Differential Diagnosis

A classification of SGA pregnancy according to cause is shown in Table 16–3. Any inference of suboptimal growth requires, by definition, serial observations. It cannot be emphasized too strongly that a pregnancy cannot be described as SGA unless the gestational age is known with certainty (see Chapter 9).

Numerous authors have differentiated between symmetric and asymmetric SGA pregnancy regarding cause and prognosis. Briefly stated, symmetric SGA infants are more likely to have an endogenous defect, which may preclude normal development. Asymmetric SGA infants are more likely to be normal but small in size owing to intrauterine deprivation. Although this classification is helpful in establishing a differential diagnosis and framework for discussion, it is not sufficiently precise to serve as a basis for decisions regarding intervention or viability.

**A. Factors Causing Decreased Growth Potential:**

**1. Genetic disorders–**Genetic disorders account for 10–15% of SGA infants. Data from the Metropolitan Atlanta Congenital Defects Program suggest that 38% of chromosomally abnormal infants are SGA and that the risk of an SGA infant having a

**Table 16–3.** Pathogenic classification of SGA pregnancy.

**Decreased Growth Potential (Endogenous, or Type I, SGA Infant)**
Genetic Disorders
    Autosomal: Trisomy 13, 18, 21; ring chromosomes; chromosomal deletions; partial trisomies
    Sex Chromosomes: Turner syndrome, multiple chromosomes (XXX, XYY)
    Neural Tube Defects
    Dysmorphic Syndromes: achondroplasia, chondrodystrophies, osteogenesis imperfecta
    Abdominal Wall Defects
    Other Rare Syndromes
Congenital Infection
    Viral: cytomegalovirus, rubella, herpes, varicella zoster
    Protozoan: toxoplasmosis, malaria
    Bacterial: listeriosis
Drugs
    Alcohol, tobacco; warfarin, folic acid antagonists (methotrexate, aminopterin), anticonvulsants
Radiation
Small maternal stature, ethnic status
Altitude
Female fetus
**Restricted Growth Potential (Exogenous, or Type II, SGA Infant)**
Placental Disorders: placenta previa, placental infarction, chronic villitis, chronic partial separation, placental malformations (circumvallate placenta, battledore placenta, placental hemangioma, twin-twin transfusion syndrome)
Co-Existent Maternal Disease: hypertension, anemia (hemoglobinopathy, decreased normal hemoglobin [especially 12 g/dL]), renal disease (hypertension, protein loss), malnutrition (inflammatory bowel disease [ulcerative colitis, regional enteritis], pancreatitis, intestinal parasites), cyanotic pulmonary disease
Multiple Pregnancy

major congenital anomaly is 8%. Infants with autosomal trisomies are more likely to be SGA, the most common being **trisomy 21 (Down's syndrome)**, with an incidence of 1.6 per 1000 live births. At term, such infants weigh an average of 350 g less than comparable normal infants and are 4 times more likely to be SGA. This decrease is apparent only in the last 6 weeks of pregnancy. A similar decrease in birth weight occurs in translocation Down's syndrome, whereas mosaic Down's syndrome is associated with an intermediate decrease in birth weight. The relative risk of a pregnancy being complicated by fetal trisomy 21 increases with progressive maternal age.

The second most common autosomal trisomy is **trisomy 18 (Edwards' syndrome)**, which occurs in 1 in 6000–8000 live births. Eighty-four percent of these infants are SGA. Ultrasound evaluation may reveal associated anomalies. There is an increased likelihood of polyhydramnios plus fetal neural tube defects and visceral anomalies. Fetuses are frequently in breech presentation. The average birth weight in trisomy 18 infants is almost 1000 g less than that of controls. In contrast to that seen in infants with trisomies 13 and 21, the placental weight in trisomy 18 infants is also markedly reduced. Trisomy 18 is also more common with older mothers.

**Trisomy 13,** the third most common autosomal trisomy, occurs in 1 in 5000–10,000 live births. Over 50% of affected infants are SGA. Birth weights average 700–800 g less than that of controls. Trisomy 13 is also more common with older mothers. As in trisomy 18, there may be associated abnormalities, including cleft lip and palate, urinary tract abnormalities, central nervous system abnormalities, and polydactyly.

Other autosomal chromosome abnormalities (eg, other trisomies, ring chromosomes, deletions, partial trisomies) are clinically uncommon but associated with an increased likelihood of the fetus being SGA. Sex chromosome abnormalities may also be associated with lower birth weight. The XYY configuration is the most common of these but is probably not associated with an increased incidence of SGA pregnancy. Extra X chromosomes (more than 2) are associated with a decrease in birth weight of 200–300 g for each extra X. **Turner's syndrome** is associated with an average birth weight of approximately 400 g below average. Fetuses with mosaic Turner's syndrome are intermediately affected.

Statistically, the growth impairment seen with fetal chromosome abnormalities occurs earlier than that which is of placental origin. However, there is considerable clinical overlap, and this observation is not always of clinical value.

Fetuses with neural tube defects are frequently SGA. Anencephalic fetuses are SGA, even considering the absent brain and skull, with average third trimester birth weights of approximately 1000–1100 g less than matched controls. Anencephaly is diagnosable by ultrasonography and alpha-fetoprotein (AFP) measurements in maternal serum or amniotic fluid. The birth weight difference is less prominent with fetal spina bifida, averaging 250 g less than that of controls. Although spina bifida may be detected by ultrasonography or AFP studies, both techniques have appreciable false-negative rates. Spina bifida is sometimes suspected on the basis of secondary mild fetal hydrocephalus. Maternal serum AFP studies, used increasingly in the USA, are effective not only in detecting neural tube defects but also in identifying multiple pregnancies and pregnancies at increased risk for small size, premature labor, or stillbirth. These studies also may improve assessment of gestational age.

Certain dysmorphic syndromes are associated with an increased incidence of SGA fetuses. Achondroplasia may be associated with low birth weight (average decrease, 300–600 g) if either parent is affected, but if spontaneous mutation is the cause, infants are generally of normal birth weight. Although achondroplasia is associated with relatively normal development, most chondrodystrophies are associated with a dismal outcome. Among the more common forms of chondrodystrophy are thanatophoric dwarfism, asphyxiating thoracic dysplasia, achondrogenesis, and osteopetrosis. Most chondrodystrophies are inherited in autosomal recessive patterns, in contrast to achondroplasia, which is usually autosomal dominant. All chondrodystrophies are frequently associated with polyhydramnios.

Osteogenesis imperfecta consists of a spectrum of diseases with different genetic transmissions and prognoses, all of which result in SGA fetuses. Shortening or fractures of the long bones help determine the diagnosis.

Infants born with abdominal wall defects are characteristically SGA, particularly those with gastroschisis.

Numerous other autosomal recessive syndromes are associated with SGA fetuses. Included among these are **Smith-Lemli-Opitz syndrome, Meckel's syndrome, Robert's syndrome, Donohue's syndrome,** and **Seckel's syndrome.** All these conditions are rare and are most likely to be diagnosed prenatally in families where a child has already been affected.

Maternal neurofibromatosis has been associated with SGA outcome.

Infants with renal anomalies of any nature are often SGA. Renal agenesis (**Potter's syndrome**) and complete urinary tract outflow obstruction are the 2 most common examples. A dysmature infant may be SGA and may have associated oligohydramnios. The presence of oligohydramnios in any infant makes prenatal diagnosis by ultrasonography or amniocentesis much more difficult. Oligohydramnios is relatively more likely to be associated with a small fundal height measurement, which may indicate that the fetus is SGA in ultrasound evaluation.

Other congenital anomalies associated with an increased incidence of SGA outcome are gastroschisis, duodenal atresia, and pancreatic agenesis.

**2. Congenital infections**–Chronic intrauterine infection may be responsible for 5–10% of SGA pregnancies (Table 16–3). The most commonly identified pathogen is cytomegalovirus. Although cytomegalovirus can be isolated from 0.5–2% of all newborns in the USA, clinically obvious infection at the time of birth affects only 0.2–2 in 1000 live births. Active fetoplacental infection is characterized by cytolysis, followed by secondary inflammation, fibrosis, and calcification. Only infants with clinically apparent infection at the time of birth are likely to be SGA due to the infection. Signs of congenital infection are nonspecific but include central nervous system involvement (eg, microcephaly), chorioretinitis, and intracranial (periventricular) calcifications. Other signs include pneumonitis, hepatosplenomegaly, and thrombocytopenia.

Congenital rubella infection also increases the likelihood of an SGA fetus. Infection during the first trimester results in the most severely affected and therefore smallest fetuses, primarily as a result of microvascular endothelial damage. Such infants are likely to have structural cardiovascular defects and central nervous system defects that include microcephaly, deafness, glaucoma, and cataracts.

The diagnosis of congenital viral infections requires serologic confirmation of elevated virus-specific IgM antibody in fetal, cord, or newborn blood specimens. Additionally, the virus may be recovered from cerebrospinal fluid, urine, stool, or nasopharyngeal secretions.

Other viruses implicated in SGA pregnancy include herpesvirus, varicella-zoster virus, influenza virus, and poliovirus. However, the number of cases is small, and it is unknown whether specific congenital syndromes can be attributed to these agents.

By virtue of their chronic, indolent nature, protozoan infections could be expected to be associated with SGA pregnancies. The most commonly associated infection is toxoplasmosis, which is caused by the tissue-bound protozoan *Toxoplasma gondii* and is transmitted by ingesting the oocyte in raw meat or the excrement of infected animals. The infection is acquired transplacentally, and only women with parasitemia (ie, primary infection) are at risk for having an affected infant. The average incidence is 1 in 1000 live births in the USA, although the incidence varies widely among locations and social populations. About 20% of newborns with congenital toxoplasmosis will be sufficiently involved to be SGA. Another protozoan infection associated with SGA pregnancy is malaria.

Although bacterial infections occur commonly in pregnancy and are frequently implicated in premature delivery, they are not commonly associated with SGA infants, because the infections are not usually chronic or subacute. Chronic infection due to *Listeria monocytogenes* is an exception. Infants are usually critically ill at the time of delivery and have encephalitis, pneumonitis, myocarditis, hepatosplenomegaly, jaundice, and petechiae.

**3. Drugs**–Since the thalidomide tragedy of the 1950s, the medical profession has become increasingly concerned about the effects of drugs on the developing fetus. Although this concern was initially related to the incidence of birth defects, concerns about effects on fetal growth have also been raised. Both socially used drugs and prescribed medications can affect fetal growth.

Alcohol has been known since ancient times to have detrimental effects on the fetus. More recently, the fetal alcohol syndrome has been described; this includes craniofacial, limb, and cardiovascular anomalies plus low birth weight. The precise incidence is unclear, but occurrence of the full syndrome seems to be dose-related and limited to women who regularly consume at least 2–3 oz of alcohol per day. However, consumption of any amount of alcohol on a regular basis during pregnancy should be considered detrimental. The syndrome is difficult to distinguish from associated problems such as genetic anomalies or problems due to poor nutrition, drug use, and cigarette smoking.

Cigarette smoking is much more common among women of childbearing age in the USA than is alcoholism. Birth weight is reduced by about 200 g in infants of smoking mothers. The amount of reduction is related to the number of cigarettes per day. Infants of smoking mothers are also shorter in length, and there is a greater risk of stillbirth or compromise in labor. Cigarette smoking is the single most common preventable cause of SGA pregnancy in the USA today.

Other socially used drugs have been associated with an increased incidence of SGA pregnancy. Heroin addicts have an increased incidence of SGA infants, but they have so many other confounding variables that it cannot be said with certainty that the increased incidence is due to heroin per se. Studies of pregnant women maintained on methadone have not shown an increased incidence of SGA newborns.

Certain pharmacologic agents have also been associated with an increased incidence of SGA pregnancies, primarily as a result of teratogenic effects. Warfarin has been associated with an increased incidence of SGA fetuses, primarily due to the sequelae of intrauterine hemorrhage. The folic acid antagonists are associated with an increased risk of spontaneous abortion and stillbirth, severe malformations, and SGA infants. Methotrexate is associated with an incidence of fetal malformations approximately 30% following first-trimester exposure. Such malformations include absence of cranial sutures, oxycephaly, absence of the frontal bone, low-set ears, hypertelorism, dextrorotation of the heart, absence of toes, and hypoplastic mandible. Although precise incidence figures are not available, multiple craniofacial, central nervous system, and extremity anomalies have also been described following first-trimester administration of aminopterin. Exposure to any of these drugs during the second and third trimesters is associated with a 40% incidence of SGA fetuses.

SGA fetuses are also more common with maternally administered immunosuppressive drugs (eg, cyclosporine, azathioprine, corticosteroids), but when controlled for the underlying maternal diseases for which these medications are indicated, the medications per se probably have little effect on fetal growth.

**4. Radiation**–Intrauterine exposure to ionizing radiation may be associated with reduced fetal growth potential, although the likelihood of this varies substantially with gestational age and amount of exposure. The human fetus is more susceptible to radiation in the first trimester than later in pregnancy. Five centigrays is the lowest amount at which teratogenic effects have been documented, even during the most vulnerable period, but it should not be assumed that no damage occurs below this level. Radiation exposure should be minimized at any time during pregnancy. The dosage at which damage would be reasonably certain to occur is approximately 100 cGy. Radiation affects primarily the central nervous system (microcephaly, microphthalmia, mental retardation), but generalized growth impairment may also occur.

**5. Small maternal stature**–A small woman may have a smaller-than-normal infant because of reduced uterine growth potential. These mothers and infants are completely normal and healthy but are small in size because of genetic variation. The infants are described by the ponderal index (PI), calculated from the following formula:

**PI = Birthweight × 1000/(crown-heel length)³**

Asymmetric SGA infants will have a low ponderal index (ie, they will be long, light-weight infants), whereas small normal infants will have a normal index. (A normal index at 28 weeks is 1.8. This increases by 0.2 every 4 weeks to reach 2.4 at 40 weeks.) Errors in cubing of the growth-heel length will skew the measurements greatly.

More recently, fetal nutritional status has also been quantified via a midarm circumference-to-head circumference ratio.

Maternal parity exerts a modest effect on birth weight. First-born infants tend to be smaller and more often categorized as SGA. This effect decreases with successive deliveries and is not seen beyond the third birth.

**6. Female fetus**–At term, female fetuses are on average 5% (150 g) smaller and 2% (1 cm) shorter than male fetuses. Female infants are more likely to be categorized as SGA unless gender-specific classifications are used.

**B. Restricted Growth Potential:** Although suboptimal intrauterine growth may be due to an intrinsic fetal abnormality, it is more likely to be the result of extrafetal restriction of growth. This has been referred to as exogenous, or type II, SGA and accounts for about 80% of cases with a definable pathologic mechanism.

**1. Placental factors**–The placenta obviously plays an important role in normal fetal growth. Several placental abnormalities are associated with an increased likelihood of SGA infants.

**Placenta previa** is associated with an increased incidence of SGA fetuses, probably owing to the unfavorable site of placental implantation. Complete placenta previa is associated with a higher incidence of SGA outcome than partial placenta previa.

Decreased functional exchange area due to **placental infarction** is also associated with an increased incidence of SGA fetuses.

**Premature placental separation** may occur at any time during pregnancy, with variable effects. When not associated with fetal death, premature labor, or exsanguination, it may be associated with an increased likelihood of SGA fetuses.

Malformations of the placenta or cord are associated with an increased incidence of SGA fetuses. Such malformations include **circumvallate placenta, placental hemangioma, battledore placenta, and twin-twin transfusion syndrome.**

Finally, **chronic villitis** is seen with increased frequency when the placentas of SGA pregnancies are examined histologically. This problem may recur in subsequent pregnancies.

Uterine anomalies are also associated with a higher risk of impaired fetal growth, primarily because of the higher likelihood of suboptimal uterine blood flow.

**2. Coexistent maternal disease**–Numerous maternal diseases are associated with suboptimal fetal growth via various mechanisms, including any that interfere with uptake or delivery of nutrients or oxygen to the fetus. Many of these diseases can be described by the **HARM** acronym (H =hypertension, A = anemia, R = renal, M = malabsorption).

**Hypertension,** either systemic or pulmonary, is the single most common maternal complication causing SGA pregnancy. With systemic hypertension, there is decreased blood flow through the spiral arterioles perfusing the placenta, resulting in decreased delivery of oxygen and nutrients to the placenta and fetus. Hypertension may also be associated with placental infarction.

Maternal **anemia** is associated with decreased fetal growth when it limits the amount of oxygen available for placental transfer. This may occur with abnormalities of either hemoglobin structure (ie, hemoglobinopathies) or hemoglobin quantity (eg, anemia due to excessive blood loss or lack of nutrient precursors).

**Renal disease** may be associated with SGA pregnancy because of resulting hypertension or significant urinary protein loss.

Maternal **malabsorption** may predispose to SGA pregnancy. The most common clinical situations are inflammatory bowel disease (ulcerative colitis, regional enteritis), pancreatitis, and intestinal parasites. Faulty or inadequate maternal nutritional intake may also predispose to SGA pregnancy.

Other diseases that affect maternal microvascular perfusion can be associated with SGA outcomes. These include collagen vascular diseases, insulin-dependent diabetes mellitus associated with microvasculopathy, and preeclampsia.

Abnormal maternal carbohydrate metabolism may be associated with SGA outcomes, in particular when a "flat" oral glucose tolerance test is associated with relative maternal hypoglycemia and hypoinsulinemia.

**3. Multiple pregnancy**–Multiple pregnancy has long been associated with premature delivery (40% of twins are delivered at 36 weeks or sooner). However, it is also associated with a 20–30% incidence of SGA fetuses. This may be due to placental insufficiency, twin-twin transfusion (only with monozygotic fetuses), or anomalies. SGA fetuses can be determined by approximately 32 weeks with twins, 30 weeks with triplets, and 28 weeks with quadruplets. Serial ultrasound estimations of fetal weights should be considered in any multiple pregnancy.

**C. General Diagnostic Considerations:** In any pregnancy at risk for SGA outcome, baseline studies should be obtained early in gestation. These should always include careful attention to gestational dating (menstrual history, serial examinations, biochemical pregnancy testing, quickening, ultrasound). An SGA outcome may also develop in pregnancies without identified risk factors. Careful attention to fundal height measurements is associated with a diagnostic sensitivity of 46–86%.

Ultrasonography should be used extensively in such pregnancies. Ultrasound examination early in pregnancy is accurate in establishing the estimated date of confinement (EDC) and may sometimes identify genetic or congenital causes of SGA pregnancy. Serial ultrasound examinations are important in documenting growth and excluding anomalies. The fetal biparietal diameter (BPD) is an unreliable predictor of fetal growth. However, the fetal head circumference is somewhat more reliable, not only of interval growth but of long-term neuropsychological prognosis as well. The fetal abdominal circumference reflects the volume of fetal subcutaneous fat as well as the size of the liver which, in turn, correlates with the degree of fetal nutrition. The femur length is not helpful in the identification of the SGA baby. Since the definition of SGA ultimately depends on birth weight and gestational age criteria, the employment of formulas that optimally predict birth weight in a given population will be the most important ultrasonographic criteria.

The role of Doppler velocimetry in the evaluation and management of the SGA pregnancy remains controversial. In fetuses already known to be SGA, umbilical artery Doppler velocimetry can estimate the likelihood of adverse perinatal outcome and may be useful in determining the intensity of fetal surveillance. However, the utility of umbilical artery Doppler velocimetry remains unproven for general population screening.

Baseline laboratory studies should also be obtained early in pregnancy. Studies vary from patient to patient, but most patients should have a complete blood count as well as tests for electrolytes, liver function, uric acid, and renal function (including serum blood urea nitrogen and creatinine), plus a 24-hour urine determination for creatinine clearance and total protein.

Maternal serum alpha-fetoprotein (MS-AFP) elevations predict increased risk for SGA outcome, regardless of maternal weight. Elevated MS-AFP also predicts an increased risk of other obstetric problems including preeclampsia, abruption, preterm labor, and stillbirth.

In some centers, severe fetal growth restriction has become an important indication for fetal blood sampling via cordocentesis. These procedures can provide useful information on fetal karyotype, acid-base balance, fetal metabolism, and possible fetal infection. Gestational age-specific values now exist for most hematologic and metabolic parameters.

If clinically indicated, studies should be done to exclude infection. Initially this usually involves determination of immune status (IgG antibodies against cytomegalovirus, rubella virus, *T gondii*). If the IgG titer is high, specific IgM antibodies should be measured. If these are present in significant quantity, primary infection may be present. A careful targeted ultrasound examination should be performed to determine the degree of fetal involvement, particularly of the central nervous system. Fetal involvement may be further investigated by direct fetal blood sampling for organism-specific IgM assays, cultures, or electron microscopy for direct visualization of viral particles.

## Complications

Numerous maternal and perinatal complications occur more frequently in SGA pregnancy. Underlying maternal disease is more likely to be present (see Table 16–3), and these women require more intensive prenatal care. Premature labor or preeclampsia is more common. SGA fetuses at any gestational age are less likely to tolerate labor well, and the need for operative delivery is increased.

Most reports suggest that perinatal mortality rates are increased in SGA pregnancies; however, many of these reports date from before the era of fetal surveillance, when SGA perinatal mortality rates were 3–5 times those of the AGA population. With the advent of fetal surveillance, the perinatal mortality rate decreased to 2–3 times that of the AGA population. With continued improvements in antenatal surveillance and neonatal care, the perinatal mortality rate for SGA pregnancies in most centers is now 1.5–2 times that of the AGA population. Unfortunately, it is unlikely that this rate will reach in the near future that of the AGA population, because of the persistent occurrence of lethal anomalies and severe congenital infections. The past decade has witnessed increased attention to minimizing the perinatal complications of surviving SGA neonates.

SGA infants are at increased risk for neonatal complications, including meconium aspiration syndrome, polycythemia, hypoglycemia, hypocalcemia, and temperature instability. All SGA infants need thorough evaluation for congenital anomalies.

## Prevention

Some SGA pregnancies are preventable (see Table 16–3). Most cases that are due to genetic causes are not preventable. However, many can be diagnosed prenatally by serum AFP screening, ultrasound scans, or amniocentesis for karyotype or AFP. In unusual situations in which a paternal chromosomal abnormality is associated with a high likelihood of abnormal fetal karyotype, donor artificial insemination is a possibility. Avoidance of factors associated with an increased likelihood of neural tube defects (eg, maternal hyperthermia at the time of neural tube closure) should be encouraged in all pregnancies.

Pregnant women should avoid close contact with individuals known to be infected or colonized with rubella virus or cytomegalovirus. Nonpregnant women of reproductive age should be tested for immunity to rubella virus and, if susceptible, should be immunized. Unfortunately, no vaccine currently exists for cytomegalovirus.

If it is clinically suspected, women of childbearing age should be tested for immunity to *T gondii*. If the woman is immune, her risk of having an affected infant is remote, but if she is susceptible, she should be cautioned to avoid animal excrement (especially that of domestic cats) and uncooked meat.

Significant alcohol ingestion and cigarette smoking represent the most common preventable causes of SGA pregnancy in the USA. It is important that all patients be made aware of the fetal risks involved.

Therapeutic medications are not a major cause of SGA pregnancy, but benefits and risks should be weighed whenever medications are prescribed. Any woman of childbearing age should be questioned about the possibility of pregnancy before receiving therapeutic or diagnostic radiation to the pelvis.

Placental factors causing SGA pregnancies are not generally preventable. However, low-dose aspirin and dipyridamole may increase prostacyclin production in certain patients and thus prevent idiopathic uteroplacental insufficiency.

Preventive measures for the maternal diseases listed in Table 16–3 are too complex to be discussed in this chapter. Treatment of many of these conditions may decrease the likelihood of SGA pregnancy. Treatment of hypertension has a positive effect on birth weight, at least in the third trimester. Although a complex issue, protein supplements for patients with significant proteinuria may increase the amount of protein available for placental transfer. Correction of maternal anemia (of whatever cause) improves oxygen delivery to the fetus and thus improves fetal growth.

Treatment of malabsorption syndrome (of whatever cause) can be expected to improve nutrient absorption and subsequent transfer to the fetus. Inflammatory bowel disease should be treated if required, but, if possible, pregnancy should be deferred until the disease has been quiescent for approximately 6 months. Intestinal parasites should be appropriately treated and negative cultures confirmed prior to pregnancy.

## Treatment

Treatment of SGA pregnancy presupposes an accurate diagnosis. Even with the history, physical examination, and ultrasound examination, diagnosis remains difficult, and some SGA pregnancies will not be detected.

All pregnant women should discontinue cigarette smoking as well as use of alcohol and all "recreational" drugs. This should be done before conception to allow time for clearance of toxins, particularly if the woman has had a previous SGA infant. Adequate nutrition must also be emphasized.

Controversy exists concerning the role of bed rest in SGA pregnancy. Its value has not been proved in women with symmetric SGA fetuses, because the most common causes are not correctable by increased uterine blood flow. However, asymmetric SGA pregnancies may benefit from the increased uterine blood flow that occurs when the patient is in the lateral recumbent position. Although bed rest may do little to prolong the duration of pregnancy, it probably is associated with increased birth weight per week of gestation, and thus is of value in asymmetric SGA pregnancy.

Low-dose aspirin may also be of value in selected cases of SGA pregnancy. This regimen decreases thromboxane $A_2$ synthesis, with resultant predominance of prostacyclin, a potent vasodilator.

Since SGA fetuses are at risk for antepartum or intrapartum compromise, they should be followed up carefully. Weekly prenatal visits should include an interview and examination with attention to frequency and intensity of fetal movements, presence or absence of contractions, and signs of spontaneous rupture of membranes. Physical examination should always include the mother's weight, fundal height, fetal heart rate, assessment of presentation, and maternal blood pressure and urinalysis. Maternal girth at the umbilicus may also be helpful in assessing uterine growth.

Electronic fetal monitoring should be performed at least weekly on all potentially viable SGA babies. The nonstress test is usually a satisfactory initial choice. Some authorities believe the nonstress test is less sensitive to fetal compromise than the contraction stress test, but if care is taken to note the baseline fetal heart rate (normal on monitoring is 110–150/min) and to allow for small variable decelerations, the 2 tests are probably equally sensitive and useful.

Ultrasound examinations to assess adequacy of fetal growth should be performed at least every 3–4 weeks. Measurements should include biparietal diameter, head circumference, and femur length, especially in those in whom an asymmetric SGA fetus is suspected. Probably the most sensitive indices of an asymmetric SGA fetus are abdominal circumference and total intrauterine volume, although both require a definite EDC for optimum interpretation. The femur length:abdominal circumference ratio is a gestational age-independent ratio, with normal being 0.20–0.24. Asymmetric SGA fetuses generally have a ratio greater than 0.24.

Amniotic fluid volume should also be assessed at least weekly in at-risk pregnancies, because the likelihood of a fetus being small because of nutritional deprivation is much less when normal amniotic fluid volume is present.

An association has recently been proposed between certain umbilical artery Doppler velocity waveforms and SGA pregnancies. In particular, increases in the systolic/diastolic ratio or absence or reversal of end-diastolic flow are thought to reflect increased placental blood flow impedance. The general sensitivity of umbilical artery doppler waveform analysis in the detection of SGA pregnancy reportedly ranges between 60% and 80%. However, the literature to date has not uniformly defined outcome parameters, and inadequate prospective randomized data exist. At this time, umbilical artery doppler waveform analysis does appear useful for distinguishing between the SGA fetus and the constitutionally small or incorrectly dated fetus. However, its ability to predict SGA outcomes remains unproven.

Ultrasonography can also be used to calculate estimated fetal weights. Although many formulas are available, the following formula of Weiner and asso-

ciates (1985) works well for gestational ages of 24–32 weeks:

**where EFW = estimated fetal weight, HC = head circumference, and AC = abdominal circumference.**

The formula of Shepard and associates (1982) works well for gestational ages beyond 32 weeks:

$$\text{Log EFW} = 0.02597 \times \text{AC} + 0.2161 \times \text{BPD} - 0.1999 \times \text{AC} \times \text{BPD}^2/1000 + 1.2659$$

where BPD = biparietal diameter. Ultrasound-derived fetal weight estimates offer higher positive predictive values than do any specific fetal measurements. Ultrasonography can also determine fetal biophysical profiles (see Chapter 13). If a nonstress test is nonreactive or if variable or spontaneous decelerations are seen, further assessment of fetal well-being is immediately indicated. Either a contraction stress test or a fetal biophysical profile can be performed. To date, there have been no randomized prospective evaluations of the relative efficacy of either procedure in an at-risk SGA population. The presence of late decelerations with more than 50% of contractions (regardless of frequency of contractions) constitutes a positive contraction stress test and is an indication to proceed with delivery unless there is an obvious, easily treatable maternal problem such as dehydration or hyperthermia. The fetal biophysical profile is discussed in more detail in Chapter 13; it provides evidence about fetal well-being and has the additional advantage of assessing fetal anatomy.

In selected cases, ultrasound-directed amniocentesis may be indicated (eg, for determination of fetal pulmonary maturity with an uncertain EDC or for assessment of fetal karyotype, certain biochemical disorders, or AFP levels). Preliminary evidence suggests that Doppler ultrasound evaluation of uterine blood flow may be of value in identifying pregnancies at risk for being SGA.

Every SGA pregnancy must be individually assessed for the optimal time of delivery (ie, the point at which the baby will do as well outside as inside the uterus). This would be whenever surveillance indicates fetal maturity, fetal compromise, or gestational age of 38 weeks (beyond which time there is no advantage to an SGA fetus remaining in utero).

SGA pregnancies are at increased risk for intrapartum problems, and, whenever possible, delivery should take place in a center where appropriate obstetric care, anesthesia, and neonatal care are readily available. Cesarean delivery may be necessary, and the presence of meconium-stained amniotic fluid or a compromised infant should be anticipated.

The type of delivery depends on the individual case. Cesarean section delivery is often indicated, especially when fetal monitoring reveals fetal compromise, malpresentation, or situations in which "traumatic vaginal delivery" might be expected.

Continuous internal electronic fetal heart rate monitoring should be performed during labor in all cases, even if recent antepartum testing has been reassuring. Scalp pH determinations (see Chapter 13) should be frequent, especially in preterm SGA pregnancies. Arteriovenous cord blood gas determinations are also useful in all cases. As many as 50% of SGA infants have some degree of metabolic acidosis. If metabolic acidosis is present, prompt evaluation by a neonatologist is necessary.

Minimization of anesthesia is generally preferable, but controlled epidural anesthesia is usually safe. Maternal hypotension or hypovolemia must be avoided.

### Prognosis

SGA pregnancy per se is not considered life-threatening for the mother. However, she may be at risk for significant morbidity or even death if she has an underlying condition that predisposes to an SGA fetus (eg, hypertension or renal disease). Most women who deliver SGA infants can be expected to have long-term prognoses equivalent to women delivering AGA infants.

Any woman who has had one SGA infant is at increased risk of having another. There is a 2-fold and 4-fold increase in risk for SGA birth after 1 and 2 SGA births, respectively. First-degree female relatives of the woman have a 2-fold increased risk of having an SGA infant.

The long-term prognosis is less benign for the SGA infant. SGA infants tend to remain physically small, particularly symmetric infants (with normal PI), since these infants are likely either to have significant intrinsic problems that will not improve following birth or to be constitutionally small infants born of constitutionally small mothers. Asymmetric infants (with low PI) tend to have accelerated growth for the first 6 months after birth, particularly if intrauterine deprivation was a major factor.

Taken as a group, SGA infants also have more neurologic and intellectual deficits than do their AGA peers. SGA infants have lower IQs as well as a higher incidence of learning and behavioral problems. Major neurologic handicaps such as severe mental retardation, cerebral palsy, and seizures are more common in SGA infants. SGA infants are more likely to have hypertension early in life, reflecting the fact that many hypertensive diseases are inheritable. In addition, the incidence of sudden infant death syndrome (SIDS) is increased in SGA infants, who account for 30% of all SIDS cases. All these problems are more frequent and more severe in infants with small head circumferences, again emphasizing that symmetrically small infants have a worse prognosis than asymmetrically small infants.

## LARGE-FOR-GESTATIONAL-AGE PREGNANCY

Although LGA pregnancy is defined according to the same concept as SGA pregnancy (LGA = heaviest 10% of newborns), LGA pregnancy has received substantially less attention. In fact, although there have been numerous reports about fetal macrosomia (usually defined as birth weight greater than 4500 g), there are no published data about LGA pregnancy as defined above. Therefore, this section will concentrate on fetal macrosomia, with additional comments regarding LGA pregnancies.

### Pathophysiology

Numerous endocrinologic changes occur during pregnancy to ensure an adequate fetal glucose supply. In the second half of pregnancy, increased concentrations of human placental lactogen, free and total cortisol, and prolactin combine to produce modest maternal insulin resistance, which is countered by postprandial hyperinsulinemia. In those who are unable to mount this hyperinsulinemic response, relative hyperglycemia may develop (ie, gestational diabetes). Because glucose crosses the placenta by facilitated diffusion, fetal hyperglycemia ensues. This in turn produces fetal hyperinsulinemia with resultant intracellular transfer of glucose, leading to fetal macrosomia.

Transplacental transfer of nutrients requires the presence of oxygen for anabolism to proceed. Optimal maternal oxygen uptake and transfer and delivery to the placental bed are important prerequisites for fetal macrosomia. In addition, adequate amounts of fetal hemoglobin must be present to deliver oxygen to fetal tissues. If any of these processes are inadequate, the likelihood of optimal fetal growth is diminished.

### Differential Diagnosis

Factors that predispose to LGA pregnancy are listed in Table 16–4. As with SGA pregnancy, diagnosis of LGA pregnancy depends on knowing with certainty the duration of the pregnancy (see Chapter 9).

**A. Maternal Diabetes:** Maternal diabetes, whether it is gestational, chemical, or insulin-dependent, is the condition classically associated with fetal macrosomia. It was long assumed that fetal macrosomia could be accounted for by the "Pedersen hypoth-

---

**Table 16–4.** Factors that may predispose to fetal macrosomia or LGA pregnancy.

**Maternal Factors**
  Diabetes (gestational, chemical, or insulin-dependent), obesity, postdatism, multiparity, advanced age, previous LGA infant, large stature
**Fetal Factors**
  Genetic or congenital disorders, male sex

esis"—ie, that the condition was due to inadequate management of diabetes during pregnancy. Initial reports suggested that careful control of blood glucose in insulin-dependent diabetic women would prevent fetal macrosomia, but recent studies have suggested that the problem is not so simple and that the incidence may correlate better with cord blood concentrations of maternally acquired anti-insulin IgG antibodies, and/or increased serum levels of free fatty acids, triglycerides, and the amino acids alanine, serine, and isoleucine.

**B. Maternal Obesity:** Maternal obesity is associated with a 4- to 12-fold increased likelihood of fetal macrosomia. This may be due in part to associated gestational or chemical diabetes, although these disorders are not present in most obese women who deliver macrosomic babies.

**C. Postdatism:** Prolonged pregnancy is more likely to result in a macrosomic fetus, presumably due to continued delivery of nutrients and oxygen to the fetus. Placental sulfatase deficiency or congenital adrenal hypoplasia should also be considered in the evaluation.

**D. Multiparity:** When controlled for gestational age and fetal gender, the average birth weight with successive pregnancies increases by 80–120 g up to the fifth pregnancy. Multiparity is also associated with other factors (eg, obesity, diabetes). Therefore, although it is not a major factor, multiparity is included as a risk factor for fetal macrosomia.

**E. Advanced Maternal Age:** Progressive maternal age contributes little to increased birth weight. As with multiparity, however, it is a frequent causative marker because of its increased association with diabetes and obesity.

**F. Previous LGA Infant:** Any woman who has delivered one LGA infant is at increased risk for delivering another.

**G. Large Maternal Stature:** Just as small women tend to have small babies, large women tend to have large babies. Birth weight correlates more closely with maternal height than with maternal weight.

**H. Genetic and Congenital Disorders:** Several genetic and congenital syndromes are associated with an increased incidence of LGA fetuses. **Beckwith-Wiedemann syndrome** is frequently associated with fetal macrosomia, usually because of pancreatic islet cell hyperplasia (nesidioblastosis). Affected infants usually have hypoglycemia, macroglossia, and omphalocele. They may also have intestinal malrotation or visceromegaly. Although usually a sporadic event, in a few families other inheritance patterns have been suggested. Other rare syndromes include **Weaver's syndrome, Sotos' syndrome, Nevo syndrome, Ruvalcaba-Myhre syndrome,** and **Marshall's syndrome. Carpenter's syndrome** and the **fragile X syndrome** may also be associated with an increased incidence of LGA infants.

**I. Male Sex:** All series addressing fetal macrosomia report an increased incidence of male fetuses, usually about 60–65%. This is because male fetuses are an average of 150 g heavier than appropriately matched female fetuses at each gestational week during late pregnancy. Appropriately defined birth weight distribution curves should control for gender, making the incidence of LGA infants equal for males and females.

## Complications

As seen in Table 16–2, there are many complications for which the LGA pregnancy is at increased risk. By far the most common indication for cesarean delivery is failure to progress in labor. Fetal distress, as determined by electronic fetal monitoring, is not more common in macrosomic pregnancies. Although not well documented, LGA pregnancy is presumably at increased risk for cesarean section.

Postpartum hemorrhage is more common in macrosomic pregnancies and presumably in LGA pregnancies as well. Both conditions are associated with a distended uterus, inadequate labor progress, and reproductive tract injury. Perineal trauma is more likely with a macrosomic pregnancy and is related to increased incidence of shoulder dystocia and operative vaginal delivery.

Although not solely a maternal complication, shoulder dystocia occurs in 6–23.6% of vaginally delivered macrosomic fetuses (compared with 0.3–1% of nonmacrosomic controls). The incidence of shoulder dystocia correlates not only with progressive fetal weight but also with increasing chest-to-head circumference. Both of these correlations suggest that shoulder dystocia should be more common in LGA pregnancy. Frequent clinical estimations of fetal weight may help to select appropriate candidates for cesarean section delivery without a trial of labor.

Although gestational diabetes and postdatism predispose to fetal macrosomia, there is no evidence that fetal macrosomia or an LGA fetus predisposes to gestational diabetes or postdatism.

The incidence of stillbirth remains higher in macrosomic fetuses than in controls of average weight. This problem has persisted even with the availability of fetal monitoring and presumably reflects the increased incidence of maternal diabetes and postdatism. This increase presumably would be seen in LGA pregnancies as well.

Many of the neonatal complications of fetal macrosomia (and presumably of LGA fetuses) are the result of underlying maternal diabetes or birth trauma and include low Apgar scores, hypoglycemia, hypocalcemia, polycythemia, jaundice, and feeding difficulties.

## Prevention

Prevention of LGA pregnancy presupposes 2 concepts: (1) LGA infants and mothers are at increased risk for complications and (2) LGA pregnancy can be accurately diagnosed. As outlined in Table 16–2, LGA pregnancy is associated with increased risks for complications. Criteria for identification of LGA pregnancy have not been specifically drawn up, although information is available on macrosomic pregnancy. History and physical examination alone can identify 28–53% of fetuses in which the birth weight will be greater than 4500 g. There is a 7–13% incidence of false-positive diagnosis in nonmacrosomic control populations, suggesting that clinical parameters alone are not overly precise. Real-time ultrasound estimation of fetal weight has continued to be fraught with questions of imprecision. Although the sonographic evaluation of the abdominal circumference seems to be the best single predictor of macrosomia, the 10–15% error rate has led some experts to the conclusion that an ultrasound EFW has to be at least 4750 g in order to predict a birth weight of 4000 g with a confidence level of 90%. Ultrasound assessments of EFW are thus better at excluding macrosomia than at confirming it.

Because LGA pregnancies cannot be accurately predicted, prevention has been difficult to achieve. Patients with the risk factors noted in Table 16–4 should be evaluated for possible fetal macrosomia with ultrasound estimates of fetal size and weight at intervals, and the EDC in each case should be confirmed both clinically and with ultrasonography. Caloric restriction during pregnancy may achieve modest decreases in birth weights of infants whose mothers are at risk, but the emphasis in management should be on avoiding excessive intake (defined as > 2400 kcal/d). Appropriate control of blood glucose in pregnant diabetics may also decrease birth weights.

Infants of women who participate in regular aerobic exercise programs have lower average birth weights than the general population, but there are no demonstrable adverse effects. To date, no studies have been done to evaluate the potential efficacy of exercise programs as a means of decreasing birth weight in women at risk for LGA pregnancy.

## Treatment

Although widely recommended, labor induction in at-risk pregnancy has been for reduction in the incidence of fetal macrosomia and/or intrapartum complications remains an unproven hypothesis. Intrapartum treatment considerations center on the increased likelihood of traumatic vaginal delivery. Although precise risk factors are not available for LGA pregnancy, the incidence of traumatic vaginal delivery for macrosomic fetuses is 6–23.6%. Most fetal trauma is the result of shoulder dystocia. Such infants are at risk for intrapartum stillbirth, fractures, and nerve injuries. These infants are more likely to have lower Apgar scores, hypoglycemia, hypocalcemia, polycythemia, jaundice, and feeding difficulties.

They are also at risk for subsequent Erb's palsy, cerebral palsy, mental retardation, and seizures.

Several published reviews of fetal macrosomia suggest routine cesarean delivery for fetuses with estimated weights of 5000 g or more. This is based in part on the data given in Table 16–2 and in part on anthropometric studies, suggesting that very macrosomic fetuses have bisacromial circumferences in excess of head circumferences. Because of current limitations in the sensitivity and specificity of ultrasound-derived fetal weight calculations, decisions regarding scheduled abdominal delivery must be partially based on clinical grounds. Such considerations are particularly warranted in women who are obese or are diabetic or in postdate pregnancies.

Abdominal delivery in cases of fetal macrosomia is performed 2–2.5 times more frequently than in nonmacrosomic controls. Women delivering macrosomic babies are also at increased risk for perineal trauma or postpartum hemorrhage.

Because of these factors, women at risk for macrosomic or LGA babies should deliver in facilities where adequate obstetric care, pediatric care, and anesthesia are present. Large-bore intravenous access must be established, and blood must be available. Delivery should take place in a setting where immediate operation can be accomplished. In many situations, this should occur in a delivery room. If vaginal delivery is contemplated, an adequate episiotomy should be performed.

## Prognosis

Any woman who delivers an LGA baby should be informed that the risk of her having another LGA baby is increased by 2.5- to 4-fold. Such women should be screened for previously undiagnosed chemical or insulin-dependent diabetes and, even if screening is negative, should be followed carefully in any subsequent pregnancy to rule out gestational diabetes. Obese women should be strongly encouraged to lose weight. Any woman who has delivered an LGA infant should also be encouraged to seek early care for any subsequent pregnancy, if for no other reason than early confirmation of the EDC, which can minimize the likelihood of subsequent postdatism. Women who deliver an LGA infant with an underlying genetic or congenital disorder should receive genetic counseling regarding recurrence risks and the feasibility of antepartum diagnosis.

Besides the many neonatal complications previously noted, infants of mothers with gestational or chemical diabetes are at increased risk for subsequent obesity, type II diabetes, or both. Infants who suffer from neonatal complications are at increased risk for subsequent neurologic or behavioral problems.

LGA infants have an increased incidence of subsequent neoplasia when compared with AGA controls. This association is not surprising, since rapidly dividing cells are prerequisites for both processes. The risk for childhood leukemia is directly related to birth weight. Likewise, Wilms' tumor and osteosarcoma are associated with increased birth weight. Other neoplasms seen with increased frequency in LGA syndromes are nephroblastoma, adrenal cortical carcinoma, and hepatoblastoma.

It is interesting that diabetic macrosomia is not associated with an increased incidence of neoplasms, probably because the macrosomia is mediated normally rather than by intrinsic cellular hyperplasia.

## FUTURE DIAGNOSIS OF SGA & LGA PREGNANCIES

Although much more is known about the risks of SGA than of LGA pregnancy, both are known to be associated with increased risks of in utero, intrapartum, neonatal, or long-term compromise. The ability to diagnose and optimally manage these pregnancies remains poor. Further effort must be directed toward precise diagnosis at a point in the pregnancy at which intervention can still be effective.

## REFERENCES

### PATHOGENESIS

Dunsted M, Moar VA, Scott A: Risk factors associated with small-for-dates and large-for-dates infants. Br J Obstet Gynaecol 1985;92:226.

Erskine RLA, Ritchie JWK: Umbilical artery blood flow characteristics in normal and growth-retarded fetuses. Br J Obstet Gynaecol 1985;66:605.

Khoury MJ et al: Congenital malformations and intrauterine growth retardation: A population study. Pediatrics 1988;82:83.

Kramer M: Determinants of low birth weight: Methodological assessment and meta-analysis. Bull WHO 1987;65:663.

Menon RK et al: Transplacental passage of insulin in pregnant women with insulin-dependent diabetes mellitus: Its role in fetal macrosomia. N Engl J Med 1990;323:309.

Snijders RJM et al: Fetal growth retardation: Associated malformations and chromosomal abnormalities. Am J Obstet Gynecol 1993;168:547.

### DIFFERENTIAL DIAGNOSIS

Benacerraff BR et al: Humeral shortening in second-trimester fetuses with Down's syndrome. Obstet Gynecol 1991;77:223.

Chang TC et al: Prediction of the small for gestational age infant: Which ultrasonic measurement is best? Obstet Gynecol 1992;80:1030.

Lang JM et al: Risk factors for small-for-gestational age birth in a preterm population. Am J Obstet Gynecol 1992;166:1374.

Patterson RM, Pouliot MR: Neonatal morphometrics and perinatal outcome: Who is growth retarded? Am J Obstet Gynecol 1987;157:691.

Sabbagha RE et al: Estimation of birthweight by use of ultrasonographic formulas targeted to large-, appropriate-, and small-for-gestational age fetuses. Am J Obstet Gynecol 1989;160:854.

Sandmire HF: Whither ultrasonic prediction of fetal macrosomia? Obstet Gynecol 1993;82:860.

Shepard MJ et al: An evaluation of two equations for predicting fetal weight by ultrasound. Am J Obstet Gynecol 1982;153:57.

Weiner CP et al: A hypothetical model suggesting suboptimal intrauterine growth in infants delivered preterm. Obstet Gynecol 1985;65:323.

Weiner CP, Williamson RA: Evaluation of severe growth retardation using cordocentesis: Hematologic and metabolic alterations by etiology. Obstet Gynecol 1989;73:225.

### COMPLICATIONS

American College of Obstetricians and Gynecologists: Technical Bulletin 159, Fetal macrosomia, Washington, DC, 1991.

Chiswick ML: Intrauterine growth retardation. Br Med J 1985;291:845.

Lockwood CJ, Weiner S: Assessment of fetal growth. Clin Perinatol 1986;13:3.

Spellacy WN et al: Macrosomia: Maternal characteristics and infant complications. Obstet Gynecol 1985;66:158.

### PREVENTION

Backe B, Nalking J: Effectiveness of antenatal care: A population based study. Br J Obstet Gynaecol 1993;100:722.

Castro LC et al: Maternal tobacco use and substance abuse; reported prevalence rates and associations with the delivery of small for gestational age neonates. Obstet Gynecol 1993;81:396.

Chamberlain G: Small for gestational age. BMJ 1991;302:1592.

### TREATMENT

Almstrom H et al: Comparison of umbilical artery velocimetry and cardiotocography for surveillance of small for gestational age fetuses. Lancet 1992;340:936.

Combs CA et al: Elective induction versus spontaneous

labor after sonographic diagnosis of fetal macrosomia. Obstet Gynecol 1993;81:492.

Launer LJ et al: The effect of maternal work on fetal growth and duration of pregnancy: A prospective study. Br J Obstet Gynaecol 1990;97:62.

## PROGNOSIS

Barker DJP: Fetal growth and adult disease. Br J Obstet Gynaecol 1992;99:275.

Lin CC et al: Comparison of associated high-risk factors and perinatal outcome between symmetric and asymmetric fetal intrauterine growth retardation. Am J Obstet Gynecol 1991;164:1535.

McCormick MC et al: The health and developmental status of very low-birth-weight children at school age. JAMA 1992;267:2204.

Sacks DA: Fetal macrosomia and gestational diabetes: What's the problem? Obstet Gynecol 1993;81:775.

# Multiple Pregnancy

# 17

*Martin L. Pernoll, MD, & Ralph C. Benson, MD*

## Essentials of Diagnosis

- Demonstration of 2 or more fetuses (eg, ultrasonography, fetal heartbeats, multiplicity of fetal parts).
- Disproportionately large uterus for dates.
- Increased fetal activity.
- Greater-than-expected maternal weight gain.
- Maternal hypochromic normocytic anemia.

Monozygotic twins ("identical twins") are the result of the division of a single fertilized ovum. Monozygotic twinning occurs in about 2.3–4 of 1000 pregnancies in all races. The rate is remarkably constant and is not influenced by heredity, age of the mother, or other factors. Dizygotic twins ("fraternal twins") are produced from separately fertilized ova. Slightly more than 30% of twins are monozygotic; nearly 70% are dizygotic. Although monozygotism is random—ie, it does not fit any discernible genetic pattern—dizygotism has hereditary determinants.

In North America, dizygotic twinning occurs about once in 83 conceptions and triplets about once in 8000 conceptions. A traditional approximation of the incidence of multiple pregnancies is as follows:

| | |
|---|---|
| **Twins** | **1:80** |
| **Triplets** | $1:80^2 = 1:6400$ |
| **Quadruplets** | $1:80^3 = 1:512,000$ |
| **(Etc)** | |

However, in a recent study (Keith, 1988) the incidence of triplets was found to be 0.37 in 1000 live births. In about two-thirds of the pregnancies, fertility-inducing agents had been used. These and other data strongly suggest that medical intervention is enhancing multiple gestation. The relative number of females increase considerably as the number of fetuses increases in multiple births.

Maternal morbidity and mortality rates are much higher in multiple pregnancy than in singleton pregnancy due to preterm labor, hemorrhage, urinary tract infection, and pregnancy-induced hypertension. Approximately two-thirds of multiple pregnancies end in a single birth; the other embryo is lost with bleeding, is absorbed within the first 10 weeks of pregnancy, or becomes mummified (fetus papyraceous). Moreover, the perinatal mortality rate of twins is 3–4 times higher—and for triplets much higher still—than in the case of singletons as a result of chromosomal abnormalities, prematurity, anomalies, hypoxia, and trauma. This is particularly true of monozygotic twins.

## Pathogenesis

**A. Monozygotic Multiple Gestation:** Monozygotic twins, resulting from the fertilization of a single ovum by a single sperm, are always of the same sex. However, the twins may develop differently depending on the time of preimplantation division. Normally, monozygotic twins have the same physical characteristics (skin, hair, eye color, body build) and the same genetic features (blood characteristics: ABO, M, N, haptoglobin, serum group; histocompatible genes; skin grafting possible), and they are often mirror images of one another (one left-handed, the other right-handed, etc). However, their fingerprints differ.

The paradox of "identical" twins is that they may be the antithesis of identical. The very earliest splits are sometimes accompanied by a simultaneous chromosomal error, resulting in heterokaryotypic monozygotes, one with Down's syndrome and the other normal.

Monozygotic triplets result from repeated twinning (also called supertwinning) of a single ovum. Trizygotic triplets develop by individual fertilization of 3 simultaneously expelled ova. Triplets may also be produced by the twinning of 2 ova and the elimination of 1 of the 4 resulting embryos. Quadruplets, similarly, may be monozygotic, paired dizygotic, or quadrizygotic; ie, they may arise from 1 to 4 ova.

**B. Dizygotic Multiple Gestation:** Dizygotic twins are the product of 2 ova and 2 sperms. The 2 ova are released from separate follicles (or, very rarely, from the same follicle) at approximately the same time. Dizygotic (fraternal) twins may be of the same or different sexes. They bear only the resemblance of brothers or sisters and may or may not have the same blood type. Significant differences usually can be identified after a time.

About 75% of dizygotic twins are the same sex. Both twins are males in about 45% of cases (a lesser preponderance of males in twins than in singletons) and both females in about 30%.

Many factors influence dizygotic twinning. Race is a factor, with multiple pregnancy most common in blacks, least common in Asians, and of intermediate occurrence in whites. The incidence of dizygotic twinning varies from 1.3 in 1000 in Japan to 49 in 1000 in western Nigeria. The rate in the USA is about 12 in 1000.

Dizygotic multiple pregnancy tends to be recurrent. Women who have borne dizygotic twins have a 10-fold increased chance of subsequent multiple pregnancy. Dizygotic twinning probably is inherited as an autosomal recessive trait via the female descendants of mothers of twins; the father's genetic contribution plays little or no part. White women who are dizygotic twins or who are siblings of dizygotic twin mothers have a higher twinning rate among their offspring than women from the general population.

Parity does not influence the incidence of dizygotic twinning, but aging does, with the rate of dizygotic twinning peaking between 35 and 40 years of age and then declining sharply. In women who are twins or daughters of twins, the twinning rate peaks at about age 35, at which time it plateaus until almost age 45 and then declines. Black women, whether or not they are twins or siblings of twins, have a prolonged period of dizygotic twinning from 35 to 45 years of age.

Height and weight have a positive influence on twinning, but the rate does not vary among social classes. Blood groups O and A are more prevalent in white mothers of twins than in the general population, for unknown reasons. Dizygotic twins are more common among unwed than among wed mothers of the same age.

High fertility (polyovulation) is associated with multiple pregnancy. Excessive production of pituitary gonadotropins, relatively high frequency of coitus, and inability of one graafian follicle to inhibit others have been postulated as reasons for a higher incidence of dizygotic twinning. Undernutrition appears to be a reductive factor. Women who conceive late in an ovulatory cycle have a greater chance of multiple pregnancy, perhaps owing to ovular "overripeness."

Dizygotic twinning is more common among women who become pregnant soon after cessation of long-term oral contraception. This may be a reflection of high "rebound" gonadotropin secretion. Induction of ovulation with human pituitary gonadotropin in previously infertile patients has resulted in many multiple pregnancies—even the gestation of septuplets and octuplets. The estrogen analog clomiphene citrate (Clomid) increases the occurrence rate of dizygotic pregnancy to about 5–10%.

**C. Other Forms of Multiple Gestation:** Other kinds of twinning are theoretically possible in humans. Dispermic mosaicism may result from fertilization of 2 ova that have not been independently released but have instead developed from the same oocyte. Another possibility is the fertilization of 1 ovum by 2 sperms. Twinning of discordant twins may be explained by meiotic abnormalities, including polar body twinning, delayed implantation of the embryo, retarded or arrested intrauterine development, or superfetation.

Superfecundation is the fertilization of 2 ova, released at about the same time, by sperm released at intercourse on 2 different occasions. The rare cases in which the fetuses are of disparate size or skin color and have blood groups corresponding to those of the mother's 2 male partners lend credence to (but do not conclusively validate) this possibility.

Superfetation is the fertilization of 2 ova released in different menstrual cycles. This is virtually impossible in humans, because the initial corpus luteum of pregnancy would have to be suppressed to allow for a second ovulation about 1 month later.

## Pathologic Factors Associated with Twinning

Although the blood volume is increased in multiple pregnancy, maternal anemia often develops because of greater demand for iron by the fetuses. However, prior anemia, poor diet, and malabsorption may precede or compound iron deficiency during multiple pregnancy. Respiratory tidal volume is increased, but the woman pregnant with twins often is "breathless" (possibly due to increased levels of progesterone).

Marked uterine distention and increased pressure on the adjacent viscera and pelvic vasculature are typical of multiple pregnancy. Lutein cysts and even ascites are the result of abnormally high levels of chorionic gonadotropin in occasional multiple pregnancies. Placenta previa develops more frequently because of the large size of the placenta or placentae.

The maternal cardiovascular, respiratory, gastrointestinal, renal, and musculoskeletal systems are especially subject to stress in multiple pregnancy, combined with greater maternal-fetal nutritional requirements. Multiple pregnancy is classified as high-risk because of the increased incidence of maternal anemia, urinary tract infection, preeclampsia-eclampsia, hemorrhage (before, during, and after delivery), and uterine inertia.

**Placental and Cord:** The placenta and membranes of monozygotic twins may vary considerably (Fig 17–1), depending on the time of initial division of the embryonic disk. Variations are noted below.

1. Division prior to the morula stage and differentiation of the trophoblast (fifth day) results in separate or fused placentas, 2 chorions, and 2 amnions. (This process grossly resembles dizygotic twinning and ac-

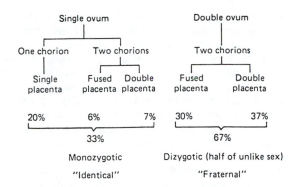

**Figure 17–1.** Placental variations in twinning. (After Potter. Reproduced, with permission, from Benson RC: *Handbook of Obstetrics & Gynecology.* 8th ed. Lange, 1983.)

counts for almost one-third of monozygotic twinning.)

2. Division after differentiation of the trophoblast but before the formation of the amnion (fifth to tenth days) yields a single placenta, a common chorion, and 2 amnions. (This accounts for about two-thirds of monozygotic twinning.)

3. Division after differentiation of the amnion (10th–14th days) results in a single placenta, 1 (common) chorion, and 1 (common) amnion. This is rare.

4. Division later than day 14 may result in incomplete twinning. Just prior to that time (day 8–14), division may result in conjoined twins.

At delivery, the membranous "T" septum or dividing membrane of the placenta between the twins must be inspected and sectioned for evidence of the probable type of twinning (Fig 17–2). Monozygotic twins most commonly have a transparent (thin) septum made up of 2 amniotic membranes only (no chorion

and no decidua). Dizygotic twins almost always have an opaque (thick) septum made up of 2 chorions, 2 amnions, and intervening decidua.

A monochorionic placenta can be identified by stripping away the amnion or amnions to reveal a single chorion over a common placenta. In virtually every case of monochorionic placenta, vascular communications between the 2 parts of the placenta can be identified by careful dissection or injection. In contrast, dichorionic placentas (of dizygotic twinning) only rarely have an anastomosis between the fetal blood vessels.

Placental and membrane examination is a certain indicator of zygosity in twins with monochorionic placentas because these are always monozygotic. Overall, approximately 1% of twins are monoamniotic and these too are monozygotic. Placental forms (single, fused, or double) do not aid in determining zygosity in individual twin pairs, because any of these forms may be found in mono- or dizygotic twins.

A single (monochorionic) placenta probably is less competent than a fused (dichorionic) placenta; as a consequence, more disease processes are noted, often as a result of placental vascular problems, in connection with the former than with the latter. Inequities of the placental circulation in one area (marginal insertion, partial infarction or thinning) may deprive or destroy one fetus while the other thrives.

The most serious problem with monochorionic placentas is local shunting of blood—also called **twin-to-twin transfusion syndrome.** This occurs because of vascular anastomoses to each twin, established early in embryonic life, probably by random growth. The possible communications are artery to artery, vein to vein, and combinations of these. Artery-to-vein communication is by far the most serious; it is most likely to cause twin-to-twin transfusion. In uncompensated cases, the twins, although genetically identical, differ greatly in size and appearance. The

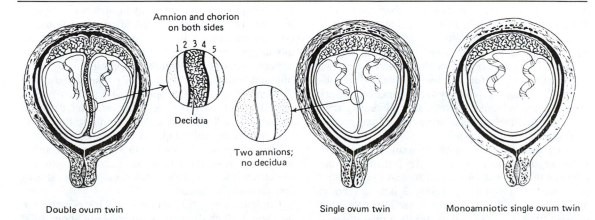

**Figure 17–2.** Amniotic membranes of twins. (Reproduced, with permission, from Benson RC: *Handbook of Obstetrics & Gynecology.* 8th ed. Lange, 1983.)

recipient twin is plethoric, edematous, and hypertensive. Ascites and kernicterus are likely. The heart, liver, and kidneys are enlarged (glomerulotubal hypertrophy). Hydramnios follows fetal polyuria. Although ruddy and apparently healthy, the recipient twin with hypervolemia may die of heart failure during the first 24 hours after birth. The donor twin is small, pallid, and dehydrated (growth retardation, malnutrition, hypovolemia). Oligohydramnios may be present. Severe anemia, due to chronic blood loss to the other twin, may lead to hydrops and heart failure.

Both twins are threatened by prolapse of the cord. The second twin may be harmed by premature separation of the placenta, hypoxia, constriction ring dystocia, operative manipulation, or prolonged anesthesia.

Velamentous insertion of the cord occurs in about 7% of twins but in only 1% of singletons. The incidence of 2-vessel cord (single umbilical artery) is 4–5 times higher in monozygotic twins than in singletons and carries the same correlation to other congenital anomalies (~17%). Whether this is due to primary aplasia or is the result of secondary atrophy is not known.

Monochorionic, monoamniotic twins (1:100 sets of twins) have less than a 50% likelihood of both surviving because of cord entanglement compromising fetal-placental blood flow. The only treatment is prompt rescue (cesarean delivery) if there is sufficient fetal maturity.

**Fetal:** Earlier and more precise sonography has revealed the incidence of multiple gestation to be 3.29–5.39% before 12 weeks (Landy, 1986). However, in over 20% of such cases one or more of the pregnancies spontaneously disappears. Although this event may be associated with vaginal bleeding, the prognosis remains good for the remaining twin. This loss has been termed the "vanishing twin."

The incidence of serious congenital anomalies is about 3 times greater in multiple than in single pregnancies. Moreover, the risk of abnormalities is greater in monozygotic than in dizygotic multiple gestations. In a collaborative project, 18% of twins had malformations (15% single and 3% multiple). Abnormalities were higher in black than white twins. Twins had more malformations of the central nervous system, musculoskeletal system, ears, respiratory system, cardiovascular system, and alimentary tract but fewer malformations of the genitourinary system and skin than singletons.

Conjoined or Siamese twins result from incomplete segmentation of a single fertilized ovum between the 8th and 14th days; if cleavage is further postponed, incomplete twinning (2 heads, 1 body) may occur. Lesser abnormalities are also noted, but these occur without regard to specific organ systems. Conjoined twins are described by site of union: pygopagus (at the sacrum—the most common conjunction); thoracopagus (at the chest); craniopagus (at the heads); and omphalopagus (at the abdominal wall). Curiously, conjoined twins usually are female. Numerous conjoined twins have survived separation.

Each twin and its placenta generally weigh less than the newborn and placenta of a singleton pregnancy after the 30th week, but near term the aggregate weight may approach twice that of a singleton. Normal twins that differ considerably in birth weight commonly have diamniotic-dichorionic placentas. This suggests independent intrauterine growth of cotwins. The converse is true of twins with fused diamniotic-dichorionic placentas. Low-birth weight monochorionic twins are the rule rather than the exception. Low birth weight in the various types of multiple pregnancy probably is evidence of growth restriction due to inadequate nutrition. This is at least partially responsible for the much higher early neonatal mortality rate of newborns from multiple births.

Monozygotic twins are smaller and succumb more often in utero than dizygotic twins. Restriction, competition for nutrition, cord compression and entanglement, prematurity, and operative delivery are responsible for a significant part of the perinatal mortality rate in multiple pregnancy.

In growth-retarded human fetuses, the brain and heart seem to be relatively less affected than the liver or peripheral musculature. Because the limits of placental growth and function are finite, hormone alterations may develop to trigger early labor. Moreover, restricted (or retarded) fetal growth has a small but lasting effect on postnatal physical and possibly mental development.

In late pregnancy, the fetus is jeopardized by the frequency of premature delivery, abnormal presentation and position, and hydramnios.

A fetus acardiacus is a parasitic monozygotic fetus without a heart. In addition to failure of the heart to develop, the growth and development of the entire body of the fetus acardiacus is distorted and rudimentary. Inexplicably, the cord may be attached to almost any part of the maldeveloped, diminutive fetus. In contrast, the other twin may appear to be normal, usually larger than average.

Fetus papyraceous (fetus compresses) is a small, blighted, mummified fetus usually discovered at the delivery of a well-developed newborn. This occurs once in 17,000–20,000 pregnancies. The cause is thought to be death of one twin, amniotic fluid loss, or reabsorption and compression of the dead fetus by the surviving twin. When one twin dies and becomes macerated, it is likely to come second, because the uterus tends to accept the smaller, more or less shapeless form in the fundus.

Collision, impaction, and interlocking of twins are accidental. Such dystocia occurs once in about 1000 twin pregnancies—usually early in the birth order, when the uterine tone is good.

## Clinical Findings

The antepartum diagnosis of multiple pregnancy is made in about 75% of cases, and often late—which is regrettable because untimely early delivery contributes to fetal jeopardy. Much can be done for the mother and the offspring if treatment is given early.

**A. Symptoms and Signs:** All of the common annoyances of pregnancy are more troublesome in multiple pregnancy. The effects of multiple pregnancy on the patient include earlier and more severe pressure in the pelvis, nausea, backache, varicosities, constipation, hemorrhoids, abdominal distention, and difficulty in breathing. A "large pregnancy" may be indicative of twinning (distended uterus). Fetal activity is greater and more persistent in twinning than in singleton pregnancy. The median weight of twins at birth is just over 2270 g in the USA. Male infants weigh slightly more than females.

Considering the possibility of multiple pregnancy is essential to early diagnosis. If one assumes that all pregnancies are multiple ones until proved otherwise, physical examination alone will identify most cases of twinning before the second trimester. Indeed, diagnosis of twinning is possible in over 75% of cases by physical examination. The following signs should alert the physician to the possibility or definite presence of multiple pregnancy:

1. Uterus larger than expected (> 4 cm) for dates.

2. Excessive maternal weight gain that is not explained by edema or obesity.

3. Polyhydramnios, manifested by uterine size out of proportion to the calculated duration of gestation, is almost 10 times more common in multiple pregnancy.

4. Outline or ballottement of more than one fetus.

5. Multiplicity of small parts.

6. Uterus containing 3 or more large parts.

7. Simultaneous recording of different fetal heart rates, each asynchronous with the mother's pulse and with each other and varying by at least 8 beats per minute. (The fetal heart rate may be accelerated by pressure or displacement.)

8. Palpation of one or more fetuses in the fundus after delivery of one infant.

Some of the common complications in early pregnancy may also occur as a result of multiple gestation. For example, maternal bleeding in the first trimester can indicate threatened or spontaneous abortion; however, the dead fetus may be one of twins, as demonstrated by real-time ultrasonography (one anechoic or hypoechoic amniotic sac and one normal sac). In the second and third trimester, a demise of one in a multiple gestation may trigger disseminated intravascular coagulation ("dead fetus syndrome"), just as may a singleton intrauterine demise. This generally becomes a problem only 3 weeks or more after fetal demise. Preeclampsia-eclampsia is a common complication of plural pregnancy.

**B. Laboratory Findings:** The majority of multiple pregnancies are currently identified by ultrasonic scanning. Indeed, identification of multiple gestation is so important for the institution of special care (to prevent prematurity) that many authorities recommend routine ultrasonic scanning at 18–20 weeks.

The hematocrit and hemoglobin values and the red cell count usually are considerably reduced, in direct relationship to the enhanced blood volume. Indeed, maternal hypochromic normocytic anemia occurs so frequently in multiple pregnancy that it has been suggested that all patients with the process be suspected of having a multiple gestation. Fetal demand for iron increases beyond the mother's ability to assimilate iron in the second trimester.

Glucose tolerance tests demonstrate that both gestational diabetes mellitus and gestational hypoglycemia are much higher in multiple gestation compared with findings in singleton pregnancy. Because perinatal death is more common in multiple pregnancy complicated by gestational (and chemical) diabetes, glucose tolerance tests should be obtained in plural pregnancy.

In multiple pregnancy, the urinary chorionic gonadotropin, estriol, and pregnanediol levels are elevated. In addition, mean serum values for cystine and leucine aminopeptidase, oxytocinase, and alkaline phosphate are elevated above those of singleton pregnancy. However, none of the previously noted determinations are augmented with sufficient uniqueness to be diagnostic of plural pregnancy. Radioimmunoassay for placental lactogen (hPL) has been suggested as a screening method, but is not widely applied (a single hPL value significantly >3 µg/mL <25 weeks' gestation, > 4 µg/mL at 25–30 weeks' gestation, or > 8 µg/mL after the 30th week) because of significant variability. Thus, the hPL assay cannot substitute for ultrasonic assessment in assessment for multiple gestation.

In twin pregnancies not accompanied by neural tube defects, the maternal serum alpha-fetoprotein (MSAFP) level will average twice the median level for singleton pregnancies, from 3–6 months of gestation. With open neural tube defects in either fetus, the MSAFP level will be significantly higher.

**C. Ultrasonography and X-Ray Findings:** Ultrasonography is the preferred imaging modality for diagnosis of multiple gestation, potentially being able to differentiate multiple gestation as early as 4 weeks (by intravaginal probe). Ultrasound examination generally reveals the presence of a septum between the fetuses and is invaluable in following growth.

Both twins present as vertex in almost 50% of cases. Twin A will be vertex and twin B a breech in slightly more than 33% of cases (Fig 17–3). Both fetuses will be breech presentations in 10% of cases, and almost that many will be single (or double) transverse presentations. Approximately 70% of first twins present by the vertex. Breech presentation oc-

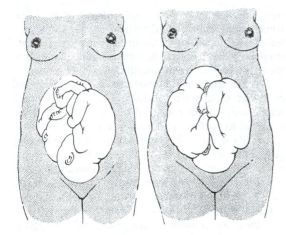

**Figure 17–3. *Left:*** Both twins presenting by the vertex. ***Right:*** One vertex and one breech presentation. (Reproduced, with permission, from Benson RC: *Handbook of Obstetrics & Gynecology.* 8th ed. Lange, 1983.)

curs in slightly more than 25%. Overall, nonvertex presentation occurs 10 times more often in multiple pregnancy than in singleton pregnancy.

## Differential Diagnosis

Multiple pregnancy must be distinguished from the following conditions:

**A. Singleton Pregnancy:** Inaccurate dates may give a false impression of the duration of the pregnancy, and the fetus may be larger than expected. However, only one fetus can be palpated and one fetal heart heard.

**B. Polyhydramnios:** Either single or multiple pregnancy may be associated with excessive accumulation of fluid. Careful examination may distinguish one or more fetuses. Use ultrasonography if the number and normality of the fetuses are still undetermined in the last trimester.

**C. Hydatidiform Mole:** Although usually easily distinguished from multiple gestation, this complication must be considered in diagnosis early in pregnancy.

**D. Abdominal Tumors Complicating Pregnancy:** Fibroid tumors of the uterus, when present in great numbers, are readily identified. Ovarian tumors are generally single, discrete, and harder to diagnose. A distended bladder or full rectum may elevate the pregnant uterus.

**E. Complicated Twin Pregnancy:** If one dizygotic twin dies early in pregnancy and the other lives, the dead fetus may become flattened and mummified (fetus papyraceous, see section on fetal pathologic factors). Its portion of a fused placenta will be pale and atrophic, but remnants of 2 sacs and 2 cords may be found. If one twin dies in late pregnancy, considerable enlargement of the uterus persists, although the

findings on palpation may be unusual and only one fetal heart will be heard. Ultrasonography generally assists in the diagnosis. The living fetus generally presents first.

## Prevention

**A. Multiple Pregnancy:** Although human pituitary gonadotropin and other ovulation induction agents result in fewer multiple pregnancies when used by experts, even in the best of hands it is inevitable that some multiple pregnancies will occur. For example, clomiphene citrate induction of multiple ovulation increases the rate of dizygotic pregnancy to 5–10%.

With many forms of assisted reproductive technology (eg, ovulation induction, in vitro fertilization), iatrogenic multiple pregnancies occur with regularity in which the number of fetuses is so great that they may preclude any being carried to the point of viability. When this occurs, many authorities recommend multifetal pregnancy reduction by transabdominal intracardiac potassium injection.

**B. Complications of Multiple Pregnancy:** To prevent the complications of multiple pregnancy, it is imperative to accomplish diagnosis as early in pregnancy as possible. Fortunately, ultrasonography can be safely used at any time during pregnancy, is highly accurate, and may be used as early as the fourth week. Later in pregnancy, ultrasonography is useful to monitor the growth status of the fetuses and to detect gross anomalies. Recall that the risk of fetal abnormality in twins is approximately 3 times that in singleton pregnancy.

There is little question that enhancing antenatal care assists in improving outcome. The most commonly used techniques are iron supplementation, vitamin and folic acid administration (an attempt to avoid anemia), a high-protein diet, more weight gain than usual (ideal weight for height and build plus about 11–13 kg), less physical exercise, and more bed rest (eg, frequent rest periods after the 24th week).In addition, more frequent antenatal visits are scheduled and several authorities recommend closely following cervical dilatation to determine whether home uterine activity monitoring (HUAM) may be necessary. Early and prompt therapy for any complications (eg, vaginal infections, preeclampsia-eclampsia) is instituted.

Whether cervical cerclage will prevent early birth in multiple pregnancy is uncertain, but tocolytic drugs may suppress premature labor and extended gestation. Treat threatened premature labor (<35–36 weeks) in the absence of complications (eg, ruptured membranes or bleeding) with first-line tocolytics. Most authorities recommend starting with intravenous magnesium sulfate. If ritodrine or a comparable beta-mimetic drug is used, very close monitoring for pulmonary edema must be accomplished, because this complication is greatly enhanced by administration of these agents in multiple gestation. Also, recall that indomethacin may influence fetal ductal constriction.

In cases of antepartum bleeding or hydramnios, try to delay the delivery until twins weigh at least 2500 g each. Increased rest periods during the second trimester may prevent premature labor.

All patients with multiple pregnancy should be delivered in a well-equipped hospital by an experienced physician who has adequate assistance. It is desirable to have a pediatrician (or neonatologist) in attendance. Generally, it is desirable to use minimal analgesia for labor (psychoprophylaxis or epidural). For delivery keep analgesia and general anesthesia to a minimum, using local anesthesia for delivery. Immaturity, trauma of manipulative delivery, and associated asphyxia are the major preventable causes of morbidity and mortality in twins, especially the second twin.

## Treatment

**Labor and Delivery:** Admit the patient to the hospital at the first sign of labor, if there is leakage of amniotic fluid, or if significant bleeding occurs. Use electronic fetal monitoring for each twin to facilitate detection of fetal compromise. Labor should be conducted so that immediate cesarean section can be performed if required. A physician-nurse team for each infant plus obstetric and anesthesiologic attendants should be present.

Type and match blood; have 2 units available for transfusion. Establish an intravenous line with a large-bore needle (> 18 gauge), and start a normal saline drip for hydration to permit drug administration or transfusion.

Limit analgesia during labor. Regional anesthesia is preferred, but meperidine in small doses may be used because the depressive effects can be negated (if necessary) by a narcotic antagonist. A reasonable choice also is pudendal block, which allows excellent patient cooperation. If primary cesarean section is indicated, epidural or spinal block may be chosen. However, if emergency cesarean section is required, rapid-induction general anesthesia may be necessary.

If either twin shows signs of persistent compromise, proceed promptly to cesarean section delivery. Other indications for primary cesarean section include (but are not limited to) both twins weighing less than 2000 g, compound or monoamniotic twins (diagnosed by ultrasonography or amniography), and probable twin-twin transfusion syndrome (gross disparity in fetal size). Nearly all (> 85%) triplets warrant cesarean section delivery.

In a woman with a previous lower-segment caesarean scar, delivery of twins does not mandate a repeat caesarean section in the absence of other complications. Management of twins that are candidates for vaginal delivery may proceed as outlined below. Intrapartum twin presentations may be classified as follows: (1) twin A and twin B vertex (slightly > 40% of all twins); (2) twin A vertex and twin B nonvertex (almost 40%); (3) twin A nonvertex and twins B vertex, breech, or transverse (about 20%).

The current treatment of twins is epitomized by Figure 17–4. For vertex-vertex presentations in labor (category 1, above), vaginal delivery of both twins may be chosen in the absence of standard indications for cesarean section delivery. Of course, if either twin develops fetal distress, cesarean section delivery should be performed.

Category 2 twins both weighing more than 2000 g usually can be managed successfully by vaginal delivery of both. This is generally accomplished by external version of twin B immediately after the delivery of twin A or by elective vaginal breech delivery. If twin B weighs less than 2000 g and external version is unsuccessful, cesarean section for this infant is warranted (as opposed to breech vaginal birth). When either twin A or both twins are nonvertex (category 3), primary cesarean section should be performed.

Vaginal delivery is facilitated by making a deep episiotomy incision just prior to vaginal delivery of twin A. Difficult forceps operation or rapid extraction should be avoided, but forceps to protect the premature head may be useful. The umbilical cord should be clamped promptly to prevent the second twin of a monozygotic twin pregnancy from exsanguinating into the firstborn.

Perform a vaginal examination immediately after delivery of twin A to note the presentation of the second twin, the presence of a second sac, an occult cord prolapse, or cord entanglement.

Cut the cord as far outside the vagina as possible so that it can hang loose to permit vaginal examination or manipulation. This eliminates inadvertent cord traction on the placenta. Tag and label the cords (twin A and B) so that they may be associated with the proper placenta or placentas.

Use external version whenever possible for conversion of twin B from breech to vertex, but try to accomplish delivery of twin B expeditiously. Do not neglect appropriate fetal heart rate monitoring of twin B after delivery of twin A. The well-being of the second twin can be assured and delivery need not be rushed unless ominous signs develop. Cautious rupture of the second sac will allow slow loss of fluid while twin B's vertex is being gently guided into the inlet.

One twin may obstruct the delivery of both fetuses in locked twins. In this circumstance twin A is always a breech and twin B a vertex presentation. The heads become impacted in the pelvis. Locked twins can be avoided by cesarean delivery in all cases in which twin A is not vertex. However, if the obstetrician is presented with a case of locked twins (Fig 17–5), having an assistant support the twin already partially delivered as a breech while pushing both heads upward out of the pelvis with rotation of both fetuses may accomplish delivery of the first. This may require deep

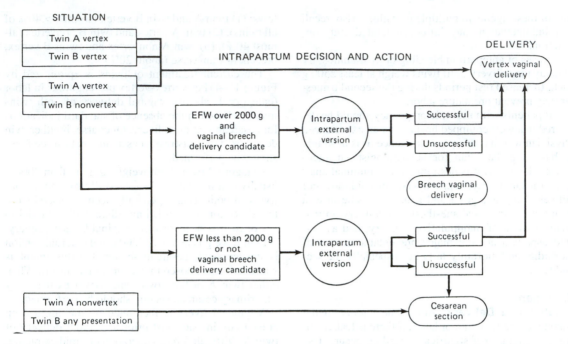

SITUATION

INTRAPARTUM DECISION AND ACTION

DELIVERY

**Figure 17–4.** Management of twin gestation, intrapartum protocol. (Modified and reproduced, with permission of the American College of Obstetricians and Gynecologists, from Chervenak FA et al: Intrapartum management of twin gestation. Obstet Gynecol 1985;65:120.)

anesthesia. If this cannot be done, cesarean with abdominal delivery of both fetuses may be the safest route. An alternative while cesarean preparations are underway is to elevate the partially delivered twin, establish an airway, and protect the cord.

Postpartum hemorrhage is common in multiple pregnancy. Increased intravenous oxytocin, elevation, and light massage of the fundus and an intravenous ergot or prostaglandin product (only after the last fetus is delivered) may be required.

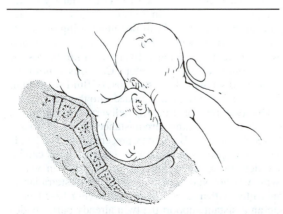

**Figure 17–5.** Locked twins. (Reproduced, with permission, from Benson RC: *Handbook of Obstetrics & Gynecology,* 4th ed. Lange, 1971.)

After delivery, if separation of the placenta is delayed or bleeding is brisk, extraction of the placenta manually may be necessary. Send the placenta, cord, and membranes to the pathology laboratory to assist in determining whether the fetuses are mono- or dizygotic after making the observations just noted.

Preeclampsia-eclampsia, premature labor and delivery, etc, are managed as outlined elsewhere in this book. If dystocia occurs, obtain x-ray films to rule out malpresentation or conjoined twins. Explore the cervical canal and the lower uterine segment vaginally for soft tissue dystocia.

## Complications

**A. Maternal:** The incidence of spontaneous abortion of at least one of several fetuses is increased in plural pregnancy. Stillbirth occurs twice as often among twins as among singleton pregnancies. Premature labor and delivery as well as premature rupture of the membranes are also greatly increased. Indeed, without aggressive preventive measures, three-fourths of all multiple pregnancies result in delivery at least 3 weeks before the estimated date of confinement.

Placenta previa may be responsible for antepartum bleeding, malpresentation, or unengagement of the first fetus. A large placenta (or placentas) and possibly, fundal scarring or tumor may lead to low implantation of the placenta. Premature separation of the placenta may occur antepartum, perhaps in association with preeclampsia-eclampsia or with rupture of the first bag of waters and the initiation of strong uterine contractions, or after the delivery of the first twin. Careless traction on the first cord may encourage early partial separation of the placenta.

Hypochromic normocytic anemia is 2–3 times more common in multiple pregnancy than in singleton pregnancy. Urinary tract infection is at least twice as frequent in multiple pregnancy as in single-fetus pregnancy due to increased ureteral dilatation secondary to higher serum progesterone and uterine pressure on the ureters. Preeclampsia-eclampsia occurs about 3 times more often in multiple pregnancy than in a singleton pregnancy.

A thinned uterine wall, secondary to unusually large uterine contents, is associated with hypotonic uterine contractions and a longer latent stage of labor. However, prolonged labor is uncommon in multiple pregnancy because rupture of the membranes generally is followed by improvements in the uterine contraction pattern. Uterine atony often is accompanied by excessive loss of blood postpartum owing to inability of the overdistended uterus to contract well and remain contracted after delivery.

If the amniotic sac of the second twin ruptures before that of the first and if the cord prolapses, cesarean section usually is indicated.

When there are 2 separate placentas, one of them may deliver immediately after the first twin. Although the second twin may not be compromised, it is best to proceed with its delivery, both for its protection and to conserve maternal blood.

Operative intervention is more likely in multiple pregnancy because of increased obstetric problems such as malpresentation, prolapsed cord, and fetal distress.

**B. Fetal:** Fetal death is about 3 times more common in multiple pregnancy than in singleton pregnancy. Death may be due to developmental anomalies, cord compression, or placental disorders. The greatest hazard from cord compression is cord entanglement of monozygotic twins with only one amniotic sac. Developmental anomalies and polyhydramnios are common in monozygotic twins.

Almost twice as many monozygotic as dizygotic twins die in the perinatal period. Attrition is even greater for triplets, quadruplets, etc. Even so, preterm delivery and intrapartum complications are the most common causes of fetal loss in multiple pregnancy. All too frequently preterm delivery is occasioned by premature rupture of the membranes, which occurs in about 25% of twin, 50% of triplet, and 75% of quadruplet pregnancies.

Abnormal and breech presentation, circulatory interference by one fetus with the other, and operative delivery all increase fetal loss. Prolapse of the cord occurs 5 times more often in multiple than in singleton pregnancy. Premature separation of the placenta

before delivery of the second twin may cause death of the second twin by hypoxia. Conjoined twins may be undetected before labor. Dystocia often occurs, and the twins may die during attempts at vaginal delivery.

Regardless of the cause, delivery before 33 weeks' gestational age (< 2000 g) is extremely hazardous for the newborns. Such premature infants account for more than 75% of the neonatal deaths in multiple pregnancies. The mortality rates for infants weighing less than 2000 g are approximately the same in twins and singletons: < 30%. Although the complications in multiple gestations are much greater, the slowing of fetal growth in the last trimester gives twin fetuses the advantage of increased maturity for weight. If delivery is delayed in cases of multiple birth until the fetuses achieve a weight of even 2000–2250 g, the overall mortality rate would be reduced at least 8-fold. Perhaps as important, the chance of residual damage in survivors would be decreased. Finally, the cost of intensive care would be greatly diminished.

It is urgent for an experienced physician to be present for resuscitation and stabilization of each infant born at high risk. Unfortunately, most multiple-birth newborns who were delivered before the 34th week and were referred to a neonatal center for care were undiagnosed before birth. Delivery before the 36th week is twice as frequent in twin pregnancies as in singleton pregnancies. Intracranial injury is more common in premature infants—even those delivered spontaneously—and often leads to death in the neonatal period.

Treatment of twin-to-twin transfusion syndrome in utero remains experimental. After delivery, therapy includes replacing blood in the donor twin to correct fluid and electrolyte imbalance. In the recipient twin, phlebotomy is necessary until normal venous pressure is restored. Often, other therapy for cardiac failure (eg, digitalis) is necessary.

**Prognosis**

The USA maternal mortality rate for multiple pregnancy is only slightly higher than for singleton. A history of previous dizygotic twins increases the likelihood of subsequent multiple pregnancy 10-fold. Hemorrhage is about 5 times as frequent in plural as in single pregnancies. The probability of abnormal presentation and of operative delivery and its complications is increased in multiple pregnancy. Premature rupture of the membranes and premature labor, often with a long prodromal phase, are common occurrences in multiple pregnancy. A gravida with a multiple pregnancy has about 5 times the likelihood of having a morbid (febrile, complicated) course as an average patient of the same parity with a single fetus.

Hydramnios is 5 times more frequent in multiple as in singleton pregnancies, principally because of fetal abnormality. "Unlike sex, generally unlike outcome" applies to twins. The greatest loss occurs when both twins are of the same sex; and male pairs succumb more readily then female pairs. Perinatal mortality and morbidity rates are increased in multiple pregnancy, mainly because of preterm delivery and its complications (ie, trauma or asphyxia).

Almost 50% of twins weigh < 2500 g, but the majority of these are of 36 weeks' gestational age or more. Directly or indirectly, multiple pregnancies are responsible for around 15% of premature births and around 9% of perinatal deaths, a rate 7-fold that of single births. Approximately 55% of twins are premature; 80% of perinatal deaths occur in those born before 31 weeks' gestation, and 93% of deaths are in those with birth weights below 1500 g. The incidence of intrauterine growth retardation is increased in multiple gestation, and multiple gestations account for 17% of infants with intrauterine growth retardation. Congenital malformations and abnormal presentation are more serious in monozygous twins. Preeclampsia-eclampsia, diabetes mellitus, and other disorders may further jeopardize the fetuses.

Good nutrition, enhanced bed rest, dietary supplementation when needed, and cessation of cigarette smoking can be expected to reduce intrauterine growth retardation and perinatal mortality rates in multiple pregnancy.

To reduce the high neonatal mortality rate in twin pregnancy, the objective should be to reduce the incidence of low-birth-weight infants rather than to perform cesarean section delivery more frequently. The critical weight level for intact survival of twins is about 1500 g. If twins weigh more than this at birth, the likelihood that they will live approximates that of a singleton of about the same gestational age. The comparative occurrence of perinatal death (per 1000) for single and multiple pregnancy are as follows: singletons, 39; twins, 152; triplets, 309; and quadruplets, 509. The rates are proportionately higher for quintuplets, etc.

The best outlook is for both twins to present by vertex. Twins and other multiple fetuses delivered by spontaneous means do better than those extracted by forceps or after version. Internal podalic version is especially dangerous. Hypoxia and trauma of operative delivery are the primary causes of death of the second twin. Central nervous system disease and hyaline membrane disease are frequently diagnosed in the surviving second twin.

Discordance noted at birth is associated with a slower weight gain during extrauterine life. A twin whose birth weight is less than 20% of that of its partner will not gain as rapidly and may never catch up with the other twin in weight and height. The IQ of the larger monozygotic twin is likely to be higher than that of the smaller twin if the weight difference is more than 300 g at birth. The female twin of a female-male pair who survives cross-transfusion is not sterile (in contrast to the situation encountered in the bovine free-martin).

Concordance of placental examination, clinical comparisons, and hematologic and serologic tests provides presumptive evidence of monozygotic twinning. The total probability of diagnosis of zygosity is over 95% using ABO, MNSs, Rh, Kell, Kidd, Duffy, and Lewis A and B antigens and approaches 100% using chromosomal analysis.

In comprehensive perinatal care centers, morbidity and mortality rates decrease greatly. In a recent report (Keith, 1988) of triplets receiving optimal care, the mean weight at delivery was 1779 g and the incidence of neonatal mortality was only 23 in 1000. First twins have about a 3% greater chance of survival than second twins. Breech presentation of the second twin carries higher mortality and morbidity rates.

## REFERENCES

Anderson RL, Goldberg JD, Golbus MS: Prenatal diagnosis in multiple gestation: 20 years' experience with amniocentesis. Prenat Diagn 1991;11:263.

Barrett JM et al: The effect of type of delivery upon neonatal outcome in premature twins. Am J Obstet Gynecol 1982;143:360.

Blumenfeld Z et al: Spontaneous fetal reduction in multiple gestations assessed by transvaginal ultrasound. Br J Obstet Gynaecol 1992;99:333.

Briauet JW, Hoorn RKJ: The use of human placental lactogen, oxytocinase and estriol in twin pregnancies with intrauterine growth retardation. Eur J Obstet Gynaecol Reprod Biol 1982;13:7.

Chervenak FA et al: Intrapartum management of twin gestation. Obstet Gynecol 1985;65:119.

Colburn DW, Pasquale SA: Monoamniotic twin pregnancy. J Reprod Med 1982;27:165.

Crane JP, Tomich PG, Kopta M: Ultrasonic growth patterns in normal and discordant twins. Obstet Gynecol 1980;55:678.

Devoe LD, Azor H: Simultaneous nonstress fetal heart rate testing in twin pregnancy. Obstet Gynecol 1981;58:450.

Dor J et al: Elective cervical suture of twin pregnancies diagnosed ultrasonically in the first trimester following induced ovulation. Gynecol Obstet Invest 1982;13:55.

Gilbert L, Saunders N, Sharp F: The management of multiple pregnancy in women with a lower-segment caesarean scar. Br J Obstet Gynecol 1988;95:1312.

Gore RM, Filly RA, Parer JT: Sonographic antepartum diagnosis of conjoined twins: Its impact on obstetric management. JAMA 1982;247:335.

Graziano EP et al: Is pulsed Doppler velocimetry useful in the management of multiple-gestation pregnancies? Am J Obstet Gynecol 1991;164:1426.

Greening DG: Vaginal delivery of conjoined twins. Med J Aust 1981;2:356.

Grennert L et al: Zygosity and intrauterine growth of twins. Obstet Gynecol 1980;55:684.

Hanna JH, Hill JM: Single intrauterine fetal demise in multiple gestation. Obstet Gynecol 1984;63:126.

Hemon D, Berger C, Lazar P: Twinning following oral contraceptive discontinuation. Int J Epidemiol 1981;10:319.

Holcberg G et al: Outcome of pregnancy in 31 triplet gestations. Obstet Gynecol 1982;59:472.

Houlton MC, Marivate M, Philpott RH: Factors associated with preterm labour and changes in the cervix before labour in twin pregnancy. Br J Obstet Gynaecol 1982; 89:190.

James FM III: Anesthetic considerations in breech or twin delivery. Clin Perinatol 1982;9:77.

Jarvis GJ, Whitfield MF: Epidural anesthesia and the delivery of twins. J Obstet Gynecol 1981;2:90.

Keith LG et al: The Northwestern University triplet study. 2. Fourteen triplet pregnancies delivered between 1981 and 1986. Acta Genet Med Gemellol (Roma) 1988; 37:65.

Keller JD et al: Northwestern University Twin Study X: Outcome of twin gestations complicated by gestational diabetes mellitus. Acta Genet Med Gemellol (Roma) 1991;40:153.

Knuppel RA et al: Intrauterine fetal death in twins after 32 weeks of gestation. Obstet Gynecol 1985;65:172.

Landy HJ et al: The "vanishing twin": Ultrasonic assessment of fetal disappearance in the first trimester. Am J Obstet Gynecol 1986;155:14.

Leveno KJ et al: Fetal lung maturation in twin gestation. Am J Obstet Gynecol 1984;148:405.

Livingston JE, Poland BJ: A study of spontaneously aborted twins. Teratology 1980;21:139.

Luke B, Keith LG: The contribution of singletons, twins and triplets to low birth weight, infant mortality and handicap in the United States. J Reprod Med 1992;37:661.

Mahony BS, Filly RA, Callen PW: Amnionicity and chorionicity in twin pregnancies: Prediction using ultrasound. Radiology 1985;155:205.

Melgar CA et al: Perinatal outcome after multifetal reduction to twins compared with nonreduced multiple gestations. Obstet Gynecol 1991;78:763.

Pergament E et al: The risk and efficacy of chorionic villus sampling in multiple gestations. Prenat Diagn 1992; 12:377.

Rayburn WF et al: Multiple gestation: Time interval between delivery and first and second twins. Obstet Gynecol 1984;63:502.

Schenker JG et al: Quintuplet pregnancies. Eur J Obstet Gynaecol Reprod Biol 1980;10:257.

Terasaki PI et al: Twins with two different fathers identified by HLA. N Engl J Med 1978;299:590.

# 18

# Diabetes Mellitus

*Sue M. Palmer, M.D.*

Diabetes mellitus may be defined as a chronic disorder of metabolism affecting carbohydrates, proteins, and fats. It is clinically recognized by a relative paucity of insulin and by hyperglycemia, glucosuria, and ketoacidosis. Over the long term, elevated glucose levels result in micro/macrovascular degenerative changes. The role of these degenerative changes in various disease states is extraordinary.

Diabetes doubles the risk for stroke, increases the risk for heart attack 2- to 3-fold with a 2-fold increase in mortality from that heart attack. Renal failure is 17 times more common and symptomatic peripheral arterial disease 3–4 times higher in diabetics. Congestive heart failure is markedly increased in diabetics, with a 2-fold increase seen in the male population and a 5-fold increase in the female population. There is a 54% higher incidence of hypertension in diabetics compared with that seen in matched nondiabetic controls. There is a high incidence of motor, sensory and autonomic impairment with a 40% rate of impotence in males. Diabetes mellitus is the third leading disease-specific cause of death in the USA today. In summation, not only is diabetes the most commonly encountered endocrinopathy, but it also possibly accounts for as much morbidity and mortality as all of the other endocrinopathies combined.

Diabetes mellitus is relatively common in most populations. Diabetes sufficient to warrant insulin or oral hypoglycemics affects 3–4 million persons in the USA. Another 3 million are treated with diet alone in addition to a possible 4 or more million with varying degrees of asymptomatic glucose intolerance. Diabetes mellitus complicates over 1% of pregnancies.

The end result of the alterations of pregnancy in diabetics is to decrease carbohydrate control reserves. Thus, pregnancy affords a unique opportunity for diabetes screening and may well be the best opportunity in a woman's life to discover (or prevent) her diabetes. In addition, for fetal well-being it is imperative to discover maternal diabetes or gestational diabetes. Ketoacidosis is an immediate threat to life. Hyperglycemia results in the developing embryo having a 6-fold increase in midline birth defects and is the leading cause of perinatal morbidity in diabetic pregnancies today, accounting for 40% of perinatal mortality.

Fortunately, through strict control of hyperglycemia beginning prior to conception, a marked decline occurs in morbidity and mortality. Twenty years ago it was not unexpected to deliver an unexplained stillbirth from a mother with insulin-dependent diabetes mellitus (IDDM). Today, this tragedy is rare, and over the last decade associated perinatal morbidity/mortality has been reduced from 60% to less than 5%. Two decades ago, most diabetics required prolonged hospitalization; whereas presently the majority are managed with only brief hospitalizations. This is partly due to the technologic improvements in home reflectance glucose monitors and the beneficial impact they have had in management of the diabetic during pregnancy.

Currently, the major challenges of caring for diabetics in pregnancy are to adequately screen pregnant women, to reduce the congenital malformations by enhancing preconceptual glucose control, and to detail the full impact of milder glucose elevations not on maternal risk for developing diabetes but on its immediate and long-term consequences to the fetus/child.

# PREGESTATIONAL DIABETES

## TYPE I OR INSULIN-DEPENDENT DIABETES MELLITUS (IDDM)

### Essentials of Diagnosis
- Hyperglycemia requiring exogenous insulin.
- Onset earlier than 30 years of age.
- Profound thirst, increased urination, weight loss.
- Ketoacidosis.

### Etiology
Type I diabetes is a chronic autoimmune disorder

that occurs in genetically susceptible persons. Major histocompatibility haplotypes (HLA) influence susceptibility. Although no genetic marker has been identified, susceptibility is noted to be increased by a gene or genes located near or within the HLA on the short arm of chromosome 6 (6p). This condition results in elevated glucose and elevated free fatty acids due to lack of sufficient insulin production in the beta islet cells of the pancreas to meet metabolic needs.

The risk to offspring of developing type I diabetes with an affected sibling is 5% if 1 haplotype is shared, 13% for 2 haplotypes, and 2% for no shared haplotypes. If both parents are affected, the incidence of type I diabetes is 33%.

## Incidence

The incidence of type I diabetes in the general population is 0.1–0.4% in various age groups under 30 years of age. Diabetes mellitus represents one of the most common maternal illnesses resulting in anomalous offspring. The incidence of major congenital anomalies among infants of diabetics mothers (with IDDM) has been estimated at 6–10%, representing a 2- to 3-fold increase over the incidence in the general population, and accounting for 40% of all perinatal deaths among these infants. The incidence of malformations is directly related to the level of glucose over the embryonic period as measured by a hemoglobin $A_{1c}$ level in the first trimester. In addition, if not well controlled, IDDM results in a comparable increase in abortions.

## Considerations

There is no data to support a shortening of the woman's lifespan or a worsening of renal disease as a result of pregnancy. Retinal complications might be worsened by pregnancy, and there should be no evidence of macular edema or proliferative retinopathy present before proceeding with a pregnancy. Persons in renal failure should be advised to undergo a transplant prior to a pregnancy because of the impact of elevated creatinine on pregnancy outcome. A history of severe or frequent maternal hypoglycemia is a major concern during pregnancy and should be addressed with the family in detail, since symptoms of hypoglycemia are blunted during pregnancy. It is especially important to establish appropriate guidelines for operating a motor vehicle by advising the patient to use proper sense (eg, taking insulin without eating) and evaluating her glucose prior to driving if level was not checked recently.

## Pathophysiology

Insulin is an anabolic hormone with crucial roles in carbohydrate, fat, and protein metabolism. It promotes uptake and utilization of amino acids, lipogenesis, glucose uptake, and storage as glycogen. Lack of insulin results in elevated levels of glucose, lipolysis with elevation of free fatty acids leading to increased formation of ketone bodies, acetoacetate and β-hydroxybutyrate. Blood glucose levels exceeding the renal capability of absorption produce an osmotic diuresis with dehydration and electrolyte loss. Ketoacidosis, a life-threatening condition for both mother and fetus, results from a paucity of insulin.

Elevated glucose levels are toxic to the developing fetus, producing an increase in serious midline defects in direct proportion to the elevation. These birth defects (Table 18–1) are fatal or seriously incapacitating to quality of life and are preventable by preconception glucose control. The presence of ketones significantly reduces the hyperglycemia necessary to produce defects. These anomalies occur within the first 8 weeks of gestation when most women are just initiating prenatal care. Hemoglobin $A_{1c}$, a particular fraction of a glycosylated hemoglobin molecule, when drawn in the first trimester can give a risk percentage for presence of anomalies (Table 18–2).

Thus, early education of all women with diabetes is crucial if reproduction is to be accomplished with optimal outcomes. *Unfortunately, due to a lack of preconception control combined with improved metabolic control during pregnancy, there are presently greater numbers of infants born today with birth defects caused by diabetes, not fewer!*

## Metabolism in Normal & Diabetic Pregnancy

Significant metabolic changes are necessary to provide proper energy delivery to the growing conceptus. The combined hormonal changes early in pregnancy lower glucose levels, promote fat deposition, and encourage appetite by raising serum levels of estrogen and progesterone, which increases insulin pro-

**Table 18–1.** Congenital anomalies of infants of diabetic mothers.*

| | |
|---|---|
| Skeletal and CNS | Caudal regression syndrome<br>Neural tube defects excluding anencephaly<br>Anencephaly with or without herniation of neural elements<br>Microcephaly |
| Cardiac | Transposition of the great vessels with or without ventricular septal defect<br>Ventricular septal defects<br>Coarctation of the aorta with or without ventricular septal defect or patent ductus arteriosus<br>Cardiomegaly |
| Renal anomalies | Hydronephrosis<br>Renal agenesis<br>Ureteral duplication |
| Gastrointestinal | Duodenal atresia<br>Anorectal atresia<br>Small left colon syndrome |
| Other | Single umbilical artery |

*Reprinted with permission from Reece EA, Hobbins JC: Diabetes embryopathy, pathogenesis, prenatal diagnosis and prevention. Obstet Gynecol Surv 1986;41:325.

**Table 18–2.** The relationship between the initial pregnancy value of glycosylated hemoglobin and the percent of major fetal congenital malformations.

| Initial Maternal Value Hb A$_1$C | Percentage of Major Congenital Malformation |
|---|---|
| 7.9 or lower | 3.2% |
| 8.9–9.9 | 8.1% |
| Greater than 10 | 23.5% |

duction and secretion, while increasing tissue sensitivity to insulin. The overall result is a lowering of the fasting glucose levels, reaching a nadir by the 12th week and remaining unchanged until delivery. The decrease is on the average 15 mg/dL; therefore, fasting values of 70–80 mg/dL are normal in a pregnant woman by the 10th week of gestation. There is a comparable decrease in postprandial values. This acts to protect the developing embryo from elevated glucose levels. Indeed, birth defects are noted at a 2- to 3-fold higher rate in women with diabetes without preconception glycemic control. In summation, human placental lactogen (HPL) and the other hormones associated with pregnancy facilitate maternal storage of energy in the first trimester and then assist in the diversion of energy to the fetus in later pregnancy as demand increases. There is marked demand on maternal glucose metabolism from the onset of pregnancy for protection of the fetus in the embryonic, organogenesis, and maturation stages.

In the second trimester, higher fasting and postprandial glucose levels are seen. This facilitates the placental transfer. Glucose transfer is via a carrier-mediated active transport system which becomes saturated at ~ 250 mg/dL. Fetal glucose levels are 80% of maternal values. In contrast, maternal amino acid levels are lowered during the second trimester by active placental transfer to the fetus. Fetal levels of amino acids are 2- to 3-fold higher than maternal levels but not as high as levels within the placenta. Lipid metabolism in the second trimester shows continued storage until midgestation; then, as fetal demands increase, there is enhanced mobilization (lipolysis).

HPL is the hormone mainly responsible for insulin resistance and lipolysis. HPL also decreases the hunger sensation and diverts maternal carbohydrate metabolism to fat metabolism in the third trimester. HPL is a single-chain polypeptide secreted by the syncytiotrophoblast and has a molecular weight of 22,308 and a half-life of 17 minutes. HPL levels are elevated during hypoglycemia to mobilize free fatty acids for energy for maternal metabolism. HPL levels are low with maternal hyperglycemia. HPL is similar in structure to growth hormone and acts by reducing the insulin affinity to insulin receptors. The effect on the fetus is to allow longer glucose elevations for placental transfer to the developing fetus and minimizing maternal use of glucose for metabolic needs.

During pregnancy, the levels of HPL rise steadily during the first and second trimesters with a plateau in the late third trimester. This plateau is the natural result of decreasing nutrient delivery to the placenta thus decreasing hormone production. It appears that this is a necessary signal to the developing fetus to initiate fetal cortisol and thyroid hormone release to in turn initiate enzyme development for maturation. In pregnancies with elevated glucose and other nutrients, there is continued placental growth with a delay in fetal organ/hormonal maturation. In short, mother and fetus communicate through nutrient delivery and utilization.

Cortisol levels rise during pregnancy and stimulate endogenous glucose production and glycogen storage and decrease glucose utilization. The "dawn phenomena" (elevated fasting glucose to facilitate brain metabolism) is marked in normal pregnancies and is even more enhanced in women with polycystic ovarian disease (PCOD) who become pregnant. Therefore, early pregnancy glucose screening is advised for the PCOD woman who becomes pregnant.

Prolactin levels are also increased 5- to 10-fold during pregnancy and may have an impact on carbohydrate metabolism. Thus, patients with hyperprolactinemia also deserve early pregnancy glucose screening.

Fetal somatic growth is associated with the anabolic properties of insulin. In that neither maternal or fetal insulin cross the placenta, it is known that the release of fetal insulin is stimulated by glucose and amino acids as well as being regulated by genetic potential. The pathophysiologic impact of elevated maternal glucose levels on the fetus is a product of the level of elevation and duration of time.

**Diagnosis**

Type I diabetes (IDDM) has an early age of onset with deficient insulin production. Profound thirst, increased urination, and weight loss or even overt diabetic ketoacidosis are the usual symptoms triggering medical evaluation.

Evaluation of the patient for possible degenerative changes in other organ systems allows a much more informed prenatal care as well as classification based on White's criteria (Table 18–3). The usual evaluation includes an ophthalmologic examination for evidence of retinopathy. Retinal hemorrhages may increase in the initial stages of improved glucose control as blood flow increases to these terminal vessels clearing atherosclerotic plaques. The negative impact of this can be controlled by frequent visits with early laser treatment as needed.

Initial evaluation, if the patient was not seen preconceptionally, includes assessment for other organ damage with 24-hour urine test, ophthalmologic examination, test for thyroid status, electrocardiogram in patients 34 or older, and hemoglobin A$_{1c}$ test for risk of fetal anomalies (this includes type II diabetic patients). The renal status is evaluated by a 24-hour

**Table 18–3.** Modified White's classification of diabetes mellitus.

| | |
|---|---|
| Class A: | Chemical diabetes diagnosed *before* pregnancy; managed by diet *alone*; any age of onset or duration. |
| Class B: | Insulin treatment necessary *before* pregnancy; onset after age 20; duration of less than 10 years. |
| Class C: | Onset at age 10–19; or duration of 10–19 years. |
| Class D: | Onset before age 10; or duration of 20 or more years; or chronic hypertension; or background retinopathy. |
| Class F: | Renal disease. |
| Class H: | Coronary artery disease. |
| Class R: | Proliferative retinopathy. |
| Class T: | Renal transplant. |

urine for creatine clearance and total protein. If protein value is less than 200 mg, a 24-hour urine test for microalbinuria should be considered, because microalbinuria is associated with increased vascular disease in the future. An electrocardiogram should be done on patients with disease duration of > 5 years or who are over the age of 30. Thyroid status should also be evaluated due to the potential multiendocrine impact of diabetes.

All patients should have a detailed ultrasound examination with fetal echocardiography at 18–20 weeks to rule out anomalies, as well as an AFP (alpha-fetoprotein) or TriScreen at 16–18 weeks' gestation due to the increased rate of congenital anomalies in the offspring of diabetics.

Fetal surveillance is increased at 32 weeks' gestation if vascular disease is present. This is accomplished with ultrasound amniotic fluid assessments until 36 weeks, then biweekly unless contraction stress tests are done weekly. Serial ultrasound testing for growth are done at 28–32 weeks and at 36 weeks. Polyhydramnios (AFI > ≅ 20) or increased abdominal girth should alert the practitioner to less than ideal glucose control. If glucose values remain labile despite all management techniques, then it is best to deliver the fetus as soon as lung maturity is established by L/S & PG by amniocentesis at 37 weeks.

## Treatment

Care of the insulin-dependent diabetic must be intensive. Support individuals should be identified and constructively involved with the therapy wherever possible. However, it is extremely important to stress that the patient herself is solely responsible for her actions. The educational focus is to develop the patient's understanding of her disease to the state that she can balance activity, diet, and insulin with guidance only as needed while assisting her in stopping self-destructive behavior or actions.

If not seen preconceptionally, prenatal vitamins should be started and additional folate, 0.5 mg given twice daily, due to the interaction of hyperglycemia with folate receptors.

## Education

The education necessary to maximize the diabetic's chance for a successful pregnancy is ideally accomplished through a team approach of health care professionals consisting of a physician trained in managing diabetes and pregnancy, a dietician, a diabetes educator, and a social worker. The education process is ongoing, taking the person who is committed to change from a dependent state to one of interdependence. Such a program will result in a successful pregnancy outcome in 96% of persons with preconception control.

A careful review of the patient's existing knowledge of diabetes and her care is necessary. This may be accomplished by any knowledgeable member of the health care team, but is ideally done by a Diabetes Educator. Each step from diet, glucose monitoring, insulin administration, exercise, and self-care during illnesses is reviewed, assessing her knowledge and correcting inappropriate information. Ideally, the patient then identifies areas that she can correct to improve glucose control. These areas are summarized, and the care goals are written in an individualized form with patient input and given to her for review at home as well as remaining in the chart so that progress on the goals can be monitored.

The patient is instructed completely on how to properly use a home glucose monitor, including running control solutions, cleaning, trouble shooting, and proper technique of sample collection. It is important not to squeeze in the area of lancet puncture since the sample becomes diluted with tissue fluids and can result in lowered values. This is so common that the care providers must constantly review the patient's techniques when values vary.

When the team approach is taken, with active patient cooperation, cesarean delivery is rarely necessary, and most patients go into spontaneous labor or are induced at 40 weeks, thus decreasing the cesarean section rate.

It is hoped that educational efforts result in a lifelong program designed to prevent the development of diabetic complications and retard the progression of complications. Indeed, the recent CDDT trials clearly indicate this to be the attainable goal. Some 20 years after the pioneering work of Karlsson and Kjeller, which showed a linear relationship between glycemic control and perinatal mortality, the same reduction in complications have been shown for those with new onset diabetes as well as those with early organ damage (eg, eye, kidney).

## Normalization of Blood Glucose

*Prevention of hyperglycemia and ketoacidosis through rigorous control of the blood glucose is mandatory in the pregnant woman with IDDM. This is best afforded by careful preconceptual analysis and counseling, achievement of normal levels of glycosylated hemoglobin before pregnancy, frequent (usually 4–5 times a day) home glucose monitoring, thoughtful control of diet (the diabetic should have the usual weight gain of pregnancy), and stabilization of exercise. Obviously this can be accomplished only by focusing the health care team's efforts on education and by including the patient as an active participant in the care of her and her fetus.*

Goal glucose levels are fasting levels of < 90, but > 70, and 1-hour postprandial values of < 130. At these levels, the normalization of glucose values increase the incidence of serious hypoglycemic reactions.

To achieve these levels, the patient must carry a reliable, portable glucose meter at all times to allow independence and to provide protection from adverse outcome. It is best if the meter has a memory of extended duration. The memory meter not only records times and values, but also allows an impersonalized review of glucoses. Unfortunately, good glucoses are invariably associated with "good person" and vice versa. The team, including the patient, must focus on the goal of glucose normalization and assist in changing behavior while always recognizing the difficulties in today's society on obtaining this goal.

All patients and significant others should be instructed on treatment of hypoglycemia and have symptoms reviewed. Nocturnal hypoglycemia episodes with nightmares, sleep walking, tossing and turning in bed, and waking with headaches are important and should be asked about on prenatal visits. After a change in the evening intermediate insulin dose, the appropriateness of the dose should be checked by a 2 AM glucose reading. If the value is below 90 in a patient with IDDM, a snack should be taken, and the health care provider should be contacted in the morning to readjust the dose. In type II insulin-dependent patients, a snack is taken if the glucose is <80.

As noted previously, women with diabetes may maximize their reproductive outcomes by normalization of glucose before pregnancy. Correction of glucose levels to normal as well as replacement of vitamin and minerals depleted during periods of diuresis result in anomaly rates similar to those of the general population. Counseling of the diabetic women must include the family and the lifestyle changes necessary to attain this goal of normalization of glucose levels.

## Diet

The patient should be instructed on an ADA diet, calories at 25–35/kg body weight but no greater than 2400 kcal nor less than 1800 kcal. Actual weight gain with confirmation of actual caloric intake will further adjust the patient's caloric needs to allow appropriate weight gain. Women who are under their ideal weight have additional weight to gain over the recommended

11-kg weight gain (a minimum of 7 kg for obese patients). The diet is 40–50% carbohydrate, 30% fat, and 20–30% protein. Women with renal disease should have protein limited to 90 g of protein to minimize impact of pregnancy on their disease. The calories are divided into 3 meals and 3 snacks with the evening snack recommended to be a half-sandwich. The protein such as a meat provides calories in the early AM hours when intermediate insulin is peaking and fetal glucose utilization is maximized due to increased movements during the lateral rest period.

The snack for hypoglycemia should be milk or peanut butter with crackers. Orange juice should be discouraged unless that is all that is available because it causes too abrupt a rise in glucose that is not sustained. Glucagon emergency kits should be given to all IDDM patients and their spouses taught how to use it in case the patient is found unresponsive.

Soluble fiber assists in satiating hunger but, more important, in reducing glycemic swings. The impact of fiber is greater in the type II diabetic or gestational diabetic but does improve insulin receptor sensitivity and glucose control in the IDDM patient. The patient should note exactly what she ate, the amount, and the mode of preparation when she has a postprandial glucose level over 130. Attention should be directed to the bedtime snack when there is elevation or lowering of the fasting glucose.

The dietitian is a crucial member in the care of an IDDM pregnant patient. Visits should occur as often as needed to obtain proper compliance. The dietitian should make a concerted effort to individualize the diet, respecting different lifestyles and ethnicity. A minimum of 2 visits is always necessary, and family involvement is encouraged for improved compliance.

## Insulin

All patients should undergo a review of insulin administration, including mixing of regular and intermediate insulin as well as injection technique. All patients are initiated on human insulin or changed from older animal products for reduction in antibody formation. Patients should be advised that regular insulin may have a more profound hypoglycemic effect due to lack of blocking antibodies, but generally a slight to no decrease in dose is necessary. Because of the increased purity of the human insulin preparations, the duration of action is shorter, and most patients require 3 injections daily for ideal glucose control, with the intermediate insulin being given at bedtime.

Initially, the injection sites should be noted, and these should be reevaluated if unexplained glucose readings are occurring. The intermediate insulin at bedtime should be given in the fatty area of the thighs for the most prolonged and even absorption. Injections with regular insulin should be given a minimum of 30 minutes prior to a meal.

Although current studies do not support an improvement in glycemic control/outcome in pregnancy using subcutaneous insulin pumps, some experienced investigators advocate their use in selected patients. Indeed, the research was not conducted using the improved pumps. Even advocates of the insulin pump note that initiation with appropriate training is tricky during pregnancy and is probably best done prior to conception.

### Severe Hyperglycemia & Ketoacidosis

*During pregnancy severe hyperglycemia and keto-acidosis are treated exactly the same as in the non-pregnant state. Insulin therapy, careful monitoring of potassium and fluid replacement are crucial for maternal survival. Fetal status and chance of survival is enhanced by: administration of maternal oxygen, lateral recumbency, and slow, but decisive lowering of the blood glucose. Fetal heart rate monitoring often demonstrates late decelerations (indicative of utero-placental insufficiency) in addition to decreased beat to beat variability (due to maternal acidosis combined with limited fetal placental clearance and buffering capabilities).*

### Postpartum

The postpartum patient should be started back on an ADA diet as soon as clinically indicated. Insulin administration should be on a reduced dose because the rapid clearing of HPL results in increased insulin receptor sensitivity. The general rule is ⅔ of the pre-pregnant dose or ⅓ to ½ of the present dose with careful observation for hypoglycemia. If the patient underwent surgery, the insulin infusion is continued until oral intake can be established. The glucose levels should be kept relatively controlled to assist the patient in healing. Infections should be aggressively treated in the postpartum patient, and she should be mobilized as soon as possible because of an increased risk of thrombotic events.

Often the patient experiences a "honeymoon" period with a significant reduction in insulin as the energy expenditure of breastfeeding increases. Breast-feeding is encouraged, and insulin is managed accordingly.

### Contraception

Use of a reliable form of contraception is necessary for the patient until she desires pregnancy or until glucose values are in the desired range. The choices are limited but should be presented to the patient. Low-dose oral contraceptives have a minimal increase in thromboembolic impact, but much less than that experienced during pregnancy. Their use offers the most complete protection from pregnancy. Barrier contraceptive methods may be useful in the properly motivated patient, but intrauterine devices in diabetics are associated with an increase in infections (especially in those with multiple partners). Indeed, if the diabetic woman is not in a monogamous relationship,

the use of both oral contraception and condoms might be advisable to decrease the possibility of being infected with other sexually transmitted diseases such as human papilloma virus, herpes, and the HIV virus.

### Prognosis

Prognosis is primarily dependent on the level of glucose control. Good control requires a motivated patient, an active management approach (education, diet, insulin and exercise) with trained health care providers and frequent patient-provider interactions. Another factor influencing prognosis is the amount of degenerative changes. With diligent antenatal care, the patient can anticipate a normal labor and delivery experience. Severe hypoglycemia and diabetic keto-acidosis can result in maternal compromise and even death. The fetus, if spared from a congenital malformation or death in utero, may suffer significant impairment in the hostile environment with poor glucose control affecting brain development as well as other organs.

## TYPE II DIABETES (NIDDM)

### Essentials of Diagnosis

- Hyperglycemia not requiring exogenous insulin.
- Onset at over 30 years of age.
- "Apple-shaped" body habitus.
- Excess appetite and weight gain, but few other symptoms.
- Delayed healing or vascular disease.

### Definition

Type II diabetes is characterized by insufficient insulin receptors to allow proper glucose control after insulin is released (insulin resistance). Those affected typically have a body habitus in which there is increased abdominal girth, often described as an "apple shape." The reason for this is that the highest concentration of insulin receptors is located in the abdominal rectus muscles and the increased layer of fat appears to impair insulin receptor sensitivity.

The patient has increased hunger due to excess insulin release as a result of elevated glucose levels. This insulin release further decreases insulin receptors due to elevated hormonal levels, and thus a vicious cycle begins of excess appetite with weight gain. Otherwise, these patients exhibit few symptoms, with the possible exception of poor wound healing and fatigue.

Type II diabetics are not ketosis-prone due to the presence of insulin but do develop a condition of hyperglycemic hyperomolarity during pregnancy generally after an episode of vomiting and diarrhea in which the patient replaced fluids with glucose solutions. This condition has a high morbidity to the fetus, but can be effectively treated with immediate fluid replacement.

Also included in this classification is "secondary diabetes." Secondary diabetes is carbohydrate intolerance secondary to pancreatic disease, excess production of certain hormones (eg, growth hormone), use of certain drugs (eg, corticosteroids), insulin receptor abnormalities, and certain genetic disorders.

## Diagnosis

The diagnosis of type II diabetes is based on hyperglycemia. In nonpregnant adults, the diagnosis is made by a fasting plasma glucose test, $> = 140$ mg/dL, on more than one occasion, 2 elevated values, $> = 200$ mg/dL, after the administration of 75 g of glucola on a 2-hour test, or a combination of an elevated fasting sugar and 1 abnormal value.

## Genetics of Inheritance

Type II diabetes is not linked to HLA or genetic markers, but evidence supports a genetic component. With type II diabetes, the risk of frank diabetes in a first-degree relative is almost 15%, and about 30% more will have impaired glucose tolerance. If both parents have type II diabetes, the incidence of diabetes in the offspring is 60–75%. Monozygous twins have a much greater propensity for type II diabetes (almost 100%) than for type I diabetes (20–50%).

## Importance

Type II diabetes has a major impact on the morbidity/mortality of the individual as well as on the quality of life (eg, amputation of extremities, blindness, strokes). Controlling glucose minimizes the onset of these complications and reduces the progression of existing ones. Education concerning glucose control has been demonstrated to have a major impact on the patient's overall health.

## Treatment

Type II diabetes is treated primarily by lifestyle modification. The level of dietary fat is decreased and the ingestion of soluble fiber stressed. Increased exercise, with particular attention to the abdominal muscles, is advised. Oral hypoglycemic agents are used in the nonpregnant, but cannot be used during pregnancy.

If weight loss can be accomplished and pregnancy delayed, maintaining a woman on oral agents can be advantageous preconceptionally to reduce insulin resistance. Preconception evaluation is the same as in type I diabetics. It is surprising that the incidence of initial renal disease detected is higher, probably due to a longer time of asymptomatic disease prior to diagnosis. Insulin is generally used during pregnancy and perhaps even during conception. Also during pregnancy, the health care team emphasizes diet and routine daily exercise.

Soluble fiber is a key in therapy for type II diabetes since it reduces the glycemic intake of the diet, thus reducing insulin release, which results in heightened sensitivity of insulin receptors. Fat intake is closely monitored because it reduces insulin sensitivity and often has been the main source of calories for these obese persons. Thus, when fat intake is decreased and portion size increased, the patient is unable to maintain weight during the increased metabolic demand of pregnancy. The dietitian must work closely with the individual and monitor actual calorie intake to allow a minimum of 15 pounds weight gain even in the massively obese patient for proper nutrition in pregnancy.

Exercise is initiated, and increased water intake prior to and during the exercise period is stressed. Swimming is the safest exercise for the massively obese to minimize trauma to joints, but walking and/or upper arm ergometrics or stationary biking are excellent alternatives.

Insulin therapy is added in small amounts with emphasis on long-acting insulin. In the past, many type II diabetics received very high doses of insulin. This was not only unnecessary, but hazardous, because it resulted in significant down-regulation of insulin receptors.

The remainder of therapy, such as glucose monitoring and evaluation of the fetus, is similar to that done in type I diabetic management. Emphasis is placed on ultrasonography to assess fetal growth due to anatomic limitations in assessing fundal growth. Unfortunately, fetal weight assessment is often inaccurate in this group of individuals, due to the fat distribution in the pannus region.

When the patient is in labor, it is extremely important to administer a controlled glucose infusion to meet the body's energy needs. Yet it is rare to need an insulin infusion due to the high metabolic demand with a limited amount of glucose. For the postpartum patient, early ambulation assists in decreasing thromboembolic risks. Often glucose control is achieved postpartum on no more than an ADA diet. If hypoglycemic agents are necessary postpartum, insulin is continued for those who are breastfeeding, whereas the oral agents may be used in the nonbreastfeeding mothers. Postpartum weight loss is encouraged (see following section on gestational diabetes). Preconception evaluation prior to the next pregnancy is stressed.

# GESTATIONAL DIABETES

## Essentials of Diagnosis

- Hyperglycemia found only during pregnancy as confirmed by a normal 75-g glucose tolerance test (GTT) postpartum.

## Definition

Gestational diabetes is carbohydrate intolerance that is present only during pregnancy. Gestational diabetes may be screened by drawing a 1-hour glucose level following a 50-g glucose load, but is definitively diagnosed only by an abnormal 3-hour GTT following a 100-g glucose load. Such persons are not within the normal (95%) for pregnancy, but have normal values when retested after pregnancy.

## Importance

The growth and maturation of the fetus are closely associated with the delivery of maternal nutrients, particularly glucose. This is most crucial in the third trimester and is directly related to the duration and degree of maternal glucose elevation. Thus, the negative impact is as highly diverse as the variety of carbohydrate intolerance that women bring to pregnancy. For example, consider the older obese, undiagnosed, type II diabetic with a fasting glucose level of 140 mg/dL in contrast to the slender young woman who gains 50 pounds or more during pregnancy on a diet consisting largely of sugar drinks and fast foods.

In those with severe abnormalities, there is an increased rate of miscarriage, congenital malformations, prematurity, pyelonephritis, preeclampsia, in utero meconium, fetal distress, cesarean section deliveries, and stillbirth.

## Incidence & Etiology

Inability to obtain glucose levels desired by the body for proper functioning is a growing health problem in the USA; thus, it is not unexpected that more women are noted during pregnancy to be unable to attain the low glucose levels desired for proper fetal growth. The incidence of gestational diabetes varies from 12% in racially heterogeneous urban regions to 1% in rural areas with a predominantly white population.

## Pathophysiology

Gestational diabetes is pathophysiologically similar to type II diabetes. Approximately 90% of the persons identified have a deficiency of insulin receptors (prior to pregnancy) or a marked increase in weight that has been placed on the abdominal region. The other 10% have deficient insulin production and will proceed to develop mature-onset insulin-dependent diabetes.

Similar to that seen in those with type II diabetes, the women most likely to develop gestational diabetes are those who are overweight with a body habitus often described as an apple shape. HPL blocks insulin receptors and increases in direct linear relation to the length of pregnancy. Insulin release is enhanced in an attempt to maintain glucose homeostasis. The patient experiences increased hunger due to the excess insulin release as a result of elevated glucose levels. This insulin release further decreases insulin receptors due to elevated hormonal levels. Thus, the vicious cycle of excess appetite with weight gain occurs. Few other symptoms mark this condition.

## Diagnosis

Glucosuria is a common finding in pregnancy due to increased glomerular filtration and is therefore unreliable as a diagnostic finding. Glucose screening should be done on every pregnant patient at or no later than 28 weeks of gestation, since risk factors are insufficient to identify all women with gestational diabetes. Ultrasound findings of a fetal weight greater than or equal to 70% for gestational age, polyhydramnios (AFI > 20), midline congenital anomalies, or an abdominal circumference measurement that exceeds the femur growth by 2 weeks merit immediate 3-hour GTT. Other clinical findings indicating possible diabetes are edema developing early in the pregnancy and excessive weight gain.

Initial screening is accomplished by ingestion of 50 g of glucose (usually chilled glucola) at any time of the day and with disregard to previous meal ingestion. The sensitivity and specificity are based on the cutoff value used to indicate a positive (Table 18–4); however, screening is not as reproducible from day to day as would be desired. If screening is positive, the patient is advised to follow a carbohydrate loading diet for 3 days and to do a full 3-hour GTT. A simple carbohydrate loading diet is all the pasta and starches she can eat at each meal and 1 candy bar per day. For the GTT, the patient is fasting and receives 100 g of glucose after a fasting glucose level is obtained. A blood sample is then taken every hour for 3 hours. The patient is advised to sit quietly during the test to minimize the impact of exercise on glucose levels.

The glucose values used to detect gestational diabetes were determined by O'Sullivan (1964) in a retrospective study designed to detect risk of developing type II diabetes in the future. The values were set using whole blood and required 2 values reaching or exceeding the value to be positive. Subsequent information has led to alteration in O'Sullivan's criteria.

**Table 18–4.** Screening glucose related to gestational diabetes.*

| Screening Test Result (mg/dl) | Incidence of Gestational Diabetes (%) |
| --- | --- |
| 135–144 | 14.6 |
| 145–154 | 17.4 |
| 155–164 | 28.6 |
| 165–174 | 20.0 |
| 175–184 | 50.0 |
| > 185 | 100.0 |

*Modified with permission from: Carpenter MW, Coustan DR: Criteria for screening tests for gestational diabetes. Am J Obstet Gynecol 1982;144:768.

For example, there is growing evidence that 1 value is sufficient to make an impact on the health of the fetus and is now the criterion used by most clinicians to initiate treatment. Whole blood glucose values are lower than plasma levels due to glucose uptake by hemoglobin. The present values used by the American College of Obstetricians and Gynecologists are based on a theoretical increase in hemoglobin and plasma with pregnancy. Recently, a study using all 3 methods of glucose determination on the same samples have disproved the theoretical values and are listed in Table 18–5.

## Treatment

The key to therapy in most patients is diet and exercise (because of the paucity of insulin receptors). This makes therapy more difficult than with the insulin-deficient patient in whom exogenous insulin may be easily administered. Therapy in the type II diabetic is based on the patient's motivation and ability to change lifestyle. Exercise of the non-weight-bearing type (noted previously) is encouraged as even small time allocations have a major benefit.

Every care provider must stress the importance of diet. Soluble fiber is invaluable to provide satiety and improve insulin receptor numbers and sensitivity. Fats must be reduced because of their negative impact on insulin receptors. Calories should be prescribed at 20–25/kcal per kilogram of present body weight (generally 1800–2400 kcal). Massively obese patients have a reduction in their metabolism rate; therefore, it is better to start low and increase the calories as needed. Food records are kept for 1 week, and the content and calories are reviewed by the dietitian with helpful suggestions on improving favorite dishes to be included in the diet. The patient is instructed to particularly note all food taken in when a 1-hour postprandial glucose value is 130 mg/dl or greater. The memory reflectance glucose meters are invaluable in assisting the patient to learn the proper diet and the impact of her actions on glucose levels. Insulin is added as needed for glucose control only after clear dietary errors are noted and attempts at correcting are done.

A minimum of 2 visits to the dietitian encourages education and interaction over dietary questions. The customization of diet to ethnic foods is often invaluable in obtaining dietary compliance. The encouragement of other family members to participate in dietary counseling assists their support for the patient and is key to making familial dietary changes. The patient often benefits from direct contact with the dietitian when glucose levels are erratic, when her weight fails to meet expected guidelines, when she is having difficulty with calorie counting, or when she increases daily calories more than 300 kcal over guidelines.

The patient checks her glucose 4 times daily (eg, fasting, and 1-hour postprandial breakfast, lunch, dinner). The desired values are a fasting of < 90 mg/dL and a 1-hour < 130 mg/dL. The average glucose levels should be ~ 90. After she has obtained a good understanding of her diet and the glucose values are in the desired range, she can decrease the frequency of testing to 3 days per week chosen randomly, preferably by a significant other without regard to social events. Monthly glycohemoglobins should reflect the level of control, showing a decline from initiation of treatment. Documentation of normal fetal growth and amniotic fluid by ultrasonography may allow continuing less frequent glucose testing.

## ANTEPARTUM CARE

Diabetics have triple the normal rate of asymptomatic bacteriuria. Therefore, a urine culture is obtained initially, and appropriate treatment initiated if it is positive. After cessation of therapy, urinary culture is again obtained to confirm elimination of the infection. Protein detected in clean-catch urine specimens should be evaluated by 24-hour urine testing and repeated as needed. In addition to routine prenatal care (see Chapter 10), the development of edema (including carpal tunnel syndrome) is closely monitored. If edema occurs, greater attention to glucose control (eg, returning to daily monitoring) and enhanced bed rest are necessities. There is an increased incidence of preeclampsia in diabetics, which is directly related to glucose control as well as to the presence of preexisting vascular and renal disease.

Assessment of the fetus by glucose memory meters combined with clinical/ultrasound assessment of fetal growth cannot be replaced by other antenatal tests. Fetuses in whom maternal glucose has been well controlled and whose mothers do not smoke or have other organ damage will tolerate pregnancy well. Patients with poor glucose control, fetal macrosomia, and/or polyhydramnios represent the patients at greatest risk for morbidity/mortality. Biweekly nonstress tests (NSTs) or weekly contraction stress tests are begun at 32 weeks for additional monitoring of poorly controlled patients, patients with complicated vascular disease, or patients who smoke. Weekly

**Table 18–5.** Oral glucose tolerance test (100g) values for the diagnosis of gestational diabetes (mg/dl).

|  | O'Sullivan (1964) | NDDG (1979) | Carpenter & Coustan (1982) | Sacks et al (1989) |
|---|---|---|---|---|
| Fasting | 90 | 105 | 95 | 96 |
| 1 Hour | 165 | 190 | 180 | 172 |
| 2 Hour | 145 | 165 | 155 | 152 |
| 3 Hour | 125 | 145 | 140 | 131 |

NSTs (also from 32 weeks' gestation) are recommended in patients with insulin-requiring gestational diabetes, with an increase to biweekly recommended after 36 weeks as well as the addition of AFI evaluation. For diet-controlled gestational diabetics, weekly NSTs are usually begun at 36 weeks. All patients should be instructed to make daily assessments of fetal movements and to alert the physician if a decrease is noted. A biophysical profile should be done if decreased movement is noted or if a nonreactive NST occurs.

In the case of abnormal fetal testing, the practitioner should assess gestational age and, if the fetus is found to be mature, should proceed to delivery. If the fetus is intermediate in maturity, amniotic fluid assessment for pulmonary maturity may assist in the decision regarding whether delivery should be effected. Lung maturity should also be assessed before elective induction if glucose control is questionable or if the fetus is less than 38 weeks unless fetal jeopardy is suspected. The lecithin/sphingomyelin ratio should be 2.5 or higher due to the higher incidence of respiratory distress in the fetus. If the fetus is immature, further testing such as contraction stress tests or hospitalization with continuous fetal heart rate monitoring is advised.

Preterm labor is increased in patients with diabetes, and they should be treated with magnesium sulfate as the initial tocolytic agent because the beta mimetics markedly influence glucose control. Corticosteroids increase maternal glucose levels, and therapy should be prescribed to keep levels into the desired range. This therapy may consist of continuous insulin infusion in certain cases.

Induction of labor is recommended at 38 weeks in patients with poor glucose control and macrosomia. Glucose control at a level < 100 mg/dL for 24 hours prior to delivery will reduce immediate neonatal hypoglycemia. Prostin gel to ripen the cervix reduces the cesarean section rate but is not advised without a negative contraction stress test if oligohydramnios is the indication for induction. Insulin-requiring diabetics should be induced at 40 weeks' gestation if spontaneous labor has not occurred. In any glucose-intolerant patient, the decision to continue pregnancy longer than 40 weeks' gestation must be carefully considered.

## NEONATAL COMPLICATIONS

Early pregnancy exposure to higher glucose levels results in enhanced rates of abortion and an increased incidence of congenital anomalies. Neonates whose mothers have higher glucose levels over a longer duration of pregnancy have higher incidences of macrosomia, hypoglycemia, hypocalcemia, polycythemia, respiratory difficulties, cardiomyopathy, and congestive heart failure. Long-term control of maternal glucose is associated with a reduction in all of these complications.

Macrosomic babies have increasing intolerance to intrauterine compromise as well as an enhanced rate of birth trauma. The original definition of neonatal hypoglycemia was glucose levels <35 mg/dL in term infants and <25 mg/dL in preterm infants. Current information suggests that hypoglycemia is present at <45 mg% in both term and preterm infants. Hypoglycemia occurs in up to 40% of the offspring of diabetic or gestational diabetic mothers. Indeed, it should be anticipated in these neonates and special monitoring initiated, since hypoglycemia may have a serious impact on fetal brain function if undetected and untreated. Hypocalcemia is defined as calcium levels <7 mg/dL and has been reported in as many as 20% of neonates with glucose-intolerant mothers. Polycythemia is a venous hematocrit >65% and increases microthrombus formation since prostacyclin production is also reduced.

Respiratory distress syndrome and transient tachypnea are increased in infants of poorly controlled diabetics. In fact, all organ maturation is delayed in direct relation to the degree of hyperglycemia. This may be compounded by impairment of maternal vascular flow to the developing fetus. Infants of inadequately controlled diabetic mothers have an increase in cardiomyopathy and congestive heart failure due to excess glycogen deposition and hypertrophy of the heart muscle as a result of intrauterine compensation for maternal hyperglycemia.

The fetal response to the intrauterine environment such as fetal pancreatic hyperplasia with increased basal insulin secretion can make an impact on the child into adulthood with an increased risk incidence of diabetes. The incidence is increased from that of the familial inheritance; for example, a recent study of Pima Indians showed that there was a greater incidence of diabetes in the offspring of women who had NIDDM during pregnancy than in the offspring of those who developed diabetes years after pregnancy (45% vs 8.6% at age 20–24 years).

## INTRAPARTUM AND POSTPARTUM MANAGEMENT

Glucose infusion (D5 Lactated Ringer's solution) is given to all patients in labor unless delivery is immediate, but care is taken to control the infusion at ~ 125 mL/hr unless the patient needs additional glucose for metabolic demands, in which case the glucose infusion is increased. It may be anticipated that women > 160 kg will require more glucose. Glucose-containing fluids should not be used for bolus prior to induction of conduction anesthesia. A bedside glucose reflectance monitor is used to follow glucose levels every 2–4 hours with the goal of maintaining levels at 70–95 mg/dL. In those requiring insulin, regular (25 U/250 mL normal saline, giving a dilution of 0.1 U/mL) is given by continuous infusion at levels of 0.5–2 U/hr.

Pitocin is given for labor induction similar to normal pregnancies. Continuous fetal monitoring is required with careful attention to decelerations. Fetal tolerance to intrauterine stress is limited in diabetic pregnancies. Early scalp pH is indicated if worrisome patterns persist. If fetal macrosomia is suspected, forceps should be used with great caution in the second stage and shoulder girdle dystocia anticipated. Additional personnel may be necessary at the time of delivery.

If repeat cesarean section or other indication for elective surgery occurs, the patient should be directed to take the evening insulin dose prior to surgery, but not her morning dose. Showering with a bacterial solution the night before delivery seems reasonable due to the increase in wound infections in this group. The patient is at increased risk of thromboembolic events due to decreased prostacyclin production on the platelets.

Breastfeeding is not affected by diabetes and is generally encouraged.

## Prognosis

Women diagnosed with gestational diabetes have an increased risk of developing diabetes mellitus in the future. If they require insulin for their pregnancy, there is a 50% risk of diabetes within 5 years. If dietary control has been sufficient, a 60% risk of developing diabetes mellitus within 10–15 years still persists. However, evidence shows that lifestyle alteration may delay or entirely prevent the onset of diabetes. Thus, these patients benefit from a reduction of their risk factors.

Postpartum, the patient should be placed back on an ADA diet (with increased soluble fiber and reduced fat). She should do a lifestyle assessment and attempt to keep her weight near ideal for her height. Weight reduction is generally necessary, and thus, if the patient is not breastfeeding, calories are reduced to 1200–1500 kcal with repeat dietary instruction, the same calorie ADA diet is continued as patient is breastfeeding. The caloric demand of breastfeeding increases with neonatal size but can reach 800–1200 kcal per day. Exercise equivalent to expend the energy is to run hard for 1 hour (900 kcal). It takes 3500 kcal expended to reduce weight by 1 pound! She should enter a regular exercise program.

All gestationally diabetic patients should have a 75-g 3-hr glucose tolerance to evaluate for preexisting diabetes. It is important to individualize a prevention program for the 98% who will have a negative test. If the 1-hr value is high, it represents decreased insulin capacity, whereas an elevated 3-hr value reflects decreased insulin receptors. With an elevated 1-hr level limiting simple sugars in the diet should become a lifetime goal. With an elevated 3-hr glucose value, weight loss with increased abdominal musculature should significantly reduce the increased risk of diabetes. Lipids should be evaluated in black and Hispanic patients because of a higher incidence of hypercholesteremia in this group. This is particularly advisable prior to initiation of oral contraceptive agents. Preconception glucose evaluation should be discussed with the patient, and she should be encouraged to have an annual fasting glucose.

## REFERENCES

Berkowitz GS, Roman SH, Lapinski RH, Alvarez M: Maternal characteristics, neonatal outcome and the time of diagnosis of gestational diabetes. Am J Obstet Gynecol 1992;167:976.

Carpenter MW, Coustan DR: Criteria for screening tests for gestational diabetes. Am J Obstet Gynecol 1982;114;768.

Coustan DR et al: A randomized clinical trial of the insulin pump vs intensive conventional therapy in diabetic pregnancies. JAMA 1986;255:631.

Datta S, Kitzmillwer JL: Anesthetic and obstetric management of diabetic pregnant women. Clin Perinatal 1982;9:153.

Dicker D, Feldberg D, Yeshaya A et al: Fetal surveillance in insulin-dependent diabetic pregnancy: Predictive value of the biophysical profile. Am J Obstet Gynecol 1988;159:800.

Dickinson J, Palmer SM: Gestational diabetes. Semin Perinatol 1990;14(1):24.

Fuhrmann K et al: Prevention of congenital malformations in infants of insulin-dependent diabetic mothers. Diabetes Care 1983;6:219.

Hollingsworth DR: Maternal metabolism in normal pregnancy and pregnancy complicated by diabetes mellitus. Clin Obstet Gynecol 1985;28:457.

Karlsson K, Kjellmer I: The outcome of diabetic pregnancies in relation to the mother's blood sugar level. Am J Obstet Gynecol 112;213.

Kinje JC, Otolorin EO, Ladipo OA: The effect of continuous subdermal levonorgestrel (Norplant) on carbohydrate metabolism. Am J Obstet Gynecol 1992;166:15.

Kitzmiller JL: Diabetes ketoacidosis and pregnancy. Contemp Obstet Gynecol 1982;20(1):141.

Kjos SL: Contraception in women with diabetes mellitus. Diabetes Spec 1993;6(2):80.

Klebe JG, Espersen T, Allen J: Diabetes mellitus and pregnancy. A seven year material of pregnant diabetics, where control during pregnancy was based on a centralized ambulant regime. Acta Obstet Gynecol Scand 1986;65(3):235.

Landon MB, Gabbe SC, Piana R et al: Neonatal morbidity in pregnancy complicated by diabetes mellitus: Predictive value of maternal glycemic profiles. Am J Obstet Gynecol 1987;156:1089.

Langer O, Brustman L, Anyaegbunam A et al: The significance of one abnormal glucose tolerance test value on adverse outcome in pregnancy. Am J Obstet Gynecol 1987;157:758.

Levenno KJ, Fortunato SJ, Raskin P et al: Continuous subcutaneous insulin infusion during pregnancy. Diabetes Res Clin Pract 1988;4(4):257.

Martin AO, Simpson JL, Ober C et al: Frequency of diabetes mellitus in mothers of probands with gestational diabetes: Possible maternal influence on the predisposition to gestational diabetes. Am J Obstet Gynecol 1985; 151:471.

Meyer BA, Palmer SM: Pregestational diabetes. Semin Perinatol 1990;14(1)12.

Mills JL: Malformations in infants of diabetic mothers. Teratology 1982;25:385.

Mimouni F, Miodovnik M, Tsang RC et al: Decreased maternal serum magnesium concentration and adverse fetal outcome in insulin-dependent diabetic women. Obstet Gynecol 1987;70:85.

National Diabetes Data Group: Classification and diagnosis of diabetes mellitus. Washington, DC: National Institutes of Health, 1986.

Ney D, Hollingsworth DR, Cousins L: Decreased insulin requirements and improved control of diabetes in pregnant women given high carbohydrate, high fiber, low fat diet. Diabetes Care 1982;5(5):529.

O'Sullivan JB, Mahan CM: Criteria for the oral glucose tolerance test in pregnancy. Diabetes 1964;13:278.

Olofsson P, Sjoberg NO, Solum T: Fetal surveillance in diabetic pregnancy. II. The nonstress test versus the oxyto-cin challenge test. Acta Obstet Gynecol Scand 1986; 65(4):357.

Rasmussen MJ, Firth R, Foley M, Stronge JM: The timing of delivery in diabetic pregnancy: A 10-year review. Aust N Z Obstet Gynaecol 1992;32(4):313.

Reece EA, Coustan DR (editors): *Diabetes mellitus in pregnancy principles and practice.* Churchill Livingstone, 1990.

Riley WJ, MaClaren NK, Krischer J et al: A prospective study of the development of diabetes in relatives of patients with insulin-dependent diabetes. N Engl J Med 1990;323:1167.

Sacks DA, Abu FS, Greenspoon JS, Fotheringham N: Do the current standards for glucose tolerance testing represent a valid conversion of O'Sullivan's original criteria? Am J Obstet Gynecol 1989;161:638.

Spirito A, Williams C, Ruggiero L et al: Psychological impact of the diagnosis of gestational diabetes. Obstet Gynecol 1989;73:562.

Stowers JM, Sutherland HW, Kerridge DF: Long range implications for the mother. The Aberdeen experience. Diabetes (Suppl 2) 1985;34:106.

Tallarigo L, Giampietro O, Penno G et al: Relation of glucose tolerance to complications of pregnancy in non-diabetic women. N Engl J Med 1986;315:989.

Tamura RK, Sabbagha RE, Dooley SL et al: Real-time ultrasound estimations of weight in fetuses of diabetic gravid women. Am J Obstet Gynecol 1985;153:57.

Teramo K, Ammala P, Ylinen K et al: Pathologic fetal heart rate associated with poor metabolic control in diabetic pregnancies. Obstet Gynecol 1983;61:559.

Wein P, Warwick MM, Beischer NA: Gestational diabetes in twin pregnancy: prevalence and long-term implications. Aust N Z Obstet Gynaecol 1992;32(4):325.

# Hypertensive States of Pregnancy

*William C. Mabie, MD, & Baha M. Sibai, MD*

Hypertensive states in pregnancy include pre-eclampsia-eclampsia, chronic hypertension (either essential or secondary to renal disease, endocrine disease, or other causes), chronic hypertension with superimposed preeclampsia, and transient hypertension (Table 19–1). **Preeclampsia** is a triad of edema, hypertension, and proteinuria occurring primarily in nulliparas after the 20th gestational week and most frequently near term. **Eclampsia** is the occurrence of seizures that cannot be attributed to other causes in a preeclamptic patient. **Chronic hypertension** is defined as hypertension that is present before conception, before 20 weeks' gestation or that persists for more than 6 weeks postpartum. Hypertension is defined as a blood pressure equal to or greater than 140/90 mm Hg. Proteinuria is defined as the excretion of 300 mg or more in a 24-hour specimen. Preeclampsia may occur in women with chronic hypertension (**superimposed preeclampsia**); the prognosis is worse for the mother and fetus than with either condition alone. The criteria for superimposed preeclampsia are worsening hypertension (30 mm Hg systolic or 15 mm Hg diastolic above the average of values before 20 weeks' gestation) together with either nondependent edema or proteinuria. **Transient hypertension** is the development of hypertension after midpregnancy or in the first 24 hours postpartum without other signs of preeclampsia or preexisting hypertension. This condition is often predictive of the later development of essential hypertension. Transient hypertension is a retrospective diagnosis and, if uncertainty exists regarding the diagnosis, these patients should be managed as if they had preeclampsia.

It is frequently difficult to determine whether a patient has preeclampsia, chronic hypertension, or chronic hypertension with superimposed preeclampsia. This is partly because blood pressure normally decreases during the second trimester, and the decrease may mask the presence of chronic hypertension. Renal biopsy studies have shown that only about 70% of primigravidas under 25 years of age with the triad of edema, hypertension, and proteinuria have **glomeruloendotheliosis,** the characteristic lesion of preeclampsia. Twenty-five percent have unsuspected renal disease. In multiparas with chronic hypertension with superimposed preeclampsia, about 3% have glomeruloendotheliosis and 21% have underlying renal disease. Renal biopsy is rarely performed in pregnancy because the benefit usually does not justify the risk. The sensitivity and specificity of biochemical markers such as uric acid, antithrombin III, serum iron, and digoxinlike immunoreactive substance are unknown.

## PREECLAMPSIA

Preeclampsia occurs in about 6% of the general population; the incidence varies with geographic location. Predisposing factors are nulliparity, black race, maternal age below 20 or over 35 years, low socioeconomic status, multiple gestation, hydatidiform mole, polyhydramnios, nonimmune fetal hydrops, diabetes, chronic hypertension, and underlying renal disease.

### Classification

There are 2 categories of preeclampsia, mild and severe. Severe and mild preeclampsia are differentiated by the following criteria: (1) blood pressure greater than 160 mm Hg systolic or 110 mm Hg diastolic; (2) proteinuria exceeding 5 g in a 24-hour period or 3–4+ on dipstick testing; (3) increased serum creatinine (> 1.2 mg/dL unless known to be elevated previously); (4) cerebral or visual disturbances; (5) epigastric pain, (6) elevated liver enzymes; (7) thrombocytopenia (platelet count <100,000/mm³); (8) retinal hemorrhages, exudates, or papilledema; and (9) pulmonary edema.

### Pathogenesis

Chesley (1978) described preeclampsia as a "disease of theories," because the cause is unknown. Some theories include (1) endothelial cell injury, (2) rejection phenomenon (insufficient production of blocking antibodies), (3) compromised placental perfusion, (4) altered vascular reactivity, (5) imbalance

**Table 19–1.** Hypertensive states of pregnancy other than preeclampsia-eclampsia.

**Chronic essential hypertension**
**Chronic hypertension due to renal disease**
  Interstitial nephritis
  Acute and chronic glomerulonephritis
  Systemic lupus erythematosus
  Diabetic glomerulosclerosis
  Scleroderma
  Polyarteritis nodosa
  Polycystic kidney disease
  Renovascular stenosis
  Chronic renal failure with treatment by dialysis
  Renal transplant
**Chronic hypertension due to endocrine disease**
  Cushing's disease and syndrome
  Primary hyperaldosteronism
  Thyrotoxicosis
  Pheochromocytoma
  Acromegaly
**Chronic hypertension due to coarctation of the aorta**

between prostacyclin and thromboxane, (6) decreased glomerular filtration rate with retention of salt and water, (7) decreased intravascular volume, (8) increased central nervous system irritability, (9) disseminated intravascular coagulation, (10) uterine muscle stretch (ischemia), (11) dietary factors, and (12) genetic factors. The relatively new theory of endothelial injury explains many of the clinical findings in preeclampsia. The theory emphasizes that there is more to preeclampsia than hypertension. The vascular endothelium produces a number of important substances including endothelial-derived relaxing factor or nitric oxide, endothelin-1, prostacyclin, and tissue plasminogen activator. Thus, endothelial cells modify the contractile response of the underlying smooth muscle cells, prevent intravascular coagulation, and maintain the integrity of the intravascular compartment. Several findings suggest endothelial injury in preeclampsia. The characteristic renal lesion of preeclampsia "glomeruloendotheliosis" is manifested primarily by swelling of the glomerular capillary endothelial cells. The hematologic changes of preeclampsia, ie, thrombocytopenia and microangiopathic hemolytic anemia, are similar to those found in thrombotic thrombocytopenic purpura or hemolytic uremic syndrome—disorders in which endothelial dysfunction is thought to be important. Activation of the clotting cascade and increased sensitivity to pressors are compatible with endothelial cell dysfunction. Biochemical evidence includes an imbalance in the prostacyclin-thromboxane ratio and high circulating concentrations of von Willebrand factor, endothelin, and cellular fibronectin. Serum from preeclamptic women, when applied to human umbilical vein endothelial cell cultures, produces no morphologic abnormalities in the cells but releases procoagulants, vasoconstrictors, and mitogens.

In summary, the current hypothesis for the patho-genesis of preeclampsia is that an immunologic disturbance causes abnormal placental implantation resulting in decreased placental perfusion. The abnormal perfusion stimulates the production of substances in the blood that activate or injure endothelial cells. The vascular endothelium provides a single target for these blood-borne products, which explains the multiple organ system involvement in preeclampsia.

### Pathophysiology

**A. Central Nervous System:** Tissues are capable of regulating their own blood flow; this process is known as **autoregulation.** Cerebral perfusion is maintained by autoregulation at a constant level of about 55 mL/min/100 g at a wide range of blood pressures (Fig 19–1). However, blood pressure may rise to levels at which autoregulation cannot function. When this occurs, the endothelial tight junctions open, causing plasma and red blood cells to leak into the extravascular space. This may result in petechial hemorrhage or gross intracranial hemorrhage. The upper limit of autoregulation varies from one person to another; eg, chronic hypertension may cause medial hypertrophy of the cerebral vessels, resulting in a shift of the curve to the right (Fig 19–1). This explains the paradox of 2 patients with equally severe hypertension who have markedly different clinical presentations. The young primigravida whose blood pressure is normally 110/70 mm Hg may convulse with a blood pressure of 180/120 mm Hg, while a chronic hypertensive may be asymptomatic or have only a headache at the same pressure.

The mechanism of the cerebral damage in eclampsia is unclear. The pathologic findings are similar to those of hypertensive encephalopathy. These abnormalities include fibrinoid necrosis and thrombosis of

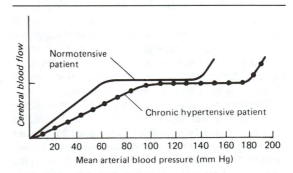

**Figure 19–1.** Representation of the relationship between cerebral blood flow and mean arterial blood pressure. Cerebral blood flow normally remains constant at mean arterial pressures of 60–140 mm Hg. In chronically hypertensive patients, medial hypertrophy causes the lower and upper limits of autoregulation to be shifted to higher blood pressure values. (Modified and reproduced, with permission from Donaldson JO: *Neurology of Pregnancy.* Saunders, 1978.)

arterioles, microinfarcts, and petechial hemorrhages. In both hypertensive encephalopathy and eclampsia, the lesions are widely distributed throughout the brain, but the brainstem is more severely affected in the former, while the cortex is more severely affected in the latter. Other differences in the two conditions are that eclampsia may be seen in the absence of hypertension and that retinal hemorrhages and infarcts are rare in eclampsia. Two theories have been proposed to explain the pathogenesis of hypertensive encephalopathy, vasospasm, and forced dilation. In the first, vasospasm causes local ischemia, arteriolar necrosis, and disruption of the blood-brain barrier. According to the second, as blood pressure rises above the limit of autoregulation, cerebral vasodilation occurs. Initially, some vessel segments dilate, and some remain constricted. Overdistension of the dilated segments results in necrosis of the medial muscle fibers and damage to the vessel wall. It is possible that both mechanisms are operant.

The presence of cerebral edema in preeclampsia-eclampsia is controversial. Sheehan and Lynch (1973) stated that cerebral edema was not present in eclamptic patients when autopsy was performed within 1 hour of death and that such edema was a late postmortem change. In contrast, Richards et al found generalized cerebral edema in some autopsy specimens and confirmed increased intracranial pressure in eclamptics with prolonged coma (>6 hours). Early studies of cerebrospinal fluid opening pressure showed elevated pressures; however, more recent studies have failed to confirm this.

Head computed tomographic (CT) scans in women with eclampsia have shown abnormalities in about one-third. By using fourth-generation equipment and with a short interval from seizure to CT scan, abnormalities may be detected in half the patients. The main findings are focal hypodensities in the white matter in the posterior half of the cerebral hemispheres with occasional lesions in the gray matter, temporal lobes, and brainstem. Brown et al suggested that these areas of radiographic hypodensity represented petechial hemorrhages accompanied by local edema. Subarachnoid or intraventricular hemorrhages may be seen in the most severe cases.

Magnetic resonance imaging (MRI) is more sensitive at demonstrating abnormalities than CT scan, but it is not as widely available. $T_2$-weighed MRI scans show high signal in the cortical and subcortical white matter. Most of the abnormalities lie in the occipital and parietal areas in watershed areas where the anterior, middle, and posterior circulations meet. Basal ganglia and brainstem abnormalities occur in more critically ill patients.

Cerebral angiography has been performed in a few patients with eclampsia, revealing diffuse arterial vasoconstriction.

Electroencephalograms (EEGs) show nonspecific abnormalities in about 75% of patients after eclamptic seizures. The pattern is usually a diffuse slowing of activity (theta or delta waves), sometimes with focal slow activity and occasional paroxysmal spike activity. These abnormalities may be seen in other conditions, such as hypoxia, renal disease, polycythemia, hypocalcemia, and water intoxication. The electroencephalographic pattern is unaffected by magnesium sulfate. It gradually returns to normal 6–8 weeks postpartum. Uncomplicated eclampsia causes no permanent neurologic deficit.

**B. Eyes:** Both serous retinal detachment and cortical blindness may occur.

**C. Pulmonary System:** Pulmonary edema may occur with severe preeclampsia or eclampsia. It may be cardiogenic or noncardiogenic and usually occurs postpartum. In some cases it may be related to excessive fluid administration or to delayed mobilization of extravascular fluid. It may also be related to decreased plasma colloid oncotic pressure from proteinuria, use of crystalloids to replace blood loss, and decreased hepatic synthesis of albumin. Pulmonary edema is particularly common in patients with underlying chronic hypertension and hypertensive heart disease, which may be manifested by systolic dysfunction, diastolic dysfunction, or both. Aspiration of gastric contents is one of the most dreaded complications of eclamptic seizures. This may result in death because of asphyxia from particulate matter plugging major airways or in chemical pneumonitis from aspirated gastric acid. Aspiration may cause various types of pneumonia, ranging from patchy pneumonitis to full-blown adult respiratory distress syndrome.

**D. Cardiovascular System:** Plasma volume is reduced in patients with preeclampsia. Normal physiologic volume expansion does not occur, possibly because of generalized vasoconstriction, capillary leak, or some other factor. Because the cause of the reduced volume is unknown, management is controversial. One theory is that the decreased volume is a primary event causing a chronic shocklike state. Hypertension is thought to be the result of release of a pressor substance from the hypoperfused uterus or of compensatory secretion of catecholamines. Proponents of this theory advocate avoidance of diuretics and use of volume expanders. Another theory is that decreased volume is secondary to vasoconstriction. Proponents of this theory advocate the use of vasodilators and warn that volume expanders may aggravate hypertension or cause pulmonary edema.

Studies using the Swan-Ganz catheter have demonstrated a spectrum of hemodynamic findings in preeclampsia ranging from a low-output, high-resistance state to a high-output, low-resistance state. The two extremes are exemplified by the studies of Wallenburg et al and Mabie et al. Wallenburg found a low wedge pressure, low cardiac output, and high systemic vascular resistance in 44 untreated nulliparous preeclamptic women, while in 22 patients who have received various therapies and were usually referred, a wide range of hemodynamics was found. He concluded that the untreated preeclamptic patient was significantly volume-depleted and that the wide spectrum of hemodynamic findings in the treated group resulted from prior therapy and the presence of other variables such as labor, multiparity, and preexisting hypertension.

Mabie et al studied the hemodynamics of 49 subjects with severe preeclampsia at a large referral center. Despite a heterogeneous population of pretreated and nonpretreated patients, a generally consistent profile emerged. Preeclampsia was in general a high cardiac output state associated with an inappropriately high peripheral resistance. Although the systemic vascular resistance was within the normal range for pregnancy, it was still inappropriately high for the elevated cardiac output. The failure of the circulation to dilate in the setting of increasing cardiac output appeared to be a characteristic feature of preeclampsia. The normal wedge and central venous pressures found in their study suggested venoconstriction with central relocation of intravascular volume if the generally accepted reports of decreased plasma volume in preeclampsia are correct. They postulated splanchnic venoconstriction as the mechanism of this volume shift.

Normal pregnant women are resistant to the vasoconstrictor effects of angiotensin II. Pregnant women require about 2½ times the amount of angiotensin II required by nonpregnant women to raise the diastolic blood pressure 20 mm Hg. Patients who will develop superimposed preeclampsia lose their refractoriness to angiotensin II many weeks before hypertension develops. These patients may be identified as early as 18–24 weeks' gestation by infusion of angiotensin II.

Normal pregnant women lose their refractoriness to angiotensin II after treatment with prostaglandin synthetase inhibitors such as aspirin or indomethacin; this suggests that prostaglandin is involved in mediating vascular reactivity to angiotensin II in pregnancy. Refractoriness to angiotensin II can be restored in patients with preeclampsia by the administration of theophylline, a phosphodiesterase inhibitor that increases intracellular levels of cAMP. Therefore, prostaglandins synthesized in the arteriole may modulate vascular reactivity to angiotensin II by altering the intracellular level of cAMP in vascular smooth muscle.

**E. Liver:** The spectrum of liver disease in preeclampsia is broad, ranging from subclinical involvement with the only manifestation being fibrin deposition along the hepatic sinusoids to rupture of the liver. Within these extremes lie the **HELLP syndrome** (Hemolysis, elevated liver enzymes, and low platelets) and hepatic infarction.

**F. Kidneys:** The characteristic lesion of preeclampsia, **glomeruloendotheliosis,** is a swelling of the glomerular capillary endothelium that causes decreased glomerular perfusion and glomerular filtration rate. Fibrin split products have been found on the basement membrane by some observers, who have suggested that intravascular coagulation may be secondary to thromboplastin released from the placenta. However, the fibrin split products are found infrequently and only in small amounts. Other investigators have detected IgM, IgG, and complement in the glomeruli of some patients and have suggested an immunologic mechanism. Serial renal biopsies have shown that the lesion is totally reversible over about 6 weeks.

**G. Blood:** Most patients with preeclampsia-eclampsia have normal clotting studies. In some, a spectrum of abnormalities may be found, ranging from isolated thrombocytopenia to microangiopathic hemolytic anemia to disseminated intravascular coagulation (DIC). Thrombocytopenia is the commonest abnormality; a count of less than 150,000/μL is found in 15–20% of patients. Fibrinogen levels are actually elevated in preeclamptic women as compared with normotensive patients. Low fibrinogen levels in preeclampsia-eclampsia are usually associated with placental abruptio or fetal demise. Elevated fibrin split products are seen in 20% of patients (usually in the range of 10–40 μL/mL). Microangiopathic hemolytic anemia without other signs of DIC may be seen in about 5% of patients, and evidence of DIC is also present in about 5%. In the past, DIC was thought to be the cause of preeclampsia; now it is regarded as a sequela of the disease. There has been considerable speculation that infants of mothers with DIC may have DIC at birth because of an immunologic factor that crosses the placenta. However, current evidence indicates that coagulation abnormalities in the newborn are more a function of associated neonatal complications such as prematurity, growth retardation, acidosis, intraventricular hemorrhage, and polycythemia.

The HELLP syndrome (Weinstein, 1982) describes patients with hemolytic anemia, elevated liver enzymes, and low platelet count. Criteria for the diagnosis at the authors' institution are schistocytes on the peripheral blood smear, lactic dehydrogenase >600 U/L, total bilirubin >1.2 mg/dL, aspartate aminotransferase >70 U/L, and platelet count <100,000/mm$^3$. This syndrome is present in about 10% of patients with severe preeclampsia-eclampsia. It is frequently seen in Caucasian patients with delay in diagnosis or delivery and in patients with abruptio placentae. The syndrome may occur remote from term (eg, at 31 weeks) and with no elevation of blood pressure. The syndrome is frequently misdiagnosed as hepatitis, gallbladder disease, idiopathic thrombocytopenic purpura, or thrombotic thrombocytopenic purpura. Most hematologic abnormalities return to normal within 2–3 days after delivery, but thrombocytopenia may persist for a week.

**H. Endocrine System:** The role of the renin-angiotensin-aldosterone system in the regulation of blood pressure during normal and hypertensive pregnancy has not been clearly defined. In normal pregnancy, estrogen's effect on the liver markedly increases production of renin substrate. This increases plasma renin activity, plasma renin concentration, and angiotensin II levels. Plasma aldosterone levels rise even higher than can be accounted for by the prevailing plasma renin activity. Despite the high plasma concentration of aldosterone, there is no blood pressure increase or hypokalemia in normal pregnancy; indeed, blood pressure falls in the midtrimester. This may be due to counterregulatory factors such as the natriuretic effect of progesterone or activation of vasodepressor systems such as kinins or prostaglandins.

Interpreting renin, angiotensin, and aldosterone levels in studies of preeclampsia is difficult because of differences in the definition of preeclampsia (parity, degree of proteinuria, early- or late-onset disease), differences in taking of blood samples (values may be affected by bed rest, sodium intake, labor, etc), and differences in assay techniques. In the majority of studies, renin, angiotensin, and aldosterone are all suppressed in preeclampsia, but they are still above nonpregnant levels. The available evidence suggests that the renin-angiotensin system is only secondarily involved in preeclampsia.

Atrial natriuretic peptide (ANP) is a volume regulatory hormone synthesized by cardiac myocytes, which has potent natriuretic, diuretic, and vasorelaxant properties. ANP secretion is stimulated by increased atrial pressure and alterations in sodium balance. Elevated concentrations of ANP accompany pathologic states characterized by fluid overload such as cirrhosis, congestive heart failure, and chronic renal failure. However, ANP is elevated in preeclampsia, a disorder supposedly characterized by hypovolemia. It is even elevated in the second trimester before the onset of clinical evidence of preeclampsia. The mechanism for the elevated is unknown. It may be that endothelin or another vasoactive peptide is stimulating release of ANP. It may also be that the widely accepted concept of central hypovolemia in preeclampsia is incorrect.

**I. Catecholamines:** Urinary and blood catecholamine levels are the same in normotensive pregnant women, women with preeclampsia, and nonpregnant controls. However, it cannot be ruled out that sympathetic activity is of pathogenetic importance for initiation or maintenance of hypertension in patients with preeclampsia. Catecholamine levels increase during labor, presumably owing to stress. The vascular refractoriness to catecholamines is lacking in preeclampsia, as is the refractoriness to other endogenous vasopressors such as antidiuretic hormone and angiotensin II.

**J. Metabolic Clearance Rate of Dehydroepiandrosterone Sulfate:** Studies of the metabolic clearance rate of dehydroepiandrosterone sulfate (DHEAS) have added to our understanding of the pathogenesis of preeclampsia. It is thought that the metabolic clearance rate of DHEAS reflects placental blood flow, though some investigators have challenged this hypothesis. Researchers have found that in patients destined to develop preeclampsia, the metabolic clearance rate of DHEAS falls before the onset of preeclampsia. This has been interpreted to mean that blood flow through the placenta decreases prior to the onset of hypertension. The metabolic clearance rate of DHEAS is also decreased by chronic thiazide, acute furosemide, and acute hydrazaline therapy in both normal and preeclamptic patients.

**K. Prostacyclin:** Prostacyclin is a prostaglandin discovered by Vane et al in 1976. It increases intracellular cyclic AMP in smooth muscle cells and platelets resulting in vasodilator and platelet antiaggregatory effects. Its half-life is about 3 minutes, breaking down in plasma to 6-keto-$PGF_{1\alpha}$, which is stable and can be measured as an indication of prostacyclin levels. These plasma levels are low, indicating that prostacyclin acts physiologically at the local level rather than as a circulating hormone.

Prostacyclin is made primarily in the endothelial cell from arachidonic acid, catalyzed by the enzyme cyclooxygenase. Cyclooxygenase can be inhibited by aspirin-like drugs. Mechanical or chemical perturbation of the endothelial cell membrane stimulated formation and release of prostacyclin. For example, pulsatile pressure or chemicals such as bradykinin or thrombin stimulate prostacyclin generation in the vessel wall.

Thromboxane $A_2$ generated by platelets from arachidonic acid via cyclooxygenase induces vasoconstriction and platelet aggregation. Thus, prostacyclin and thromboxane have opposing roles in regulating platelet-vessel wall interaction.

Aspirin irreversibly inhibits cyclooxygenase. Cyclooxygenase must be produced continuously by endothelial cells, because they recover their ability to synthesize prostacyclin within a few hours after a dose of aspirin. On the other hand, platelets do not have a nucleus and therefore cannot make fresh cyclooxygenase. Thromboxane synthesis recovers only as new platelets enter the circulation. Platelet life span is about 1 week. Thus, daily treatment with low-dose aspirin results in chronic inhibition of thromboxane metabolites and decreased excretion of prostacyclin metabolites in preeclamptic patients. Low-dose aspirin therapy is aimed at restoring the presumed thromboxane-prostacyclin imbalance in preeclampsia.

**L. Endothelium-Derived Relaxing Factor:** First described in 1980, endothelium-derived relaxing factor (EDRF) is an endogenous nitrovasodilator thought to be identical to nitric oxide. EDRF is produced by endothelial cells from L-arginine. It relaxes vascular smooth muscle and inhibits platelet aggregation by elevating the intracellular level of cyclic GMP. Synthesis can be inhibited by arginine analogs such as $N^G$-monomethyl-L-arginine and $N^G$-nitro-L-arginine. Intravenous injection of one of these inhibitors into rats, rabbits, or guinea pigs causes an immediate rise in blood pressure that is reversed by L-arginine. This indicates that continual basal release of EDRF from endothelial cells keeps the vasculature in a dilated state. EDRF acts only in the immediate vicinity of the cell that releases it. Any that escapes into the bloodstream decays chemically to form nitrite or is immediately inactivated by hemoglobin.

EDRF plays an important role in several pathologic processes. It is one of the mediators of hypotension in septic shock. A deficiency of EDRF contributes to the cause of hypertension and atherosclerosis. Currently it is thought that the EDRF system may be more important than the prostaglandins in the pathogenesis of preeclampsia. In the genetically hypertensive spontaneously hypertensive rate, increased EDRF production is responsible for the profound antihypertensive effect of gestation. Chronic blockade of the endogenous EDRF system produces a model of hypertension and renal damage in pregnant and nonpregnant rats.

**M. Endothelin-1:** In addition to the relaxing factors prostacyclin and EDRF, the vascular endothelium releases vasoconstrictor substances. The vasoconstrictor endothelin was discovered in 1988. There are 3 different isopeptides: endothelin 1,2, and 3. Endothelin-1 is the only endothelin manufactured by endothelial cells. Endothelins are also synthesized by kidney cells and nervous tissue. There are widespread endothelin binding sites including those in the brain, lung, kidney, adrenal, spleen, intestine, and placenta. It is thought that endothelins act as endogenous agonists of dihydropyridine—sensitive calcium channels. The most striking property of endothelin-1 is its long-lasting vasoconstrictor action. It is 10 times more potent than angiotensin II. Endothelin may play a role in constriction of placental vessels after delivery and may regulate closure of the ductus arteriosus in the newborn. The mitogenic effects of endothelin-1 may cause vascular wall hypertrophy in atherosclerosis and hypertension. Endothelin-1 may play a role in renal vasoconstriction in acute renal failure. A 3-fold elevation of plasma endothelin 1 and 2 has been found in women with preeclampsia compared with gestation-matched controls.

The current working hypothesis of Vane and Botting is that prostacyclin is an antiplatelet and vasodilator mechanism held in reserve to reinforce the EDRF system when endothelial damage occurs. Lack of EDRF may be a causative factor in hypertension. Endothelin-1 is released by endothelial cells to constrict the underlying smooth muscle in an emergency such as laceration. Excess endothelin-1 may also be involved in the genesis of hypertension.

**N. Placenta:** In normal pregnancy, the proliferating trophoblast invades the decidua and the adjacent myometrium in 2 forms: interstitial and endovascular. The role of the interstitial form is not clear but it may serve to anchor the placenta. The endovascular trophoblastic cells invade the maternal spiral arteries, where they replace the endothelium and destroy the medial elastic and muscular tissue of the arterial wall. The arterial wall is replaced by fibrinoid material. This process is complete by the end of the first trimester, at which time it extends to the deciduomyometrial junction. There appears to be a resting phase in the process until 14 to 16 weeks' gestation, when a second wave of trophoblastic invasion extends down the lumen of the spiral arteries to their origin from the radial arteries deep in the myometrium. The same process is then repeated ie, replacement of the endothelium, destruction of the medial musculoelastic tissue, and fibrinoid change in the vessel wall. The end result is that the thin-walled, muscular spiral arteries are converted to saclike, flaccid uteroplacental vessels, which passively dilate to accommodate the greatly augmented blood flow required in pregnancy (Fig 19–2).

Preeclampsia develops following a partial failure in the process of placentation. First, not all the spiral arteries of the placental bed are invaded by trophoblast. Second, in those arteries that are invaded, the first phase of trophoblastic invasion occurs normally, but the second phase does not occur, and the myometrial portions of the spiral arteries retain their reactive musculoelastic walls.

In addition, acute atherosis (a lesion similar to atherosclerosis) develops in the myometrial segments of the spiral arteries of patients with preeclampsia. The lesion is characterized by fibrinoidnecrosis of the arterial wall, the presence of lipid and lipophages in the damaged wall, and a mononuclear cell infiltrate around the damaged vessel. Acute atherosis may progress to vessel obliteration with corresponding areas of placental infarction.

Thus, in preeclampsia there is an area of vascular resistance in the spiral artery because of failure of the second wave of trophoblastic invasion. In addition, acute atherosis further compromises the vascular lumen. Consequently, the fetus is subjected to poor intervillous blood flow from the time of early gestation; this may result in intrauterine growth retardation or stillbirth. Antihypertensive therapy may be detrimental because peripheral vasodilatation may further reduce the already compromised placental blood flow.

### Clinical Findings

#### A. Symptoms and Signs:

**1. Edema—**Dependent edema is a normal finding in pregnancy, but nondependent edema of the hands and face present upon morning arising is considered pathologic. Weight gain in excess of 2 lb/week or particularly sudden weight gain over 1 or 2 days should raise the suspicion of preeclampsia. Preeclampsia may occur without edema; 39% of eclamptic patients in one series had no edema.

**2. Hypertension—**Hypertension is the most im-

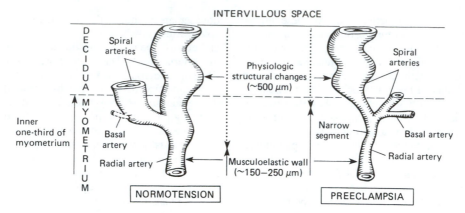

INTERVILLOUS SPACE

**Figure 19–2.** The placental bed in normal and preeclamptic pregnancy. In preeclampsia, the physiologic changes in the uteroplacental arteries do not extend beyond the deciduomyometrial junction, leaving a constricting segment between the radial artery and the decidual portions. (Reproduced, with permission, from Brosens IA: Morphological changes in the uteroplacental bed in pregnancy hypertension. Clin Obstet Gynaecol 1977;4:573.)

portant criterion for the diagnosis of preeclampsia. This too may occur suddenly. Many young primigravidas have blood pressure readings of 100–110/60–70 mm Hg during the second trimester. An increase of 15 mm Hg in the diastolic or 30 mm Hg in the systolic pressure should be considered ominous. Thus, in these patients, blood pressures of 120/80 mm Hg may be relative hypertension. The blood pressure is often quite labile. It usually falls during sleep in patients with mild preeclampsia and chronic hypertension, but in patients with severe preeclampsia, blood pressure may increase during sleep, eg, the most severe hypertension may occur at 2:00 AM.

**3. Proteinuria–**Proteinuria is the last sign to develop. Eclampsia may occur without proteinuria. Sibai (1982) and associates found no proteinuria in 29% of one series of eclamptic patients. Most patients with proteinuria will have glomeruloendotheliosis on kidney biopsy. Proteinuria in preeclampsia is an indicator of fetal jeopardy. The incidence of SGA infants and perinatal mortality is markedly increased in patients with proteinuric preeclampsia.

**4. Differing clinical picture in preeclampsia crises–**Preeclampsia-eclampsia is a multisystem disease with varying clinical presentations. One patient may present with eclamptic seizures, another with liver dysfunction and intrauterine growth retardation, another with pulmonary edema, still another with abruptio placenta and renal failure, and another with ascites and anasarca.

**B. Laboratory Findings:** The hemoglobin and hematocrit may be elevated due to hemoconcentration, or in more severe cases, there may be anemia secondary to hemolysis. Thrombocytopenia is often present. Fibrin split products and decreased coagulation factors may be detected. Uric acid is usually elevated above 6 mg/dL. Serum creatinine is most often normal (0.6–0.8 mg/dL) but may be elevated in se-

vere preeclampsia. Although hepatic abnormalities occur in about 10% of patients, the bilirubin is usually below 5 mg/dL and the aspartate aminotransferase (AST) below 500 IU. Alkaline phosphatase may increase 2- to 3-fold. Lactate dehydrogenase may be quite high (because of hemolysis or liver injury). Blood glucose and electrolytes are normal. Urinalysis reveals proteinuria and occasional hyaline casts.

### Differential Diagnosis
See Table 19–1.

### Complications
Preeclampsia may be associated with early delivery and fetal complications due to prematurity. Fetal risks include acute and chronic uteroplacental insufficiency. In the most severe cases, this may result in intrapartum fetal distress or stillbirth. Chronic uteroplacental insufficiency increases the risk of an asymmetric (cranial-sparing) or symmetric SGA fetus.

### Prevention
More than 100 clinical, biophysical, and biochemical tests have been reported to predict preeclampsia. Unfortunately, most suffer from poor sensitivity, and none are suitable for routine use as a screening test in clinical practice. As a result, most studies of prevention have used patients with various risk factors for preeclampsia.

**A. Calcium Supplementation:** Several authors have reported reduced urinary excretion of calcium during preeclampsia and for several weeks prior to the onset of clinically apparent disease. In addition, abnormal intracellular calcium metabolism in platelets and red blood cells has been demonstrated in women with preeclampsia as compared with normotensive pregnant women. Moreover, Belizan and associates reported an inverse association between calcium intake and maternal blood pressure and the incidences of preeclampsia and eclampsia.

There are 8 clinical studies comparing the use of calcium with no treatment or with placebo in pregnancy. Two of these studies compared calcium with no treatment. One study used 156 mg of elemental calcium and reported a significant reduction in the incidence of preeclampsia (4.5% in the calcium group versus 21.2% in the untreated group). The other study compared the use of 375 mg of calcium plus 1200 IU/day of vitamin D with no supplementation. The incidence of preeclampsia in the supplemented group was 6%, which was similar to the incidence in the nonsupplemented group, ie, 9%.

Six other trials were placebo-controlled, and the dose of calcium was 1500–2000 mg/day. The results of these studies suggest that calcium supplementation reduces the incidence of transient hypertension with a trend toward reducing the incidence of preeclampsia. Currently, a large multicenter study sponsored by the National Institute of Child Health and Human Development is underway to address the issue.

**B. Aspirin:** There is evidence to suggest that thromboxane $A_2$ production is markedly increased, while prostacyclin production is reduced in women with well-established preeclampsia and prior to the onset of preeclampsia. In addition, placental infarcts and thrombosis of the spiral arteries have been demonstrated in pregnancies complicated by preeclampsia, particularly in those with severe fetal growth retardation or fetal demise. As a result of these findings, several authors have used various antithrombotic agents in an attempt to prevent preeclampsia.

There have been several randomized trials comparing the use of low-dose aspirin with or without dipyridamole versus placebo in women at risk for preeclampsia. The dose of aspirin ranged from 50 mg to 150 mg daily. Gestational age at enrollment ranged from 12 to 29 weeks' gestation. It is important to note that all these studies had a limited sample size and included patients with various risk factors for preeclampsia. The initial results were promising and were confirmed by meta-analysis. However, two larger trials failed to confirm the benefits (Sibai et al, 1993; Italian Study of Aspirin in Pregnancy, 1993). Both differed from the earlier trials in that low-risk women were recruited. So the place of aspirin in preeclampsia prevention is uncertain. It may be that the benefits are confined to high-risk women. A further matter of concern is the higher incidence of abruptio placenta in the aspirin-treated patients in the study of Sibai and colleagues.

**C. Fish Oil Supplementation:** There are no randomized controlled trials describing the efficacy of fish oil supplementation in preventing preeclampsia. However, there are a few reports describing an association between consumption of diets rich in fish oil and lower incidences of preeclampsia and fetal growth retardation. There is some evidence from a 50-year-old uncontrolled trial suggesting that nutritional supplementation with several nutrients and vitamins including fish oil resulted in a lower incidence of preeclampsia in 1530 nulliparous women. This trial demonstrated no reduction in the incidence of transient hypertension or preeclampsia in 980 multiparous women receiving such supplementation. It is important to note that the patients receiving supplementation had different prenatal follow-up than those in the control group. In addition, the diagnoses of transient hypertension and preeclampsia were not well defined. A trial is currently being conducted in a large population of pregnant women in Denmark.

There is currently no proven way to prevent preeclampsia, but good prenatal care and regular visits to the physician will allow for early diagnosis before the condition becomes severe. The physician must have full knowledge of the patient profile and must maintain a high index of suspicion throughout the pregnancy. Eclampsia cannot always be prevented. Patients may deteriorate suddenly and without warning.

## Treatment

### A. Mild Preeclampsia:

**1. Treatment of mother**—The treatment of preeclampsia is bed rest and delivery. The patient is usually hospitalized upon diagnosis, since this diminishes the possibility of convulsions and enhances the chance of fetal survival. Hospitalization to prevent premature delivery in preeclampsia is far less expensive than the cost of caring for a premature infant.

Women with mild preeclampsia who can be relied on to follow the physician's instructions may be treated as outpatients. A typical home regimen consists of bed rest, daily urine dipstick measurements of proteinuria, and blood pressure monitoring. Patients are seen at least twice weekly for antepartum fetal heart rate testing and periodic 24-hour urine protein measurements. Patients must be warned of danger signals such as severe headache, epigastric pain, or visual disturbances. The occurrence of these signals, increasing blood pressure, or proteinuria mandates communication with the physician and probable hospitalization.

Hospitalized patients are allowed to be up and around as they feel comfortable. The blood pressure is measured every 4 hours, and patients are weighed daily. Urine dipstick testing for protein is performed daily. Twenty-four-hour urine studies for creatinine clearance and total protein are obtained twice weekly. Liver function, uric acid, electrolytes, and serum albumin are determined on admission and weekly. Coagulation studies such as prothrombin clotting time, partial thromboplastin time, fibrinogen, and platelet count should be measured in patients with severe preeclampsia. Assessments of gestational age and estimated fetal weight are performed by ultrasonic examination on admission and thereafter as indicated (usually every 2 weeks).

Antihypertensive medications are usually withheld unless the diastolic blood pressure exceeds 100 mm Hg and the gestational age is 30 weeks or less. (Long-term antihypertensive therapy is discussed later under Chronic Hypertension.) Sedatives were used in the past but have become disfavored because they interfere with fetal heart rate testing and because one of them—phenobarbital—impaired vitamin K-dependent clotting factors in the fetus. The usual indications for delivery of patients with preeclampsia are summarized in Table 19–2.

**2. Assessment of fetal status**—Fetal status is evaluated by twice-weekly nonstress testing and ultrasound assessment of amniotic fluid volume. Nonreactive nonstress tests require further evaluation with either a biophysical profile or an oxytocin challenge test. Amniocentesis to determine the lecithin:sphingomyelin (L:S) ratio is not frequently used in preeclampsia, since early delivery is usually for maternal indications but may be useful as the fetus approaches maturity. Corticosteroids may be used to accelerate fetal lung maturity in patients with preeclampsia when there is an immature L:S ratio if it is thought that delivery may occur in the next 2–7 days. With rapidly worsening preeclampsia, fetal monitoring should be continuous because of the risk of abruptio placentae and uteroplacental insufficiency.

**B. Severe Preeclampsia:** The goals of management of severe preeclampsia are (1) prevention of convulsions, (2) control of maternal blood pressure, and (3) initiation of delivery. Delivery is the definitive mode of therapy if severe preeclampsia develops at or beyond 36 weeks' gestation or if there is evidence of fetal lung maturity or fetal jeopardy. If delivery of a preterm infant (<36 weeks' gestation) is anticipated, maternal transfer to a tertiary care center is advised to ensure proper neonatal intensive care.

Management of patients with severe preeclampsia occurring earlier in pregnancy is controversial. Some institutions use diuretics or other antihypertensive drugs to control maternal blood pressure until fetal

**Table 19–2.** Indications for delivery in patients with preeclampsia.

Blood pressure consistently higher than 100 mm Hg diastolic in a 24-hour period or confirmed higher than 110 mm Hg.
Rising serum creatinine.
Persistent or severe headache.
Epigastric pain.
Abnormal liver function tests.
Thrombocytopenia.
HELLP syndrome.
Eclampsia.
Pulmonary edema.
Abnormal antepartum fetal heart rate testing.
SGA fetus with failure to grow on serial ultrasound examinations.

lung maturity is reached. Corticosteroids may also be used to accelerate lung maturity; however, most studies supporting the use of corticosteroids are not convincing, because they do not include data on pulmonary maturity or do not use a control group.

**C. Goals of Management:** If the pregnancy has advanced beyond 28 weeks and a tertiary nursery is available, delivery is the treatment of choice. Severe preeclampsia occurring prior to 28 weeks is a difficult management problem. No single institution has enough patients to study conservative management versus immediate delivery. One review of conservative management in 60 patients over a 7-year period (Sibai, 1985) revealed several maternal complications, including abruptio placentae (22%), eclampsia (17%), coagulopathy (8%), renal failure (5%), hypertensive encephalopathy (3%), and hepatic rupture (1%). Perinatal mortality was 87%.

In a subsequent study of 109 patients at less than 28 weeks' gestation managed between 1985 and 1989 (Sibai, 1990), results with conservative management were better. Maternal complications included abruptio placenta (5.6%), eclampsia (5.6%), and HELLP syndrome (13.6%). Perinatal mortality was only 24.6%. In 78% of conservatively managed patients, delivery was for fetal indications. They attributed the improved outcome during the latter period to more aggressive monitoring of maternal and fetal status and to early referral to their tertiary care center. In the earlier report, most patients had not been referred until the onset of maternal complications. If the gestational age is less than 24 weeks, patients should be offered induction of labor with prostaglandin $E_2$ suppositories. For gestations between 24 and 28 weeks, conservative management may be attempted; however, maternal complications, intrauterine asphyxia, or abruptio placentae may result.

## Prognosis

See Eclampsia, later.

## ECLAMPSIA

Eclampsia occurs in 0.2–0.5% of all deliveries, with occurrence being influenced by the same factors as in preeclampsia. In rare instances, eclampsia develops before 20 weeks' gestation. About 75% of eclamptic seizures occur before delivery. About 50% of postpartum eclamptic seizures occur in the first 48 hours after delivery, but they may occur as late as 6 weeks postpartum.

## Pathophysiology

The pathogenesis of eclamptic seizures is poorly understood. Seizures have been attributed to platelet thrombi, hypoxia due to localized vasoconstriction, and foci of hemorrhage in the cortex. There is also a mistaken tendency to equate eclampsia with hypertensive encephalopathy. There is a poor correlation between occurrence of seizures and severity of hypertension. Seizures may occur with insignificant blood pressure elevations that are only slightly higher than readings recorded 24 hours previously. The hallmarks of hypertensive encephalopathy (retinal hemorrhages, exudates, and papilledema) are very infrequent in eclampsia, where funduscopic changes are minimal.

## Clinical Findings

There is usually no aura preceding the seizure, and the patient may have one, 2, or many seizures. Unconsciousness lasts for a variable period of time. The patient hyperventilates after the tonic-clonic seizure to compensate for the respiratory and lactic acidosis that develops during the apneic phase. Fever is rare but is a poor prognostic sign. Seizure-induced complications may include tongue biting, broken bones, head trauma, or aspiration. Pulmonary edema and retinal detachment have also been noted following seizures.

## Treatment

### A. Prenatal Treatment:

**1. Control of seizures**–In many centers outside the USA, anticonvulsants are not used prophylactically. In the United Kingdon, eg, it is thought that the maternal risk of eclampsia, although variable, can be predicted. Anticonvulsant drugs such as diazepam, phenytoin, and chlormethiazole are used sparingly. In the USA, obstetricians believe the risk of eclampsia to be unpredictable and not correlated with symptoms of preeclampsia, blood pressure readings, deep tendon reflexes, or the degree of proteinuria. Most authorities recommend giving anticonvulsants to all patients in labor who have hypertension with or without proteinuria or edema. Since many women will be treated who are at low risk for seizures, the drug must be safe for mother and fetus. Fifty years of experience with magnesium sulfate has shown it to be effective and safe. The mechanism of the anticonvulsant action of magnesium sulfate is unknown. Its use has been criticized on the grounds that it does not cross the blood-brain barrier and does not have a central nervous system inhibitory effect. While early studies failed to show a significant increase in cerebrospinal fluid (CSF) magnesium concentrations during therapy, more recent studies have shown about a 20% increase in CSF magnesium levels, and these levels parallel those in the serum. Magnesium sulfate decreases the amount of acetylcholine released at the neuromuscular junction resulting in peripheral neuromuscular blockade at high magnesium concentrations; however, this does not account for its anticonvulsant effect. Recent work by Cotton et al demonstrated that magnesium sulfate had a central anticonvulsant effect on electrically stimulated hippocampal seizures in rats. They speculated that since

magnesium ion blocks calcium entry into neurons through the N-methyl-D-aspartate (NMDA) receptor-operated calcium channel, magnesium sulfate might be acting through this mechanism. On the other hand, Link et al found that magnesium sulfate was ineffective in altering seizure discharge in pentylentetrazole-induced status epilepticus in rats. They argued that because magnesium blocks calcium entry through the NMDA receptor-operated calcium channel in a voltage-dependent manner, it would be ineffective in neurons that are continuously depolarizing as in status epilepticus. Finally, Doppler studies of brain blood flow in preeclamptic women suggest that magnesium sulfate vasodilates the smaller diameter intracranial vessels distal to the middle cerebral artery and may exert its main effect in the prophylaxis and treatment of eclampsia by reversing vasospastic cerebral ischemia (Belfort et al, 1992).

Other actions are transient mild hypotension during intravenous loading, transient mild decrease in uterine activity during active labor, tocolytic effect in premature labor, and potentiation of depolarizing and nondepolarizing muscle relaxants. Magnesium sulfate has unpredictable effects on fetal heart rate variability (increased, decreased, unchanged).

Maternal dose-related effects at various serum levels are 10 mg/dL, loss of deep tendon reflexes; 15 mg/dL, respiratory paralysis; and 25 mg/dL, cardiac arrest. The therapeutic level is between 4.8 and 8.4 mg/dL. This range is empiric based on levels obtained with an intramuscular dose usually found to be effective. Magnesium sulfate is usually given intravenously as a loading dose of 6 g over 20 minutes followed by a constant infusion of 2 g/h. If plasma levels are less than 5 mg/dL, the maintenance dose is increased to 3 g/h.

Patients may have seizures while receiving magnesium sulfate. If a seizure occurs within 20 minutes after the loading dose, the convulsion is usually short, and no treatment is indicated. If the seizure occurs more than 20 minutes after the loading dose, an additional 2–4 g of magnesium sulfate may be given. Usually a magnesium level drawn acutely reveals subtherapeutic levels, but occasionally this is not so. In such cases, diazepam, 5–10 mg given intravenously, or amobarbital, up to 250 mg given intravenously, may be used. The patient should be checked every 4 hours to be sure that deep tendon reflexes are present, respirations are at least 12/min, and urine output has been at least 100 mL during the preceding 4 hours. The antidote for magnesium sulfate over dose is 10 mL of 10% calcium chloride or calcium gluconate given intravenously. The remedial effect occurs within seconds.

Phenytoin is receiving consideration as an alternative to magnesium sulfate for several reasons: (1) Its central anticonvulsant effect is known; (2) it has proven to be a safe and effective anticonvulsant in other areas of medicine; (3) it can be continued orally for several days postpartum until the risk of eclamptic convulsions has subsided; (4) therapeutic serum levels are known, and testing is widely available; and (5) there are no known neonatal side effects associated with short-term usage. A study of 105 patients by Friedman et al comparing magnesium sulfate with phenytoin found fewer side effects, a short active phase of labor, and a smaller blood loss in the phenytoin group. They estimated that, because eclamptic seizures are relatively uncommon, it would take 1750 patients in each arm of a randomized trial to show a 2-fold difference in anticonvulsant effect between the two drugs. Other studies comparing phenytoin with magnesium sulfate have shown that there will be failures with either agent. Several regimens for administration of phenytoin have been proposed. Ryan et al found that a 10 mg/kg loading dose infused no faster than 50 mg/min followed 2 hours later by 5 mg/kg obtained satisfactory serum levels with few side effects. The main problems during intravenous loading of phenytoin are bradycardia, hypotension, and burning at the intravenous site.

Diazepam causes respiratory depression, hypotonia, poor feeding, and thermoregulatory problems in the newborn. Also, the sodium benzoate preservative competes with bilirubin for albumin binding, thus predisposing the infant to kernicterus.

**2. Control of hypertension**—There is controversy about whether or not uteroplacental blood flow is autoregulated. Most evidence indicates that the uterine vasculature is maximally vasodilated at all times. Therefore, most physicians believe that reductions in maternal blood pressure tend to decrease uteroplacental perfusion and caution against treatments that will cause large, precipitate drops in mean arterial pressure. Antihypertensive drugs are usually given if the diastolic blood pressure exceeds 110 mm Hg. The goal is to bring the diastolic blood pressure into the 90–100 mm Hg range.

**a. Hydralazine**—The drug of choice is hydralazine, a direct arteriolar vasodilator that causes a secondary baroreceptor-mediated sympathetic discharge resulting in tachycardia and increased cardiac output. This latter effect is important because it increases uterine blood flow and blunts the hypotensive response, making it difficult to give an overdose. If late decelerations of fetal heart rate do occur after hydralazine administration, they usually respond to fluid-loading, administration of oxygen, turning the patient on her side, and discontinuing oxytocin. Hydralazine is metabolized by the liver, and in patients with slow acetylation, it has a longer duration. The dose is 5 mg given intravenously every 15–20 minutes. The onset of action is 15 minutes, the peak effect occurs within 30–60 minutes, and the duration of action is 4–6 hours. Side effects include flushing, headache, dizziness, palpitations, angina, and an idiosyncratic lupuslike syndrome in patients taking more than 200 mg/d chronically. In more than 95% of cases of pre-eclampsia, hydralazine will be effective in controlling blood pressure. Recently the production of parenteral hydralazine had been discontinued while the manufacturer reformulates it in a lyophilized form. Other agents have been substituted to hydralazine, most commonly labetalol, nifedipine, and diazoxide.

**b. Labetalol**—Labetalol is a nonselective beta blocker and a postsynaptic $\alpha_1$-adrenergic blocking agent available for both oral and intravenous administration. Intravenous labetalol is given every 10 minutes as follows: the first dose is 20 mg, the second is 40 mg, and subsequent doses are 80 mg—to a maximum cumulative dosage of 300 mg or until blood pressure is controlled. It may also be given as a constant infusion. Onset of action is in 5 minutes, peak effect is in 10–20 minutes, and duration of action ranges from 45 minutes to 6 hours. Uteroplacental blood flow appears to be unaffected by intravenous labetalol. Initial experience indicates it to be well-tolerated by mother and fetus, but more experience with this agent is needed.

**c. Nifedipine**—Nifedipine, a calcium channel blocker, can be administered in a bite-and-swallow technique to lower blood pressure acutely. It is a powerful arteriolar vasodilator with the main problem being overshoot hypotension. For this reason, it probably should not be used in patients with intrauterine growth retardation or abnormal fetal heart rate patterns. Profound hypotension may be reversed by volume administration or intravenous calcium. Although nifedipine appears to have much potential, it requires further assessment of its use in pregnancy.

**d. Diazoxide**—Diazoxide is another direct arteriolar vasodilator. It is more powerful and has a more rapid onset of action than hydralazine. It is given in small boluses of 30–75 mg until satisfactory control of blood pressure is achieved. The main difficulty with diazoxide usage is overshoot hypotension, particularly when diazoxide is used as a second agent after hydralazine failure. Labor ceases in about 50% of patients, and the agent may cause sodium and water retention, hyperglycemia, and late decelerations in fetal heart rate during labor. Diazoxide is the drug of choice in many centers in Australia but has not gained popularity in the USA.

**e. Sodium nitroprusside**—Sodium nitroprusside causes equal degrees of vasodilatation in arteries and veins without autonomic or central nervous system effects. Its onset of action is 1.5–2 minutes, the peak effect occurs in 1–2 minutes, and the duration of action is 3–5 minutes. It is an excellent drug for minute-to-minute control in an intensive care unit setting. It may be titrated against a segmental epidural block for labor or cesarean section. It is recommended that the drug not be administered intravenously over a period longer than 30 minutes in the undelivered mother because of the risk of cyanide and thiocyanate toxicity in the fetus.

**f. Trimethaphan**—Trimethaphan, a ganglionic

blocker, is used acutely by anesthesiologists to lower blood pressure prior to laryngoscopy and intubation for general anesthesia. A reported fetal side effect is meconium ileus.

**g. Nitroglycerin**–Nitroglycerin given intravenously is a predominantly venular vasodilator that appears to be safe for the fetus. It is only a moderately powerful antihypertensive agent.

**B. Management of Labor and Delivery:** A 4- to 8-hour trial of labor is indicated for most patients with preeclampsia-eclampsia. If neither effacement nor dilatation of the cervix has occurred and does not occur significantly over this period, cesarean section is performed. With severe preeclampsia, fetal gestational age less than 32 weeks, and an unfavorable cervix, cesarean section is performed without a trial of labor. Internal fetal monitoring is used as soon as sufficient cervical dilatation permits. Fluids such as 5% dextrose in Ringer's lactate, 125–150 mL/h, are given intravenously. A Swan-Ganz catheter is helpful in patients with pulmonary edema, massive hemorrhage, or oliguria unresponsive to a 1000-mL fluid challenge. Analgesia with intravenous meperidine or butorphanol is given in small doses every 1–2 hours. Local anesthesia with or without pudendal block is used in most cases for vaginal delivery.

The use of epidural anesthesia in patients with preeclampsia is somewhat controversial. The problem is sudden hypotension due to pooling of blood in the venous capacitance vessels secondary to sympathetic blockade. However, with the almost universal use of epidural anesthesia for cesarean section, it has been widely used in preeclamptic patients. If there is no evidence of fetal compromise (by fetal heart rate criteria), if there is no coagulopathy present, if the patient is prehydrated, and if a segmental activation technique is used by an experienced anesthesiologist, epidural anesthesia may be used for labor and delivery or for cesarean section. If these criteria are not met, then balanced general anesthesia is preferred for cesarean section. Spinal anesthesia should be avoided.

**C. Postpartum Treatment:** Some of the constraints of therapy no longer apply once delivery has occurred, eg, sodium nitroprusside or diuretics may be used. Since 25% of eclamptic seizures occur postpartum, patients with severe preeclampsia are maintained on magnesium sulfate for 24 hours after delivery. Patients with mild preeclampsia who have diuresis and controlled blood pressure may be withdrawn from magnesium sulfate 8–12 hours postpartum. Phenobarbital, 120 mg/ d, is sometimes used in patients with persistent hypertension in whom spontaneous postpartum diuresis does not occur or in whom hyperreflexia persists after 24 hours of magnesium sulfate. Alternatively, magnesium sulfate may not be continued for 36–48 hours. Hypertension may not resolve until 6 weeks postpartum. If the diastolic blood pressure remains consistently above 100 mm Hg for 24 hours postpartum, any number of antihypertensive agents could be given including a diuretic, calcium-channel blocker, ACE inhibitor, central alpha agonist, or beta-blocker. The blood pressure should be checked in the standing position to avoid the possibility of orthostatic hypotension. At follow-up after 1 week, the need for continuing antihypertensive therapy may be reevaluated.

## Prognosis

Maternal deaths due to preeclampsia-eclampsia are rare in the USA, but death may be caused by cerebral hemorrhage, aspiration pneumonia, hypoxic encephalopathy, thromboembolism, hepatic rupture, renal failure, or anesthetic accident. It is important to stress that iatrogenic complications increase if multiple drugs are given. If the patient truly had preeclampsia, the risk of recurrence is less likely (33%) than if she had chronic hypertension mistaken for preeclampsia. In the latter situation, the risk of recurrence is quite high (70%). In studies that include multiparas with preeclampsia, the recurrence rate in the next pregnancy is as high as 70%. In Chesley's study of primigravidas with eclampsia (1978), only 33% had some hypertensive disorder in any subsequent pregnancy; in most cases, the condition was not severe, but 2% did have recurrence of eclampsia.

The effect of preeclampsia-eclampsia on subsequent development of chronic hypertension is debatable. According to Chesley, confusion may result from a mistaken diagnosis of preeclampsia in women with underlying renal disease or chronic hypertension. In women with eclampsia during their first pregnancy who were followed for more than 40 years, he found no increase in the incidence of hypertension or deaths due to cardiovascular disease or other causes. Multiparas with eclampsia had a much higher incidence of subsequent hypertension and deaths due to cardiovascular disease and other causes. It seems reasonable to conclude that the risk of recurrent eclampsia in subsequent pregnancies is not high enough to recommend against future pregnancies. Preeclampsia does not cause permanent damage, predispose to chronic hypertension, or adversely affect the long-term health of the mother.

## CHRONIC HYPERTENSION

The incidence of chronic hypertension varies among different populations, ranging from 0.5 to 4% and averaging 2.5%. Chronic hypertension in pregnancy is usually idiopathic (80%) or due to renal disease (20%), though these figures may reflect insufficient investigation. A number of renal diseases may be causative, the most common being chronic glomerulonephritis, interstitial nephritis, diabetic glomerulosclerosis, IgA nephropathy, and renal artery stenosis.

## Clinical Findings

**A. Symptoms and Signs:** Patients with chronic hypertension tend to be over 30 years of age, obese, and multiparous, with associated medical problems such as diabetes or renal disease. The incidence is higher in black women and in women with a family history of hypertension. A woman who has delivered one or more infants and has hypertension in this pregnancy most likely has chronic hypertension. The typical patient has hypertension without other signs of preeclampsia (eg, proteinuria or nondependent edema). The diagnosis is made on the basis of documented hypertension before conception or before 20 weeks' gestation or of persistence of hypertension after the puerperium (6 weeks). Whether worsening hypertension represents superimposed preeclampsia or hypertension associated with renal disease is sometimes difficult to determine. Preexisting renal disease alone may have all the manifestations of preeclampsia (hypertension, edema, proteinuria, and hyperuricemia). Renal biopsy would confirm the diagnosis but is usually not necessary, because the decision to deliver can be based on difficulty of blood pressure control, renal function, and fetal well-being. For the same reasons, renal biopsy is usually not performed for the work-up of proteinuria or elevated serum creatinine in pregnancy.

**B. Laboratory, X-Ray, and Electrocardiographic Findings:** The ECG may show left ventricular hypertrophy in 5–10% of patients. Elevated serum creatinine, decreased creatinine clearance, and proteinuria are also present in about 5–10% of patients with chronic hypertension. The chest x-ray is usually normal, though it may reveal cardiomegaly. Patients with left ventricular hypertrophy or elevated serum creatinine are at increased risk for developing superimposed preeclampsia. Patients with cardiomegaly due to either hypertensive cardiovascular disease or congestive cardiomyopathy are at increased risk for superimposed preeclampsia, pulmonary edema, and arrhythmias.

## Complications

**A. Maternal Complications:** The main complication of chronic hypertension is superimposed preeclampsia, which occurs in about one-third of patients. Patients tend to deteriorate faster with superimposed preeclampsia than with preeclampsia alone. While maternal death is rare today, older studies of hypertension show that the mortality rate was high in elderly multiparas with chronic hypertension and superimposed preeclampsia. The mechanism of death was stroke and heart failure. There is an increased risk of abruptio placentae with chronic hypertension (0.4–10%). Associated with this condition is the risk of disseminated intravascular coagulation, acute tubular necrosis, or renal cortical necrosis.

The effect of pregnancy on chronic renal disease is uncertain. Although there are few data for patients with severe disease, limited evidence suggests that if renal function is well preserved (creatinine <1.5 mg/dL), pregnancy does not change the course of renal disease, but if renal insufficiency exists prior to pregnancy (creatinine >1.5 mg/dL), the decline in renal function may be more rapid than expected.

**B. Fetal Complications:** The fetus has a 25–30% risk of prematurity and a 10–15% risk of being SGA. Preeclampsia tends to occur after 34 weeks' gestation, so that prematurity is not a great concern. Preeclampsia superimposed on chronic hypertension frequently occurs earlier (at 26–34 weeks), and in such cases, fetuses are at double jeopardy for prematurity and IUGR. In addition, there is a risk of still birth or intrapartum fetal distress due to abruptio placentae or chronic intrauterine asphyxia.

## Prevention

There are no absolute criteria for blood pressure or renal function on which to base recommendations for therapeutic abortion or sterilization in patients with chronic hypertension. Though data are few in patients with severe hypertension, in one group there was a maternal survival rate of 100% and a perinatal survival rate of 75% in 44 patients with diastolic pressure of more than 110 mm Hg in the first trimester. There have been occasional reports of successful pregnancies in patients on chronic dialysis, and more than 1200 pregnancies have been successful in women who have undergone renal transplantation.

## Treatment

**A. Control of Hypertension:** Most authorities agree that antihypertensive therapy will decrease the incidence of stroke and heart failure in pregnant patients with diastolic blood pressures exceeding 110 mm Hg. The real controversy concerns the value of antihypertensive therapy of mild hypertension (approximately 95% of pregnant patients with chronic hypertension have mild hypertension). The Veterans Administration Cooperative Study demonstrated that treatment of diastolic blood pressures of 104–115 mm Hg in men decreased cardiovascular morbidity (myocardial infarction, congestive heart failure, and stroke) in just 10 months. Patients with diastolic pressures of 94–104 mm Hg showed benefits of therapy only after 5 years had elapsed. Therefore, no benefits of antihypertensive therapy for mild chronic hypertension could be expected during the 9 months of pregnancy, and therapy cannot be justified by the same arguments used in general internal medicine. Some authors claim that antihypertensive therapy for mild chronic hypertension will decrease the incidence or delay the onset of superimposed preeclampsia, thus lowering perinatal mortality and morbidity rates. Others claim there is no benefit and considerable risk. Since this issue is still unresolved, a review of some of the recent clinical studies is helpful (see references).

Several oral agents may be considered if hypertension is to be treated.

**1.  Thiazide diuretics–**Thiazide diuretics have been reported to cause a number of harmful maternal and fetal side effects, the main one being plasma volume contraction. Studies in nonpregnant patients show that thiazides have acute and chronic effects. Acutely, they cause a 5–10% decrease in plasma volume, which lowers cardiac output and blood pressure in the first 3–5 days. Over the next 4–6 weeks, renal compensatory mechanisms return the plasma volume toward normal but not to pretreatment levels. At the same time, cardiac output returns to pretreatment levels, but total peripheral resistance stays low. Thus, the acute blood pressure-lowering effect of thiazides is due to volume contraction. The sustained antihypertensive effect is thought to involve mobilization of excess sodium from the arterial wall. This leads to widening of the vascular lumen and possibly to a decrease in the vascular responsiveness to endogenous catecholamines. Sibai and associates have recently shown that plasma volume contraction occurs in early pregnancy in hypertensive patients on chronic thiazide therapy. When the thiazide was stopped, normal physiologic volume expansion occurred; if the thiazide was continued, plasma volume expansion was minimal (18% mean increase in patients taking thiazides versus 52% mean increase in patients in whom diuretics were discontinued early in pregnancy). Perinatal outcome was the same in both groups. Another consideration is the volume expansion caused by antihypertensive agents. It may be that the sodium and water retention produced by antihypertensive agents offsets the volume contraction caused by the thiazide. In summary, diuretics do not prevent preeclampsia or eclampsia. Thiazide diuretics are contraindicated in patients with pure preeclampsia. They may have a place in the treatment of patients with chronic hypertension; however, with the availability of more powerful antihypertensive agents such as nifedipine and labetalol, their use is declining.

**2.  Methyldopa–**Methyldopa, a central α-adrenergic agonist, is the only antihypertensive drug whose long-term safety for mother and fetus has been adequately assessed. It reduces total peripheral resistance without causing physiologically significant changes in heart rate or cardiac output. If methyldopa is used alone, fluid retention and loss of antihypertensive effect are frequent. For this reason, methyldopa is usually combined with a diuretic for treatment of nonpregnant patients. It is usually started at a dose of 250 mg 3 times a day and increased to 2 g/d. Peak plasma levels occur 2–3 hours after administration; the plasma half-life is about 2 hours, and the maximum effect occurs 4–6 hours after an oral dose. Most of the agent is excreted via the kidney. The most commonly reported side effects are sedation and postural hypotension. With prolonged therapy, 10–20% of patients develop a positive direct Coombs' test, usually after 6–12 months of therapy. Hemolytic anemia occurs in fewer than 5% of these patients and is an indication to stop the drug. Fever, liver function abnormalities, granulocytopenia, and thrombocytopenia have occurred rarely.

**3.  Clonidine–**Clonidine is another central α-adrenergic agonist. Treatment is usually started at 0.1 mg twice daily and increased in increments of 0.1–0.2 mg/d up to 2.4 mg/d. Blood pressure declines 30–60 mm Hg with use of clonidine, with a maximum effect in 2–4 hours and a duration of action of 6–8 hours. Renal blood flow and the glomerular filtration rate are preserved, but cardiac output falls. This is attributable to a decrease in venous return secondary to systemic vasodilatation and bradycardia. Cardiac output responds normally to exercise. Xerostomia and sedation are the most frequently encountered side effects. Withdrawal of clonidine produces a hypertensive crisis that responds well to reinstitution of the drug. There is not as much information on clonidine in pregnancy as there is on methyldopa; one large study found it to be equivalent to methyldopa.

**4.  Calcium channel blockers–**Currently available calcium channel blockers include nifedipine, verapamil, ditiazem, nicardipine, isradipine, amlodipine, and felodipine. They cause direct arteriolar vasodilation by selective inhibition of slow inward calcium channels in vascular smooth muscle. Since calcium channel blockers affect such a fundamental cellular response, their therapeutic applications are wide-ranging from angina pectoris to premature labor. Nifedipine is the calcium blocker most widely used in pregnancy. Ninety percent of oral nifedipine is absorbed from the gastrointestinal tract. After moderate first-pass liver metabolism, the bioavailability is 65–70%. Onset of action after bite-and-swallow administration is in about 3 minutes. The drug has an initial fast half-life of 2.5–3 hours and a terminal slow half-life of 5 hours. It is almost completely metabolized by the liver and excreted 90% by the kidney and 10% by the liver. Side effects include hypotension, headache, flushing, tachycardia, and ankle edema. Since magnesium sulfate is also a calcium channel blocker, the use of both nifedipine and magnesium sulfate together could be potentially hazardous (eg, hypotension). There is controversy in the literature about the effects of nifedipine on uteroplacental blood flow in animals, to differences in the uteroplacental vasculature of various animal species, or to the dosage of nifedipine and whether maternal hypotension occurred. Nifedipine has been used in several human studies comparing its tocolytic effect with ritodrine. It has also been used both acutely and chronically as an antihypertensive agent in pregnancy. In the largest study to date, Sibai et al randomly treated 200 preeclamptic patients with nifedipine and bed rest or bed rest alone. There was no prolongation of pregnancy or improved perinatal outcome in the nifedipine group, but uncontrolled hypertension as an indication for delivery was reduced. Because it is such a powerful and dependable agent, nifedipine is becoming increasingly popular for antihypertensive therapy in pregnancy.

**5. Prazosin–**Prazosin is a competitive blocker of the postsynaptic $\alpha_1$-adrenergic receptor. It causes vasodilatation of both the resistance and capacitance vessels, reducing cardiac preload and afterload. It lowers blood pressure without significantly lowering heart rate, cardiac output, renal blood flow, or the glomerular filtration rate. It is almost exclusively metabolized in the liver. Approximately 90% of the drug is excreted via bile into the feces. It appears to be more slowly absorbed and its half-life slightly prolonged during pregnancy. In one study, the median time to peak concentration was 165 minutes in pregnant women and 120 minutes in men of similar age. The mean elimination half-life was 171 minutes in pregnant women and 130 minutes in men. Prazosin may cause a first-dose phenomenon characterized by sudden hypotension 30–90 minutes after the initial dose. This can be avoided by limiting the first dose to 1 mg given just prior to bedtime. Animal studies have demonstrated no teratogenic effects. Prazosin is not a very powerful agent and has usually been combined with the beta blocker oxprenolol in obstetric studies. Lubbe and Hodge used prazosin alone or in combination with oxprenolol in 44 pregnant women. No fetal abnormalities or adverse effects were noted. Dommissee and coworkers used prazosin with or without oxprenolol to treat pregnancy hypertension beginning before 34 weeks' gestation. None of the 22 patients had significant maternal or fetal side effects attributable to drug therapy. Although available since 1976, prazosin had not been widely used in pregnancy.

**6. Hydralazine–**Hydralazine is an excellent drug for intravenous therapy of hypertension in pregnancy. It is an arteriolar vasodilator that causes a secondary baroreceptor-mediated sympathetic response, increasing heart rate, and cardiac output. However, it is poorly tolerated orally as a single agent. Prominent side effects are headache, tachycardia, palpitations, fluid retention, and a lupuslike syndrome when chronic dosage exceeds 200 mg/d. Many of the unwanted side effects are minimized when it is used with a diuretic, methyl-dopa, or a beta blocker; however, use of multiple agents is discouraged in pregnancy. Dosage is initiated at 10 mg 4 times daily and increased to 200 mg/d.

**7. Beta blockers–**Beta blockers were introduced in the 1960s and have been used in pregnancy to treat migraine headache, hypertrophic obstructive cardiomyopathy, mitral valve prolapse, Graves' disease, and hypertension. Beta blockers are usually not adequate to control severe hypertension and are frequently combined with a diuretic, a vasodilator, or both. Beta blockers have been associated with neonatal bradycardia, hypoglycemia, hyperbilirubinemia, intrauterine growth retardation, respiratory depression, blocking of tachycardiac response to hypoxia, and increase in uterine muscle tone causing decreased uterine blood flow. The frequency of these side effects is unknown. Though clinical experience is accumulating, the safety of beta blockers in pregnancy has not yet been clearly established. Their use requires thoughtful risk-benefit analysis and clinical judgment. Infants of mothers taking beta blockers should be placed in an intermediate care unit after delivery to be monitored for side effects.

**8. Labetalol–**The low incidence of side effects, lack of teratogenicity, maintenance of uterine blood flow, and low propensity to cross the placenta make labetalol attractive for treatment of pregnant women. One randomized study found it offered no advantages over methyldopa in hypertensive pregnancy. Another study compared the use of labetalol plus hospitalization versus hospitalization alone in the management of 200 mildly preeclamptic women. No benefit was demonstrated in the labetalol-treated group; in addition, the incidence of SGA infants was higher in that group. Labetalol is started at 100 mg 3–4 times daily and increased to a maximum dosage of 2400 mg/d. Side effects are minor and include tremulousness and headache.

**9. ACE inhibitors–**The FDA-approved angiotensin-converting enzyme inhibitors include captopril, enalapril, lisinopril, fosinopril, ramipril, benazepril, and quinapril. They are widely used as first-line therapy for hypertension because they decrease systemic vascular resistance and have few side effects. Most of the reported experiences with ACE inhibitors in pregnancy are with captopril or enalapril. In human pregnancy these agents have been associated with several fetal and neonatal complications including hypotension, growth retardation, oligohydramnios, anuria, renal failure, malformations, stillbirth, and neonatal death. Although they have been successfully used in pregnancy, (Kreft-Jais, 1988), they should be avoided in pregnant women.

**B. Effects of Antihypertensives on Breast-Feeding:** Little is known about the pharmacokinetics of antihypertensive drugs in human breast milk. In general, drugs that are lipid-soluble, unionized, and not protein bound are found in significant levels in breast milk. Specific recommendations concerning some of the more important agents are as follows: Thiazide diuretics should be avoided, since they decrease milk production and have been used in the past to suppress lactation. However, no electrolyte abnormalities have been found in infants of mothers taking thiazides. Methyldopa is probably safe during breast-feeding, since low plasma levels are found in the infants. Except for propranolol, the other beta-blocking agents are found in higher concentrations in breast milk than in maternal plasma. Therefore, propranolol would probably be the drug of choice if a beta blocker was needed. Nevertheless, accumulated experience with various beta blockers has shown only very low drug concentrations in breast milk. Clonidine is found in very small amounts in breast milk. Captopril appears to be safe during breast-feeding because only small amounts are found in breast milk. Data on the other drugs are too few to serve as a basis for recommendations.

**C. General Obstetric Management:** In taking the medical history of the hypertensive pregnant patient, particular attention should be paid to the duration of hypertension, use of antihypertensive medications, history of renal or heart disease, and the outcome of previous pregnancies. Physical examination should include a careful funduscopic examination, listening for renal artery bruit, and checking the dorsalis pedis pulses for coarctation of the aorta. The blood pressure should be measured in the sitting position. If the bladder of the blood pressure cuff does not completely encircle the arm, a falsely high blood pressure reading may be obtained. In this situation, a thigh cuff should be used.

At the first prenatal visit, baseline laboratory studies should be obtained for organ systems likely to be affected by chronic hypertension or to deteriorate during pregnancy. Tests should include (but are not limited to) urinalysis; complete blood count; measurements of blood urea nitrogen, creatinine, serum electrolytes, uric acid, calcium, and phosphorus; liver function tests; ECG; and 24-hour urine collection for creatinine clearance and total protein. If significant heart disease is suspected, a chest x-ray (with the abdomen shielded) or echocardiogram should be obtained. A 3-hour oral glucose tolerance test is desirable, since as many as one-fourth of patients may have unrecognized diabetes. If hyperglycemia or wide blood pressure swings are evident, 24-hour urine testing for vanillylmandelic acid and metanephrines is recommended to rule out pheochromocytoma. The patient may be given a regular diet without salt restriction and should be followed every 2–3

weeks until 30 weeks' gestation and then weekly thereafter. Gestational age can be documented and an SGA infant detected with serial ultrasound examinations started early in pregnancy. Fetal well-being may also be assessed with the nonstress test and amniotic fluid index starting at 34 weeks or whenever the patient develops superimposed preeclampsia. Superimposed preeclampsia is diagnosed on the basis of worsening hypertension (30 mm Hg systolic or 15 mm Hg diastolic rise) together with either nondependent edema or proteinuria. Some of the more frequent indications for early delivery include superimposed preeclampsia, underlying medical problems such as diabetes or renal insufficiency, abnormal antepartum fetal heart rate, and an SGA fetus. A patient with worsening hypertension may be given beta methasone to accelerate fetal lung maturity if the L:S ratio is less than 2 and if delivery can be delayed for 48–72 hours after the first dose.

## Prognosis

Pregnancy outcome is usually favorable in patients with mild chronic hypertension, and perinatal survival rates of 95–97% can be expected. The main complications are superimposed preeclampsia, abruptio placentae, prematurity, and SGA fetus. If the patient has severe hypertension in the first trimester, onset of superimposed preeclampsia before 28 weeks' gestation, renal insufficiency prior to pregnancy, hypertensive cardiovascular disease, or congestive cardiomyopathy, the prognosis is more guarded. These patients require close follow-up of multiple clinical and laboratory parameters. The physician must be certain that they can be relied on to take their medication. They may require a long period of hospitalization and are likely to require cesarean delivery. Their fetuses are at significant risk for prematurity, growth retardation, and death.

## REFERENCES

Arias F, Zamora J: Antihypertensive treatment and pregnancy outcome in patients with mild-chronic hypertension. Obstet Gynecol 1979;53:489.

Barton JR, Sibai BM: Cerebral pathology in eclampsia. Perinatal 1991;18:871.

Beaufils M et al: Prevention of preeclampsia by early antiplatelet therapy. Lancet 1985;1:840.

Beer AE: Possible Immunologic bases of preeclampsia/eclampsia. Semin Perinatal 1978;2:39.

Belfort MA, Moise KJ: Effects of magnesium sulfate on maternal brain blood flow in preeclampsia: A randomized, placebo-controlled study. Am J Obstet Gynecol 1992;167:661.

Beneditti TJ et al: Hemodynamic observations in severe preeclampsia with flow-directed pulmonary artery catheter. Am J Obstet Gynecol 1980;136:465.

Brosens IA: Morphological changes in the uteroplacental bed in pregnancy hypertension. Clin Obstet Gynecol 1977;4:573.

Brown CEL, Purdy P, Cunningham FG: Head tomographic scans in women with eclampsia. Am J Obstet Gynecol 1988;159:915.

Chesley LC: *Hypertensive Disorders in Pregnancy.* Appleton-Century-Crofts, 1978.

Chester EM et al: Hypertensive encephalopathy: A clinico-pathologic study of 20 cases. Neurology 1978;28:928.

Cockburn J et al: Final report of study on hypertension during pregnancy: The effects of specific treatment of the growth and development of the children. Lancet 1982;1:647.

Cotton DB, Janusz CA, Berman RF: Anticonvulsant effects of magnesium sulfate on hippocampal seizures: Therapeutic implications in preeclampsia-eclampsia. Am J Obstet Gynecol 1992;166:1127.

Cotton DB et al: Hemodynamic profile of severe pregnancy-induced hypertension. Am J Obstet Gynecol 1988;158:523.

Cunningham FG, Lindheimer MD: Hypertension in pregnancy. New Engl J Med 1992;326:927.

Curet LB, Olson RW: Evaluation of a program of bed rest in treatment of chronic hypertension in pregnancy. Obstet Gynecol 1979;53:336.

Dahmus MA, Barton JR, Sibai BM: Cerebral imaging in eclampsia: Magnetic resonance imaging versus computed tomography. Am J Obstet Gynecol 1992;167:935.

Davison JM. Renal transplantation and pregnancy. Am J Kidney Dis 1987;9:374.

Fidler J et al: Randomized controlled comparative study of methyldopa and oxprenolol in treatment of hypertension in pregnancy. Br Med J 1983;286:1927.

Fisher KA et al: Hypertension in pregnancy: Clinical-pathological correlations and remote prognosis. Medicine 1981;60:267.

Friedman SA et al: Phenytoin versus magnesium sulfate in preeclampsia: A pilot study. Am J Perinatal 1993;10:233.

Gallery EDM et al: Randomized comparison of methyldopa and oxprenolol for treatment of hypertension in pregnancy. Br Med J 1979;1:1591.

Goodlin RC: Severe preeclampsia: Another great imitator. Am J Obstet Gynecol 1976;125:747.

Goodlin RC, Cotton DB, Haesslein HC: Severe edema-proteinuria-hypertension gestosis. Am J Obstet Gynecol 1978;2:595.

Groenendijk KR, Trimbos JBMJ, Wallenburg HCS: Hemodynamic measurements in preeclampsia: Preliminary observations. Am J Obstet Gynecol 1984;150:232.

Habib A, McCarthy JS: Effects on the neonate of propranolol administered during pregnancy. Pediatrics 1977;91:808.

Hankins GD et al: Longitudinal evaluation of hemodynamic changes in preeclampsia. Am J Obstet Gynecol 1984; 150:506.

Horvath JS et al: Clonidine hydrochloride: A safe and effective antihypertensive agent in pregnancy. Obstet Gynecol 1985;66:634.

Italian Study of Aspirin in Pregnancy. Low-dose aspirin in prevention and treatment of intrauterine growth retardation and pregnancy-induced hypertension. Lancet 1993; 341:396.

Kawasaki N et al: Effects of calcium supplementation on the vascular sensitivity to angiotensin II in pregnant women. Am J Obstet Gynecol 1985;153:576.

Keefer JR et al: Noncardiogenic pulmonary edema and invasive cardiovascular monitoring. Obstet Gynecol 1981; 58:46.

Kreft-Jais C et al: Angiotensin converting enzyme inhibitors in pregnancy: A survey of 22 patients given captopril and 9 given enalapril. Br J Obstet Gynecol 1988;94:420.

Lindheimer MD, Katz AI: Sodium and diuretics in pregnancy. N Engl J Med 1973;288:891.

Link MJ, Anderson RE, Meyer FB: Effects of magnesium sulfate on pentylenetetrazole-induced status epilepticus. Epilepsia 1991;32:543.

Lubbe WF, Hodge JV. Combined alpha and beta adrenoceptor antagonism with prazosin and oxprenolol in control of severe hypertension in pregnancy. NZ Med J 1981; 94:169.

Mabie WC, Ratts TE, Sibai BM: The central hemodynamics

of severe preeclampsia. Am J Obstet Gynecol 1989; 161:1443.

Mabie WC, Hackman BB, Sibai BM: Pulmonary edema associated with pregnancy: Echocardiographic insights and implications for treatment. Obstet Gynecol 1993;81:227.

Mallee MP et al: Increase in plasma atrial natriuretic peptide concentration antedates clinical evidence of preeclampsia. J Clin Endocrinol Metab 1992;74:1095.

Mitchell M: Endothelins in perinatal biology. Semin Perinatal 1991;15:79.

National High Blood Pressure Education Working Group Report on High Blood Pressure in Pregnancy. Am J Obstet Gynecol 1990;163:1689.

Phelan JP, Yurth DA: Severe preeclampsia. I. Peripartum hemodynamic observations. Am J Obstet Gynecol 1982; 144:17.

Pritchard JA, Cunningham MG, Pritchard SA: The Parkland Memorial Hospital protocol for treatment of eclampsia: Evaluation of 245 cases. Am J Obstet Gynecol 1984; 148:951.

Pritchard JA, MacDonald PC, Gant NF: *Williams Obstetrics,* 17th ed. Appleton-Century-Crofts, 1985.

Redman CWG: A controlled trial of treatment of hypertension in pregnancy: Labetalol compared with methyldopa. Pages 101–110 in: *The Investigation of Labetalol in the Management of Hypertension in Pregnancy.* Riley A, Symonds EM (eds). Amsterdam Excerpta Medica, 1982.

Redman CWG et al: Fetal outcome in trial of antihypertensive treatment in pregnancy. Lancet 1976;2:753.

Richards AM et al: Active management of the unconscious eclamptic patient. Br J Obstet Gynecol 1986;93:554.

Richards A, Graham D, Bullock R: Clinicopathological study of neurological complications due to hypertensive disorders of pregnancy. J Neurol Neurosurg Psychiatry 1988;51:416.

Ricke PS, Elliott JP, Freeman RK: Use of corticosteroids in pregnancy-induced hypertension. Obstet Gynecol 1980; 55:206.

Roberts JM, Redman CWG: Preeclampsia: More than pregnancy-induced hypertension. Lancet 1993;341:1447.

Roberts JM, Redman CWG: Management of preeclampsia. Lancet 1993;341:1451.

Roberts JM, Taylor RN: Preeclampsia: An endothelial cell disorder. Am J Obstet Gynecol 1989;161:1200.

Rubin PC: Current concepts: Beta Blockers in pregnancy. N Engl J Med 1981;305:1323.

Rubin PC (ed): Handbook of Hypertension. Vol. 10: *Hypertension in Pregnancy.* Elsevier, 1988.

Rubin PC et al: Clinical pharmacological studies with prazosin during pregnancy complicated by hypertension. Br J Clin Pharmacol 1983;16:543.

Rubin PC et al: Placebo-controlled trial of atenolol in treatment of pregnancy-associated hypertension. Lancet 1983;1:431.

Ryan G, Lange JR, Naughler MA: Clinical experience with phenytoin prophylaxis in severe preeclampsia. Am J Obstet Gynecol 1989;161:1297.

Shoenberger JA: Mild hypertension: The rationale for treatment. Am Heart J 1986;112:872.

Sibai BM, Abdella TN, Anderson GD: Pregnancy outcome in 211 patients with mild-chronic hypertension. Obstet Gynecol 1983;61:571.

Sibai et al: A protocol for managing severe preeclampsia in the second trimester. Am J Obstet Gynecol 1990; 163: 733.

Sibai BM, Anderson GD, Intensive management of severe hypertension in the first trimester. Obstet Gynecol 1986;67:517.

Sibai BM, Anderson GD, McCubbin JH: Eclampsia. 2. Clinical significance of laboratory findings. Obstet Gynecol 1982;59:153.

Sibai BM et al: A comparison of labetalol plus hospitalization versus hospitalization alone in the management of preeclampsia remote from term. Obstet Gynecol 1987;70:323.

Sibai BM et al: Eclampsia. 1. Observations from 67 recent cases. Obstet Gynecol 1981;58:609.

Sibai BM et al: Eclampsia. 4. Neurological findings and future outcome. Am J Obstet Gynecol 1985;152:184.

Sibai BM et al: Maternal and perinatal outcome of conservative management of severe preeclampsia in mid trimester. Am J Obstet Gynecol 1985;152:32.

Sibai BM et al: Pregnancy outcome of 303 cases with severe preeclampsia. Obstet Gynecol 1984;64:319.

Sibai BM et al: Prevention of preeclampsia: Low-dose aspirin in nulliparous women, a double-blind, placebo-controlled trial. Am J Obstet Gynecol 1993;167:286.

Sibai BM et al: A randomized prospective comparison of nifedipine and bed rest versus bed rest alone in the management of preeclampsia remote from term. Am J Obstet Gynecol 1992;167:879.

Strauss RG et al: Hemodynamic monitoring of cardiogenic pulmonary edema complicating toxemia of pregnancy. Obstet Gynecol 1980;55:170.

Tuffnell DJ et al: Randomized controlled trial of daycare for hypertension in pregnancy. Lancet 1992;339:224.

Vane JR, Botting RM: Endothelium-derived vasoactive factors and the control of the circulation. Semin Perinatal 1991;15:4.

Villar J et al: Calcium supplementation reduced blood pressure during pregnancy: Results from a randomized controlled clinical trial. Obstet Gynecol 1987;70:317.

Wallenburg HCS: Hemodynamics in hypertensive pregnancy. Pages 73–101 in: *Hypertension in Pregnancy*. Rubin PC (ed). Elsevier Publishers, 1988.

Wallenburg HCS et al: Low-dose aspirin prevents pregnancy-induced hypertension and preeclampsia in angiotensin-sensitive primigravidae. Lancet 1986;1:1.

Walters NJ, Redman CWG: Treatment of severe pregnancy-associated hypertension with the calcium antagonist nifedipine. Br J Obstet Gynecol 1984;91:330.

Watson DL et al: Late postpartum eclampsia: An update. South Med J 1983;76:1487.

Weinstein L: Syndrome of hemolysis, elevated liver enzymes, and low platelet count: A severe consequence of hypertension in pregnancy. Am J Obstet Gynecol 1982;142:159.

White WB: Management of hypertension during lactation. Hypertension 1984;6:297.

Zuspan FP: Problems encountered in the treatment of pregnancy-induced hypertension: A point of view. Am J Obstet Gynecol 1978;131:591.

Zuspan FP, O'Shaughnessy R: Chronic Hypertension in Pregnancy. Year Book, 1979.

# 20

# Third-Trimester Hemorrhage

*Martin L. Pernoll, MD*

Third-trimester hemorrhage continues to be one of the most ominous complications of pregnancy. Bleeding in late pregnancy is common; it requires medical evaluation in 5–10% of pregnancies. The seriousness and frequency of obstetric hemorrhage make it one of the 3 leading causes of maternal death and also a major cause of perinatal morbidity and mortality in the USA. Fortunately, most patients have only slight blood loss. However, even minor bleeding may be caused by a life-threatening disorder.

Differentiation must be made between obstetric causes of bleeding (usually more hazardous) and nonobstetric causes (usually less hazardous) (Table 20–1). Nonobstetric causes usually result in relatively little blood loss and little threat to mother or fetus. An exception is invasive carcinoma of the cervix. Obstetric causes are of more concern. Most serious hemorrhages (2–3% of pregnancies) lose more than 800 mL of blood and are due to premature separation of the placenta or placenta previa. Less common but still dangerous causes of bleeding are circumvallate placenta, abnormalities of the blood-clotting mechanism, and uterine rupture. Bleeding from the peripheral portion of the intervillous space, or marginal sinus rupture, is a debatable cause of bleeding. Extrusion of cervical mucus ("bloody show") is the most common cause of bleeding in late pregnancy. Enough blood may be lost to cause concern to the mother, but medical intervention is almost never necessary.

This chapter will focus on 3 major causes of hemorrhage: premature separation of the placenta, placenta previa, and uterine rupture. Circumvallate placenta (uncommon in late pregnancy but a major cause of second-trimester hemorrhage and fetal death) and marginal sinus rupture (usually self-limited) will be considered variants of premature separation of the placenta.

Although almost all of the blood loss from placental accidents is maternal, some fetal loss is also possible, particularly if the substance of the placenta is traumatized. Bleeding from vasa praevia is the only cause of pure fetal hemorrhage. Fortunately, this is rare. If fetal bleeding is suspected, the presence of nucleated red cells in the vaginal blood may be seen or the presence of fetal hemoglobin may be confirmed by elution or electrophoretic techniques.

## INITIAL EVALUATION

### Principles of Management

There are 2 principles that must be followed in investigation of third-trimester hemorrhage. (1) Any woman experiencing vaginal bleeding in late pregnancy must be evaluated in a hospital capable of dealing with maternal hemorrhage and a compromised perinate. (2) A vaginal or rectal examination must not be performed until placenta previa has been ruled out and until preparations are complete for management of massive hemorrhage and maternal or perinatal complications. Vaginal or rectal examination is extremely hazardous because of the possibility of provoking an uncontrollable, catastrophic hemorrhage.

### Life-Threatening Hemorrhage Associated With Hypovolemic Shock

Signs and symptoms of acute blood loss (hypovolemic shock) must be quickly noted. These include pallor, clammy skin, syncope, thirst, air hunger (dyspnea), restlessness, agitation, anxiety, confusion, falling blood pressure, increased or thready pulse (tachycardia), and oliguria (or anuria).

*Hypovolemic shock requires immediate treatment!* First, general antishock measures must be undertaken. Place the patient in the Trendelenburg position (but not in a position that would interfere with breathing). Guarantee an adequate airway (usually with a plastic oral airway.) Keep the patient warm, and provide fluid replacement with dextrose 5% and saline or lactated Ringer's injection while blood components are being obtained.

**A. Blood Transfusion:** Blood (whole or packed red blood cells), Plasmanate, or other plasma expanders should be administered rapidly, but cardiac overload must be carefully avoided. In extraordinary cases (severe blood loss, complicating maternal medical conditions), hemodynamic monitoring may be necessary. Correction of bicarbonate deficit and ad-

**Table 20–1.** Nonobstetric and obstetric causes of third-trimester bleeding.

**Nonobstetric causes**
    Cervicitis; cervical eversion, erosion, polyps and other benign neoplasms, malignant neoplasms
    Vaginal lacerations, varices, benign and malignant neoplasms (rare)
**Obstetric causes**
    Extrusion of cervical mucus ("bloody show")
    Premature separation of placenta
    Circumvallate placenta
    Marginal sinus rupture
    Placenta previa
    Uterine rupture
    Abnormal blood-clotting mechanism

justment of electrolyte imbalance may be necessary secondary steps.

**B. Vasoactive Drugs:** Vasoactive drugs should be used only when specific pharmacologic effects are desired (eg, increasing myocardial contractility), when volume expanders are not available, or when volume expansion and other measures are ineffective. Even in these cases, efficacy may be questioned; these agents should be used only when their benefit clearly outweighs the potential risk. The most commonly used agent is dopamine (a mixed alpha- and beta-adrenergic stimulant), 200 mg in 500 mL sodium chloride injection, USP, starting at 2–5 mcg/kg/min and increasing gradually in 5–10 mcg/kg/min up to 20–50 g/kg/min. Other agents that might be given by experienced personnel include levarterenol bitartrate, isoproterenol, metaraminol bitartrate, and phenylephrine.

### Nonemergency Bleeding

**A. History and Abdominal Examination:** If fulminant hemorrhage is not present, the usual plan of action for third-trimester bleeding is implemented. Obtain information about the acute episode and (briefly) the obstetric history, and record the patient's vital signs.

Abdominal examination is often the key in determining the next steps in immediate management. The upper extent of the uterus should be indicated with a ballpoint pen or other indelible ink mark on the patient's abdomen and measured in centimeters. This aids in determining gestational age and, later, in ascertaining if the uterus is rapidly expanding from concealed hemorrhage due to abruptio placentae. Leopold's maneuvers assist in determination of fetal size, presentation, position, and engagement. It is crucial to determine whether the presenting part is well engaged in the pelvis. When there is engagement, total placenta previa is unlikely. Palpation for uterine contractions, tone, and tenderness should be conducted. It should be determined whether the palpations evoke contractions (ie, ascertain uterine irritability). The fetal heart tones (or their absence) must be ascertained and appropriate monitoring initiated.

**B. Intravenous Fluids and Laboratory Evaluation:** Intravenous infusion (usually dextrose 5% in lactated Ringer's injection) is started with a large-gauge catheter (18-gauge minimum), and an appropriate laboratory workup is initiated. A typical laboratory evaluation for third-trimester bleeding includes a complete blood count (hemoglobin, hematocrit, and white blood count with differential), blood typing and cross-matching for whole blood or packed red cells (2-6 or more units may be needed, depending on the hemodynamic status), fibrinogen, prothrombin time, partial thromboplastin time, platelet count, and, possibly, peripheral smear for morphology. Additionally, a tube of blood sample retained at the bedside assists in clot observation. Urinary output monitoring is initiated. This usually requires an indwelling urinary catheter.

**C. Vaginal Examination:** If the patient is in active labor and the presenting part is unquestionably engaged, there is no merit in further delaying vaginal examination. Indeed, vaginal delivery may be imminent. Both a speculum and a manual vaginal examination should be performed. If possible, the membranes should be ruptured. The diagnosis will probably be either "bloody show" or partial premature separation of the placenta. If delivery is not imminent, preparations for ultrasonic study are completed.

**D. Ultrasound Examination:** When the patient's status permits, ultrasound scan is useful in diagnosis of placenta previa and placental separation. If the presentation is unengaged (whether or not the patient is in labor), vaginal or rectal examination should be delayed until (1) blood for possible transfusion is available and (2) ultrasonic scan has shown the placement of the placenta and whether or not a retroplacental clot exists. Ultrasonic evaluation should also include assessment of fetal well-being, estimation of gestational age, and localization of amniotic fluid. Ultrasonic evaluation is best done in the labor and delivery area, and fetal heart rate monitoring should continue at reasonable intervals throughout the procedure. Fetal maturity determination by amniocentesis and subsequent amniotic fluid evaluation may be necessary. Should this be the case, this is often the best time to perform amniocentesis. If the presenting part subsequently descends into the pelvis, vaginal examination is indicated, as noted above.

**E. Management of Bleeding:** At this point, findings regarding the status of the mother, fetus, and placenta and evaluation of labor should be combined to provide a diagnosis and to plan the course of management. The 3 general management options are immediate delivery, continued labor, or "expectant management," depending on the diagnosis.

If the fetus is not mature, the patient should be treated expectantly unless additional complications appear, eg, continuing bleeding, fetal distress, labor, or spontaneous rupture of the membranes. In about 90% of cases, third-trimester bleeding will subside within 24 hours. If placental studies signify a high placental implantation and bleeding stops, vaginal examination is indicated prior to discharge of the patient to exclude nonobstetric causes of bleeding.

In the past, a **"double setup examination"** was frequently employed for diagnosis of third-trimester bleeding. All preparations were made for cesarean section, except for administering the anesthetic. A careful vaginal examination with a speculum was then conducted. If the placenta was not visualized, it was thought that placenta previa could be ruled out. This proved to be a highly inaccurate, dangerous method of diagnosis as compared with ultrasonic localization of the placenta and cesarean delivery without vaginal examination for placenta previa. Therefore, the double setup examination has largely been abandoned.

Nonobstetric causes of bleeding in late pregnancy usually result only in spotting that does not increase with activity. There are no uterine contractions, and the definitive diagnosis is usually made by speculum examination, Papanicolaou smear, culture, or colposcopy. Only in advanced cancer is there a poor maternal prognosis. Vaginal lacerations and varices may require repair but have a good prognosis. Most infections causing bleeding clear readily when treated with appropriate agents. Benign neoplasias and eversions require simple treatment and have a good prognosis.

## PREMATURE SEPARATION OF THE PLACENTA
### (Abruptio Placentae, Ablatio Placentae, Accidental Hemorrhage)

### Essentials of Diagnosis
- Unremittent abdominal (uterine) or back pain.
- Irritable, tender, and often hypertonic uterus.
- Visible or concealed hemorrhage.
- Evidence of fetal distress may or may not be present depending on the severity of the process.

### General Considerations

Premature separation of the placenta is defined as separation from the site of uterine implantation before delivery of the fetus (about 1 in 77–89 deliveries). The severe form (resulting in fetal death) has an incidence of about 1 in 500–750 deliveries. Two principal forms of premature separation of the placenta may be recognized depending on whether the resulting hemorrhage is external or concealed (Fig 20–1). In the **concealed form** (20%), the hemorrhage is confined within the uterine cavity, detachment of the placenta may be complete, and the complications are often severe. Five to 8% develop coagulopathies, and fetal demise is far more likely. In the **external form** (80%), the blood drains through the cervix, placental detachment is more likely to be incomplete, and the

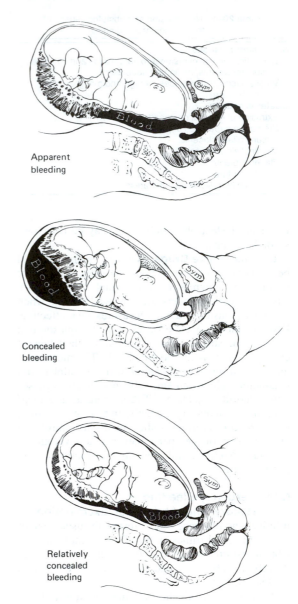

**Figure 20–1.** Types of premature separation of the placenta. (Redrawn and reproduced, with permission, from Beck AC, Rosenthal AH: Obstetrical Practice, 7th ed. Williams & Wilkins, 1957.)

complications are fewer and less severe. Hemorrhage from an incompletely detached placenta may sometimes be concealed by intact membranes, in which case it is said to be **relatively concealed.** Occasionally, the placental detachment involves only the margin or placental rim. Here, the most important complication is the possibility of premature labor.

Approximately 30% of cases of third-trimester bleeding are due to placental separation, with the initial hemorrhage usually encountered after the 26th week. Placental separation in early pregnancy cannot be distinguished from other causes of abortion. About 50% of separations occur before the onset of labor, and 10-15% are not diagnosed before the second stage of labor.

## Etiology

The exact causes of placental separation are often difficult to ascertain, although there are a number of predisposing and precipitating factors. A common predisposing factor is previous placental separation. Following one episode, the incidence of recurrence is 10–17%. Following 2 previous episodes, the incidence of recurrence exceeds 20%. The hypertensive states of pregnancy are associated with 2.5–17.9% incidence of placental separation. However, in abruptio placentae extensive enough to cause fetal death, about 50% of cases are associated with hypertensive states of pregnancy. Approximately half of these cases have chronic hypertension and half pregnancy-induced hypertension. Other predisposing factors include advanced maternal age, multiparity, uterine distention (eg, multiple pregnancy, hydramnios), vascular deficiency or deterioration (eg, diabetes mellitus, collagen diseases complicating pregnancy), uterine anomalies or tumors (eg, leiomyoma), cigarette smoking, alcohol consumption (> 14 drinks per week), and possibly maternal type O blood.

Precipitating causes of premature separation of the placenta, although more direct and definable, are no less diverse. All are rare. Included in this category are circumvallate placenta, trauma (eg, external or internal version, automobile accident, abdominal trauma directly transmitted to an anterior placenta), sudden reduction in uterine volume (eg, rapid amniotic fluid loss, delivery of a first twin), abnormally short cord (usually only a problem during delivery, when traction is exerted on the cord as the fetus moves down the birth canal), and increased venous pressure (usually only problematic with abrupt or extreme alterations).

## Pathophysiology & Pathology

Several mechanisms are thought to be important in the pathophysiology of premature placental separation. One mechanism is local vascular injury that results in vascular rupture into the decidua basalis, bleeding, and hematoma formation. The hematoma shears off adjacent denuded vessels, producing further bleeding and enlargement of the area of separation. Another mechanism is initiated by an abrupt rise in uterine venous pressure transmitted to the intervillous space. This results in engorgement of the venous bed and the separation of all or a portion of the placenta. Conditions predisposing to vascular injury and known to be associated with an increased incidence of placental separation are preeclampsia-eclampsia, chronic hypertension, diabetes mellitus, and chronic renal disease. Factors that may predispose to a disturbed vascular equilibrium and the possibility of

passive congestion of the venous bed in response to an abrupt rise in uterine venous pressure are vasodilatation secondary to shock, compensatory hypertension as a result of aortic compression, and the paralytic vasodilatation of conduction anesthesia.

Mechanical factors causing premature separation are rare (1–5%). They include transabdominal trauma, sudden decompression of the uterus such as with the delivery of a first twin or rupture of the membranes in hydramnios, or traction on a short umbilical cord.

Another possible mechanism is initiation of the coagulation cascade. This may occur, for example, with trauma causing release of tissue thromboplastin. These activated coagulation factors in turn may act to initiate clot formation in the relative hemodynamic stasis occurring in the placental pool.

Anatomically, placental abruption may occur by hemorrhage into the decidual basalis, which splits, leaving a thin layer adjacent to the myometrium. This decidual hematoma leads to separation, compression, and further bleeding. Alternatively, a spiral artery may rupture, creating a retroplacental hematoma. In either case, bleeding occurs, a clot forms, and the placental surface can no longer provide metabolic exchange between mother and fetus.

The clot depresses the adjacent placenta. Nonclotted blood courses from the site of injury. In concealed hemorrhage, this effusion may be totally retained behind the placental margins, behind the membrane attachment to the uterine wall, or behind a closely applied fetal presenting part. The blood may rupture through the membranes or placenta and gain access to the amniotic fluid (and vice versa). The tissue disruption by bleeding may allow maternal-fetal hemorrhage, fetomaternal hemorrhage, maternal bleeding into the amniotic fluid, or amniotic fluid embolus, depending on the areas disrupted and their relative pressure differences.

Concealed hemorrhage is more likely to be associated with complete placental detachment. If the placental margins remain adherent, central placental separation may result in hemorrhage that infiltrates the uterine wall. Uterine tetany follows. Occasionally, extensive intramyometrial bleeding results in uteroplacental apoplexy—so-called **Couvelaire uterus,** a purplish and copper-colored, ecchymotic, indurated organ that all but loses its contractile power because of disruption of the muscle bundles.

In the more severe cases of separation, there may be a clinically significant amount of disseminated intravascular coagulation associated with depletion of fibrinogen and platelets as well as other clotting factors. The mother may then develop a hemorrhagic diathesis that is manifested by widespread petechiae, active bleeding, hypovolemic shock, and failure of the normal clotting mechanism. In addition, fibrin deposits in small capillaries (along with the hypoxic vascular damage of shock) can result in potentially lethal complications, including acute cor pulmonale, renal cortical and tubular necrosis, and anterior pituitary necrosis (Sheehan's syndrome).

The likelihood of fetal hypoxia and fetal death depends on the amount and duration of placental separation and, in severe cases, the loss of a significant amount of fetal blood.

### Clinical Findings

**A. Symptoms and Signs:** In general, the clinical findings correspond to the degree of separation. About 30% of separations are small, produce few or no symptoms, and usually are not noted until the placenta is inspected. Larger separations are accompanied by abdominal pain and uterine irritability. Hemorrhage may be visible or concealed. If the process is extensive, there may be evidence of fetal distress, uterine tetany, disseminated intravascular coagulation, or hypovolemic shock. Increased uterine tonus and frequency of contractions reflected by fetal heart rate monitoring may provide early clues of abruption.

About 80% of patients will present with vaginal bleeding, and two-thirds will have uterine tenderness and abdominal or back pain. One-third will have abnormal contractions; about half of these will have high-frequency contractions and half hypertonus. More than 20% of patients with abruptio placentae will be diagnosed erroneously as having idiopathic premature labor. Fetal distress will be present in more than 50% of cases, and 15% will present with fetal demise.

If the placental separation is marginal, there will be only minimal irritability and no uterine tenderness or fetal distress. There may be a limited amount of external bleeding (50–150 mL), either bright or dark red depending on the rapidity of its appearance.

**B. Laboratory Findings:** The degree of anemia will probably be considerably less than the amount of blood loss would seem to justify, because changes in hemoglobin and hematocrit are delayed during acute blood loss until secondary hemodilution has occurred. A peripheral blood smear may show a reduced platelet count; the presence of schistocytes, suggesting intravascular coagulation; and fibrinogen depletion with release of fibrin split products. If serial laboratory determinations of fibrinogen levels are not available, the clot observation test, a simple but invaluable bedside procedure, can be performed. A venous blood sample is drawn every hour, placed in a clean test tube, and observed for clot formation and clot lysis. Failure of clot formation within 5–10 minutes or dissolution of a formed clot when the tube is gently shaken is proof of a clotting deficiency that is almost surely due principally to a lack of fibrinogen and platelets.

More sophisticated studies should be available on an emergency basis in most hospitals. The following will assist in determination of coagulation status: prothrombin time, and partial thromboplastin time, platelet count, fibrinogen, and fibrin split products.

Ultrasonography may be useful but is not totally reliable, because it may not reveal the retroplacental clot in most cases.

### Treatment

**A. Emergency Measures:** If the patient exhibits clinical findings that become progressively more severe or if a major placental separation has already occurred as manifested by hemorrhage, uterine spasm, or fetal distress, an acute emergency exists.

As the first step toward delivery and in an effort to minimize the possibility of disseminated intravascular coagulation or amniotic fluid embolus, the membranes should be artificially ruptured to release as much amniotic fluid as possible. Internal monitoring will provide useful information about uterine tonus and contractions as well as the status of the fetus.

At the same time, blood should be drawn for laboratory studies and at least 4 units of blood made ready for possible transfusion. An infusion apparatus with an 18-gauge needle or cannula is advisable. A solution of lactated Ringer's injection should be administered, and additional antishock measures should be instituted as necessary.

**B. Expectant Therapy:** Expectant therapy is appropriate when the fetus is immature; bleeding is not extensive; uterine irritability is absent or minimal; and there is no fetal distress. The presumptive diagnosis, if placenta previa can be ruled out, is probably a small marginal placental separation. The patient should be hospitalized, typed and crossmatched, and observed for a period of 24–48 hours until one is certain that further placental separation is not occurring, premature labor is not likely, and placenta previa is not present.

**C. Vaginal Delivery:** An attempt at vaginal delivery is indicated if the degree of separation appears to be limited and if the fetus can be monitored for signs of fetal distress. When placental separation is extensive but the fetus is dead or of dubious viability vaginal delivery is also indicated. The exception to vaginal delivery occurs when hemorrhage is rapid and uncontrollable and operative delivery is necessary to save the mother's life.

Induction of labor with an oxytocin infusion should be instituted if active labor does not begin shortly after amniotomy. In practice, augmentation is not often needed, because the uterus usually is already excessively irritable. If the uterus is extremely spastic, uterine contractions cannot be clearly identified unless an internal monitor is used, and the progress of labor must be judged by observing cervical dilatation. Progress in labor is usually so rapid that forceps are not needed to shorten the second stage of labor. Pudendal block anesthesia is recommended.

Conduction anesthesia is to be avoided in the face of significant hemorrhage because profound, persistent hypotension may result.

**D. Cesarean Section:** The indications for cesarean section are both fetal and maternal. Abdominal delivery should be selected whenever delivery is not imminent for a fetus with a reasonable chance of survival who exhibits persistent evidence of distress. Cesarean section is also indicated if the fetus is in good condition but the situation is not favorable for rapid delivery in the face of progressive or severe placental separation. This includes most nulliparous patients with less than 3–4 cm of cervical dilatation. Maternal indications for cesarean section are uncontrollable hemorrhage from a contracted uterus, a rapidly expanding uterus with concealed hemorrhage (with or without a live fetus) when delivery is not imminent, uterine apoplexy as manifested by hemorrhage with secondary relaxation of a previously spastic uterus, or refractory uterus with delivery necessary (20%).

**Complications**

**A. Defibrination Syndrome:** The mother must be continuously monitored well into the postpartum period for evidence of a clotting deficiency. There may be depletion not only of fibrinogen but also of platelet and of factors II, V, VIII, and X. Treatment will depend not only on the demonstration of hematologic deficiencies but also on the amount of active bleeding and the anticipated route of delivery.

**1. Fresh whole blood**–Fresh whole blood, although often difficult to obtain, is superior for treating clotting deficiencies and replacing blood loss because all the necessary factors will be present.

**2. Packed red blood cells**–Packed red blood cells are satisfactory for immediately replacing blood loss, but they do not contain clotting factors.

**3. Cryoprecipitate packs**–Cryoprecipitate packs contain all the necessary labile coagulation factors and are free of hepatitis B virus.

**4. Platelets**–During active bleeding, the transfusion of platelets is often the best practical means of counteracting a clotting deficiency. A platelet pack contains about 20% fewer platelets than 1 unit of fresh blood.

**5. Fibrinogen**–Fibrinogen is rarely indicated. *Do not administer fibrinogen solely on the basis of laboratory tests.* In the absence of active bleeding, fibrinogen deficiency may be corrected spontaneously in a matter of hours. To administer fibrinogen under these circumstances is both unnecessary and likely to make matters worse because the excess fibrinogen may be converted to fibrin emboli. The best source of fibrinogen other than fresh blood is a cryoprecipitated preparation. Concentrated plasma can also be used. Quadruple-strength plasma contains about 4.4 g of fibrinogen per unit. The initial dose of fibrinogen is 4–6 g, but as much as 20–24 g may be required depending on the response.

**6. Heparin**–The prophylactic administration of heparin to block conversion of prothrombin to thrombin (and thereby reduce the consumption of coagulation factors) has been successfully employed in the management of the defibrination associated with fetal death ("dead fetus syndrome"). The value of heparin in the treatment of acute placental separation has never been established; its use cannot be recommended, because of the risks of operative and postoperative hemorrhage if cesarean section is required.

**7. Fibrinolysins**–Fibrinolysins such as aminocaproic acid (Amicar) should not be given. This drug will complicate the problem by interfering with the mechanism of fibrinolysis.

**8. Preparation for surgery**–Preparation for surgery must be completed quickly. If cesarean section is indicated, materials to control a clotting deficiency must be on hand before an operation is undertaken, and treatment with coagulants should be underway if a clotting deficiency is already present. Although control of a clotting deficiency before surgery is started is desirable, a rapid rate of blood loss may require earlier intervention. In rare instances, removal of an extensively damaged uterus has been necessary to control hemorrhage—or even the clotting deficiency.

**B. Acute Cor Pulmonale:** Acute cor pulmonale is always a possibility because of emboli in the pulmonary microcirculation as a result of either defibrination or the escape of amniotic cellular debris into maternal veins. The most important aspect of the immediate treatment of this life-threatening complication is the use of a volume respirator.

**C. Renal Cortical and Tubular Necrosis:** The possibility of renal cortical or tubular necrosis must be considered if oliguria persists after an adequate blood volume has been restored. An attempt should be made to improve renal circulation and promote diuresis by increasing fluid volume (with the aid of monitoring). If oliguria or anuria persists, renal necrosis is probable and fluid intake and output must be carefully monitored. Continuing impairment of renal function may require peritoneal dialysis or hemodialysis.

**D. Transfusion Hepatitis:** The risk of post transfusion hepatitis has been reduced an estimated 25–40% by hepatitis antigen (HAA) screening tests. However, there is no evidence that prophylactic gamma globulin will reduce either the incidence or the severity of hepatitis.

**E. Uterine Apoplexy:** Extensive infiltration of the myometrial wall with blood may result in loss of myometrial contractility. If, as a result, bleeding from the placental bed is not controlled, hysterectomy may be necessary. If future childbearing is an important consideration, bilateral ligation of the ascending branches of the uterine arteries should be accomplished before resorting to hysterectomy. Not only will blood flow be reduced, but the relative ischemia produced may result in a satisfactory contraction of the damaged uterus. If ligation of the uterine vessels proves ineffective, bilateral ligation of the hypogastric arteries, reducing arterial pressure within the uterus to venous levels, may effect hemostasis. Following ligation of either the uterine or hypogastric arteries, collateral circulation should be adequate to preserve uterine function, including subsequent pregnancies.

## Prognosis

External or concealed bleeding, excessive blood loss, shock, nulliparity, a closed cervix, absence of labor, and delayed diagnosis and treatment are unfavorable prognostic factors. Maternal mortality rates ranging from 0.5% to 5% are currently reported from various parts of the world. Most women die of hemorrhage (immediate or delayed) or cardiac or renal failure. A high degree of suspicion, early diagnosis, and definitive therapy should reduce the maternal mortality rate to 0.5–1%.

With severe abruption reported fetal mortality rates range from 50% to 80%. In about 15% of cases, no fetal heart-beat can be heard on admission to the hospital, and in another 50%, fetal distress is noted early. The fetal distress has several possible causes, eg, decreased metabolic exchange from decreased

placental surface, maternal hemorrhage with decreased uterine perfusion, fetal hemorrhage, uterine hypertonus interfering with proper metabolic exchange. In cases in which transfusion of the mother is urgently required, the fetal mortality rate will probably be at least 50%. Liveborn infants have a high rate of morbidity resulting from predelivery hypoxia, birth trauma, and the hazards of prematurity (40–50%).

## PLACENTA PREVIA

### Essentials of Diagnosis

- Spotting during first and second trimesters.
- Sudden, painless, profuse bleeding in third trimester.
- Initial cramping in 10% of cases.

### General Considerations

In placenta previa, the placenta is implanted in the lower uterine segment within the zone of effacement and dilatation of the cervix, thus constituting an obstruction to descent of the presenting part (Fig 20–2). Placenta previa is encountered in approximately one in 200 births, but only 20% are total (placenta over the entire cervix). About 90% of patients will be parous. Among grand multiparas the incidence may be as high as 1 in 20. Placenta previa may also be in-

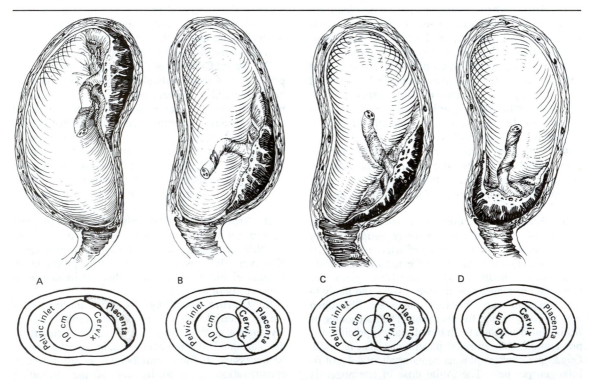

**Figure 20–2. A:** Normal placenta. **B.** Low implantation. **C:** Partial placenta previa. **D:** Complete placenta previa.

volved in up to 5% of spontaneous abortions, although its presence usually is not recognized.

## Etiology

The incidence of placenta previa is increased by advancing age, multiparity, and previous cesarean delivery. Thus, possible etiologic factors include scarred or poorly vascularized endometrium in the corpus, a large placenta, and abnormal forms of placentation such as succenturiate lobe or placenta diffusa. A large placenta probably accounts for the observation that the incidence of placenta previa is doubled in multiple pregnancy. A low cervical cesarean section scar triples the incidence of placenta previa. Another contributory factor is an increased average surface area of a placenta implanted in the lower uterine segment, possibly because these tissues are less well suited for nidation.

Bleeding in placenta previa may be due to any of the following causes: (1) Mechanical separation of the placenta from its implantation site, either during the formation of the lower uterine segment or during effacement and dilatation of the cervix in labor, or as a result of intravaginal manipulation. (2) Placentitis. (3) Rupture of poorly supported venous lakes in the decidua basalis that have become engorged with venous blood.

## Classification

A number of different clinical classifications of placenta previa have been proposed, all of which are based on the relationship of the placenta to the cervix either prior to the onset of labor or at various stages of cervical effacement and dilatation. As a practical matter, a precise clinical classification of placenta previa is not of great importance.

## Diagnosis

Every patient suspected of placenta previa should be hospitalized, and at least 3 units of cross-matched blood should be at hand. Unless these precautions are taken, there is always the danger that vaginal manipulation may provoke an uncontrollable, fatal hemorrhage.

**A. Symptoms and Signs:** Painless hemorrhage is the cardinal sign of placenta previa. Although spotting may occur during the first and second trimesters of pregnancy, the first episode of hemorrhage usually begins at some point after the 28th week and is characteristically described as being sudden, painless, and profuse. With the initial bleeding episode, clothing or bedding is soaked by an impressive amount of bright red, clotted blood, but the blood loss usually is not extensive, seldom produces shock, and is almost never fatal. In about 10% of cases there is some initial pain because of coexisting placental abruption, and spontaneous labor may be expected over the next few days in 25% of patients. In a small minority of cases, bleeding will be less dramatic or will not begin until after spontaneous rupture of the membranes or the onset of labor. A few nulliparous patients even reach term without bleeding, possibly because the placenta has been protected by an uneffaced cervix.

The uterus usually is soft, relaxed, and nontender. A high presenting part cannot be pressed into the pelvic inlet. The infant will present in an oblique or transverse lie in about 15% of cases. No evidence of fetal distress is likely unless there are complications such as hypovolemic shock, abruption, or a cord accident.

**B. Ultrasonography:** Prior to vaginal examination, an effort should be made to confirm or rule out placenta previa by means of sonography, unless immediate delivery is either desirable or made necessary by hemorrhage, labor, or fetal distress (Fig 20–3). The real-time scanner is ideal for screening purposes, because the equipment is portable, the test is rapidly and easily performed, and the accuracy rate is over 95%. During the middle of the second trimester, the placenta will be observed by ultrasound to cover the internal cervical os in about 30% of cases. With development of the lower uterine segment, most of these low implantations will be carried to a higher station. An early ultrasonic diagnosis of placenta previa will require the confirmation of an additional study before definitive action is taken. A second source of error is a blood clot in the lower uterine segment that can be mistaken for placenta if the test has not been carefully performed.

Ultrasonography is an excellent means of identifying those patients who clearly do not have placenta previa and who can thereafter be examined vaginally with impunity. Ultrasonography is also an important method of identifying the low-lying posteriorly implanted placenta. Knowledge of this condition is important for the placenta lying over the sacral promin-

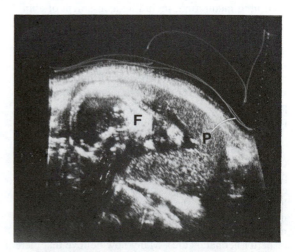

**Figure 20–3.** Ultrasonogram showing complete placenta previa. The placenta (P) is clearly shown implanted on the lower uterine segment. F, fetus.

tory may preclude the fetal presenting part from entering the pelvis. Additionally, with long labors or particularly strong contractions the placenta may be traumatized enough to initiate bleeding.

### Differential Diagnosis

Placental causes of bleeding other than placenta previa include partial premature separation of the normally implanted placenta or circumvallate placenta.

### Treatment

The type of treatment given depends on the amount of uterine bleeding; the duration of pregnancy and viability of the fetus; the degree of placenta previa; the presentation, position, and station of the fetus; the gravidity and parity of the patient; the status of the cervix; and whether or not labor has begun. The patient must be admitted to the hospital to establish the diagnosis and ideally should remain in the hospital once the diagnosis is made. Two or more units of bank blood should be typed, cross-matched, and ready for transfusion.

**A. Expectant Therapy:** The initial hemorrhage of placenta previa may occur before pulmonary maturation is established. In such cases, fetal survival can often be enhanced by expectant therapy. Early in pregnancy, transfusions to replace blood loss and the use of tocolytic agents to prevent premature labor are indicated to prolong pregnancy to at least 36 weeks. After 36 weeks, the benefits of additional maturity must be weighed against the risk of major hemorrhage. The possibility that repeated small hemorrhages may be accompanied by intrauterine growth retardation must also be considered. About 75% of cases of placenta previa are now terminated at between 36 and 40 weeks.

In selecting the optimum time for delivery, tests of fetal lung maturation, including assessment of amniotic fluid surfactants and ultrasonic growth measurements, are invaluable adjuvants.

Because of the costs of hospitalization, patients with a presumptive diagnosis of placenta previa are somtimes sent home after their condition has become stable under ideal, controlled circumstances. Such a policy is always a calculated risk in view of the unpredictability of further hemorrhage.

**B. Delivery:**

**1. Cesarean section–**Cesarean section has become the delivery method of choice with placenta previa. Perinatal mortality rates are lower with cesarean delivery for every type of placenta previa (even lesser degrees). Cesarean section has proved to be the most important factor in lowering maternal and perinatal mortality rates (more so than blood transfusion or better neonatal care). Many now believe that there is almost no indication for vaginal delivery in these cases.

Hypovolemic shock should be corrected by intravenous fluids and blood before the operation is started. Not only will the mother be better protected, but a jeopardized fetus will also recover more quickly in utero than if born while the mother is still in shock.

The choice of anesthesia depends on current and anticipated blood loss. A combination of rapid induction, endotracheal intubation, succinylcholine, and nitrous oxide is a suitable way to proceed in the presence of active bleeding.

The choice of operative technique is of importance because of the placental location and the development of the lower uterine segment. If the incision passes through the site of placental implantation, there is a strong possibility that the fetus will lose a significant amount of blood—even enough to require subsequent transfusion. With posterior implantations of the placenta, a low transverse incision may be best if the lower uterine segment is well developed. Otherwise, a classic incision may be required to secure sufficient room and to avoid incision through the placenta.

Preparations should be made for care and resuscitation of the infant if it becomes necessary. In addition, the possibility of blood loss should be monitored in the newborn if the placenta has been incised. A fall in hemoglobin to 12 g/dL within 3 hours or to 10 g/dL within 24 hours requires urgent transfusion.

In a small percentage of cases, hemostasis in the placental bed will not be satisfactory, because of the poor contractility of the lower uterine segment. Mattress sutures or packing may be required in addition to the usual oxytocin, prostaglandins and methergine. If placenta previa increta is found, hemostasis may necessitate a total hysterectomy.

Puerperal infection and anemia are the most likely postoperative complications.

**2. Vaginal delivery–**Vaginal delivery is usually reserved for patients with a low-lying implantation and a cephalic presentation or a greater degree of placenta previa when there is little or no prospect of salvaging the fetus. If vaginal delivery is elected, the membranes should be artifically ruptured prior to any attempt to stimulate labor (oxytocin given before amniotomy is likely to cause further bleeding). Tamponade of the presenting part against the placental edge usually reduces bleeding as labor progress.

If labor does not follow rupture of the membranes within 6–8 hours, cautious stimulation with intravenous oxytocin (Pitocin, Syntocinon), 5 units (0.5 mL) in 1 L of 5% glucose, may be given at a rate of 1–2 mL/min (or better given by an infusion pump).

Because of the possibility of fetal hypoxia either due to placental separation or to a cord accident (as a result of either prolapse or compression of low insertion of the cord by the descending presenting part), internal fetal monitoring must be employed. If fetal distress develops, a rapid cesarean section should be performed unless vaginal delivery is imminent.

Deliver the patient in the easiest and most expeditious manner as soon as the cervix is fully dilated and the presenting part is on the perineum. For this purpose, a vacuum extractor is particularly valuable because it expedites delivery without risking rupture of the lower uterine segment. Operative vaginal manipulations such as forceps rotation, breech extraction, and version should be undertaken with caution because of the danger of uterine rupture.

## Complications

**A. Maternal:** Maternal hemorrhage, shock, and death may follow severe antepartum bleeding resulting from placenta previa. Death may also occur as a result of intrapartum and postpartum bleeding, operative trauma, infection, or embolism.

Premature separation of a portion of a placenta previa occurs in virtually every case and causes excessive external bleeding without pain; however, complete or wide separation of the placenta before full dilatation of the cervix is not common.

Placenta previa accreta is a rare but serious abnormality in which the sparse endometrium and the myometrium of the lower uterine segment are penetrated by the trophoblast in a manner similar to placenta acreta higher in the uterus.

**B. Fetal:** Prematurity (gestational age less than 36 weeks) due to placenta previa accounts for 60% of perinatal deaths. The fetus may die as a result of intrauterine asphyxia or birth injury. Fetal hemorrhage due to tearing of the placenta occurs with vaginal manipulation and especially upon entry into the uterine cavity as cesarean section done for placenta previa. About half of these cesarean babies lose some blood. Fetal blood loss is directly proportionate to the time that elapses between laceration of cotyledon and clamping the cord.

## Prognosis

**A. Maternal:** With antibiotics, a blood bank, expertly administered anesthesia, and cesarean section, the maternal prognosis in placenta previa is excellent. This has been particularly true since the almost total abandonment of vaginal examination and the double setup examination. The total abandonment of hazardous vaginal maneuvers such as internal podalic version and the hydrostatic bag, the recognition of the dangers of injudicious vaginal and rectal examinations, and the hospitalization of mothers at risk have decreased the principal maternal hazard, hypovolemic shock.

**B. Fetal:** The perinatal mortality rate associated with placenta previa in most medical centers has been 15–20%, or at least 10 times that of normal pregnancy. Although premature labor, placental separation, cord accidents, and uncontrollable hemorrhage cannot be avoided, the mortality rate can be greatly reduced if ideal obstetric and newborn care is given.

# RUPTURE OF THE UTERUS

## Essentials of Diagnosis

- Increased suprapubic pain and tenderness with labor.
- Sudden cessation of uterine contractions with a "tearing" sensation.
- Vaginal bleeding (or bloody urine).
- Recession of the fetal presenting part.
- Disappearance of fetal heart tones.

## General Considerations

Rupture of the pregnant uterus is a potential obstetric catastrophe and a major cause of maternal death. The incidence of uterine rupture is approximately one in 1500 deliveries.

Complete rupture includes the entire thickness of the uterine wall and, in most cases, the overlying serosal peritoneum (Fig 20–4). "Occult" or "incomplete rupture" is a term usually reserved for dehiscence of a uterine incision from previous surgery. Such defects are usually asymptomatic unless converted to complete rupture during the course of pregnancy or labor.

Complete ruptures usually occur during the course of labor. One notable exception is the scar of a classic cesarean section (or hysterotomy) that typically ruptures during the third trimester before term and before the onset of labor. Other causes of rupture without labor are placenta percreta, invasive mole, choriocarcinoma, and cornual pregnancy.

Complete ruptures may be classified as traumatic or spontaneous. Traumatic ruptures occur most commonly as a result of motor vehicle accidents, improper administration of an oxytocic agent, or an inept attempt at operative vaginal delivery. Breech extraction through an incompletely dilated cervix is

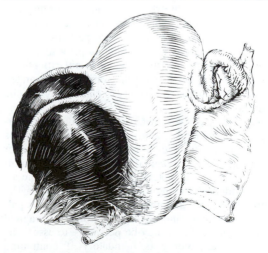

**Figure 20–4.** Rupture of lower uterine segment into broad ligament.

the type of operative vaginal delivery most likely to produce uterine rupture. Other maneuvers that impose risk of rupture are internal podalic version and extraction, difficult forceps, destructive operations, and maneuvers to relieve shoulder dystocia. Tumultuous labor, excessive fundal pressure or violent bearing-down efforts, and neglected obstructed labor may also be responsible for rupture of the uterus. Causes of obstructed labor include contracted pelvis, fetal macrosomia, brow or face presentation, hydrocephalus, or tumors involving the birth canal. Direct violence to the abdomen is a rare cause of rupture but is occasionally encountered in automobile accidents, particularly if the victim was wearing a lap-type seat belt.

Spontaneous rupture is somewhat of a misnomer because most such patients either have a uterine scar or give a history compatible with previous trauma that may have resulted in permanent uterine damage. Previous uterine surgery includes both classic and low cervical section, intramural or submucuous myomectomy, resection of the uterine cornu, metroplasty, and trachelectomy. Other operative procedures that may have damaged the uterus are vigorous curettage, induced abortion, and manual removal of the placenta. In contrast, some patients give no history of surgery but may be suspected of having a weakened uterus because of multiparity. Such patients are particularly at risk if they have an old lateral cervical laceration that could extend to involve a uterine artery.

### Clinical Findings

There are no reliable signs of impending uterine rupture, although the sudden appearance of gross hematuria is suggestive.

Prior to the onset of labor, a beginning rupture may produce local pain and tenderness associated with increased uterine irritability and, in some cases, a small amount of vaginal bleeding. Premature labor may follow. As the extent of the rupture increases, there will be more pain, more bleeding, and perhaps signs of hypovolemic shock. Exsanguination prior to surgery is unlikely because of the reduced vascularity of scar tissue, but the placenta may be completely separated and the fetus extruded partially or completely into the abdominal cavity.

Rupture of a low cervical scar usually occurs during labor, but clearly identifiable signs and symptoms are often lacking. Thus, it is quite possible that labor will progress to the vaginal birth of an unaffected infant. Even so, the rupture may lacerate a uterine artery, producing exsanguination, or the fetus may be extruded into the abdominal cavity. If a defect is palpated in the lower uterine segment following vaginal delivery, laparotomy may be necessary to assess the damage. Laparotomy is mandatory if continuing hemorrhage is present.

The classic findings of spontaneous rupture during labor are suprapubic pain and tenderness, cessation of uterine contractions, disappearance of fetal heart tones, recession of the presenting part, and vaginal hemorrhage—followed by the signs and symptoms of hypovolemic shock and hemoperitoneum. X-ray examination might confirm an abnormal fetal position or extension of the fetal extremities. Hemoperitoneum can easily be confirmed by paracentesis.

Uterine rupture due to obstetric trauma is usually not diagnosed until after the infant's birth. The clinical picture dpends on the site and extent of rupture. Unfortunately, valuable time is often lost because the rupture was not diagnosed at the time of the initial examination. Whenever a newly delivered patient exhibits persistent bleeding or shock, the uterus must be carefully reexamined for signs of a rupture that may have been difficult to palpate because of the soft, irregular tissue surfaces. Whenever an operative delivery is performed—especially if the past history includes events or problems that increase the likelihood of uterine rupture—the initial examination of the uterus and birth canal must be diligent.

### Treatment

Hysterectomy is the preferred treatment for most cases of complete uterine rupture. Either total hysterectomy or the subtotal operation can be employed, depending on the site of rupture and the patient's condition. The most difficult cases are lateral ruptures involving the lower uterine segment and a uterine artery with hemorrhage and hematoma formation obscuring the operative field. These patients may be better saved by ligation of the ipsilateral hypogastric artery for hemostasis, thus avoiding the risk of ureteral drainage by blind suturing at the base of the broad ligament. If there is a question of ureteral occlusion by a suture, it is best to perform cystotomy to observe the bilateral appearance of an intravenously injected dye, eg, indigo carmine. If doubt still exists, a retrograde ureteral catheter should be passed upward through the cystotomy wound.

If childbearing is important and the risks—both short- and long-term—are acceptable to the patient, rupture repair can be attempted. Many ruptures can be repaired.

In long-neglected and badly infected cases, survival may be improved by limiting the surgical procedure to repair of the rupture and by antibiotic therapy.

Occult ruptures of the lower uterine segment encountered at repeat section may be treated by freshening the wound edges and secondary repair, but the newly repaired incision will probably be weak.

### Prevention

Most of the causes of uterine rupture can be avoided by good obstetric assessment and technique. Probably the most common error in judgment leading to rupture is underestimation of fetal weight, resulting in traumatic delivery. The most common technical error is the poorly supervised administration of oxytocin during labor. A frequent deficiency in operative technique is poor closure of a cesarean section incision.

## Complications

The complications of ruptured uterus are hemorrhage, shock, postoperative infection, ureteral damage, thrombophlebitis, amniotic fluid embolus, disseminated intravascular coagulation, pituitary failure, and death. If the patient survives, infertility or sterility may result.

## Prognosis

The maternal mortality rate is 10–40%, and deaths are about equally divided among cases of oxytocic augmentation of labor, delivery trauma, and previous obstetric or surgical uterine scars. Only about 25% of delivered patients who die are correctly diagnosed at the time of initial postdelivery vaginal examination. The perinatal mortality rate exceeds 50%.

## REFERENCES

Adams DM, Druzin ML, Cederqvist LL: Intrapartum uterine rupture. Obstet Gynecol 1989;73:471.

Arias F: Cervical cerclage for the temporary treatment of patients with placenta previa. Obstet Gynecol 1988; 71:545.

Barrett JM, Boehm FH, Killiam AP: Induced abortion: A risk factor for placenta previa. Am J Obstet Gy 1981; 141:769.

Bond AL: Expectant management of abruptio placenta before 35 weeks gestation. Am J Perinatol 1989;6:123.

Brenner WE, Edelman DA, Hendricks CH: Characteristics of patients with placenta previa and results of "expectant management." Am J Obstet Gynecol 1978;132:180.

Carp HJA, Mashiach S, Serr DM: Vasa previa: A major complication and its management. Obstet Gy 1979; 53:273.

Clark SL: Rupture of the scarred uterus. Obstet Gynecol Clin North Am 1988;15:737.

Crenshaw C Jr, Darnell J, Parker RT: Placenta previa: A survey of twenty years' experience with improved perinatal survival of expectant therapy and cesarean section. Obstet Gynecol Surv 1973;28:461.

Crosby WM, Costiloe JP: Safety of lap-belt restraint for pregnant victims of automobile collisions. N Engl J Med 1971;284:632.

Darby MJ, Caritis SN, Shen-Schwarz S: Placental abruption in the preterm gestation: An association with chorioamnionitis. Obstet Gynecol 1989;74:88.

DeValera E: Abruptio placentae. Am J Obstet Gynecol 1968;100:999.

Dunster GD et al: Placental localization: A comparison of isotopic and ultrasonic placentography. Br J Radiol 1976;49:940.

Eden RD, Parker RT, Gall SA: Rupture of the pregnant uterus: A 53-year review. Obstet Gynecol 1986;68:671.

Farine D, et al: Vaginal ultrasound for diagnosis of placenta previa. Am J Obstet Gynecol 1988;159:566.

Fedorkow DM, Nimrod CA, Taylor PJ: Ruptured uterus in pregnancy: A Canadian hospital's experience. Can Med Assoc J 1987;137:27.

Fuchs AR, Fuchs F, Stubblefield PG: *Preterm Birth,* Second Edition. McGraw-Hill, New York, 1993.

Goldberg BB: The identification of placenta previa. Radiology 1978;128:255.

Goujard J, Rumeau C, Schwartz D: Smoking during pregnancy, stillbirth and abruptio placentae. Biomedicine [Express] 1975;23:20.

Hertig AT, Rock J: On the development of the early human ovum with special reference to the trophoblast of the previlous stage: A description of 7 normal and 5 pathologic ovarian ova. Am J Obstet Gynecol 1944;47:149.

Hurd WW et al: Selective management of abruptio placentae: A prospective study. Obstet Gynecol 1983;61:467.

Jaffe MH et al: Sonography of abruptio placentae. AJR 1981;137:1049.

Jeffrey RB, Laing FC: Sonography of the low-lying placenta: Value of Tredelenburg and traction scans. AJR 1981;137:547.

Kohler HG, Iqbal N, Jenkins DM: Chorionic haemangiomata and abruptio placentae. Br J Obstet Gynaecol 1976;83:667.

Meehan FP, Magani IM: True rupture of the ceasarean scar: A 15 year review, 1972-1987. Eur J Obstet Gynecol Reprod Biol 1989;30:129.

Naeye RL: Abruptio placentae and placenta previa: Frequency, perinatal mortality, and cigarette smoking. Obstet Gynecol 1980;55:701.

Naeye RL, Harkness WL, Utts J: Abruptio placentae and perinatal death: A prospective study. Am J Obstet Gynecol 1977;128:740.

Paterson MEL: The aetiology and outcome of abruptio placentae. Acta Obstet Gynecol Scand 1979;58:31.

Pritchard JA et al: Genesis of severe placental abruption. Am J Obstet Gynecol 1970;108:22.

Rizos N et al: Natural history of placenta previa ascertained by diagnostic ultrasound. Am J Obstet Gy 1979;133:287.

Sher G: Pathogenesis and management of uterine inertia complicating abruptio placentae with consumption coagulopathy. Am J Obstet Gynecol 1977;129:164.

Smith JJ, Schinfeld J, Schulman H: Placenta previa: Reappraisal and new therapeutic classification (HALO). NY State J Med 1982;82:1037.

Tucker SM: Perinatal protocol. Second or third trimester bleeding. J Perinatol 1988;8:174.

Wexler P, Gottesfeld KR: Early diagnosis of placenta previa. Obstet Gynecol 1979;54:231.

# Malpresentation & Cord Prolapse

*Joseph V. Collea, MD*

## BREECH PRESENTATION

Breech presentation occurs when the fetal pelvis or lower extremities engage in the maternal pelvic inlet. Three types of breech are distinguished, according to fetal **attitude** (Fig 21–1). (1) In **frank breech,** the thighs are flexed on the abdomen and both legs are extended at the knee. (2) In **complete breech,** both thighs are flexed on the abdomen and both legs are flexed at the knee. (3) In **footling breech,** one (single footling breech) or both (double footling breech) legs are extended below the level of the buttocks.

In singleton breech presentations in which the infant weighs less than 2500 g, 40% are frank breech, 10% complete breech, and 50% footling breech. With birth weights of more than 2500 g, 65% are frank breech, 10% complete breech, and 25% footling breech.

The incidence of singleton breech presentations is shown in Table 21–1.

Fetal **position** in breech presentation is determined by using the sacrum as the fetal point of reference to the maternal pelvis. This is true for frank, complete, and footling breeches (Fig 21–2). Eight possible positions are recognized: sacrum anterior (SA), sacrum posterior (SP), left sacrum transverse (LST), right sacrum transverse (RST), left sacrum anterior (LSA), left sacrum posterior (LSP), right sacrum anterior (RSA), and right sacrum posterior (RSP).

The **station** of the breech presenting part is the location of the fetal sacrum with regard to the maternal ischial spines.

## Causes

Before 28 weeks, the fetus is small enough in relation to intrauterine volume to rotate from cephalic to breech presentation and back again with relative ease. As gestational age and fetal weight increase, the relative decrease in intrauterine volume makes such changes more difficult. In most cases, the fetus spontaneously assumes the cephalic presentation to better accommodate the bulkier breech pole in the roomier fundal portion of the uterus.

Breech presentation occurs when spontaneous version to cephalic presentation is prevented as term approaches or if labor and delivery occur prematurely before cephalic version has taken place. Some causes include oligohydramnios, uterine anomalies such as bicornuate or septate uterus, pelvic tumors obstructing the birth canal, multiple gestation, and fetal congenital malformation.

Multiple fetuses may prevent each other from turning. In twin gestation, the incidence of breech for the first twin is 25% and for the second twin nearly 50%. The percentage is increased with additional fetuses. Congenital malformations of the fetus commonly associated with breech presentation include congenital hip dislocation, hydrocephalus, anencephalus, familial dysautonomia, spina bifida, meningomyelocele, and chromosomal trisomies 18 and 21 (Down's syndrome). Chromosomal, neuromuscular, and skeletal malformations that affect the form, function, and movement of the fetus may prevent turning. The incidence of congenital fetal malformations in singleton breech presentation exceeds 6%, while that for cephalic presentation is only 2-3%.

Once a fetus assumes frank breech presentation, it may not be able to revert to cephalic presentation, because the lower extremities essentially act as a splint for the body. Advanced multiparity, contracted maternal pelvis, placenta previa, and hydramnios are no longer considered causative factors in breech presentation.

## Diagnosis

**A. Palpation and Ballottement:** Performance of Leopold's maneuvers and ballottement of the uterus may confirm breech presentation. The softer, more ill-defined breech may be felt in the lower uterine segment above the pelvic inlet. Diagnostic error is common, however, if palpation and ballottement alone are used to determine presentation.

**B. Pelvic Examination:** During vaginal examination, the round, firm, smooth head in cephalic presentation can easily be distinguished from the soft,

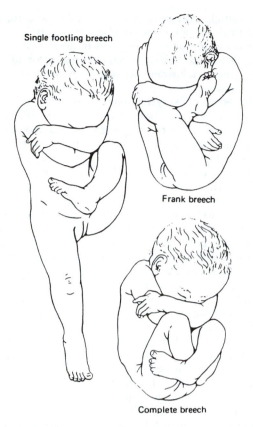

Single footling breech

Frank breech

Complete breech

**Figure 21–1.** Types of breech presentations. (Reproduced, with permission, from Benson RC: *Handbook of Obstetrics & Gynecology*, 8th ed. Lange, 1983.)

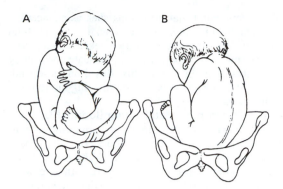

**Figure 21–2.** Breech presentation. A: Right sacrum posterior (RSP) position. B: Left sacrum anterior (LSA) position. (Redrawn and reproduced, with permission, from Bumm E: *Grundriss zum Studium der Geburtshilfe.* Bergmann, 1922.)

irregular breech presentation if the presenting part is dipping into the maternal pelvis. However, if no presenting part is palpable, further studies are necessary.

**C. Ultrasound:** Ultrasonographic scanning by an experienced examiner will document fetal presentation, attitude, and size; multiple gestation; location of the placenta; and amniotic fluid volume. Ultrasound will also reveal skeletal and soft tissue malformations of the fetus. Ultrasonographic measurements of the biparietal diameter, abdominal circumference, and femur length will provide a good estimate of weight and gestational age.

**D. X-Ray Studies:** X-ray studies will differentiate breech and cephalic presentations and also the type of breech by locating the position of the lower extremities. X-ray will also reveal multiple gestation and skeletal defects. Fetal attitude may be seen, but fetal size cannot readily be determined by x-ray. Because of the risks of radiation exposure to the fetus with this technique, ultrasonography is now often used instead to determine fetal presentation or malformations.

## Management

**A. Antepartum Management:** Following confirmation of breech presentation, the mother must be closely followed to see if spontaneous version to cephalic presentation occurs. If breech presentation persists beyond 36 weeks, external cephalic version should be considered (see below). The mother should be informed of the presentation and of management options.

X-ray pelvimetry should be done to rule out women with a borderline or contracted pelvis. Accurate pelvic examination may also be obtained by computed tomographic techniques or by MRI. Attempts at vaginal delivery with an inadequate pelvis are associated with a high rate of difficult delivery and significant trauma to mother and fetus. Difficult vaginal delivery may still occur in women with adequate pelvic measurements.

**B. Management During Labor:**

**1. Examination**–Patients with singleton breech presentations are admitted to the hospital as soon as labor begins or spontaneous rupture of membranes occurs because of the possibility of umbilical cord complications. Upon admission, a repeat ultrasonographic or x-ray study is obtained to confirm the type of breech presentation and to ascertain whether the head is deflexed. The fetus is again scrutinized for

**Table 21–1.** Incidence of singleton breech presentations by birth weight and gestational age.

| Birth Weight (g) | Gestational Age (weeks) | Incidence (%) |
|---|---|---|
| 1000 | 28 | 35 |
| 1000–1499 | 28–32 | 25 |
| 1500–1999 | 32–34 | 20 |
| 2000–2499 | 34–36 | 8 |
| 2500 | 36 | 2–3 |
| All weights | | 3–4 |

lethal congenital malformations such as anencephalus, which would preclude cesarean delivery for fetal indications. A thorough history is taken, and a physical examination is performed to evaluate completely the status of mother and fetus. Based on these findings, a decision must be made regarding the route of delivery (see below).

**2. Electronic fetal monitoring**–Electronic monitoring of fetal heart rate and uterine contractions should continue throughout labor. Whenever possible, the fetal ECG electrode should be carefully attached to the breech presenting part, with care taken to avoid injury to the fetal anus, perineum, and genitalia. The transcervical catheter for direct recording of intrauterine pressure should be used to determine accurately the frequency, strength, and duration of uterine contractions. Fetal distress or dysfunctional labor often requires cesarean section rather than vaginal delivery for optimal fetal outcome.

**3. Oxytocin**–The use of oxytocin in the management of dysfunctional breech labor is controversial. Although some obstetricians condemn its use, others employ oxytocin with benefit and without complications. Oxytocin should be administered only if uterine contractions are insufficient to sustain normal progress in labor. A continuous intravenous infusion of a very dilute solution should always be used to prevent hyperstimulation or tetany of the uterus. Continuous electronic monitoring of the fetal heart rate and uterine contractions should be employed whenever oxytocin is administered.

**C. Delivery:** The decision regarding route of delivery must be made carefully on an individual basis. Criteria for vaginal or cesarean delivery are outlined in Table 21–2.

Prior to 1975, virtually all viable singleton breech presentations were delivered vaginally. Cesarean section was reserved for specific fetal indications such as unremitting distress or prolapsed umbilical cord, or maternal indications such as placenta previa, abruptio placentae, or failure of progress in labor. However, breech infants delivered vaginally had a 5-fold increase in mortality rate over comparable cephalic presentations.

Cesarean delivery has now become much more common in breech presentation, with significantly lower rates of perinatal morbidity and mortality. Complications of traumatic vaginal delivery are avoided (eg, umbilical cord prolapse, difficult delivery of aftercoming head, nuchal arms). However, not all breech presentations require cesarean delivery. Many can be safely delivered vaginally without significant risk of injury or death. Risks to the mother with cesarean section (anesthesia, blood loss, infection) must be weighed against risks to the fetus with vaginal delivery (asphyxia, trauma). Decisions must be made with the utmost care to prevent unnecessary cesarean section or inadvertent vaginal delivery. Only obstetricians skilled in breech techniques should attempt any breech delivery, whether vaginal or cesarean.

Obstetricians have long believed that primigravid women have longer labors, more difficult breech extractions, and higher perinatal mortality rates than multiparas. As a result, multiparous women with previously proved adequate pelves were allowed a trial of labor and vaginal delivery, whereas primigravid patients were more often delivered by cesarean section. However, data regarding vaginal delivery in multiparous versus primigravid women demonstrate no benefit in perinatal outcome. Rates of difficult breech extraction, birth trauma, and perinatal death are not influenced by maternal parity. With any type of delivery, the fetus must be handled with great care.

**1. Cesarean delivery**–The type of incision chosen is extremely important. If the lower uterine seg-

**Table 21–2.** Criteria for vaginal or cesarean delivery in breech presentation.

| Vaginal Delivery | Cesarean Delivery |
|---|---|
| **Frank breech presentation.** | **Estimated fetal weight of 3500 g or more.** |
| **Gestational age of 34 weeks or more.** | **Contracted or borderline maternal pelvic measurements.** |
| Estimated fetal weight of 2000–3500 g. | Deflexed fetal head. |
| Flexed fetal head. | Prolonged rupture of membranes. |
| Adequate maternal pelvis as determined by x-ray pelvimetry (pelvic inlet with transverse diameter of 11.5 cm and anteroposterior diameter of 10.5 cm; midpelvis with transverse diameter of 10 cm and anteroposterior diameter of 11.5 cm). | Unengaged presenting part. |
| | Dysfunctional labor. |
| | Elderly primigravida. |
| No maternal or fetal indications for cesarean section. | Mother with infertility problems or poor obstetric history. |
| Previable fetus (gestational age < 25 weeks and weight <700 g). | Premature fetus (gestational age of 25–34 weeks). |
| Documented lethal fetal congenital anomalies. | Most cases of complete or footling breech over 25 weeks gestation without detectable lethal congenital malformations (to prevent umbilical cord prolapse). |
| Presentation of mother in advanced labor with no fetal or maternal distress, even if cesarean delivery was originally planned (a carefully performed, controlled vaginal delivery is safer in such cases than a hastily executed cesarean section). | Fetus with variable heart rate decelerations on electronic monitoring. |
| Some carefully selected cases of complete or footling breech (continuous electronic monitoring must be done to detect variable fetal heart rate decelerations due to umbilical cord prolapse; if this occurs, perform immediate cesarean delivery). | |

ment is well developed (generally the case in women at term who have experienced labor), or if the presenting part is not well down in the uterus, a longer transverse "lower segment" incision is adequate for easy delivery. In premature gestations, the lower uterine segment may be quite narrow, and a low vertical incision is almost always required for atraumatic delivery.

**2. Vaginal delivery**–Obstetricians who contemplate performing a vaginal breech delivery should be experienced in the maneuver and should be assisted by 3 physicians: (1) an experienced obstetrician who will assist with delivery; (2) an anesthesiologist, to ensure that the patient is comfortable and cooperative during labor and delivery; and (3) a pediatrician capable of providing total resuscitation of the newborn, should it be required.

**a. Anesthesia**–The type of anesthesia required depends on the type of breech delivery. Multiparous women undergoing spontaneous breech delivery may require only analgesia for pain relief during labor and a pudendal anesthetic during delivery. A continuous "segmental" epidural anesthetic may also be administered during labor or during partial breech extraction, including application of Piper forceps to the aftercoming head.

In emergency circumstances when total breech extraction is performed in lieu of cesarean section, complete relaxation of the perineum and uterus is essential for a successful outcome. This is accomplished by immediate induction of inhalation anesthesia using halothane. This technique may also be used in partial breech extraction, when complete perineal relaxation is necessary for optimal delivery of the aftercoming head.

**b. Spontaneous vaginal delivery**–During spontaneous delivery, delivery occurs without assistance, and no obstetric maneuvers are applied to the body. The fetus negotiates the maternal pelvis as outlined below, while the operator simply supports the body as it delivers.

The transverse (bitrochanteric) diameter of the fetal pelvis is wider than the anteroposterior diameter is deep. During labor, the breech usually engages the pelvis in the sacrum anterior position. As the fetus descends into the pelvis (Fig 21–3), it continues in the sacrum anterior position or rotates slightly to a left or right sacrum anterior position, until the buttocks reach the levator ani muscles of the maternal pelvis. At this point, internal rotation occurs, whereby the anterior hip rotates beneath the pubic symphysis, resulting in a sacrum transverse position. The bitrochanteric diameter of the fetal pelvis is now in an anteroposterior position within the maternal pelvis. The anterior hip then descends below the pubic symphysis, and the buttocks begin to distend the perineum. As this occurs, the shoulders enter the pelvic inlet with the bisacromial diameter in the transverse position. As descent occurs, the bisacromial diameter ro-

tates to an oblique or anteroposterior diameter, until the anterior shoulder rests beneath the pubic symphysis. Delivery of the anterior shoulder occurs as it slips beneath the pubic symphysis. Upward flexion of the body allows for easy delivery of the posterior shoulder over the perineum.

As the shoulders descend, the head engages the pelvic inlet in a transverse or oblique position. Rotation of the head to the occiput anterior position occurs as it enters the midpelvis. The occiput then slips beneath the pubic symphysis, and the remainder of the head is delivered by flexion as the chin, mouth, nose, and forehead slip over the maternal perineum.

As delivery of the breech occurs, increasingly larger diameters (bitrochanteric, bisacromial, biparietal) of the body enter the pelvis, whereas in cephalic presentation, the largest diameter (biparietal diameter) enters the pelvis first. Particularly in preterm labors, the head is considerably larger than the body and provides a better "dilating wedge" as it passes through the cervix and into the pelvis. The breech is a much poorer "dilating wedge." The smaller bitrochanteric and bisacromial diameters may descend into the pelvis through a partially dilated cervix, but the larger biparietal diameter may be trapped. Delivery in these cases is described below.

**c. Partial breech extraction**–Partial breech extraction (assisted breech extraction) is employed when the operator discerns that spontaneous delivery will not occur or that expeditious delivery is indicated for fetal or maternal reasons. The body is allowed to deliver spontaneously up to the level of the umbilicus (Fig 21–4). The operator then assists in delivery of the shoulders, arms, and head (Fig 21–5).

The body is supported by an assistant while the operator rotates the spine as necessary until it rests directly under the pubic symphysis. The operator applies gentle downward pressure on the body until both scapulas are visible. The body is then rotated until the right shoulder is beneath the pubic symphysis. Reaching up with the right hand, the operator locates the right humerus and applies gentle downward pressure until the right arm is delivered. The body is rotated until the left shoulder is beneath the pubic symphysis, and the left arm is delivered in like fashion. Rotating the spine again to a position below the pubic symphysis, the operator begins to deliver the head. As the body is lifted gently upward and as fundal pressure is applied from above to keep the head in a flexed position, the head may be delivered spontaneously over the perineum. The operator may elect to manually assist in delivery of the head by performing the **Mauriceau-Smellie-Veit maneuver** (Fig 21–6). In this procedure, the index and middle fingers of one of the operator's hands are applied over the maxilla as the body rests on the palm and forearm of the operator. Two fingers of the operator's other hand are applied on either side of the neck with gentle downward traction. At the same time, the body is ele-

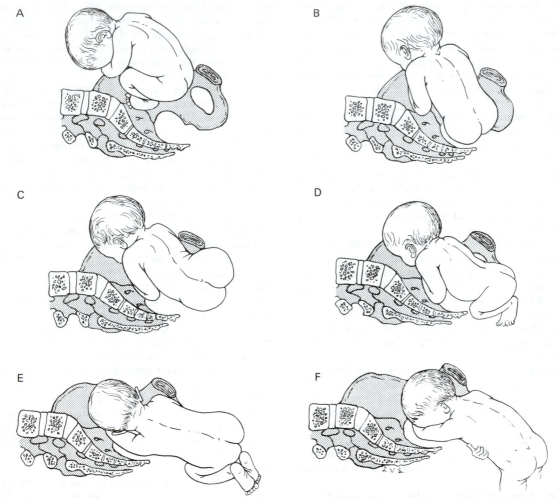

**Figure 21–3.** Mechanism of labor in breech delivery. A: Mechanism of breech delivery. RST at the onset of labor; engagement of the buttocks usually occurs in the oblique or transverse diameter of the pelvic brim. B: Early second stage. The buttocks have reached the pelvic floor and internal rotation has occurred so that the bitrochanteric diameter lies in the AP diameter of the pelvic outlet. C: Late second stage. The anterior buttock appears at the vulva by lateral flexion of the trunk around the pubic symphysis. The shoulders have not yet engaged in the pelvis. D: The buttocks have been born, and the shoulders are adjusting to engage in the transverse diameter of the brim. This movement causes external rotation of the delivered buttocks so that the fetal back becomes uppermost. E: The shoulders have reached the pelvic floor and have undergone internal rotation so that the bisacromial diameter lies in the AP diameter of the pelvic outlet. Simultaneously, the buttocks rotate anteriorly through 90 degrees. This is called restitution. The head is engaging in the pelvic brim, and the sagittal suture is lying in the transverse diameter of the brim. F: The anterior shoulder is born from behind the pubic symphysis by lateral flexion of the delivered trunk. (Redrawn and reproduced, with permission, from Llewellyn-Jones D: *Fundamentals of Obstetrics and Gynecology.* Vol 1. Faber & Faber, 1969.)

vated toward the pubic symphysis, allowing for controlled delivery of the mouth, nose, and brow over the perineum.

During partial breech extraction, the anterior shoulder may be difficult to deliver if it is impacted behind the pubic symphysis. In this event, the body is gently lifted upward toward the pubic symphysis, and the operator inserts one hand along the hollow of the maternal pelvis and identifies the posterior humerus

of the fetus. By gentle downward traction on the humerus, the posterior arm can be easily delivered, thus allowing for easier delivery of the anterior shoulder and arm.

**d. Total breech extraction**–In total breech extraction (Fig 21–7), the entire body is manually delivered. This procedure is employed only occasionally when fetal distress is encountered and an expeditious delivery is indicated. Total breech extraction has

A

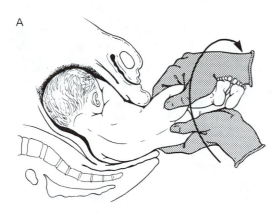

B

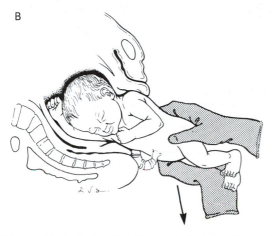

**Figure 21–4.** Assisted delivery of the shoulders. A: Shoulders engaged, posterior (left) shoulder at lower level in pelvis than anterior shoulder. B: Rotation of trunk causing posterior shoulder to rotate to anterior and stem beneath the pubic symphysis. (Redrawn and reproduced, with permission, from Lovset J: Shoulder delivery by breech presentation. J Obstet Gynaecol Br Commonw 1937;44:696.)

been virtually replaced by cesarean delivery in modern obstetrics.

For complete or footling presentation, total breech extraction is accomplished by initially grasping both feet and applying gentle downward pressure until the buttocks are delivered. A generous midline or mediolateral episiotomy is then performed. The operator gently grasps the fetal pelvis, with both thumbs placed directly on either side of the sacrum. The spine is rotated, if necessary, until it rests under the pubic symphysis. Gentle, firm downward pressure is applied to the body until both scapulas are visible. The shoulders, arms, and head are delivered as in partial breech extraction.

If the fetus is in frank breech presentation, the index finger of the right hand must initially be placed

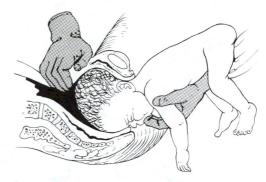

**Figure 21–5.** Maneuver for delivery of the head. The fingers of the left hand are inserted into the infant's mouth or over mandible; the right hand exerts pressure on the head from above. (Modified and reproduced, with permission, from Benson RC: *Handbook of Obstetrics & Gynecology,* 8th ed. Lange, 1983.)

into the anterior groin of the fetus and gentle downward pressure applied (Fig 21–8). As the fetus descends further into the birth canal, the left index finger is inserted into the posterior groin, and additional gentle downward traction is applied, until the buttocks are delivered through the vaginal introitus (Fig 21–9). The fetus is gently rotated until the spine rests directly under the pubic symphysis. To deliver the extended legs from the birth canal, the operator places the index finger in the popliteal fossa of one leg and applies pressure upward and outward, causing the knee to flex. As the knee flexes, the foot is often seen

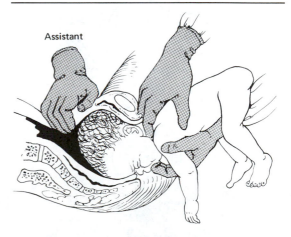

**Figure 21–6.** Mauriceau-Smellie-Veit maneuver for delivery of the head. The fingers of the left hand are inserted into the infant's mouth or over the mandible; the fingers of the right hand curve over the shoulders. An assistant exerts suprapubic pressure on the head. (Reproduced, with permission, from Benson RC: *Handbook of Obstetrics & Gynecology,* 8th ed. Lange, 1983.)

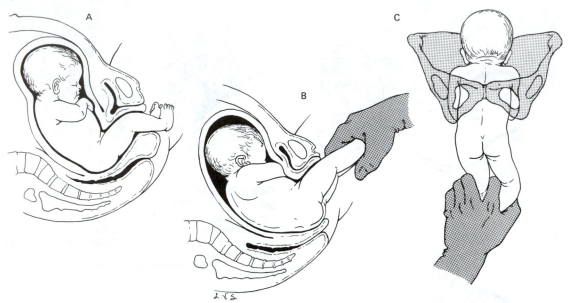

**Figure 21–7.** Extraction of breech. A: Buttocks brought to hollow of sacrum. B: Traction on anterior leg causes buttocks to advance and rotate into direct AP diameter of pelvis. Continued downward traction causes the back to rotate anteriorly. C: Further downward traction causes the shoulders to engage in the transverse diameter of the inlet. (Redrawn and reproduced, with permission, from Caldwell WE, Studdiford WE: A review of breech deliveries during a 5-year period at the Sloane Hospital for Women. Am J Obstet Gynecol 1929;18:623.)

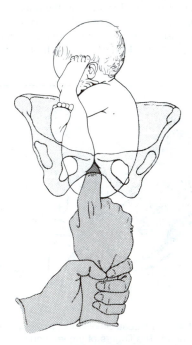

**Figure 21–8.** Delivery of breech with one finger in the groin. The wrist is supported with the other hand. When the posterior groin is accessible, the index finger of the other hand is placed in it to complete delivery of the breech. (Redrawn and reproduced, with permission, from Greenhill JP: *Obstetrics,* 12th ed. Saunders, 1960.)

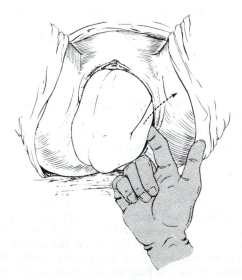

**Figure 21–9.** Flexion and abduction of thigh to deliver extended leg. (Redrawn and reproduced, with permission, from Llewellyn-Jones D: *Fundamentals of Obstetrics and Gynecology.* Vol 1. Faber & Faber, 1969.)

or easily palpated. The lower leg is grasped firmly and gently delivered (Fig 21–10), and the opposite leg is then delivered. The rest of the body is extracted as previously described for footling presentation.

Occasionally during partial breech extraction and more often during total breech extraction, excessive downward traction on the body to effect delivery of the scapulas results in a single or double **nuchal arm.** Because the body descends too rapidly through the birth canal, one or both arms are extended upward from their normal flexed position against the chest and become lodged behind the neck (Fig 21–11).

A single or bilateral nuchal arm is suspected when delivery of the shoulder is difficult to accomplish. To dislodge an impacted nuchal arm, the operator rotates the body in a half circle to bring the elbow toward the face. The humerus can then be readily identified by palpation and delivered as previously described. For bilateral nuchal arms, the fetus is rotated counterclockwise to deliver the right arm and often clockwise to dislodge and deliver the left arm. If rotation does not dislodge a nuchal arm, the operator must insert a finger into the maternal pelvis, identify the fetal humerus, and possibly extract the arm. Fractures of the humerus or clavicle may result.

**e.  Delivery of the aftercoming head**–Following delivery of the shoulders and arms, the body is

rotated as necessary until the spine rests beneath the pubic symphysis and the head is in the occiput anterior position. At this point, the aftercoming head may be delivered spontaneously or by the Mauriceau-Smellie-Veit maneuver.

**(1) Piper forceps**–Piper forceps may be used electively or when the Mauriceau-Smellie-Veit maneuver fails to deliver the aftercoming head in an expeditious manner. Use of Piper forceps has improved the neonatal outcome in infants with birth weights of 1000–3000 g.

Prerequisites for use of Piper forceps in delivery of the aftercoming head include a completely dilated cervix and engagement of the head in the pelvis. Preferably, the head should be in the direct occiput anterior position for best application of the forceps, but the left or right occiput anterior position is acceptable. Piper forceps application should not be attempted in the occiput transverse positions, because significant fetal or maternal injury may result. Although some obstetricians use the Piper forceps in the direct occiput posterior positions, better perinatal results are obtained if the body is rotated to an occiput anterior position. An obstetric assistant supports the fetal body as the operator gently inserts the Piper forceps into the birth canal. As the assistant elevates the body slightly, the operator places each forceps blade alongside the head. After proper placement of both

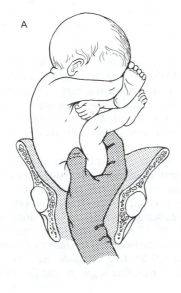

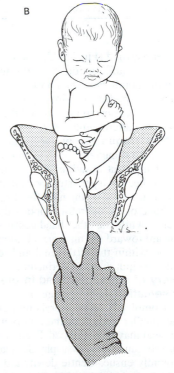

**Figure 21–10.** Extraction of breech. A: Abduction of thigh and pressure in popliteal fossa causes the knee to flex and become accessible. B: Delivery of leg by traction on the foot.

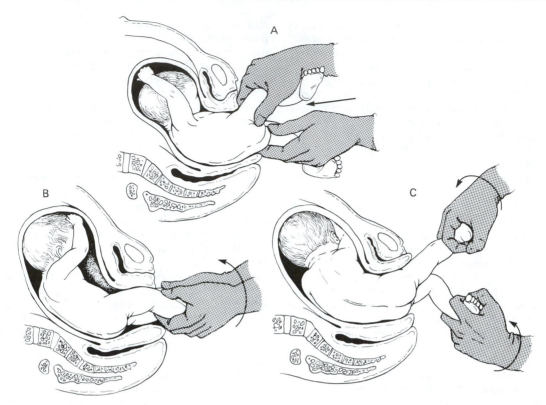

**Figure 21–11.** Method of dealing with sacrum posterior that results from permitting the breech to advance too far without rotation. A: and B: Fetus is pushed back until the buttocks are in the hollow of the sacrum, causing the shoulders to disengage. C: Rotation is accomplished by traction on anterior leg, as in Figure 21. (Redrawn and reproduced, with permission, from Piper EG, Bachman C: The prevention of fetal injuries in breech delivery. JAMA 1929;92:217.)

blades has been verified (Fig 21–12), the forceps are locked in position, and traction is gently applied to deliver the chin, mouth, nose, and brow over the perineum. A generous midline episiotomy is often indicated to allow for easier application of the forceps and delivery of the aftercoming head.

**(2) Modified Prague maneuver**–If, after delivery of the body, the spine remains in the posterior position and attempts at rotation are unsuccessful, extraction of the head in a persistent occiput posterior position may be achieved by the modified Prague maneuver. One hand of the operator supports the shoulders from below while the other hand gently elevates the body upward toward the maternal abdomen. This flexes the head within the birth canal and results in delivery of the occiput over the perineum.

**(3) Delivery of entrapped head in premature breech presentation**–In premature breech presentations, the incompletely dilated cervix may allow delivery of the smaller body, but the relatively larger aftercoming head may be entrapped. Prompt delivery is mandatory because severe asphyxia leading to death may rapidly ensue. Gentle downward traction on the shoulders combined with fundal pressure ap-

plied by an assistant may effect delivery. If this fails, the anesthesiologist should administer deep inhalation anesthesia (halothane may be useful) to obtain complete relaxation of the lower uterine segment and pelvic floor. Gentle downward traction on the shoulders will then often successfully deliver the aftercoming head.

If delivery is still not accomplished, a **hysterostomatomy (Dührssen's incision)** must be considered to preserve fetal life. Incisions are made in the posterior cervix at 6 o'clock to loosen the entrapped head. Occasionally, additional incisions are necessary at 2 and 10 o'clock. Hysterostomatomy invariably releases the head, but the maternal consequences may be severe because incisions may extend upward into the lower uterine segment, causing severe hemorrhage.

Hysterostomatomy should be performed rarely today (if at all). Viable premature breech gestations should usually be delivered by cesarean section. Previable gestations delivered vaginally may become entrapped, but the maternal risks of Dührssen's incisions or cesarean section performed to release the entrapment outweigh any potential benefit to the im-

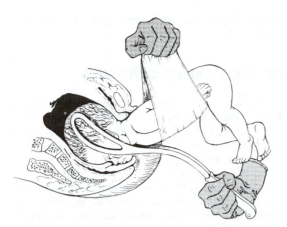

**Figure 21–12.** Application of Piper forceps, employing towel sling support. The forceps are introduced from below, left blade first, aiming directly at intended positions on sides of the head. (Reproduced, with permission, from Benson RC: *Handbook of Obstetrics & Gynecology,* 8th ed. Lange, 1983.)

mature fetus. Continued labor and gentle downward pressure will release the aftercoming head but generally not without fetal death from asphyxia.

## Complications of Breech Delivery

**A. Birth Anoxia:** Umbilical cord compression and prolapse may be associated with breech delivery, particularly in complete (5%) and footling (15%) presentations. This is due to the inability of the presenting part to fill the maternal pelvis, either due to prematurity or poor application of the presenting part to the cervix, so that the umbilical cord is allowed to prolapse below the level of the breech. Frank breech presentation (thighs flexed against the abdomen) offers a contoured presenting part, which accommodates better to the maternal pelvis and is usually well applied to the cervix. The incidence of cord prolapse in frank breech is only 0.5% (the same as for cephalic presentations).

Compression of the prolapsed cord may occur during uterine contractions, causing moderate to severe variable decelerations in the fetal heart rate. Fetal anoxia or death may occur. Continuous electronic monitoring is mandatory during labor in these cases to detect ominous decelerations. If they occur, immediate cesarean delivery must be performed.

**B. Birth Injury:** The incidence of birth trauma during vaginal breech delivery is 6.7%, 13 times that of cephalic presentations (0.51 per 1000 deliveries). Only high forceps and internal version and extraction procedures have higher rates of birth injury than vaginal breech deliveries. The types of perinatal injuries reported in breech delivery include tears in the tentorium cerebellum, cephalohematomas, disruption of

the spinal cord, brachial palsy, fracture of long bones, and rupture of the sternocleidomastoid muscles. Vaginal breech delivery is also the main cause of injuries to the fetal adrenal glands, liver, anus, genitalia, spine, hip joint, sciatic nerve, and musculature of the arms, legs, and back.

Factors contributing to difficult vaginal breech delivery include a partially dilated cervix, unilateral or bilateral nuchal arms, and deflexion of the head. The type of procedure used may also affect the neonatal outcome.

**1. Partially dilated cervix**–Delivery of a breech fetus may progress even though the cervix is only partially dilated, since the bitrochanteric and bisacromial diameters are smaller than the biparietal diameter. This is true especially in prematurity. The hips and shoulders may negotiate the cervix, but the aftercoming head becomes entrapped, resulting in difficult delivery and birth injury.

**2. Nuchal arms**–Nuchal arms hinder delivery of the aftercoming head, causing delay in delivery and an increased incidence of birth asphyxia. Fractures of the humerus and trauma to the musculature of the shoulders and arms may occur as the operator attempts to free the nuchal arm and deliver the head.

**3. Deflexion of the head**–Hyperextension of the head is defined as deflexion or extension of the head posteriorly beyond the longitudinal axis of the fetus (5% of all breech deliveries). Causes of hyperextension include neck cysts, spasm of the neck musculature, and uterine anomalies, but over 75% have no known cause. Although deflexion may be documented by ultrasonographic or x-ray studies weeks before delivery, there is little apparent risk to the fetus until vaginal delivery is attempted. At that time, deflexion causes impaction of the occipital portion of the head behind the pubic symphysis, which may lead to fractures of the cervical vertebrae, lacerations of the spinal cord, epidural and medullary hemorrhages, and perinatal death. If head deflexion is diagnosed prior to delivery, cesarean section should be performed to avert injury. Cesarean section cannot prevent injuries such as minor meningeal hemorrhage or dislocation of the cervical vertebrae; these may develop in utero secondary to long-standing head deflexion.

**4. Type of delivery**–More complex delivery procedures have a higher rate of birth trauma. While few infants are injured during spontaneous breech births, as many as 6% are injured during partial breech extraction and 20% during total breech extraction. Injuries associated with total breech extraction are usually extensive and severe, and this procedure should never be attempted unless fetal survival is in jeopardy and cesarean section cannot be immediately performed.

An additional important factor in breech injury and perinatal outcome is the experience of the operator.

Inexperience may lead to hasty performance of obstetric maneuvers. Delay in delivery may result in birth asphyxia due to umbilical cord compression, but haste in the management of breech delivery results in application of excessive pressure on the fetal body, causing soft tissue damage and fracture of long bones. Too-rapid extraction of the body from the birth canal causes the arms to extend above the head, resulting in unilateral or bilateral nuchal arms and difficult delivery of the aftercoming head. All breech deliveries should be carried out slowly and methodically by experienced obstetricians who execute the maneuvers with gentleness and skill—not speed.

## Prognosis

The incidence of cesarean section for breech delivery has been steadily increasing, from approximately 30% in 1970 to 75% in 1990. Rates of perinatal death have not decreased to those associated with cephalic presentations, mainly because many breech fetuses are very premature or have lethal congenital malformations. Cesarean section for the immature or malformed fetus does not improve chances for perinatal survival; vaginal delivery should be performed in these cases.

The route of delivery for term breech infants does not seem to affect neonatal mortality rates. For infants with birth weights of 2000–3500 g, neonatal mortality rates approach zero regardless of the route of delivery. However, the impact of cesarean section on perinatal outcome is clearly seen in singleton breech presentations with extremes in birth weight. The premature breech fetus (25–34 weeks with birth weight of 700–2000 g) and large term breech fetus (birth weight > 3500 g) have significantly better neonatal outcomes when delivered by cesarean section. For a tiny premature fetus, cesarean delivery avoids umbilical cord prolapse, entrapment of the aftercoming head by a partially dilated cervix, and birth trauma. For a large fetus, cesarean section avoids prolonged labor and difficult, traumatic breech extraction.

# VERSION

Version is a procedure used for turning the fetal presenting part from breech to cephalic presentation (cephalic version) or from cephalic to breech presentation (podalic version). Because cephalic version is performed by manipulating the fetus through the abdominal wall, the maneuver is known as **external cephalic version.** Podalic version is performed by means of internal maneuvers and is known as **internal podalic version.** External cephalic version is re-gaining popularity, but internal podalic version is rarely used.

## EXTERNAL CEPHALIC VERSION

External cephalic version is used in the management of singleton breech presentations. Before tocolytic agents were available to suppress uterine contractions, the procedure was performed at 28–32 weeks. There were some reports of success, but others reported that nearly half the versions reverted to breech presentation before the onset of labor. In addition, the maternal and fetal complications of the procedure, including intrauterine fetal demise secondary to umbilical cord entanglement, abruptio placentae, premature rupture of membranes, premature labor, umbilical cord prolapse, transplacental fetomaternal hemorrhage, and uterine rupture, led to less frequent use of this procedure. External cephalic version is now regaining popularity because safe tocolytic agents are available to suppress uterine activity during the procedure, fetal heart rate monitors can document fetal well-being, and real-time ultrasonography is used to guide the maneuver.

### Indications

Patients with unengaged singleton breech presentations at 37–42 weeks' gestation are candidates for external cephalic version. The procedure is usually successful in multigravidas with lax abdominal walls, in pregnancies with a sufficient quantity of amniotic fluid to facilitate version, and in unengaged complete and footling breech presentations.

### Contraindications

Contraindications to external cephalic version include engagement of the presenting part in the pelvis, marked oligohydramnios, placenta previa, premature rupture of membranes, previous uterine surgery (including cesarean section, myomectomy, or metroplasty), and suspected or documented congenital malformations or abnormalities (including intrauterine growth retardation). Additional contraindications include maternal cardiac disease, diabetes mellitus, or thyroid disorders, all of which may preclude the administration of tocolytic agents. The patient's informed consent should be obtained before the procedure is done.

Frank breech presentations with both extremities flexed on the abdomen are difficult to turn because the lower extremities act as a splint and prevent the necessary flexion. Any presentation engaged in the pelvis is impossible to turn. Attempts to perform version in such cases may lead to fetal or maternal injury and are contraindicated.

### Complications

**A. Fetal Cardiac Abnormalities:** Fetal cardiac

abnormalities may be readily documented during external cephalic version by continuous ultrasonographic surveillance. Normal cardiac activity will usually return if the procedure is stopped for a short time. In most cases, the procedure may be continued without further cardiac difficulties. If significant unremitting fetal cardiac alterations occur, the attempt at version is discontinued, and cesarean delivery is performed immediately. Although cesarean delivery is rarely needed for this purpose, it is important that the procedure be performed in a hospital setting in case emergency operation is needed.

**B. Fetomaternal Transplacental Hemorrhage:** Fetomaternal transplacental hemorrhage may occur during version. The **Kleihauer-Betke acid elution test** should be performed if this is suspected. Minor hemorrhages are unimportant except in women at risk for Rh isoimmunization; in such cases, Rh IgG is administered for prophylaxis. If significant fetomaternal hemorrhage is detected, the fetal heart rate should be closely monitored following the procedure. Any signs of fetal distress are an indication for prompt cesarean delivery.

## Technique

External cephalic version is performed as follows:

(1) Perform an ultrasound examination to verify presentation and rule out fetal congenital anomalies or uterine abnormalities.

(2) Perform a nonstress test. Results must be reactive.

(3) Perform a Kleihauer-Betke acid elution test to rule out fetomaternal transplacental hemorrhage.

(4) Administer ritodrine hydrochloride, 0.15 mg/min intravenously for 15 minutes, to relax the uterine muscles and prevent contractions or irritability.

(5) Do not give analgesia or anesthesia. Ask the patient to inform the operator if maneuvers are excessively forceful or painful.

(6) Perform external cephalic version. Place both hands on the patient's abdomen, and locate each pole of the fetus by palpation. Gently but firmly displace the breech upward and lateralward while moving the head downward toward the pelvic inlet (forward somersault).

(7) Use real-time ultrasonographic scanning throughout the procedure to monitor fetal well-being and document version. (As a precaution, the procedure should always be done in or near a hospital in case immediate cesarean delivery is required.)

(8) Following the procedure, repeat the nonstress and the Kleihauer-Betke tests. If the Kleihauer-Betke test is positive and the mother is Rh-negative, she should be given Rh IgG to prevent sensitization. If there are indications of massive fetomaternal transfusion, immediate cesarean delivery should be considered to prevent fetal damage or death.

External cephalic version is safe for both mother and fetus if the procedure is done as outlined above. Version is successful in up to 75% of cases, and over 90% of these remain in cephalic presentation until delivery. If version is successful and the Kleihauer-Betke test and nonstress test are normal, the mother may be sent home to await the normal onset of labor. Studies show a significant reduction in the incidence of breech presentation in labor as a result of external cephalic version, with few or no complications.

If version is unsuccessful and there are no complications, the patient may be scheduled for elective cesarean delivery. In some cases, a trial of labor and vaginal delivery may be planned.

## INTERNAL PODALIC VERSION

Internal podalic version is now used rarely because of the many associated risks to mother and fetus. It is occasionally performed as a lifesaving procedure (eg, second twin with fetal distress, prolapsed umbilical cord, or significant maternal hemorrhage owing to premature separation of the placenta). (See Chapter 17 for delivery of a second twin.)

### Indications

A life-threatening condition as described above is the only indication for internal podalic version. The cervix must be completely dilated, and the membranes must be intact. A skilled operator is crucial for safe performance of this procedure.

### Contraindications

Internal podalic version is contraindicated in cases where the membranes are ruptured or oligohydramnios is present, precluding easy version. This procedure should not be performed through a partially dilated cervix or if the uterus is firmly contracted down on the fetal body.

### Complications

Internal podalic version is associated with considerable risk of traumatic injury to both fetus and mother. Prior to 1950, when this procedure was performed much more frequently than it is today, associated uterine rupture and hemorrhage caused 5% of all maternal deaths. Perinatal mortality rates were 5–25% (primarily due to traumatic intracerebral hemorrhage and birth asphyxia). Considerable birth trauma, eg, long bone fractures, dislocations, epiphyseal separations, and central nervous system deficits, was also linked to this procedure. For these reasons, internal podalic version has been abandoned with rare exceptions in favor of cesarean section.

### Technique

Internal podalic version is performed as follows:

(1) Establish an intravenous line for administration

of parenteral fluids, including blood. Cross-matched blood should be available in the hospital blood bank.

(2) Administer deep inhalation anesthesia (halothane) to achieve relaxation of the uterus.

(3) Place the patient in the dorsolithotomy position. Insert a hand through the fully dilated cervix along the fetal body until both feet are identified. Grasp both feet firmly. Perform an amniotomy. Apply dorsal traction on both lower extremities until both feet are delivered through the vagina. Then, perform a total breech extraction for delivery of the body (Fig 21–13).

## COMPOUND PRESENTATION

Compound presentation is prolapse of a fetal extremity into the lower uterine segment alongside the presenting part. Prolapse of the hand in cephalic presentation is most common, followed by prolapse of an upper extremity in breech presentation. Prolapse of a lower extremity in cephalic presentation is relatively rare.

Compound presentations are uncommon (1 in 1200 pregnancies; birth weight > 1500 g, 1 in 1600 pregnancies).

### Causes

Obstetric factors that prevent descent of the presenting part into the pelvic inlet predispose to prolapse of an extremity alongside the presenting part (ie, prematurity, cephalopelvic disproportion, multi-ple gestation, grand multiparity, and hydramnios). Prematurity occurs in over 50% of compound presentations. In twin gestations, over 90% of compound presentations are associated with the second twin.

Because of poor application of the presenting part to the cervix found in compound presentations, umbilical cord prolapse is common and a major contributor to fetal loss during labor.

### Diagnosis

The diagnosis of compound presentation is made by palpation of a fetal extremity adjacent to the presenting part. The diagnosis is usually made during labor; as the cervix dilates, the prolapsed extremity is more easily palpated alongside the vertex or breech. Compound presentation may be suspected if poor progress in labor is noted, particularly when the presenting part fails to engage during the active phase. If the diagnosis of compound presentation is suspected but uncertain, ultrasound or x-ray may be used to locate the position of the extremities and search for malformations.

### Management

Management of compound presentation depends on gestational age, type of presentation, and whether it is the hand or foot that is prolapsed. Since 50% of compound presentations are associated with prematurity, viability of the fetus should be documented prior to delivery. If the fetus is considered nonviable (< 25 weeks' gestation), labor should be permitted and vaginal delivery anticipated. The small size of the fetus makes dystocia or difficult vaginal delivery uncommon.

Prolapse of a foot in cephalic presentation is associated with prolonged labor, poor descent of the pre-

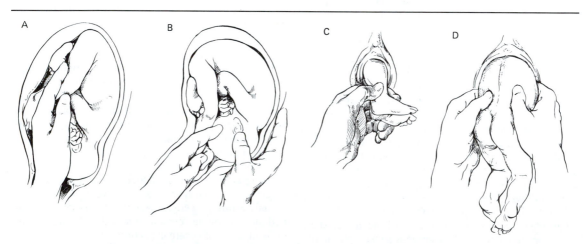

**Figure 21–13.** Internal podalic version and extraction. A: Feet are grasped. B: Baby is turned; hand on abdomen pushes head toward uterine fundus. C: Feet are extracted. D: Torso is delivered. From this point onward, procedure is same as for uncomplicated breech delivery. (Reproduced, with permission, from DeCosta EL: *Cesarean section and other obstetric operations.* In: *Textbook of Obstetrics and Gynecology,* 2nd ed. Danforth DN [editor]. Harper & Row, 1972.)

senting part, and traumatic vaginal delivery. If the fetus is viable (> 25 weeks) and the presentation is cephalic compounded by a foot or a hand and a foot, cesarean delivery is indicated.

Compound breech presentations frequently occur in premature pregnancies. Perinatal outcome is better with cesarean section than with vaginal delivery. In such cases, version and extraction and total breech extraction are extremely traumatic to the fetus and should never be performed.

Labor may be allowed and vaginal delivery anticipated in viable cephalic presentations with a prolapsed hand. At term, these cases generally pose no difficulty in labor or delivery, since the hand moves upward into the lower uterine segment as the vertex descends into the birth canal. In premature cephalic presentations with a prolapsed hand, if the hand does not spontaneously retract, gentle replacement of the extremity may be attempted. Forceful repositioning may lead to fetal and maternal injury and should be avoided.

Umbilical cord prolapse is a risk in all cases of compound presentation, and internal electronic monitoring should be done to detect fetal distress or changes in the fetal heart rate. Umbilical cord complications should be managed by immediate cesarean delivery.

### Prognosis

Compound presentations are associated with perinatal mortality rates approaching 25%. Contributing significantly to this persistent loss are prematurity, prolapsed umbilical cord complications, and traumatic vaginal delivery.

# SHOULDER DYSTOCIA

Shoulder dystocia is defined as an inability to deliver the shoulders after the head has delivered despite the performance of routine obstetric maneuvers. Characteristically, after the head is delivered, the chin applies tightly against the perineum as the anterior shoulder becomes impacted behind the pubic symphysis. Shoulder dystocia is relatively infrequent with cephalic presentation. It is an acute obstetric emergency requiring prompt, skillful management in order to avoid significant fetal damage or death.

The incidence of shoulder dystocia is 0.15% in pregnancies with birth weights over 2500 g, increasing to 1.7% with birth weights over 4000 g. The incidence is 4.6% in attempted midforceps delivery after a prolonged second stage of labor (for infants > 4000 g, 23%).

### Causes

Obese women (> 180 lb) and women with gestational or overt diabetes mellitus tend to have large infants and are therefore at greater risk for shoulder dystocia. Multiparas who have previously delivered a large infant are also at increased risk.

Women at risk for shoulder dystocia should be carefully assessed before labor begins. Ultrasonographic examinations should be performed to evaluate fetal morphology, biparietal diameter, and abdominal circumference in order to estimate fetal weight.

### Complications

Immediate neonatal complications (up to 50% of cases) occur when delivery is delayed or inappropriately performed, resulting in birth asphyxia or traumatic injury. Birth asphyxia may result in fetal death during delivery, neonatal death, or neurologic damage. Short-term neonatal complications of birth asphyxia include metabolic acidosis, shock, renal failure, central nervous system depression, and seizures. Long-term complications include central nervous system damage resulting in mental retardation, cerebral palsy, learning disabilities, seizure disorders, and speech defects.

Traumatic birth injuries include fractures of the humerus or clavicle and injury to the brachial plexus of the anterior shoulder **(Erb's palsy).** Fractures of the humerus and clavicle generally heal without incident, and most traumatic injuries to the brachial plexus resolve with minimal or no neurologic deficit detectable during the neonatal period. However, traumatic injury to the brachial plexus severe enough to cause evulsion of the brachial nerve roots may result in permanent neurologic deficit.

Maternal complications of shoulder dystocia include those commonly seen in any traumatic delivery (eg, lacerations of the cervix, vagina, and perineum and excessive blood loss).

### Prevention

Accurate assessment of fetal weight, attention to risk factors associated with shoulder dystocia, and avoidance of midpelvic deliveries in patients with a prolonged second stage of labor should minimize the occurrence of shoulder dystocia. Patients at risk for shoulder dystocia should be delivered by cesarean section.

In deliveries of large infants, suprapubic pressure applied by an assistant as the head delivers may prevent this complication. In unavoidable cases, careful, methodical performance of maneuvers to dislodge the shoulder from behind the pubic symphysis should result in a successful, atraumatic outcome.

### Management

Shoulder dystocia should be anticipated when there are any indications of macrosomia. The diagnosis is confirmed when gentle downward pressure on the head fails to deliver the anterior shoulder from behind the pubic symphysis. At this point, the fetus is at risk for asphyxiation, since it cannot expand its chest to breathe, and umbilical cord circulation is compressed within the birth canal. Confronted with this terrifying dilemma, the inexperienced operator often continues to apply downward pressure on the head in a vain attempt to deliver the anterior shoulder. Such action should be avoided, because it is not only ineffective but also potentially damaging to the brachial plexus and may result in permanent Erb's palsy. The following obstetric procedures should be rapidly and skillfully performed to prevent birth anoxia and trauma.

The operator places a hand within the birth canal and examines the anterior and posterior surfaces of the fetus as well as the lateral walls of the vagina for soft tissue tumors that may be impeding the progress of birth. At the same time, assistants are summoned to aid in the delivery, including a second obstetrician, an anesthesiologist or nurse anesthetist to administer rapid-inhalation anesthesia for pain relief and relaxation, and a pediatric team for immediate resuscitation of the newborn.

A proctoepisiotomy is performed, and gentle downward pressure on the head is applied at the same time that suprapubic pressure is applied by an assistant to dislodge the anterior shoulder. If these maneuvers are successful, the anterior shoulder slips beneath the pubic symphysis, and delivery is accomplished. If they are unsuccessful, the examiner attempts to rotate the bisacromial diameter of the fetus from the anteroposterior to an oblique diameter of the pelvis. This is accomplished by placing 2 fingers against the anterior surface of the posterior shoulder and applying gentle but firm pressure until rotation occurs. Suprapubic pressure is again applied to relieve the anterior shoulder impaction.

If the maneuvers to this point fail to accomplish delivery, delivery of the posterior arm is indicated. The obstetrician's hand is inserted posteriorly into the hollow of the maternal sacrum, and the posterior arm of the fetus is identified. Gentle pressure by the examiner's forefinger on the fetal antecubital fossa will cause flexion of the arm. As the arm flexes across the chest, the forearm is gently grasped, and the hand and forearm are gently delivered from the birth canal. Combined suprapubic and fundal pressure will deliver the posterior shoulder.

The **McRoberts maneuver** may also be used. The mother's legs are flexed over the abdomen in an attempt to rotate the pubic symphysis cephalad. Rotation of the pubic symphysis superiorly frees the impacted shoulder without manipulation of the fetus. This simple technique has proved so effective that it is recommended for anticipated cases of shoulder dystocia as well as when it has already become apparent.

# UMBILICAL CORD PROLAPSE

Umbilical cord prolapse is defined as descent of the umbilical cord into the lower uterine segment, where it may lie adjacent to the presenting part (**occult cord prolapse**) or below the presenting part (**overt cord prolapse**) (Fig 21–14). Funic presentation is characterized by prolapse of the umbilical cord below the level of the presenting part before rupture of the membranes occurs. In occult prolapse, the umbilical cord cannot be palpated during pelvic examination, whereas in funic presentation, the cord often can be easily palpated through the membranes if the

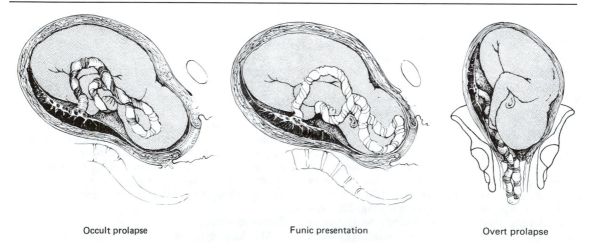

Occult prolapse      Funic presentation      Overt prolapse

**Figure 21–14.** Types of prolapsed cords.

cervix is patulous. Overt cord prolapse is associated with rupture of the membranes and displacement of the umbilical cord into the vagina, often through the introitus.

Prolapse of the umbilical cord to a level at or below the presenting part exposes the cord to intermittent compression between the presenting part and the pelvic inlet, cervix, or vaginal canal. Compression of the umbilical cord compromises fetal circulation and, depending on the duration and intensity of compression, may lead to fetal hypoxia, brain damage, and death. In overt cord prolapse, exposure of the umbilical cord to air causes irritation and cooling of the cord, resulting in further vasospasm of the cord vessels.

The incidence of overt umbilical cord prolapse in cephalic presentations is 0.5%; frank breech, 0.5%; complete breech, 5%; footling breech, 15%; and transverse lie, 20%. The incidence of occult prolapse is unknown because it can be detected only by fetal heart rate changes characteristic of umbilical cord compressions. However, some degree of occult prolapse appears to be common, since as many as 50% of monitored labors demonstrate fetal heart rate changes compatible with umbilical cord compression. In most cases, the compression is transient and may be rectified simply by changing the position of the patient.

Whether occult or overt, umbilical cord prolapse is associated with significant rates of perinatal morbidity and mortality because of intermittent compression of blood flow and resultant fetal hypoxia. Perinatal mortality rate associated with all cases of overt umbilical cord prolapse approach 20%. Prematurity, itself a contributor to the incidence of umbilical cord prolapse, accounts for a considerable portion of this perinatal loss.

## Causes

Any obstetric condition that predisposes to poor application of the fetal presenting part to the cervix may result in prolapse of the umbilical cord. Cord prolapse is associated with prematurity (< 34 weeks' gestation), abnormal presentations (breech, brow, compound, face, transverse), occiput posterior positions of the head, pelvic tumors, placenta previa, low-lying placenta, and cephalopelvic disproportion. In addition, cord prolapse may occur with hydramnios, multiple gestation, or premature rupture of the membranes occurring before engagement of the presenting part.

## Clinical Findings

**A. Overt Cord Prolapse:** Overt cord prolapse may be diagnosed simply by visualizing the cord protruding from the introitus or by palpating loops of cord in the vaginal canal.

**B. Funic Presentation:** The diagnosis of funic presentation is also made by pelvic examination if loops of cord are palpated through the membranes.

**C. Occult Prolapse:** Occult prolapse is rarely palpated during pelvic examination. This condition may be inferred only if fetal heart rate changes (variable decelerations, bradycardia, or both) associated with intermittent compression of the umbilical cord are detected during monitoring.

**D. Fetus:** The fetus in good condition whose well-being is jeopardized by umbilical cord compression may exhibit violent activity readily apparent to the patient and the obstetrician. Variable fetal heart rate decelerations will occur during uterine contractions, with prompt return of the heart rate to normal as each contraction subsides. If cord compression is complete and prolonged, fetal bradycardia occurs. Persistent, severe, variable decelerations and bradycardia lead to development of hypoxia, metabolic acidosis, and eventual damage or death. As the fetal status deteriorates, activity lessens and eventually ceases. Meconium staining of the amniotic fluid may be noted at the time of membrane rupture.

## Complications

**A. Maternal:** Cesarean section is a major operative procedure with known anesthetic, hemorrhagic, and operative complications. These risks must be weighed against the real risk to the fetus of continued hypoxia if labor were to continue.

Maternal risks encountered at vaginal delivery include laceration of the cervix, vagina, or perineum resulting from a hastily performed delivery.

**B. Neonatal:** The neonate at delivery may be hypoxic, acidotic, or moribund. A pediatric team should be present to effect immediate resuscitation of the newborn.

## Prevention

Patients at risk for umbilical cord prolapse should be treated as high-risk patients. Patients with malpresentations or poorly applied cephalic presentations should be considered for ultrasonographic examination at the onset of labor to determine fetal lie and cord position within the uterine cavity. Because most prolapses occur during labor as the cervix dilates, patients at risk for cord prolapse should be continuously monitored to detect abnormalities of the fetal heart rate. Artificial rupture of membranes should be avoided until the presenting part is well applied to the cervix. At the time of spontaneous membrane rupture, a prompt, careful pelvic examination should be performed to rule out cord prolapse. Should amniotomy be required and the presenting part remains unengaged, careful needling of the membranes and slow release of the amniotic fluid may be performed until the presenting part settles against the cervix.

## Management

**A. Overt Cord Prolapse:** The diagnosis of overt cord prolapse demands immediate action to preserve the life of the fetus. An immediate pelvic examination should be performed to determine cervical effacement and dilatation, station of the presenting part, and the strength and frequency of pulsations within the cord vessels. If the fetus is viable (> 25 weeks' gestation and normal cardiac activity), the patient should be placed in the knee-chest position, and the examiner should apply continuous upward pressure against the presenting part to lift and maintain the fetus away from the prolapsed cord until preparations for cesarean delivery are complete. Oxygen should be given to the mother until the anesthesiologist is prepared to administer a rapid-inhalation anesthetic for delivery. Attempts to replace the cord within the uterine cavity during this time are impractical and ineffectual. Abdominal delivery should be accomplished as rapidly as possible through a generous midline abdominal incision, and a pediatric team should be standing by for immediate resuscitation of the newborn.

**B. Occult Cord Prolapse:** If cord compression patterns (variable decelerations) of the fetal heart rate are recognized during labor, an immediate pelvic examination should be performed to rule out overt cord prolapse. If occult cord prolapse is suspected, the patient should be placed in the lateral Sims or Trendelenburg position in an attempt to alleviate cord compression. If the fetal heart rate returns to normal, labor may be allowed to continue, provided no further fetal insult occurs. Oxygen should be administered to the mother, and the fetal heart rate should be continuously monitored electronically. If the cord compression pattern persists or recurs to the point of fetal jeopardy (moderate to severe variable decelerations or bradycardia), a rapid cesarean section should be accomplished.

**C. Funic Presentation:** The patient at term with funic presentation should be delivered by an expeditiously performed cesarean section prior to membrane rupture. If the fetus is premature, however, the patient should be hospitalized at bedrest in the Sims or Trendelenburg position in an attempt to reposition the cord within the uterine cavity. Serial ultrasonographic examinations should be performed to ascertain cord position, presentation, and gestational age.

**D. Route of Delivery:** Vaginal delivery may be successfully accomplished in cases of overt or occult cord prolapse if, at the time of prolapse, the cervix is fully dilated, cephalopelvic disproportion is not anticipated, and an experienced physician determines that delivery is imminent. Internal podalic version, midforceps rotation, or any other operative technique is generally more hazardous to mother and fetus in this situation than is a judiciously performed cesarean delivery. Cesarean section is the preferred route of delivery in most cases. Vaginal delivery is the route of choice for an immature or dead fetus.

**Prognosis**

**A. Maternal:** Maternal complications include those related to anesthesia, blood loss, and infection following cesarean section or operative vaginal delivery. Maternal recovery is generally complete.

**B. Neonatal:** Fetal mortality and morbidity rates are high, and the prognosis depends on the degree and duration of umbilical cord compression occurring before the diagnosis is made and neonatal resuscitation begun. If the diagnosis is made early and the duration of complete cord occlusion is less than 5 minutes, the prognosis is good. Gestational age and trauma at delivery also affect the final neonatal outcome. If complete cord occlusion has occurred for longer than 5 minutes or if intermittent partial cord occlusion has occurred over a prolonged period of time, fetal damage or death may be inevitable.

# REFERENCES

## BREECH PRESENTATION

Alexopoulos KA: The importance of breech delivery in the pathogenesis of brain damage: End results of a long-term follow-up. Clin Pediatr 1973;12:248.

Bingham P, Lilford RJ: Management of the selected term breech presentation: Assessment of the risks of selected vaginal delivery versus cesarean section for all cases. Obstet Gynecol 1987;69:965.

Bock JE: The influence of prophylactic external cephalic version on the outcome of breech delivery. Acta Obstet Gynecol Scand 1969;48:215.

Braun FH, Jones KL, Smith DW: Breech presentation as an indicator of fetal abnormality. J Pediatr 1975; 86:419.

Brenner WE, Bruce RD, Hendricks CH: The characteristics and perils of breech presentation. Am J Obstet Gynecol 1974;118:700.

Caterini H et al: Fetal risk in hyperextension of the fetal head in breech presentation. Am J Obstet Gynecol 1975;123:632.

Collea JV: *Complications and Management of Breech Presentations.* Vol 1 in: *Advances in Perinatal Medicine.* Milunsky A, Friedman E, Gluck L (editors). Plenum Press, 1981.

Collea JV, Chein C, Quilligan EJ: The randomized management of term frank breech presentation: A study of 208 cases. Am J Obstet Gynecol 1980;137:235.

Collea JV et al: The randomized management of term frank breech presentation: Vaginal delivery vs. cesarean section. Am J Obstet Gynecol 1978;131:186.

Gimovsky ML, Paul RH: Singleton breech presentation in labor: Experience in 1980. Am J Obstet Gynecol 1982;143:733.

Hage ML et al: Changing rates of cesarean delivery: The Duke experience, 1978–1986. Obstet Gynecol 1988;72:98.

Kauppila O: The perinatal mortality in breech deliveries and observations on affecting factors: A retrospective study of 2227 cases. Acta Obstet Gynecol Scand [Suppl] 1975;39:9.

Mahomed K: Breech delivery: A critical evaluation of the mode of delivery and outcome of labor. Int J Gynaecol Obstet 1988;27:17.

Milner RDG: Neonatal mortality of breech deliveries with and without forceps to the aftercoming head. Br J Obstet Gynaecol 1975;82:783.

Minogue M: Vaginal breech delivery in multiparae: A review of perinatal mortality, National Maternity Hospital, 1967–1971. J Jr Med Assoc 1974;67:117.

Moore MM, Shearer DR: Fetal dose estimates for CT pelvimetry. Radiology 1989;171:265.

Perkins RP: Fetal dystocia. Clin Obstet Gynecol 1987; 30:56.

Rayburn W, et al: Routine preoperative ultrasonography and cesarean section. Am J Perinatol 1988;5:297.

Rubin A, Grim G: Results in breech presentation. Am J Obstet Gynecol 1963;86:1048.

Stank DD, McCarthy SM, Filly RA, et al: Pelvimetry by magnetic resonance imaging. Am J Radiol 1985; 144:947.

Strong C: Ethical conflicts between mother and fetus in obstetrics. Clin Perinatol 1987;14:313.

Tank ES et al: Mechanisms of trauma during breech delivery. Obstet Gynecol 1971;38:761.

Thurnau GR, Morgan MA: Efficacy of the fetal-pelvic index as a predictor of fetal-pelvic disproportion in women with abnormal labor patterns that require labor augmentations. Am J Obstet Gynecol 1988;159:1168.

Van Dorsten JP, Schifrin BS, Wallace RL: Randomized control trial of external cephalic version with tocolysis in late pregnancy. Am J Obstet Gynecol 1981; 141:417.

## VERSION

Brocks V, Philipsen T, Secher NJ: A randomized trial of external cephalic version with tocolysis in late pregnancy. Br J Obstet Gynaecol 1984;91:653.

Chapman K: Internal version: Review of 118 cases. J Obstet Gynaecol India 1967;17:368.

Kasule J, Chimbira TH, Brown IM: Controlled trial of external cephalic version. Br J Obstet Gynaecol 1985;92:14.

Potter MG: The pitfalls of podalic version and extraction. Am J Obstet Gynecol 1939;37:675.

Rosensohn M: Internal podalic version at New York Lying-In Hospital (1932–1950). Am J Obstet Gynecol 1954;68:916.

Stine LE et al: Update on external cephalic version performed at term. Obstet Gynecol 1985;65:642.

Westgren M et al: Spontaneous cephalic version of breech presentation in the last trimester. Br J Obstet Gynaecol 1985;92:19.

## COMPOUND PRESENTATION

Weissberg SM, O'Leary JA: Compound presentation of the fetus. Obstet Gynecol 1973;41:60.

## SHOULDER DYSTOCIA

Benedetti TJ, Gabbe SG: Shoulder dystocia: A complication of fetal macrosomia and prolonged second stage of labor with midpelvic delivery. Obstet Gynecol 1978;52:526.

Golditch IM, Kirkman K: The large fetus: Management and outcome. Obstet Gynecol 1978;52:26.

Hardy AE: Birth injuries of the brachial plexus: Incidence and prognosis. J Bone Joint Surg [Br] 1981; 63:98.

Hopwood HG Jr: Shoulder dystocia: Fifteen years' experience in a community hospital. Am J Obstet Gynecol 1982;144:162.

Modanlou HD et al: Large-for-gestational age neonates: Anthropometric reasons for shoulder dystocia. Obstet Gynecol 1982;60:417.

Morris WIC: Shoulder dystocia. J Obstet Gynaecol Br Emp 1955;62:302.

Resnick R: Management of shoulder girdle dystocia. Clin Obstet Gynecol 1980;23:559.

Swartz DP: Shoulder girdle dystocia in vertex delivery. Obstet Gynecol 1960;15:194.

Woods CE: A principle of physics as applicable to shoulder delivery. Am J Obstet Gynecol 1943;45:769.

## UMBILICAL CORD PROLAPSE

Ekwempu CC: Cord prolapse through a fenestration in a cesarean section scar. East Afr Med J 1977;54:692.

Katz Z, Lancet M, Borenstein R: Management of labor with umbilical cord prolapse. Am J Obstet Gynecol 1982;142:239.

Lange IR et al: Cord prolapse: Is antenatal diagnosis possible? Am J Obstet Gynecol 1985;151:1083.

Tchabo JG: The use of the contact hysteroscope in the diagnosis of cord prolapse. Int Surg 1988;73:57.

Tejani NA et al: The association of umbilical cord complications and variable decelerations with acid-base findings. Obstet Gynecol 1977;49:159.

# Cardiac, Hematologic, Pulmonary, Renal & Urinary Tract Disorders In Pregnancy

*Manoj K. Biswas, MD, FACOG, FRCOG, & Dorothee Perloff, MD*

## CARDIOVASCULAR DISORDERS*

### CARDIOVASCULAR CHANGES IN NORMAL PREGNANCY

The major cardiocirculatory changes that occur during normal pregnancy include an increase in cardiac output and blood volume and a decrease in peripheral resistance (Table 22–1). In patients with twin or multiple pregnancy, these changes are exaggerated. During normal pregnancy, 6–8.5 L of fluid and 500–900 mmol of sodium are retained because of the action of progesterone, renin, aldosterone, and prolactin. Because the increase in red cell mass lags behind the increase in plasma volume, a dilutional anemia is common. Renal blood flow increases by 30%, the glomerular filtration rate increases by 50%, and uterine blood flow reaches 500 mL/min at term. Hormonal changes include a rise in levels of estrogen and progesterone, renin, angiotensinogen, angiotensin II, and aldosterone and a decreased sensitivity to infused angiotensin II.

Myocardial contractility increases as do heart rate and atrial and ventricle chamber size (Table 22–1). Late in pregnancy, a decrease in cardiac output has been reported when measurements are made with the patient in the supine rather than the lateral recumbent position. This apparent decrease is due to interference with venous return resulting from compression of the inferior vena cava by the gravid uterus. If marked, this may result in the **supine hypotensive syndrome,** which is characterized by dizziness and even syncope on recumbency. However, the profound hypotension may represent a failure of the normal baroreceptor-mediated reflex adaptation to a fall in pressure, inad-

equate collateral venous circulation, and exaggerated parasympathetic response.

Additional hemodynamic changes occur during the various stages of labor and delivery and depend on the patient's position, the degree of sedation, and the type of anesthesia used. Cardiac output increases by about 20% with each uterine contraction as 300–500 mL of blood is expelled from the contracting uterus. Systolic blood pressure also rises with each contraction, increasing the load on the left ventricle by 10%, while the heart rate falls. Pain, fear, and anxiety contribute further to an increase in cardiac output. These changes are less marked if the patient is in the lateral decubitus position during labor or receiving epidural anesthesia. Following delivery, depending on the amount of blood lost—usually 500 mL during vaginal delivery and 1000 mL or more with cesarean section—the cardiac output and plasma volume increase by 20–60% because of a shift of blood from the uterus and placenta into the vascular space as well as resorption of interstitial fluid. Oxytocic drugs can produce further hemodynamic changes. The hemodynamic changes of pregnancy begin to regress shortly after delivery, and pre-pregnancy levels are usually reached within 2 weeks postpartum, but may take longer.

The hemodynamic changes of normal pregnancy can result in symptoms and signs that mimic those of heart disease, often making it difficult to differentiate the two (Table 22–2). It is the severity and persistence of symptoms that suggest underlying organic heart disease (Table 22–3).

### HEART DISEASE

Cardiovascular disease is the most important non-obstetric cause of disability and death in pregnant women, occurring in 0.4–4% of pregnancies. The reported maternal mortality rate ranges from 0.4% in patients with New York Heart Association classifications I and II to 6.8% or higher among patients with

---

*See also Chapter 19, Hypertensive States of Pregnancy.

Table 22–1. Hemodynamic and respiratory changes of normal pregnancy.[1]

| Physiologic Variable | Direction and Percent of Change | | Time of Onset (Weeks) | Time of Peak Effect (Weeks) |
|---|---|---|---|---|
| Cardiac output | Increased | 30–50 | ± 10 | 20–30 |
| Heart rate | Increased | 10–25 | 10–14 | 40 |
| Blood volume | Increased | 25–50 | 6–10 | 32–36 |
| Plasma volume | Increased | 40–50 | 6–10 | 32 |
| Red cell mass | Increased | 20–40 | 6–10 | 40 |
| Blood pressure | Decreased early; increased late | No net change | First trimester | 20 |
| | | | Third trimester | 40 |
| Pulmonary and peripheral vascular resistance | Decreased | 40–50 | 6–10 | 20–24 |
| Oxygen consumption | Increased | 15–30 | 12–16 | 40 |
| Respiratory rate | Increased | 40–50 | 6–10 | 40 |

[1]Greater increase with twin or multiple pregnancy.

class III and IV severity. It is not surprising that the added hemodynamic burden of pregnancy, labor, and delivery can aggravate symptoms and precipitate complications in a woman with preexisting cardiac disease. However, even a previously healthy woman may develop cardiovascular problems specifically related to pregnancy, such as preeclampsia, varicose veins, thromboembolic complications such as pulmonary emboli, aortic dissection, or shock due to hemorrhage, amniotic fluid emboli, disseminated intravascular coagulation, or sepsis. Furthermore, any woman in the child bearing years may develop incidental myocarditis, pericarditis, or infective endocarditis while she is pregnant. Drugs used for obstetric complications such as preterm labor may have adverse effects on the woman with heart disease, and drugs used for the treatment of maternal heart disease may have adverse effects on the fetus.

Heart disease can be classified as congenital (operated or unoperated) or acquired. Acquired diseases can be infectious, autoimmune, degenerative, malignant or idiopathic. The patient can be further classified as having mild or severe disease, compatible with a normal pregnancy, or posing a serious risk to either mother or baby.

Ideally, the patient with known heart disease should consult her physician before becoming pregnant in order to determine the advisability and optimum timing for pregnancy, the need for and timing of diagnostic procedures, the prospects for corrective or palliative cardiac surgery, the type of prosthetic valve to be used, and the need for discontinuing certain drugs during pregnancy. If a woman with heart disease presents for medical care after she has become pregnant, the obstetrician must be able to recognize the presence of preexisting cardiac disease, assess the degree of disability, and understand the impact of the added hemodynamic changes of pregnancy.

Pre-pregnancy planning might, for instance, include performance of an exercise tolerance test to de-

termine if the woman with severe heart disease can tolerate the added hemodynamic burden of pregnancy. The obstetrician must also be able to anticipate, prevent, diagnose, and treat complications such as arrhythmias or congestive heart failure when they arise and advise the patient regarding discontinuation or continuation of the pregnancy and the risk of future pregnancies. Management of an obstetric patient with heart disease should be carried out by a team consisting of the obstetrician and obstetric nurse or midwife, as well as the cardiologist/internist and, at the time of labor, the anesthesiologist and neonatologist.

Rheumatic heart disease has historically been the most common type of heart disease in pregnant women. However, in countries where infectious causes of heart disease are generally under good control, congenital heart disease now represents a larger percentage of diseases encountered. It is therefore especially important that obstetricians understand the late complications of surgically corrected or uncorrected congenital heart disease that are likely to occur during pregnancy, labor, delivery, and lactation. In addition, degenerative diseases such as ischemic heart disease are encountered more frequently due to the longer survival of patients with diabetes mellitus and chronic renal disease, the prevalence of tobacco addiction, cocaine use, and delayed childbearing.

In patients with limited ability to increase cardiac output due to valvular or intrinsic myocardial disease, the added hemodynamic burden leads to symptoms early in pregnancy (often by 16–20 weeks), when blood volume has increased considerably. The normal increase in blood flow to the uterus is limited, resulting in increased incidence of spontaneous abortion, prematurity, and intrauterine growth retardation. In women with cyanotic heart disease, the incidence of spontaneous abortion may be as high as 60%, and preterm delivery and fetal growth retardation are common. Maternal risks increase with increasing age and parity and are greatest after 30 weeks' gestation.

**Table 22–2.** Symptoms and signs of normal pregnancy mimicking heart disease.

| Clinical Manifestations | Mechanisms |
|---|---|
| **Symptoms** | |
| Palpitations/cardiac awareness | Increased heart rate; increased stroke volume, increased ectopy |
| Nasal stuffiness | Vasodilatation, increased cutaneous blood flow |
| Dyspnea, shortness of breath; orthopnea | Increased progesterone causing hyperventilation; low alveolar $CO_2$ tension: upward displacement of diaphragm |
| Decreased exercise tolerance; easy fatigability | Weight gain; lack of exercise; ungainliness; increased cardiac output at rest, limiting maximum cardiac output increase with exercise |
| Dizziness; lightheadedness; syncope | Decreased venous return due to compression of inferior vena cava by enlarged uterus and increased venous capacitance |
| Epigastric or subxiphoid pain; bloating, heartburn | Displacement of diaphragm, stomach, and liver by large uterus; decreased gastrointestinal motility |
| Heat intolerance, sweating and flushing | Increased cutaneous blood flow and increased metabolic rate |
| **Signs** | |
| Sinus tachycardia; ectopic beats (ventricular, atrial) | Increased cardiac output; increased $O_2$ demand; decreased threshold for ectopic beats and arrhythmias |
| Bounding pulses and capillary pulsations | Increased cardiac output; decreased total peripheral resistance; widened pulse pressure; increased cutaneous blood flow; placenta acts as arteriovenous fistula |
| Prominent jugular venous pulsations | Increased cardiac output; decreased venous tone; right ventricular volume overload |
| Plethoric facies | Increased cutaneous blood flow |
| Lateral displacement of cardiac apex | Mechanical, high diaphragm; right and left ventricular volume overload |
| Widely split $S_1$ and $S_2$ heart sounds | Increased cardiac output; increased venous return; delayed right ventricular emptying |
| Third heart sound | Increased cardiac output; rapid filling of ventricles |
| Systolic murmur (left sternal edge or precordial) | Increased cardiac output; turbulent flow, through pulmonary valve; increased venous return; increased mammary flow. |
| Continuous murmurs | Venous hum; mammary souffle; increased venous distensibility |
| Varicose veins | Obstruction of inferior vena cava by uterus; increased venous distensibility |
| Capillary telangiectases | Increased estrogen level and increased venous distensibility |
| Pulmonary rales | Atelectasis due to hypoventilation of lung bases because of displacement of diaphragm |
| Edema (legs, occasionally hands and face) | Mechanical obstruction of inferior vena cava by uterus; increased venous pressure in legs |
| Ectopic beats; supraventricular tachycardias | Decreased threshold for ectopic beats and arrhythmias |
| **Electrocardiogram** | |
| Leftward or rightward axis shift; nonspecific ST-T wave changes | Mechanical displacement of diaphragm; right ventricular volume overload; altered sympathetic tone and altered repolarization sequence |
| **Echocardiogram/Doppler ultrasound** | |
| Increased left and right ventricular end diastolic dimensions | Increased blood volume; increased cardiac output |
| Increased velocity of circumferential fiber shortening increased ejection fraction, hyperdynamic function | Increased myocardial contractility, increased cardiac output, increased sympathetic tone |

The major clinical complications of heart disease that may be precipitated or aggravated by pregnancy include atrial and ventricular arrhythmias, right- and left-sided congestive heart failure, acute pulmonary edema, low cardiac output, hypotension or hypertension, myocardial ischemia, cerebral ischemia, syncope, thromboembolic disease, infective endocarditis, and death.

### Evaluation of the Patient With Heart Disease

Evaluation of the pregnant woman in whom heart disease is suspected should include a careful medical

**Table 22–3.** Symptoms and signs suggesting significant cardiovascular disease.

Severe or progressive dyspnea and orthopnea, especially at rest.

Paroxysmal nocturnal dyspnea; signs of pulmonary edema; cough, frothy pink sputum

Effort syncope or chest pain.

Chronic cough, hemoptysis.

Clubbing, cyanosis, or persistent edema of extremities.

Increased jugular venous pressure, abnormal venous pulsations.

Accentuated or barely audible first heart sound.

Fixed or paradoxic splitting of $S_2$; single $S_2$.

Ejection click or late systolic click, opening snap

Friction rub.

Systolic murmur of grade III or grade IV intensity or palpable thrill.

Any diastolic murmur.

Cardiomegaly with diffuse sustained right or left ventricular heave.

Electrocardiographic evidence of significant arrhythmias.

history, complete physical examination, and noninvasive laboratory tests in order to establish a diagnosis and to determine the severity of the disease in order to facilitate planning the patient's management. The degree of functional disability is graded according to the following New York Heart Association classification:

Class I: No symptoms limiting ordinary physical activity.

Class II: Slight limitation with mild to moderate activity but no symptoms at rest.

Class III: Marked limitation with less than ordinary activity; dyspnea or pain on minimal activity.

Class IV: Symptoms at rest or with minimal activity and symptoms of frank congestive heart failure.

However, such a classification, which is based on symptoms is only a rough guideline and may not accurately reflect the severity of disease, and sudden and unpredictable changes in classification can occur during pregnancy.

**A. Medical History:** In patients with a previous diagnosis of heart disease or hypertension, the following information should be obtained: age at diagnosis and circumstances of diagnosis; previous symptoms and complications; previous diagnostic procedures, including cardiac catheterization, exercise testing, echocardiography; prior drug treatment; timing and exact nature of operative procedures and degree of improvement achieved; residual defects, symptoms, and limitations; current medications and diet; and previously imposed prohibitions regarding activity. Medical records from previous physicians regarding previous hospitalizations, diagnostic and therapeutic procedures, and complications should be obtained.

In patients without an established diagnosis of heart disease, the intake health provider should routinely inquire about a history of rheumatic fever and other illnesses that may be related to heart disease,

such as scarlet fever, systemic lupus erythematosus, pulmonary disease, renal disease, diphtheria, or pneumonia, as well as prior hospitalizations, accidents, and major operations. The physician should elicit a history of signs and symptoms such as cyanosis at birth or with exertion, squatting in childhood, multiple respiratory infections in childhood, prior arrhythmias, dyspnea at rest or on exertion, chronic cough, hemoptysis, asthma, exercise intolerance, headache, dizziness, effort syncope, chest pain, and peripheral edema. Activities or events precipitating these symptoms should be assessed. Finally, the family history of cardiovascular disease or other congenital anomalies should be ascertained, together with a history of prior fetal abnormalities. In patients from developing countries, a history of exposure to tuberculosis, hepatitis rickettsial, and parasitic infections should also be obtained.

**B. Physical Examination:** On physical examination, note should be made of height, weight, and body build; any facial, digital, or skeletal abnormalities that suggest congenital anomalies; and skin changes such as cyanosis, pallor, angiomas, pigmentation, xanthelasmas, and xanthomas. The blood pressure should be carefully measured with an appropriately sized cuff and, if elevated, repeated measurements should be made in both arms and in several positions. The radial pulses should be carefully palpated. A collapsing pulse of aortic insufficiency, a diminished pulse of low cardiac output, or the absence of a pulse due to prior surgery or thrombosis should be noted.

Inspection of the head should focus on congenital abnormalities such as low hairline or low-set ears, nasal deformities, and high-arched palate, as well as gingival overgrowth, dental caries, or cyanosis. The jugular venous pressure and venous waves in the neck should be inspected with the patient's head elevated at a 30-degree angle above the table, and the carotid pulse and thyroid gland should be palpated. A venous hum should be differentiated from a cardiac murmur or bruit.

Inspection and palpation of the chest should identify the presence of scars and skeletal abnormalities such as pectus excavatum deformity, precordial bulge, left or right ventricular heave, or thrill. The cardiac rhythm (regular or irregular, fast or slow) should be assessed. The first heart sound is often widely split in pregnant women, when listening with the diaphragm. Increased intensity of the first heart sound is the hallmark of mitral stenosis, and decreased intensity suggests first-degree heart block. Fixed splitting of the second heart sound suggests atrial septal defect or right bundle branch block, while paradoxic splitting suggests advanced left ventricular hypertrophy or left bundle branch block. A third heart sound is commonly heard, especially late in pregnancy. However, a fourth heart sound, an opening snap, an ejection click, or a mid- or late systolic click should suggest heart disease. In patients with prosthetic valves, the opening and closing of the valve may produce characteristic metallic clicking sounds.

The systolic murmurs of normal pregnancy must be differentiated from those of underlying heart disease. The murmurs of right or left ventricular outflow tract obstruction may be initiated by an ejection click and are characteristically crescendo-decrescendo, ending before the closing sound of the valve involved, and are usually grade III or IV/VI in intensity, as opposed to the grade II murmurs heard in normal pregnancy. Regurgitant murmurs of the semilunar valves (aortic and pulmonary) are diastolic and decrescendo and are well heard along the left sternal edge when the patient is sitting with held expiration.

Diastolic murmurs are not heard in normal pregnancy. The diastolic murmur of mitral stenosis is characteristically associated with a loud first heart sound and an opening snap, a high-frequency sound that follows the aortic valve closure by 0.07–0.12 second. This low-frequency diastolic rumble of mitral stenosis is best heard when the patient is positioned in the left lateral decubitus position, with the bell of the stethoscope lightly placed upon the skin. The mitral regurgitation murmur is a long holosystolic murmur, which is best heard at the apex radiating into the left axilla, whereas the tricuspid regurgitation murmur is best heard at the lower left sternal edge and increases markedly with inspiration. The murmur of mitral valve prolapse may be musical, and both murmur and click are often inaudible late in pregnancy unless the patient is sitting up or standing.

Patients with atrial septal defect have a pulmonary systolic ejection murmur, often a low-frequency diastolic rumble, which represents a tricuspid flow murmur, and a characteristic widely split second heart sound, which remains widely split even in expiration. Those with a ventricular septal defect have a pansystolic, loud, harsh murmur resembling that of mitral regurgitation, which is heard best along the lower left sternal edge. The systolic murmur of coarctation of the aorta is best heard in the left second interspace and between the scapulae. Patients with an extracardiac shunt (patent ductus arteriosus) usually have a continuous systolic and diastolic murmur.

Examination should continue with percussion and auscultation of the lungs and palpation and auscultation of the abdomen to ascertain the presence of hepatosplenomegaly, aortic aneurysm, masses, or bruits. The peripheral pulses should be carefully palpated and the extremities examined for the presence of varices, cyanosis, edema, stasis changes, clubbing, "splinter" hemorrhages, joint deformities, muscle wasting, or skeletal deformities such as arachnodactyly or brachydactyly, which suggest multiple congenital anomalies.

Funduscopic examination should be performed in patients with hypertension to determine the presence of arteriolar narrowing, sclerosis, and arteriovenous compression; these imply long-standing hypertension. The presence of retinal edema, cotton-wool patches, and papilledema suggests preeclampsia or accelerated hypertension. A brief neurologic examination, including examination of the cranial nerves, muscle strength, sensation, and reflexes, should be performed when indicated.

**C. Laboratory Tests:** In addition to routine laboratory tests, patients with suspected cardiac disease may need the following noninvasive diagnostic procedures:

**1. Electrocardiogram**–The electrocardiogram (ECG) is useful for determining abnormalities of rhythm and the presence of conduction defects, evidence of chamber enlargement, and signs of myocardial or pericardial disease, ischemia, or infarction. The Holter monitor (24-hour continuous ECG) is occasionally useful for documenting the presence and nature of recurring arrhythmias or heart blocks and for correlating symptoms of palpitations, near syncope or syncope with concurrent cardiac rhythm.

**2. Phonocardiogram**–Phonocardiography is no longer performed routinely but can be a useful adjunct to echocardiography and is a useful teaching tool.

**3. Echocardiogram**–The transthoracic (TTE) echocardiogram (both M mode and 2-dimensional sector scan) is a rapid, safe, and reliable tool for differentiating the physiologic murmurs resulting from the increased cardiac output of a normal pregnancy from the murmurs of congenital or acquired heart disease. The echocardiogram can provide information about abnormalities of anatomy and function of the chambers, valves, and pericardium. By inspection of the collapsibility of the inferior vena cava, the echocardiogram can provide information about the patient's volume status and differentiate cardiac from noncardiac causes of pulmonary edema that are important for diagnosis and treatment. The presence, location, and magnitude of intracardiac left-to-right and right-to-left shunts can be approximated by injecting 1–2 mL of normal saline shaken with 1 cc of air into a peripheral vein to produce microbubbles. The microbubbles magnify the reflected echo signal, and the presence of bubbles on the left side or an area of "negative contrast" in the right atrium or ventricle suggest an intracardiac shunt. Echocardiography can also be used to diagnose aortic dissection and coarctation. Transesophageal echocardiography (TEE) has added a new dimension to the evaluation especially of posterior structures such as the left atrium and the mitral valve. Transesophageal echocardiography, because of its better resolution, is particularly useful for the detection of left atrial thrombi and evaluation of prosthetic valves, and has been used in the place of fluoroscopy for insertion of a pacemaker or even for performing valvuloplasty. TEE is also useful in the operating room and intensive care unit when TTE does not provide adequate resolution.

**4. Doppler echocardiography**–Pulsed, continuous-wave, and color Doppler echo-cardiography is combined with 2-dimensional echocardiography for determination of blood flow and velocity, quantitation of pressure gradients and the degree of regurgitation as well as for measuring intracardiac shunts, and estimation of pulmonary pressure.

**5. Exercise tolerance test**–Exercise studies such as the treadmill test are normally not used during pregnancy, since pregnancy itself is a form of stress test. However, they may be useful in a woman contemplating pregnancy or in early pregnancy if the degree of compensation and ability to carry a pregnancy to term are in doubt, or to investigate the cause of chest pain and certain arrhythmias. In a woman with a prior myocardial infarct who is contemplating becoming pregnant, an exercise study with radionuclide myocardial perfusion would be a useful test to perform to determine the amount of fixed myocardial damage and the presence of reversible ischemia.

**6. Miscellaneous**–Additional studies for specific conditions include a throat culture to diagnose the presence of beta-hemolytic streptococcal infection and a C-reactive protein and antistreptolysin titer if antecedent streptococcal infection is suspected. Serial blood cultures are indicated if infective endocarditis is suspected. Chest x-rays, cardiac catheterization, and radio nuclide scans are generally avoided during pregnancy, since the radiation can be harmful to the fetus, especially early in gestation. However, these tests can be performed with careful shielding of the abdomen and pelvis, if the mother's condition requires it.

## RHEUMATIC HEART DISEASE

In developed countries, the incidence and the severity of rheumatic fever have declined progressively since the 1960s because of the widespread, prompt use of penicillin in the treatment of group A beta-hemolytic streptococcal upper respiratory tract infections and because of an apparent decrease in virulence of the organism. However, in Asia and Central and South America, rheumatic heart disease is still prevalent, and valvular abnormalities are common in women of child-bearing age.

Active rheumatic carditis, although rare during pregnancy, can be a serious and potentially fatal complication. The diagnosis is based on the Jones Criteria: evidence of a preceding group A streptococcal infection (positive throat culture, scarlet fever, or elevated antistreptolysin titer), carditis, chorea, subcutaneous nodules, erythema marginatum, and polyarthritis. The minor criteria included fever, arthralgias, elevated sedimentation rate, and first-degree heart block. Carditis may result in acute congestive heart failure or may aggravate established rheumatic valvular disease. Treatment should consist of specific anti-

streptococcal antibiotics as well as salicylates and corticosteriods when indicated. Sodium restriction and bed rest are general nonspecific measures.

Continuous prophylaxis against recurring rheumatic fever (secondary prevention) is advised until at least age 30 years in any patient with a history of rheumatic fever or rheumatic heart disease. In areas where rheumatic fever is prevalent, prophylaxis probably should be continued for patients with rheumatic heart disease, especially if they have small or school aged children. The American Heart Association regimen is as follows:

Benzathine penicillin G, 1.2 million units intramuscularly at monthly intervals; or

Penicillin V, 250 mg orally twice daily for compliant patients; or

Sulfadiazine, 0.5–1 g orally once a day (contraindicated late in pregnancy because of transplacental passage); or

Erythromycin, 250 mg orally twice daily.

Allergic reactions to penicillin include urticaria, angioneurotic edema, and, rarely, a serum sickness-like reaction characterized by fever and joint pains, which may be mistaken for acute rheumatic fever.

## 1. MITRAL VALVE DISEASE

**Mitral stenosis** is the most common lesion in young women with rheumatic heart disease, although mitral stenosis can result from Libman Sacks endocarditis in patients with lupus and can be congenital, especially in association with atrial septal defect (Lutembacher's syndrome). Most patients with mild to moderate stenosis who are in sinus rhythm tolerate pregnancy well, although the risk for superimposed infective endocarditis, on the abnormal valve, is ever present even in hemodynamically mild disease. Those with moderate to severe disease are more likely to develop complications such as pulmonary venous congestion or frank pulmonary edema, right ventricular failure, pulmonary vascular hypertension, hemoptysis, atrial fibrillation, and systemic or pulmonary emboli. However, sudden and unexpected deterioration can occasionally occur during pregnancy in patients with any degree of mitral stenosis. New onset of atrial fibrillation in a previously asymptomatic woman can precipitate acute pulmonary edema, which occasionally requires emergency commissurotomy.

The normal hemodynamic changes of pregnancy put patients with mitral stenosis at special risk for developing pulmonary congestion. The increased heart rate with consequent shortening of the diastolic filling period, augmented cardiac output and blood volume, and increased pulmonary venous pressure all contribute to raising left atrial pressure. The increased atrial irritability and increased sympathetic tone predispose to the onset of atrial fibrillation. The pregnant cardiac patient is also at risk for the development of thromboembolic complications, because of the hypercoagulable state of the blood during pregnancy as well as venous stasis in the legs. When right ventricular failure is associated with increased pulmonary vascular resistance, fluctuations in venous return can result in decreased cardiac output, even syncope. The risk for developing heart failure increases progressively throughout pregnancy and is further increased during labor and delivery and immediately postpartum. Symptoms can also be aggravated by associated anemia, thyrotoxicosis, fever, respiratory infections, and tachycardia resulting from anxiety, stress, and unusual physical exertion as well as a hot, humid environment. The risk of infective endocarditis remains throughout pregnancy, delivery, and the early puerperium.

Labor imposes an additional load on the pregnant cardiac patient, but congestive failure rarely occurs for the first time during labor in a previously well-controlled patient with mitral stenosis. Postpartum pulmonary edema occurs more frequently, however, because of the abrupt redistribution of blood volume. The mortality rate in women with rheumatic mitral valve disease is 1% overall and reaches 3–4% in women with class III and class IV severity.

## Clinical Findings

The symptoms of mitral valve disease are those of pulmonary venous congestion; dyspnea on exertion and, later, at rest; right ventricular failure; atrial arrhythmias; and occasionally, hemoptysis. Fatigue and decrease in exercise tolerance are more often manifestations of mitral insufficiency. The characteristic findings on physical examination include a right ventricular lift, a loud first heart sound (S-1), accentuated pulmonic component of the second heart sound (P-2), a widely heart opening snap (OS), and a low frequency diastolic rumble at the apex with presystolic accentuation (if the patient is in sinus rhythm). The murmur is best heard with the bell and should be carefully listened for when the characteristic cadence of S-1, P-2, OS is appreciated. The electrocardiogram is often normal but may indicate left atrial enlargement, right axis deviation, or even right ventricular hypertrophy. The echocardiogram is particularly useful for defining the anatomy of the valve and intravalvular structures, quantitating the degree of stenosis and associated regurgitation, and identifying the presence of abnormalities in other valves and pulmonary artery pressure.

## Treatment

The goals of treatment for the patient with mitral stenosis should be to prevent or treat tachycardia and atrial fibrillation, to avoid fluid overload, and to avoid unnecessary increases in oxygen demand such as occur with anxiety or physical activity. Digitalis, quinidine, occasionally beta adrenergic blocking agents, sodium restriction, and diuretics may be necessary for treating congestive failure and atrial arrhythmias. Patients with chronic atrial fibrillation should be anticoagulated with subcutaneous heparin. Anemia, intercurrent infection, and thyrotoxicosis should be corrected. Large fluctuations in hemodynamics due to venous pooling in the legs should be avoided by the use of elastic support hose, especially late in pregnancy.

Cardiac surgery or balloon valvuloplasty, although rarely necessary as an adjunct to careful medical management of patients with chronic rheumatic heart disease, occasionally becomes necessary as a lifesaving maneuver. In patients with severe mitral stenosis, especially if manifested in childhood, mitral valvotomy has often been performed for relief of symptoms before the patient becomes pregnant. Closed surgical mitral commissurotomy can be performed at any time during pregnancy but is rarely necessary as a lifesaving procedure until cardiac output has increased significantly in the late second or early third trimester. Balloon valvuloplasty has become a preferred, less invasive procedure, especially for patients with a noncalcified, pliable valve. In an occasional patient, mitral valve replacement may be necessary as an emergency procedure during pregnancy, as, for instance, in a patient with prior valve replacement whose valve becomes obstructed by pannus or thrombus. Recent reports indicate a low mortality rate for both mother and fetus with cardiopulmonary bypass. However, open heart surgery should be deferred until after the first trimester, if possible.

Patients who have had a valve replaced with a prosthetic valve require anticoagulation and need to be switched from coumadin to heparin during the pregnancy. The teratogenic and fetotoxic effects of warfarin and the risks of bleeding for the mother and fetus during labor and delivery must be balanced against the risks of thromboembolic episodes, especially in patients with earlier-model prosthetic valves. The use of tissue valves obviates the need for anticoagulants, but the lifespan of bioprosthetic valves is only 8–10 years, and, if the patient is in atrial fibrillation, anticoagulation is still required.

Patients with rheumatic valvular disease should be delivered vaginally at term unless cesarean section is indicated for obstetric reasons. Appropriate analgesia should be given during labor, and epidural anesthesia without epinephrine should be used for delivery. Fluid loading for epidural anesthesia must be done gradually. To avoid the added exertion of bearing down during the third stage of labor, outlet forceps may be used. Careful hemodynamic monitoring during labor and delivery is indicated in patients with compromised circulation. Postpartum oxytocics should be given cautiously and blood loss carefully monitored. Redistribution of fluid from the interstitial to the intravascular space immediately postpartum can precipitate pulmonary edema in compromised patients.

## 2. MITRAL REGURGITATION

Patients with isolated or predominant **mitral regurgitation** tolerate the physiologic consequences of pregnancy better than do patients with predominant mitral stenosis. The fall in systemic vascular resistance decreases the left ventricular afterload and actually reduces the regurgitant fraction, thus reducing the risk of pulmonary congestion. The risk of atrial fibrillation and of endocarditis, however, is no less in patients with predominant mitral insufficiency. Although mitral regurgitation is frequently the result of rheumatic disease, other causes include: genetic defects in collagen synthesis (such as occur in Marfan's syndrome and Ehlers-Danlos syndrome) or following endocarditis on a previously abnormal valve, late complication of mitral valve prolapse, or papillary muscle infarction or rupture. The clinical course and findings are similar to those of rheumatic mitral insufficiency. The characteristic finding on physical examination is a long systolic murmur that ends with the second heart sound and is best heard at the apex with radiation into the axilla. An associated third heart sound is often present, and in rheumatic mitral valve disease the loud first heart sound and opening snap are generally present.

## 3. RHEUMATIC DISEASE IN OTHER VALVES

The aortic, pulmonary, and tricuspid valves may also be involved by the rheumatic process, usually in association with mitral valve disease. Involvement of multiple valves compounds the problems of management in these patients. In patients with aortic or pulmonary stenosis who have fixed ventricular outflow obstruction, the gradient across the valve increases with progressive increase in cardiac output during pregnancy, leading to an increased systolic pressure load on the ventricle. Although left ventricular failure is rare, post-exertion syncope and angina due to inadequate cardiac output reserve may develop for the first time during pregnancy, especially in the last trimester, when venous return may be abruptly reduced due to compression of the inferior vena cava by the uterus. Patients with severe aortic stenosis should be advised to undergo surgical correction before becoming pregnant. Because patients with high-grade aortic stenosis are unable to maintain normal cardiac output, hypotension, hypertension, and increased cardiac work must be avoided by restricting physical activity and carefully replacing intrapartum blood loss.

Patients with aortic insufficiency—like those with mitral regurgitation—tolerate pregnancy well, since the fall in peripheral resistance favors blood flow and decreases the regurgitant fraction. The risk of endocarditis is present in both stenotic and insufficient valves regardless of severity, and antibiotic prophylaxis during delivery is recommended. Patients with elevated left ventricular end-diastolic pressure, however, are more likely to develop left ventricular failure during pregnancy.

Corrective surgical procedures for rheumatic valve disease include balloon valvuloplasty, surgical commissurotomy, and valve replacement. Two types of valves are available. Heterograft or homograft tissue valves do not require systemic anticoagulation but tend to deteriorate in 8–10 years. Prosthetic valves such as the tilting disc or caged ball valves may last 20 years or longer but always require anticoagulation, complicating the management of pregnancy.

## INFECTIVE ENDOCARDITIS

Endocarditis is an acute or subacute inflammatory process resulting from blood-borne infection with *Streptococcus viridans* or other streptococci such as enterococcus (eg, Streptococcus faecalis), staphylococci, gram-negative organisms, or fungi. Abnormal heart valves and the endocardium in the proximity of congenital anatomic defects are preferential sites for involvement by blood-borne infections. Progressive involvement of the valve leaflets may result in acute aortic, mitral, or tricuspid valvular regurgitation, which may precipitate cardiac failure. Infected material from vegetations can embolize from right-sided lesions such as the tricuspid valve to the lungs, and from left-sided lesions to the systemic circulation. A focal embolic or immune complex glomerulonephritis may also develop. Untreated endocarditis carries a high mortality rate. Patients with endocarditis often give a history of recent extensive dental work, intravascular or urologic procedures, cardiac surgery, or intravenous illicit drug abuse. Intravenous drug users are at particular risk for developing acute endocarditis, often due to unusual pathogens and often on previously normal valves. Aseptic endocarditis occasionally occurs with rheumatoid arthritis, systemic lupus erythematosus (Libman-Sacks disease), and hypereosinophilic states (Löffler's endocarditis).

### Clinical Findings

The diagnosis is based on symptoms such as persistent fever, malaise, chills, sweats, weakness, and embolic phenomena, both to the lungs and to the periphery in an individual with risk factors for endocarditis. Physical findings include petechial hemorrhages, clubbing of the fingers and toes, splenomegaly, Osler's nodes, (septic emboli to the finger tips), the appearance of new murmurs or change in existing murmurs, and manifestations of congestive heart failure. The diagnosis is confirmed by the finding of a positive blood culture or demonstration of vegetations on the valves by echocardiography.

## Prevention

Patients at risk for developing infective endocarditis include those with underlying congenital or acquired valvular heart disease and intravenous drug abusers (Table 22–4). Table 22–5 lists the types of procedures for which endocarditis prophylaxis is recommended or discretionary. The currently recommended antibiotic regimens for both upper respiratory tract and gynecologic or urologic procedures are listed in Table 22–6. Patients with underlying heart disease should be advised to maintain good oral hygiene and attend promptly to any infections.

## PERICARDIAL DISEASE

Pericardial disease, which is rare, during pregnancy occurs in various forms: as an acute infective process, usually due to a virus; as tamponade due to hemorrhage from trauma, aortic dissection, tumor, or effusion complicating collagen vascular disease, acquired immune deficiency syndrome (AIDS), or uremia; or as chronic pericardial constriction secondary to infection, irradiation, or infiltrative process. The symptoms and physical findings, diagnostic approach, and management are the same in the pregnant

**Table 22–4.** Cardiac conditions for which endocarditis prophylaxis should be considered.[1]

**Endocarditis prophylaxis recommended**
Prosthetic cardiac valves, including bioprosthetic and homograft valves
Previous bacterial endocarditis, even in the absence of heart disease
Most congenital cardiac malformations
Rheumatic and other acquired valvular dysfunction, even after valvular surgery
Hypertrophic cardiomyopathy
Mitral valve prolapse with valvular regurgitation
**Endocarditis prophylaxis not recommended**
Isolated secundum atrial septal defect
Surgical repair without residua beyond 6 mo of secundum atrial septal defect, ventricular septal defect, or patent ductus arteriosus
Previous coronary artery bypass graft surgery
Mitral valve prolapse without valvular regurgitation[2]
Physiologic, functional, or innocent heart murmurs
Previous Kawasaki disease without valvular dysfunction
Previous rheumatic fever without valvular dysfunction
Cardiac pacemakers and implanted defibrillators

[1]Reproduced, with permission, from Dajani AS et al: Prevention of bacterial endocarditis. JAMA 1990;264:2919. This table lists selected conditions but is not meant to be all-inclusive.
[2]Individuals who have a mitral valve prolapse associated with thickening and/or redundancy of the valve leaflets may be at increased risk for bacterial endocarditis, particularly men who are 45 years of age or older.

**Table 22–5.** Dental or surgical procedures for which endocarditis prophylaxis should be considered.[1]

**Endocarditis prophylaxis recommended**
Dental procedures known to induce gingival or mucosal bleeding, including professional cleaning
Tonsillectomy and/or adenoidectomy
Surgical operations that involve intestinal or respiratory mucosa
Bronchoscopy with a rigid bronchoscope
Sclerotherapy for esophageal varices
Esophageal dilatation
Gallbladder surgery
Cystoscopy
Urethral dilatation
Urethral catheterization if urinary tract infection is present[2]
Urinary tract surgery if urinary tract infection is present[2]
Prostatic surgery
Incision and drainage of infected tissue[2]
Vaginal hysterectomy
Vaginal delivery in the presence of infection[2]
**Endocarditis prophylaxis not recommended**[3]
Dental procedures not likely to induce gingival bleeding, such as simple adjustment of orthodontic appliances or fillings above the gum line
Injection of local intraoral anesthetic (except intraligamentary injections)
Shedding of primary teeth
Tympanostomy tube insertion
Endotracheal intubation
Bronchoscopy with a flexible bronchoscope, with or without biopsy
Cardiac catheterization
Endoscopy with or without gastrointestinal biopsy
Ceasarean section
In the absence of infection for urethral catheterization, dilatation and curettage, uncomplicated vaginal delivery, therapeutic abortion, sterilization procedures, or insertion or removal of intrauterine devices

[1]Reproduced, with permission, from Dajani AS et al: Prevention of bacterial endocarditis. JAMA 1990:264:2919. This table lists selected procedures but is not meant to be all-inclusive.
[2]In addition to prophylactic regimen for genitourinary procedures, antibiotic therapy should be directed against the most likely bacterial pathogen.
[3]In patients who have prosthetic heart valves, a previous history of endocarditis, or surgically constructed systemic-pulmonary shunts or conduits, physicians may choose to administer prophylactic antibiotics even for low-risk procedures that involve the lower respiratory, genitourinary, or gastrointestinal tracts.

as in the nonpregnant patient and are well described in standard texts. However, the peripheral edema and increased jugular venous pulsations of normal pregnancy may mask the signs of both tamponade and chronic constrictive pericarditis, leading to frequent delays in diagnosis. Diagnosis can be suspected from the presence of a friction rub, a positive Kussmaul sign (increased jugular venous pressure with inspiration), a pulsus paradoxus (decreased systolic pressure with inspiration), and confirmed by electrocardiography, echocardiography, and pericardiocentesis. *Acute tamponade is a medical emergency requiring rapid pericardiocentesis or surgical decompression.* Symptomatic treatment with salicylates and corticosteroids may be indicated for acute viral infections. In chronic

**Table 22–6.** Regimens for genitourinary/gastrointestinal procedures.[1]

| Drug | Dosage Regimen |
|---|---|
| **Standard regimen** | |
| Ampicillin, gentamicin, and amoxicillin | Intravenous or intramuscular administration of ampicillin, 2.0 g, plus gentamicin, 1.5 mg/kg (not to exceed 80 mg), 30 min before procedure; followed by amoxicillin, 1.5 g, orally 6 h after initial dose; alternatively, the parenteral regimen may be repeated once 8 h after initial dose |
| **Ampicillin/amoxicillin/penicillin-allergic patient regimen** | |
| Vancomycin and gentamicin | Intravenous administration of vancomycin, 1.0 g, over 1 h plus intravenous or intramuscular administration of gentamicin, 1.5 mg/kg (not to exceed 80 mg), 1 h before procedure; may be repeated once 8 h after initial dose |
| **Alternate low-risk patient regimen** | |
| Amoxicillin | 3.0 g orally 1 h before procedure; then 1.5 g 6 h after initial dose |

[1]Reproduced, with permission, from Dajani AS et al: Prevention of bacterial endocarditis. JAMA 1990;264:2919.

constrictive pericarditis, surgical decortication may be indicated, but is rarely necessary during pregnancy.

## MYOCARDIAL DISEASE

### 1. MYOCARDITIS

Acute inflammation of the myocardium may be due to rheumatic fever, diphtheria, or viral diseases such as infection with group B coxsackie viruses or protozoal diseases such as toxoplasmosis. Other infectious causes include many other viruses including the human immunodeficiency virus (HIV), rickettsia (Q fever, Rocky Mountain spotted fever and scrub typhus), trichinosis, and spirochetal infections (leptospirosis, Lyme disease). In South America, Chagas' disease due to *Trypanosoma Cruzi* is common. The myocarditis may be acute or subacute, may be associated with symptoms of systemic illness, and may occur at any time during pregnancy. The clinical manifestations are those of chest pain, fever, pulmonary rales, tachycardia, edema, and systolic murmurs and gallops on physical examination; and cardiomegaly, reduced ventricular function, conduction defects, and arrhythmias on electrocardiography and echocardiography. Specific serologic and bacteriologic tests may reveal the identity of the initiating organism. The clinical course is variable, depending on the severity of the infection and the extent of myocardial inflammation. The acute phase of the disease may be subclinical and hence is probably often not recognized as such. The disease may run an acute, subacute, or chronic course; be self-limited with complete recovery; or lead to progressive myocardial fibrosis and eventually to cardiomyopathy. The relationship to peripartum cardiomyopathy is unknown.

Treatment consists of bed rest, digitalis, diuretics, antiarrhythmic agents, and appropriate antibiotics if a specific organism has been identified. Salicylates and corticosteroids are effective in patients with active rheumatic carditis. The incidence of spontaneous abortions in patients with persistent infection is high.

### 2. CARDIOMYOPATHY

Cardiomyopathy is a rare primary disease of cardiac muscle that presents clinically as heart failure and myocardial dysfunction that probably represent the end stage of various processes that affect the myocardium. Cardiomyopathy is classified broadly as **dilated, restrictive/infiltrative**, or **hypertrophic**. Restrictive cardiomyopathy is seen as the end stage of amyloidosis, scleroderma, sarcoid, hemochromatosis, or endomyocardial fibroelastosis. Dilated cardiomyopathy may result from excess alcohol (beriberi), thyrotoxicosis, excessive catecholamine levels (pheochromocytoma), cocaine, and cytotoxic drugs such as doxorubicin. Infectious causes for cardiomyopathy include rheumatic fever, diptheria, rickettsia (scrub typhus) protozoa (Chaga's disease), spirochetes (Lyme disease) toxoplasmosis, and viral diseases. Lupus erythematosus, hypereosinophilia (Löffler's), ischemia, multiple infarction, and sickle cell disease can also cause a diffuse myocardial process that can lead to congestive heart failure.

### Peripartum cardiomyopathy

**Peripartum cardiomyopathy** is used to describe this form of cardiac failure when the onset occurs in the last months of pregnancy or within 6 months postpartum, and no specific etiology or prior heart disease is identified. The assumption is that the pregnant condition has somehow predisposed the woman to develop myocardial disease, but the mechanism remains unexplained. It is not understood why the symptoms usually appear following parturition rather than during the late second and third trimesters, when the hemodynamic burden is greatest. It may also be that symptoms of congestive failure are overlooked or misinterpreted as complaints often seen normally late in a normal pregnancy. The incidence appears to be higher in women of African descent, perhaps due to the high prevalence of hypertension, and in women living in warm climates, in twin gestations, and in women with preeclampsia. Cardiomegaly and heart failure may persist or regress postpartum and recur in subsequent pregnancies. The incidence varies from one in 1300 to one in 4000 deliveries, although among the Hausa people in Zaria in northern Nigeria, the incidence may be as high as one in 100–400 deliveries, probably because of the traditional high postpartum salt intake among these women.

## Clinical Findings

The clinical manifestations are those of right and left ventricular failure with pulmonary congestion, hepatomegaly, low cardiac output, chest pain, hemoptysis and cough, fatigue, dyspnea, decreased exercise tolerance, edema, systolic murmurs, third heart sound, elevated jugular venous pressure, pulmonary rales, and cardiomegaly. Arrhythmias and pulmonary as well as systemic emboli are common. The electrocardiographic changes are nonspecific but include arrhythmias, low QRS voltage, left ventricular hypertrophy, abnormal Q waves, nonspecific ST-T wave changes, and conduction defects. On echocardiography, there is evidence of enlargement of all chambers, generalized decrease in wall motion, reduced ejection fraction, and often mural thrombi.

## Treatment & Prognosis

The prognosis depends on the degree to which the cardiomegaly is reversible with standard treatment for congestive heart failure, such as digitalis, diuretics, salt restriction, and prolonged bed rest. Afterload reduction with vasodilators, but not converting enzyme inhibitors that are contraindicated in pregnancy, and use of anticoagulants are indicated for patients with intractable heart failure and repeated embolic episodes. Mortality rates of 25–50% have been reported. Patients with persistent cardiomegaly following standard therapy or 6 months after the onset of symptoms, have a high incidence of recurrence, progression, and even mortality with subsequent pregnancies and should be cautioned not to become pregnant again.

## Hypertrophic Cardiomyopathy

Hypertrophic cardiomyopathy with or without left ventricular outflow tract obstruction (subaortic stenosis) is a developmental abnormality of cardiac muscle inherited as an autosomal dominant abnormality, although occasionally sporadic, that may result in symptoms within the first 3 decades of life. The asymmetrically hypertrophied septum encroaches on the left ventricular outflow tract, producing an intraventricular pressure gradient and outflow tract obstruction, as well as systolic anterior motion for dis-

tortion of the mitral valve with mitral insufficiency. The thickened, distorted, abnormally developed, noncompliant muscle causes impaired left ventricular diastolic filling. Decreased cardiac output, atrial, and ventricular arrhythmias, and post-exertion syncope are common complications.

The diagnosis is suspected on physical examination and must be differentiated from valvular aortic stenosis. Physical findings include a left ventricular heave, an aortic ejection murmur along the sternal edge, and a mitral insufficiency murmur at the apex. A fourth heart sound is common. With increased sympathetic stimulation, the left ventricular outflow gradient, and hence the murmur, increase. A definitive diagnosis is made by echocardiography. The electrocardiogram usually shows left ventricular hypertrophy with septal hypertrophy, but the axis and prominent Q waves are often suggestive of prior infarction. Management includes use of beta-adrenergic blockers and calcium entry blockers to decrease the vigor of ventricular contraction as well as to manage tachyarrhythmias. Care must be taken to avoid volume depletion. Sympathomimetics should not be used. Careful hemodynamic monitoring during labor and delivery is indicated in symptomatic patients.

## ISCHEMIC CORONARY ARTERY DISEASE

The diagnosis of myocardial ischemia due to occlusive coronary artery disease is rarely made in women of childbearing age and is even less frequently made during pregnancy. Nonatherosclerotic causes, such as congenital malformations, Kawasaki disease, vasculitis, endocarditis, emboli, and coronary artery spasm as may occur with cocaine use, excessive levels of catecholamines, or bromocriptine used for postpartum suppression of lactation, predominate in young women.

However, the presence of risk factors for accelerated arteriosclerosis such as diabetes mellitus, hyperlipidemia, cigarette smoking, chronic hypertension, and a family history of premature coronary artery disease may combine with delayed childbearing to produce atherosclerotic coronary artery disease in even relatively young pregnant women. In addition, angina pectoris can occur in women with high-grade aortic stenosis, hypertrophic cardiomyopathy, thyrotoxicosis, profound anemia, and increased levels of circulating catecholamines. Myocardial ischemia or reversible ischemia, manifested by chest pain and transient electrocardiographic changes, may also occur during tocolytic therapy for premature labor and in a patient with high levels of circulating catecholamines.

The increases in myocardial oxygen consumption, heart rate, cardiac output, and total blood volume of pregnancy are poorly tolerated by patients with limited coronary artery reserve. Symptoms of ischemia occur at lower levels of exertion than in nonpregnant patients, especially as pregnancy advances. In patients with infarction during pregnancy, the outcome for both mother and fetus depends on the size of the infarct and the presence of complications. Risk to the mother and therefore to the fetus increases near term and especially with the stress of labor and delivery.

In addition to controlling precipitating or aggravating factors, the principles of management of angina pectoris and of myocardial infarction in pregnant women do not differ from those in nonpregnant patients. Patients with angina pectoris should be treated with restriction of activity, avoidance of stress (to reduce oxygen demand) and coronary vasodilators to improve oxygen supply. Nitrates, beta-adrenergic blocking drugs, and calcium channel antagonists should be given. Smoking should be forbidden and other risk factors meticulously controlled. Acute myocardial infarction can be a catastrophic event during pregnancy, especially near term when the hemodynamic load is maximal. Standard therapy to reduce oxygen demands and to improve myocardial perfusion include bed rest, oxygen by nasal canula, control of hypertension, treatment of hypotension, cautious afterload reduction, intravenous nitroglycerin or other coronary vasodilators, beta receptor antagonists for treatment of tachycardia, and, when indicated, thrombolysis and angioplasty. However, there is as yet no experience with use of thrombolytic agents in the acute phase of infarction in pregnancy. Women who have had a myocardial infarction before or during pregnancy should be delivered vaginally, if possible, with epidural anesthesia and outlet forceps to shorten the second stage of labor. Careful intrapartum hemodynamic monitoring may be indicated, especially if infarction has occurred in the third trimester.

## AORTIC DISSECTION

Aortic dissection is a rare catastrophic event that occurs occasionally during the third trimester of pregnancy or postpartum. It is rare in normotensive patients under age 40. However, chronic hypertension and the effects of estrogen and relaxin may cause degeneration of the arterial media and disruption of elastic tissue in the aorta thus contributing to the risk of dissection especially late in pregnancy. Aortic dissection is a much feared potential complication in patients with Marfan's syndrome, unoperated coarctation of the aorta, aortic aneurysm, Ehlers-Danlos syndrome, and myxomatous degeneration and dilatation of the ascending aorta or aortic root.

The diagnosis should be suspected in a woman who has a sudden cardiovascular catastrophe in the third trimester, typically with severe crushing or searing pain in the chest or back, pulmonary edema, neurologic symptoms, evidence of cardiac tamponade, acute aortic insufficiency, and shock. Diagnostic radiologic and echocardiographic studies should be initiated immediately. In patients with a proximal intimal tear (Type A), immediate operative intervention, occasionally with aortic valve replacement, can be lifesaving. In patients with more distal intimal tear (Type B), if aortic rupture is not imminent, medical treatment is indicated. This consists of rapid and sustained reduction of blood pressure with intravenous nitroprusside and reduction of the shearing forces on the aortic wall with beta-adrenergic blocking agents. The risk to the fetus is unavoidably high in either case.

Pregnant patients with Marfan's syndrome (a hereditary connective tissue disorder) are at an especially increased risk for aortic dissection. Because of the high risk, many obstetricians counsel these women not to become pregnant. However, in women without aortic root dilatation (less than 4 cm in diameter measured just above the aortic valve by echocardiography), the risk of aortic rupture or dissection is acceptably low.

## CONGENITAL HEART DISEASE

Patients with congenital heart disease are surviving to childbearing age in increasing numbers because of the early recognition and treatment of complications that develop in infancy and the availability of palliative and curative operative procedures. Congenital heart disease occurs in approximately 0.9% of liveborn infants in the USA. The prevalence in the population of bicuspid aortic valve, mitral valve prolapse, hypertrophic cardiomyopathy, and ventricular pre-excitation (Wolff-Parkinson-White syndrome)—all congenital lesions that usually do not become manifest until later in life—is unknown but may be as high as 2%. Congenital cardiac defects may occur as isolated lesions, as part of a syndrome, associated with other congenital anomalies, and possibly inherited as mendelian dominant or recessive characteristic. The common congenital cardiac anomalies can be broadly grouped under various categories such as cyanotic or acyanotic, simple or complex, mild or severe, compatible with a normal pregnancy or a contraindication for pregnancy. The following is a simplified classification:

**(1) Obstructive lesions of the right or left ventricular outflow tract** that result in pressure overload of the ventricle, such as pulmonary stenosis, aortic stenosis, hypertrophic subaortic stenosis, or coarctation of the aorta.

**(2) Left-to-right shunts** resulting in ventricular volume overload and increased pulmonary blood flow, such as atrial septal defect, AV canal, ventricular septal defect, or endocardial cushion defect, patent ductus arteriosus, and truncus arteriosus.

**(3) Cyanotic or hypoxic congenital heart disease** in which unoxygenated venous blood enters the systemic circulation, such as tetralogy of Fallot,

Eisenmenger's complex, tricuspid atresia, pulmonary atresia, single ventricle, transposition of the great arteries, and Ebstein's anomaly. Complex lesions may combine several of these features.

Operative procedures for correction or palliation are now available for almost all of these defects and are performed even in small infants. However, problems persist in most patients because of residual inoperable lesions, conduction defects, arrhythmias, irreversible pulmonary hypertension, valvular incompetence, ventricular failure, deterioration of prosthetic materials such as valves and conduits, and the need for anticoagulation (Table 22–7). Susceptibility to infective endocarditis persists in all patients except those with corrected uncomplicated secundum atrial septal defects, completely closed ventricular septal defects, and patent ductus arteriosus.

Patients with acyanotic congenital heart disease tolerate pregnancy well, whether the heart disease has been surgically corrected or not, and have a low incidence of spontaneous abortions and premature labor. Induced abortion is rarely indicated for cardiac causes in patients with class I or class II severity. However, patients with class III or class IV severity at the onset of pregnancy have a high incidence of spontaneous abortions and still births, and interruption of pregnancy or postponement until a corrective or palliative procedure can be performed for cardiac indications may be required. In patients with congestive heart failure or large intracardiac shunts, pregnancy is not well tolerated.

### Atrial Septal Defect

**Ostium secundum atrial septal defect,** one of the commonest forms of congenital heart disease, is well tolerated by most women, although secondary pulmonary hypertension and right ventricular failure can develop especially in women with large left-to-right shunts. The characteristic findings on physical examination include a right ventricular lift; a widely split and accentuated second heart sound that does not change with respiration; and a pulmonic systolic ejection murmur, usually considerably louder than the systolic murmur of normal pregnancy. A diastolic tricuspid rumble is often present with large shunts. The electrocardiogram shows an incomplete right bundle branch block and right-axis deviation. The presence, location, and size of the shunt can be identified by echocardiography and color flow Doppler studies. If significant pulmonary hypertension has developed, patients are characterized as having Eisenmenger's syndrome, and the risk of pregnancy rises steeply, (see later). Atrial arrhythmias are more likely to occur with advancing age. The risk of infectious endocarditis is low, and paradoxic emboli occur rarely.

Patients with **ostium primum atrial septum defects** (one end of the spectrum of atrioventricular canal defect), who have associated cleft mitral or tricuspid valves with insufficiency, tolerate pregnancy less well because of the increased risk of both left or right ventricular failure. If the mitral insufficiency is severe, a mitral prosthesis may have been previously implanted, raising the issue of anticoagulation for a mechanical valve and the risk of deterioration of a tissue valve. Due to the presence of mitral regurgitation, the risk for endocarditis is correspondingly higher, as is the risk for developing atrial arrhythmias. In ostium primum septal defect, the clinical findings include a right ventricular lift and often a left ventricular heave as well, a widely split second heart sound, and a pulmonic ejection murmur as well as the long pansystolic murmur of mitral insufficiency at the apex and occasionally of tricuspid insufficiency at the lower end of the sternum. The electrocardiogram is more likely to show left ventricular hypertrophy and, characteristically, left axis deviation, although the incomplete right bundle branch block may be present as well. The echocardiogram and color flow Doppler studies are used to define the location of the atrial septal and the degree of involvement of the mitral and tricuspid valves. Transesophageal echocardiography may be needed to evaluate a prosthetic valve.

### Ventricular Septal Defect

Isolated **ventricular septal defect,** although common in infancy, is seen less frequently among pregnant women because the ventricular septal defect tends to close spontaneously before the woman reaches adulthood. Women with small to moderate-sized ventricular septal defects tolerate pregnancy well, although they are at risk for developing secondary infectious endocarditis and heart failure. With large ventricular septal defects, the risk of secondary pulmonary hypertension (Eisenmenger's syndrome) increases progressively (see later). Ventricular septal defects are often associated with other intracardiac defects, but large, complicated ones are likely to have been surgically corrected before the age of puberty. Important late complications of ventricular septal defect, operated or unoperated, include ventricular arrhythmias and aortic valve insufficiency. The characteristic findings on examination include a palpable systolic thrill along the left sternal border and a loud pansystolic murmur best heard at the same location. There may be both a left and right ventricular heave or lift. When aortic insufficiency has developed, the presence of a systolic and diastolic murmur can be mistaken for a patent ductus arteriosus. Small ventricular septal defects, such as maladie de Roger may be very noisy but hemodynamically unimportant. The electrocardiogram may appear normal or show biventricular hypertrophy. The echocardiogram and Doppler studies readily identify the location and size of the defect, as well as associated lesions.

**Patent ductus arteriosus** is now rarely seen in adults because the condition is so readily diagnosed and in childhood. Small defects are well tolerated, al-

**Table 22–7.** Late problems to be anticipated in patients with common congenital heart defects.

| Defect | Prevalence[1] (Percent) | Surgical Repair | Late Complications |
|---|---|---|---|
| Tetralogy of Fallot | 5 | Blalock-Taussig, Waterston, or Potts extracardiac shunt, or complete intracardiac repair. | Residual right ventricular outflow obstruction; pulmonary valve insufficiency; conduction defects; right bundle branch block and complete heart block; arrhythmias; late sudden death; ventricular aneurysm; recurring ventricular septal defect; endocardial fibroelastosis. |
| Transposition of great vessels | 5 | Mustard or Senning intra-atrial baffle; redirection of venous inflow to ventricles or arterial switch with reimplantation of coronary arteries (Jatene). | Ventricular inflow or outflow obstruction; tricuspid valve insufficiency; decreased right ventricular function; arrhythmias; conduction defects; late sudden death; sinus node dysfunction; calcification, degeneration, or progressive proliferative fibrosis of synthetic or heterograft valves or conduits. Complete heart block, need for pacemaker revision. |
| Ebstein's anomaly | < 1 | Usually not surgically corrected, but occasionally right atrium to pulmonary artery conduit or tricuspid valve replacement with closure of atrial septal defect. | Right ventricular failure; right bundle branch block; recurring supraventricular tachycardia or atrial fibrillation; paradoxic embolization; sudden death; preexcitation (Wolff-Parkinson-White syndrome); intermittent cyanosis. |
| Atrial septal defect | 7 | Patch repair potentially "curative" for ostium secundum. Mitral valve replacement may be needed for ostium primum. | Atrial arrhythmias; persistent right ventricular enlargement; persistent or progressive pulmonary vascular hypertension; mitral valve prolapse and mitral regurgitation. Mitral regurgitation in ostium primum defect with cleft mitral valve. Tricuspid regurgitation. |
| Ventricular septal defect | 30 | Spontaneous closure common; patch repair potentially "curative." | Persistent or progressive pulmonary vascular disease with hypertension; conduction defects; heart block; aortic insufficiency; persistent or recurring ventricular septal defect; late sudden death; arrhythmias. |
| Patent ductus arteriosus | 9 | Ligation and division of ductus potentially "curative." | Persistent or progressive pulmonary vascular disease; associated unoperated intracardiac defects; recanalization of ductus; persistent left ventricular hypertrophy. |
| Aortic stenosis | 5 | Valvotomy or valve replacement. | Persistent or recurring stenosis; aortic insufficiency; conduction defects; left ventricular failure; calcification; degeneration, progressive proliferative fibrosis, thrombosis, or dehiscence of synthetic or heterograft valves. |
| Pulmonic stenosis | 7 | Valvotomy and infundibulectomy; rarely, valve replacement, balloon valvotomy | Persistent right ventricular outflow gradient; pulmonary valve insufficiency; atrial arrhythmias; right ventricular failure. |
| Coarctation of aorta | 6 | Segmental resection with reanastomosis with or without synthetic graft. | Persistent or recurrent gradient, bicuspid aortic valve with insufficiency; cerebral hemorrhage due to rupture of berry aneurysm; proximal aortic dissection or rupture, hypertension. |
| Complex cyanotic lesions, single ventricle, tricuspid or pulmonary atresia, etc. | | Various shunts from systemic venous to pulmonary circulation, Fontan, Glenn, Rastelli, etc. | Inadequate pulmonary perfusion, cyanosis, enlarging bronchial collaterals. |

[1]Prevalence in patients with common congenital heart defects.

though patients are at risk for endocarditis, but with large defects, the risk of secondary pulmonary hypertension with shunt reversal and left ventricular failure increases. Patients with a patent ductus characteristically have a palpable left ventricular heave, a loud pulmonic component of the second heart sound, and a systolic/diastolic murmur that is often described as a machinery murmur. However, as pulmonary hypertension develops, secondary to a large pulmonary flow, the duration and intensity of the diastolic component decrease. The electrocardiogram may be normal or show left ventricular hypertrophy, while the echocardiogram and Doppler studies identify the magnitude of the shunt and size of the ductus, as well as the degree of ventricular hypertrophy.

## Pulmonic Valve Stenosis

**Pulmonic valve stenosis** is another relatively common congenital cardiac lesion that is well tolerated if the gradient across the pulmonary valve is less than 80 mm Hg, since the valve continues to enlarge in relation to body mass. However, the added hemodynamic load of pregnancy can lead to right ventricular failure in patients with larger gradients. The stenosis can be at the valve, subvalvular, or occasionally supravalvular level. The characteristic physical findings include a right ventricular heave, often with a palpable thrill and a crescendo/decrescendo murmur best heard in the left second intercostal space, radiating to the left side of the neck, initiated by an ejection click, and ending before a delayed and diminished pulmonic component of the second heart sound. The electrocardiogram show increasing degrees of right ventricular hypertrophy depending on the magnitude of the shunt, which can be quantitated by echo/doppler. The risk of endocarditis is present, and antibiotic prophylaxis is recommended during delivery. In women with a high transvalvular gradient and right ventricular hypertrophy, the risk of right ventricular failure and atrial arrhythmias is increased, and assisted delivery is recommended. Although pulmonary valvotomy has been successfully carried out during pregnancy, this is rarely necessary. Patients who have previously undergone balloon or operative valvuloplasty often have resulting mild pulmonary valve insufficiency (a high-frequency decrescendo diastolic blow along the left sternal border); this is well tolerated.

## AORTIC VALVE DISEASE

Patients with left ventricular outflow obstruction, such as congenital **aortic stenosis,** tolerate pregnancy less well and are more likely to develop left ventricular failure with dyspnea, postexertion syncope, and angina resulting from decreased coronary reserve. They are also at high risk for developing infectious endocarditis. The increased afterload resulting from the hypertension of preeclampsia in poorly tolerated and can contribute to left ventricular failure. The incidence of congenital anomalies is the fetus is rela-

tively high. The physical findings include a diminished carotid pulse with delayed upstroke, a left ventricular heave with lateral displacement of the apex, often a diminished aortic component of the second heart sound, and a crescendo/decrescendo murmur, initiated by an ejection click radiating to the neck. The electrocardiogram is likely to show left ventricular hypertrophy and left atrial enlargement, and the echocardiogram/Doppler studies can define the magnitude of the transvalvular gradient, the degree of left ventricular hypertrophy, and adequacy of left ventricular function. Balloon valvuloplasty or even valve surgery is rarely necessary during pregnancy as an emergency measure. Eventually the need for valve replacement must be considered, raising the issue of the choice of valve and the need for anticoagulation and the risk of future pregnancies.

Patients with **bicuspid aortic valve** require no special management during pregnancy except for prophylaxis at the time of delivery, because of their susceptibility for developing infective endocarditis, which can lead to aortic insufficiency. The incidence of congenital bicuspid aortic valve in the population is estimated to be 2%. The murmur of a bicuspid aortic valve can be differentiated from the systolic murmur normally heard in pregnancy in that it is heard better to the right of the sternum in the second interspace, radiating to the right carotid artery, and is usually initiated by an ejection click well heard at the lower left sternal edge and apex.

**Aortic insufficiency** can be due to rheumatic heart disease, usually in association with mitral valve disease, as an isolated congenital lesion, or it can occur as a manifestation of a dilated aortic ring or myxomatous degeneration of the valve, as a complication of Marfan's syndrome. It may also result from infective endocarditis in a patient with underlying aortic valve disease or secondary to balloon or surgical commissurotomy of a stenotic valve or aortic dissection. In patients with acute infective endocarditis or aortic dissection and acute development of aortic insufficiency, left ventricular failure occurs rapidly and operation is often lifesaving. Chronic aortic insufficiency, however, is well tolerated in pregnancy, because of the reduced peripheral resistance and hence reduced afterload of pregnancy. However, antibiotic prophylaxis is recommended at the time of delivery. The characteristic clinical findings include a wide pulse pressure, sometimes with an elevated systolic pressure, readily collapsing peripheral pulses, prominent carotid arterial pulsations, a left ventricular heave and lateral displacement of the apex, and a high-frequency decrescendo diastolic murmur best heard along the left sternal edge with the patient sitting up and leaning forward. A short aortic systolic murmur is often present. The electrocardiogram is likely to show the voltage criteria for left ventricular hypertrophy, and the regurgitant volume and left ventricular size and function can readily be determined by echocardiogram/Doppler. The presence of early closure of the mitral valve on echocardiogram is a sign of acute massive regurgitation and imminent decompensation.

## Coarctation of the Aorta

**Coarctation of the aorta** results in hypertension of the arms with lower pressures in the legs. Pregnant patients are at increased risk for aortic dissection or rupture and congestive heart failure. The frequently associated bicuspid aortic valve increases the risk of infective endocarditis even in operated patients, and aneurysms in the circle of Willis may lead to subarachnoid hemorrhage, especially if the blood pressure rises during pregnancy. Up to 20% of patients with operated coarctation have some residual hypertension and left ventricular hypertrophy. The physical findings include elevated blood pressures in both arms, with diminished and delayed pulses in the lower extremities, bounding arterial pulsation in the neck, usually a systolic aortic murmur of a bicuspid aortic valve, and a characteristically late systolic murmur, which sounds extracardiac and is best heard in the left second intercostal space and between the scapulae in the back. Endocarditis prophylaxis is required for delivery, even in operated cases, and blood pressure control must be carefully maintained.

## Mitral Valve Prolapse

Prolapse of the leaflets of the mitral valve into the left atrium during systole is estimated to occur in 5–8% of young women. In some patients, this is due to valvuloventricular disproportion and superior displacement of the mitral valve, a benign variation of normal mitral valve architecture. At the other end of the spectrum are patients with a generalized connective tissue abnormality inherited as an autosomal dominant and characterized by myxomatous degeneration and attenuation of the valve and chordae tendineae, mitral and tricuspid valve insufficiency, dysautonomia, potentially fatal arrhythmias, and transient cerebral ischemic attacks possibly due to platelet emboli. Mitral valve prolapse may be associated with atrial septal defect, hypertrophic subaortic stenosis, Marfan's syndrome, or may result from papillary muscle infarction. A rare patient with mitral valve prolapse develops sudden rupture of the myxomatous chordae, resulting in acute mitral valve insufficiency and pulmonary edema. Urgent surgical therapy (eg, valve plication or replacement) may be required in these patients. Mitral valve prolapse is the usual cause of the nonrheumatic chronic mitral regurgitation that is seen in older patients.

The diagnosis is suspected on the basis of a characteristic body habitus (long tapered fingers; high, narrow, arched palate; pectus excavatum; scoliosis) and the presence of an apical late systolic murmur or one or more clicks. The diagnosis is confirmed by echocardiography. The auscultatory findings tend to disappear during pregnancy as the augmented cardiac output increases the left ventricular chamber size, resulting in maximal stretching of the mitral valve chordae throughout systole.

Symptoms of mitral valve prolapse are usually nonspecific, including palpitations due to atrial and ventricular ectopic beats and tachyarrhythmias, atypical nonanginal chest pain, vasomotor instability with postural hypotension, and, rarely, transient cerebral ischemic attacks. These symptoms also tend to diminish as pregnancy progresses.

Specific therapy is rarely necessary except for treatment of symptomatic tachyarrhythmias. Although patients with mitral valve prolapse are at increased risk for development of infective endocarditis, the routine use of prophylactic antibiotics, during uncomplicated vaginal delivery, is unnecessary, in patients who have only a click but no evidence of valvular insufficiency or valvular thickening.

## Cyanotic Congenital Heart Disease

In women with cyanotic congenital heart disease, both maternal and fetal morbidity and mortality rates are high. The incidence of spontaneous abortions, stillbirths, prematurity, and low birth weight is high. The incidence of congenital heart disease in the offspring is also high. Mothers with congenital heart disease are at particular risk for thromboembolic complications, brain abscess, syncope, and even sudden death.

## Tetralogy of Fallot

The commonest form of cyanotic congenital heart disease in adults is Tetralogy of Fallot, which consists of right ventricular outflow obstruction, right ventricular hypertrophy, large ventricular septal defect, and overriding aorta. The increased cardiac output and decreased peripheral resistance of pregnancy increase the right-to-left shunt and hence the degree of cyanosis, desaturation, and secondary polycythemia. These patients tolerate sudden hemodynamic changes (such as occur during labor, parturition, or with positional changes late in pregnancy) poorly and are also at high risk for infective endocarditis. Although spontaneous abortion and premature delivery of small babies are common in women with marked cyanosis, the fetal lungs are often more mature than expected for gestational age because they have adapted to chronic anoxia. In the past, various palliative operative procedures were performed in infants with tetralogy, which were designed to connect a systemic artery to the pulmonary artery, including the Blalock-Taussig, Potts, and Waterston shunts. These are rarely performed now, and most patients undergo a complete repair with closure of the ventricular septal defect and reconstruction of the right ventricular outflow tract. In uncorrected patients the physical findings include cyanosis; clubbing; a right ventricular heave; and loud, long harsh systolic murmur heard over the entire precordium and also over the back (representing bronchial anastomoses). Because of the pulmonary atresia or stenosis, the second heart sound has only an aortic component.

### Tricuspid Atresia, Pulmonary Atresia, and Transposition of the Great Arteries

**Tricuspid atresia, pulmonary atresia,** and **transposition of the great arteries** are other cyanotic congenital lesions for which various palliative or switch operations are now available in infancy. An increasing number of these infants are maturing to the child-bearing age. Decisions about the advisability of pregnancy must be made individually and depend on the degree of residual cyanosis and adequacy of pulmonary blood flow.

### Ebstein's anomaly

**Ebstein's anomaly** consists of downward displacement of the tricuspid valve, leading, in some cases, to obstruction of the right ventricular outflow. In milder forms, in the absence of an atrial septal defect, there is no cyanosis, only a flair septal leaflet of the tricuspid valve resulting in tricuspid insufficiency, and "atrialization" of a large part of the right ventricle. This form is generally well tolerated, except for the development of atrial arrhythmias, the frequent coexistence of an accessory bypass tract (Wolff-Parkinson-White syndrome) and atrioventricular conduction defects. The condition may be hereditary and the manifestations in the offspring more severe than in the mother. The physical findings include prominent jugular venous pulsations with a large V wave, a murmur of tricuspid insufficiency, and often an early diastolic sound from the motion of the displaced tricuspid leaflet.

### Pulmonary Hypertension

The common causes of pulmonary hypertension are as follows: (1) Increased resistance to pulmonary blood flow at any of several sites in the pulmonary vascular bed. This may be due to multiple pulmonary emboli, primary pulmonary vascular disease, Takayasu's arteritis, or infestation with schistosomes or filariae. (2) Increased pulmonary blood flow, as in left-to-right intra- or extracardiac shunts with the development of secondary pulmonary vascular disease. (3) Increased resistance to pulmonary venous drainage, as in increased left ventricular end-diastolic pressure, left ventricular failure, or mitral stenosis. (4) Pulmonary parenchymal disorders such as sarcoid or chronic fibrosis. (5) Hypoventilation syndromes. (6) Chronic hypoxia, as in high-altitude dwellers or heavy cigarette smokers.

Patients with large intracardiac left-to-right shunts eventually develop irreversible structural changes and obliterative pulmonary vascular disease in response to the increased pulmonary flow. In these persons, pressure in the right ventricle approaches systemic levels, and reversal of the shunt may occur, with resulting cyanosis (**Eisenmenger's syndrome**). The term **Eisenmenger's complex** is used specific-

ally for patients with a large ventricular septal defect and with pulmonary hypertension manifest at birth. These patients are considered inoperable because correction of the cardiac defect does not relieve the pulmonary hypertension and because there is a high rate of operative and postoperative mortality due to right ventricular failure. Patients in whom no cardiac or pulmonary cause for pulmonary hypertension is found are considered to have **primary pulmonary hypertension.**

In patients with pulmonary hypertension, either primary or secondary, the right ventricle tends to fail early in pregnancy because of the added hemodynamic load. Later in pregnancy, rapid hemodynamic changes such as postural hypotension (due to the fall in systemic vascular resistance) or decrease in venous return, result in a sudden decrease in cardiac output with syncope and decreased coronary perfusion, potentially deteriorating to ventricular fibrillation and death. The risk of spontaneous abortion is also high. These patients are at particularly high risk in the last trimester and during parturition.

Patients present clinically with increasing dyspnea, chest pain, edema, and, often, syncope. On physical examination patients they may be cyanotic at rest or with exercise, and have clubbed fingers and toes and a loud pulmonic component of the second heart sound. The murmur of the primary left-to-right shunt, if present, may be only faint due to reversal of flow through the defect. Because maternal mortality rates as high as 50% have been reported, patients with pulmonary hypertension should be counseled against becoming pregnant or should be advised to have an early induced abortion.

When pregnancy occurs and is continued, patients should avoid all unnecessary exertion, especially in the third trimester, when the risk of complications is highest. Prolonged bed rest, sodium restriction, digitalis, oxygen, maintenance of blood pressure, and close supervision in a hospital setting are mandatory. Close hemodynamic monitoring, meticulous avoidance of hypotension and volume depletion, and maintenance of adequate preload are important concerns in the management. Patients should be delivered vaginally under epidural anesthesia, with close and continued hemodynamic monitoring in an intensive care unit. Close observation must continue for at least 3–5 days postpartum, although complications and even death can occur as late as 2–3 weeks after delivery, as the normal postpartum hemodynamic changes occur.

### ARRHYTHMIAS

Rhythm disturbances are common in pregnancy, and most are well tolerated in the absence of underlying heart disease unless the ventricular rate is ≥ 180/min and the episodes are prolonged. In patients with heart disease, especially those with mitral stenosis and hypertrophic cardiomyopathy, tachycardia is poorly tolerated and can lead to rapid decompensation. Cardiac arrhythmias may also be the first manifestation of serious cardiac problems in patients in whom heart disease was not previously suspected. The diagnosis can be readily made with an electrocardiogram or, if intermittent, with a Holter monitor or event recorder. Life-threatening arrhythmias should be treated promptly with standard therapy. *Diagnosis and treatment of arrhythmias may require the attention of a skilled internist or cardiologist.*

## Sinus Tachycardia

Sinus tachycardia is a common finding in pregnancy. There is a 10–25% increase in heart rate during normal pregnancy and a greater increase during twin gestations. Conditions such as anxiety, pain, exercise, anemia, fever, and thyrotoxicosis further increase the heart rate. Treatment is usually not necessary other than that directed at underlying or complicating conditions.

## Premature Beats

Premature beats, both atrial and ventricular, are common in nonpregnant patients but appear to occur more frequently during pregnancy. Unless associated with underlying heart disease or tachyarrhythmias, treatment is generally not required. Digitalis or beta-adrenergic blocking agents may be effective in suppressing premature beats if the patient is particularly symptomatic or anxious.

## Atrial Arrhythmias

Atrial arrhythmias are common in young women, and during pregnancy there is increased atrial irritability. A wandering or shifting atrial pacemaker or accelerated junctional rhythm usually requires no specific intervention if the rate is under 100/min. More serious atrial arrhythmias such as supraventricular tachycardia (reentrant or from an ectopic focus), atrial fibrillation, and atrial flutter occur in patients with atrial septal defects, accessory bypass tracts as in Wolff-Parkinson-White syndrome, AV-node re-entrant tachycardia, and rheumatic heart disease. Profound hemodynamic alteration may result. Atrial arrhythmias are identified by electrocardiography and should be treated promptly. Maneuvers that stimulate the vagus nerve, such as carotid sinus massage or the Valsalva maneuver, should be tried first. If these are not effective, verapamil, 5 mg given intravenously (cautiously) over 1–5 minutes, is often effective in converting the rhythm to a sinus rhythm. This dose may be repeated. Because of the potential for hypotension with intravenous verapamil, intravenous adenosine, which has a very brief duration of action, has been used with increasing frequency. The initial dose is 6 mg given rapidly intravenously; rarely is repeat dose of 12 mg necessary. When given through a central venous line, a starting dose of 3 mg is recommended. Digoxin, 0.25 mg given orally or intravenously, may also be effective. DC cardioversion is re-

served for refractory cases. In patients with Wolff-Parkinson-White syndrome with atrial fibrillation and conduction over the bypass tract (broad complex rhythm), both digitalis and verapamil are contraindicated, and DC cardioversion may be required. Digitalis, quinidine, and verapamil have all been used to prevent recurring tachyarrhythmias. In patients with recurring, incapacitating episodes of supraventricular tachycardia, it is often possible to ablate the accessory bypass tract or intranodal reentry with radiofrequency waves delivered via a catheter. The electrophysiologic testing, however, requires fluoroscopy and hence is best deferred until after pregnancy, but can be performed in critical situations with careful abdominal and pelvic shielding.

## Ventricular Tachycardia

Ventricular tachycardia is a rare but usually serious tachyarrhythmia that results in rapid hemodynamic deterioration. Prompt recognition and specific therapy, including intravenous lidocaine or procainamide, and occasionally even DC cardioversion, are indicated; a cardiologist should be consulted. Procainamide, quinidine, disopyramide, and amiodarone have all been used to prevent recurring ventricular tachycardia, although they may all have pro-arrhythmic effects. Patients with congenital (Romano-Ward or Jervelle and Lange-Nielson syndromes) or acquired long QT syndrome are particularly prone to recurring attacks of syncope and sudden death because of a peculiar form of ventricular tachycardia known as **torsade de pointes.** These patients may be controlled with beta-adrenergic blocking drugs but may require an automatic implantable defibrillator. Ventricular tachycardia may be a late complication from scars in the myocardium such as occur in operated congenital heart disease, especially in patients with tetralogy of Fallot or right ventricular dysplasia. In some of these situations, ablation of the ectopic focus can be accomplished via a catheter electrode. An occasional patient may have a repetitive ventricular tachycardia (recurring short runs of 5–10 ventricular beats) in the absence of underlying heart disease. This is a relatively benign condition that does not require therapy unless the patient is frightened by the symptoms.

## Heart Block

**First-degree heart block** is a benign condition, diagnosed by the presence of diminished intensity of the first heart sound on physical examination and confirmed by electrocardiogram. It may, however, be associated with acute carditis. **Second-degree heart block** is classified as Mobitz type I or Mobitz type II block. Type I may indicate digitalis intoxication or increased vagal tone, whereas type II usually indicates serious underlying heart disease. Complete heart block may be congenital or acquired, especially after surgery for congenital heart disease. The diagnosis is suspected in the presence of a slow heart rate (30–40/min), cannon venous waves in the neck, and variable intensity of the first heart sound, and is confirmed by electrocardiography. In occasional patients, continuous electrocardiographic (Holter) monitoring is required if the heart block is intermittent. Decisions regarding the need for pacemaker insertion and maintenance should be referred to a cardiologist. Successful pregnancies have been reported in patients with implanted artificial pacemakers, and emergency implantation during pregnancy can be accomplished with echocardiographic guidance.

## CARDIOVASCULAR DRUGS IN PREGNANCY

Since many drugs cross the placenta, their use during pregnancy has potential for being teratogenic or directly harmful to the fetus. Table 22–8 lists the drugs most commonly used for the treatment of cardiac disease and their potential side effects. Several newer drugs have been used in pregnant women, including the calcium channel entry blockers and the antiarrhythmic drug amiodarone.

**Tocolytic agents,** including the sympathomimetic $\beta_2$ agonists, terbutaline, ritodrine, salbutamol, and fenoterol, are used as uterine relaxants in the treatment of premature labor. These are often given in conjunction with glucocorticoids such as betamethasone or dexamethasone, which accelerate maturation of fetal lungs. The use of sympathomimetics alone—but especially together with glucocorticoids given in large volumes of fluid—has resulted in pulmonary edema in a small percentage of women with normal hearts. Furthermore, although these drugs are primarily $\beta_2$ agonists, they do produce some $\beta_1$ stimulation, leading to increased heart rate, cardiac output, cardiac work, increase in systolic blood pressure, and decreased diastolic pressure and systemic vascular resistance. These drugs can also cause a rise in serum glucose, free fatty acids, and lactate, as well as a fall in serum potassium. Experience with the calcium-channel antagonists verapamil and nifedipine is growing, and these drugs also have cardiovascular effects. In patients with underlying heart disease, the likelihood of precipitating myocardial ischemia or pulmonary edema with the use of tocolytics is increased, especially in patients with aortic stenosis, hypertrophic subaortic stenosis, or mitral stenosis. Therefore tocolytics must be used with great caution in patients with underlying heart disease, especially in those conditions where tachycardia is not well tolerated.

## GENERAL MANAGEMENT OF HEART DISEASE IN PREGNANCY

General principles for management of patients with heart disease can be summarized as follows:

(1) Establish a diagnosis of heart disease, and assess the severity and functional status with appropriate noninvasive diagnostic studies that preferably do not involve ionizing radiation.

(2) Establish a method of regular follow-up, close surveillance, and consultation with a cardiologist and other supporting personnel.

(3) Reduce unnecessary cardiac work by ensuring regular rest and by avoidance of excess exertion, heat, and humidity.

(4) Make certain that the patient receives an adequate diet, avoids excessive weight gain, and complies with a regimen of moderate sodium restriction when indicated.

(5) Treat intercurrent infections, anemia, fevers, thyrotoxicosis, etc.

(6) Treat paroxysmal arrhythmias with appropriate drugs or DC cardioversion; prevent recurring arrhythmias with approved antiarrhythmic drugs.

(7) In patients with chronic atrial fibrillation, large left atrium, prosthetic valves, or recurring thromboembolism who require anticoagulant therapy, switch from oral anticoagulants with coumarin type drugs to subcutaneous heparin.

(8) Treat chronic venous insufficiency with well-fitting elasticized support hose.

(9) Treat congestive heart failure with bed rest, digitalis, and diuretics, and treat precipitating factors if recognized.

(10) Provide prophylaxis against infective endocarditis at the time of delivery.

(11) In women with compromised cardiac function, provide careful hemodynamic monitoring of both the mother and the fetus during labor and delivery and in the postpartum period. In patients with pulmonary hypertension, heart failure, or major arrhythmias, continue postpartum monitoring for 4–5 days to avoid late complications.

(12) To decrease the work of bearing down and associated pain and anxiety, provide caudal or epidural anesthesia for delivery and use outlet forceps to shorten the third stage of labor.

(13) Operative valvotomy or valve replacement is rarely necessary during pregnancy and may be forestalled with the less invasive technique of balloon valvotomy, but should be considered at any time during pregnancy (in consultation with a cardiologist and cardiac surgeon) if rapid deterioration occurs, if a prosthetic valve fails, or if an emergency complication develops.

Fetal echocardiography after 20 weeks of gestation is a useful technique for detecting fetal cardiac abnormalities, especially in women with congenital heart disease or prior offspring with anomalies. The finding of an abnormality can be helpful in planning perinatal management of the fetus, while the assurance of a normal offspring provides great peace of mind to a woman who has cardiac problems.

**Table 22–8.** Use of cardiovascular drugs in pregnancy.

| Drug | Maternal Indications | Maternal Complications | Fetal Complications |
|---|---|---|---|
| Beta-adrenergic blocking agents | Arrhythmias, thyrotoxicosis, hypertrophic cardiomyopathy, angina pectoris. Widely used for treatment of hypertension and mitral stenosis with tachycardia. | Bradycardia, asthma, congestive heart failure, hyperglycemia, and hypoglycemia (in insulin-dependent diabetics). | Fetal bradycardia, rarely heart block neonatal hypoglycemia, and hyperbilirubinemia. |
| Coumarin derivatives | Anticoagulant contraindicated in pregnancy because of teratogenic effects. | Hemorrhage. | Teratogenic: causes fetal warfarin syndrome. First trimester: nasal hypoplasia, chondrodysplasia punctata, brachydactyly. Second trimester: optic nerve atrophy, mental retardation, microcephaly. High incidence of spontaneous abortion, stillbirths, deformed offspring. Fetal hemorrhage. |
| Digoxin | Congestive heart failure, atrial fibrillation or flutter, paroxysmal atrial tachycardia. Prevention of atrial arrhythmias. | Avoid in patients with Wolff-Parkinson-White syndrome and atrial fibrillation. Obtain plasma levels for titration of dosage. Reduce dosage when given with verapamil or quinidine and postpartum. | Negligible. |
| Disopyramide | Ventricular arrhythmias. | Probably safe, although little experience reported. May be oxytocic and negative inotrope. | Probably safe. |
| Diuretics (oral) | Hypertension and congestive heart failure. Should not be started after 20 weeks gestation unless required for treatment of heart failure. May be continued in hypertensive patients if used before onset of pregnancy. | Hypercalcemia, hyperuricemia, hyperglycemia, hypokalemia, hyponatremia, hypotension, alkalosis may occur. | Rarely, fetal distress due to abrupt profound volume depletion and blood pressure reduction. Risk of neonatal hypoglycemia and hyperbilirubinemia. |
| Heparin | Anticoagulant of choice in patients with prosthetic valves, thromboembolic disease, or mitral stenosis with atrial fibrillation. | Hemorrhage. | Does not cross placenta. No teratogenic effects. Risks of premature labor, stillbirths, and hemorrhage during labor and delivery persist. |
| Phenytoin | Antiepileptic, antiarrhythmic. (Contraindicated in pregnancy because of teratogenic effects). | Drowsiness, gingival overgrowth, diplopia, ataxia. | Teratogenic: causes fetal hydantoin syndrome: intrauterine growth retardation, microcephaly, mental retardation, ptosis, depressed nasal bridge. |
| Procainamide | Ventricular arrhythmias. | May cause positive antinuclear antibody reaction and hypotension. Obtain plasma levels for titration of dosage. | Relatively safe. |
| Quinidine | Atrial or ventricular arrhythmias. | Hypotension and premature labor may occur. Obtain blood levels for titration of dosage. Potentially pro-arrhythmic, ie torsade de pointes. | Relatively safe. |
| Verapamil | Supraventricular tachycardias, hypertrophic cardiomyopathy, and hypertension. | Heartblock, hypotension, acceleration of rate in Wolff-Parkinson-White syndrome with atrial fibrillation. | No major abnormalities reported. |
| Nifedipine | Preterm labor and hypertension. | Headache, flushing, tachycardia, hypotension, edema. | None reported. |
| Amiodarone | Antiarrhythmic, atrial fibrillation, ventricular tachycardia. | Pulmonary fibrosis, hyper- or hypothyroidism. | Fetal or neonatal hypothyroidism. |
| Adenosine | Antiarrhythmic, supraventricular tachycardia. | Fleeting flush, hypotension. | None reported. |

## VARICOSE VEINS

Varicosities are particularly a problem of the multipara and may cause severe complications. They are caused by congenital weakness of the vascular walls, with superimposed increased venous stasis in the legs because of the hemodynamics of pregnancy, extensive collateral circulation in the pelvis, inactivity and poor muscle tone, and obesity.

The vulvar, vaginal, and even the inguinal veins may be markedly enlarged during pregnancy. Damaged vulvovaginal vessels give rise to hemorrhage at delivery. Large vulvar varices cause pudendal discomfort. A vulvar pad wrapped in plastic film, snugly held by a menstrual pad belt or T-binder, and elastic leotards are helpful.

Injection treatment of varicose veins during pregnancy is futile and hazardous. Varicose veins secondary to causes other than pregnancy, eg, deep vein thrombosis, congenital arteriovenous fistula, are difficult to control.

Vascular surgery can be performed during the first or second trimester, but vein stripping is best delayed until after the puerperium. In all other respects, management is the same as in nonpregnant women.

# HEMATOLOGIC DISORDERS

## ANEMIA

Anemia is a significant maternal problem during pregnancy. A hemoglobin of less than 11 g/dL or a hematocrit of less than 33% should be investigated and treated to avoid blood transfusion and its related complications. A pregnant woman will lose blood during delivery and the puerperium, and an anemic woman is therefore at increased jeopardy. During pregnancy, the blood volume increases by about 50% and the red blood cell mass by about 25%. This physiologic hydremia of pregnancy will lower the hematocrit but does not truly represent anemia.

Nutritional anemia is the most common form. It results from deficiency of iron, folic acid, or vitamin $B_{12}$. Pernicious anemia due to vitamin $B_{12}$ deficiency almost never occurs during pregnancy. Other anemias occurring during pregnancy are aplastic anemia and drug-induced hemolytic anemia.

## 1. IRON DEFICIENCY ANEMIA

Iron deficiency is responsible for about 95% of the anemias during pregnancy, reflecting the increased demands for iron. The total body iron consists mostly of (1) iron in hemoglobin (about 70% of total iron; about 1700 mg in a 56-kg woman) and (2) iron stored as ferritin and hemosiderin in reticuloendothelial cells in bone marrow, the spleen, and parenchymal cells of the liver (about 300 mg). Small amounts of iron exist in myoglobin, plasma, and various enzymes. Hemosiderin contains 37% more iron than does ferritin. Absence of hemosiderin in the bone marrow indicates that iron stores are exhausted. This is both diagnostic of anemia and one of the earliest signs of iron deficiency. This will be followed by a decrease in serum iron and an increase in serum total iron-binding capacity and anemia.

During the first half of pregnancy, iron requirements may not be increased significantly, and iron from food (10–15 mg/d) is sufficient to cover the basal loss of 1 mg/d. However, in the second half of pregnancy, iron requirements increase owing to expansion of red blood cell mass and rapid growth of the fetus. Increased numbers of red blood cells and a greater hemoglobin mass require about 500 mg of iron. The iron needs of the fetus average 300 mg. Thus, the total amount of iron necessary over the course of a normal pregnancy is approximately 800 mg; this cannot be supplied in the diet, and iron supplementation must be given. Data published by the Food and Nutrition Board of the National Academy of Sciences show that pregnancy increases a woman's iron requirements to approximately 3.5 mg/d. This need can be met by iron supplements exceeding 40 mg/d of elemental iron.

Iron deficiency anemia normally does not endanger the pregnancy unless it is severe, in which case intrauterine growth retardation and preterm labor may result.

### Clinical Findings

**A. Symptoms and Signs:** The symptoms may be vague and nonspecific, including pallor, easy fatigability, palpitations, tachycardia, and dyspnea. Angular stomatitis, glossitis, and koilonychia may be present in long-standing severe anemia.

**B. Laboratory Findings:** The hemoglobin may fall as low as 3 g/dL, but the red cell count is rarely below 2.5 million/L. The red cells are usually microcytic, with mean corpuscular volumes of less than 79 fL, and hypochromic. The reticulocyte count is low for the degree of anemia. Platelet counts are frequently increased, but white cell counts are normal. Occasional hypersegmented neutrophils are seen. Serum iron levels are usually less than 60 μg/dL. The total iron-binding capacity is elevated to 350–500 μ/dL, transferrin saturation is less than 16%, and the serum ferritin concentration is less than 10 μg/dL. The amount of stainable iron (hemosiderin) in the marrow aspirate is a reasonably accurate indication of stored iron.

## Differential Diagnosis

Anemia due to chronic disease or an inflammatory process (eg, rheumatoid arthritis) may be hypochromic and microcytic. A similar type of anemia in thalassemia trait can be differentiated from iron deficiency anemia by normal serum iron levels, the presence of stainable iron in the marrow, and elevated levels of hemoglobin $A_2$.

## Complications

Angina pectoris or congestive heart failure may develop as a result of marked iron deficiency anemia. **Sideropenic dysphagia (Paterson-Kelly syndrome, Plummer-Vinson syndrome)** due to long-standing severe iron deficiency anemia is rare in women of child-bearing age.

## Prevention

During the course of pregnancy and the puerperium, at least 60 mg/d of elemental iron should be prescribed to prevent anemia.

## Treatment

In an established case of anemia, prompt adequate treatment is necessary.

**A. Oral Iron Therapy:** Ferrous sulfate, 300 mg containing 60 mg of elemental iron of which about 10% is absorbed), should be given 3 times a day. If this is not tolerated, ferrous fumarate or gluconate should be prescribed. Therapy should be continued for about 3 months after hemoglobin values return to normal in order to replenish iron stores. Hemoglobin levels should increase by at least 0.3 g/dL/wk if the patient is responding to therapy.

**B. Parenteral Iron Therapy:** The indication for parenteral iron is intolerance of or refractoriness to oral iron. In most cases of moderate iron deficiency anemia, the total iron requirements equal the amount of iron needed to restore hemoglobin levels to normal or near normal plus 50% of that amount to replenish iron stores.

Imferon is a mixture of ferric hydroxide in a 0.9% sodium chloride solution for injection. It contains the equivalent of 50 mg/mL of elemental iron as an iron dextran complex. Imferon may be given intramuscularly or intravenously. Intramuscular injection must always be given into the muscle mass of the upper outer quadrant of the buttock with a 2-inch, 20-gauge needle, using the **Z technique** (ie, pulling the skin and superficial musculature to one side before inserting the needle to prevent leakage of the solution and subsequent tattooing of the skin). A test dose of 0.5 mL is administered and the patient watched carefully for anaphylactic reactions. After an hour or longer, 2.5 mL of dextran is given in each buttock for a total of 5 mL (total dose of 250 mg of elemental iron). This should be repeated every week until the total dosage has been given. Imferon may also be given intravenously after testing for anaphylaxis has been done with 0.5 mL of dextran. Excessive dosage must be avoided to prevent hemosiderosis.

## 2. FOLIC ACID DEFICIENCY ANEMIA (Megaloblastic Anemia of Pregnancy)

Megaloblastic anemia of pregnancy is caused by folic acid deficiency and is common where nutrition is inadequate. Based on bone marrow studies, the incidence is 25–60%, depending upon the population studied; peripheral blood examination shows a much lower incidence. The incidence of folate deficiency in the USA is 0.5–15%, depending on the population studied and the diagnostic methods used.

The minimum daily intake of folate necessary to maintain stores and adequate hematopoiesis is 50 μg. This is increased during pregnancy (National Academy of Sciences recommendation) to 800 μg. Folic acid deficiency anemia is more common in multiple pregnancy and in multigravid patients. It may recur in subsequent pregnancies.

Folic acid absorption or metabolism may be impaired during use of oral contraceptives, pyrimethamine, trimethoprim-sulfamethoxazole, primidone, phenytoin, or barbiturates. Jejunal bypass surgery for obesity or the malabsorption syndrome (sprue) may also impair folic acid absorption. Folic acid is necessary for the DNA synthesis of erythropoiesis; thus, sickle cell anemia, a chronic hemolytic state, requires increased folate. Other hemolytic states are also commonly complicated by folic acid deficiency, including hereditary spherocytosis and malarial infestation. Alcohol consumption has been known to interfere with folate metabolism.

Megaloblastic anemia should be suspected if iron deficiency anemia fails to respond to iron therapy. Diagnosis of folic acid deficiency anemia is usually made late in pregnancy or in the puerperium. Low birth weight as well as fetal neural tube defects are known to be associated with maternal folic acid deficiency; however, an association with placental abruption, spontaneous abortion, and preeclampsia-eclampsia is not universally accepted.

## Clinical Findings

**A. Symptoms and Signs:** The symptoms are nonspecific (eg, lassitude, anorexia, nausea and vomiting, diarrhea, and depression). Pallor often is not marked. Rarely, a sore mouth or tongue may be present. An accompanying urinary tract infection is common. Occasionally, purpura may be a clinical manifestation.

**B. Laboratory Findings:** Folic acid deficiency results in a hematologic picture similar to that of true pernicious anemia (due to vitamin $B_{12}$ deficiency), which is extremely rare in women of child-bearing age. Indeed, megaloblastic anemia in pregnancy almost always implies folate deficiency. The hemoglobin may be as low as 4–6 g/ dL, and the red cell count may be less than 2 million/μL in severe cases. Extreme anemia often is associated with leukocytopenia and thrombocytopenia. The red cells are macrocytic (mean corpuscular volume usually > 100 fL), and megaloblastic changes are present in the marrow. However, in pregnancy, macrocytosis may be concealed by accompanying iron deficiency or thalassemia. Serum folate levels of less than 4 ng/mL are suggestive of folic acid depletion in nonpregnant patients, but in otherwise normal pregnant patients, folate tends to fall slowly to low levels (3–6 ng/ mL) with advancing gestation. The red cell folate level in megaloblastic patients is lower, but in 30% of patients the values overlap. The peripheral white blood cells are hypersegmented. Seventy-five percent of folate-deficient patients have more than 5% of neutrophils with 5 or more lobes, but this may also be true for 25% of normal pregnant patients.

Urinary excretion of formiminoglutamic acid (Figlu) has been used to diagnose folate deficiency, but levels are abnormal only in severe megaloblastic anemia. Bone marrow aspirate will be helpful in the diagnosis, as well as a positive hematologic response to folate. Serum iron and vitamin $B_{12}$ levels should be normal.

### Treatment

Folic acid, 1–5 mg/d orally or parenterally, continued for several weeks after delivery or for several weeks in patients diagnosed in the puerperium, produces the maximum hematologic response, replaces body stores, and provides the minimum daily requirements. The hematocrit should rise about 1% each day beginning at day 5–6 of therapy. The reticulocyte count should elevated after 3–4 days of therapy and is the earliest morphologic sign of remission. Iron should be administered orally or parenterally as indicated.

### Prognosis

Megaloblastic anemia due to folate deficiency during pregnancy carries a good prognosis if adequately treated. The anemia is usually mild unless associated with multifetal pregnancy, systemic infection, or hemolytic disease (eg, sickle cell anemia). The disorder usually disappears after delivery and is likely to recur only when the patient becomes pregnant again. For complete hematologic response during pregnancy, both folic acid and iron must be given because 70% of folate-deficient patients also lack iron stores.

### 3. APLASTIC ANEMIA

Aplastic anemia with primary bone marrow failure during pregnancy is fortunately rare. The anemia may be secondary to exposure to known marrow toxins such as chloramphenicol, phenylbutazone, mephenytoin, alkylating chemotherapeutic agents, and insecticides. In most cases, no obvious cause is detected. Idiopathic aplastic anemia in pregnancy may have a spontaneous remission following delivery but may recur in subsequent pregnancies. This suggests that the cause is a disorder of the immune mechanism.

### Clinical Findings

The rapidly developing anemia causes pallor, fatigue, tachycardia, painful ulceration of the throat, and fever. The diagnostic criteria are pancytopenia and empty bone marrow on biopsy examination. Patients with aplastic anemia are at increased risk for infection and hemorrhage.

### Complications

Aplastic anemia in pregnancy may cause increased fetal wastage, prematurity, intrauterine fetal demise, and increased maternal morbidity and death.

### Treatment

The patient must avoid any toxic agents known to cause aplastic anemia. Prednisolone should be given, 10–20 mg 4 times daily. A transfusion of packed red blood cells and platelets may be needed. In some cases, termination of pregnancy may be necessary. Bone marrow transplantation is performed if remission does not occur following delivery or termination of pregnancy. Infection must be treated aggressively with appropriate antibiotics, but most authorities do not recommend giving prophylactic antibiotics.

### 4. DRUG-INDUCED HEMOLYTIC ANEMIA

Drug-induced hemolytic anemia often occurs in individuals with inborn errors of metabolism. In the USA, blacks are frequently affected. Glucose-6-phosphate dehydrogenase (G6PD) deficiency in erythrocytes is the most common cause, but catalase and glutathione deficiency may also be associated with this disorder. The traits are X-linked. About 12% of black males and 3% of black females are affected.

### Clinical Findings

There is decreased G6PD activity in one-third of patients in the third trimester, causing an increased risk of hemolytic episodes. About two-thirds of pregnant patients with this disorder will have a hematocrit of less than 30%. Urinary tract infections are more common in these patients; use of sulfonamides will precipitate hemolysis. Overexposure of the G6PD-deficient fetus to maternally ingested oxidant drugs (eg, sulfonamides) may produce fetal hemolysis, hydrops fetalis, and fetal death. A black pregnant woman should probably be screened for G6PD deficiency before starting sulfonamide therapy for urinary tract infection.

The red blood cell count and morphology are normal until challenged by noxious drugs. Over 40 substances toxic to susceptible people are recognized, including sulfonamides, nitrofurans, antipyretics, some analgesics, sulfones, vitamin K analogues, uncooked fava beans, some antimalarials, naphthalene, and nalidixic acid.

Specific laboratory tests to identify susceptible individuals include a glutathione stability test and cresyl blue dye reduction test.

## Treatment

Management includes immediate discontinuation of any suspected medications, treatment of intercurrent illness, and blood transfusion where indicated.

## SICKLE CELL DISEASE

Sickle cell disease is a genetic disorder almost always occurring in blacks. It is characterized by an abnormal hemoglobin molecule, hemoglobin S, which causes red blood cells to become sickle-shaped. Sickle cell hemoglobin results from a genetic substitution of valine for glutamic acid in the sixth position from the N-terminal end of beta chains. The autosomal recessive sickle cell gene is passed to both sexes. Patients homozygous for the hemoglobin S gene have **sickle cell anemia,** and those who are heterozygous have **sickle cell trait**. About 10% of blacks in the USA carry sickle cell trait, and 1 in 500 has sickle cell anemia. Women who are heterozygous for both the S and C genes have **hemoglobin S/C disease;** maternal mortality rates are as high as 2–3%. Hemoglobin S/C disease is peculiarly associated with embolization of necrotic fat and cellular bone marrow with resultant respiratory insufficiency. Neurologic symptoms from fat embolism have also been reported with sickle cell disease. In **hemoglobin S/beta thalassemia disease,** the patient is heterozygous for both hemoglobin S and beta thalassemia; the severity of complications during pregnancy is related to hemoglobin S concentrations in this particular trait.

Prenatal genetic counseling is of great importance. If both partners have the gene for S hemoglobin, their offspring have a 1 in 4 chance of having sickle cell anemia. Restrictive nuclease techniques using DNA isolated from amniotic fluid cells are most useful for prenatal diagnosis of hemoglobinopathy in cases at risk.

## Clinical Findings

Sickle cell disease is characterized by chronic hemolytic anemia and intermittent crises of variable frequency and severity. While persons with sickle cell trait are not anemic and are usually asymptomatic, they have twice as many urinary tract infections as normal women. Additionally, their red blood cells tend to sickle when oxygen tension is significantly lowered; thus, hypoventilation during general anesthesia may be fatal.

**A. Symptoms and Signs:**

**1. Chronic anemia**–Chronic anemia results from the shortened survival time of the homozygous S red blood cells due to circulation trauma and intravascular hemolysis or phagocytosis by reticuloendothelial cells in the spleen and liver.

**2. Sickling of red blood cells**–Intravascular sickling leads to vaso-occlusion and infarction. Small blood vessels supplying various organs and tissues can be partially or completely blocked by sickled erythrocytes, resulting in ischemia, pain, necrosis, and organ damage.

**3. Crises**–Crises of variable frequency and severity occur. **Pain crises** involve the bones and joints. These are usually precipitated by dehydration, acidosis, or infection. An **aplastic crisis** is characterized by rapidly developing anemia. The hemoglobin is 2–3 g/dL due to cessation of red blood cell production. An **acute splenic sequestration** crisis is associated with severe anemia and hypovolemic shock, resulting from sudden massive trapping of red blood cells within the splenic sinusoids.

**4. Other manifestations**–Other manifestations include increased susceptibility to bacterial infection; bacterial pneumonia, segmental bronchopneumonia, and pulmonary infarction; myocardial damage and cardiomegaly; and functional and anatomic renal abnormalities in the form of sickle cell nephropathy or papillary renal necrosis, resulting in hematuria. Central nervous system manifestations include headache, convulsions, hemorrhage, or thrombosis (from vaso-occlusion). Ophthalmologic abnormalities include anoxic retinal damage, retinal detachments, vitreous hemorrhages, and proliferative retinopathy. Hepatosplenomegaly or cholelithiasis may also occur.

**B. Laboratory Findings:** Sickle cell anemia is associated with high risks for mother and fetus. Screening for abnormal hemoglobin is imperative in the population at risk. Two screening tests are in common use. The sodium metabisulfite test uses 1 drop of fresh 2% reagent mixed on a slide with 1 drop of blood. Sickling of most red cells will occur in a few minutes with both sickle cell trait and sickle cell disease. The Sickledex test is a simple solubility test that uses 20 µL of blood mixed with 2 mL of sodium dithionite reagent. Clouding of the solution indicates the presence of hemoglobin S. If the test is positive, the homozygous and heterozygous states must be differentiated by hemoglobin electrophoresis.

**C. Effects on Pregnancy:** Pregnancy has deleterious effects on sickle cell disease. There are increased rates of maternal mortality and morbidity from hemolytic and folic acid deficiency anemias, frequent crises, pulmonary complications, congestive heart failure, infection, and preeclampsia-eclampsia. It is encouraging, however, that the maternal mortality has decreased to 1% since 1972 as reported by

Powers and colleagues. There is an increased incidence of early fetal wastage, stillbirth, preterm delivery, and intrauterine growth retardation.

## Treatment

Good prenatal care, avoidance of complications, and prompt effective treatment for complications are necessary for a good outcome of pregnancy. Folic acid, 1 mg/d, will prevent megaloblastic anemia. Ultrasonic evaluations adequately assess fetal growth, but biophysical monitoring is necessary for antepartum fetal surveillance. Adequate pain relief must be given during labor. Close intrapartum electronic monitoring of labor is indicated. Prevent hypoxia during general anesthesia by maintaining adequate oxygenation and ventilation. Cesarean section should be done at the earliest sign of fetal compromise for the best perinatal outcome.

In the management of crises, predisposing factors should be searched for and eliminated, if possible. Symptomatic treatment for pain crisis consists of intravenous fluid and adequate analgesics (eg, meperidine or codeine). Bacterial pneumonia or pyelonephritis must be treated rigorously with blood culture and intravenous antibiotics. Streptococcal pneumonia is common and is an ominous complication. Pneumococcal polyvalent vaccine has been shown to reduce the incidence of pneumoncoccal infection in adults with sickle disease, and therefore it is highly recommended. This vaccine is not contraindicated in pregnancy. In all cases, adequate oxygenation must be maintained by face mask as necessary.

The concentration of hemoglobin S should be less than 50% of the total hemoglobin to prevent crisis. Blood transfusion should be considered in cases of a fall in hematocrit to less than 25%; repeated crisis; symptoms of tachycardia, palpitation, dyspnea, or fatigue; or evidence of inadequate or retarded intrauterine growth.

The immediate risk of transfusion (eg, congestive cardiac failure) must be avoided. Prophylactic hypertransfusion or exchange transfusion to prevent maternal complications, improve uteroplacental perfusion, and achieve a better perinatal outcome has been advocated by some, but these methods are not universally accepted. Transfusion always carries a risk of allergic reaction, delayed hemolytic reaction with rapid fall in hemoglobin A, and transmission of hepatitis virus or the AIDS virus. Isoimmunization may also occur. The antibodies most commonly found are Rh, Kell, Duffy, and Kidd; all pregnant patients with sickle cell trait or disease should be tested for these antigens plus ABO type. Hemolytic disease of the newborn or transfusion reactions due to improper cross-matching of blood may occur if careful blood typing is not done. The use of fresh buffy coat-poor washed packed cells for exchange transfusion will help in avoiding transfusion reactions. (See also Chapter 15.) Inducing of nonsickling red blood cells

(RBC) from bone marrow has been considered. The use of erythropoietin was found to increase production of hemoglobin F in baboons, however, it stimulated hemoglobin S production in humans. Hemoglobin F synthesis by stimulating Y-Chain production appears to be a promising forum of therapy for the sickle cell disease and thalassemia syndrome. Y-chains of hemoglobin F inhibit polymoriration of hemoglobin S and therefore inhibit sickling. Recombinant erythropoietin and hydroxyurea have been used together recently with elevation of hemoglobin F. More recently intravenous arginine butyrate has been used with the increase in fetal globin synthesis, production of F reticulocytes, and the level of Y-globin. Bone marrow transplant has been limited by the complication of infection and graft versus host disease. Prenatal diagnosis of sickle cell disease might encourage in utero stem cell therapy with normal hemoglobin stem cells.

Sterilization should be considered if maternal complications are too threatening. Oral contraceptives are avoided because of the risk of thromboembolism.

## THALASSEMIA

The thalassemias are genetically determined disorders of reduced synthesis of one or more of the structurally normal globin chains in hemoglobin. Thalassemia is found throughout the world but is concentrated in the Mediterranean coastal areas, central Africa, and parts of Asia. The high incidence in these regions may represent a balanced polymorphism due to heterozygous advantage.

All thalassemias are inherited as an autosomal recessive trait. The 2 major groups are the alpha and beta thalassemias, both of which affect the synthesis of hemoglobin A, which contains 2 alpha and 2 beta chains. The severity of the anemia varies with the type of hemoglobin abnormality. In beta thalassemia, the beta hemoglobin chains are defective, but the alpha chains are normal; in alpha thalassemia, the reverse is true. The unbalanced synthesis results in precipitation of the normal chains. If the beta chains are impaired, the alpha chains are produced at a normal rate but in relative excess. The alpha chains then form tetrameres that precipitate within red blood cell precursors in the bone marrow, resulting in ineffective erythropoiesis, red cell sequestration and destruction, and hypochromic anemia. The most severe forms of this disorder may cause intrauterine or childhood death. A person who is heterozygous, or a carrier, for a thalassemia trait may be asymptomatic.

The most severe form of alpha thalassemia compatible with extrauterine life is **hemoglobin H (beta4) disease,** which results from deletion of 3 genes. In patients with this disease, abnormal quantities of both hemoglobin H and hemoglobin Barts accumulate. In **alpha thalassemia minor,** 2 genes are deleted, causing a mild hypochromic, microcytic anemia that must be differentiated from iron deficiency anemia.

In beta thalassemia, no gene deletions have been demonstrated. There are 2 forms of beta thalassemia, beta$^+$ and beta$^0$, depending on whether beta chain production is reduced or entirely absent. **Beta thalassemia major** is the homozygous state, in which there is little or no production of beta chains. **Beta thalassemia minor,** the heterozygous state, is frequently diagnosed only after the patient fails to respond to iron therapy or delivers a baby with homozygous disease. Such patients usually suffer from hypochromic microcytic anemia, with increased red blood cell count, elevated hemoglobin A2 concentrations, increased serum iron levels, and iron saturation greater than 20%.

The fetus is protected from severe disease because fetal hemoglobin (alpha22) contains no beta globin chain. However, this protection disappears at birth, when fetal hemoglobin production terminates. At about 1 year of age, a baby with defective beta globin production usually begins to show signs of thalassemia (anemia, hepatosplenomegaly) and requires frequent blood transfusions. Victims of severe thalassemia often die in their late teens or early twenties because of congestive heart failure, often related to myocardial hemosiderosis, liver failure, or diabetes mellitus. During pregnancy, iron supplementation should be given only following assessment of iron stores to prevent hemosiderosis. Suspected cases of thalassemia must be diagnosed by means of hemoglobin electrophoresis.

Antenatal diagnosis of thalassemia is now possible. A technique known as molecular hybridization measures the number of intact alpha globin structural genes in fetal cells obtained by amniocentesis. In antepartum diagnosis of beta thalassemia, hemoglobin A is measured in fetal blood obtained via fetoscopy or sonographically directed placental aspiration of fetal blood.

## LEUKEMIA & LYMPHOMA

Leukemia is a neoplastic process affecting the leukopoietic tissues of the body. Acute leukemia has a short and fulminant clinical course, whereas chronic leukemia may have a prolonged course lasting several years. Depending upon the type of leukocyte affected, leukemia may be lymphatic, myeloid, or monocytic. Lymphomas result from proliferation of cells of the lymphoreticular system. Two types are known: **Hodgkin's disease** and **non-Hodgkin's lymphoma.** Fortunately, these diseases are uncommon in pregnancy. The peak incidence of chronic lymphocytic leukemia and non-Hodgkin's lymphoma occurs after childbearing age, so the association of pregnancy with these diseases is extremely rare.

### Clinical Findings

Pregnancy does not affect the course of these diseases, but several complications should be anticipated. Chemotherapy may cause fetal death or malformation or intrauterine growth retardation. The teratogenic and mutagenic effects of ionizing radiation in the first trimester have long been known. More than 10 rads of irradiation to the pelvis during the first trimester in Hodgkin's disease can have deleterious effects on the fetus. The carcinogenic potential and alteration in intelligence and behavior in fetuses exposed to chemotherapy and radiation in utero are uncertain. Intrauterine growth retardation and preterm labor, both iatrogenic and spontaneous, are not uncommon in maternal leukemia. Perinatal mortality rates are increased considerably. Several cases of possible transfer of leukemia and Hodgkin's disease to offspring have been reported.

Splenomegaly, a common manifestation, may cause abdominal discomfort. Severe anemia may cause marked weakness and heart failure. The patient may need multiple blood transfusions. Thrombocytopenia may lead to bruising of the skin and bleeding from the mucous membranes, necessitating platelet transfusion. Postpartum hemorrhage occurs in about 20% of cases. In acute leukemia, severe infection with organisms of usually low virulence is common. Patients with Hodgkin's disease may have complications of irradiation, including pneumonitis causing restrictive lung disease, pericarditis leading to congestive heart failure, various neurologic symptoms, nephritis and ovarian failure. The risk of a second cancer is substantially increased in patients with Hodgkin's disease. The risk for leukemia has been reported to have increased almost 100-fold if chemotherapy has been given.

### Treatment

Management is difficult. Therapy must be individualized if pregnancy is allowed to continue. The obstetrician and a hematologic oncologist should work together. Treatment will require chemotherapy, correction of anemia, and prevention of, or aggressive therapy for, infection. Induced abortion should be considered if chemotherapy is given early in pregnancy.

Effective agents in acute leukemia include prednisone, vincristine, asparaginase, daunorubicin, doxorubicin, mercaptopurine, methotrexate, cyclophosphamide, and cytarabine. Major drugs for chronic leukemia include busulfan, hydroxyurea, and cyclophosphamide. Although chemotherapy entails a risk to the fetus, it often cannot be deferred. In acute leukemia, the median maternal survival rate is only 2.5 months without chemotherapy.

Termination of pregnancy does not seem to affect the course of Hodgkin's disease or the length of survival. Interruption of the pregnancy is recommended if irradiation or chemotherapy is given early in pregnancy. However, neither chemotherapy during second and third trimesters nor irradiation to the mediastinum and neck appeared to affect adversely the fetus or neonate. The chemotherapeutic agents normally used in Hodgkin's disease include mechlorethamine, vincristine, procarbazine, and prednisone. If local radiation therapy to the liver, spleen, or lymph nodes is indicated, the uterus should be shielded. Agents used in non-Hodgkin's lymphoma include cyclophosphamide, doxorubicin, vincristine, and prednisone.

Fetal status should be monitored with periodic ultrasonic examination and biophysical monitoring. Delivery should be accomplished when fetal lung maturation is evident on amniotic fluid phospholipid study, and, ideally, the mother is in complete remission.

### Prognosis

The prognosis of pregnant patients with these disorders is not significantly different from that for nonpregnant patients. However, since 85% of relapses in Hodgkin's disease occur within 2 years, it is generally accepted that pregnancy should be deferred for 2 years following remission.

The newborn should be carefully evaluated periodically to note any immediate or delayed toxic effects of maternal chemotherapy.

## HEMORRHAGIC DISORDERS

Although hemorrhagic disorders (eg, immune thrombocytopenic purpura, disseminated intravascular coagulation, circulating anticoagulants) are not common during pregnancy, these conditions could cause significant risks for both mother and fetus.

### Immune Thrombocytopenic Purpura

In immune thrombocytopenic purpura, platelet destruction is secondary to a circulating IgG antibody that crosses the placenta and may also affect fetal platelets. The maternal clinical picture varies from asymptomatic to minor bruises or petechiae, bleeding from mucosal sites, or fatal intracranial bleeding. There may be splenomegaly. The marrow aspirate demonstrates hyperplasia of megakaryocytes. In the peripheral circulation, the platelet count will be 80,000–160,000/$\mu$L.

Maternal morbidity and mortality rates are low, but the perinatal mortality rate is around 20%, mostly related to intracranial bleeding. Differences of opinion exist regarding antepartum and intrapartum management of the pregnant woman. Steroids should be given. In refractory cases, splenectomy should be performed in the second trimester, if possible. Immunosuppressive agents should be used with great caution and only in extraordinary cases of immune thrombocytopenic purpura in pregnancy. Transfusion of platelets and whole blood may be necessary to restore losses from acute hemorrhage or to normalize low perioperative platelet counts (<50,000 mL). More recently, maternal infusion of gamma globulin during pregnancy has been used in an attempt to block placental transfer of maternal IgG.

Fifty percent of thrombocytopenic mothers have babies with low platelet counts during the first week of neonatal life. Maternal levels of circulating IgG correlate well with the presence of neonatal thrombocytopenia.

Intrapartum management includes avoidance of traumatic vaginal delivery and maternal soft tissue injury. However, delivery by cesarean section is not universally accepted. Fetal scalp blood sampling done as soon as possible during labor will determine the fetal platelet count. If the count is below 50,000/$\mu$L, cesarean section should be performed to avoid fetal birth trauma that may cause intracranial bleeding.

### Circulating Anticoagulants

Circulating anticoagulants, mainly inhibitors of factor VIII, an IgG immunoglobulin, can cause minor to severe bleeding from various sites. Bleeding may be spontaneous or due to trauma, surgery, or, sometimes, delivery. Treatment may include exchange transfusion with replacement of specific factors or use of corticosteroids or immunosuppressive agents.

## THROMBOEMBOLIZATION

Thromboembolization denotes all vascular occlusive processes, including thrombophlebitis, phlebothrombosis, septic pelvic thrombophlebitis, and embolization of venous clots to the lungs. The incidence of thromboembolism is 0.2% in the antepartum period and 0.6% in the postpartum period. Cesarean section increases the incidence to 1–2%. Pulmonary embolism, with a mortality rate of 15%, occurs in 50% of patients with documented deep vein thromboses; only 5–10% of these are symptomatic. Early diagnosis and adequate treatment drastically reduce the incidence of pulmonary embolism and death.

### Pathophysiology

Vascular clotting develops mainly due to circulatory stasis, infection, vascular damage, or increased coagulability of blood. All the elements of **Virchow's triad** (circulatory stasis, vascular damage, and hypercoagulability of blood) are present during pregnancy. Increase in caliber of capacitance vessels produces vascular stasis, and blood hypercoagulibility is due to increased amounts of factors VII, VIII, and X. Thrombin-mediated fibrin generation is increased many times during pregnancy. Significant vascular damage occurs during delivery. Venous return from the lower extremities is reduced by the pressure of the gravid uterus on both the iliac veins and the inferior vena cava. Other important predisposing factors include heavy cigarette smoking, obesity, previous thromboembolism, anemia, hemorrhage, heart disease, hypertensive disorders, prolonged labor, operative delivery, and postpartum endomyometritis.

The venous thrombi may develop first in the relatively small veins of the calf muscle and extend proximally as far as the femoral or iliac veins or, rarely, even into the inferior vena cava. Another common site of postpartum thrombosis is the pelvic veins due to diminished blood flow in the hypertrophied uterine veins. Thrombi may extend into the iliac veins and may produce pelvic venous thrombosis. Fatal pulmonary embolism may follow. Septic emboli are usually from the uterine, ovarian, or iliac veins. Partial liquefaction of the infected thrombus allows showers of bacteria-laden emboli. Although the lungs are almost always involved, secondary abscesses may occur in the brain or the heart, or a mycotic aneurysm may develop in one of the great vessels.

**Phlebothrombosis** is coagulation of blood in the veins without apparent antecedent inflammation. The clot is usually loosely adherent and causes incomplete occlusion. When thrombosis of a vein is secondary to inflammation of the wall of the vein, the condition is known as **thrombophlebitis.** This pathologic difference has little significance so far as the management is concerned because both disorders can cause pulmonary embolism. Superficial thrombophlebitis is the most common venous thrombosis associated with pregnancy. It usually occurs in varicose veins in the calf and is most frequent after delivery. Deep vein thrombophlebitis may be a sequela of the superficial form; this is an ominous condition. It is more common during the third trimester and the first few days of the puerperium.

## Clinical Findings

**A. Symptoms and Signs:** Superficial thrombophlebitis is suspected when an erythematous tender, firm cordlike superficial vein is palpated. Clinical diagnosis of deep vein thrombophlebitis is neither sensitive nor specific; the false-positive rate is as high as 50%. Most deep vein thrombi are completely asymptomatic. Symptoms may be subtle or classic depending upon the site and extent of the thrombus and the status of the collateral venous circulation. Classic features include swelling of the affected site of the legs, pain, tenderness, local cyanosis, and fever. These features are common if the proximal veins are involved. Pain in the calf muscle with dorsiflexion of the foot on the affected leg **(Homans' sign)** has little value in diagnosis. Moreover, embolic risk cannot be correlated with the severity of the pain. Most patients with pulmonary emboli do not have prior evidence of ve-

nous thrombosis. Iliofemoral venous thrombophlebitis causes acute swelling in the leg, pain above the hip, tenderness over the femoral triangle, and vaginal bleeding.

**B. Diagnostic Studies:** Ideally, the diagnosis should be objectively confirmed prior to initiation of treatment. Objective tests may be noninvasive (eg, doppler ultrasound) or invasive (eg, venography). There are limitations to both the performance and interpretation of the objective tests, eg, an antepartum venogram exposes the fetus to radiation. The safest method of diagnosing venous thrombosis in pregnancy is use of impedance plethysmography, doppler ultrasonography, and limited venography.

**1. Impedance plethysmography**–Impedance plethysmography measures the volume changes within the veins of the leg. Thrombotic and nonthrombotic occlusions cannot be differentiated by this method. The pressure by the gravid uterus on the common iliac vein or inferior vena cava (particularly after 20 weeks' gestation) can produce false-positive results. A normal result excludes proximal venous thrombosis but does not exclude calf vein thrombosis.

**2. Directional doppler ultrasound**–Directional doppler ultrasound can detect the presence or absence of venous flow. Damping of pulsatile flow is consistent with nonocclusive thrombus. This test is also insensitive to calf vein thrombosis and could be influenced by the pressure of the gravid uterus on the pelvic veins. Real-time sonography coupled with duplex and color Doppler ultrasound have been found to be useful in the diagnosis of deep venous thrombosis of the lower extremities, but its role in the evaluation of pelvic vein thrombosis is less clear. During pregnancy thrombosis frequently originates in the iliac veins. Magnetic resonance imaging allows for excellent delineation of anatomical detail above the inguinal ligaments, and phase images can be used to diagnose the presence or absence of flow in the pelvic veins. Computed tomographic scanning requires contrast agent and ionizing radiation, which is therefore avoided in favor of magnetic resonance imaging.

**3. Venography**–Venography allows the entire lower extremity, including the external and common iliac veins, to be evaluated. It is the most definitive method for diagnosis of venous thrombosis. Unfortunately, 1–2% of patients develop clinically significant phlebitis following venography. This risk can be minimized by flushing the dye with saline and elevating the legs. If the pelvic veins are not well visualized by ascending venography, femoral venography should be done. The abdomen must be shielded during venography.

**4. $^{125}$I-fibrinogen scanning**–$^{125}$I-fibrinogen will be absorbed by the thrombus following intravenous injection. A hand-held probe is placed over the affected area. Unbound $^{125}$I-fibrinogen scanning is contraindicated during pregnancy and breast-feeding.

Leg scanning should not be used when proximal vein thrombosis (iliac or femoral vein) is suspected.

## Prevention

The indications for preventive therapy include previous documented deep vein thrombosis or pulmonary embolism or antithrombin III deficiency. Heparin is the drug of choice; give 5000–7500 units subcutaneously twice a day during the first and second trimesters. Around the beginning of the third trimester, increase the dosage by approximately one-third to provide additional anticoagulation for the increased coagulation factors in late pregnancy. Prophylaxis should be stopped with the onset of labor and started again following delivery and continued for at least 2 weeks.

## Treatment

**A. Superficial Venous Thrombophlebitis:** Treatment of superficial venous thrombophlebitis consists of elevation of the involved leg and local application of moist heat. In resistant cases in nonpregnant patients, nonsteroidal anti inflammatory agents (eg, phenylbutazone) may be used, but these should be avoided in pregnant women because they may cause premature closure of the ductus arteriosus in the fetus. In high-risk patients with varicose veins, custom-made support panty hose should be worn.

**B. Deep Vein Thrombosis:**
**1. Heparin–**Heparin is the drug of choice. It is a naturally occurring, negatively charged polysaccharide with an average molecular weight of 16,000 found in the mast cells of most mammals. It is effective intravenously or subcutaneously. It exerts its anticoagulant effect in the presence of a plasma cofactor, antithrombin III. The activity of antithrombin III is markedly increased by heparin.

Heparin may be given by continuous intravenous infusion; an initial loading dose of 5000 units is followed by 25,000–30,000 units given over a 24-hour period. Heparin may also be given subcutaneously, 15,000 units twice daily. With intermittent intravenous infusion, 5000 units is given every 4 hours. For prevention of postoperative thrombosis, 5000 units of heparin is given subcutaneously 2 hours before surgery; this dose should be repeated 12 hours after operation and then twice daily until the patient is ambulatory. The anticoagulant action of heparin occurs within 10–15 minutes of injection, but the effect disappears in about 2 hours.

Tests used to monitor heparin therapy include coagulation time, activated partial thromboplastin time, thrombin clotting time, and heparin assay. Heparin should not be given if the platelet count is below $50,000/\mu L$. The partial thromboplastin time should be 1.5–2 times the control value during heparin therapy.

The major side effect is bleeding in about 5% of cases. Other complications include thrombocytopenia, osteoporosis, and fat necrosis. Protamine sulfate is the antidote for heparin. Protamine, 1 mg per 100 units of heparin, will quickly shorten the partial thromboplastin time. Care must be taken not to give too much protamine, since it can induce bleeding.

**2. Oral anticoagulants–**Oral anticoagulants such as warfarin, a coumarin derivative, are usually contraindicated during pregnancy and breast-feeding. The teratogenic effects of warfarin (warfarin embryopathy) include nasal hypoplasia, skeletal abnormalities, and multiple central nervous system abnormalities. Fetal and placental bleeding leading to intrauterine fetal demise has been described with the use of warfarin. Its therapeutic effect depends on its ability to inhibit the action of vitamin K. The usual dose of warfarin is 10–15 mg/d until the therapeutic level of prothrombin time is achieved (1.5–2.5 times the control value). Thereafter, a maintenance dose is given based on prothrombin time, which should be checked twice daily. Vitamin $K_{1/}$ (phytonadione), 5 mg given intravenously, is the specific antidote for warfarin.

## SEPTIC PELVIC THROMBOPHLEBITIS

Septic pelvic thrombophlebitis is clotting in the veins of the pelvis due to infection. This may occur following vaginal or cesarean delivery. Predisposing factors include cesarean section after a long labor, premature rupture of the membranes, difficult delivery, anemia, malnourishment, and systemic disease. Septic pelvic thrombophlebitis occurs in 1 in 2000 deliveries. The pathologic process involves bacterial invasion of the intimal lining of the veins. The clotting process is initiated by the damaged intima, and the clot is invaded by microorganisms. Suppuration follows, with liquefaction, fragmentation, and, finally, septic embolization. Thirty to 40% of untreated patients will have septic pulmonary emboli.

### Clinical Findings

Both the uterine and ovarian veins are involved, as well as the common iliac, hypogastric, and vaginal veins and the inferior vena cava. The ovarian vein is the most common site (40% of cases). The onset may be as early as 2–3 days postpartum or as late as 6 weeks following delivery. The condition is suspected when fever persists in the puerperium in spite of adequate antibiotic therapy for aerobic and anaerobic organisms and there is no other discernible cause of fever. A picket-fence fever curve with wide swings from normal to as high as 41 °C (105.8 °F) is seen in 90% of cases. The pulse rate is rapid and sustained in most cases. The respiratory rate is increased, but there is no indication of pulmonary disease. There are no typical x-ray signs, because the emboli are small, multiple, and infected, but around 46% of cases show some x-ray abnormality due to abscess or infarct. The pelvic examination may be normal; however, hard, tender, wormlike thrombosed veins are palpable in the vaginal fornices or in one or both parametrial areas in about 30% of cases. Abdominal examination may occasionally reveal thrombosed ovarian veins. A temperature spike may be noted following examination because of disturbance of infected pelvic veins; this may be considered one diagnostic indication. Resolution of fever with heparin anticoagulation will help in the presumptive diagnosis. Blood for culture should be drawn during fever spikes; cultures are positive more than 35% of the time.

### Differential Diagnosis

The differential diagnosis includes pyelonephritis, meningitis, systemic lupus erythematosus, tuberculosis, malaria, typhoid, sickle cell crisis, appendicitis, and torsion of the adnexa.

### Treatment

Heparin and broad-spectrum antibiotics should be given (eg, penicillin and gentamicin with clindamycin or metronidazole; ampicillin may be added to clindamycin and gentamicin to cover enterococci). Within 48–72 hours of initiation of heparin therapy, fever should resolve. Heparin should be continued for 7–10 days.

Surgery is indicated in the following cases: (1) medical management fails, (2) septic emboli occur during therapy, (3) the patient is admitted to the hospital with puerperal sepsis and pulmonary infarction. Ligation of the major venous tributaries from the pelvis is performed (ie, the vena caval or ovarian veins). Such aggressive management will lower the maternal mortality rate to less than 10%. Ligation of the veins should not have significant side effects; resultant pedal edema should resolve within 6 weeks. Ovarian function and fertility usually are not affected. Collateral circulations between the vertebral azygos vein and the portal system veins will be established; this will prevent any complications related to ligation of the pelvic veins.

# PULMONARY DISORDERS

## ASPIRATION PNEUMONITIS

Aspiration of gastric contents is the commonest cause of maternal death due to anesthetic complications. With superimposed infection, mortality rates are even higher. In 1946, Curtis Mendelson showed that 96% of 66 cases of aspiration involved acidic gastric contents. The primary causative factor in aspiration pneumonitis is the acidity of the aspirate; a pH less than 2.5 is required to produce clinical manifestations.

Predisposing factors for aspiration include recent ingestion of food, delayed gastric emptying, relaxation of the gastroesophageal sphincter, raised intragastric pressure, use of general anesthesia, and a less experienced anesthesiologist.

### Clinical Findings

The pathologic mechanism and clinical manifestations of aspiration pneumonitis will depend upon the volume and composition of the aspirate. Aspiration of solid particulate matter may occlude parts of the tracheobronchial tree, causing collapse of the lungs. Aspiration of liquid material will produce cyanosis, tachycardia, dyspnea, and expiratory wheezing. The patient will be hypoxic, hypercapnic, and acidotic. The chest x-ray reveals interstitial pulmonary edema. With aspiration of acidic material, such a clinical picture may be delayed.

### Prevention

If one consider the high rate of maternal death associated with aspiration pneumonitis, every effort should be made to prevent this catastrophic condition. Oral intake during labor must be prohibited. All anesthetized obstetric patients should be intubated, and regional anesthesia should be used as often as possible during labor and delivery. Any method that effectively reduces the volume of gastric contents to less than 25 mL or raises the gastric pH to more than 2.5 reduces the risk. Antacids must be given for resorption and buffering of acids and to inhibit further gastric acid production. Thirty milliliters of nonparticulate systemic alkalizer, a mixture of sodium citrate and citric acid, effectively neutralizes gastric acidity. It should be given every 3 hours and 1 hour prior to elective cesarean section. The physician administering a regional block should also have expertise in intubation and ventilation.

### Treatment

If aspiration occurs during anesthesia, immediate intubation and suction of the trachea should be carried out, followed at once by ventilation with oxygen. The patient should be turned onto her right side. Bronchoscopic suction should be done as soon as possible if solid material has been aspirated. A chest x-ray should be taken and blood gas determinations made; these may be repeated periodically. Arterial oxygenation is improved by decreasing the intrapulmonary shunt, and ventilation-perfusion inequalities are improved with positive end-expiratory pressure, which expands collapsed and fluid-filled airways, thereby increasing the functional residual capacity. If the gastric fluid sample has a pH of less than 3.0, the patient should be treated with endotracheal intubation, sedatives, muscle relaxants, and ventilation. If the gastric fluid pH is more than 3.0

and the patient appears to be well oxygenated, she may be followed carefully with periodic chest x-rays and blood gas determinations. The use of corticosteroids and prophylactic broad-spectrum antibiotics is debatable. Gram-stained smears and cultures of the tracheal aspirate should be taken daily, and antibiotics should be given when clinical evidence and culture indicate bacterial pneumonitis.

## BRONCHIAL ASTHMA

Asthma is obstructive disease of the large or small airways. It may reverse spontaneously or may require treatment. It is the most common form of obstructive lung disease in pregnancy (0.4–1.3% of pregnancies). Fortunately, severe asthma (status asthmaticus, persistent or recurring asthma) occurs in only a few pregnancies.

### Etiology
Based on the etiology, there are several types of asthma.

**A. Extrinsic Asthma:** Extrinsic asthma is IgE-mediated. The symptoms of bronchospasm are triggered shortly after inhalation of a specific allergen (eg, ragweed pollen).

**B. Intrinsic Asthma:** Intrinsic asthma occurs when no specific allergens can be detected.

**C. Mixed Asthma:** Mixed asthma occurs when both IgE-mediated and non-IgE-mediated factors are present.

**D. Aspirin-Intolerant Asthma:** Aspirin-intolerant asthma occurs when aspirin and other nonsteroidal anti inflammatory drugs inhibit prostaglandin synthesis, thereby precipitating bronchospasm.

**E. Exercise-Induced Asthma:** Asthma induced by exercise occurs when patients who are asymptomatic develop bronchospasm soon after a period of exercise.

**F. Occupational Asthma:** Persons exposed to allergens on the job may develop occupational asthma.

The course of asthma in pregnancy is unpredictable; disease may improve, remain the same, or worsen. Increased circulating free cortisol, decreased bronchomotor tone and airway resistance, and increased serum levels of cyclic AMP could each be responsible for the improvement of asthma in pregnancy. Exposure to fetal antigens, alterations in cell-mediated immunity (with an increase in viral upper respiratory tract infections), and hyperventilation could precipitate or worsen bronchospasm. In a study of more than 1000 pregnant asthmatics, 48% had no change, 29% improved, and 23% deteriorated. A patient with severe asthma before pregnancy tends to become worse during pregnancy. The changes in the course of asthma that women attribute to pregnancy generally revert toward the pregnancy course

in the 3 months postpartum. It is also interesting to note that the similar course in a particular patient during a pregnancy tends to repeat in her future pregnancy. Upper respiratory tract infection appears to be the most common precipation factor of severe asthma during pregnancy.

Mild asthma imposes little, if any, risk to the mother and fetus. Severe asthma is associated with increased perinatal mortality and morbidity rates related to hypoxemia, alkalosis, reduced uterine blood flow, and teratogenic effects of drugs used for treatment. A slightly increased incidence of prematurity and low birth weight has been suggested in severe cases of asthma, but the cause-and-effect relationship is not clear.

### Complications
Acute complications include physical exhaustion, progressive hypoxemia or hypercarbia, atelectasis, pneumothorax, pneumomediastinum, pulsus paradoxus, and drug hypersensitivity reactions. Chronic complications are pulmonary emphysema and cor pulmonale.

### Treatment
**A. General Measures:** The general principles of management for pregnant asthmatic patients are similar to those for nonpregnant patients. The following steps should be taken:

1. Prevent exposure to known allergens.
2. Treat sinusitis.
3. Avoid antiprostaglandin drugs (eg, aspirin) in aspirin-intolerant asthma.
4. Avoid strenuous exercise and exposure to cold.
5. Treat viral infections rigorously.
6. Treat reflux esophagitis to avoid induction of bronchospasm.
7. Stop cigarette smoking.
8. Give a prophylactic short course of prednisone, 30-50 mg/d for 4–7 days, at the onset of a viral upper respiratory tract infection. This often prevents the need for emergency management of asthma.

**B. Status Asthmaticus or Severe Attacks of Asthma:** The patient must be hospitalized. Oxygen may be administered by mask or nasal catheter. Correction of dehydration and electrolyte imbalance is achieved by adequate intravenous fluids. Blood gas determinations are mandatory. Aminophylline, 0.25–0.5 g in 30 mL of saline, is given slowly intravenously and followed with continuous intravenous infusion of 0.9 mg/kg/h. Hydrocortisone sodium succinate or equivalent, 100–200 mg, is given intravenously every 2–4 hours as necessary. If the patient fails to improve clinically with the previous measures and there is evidence of progressive hypoxemia and hypercapnia, intubation and controlled ventilatory assistance may be required.

**C. Mild or Moderate Attacks of Asthma:** Epinephrine injection (1:1000), 0.2–0.5 mL given subcutaneously, will often stop the attack. For moderately severe attacks, it may be repeated every 1–2 hours. Inhalation of epinephrine or isoproterenol (1/200 in aqueous solution) or use of a nebulizer, 1 or 2 inhalations every 30–60 minutes as necessary, may suffice for mild attacks. If the attack is not controlled by epinephrine or isoproterenol, give aminophylline, 0.25–0.5 g in 10–20 mL of saline slowly intravenously. Aminophylline may also be given rectally in solution or as a suppository. Epinephrine (sulfate or hydrochloride), 25–50 mg orally 2–3 times daily, may relieve mild attacks. Oral theophylline is also useful. Phenobarbital, 30 mg orally 3–4 times a day, may be used to counteract overstimulation by bronchodilator drugs. Heavy sedation must be avoided.

**D. Interim Therapy:** The main drugs used in long-term management of asthma include methyl xanthines, beta-adrenergic agonists, glucocorticoids, and cromolyn sodium. The methylxanthines, anhydrous theophylline and aminophylline, are widely used drugs. Beta-adrenergic agonists such as terbutaline can be used for asthma uncontrolled with chronic theophylline. If wheezing persists despite these medications and other explanations are not likely, a short course of prednisone may be indicated to reverse ongoing asthma. Cromolyn sodium or beclomethasone dipropionate by inhalation or terbutaline inhalation may be instituted to supplement theophylline once the acute episode has resolved.

Medication should generally be added one by one until adequate control is achieved. It is important to maintain a high index of suspicion for bacterial respiratory infections during pregnancy, particularly for bacterial sinusitis, which has been estimated to be six times more common during pregnancy.

Allergic immunotherapy is effective for allergic rhinitis and possibly for allergic asthma. It may be continued during pregnancy, but caution should be exercised to reduce the risk of anaphylaxis.

Cough preparations with iodides and dextromethorphan should be avoided because of the risks of fetal goiter and malformation, respectively. Antihistamines should be avoided during the first trimester. Pseudoephedrine decongestants can be used when necessary.

**E. Management of Labor and Delivery:** Vaginal delivery is best for asthmatic patients unless obstetric indications demand cesarean section. During normal labor, minute ventilation can approach or exceed 20 L/min; therefore, the therapeutic goal should be stable pulmonary function without bronchospasm. For patients who have received systemic or inhaled corticosteroids during pregnancy, hydrocortisone, 100 mg intravenously, is given immediately and every 8 hours until delivery has occurred. Paracervical, pudendal, or epidural block is preferable to general anesthesia. Meperidine, 50–100 mg given intramuscularly, usually will relieve bronchospasm while providing adequate pain relief.

## TUBERCULOSIS

Tuberculosis in adults is a disease of the pulmonary parenchyma caused by *Mycobacterium tuberculosis,* a nonmotile, acid-fast aerobic rod. Foci of infection are usually widespread, with dissemination occurring early in the course of disease, before sites are walled off by granulomatous inflammation. In the early 1900s, tuberculosis was the leading cause of death in the USA (200 deaths per 100,000 persons per year). As therapy has steadily improved, the incidence of disease progressively declined until recently when the disease made a startling comeback in the underprivileged.

### Clinical Findings

Most cases of tuberculosis (77%) can be diagnosed on the basis of a history of cough and weight loss, positive tuberculin skin test, and chest x-ray.

**A. Symptoms and Signs:** Typical symptoms include cough, weight loss, fatigue, and anorexia. Occasionally, patients are asymptomatic.

**B. Laboratory Findings:** Laboratory studies are needed for definitive diagnosis. Ziehl-Neelsen staining should be performed. *M tuberculosis* can be distinguished from other organisms by culture (production of niacin in vitro).

**C. Tuberculin Skin Test:** The tuberculin skin test is the most important screening test for tuberculosis. It should be performed early in pregnancy, especially in high-risk populations. The test is positive with induration at the test site of 10 mm or more.

**D. Chest X-Ray:** Chest x-ray is not done routinely in pregnancy because of risk to the fetus. With the abdomen shielded, a chest x-ray should be taken in patients in whom skin testing is positive following an earlier negative test and in patients with a suggestive history or physical examination even though skin testing is negative.

**E. Congenital Tuberculosis:** Congenital tuberculosis is rare. The criteria for diagnosis include positive bacteriologic studies, primary disease complex in the liver, disease occurring within the first few days of life, and exclusion of extrauterine infection. The most common signs are nonspecific, including fever, failure to thrive, lymphadenopathy, hepatomegaly, and splenomegaly. Disease is usually miliary or disseminated. Effective treatment depends on early diagnosis.

### Treatment

**A. Medical Therapy:** Treatment of active tuberculosis during pregnancy is only slightly different from that in nonpregnant patients. A year-long course of isoniazid is given to those with a positive skin test and no radiologic or symptomatic evidence of active disease. Such therapy perhaps could be withheld during pregnancy and started in the postpartum period, although most studies have shown no teratogenic effects of isoniazid. Immigrants and refugees who have received bacillus Calmette-Guaaerin (BCG) vaccine for prevention of tuberculosis still need chemoprophylaxis if the skin test is positive.

Active tuberculosis should be treated with a 2-drug regimen, usually isoniazid, 5 mg/kg/d (total of 300 mg/d), and ethambutol, 15 mg/kg/d, continued for at least 18 months to prevent relapse. Two-drug regimens are not recommended if isoniazid resistance is suspected. If a third drug or a more potent drug is necessary due to extensive or severe disease, rifampin could be added. Because of the risk of ototoxicity, streptomycin should not be used. Isoniazid has many therapeutic advantages (eg, high efficacy, patient acceptability, and low cost) and appears to be the safest drug during pregnancy.

The major side effects of isoniazid are hepatitis, hypersensitivity reactions, peripheral neuropathy, and gastrointestinal distress. A baseline liver function test should be obtained and then repeated periodically. *Pyridoxine, 50 mg/d, should be administered to prevent isoniazid-induced neuritis due to vitamin $B_6$ deficiency.* Optic neuritis has been the rare complication described with use of ethambutol. Rifampin may cause hepatitis, hypersensitivity reactions, occasional hematologic toxicity, a flulike syndrome, abdominal pain, acute renal failure, and thrombocytopenia. The role of rifampin in congenital malformations is not clear. Limb reduction defect in the neonate has been suspected, but the number of pregnancies studied is too small for any conclusions to be drawn.

**B. Obstetric Management:** Routine antepartum obstetric management includes adequate rest, nutritious diet, family support, correction of anemia, and appropriate follow-up.

Immediate neonatal contact is allowed if the mother has received treatment for inactive disease and there is no evidence of reactivation. In cases of inactive disease for which prophylactic isoniazid was not given or of active disease for which adequate treatment was given, early neonatal contact may be allowed, provided the mother is reliable in continuing therapy. A mother with active disease should receive at least 3 weeks of treatment before coming into contact with her baby, and the baby must also receive prophylactic isoniazid.

There are no absolute contraindications to breastfeeding once the mother is noninfectious. Although antituberculosis drugs are found in breast milk, the concentrations are so low that the risk of toxicity in the infant is minimal. However, each case should be judged individually if the mother wishes to breastfeed her infant.

Immunization of the newborn with BCG vaccine remains controversial. If prompt use of isoniazid as prophylaxis is unlikely or if the mother has isoniazid-resistant disease, BCG vaccination of the infant should be considered.

## Prognosis

If the pregnant patient is adequately treated with antitubercular chemotherapy for active disease, tuberculosis generally has no deleterious effect on the course of pregnancy or the puerperium or on the fetus. Pregnant women have the same prognosis as nonpregnant women. Therapeutic abortion is no longer recommended for most tuberculosis patients.

# RENAL & URINARY TRACT DISORDERS

For a discussion of renal and urinary tract function in normal pregnancy, see Chapter 7.

## URINARY TRACT INFECTION

Asymptomatic bacteriuria, acute cystitis, and acute pyelonephritis are common renal disorders in pregnancy.

### Asymptomatic Bacteriuria

Asymptomatic bacteriuria is defined as the presence of actively multiplying bacteria in the urinary tract excluding the distal urethra in a patient without any obvious symptoms. The incidence during pregnancy is 2–7%. Asymptomatic bacteriuria is twice as common in pregnant women with sickle cell trait and 3 times as common in pregnant women with diabetes as in normal pregnant women. If asymptomatic bacteriuria is untreated in pregnancy, about 25–30% of women will develop acute pyelonephritis. With treatment, the rate is only 10%. The diagnosis of asymptomatic bacteriuria is based upon isolation of microorganisms with a colony count of more than $10^5$ organisms per milliliter of urine in 2 consecutive clean-catch specimens. The patient should be instructed to clean the vulvar area from front to back to avoid contamination of the urine sample. *Escherichia coli* is the most common offending organism for asymptomatic bacteriuria (about 80% of cases). The *Klebsiella-Enterobacter-Serratia* family and Proteus family are responsible for the remainder of cases. Acute cystitis is rare in pregnancy (about 1%).

### Acute Cystitis

The bacterial flora in acute cystitis are similar to those in asymptomatic bacteriuria. Clinically, the patient will present with symptoms of urinary frequency, urgency, dysuria, and suprapubic discomfort. An acute febrile illness with nausea, vomiting, and chills is usually absent. The characteristic cloudy, malodorous urine should be cultured for confirmation of the diagnosis.

## Acute Pyelonephritis

Acute pyelonephritis occurs in 1–2% of all pregnant women (usually, although not invariably, in those with previous asymptomatic bacteriuria) and is associated with risk to the mother and fetus. Maternal effects include fever, bacterial endotoxemia, endotoxic shock, renal dysfunction leading to acute renal failure, leukocytosis, thrombocytopenia, and elevated fibrin split products. There is an increased incidence of anemia; this may be due to marrow suppression, increased erythrocyte destruction, or diminished red cell production. More recently, pulmonary dysfunction has been described in association with acute pyelonephritis; symptoms and signs may range from minimal (mild cough and slight pulmonary infiltrate) to severe (adult respiratory distress syndrome requiring intensive therapy). Neonatal effects include prematurity and small-for-gestational-age babies.

Clinical manifestations of acute pyelonephritis include fever, shaking chills and flank pain, nausea and vomiting, headache, increased urinary frequency, and dysuria. Urine examination will reveal significant bacteriuria, with pyuria and white blood cell casts in the urinary sediment. A count of 1–2 bacteria per high-power field in unspun urine or more than 20 bacteria in the sediment of a centrifuged specimen of urine collected by bladder catheterization will help in the bedside diagnosis. The diagnosis should be confirmed by culture of urine. Associated hematuria may indicate urinary calculi.

## Treatment

A midstream urine specimen should be collected for culture at the initial prenatal visit and repeated later in pregnancy. At each prenatal visit, dipstick testing should be done, and if proteinuria is present, urinalysis, culture, or both should be done. A pregnant woman with sickle cell trait should have urine culture and sensitivity testing every 4 weeks. Pregnant women should be encouraged to maintain adequate fluid intake and to void frequently.

The initial antibiotic selection should be empiric. Based on the fact that the most common offending pathogen is *E coli,* sulfonamides, nitrofurantoin, ampicillin, or cephalosporins could be selected. These antibiotics should be safe for the mother and fetus, with minimal side effects. A 10- to 14-day course of one of these agents will effectively eradicate asymptomatic bacteriuria in about 65% of pregnant patients. Culture of urine should be done 1–2 weeks after therapy is begun and then monthly for the remainder of pregnancy.

Sulfa drugs must be avoided in mothers with glucose-6-phophatase deficiency. Additionally, sulfa drugs are best avoided late in pregnancy because of the increased likelihood of neonatal hyperbilirubinemia. Trimethoprim is a folic acid antagonist, so trimethoprim-sulfamethoxazole should be avoided in pregnancy. Nitrofurantoin should be avoided in the last trimester because it may induce hemolytic anemia in the newborn.

Any woman with acute pyelonephritis in pregnancy should be admitted to the hospital for therapy. Antibiotics should be given parenterally and dehydration corrected. Antipyretic agents are given where indicated, and vital signs and urinary output are closely monitored. Ampicillin or a cephalosporin is usually administered intravenously in doses of 1–2 g every 6 hours.

If there is no appropriate response in 48–72 hours, an aminoglycoside (eg, gentamicin or tobramcyin, 3–5 mg/kg/24 h in 3 divided doses) is administered. If there is no improvement, further evaluation should be considered. The most helpful study at this time is an intravenous pyelogram. A preliminary film and a 15-minute film are usually adequate for the diagnosis of urinary tract obstruction. With persistent flank pain and fever despite proper therapy, perinephric abscess must be ruled out with ultrasound examination. This is generally a complication of obstruction associated with infection. With confirmation of the diagnosis, the abscess must be drained to avoid maternal death. In selected cases of persistent infection, cystoscopy and retrograde pyelographic studies may be useful.

Cunningham noted that 28% of women with pyelonephritis developed recurrent bacteriuria and 10% had recurrent acute pyelonephritis during the same pregnancy. Such women should be given long-term prophylactic treatment. Nitrofurantoin, 100 mg every night, has been suggested, although the efficacy of such therapy is questionable.

Periodic culture of the urine will assist in detecting recurrence. Relapse is defined as recurrent infection due to the same species and type-specific strain of organism present before treatment; this represents a treatment failure. Most relapses occur less than 2 weeks after completion of therapy. Reinfection is recurrent infection due to a different strain of bacteria following successful treatment of the initial infection, occurring more than 3 weeks after completion of therapy.

## URINARY CALCULI

The incidence of urinary calculi is not altered by pregnancy (overall incidence is 0.24% [1 in 425 persons]). This condition predisposes pregnant women to urinary tract infection, recurrent hospitalization, premature labor, and operative intervention. The cause of urinary calculi in pregnant women is the same as in nonpregnant women, ie, chronic urinary tract infection, hyperparathyroidism, congenital or familial cystinuria (or oxaluria), gout, and obstructive uropathy. Most stones are composed of calcium and less frequently in multiparous women. They are more common as pregnancy progresses, being rare during the first trimester. Although physiologic hydroureter is more pronounced on the right side, stones occur with equal frequency in both tracts.

## Clinical Findings

Patients may present with a variety of symptoms, including classic renal or ureteric colic or vague abdominal or back pain. The differential diagnosis must include other acute abdominal conditions, ie, acute appendicitis, biliary colic, adnexal torsion, preterm labor, and placental abruption. The patient may present with fever, bacteriuria, flank pain, and nausea and vomiting suggestive of acute pyelonephritis. The persistence of fever after 48 hours of parenteral antibiotics is strongly suggestive of urinary tract obstruction with calculus. Although hematuria (varying from gross to microhematuria) may be present, it is not always pathognomonic of calcular disease. A high index of suspicion will help in the diagnosis, particularly in cases with negative culture of urine in suspected pyelonephritis, persistent hematuria, and recurrent urinary tract infection.

Clinical diagnosis may be difficult. In most cases, diagnostic imaging is necessary. For preliminary screening, an ultrasonic examination could be useful. In selected cases, excretory urography (a single film taken 20 minutes after infusion) should be done. This exposes the fetus to only 0.2 rad.

## Treatment

Treatment consists of admission to the hospital, hydration, culture of urine, appropriate intravenous antibiotic therapy, correction of electrolyte imbalance, and analgesics. Fortunately, most stones are passed spontaneously. Surgical intervention (ureteral stunting, cystoscopic extraction, open surgery) will be needed in a few cases with persistent severe pain, infection not responding to antibiotics, and obstructive uropathy.

## ACUTE RENAL FAILURE

Acute renal failure in pregnancy is rare but carries a high mortality rate and therefore must be prevented where possible and treated aggressively. Most cases are due to acute hypovolemia. Clinically, acute renal failure is a condition in which the kidneys are temporarily unable to perform their excretory and regulatory functions. Urine output is usually less than 40 mL/24 h, and blood urea nitrogen and serum creatinine levels are elevated. Acute renal failure during pregnancy may result in abortion, low birth weight, premature labor and stillbirth. Hypotension and vaginal hemorrhage may occur during dialysis, although successful outcomes without adverse effects have been reported.

Based on the cause, acute renal failure may be classified as prerenal, renal, or postrenal. In the prerenal type, acute renal failure occurs due to renal hypoperfusion secondary to maternal hypovolemia (eg, hemorrhage, dehydration, abruptio placentae, septicemia, circulating nephrotoxins (eg, aminoglycosides), mismatched blood transfusion, preeclampsia-eclampsia, disseminated intravascular coagulation, and hypoxemia (eg, chronic lung disease and heart failure). In the renal type, a variety of intrinsic renal diseases such as acute glomerulonephritis, acute pyelonephritis, and amyloidosis are responsible for acute renal failure. The postrenal type is caused by urinary obstruction from ureteric stone, retroperitoneal tumor, or other diseases. Bilateral ureteral obstruction due to polyhydramnios is fortunately rare.

The state of renal hypoperfusion is reversible within 24–36 hours with volume restoration and treatment of the precipitating factors. Acute tubular necrosis may develop following reduction of the outer cortical blood flow in the absence of such treatment. The most serious condition arising secondary to acute renal failure is **acute cortical necrosis** in damaged glomerular capillaries and small kidney vessels. Acute cortical necrosis is rare but carries a poor prognosis; partial recovery may be anticipated in patients with patchy lesions.

## Clinical Findings

The clinical course has been divided into an oliguric phase, a diuretic phase, and a recovery phase. In the oliguric phase, urine output drops below 30 mL/h, with accumulation of blood urea nitrogen and potassium. The patient becomes acidotic with the increase in hydrogen ion and loss of bicarbonate. In the diuretic phase, large volumes of dilute urine are passed, with loss of electrolytes due to absence of function of the renal tubules. As tubular function returns to normal in the recovery phase, the normal volume and composition of urine returns. Clinical manifestations and complications include anorexia, nausea and vomiting, lethargy, cardiac arrhythmia (secondary to electrolyte disturbance), anemia, renal or extrarenal infection, thrombocytopenia, metabolic acidosis, and electrolyte imbalance (hyperkalemia, hyponatremia, hypermagnesemia, hyperphosphatemia, hypocalcemia).

Infection in an operative site or the respiratory or urinary tract remains the main cause of death. Other causes of death include azotemia, pulmonary edema, and cardiac arrhythmia (induced by hyperkalemia).

## Treatment

In obstetric practice, prevention of acute renal failure should be the aim, with appropriate volume replacement to maintain urine output of 60 mL/h or more. Proper management of high-risk obstetric conditions (eg, preeclampsia-eclampsia, abruptio placentae, chorioamnionitis), careful typing and cross-matching of blood, and avoidance of nephrotoxic antibiotics are also important.

Specific treatment includes the following:

**A. Emergency Treatment:** Underlying causes of acute renal failure (eg, hemorrhagic shock) may require emergency treatment.

**B. Surgical Measures:** Surgical measures include determination of any obstructive uropathy or sepsis due to infected products of conception. Such problems should be treated appropriately.

**C. Routine Measures:** Routine measures include achieving fluid and electrolyte balance. Fluid intake may be calculated from the urinary output, loss of fluid from other sources (eg, diarrhea, vomiting), and insensible loss of about 500 mL/d (correcting for fever may be necessary). Intake and output must be recorded carefully. The patient should be weighed daily and should maintain a constant weight or lose weight slowly (250 g/d, if one assumes a room temperature of 22–23 °C[71-73 °F]). Hyperkalemia is a significant problem that can be controlled by giving glucose and insulin. The diet should be high in calories, low in protein and electrolytes, and high in carbohydrates. Parenteral feeding may be given in cases of nausea and vomiting. Prophylactic antibiotics should not be used, but infections may be treated with antibiotics without renal toxicity. Indwelling bladder catheters are to be avoided.

**D. Dialysis:** Dialysis is indicated if serum potassium levels rise to 7 meq/L or more, serum sodium levels are 130 meq/L or less, the serum bicarbonate is 130 meq/L or less, blood urea nitrogen levels are more than 120 mg/dL or there are daily increments of 30 mg/dL in patients with sepsis, and dialyzable poisons or toxins are present.

## GLOMERULONEPHRITIS

Acute glomerulonephritis during pregnancy is rare. There is increased perinatal loss with this condition. The clinical course is variable during pregnancy. In some patients, the condition may resolve early in pregnancy, with return to normal renal function. These cases may be mistaken for preeclampsia. Microscopic hematuria with red blood cell casts, low serum complement, and a rising antistreptolysin O titer indicate acute glomerulonephritis. Treatment consists of control of blood pressure, prevention of congestive heart failure, administration of fluids and electrolytes, and close follow-up.

The outcome of pregnancy with chronic glomeru-lonephritis will depend on the degree of functional impairment of the kidneys, blood pressure levels prior to conception, and the exact histology of the glomerulonephritis. Patients are more likely to develop superimposed preeclampsia or hypertensive crisis earlier in pregnancy. Successful pregnancy should be anticipated, although renal function is expected to decrease. The incidence of fetal intrauterine growth retardation, premature labor, abruptio placentae, and intrauterine fetal demise is significantly high. Routine prenatal care must include periodic renal function tests, control of blood pressure, ultrasonic evaluation of fetal growth, and biophysical monitoring of fetal well-being. Early delivery is indicated after evaluation of pulmonary maturity with lecithin:sphingomyelin ratios and phosphatidylglycerol levels in amniotic fluid. Nephrotoxic drugs must be avoided, and acute renal failure should be anticipated, particularly during the postpartum period.

## SOLITARY KIDNEY

A solitary kidney may be the result of developmental aberration or disease requiring removal of one kidney. A single kidney may be abnormally developed or it may be placed low, perhaps even within the true pelvis. A second small, virtually functionless kidney may not be discovered by the usual diagnostic tests. Anatomic and functional hypertrophy of the kidney usually occurs and is augmented by pregnancy. There is no medical contraindication to pregnancy with a solitary kidney. However, if infection occurs in a solitary kidney and does not respond to antibiotics quickly, consideration must be given to termination of the pregnancy to preserve renal function.

## RENAL TRANSPLANTATION

Successful renal transplantation has not prevented pregnancy in the limited number of cases to date. Patients with adequate renal function prior to pregnancy will experience little if any deterioration in graft function during pregnancy. The likelihood of graft rejection during pregnancy remains the same as in nonpregnant graft recipients. The spontaneous abortion rate is not increased, but many patients choose to terminate the pregnancy. Pregnancy-induced hypertension occurs in about 30% of patients with renal transplant, and there is a 60% incidence of proteinuria in the third trimester.

The risk of infection is considerably higher during pregnancy in renal transplant patients. Primary or reactivated herpesvirus infection is a significant risk. The incidence of hepatitis B surface antigenemia has been noted to be about 50% among patients receiving dialysis.

Prematurity with its related complications, intrauterine growth retardation, and fetal abnormalities caused by immunosuppressive agents taken by the mother may occur. The route of delivery depends primarily on obstetric indications. A transplanted kidney in the false pelvis does not usually cause obstruction leading to dystocia. In patients with aseptic necrosis of the hip joints or other bony dystrophy secondary to long-term use of immunosuppressive agents, cesarean section may be required.

## ECTOPIC KIDNEY

An ectopic kidney in the true pelvis with an aberrant blood supply may cause obstruction interfering with delivery. Cesarean section should be done in this situation with great caution to avoid injury to the kidney or its blood supply.

## REFERENCES

### CARDIOVASCULAR DISORDERS

Abdalla MY, el Din Mostafa E: Contraception after heart surgery. Contraception 1992;45:73.

al Kasab SM et al: Beta-adrenergic receptor blockade in the management of pregnant women with mitral stenosis. Am J Obstet Gynecol 1990;163:37.

Austin DA, Davis PA: Valvular disease in pregnancy. J Perinat Neonatal Nurs 1991;5:13.

Brady K, Duff P: Rheumatic heart disease in pregnancy. Clin Obstet Gynecol 1989;32:21.

Burlew BS: Managing the pregnant patient with heart disease. Clin Cardiol 1990;13:757.

Clark SL: Cardiac disease in pregnancy. Obstet Gynecol Clin North Amer 1991;18:237.

Cole PL, Sutton MS: Normal cardiopulmonary adjustments to pregnancy: Cardiovascular evaluation. Cardiovasc Clin 1989; 19:37.

Copel JA, Pilu, G, Kleinman CS: Extracardiac anomalies and congenital heart disease. Semin Perinatol 1993; 17:89.

Cowles T, Gonik B: Mitral valve prolapse in pregnancy. Semin Perinatol 1990;14:34.

Dajani AS et al: Prevention of bacterial endocarditis. Recommendations by the American Heart Association. JAMA 1990;264:2919.

Derksen RH: Systemic lupus erythematosus and pregnancy. Rheumatol Int 1991;11:121.

Donnelly JE, Brown JM, Radford DJ: Pregnancy outcome and Ebstein's anomaly. Br Heart J 1991; 66:368.

Drummond SB: Cardiac disease in pregnancy: Intrapartum considerations. Crit Care Nurs Clin North Am 1992;4:659.

Ducey JP, Ellsworth SM: The hemodynamic effects of severe mitral stenosis and pulmonary hypertension during labor and delivery. Intensive Care Med 1989; 15:192.

Esteves CA et al: Effectiveness of percutaneous balloon mitral valvotomy during pregnancy. AM J Cardiol 1991;68:930.

Faidley CK et al: Electrocardiographic abnormalities during ritodrine administration. South Med J 1990; 83:503.

Frenkel Y et al: Pregnancy after myocardial infarction: Are we playing safe? Obstet Gynecol 1991;77:822.

Friedman AH, Copel JA, Kleinman CS: Fetal echocardiography and fetal cardiology: indications, diagnosis and management. Semin Perinatol 1993; 17:76.

Friedman SA, Berstein MS, Kitzmiller JL: Pregnancy complicated by collagen vascular disease. Obstet Gynecol Clin North Am 1991;18:213.

Hands ME et al: The cardiac, obstetric, and anesthetic management of pregnancy complicated by acute myocardial infarction. J Clin Anesthiol 1990;2:258.

Heller MB, Verdile VP: Ultrasonography in emergency medicine. Emerg Med Clin North Am 1992;10:27.

Henderson CE et al: Cardiac screening for pregnant intravenous drug abusers. Am J Perinatol 1989;6: 397.

Hess DB, Hess LW: Management of cardiovascular disease in pregnancy. Obstet Gynecol Clin North Am 1992;19:679.

Hyers TM: Heparin therapy. Regimens and treatment considerations. Drugs 1992;44:738.

Kain ZN, Kain TS, Scarpelli EM: Cocaine exposure in utero: Perinatal development and neonatal manifestations—review. J Toxicol Clin Toxicaol 1992; 30:607.

Lampert MB et al: Peripartum heart failure associated with prolonged tocolytic therapy. Am J Obstet Gynecol 1993;168:493.

Lee W: Clinical management of gravid women with peripartum cardiomyopathy. Obstet Gynecol Clin North Am 1991;18:257.

Mabie WC, Hackman BB, Sibai BM: Pulmonary edema associated with pregnancy; Echocardiographic insights and implications for treatment. Obstet Gynecol 1993;81:227.

Mansur AJ et al; The complications of infective endocarditis. A reappraisal in the 1980's. Arch Intern Med 1992;152:2428.

Mason BA, Ricci-Goodman J, Koos BJ: Adenosine in the treatment of maternal paroxysmal supraventricular tachycardia. Obstet Gynecol 1992;80:478.

Mishra M, Chambers, Jackson G: Murmurs in pregnancy: An audit of echocardiography. BMJ 1992; 304:1413.

Moller JH, Anderson RC: 1,000 consecutive children with cardiac malformation with 26- to 37-year follow-up. Am J Cardiol 1992;70:661.

Moodie DS et al: Aortic valve replacement in young patients: Long-term follow-up. Cleve Clin J Med 1992; 59:473.

Murphy JG et al:Long-term outcome in patients undergoing surgical repair of Tetralogy of Fallot. New Engl J Med 1993;329:593.

Nienaber CA et al: Diagnosis of thoracic aortic dissection: Magnetic resonance imaging versus transesophageal echocardiography. Circulation 1992;85:434.

Patel JJ et al: Percutaneous balloon mitral valvotomy in pregnant patients with tight pliable mitral stenosis. Am Heart J 1993;125:1106.

Patton DE et al: Cyanotic maternal heart disease in pregnancy. Obstet Gynecol Surv 1990;45:594.

Penkala M, Hancock EW: Wide-complex tachycardia in pregnancy. Hosp Pract (Off Ed) 1993;28:63.

Perloff JK: 22nd Bethesda Conference. Congenital heart disease after childhood: An expanding patient population. October 18–19, 1990. J Am Coll Cardiol 1991; 18:311.

Pitkin RM et al: Pregnancy and congenital heart disease. Ann Intern Med 1990;112:445.

Plomp TA, Vulsma T, de Vijlder JJ: Use of amiodarone during pregnancy. Eur J Obstet Gynecol Reprod Biol 1992;43:20.

Podolsky SM, Varon J: Adenosine use during pregnancy. Ann Emerg Med 1991;20:1027.

Reed KL: Fetal arrhythmias: Etiology, diagnosis, pathophysiology, and treatment. Semin Perinatol 1989; 13:294.

Resnekov L: Aortic valve stenosis. Management in children and adults. Postgrad Med 1993;93:107.

Ribeiro PA et al: Balloon valvotomy for pregnancy patients with severe pliable mitral stenosis using the Inoue technique with total abdominal and pelvic shielding. Am Heart J 1992;124:1558.

Sadaniantz A et al: Cardiovascular changes in pregnancy evaluated by two-dimensional and Doppler echocardiography. J Am Soc Echocardiogr 1992; 5:253.

Saenger JS et al: Ductus-dependent fetal cardiac defects contraindicate indomethacin tocolysis. J Perinatol 1992; 12:41.

Shulman ST et al: Prevention of rheumatic fever, a statement for health professionals by the Committee on Rheumatic fever and Infective Endocarditis of the Council on Cardiovascular Disease in the Young. Circulation 1984;70:1118A.

Sugrue DD et al: The clinical course of idiopathic dilated cardiomyopathy: A population-based study. Ann Intern Med 1992;118:117.

Uren NG, Oakley CM: The treatment of primary pulmonary hypertension. Br Heart J 1991;66:119.

Ward RM: Maternal drug therapy for fetal disorders. Semin Perinatol 1992;16:12.

Widerhorn J et al: Fetal and neonatal adverse effects profile of amiodarone treatment during pregnancy. Am Heart J 1991;122:1162.

Widerhorn J et al: WPW syndrome during pregnancy: Increased incidence of supraventricular arrhythmias. Am Heart J 1992;123:796.

Wong V, Cheng CH, Chan KC: Fetal and neonatal outcome of exposure to anticoagulants during pregnancy. Am J Med Genet 1993;45:17.

Wong MC, Giuliani MJ, Haley EC Jr: Cerebrovascular disease and stroke in women. Cardiology 1990; 77(Suppl 2):80.

Wooley CF, Sparks EH: Congenital heart disease, heritable cardiovascular disease, and pregnancy. Prog Cardiovasc Dis 1992;35:41.

Zeldis SM: Dyspnea during pregnancy. Distinguishing cardiac from pulmonary causes. Clin Chest Med 1992; 13:567.

## HEMATOLOGIC DISORDERS

Alger LS, Golbus MS, Laros RK Jr: Thalassemia and pregnancy: Results of an antenatal screening program. Am J Obstet Gynecol 1979;134:662.

Banks PM: Pregnancy and lymphoma. (Editorial.) Arch Pathol Lab Med 1985;109:802.

Brumfield CG et al: A delayed hemolytic transfusion reaction after partial exchange transfusion for sickle cell disease in pregnancy. Obstet Gynecol 1984;63(Suppl 3):13S.

Cantini E, Yanes B: Acute myelogenous leukemia in pregnancy. South Med J 1984;77:1050.

Catanzarite VA, Ferguson JE II: Acute leukemia and pregnancy: A review of management and outcome, 1972-1982. Obstet Gynecol Surv 1984;39:663.

Cefalo RC et al: Maternal and fetal effects of exchange transfusion with a red blood cell substitute. Am J Obstet Gynecol 1984;148:859.

Chanarin I: Folate and cobalamin. Clin Haematol 1985; 14:629.

Charache S et al: Management of sickle cell disease in pregnant patients. Obstet Gynecol 1980;55:407.

Cohen MB et al: Septic pelvic thrombophlebitis. An update. Obstet Gynecol 1983;62:83.

Cunningham FG, Pritchard JA, Mason R: Pregnancy and sickle cell hemoglobinopathies: Results with and without prophylactic transfusion. Obstet Gynecol 1983;62:419.

Cunningham FG et al: Prophylactic transfusions of normal red blood cells during pregnancies complicated by sickle cell hemoglobinopathies. Am J Obstet Gynecol 1979;135:994.

Garg A, Kochupillai V: Non-Hodgkin's lymphoma in pregnancy. South Med J 1985;78:1263.

Gililland J, Weinstein L: The effects of cancer chemotherapeutic agents on the developing fetus. Obstet Gynecol Surv 1983;38:6.

Gounder MP et al: Intravenous gammaglobulin therapy in the management of a patient with idiopathic thrombocytopenic purpura and a warm autoimmune erythrocyte panagglutinin during pregnancy. Obstet Gynecol 1986;67:741.

Ioachim HL: Non-Hodgkin's lymphoma in pregnancy. Three cases and review of the literature. Arch Pathol Lab Med 1985;109:803.

Kelton JG et al: The prenatal prediction of thrombocytopenia in infants of mothers with clinically diagnosed immune thrombocytopenia. Am J Obstet Gynecol 1982;144:449.

Laros RK Jr, Kagan R: Route of delivery for patients with immune thrombocytopenic purpura. Am J Obstet Gynecol 1984;148:901.

Lavery JP et al: Immunologic thrombocytopenia in pregnancy: Use of antenatal immunoglobulin therapy. Case report and review. Obstet Gynecol 1985; 66 (Suppl 3):41S.

Levin J: Hematologic disorders of pregnancy. Chap 3, pp 62-87, in: *Medical Complications During Pregnancy,* 2nd ed. Burrow MD, Ferris TF (editors). Saunders, 1982.

Levine AM, Collea JV: When pregnancy complicates chronic granulocytic leukemia. Contemp Obstet Gynecol 1979;13:47.

McFee JG: Iron metabolism and iron deficiency during pregnancy. Clin Obstet Gynecol 1979;22:799.

Miller JM Jr: Alpha thalassemia minor in pregnancy. J Reprod Med 1982;27:207.

Miller JM Jr et al: Management of sickle hemoglobinopathies in pregnant patients. Am J Obstet Gynecol 1981;141:237.

Milner PF, Jones BR, Dobler J: Outcome of pregnancy in sickle cell anemia and sickle cell-hemoglobin C disease: An analysis of 181 pregnancies in 98 patients, and a review of the literature. Am J Obstet Gynecol 1980;138:239.

Morrison JC et al: Fetal health assessment in pregnancies complicated by sickle hemoglobinopathies. Obstet Gynecol 1983;61:22.

Noriega-Guerra L et al: Pregnancy in patients with autoimmune thrombocytopenic purpura. Am J Obstet Gynecol 1979;133:439.

Powars DR et al: Pregnancy in sickle cell disease. Obstet Gynecol 1986;67:217.

Scott JR, Rote NS, Cruikshank DP: Antiplatelet antibodies and platelet counts in pregnancies complicated by autoimmune thrombocytopenic purpura. Am J Obstet Gynecol 1983;145:932.

Tawil E, Mercier JP, Dandavino A: Hodgkin's disease complicating pregnancy. J Can Assoc Radiol 1985; 36:133.

Transfusion therapy in pregnant sickle cell disease patients. (Editorial.) Am J Obstet Gynecol 1979; 134:851.

White JM et al: Thalassaemia and pregnancy. J Clin Pathol 1986;38:810.

## PULMONARY DISORDERS

Corkey CWB et al: Pregnancy in cystic fibrosis: A better prognosis in patients with pancreatic function. Am J Obstet Gynecol 1981;140:737.

Dunlap NE, Fulmer JD: Corticosteroid therapy in asthma. Clin Chest Med 1984;5:669.

Good JT Jr et al: Tuberculosis in association with pregnancy. Am J Obstet Gynecol 1981:140:492.

Greenberger PA: Asthma in pregnancy. Clin Peri 1985;12:571.

Greenberger PA: Pregnancy and asthma. Chest 1985; 87:85S.

Greenberger PA, Patterson R: Management of asthma during pregnancy. N Engl J Med 1985;312:897.

Harman EM: Pulmonary problems of pregnancy. Compr Ther 1985;11:26.

McCormack JG: Drug therapy of tuberculosis. Ir Med J 1984;77:88.

Mendelson's syndrome. (Editorial.) Br J Anaesth 1978; 50:81.

Nemir RL, O'Hare D: Congenital tuberculosis: Review and diagnostic guidelines. Am J Dis Child 1985; 139:284.

Roberts RB, Shirley MA: The obstetrician's role in reducing the risk of aspiration pneumonitis: With particular reference to the use of oral antacids. Am J Obstet Gynecol 1976;124:611.

Snider D: Pregnancy and tuberculosis. Chest 1984;8 6:10S.

Snider DE Jr et al: Treatment of tuberculosis during pregnancy. Am Rev Respir Dis 1980;122:65.

Stablein JJ, Lockey RF: Managing asthma during pregnancy. Compr Ther 1984;10:45.

Summer WR: Status asthmaticus. Chest 1985;87:87S.

Sutherland AM: Surgical treatment of tuberculosis of the female genital tract. Br J Obstet Gynaecol 1980; 87:610.

Weinberger SE: Pulmonary diseases. Chap 17, pp 405-434, in: *Medical Complications During Pregnancy,* 2nd ed. Burrow MD, Ferris TF (editors). Saunders, 1982.

## RENAL & URINARY TRACT DISORDERS

Beydoun SN: Morphologic changes in the renal tract in pregnancy. Clin Obstet Gynecol 1985;28:249.

Davison JM: The physiology of the renal tract in pregnancy. Clin Obstet Gynecol 1985;28:257.

Davison JM, Katz Al, Lindheimer MD: Kidney disease and pregnancy: Obstetric outcome and long-term renal prognosis. Clin Perinatol 1985;12:497.

Davison JM, Lindheimer MD: Pregnancy in women with renal allografts. Semin Nephrol 1984;4:240.

Drago JR, Rohner TJ Jr, Chez RA: Management of urinary calculi in pregnancy. Urology 1982;20:578.

Ferris TF: Renal diseases. Chap 10, pp 235-259, in: *Medical Complications During Pregnancy,* 2nd ed. Burrow MD, Ferris TF (editors). Saunders, 1982.

Foley ME et al: Urinary tract infection in pregnancy. Ir Med J 1982;75:188.

Gilstrap LC et al: Renal infection and pregnancy outcome. Am J Obstet Gynecol 1981;141:709.

Grauunfeld J-P, Ganeval D, Bournaaerias F: Acute renal failure in pregnancy. Kidney Int 1980;18:179.

Hankins GDV, Whalley PJ: Acute urinary tract infections in pregnancy. Clin Obstet Gynecol 1985; 28:266.

Harris RE, Gilstrap LC III, Pretty A: Single-dose antimicrobial therapy for asymptomatic bacteriuria during pregnancy. Obstet Gynecol 1982;59:546.

Horowitz E, Schmidt JD: Renal calculi in pregnancy. Clin Obstet Gynecol 1985;28:324.

Klein EL: Urologic problems of pregnancy. Obstet Gynecol Surv 1984;39:605.

Knuppel RA, Montenegro R, O'Brien WF: Acute renal failure in pregnancy. Clin Obstet Gynecol 1985; 28:288.

Lattanzi DR, Cook WA: Urinary calculi in pregnancy. Obstet Gynecol 1980;56:462.

MacCarthy EP, Pollak VE: Maternal renal disease: Effect on the fetus. Clin Perinatol 1981;8:307.

Meier PR, Makowski EL: Pregnancy in the patient with a renal transplant. Clin Obstet Gynecol 1984;27:902.

Perreault J-P et al: Urinary calculi in pregnancy. Can J Surg 1982;25:453.

The Registration Committee of the European Dialysis and Transplant Association (St. Thomas Hospital, London): Successful pregnancies in women treated by dialysis and kidney transplantation. Br J Obstet Gynaecol 1980;87:839.

Rehm M, Nilsson CG, Hankkamaa M: Significant bacteriuria in the puerperium: A prospective study of the risk factors. Ann Clin Res 1980;12:112.

Robertson EG: Assessment and treatment of renal disease in pregnancy. Clin Obstet Gynecol 1985; 28:279.

Verco CJ, Hawkins DF: Pregnancy after renal transplantation. J Obstet Gynecol 1982;3:29.

Warren SE, Mitas JA II, Evertson LR: Pregnancy after renal transplantation: Reversible acidosis and renal dysfunction. South Med J 1981;74:1139.

# 23

# General Medical Disorders During Pregnancy

*L. Wayne Hess, MD, & John C. Morrison, MD, & Darla B. Hess, MD*

Medical complications of pregnancy may have adverse effects on the mother, fetus, and newborn. The physiologic changes that occur during a normal gestation may aggravate a maternal disease process. The diagnostic and therapeutic acumen of the physician, the severity of the disease, and the stage of gestation at which the complication occurs all have an impact on the outcome of pregnancy. The sum of these variables may cause the complication to improve, equilibrate, or deteriorate during pregnancy. Most of the common medical complications of pregnancy (such as anemia, which affects ~ 50% of all gestations in the USA) are relatively mild, do not usually affect the pregnancy, and can be managed by the obstetrician-gynecologist.

## DISORDERS OF THE NERVOUS SYSTEM

### CEREBROVASCULAR DISORDERS

The causes of cerebrovascular disease include insufficiency **(arteriosclerosis, cerebral embolism, vasospasm from hypertensive disease)** and disorders associated with bleeding into the cerebral cortex **(arteriovenous malformation, ruptured aneurysm).** The brain becomes infarcted from lack of blood flow, or intracranial bleeding results in a space-occupying lesion. The severity of such disorders can be affected by blood pressure, oxygen saturation (anemia or polycythemia), hypoglycemia, and adequacy of collateral circulation.

The overall incidence of ischemic cerebrovascular accidents in pregnancy is approximately 1 in 20,000 births, with most occurring in the last trimester or immediately postpartum. Predisposing factors can be found in approximately one-third of cases (eg, arteriosclerosis, hypertension), but maternal age is usually not a factor, since most of the affected patients

are under 35 years of age. Although cerebral ischemic disease can occur in either the arterial or venous system, approximately 75% of occlusive cerebral disease is on the arterial side.

Cerebrovascular accidents involving cortical hemorrhage are slightly more common (1 in 15,000 births) and are usually associated with aneurysms, arteriovenous malformations, or hypertension. The most common aneurysm is the saccular (berry) variety, which protrudes from the major arteries in the circle of Willis, particularly at its bifurcations. The incidence of rupture of an aneurysm is approximately 1 in 10,000 births and usually affects multiparous women over age 30 in the last half of gestation; the risk of rupture is not increased by pregnancy. Arteriovenous malformations, on the other hand, usually rupture in the first half of pregnancy and are noted in younger women (20–25 years). Rupture of the malformation does appear to be more frequent during pregnancy. Pregnancy-induced hypertension or malignant exacerbation of chronic hypertension can also cause intracerebral bleeding but is not commonly associated with cortical hemorrhage unless the diastolic blood pressure exceeds 110–120 mm Hg for an extended period.

### Clinical Findings

Headaches, visual disturbances, syncope, dysphasia, and coma are present in up to 40% of patients, but seizures are rare. Hemiplegia, the most common presenting symptom, has an abrupt onset in 70% of cases.

### Diagnosis

The pattern of clinical signs and symptoms generally allows recognition of the area of the brain involved. CT scan and MRI can be employed in pregnancy to increase the delineation of cerebrovascular involvement. Ultrasonography may be helpful, particularly in hemorrhagic lesions. Arteriography is considered definitive if surgical intervention is being considered, since it can more precisely localize the involved area. Because coagulopathies can also cause intracranial bleeding or may be secondary to the cerebrovascular lesion itself; a coagulation profile should be performed. Additionally, ANA, anticardiolipin, proteins C and S, antithrombin 3, and plasminogen levels should be considered with thrombolic cerebral events.

## Treatment

The treatment of ischemic or hemorrhagic cerebrovascular disease is best managed supportively; however, surgery is indicated for the treatment of some aneurysms and arteriovenous malformations. Normalization of blood pressure, adequate respiratory support, therapy for metabolic complications, and treatment of coagulopathies or cardiac abnormalities are crucial. Dexamethasone, 10 mg intravenously initially followed by 5 mg every 6 hours for 24 hours, may decrease cerebral edema and be of some assistance prior to surgery or in recovery. Additionally, hyperventilation, mannitol infusions, phenobarbital coma, and intracerebral pressure monitoring may be helpful with severe cerebral edema. Other treatment modalities, such as osmotic diuretics, volume expanders, and vasodilators, have not been helpful during pregnancy. Anticoagulants are usually not helpful except in the rare patient with a superior sagittal sinus thrombosis and nonbloody cerebrospinal fluid. Once the patient has been stabilized, physical therapy and rehabilitation should begin as soon as possible.

Appropriate surgery for aneurysms and arteriovenous malformations should be carried out with the pregnancy undisturbed unless fetal maturity allows for cesarean birth just prior to the neurosurgical procedure. On the other hand, inoperable lesions during pregnancy are managed by pregnancy conservation until fetal maturity is sufficient to allow abdominal birth. In addition, therapeutic abortion is an option in the first or second trimester. Once a lesion has been surgically corrected, vaginal delivery can be attempted. However, the second stage of labor should be modified by regional anesthesia and forceps delivery to reduce cerebral pressures associated with the Valsalva maneuver.

## Complications & Prognosis

For patients with cerebral occlusive disease, venous occlusion has a poor initial prognosis because of infection. On the other hand, the percentage of patients with venous occlusion who recover from the initial episode without neurologic sequelae during rehabilitation is equal to that of patients with arterial occlusion. Thrombosis of the superior sagittal sinus is a rare complication, but its incidence is increased during pregnancy, and it has a grave prognosis (~ 70% mortality rate). If the cerebral hemorrhagic disorder is operable, the prognosis is quite favorable, with few long-term neurologic deficits. In inoperable lesions or when severe maternal cerebral hemorrhage has occurred, the prognosis—while unfavorable—is better for those with aneurysms than for those with arterio-

venous fistulas. If a neurosurgical procedure takes place during pregnancy, the fetus is usually not adversely affected, despite the induced hypotension that is often necessary. The prognosis for the mother and fetus is the same as that in a normal gestation once the condition has been corrected.

## CEREBRAL NEOPLASMS

Cerebral neoplasms occur primarily at the extremes of life; thus, primary cancer or even metastatic tumors are uncommon during the childbearing years. Although brain tumors are not specifically related to gestation, meningiomas, angiomas, and neurofibromas are thought to grow more rapidly with pregnancy. Of the primary neoplasms (half of all brain tumors), gliomas are the most common (50%), with meningiomas and pituitary adenomas accounting for 35%. Of the metastatic cerebral tumors, lung and breast tumors account for 50%. **Choriocarcinoma** (see Chapter 50) commonly metastasizes to the cerebrum.

## Clinical Findings

The clinical manifestations, while dependent on the type and location of the tumor, are generally characterized by a slow progression of neurologic signs with evidence of increased intracranial pressure. One of the most frequent signs is headache, which must be differentiated from that occurring in tension and in vascular or inflammatory conditions. Pain that is not relieved by analgesics or muscle relaxants (as a tension headache would be), the absence of a history of migraine headaches, and the lack of signs of infection or meningeal inflammation all point to increased intracranial pressure as the cause of the headache. Tumors in the pituitary gland or occipital region may be associated with visual deficits.

## Diagnosis

CT scan and MRI are of greatest assistance in revealing space-occupying lesions. If the cerebrospinal fluid glucose and protein levels are normal, inflammation or infection of the central nervous system are unlikely. Similarly, an increase in the cerebrospinal fluid hCG titer raises the suspicions of metastatic choriocarcinoma. Pleocytosis may be present with cerebral neoplasia, but it is usually lymphocytic or monocytic, without an increase in the number of polymorphonucleocytes. Finally, failure to find blood or xanthochromic fluid in the cerebrospinal fluid helps in differentiating a neoplasm from a hemorrhagic lesion, unless the tumor has undergone hemorrhagic necrosis.

## Treatment

The treatment of cerebral neoplasms during pregnancy depends on the type of tumor, its location, and the stage of gestation. In early pregnancy and with life-threatening tumors, therapeutic abortion is an option. Later in gestation, delivery is usually effected by cesarean section or induction of labor so that maternal therapy (eg, surgery of chemotherapy) can be implemented. During the second trimester, therapy may be initiated using radiation therapy or cytotoxic agents with the pregnancy allowed to continue. However, this course of action is controversial and requires individual judgment, consultation, and informed consent.

## Complications & Prognosis

Brain tumors usually do not affect pregnancy or the fetus unless the neoplasm leads to early delivery or maternal death. When diagnosed in the second or third trimester, the outcome for the fetus is excellent, with 95% surviving even though therapy may be initiated during the course of the pregnancy.

## MIGRAINE HEADACHE

Chronic migraine headaches decrease during pregnancy in 50–80% of affected patients. Even hemiplegic migraine is not altered adversely. Very few women experience initial onset during pregnancy, and history of migraine does not predispose to pregnancy-induced hypertension.

## Clinical Findings

Most often, the patient has a history of migraine headaches, which are usually described as "pounding" and may settle in the eyes or the temporal region. Frequently, migraines are associated with gastrointestinal complaints (eg, nausea, vomiting, and diarrhea) or with systemic symptoms (eg, vertigo or syncope). An aura may or may not precede the headache, but vision is not usually impaired.

## Diagnosis

Migraine headaches are rarely relieved by analgesics and muscle relaxants, a fact that helps differentiate them from tension headaches. If vertigo is associated with migraine headaches, it is important to rule out Meniere's disease (labyrinthitis). In the latter, vertigo is accompanied by tinnitus, a fluctuating sensorineural hearing loss, and nystagmus. On the other hand, if vertigo is associated with ataxia of gait, it is almost always central, in which case head trauma, brain tumors, seizure disorders, and multiple sclerosis need to be excluded. Syncope (fainting) may occur with migraine or vascular headaches and is very common during pregnancy. However, when syncope occurs with migraine headache, it usually is associated with vertigo. Rarely, ocular nerve palsy develops in association with migraine headaches; the third cranial nerve is the most commonly involved, and the palsy usually disappears with abatement of the migraine. It is important to visualize the optic disk to ensure that cerebrospinal fluid pressure is not increased. In cases in which the disk borders are not sharp, **pseudotumor cerebri** should be considered. In this disorder the headache and the pressure on the optic disk are usually self-limited, and in most patients the condition improves after delivery. Pseudotumor cerebri usually responds to corticosteroids, bed rest, and diuretics, thus differentiating the disorder from migraine headache with questionable papilledema. When migraine headaches are accompanied by papilledema, visual fields should be assessed.

## Treatment

Treatment of migraine headaches initially includes identification of any factor that precipitates attacks, followed by avoidance of those factors. Factors known to precipitate some migraines include the following: cheese, sausage, chocolate, citrus fruit, wine, monosodium glutamate, odors, lights, inadequate sleep, etc. When this environmental manipulation fails to control migraines, drug therapy is indicated. Migraine therapy is either abortive or prophylactic. Abortive medications include isometheptene (Midrin), aspirin, naproxen, ibuprofen, ergotamine, or sumatriptan. Prophylactic medications include beta mimetic blockers, tricyclic antidepressants, calcium channel blockers, and aspirin. Some of these medications should be avoided during pregnancy unless the benefits clearly outweigh their theoretical risks.

## Complications & Prognosis

Migraine headaches usually have no deleterious long-term effect on mother or fetus, and treatment for acute exacerbation is usually successful.

## SEIZURE DISORDERS

Seizure disorders during pregnancy are most often generalized and can be either convulsive (tonic-clonic or grand mal) or nonconvulsive (petit mal). Focal motor, sensory, or autonomic seizures are relatively rare during pregnancy. The onset of seizure disorders is not increased during pregnancy. More than 95% of patients who have seizures during pregnancy have a history of a seizure disorder or have been receiving anticonvulsant therapy. Patients whose seizures are adequately controlled are not likely to experience a deterioration of their condition during pregnancy. On the other hand, patients who have had frequent and uncontrolled seizures before pregnancy will likely experience the same pattern, particularly during early pregnancy.

## Clinical Findings

It is imperative to distinguish true seizures from other forms of loss of consciousness such as syncopal episodes, hysteric attacks, or hyperventilation. These problems do not commonly involve a postictal state, nor do they usually involve loss of bladder or bowel control. Non-central nervous system causes, such as hypoxia, hypoglycemia, hypocalcemia, and hyponatremia, also must be excluded. Finally, seizures may result from drug withdrawal, medications, or exposure to toxic substances; thus, appropriate physical examination and screening for toxic substances is important in patients suffering an apparent first seizure during pregnancy.

### Diagnosis

Detailed neurologic work-up is required in patients whose first seizure occurs during pregnancy. Skull x-rays, electroencephalogram, CT scan or MRI, and lumbar puncture are useful in detailing the cause of the seizure and are not contraindicated during pregnancy.

### Treatment

During pregnancy, the plasma level of anticonvulsants decreases because of increased protein binding. In addition, phenytoin, phenobarbital, and carbamazepine have an increased plasma clearance that is probably related to high hepatic metabolism. Therefore, blood level measurements of antiseizure medications are used to document a therapeutic range. Phenytoin, 300–400 mg/d in divided doses, is recommended for most generalized seizure disorders. Two weeks of therapy are generally needed to achieve a therapeutic blood level (10–20 mg/mL). If seizure control is inadequate, a second anticonvulsant (eg, phenobarbital) can be added. The therapeutic range of phenobarbital is 25–30 μg/dL, and the small doses necessary to reach this level (5–10 mg twice daily) do not usually sedate the patient. For petit mal seizures, ethosuximide, 250–500 mg 3 or 4 times a day, is given instead of trimethadione.

In patients with status epilepticus, control of seizures is mandatory. If delivery is not imminent, 10 mg intravenous doses of diazepam can be slowly administered. If seizures continue, phenytoin (750–1000 mg slow IV push at a rate of 25mg/min) or amobarbital sodium (500 mg) may be given intravenously. Paraldehyde and general anesthesia may be considered if seizures persist. In these cases, cerebral edema is almost invariably present and may be reduced with dexamethasone, mannitol, or hyperventilation. Many cases of status epilepticus in pregnancy are due to inadequate treatment with antiepileptic drugs, because of either noncompliance or failure to monitor serum levels.

### Complications & Prognosis

All therapeutic anticonvulsants cross the placenta, equilibrate rapidly in cord blood, and may have teratogenic effects. The risk of anomalies among infants exposed to anticonvulsants is approximately 3-fold greater than in the general population. The **fetal hydantoin syndrome** (associated with phenytoin) has been well described and affects 3–5% of exposed offspring. It is characterized by mental retardation, small size for gestational age, craniofacial anomalies, and limb defects. A milder phenytoin-associated syndrome may be present at a greater frequency (8–15%) but is detectable only by careful assessment during the first 3 years of life.

Anomalies associated with trimethadione are similar to those in fetal hydantoin syndrome but are twice as frequent (up to 30%). Affected infants have growth delays, cardiac and ocular defects, microcephaly, hypospadias, low-set ears, and palatal anomalies. No fetal abnormalities have been noted in humans exposed to carbamazepine or ethosuximide. There are conflicting data concerning the teratogenesis of primidone. Phenobarbital has been used for many years and appears to be safe for the fetus. Valproic acid has been used for major as well as focal seizures, but several reports have described birth defects (especially neural tube defects [1–2%]) related to use of valproic acid during pregnancy; thus, it should be avoided if possible.

Women with existing seizure disorders who are contemplating pregnancy should be tested to see whether they still require anticonvulsant therapy— particularly if anticonvulsants were begun during childhood or if the patient has been seizure-free for an extended period. If a pregnant woman requires seizure medication, she should be informed of the likelihood of fetal anomalies associated with each drug (eg, phenytoin, 10%; valproic acid, primidone, and carbamazepine; 3–5%; trimethadione, 25–30%), and informed consent should be obtained.

## MULTIPLE SCLEROSIS

Multiple sclerosis is a demyelinating process in the white matter of the central nervous system. It affects males and females equally and usually has its onset between the ages of 20 and 40. People in the northern hemisphere are more commonly affected. The cause is not known, but it is more likely environmental or viral than genetic.

### Clinical Findings

Findings include weakness in the extremities, difficulty with coordination, and visual problems. Myasthenia gravis should be ruled out with an anticholinesterase (neostigmine) challenge, and a history of recent viral infection may make it important to rule out Guillain-Barré syndrome.

### Diagnosis

The appropriate laboratory test is a lumbar puncture. The cerebrospinal fluid IgG level is elevated (40–60% of the total protein, in contrast to 15% in normal cerebrospinal fluid). The oligo-clonal band of IgG is particularly diagnostic.

### Treatment

There is no specific therapy, but short courses of corticosteroids may be helpful if the patient has optic neuritis. Immunosuppressant therapy has not been effective.

### Complications & Prognosis

The disease is characterized by exacerbations and remissions, with 70% of patients experiencing slow progression over a number of years. Pregnancy does not appear to exert any deleterious effect on multiple sclerosis, and its initial occurrence is not increased during pregnancy. The disease itself may not be an indication for therapeutic abortion or sterilization, but since it is a progressive neurologic disease, the patient's participation in long-term child-rearing may be impossible. Average life expectancy after diagnosis is 15–25 years, with death usually resulting from infection. Approximately 50% of patients are still functional after 10 years and 35% after 15 years.

## CHOREIC DISORDERS

Chorea is characterized by involuntary movements of the limbs, face, and trunk with muscular weakness and incoordination. Pathologic changes occur in the caudate nucleus, corpus striatum, and putamen of the brain. It may be familial, occur with other neurologic disorders, or be associated with infectious disease. Acute chorea, also known as Sydenham's chorea, occurs most often in childhood following viral or bacterial encephalitis. **Chorea gravidarum** is a rare disorder first identified in patients with rheumatic fever. It probably represents the onset of acute chorea during pregnancy and usually occurs in adolescents. Huntington's chorea is a degenerative disorder of the basal ganglia and cerebral cortex that is inherited as an autosomal dominant trait.

### Clinical Findings

The most striking feature of patients with different varieties of chorea is involuntary movements. These movements may be of the trunk, face, tongue, hands, or limbs. Symptoms at initial onset (clumsiness, irritability, and an ataxic gait) may be subtle or may appear abruptly.

### Diagnosis

The diagnosis of chorea is usually suspected in an individual with the above signs and symptoms in whom the movements can be documented as involuntary. Occasionally the movements may appear coordinated but on further observation are noted to be purposeless. Facial grimacing and difficulty chewing, swallowing, and speaking are also noted. A particu-larly important diagnostic point is that the involuntary movements usually occur at rest and disappear during sleep. They are usually made worse by attempts at control of the movements. Acute chorea is rarely noted in pregnancy since it is not common after age 15, but it may be seen following viral encephalitis. A family history of chorea is helpful in diagnosing Huntington's chorea.

### Treatment

In most of the choreic disorders, rest and sedation is the only treatment available. Chlorpromazine may be helpful in some cases. In Huntington's chorea, genetic counseling is mandatory.

### Complications & Prognosis

The fetus is not affected except by the possibility of inheriting a genetic degenerative disorder. As many as one-fourth of women with a history of chorea in childhood may notice an exacerbation during pregnancy. While most choreic disorders are permanent, chorea gravidarum may disappear several months after pregnancy.

## ORGANIC MENTAL SYNDROMES

Disorders of mentation during pregnancy are rare, although organic brain syndromes (more common in older people) may appear during pregnancy in extremely stressful situations.

### Diagnosis

Other disorders of mental function to be considered in the differential diagnosis are overuse of vitamins (particularly A and D), postictal confusion, brain tumors, cerebrovascular accidents, infections of the central nervous system, and chronic intoxication. The work-up involves psychiatric evaluation and neurologic assessment.

### Treatment

Treatment of severe mental dysfunction is usually not altered by pregnancy. Lithium carbonate (for manic depressive patients) has teratogenic effects (Ebstein's anomaly of the fetal heart); therefore, it is not recommended during pregnancy if the patient can be treated with any other drug. Fetal echocardiography is recommended in pregnant patients who have taken lithium. Lithium is concentrated in breast milk; thus, breastfeeding is contraindicated. The use of tricyclic antidepressants is controversial. At this time, their use during pregnancy is best avoided.

### Complications & Prognosis

Hypoglycemic shock in the treatment of severe mental dysfunction should be avoided, because it can adversely affect both mother and fetus. Other complications of lithium carbonate include an increased frequency of growth retardation, prematurity, hypothermia, neonatal goiter, and renal disorders. Phenothiazines cross the placenta, but their extensive use in pregnancy indicates they are relatively safe drugs. Nevertheless, the smallest therapeutic dose of even these agents should be used.

## MYASTHENIA GRAVIS

Myasthenia gravis is a chronic disorder of unknown cause occurring more commonly in females than in males. Its peak occurrence is in the third decade of life. It is characterized by abnormal voluntary muscle function with muscle weakness after repeated effort. Antibodies to muscle and acetylcholine receptors are present, but levels do not correlate with the severity of disease. Although some cases of myasthenia gravis appear to be hereditary, most adult cases appear to be acquired.

### Clinical Findings
The most common symptom is easily fatigued small muscles, most frequently the ocular muscles. Weakness usually increases as the muscles are used repeatedly, and patients who may not have noticeable symptoms in the morning may be easily diagnosed in the afternoon. Difficulties with swallowing and speech are not uncommon, and the facial muscles are almost always affected.

### Diagnosis
The diagnosis may be confirmed by administration of edrophonium (the Tensilon test). A parenteral solution of 10 mg should result in improvement of muscular weakness. This disorder must be differentiated from other neurologic conditions that cause general fatigue, including infections such as botulism, several inflammatory myopathies, and amyotrophic lateral sclerosis. The greatest challenge is to distinguish patients with myasthenia gravis from those with neurosis and chronic fatigue. Distinction is difficult during pregnancy, particularly during the first and early second trimester, when fatigue is almost universal.

### Treatment
Treatment with anticholinesterases (eg, neostigmine) is the same as in the nonpregnant state, although dosages need to be administered more frequently during pregnancy. During labor, anticholinesterases should be administered parenterally rather than orally. Curare-like agents, magnesium sulfate, as well as the older general anesthetics such as ether and chloroform, should be avoided. Meperidine and pudendal analgesia or anesthesia are usually employed for delivery, but regional techniques (spinal or epidural anesthesia) are not contraindicated. Women taking anticholinesterase drugs are advised not to breast-feed.

### Complications & Prognosis
One-third of pregnant patients with myasthenia experience exacerbation, one-third do not change, and one-third have a remission. Exacerbations are most common during the postpartum period. Placental transfer of the acetylcholine receptor antibodies will cause 12–15% of newborns to be affected with transient neonatal myasthenia gravis. However, a few neonates will not show symptoms until several days after delivery. Thus, it is important to observe the infant for at least 4–5 days prior to discharge.

## PORPHYRIA

In its most severe form, this hereditary disease involves rapid appearance of peripheral neuropathies and associated nerve palsies coexistent with acute abdominal pain. Rapid respiratory arrest necessitating intubation or tracheostomy is frequent. Acute intermittent porphyria is the most dangerous variety during pregnancy. In more than one-third of patients, porphyria first occurs during pregnancy, and up to 75% of patients experiencing exacerbations during pregnancy. Only 15% go into remission during pregnancy.

### Clinical Findings
Most frequently, patients present with recurrent bouts of abdominal pain. Patients may also present with neurologic symptoms ranging from organic mental syndromes with confusion and coma to asymmetric peripheral neuropathies, particularly those associated with the cranial nerves.

### Diagnosis
A personal or family history of porphyria can be crucial in patients seen for the first time with an attack of acute intermittent porphyria. Likewise, a history of ingestion of an offending drug, such as barbiturates, sulfonamides, or thiopental, is helpful. The differential diagnosis of abdominal pain must include acute surgical emergencies such as appendicitis, cholecystitis, abruptio placentae, and ectopic pregnancy. Quantitative determination of porphobilinogen levels in the urine is specific. Porphyrin metabolism tests also are helpful.

### Treatment
The treatment for acute intermittent porphyria is supportive, particularly for respiratory failure. Anticonvulsants and sedatives, excluding barbiturates, may be helpful, and hypertension (frequently present) is best treated with beta-blocking agents such as propranolol. Infusion of hematin to control enzyme deficiency has not proved helpful. In early pregnancy, there is no benefit from therapeutic abortion, and the procedure is contraindicated during an acute attack.

## Complications & Prognosis

There is significant fetal risk with acute exacerbations of porphyria. A spontaneous abortion rate of about 30% and a fetal loss rate of 40% have been described. The maternal mortality rate is approximately 20%, particularly if the initial attack occurs during pregnancy. If the pregnancy proceeds to term, labor and delivery are usually not affected. Barbiturates and sulfonamides should be avoided, since they may precipitate attacks. There are no known neonatal effects despite passive placental transfer of porphyrins.

## SPINAL CORD DISORDERS

Spinal cord lesions that are caused by trauma, tumor, infection, or vascular disorders usually do not prevent conception. Diagnosis and therapy should be carried out without regard to pregnancy. In general, pregnancy coexisting with trauma to the spinal cord from any cause, even paraplegia, proceeds unremarkably with the exception of an increased frequency of urinary tract infections and sepsis from pressure necrosis of the skin. Fetal growth usually is unimpeded even though initial maternal weight is frequently less than 100 pounds because of muscular wasting. Radiographs to assess pelvic deformities may be helpful, but generally labor proceeds without evidence of fetopelvic disproportion. Women whose paraplegia is related to anterior horn cell damage or to cord lesions below the tenth thoracic level have appropriate perception of labor contractions and may need analgesia or anesthesia. In most patients, rapid, painless labors are the rule with the only abnormality being a prolonged second stage because of decreased muscular effort. Autonomic dysfunction may lead to severe hypotension during labor. This may be avoided with adequate fluid regulation and avoidance of the supine hypotensive syndrome.

## AMYOTROPHIC LATERAL SCLEROSIS

Patients with amyotrophic lateral sclerosis are usually beyond childbearing age, but an occasional pregnancy has been reported. Pregnancy is not usually adversely affected, and the offspring are generally normal; thus, termination of pregnancy gives no maternal benefit. However, decreased longevity characterized by progressive weakness may make family planning and avoidance of future pregnancies desirable.

## WILSON'S DISEASE

Wilson's disease is an autosomal recessive disorder involving degeneration of the hepatolenticular system and is an inborn error of copper metabolism.

Treatment with penicillamine has allowed women who otherwise would have died before reaching childbearing age to become pregnant. Although the effect of penicillamine therapy on the fetus is controversial, most authors believe both pregnancy and infant outcome are normal. Pregnancy has no adverse effects on the disease as long as penicillamine therapy is continued.

## DISORDERS OF CRANIAL & PERIPHERAL NERVES

Palsies of the facial nerve due to inflammation are called **Bell's palsy.** Although patients may complain of paresthesia over the area of paralysis, this is strictly a motor disorder involving paralysis of the facial nerve. Since approximately one-fifth of cases of Bell's palsy occur during pregnancy or shortly thereafter, it has been suggested that pregnancy increases the frequency of this disorder, although viral infections have also been causally related. Treatment with corticosteroids (prednisone, 40–60 mg/d) is helpful if given within 1 week of onset. However, Bell's palsy is usually self-limited, and simple therapy such as closure of the affected eye suffices during the 1- to 5-week course. Rarely is surgical decompression of the nerve indicated.

## GUILLAIN-BARRÉ SYNDROME

Guillain-Barré syndrome is related to a viral respiratory infection and causes a relapsing idiopathic polyneuritis of unusually rapid onset. Most frequently, weakness of the face and extremities and respiratory depression occur, and supportive treatment aimed at preventing respiratory failure is mandatory. Hospitalization is required, and if the vital respiratory capacity falls to 800 mL or below, tracheostomy should be performed. Although the role of corticosteroids is not clear, prednisone, 60 mg/d for 5–7 days in the early course of the disease, is recommended. Immunosuppressants are not helpful. Most patients progress normally through pregnancy and deliver at term; thus, abortion is not mandated. On the other hand, if respiratory paralysis occurs near term, cesarean delivery may be indicated to improve ventilation.

## PERIPHERAL NEUROPATHIES

**Carpal tunnel syndrome** is a neuropathic disorder related to median nerve compression by swelling of the tissue in the synovial sheaths at the wrist. Symptoms are usually limited to paresthesia over the thumb, index, and middle fingers and the medial portion of the ring finger. Most commonly, symptoms are noted at night and are usually best treated conservatively with elevation of the affected wrist and splinting. The syndrome usually abates postpartum. Surgery and corticosteroids are rarely indicated.

**Compression of the obturator nerve** is characterized by adduction weakness of the thigh and minimal sensory loss over the medial aspect of the affected limb. This can occur from retraction at the time of cesarean delivery or hysterectomy, but it is most commonly related to pressure of the fetus just before and during vaginal delivery.

**Peroneal neuropathy** reveals footdrop and weakness on dorsiflexion of the foot, occasionally with paresthesia in the foot and second toes. This disorder usually appears 1–2 days postpartum and may be related to prolonged episiotomy repair and to pressure on the nerve from knee stirrups. Women at risk include small women with relatively large babies, those who have had midforceps rotations, and those who have had prolonged labor, especially with abnormally large infants (owing to compression of L4–5 lumbosacral nerve trunk). The prognosis is excellent with conservative therapy, but occasionally a short leg brace may be necessary.

**Brachialgia** or the **thoracic outlet syndrome** occurs when the brachial plexus and subclavian artery are compressed by the clavicle and first rib. Occurrence in pregnancy is increased because of the greater weight of the breasts and abdomen. The pain is referred to the lateral aspect of the hand and forearm, although motor symptoms are rare. Blanching of the fingers and exacerbation of symptoms when the hands are elevated are diagnostic. The syndrome is usually self-limited; posture instruction and strengthening of shoulder suspension muscles are helpful. Surgical removal of the rib may very occasionally be necessary (as in the nonpregnant patient).

**Herniation of intervertebral disks** occurs more commonly in the lumbar than the cervical region. There are both motor and sensory findings along the distribution of the sciatic nerve. It is limited to one extremity and must be differentiated from more serious disorders such as spinal cord tumors and hemorrhage. Diagnosis can usually be made by physical examination and history. MRI of the spine is the best diagnostic modality. Conservative management with bed rest and pelvic traction is helpful. The process should cause no problems during pregnancy or vaginal delivery unless there is cervical disk disease. In that event, cesarean delivery is advised to prevent herniation and paralysis. Surgical correction should be avoided during pregnancy if possible.

## DISORDERS OF THE SKIN

Many physiologic changes that occur during pregnancy can be noted in the integumentary system and may be confused with disease processes. For example, the impressive vascular changes during pregnancy lead to **erythema** early in gestation, particularly in the midpalmar and thenar areas. Although this sign could be diagnostic of hyperthyroidism, cirrhosis of the liver, or systemic lupus erythematosus, other signs of disease are not present. Palmar erythema usually vanishes postpartum, as do vascular spiders (spider angiomas) and pregnancy-related congestion of the vaginal mucosa.

Although edema in dependent areas is common because of venostasis, **varicosities** of significant size rarely occur unless hereditary valvular incompetence is present. Vascular proliferations such as **capillary hemangiomas** are most commonly seen around the gums, tongue, upper lip, and eyelids, and there is usually a history of preexisting lesions. These usually do not recede completely after pregnancy.

**Striae** are normal findings during pregnancy but also may be observed with adrenocortical hyperactivity (eg, Cushing's syndrome, exogenous corticosteroid administration). Increased activity of the adrenal gland during pregnancy may increase their occurrence, but most physicians think heredity is the most common predictor of the development of these pinkish or purplish lines on the abdomen, buttocks, and breasts. After pregnancy, striae usually becomes silvery-white and sunken, but they rarely disappear. Many remedies have been proposed (vitamin E oil, lubricants, lotions, etc), but none are effective.

**Hyperpigmentation** is common in pregnancy and occurs most frequently in the localized areas of hyperpigmentation (eg, nipples, areolae, and axillas) of dark-skinned persons. Hyperpigmentation is probably related more to the hormones associated with pregnancy (estrogen and progesterone) than to melanocyte-stimulating hormone (MSH). Melasma gravidarum ("mask of pregnancy") has a similar cause but usually develops on the forehead and across the cheeks and nose. It tends to recur and worsen with successive pregnancies. There is no effective treatment during pregnancy, although topical application of hydroquinone 2% after delivery may assist in lightening areas of hyperpigmentation. Preexisting nevi or freckles may increase in pigmentation during pregnancy but usually regress afterward. Hyperpigmentation also occurs in nonpregnant individuals without excess sources of estrogen and progesterone, and it often occurs in women taking oral contraceptives.

Changes in distribution and amount of **hair** are common during pregnancy. Increased hair growth in facial areas and around the breasts is common, particularly during the second and third trimesters. Importantly, there are no signs of virilization, and hirsutism regresses slightly or remains unchanged postpartum. Postpartum loss of hair is fairly common. During pregnancy, the number of hair follicles in the resting phase (telogen) is decreased by about half and then nearly doubles in the first few weeks postpartum. This increased hair loss usually stops in 2–6 months as the hair follicles enter the growing phase (anagen).

Thus, no therapy other than reassurance is required. In women who will subsequently develop female-pattern baldness, there is no increased tendency to lose hair during pregnancy, and the process is not thought to be accelerated.

## PAPULAR DERMATITIS OF PREGNANCY

Papular dermatitis of pregnancy is a rare disorder with an incidence of 3 in 10,000 births; it does not tend to recur with subsequent pregnancies. In some patients, intradermal skin testing with placental extracts from their own delivery has suggested an allergic reaction. Many dermatologists consider this disorder to be a variant of pruritic urticarial papules and plaques of pregnancy (PUPPP), although it is less common.

### Clinical Findings
Papular dermatitis of pregnancy presents as an intensely pruritic eruption of diffuse erythematous papules. Because of the severe pruritus, most lesions are excoriated and then heal after 1 week, leaving a hyperpigmented spot.

### Diagnosis
The level of hCG is high in the few patients in whom it has been measured. Prurigo of pregnancy is difficult to exclude because the lesions are similar to those of papular dermatitis, except that they are located predominantly on the proximal portion of the limbs, and the pruritus is less intense. Also, prurigo of pregnancy most often appears in the third trimester and is not associated with an increased fetal loss rate.

### Treatment
Treatment of papular dermatitis of pregnancy is symptomatic (oral trimeprazine and topical calamine lotion), but oral corticosteroids are required in some cases. Corticosteroids given at a high dosage with rapid tapering are effective in most cases. Sulfapyridine and diethylstilbestrol should be avoided as they are clinically ineffective and have teratogenic effects. When symptoms do not resolve spontaneously following delivery, D&C including removal of retained placental tissue is usually curative.

### Complications & Prognosis
The effect on pregnancy is difficult to ascertain because of the small number of reported cases. A high fetal loss rate (up to 27%) may occur; however, losses after the disorder is diagnosed are uncommon. In addition, a large percentage of the reported patients were Rh-isoimmunized; this factor may have been responsible for some of the fetal losses. Nevertheless, fetal prognosis is guarded.

## PRURITIC URTICARIAL PAPULES AND PLAQUES OF PREGNANCY

Pruritic urticarial papules and plaques of pregnancy (PUPPP syndrome) may be the most common of all the pruritic skin conditions that occur during pregnancy. The lesions usually appear during the third trimester and disappear completely within 2 weeks after delivery.

### Clinical Findings
The pruritic papules are generally red, unexcoriated, and found principally on the abdomen and thighs. In most lesions a marked halo surrounds the small papules and plaques. Focal lesions are rare and never appear on the face or distal extremities. The lesions may be indistinguishable from those of papular dermatitis of pregnancy or herpes gestationis.

### Diagnosis
Human chorionic gonadotropin levels are normal, and immunofluorescence reveals no immunoglobulin or complement, unlike the case with papular dermatitis of pregnancy.

### Treatment
Symptomatic treatment with antihistamines and antipruritic medications is usually curative. Occasionally, corticosteroid therapy is necessary.

### Complications & Prognosis
This disorder appears to have no ill effect on the mother or the fetus and is self-limiting.

## HERPES GESTATIONIS

Herpes gestationis has an incidence of 2 per 10,000 gestations and usually appears in the second and third trimester. Despite its name, the herpes virus is not the causative agent, and the etiology remains unknown. It is suspected that elevated hormone levels during pregnancy are causative since progestins can induce exacerbations. Radioimmunoassay classifies the typical lesion as an immunologic reaction localized in the lamina lucida of the basement membrane where IgG, C3, and a circulating immunoglobulin G (known as HG factor) are found.

### Clinical Findings
Systemic signs of herpes gestationis may be severe and include malaise, fever, and chills. The lesion appears as erythematous plaques with vesicles that soon form bullae in the periphery of the lesion. The typical blistering eruption has a herpetiform appearance, but the vesicles are not clustered and are more peripheral than herpes. Lesions usually begin on the trunk and spread to the entire body, including the distal extremities. Lesions on mucous membranes are uncommon.

### Diagnosis

Most patients with herpes gestationis have circulating IgG that will fix C3 complement. The pattern of immunofluorescence suggests a relationship to bullous pemphigoid. Pathologically, a distinct immunofluorescent change between normal and affected skin is noted. Immunofluoresence testing of bullous lesions aids in establishing the diagnosis. Pemphigus vulgaris can be differentiated by histologic examination, while the pustules, fever, and hypocalcemia of impetigo herpetiformis are not present in herpes gestationis. Dermatitis herpetiformis is excluded because, while it is pruritic, the clusters of vesicles do not form bullae, and there are no plaques. In herpes gestationis a crust forms, and after the lesion heals there is a hyperpigmented area but little or no scarring.

### Treatment

Corticosteroids, administered orally, are the treatment of choice.

### Complications & Prognosis

Unlike most of the dermatologic conditions discussed thus far, herpes gestationis is characterized by exacerbations and remissions during pregnancy. While significant exacerbations can occur postpartum, the condition usually abates by the sixth week postpartum. Recurrence is frequent in subsequent pregnancies, and the disorder may appear earlier in pregnancy than the other disorders discussed. Its effect on maternal and fetal morbidity is not clear because it is so rare, but an increase in stillbirths and premature births has been reported.

## IMPETIGO HERPETIFORMIS

Impetigo herpetiformis (also called pustular psoriasis, von Zumbusch's type) is a pustular eruption on an erythematous base with total body distribution. It is rare and probably represents an acute form of psoriasis occurring during pregnancy. Pregnancy may precipitate this acute manifestation, but the disease is not restricted to gestation since it has been documented in nonpregnant women and in males. Most patients with this disease also have chronic psoriasis or a family history of psoriasis.

### Clinical Findings

Generalized erythematous patches covered with sterile pustules allow a presumptive diagnosis. Fever and malaise often accompany this symptom complex.

### Diagnosis

Spongiform pustules noted in the epidermis on biopsy distinguish this disorder from pustular dermatosis or infection. The pustules are usually sterile, but they may become secondarily infected. In addition, pruritus is not a prominent symptom. The disorder is almost always associated with hypocalcemia, and this helps to distinguish it from other types of dermatologic problems that may occur during pregnancy.

### Treatment

Treatment is usually limited to supportive measures, occasional corticosteroids, and appropriate antibiotics for superimposed infection. Methotrexate and tetracycline have been recommended for nonpregnant patients but probably should not be used during pregnancy, because their efficacy in this disorder is questionable and does not outweigh the risk of these drugs to the fetus.

### Complications & Prognosis

There are inadequate data on the fetal effects of this disorder. There have been reports of increased maternal and perinatal mortality, but reports of such problems may have been related to secondary infection and sepsis.

## DISORDERS OF THE GASTROINTESTINAL TRACT PEPTIC ULCER DISEASE

Pregnancy usually ameliorates extension of ulceration, and an initial attack rarely occurs during pregnancy. The salutary effect of pregnancy may be related to progesterone's ability to inhibit motility, because acid secretion remains unchanged. The incidence of peptic ulcer disease in pregnancy is rare (1 in 4000 deliveries); it seems to be more common when there is associated preeclampsia. If activation of previously dormant ulcer disease does occur, it is usually in the puerperium.

### Clinical Findings

The classic signs of gastric or duodenal ulcer are related to a burning epigastric pain that is relieved by meals or antacids. Peptic ulcer disease must be differentiated from reflex esophagitis or simple heartburn, which commonly occurs during pregnancy. Patients with a gastric or duodenal ulcer most often report discomfort rather than pain and describe this feeling as "acid" or burning or indigestion.

### Diagnosis

The above symptoms of peptic ulcer disease are relieved by food and return approximately 1–2 hours later, paralleling gastric acidity. Likewise, antacids may relieve the pain and help confirm the diagnosis. Most commonly, the diagnosis is confirmed by endoscopic visualization of the ulcer crater in the stomach or duodenum. Although gastric carcinoma is rare, many physicians recommend biopsy during the endoscopic procedure. Upper gastrointestinal x-rays with barium studies are usually avoided because of radiation exposure and because endoscopy is a more direct diagnostic method. Gastric analysis or serum pepsinogen levels are not used in establishing the diagnosis of peptic ulcer disease during pregnancy.

### Treatment

Documented peptic ulcer disorders are treated symptomatically during pregnancy by avoidance of symptom-provoking foods and by antacids. Supportive advice may be given regarding cessation of smoking, bed rest, avoidance of stress, and so on. Patients who require additional therapy can be given $H_2$-receptor antagonists such as cimetidine. Newer drugs such as ranitidine (Zantac) should not be used during the first trimester, as animal studies have revealed possible teratogenicity. Sucralfate should be avoided, because it has not been adequately studied during pregnancy. Carbenoxolone is best avoided during pregnancy, because it may cause fluid retention and electrolyte imbalance.

### Complications & Prognosis

In general, the fetus is not adversely affected by peptic ulcer disease unless maternal compromise, such as perforated ulcer with bleeding, occurs. Particular vigilance in the postpartum period is necessary because ulcers become active again during this time and can become penetrating.

## INFLAMMATORY BOWEL DISEASE

Inflammatory bowel disease encompasses regional enteritis (Crohn's disease), ulcerative colitis, and granulomatous colitis. In general, inflammatory bowel disease has no effect on fertility unless colonic disease has resulted in pelvic abscesses. Recurrences are more frequent in the first trimester and postpartum but are usually easily treated. Relapse rates are not significantly different (by age) from those in nonpregnant women. Subsequent pregnancies will not necessarily have the same course.

### Clinical Findings

In these conditions, cramping, lower abdominal pain, and diarrhea are the main complaints. Weight loss and anorexia, even during pregnancy, may occur, as may electrolyte imbalance with severe diarrhea.

### Diagnosis

Infectious disorders that would cause diarrhea and abdominal pain must be ruled out. A personal or family history of inflammatory bowel disease is helpful in confirming the diagnosis. If the lower intestine is involved, proctoscopy or colonoscopy may be helpful. However, in some cases a small bowel series and barium enema are needed to make the diagnosis. Malignancy and infectious disease such as tuberculosis of the small intestine also must be considered because they have appearances similar to inflammatory bowel

disease on x-ray. Finally, a response to trials of medication and a change in diet may be helpful in confirming the diagnosis.

### Treatment

Treatment for inflammatory bowel disease usually involves dietary management and use of corticosteroids. Sulfasalazine inhibits prostaglandin synthesis, which is thought to be important in bowel disease. Although sulfasalazine and corticosteroids cross the placenta, their use during pregnancy may be preferable to acute exacerbations of disease. If sulfasalazine is used, maternal folic acid should be given daily. Other immunosuppressant drugs have not been shown to be helpful and should not be used during pregnancy.

### Complications & Prognosis

Complications during pregnancy are similar to those in the nonpregnant state, eg, abdominal pain, cramping, and rectal bleeding. Women with ulcerative colitis have a normal abortion rate (15–18%), whereas the rate for those with Crohn's disease is increased to 25%. In later pregnancy, there is no greater risk in either condition of premature delivery, congenital malformation, or fetal loss. Thus, pregnancy is not contraindicated with inflammatory bowel disease, but when possible the disorder should be controlled by surgery or medication prior to conception. Pregnancy does not exert an adverse effect on inflammatory bowel disease. Approximately half of women with ulcerative colitis have flare-ups during pregnancy, but when the disease is under control, these women have fewer relapses than those who have active disease at the time of conception.

## CHOLECYSTITIS

**Cholecystitis** occurs rarely during pregnancy (0.3%) because the gallbladder and biliary duct smooth muscle is relaxed by progesterone. Acute inflammation during pregnancy is treated with intravenous fluids and nasogastric suction. If acute cholecystitis does not resolve or if pancreatitis develops, cholecystectomy should be considered. If this operation can be performed in the second trimester, the fetal loss rate is not increased. Abortion during the first trimester is not increased, but in the third trimester, the uterus frequently must be emptied before the gallbladder can be surgically exposed. In this situation, prolonged IV hyperalimentation may be required to avoid preterm delivery.

## INTRAHEPATIC CHOLESTASIS

Intrahepatic cholestasis is a condition characterized by accumulation of bile acids in the liver with subsequent accumulation in the plasma, causing pruritus and jaundice. It is similar to the cholestasis that occasionally occurs during oral contraceptive therapy. Estrogen and progesterone are therefore considered to play a role in its etiology. Ultrasound examination of the gallbladder helps rule out cholelithiasis. If hepatitis is not present, the most likely diagnosis is cholestasis associated with pregnancy. The disease is usually self-limited, and maternal serum bilirubin levels are only modestly elevated. Considerable controversy surrounds the fetal effects of this condition but most data indicate a slight increase in preterm births and stillbirth and maternal postpartum hemorrhage. Treatment is symptomatic; cholestyramine is the drug most frequently used. Since this drug decreases absorption of fat-soluble vitamins, vitamin K supplementation of the mother and newborn is necessary.

## ACUTE FATTY LIVER OF PREGNANCY

Acute fatty liver of pregnancy is a rare complication (1 in 13,000), which in the past had maternal and fetal mortality rates of 75–85%. Early recognition and termination of the pregnancy (delivery) and extensive supportive therapy have reduced the mortality rate to approximately 20%. This condition usually occurs late in pregnancy (> 35 weeks). There is no increased risk of recurrence in subsequent pregnancies. Signs and symptoms are protean, but elevated serum transaminase levels assist in diagnosis. Although liver necrosis is not extensive, pathologically there is an increase in cytoplasmic fat within hepatocytes and liver changes are similar to those seen in Reye's syndrome. Parenteral tetracycline administration has been incriminated in this disorder, although most cases occur spontaneously.

## HELLP SYNDROME

A disorder that mimics acute fatty liver of pregnancy is the HELLP (*h*emolysis, *l*iver dysfunction, *l*ow *p*latelets) syndrome. Typically, this liver derangement occurs with severe preeclampsia and eclampsia. Symptoms are similar to those of fatty liver of pregnancy, but intrahepatic and subcapsular hemorrhage are more common. The disorder occurs in the last trimester of pregnancy and is characterized by vomiting, upper quadrant pain, and progressive nausea. Liver function deteriorates rapidly, and delivery is essential in treatment. Stillbirth is frequent (10–15%), with a high neonatal loss (20–25%) usually due to prematurity. (See also Chapter 19.)

## VIRAL HEPATITIS

Viral hepatitis complicates 0.2% of all pregnancies. Hepatitis may be caused by numerous viruses, drugs, or toxic chemicals; the clinical manifestations of all forms are similar. The development of specific serologic markers has improved the accuracy of the diagnosis. The most common viral agents causing hepatitis in pregnancy are hepatitis A virus, hepatitis B virus, hepatitis C (non-A, non-B hepatitis virus), and Epstein-Barr virus. Delta agent hepatitis has also received increasing attention as a cause of hepatitis.

**A. Hepatitis A:** Hepatitis A may occur sporadically or in epidemics. A generalized viremia occurs with the infection that is predominantly hepatic. The primary mode of transmission is the fecal-oral route. Excretion of the virus in stool normally begins approximately 2 weeks prior to the onset of clinical symptoms and is complete within 3 weeks following onset of clinical symptoms. No known carrier state exists for the virus. Both blood and stool are infectious during the 2–6 week incubation period.

The hepatitis A virus belongs to the picornavirus group, which also includes poliomyelitis virus and coxsackievirus. It is a 27-nm RNA virus that is readily deactivated by ultraviolet light or heat.

**B. Hepatitis B:** Hepatitis B is usually transmitted by inoculation of infected blood or blood products, or sexual intercourse. The virus is contained in most body secretions. Infection by oral and sexual contact has been well documented. The virus is frequently present in intravenous drug abusers and homosexuals. Other groups at risk for hepatitis B infection are medical, hemodialysis, blood bank, and medical laboratory personnel; spouses of hepatitis carriers; prostitutes and others with multiple sexual partners; and Southeast Asian emigrants. Approximately 5–10% of people infected with hepatitis B virus become chronic carriers of the virus. The incubation period of hepatitis B is 6 weeks to 6 months. The clinical features of hepatitis A and B are similar, although hepatitis B is more insidious. Additionally, fulminant hepatitis is very rare with hepatitis A but occurs in approximately 1% of patients infected with hepatitis B.

The hepatitis B virus is a DNA hepadnavirus. It is pleomorphic, occurring in spherical and tubular forms of different sizes. The largest of these, the 42-nm Dane particle, is the complete infectious agent, which is composed of a surface coat and a 27-nm central core. The surface antigen (HBsAg) of the Dane particle is the marker usually measured in blood. The presence of HBsAg is the first manifestation of viral infection; it usually appears before clinical evidence of the disease and lasts throughout the infection. Persistence of HBsAg after the acute phase of hepatitis is usually associated with clinical and laboratory evidence of chronic hepatitis. The core antibody (HBcAb) is produced against the 27-nm core of the

Dane particle. Core particles and antigen are not normally present in blood except in overwhelming infections. HBcAb occurs with acute hepatitis B infection at the onset of clinical illness. Hepatitis B e antigen (HBeAg) is a soluble, nonparticulate antigen that is found only when HBsAg is present. HBeAg probably serves as an accurate indicator of viral replication and infectivity. Pregnant women who are HBeAg-positive in the third trimester frequently transmit this infection to the fetus, whereas those who are negative rarely infect the fetus. DNA polymerase activity is usually transient, occurring with peak HBsAg positivity; however, its persistence usually suggests continued infectivity.

**C. Hepatitis C (Non-A, Non-B Hepatitis):** Hepatitis C is probably caused by 2 or more viral agents, which are currently poorly defined. About 90% of posttransfusion hepatitis is now caused by hepatitis C. The incubation period is usually 7–8 weeks but may vary from 3–21 weeks. A chronic carrier state for hepatitis C exists. The course of infection is similar to that of hepatitis B. Hepatitis C antibody is present in approximately 90% of these patients.

**D. Epstein-Barr Virus:** Epstein-Barr virus causes the clinical picture of infectious mononucleosis with hepatitis. Serologic testing for this agent involves determining antibody titers to latently infected (anti-EGNA), early replication cycle (anti-EA), or late replication cycle (anti-VCA) viral proteins.

**E. Delta Agent:** Hepatitis delta virus is an RNA virus that is smaller than all other known RNA viruses. The agent can cause infection only when HBsAg positivity exists. Delta agent is isolated in up to 50% of cases of fulminant hepatitis B infection. HDAg (hepatitis delta antigen) and HDAb (hepatitis delta antibody) are serologic markers for the disease.

## Clinical Findings

The clinical picture of hepatitis is highly variable; most patients have asymptomatic infection, while a few may present with fulminating disease and die within a few days. General malaise, myalgia, arthralgia, easy fatigability, and severe anorexia are frequent symptoms, as are nausea, vomiting, and low-grade fever. Mild hepatomegaly occurs in over 50% of cases; splenomegaly occurs in an additional 15%. The white blood cell count is depressed and mild proteinuria and bilirubinuria occur early in the course of the disease. AST (SGOT), ALT (SGPT), bilirubin, and alkaline phosphatase are usually elevated. Prothrombin and partial thromboplastin times may also be prolonged with severe liver involvement.

## Diagnosis

The diagnosis is made using the previously described serologic markers. The differential diagnosis of viral hepatitis should include viruses A, B, C, and delta, Epstein-Barr virus, cytomegalovirus infection, TORCH infections, secondary syphilis, Q fever, and toxic or drug-induced hepatitis. Additionally, intra- or extra hepatic bile duct obstruction should be included.

## Treatment

Bedrest should be instituted during the acute phase of the illness. If nausea, vomiting, or anorexia is prominent, intravenous hydration and general supportive measures are instituted. All hepatotoxic agents should be avoided. Antepartum fetal assessment should be instituted in the third trimester because of the increased risks of premature delivery and stillbirth. Gamma globulin prophylaxis should be given to pregnant women exposed to hepatitis A or non-A, non-B hepatitis. Hepatitis B immunoglobulin may be given to those parenterally exposed to blood or secretions from hepatitis B-infected individuals. Hepatitis B vaccine should be administered to an HBsAg-negative patient whose spouse is HGsAg-positive. Hepatitis B immunoglobulin, 0.5 mL intramuscularly with a repeat dose at 3 and 6 months, should be administered to neonates born of HBsAg-positive mothers, to decrease the risk of vertical transmission. These infants should also receive hepatitis B vaccine.

## Complications & Prognosis

The acute illness usually resolves rapidly in 2–3 weeks with complete recovery usually occurring within 8 weeks. In 10% of cases of type B & C hepatitis, chronic persistent or chronic active hepatitis develops. Additionally, 1–3% of patients develop acute fulminant hepatitis.

The maternal course of viral hepatitis is unaltered by pregnancy, but prematurity may be increased. In general, with severe liver disease, infertility results. Chronic active hepatitis does not mandate therapeutic abortion, but there is an increase in fetal loss. All pregnant women should routinely be tested for HBsAg during an early prenatal visit in each pregnancy. Women with cirrhosis of the liver from other causes have an outcome related to the extent of maternal disease, but perinatal loss rates are usually high with a poor maternal prognosis, particularly with poor liver function or esophageal varices. Pregnancy in women with liver transplants has been reported and, in general, has an uncomplicated prenatal and delivery course. Treatment with immunosuppressants and corticosteroids usually does not interdict pregnancy. Interferon therapy improves the prognosis for chronic active hepatitis.

The effect of chronic active hepatitis on the fetus and newborn depends on the extent of maternal disease. Fetal infection in utero is rare, but the neonate may be exposed to the virus at delivery and the virus may be spread by breast-feeding. The pediatrician should be notified at delivery of a mother with hepatitis B, since the infant needs to be followed closely for liver function and for antigen-antibody status.

# DISORDERS OF THE THYROID

In pregnancy, the diagnosis of thyroid disease is difficult because of both normal gravid physiologic changes and the hypertrophy of the thyroid gland encountered in pregnancy. Triiodothyronine ($T_3$) is the active thyroid hormone resulting from peripheral metabolism of thyroxine ($T_4$). Thyroid-binding globulin (TBG; the major protein fraction responsible for carrying bound thyroxine), albumin, and prealbumin increases with pregnancy, thus increasing both total $T_4$ and $_3$. These alterations are thought to be secondary to the increase in total and free estrogen.

This hormonal milieu of pregnancy complicates interpretation of thyroid function studies. The $T_3$ resin uptake ($T_3RU$) decreases secondary to an increase in carrier proteins. The functional (free) $T_4$ can be estimated by creating a fraction of the normal for $T_3RU$ (measured $T_3RU$ over the mean of normal) and multiplying by the level of $T_4$. This can also be done for $T_3$. An example of this is as follows: If the normal range of $T_3RU$ is 25–35%, then 30% is the mean. If the $T_3RU$ is 15%, then 15 is divided by 30 and multiplied by the $T_4$ level (16 µmg/dL); the result is 8 µmg/dL; a level that is within normal limits for $T_4$. For a $T_3RIA$ (normal, 80–200 ng/dL), a value of 250 ng/dL is reduced to 125 ng/dL. Such calculations are necessary to evaluate any patient with an increased estrogenic state, whether due to pregnancy or to exogenous estrogen therapy. Tests that are the most important in diagnosing the various disease states are $T_3RU$, $T_4$, $T_7$ (or free thyroid index, which is a multiple of $T_3RU$ and $T_4$, and eliminates hormonal influence), and thyroid-stimulating hormone (TSH; a pituitary hormone that is not altered by changes in pregnancy hormone levels or carrier protein levels). TSH is most important in diagnosing and following hypothyroidism, whereas $T_3RIA$ is most important in diagnosing hyperthyroidism.

## HYPOTHYROIDISM

Hypothyroidism is generally thought to be an immunologic disease with a multifactorial inheritance; it is found predominantly in females. One of the more common causes is iatrogenic, ie, patients are told to stop thyroid replacement medications to observe for possible resolution of the condition. The primary condition is usually associated with a goiter (due to the gland's inability to produce $T_4$ and $T_3$, which results

in hypertrophy of the organ). The goiter is generally multinodular and can reach such size as to cause local symptoms and potential airway obstruction. Primary hypothyroidism is usually secondary to chronic thyroiditis, prior radioactive iodine therapy, thyroidectomy, or the ingestion of goitrogens (eg, thiocyanates, lithium carbonate, amiodarone). Secondary hypothyroidism due to chromophobe adenoma of the pituitary gland, or Sheehan's syndrome, is very rare.

### Clinical Findings

General complaints include skin dryness, weakness, fatigue, hoarseness, yellowing of the skin (especially in the periorbital area), hair loss, cold intolerance, constipation, and sleep disturbances. Physical examination of hypothyroid patients usually reveals a goiter and delayed relaxation of deep tendon reflexes. Anemia, low $T_4$, and elevated TSH are characteristic in laboratory findings.

### Treatment

Most patients with early hypothyroidism may be started on 50–100 µm/d of levothyroxine. The dosage is increased by 25 µmg/d per week until the patient is euthyroid. Most patients will require 100–200 µmg/d of thyroxine for maintenance therapy. Optimal maintenance therapy can be determined by clinical symptoms, TSH levels, and free thyroxine index.

### Complications & Prognosis

Congestive heart failure is the most serious complications of hypothyroidism. Megacolon, adrenal crisis, organic psychosis, and myxedema coma are other complications of hypothyroidism. Hyponatremia secondary to the syndrome of inappropriate secretion of antidiuretic hormone (SIADH) may also occur. Prognosis for both mother and fetus is excellent when hypothyroidism is corrected in pregnancy. Antepartum fetal assessment in the third trimester is indicated because of a small increase in the stillbirth rate.

## THYROIDITIS

Thyroiditis has been diagnosed with increasing frequency in recent years. This disorder is most commonly autoimmune in etiology; viral infection of the thyroid is the second most common cause.

### Clinical Findings
**A. Hashimoto's Thyroiditis:** Hashimoto's disease (struma lymphomatosa) is a chronic inflammatory disease of the thyroid that is believed to be due to the generation of antibodies directed against several components of thyroid tissue. It is the most common thyroid disorder and the most common cause of hypothyroidism. This disorder has a high association with other autoimmune diseases (Sjögren's syndrome, systemic lupus erythematosus, rheumatoid arthritis, dia-

betes, and Graves' disease), and other family members frequently have the condition. Glandular lymphocytic infiltration results in a uniform goiter with a rubbery consistency on palpation. Early in the disease, the patient may be metabolically normal with goiter as the only symptom. The diagnosis is confirmed by biopsy and from a positive tanned erythrocyte agglutination test revealing antibodies to thyroglobulin. Eventually, hypothyroidism develops, and treatment with thyroxine is indicated.

**B. Acute or Subacute Nonsuppurative Thyroiditis:** Nonsuppurative thyroiditis is usually acute in onset with painful enlargement of the thyroid, dysphagia, and pain radiating to the ears. The disease may be associated with either hyper- or hypothyroidism. Viral infection has been implicated as the most common cause.

**C. Lymphocytic Subacute Thyroiditis:** Lymphocytic subacute thyroiditis is characterized by insidious, painless enlargement of the thyroid gland with associated hyperthyroidism. The hyperthyroidism is transient and secondary to release of stored thyroxin owing to glandular inflammation. Therapy for hyperthyroidism is not required. The etiology of the disorder remains unclear and thyroid biopsy may be required to establish the diagnosis.

**D. Postpartum Thyroiditis:** Postpartum thyroiditis is an' autoimmune disorder occurring in patients shortly after parturition. Transient hyperthyroidism is usually followed by hypothyroidism. Spontaneous recovery is generally anticipated, but recurrence during future pregnancies is common.

**E. Riedel's Thyroiditis:** Riedel's thyroiditis is the rarest form of thyroiditis and occurs only in middle-aged gravidas. The gland is enlarged, adherent, asymmetrical, and stony hard.

## Diagnosis

The $T_3RU$ and $T_4$ are usually elevated in acute forms of thyroiditis but are usually normal or decreased in chronic forms. Thyroid antibodies occur most commonly with Hashimoto's disease but also may be elevated with other forms of thyroiditis.

## Treatment

**A. Subacute or Acute Thyroiditis:** The drug of choice is aspirin, which decreases pain, inflammation, and swelling of the thyroid gland. Prednisone in doses of 20–30 mg/d for 1–2 weeks may also decrease pain, inflammation, and swelling. The disease is usually self-limited.

**B. Lymphocytic Thyroiditis:** Hyperthyroidism associated with this disorder is usually self-limited and transient. No therapy is required. If symptoms are severe, they may be relieved with short-term propranolol therapy. Late-occurring hypothyroidism usually requires thyroid hormone replacement as described above for hypothyroidism.

**C. Hashimoto's Disease.** Levothyroxine therapy (0.1–0.2 mg/d) is indicated in the presence of hypothyroidism or in the presence of a large goiter. The dosage should be adjusted by the clinical response and the $T_4$ and TSH levels. If no goiter exists or the patient is euthyroid, no specific therapy is indicated.

## Complications & Prognosis

Hashimoto's thyroiditis frequently leads to clinical hypothyroidism. Hashimoto's disease may also be associated with Addison's disease, hypoparathyroidism, diabetes, pernicious anemia, collagen vascular disease, and other immune disorders. The incidence of mitral valve prolapse is also increased in patients with thyroiditis.

Spontaneous remissions and exacerbations are common with most forms of thyroiditis. Rarely, lymphoma or carcinoma of the thyroid gland develops. Autoantibodies (IgG variety) rarely cross the placenta to cause thyroiditis in the fetus. In general, the prognosis for mother and fetus is very good in the presence of thyroiditis.

## HYPERTHYROIDISM

The incidence of maternal hyperthyroidism ranges from 0.05% to 0.2% during pregnancy. The most frequent etiologies, in order of frequency, are Graves' disease, acute (subacute) thyroiditis, toxic nodular goiter, and toxic adenoma.

**Graves' disease** is more frequent in women and is found most frequently in the third and fourth decades. In non-iodide-deficient geographic regions, the ratio of predominance in women may be as high as 7:1. The cause of Graves' disease is unknown, but it appears to be an autoimmune disorder that develops in genetically susceptible individuals. Sera of patients with Graves' disease reveal IgG elaborated by long-acting thyroid stimulator (LATS). The diagnostic triad for Graves' disease includes hyperthyroidism with diffuse goiter, ophthalmopathy, and dermopathy. However, these 3 major manifestations may not appear together. The disease is characterized by unpredictable intervals of exacerbation and remission but appears to be precipitated by emotional trauma or by metabolic stress. It may also be associated with other systemic autoimmune disorders such as pernicious anemia, myasthenia gravis, and diabetes mellitus. Graves' disease has a familial·tendency with a propensity to occur in individuals with HLA-B8 and -DW3 haplotypes.

**Acute (subacute) thyroiditis** appears to be viral in origin, with symptoms (asthenia, malaise, and pain due to stretching of the thyroid capsule) usually following an upper respiratory infection. Additionally, pain over the thyroid or, more commonly, referred to the lower jaw or ear is perceived. These symptoms may be present for many weeks before the diagnosis is clear. Less commonly, the onset is acute with severe pain over the thyroid accompanied by fever and occasionally by symptoms of thyrotoxicosis.

**Toxic nodular goiter** appears to be an infrequent consequence of long-standing simple goiter. Viral toxicosis may develop spontaneously in multinodular goiters (Plummer's disease) or in single nodular goiters. The syndrome may also be the consequence of exogenous iodide in patients with nodular goiters. Affected individuals are usually more than 40 years of age.

True **toxic adenomas** of the thyroid are encapsulated and usually compressed contiguous tissues. They vary greatly in size, histologic characteristics, and ability to concentrate radioiodine. They may be classified into 3 major types: papillary, follicular, and those with Hauurthle cells. Adenoma function is independent of TSH stimulation. Clinically, they usually present as a solitary nodule. In time, nodular function increases, with subsequent atrophy and decrease of function in the remainder of the gland. Initially, the patient may not be thyrotoxic, but frank thyrotoxicosis usually develops (thus the term *toxic adenoma*).

### Clinical Findings

Restlessness, nervousness, fatigue, unexplained weight loss, loose stools, and night sweats are frequent signs and symptoms of hyperthyroidism, as are excess sweating, heat intolerance, a rapid pulse, warm, moist skin, and trembling hands. Goiter and spider angiomas are usually present on physical examination. Cardiac manifestations vary from mild sinus tachycardia to paroxysmal atrial fibrillation and high-output congestive heart failure.

The $T_4$ and $T_3RU$ are usually increased. The T4 is frequently higher than 16 $\mu$mg/dL in patients with accompanying hyperthyroidism. In patients with Graves' disease, antithyroid antibodies (antimicrosomal and antithyroglobulin) are frequently positive. TSH is usually very low.

### Treatment

All therapies of hyperthyroidism initially concentrate on slowing release or stopping conversion of $T_4$ to $T_3$. Management is separated into 4 physiologic stages: (1) therapy against the thyroid gland; (2) therapy to avoid decompensation of normal homeostatic mechanisms; (3) therapy against peripheral conversion of $T_4$ to $T_3$; and (4) therapy against the coexistent illness. Therapy against the hyperactive thyroid gland is directed at inhibiting the new synthesis of additional $T_3$ and $T_4$; in pregnancy, propylthiouracil is probably the drug of choice. In severe hyperthyroidism, doses of 100–200 mg 4 times a day may be required. Mild hyperthyroidism will usually respond to 100 mg 3 times a day. Symptoms of hyperthyroidism will usually decrease 2–3 weeks after the institution of propylthiouracil therapy. After the hyperthyroidism is controlled, propylthiouracil should be de-

creased to the lowest effective dose to maintain the $T_4$ at approximately 14 $\mu$mg/dL, usually a dose of less than 200 mg/d.

In the face of impending thyroid storm, therapy to avoid decompensation of normal homeostatic mechanisms should also be rapidly undertaken. Treatment of hyperthermia with acetaminophen suppositories (aspirin should be avoided as it can cause displacement of thyroxine from TBG), and cooling blankets can be effective. General therapy should also include the use of intravenous multivitamin preparations, glucose, and fluids and electrolytes. Oxygen therapy, vasopressor agents to correct hypotension, and diuretics for cardiac decompensation are indicated as needed. Because this condition could be secondary to an immunologic dysfunction, the use of 100 mg of hydrocortisone intravenously every 6–8 hours is also indicated. Corticosteroids have the additional benefit of blocking conversion of $T_4$ to $T_3$.

Therapy directed against the conversion of $T_4$ to $T_3$ is an important aspect of the care of patients with impending thyroid storm. Again, propylthiouracil is especially important in this regard; methimazole does not possess the ability to block conversion of $T_4$ to $T_3$, limiting its usefulness. The dosage of propylthiouracil should be less than 250 mg every 4 hours with a maximum total dose of 1500 mg/d. No parenteral formulation exists for this agent; therefore, B-adrenergic blockade has become the most important therapeutic modality in the acute phases of treatment. Propranolol has been the standard beta-blocking agent employed because of its physiologic role in controlling heart rate as well as blocking peripheral conversion of $T_4$ to $T_3$. The dosage of propranolol for the patient in thyroid storm is 60–120 mg orally every 6 hours until the pulse rate falls below 90 beats/min, at which time the dosage can be halved. In patients who will need emergent cesarean section, the use of the intravenous formulation for rapid control is preferred. It is of utmost importance to remember that the intravenous preparation is extremely potent: The starting dose of propranolol is 0.5–1 mg followed by 2–3 mg every 10–15 minutes. Again, a heart rate less than 90 beats/min is the desired endpoint. Another option for IV use has been a newer short-acting beta blocker, esmolol. If the patient has a history of bronchospasm, the use of propranolol is contraindicated; metoprolol tartrate (Lopressor), a $B_1$-adrenergic blocking agent, should be substituted. The dosage for metoprolol is 5 mg every 2 minutes to a maximum dose of 15 mg. The $B_1$-selective blocking agents still carry a possibility of bronchospasm (1%), making frequent physical examinations mandatory. In the patient with mild congestive heart failure secondary to hyperthyroidism, beta blockers are helpful. By increasing ventricular filling time, congestive heart failure can be reversed by allowing larger stroke volumes. In this clinical situation, a pulmonary artery catheter should be placed to monitor pulmonary wedge pressures.

The last therapy for thyroid storm relates to treatment of the underlying disease. If the patient presents with cardiovascular decompensation, use of a pulmonary artery catheter for volume and fluid management should be considered early. Volume replacement can be as high as 5 L or more per day, making pulmonary edema a potential complication. Plasma exchange may be considered, since success has been reported in several cases with severe thyrotoxicosis refractory to medical management.

## Complications & Prognosis

The ocular and cardiac disturbances are generally the most serious complications of hyperthyroidism. Periodic paralysis and hypokalemia following exercise or carbohydrate ingestion may rarely complicate hyperthyroidism. Hypercalcemia or thyroid storm occur rarely but carry substantial mortality rates. Exophthalmos may require surgical decompression to prevent corneal ulceration.

Graves' disease is a cyclic disease and may subside spontaneously. With adequate treatment and follow-up, the long-term maternal prognosis is excellent. Fetal prognosis with well-controlled hyperthyroidism is also excellent. However, 2 fetal precautions are necessary: A few studies have reported an increased stillbirth rate with maternal hyperthyroidism; thus, antepartum fetal assessment is probably indicated in the third trimester. A fetal goiter rarely may lead to extension of the head at delivery, necessitating operative delivery. Skilled resuscitation of the newborn after delivery may be needed if the airway is obstructed by a goiter.

---

# DISORDERS OF THE PARATHYROID

---

During normal pregnancy, the maternal parathyroid undergoes hyperplasia and increased hormone production. Serum levels of parathyroid hormone (PTH) rise progressively throughout pregnancy, but there is no correlation between total serum calcium and serum PTH levels. The total serum calcium begins to fall during the second or third month of gestation and reaches a nadir at 28–32 weeks (5 meq/L, nonpregnant level; 4.6 meq/L at term). This decrease in serum calcium is attributed to the dilutional hypoalbuminemia (4.3–3.4 g/dL) of pregnancy without alteration in the protein binding of calcium. The serum ionized calcium level remains unchanged during pregnancy (2.3 meq/L), implying no significant change in parathyroid function. Serum calcitonin is inconsistently elevated during pregnancy (220 ± 60 pg/mL). Calcitonin is important in inhibiting PTH-in-

duced bone resorption and thus conserving skeletal calcium. Maternal 1,25-dihydroxy-vitamin $D_3$ levels are elevated, with a resultant increase in intestinal absorption of calcium. The significant changes in secretion, absorption, and turnover of calcium occur well in advance of fetal skeletal mineralization and do not appear to be reduced by high doses of estrogen and progesterone. The normal woman requires 1–2 g/d of calcium in the last half of pregnancy to maintain calcium balance, in contrast to the 0.5 g/d required in the nonpregnant stage. The fetus requires a total of 25–30 g of calcium in the latter half of gestation. Thus, changes during pregnancy generate increased absorption of calcium for deposition to the fetus while maintaining normal maternal skeletal calcium.

## HYPERPARATHYROIDISM

**Primary hyperparathyroidism** is a generalized disorder, usually chronic in nature, that results from increased PTH secretion. The excessive concentration of PTH leads to hypercalcemia and hyperphosphatemia, which usually result in recurrent nephrolithiasis, peptic ulcers, mental changes, and excessive bone absorption. The incidence peaks between ages 30 and 40. In more than 80% of patients, primary hyperparathyroidism results from a neoplastic transformation of one parathyroid gland; other causes are benign adenomas and a familial pattern of hyperparathyroidism that may occur without other endocrinologic abnormalities. The tumor is usually located in the inferior parathyroid gland.

### Clinical Findings

Signs and symptoms are those of hypercalcemia and characteristically involve the kidneys and skeletal system. Renal involvement is present in 60–70% of patients with overt hyperparathyroidism. Bone involvement can cause osteitis fibrosa cystica, but in milder forms skeletal involvement can be detected only by x-rays of the hands and skull. Phalangeal tips may resorb, and an irregular outline replaces the normally sharp cortical outline of the bones in the digits (subperiosteal resorption). The skull exhibits tiny "punched out" lesions with a "salt and pepper" appearance.

### Diagnosis

Hypercalcemia is the most common manifestaton, and radioimmunoassay for PTH is diagnostic. In pregnancy coexisting with hyperparathyroidism, serum calcium levels are generally greater than 12 mg/dL.

### Treatment

The recommended therapy for moderate to severe hyperparathyroidism during pregnancy is surgical removal of 3 or 4 of the parathyroid glands. Total parathyroidectomy with transplantation of functioning parathyroid tissue in the forearm is an experimental approach, which minimizes the common risk of hypocalcemia following partial parathyroidectomy. Mild hyperparathyroidism may be managed by forcing fluids, increasing oral phosphate intake, and decreasing oral calcium intake. If symptoms occur during medical therapy, surgical therapy is indicated.

### Complications & Prognosis

Maternal hyperparathyroidism has high fetal morbidity and variable mortality rates. Neonatal effects can be summarized as a high incidence (> 50%) of neonatal tetany due to increased active placental transport of calcium has a detrimental effect on the fetus, and an inhibition of fetal parathyroid hormone. In addition, neonates of mothers with hyperparathyroidism have immature kidneys and parathyroid glands. Neonatal tetany may not become manifest for 5–14 days postpartum, probably owing to limited ability to handle the increased phosphorus of cow's milk; thus, close observation of the infant in the first weeks is important. Hypomagnesemia may also occur in conjunction with neonatal hypocalcemia. Neonatal tetany is usually transient, and complete recovery often occurs without treatment.

Maternal complications of hyperparathyroidism involve the cardiac, renal, gastrointestinal, and skeletal systems. Pathologic fractures are common in severe hyperparathyroidism. Urinary tract infection due to stones and obstruction may (rarely) lead to uremia. With severe hypercalcemia, severe hypertension with acute cardiac or renal failure and intractable pancreatitis may occur.

## HYPOPARATHYROIDISM

Normal maintenance of calcium balance depends on adequate PTH levels, and significant hypocalcemia occurs in its absence. The characteristics of maternal **hypoparathyroidism** are tetany, seizures, weakness, fatigue, and mental aberrations. The most common cause of hypoparathyroidism is iatrogenic ablation during thyroid surgery, but idiopathic hypoparathyroidism may also be autoimmune in nature. This condition must be distinguished from pseudohypoparathyroidism, in which the parathyroid glands are normal but there is end-organ unresponsiveness.

### Clinical Findings

Patients usually report an increased level of excitability, with numbness and tingling in the extremities, cramps, and carpopedal spasms. Tetany can be induced either by alkalosis, which increases calcium binding, or by a measurable decrease in total serum calcium.

### Diagnosis

Diagnosis is by confirmation of low ionized calcium and PTH levels and by measurement of urinary cyclic AMP excretion after administration of PTH.

### Treatment

The chief therapeutic goal is to restore normal calcium levels with supplementary dietary calcium and vitamin D, thus relieving symptoms of neuromuscular irritability.

### Complications & Prognosis

The fetal effect of decreased calcium transport across the placenta is increased fetal PTH release and resultant parathyroid hyperplasia and signs of osteitis fibrosa cystica. In general, however, hypoparathyroidism causes no deleterious effects on pregnancy or the newborn. Breast-feeding is discouraged, since calcium replacement to meet breast milk loss is difficult. Since idiopathic hypoparathyroidism may have an inherited autosomal recessive basis, the neonate needs to be evaluated.

Maternal complications of hypoparathyroidism relate predominantly to the degree of hypocalcemia. Acute tetany with stridor may lead to respiratory obstruction requiring tracheostomy. Severe hypocalcemia rarely leads to cardiac dilatation and failure or to cardiac arrhythmias resistant to antiarrhythmic agents. Permanent brain damage with convulsions or psychosis rarely occurs.

## DISORDERS OF ADRENOCORTICAL FUNCTION

The weight of the adrenal gland does not change significantly in pregnancy, although there is a suggestion of increased thickness of the zona fasciculata. There is an increase in both bound and free cortisol levels throughout gestation.

## ADRENOCORTICAL INSUFFICIENCY

Adrenocortical hypofunction is of 2 types: that associated with primary inability of the adrenal gland to elaborate hormones, and that secondary to primary failure in the elaboration of ACTH by the pituitary gland.

**Addison's disease** (primary adrenocortical deficiency) is relatively rare, may occur at any age, and affects both sexes with equal frequency. Because of the increasing use of exogenous steroids and subsequent withdrawal, secondary adrenocortical insufficiency is seen with increasing frequency.

## Clinical Findings

Signs and symptoms include slowly progressive fatigue, weakness, anorexia, nausea, weight loss, cutaneous pigmentation, hypotension, and hypoglycemia. Some of these symptoms are common complaints during pregnancy; therefore, the most reliable signs of adrenocortical insufficiency in pregnancy are persistent nausea and vomiting and weight loss.

## Diagnosis

Laboratory diagnosis of adrenal insufficiency during pregnancy is difficult, since the increase in plasma cortisol may be within the normal nonpregnant range. The diagnosis of Addison's disease rests on the lack of rise in plasma cortisol concentration after cosyntropin infusion (250 μmg intravenously). Urinary 17-hydroxycorticosteroid excretion, although decreased in pregnancy, should increase after cosyntropin stimulation if adrenal function is intact.

## Treatment

The treatment of chronic primary adrenocortical insufficiency requires both glucocorticoid and mineralocorticoid replacement, whereas the chronic secondary form usually requires only glucocorticoid replacement. For both the primary and secondary forms of the disease, the dose of oral cortisol is 15–20 mg in the morning and 5–10 mg in the evening. Primary adrenocortical insufficiency also requires 0.05–0.1 mg of oral 9αa-fluorocortisol each morning. The cortisol dose should be increased during times of stress. Adequacy of therapy can be assessed by evaluation of electrolytes and blood pressure.

If addisonian crisis is suspected, treatment should begin immediately, without waiting for a plasma cortisol determination to verify the diagnosis. Treatment includes administration of hydrocortisone sodium succinate (usually 200 mg as an intravenous bolus followed by 100 mg every 8 hours) and fluid replacement with isotonic saline (5–6 L may be required for full hydration). The patient should also be given glucose (50 g) to decrease the incidence of hypoglycemic attacks.

The therapeutic use of glucocorticoids has expanded over the past 15 years in the therapy of many medical diseases. Because of this, and because adrenal suppression can last as long as 9 months to 1 year after therapy, the prudent physician should consider preoperative glucocorticoid therapy in patients undergoing cesarean delivery. Treatment may be eliminated if the patient has had a normal cosyntropin stimulation test since withdrawal of supraphysiologic steroids. However, in the absence of this stimulation test, all patients who have been on steroids on any basis except alternate-day therapy in the year prior to surgery should be treated perioperatively.

Therapy to prevent the complications secondary to adrenal insufficiency can usually be accomplished very simply. Hydrocortisone is supplied in 100-mg vials and has the equivalence of 25 mg of prednisone (4:1 ratio). Approximately 200 mg of hydrocortisone is needed per day with surgical stress. It is recommended that 100 mg be given intravenously 3 times daily in the first 24 hours, followed by the same dose twice daily in the second 24 hours. On the third postoperative day, either 20 mg of prednisone or a single 100-mg intravenous dose of hydrocortisone can be given. On the fourth day, 10 mg of prednisone is given and then discontinued on the following (fifth) day. The shorter tapering schedule noted above maximizes wound healing. If the patient was on therapeutic doses of glucocorticoids prior to surgery, then the tapering should be stopped and the patient maintained on 10 mg/d. If the patient has postoperative problems such as sepsis, or if reexploration is required, then the high-dose schedule (100 mg three times daily) should be repeated and the tapering should progress over 10–14 days.

## Complications & Prognosis

The metabolic effects of insufficient mineralocorticoids are expressed by an inability to retain sodium and to excrete potassium, resulting in a decrease in extracellular electrolytes, renal perfusion, and cardiac output. Rarely, a decrease in intravascular volume with poor vascular tone and, ultimately, vascular collapse occurs. Most of these rare cases develop insidiously, but a few are characterized by acute onset with symptoms of anorexia rapidly progressing to nausea and vomiting, diarrhea, and abdominal pain. In these patients, blood pressure soon plummets, temperature elevates, and severe shock occurs.

In general, however, maternal prognosis is excellent with adequate adrenal steroid replacement therapy. Fetal and neonatal effects are few, and a reported increase in low birth weight is perhaps attributable to fetal hypoglycemia. It is rare for the newborn to have adrenal insufficiency.

## CUSHING'S SYNDROME

Cushing's syndrome is characterized by excessive secretion of adrenocorticotropic hormone (ACTH). Symptoms and signs include truncal obesity, hypotension, fatigue, weakness, amenorrhea, hirsutism, purplish abdominal striae, edema, glycosuria, and osteoporosis. Most cases are due to bilateral adrenal hyperplasia secondary to adrenocortical stimulation from hypersecretion of pituitary ACTH or the production of ACTH by nonendocrine tumors. The classic features of Cushing's syndrome include a round face with full cheeks ("moon face") and increased fat deposition over the upper doral vertebrae ("buffalo hump") and in the supraclavicular bursa. Striae are usually broader than those in pregnancy and purple in color. Tinea versicolor is common. The diagnosis of Cushing's syndrome in pregnancy is made difficult because weight gain, hypertension, striae, edema, and increased pigmentation may all normally occur. The laboratory diagnosis includes demonstration of increased cortisol production, absence of normal diurnal rhythmicity of cortisol secretion, and failure to suppress cortisol secretion. Adrenal exploration is performed, with excision of the tumor when adenoma or carcinoma is suspected. However, with bilateral adrenal hyperplasia, the most likely diagnosis is a small pituitary adenoma. Therapy includes medical suppression by bromocriptine therapy or surgical transsphenoidal hypophysectomy. Pregnancy is an unusual occurrence in Cushing's syndrome, but there is a reported increase in fetal loss from spontaneous abortion, stillbirth, and preterm labor. Neonates may demonstrate adrenal insufficiency.

## CONGENITAL ADRENAL HYPERPLASIA

Congenital adrenal hyperplasia is an inherited enzymatic defect of steroid biosynthesis that interferes with the production of cortisol. Although defective enzymatic activity may occur in each step of cortisol biosynthesis, approximately 95% of patients have 21-hydroxylase deficiency. Deficiency in this specific enzymatic activity results in increased cortisol level and ACTH secretion. The hyperplastic adrenal cells may secrete sufficient cortisol for normal life, but overproduction of other adrenal steroids, usually androgens, cause the characteristic hirsutism and acne. Pregnancy is rare in untreated patients, but with adequate corticosteroid replacement, pregnancy appears to proceed normally, although maternal hypertension may occur. Potential adverse effects on the fetus include masculinization of the female fetus. Since congenital adrenal hyperplasia is inherited as a recessive trait, the parents of affected children have a 25% risk of having another affected child. A patient who is treated for the disease has a 1 in 100 to 1 in 200 chance of producing an affected infant.

## PHEOCHROMOCYTOMA

Pheochromocytomas are catecholamine-producing tumors of neuroectodermal tissue. They are an uncommon cause of hypertension and are amenable to surgical therapy. The frequency of pheochromocytoma is greater at autopsy (1 in 1000) than clinical recognition of the disorder, emphasizing the problem in making the diagnosis. They are predominantly singular and benign, but 10% are malignant, 10% are extra-adrenal, and 10% are bilateral or multiple. All races are affected, and peak occurrence is in the fourth decade, although a few occur in the newborn.

Ten percent are familial and usually associated with neurofibromatosis. During pregnancy, the maternal mortality rate approximates 50%, with death usually due to pulmonary edema or cerebral hemorrhage. The clinical manifestations are predominantly those associated with excessive catecholamine secretion and include severe headache, profuse sweating, palpitation, nausea and vomiting, blurred vision, vertigo, tremulousness, seizures, and general weakness. On physical examination, hypertension is noted, and there may be signs of hypothyroidism (eg, tachycardia, lid lag, and fine tremor). The treatment is surgical removal of the tumor. Fetal and neonatal effects due to excessive catecholamine secretion include intrauterine growth retardation, stillbirth, and increased abortion rate.

## DISORDERS OF THE PITUITARY

The pituitary gland in normal pregnancy shows a 2- to 3-fold increase in size of anterior lobe from an increase in prolactin-secreting cells. Serum prolactin concentration increases from the fifth to eighth weeks of gestation from a level of 10 ng/ mL to 200 ng/mL at term. Serum FSH and LH concentrations are reduced because of high estrogen levels. Growth hormone levels are difficult to measure in the first 2 trimesters, but a sample obtained 1 hour after nocturnal sleep should be greater than 5 ng/mL. Posterior pituitary function demonstrates an increase in neurophysins, which act as intraneuronal carrier proteins for oxytocin and vasopressin.

## PITUITARY TUMORS

Most pregnancies with pituitary tumor involvement are the result of bromocriptine therapy used for ovulation induction. The adenomas may be estrogen-dependent and, thus, at potential risk of enlargement. It is recommended that the patient be monitored closely throughout pregnancy for visual changes and increased number of headaches. Perinatal risk is not established, but most patients have carried to term without significant complications.

## ACROMEGALY

Acromegaly may occur during pregnancy and is characterized by excessive growth due to a growth hormone-secreting tumor. Acromegaly occurs equally in men and women. Clinical signs are enlargement of the feet, hands, mandible, nose, and lips (which gives the characteristic course facial appearance). Hypertension is present in 25% of patients. Cardiac enlargement may be present. Glucose intolerance is noted in approximately 50% of patients. Pregnancy has occurred in a small number of patients without complications.

## SHEEHAN'S SYNDROME

Sheehan's syndrome (postpartum pituitary necrosis) is the most common cause of anterior pituitary insufficiency in adult females. Symptoms appear after 75% destruction of the pituitary gland. The cause is believed to be insufficient blood flow to the pituitary, usually as a result of postpartum blood loss and subsequent hypotension. Onset of symptomatology depends on the degree of pituitary necrosis. It may begin early as failure to lactate, with rapid breast involution after delivery, or take several years, at which time the patient will have menstrual irregularities or symptoms of decreased thyroid or adrenal function. Treatment of pituitary hypofunction during pregnancy includes careful balancing of replacement adrenal corticosteroid therapy and thyroid hormone. Generally, patients carry pregnancy well and without complication once treatment is given. However, a few patients with diabetes and hypopituitarism develop severe headache, and maternal death occurs in 30% of these patients.

## DIABETES INSIPIDUS

Posterior pituitary hypofunction usually is the result of trauma or tumor that has damaged the hypothalamic-hypophyseal region, but one-third of cases may be idiopathic and less than 1% inherited as an autosomal dominant trait. Symptoms and signs include polydipsia and polyuria with a specific gravity below 1.005. Diagnosis is made by water deprivation followed by increasing serum osmolality but continued low urine osmolality. Treatment is by administration of the synthetic analogue of arginine vasopressin, which can be given intranasally. The disease does not adversely affect pregnancy, nor does pregnancy adversely affect the disease.

# AUTOIMMUNE DISORDERS

## RHEUMATOID ARTHRITIS

Rheumatoid arthritis is a chronic disease of unknown cause (probably autoimmune). It is manifested by inflammatory arthritis of peripheral joints in a symmetric distribution. Systemic manifestations include hematologic, pulmonary, neurologic, and cardiovascular abnormalities. The prevalence in North America is 0.5–3.8%, and it occurs 3 times more frequently in women. Symptoms of rheumatoid arthritis are insidious, with a prodrome of fatigue, weakness, generalized joint stiffness, and myalgias preceding the appearance of joint swelling. The course is variable and unpredictable, with spontaneous remissions and exacerbations. Laboratory findings are mild leukocytosis, elevated erythrocyte sedimentation rate (which may not always reflect the activity of the disease), and a positive rheumatoid factor (in the majority of patients).

Treatment is rest, antiinflammatory drugs, splints, physical therapy, a well-balanced diet, and adequate movement of all joints. The course of arthritis in pregnancy is basically unaltered: Approximately one-third will improve, one-third will not change, and one-third will worsen. The activity of the disease during pregnancy is best followed by assessment of duration of morning stiffness and the number of joints involved. There is no effect of rheumatoid arthritis on pregnancy with the exception of possible prolongation of pregnancy due to the antiprostaglandin medications administered. Additionally, $Ro(SS_A)$ and $LA(SS_B)$ antibodies should be obtained to determine the fetal risk for complete heart block.

## SYSTEMIC LUPUS ERYTHEMATOSUS

Systemic lupus erythematosus (SLE) is an autoimmune disorder having a multiorgan effect. It predominantly affects females (8:1) between the ages of 20 and 30 and has a higher incidence among blacks. The clinical presentation includes arthritis and arthralgias, cutaneous manifestations, nephritis, fever, central nervous system manifestations, Raynaud's phenomenon, pleurisy, pericarditis, hemolytic anemia, leukopenia, and thrombocytopenia. Diagnosis is made by the presence of a positive antinuclear antibody and the presence of 4 or more of the above signs. The fertility rate of patients with SLE is normal, with the exception that amenorrhea has been associated with corticosteroid therapy. Patients in the quiescent disease state do best during pregnancy, but an increased risk of premature birth is likely if there is increased activity of the disorder or if it is newly diagnosed.

Management during pregnancy includes a careful history, physical examination, and laboratory evaluation for evidence of cardiac or renal disease. The patient should be advised to maintain a lifestyle of minimal emotional disruption and increased rest. Antiinflammatory medications previously given to the patient should be continued and not reduced throughout pregnancy. Antepartum management should include monthly measurement of serum C3 and C4 levels, since sharp declines appear to herald exacerbations, thus allowing therapeutic intervention. Renal status should be serially evaluated throughout pregnancy, and fetal growth should be frequently assessed. Antenatal testing usually begins at 32 weeks.

The possible effects of SLE on pregnancy and vice versa have been the subject of controversy mainly because all reported studies are retrospective. However, it is generally accepted that 30–50% of patients have an exacerbation of SLE during pregnancy and that pregnancy does not alter the long-term course of the disease but may lead to maternal death if not properly treated. The frequency of spontaneous abortion is double that in the general population. The risk of preterm delivery in gravidas with SLE approximates 50%. Total fetal loss in patients with SLE is 25–30%. Gravidas with SLE have a 25% chance of having

newborns that are small for gestational age. Fetuses of SLE mothers have a 1–2% incidence of complete heart block in utero (mothers are usually $Rh_o[SS_A]$ positive).

## SCLERODERMA AND DERMATOMYOSITIS

Pregnancy in patients with scleroderma is rare, since the disorder occurs most frequently in patients beyond reproductive age. The course remains unaltered in pregnancy, but there is an apparent increase in preeclampsia and fetal loss. The course of dermatomyositis follows a similar pattern without associaton with preeclampsia.

## REFERENCES

### DISORDERS OF THE NERVOUS SYSTEM

Albert JR, Morrison JC: Neurologic diseases in pregnancy. Obstet Gynecol Clin North Am 1992;19:765.

Carr SR, Gilchrist JM, Abuelo DN, Clark D: Treatment of antenatal myasthenia gravis. Obstet Gynecol 1992;78:485.

Charlifue SW, Gerhart KA, Menter RR, Whitenech GG, Manley MS: Sexual issues of women with spinal cord injuries. Paraplegia 1992;30:192.

Colachis SC: Autonomic hyperreflexia with spinal cord injury. J Am Paraplegia Soc 1992;15:171.

Cross LL, Meythaler JM, Tuel SM, Cross AL: Pregnancy, labor and delivery post spinal cord injury. Paraplegia 1992;30:890.

Davis RK, Maslow AS: Multiple sclerosis in pregnancy: A review. Obstet Gynecol Surv 1992;47:290.

Deshpande AD: Recurrent Bell's palsy in pregnancy. J Laryngol Otol 1990;104:713.

Dias MS, Sekhar LN: Intracranial hemorrhage from aneurysms and arteriovenous malformations during pregnancy and the puerperium. Neurosurgery 1990;27:855.

Ditmars DM Jr: Patterns of carpal tunnel syndrome. Hand Clin 1993;9:241.

Donaldson JO: Neurologic emergencies in pregnancy. Obstet Gynecol Clin North Am 1991;18:199.

Duquette P, Girard M: Hormonal factors in susceptibility to multiple sclerosis. Curr Opin Neurol Neurosurg 1993;6:195.

Enevodson TP, Russell RW: Cerebral venous thrombosis: new causes for an old syndrome? Q J M 1990;77:1255.

Feyi-Waboso PA: An audit of five years' experience of pregnancy in spinal cord damaged women. A regional unit's experience and a review of the literature. Paraplegia 1992;30:631.

Fox MW, Harms RW, Davis DH: Selected neurologic complications of pregnancy. Mayo Clin Proc 1990;65:1595.

Gaughan RK, Harner SG: Acoustic neuroma and pregnancy. Am J Otol 1993;14:88.

Gautier PE, Hantson P, Vekemans MC, Fievez P, Lecart C, Sindic C, Mahieu P: Intensive care management of Guillain-Barre syndrome during pregnancy. Intensive Care Med 1990;16:460.

Gilman S: Advances in neurology part I. N Eng J Med 1992;326:1608.

Gilman S: Advances in neurology part II. N Eng J Med 1992;326:1671.

Goldberg M, Rappaport ZH: Neurosurgical, obstetric and endocrine aspects of meningioma during pregnancy. Isr J Med Sci 1987;23:825.

Havard CW, Fonseca V: New treatment approaches to myasthenia gravis. Drugs 1990;39:66.

Horton JC, Chambers WA, Lyons SL, Adams RD, Kjellberg RN: Pregnancy and the risk of hemorrhage from cerebral arteriovenous malformations. Neurosurgery 1990;27:867.

Hurley TJ, Brunson AD, Archer RL, Lefler SF, Quirk JG Jr: Landry Guillain-Barre Strohl syndrome in pregnancy: Report of three cases treated with plasmapheresis. Obstet Gynecol 1991;78:482.

Katz VL, Peterson R, Cefalo RC: Pseudotumor cerebri and pregnancy. Am J Perinatol 1989;6:442.

Kibria EM: Pregnancy and epilepsy. J Fla Med Assoc 1992;79:756.

Laidler JA, Jackson IJ, Redfern N: The management of ceasarean section in a patient with an intracranial arteriovenous malformation. Anaesthesia 1989;44:490.

Laughey WF, MacGregor EA, Wilkinson MI: How many different headaches do you have? Cephalalgia 1993;13:136.

Lisovoski F, Rousseaux P: Cerebral infarction in young people. A study of 148 patients with early cerebral angiography. J Neurol Neurosurg Psychiatry 1991;54:576.

Mitchell PJ, Bebbington M: Myasthenia gravis in pregnancy. Obstet Gynecol 1992;80:178.

Nygaard IE, Saltzman CL Whitehouse MB, Hankin FM:

Hand problems in pregnancy. Am Fam Physician 1989;39:123.

Paonessa K, Fernand R: Spinal cord injury and pregnancy. Spine 1991;16:596.

Plauche WC: Myasthenia gravis in mothers and their newborns. Clin Obstet Gynecol 1991;34:82.

Pryse-Phillips W, Findlay H, Tugwell P, Edmeads J, Murray TJ, Nelson RF: A Canadian population survey on the clinical, epidemiologic and societal impact of migraine and tension-type headache. Can J Neurol Sci 1992;19:333.

Roelvink NC, Kamphorst W, Van-Alphen HA, Rao BR: Pregnancy-related primary brain and spinal tumors. Arch Neurol 1987;44:209.

Sadasivan B, Malik GM, Lee C, Ausman JI: Vascular malformations and pregnancy. Surg Neurol 1990; 33:305.

Simolke GA, Cox SM, Cunningham FG: Cerebrovascular accidents complicating pregnancy and the puerperium. Obstet Gynecol 1991;78:37.

So EL: Update on epilepsy. Med Clin North Am 1993; 77:203.

Stevens JC, Beard CM, OFallon WM, Kurlant LT: Conditions associated with carpal tunnel syndrome. Mayo Clin Proc 1992;67:541.

Stewart WF, Lipton RB: Migraine headache: Epidemiology and health care utilization. Cephalalgia 1993;13 (suppl 12):41.

Toddle RC et al: Pregnancy-induced changes in prolactinomas as assessed with computed tomography. J Rep Med 1988;33:821.

Walling AD: Bell's palsy in pregnancy and the puerperium. J Fam Pract 1993;36:559.

Wan WL, Geller JL, Feldon SE, Sadun AA: Visual loss caused by rapidly progressive intracranial meningiomas during pregnancy. Ophthalmology 1990; 97:18.

Wand JS: Carpal tunnel syndrome in pregnancy and lactation. J Hand Surg [Br] 1990;15:93.

Wong MC, Giuliani MJ, Haley EC Jr: Cerebrovascular disease and stroke in women. Cardiology 1990;77 (suppl 2):80.

## DISORDERS OF THE SKIN

Dacus JV, Muram D: Pruritis in pregnancy. South Med J 1987;80:614.

Kanaan C, Veille JC, Lakin M: Pregnancy and acute intermittent porphyria. Obstet Gynecol Surv 1989; 44:244.

Kaplan RP, Callen JP: Pemphigus associated diseases and induced pemphigus. Clin Dermatol 1983;1:42.

Milo R, Neuman M, Klein C, Caspi E, Arlzoroff A: Acute intermittent porphyria in pregnancy. Obstet Gynecol 1989;73:450.

Winton GB, Lewis CS: Dermatoses of pregnancy. J Am Acad Dermatol 1982;6:977.

## DISORDERS OF THE GASTROINTESTINAL TRACT

Abell TL, Riely CA: Hyperemesis gravidarum. Gastroenterol Clin North Am 1992;21:835.

Anday, EK, Cohen A: Liver disease associated with pregnancy. Ann Clin Lab Sci 1990;20:233.

Back N, Boden-Heimer HC Jr: Transmission of hepatitis C: sexual, vertical or exclusively blood-borne? Hepatology 1992;16:1497.

Block GE, Michelassi F, Tanaka M, Riddell RH, Hanauer SB: Crohn's disease. Curr Probl Surg 1993;30:173.

Dupont P, Irion O, Beguin F: Pregnancy in a patient with treated Wilson's disease: A case report. Am J Obstet Gynecol 1990;163:1527.

Elerding SC: Laparoscopic cholecystectomy in pregnancy. Am J Surg 1993;165:625.

Fedorkow DM, Persaud D, Nimrod CA: Inflammatory bowel disease: A controlled study of late pregnancy outcome. Am J Obstet Gynecol 1989;160:998.

Korelitz BI: Inflammatory bowel disease in pregnancy. Gastroenterol Clin North Am 1992;21:827.

Lee WM: Pregnancy in patients with chronic liver disease. Gastroenterol Clin North Am 1992;21:889.

Mabie WC: Acute fatty liver of pregnancy. Gastroenterol Clin North Am 1992;21:951.

Mabie WC: Obstetric management of gastroenterologic complications of pregnancy. Gastroenterol Clin North Am 1992;21:923.

Medhat A, Sharkawy MM, Shaaban MM, Makhlouf MM: Acute viral hepatitis in pregnancy. Int J Gynecol Obstet 1993;40:25.

Mishra L, Seeff LB: Viral hepatitis, A through E, complicating pregnancy. Gastroenterol Clin North Am 1992;21:873.

Morrell DG, Mullins JR, Harrison PB: Laparoscopic cholecystectomy during pregnancy in symptomatic patients. Surgery 1992;112:856.

Olsson R, Tysk C, Aldenborg F, Holm B: Prolonged postpartum course of intrahepatic cholestasis of pregnancy. Gastroenterology 1993;105:267.

Reyes H: The spectrum of liver and gastrointestinal disease seen in cholestasis of pregnancy. Gastroenterol Clin North Am 1992;21:905.

Samuels P, Cohen AW: Pregnancies complicated by liver disease and liver dysfunction. Obstet Gynecol Clin North Am 1992;19:745.

Schoen RE, Sternlieb I: Clinical aspects of Wilson's disease [clinical conference]. Am J Gastroenterol 1990;85:1453.

Scott LD: Gallstone disease and pancreatitis in pregnancy. Gastroenterol Clin North Am 1992;21:803.

Selby W: Current management of inflammatory bowel disease. J Gastroenterol Hepatol 1993;8:70.

Wang LR, Jeng CJ, Chu JS: Pregnancy associated with primary hepatocellular carcinoma. Obstet Gynecol 1993;81:811.

Watson WJ, Seeds JW: Acute fatty liver of pregnancy. Obstet Gynecol Surv 1990;45:585.

## DISORDERS OF THE THYROID

Buckshee K, Kriplani A, Kapil A, Bhargava VL, Takkar D: Hypothyroidism complicating pregnancy. Aust NZ J Obstet Gynecol 1992;32:240.

Burrow GN: Thyroid function and hyperfunction during gestation. Endocr Rev 1993;14:194.

Hamburger JI: Diagnosis and management of Graves' disease in pregnancy. Thyroid 1992;2:219.

Lazarus JH: Treatment of hyper-and hypothyroidism in pregnancy. J Endocrinol Invest 1993;16:391.

Leung AS, Millar LK, Koonings PP, Montoro M, Mestman JH: Perinatal outcome in hypothyroid pregnancies. Obstet Gynecol 1993;81:349.

Sipes SL, Malee MP: Endocrine disorders in pregnancy. Obstet Gynecol Clin North Am 1992;19:655.

## DISORDERS OF THE PARATHYROID

Along U, Chan JC: Hypocalcemia from deficiency of and resistance to parathyroid hormone. Adv Pediatr 1985;32:439.

Fitzpatrick LA, Bilezikian JP: Acute primary hyperparathyroidism. Am J Med 1987;82:275.

Furui T, Imai A, Tamaya T: Successful outcome of pregnancy complicated with thyroidectomy-induced hypoparathyroidism and sudden dyspnea. A case report. Gynecol Obstet Invest 1993;35:57.

Savani RC, Mimouni F, Tsang RC: Maternal and neonatal hyperparathyroidism as a consequence of maternal renal tubular acidosis. Pediatrics 1993;91:661.

Zaloga GP, Chernow B: Hypocalcemia in critical illness. JAMA 1986;256:1924.

## DISORDERS OF ADRENOCORTICAL FUNCTION

Byyny RL: Preventing adrenal insufficiency during surgery. Postgrad Med 1980;65:219.

Easterling TR, Carlson K, Benedetti TJ, Mancuso JJ: Hemodynamics associated with the diagnosis and treatment of pheochromocytoma in pregnancy. Am J Perinatol 1992;9:464.

Goldman DR: Surgery in patients with endocrine dysfunction. Med Clin North Am 1987;71:499.

Samaan NA, Hickey RC: Pheochromocytoma. Semin Oncol 1987;14:297.

Seckl JR, Dunger DB: Diabetes insipidus. Current treatment recommendations. Drugs 1992;44:216.

## DISORDERS OF THE PITUITARY

Burrow GN et al: DDAVP treatment of diabetes insipidus during pregnancy and the postpartum period. Acta Endocrinol 1981;97:23.

Coyne TJ, Atkinson RL, Prins JB: Adrenocorticotropic hormone-secreting pituitary tumor associated with pregnancy: Case report. Neurosurgery 1992;31:953.

Ezzat S: Living with acromegaly. Endocrinol Metab Clin North Am 1992;21:753.

Golan A, Abramov L, Yedwab G, David MP: Pregnancy in panhypopituitarism. Gynecol Obstet Invest 1990;29:232.

Grimes HG, Brooks MA: Pregnancy in Sheehan's syndrome: Report of a case and review. Obstet Gynecol Surv 1980;35:481.

Loucopolo A, Jewelewicz R: Prolactinomas and pregnancies. Sem Reprod Endocrinol 1984;2:83.

Molitch ME: Endocrine emergencies in pregnancy. Baillieres Clin Endocrinol Metab 1992;6:167.

Nader S: Pituitary disorders and pregnancy. Semin Perinatol 1990;14:24.

Uhiara JE, Narayan R, Kumar S:Sheehan's syndrome following eclampsia: A case report. Asia Oceania J Obstet Gynecol 1992;18:121.

Yap AS, Clouston WM, Mortimer RH, Drake RF: Acromegaly first diagnosed in pregnancy: The role of bromocriptine therapy. Am J Obstet Gynecol 1990; 163:477.

## AUTOIMMUNE DISORDERS

Avrech OM, Golan A, Pansky M, Langer R, Caspi E: Raynaud's phenomenon and peripheral gangrene complicating scleroderma in pregnancy—diagnosis and management, Br J Obstet Gynecol 1992;99:850.

Ben-Chetrit E: Target antigens of the SSA/Ro and SSB/La sysytem. Am J Reprod Immunol 1992;28: 256.

Birdsall M, Pattison N, Chamley L: Antiphospholipid antibodies in pregnancy. Aust NZ J Obstet Gynaecol 1992;32:328.

Branch DW: Antiphospholipid antibodies and pregnancy: Maternal implications. Semin Perinatol 1990; 14:139.

Buchanan NM, Khamashta MA, Morton KE, Kerslake S, Baguley EA, Hughes GR: A study of 100 high risk lupus pregnancies. Am J Reprod Immunol 1992;28: 192.

Carpenter AB, Medsger TA Jr:Previous pregnancy outcome is an important determinant of subsequent pregnancy outcome in women with systemic lupus erythematosus. Am J Reprod Immunol 1992;28:195.

Englert H, Brennan P, McNeil D, Black C, Silman AJ: Reproductive function prior to disease onset in women with scleroderma. J Rheumatol 1992;19:1575.

Floyd RC, Roberts WE: Autoimmune diseases in pregnancy. Bostet Gynecol Clin North Am 1992;19:719.

Giacoia GP, Azubuike K: Autoimmune diseases in pregnancy: Their effect on the fetus and newborn. Obstet Gynecol Surv 1991;46:732.

Hayslett JP: The effect of systemic lupus erythematosus on pregnancy and pregnancy outcome. Am J Reprod Immunol 1992;28:199.

Julkunen H, Kaaja R, Palosuo T, Gronhagen Riska C, Teramo K: Pregnancies in lupus neuropathy. Acta Obstet Gynecol Scand 1993;72:258.

Lansink M, DeBoer A, Dikmans BA, Vandenbroucke JP, Hazes JM: The onset of rheumatoid arthritis in relation to pregnancy and childbirth. Clin Exp Rheumatol 1993;11:171.

Lockshin MD: Antiphospholipid antibody and antiphospholipid antibody syndrome. Curr Opin Rheumatol 1991;3:797.

Lockshin MD: Overview of lupus pregnancies. Am J Reprod Immunol 1992;28:181.

Morgan GJ Jr, Chow WS: Clinical features, diagnosis, and prognosis in rheumatoid arthritis. Curr Opin Rheumatol 1993;5:184.

Nieuwenhuis HK, Derksen RH: A prospective, controlled multicenter study on the obstetric risks of pregnant women with antiphospholipid antibodies. Am J Obstet Gynecol 1992;167:26.

Ostensen M: The effect of pregnancy on ankylosing spondylitis, psoriatic arthritis, and juvenile rheumatoid arthritis. Am J Reprod Immunol 1992;28:235.

Petri M, AllbrittonK: Fetal outcome of lupus pregnancy: A retrospective case-control study of the Hopkins Lupus Cohort. J Rheumatol 1993;20:650.

Petri M, Howard D, Repke J, Goldman DW: The Hopkins Lupus Pregnancy Center. 1987–1991 update. Am J Reprod Immunol 1992;28:188.

Pinheiro G da R, Goldenberg J, Atra E, Pereira RB, Camano L, Schmidt B: Juvenile dermatomyositis and pregnancy: report and literature review. J Rheumatol 1992;19:1798.

Rubbert A, Pirner K, Wildt L, Kalden JR, Manger B: Pregnancy course and complications in patients with systemic lupus erythematosus. Am J Reprod Immunol 1992;28:205.

Samuels P, Pfeifer SM: Autoimmune diseases in pregnancy. The obstetrician's view. Rheum Dis Clin North Am 1989;15:307.

Silman AJ: Pregnancy and scleroderma. Am J Reprod Immunol 1992;28:238.

Silver RM, Branch DW: Autoimmune disease in pregnancy. Baillieres Clin Obstet Gynaecol 1992;6:565.

Spector TD, DaSilva JA: Pregnancy and rheumatoid arthritis: an overview. Am J Reprod Immunol 1992;28:222.

Varner MW: Autoimmune disorders and pregnancy. Semin Perinatol 1992;15:238.

# Surgical Diseases & Disorders in Pregnancy

# 24

*Rick W. Martin, MD, Kenneth G. Perry, MD, & John Morrison, MD*

Surgical interventions other than cesarean section are performed in 0.2–2.2% of all pregnancies (50,000 per year), and the incidence is rising. Altered anatomy and physiology and potential risks to the mother and fetus make diagnosis and management of surgical disorders more difficult. Generally, the interests of mother and fetus are best served by active participation of the obstetrician throughout the mother's course of diagnosis and management with a nonobstetric surgical disorder, although the responsibility is usually shared with other specialists. It is imperative that the obstetrician be well informed concerning the ways in which surgical disorders influence pregnancy and vice versa, the risks of diagnostic and therapeutic procedures to the fetus, and appropriate management of preterm labor in the immediate postoperative period.

Surgical disorders may be either incidental to or directly related to the pregnancy. Diagnostic evaluation requires gentle, sensitive elicitation of physical signs, often without resort to sophisticated diagnostic aids that involve risk to the developing fetus. Experienced judgment is important regarding the timing, methods, and extent of treatment. In the absence of peritonitis or perforation, surgical disorders during gestation generally have little effect on placental function and fetal development.

## MATERNAL CONSIDERATIONS

Pregnancy is accompanied by physiologic and anatomic changes that alter the evaluation and management of the surgical patient. The 50% increase in plasma volume during pregnancy affects drug distribution and may alter laboratory tests. Red cell mass increases but not as much as the plasma volume, resulting in a slight fall in the hematocrit. Colloid osmotic pressure is decreased during pregnancy. Increased interstitial fluid is seen as mild edema particularly in the lower extremities. Cardiac output rises. Lung tidal volume increases and a compensated mild respiratory alkalosis exists. Increased renal blood flow is evidenced by increased glomerular filtration rate and decreased creatinine and blood urea nitrogen values. Gastric motility is diminished resulting in delayed gastric emptying and constipation. The enlarging uterus may alter the anatomic relation among the different organs. In the supine position the enlarged uterus may compress the vena cava and result in the supine hypotensive syndrome.

## FETAL CONSIDERATIONS

Optimal care of the pregnant surgical patient requires that potential hazards to the fetus be minimized. This includes risks associated with anesthesia, therapeutic drugs, diagnostic radiation, and maternal disease and surgery. It is relatively easy to assess risks and benefits to the mother but less so for the fetus because of its relative inaccessibility.

Presently, it is unclear whether surgery or anesthesia has a teratogenic effect on the developing human embryo or fetus. Short exposure increases rate of congenital malformations, although spontaneous abortion may be more likely if the exposure occurs during the first trimester of pregnancy. Alterations in perioperative arterial oxygen tension have not been shown to have untoward effects on humans, in contrast to that which occurs in some laboratory animals.

Postoperative use of analgesic agents generally appears to produce no adverse effects. Because an increased risk of congenital anomalies has been related to codeine administration, it is suggested that this analgesic be avoided in the first trimester. Although brief use of aspirin probably has no adverse effect on the fetus, long-term or high-dose use should be discouraged. Acetaminophen should be substituted, since therapeutic doses of this agent are apparently safe. In very large doses, acetaminophen may cause fetal liver or renal damage. Tetracyclines and sulfonamides are generally to be avoided; cephalosporins, penicillins, and erythromycin are preferable. Aminoglycosides may cause fetal ototoxicity and nephrotoxicity but are not likely to do so when given for short periods.

Diagnostic x-ray procedures are often performed

prior to surgical intervention. Abdominal shielding should be used when possible to reduce fetal exposure. In experimental animals, gestational exposures below 10–20 cGy do not produce detectable increases in the incidence of congenital anomalies or microcephaly. For humans, the National Council on Radiation Protection considers the risk of malformations with exposure to 5 cGy or less to be negligible when compared with the other risks of pregnancy. A number of investigators have estimated the doses of ionizing radiation received by the fetus during a variety of x-ray projections for clinical studies and have noted that, even when multiple fluoroscopic studies are performed, a dose exceeding 5 cGy would be exceptional. From a clinical standpoint, therefore, human fetal exposure to less than 5 cGy is conservatively considered insufficient reason to recommend pregnancy termination. Doubling this exposure to 10 cGy is probably safe.

Because intrauterine asphyxia is a major risk to the fetus consequent to maternal surgery, it is important to monitor and maintain maternal oxygen-carrying capacity, oxygen affinity, arterial $PO_2$, and placental blood flow throughout the preoperative, operative, and postoperative periods. Attention should be given to providing uterine displacement to prevent venocaval compression in the supine position. Supplemental oxygen administration and maintenance of circulating volume also assist fetal oxygenation. A reduction in maternal blood pressure can lead directly to fetal hypoxia. Greater reductions in uteroplacental perfusion by direct vascular constriction and an increase in uterine tonus are noted in association with the use of vasopressors, especially those with predominantly alpha-adrenergic activity. To defect fetal hypoxia, continuous electronic fetal heart rate monitoring should be used when maternal surgery is performed in the latter half of gestation as long as the monitoring device can function outside the sterile surgical field.

The severity of the inflammatory response associated with the surgical disease appears to be more important in determining pregnancy outcome than is the use of anesthesia or the surgical procedure itself. Premature labor does not appear to be a common result of procedures such as exploratory celiotomy unless perforation or peritonitis is encountered. If possible, uterine activity should be monitored following surgery to detect preterm labor and allow for early intervention.

## DIAGNOSTIC CONSIDERATIONS

### Pain

Pain is the most prominent symptom encountered with acute abdominal conditions complicating pregnancy. Generalized abdominal pain strongly suggests peritonitis secondary to bleeding, exudation, or leakage of intestinal contents. Cramping lower central abdominal pain suggests a uterine disorder. Lower abdominal pain to either side suggests torsion, rupture, or hemorrhage of an ovarian cyst or tumor. Disorders of the descending and sigmoid colon with left lower-quadrant pain are infrequently encountered because of the relative young age of patients. Midabdominal pain early in gestation suggests an intestinal origin. Upper abdominal pain is often related to the liver, spleen, gallbladder, stomach, duodenum, or pancreas. Constipation is a common problem but is rarely associated with other symptoms.

### Other Symptoms

When abdominal pain is associated with nausea and vomiting after the first trimester, it usually suggests an upper intestinal disorder. Constipation more frequently is associated with lower intestinal obstruction. Diarrhea is seldom encountered in association with acute surgical problems except as a symptom of recurrent ulcerative colitis.

Syncope associated with pain and signs of peritoneal irritation usually indicates an acute abdominal emergency with rupture of a viscus or hemorrhage. A temperature of over 38°C (100°F) suggests infection, which may be localized by other clinical findings. Vaginal bleeding usually points to an intrauterine problem. Urinary tract infection is often accompanied by urinary frequency and urgency.

### History Taking & Examination

Clues to the cause of surgical disorders in pregnancy are often found in a careful review of the medical history. The stage and status of pregnancy are also relevant (the second trimester is the safest time to perform surgery). The patient with an acute abdomen should undergo careful assessment of the reproductive organs, and her vital signs and general condition should be noted as well as the presence or absence of peristalsis, abdominal rigidity, and rebound tenderness, and the presence or absence of a mass. The fewest possible number of abdominal examinations should be gently performed without haste and with adequate explanation, using the flat of the hand and starting in an asymptomatic area.

### Laboratory Studies

Several laboratory studies routinely used in the evaluation of surgical disease have altered values during gestation. The white blood cell count is considered elevated if it is above 16,000/µL in any trimester. An interval of several hours usually passes between onset of hemorrhage and detection of lowered hematocrit values.

## PRINCIPLES OF SURGICAL MANAGEMENT

Delay in diagnosis and performance of operation is the factor primarily responsible for increased maternal morbidity rates and perinatal loss, especially with maternal abdominal trauma. When operation is not urgent and can be delayed, it is best deferred until the second trimester or puerperium. Surgical techniques usually are not altered because of the pregnancy. In subacute conditions, caution should be used in deciding to proceed with operation. However, with unmistakable signs of peritoneal irritation, evidence of strangulating intestinal obstruction with possible gangrene, or a probable diagnosis of cancer, immediate surgical exploration generally is indicated. Essentials of good preoperative care include adequate hydration, availability of blood for transfusion, and appropriate preoperative medication that will not decrease oxygenation for mother and fetus.

Stage of gestation, uterine size, the specific surgical disorder, and the anticipated type of surgery to be performed are important factors in the selection of abdominal incision. During the first trimester, a lower midline incision or a transverse incision is usually used. Later on, as the uterus enlarges, a higher vertical or transverse incision at the level of the umbilicus is usually preferred. For the very obese patient, a paramedian incision above and below the umbilicus (Wiser incision) allows for adequate operative exposure yet minimizes incisional depth, potential for infection, and operative closure time. At operation, the least extensive procedure necessary should be performed with as little manipulation of the uterus as possible. Unless there is an obstetric indication or the uterus interferes with performance of a procedure, it is usually best not to perform a cesarean delivery during an abdominal operation. Primary concerns related to anesthesia are maintenance of maternal and fetal oxygenation, prevention of maternal hypotension by avoiding the supine position, and minimizing of uterine irritability by using appropriate anesthetic agents. Following endotracheal intubation for anesthesia, the oxygen concentration is maintained at 35% or greater in the anesthetic mixture.

Postoperative care depends on the stage of pregnancy and the operation performed. For patients in the last half of gestation, continuous electronic monitoring of the fetus or intermittent auscultation by fetal stethoscope should be continued in the immediate postoperative period. Electronic monitoring is preferable because uterine contractions as well as fetal heart rate can be monitored accurately and easily over time to provide early, definitive evidence of preterm labor or fetal hypoxia. Oversedation and fluid or electrolyte imbalance are to be avoided. Encouragement of early maternal activity and resumption of normal food intake are recommended.

## UPPER ABDOMINAL DISEASES & DISORDERS

Early, accurate diagnosis of serious abdominal surgical disease during pregnancy is compromised for the following reasons: (1) altered anatomic relationships, (2) impaired palpation and detection of nonuterine masses, (3) depressed symptoms, (4) symptoms that mimic the normal discomforts of pregnancy, and (5) difficulty in differentiating surgical and obstetric disorders. In general, elective surgery should be avoided during pregnancy, but operation should be performed promptly for definite or probable acute disorders. The approach to surgical problems in pregnant or puerperal patients should be the same as in nonpregnant patients, with prompt surgical intervention when indicated. The risk of inducing labor with diagnostic laparotomy is low, provided unnecessary manipulation of the uterus and adnexa is avoided. Spontaneous abortion is most likely to occur if surgery is performed before 16 weeks' gestation or when peritonitis is present.

### APPENDICITIS

Acute appendicitis is the most common extrauterine complication of pregnancy for which laparotomy is performed. Suspected appendicitis accounts for nearly two-thirds of all nonobstetric exploratory celiotomies performed during pregnancy; most cases occur in the second and third trimesters.

Appendicitis occurs in 0.4–1.4 per 1000 pregnancies. Although the incidence of disease is not increased during gestation, rupture of the appendix occurs 2–3 times more often during pregnancy secondary to delays in diagnosis and operation. Maternal and perinatal mortality and morbidity rates are greatly increased when appendicitis is complicated by peritonitis.

#### Clinical Findings

**A. Symptoms and Signs:** Diagnostic delays occur because symptoms are often atypical and not dramatic. Right lower- or middle-quadrant pain is almost always present when acute appendicitis occurs in pregnancy but may be ascribed to so-called round ligament pain or urinary tract infection. In nonpregnant women, the appendix is located in the right lower quadrant (65%), the pelvis (30%), or retrocecally (5%), but in pregnancy, there is upward displacement of the appendix (Fig 24–1). After the first trimester, the appendix is gradually displaced above McBurney's point, with horizontal rotation of its base. The migration continues until the eighth month

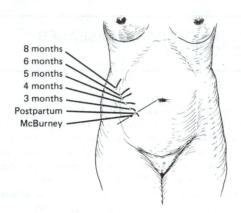

8 months
6 months
5 months
4 months
3 months
Postpartum
McBurney

**Figure 24–1.** Changes in position of the appendix as pregnancy advances.

of gestation, when more than 90% of appendices lie above the iliac crest and 80% rotate upward and toward the right subcostal area.

The most consistent clinical symptom encountered in pregnant women with appendicitis is vague pain in the right side of the abdomen, although atypical pain patterns abound. Muscle guarding and rebound tenderness are much less demonstrable as gestation progresses. Rectal and vaginal tenderness are present in 80% of patients, particularly in early pregnancy. Nausea, vomiting, and anorexia are usually present, as in the nonpregnant patient. During early appendicitis, the temperature and pulse rate are relatively normal. High fever is not characteristic of the disease, and 25% of pregnant women with appendicitis are afebrile.

**B. Laboratory Findings:** The relative leukocytosis of pregnancy (normal = 12,500–16,000/μL) clouds interpretation of infection. Although not all patients with appendicitis have white blood cell counts above 16,000/μL, at least 75% show indications of a left shift in the differential. Urinalysis may reveal significant pyuria (20%) as well as microscopic hematuria. This is particularly true in the latter half of pregnancy, when the appendix migrates closer to the retroperitoneal ureter.

### Differential Diagnosis

The differential diagnosis of appendicitis includes ruptured corpus luteum cyst, adnexal torsion, ectopic pregnancy, abruptio placentae, early labor, round ligament syndrome, chorioamnionitis, degenerating myoma, salpingitis, pyelonephritis, cholangitis, mesenteric adenitis, neoplasm, diverticulitis, parasitic infection of the intestine, and Meckel's diverticulum.

### Treatment

The difficult clinical problem in treating appendicitis during pregnancy is making the decision to oper-

ate. Treatment of nonperforated acute appendicitis complicating pregnancy is appendectomy. Antibiotic therapy is not of value unless rupture has occurred, but intravenous antibiotics are appropriate when there has been perforation, peritonitis, or abscess formation. Induced abortion is rarely indicated. If drainage is necessary for generalized peritonitis, drains should be placed transabdominally and not transvaginally. During the first trimester, a vertical midline or paramedian incision on the right side is generally considered appropriate. In the second or third trimester, a muscle-splitting incision centered over the point of maximal tenderness usually provides optimal appendiceal exposure. As a rule, appendiceal disease is managed and the pregnancy is left alone. A Smead-Jones closure with secondary wound closure 72 hours later may be advisable when the appendix is gangrenous or perforated or if there is peritonitis or abscess formation.

In the late third trimester, abdominal delivery occasionally is performed when there is perforation or peritonitis and if expert neonatal care is available. Cesarean delivery and hysterectomy may be indicated for appendiceal abscess with peritonitis. Prelabor cesarean section is also indicated if appendicitis has created a cul-de-sac abscess (usually discernible by ultrasonic examination). It appears that tocolytic therapy is unnecessary in uncomplicated appendicitis but may be efficacious with advanced disease. If labor follows shortly after surgery in the late third trimester, it should be allowed to progress, because it is not associated with a significant risk of wound dehiscence.

### Prognosis

Better fluid and nutritional support, use of antibiotics, safer anesthesia, and improved surgical technique have been important elements in the significant reduction of maternal mortality from appendicitis during pregnancy. Perinatal loss may occur in association with preterm labor and delivery or with generalized peritonitis and sepsis; it occurs infrequently in uncomplicated appendicitis. Fetal loss appears to be more closely associated with severity of appendicitis than with surgical intervention.

## CHOLECYSTITIS & CHOLELITHIASIS

Gallbladder disease represents one of the most common medical conditions and the second most common visceral complication of pregnancy (1–6 per 1000 pregnancies). It has been estimated that at least 3.5% of pregnant women harbor gallstones. Parity is an important risk factor, and the rate of gallbladder disease in women who have taken oral contraceptives in the past is almost double that of those who have not. Both an increase in lithogenicity of the bile and changes in gallbladder function are seen during pregnancy. During the second and third trimesters, the volume of the gallbladder increases almost 2-fold and its ability to empty efficiently is reduced.

## Clinical Findings

**A. Symptoms and Signs:** These are similar to those expected in the nonpregnant state, but the anatomic changes associated with pregnancy make diagnosis of appendicitis difficult. In addition to displacement of the cecum and ascending colon, the liver and diaphragm become elevated during gestation and the gallbladder is well under the right costal arch. The appendix may also occupy the right upper quadrant. Cholecystitis may cause epigastric, right scapular, and even left upper-quadrant or lower-quadrant pain that tends to be episodic in nature. Attacks are seemingly triggered by meals and may last from a few minutes to several hours. Fever and right upper-quadrant tenderness may be accompanied by nausea and vomiting. Right upper-quadrant tenderness and severe pain under the liver with deep inspiration (Murphy's sign) is often noted on physical examination. It is uncommon to encounter a palpable gallbladder.

**B. Laboratory Findings:** An increased white blood cell count with an increase in immature forms may occur. Abnormalities of liver function tests are often encountered, eg an increase in AST (alanine aminotransferase [SGOT]) and ALT (aspartate aminotransferase [SGPT]) with modest increases in the alkaline phosphatase and bilirubin levels are anticipated very early in cholecystitis or common duct obstruction. However, a more characteristic pattern of relatively normal AST and ALT with elevated alkaline phosphatase and bilirubin is generally found after the first day of the attack. These changes are not diagnostic and do not signify common bile duct stone or obstruction but when present serve to support the diagnosis.

**C. Ultrasound Findings:** Ultrasound findings of stones in the gallbladder, a thickened gallbladder wall, or even swelling in the pancreas are suggestive of cholelithiasis and cholecystitis. Failure to demonstrate existing gallstones is estimated to occur in 10%, with technical inadequacy occasionally a factor, particularly in the acutely ill patient who has a paralytic ileus and excess gas in the small intestine. If documentation is needed to establish the presence of a common duct stone, consideration can be given to the use of HIDA scanning with its very low radiation dose to the fetus (substantially less than 1 cGy).

## Differential Diagnosis

The major diagnostic difficulty that pregnancy imposes is differentiating between cholecystitis and appendicitis. In addition to gallstones, cholecystitis can be infectious secondary to *Salmonella typhi* or parasites. A number of other lesions of the biliary tract occur rarely during gestation, including choledochal

cysts seen as a spherical dilatation of the common bile duct with a very narrow or obstructed distal end. Associated pancreatitis may be present. Severe pre-eclampsia with associated right upper-quadrant abdominal pain and abnormal liver function tests, often with thrombocytopenia, can be confused with acute cholecystitis. The presence of proteinuria, pedal edema, hypertension, and sustained increases in AST and ALT compared with alkaline phosphatase are clinical and laboratory features usually associated with preeclampsia.

## Complications

Pancreatitis may frequently accompany cholecystitis during pregnancy. Removal of the gallbladder and gallstones may be preferred over conservative medical therapy when there is concurrent pancreatitis. Other uncommon complications of cholecystitis during gestation include retained intraductal stones, cholangitis, and rupture of the cystic duct.

## Treatment

Most authorities advise initial nonoperative medical management of cholecystitis during pregnancy, especially during the first trimester, because surgery at that time is associated with an increased incidence of fetal loss. Gravidas with intractable symptoms and multiple hospital admissions and those with associated pancreatitis are best managed surgically. When operative therapy for cholecystitis is effected during the second and third trimesters, there does not appear to be an appreciable increase in morbidity and mortality rates or fetal loss.

## Prognosis

The outcome for mother and fetus following uncomplicated gallbladder surgery is excellent. Morbidity and mortality rates increase with maternal age and extent of disease.

## ACUTE PANCREATITIS

The true incidence of acute pancreatitis in pregnancy is unknown but is probably lower than the 0.5% incidence reported in the nonpregnant patient. However, the mortality rate associated with acute pancreatitis may be higher during pregnancy because of delay in diagnosis. The ultimate cause of pancreatitis is the presence of activated digestive enzymes within the pancreas. Similar to that seen in the nonpregnant state, cholelithiasis is the most commonly identified cause. There often is no identifiable cause, however. Second in importance is hypertriglyceridemia and drug-induced pancreatitis (tetracycline, thiazide diuretics), familial pancreatitis, structural abnormalities of the pancreas or duodenum, infections, severe abdominal trauma, and vascular disease. Some authors have suggested that pregnancy-induced hypertension may lead to pancreatitis. Probably the only proven circumstance in which pregnancy per se causes pancreatitis is the parturient with hyperlipidemia.

## Clinical Findings

**A. Symptoms and Signs:** Gravidas with pancreatitis usually present with severe, steady epigastric pain that often radiates to the back in general approximation to the retroperitoneal location of the pancreas. Often exacerbated by food intake, its onset may be gradual or acute and frequently accompanied by nausea and vomiting. During gestation, patients may present primarily with vomiting with little or no abdominal pain. Although physical examination is rarely diagnostic, several findings of note may be present, including a low-grade fever, tachycardia, and orthostatic hypertension. The latter finding may be present with hemorrhagic pancreatitis in addition to Cullen's sign (periumbilical ecchymosis) and Turner's sign (flank ecchymosis). Epigastric tenderness and ileus may also be present.

**B. Laboratory Findings:** The cornerstone of diagnosis is the determination of serum amylase. A laboratory value of serum amylase that is several times above the upper limit of normal suggests pancreatitis or another pathologic process. Because serum amylase levels usually return to normal within a few days of an attack of uncomplicated acute pancreatitis, a timed 2-hour measurement of urinary amylase helps to support the clinical diagnosis. The ratio of renal clearance of amylase to creatinine may be of value for the diagnosis of acute pancreatitis. Serum lipase determinations are of uncertain help in the diagnosis of acute pancreatitis. ALT values tend to be elevated with gallstone pancreatitis.

**C. Ultrasound Diagnosis:** Although sonographic examination is unable to define efficiently an edematous pancreas, it is excellent as an aid in detecting complications of pancreatitis such as the presence of peritoneal fluid, peripancreatic blood, or abscess, or pseudocyst formations. Ultrasonography is especially helpful because it can help rule out such differential diagnostic considerations as ectopic pregnancy. It is also very helpful in facilitating the diagnosis of cholelithiasis, which may be etiologic for pancreatitis. The mere presence of gallstones does not imply etiologic relevance.

## Differential Diagnosis

Especially pertinent in the differential diagnosis of pancreatitis in pregnancy is hyperemesis gravidarum, preeclampsia, ruptured ectopic pregnancy (often with elevated serum amylase levels), perforated peptic ulcer, acute cholecystitis, ruptured spleen, liver abscess, and perinephric abscess.

## Complications

Although all of the usual complications of pancre-atitis can occur in parturients, there is no special predisposition to complications during pregnancy. Acute complications include hemorrhagic pancreatitis with severe hypotension and hypocalcemia, respiratory distress syndrome, pleural effusions, pancreatic ascites, abscess formation, and liponecrosis.

## Treatment

Treatment of acute pancreatitis is primarily medical and supportive, with intravenous fluids and colloids, nasogastric suction, and restricting alimentation. Parenteral analgesics for pain relief are often necessary. Prophylactic antibiotics are unnecessary and pancreatic enzyme inhibitors have not been successful. Surgical exploration is reserved for patients with pancreatic abscess, ruptured pseudocyst, or severe hemorrhagic pancreatitis, and for those with pancreatitis secondary to a surgically remediable lesion. A decision to terminate pregnancy should be based on nonobstetric factors since the continuation of pregnancy does not influence the course of pancreatitis. Pancreatitis in pregnancy is managed as it is in the nonpregnant state, except that parenteral nutritional supplementation is considered at an earlier point in treatment to protect the fetus.

## Prognosis

Maternal mortality rates as high as 37% were reported prior to the era of modern medical and surgical management. Perinatal losses are few, although preterm labor appears to occur in a high proportion of later gestations. Most recent single-institution series reflect a maternal mortality rate of only 3.4% and a fetal salvage rate of 89%.

# PEPTIC ULCER DISEASE

Pregnancy appears to be somewhat protective against the development of gastrointestinal ulcers. Thus, peptic ulcer disease occurring as a complication of pregnancy or diagnosed during gestation is encountered infrequently, although the exact incidence is unknown. The apparent protection afforded by pregnancy against peptic ulcer disease remains unexplained. High levels of estrogen are considered to be the most likely explanation.

## Clinical Findings

Signs and symptoms of ulcer disease in pregnancy can be mistakenly dismissed as being a normal part of the gravid state. Dyspepsia is the major symptom of ulcers during gestation, although reflux symptoms and nausea are common. Epigastric discomfort that is chronologically unrelated to meals is often reported. Abdominal pain might suggest a perforated ulcer, especially in the presence of peritoneal signs and systemic shock. Flexible endoscopy is preferred to radiologic techniques for diagnosis because the use of endoscopy does not carry the risk of exposing the fetus to radiation.

### Differential Diagnosis

The signs and symptoms of ulcer disease in pregnancy can be mistakenly dismissed as being a normal part of the gravid state. Reflux esophagitis, a common occurrence in pregnancy, and Mallory-Weiss tears may have symptoms very similar to those of peptic ulcer disease. Gastritis and the irritable bowel syndrome must be ruled out.

### Treatment

Currently, antacids are clearly the favorite first agent of therapy for peptic ulcer, since they have the distinct advantages of local action and the absence of major systemic side effects. The best choice appears to be a magnesium-aluminum combination antacid taken at frequent intervals in high doses for 6–8 weeks. Cimetidine has proven efficacious in the healing of both gastric and duodenal ulcers, but its safety during gestation is of theoretic concern. In the patient unresponsive to antacid therapy, cimetidine should be considered as well as the $H_2$ blocker ranitidine. The role of cimetidine and other histamine blockers remains to be defined; they continue to be reserved for gravidas with complicated disease refractory to the first-line agents.

### Complications

Fewer than 100 parturients have been reported with complications of peptic ulceration such as perforation, bleeding, and obstruction. Most of these have occurred in the third trimester of pregnancy. Gastric perforation during pregnancy has an exceedingly high mortality rate, partly because of the difficulty in establishing a proper diagnosis. Other causes for upper gastrointestinal bleeding in pregnancy are reflux esophagitis and Mallory-Weiss tears. Surgical intervention is indicated for significant bleeding ulcerations. Obstruction usually resolves with conservative measures, and surgery is rarely needed for these patients. In patients requiring surgery for complicated peptic ulcers late in the third trimester, concurrent cesarean delivery may be indicated to enhance operative exposure of the upper abdomen and to prevent potential fetal death or damage from maternal hypotension and hypoxemia.

## ACUTE INTESTINAL OBSTRUCTION

Intestinal obstruction is an infrequently encountered complication of pregnancy that is estimated to occur in about 1–3 of every 10,000 pregnancies. It results most often from pressure of the growing uterus on intestinal adhesions subsequent to previous abdominal surgery. Incarcerated hernias and bowel neoplasms are the next most common causes of intestinal obstruction in nonpregnant women, but volvulus and intussusception are the next most common causes for gestational intestinal obstruction. Appendectomy and gynecologic procedures are the most common antecedents predisposing to adhesion formation.

### Clinical Findings

The same classic triad of abdominal pain, vomiting, and obstipation is observed in pregnant and nonpregnant women with intestinal obstruction. Pain may be diffuse, constant, or periodic, occurring every 4–5 minutes with small bowel obstruction or every 10–15 minutes with large bowel obstruction. Small bowel obstruction usually produces more pain than the milder discomfort of volvulus and intussusception. Bowel sounds are of little value in making an early diagnosis of obstruction, and tenderness to palpation is typically absent with early obstruction. Vomiting occurs early with small bowel obstruction, while guarding and rebound tenderness are observed in association with strangulation. Late in the course of disease, fever, oliguria, and shock occur as manifestations of massive fluid loss into the bowel, acidosis, and infection. The diagnosis is usually confirmed by radiologic studies, which should be obtained despite the slight risk to the fetus. A simple x-ray of the abdomen is nondiagnostic in about 50% of early cases, but serial films obtained at 4–6-hour intervals usually reveal progressive changes that confirm the diagnosis. Volvulus should be suspected when there is a single, grossly dilated loop of bowel.

### Differential Diagnosis

Volvulus of the colon is the second most common cause of gestational bowel obstruction accounting for about 25% of cases. The primary area of obstruction is usually cecal due to inadequate fixation in the right lumbar gutter. Radiographs can be diagnostic of sigmoid volvulus; with cecal volvulus the cecum is massively distended and kidney-shaped. Intussusception is an infrequent cause of gestational bowel obstruction and is difficult to diagnose because the obstruction may be intermittent and typical radiologic features may be absent. Pseudo-obstruction during pregnancy is a diagnosis of exclusion and is rarely seen.

### Treatment

Enemas that are repeatedly nonproductive may be helpful in diagnosing intestinal obstruction. After the diagnosis is made, the only definitive treatment for intestinal obstruction is surgical. The patient must be rapidly stabilized, since the maternal fluid deficit may be 1–6 L by the time obstruction can be identified on a scout film. With advanced obstruction, the patient must be rapidly and aggressively hydrated to support both her and the fetus. A large vertical incision on the abdomen provides the best operative exposure. Surgical principles for intraoperative management apply similarly to pregnant and nonpregnant patients. Cesarean delivery is performed first, if, later in gestation the large uterus prevents adequate exposure of the bowel.

## Prognosis

Intestinal obstruction in pregnancy is associated with a maternal mortality rate of 10–20%, with losses occurring secondary to infection and irreversible shock. Early diagnosis and treatment are essential for an optimal outcome because perinatal mortality is even higher than maternal mortality and usually results from maternal hypotension and resultant fetal hypoxia and acidosis.

## SPONTANEOUS HEPATIC & SPLENIC RUPTURE

Spontaneous intra-abdominal hemorrhage during pregnancy has diverse causes, including trauma, preexisting splenic disease, and preeclampsia-eclampsia. Often, the exact cause can not be determined. Spontaneous hepatic rupture associated with severe preeclampsia-eclampsia may be manifested by severe abdominal pain and shock, with thrombocytopenia and low fibrinogen levels. Exploratory celiotomy should be undertaken immediately because early diagnosis, blood transfusion, and prompt operation have been associated with improved survival rates.

Bleeding from a lacerated or ruptured spleen does not cease spontaneously and requires immediate surgical attention. Peritoneal tap or peritoneal lavage in association with a falling hematocrit and abdominal pain are often helpful in establishing the presence of a hemoperitoneum.

## SPLENIC ARTERY ANEURYSM

Autopsy data suggest that splenic artery aneurysm occurs in 0.1% of adults, with a 100-fold increase in elderly people. Nearly 1% of patients undergoing abdominal arteriographic studies are found incidentally to have the lesion. It is estimated that 6–10% of lesions will rupture. Twenty-five to 40% of ruptures occur during gestation, especially in the last trimester. Pregnant women who develop ruptured splenic artery aneurysm have a 75% mortality rate (as do their fetuses) because the cause is often unsuspected and preoperative or intraoperative treatment is delayed. Most patients with this condition are thought to have placental abruption or uterine rupture.

Spontaneous rupture of a splenic artery aneurysm has been reported as a major cause of intraperitoneal hemorrhage during late gestation. Prior to rupture, the presenting symptoms may be completely absent or vague, with the most common symptom being vague epigastric or left upper-quadrant pain. The induction of epigastric pain by bending or stooping is an important symptom. Although splenomegaly is often present, a mass often cannot be detected, especially late in gestation. A bruit may be audible. A highly diagnostic finding on flat x-ray film of the abdomen is the demonstration in the upper left quadrant of an oval calcification with a central lucent area. In stable clinical situations, angiography can provide positive confirmation.

Whenever disease is suspected, the obstetrician must undertake immediate laparotomy, often with general surgical assistance, to manage the problem and maximize maternal and fetal survival rates. Following ligation of the splenic artery and resection of the aneurysm, the surgeon can choose to retain the spleen if adequate collateral arterial blood supply can be demonstrated, but more usually splenectomy is performed.

# PELVIC DISEASES & DISORDERS

## OVARIAN MASSES

Complications of ovarian cysts during pregnancy and the puerperium are second to appendicitis in overall incidence when all abdominopelvic conditions are considered. Found in 0.1% of all pregnant women, ovarian masses are usually asymptomatic unless rupture or torsion occurs. Only 2% of such masses will rupture during gestation; however, it is much more likely that torsion will occur (50–60%).

The most common adnexal mass palpable early in pregnancy is the corpus luteum of gestation, which rarely exceeds 6 cm in diameter. The most common pathologic ovarian neoplasms during pregnancy are benign cystic teratoma (21%), serous cystadenoma (21%), cystic corpus luteum (18%), and mucinous cystadenoma.

Ultrasonography usually facilitates delineation of the size and consistency of adnexal masses. If the mass is unilateral, mobile, and cystic, anaplastic elements are less likely and operation can be deferred until the second trimester. Ovarian enlargement must be differentiated from lesions of the colon, pedunculated leiomyomas, pelvic kidneys, and congenital abnormalities of the uterus. Any adnexal lesion present after 15 weeks or larger than 6 cm in diameter, especially if it contains solid or septate components, contains internal vegetations, shows evidence of fixation, or is present in association with abdominal ascites, warrants surgical exploration and pathologic diagnosis. Asymptomatic ovarian masses that are initially noted in the third trimester of pregnancy may be followed until the onset of labor, because the size of the uterus may present problems of access during laparotomy and because labor may be inadvertently induced.

### Solid Ovarian Tumors

Solid ovarian tumors discovered during pregnancy generally should be treated surgically because of the low but significant incidence of cancer (2–5%) and to prevent torsion, rupture, and soft tissue dystocia at the time of labor. Because of these potential hazards, persistent solid or cystic ovarian masses discovered in the first trimester should ideally be removed in the second trimester.

### Torsion of Ovarian Pedicle

Torsion of an ovarian pedicle, uterine tube, and broad ligament can produce an acute surgical disorder with shock and peritonitis. Other causes are often considered, and the diagnosis of torsion is usually made at surgery. Prompt operation is necessary to prevent tissue necrosis, preterm labor, and potential perinatal or maternal death. Most patients with adnexal torsion complain of pain that is initially slow in onset, intermittent, and progressively more severe. The right ovary is involved more frequently than the left. Although more commonly noted in the first trimester, torsion does occur in the second trimester. Benign cystic teratomas and cystomas are the most common histologic findings in ovaries that have undergone torsion. Surgical removal of ovarian benign cystic teratomas is recommended to avert torsion and rupture with severe generalized peritonitis. Ovarian cysts that have undergone torsion must not be untwisted prior to pedicle clamping, because of potential fatal pulmonary embolization.

### Carcinoma of Ovary

Carcinoma of the ovary occurs in less than 0.1% of all gestations and has been encountered in all trimesters. Between 2% and 5% of all ovarian tumors complicating pregnancy are malignant. Many are germ cell tumors (dysgerminoma, endodermal sinus tumor, malignant teratoma, embryonal carcinoma, choriocarcinoma) and papillary serous cystadenocarcinomas. Approximately 50% are discovered by routine prenatal pelvic examination.

The treatment for gestational ovarian cancer is no different from that for the nonpregnant patient. Surgical removal of as much of the cancer as possible is indicated. A generous surgical incision is important not only to remove the tumor but also to properly explore the abdomen, to perform at least a partial omentectomy, and to reduce uterine manipulation until the definitive surgical course of management is determined. Staging is accomplished and adequate tissue obtained for histologic diagnosis. Conservative surgery may be considered for a low-grade encapsulated tumor if there is no evidence of peritoneal disease or other spread (on cytologic examination and exploration) and if the contralateral ovary proves normal on wedge resection.

If the tumor is benign, residual ovarian tissue is conserved if possible. The opposite ovary must always be carefully inspected, incised, or biopsied to rule out disease. Salpingectomy should be avoided if possible. Regardless of the stage of gestation, ovarian cancer is usually managed aggressively, with surgical extirpation of all pelvic generative organs. The implications of the disease must be fully and frankly discussed with the patient prior to operation.

## LEIOMYOMAS

Uterine leiomyomas (0.3–2.6% of pregnancies) may complicate pregnancy by tumor degeneration, torsion, or mechanical obstruction of labor. Red degeneration or necrobiosis of leiomyomas is clinically similar to visceral infarction. Pathologic examination of this tissue reveals loss of normal structure and presence of capillaries congested with red cells. Degeneration may be focal or diffuse. A degenerating leiomyoma or one undergoing torsion is characterized by acute abdominal pain with point tenderness over the site of the leiomyoma. Conservative treatment with analgesia, reassurance, and supportive therapy is almost always adequate. The 2 usual indications for surgery during pregnancy include torsion of an isolated, pedunculated leiomyoma and obstruction of labor. Myomectomy should never be performed during pregnancy because of the risk of uncontrollable hemorrhage. Disseminated intravascular coagulation has been reported as a complication of leiomyoma degeneration. Although this is certainly a rare occurrence, a coagulation profile may prove useful in cases of degeneration.

The onset of pain is typically rapid, localized, and severe with minimal or absent gastrointestinal symptoms. Clinical or laboratory evidence of hemorrhage is absent. Smooth muscle enzymes such as SGOT (AST), LDH (lactic dehydrogenase), and CPK (creatine phosphokinase) may be elevated. Ultrasonography is of great value to document the location, size, and consistency of leiomyomas in a pregnant uterus. Cystic changes in leiomyomas are often visualized when there are clinical signs of degeneration. Early in pregnancy, diagnostic laparoscopy may be of value to differentiate leiomyoma from ovarian tumor, especially when ultrasonography is inadequate.

## OTHER PELVIC DISORDERS

Other nonobstetric pelvic conditions that may require operative intervention during pregnancy include spontaneous rupture of utero-ovarian vessels, abnormal uterine fixation, and uterine torsion.

# BREAST CANCER

Breast cancer is the most common cancer affecting women. One of every 6 cases occurs in women under 45 years of age; this means that the disease can occur during pregnancy (3 in 10,000). For this reason, breast examination should be performed at regular intervals (usually each trimester) during the prenatal and postnatal visits. Any mass found by the woman or the obstetrician should be satisfactorily explained physiologically or surgically without undue delay.

Management of the pregnant woman with breast carcinoma is especially difficult because it requires careful consideration of both mother and fetus. In general, initial management does not differ from that for nonpregnant women. When a localized lesion is present, needle aspiration and needle biopsy may be appropriate, and risks of radiation exposure from mammography can be deferred. Surgical biopsy with the patient under general anesthesia may be more appropriate for a less well-defined lesion. Cystic lesions should be aspirated and the fluid examined for abnormal cytologic characteristics. Malignant cells are rarely found in nonbloody fluid. Despite pregnancy, all presumed fibroadenomas and lesions found to be equivocal on cytologic study should be excised using local anesthesia. The increased vascularity of the breasts does not appear to interfere with excisional biopsy in an outpatient setting.

The general approach to treatment for breast cancer should be similar in pregnant and nonpregnant patients. Termination of pregnancy has not been shown to improve survival rates. Cancerous lesions occurring during pregnancy have traditionally been promptly treated by mastectomy. Most clinicians recommend termination of pregnancy only if the diagnosis is made in the first trimester. Because there have been reports of improved survival rates in breast cancer patients who have had subsequent pregnancies compared with those who have not, subsequent pregnancies need not necessarily be discouraged after a suitable period of recuperation and observation. Radical mastectomy is well tolerated during pregnancy, and the results of treatment are much the same stage-for-stage as they are otherwise. Many authorities recommend radical mastectomy for stage I or stage II disease. Several studies have shown that prophylactic oophorectomy does not alter the course of the disease. Breastfeeding is usually discouraged to avoid vascular enrichment in the opposite breast.

# BONE TUMORS

Benign bone tumors rarely cause problems in pregnancy. The natural history of malignant bone tumors is not affected by pregnancy, but treatment can be complicated. The most frequently encountered malignant tumors are Ewing's sarcoma and osteogenic sarcoma. Sites in such areas as the clavicle, sternum, spine, humerus, and femur initially appear as a lump or mass with local pain and disability. Osteogenic sarcoma is treated with wide surgical excision. Although highly effective, chemotherapy often is delayed until the postpartum period, especially if the lesion is diagnosed near term. Because adjuvant combination chemotherapy considerably enhances the outcome of osteogenic sarcoma, pregnancy should not delay optimum therapy for more than a few weeks. An excellent outcome usually follows wide local excision of giant cell bone tumors. In general, pregnancy considerations should not be reason for postponement of surgery for biopsy and treatment of malignant bone tumors.

# CARDIAC DISEASE

Most cardiac problems in pregnant women can be managed medically. In the few patients requiring it, cardiac surgery can be performed with excellent results, although there is maternal and fetal risk. The risk for the mother is probably no greater than for the nonpregnant patient. Fetal risk can be minimized with careful surveillance. Closed cardiac techniques in general are associated with better fetal outcome than open cardiac techniques. When valve replacement is required, tissue valves rather than artificial valves are recommended, so that anticoagulation is not needed. Congenital heart defects usually do not require surgery unless cyanotic heart disease is present. Pulmonary hypertension secondary to fixed pulmonary vascular resistance and right-to-left shunting is associated with increased maternal and perinatal mortality rates. If pulmonary artery hypertension is demonstrated on cardiac catheterization early in pregnancy and is not reactive to oxygen administration, therapeutic abortion is strongly indicated.

Close fetal surveillance by electronic heart rate and uterine contraction monitoring is essential during any cardiac surgical procedure whether or not cardiopulmonary bypass is used. During bypass, blood flow to the uterus can be assessed indirectly by changes in the fetal heart rate, and alterations in flow can be made accordingly. Operations should generally be performed early in the second trimester when organogenesis is complete and there is comparatively less hemodynamic burden and less risk of preterm labor than later in gestation. Fetal bradycardia and increased uterine contractions often occur during and shortly after bypass but usually abate soon thereafter. If contractions persist and preterm labor ensues, carefully monitored tocolytic therapy is recommended.

## NEUROLOGIC DISEASE

The anesthetic management of a pregnant woman with intracranial aneurysm requires induced, carefully controlled hypotension for surgery to be properly performed. Judicious use of sodium nitroprusside with primary attention to the mother's status is unlikely to compromise the fetus. Operation is safer earlier in pregnancy, when the blood flow and metabolic needs of the developing fetus are less than those closer to term.

Systemic arterial hypertension associated with endotracheal intubation has been shown to increase cerebral blood flow and elevate intracranial pressure, with resultant rupture of intracerebral aneurysms. Inadequate skeletal muscle relaxation during and after tracheal intubation may raise venous pressure and cause significantly increased intracranial pressure with proportionately decreased cerebral perfusion pressure.

Controlled hyperventilation for neuroresuscitation can lead to fetal compromise, especially in the presence of maternal hypovolemia. Maintenance of adequate intravascular volume, with minimal mean airway pressures should lessen any adverse fetal effects. Diuresis with high doses of mannitol can have deleterious effects on the fetus; lower doses may or may not be hazardous. Controlled hypothermia is safe during pregnancy and is probably especially useful for optimal cerebrovascular surgery without adverse maternal or fetal effects. Oxytocin probably has no deleterious neurologic effects.

## AORTIC ANEURYSM

Because a substantial period of cardiopulmonary bypass is required to repair aortic dissection involving the ascending aorta, delivery of the fetus before the bypass procedure appears advantageous. Proportionately better results are obtained later in gestation. Maternal risk for cardiopulmonary bypass is not increased during pregnancy, but the fetal mortality rate generally exceeds 15%. Episodes of fetal bradycardia have been recorded during open heart surgery and normothermic bypass. Emergency cesarean delivery followed by repair of the dissection appears to be optimal management, especially since fetal viability becomes more likely late in gestation.

## PHEOCHROMOCYTOMA

Deliberate, nonemergency operative removal of a pheochromocytoma is a lifesaving procedure, especially during pregnancy. The tumor is best removed when the patient is optimally prepared and in a stable cardiovascular condition. Removal prior to the stressful period of labor and delivery has been recommended. Even in young, generally healthy women with known pheochromocytoma who have been carefully studied and managed with medication, fetal mortality rates are high, and vaginal delivery is usually considered only after tumor resection. After careful preparation, tumor resection has been performed in the second trimester with subsequent progression of the pregnancy to term and with the mode of delivery dependent on obstetric considerations. Later in gestation, the treatment of choice is a combined procedure of tumor resection and cesarean delivery. Despite careful preparations, surgical technique, and timing, the risk of death for the mother and fetus still remains high.

## HEMORRHOIDS

Pregnancy is the most common cause of symptomatic hemorrhoids. Venous congestion secondary to portal vein obstruction by the enlarging uterus is probably the culprit. Medical therapy with stool softeners and hemorrhoidal analgesics often is the only requirement for nonthrombosed hemorrhoids.

Thrombosis or clots in the vein lead to severe symptoms. The current surgical approach to hemorrhoid disease is conservative, with simple outpatient treatment preferred, particularly during pregnancy and the puerperium. If thrombosed external hemorrhoids remain tender and resist conservative treatment, they can be infiltrated with 1% lidocaine and a small incision made to extract the clot. This is rarely needed if the patient follows all directions for conservative treatment. In the immediate puerperium, thrombosis of external or prolapsing internal hemorrhoids may require hemorrhoidectomy. This is best accomplished by the Lord procedure, in which the perianal region and sphincter are anesthetized using either 1% lidocaine or 0.25% bupivacaine, occasionally with 150 units of hyaluronidase mixed with each 10 mL of anesthetic. The sphincter is gently dilated digitally, after which spasm is relieved and the hemorrhoids recede.

# TRAUMA

Approximately 7% of pregnancies are complicated by trauma. Automobile accidents are the most common nonobstetric cause of death during pregnancy. The most common cause of fetal death is death of the mother. The second cause of fetal death is abruptio placentae. Evaluating the pregnant patient during the early weeks of gestation involves procedures similar to those for other surgical conditions. Emphasis is placed on protecting the fetus from unnecessary drug and x-ray exposure. After fetal viability is reached, fetal monitoring is used. It appears that the fetus should be monitored at least 4 hours with significant trauma, although cases of fetal death have been reported even 24 hours after trauma. A rising baseline fetal heart rate or late decelerations may not only indicate fetal distress from a placental abruption or fetal injury, but also may indicate reduced uterine blood flow from a deterioration of maternal status. Kleihauer-Betke test may indicate fetomaternal hemorrhage.

During pregnancy the enlarging uterus displaces bowel and other structures upward within the abdomen. Injury from a stab wound or bullet is more likely to involve the uterus in such cases. Exploratory laparotomy is usually indicated. Pregnant women with traumatic injuries may be victims of physical abuse. A pregnancy may increase family stress and the practitioner should, therefore be alert for signs of abuse.

# REFERENCES

## GENERAL

Allen JR, Helling TS, Langenfeld M: Intraabdominal surgery during pregnancy. Obstet Gynecol Surv 1990; 45:537.

Barron WM: The pregnant surgical patient: Medical evaluation and management. Ann Intern Med 1984; 101:683.

Brent RL: Ionizing radiation. Contemp OB/GYN 1987:20.

Clark SL et al: Central hemodynamic assessment of normal term pregnancy. Am J Obstet Gynecol 1989; 161:1439.

Hunt MG et al: Perinatal aspects of abdominal surgery for nonobstetric disease. Am J Perinatol 1989;6:412.

Lione A: Ionizing radiation and human reproduction. Reprod Toxicol 1987;1:3.

Niebyl JR: Drugs with potential fetal toxicity. Contemp OB/GYN 1991;36:68.

Rustgi VK, Cooper JN (editors): *Gastrointestinal and Hepatic Complications in Pregnancy.* Wiley, 1986.

Sorensen VJ et al: Management of general surgical emergencies in pregnancy. Am Surg 1990;56:245.

## ANESTHESIA

Duncan PG et al: Fetal risk of anesthesia and surgery during pregnancy. Anesthesiology 1986;64:790.

James FM III: Anesthesia for nonobstetric surgery during pregnancy. Clin Obstet Gynecol 1987;30:621.

## APPENDICITIS

Baily LE et al: Acute appendicitis during pregnancy. Am Surg 1986;52:218.

Hansen GC, Toot PJ, Lynch CO: Subtle ultrasound signs of appendicitis in a pregnant patient: A case report. J Reprod Med 1993;38:223.

Hunt MG et al: Perinatal aspects of abdominal surgery for nonobstetric disease. Am J Perinatol 1989;6:412.

Mazze RI, Kallen B: Appendectomy during pregnancy: A Swedish registry study of 778 cases. Obstet Gynecol 1991;77:835.

Thurnau GR, Hales KA: Appendicitis in pregnancy. Female Patient 1992;17:81.

## BREAST DISEASE

Cobleigh MA, Kiel K, Witt TR: Breast cancer, pp. 1148–1157. In: *Principles and Practice of Medical Therapy in Pregnancy.* Gleicher N (editor). Appleton & Lange, 1992.

Novotny DB et al: Fine needle aspiration of benign and malignant breast masses associated with pregnancy. Acta Cytol 1991;35:676.

Papatestas AE: Breast disease in pregnancy. Contemp OB/GYN 1989;34:79.

Petrek JA, Dukoff Ruth, Rogatko A: Prognosis of pregnancy-associated breast cancer. Obstet Gynecol Surv 1991;46:602.

Zemlickis D et al: Maternal and fetal outcome after

breast cancer in pregnancy. Am J Obstet Gynecol 1992;166:781.

## CHOLECYSTITIS

Elerding SC: A Laparoscopic cholecystectomy in pregnancy. Am J Surg 1993;165:625.

Bateson MC: Gallstone disease—present and future. Lancet 1986;2:1265.

Dixon NP, Faddis DM, Silberman H: Aggressive management of cholecystitis in pregnancy. Am J Surg 1987;154:292.

Landers D et al: Acute cholecystitis in pregnancy. Obstet Gynecol 1987;69:131.

Morrell DG, Mullins JR, Harrison PB: Laparoscopic cholecystectomy during pregnancy in symptomatic patients. Surgery 1992;112:856.

## PANCREATITIS

Hyder SA, Barkin JS: Pancreatic disease, pp. 981–986. In: *Principles and Practice of Medical Therapy in Pregnancy.* Gleicher N (editor). Appleton & Lange, 1992.

Scott LD: Gallstone disease and pancreatitis in pregnancy. Gastroenterol Clin North Am 1992;21:803.

Wilkinson EJ: Acute pancreatitis in pregnancy: A review of 98 cases and a report of 8 new cases. Obstet Gynecol Surv 1973;28:281.

## PEPTIC ULCER DISEASE

Fullman H, Ippoliti A: Acid peptic disease in pregnancy, pp. 87–103. In: *Gastrointestinal and Hepatic Complications in Pregnancy.* Rusti VK, Cooper JN (editors). Wiley, 1986.

Michaletz-Onody PA: Peptic ulcer disease in pregnancy. Gastroenterol Clin North Am 1992;21:817.

## INTESTINAL TRACT

Anderson JB, Turner GM, Williamson RCN: Fulminant ulcerative colitis in late pregnancy and the puerperium. J R Soc Med 1987;80:492.

Perdue PW, Johnson HW Jr, Stafford PW: Intestinal obstruction complicating pregnancy. Am J Surg 1992; 164:384.

## ADNEXAL DISEASE

Hess LW et al: Adnexal mass occurring with intrauterine pregnancy: Report of fifty-four patients requiring laparotomy for definitive management. Am J Obstet Gynecol 1988;158:1029.

Hogston P, Lilford RJ: Ultrasound study of ovarian cysts in pregnancy: Prevalence and significance. Br J Obstet Gynaecol 1986;93:625.

Hopkins MP, Duchon MA: Adnexal surgery in pregnancy. J Reprod Med 1986;31:1035.

Johnson TRB Jr, Woodruff JD: Surgical emergencies of the uterine adnexae during pregnancy. Int J Gynaecol Obstet 1986;24:331.

Koonings PP, Platt LD, Wallace R: Incidental adnexal neoplasms at cesarean section. Obstet Gynecol 1988; 72:767.

Lavery JP et al: Sonographic evaluation of the adnexa during early pregnancy. Surg Gynecol Obstet 1986; 163:319.

Lizzi L, Bolognese RJ: Ovarian masses in pregnancy. Postgrad Obstet Gynecol 1988;8:1.

## TRAUMA

McFarlane J et al: Assessing for abuse during pregnancy: Severity and frequency of injuries and associated entry into prenatal care. JAMA 1992;267:3176.

Fildes J et al: Trauma: The leading cause of maternal death. J Trauma 1992;32:643.

Pearlman MD, Tintinallli JE, Lorenz RP: A prospective controlled study of outcome after trauma during pregnancy. Am J Obstet Gynecol 1990;162:1502.

Sherman HF, Scott LM, Rosemurgy AS: Changes affecting the initial evaluation and care of the pregnant trauma victim. J Emerg Med 1990;8:575.

Williams JK, McClain L, Alexander SR, Colorado, NM: Evaluation of blunt abdominal trauma in the third trimester of pregnancy: Maternal and fetal considerations. Obstet Gynecol 1990;75:33.

## MISCELLANEOUS

Asher S et al: Carcinoma of the colon during pregnancy. Obstet Gynecol Surv 1992;47:222.

Burton CA, Grimes DA, March CM: Surgical management of Leiomyomata during pregnancy. Obstet Gynecol 1989;74:707.

Catanzarite VA et al: Management of pregnancy subsequent to rupture of an intracranial arterial aneurysm. Am J Perinatol 1984;1:174.

Gawly RM: Ruptured intracranial aneurysm in pregnancy: A case report and review of the literature. Eur J Obstet Gynecol Reprod Biol 1992;46:150.

Geelhoed GW: Surgery of the endocrine glands in pregnancy. Clin Obstet Gynecol 1983;26:865.

Katz NM et al: Aortic dissection during pregnancy: Treatment by emergency cesarean section immediately followed by operative repair of the aortic dissection. Am J Cardiol 1984;54:699.

Kofke WA, Wuest HP, McGinnis LA: Cesarean section following ruptured cerebral aneurysm and neuroresuscitation. Anesthesiology 1984;60:242.

Lennon RL, Sundt TM Jr, Gronert GA: Combined cesarean section and clipping of intracerebral aneurysm. Anesthesiology 1984;60:240.

Shushan A et al: Carcinoma of the colon during pregnancy. Obstet Gynecol Surv 1992;47:222.

Simon MA, Phillips WA, Bonfiglio M: Pregnancy and aggressive or malignant primary bone tumors. Cancer 1984;53:2564.

Smith LG Jr et al: Spontaneous rupture of liver during pregnancy: current therapy. Obstet Gynecol 1991; 77:171.

Ueland K: Cardiovascular surgery and the ob patient. Contemp OB/GYN 1984;24:117.

# Complications of Labor & Delivery

*Eduardo Herrera, MD, & Martin L. Pernoll, MD*

## FETAL BLOOD LOSS IN PREGNANCY

Most blood loss occurring in late pregnancy is of maternal origin, but fetal blood may be lost either from trauma to the placenta or from vasa previa.

## TRAUMA TO THE PLACENTA

Trauma to the placenta most commonly occurs in low placental implantation or abruptio placentae with retroplacental clot formation. Since special studies are necessary for detection, fetal blood is almost never found in maternal vaginal, and unless the clinical finding of fetal tachycardia triggers special analysis (see below). Whenever vaginal bleeding occurs in late pregnancy in combination with fetal tachycardia, the physician must quickly determine whether significant fetal bleeding is present. The vascular volume of a term fetus is usually no more than 250 mL, so that what appears to be minor vaginal bleeding could be life-threatening to the fetus. The Apt test and the Kleihauer-Betke test can detect fetal hemoglobin; hemoglobin electrophoresis is also possible but so time-consuming that it is usually of little value. When fetal bleeding is present, delivery must be accomplished as quickly as possible if the infant is to be saved.

## VELAMENTOUS CORD INSERTION & VASA PREVIA

### Velamentous Cord Insertion

In velamentous cord insertion, the umbilical cord does not insert on the chorionic plate but rather at some point on the fetal membranes. This happens in about 1 in 5000 deliveries, but the incidence is 6–9 times higher in twin placentas than in singletons, and an even greater incidence is noted in higher orders of multiple birth. In multiple gestations, the vessels often lie within the membranes dividing the fetuses. The possibility of velamentous cord insertion in multiple gestations must always be kept in mind.

Abnormal insertion of the cord and distribution of vessels appear to cause no physiologic difficulty, but as the vessels pass through the membranes, the nonvascular matrix of the umbilical cord (Wharton's jelly) and the epithelial surface of the cord are lost. This leaves the vessels vulnerable to rupture, shearing, or laceration.

### Vasa Previa

In vasa previa, the fetal vessels associated with velamentous insertion of the cord traverse the lower uterine segment and present in advance of the fetal presenting part. In this location, the vessels are likely to be disrupted by labor or rupture of membranes, with resulting rapid bleeding and a high risk of fetal exsanguination.

### Diagnosis & Treatment

The diagnosis of vasa previa or velamentous cord insertion is rarely made before rupture of the membranes. The usual presentation is onset of bleeding with fetal tachycardia occurring soon after rupture of the membranes. The diagnosis can potentially be made by ultrasonography, but it is most frequently accomplished by palpation (through the partially or fully dilated cervix) of fetal vessels in the membranes overlying the presenting part. Sinusoidal fetal heart rate patterns on electronic fetal monitoring may be another indication of fetal bleeding or severe anemia. Finally, if fetal scalp blood sampling can be done, a fetal scalp blood hematocrit indicating anemia may aid in the diagnosis.

If the diagnosis is made before rupture of the membranes or fetal exsanguination occurs, delivery should be by cesarean section. If the diagnosis is made at the time of rupture of the membranes, delivery should be accomplished by the most expeditious method (usually, emergency cesarean section).

# DYSTOCIA

## DEFINITION & CLASSIFICATION

Dystocia is defined as difficult labor. It may be associated with various abnormalities that prevent or deviate from the normal course of labor and delivery. These abnormalities are classified into 3 general categories that are often interrelated; eg, a contracted pelvis may increase the likelihood of fetal malpresentation. Malpresentation or excessive fetal size may be related to ineffective uterine action. Disproportion between pelvic architecture and the presenting part often accompanies uterine dysfunction.

### Abnormalities of the Passage

Abnormalities of the passage constitute pelvic dystocia, ie, aberrations of pelvic architecture and its relationship to the presenting part. Such abnormalities may be related to size or configurational alterations of the bony pelvis, soft tissue abnormalities of the birth canal, reproductive tract masses or neoplasia, or aberrant placental location.

### Abnormalities of the Passenger

Abnormalities of the passenger are known as fetal dystocia, ie, that are caused by abnormalities of the fetus. Common fetal abnormalities leading to dystocia include excessive fetal size, malpositions, congenital anomalies, and multiple gestation.

### Abnormalities of the Powers

Abnormalities of the "powers" constitute uterine dystocia, ie, uterine activity that is ineffective in eliciting the normal progress of labor. Hypertonic, hypotonic, or discoordinated uterine activity is characteristic of ineffective uterine action. Lack of voluntary expulsive effort during the second stage may also impede the normal course of delivery.

## INCIDENCE

Since 1970, the trend in the USA has been to diagnose dystocia more frequently and to perform cesarean section more often as a means of treatment. Cesarean section has thereby become a major concern because of its impact on both maternal morbidity and the cost of medical care. In 1980, the NIH Consensus Development Task Force on Cesarean Childbirth reported a 3-fold increase in the cesarean birth rate: from 5.5% in 1970 to 15.2% in 1978. By 1984, the incidence of cesarean delivery reached 21.1%. A similar increase was noted in Canada. A trend toward increasing use of cesarean section was also noted in northern European nations, but rates were considerably lower than in the USA. Thirty-one percent of cesarean sections performed in the USA in 1978 were performed for dystocia; 12% of cesarean sections were performed for breech presentation.

Of particular concern to the NIH Task Force was the marked increase in cesarean sections performed for abnormal labors with the fetus in a vertex presentation. Most of the infants delivered operatively in this category weighed more than 2500 g, and there was no evidence of increased infant survival compared with vaginal births. The task force urged further study into the differential diagnosis of dystocia and alternative therapy in selected cases.

The overall incidence of dystocia in women in labor is difficult to determine, perhaps because of unclear generally applied definitions. In nulliparous patients the incidence of labor disorders is less than 10%. Since the incidence of malpresentation or forceps delivery is more easily defined, the diagnosis of dystocia in a vertex presentation is often retrospective; if the outcome is uneventful, spontaneous vaginal delivery, the diagnosis may go unreported. Few confirmatory laboratory tests are of value in the clinical diagnosis of dystocia.

Although fetal malposition, congenital anomalies, maternal soft tissue dystocia, and neoplasms are easily diagnosed by physical examination, ultrasonography, and roentgenography, they occur in a minority of cases. X-ray pelvimetry has generally not been found helpful in the diagnosis of the most commonly diagnosed conditions ("failure to progress," cephalopelvic disproportion) or in other causes of dystocia with the fetus in a vertex presentation. These diagnoses must be made after clinical identification of an abnormal labor pattern.

## ABNORMAL PATTERNS OF LABOR

Labor is a dynamic process characterized by uterine contractions that increase in regularity, intensity, and duration to cause progressive dilatation and effacement of the cervix and permit descent of the fetus through the birth canal.

Estimates of cervical dilatation and of descent of the fetal presenting part have been used to evaluate the progress of labor. Normal labor patterns in primigravidas and multiparas have been described in detail by Friedman and others (see Figs 10–7, 10–8, and 10–9). Using the 95th percentile value as the upper limit of normal, Friedman has also described 4 abnormal patterns of labor (see Fig 10–10). These abnormal labor patterns are prolonged latent phase, the 2 protraction disorders (protracted active-phase dilatation and protracted descent), the 4 arrest disorders (prolonged deceleration phase, secondary arrest of dilatation, arrest of descent, and failure of descent), and precipitate labor disorders.

## 1. PROLONGED LATENT PHASE

### Definition

The latent phase of labor begins with the onset of regular uterine contractions and extends to the beginning of the active phase of cervical dilatation. The duration of the latent phase averages 6.4 hours in nulliparas and 4.8 hours in multiparas. The latent phase is abnormally prolonged if it lasts more than 20 hours in nulliparas or 14 hours in multiparas.

### Causes

1. Excessive sedation or sedation given before the end of the latent phase.

2. The use of conduction or general anesthesia before labor enters the active phase.

3. Labor that begins with an unfavorable or unripe cervix, ie, one that is long, closed, rigid, and thick (a low Bishop score; see Chapter 10).

4. Uterine dysfunction characterized by weak, irregular, uncoordinated, and ineffective uterine contractions.

5. Fetopelvic disproportion.

### Treatment

Treatment should acknowledge that these patients tend to be physically exhausted and emotionally discouraged by their lack of progress and that they are suffering from fluid and electrolyte imbalances. A regimen of rest is therefore recommended in the absence of any risk factors (eg, premature rupture of the membranes, amnionitis, preeclampsia-eclampsia).

**A. Therapeutic Rest Regimen:** A narcotic agent such as morphine sulfate is given in doses large enough to arrest uterine contractions temporarily and provide from 6 to 12 hours of rest. An initial dose of 8–12 mg (depending on the patient's weight) is given subcutaneously. If uterine contractions persist after 20 minutes, no cervical changes have occurred (ie, the active phase of labor has not begun unexpectedly), and maternal respiration is not depressed, an additional 4 mg of morphine may be given. Hydration (See Chapter 15) may also be of benefit.

After 6–12 hours of rest, most patients (85%) will have entered the active phase of labor, and further progression in dilatation and effacement may be expected. Ten percent of patients will have been in false labor, as shown by the response to therapy. As soon as these patients are ambulatory and fetal monitoring reveals fetal reactivity, they may be allowed to return home to await the onset of true labor. In the remaining 5% of patients, uterine contractions that are ineffective in producing dilatation resume; in the absence of any contraindication, active stimulation of labor with oxytocin infusion may be effective in terminating the latent phase of labor.

**B. Oxytocin Infusion:** As an alternative to sedation (and possible hydration), some authorities recommend oxytocin infusion as the primary treatment

for all patients with a prolonged latent phase. Although it is probably as effective as bed rest, it decreases the time available to correct fluid and electrolyte imbalances and to meet the patient's psychologic needs. There is also no opportunity to identify patients who are in false labor.

If immediate delivery is required for clinical reasons (eg, severe preeclampsia or amnionitis), oxytocin infusion is the treatment of choice.

### Prognosis

The prognosis for vaginal delivery after these therapeutic measures is excellent. Patients with a prolonged latent phase of labor who respond to rest can be expected to deliver vaginally in nearly all cases. After abnormalities in the latent phase have been corrected, patients are not at any greater risk of developing subsequent labor disorders than are patients who have experienced a normal latent phase.

## 2. PROTRACTION DISORDERS

### Definition

Protracted cervical dilatation in the active phase of labor and protracted descent of the fetus constitute the protraction disorders, which share some common characteristics outlined below.

Protracted active-phase dilatation is characterized by an abnormally slow rate of dilatation in the active phase, ie, less than 1.2 cm/h in nulliparas or less than 1.5 cm/h in multiparas. Protracted descent of the fetus is characterized by a rate of descent under 1 cm/h in nulliparas or under 2 cm/h in multiparas.

### Causes

The underlying pathogenesis is probably multifactorial; several common factors have been implicated, including fetopelvic disproportion, which is encountered in about one-third of patients. Other factors include minor malpositions (occiput posterior), improperly administered conduction anesthesia (eg, epidural anesthesia administered above dermatome T10 or given before the onset of the active phase or in the presence of other inhibitory factors), excessive sedation, and pelvic tumors obstructing the birth canal. Electronic monitoring using an intrauterine catheter to assess both uterine contractions and fetal heart rate is imperative, since the choice of treatment depends partly on the efficiency of contractions (ie, occurring every 3–4 minutes and showing a rise in pressure of more than 25 mm Hg lasting for more than 30 seconds).

### Treatment

Treatment of protraction disorders is not clearly established except in cases of documented fetopelvic disproportion. Definitive evaluation of fetopelvic relationships by physical examination and possibly by x-ray examination is important in these patients. Cesarean section is indicated in the presence of confirmed fetopelvic disproportion.

If fetopelvic disproportion has been ruled out in a patient with adequate labor who is still experiencing a protraction disorder, supportive measures are necessary. Although inhibitory factors should be avoided, it is relatively easy to inhibit further progress or even to cause secondary arrest by administering excessive sedation or regional block anesthesia. Patients experiencing protraction disorders generally do not respond to oxytocin infusion or other forms of stimulation of labor if their contractions are already adequate. Special attention should be paid to fluid and electrolyte balance and to the patient's emotional and physical needs, because a prolonged labor may be anticipated. Even though it is possible to enhance uterine contractility, progression of dilatation may not improve.

Conservative management, consisting of support and close observation, carries a good prognosis for vaginal delivery (approximately two-thirds of patients) if continued progress occurs and there is no fetal compromise. Other authorities recommend active intervention with oxytocin in nulliparas with protraction disorders, and equally successful outcomes are reported. Cesarean section is likely if disproportion exists: vaginal delivery can often be achieved if disproportion is absent and there are no other complications.

## Prognosis

The prognosis for women with protraction disorders depends on the presence or absence of fetopelvic disproportion. The prognosis for the fetus is closely related to the quality of delivery. These infants seem particularly sensitive to instrumental vaginal delivery. Spontaneous vaginal delivery or one achieved with minimal manipulation is the most crucial factor favoring a good outlook for the fetus, and its importance cannot be overemphasized.

## 3. ARREST DISORDERS

### Definition

The 4 patterns of arrest in labor may be characterized as follows:

1. In prolonged deceleration phase, the deceleration phase lasts more than 3 hours in nulliparas or more than 1 hour in multiparas.

2. With secondary arrest of dilatation, there is no progressive cervical dilatation in the active phase of labor for 2 hours or more.

3. With arrest of descent, descent fails to progress for 1 hour or more.

4. In failure of descent, descent fails to occur during the deceleration phase of dilatation and during the second stage.

### Causes

About 50% of patients with arrest disorders demonstrate fetopelvic disproportion. Other causative factors include various fetal malpositions (eg, occiput posterior, occiput transverse, face, or brow), inappropriately administered anesthesia, or excessive sedation.

### Treatment

When an arrest disorder is diagnosed, thorough evaluation of fetopelvic relationships before treatment is begun is crucial. Evaluation should include a careful clinical pelvic examination for pelvic adequacy and, possibly, x-ray pelvimetry. If documented fetopelvic disproportion and an arrest disorder exist, cesarean section is clearly warranted, since considerable trauma to both mother and baby could otherwise occur.

If no documented fetopelvic disproportion is present, oxytocin stimulation may be of benefit. In certain cases, it may also be helpful to permit the effects of excessive sedation or conduction anesthesia to wear off. Oxytocin stimulation is generally effective in producing further progress, provided there are no contraindications to its use.

### Prognosis

The arrest disorders generally carry a poor prognosis for vaginal delivery. If a postarrest slope of dilatation or descent can be established that is equal to or greater than the prearrest slope, however, the prognosis for vaginal delivery is excellent. If the postarrest slope develops at a rate that is less than the prearrest slope, the outlook is not as optimistic, because it suggests that significant disproportion may have been overlooked and points to the need for reevaluation of fetopelvic relationships.

Arrest disorders are associated with increased perinatal morbidity even if midforceps are not used. It is therefore essential to monitor the fetal heart rate and uterine contractions during labor in all patients with arrest disorders.

## 4. PRECIPITATE LABOR DISORDERS

Precipitate dilatation in a primigravida is a maximum slope of 5 or more centimeters per hour and in a multigravida a maximum slope of 10 cm or more per hour. Precipitate descent for a primigravida is descent of the fetal presenting part of 5 cm or more per hour and for multiparas as descent of 10 cm or more per hour.

### Causes

Precipitate labor may result from either extremely strong uterine contractions or low birth canal resistance. Although the initiating mechanism for extraordinarily forceful uterine contractions is usually not known, occasionally abnormal contractions are associated with administration of oxytocin. Strong uterine contractions (both in force and increased basal tone) may also accompany abruptio placentae. Little is known about the cause of low birth canal resistance.

## Treatment

Oxytocin has a brief half-life. Thus, if oxytocin administration is the cause of abnormal contractions it may simply be stopped and the problem should resolve in less than 5 minutes. Although parenteral epinephrine, magnesium sulfate, and various tocolytic agents have been recommended to decrease the uterine contractions, the evidence for their use remains unsubstantiated. Anesthesia and analgesia are relatively contraindicated, given the already compromised fetus. Physical attempts to retard delivery are absolutely contraindicated.

## Complications

Maternal complications are rare if the cervix and birth canal are relaxed, but precipitate labor is one of the known antecedents of maternal amniotic fluid embolism. Thus, enhanced maternal monitoring for this complication is imperative (see Chapter 59). In addition, the uterus that has been hypertonic with labor tends to be hypotonic postpartum, thereby predisposing to postpartum hemorrhage (see Chapter 28).

When the birth canal is rigid and extraordinary contractions occur, uterine rupture may result (see Chapter 20). Even in cases in which uterine rupture does not occur, there are likely to be lacerations of the birth canal (see Chapter 28).

Perinatal mortality is enhanced because of hypoxia, possible intracranial hemorrhage, and the risks associated with unattended delivery. Impeded placental exchange (with resultant hypoxia) created by decreased uteroplacental blood flow as a result of the more frequent and more forceful contractions is often further complicated by enhanced basal uterine tone. Perinatal intracranial hemorrhage may result from the presenting part literally serving as a battering ram against unyielding maternal tissue. Unattended delivery may result in direct injury from ill-directed efforts, resuscitation may not be available, and the fetus is likely to be chilled.

## PATHOGENESIS & TREATMENT

### Abnormalities of the Passage

Abnormalities of the passage are a diagnostic consideration in every patient with active dystocia. Causes of these abnormalities include bony abnormalities (pelvic dystocia), soft tissue obstruction of the birth canal, and abnormal placental location. Pelvic dystocia, particularly that due to small bony architecture, is the most common cause of passage ab-

normalities. The etiology and diagnosis of pelvic abnormalities begins with the shape, classification, and clinical assessment of the adult female pelvis.

**A. Pelvic Types:** Using roentgenographic studies, Caldwell and Maloy (1933) classified the 4 major types of adult pelves (see Table 10–1). Pure forms of the pelvic types are rare; mixed elements are more often present in each type of pelvis. A line is drawn through the greatest transverse diameter of the inlet, dividing the inlet into posterior and anterior segments.

**1. Gynecoid pelvis–**The gynecoid pelvis is considered the most typically "female" type and is the most favorable for uncomplicated vaginal delivery. This pelvic type can be found in about 50% of all women. The inlet has an oval configuration with a transverse diameter slightly greater than the anteroposterior diameter. The side walls of the pelvis are straight. The ischial spines are not prominent. The subpubic arch is wide, and the sacrum is concave.

**2. Android pelvis–**The android, or male, type of pelvis is found in about 33% of white women and about 15% of black women. The inlet is wedge-shaped, and the pelvic side walls are convergent. The ischial spines are prominent, the subpubic arch is narrowed, and the sacrum is inclined anteriorly in its lower third. The android pelvis is associated with persistent occiput posterior position and deep transverse arrest dystocia.

**3. Anthropoid pelvis–**Anthropoid pelves are reportedly present in about 85% of black women and 20% of white women. The inlet is oval, with an anteroposterior diameter greater than the transverse diameter. The pelvic side walls are divergent, and the sacrum is inclined posteriorly. This pelvic type is most often associated with persistent occiput posterior dystocia.

**4. Platypelloid pelvis–**The platypelloid pelvis is a rare type more common in white than in black women and present in fewer than 3% of all women. This pelvis is characterized by a transverse diameter that is wide with respect to the anteroposterior diameter. Deep transverse arrest patterns of labor are commonly associated with this pelvic type.

**B. Pelvimetry:** Disruption of the normal female pelvic architecture is an infrequent consideration in the differential diagnosis of abnormal pelves. Traumatic pelvic fractures are the most common abnormalities; other possibilities include rachitic pelves, chondrodystrophic dwarf pelves, kyphotic and scoliotic pelves, exostoses, and bony neoplasms. In such unusual cases, pelvimetry (particularly x-ray pelvimetry) is often helpful in predicting the prognosis.

**1. X-ray pelvimetry–**Although both ultrasonography and magnetic resonance imaging (MRI) have been used to investigate pelvic size and shape for evidence of pelvic contraction obstructing the normal progress of labor, roentgenographic techniques have been the most widely used pelvimetric method. X-ray pelvimetry has now fallen into limited use, however, since accumulating evidence suggests that the measurements obtained do not influence the management of labor and that radiation exposure subjects the fetus to an increased risk of oncogenesis.

Current thinking is that in an era of continuous fetal monitoring and safe protocols for the use of dilute oxytocin to induce labor, a trial of labor is indicated. The diagnosis of fetopelvic disproportion must generally be a diagnosis of exclusion after fetal factors and uterine dysfunction have been ruled out. However, x-ray pelvimetry is useful in a few selected instances, eg, to evaluate a pelvis for the feasibility of vaginal breech delivery and to assess gross bony distortion such as previous pelvic fracture or rachitic deformity.

Three techniques of x-ray pelvimetry are in general use.

**a. Colcher-Sussman system–**The Colcher-Sussman system is the most widely used and compares the anteroposterior and transverse diameters of a given pelvis with the average and lower limit of normal values shown in Table 25–1.

**b. Mengert's method–**Mengert's system uses measurements derived from pelvimetry films to calculate the areas of the inlet and midpelvic planes. Values under 85% of the average measurement are associated with a 58% incidence of cesarean section. The average for the inlet is 145 $cm^2$, and the lower statistical limit (85%) is 123 $cm^2$. The average for the midplane is 125 $cm^2$, and the 85% limit is 106 $cm^2$.

**c. Ball method–**The Ball technique uses anteroposterior and transverse diameters corrected for the x-ray beam divergence to calculate the volume capacities of the maternal pelvis and the fetal skull. This technique determines disproportion based on the deficit of maternal pelvic capacity expressed in $cm^3$.

**2. Clinical pelvimetry–**(Chapter 10) Clinical pelvimetry has largely supplanted x-ray pelvimetry in the routine evaluation of most obstetric patients. Estimation of the diagonal conjugate has been particularly helpful. If the diagonal conjugate is greater than 12.5 cm, the obstetric conjugate is rarely less than 10 cm, and the incidence of operative delivery is significantly decreased.

**C. Pelvic Contractions:** Contractions of the

pelvis are generally classified as contractions of the inlet, midpelvis, or outlet or as a combination of 2 or more elements.

**1. Inlet contraction–**Inlet contraction is suspected if the anteroposterior diameter of the pelvis is less than 10 cm, the transverse diameter is under 12 cm, or both. Inlet contraction may be detected clinically by x-ray pelvimetry, clinical estimation of the diagonal conjugate, or inability to perform the Müller-Hillis maneuver (manually pushing the fetal head into the pelvis with gentle fundal pressure). This pelvic contraction may present as a floating vertex presentation with no descent during labor; an abnormal presentation such as breech, oblique, transverse lie, or face presentation; or a prolapsed cord, prolapsed extremity or both. The floating presenting part is usually not well applied to the cervix, and contraction of the inlet is also associated with poor progress in labor and uterine dystocia.

In prolonged labors complicated by inlet contraction, considerable molding of the fetal head, caput succedaneum formation, and prolonged rupture of the membranes are common. In addition, with prolonged labor, abnormal thinning of the lower uterine segment may develop, and a Bandl's pathologic retraction ring or ridge at the junction of the lower uterine segment and fundus may develop, signifying impending uterine rupture.

In modern practice, in which the patient's progress is compared with known labor curves and possible inlet contraction is suspected on the basis of clinical examination, neglected cases of inlet contraction are rare and the prognosis is excellent. With continuous fetal monitoring in these cases, fetal well-being may be ensured, even with concurrent use of dilute oxytocin. Cesarean section is the treatment of choice in true inlet contraction.

**2. Midpelvic-outlet contraction–**The obstetric midpelvis is defined as that area bounded by an anteroposterior diameter extending from the inferior border of the symphysis pubis through the ischial spines to the sacrum at approximately the junction of the fourth and fifth sacral vertebrae, combined with the transverse diameter between the ischial spines. The intersection of these 2 lines at the same point of the sacrum constitutes the posterior sagittal diameter of the midplane; the intersection of these 2 lines at the inferior border of the symphysis pubis constitutes the anterior sagittal diameter of the midplane. Critical values for these diameters are 11.5 cm for the anterior sagittal diameter, 9.5 cm for the interspinous diameter, and 5 cm for the posterior sagittal diameter. Techniques for estimating midpelvic adequacy include the sum of the posterior sagittal diameter and interspinous diameter, which should be greater than 13.5 cm. Mengert's criteria (see previous text) have also been widely used.

The dimensions of the **pelvic outlet** are defined by the anteroposterior diameter of the outlet from the

**Table 25–1.** Average and lower limit of normal pelvic diameters.

| Diameters | Average (cm) | Lower Limit of Normal (cm) |
|---|---|---|
| **Inlet** | | |
| Anteroposterior | 12.5 | 10 |
| Transverse | 13.0 | 12 |
| **Midplane** | | |
| Anteroposterior | 11.5 | Not critical |
| Transverse | 10.5 | 9.5 |

lower margin of the symphysis pubis to the end of the sacrum and by the intertuberous diameter (the distance between the 2 ischial tuberosities). The posterior sagittal diameter of the outlet is measured from the midpoint of the intertuberous diameter to the end of the sacrum. The intertuberous diameter is the most critical measurement and should be greater than 8 cm. The sum of the intertuberous diameter and the anteroposterior diameter of the outlet should be more than 15 cm.

Kaltreider discussed the impracticality of separating the midplane from the outlet and the clinical difficulties of distinguishing the contracted states of each. The anteroposterior diameter of the outlet is only 1–2 cm from the anterior sagittal diameter of the inlet and often involves a smaller diameter. Small intertuberous and interspinous diameters generally occur together. In women with interspinous diameters that are on the borderline of normal values, the fetal head is forced posteriorly, and the prognosis for delivery depends in part on the roominess of the posterior sagittal diameter of the outlet. In view of these relationships, it is easy to understand that midplane and outlet contractions only rarely occur in isolation, and they are considered here as "midpelvic-outlet contractions."

Midpelvic-outlet obstruction is detected clinically on the basis of convergent side walls, prominent ischial spines, or a narrow pelvic arch. In the case of the last-named abnormality, midpelvic-outlet obstruction may present as a prolonged second stage, persistent occiput-posterior position, or deep transverse arrest. Uterine dystocia may develop secondarily. Molding of the fetal head and caput succedaneum formation are common. Neglected labors may cause vesicovaginal or rectovaginal fistula due to pressure necrosis of the surrounding tissues of the birth canal. In neglected cases, eventual uterine rupture may occur because of the same mechanism as in inlet disproportion.

A poor prognosis is typical in midpelvic-outlet contraction, partly due to difficult midforceps rotation and difficult vaginal deliveries. Cesarean section is therefore the delivery method of choice in this complication.

**D. Soft-Tissue Dystocia:** Other anatomic abnormalities of the reproductive tract may cause dystocia. So-called soft tissue dystocia may be caused by congenital anomalies, scarring of the birth canal, pelvic masses, or low implantation of the placenta.

**1. Congenital anomalies**–Congenital anomalies of note include bicornuate uterus (which generally causes malpresentation) and longitudinal and transverse vaginal septa that may prevent fetal descent. A longitudinal septum is usually pushed aside or spontaneously lacerated during labor; however, transverse septa may require incision to permit vaginal delivery.

Conglutination of the external cervical os is of un-

certain etiology and may be either congenital or acquired following previous injury. It is manifested as a small external os that fails to dilate after full effacement. Mechanical dilatation is usually required and is often easily accomplished with just the examining digit.

**2. Scarring of the birth canal**–Previous scarring from injury to the birth canal may cause tissue rigidity and dystocia. This problem may arise from previous birth laceration, conization, cauterization, rape injury in a small child, or caustic abortifacient injury to the vaginal vault and cervix. Episiotomy, repair of extensive laceration, or cesarean section may occasionally be required to treat these rare occurrences. **Incarceration of the fundus** of the uterus from scarring secondary to endometriosis may cause sacculation of the uterus, elevation of the cervix out of the pelvis, and incomplete dilatation; cesarean section is generally required. **Diastasis recti abdominis** from previous pregnancies may cause acute anteflexion of the uterus, preventing descent of the presenting part into the pelvic cavity; abdominal binders provide adequate correction.

**3. Pelvic masses**–Pelvic masses may rarely complicate the progress of labor; these include carcinoma of the cervix, leiomyomas of the cervix or lower uterine segment, and distended bladder. Ovarian neoplasms may be diagnosed before delivery in the course of prenatal care, but they have been first discovered when they obstructed labor; cesarean section and removal of the neoplasm may be required. A transplanted pelvic kidney may similarly necessitate cesarean section delivery.

**4. Low-lying placenta**–A marginal or low-lying placenta may prevent normal fetal descent in labor. (See Chapter 20.)

### Abnormalites of the Passenger

Fetal dystocia is abnormal labor caused by malposition or malpresentation, excessive size of the fetus, or fetal malformation.

**A. Malposition and Malpresentation:** Fetal malpresentations are essentially abnormalities of fetal position, presentation, attitude, or lie; they collectively constitute the most common cause of fetal dystocia, occurring in approximately 5% of all labors. Included in this category are persistent occiput posterior and occiput transferse positions, sinciput and brow presentation, face presentation, transverse or oblique lies, and breech and compound presentation.

**1. Vertex malpositions**–

**a. Occiput posterior**–The occiput posterior position may be normal in early labor. When it persists, it may cause dystocia. Generally, the head rotates to the occiput anterior position when it reaches the pelvic floor. If no rotation occurs (about 5–10% of cases), dystocia may result. The mechanism of this fetopelvic disproportion is partial deflexion of the fetal head. The fetal vertebral column lies directly on the maternal vertebral column in the direct occiput posterior position, and some extension occurs when the fetal head enters the pelvic cavity. This partial deflexion increases the diameter that must engage in the pelvis. Lack of spontaneous rotation from the occiput posterior to the occiput anterior position generally prolongs the deceleration phase and the second stage of labor and may be caused by a contracted, anthropoid, or android pelvis or insufficient uterine action.

The diagnosis of occiput posterior position is generally easily made by manual vaginal examination of the orientation of the fetal cephalic sutures and may be confirmed by palpating the configuration of the fetal ear. Clinical pelvimetry should be attempted. If no gross pelvic contraction is documented and uterine contractions are inadequate, cautious infusion of oxytocin may be tried. Depending on the clinical findings, the following modes of delivery are available: (1) spontaneous vaginal delivery; (2) outlet forceps delivery of a direct occiput posterior presentation; (3) manual rotation to the occiput anterior position, followed by spontaneous or outlet forceps delivery; (4) midforceps rotation and extraction; (5) vacuum extraction for rotation, extraction, or both; and (6) cesarean section.

A few authorities advocate midforceps rotation from the occiput posterior to the occiput anterior position and delivery in selected cases when macrosomia and gross fetopelvic disproportion have been excluded, other criteria for forceps delivery have been met, and the operator is sufficiently skilled. The prognosis for the infant is excellent when these guidelines are followed; however, great care and skill must be exercised. Maternal morbidity, including extension of episiotomies and other birth canal lacerations, occurs more frequently in occiput posterior deliveries.

**b. Occiput transverse**–Occiput transverse (like occiput posterior) is frequently a transient position, and in most labors the fetal head spontaneously rotates to the occiput anterior position. Persistent occiput transverse is frequently associated with pelvic dystocia, uterine dystocia, and platypelloid or android pelves. Diagnosis, management, and prognosis are similar to those of persistent occiput posterior presentation. When the fetal head engages but for various reasons does not rotate spontaneously in the midpelvis as in normal labor, midpelvic transverse arrest is diagnosed. Deep transverse arrest occasionally occurs at the inlet, with molding and caput succedaneum formation falsely indicating a lower descent. Cesarean section is required.

**2. Sinciput and brow presentation**–Sinciput and brow presentations usually are transient fetal presentations with various degrees of deflexion of the fetal head. During the normal course of labor, conversion to face or vertex presentation generally occurs. If no conversion takes place, dystocia is likely. The anteroposterior diameter of the deflexed fetal head exceeds the average 9.5 cm of the suboccipitobregmatic diameter in vertex presentation. The average value for the occipitofrontal diameter in the sinciput position is 12 cm and for the occipitomental diameter in the brow position, 13.5 cm.

**a. Sinciput presentation**–Sinciput presentation is most easily diagnosed by vaginal examination; the bregmatic fontanelle and lambdoid suture are equally prominent. In this position, also called the **military attitude,** no flexing or extension of the fetal head is present with respect to the trunk. As previously mentioned, spontaneous conversion to face, brow, or vertex presentation is common as labor progresses; therefore, expectant management is recommended. However, cephalopelvic disproportion, uterine inertia, and arrested progress may occur, in which case cesarean section is recommended.

**b. Brow presentation**–Brow presentation occurs in approximately 0.06% of deliveries and is associated with the same causative factors as face presentation. In approximately 60% of cases, pelvic contraction, prematurity, and grand multiparity are associated findings. The diagnosis is made by vaginal examination, and management is expectant. Spontaneous conversion occurs in more than one-third of all brow presentations. Arrest patterns and uterine inertia are common sequelae because pelvic contraction is so often associated with this presentation. Oxytocin is not recommended, and continuous electronic fetal monitoring is necessary. Liberal use of cesarean section should be made for delivery in cases complicated by a poor outlook for labor. Perinatal mortality rates are low when corrected for congenital anomaly, prematurity, and manipulative vaginal delivery.

**3. Face presentation**–In face presentation, the fetal head is fully deflexed from the longitudinal axis; this presentation occurs in about 0.2% of all deliveries. Causative factors include grand multiparity; advanced maternal age; pelvic masses; pelvic contraction; multiple gestation; polyhydramnios; macrosomia; congenital anomalies, including anencephaly and hydrocephaly; prematurity; cornual implantation of the placenta; placenta previa; and premature rupture of the membranes. The most common causes are congenital malformations (particularly anencephaly), cephalopelvic disproportion, prematurity, and grand multiparity.

The diagnosis of face presentation may be made by the fourth maneuver of Leopold but is most often accomplished by vaginal examination and confirmed by radiography. Face presentation may be distinguished from breech presentation by identification of the mouth and both malar eminences in a triangular configuration.

The prognosis for vaginal delivery is guarded for face presentation. The submentobregmatic diameter is only slightly larger than the 9.5-cm suboccipitobregmatic diameter, but complications generally arise with simultaneously occurring pelvic contraction or a persistent mentum posterior position. Mentum posterior positions in average-size fetuses are not deliverable vaginally as they are unable to extend. Arrested labor is typical when spontaneous rotation to the mentum anterior position fails to occur. Management should include continuous electronic fetal monitoring. With mentum anterior presentation, oxytocin augmentation may be used for arrested labor if cephalopelvic disproportion can be ruled out. Delivery may be accomplished by spontaneous vaginal delivery, use of low forceps to rotate to the mentum anterior position, or cesarean section for arrested labor. There is little or no place for manual flexion of the fetal head or manual rotation from the mentum posterior position to the mentum anterior position.

**4. Abnormal fetal lie**—Fetal dystocia may be caused by abnormalities of fetal lie. In transverse or oblique lie, the long axis of the fetus is perpendicular to or at an angle to the maternal longitudinal axis. Abnormalities in axial lie occur overall in about 0.33% of all deliveries but may occur 6 times more frequently than normally in premature labors. The most frequently associated causative factors include grand multiparity, prematurity, pelvic contraction, and abnormal placental implantation. The diagnosis is suggested by Leopold's maneuvers and the absence of a presenting part in the pelvis. These findings may be confirmed by real-time ultrasound scanning or x-ray.

When the diagnosis is made in the third trimester prior to labor, carefully performed external cephalic version enables a greater number of these patients to undergo vaginal delivery or low transverse cesarean section. Abnormal axial lies have a 20 times greater incidence of cord prolapse than vertex presentations. Thus, with onset of labor or when the membranes rupture, prompt low vertical cesarean delivery is mandatory. The prognosis for the infant is good when these management guidelines are followed. Increased perinatal mortality is associated mainly with prematurity, cord prolapse, and manipulative vaginal delivery.

A prolapsed extremity alongside the presenting part constitutes **compound presentation.** Most commonly a hand is palpated beside the vertex. The average incidence is 0.1% of deliveries. Prematurity and a large pelvic inlet are associated clinical findings. Compound presentations are often diagnosed during physical examination and investigation for failure to progress in labor. Labor in most of these patients will end in uncomplicated vaginal delivery, but cesarean section is frequently used in the presence of dystocia or cord prolapse. Attempts to reposition the fetal extremity are discouraged, except perhaps for gentle pinching of the digits to determine whether the fetus will retract the extremity.

Increased perinatal mortality rates have been consistently reported secondary to internal podalic version, other birth trauma associated with manipulation, and cord prolapse (11–20% of cases of the latter).

**5. Breech presentation**—Breech presentation is a longitudinal lie with the fetal head occupying the fundus. A **frank breech** describes a breech presentation with flexed hips and extended knees. A **complete breech** describes flexion at both hips and knees. An **incomplete (footling) breech** describes extension of one or both hips. Breech presentation at term occurs in about 3–4% of all deliveries. The incidence increases with the degree of prematurity; the incidence at 32 weeks is 7% and at under 28 weeks, the incidence is 25%. Breech presentation is associated with all of the causative factors associated with face presentation and is particularly associated with previous breech presentation, congenital anomalies, and any anomaly that alters the normal piriform shape of the uterus. The diagnosis is generally made by Leopold's maneuvers, vaginal examination, ultrasonography, or abdominal x-ray. Breech may be distinguished from face presentation by the linear alignment of the anus with the ischial tuberosities.

Management of breech presentation is controversial. High perinatal mortality rates have been clearly demonstrated for all breech presentations but in particular for footling breech and for breech presentations associated with congenital anomalies, hyperextended vertex, and weight under 1500 g. Other indications for cesarean section are contracted pelvis as demonstrated by x-ray pelvimetry, secondary arrest of dilatation, fetal weight over 3500 g, primigravidity, floating station, and inexperienced practitioner.

Prospective studies have identified a subgroup of breech presentations that may be safely delivered vaginally—specifically, near-term frank breeches weighing between 2500 and 3500 g with flexed head and no concurrent congenital anomalies; maternal pelvis of adequate dimensions as demonstrated by x-ray pelvimetry; and a normal labor pattern without fetal distress. Continuous electronic fetal monitoring is essential, and immediate cesarean section should be available.

An alternative to cesarean section advocated by some authors is external cephalic version, which is performed after 34 weeks with constant fetal heart rate monitoring and no anesthesia. It may significantly reduce both the incidence of breech presentation in labor and the number of cesarean sections. A more detailed discussion of breech presentation may be found in Chapter 21.

**B. Fetal Macrosomia:** Excessive fetal size, or macrosomia, is defined as fetal size over 4000 g, which occurs in about 5% of deliveries. Associated factors include maternal obesity, maternal diabetes (gestational or overt), midforceps deliveries, prolonged second stage of labor, postdate pregnancies, multiparity, and previous delivery of a macrosomic infant. Diagnosis by abdominal palpation is notoriously inaccurate. Recent work indicates that diagnosis may be possible with ultrasonography. A difference of 1.6 cm between chest and head circumferences, or of 4.8 cm between shoulder and head circumferences, identifies macrosomic infants. Perinatal mortality for fetuses weighing more than 4500 g is about 5-fold higher than in normal term infants, and the incidence of shoulder dystocia is at least 10% in this group.

**Shoulder dystocia** (see Chapter 21), or difficult delivery of the shoulders after delivery of the fetal head, is an obstetric emergency that is usually managed first by rotation of the symphysis pubis in McRobert's maneuver. The patient's legs are sharply flexed against her abdomen, a movement that tends to free the fetus's anterior shoulder. Other management maneuvers (application of suprapubic pressure or Wood's screw maneuver) essentially rotate the shoulder so that it occupies a transverse or oblique (rather than an anteroposterior) diameter of the pelvis. Eventually, delivery of the posterior arm or intentional fracture of the clavicle may be required to prevent further neonatal hypoxia. Further discussion of fetal macrosomia can be found in Chapter 16.

**C. Fetal Malformation:** Fetal malformation may also cause dystocia, mainly through fetopelvic disproportion. The most common malformation is hydrocephalus, with an incidence of 0.05%. In addition to ultrasound measurements of the lateral ventricles, hydrocephalus may also be suspected on the basis of abdominal or vaginal examination showing an enlarged globular fetal head in breech or transverse lie or overriding the symphysis pubis. Management is determined by the severity of the disorder and its prognosis.

Other fetal anomalies that may prevent the normal progress of labor include enlargement of the fetal abdomen caused by distended bladder, ascites, or abdominal neoplasms; or other fetal masses, including meningomyelocele or cystosarcoma. Other rare problems such as incomplete twinning and locked twins should be considered in the differential diagnosis of fetal dystocia.

## Abnormalities of the Powers

Uterine dysfunction, along with inadequate voluntary expulsive efforts during the second stage of labor, constitutes a dysfunction of the powers of the labor process (Chapter 10). Uterine dystocia denotes any abnormality in the force or coordination of uterine contractility that prevents the normal progress of labor.

**A. Normal Uterine Activity in Labor:** Studies of uterine activity during labor have revealed the following characteristics:

(1) The relative intensity of contractions is greater in the fundus than in the midportion or lower uterine segment (this is termed **fundal dominance**).

(2) The average value of the intensity of contractions is more than 24 mm Hg. In the active phase of labor, pressures often increase to 40–60 mm Hg.

(3) Contractions are well synchronized in different parts of the uterus.

(4) The basal resting pressure of the uterus is between 12 and 15 mm Hg.

(5) The frequency of contractions progresses from 1 every 3–5 minutes to 1 every 2–3 minutes during the active phase.

(6) The duration of effective contraction in active labor approaches 60 seconds.

(7) The rhythm and force of contractions are regular.

**B. Methods of Measurement:** Quantification of uterine activity during labor uses one of two readily available techniques: an external tocodynamometer or an intrauterine pressure catheter.

**1. External tocodynamometer**–The external tocodynamometer is a pressure sensor placed over the fundal prominence of the uterus that gives an accurate determination of the frequency and duration of uterine contractions. This technique is not adequate for assessment of the resting tone of the uterus or the intensity of contractions.

**2. Intrauterine pressure catheter**–An internal uterine pressure catheter measures intra-amniotic pressure, which is transmitted through the noncompressible fluid within the catheter to a pressure sensor and recorded as millimeters of mercury. The pressure sensor is calibrated at the level of the midportion of the uterus. This technique shows baseline uterine resting pressure, contraction intensity and duration, and frequency of uterine activity. It is the most accurate method of diagnosing uterine dysfunction and evaluating treatment.

There are 4 basic techniques of quantifying uterine activity, and each depends on use of an intrauterine pressure catheter. The **Montevideo unit** is the most universally accepted and is defined as the product of the average intensity of uterine contractions (measured from the baseline resting pressure) multiplied by the number of contractions in a 10-minute interval. This method cannot quantify the duration of contractions. The **Alexandria unit** is the product of the average intensity of contractions multiplied by the average duration multiplied by the frequency of contractions in a 10-minute interval. The **uterine activity unit** measures the area under the pressure curve above uterine diastole for a 10-minute interval and is expressed in millimeters of mercury per minute. **Online total planimetry** measures the entire area under the pressure curve, including resting pressure, and is expressed as average pressure in millimeters of mercury.

**C. Abnormal Uterine Activity:** Uterine dysfunction generally comprises 3 categories: hypotonic dysfunction, hypertonic dysfunction, and uncoordinated dysfunction.

**1. Hypotonic dysfunction**–Hypotonic dysfunction is uterine activity characterized by contraction of the uterus with insufficient force (< 24mm Hg), irregular or infrequent rhythm, or both. Hypotonic dysfunction is seen more often in primigravidas in the active phase of labor. It may be caused by excessive sedation, early administration of conduction anesthesia, twins, polyhydramnios, or overdistention of the uterus. Hypotonic dysfunction responds well to oxytocin; however, care must be taken to first rule out cephalopelvic disproportion and malpresentation, which commonly accompany this type of dysfunction.

Treatment must first eliminate coexisting disorders. Physical examination, ultrasonography, and sometimes x-ray are used to rule out abnormalities of the passage or passenger requiring cesarean section. Pure hypotonic patterns may be effectively treated with oxytocin augmentation of labor. Intravenous administration of a dilute oxytocin solution through an infusion pump is the procedure of choice. A frequently used dilution is 10 U of oxytocin per liter of balanced salt solution. The in vivo half-life of oxytocin is about 5 minutes. With intravenous administration, a steady-state plasma level is achieved in 40–60 minutes. The response of each patient to a given dosage is unpredictable and must be titrated. Overzealous administration may lead to hypertonic uterine action, precipitate labor, fetal distress or hypoxia, or uterine rupture (particularly in multiparas).

Protocols for administration of oxytocin generally recommend a starting dose of 1–2 mU/min increasing in fractional fashion every 15 minutes to achieve the desired response. Seitchik and Castillo (1983) recommend a lower dosage of oxytocin and report similar efficacy when starting doses of 1 mU/min are increased at intervals of not less than 30 minutes. They report satisfactory cervical dilatation in more than 90% of patients at a dosage of 4 mU/min or less, with fewer adjustments for hypertonic patterns of fetal distress.

Treatment for abnormal uterine activity remains controversial. The efficacy of oxytocin in hypotonic labor may depend on the type of dysfunctional pattern; for example, protraction disorders are generally not affected by the administration of oxytocin. Arrest disorders are accompanied by a 50% incidence of cephalopelvic disproportion and an increase in perinatal mortality; therefore, pelvic dystocia should be ruled out before the cautious administration of oxytocin is attempted. O'Driscoll and coworkers (1984) think that in the absence of gross pelvic dystocia or other contraindications to labor, "active management of labor" should be undertaken. They recommend oxytocin augmentation up to a dosage of 40 mU/min for failure to dilate at least 1 cm/h in the first stage of labor in nulliparas. O'Driscoll reported a cesarean section rate of 4.8% in 1980, which was not significantly increased over that of the previous 15 years. He noted a concomitant decrease in the perinatal mortality rate in the same time period.

**2. Hypertonic and uncoordinated dysfunction**—Hypertonic uterine contractions and uncoordi-nated contraction often occur together and are characterized by elevated resting tone of the uterus, dyssynchronous contractions with elevated tone in the lower uterine segment, and frequent intense uterine contractions. The patient usually describes constant pain when the resting tone of the uterus is 25 mm Hg or more, and the uterus is generally painful to palpation. A constriction ring may develop at the level of the isthmus and further obstruct the progress of labor.

Hypertonic or uncoordinated uterine action is less common than hypotonic dysfunction and is generally associated with abruptio placentae, overzealous use of oxytocin, cephalopelvic disproportion, fetal malpresentation, and the latent phase of labor. Treatment may require tocolysis, amyl nitrite, decrease in oxytocin infusion, or cesarean section as indicated for concomitant malpresentation, cephalopelvic disproportion, or fetal distress. Oxytocin administration is generally of no value. When these patterns occur in the latent phase of labor, sedation is generally effective in converting hypertonic contractions to normal labor patterns.

Hypertonic labor may also cause precipitate labor disorders, which constitute Friedman's fourth pattern of labor aberration. This pattern may result in fetal intracranial hemorrhage, fetal distress, neonatal injury or depression, and birth canal lacerations from rapid delivery.

**D. Inadequate Expulsive Efforts:** Inadequate pushing in the second stage of labor is common and may be caused by conduction anesthesia, oversedation, exhaustion, or neurologic dysfunction such as paraplegia or hemiplegia of various causes or psychiatric disorders. Mild sedation or a waiting period to permit analgesic or anesthetic agents to wear off may improve expulsive efforts, and outlet forceps delivery may be effected in selected cases.

# FETAL COMPROMISE

Fetal distress may be defined as a complex of signs indicating a critical response to stress. It implies metabolic derangements—notably hypoxia and acidosis—that affect the functions of vital organs to the point of temporary or permanent injury or death. Fetal distress may be acute or chronic.

Unfortunately, the contemporarily detectable signs of fetal compromise do not indicate the lasting degree to which that compromise is affecting the fetus. Thus, to discuss fetal distress in any save a retrospective is nearly impossible. Therefore, it has become more common to designate the "real time" detectable changes not as fetal distress, but as fetal compromise.

This alteration is more than semantic, for it more accurately portrays our current state of information.

Skillful monitoring (Chapter 13) will detect some degree of fetal compromise (perinatal jeopardy) in at least 20% of all obstetric patients. Prompt recognition of the symptoms of fetal compromise and, when necessary, decisive, well-planned intervention are imperative for the reduction of perinatal mortality and morbidity—especially to prevent permanent damage to the central nervous system. However, the diagnostic criteria for fetal compromise must consider a continuum of several possibilities.

## CHRONIC FETAL COMPROMISE

Chronic fetal compromise implies an interval of fetal deprivation that affects growth and development. The compromise may be caused by a reduction of placental perfusion, by a placental abnormality, or by deficient fetal metabolism. Decreased placental perfusion may reflect any of the following conditions in the mother: (1) vascular abnormality, as in hypertensive disease, preeclampsia-eclampsia, or diabetes with pelvic vascular complications; (2) inadequate systemic circulation, as in congenital or acquired heart disease; and (3) inadequate oxygenation of the blood, as in emphysema or by reason of residence at high altitude. Chronic fetal compromise due to placental abnormality includes "premature placental aging" and diabetes mellitus. Possible fetal causes of jeopardy include multiple gestations, with possible overdistention of the uterus and risk of premature delivery, as well as the risk of twin-to-twin transfusion. Other fetal causes are postmaturity, congenital anomalies, congenital infections, and erythroblastosis fetalis.

The earliest studies that made possible the diagnosis of chronic fetal compromise are simple serial measurements of the height of the uterus or the patient's girth at each antenatal visit. These are at best very gross measurements of fetal growth, and ultrasonic measurement of the skull, thorax, and placenta provides a more accurate means of determining a decreased fetal growth rate. In the latter half of pregnancy, the various fetal tests outlined previously may be useful.

## ACUTE FETAL COMPROMISE

The differential diagnosis of acute fetal compromise involves 3 possibilities: possible fetal compromise, probable fetal compromise, and certain fetal compromise (see Table 13–11). Because the recommended treatment is different for each, the causes and diagnostic criteria of each must be considered. No fetal compromise is present when there is absence of any abnormality of fetal heart rate (FHR) or rhythm and no response to uterine contractions other than early deceleration.

### Possible Compromise

Transient acceleration of FHR, in conjunction with uterine contractions, may indicate mild cord occlusion (venous only) or slight fetal hypercapnia and hypoxia, if normal FHR variability is retained. Variable FHR decelerations in relation to uterine contractions are thought to be due to more severe cord compression. There may be violent fetal movements, and the pH of the fetal scalp blood (see Chapter 13) may be slightly reduced. If the variable deceleration is transient and not severe, permanent damage is unlikely.

### Probable Fetal Compromise

Lack of FHR short-term variability may be associated with a number of factors (eg, fetal immaturity, effect of drugs) that do not indicate fetal compromise. However, the absence of FHR short-term variability may be an indication of the state of the neural mechanisms controlling the heart. For this reason, changes (decreasing variability) indicating a lessening of central nervous system control are worrisome. If lack of short-term variability of the FHR is coupled with acceleration in relation to uterine contractions, it is even more serious.

Prolonged or increasingly more severe variable deceleration is another warning sign. Late deceleration of the FHR, which may or may not be coupled with accelerations, is of great importance because the presumed cause of this pattern is the inability of the placenta to provide necessary exchange for normal fetal metabolism (uteroplacental insufficiency). Meconium may be passed during this fetal insult, but unfortunately it is also seen in uncompromised fetuses. Under these circumstances, one should expect the pH of the fetal scalp blood to be 7.10–7.24, and abnormally active fetal movements may occur.

Maternal causes of fetal compromise include diverse problems such as decreased uterine blood flow (hypotension, shock, sudden heart failure), decreased blood oxygenation (hypoxia-hypercapnia), and uterine hypertonia (injudicious use of oxytocin, tetanic contractions, abruptio placentae). Placenta and cord problems include abruptio placentae, placenta previa, umbilical cord compression (knots, prolapse, or entanglement), lack of sufficient placental reserve to tolerate labor (postmaturity, premature placental aging), and ruptured vasa previa.

### Certain Fetal Compromise

If tachycardia, lack of FHR short-term variability, and late FHR deceleration occur and are confirmed as an ensemble characteristic of the uterine contraction and FHR patterns, then fetal compromise is thought to exist. Another exceedingly critical combination is severe and prolonged variable deceleration and the development of late deceleration. If severe variable deceleration persists for 30 minutes or more or if any degree of late deceleration persists despite attempted therapy, fetal compromise is present. Concomitantly, the fetal scalp blood pH will probably be 7.20 or less, and meconium most likely will be passed. Prompt treatment is mandatory.

## MANAGEMENT OF FETAL COMPROMISE

### Specific Considerations

**A. Position of the Patient:** A change of the mother's position may relieve pressure on the umbilical cord. Uterine function may also be improved with the patient in a lateral position—certainly, uterine blood flow is increased. Therefore, labor should be conducted largely with the patient on her side.

**B. Hypotension:** The position change discussed above usually corrects the supine hypotensive syndrome. If it fails to, shifting the uterus off the great vessels by manual pressure may be necessary. Additional measures may include elevation of the legs, application of elastic leg bandages, and rapid administration of fluids intravenously. These help to restore the gravida's arterial pressure and increase the blood flow in the intervillous space. If drugs are required, cardiotonics (eg, ephedrine) are preferred.

**C. Decreasing Uterine Activity:** One of the more common causes of late deceleration of the FHR is overzealous use of oxytocin. Therefore, discontinue the administration of oxytocin if stimulation is in progress. Moreover, oxytocin should only be given intravenously. Decreased uterine activity permits better placental perfusion, and the stress of violent uterine contractions will be reduced.

**D. Hyperoxygenation:** The administration of high concentrations of oxygen (6–7 L/min by mask) will raise the maternal-fetal $PO_2$ gradient and will increase maternal-fetal oxygen transfer. This may be helpful when fetal hypoxia occurs.

**E. Acid-Base Balance:** Although attempts may be made to correct acid-base balance by administering sodium bicarbonate to the mother during labor, the transfer of fixed alkali is relatively slow, and treatment is therefore unlikely to be of use when given to the mother whose fetus is hypoxic and acidotic. If the acidosis is severe, the infant should be promptly delivered for primary corrective therapy. Nevertheless, if maternal acidosis is the cause of fetal acidosis, administering bicarbonate to the mother may benefit both patients.

Hypertonic glucose (usually 50 g intravenously) may be administered when there is maternal deprivation acidosis or hypoglycemia, although there may be only an indirect relationship between the level of fetal blood glucose and the base deficit.

### Summary of Treatment

In cases of possible fetal compromise, change the position of the mother, correct maternal hypotension, decrease uterine activity by stopping the administration of oxytocin, and administer oxygen at 6–7 L/min by face mask.

If the situation worsens, if the signs of probable fetal distress persist for 30 minutes, or if there is fetal distress despite conservative treatment, immediate delivery is mandatory. Obstetric judgment must dictate how the delivery will be accomplished in accordance with the presentation, station, position, dilatation of the cervix, and presumed fetal status. If cesarean section is chosen, it must be done rapidly. This implies the desirability of maintaining facilities for cesarean delivery in the labor-delivery suite and the constant availability of support services for the delivery area (ie, anesthesia, laboratory, blood bank, and neonatology). The indications for cesarean section have been broadened with its increased safety. Thus, the use of cesarean section may be justifiably increased for fetal distress, diabetes mellitus, isoimmunization, cord accidents, herpes genitalis, fetopelvic disproportion, previous uterine operation (including cesarean section), placenta previa, abruptio placentae, uterine inertia, abnormal presentations, hypertensive states of pregnancy, and maternal complications (eg, vesicovaginal fistula, invasive cervical carcinoma, and functional class IV cardiac disease).

## REFERENCES

### VELAMENTOUS INSERTION OF THE CORD & VASA PREVIA

Antoine C et al: Sinusoidal fetal heart rate pattern with vasa previa in twin pregnancy. J Reprod Med 1982; 27:295.

Kouyoumdjian A: Velamentous insertion of the umbilical cord. Obstet Gynecol 1980;56:737.

### DYSTOCIA

Anderson N: X-ray pelvimetry: Helpful or harmful? J Fam Pract 1985;17:405.

Caldwell WE, Moloy HC: Anatomical variations in the female pelvis and their effect in labor with a suggested classification. Am J Obstet Gynecol 1933;26:479.

Campbell S (editor): Ultrasound in obstetrics and gynecology: Recent advances. Clin Obstet Gynaecol 1983; 10:369.

Cardozo LD et al: Should we abandon Kielland's forceps? Br Med J [Clin Res] 1983;287:315.

Crosby WM: Difficult vaginal deliveries and how to avoid them. J Okla State Med Assoc 1982;75:144.

Cunningham FG, MacDonald PC, Gant NF, et al: *Williams Obstetrics,* 19th ed. Appleton & Lange, 1993.

Drife JO: Kielland or Caesar? (Editorial.) Br Med J [Clin Res] 1983;287:309.

Fine EA, Bracken M. Berkowitz RL: An evaluation of the usefulness of x-ray pelvimetry: Comparison of the Thoms and modified Ball methods with manual pelvimetry. Am J Obstet Gynecol 1980;137:15.

Friedman EA: *Labor: Clinical Evaluation and Management,* 2nd ed. Appleton-Century-Crofts, 1978.

Friedman EA: The labor curve. Clin Perinatol 1981;8:15.

Freidman EA: Midforceps delivery: Yes? Clin Obstet Gynecol 1987;30:93

Friedman EA: The therapeutic dilemma of arrested labor. Contemp Obstet Gynecol (March) 1978;11:34.

Gonik B, Stringer CA, Held B: An alternate maneuver for management of shoulder dystocia. Am J Obstet Gynecol 1983;145:882.

Hayashi RH: Midforceps Delivery: No? Clin Obstet Gynecol 1987;30:90.

Hernandez C, Wendel, GD: Shoulder dystocia. Clin Obstet Gynecol 1990;33:526.

Jacobs JB: Solving the problem of cervical dystocia and prolonged labor. (Letter.) Am J Obstet Gynecol 1983;145:650.

Kaltreider DF: The pelvic outlet. JAMA 1954;154:824.

Manzke H: Morbidity among infants born in breech presentation. J Perinat Med 1978;6:127.

Nakano H: Assessment of dystocia pelvis by ultrasound pelvimetry. Acta Obstet Gynecol Jpn 1981;33:1077.

Niswander KR, Gordon M: *The Women and Their Pregnancies.* (The Collaborative Perinatal Study of the National Institute of Neurological Diseases and Stroke.) Saunders, 1972.

O'Brien WF, Cefalo RC: Evaluation of x-ray pelvimetry and abnormal labor. Clin Obstet Gynecol 1982;25:157.

O'Driscoll K, Foley M, MacDonald D: Active management of labor as an alternative to cesarean section for dystocia. Obstet Gynecol 1984;63:485.

Philpott RH: Obstructed labour. Clin Obstet Gynaecol 1982;9:625.

Philpott RH: The recognition of cephalopelvic disproportion. Clin Obstet Gynaecol 1982;9:609.

Prasad B, Sharma D, Sinha GR: Dystocia due to foetal ascites. J Indian Med Assoc 1983;80:106.

Rodrigues C, Singh PM, Gupta AN: Kielland's forceps for deep transverse arrest. Asia Oceania J Obstet Gynaecol 1983;9:159.

Schramm M: Impacted shoulders: A personal experience. Aust NZ J Obstet Gynaecol 1983;23:28.

Sehgal NN: Early detection of abnormal labor using the Friedman labor graph. Postgrad Med 1980;68:189.

Seitchik J, Castillo M: Oxytocin augmentation of dysfunctional labor. 2. Uterine activity data. Am J Obstet Gynecol 1983;145:526.

Seitchik J, Castillo M: Oxytocin augmentation of dysfunctional labor. 3. Multiparous patients. Am J Obstet Gynecol 1983;145:777.

Toppozada HK: Subcutaneous partial symphysiotomy. (Letter.) Am J Obstet Gynecol 1983;146:344.

## FETAL DISTRESS

Cohen WR, Schifrin BS: Diagnosis and management of fetal distress during labor. Semin Perinatol 1978;2:155.

Heill LM: Diagnosis and management of fetal distress. Mayo Clin Proc 1979;54:784.

Hon EH, Quilligan EJ: Classification of fetal heart rate. 2. A revised working classification. Conn Med 1967;31:779.

Huddleston JF: Management of acute fetal distress in the intrapartum period. Clin Obstet Gynecol 1984;27:84.

Intrapartum Fetal Heart Rate Monitoring. Technical Bulletin No. 132. American College of Obstetrics and Gynecologists, 1989.

Katz M et al: Clinical significance of sinusoidal fetal heart rate pattern. Br J Obstet Gynaecol 1983;90:832.

Martin CB Jr: Regulation of the fetal heart rate and genesis of FHR patterns. Semin Perinatol 1978;2:131.

Paul RH et al: Clinical fetal monitoring. 7. The evaluation and significance of intrapartum baseline FHR variability. Am J Obstet Gynecol 1975;123:206.

Sibai BM et al: Sinusoidal fetal heart rate pattern. Obstet Gynecol 1980;55:637.

Tejani NA et al: Terbutaline in the management of acute intrapartum fetal acidosis. J Reprod Med 1983; 28:857.

Wood C: Fetal scalp sampling: Its place in management. Semin Perinatol 1978;2:169.

# 26

# Obstetric Analgesia & Anesthesia

*John S. McDonald, MD, & Ralph W. Yarnell, MD, FRCPC*

**Analgesia** is the loss or modulation of pain perception. It may be local and affect only a small area of the body; regional and affect a larger portion; or systemic. Analgesia is achieved by the use of hypnosis (suggestion), systemic medication, regional agents, or inhalation agents.

**Anesthesia** is the total loss of sensory perception, and may include loss of consciousness. It is induced by various agents and techniques. In obstetrics, **regional anesthesia** is accomplished with local anesthetic techniques (epidural, spinal) and **general anesthesia** with systemic medication and endotracheal intubation.

The terms analgesia and anesthesia are sometimes confused in common usage. Analgesia denotes those states in which only modulation of pain perception is involved. Anesthesia denotes those states in which mental awareness and perception of other sensations are lost. Attempts have been made to divide anesthesia into various components, including analgesia, amnesia, relaxation, and loss of reflex response to pain. Analgesia can be regarded as a component of anesthesia if viewed in this way.

The use of techniques and medications to provide pain relief in obstetrics requires an expert understanding of their effects to ensure the safety of both mother and fetus.

## ANATOMY OF PAIN

It may be academic to argue that pain should be defined as the parturient's response to the stimuli of labor, since agreement on a definition of pain has eluded scholars for centuries.

Nevertheless, it should be appreciated that the "pain response" is a response of the total personality and cannot be dissected systematically and scientifically. Physicians are obligated to provide a comfortable or at least tolerable labor and delivery. Many patients are tense and apprehensive at the onset of labor, although there may be little or no discomfort. The physician must be knowledgeable of the options for pain relief and respond to the patient's needs and wishes.

The evolution of the pain in the first stage of labor was originally described as involving spinal segments T11 and T12 (Cleland J). Subsequent research has determined that segments T10–L1 are involved (Bonica, 1972). Discomfort is associated with ischemia of the uterus during contraction as well as dilatation and effacement of the cervix. Sensory pathways that convey nociceptive impulses of the first stage of labor include the uterine plexus, the inferior hypogastric plexus, the middle hypogastric plexus, the superior hypogastric plexus, the lumbar and lower thoracic sympathetic chain, and the T10–L1 spinal segments.

Pain in the second stage of labor undoubtedly is produced by distention of the vagina and perineum. Sensory pathways from these areas are conveyed by branches of the pudendal nerve via the dorsal nerve of the clitoris, the labial nerves, and the inferior hemorrhoidal nerves. These are the major sensory branches to the perineum and are conveyed along nerve roots S2, S3, S4. Nevertheless, other nerves may play a role in perineal innervation; the ilioinguinal nerves, the genital branch of the genitofemoral nerves, and the perineal branch of the posterior femoral cutaneous nerves.

Although the major portion of the perineum is innervated by the 3 major branches of the pudendal nerve, innervation by the other nerves mentioned may be important in some patients. The type of pain reported may be an ache in the back or loins (referred pain, perhaps from the cervix), a cramp in the uterus (due to fundal contraction), or a "bursting" or "splitting" sensation in the lower vaginal canal or pudendum (due to dilatation of the cervix and vagina).

Dystocia, which is usually painful, may be due to fetopelvic disproportion; tetanic, prolonged, or dysrhythmic uterine contractions; intrapartal infection; or many other causes (see Chapter 25).

Substantial advances in the quality and safety of obstetric anesthesia have been made in the past 3 decades. Outdated techniques such as "twilight sleep" and mask anesthesia have been recognized as ineffective or unsafe and have been replaced by epidural infusion of narcotic/local anesthesia mixtures, patient-controlled analgesic during labor, and postoperatively. When required, general anesthesia is provided using short-acting drugs with well-known fetal effects, and careful attention is focused on airway management.

Maternal mortality relating to anesthesia has reduced 10-fold since the 1950s, largely due to an enhanced appreciation of special maternal risks associated with anesthesia. Ideally, obstetric deliveries today should be conducted only in hospitals where equipment and specially trained personnel are available.

## TECHNIQUES OF ANALGESIA WITHOUT THE USE OF DRUGS

### Psychophysical Methods
### (See also Chapter 10.)

Three distinct psychologic techniques have been developed as a means of facilitating the birth process and making it a positive emotional experience: "natural childbirth," psychoprophylaxis, and hypnosis. So-called natural childbirth was developed by Grantly Dick-Read in the early 1930s and popularized in his book *Childbirth Without Fear*. Dick-Read's approach emphasized the reduction of tension to induce relaxation. The psychoprophylactic technique was developed by Velvovski, who published the results of his work from Russia in 1950. In Russia in the mid-1950s, it became evident that obstetric psychoprophylaxis was a useful substitute for poorly administered or dangerously conducted anesthesia for labor and delivery. This method was later introduced in France by Lamaze. Hypnosis for pain relief has achieved periodic spurts of popularity since the early 1800s and depends on the power of suggestion.

Many obstetricians argue that psychoprophylaxis can largely eliminate the pain of childbirth by diminishing cortical appreciation of pain impulses rather than by depressing cortical function, as occurs with drug-induced analgesia. Relaxation, suggestion, concentration, and motivation are factors that overlap other methods of preparation for childbirth. Some of them are closely related to hypnosis.

These techniques can significantly reduce anxiety, tension, and fear. They also provide the parturient with a valuable understanding of the physiologic changes that occur during labor and delivery. In addition, they serve as an occasion for closer understanding and communication between the patient and her spouse, who may be an important source of comfort to the patient during the stressful process of birth. If psychophysical techniques do no more than this, they deserve the commendation of the obstetrician.

Studies undertaken to assess the effectiveness of psychophysical techniques have reported widely divergent results, ranging from as low as 10–20% effective to as high as 70–80% effective. It is clear that the overall benefit is best judged by the parturient herself, with validation by the observations of attendants. As is no doubt true in other aspects of medical practice where emotional overlay and subjective reporting play a role in the evaluation of specific types of therapy, the personality and enthusiasm of the doctor have a lot to do with what the patient will think and say about what has just happened. Practitioners who are skeptical of psychophysical techniques cannot expect to accomplish very much using them.

It should be obvious that none of the psychophysical techniques should be "forced" on a patient, even by a skillful practitioner. The patient must not be made to feel that she will fail if she does not choose to complete her labor and delivery without analgesic medication. It must be made clear to her from the outset that she is expected to ask for help if she feels she wants or needs it. All things considered, psychophysical techniques should be viewed as adjuncts to other analgesic methods rather than substitutes for them.

The effectiveness of hypnosis is partially due to the well-known although incompletely understood mechanisms by which emotional and other central processes can influence a person's total responses to the pain experience. Verbal suggestion and somatosensory stimulation may help to alleviate discomfort associated with the first stage of labor. In addition, hypnotic states may provide apparent analgesia and amnesia for distressing, anxiety-provoking experiences. Finally, hypnotic techniques may substantially improve the parturient's outlook and behavior by reducing fear and apprehension. However, there are certain practical points to consider in regard to hypnosis because the time needed to establish a suitable relationship between physician and patient is often more than can be made available in the course of a busy medical practice.

### Psychoprophylaxis

A currently popular technique of "psychophysiologic preparation" involves educating the patient about her body functions and the physiology of labor. Positive attitudes and the need for good medical care are stressed. The goal of this technique is to use few if any drugs during the first and second stages of labor. Under optimal circumstances the need for narcotic drugs in the first stage of labor is reduced or eliminated altogether. When combined with certain analgesic "regional techniques" for late first-stage pain relief and second-stage analgesia, it approaches the ideal in management of pain relief for the childbirth experience. For maximum effectiveness, the husband should be instructed and included in the management of pain of the first and second stages of labor. His presence alone is reassuring, and as the "coach," he can direct and encourage his wife in proper breathing and bearing-down efforts; this will limit and reduce pain.

## ANALGESIC, AMNESTIC, & ANESTHETIC AGENTS

### General Comments & Precautions

1. If the patient is prepared psychologically for her experience, she will require less medication. Anticipate and dispel her fears during the antenatal period and in early labor. Never promise a painless labor.

2. Individualize the treatment of every patient, because each one reacts differently. Unfavorable reactions to any drug can occur.

3. Know the drug you intend to administer. Be familiar with its limitations, dangers, and contraindications as well as its advantages.

4. All analgesics given to the mother will cross the placenta. Systemic medications produce higher maternal and fetal blood levels than regionally administered drugs. Many drugs have central nervous system depressant effects. Although they may afford the desired effect on the mother, they may exert a mild to severe depressant effect on the fetus or newborn.

The ideal drug will have an optimal beneficial effect on the mother and a minimal depressant effect on the offspring. None of the presently available narcotic and sedative medications used in obstetrics has selective maternal effects. The regional administration of local anesthetics accomplished this goal to a large extent because the low maternal serum levels that are produced expose the fetus to insignificant drug mass.

### Pharmacologic Aspects

**A. Route of Administration:** Systemic techniques of analgesia and anesthesia include both oral and parenteral routes of administration. Parenteral administration includes subcutaneous, intramuscular, and intravenous injection. Sedatives, tranquilizers, and analgesics are usually given by intramuscular injection. In some cases, the intravenous route is preferred.

The advantages of intravenous administration may be listed as follows: (1) avoidance of variable rates of uptake due to poor vascular supply in fat or muscle; (2) prompt onset of effect; (3) titration of effect, avoiding the "peak effect" of an intramuscular bolus; and (4) smaller effective doses because of earlier onset of action.

The disadvantages of intravenous injection are inadvertent arterial injection and the depressant effect of overdosage. The advantage of smaller dosage overshadows the disadvantages.

Always administer the lowest concentration and the smallest dose to obtain the desired effect.

**B. Physical and Chemical Factors:** Anesthetics penetrate body cells by passing a lipid membrane

**Figure 26–1.** Local anesthetics are weak bases coexisting as undissociated free base and dissociated cation. Their proportion can be calculated by means of the Henderson-Hasselbalch equation.

boundary. This membrane is not receptive to charged (ionized) drugs but is permeable to un-ionized forms of drugs. Much of the total drug transfer is dependent on the degree of lipid solubility. Therefore, local anesthetics are characterized by aromatic rings that are lipophilic. Hence, all local anesthetics are lipid-soluble. In addition, the intermediate amine radical of a local anesthetic is a weak base that in aqueous solutions exists partly as undissociated free base and partly as dissociated cation. Fig 26–1 shows the equilibrium for such an existence and the Henderson-Hasselbalch equation, with which the proportion of the anesthetic in the charged and uncharged form can be determined. The ratio of the cation to the base form of the drug is important, because the base form is responsible for penetration and tissue diffusion of the local anesthetic, whereas the cation form is responsible for local analgesia when the drug contacts the nerve structure.

The $pK_a$ of a drug is the pH at which equal proportions of the free base and cation form occur. Most local anesthetics used in obstetric analgesia have $pK_a$ values ranging from 7.7 to 9.1 (Table 26–1). Since the pH of maternal blood is equal to or greater than 7.4, the $pK_a$ of local anesthetics is so close that significant changes in maternal and fetal acid-base balance may result in fluxes in the base versus the cation forms of the drug. For example, a rising pH shifts a given amount of local anesthetic cation to the base form, and, conversely, a fall in pH will generate more of the cationic form.

Physical factors are also important in drug transfer. Drugs with molecular weights under 600 cross the placenta without difficulty, whereas those with molecular weights of over 1000 do not. A molecule such as digoxin (MW 780.95) crosses the ovine placenta very poorly. Molecular weights of most local anes-

**Table 26–1.** $pK_a$s of the more commonly used local anesthetics.

| Drug | Brand Name | $pK_a$ |
|------|-----------|------|
| Bupivacaine | Marcaine | 8.1 |
| Chloroprocaine | Nesacaine | 8.7 |
| Etidocaine | Duranest | 7.7 |
| Lidocaine | Xylocaine | 7.9 |

thetics are in the 200–300 range. From the physical aspect, most local anesthetics cross the maternal-fetal barrier by simple diffusion according to the principles of Fick's law (Fig 26–2), which states that the rate of diffusion of a drug depends on the concentration gradient of the drug between the maternal and fetal compartments and the relationship of the thickness and total surface available for transfer.

**C. Placental Transfer:** Factors other than the physical or chemical properties of a drug may affect its transfer across the placenta. These factors include the rate and route of drug administration and the distribution, metabolism, and excretion of the drug by the mother and fetus. Fick's law may appear to be a simple method of determining drug transfer, but other complexities exist: differential blood flow on either side of the placenta; volume of maternal and fetal blood; and various shunts in the intervillous space that are important determinants of the final amount of drug a fetus may receive. Certain maternal disorders such as hypertensive cardiovascular disease, diabetes, and preeclampsia-eclampsia may alter placental blood flow and may in some way affect the extent of drug distribution.

As the placenta matures, there is a progressive reduction in the thickness of the epithelial trophoblastic layer. This may cause the thickness of the tissue layers between the maternal and fetal compartments to decrease 10-fold (from as much as 25 μm in early gestation to 2 μm at term in some species). As gestation progresses, the surface area of the placenta increases also. At term, these changes in physical structure tend to favor improved transfer of drugs across the placenta.

Uterine blood flow alterations may be induced by spontaneous labor, oxytocic drugs, hypotension, or aortocaval obstruction. All of these, although quite different etiologically, affect drug transfer and bring about a transient reduction in intervillous space perfusion. For example, placental transfer of thiobarbiturates may be reduced by mechanical aortic compression or by reduction of end-artery perfusion secondary to a hypertonic uterine contraction. In either case, reduction in placental transfer may be expected because maternal cardiac output to the end organs, eg, the uterus, placenta, and fetus, is altered. In contrast, venous obstruction with intervillous sequestration may increase the interval over which a given drug comes in contact with the diffusing membrane, so that the total amount of drug transferred may be

facilitated instead of reduced. At the same time, fetal cardiac output is important, since drugs that reduce it may also tend to reduce the uptake of other drugs because of depressed fetal circulation.

Placental transfer is also affected by the pH of the blood on both sides of the placenta. The pH of the blood on the fetal side of the placenta is normally 0.1–0.2 U lower than that on the maternal side. Therefore, passage of drug to the fetal unit results in a tendency for more of the drug to exist in the ionized state. Because the maternal/fetal equilibrium is established only between the un-ionized fraction of the drug on either side of the barrier, this physiologic differential will expedite maternal-fetal transfer of drug. With more drug in the ionized form in the fetal unit, the new equilibrium that arises results in a greater total (ionized plus un-ionized) drug load in the fetus. Because the $pK_a$ values of commonly used local anesthetics are closer to the maternal blood pH, these agents tend to accumulate on the fetal side of the placenta. This is also true of other basic drugs such as morphine, meperidine, and propranolol. Further decreases in the fetal pH lead to additional drug entrapment in the fetus. For acidic drugs (eg, thiopental) the shift in total drug concentration is in the opposite direction, ie, toward the maternal side of the placenta.

In summary, the rate of transfer of a drug is governed mainly by (1) lipid solubility, (2) degree of drug ionization, (3) placental blood flow, (4) molecular weight, (5) placental metabolism, and (6) protein binding.

**D. Fetal Distribution:** After a drug deposited in the maternal compartment passes through the maternal-fetal barrier, the drug must reach the fetus and be distributed (Fig 26–3). The response of the fetus and newborn depends on drug concentration in vessel-rich organs, eg, the brain, heart, and liver. Drugs transferred from the maternal to the fetal compartment of the placenta are then diluted before distribution to the various fetal vital organs. About 85% of the blood in the umbilical vein, which passes from the placenta to the fetus, passes through the fetal liver and then into the inferior vena cava. The remainder bypasses the liver and enters the vena cava primarily via the ductus venosus. The drug concentration is further reduced by an admixture of blood coming from the lower extremities, the abdominal viscera, the upper extremities, and the thorax. Blood from the right atrium shunts from right to left through the foramen ovale into the left atrium, resulting in a final concentration on the left side of the heart, which is only slightly lower than that in the vena cava.

The amount of drug ultimately reaching a vital organ is related to that organ's blood supply. Since the central nervous system is the most highly vascularized fetal organ, it receives the greatest amount of drug. Once the drug reaches the fetal liver, it may either be bound to protein or metabolized.

The uptake of drug by fetal tissues can be very

$$Q/T = K \left[ \frac{A(C_M - C_F)}{D} \right]$$

**Figure 26–2.** Fick's law. Q/T is rate of diffusion. A, the surface area available for drug transfer; $C_M$, maternal drug concentration; $C_F$, fetal drug concentration; D, membrane thickness; K, the diffusion constant of the drug.

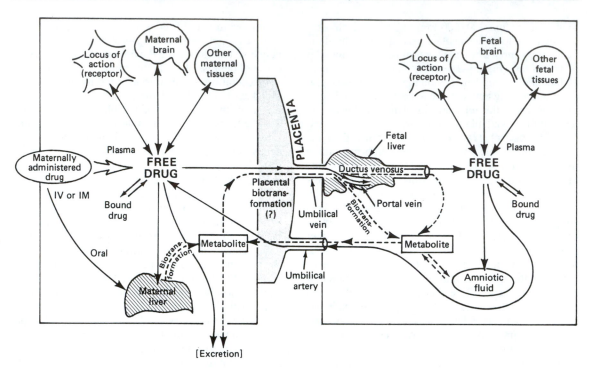

**Figure 26–3.** Relationship between maternal and fetal compartments and distribution of drugs between them. Drug is passed from the maternal compartment, via the placenta (a partial barrier), to the fetal compartment, where the principles of drug dynamics, ie, distribution, biotransformation, and excretion, determine the eventual specific organ tissue levels. One purely mechanical barrier exists between the maternal and fetal compartments, which attains importance in the late first and second stage of labor—the umbilical cord, which is susceptible to partial and total occlusion. (Reproduced, with permission, from Mirkin BL: Drug distribution in pregnancy. In: *Fetal Pharmacology.* Boreus L [editor]. Raven Press, 1973.)

rapid after either intravenous or epidural administration. Measurable concentrations of local anesthetics have been found in fetal tissues as early as 1–2 minutes after injection. Lipid solubility of a drug is important in developing concentrations in certain organs with high lipid content such as the adrenal, ovary, liver, and brain.

Drug metabolism and excretion are the final features of the fetal distribution picture. The fetal liver is able to metabolize drugs and numerous substrates as early as the second trimester, an ability that improves to term. Narcotics and sedatives are metabolized much more slowly by the fetal liver, producing a prolonged effect of these drugs in the newborn who is exposed in utero. Finally, the ability of the fetus to excrete drugs is also reduced by reduced renal function.

## Specific Types of Analgesic, Amnestic, & Anesthetic Agents

**A. Inhalant Anesthetics and Analgesics:** A number of potent agents that are often used for major operative procedures are included in this group. Nitrous oxide is the most commonly used inhalation agent. Halothane and isoflurane are volatile anesthet-

ics used in low concentration (0.5–0.7%) to supplement nitrous oxide for general endotracheal anesthesia. Nitrous oxide is the only inhalation anesthetic presently available with analgesic effects in subanesthesia concentrations 50% $N_2O$ in oxygen; it is used in Great Britain to provide pain relief in labor, however, its use is unsafe in unexperienced hands. Familiarity with the physicochemical features of all inhalant agents is necessary; it is a mistake to allow a novice to administer these agents in the belief that no harm can be done. Administration of any potent inhalation anesthetic can result in serious complications if adequate supervision is not available.

Methoxyflurane, cyclopropane, and trichloroethylene all have inherent disadvantages and are no longer used as inhalant analgesics.

**B. Sedatives (Hypnotics):** The principal use of sedative-hypnotic drugs is to produce drowsiness. For many years, these drugs were the only ones available to reduce anxiety and induce drowsiness. The latent phase of the first stage of labor may be managed by either psychologic support alone or utilization of sedative-hypnotic compounds. Psychologic support may be complemented by the use of sedatives. When properly utilized, these drugs induce tranquility and an enhanced feeling of well-being. They are poor analgesics and do not raise the pain threshold appreciably in conscious subjects. Amnesia does not occur. Labor may be slowed by large doses of sedatives, especially when given too early in the first stage.

The use of barbiturates alone for obstetric analgesia is not common practice and should be discouraged. The required dosage is dangerous to the fetus, which is extremely sensitive to central nervous system depression by these drugs. Periodic apnea and even abolition of all movements outlast the effects of the barbiturates on the mother.

**C. Tranquilizers and Amnestics:** These drugs are used principally to relieve apprehension and anxiety and produce a calm state. Additionally, they may potentiate the effects of other sedatives. An analgesic-potentiating effect is often claimed for this group of agents, but it has not been definitely demonstrated. Hydroxyzine (Atarax, Vistaril) and diazepam (Valium) are popular tranquilizer-amnestics. Scopolamine, which was widely popular in obstetrics in the past, produces no analgesia but has a mild sedative and marked amnestic effect. Scopolamine is no longer used because the amnesia produced is excessive and prolonged. Diazepam should also be avoided during labor because it has a long chemical half-life, which is even more prolonged in the neonate. Diazepam readily crosses the placenta and is found in significant concentrations in fetal plasma. At present, diazepam is not recommended if the neonate is premature, because of the threat of kernicterus. Other potential side effects related to the use of diazepam are fetal hypotonia, hypothermia, and a loss of beat-to-beat variability in the fetal heart rate.

One of the controversies over diazepam concerns the content of sodium benzoate and benzoic acid buffers. Both compounds are potent uncouplers of the bilirubin-albumin complex, and some investigators have suggested that the neonate may be more susceptible to kernicterus because of an increase in free circulating bilirubin. However, because injectable diazepam is effective in the treatment of human newborn seizure disorders, opiate withdrawal, and tetanus, and since it is regarded as a useful adjunct in obstetric analgesia, a study was undertaken in animals in which comparable quantities of sodium benzoate were injected to determine whether significant amounts of bilirubin would be made available to the circulation. Midazolam, a short-acting water-soluble benzodiazepine appears to be devoid of the neonatal effects seen with diazepam and is more rapidly cleared. Midazolam is a relatively new agent with minimal clinical use to date in obstetrics, but in small doses could conceivably become a useful anixolytic for the laboring patient. Midazolam is 3–4 times more potent than diazepam, and there is a mild delay in the onset of its sedative effect after intravenous injection. Doses should be kept below 0.075 mg/kg to avoid excessive anterograde amnesia.

**D. Narcotic Analgesics:** Systemic analgesic drugs (including narcotics) are commonly used in the first stage of labor because they produce both a state of analgesia and mood elevation. The favored drugs are codeine, 60 mg intramuscularly, or meperidine (Demerol), 50–100 mg intramuscularly or 25–50 mg (titrated) intravenously. The combination of morphine and scopolamine was once popular for its "twilight sleep" effect but is rarely used now. Common undesirable effects of this combination of drugs are nausea and vomiting, cough suppression, intestinal stasis, and diminution in frequency, intensity, and duration of uterine contractions in the early first stage of labor. Also, amnesia is excessive for these patients.

Morphine is not used in laboring patients because of the excessive respiratory depression seen in the neonate compared with equipotent doses of other narcotics. Fetuses who are of young gestational age or are small-for-dates or those who have undergone trauma or long labor are more susceptible to narcosis.

Fentanyl is a popular synthetic narcotic that has been used in obstetrics in both the systemic and epidural compartments. Its use in the epidural compartment has met with good success when combined with small quantities and low concentrations of bupivacaine. Data supporting its use come from both Europe and the USA.

**E. Thiobarbiturates:** Intravenous anesthetics such as thiopental (Pentothal) and thiamylal (Surital) are widely used in general surgery. However, in less than 4 minutes after injection of a thiobarbiturate into the mother's vein, the concentrations of the drug in the fetal and maternal blood will be equal. The mother will lose consciousness and airway protective reflexes with a pentothal dose of 1.5–2 mg/kg and therefore should be used only in association with general endotracheal anesthesia.

**F. Potentiating Drugs:** Phenothiazine drugs potentiate the tranquilizing effects of the analgesics, amnestics, and general anesthetics.

**G. Ketamine:** The phencyclidine derivative ketamine produces anesthesia by a dissociative interruption of afferent pathways from cortical perception. It has become a useful and widely used adjunctive agent in obstetrics, because maternal cardiovascular status and uterine blood flow are well maintained. In low doses of 0.25–0.5 mg/kg intravenously, effective maternal analgesia results but without loss of consciousness or protective reflexes. The margin of safety is narrow, however, and therefore should be used only by physicians able to easily secure and protect the airway if loss of consciousness occurs. For cesarean section delivery, general anesthetic induction can be produced with 1–2 mg/kg intravenously and is followed in rapid sequence with muscle relaxant and endotracheal intubation. Ketamine is therefore useful in the setting of major blood loss, when rapid induction of general anesthesia is required. It has significant hallucinogenic effects which otherwise limit its appeal in obstetrics.

Ketamine stimulates the cardiovascular system to maintain heart rate, blood pressure, and cardiac output and therefore is useful in complicated situations of maternal hypotension/hemorrhage.

## REGIONAL ANESTHESIA

Regional anesthesia is achieved by injection of a local anesthetic (Table 26–2) around the nerves that pass from spinal segments to the peripheral nerves responsible for sensory innervation of a portion of the body. More recently, narcotics have been added to local anesthetics to improve analgesia and reduce some side effects of local anesthetics. Regional nerve blocks used in obstetrics include the following: (1) lumbar epidural and caudal epidural block, (2) subarachnoid (spinal)block, and (3) pudendal block.

Infiltration of a local anesthetic drug and pudendal block analgesia carry minimal risks. The hazards increase with the amount of drug used. The safety and suitability of regional anesthesia depend on the proper selection of the drug and the patient and the obstetrician-gynecologist's knowledge, experience, and expertise in the diagnosis and treatment of possible complications. Major conductive anesthesia and general anesthesia in obstetrics requires specialized knowledge and expertise in conjunction with close maternal and fetal monitoring. This field of expertise has indeed developed as a subspecialty within anesthesia, reflecting the need for specialized understanding of the obstetric patient and her response and the fetal responses to anesthesia.

### Patient Selection

Good candidates for regional anesthesia are healthy, mature women; poor candidates include young, emotionally unstable, or medically compromised women, ie, those with preeclampsia-eclampsia, hypotension, or hypovolemia. Tense, fearful, psychoneurotic, or psychotic patients may require general anesthesia for surgical procedures, and the physician should not try to coerce such women to accept regional anesthesia.

Patients with severe obstetric, gynecologic, cardiac, or pulmonary disorders may do well with regional block anesthesia, but general anesthesia may be less hazardous if a prolonged procedure is anticipated. Large amounts of local anesthetics may jeopardize the patient. Moreover, the anxiety and discomfort during administration of the local anesthetic and surgery increase epinephrine secretion and oxygen consumption. This usually imposes a greater threat of cardiorespiratory decompensation than with a well-managed general anesthetic. The anesthesiologist will assess the patient to determine the relative risks of general versus regional anesthesia. Some forms of valvular heart disease, for example, may contraindicate regional block and general anesthesia may be considered more appropriate.

### Patient Preparation

The woman who is well informed and has good rapport with her physician generally is a calm and co-

**Table 26–2.** Drugs used for local anesthesia.

|  | Tetracaine (Pontocaine) | Lidocaine (Xylocaine) | Bupivacaine (Marcaine) |
|---|---|---|---|
| Potency (compared to procaine) | 10 | 2–3 | 9–12 |
| Toxicity (compared to procaine) | 10 | 1–1.5 | 4–6 |
| Stability at sterilizing temperature | Stable | Stable | Stable |
| Total maximum dose | 50–100 mg | 500 mg | 175 mg |
| Infiltration<br>　Concentration<br>　Onset of action<br>　Duration | <br>0.05–0.1%<br>10–20 min<br>1½–3h | <br>0.5–1%<br>3–5 min<br>30–60 min | <br>0.25%<br>5–10 min<br>90–120 min |
| Nerve block and epidural<br>　Concentration<br>　Onset of action<br>　Duration | <br>0.1–0.2%<br>10–20 min<br>1½–3 h | <br>1–2%<br>5–10 min<br>1–1 1/2 h | <br>0.5%<br>7–21 min<br>2–6 h |
| Subarachnoid<br>　Concentration<br>　Dose<br>　Onset of action<br>　Duration | <br>0.1–0.5%<br>5–20 mg<br>5–10 min<br>1½–2 h | <br>5%<br>40–100 mg<br>1–3 min<br>1–1½ h | <br>. . .<br>. . .<br>. . .<br>. . . |

Modified and reproduced, with permission, from Guadagni NP, Hamilton WK: Anesthesiology. In: *Current Surgical Diagnosis & Treatment*, 4th ed. Dunphy JE, Way LW (editors). Lange, 1979.

operative candidate for regional or general anesthesia. The patient and her partner should be well informed early in her pregnancy of the options for labor anesthesia as well as for cesarean section if that circumstance arises. The anesthesiologist can be involved early in pregnancy if the patient has special concerns about anesthesia (family history of anesthetic risk, previous back surgery, coagulation problems). Some hospitals have obstetric anesthesia preassessment clinics organized to deal with these patient concerns.

## Local Anesthetic Agents

A local anesthetic drug blocks the action potential of nerves when their axons are exposed to the medication. Local anesthetic agents act by modifying the ionic permeability of the cell membrane to stabilize its resting potential. The smaller the nerve fiber, the more sensitive it is to local anesthetics because the susceptibility of individual nerve fibers is inversely proportional to the cross-sectional diameters of the fibers. Hence, with regional anesthesia, the patient's perception of light touch, pain, and temperature, and her capacity for vasomotor control, are obtunded sooner and with a smaller concentration of the drug than is the perception of pressure or the function of motor nerves to striated muscles. The exception to this rule is the sensitivity of autonomic nerve fibers that are blocked by the lowest concentration of local anesthetic—this, despite being larger than some sensory nerves.

Only anesthetic drugs that are completely reversible and nonirritating and that cause minimal toxicity are clinically acceptable. Other desirable properties of regional anesthetic agents include rapidity of onset, predictability of duration, and ease of sterilization. Table 26–2 summarizes the local anesthetics commonly used in obstetrics and gynecology patients together with their uses and doses.

All local anesthetics have certain undesirable dose-related side effects when absorbed systemically. All these drugs are capable of stimulating the central nervous system and may cause bradycardia, hypertension, or respiratory stimulation at the medullary level. Moreover, they may produce anxiety, excitement, or convulsions at the cortical or subcortical levels. This response stimulates grand mal seizures because it is followed by depression, loss of vasomotor control, hypotension, respiratory depression, and coma. Such an episode of indirect cardiovascular depression often is accentuated by a direct vasodilatory and myocardial depressant effect. The latter is comparable to the action of quinidine. This is why lidocaine is useful for the treatment of certain cardiac arrhythmias.

Chloroprocaine (Nesacaine) is an ester derivative that was popular in the mid-1960s but fell into disuse clinically. In the 1970s, it enjoyed a resurgence in popularity primarily because of its rapid onset and short duration of action and its low toxicity to the fetus. Its physicochemical properties are imparted by the chloro substitution of the 2-position in the benzene ring of procaine. It is metabolized by plasma cholinesterase and therefore does not demand liver enzyme degradation, as do the more complex and longer-acting amide derivatives. Chloroprocaine has a half-life of 21 seconds in adult blood and 43 seconds in neonatal blood. Direct toxic effects on the fetus are minimized, since less drug is available for transfer in the maternal compartment.

The potency of chloroprocaine is comparable to that of lidocaine and mepivacaine, and the drug is 3 times more potent than procaine. Its average onset of action ranges from 6 to 12 minutes and persists for 30–60 minutes, depending on the amount used. Its use has been severely curtailed because of recent reports of toxicity that include arachnoiditis and associated neuropathies. The new 3% chloroprocaine is less acidic and has a reduced concentration of sodium metabisulfate (0.5 mg/mL) and is safe for epidural use.

Bupivacaine, the amide local anesthetic, is related to lidocaine and mepivacaine but has some very different physicochemical properties. It has a much higher lipid solubility, a higher degree of binding to maternal plasma protein, and a much longer duration of action. More than with other local anesthetics, the concentration of bupivacaine can be reduced to produce sensory block with minimal motor block. Since injection of bupivacaine for labor pain relief is now mostly in the form of continuous small volume and minimal concentration administration via a pump mechanism, the complications previously of concern such as hypotension and convulsions are now rare. Zador and associates were among the first to study the effects of continuous infusion of local anesthetics on uterine activity as measured electronically. Abboud and associates also used tokodynamometer measurements in 61 parturients at term who received continuous infusion epidural analgesia. They noted no statistically significant effect on the uterine activity produced by continuous epidural infusion of 0.125% bupivacaine at a rate of 14 mL/hr, 0.75% chloroprocaine at a rate of 27 mL/hr, and 0.75% lidocaine at a rate of 14 mL/hr. Consequently, the progress of cervical dilatation and duration of the first stage of labor was not influenced by the continuous infusion of the local anesthetics.

In view of the increasing use of continuous epidural infusion of dilute solutions of local anesthetic combined with opioids, Baxin also was prompted to study 40 parturients given segmental epidural block with 0.375% bupivacaine. Chestnut and associates also reported that a continuous infusion of 0.0625% bupivacaine–0.0002% fentanyl given to primiparas did not prolong, but tended to decrease the duration of the active phase of the first stage of labor compared to the general obstetric population. McDonald and colleagues at OSU have used the most dilute concentration of sufentanil and bupivacaine (0.0625%) for nearly 4 years and have collected impressive clinical results in close to 1,000 parturients. The solution is made up by placement of 60 mcg of sufentanil, 75 mg of bupivacaine, and 200 mcg of epinephrine (making up a 30 mL volume) into a 120 mL saline bag, which has had 30 mL extracted, then the final volume in the bag is still 120 mL. The final dosing solution contains 0.5 mcg sufentanil, 0.625 mg bupivacaine, and 1.6 mcg of epinephrine. In addition, since bupivacaine is well bound to maternal protein, it has a low fetal-maternal concentration ratio (0.3) compared with that of lidocaine (0.5). In behavior studies, bupivacaine did not decrease newborn muscle tone, as do lidocaine and mepivacaine. Thus, bupivacaine is the most popular local anesthetic drug used for regional anesthesia today.

A word of caution must be added regarding the administration of bupivacaine for cesarean section delivery. This drug has been implicated in certain cardiovascular catastrophes associated with initial drug injection; eg, cardiac arrests have been refractory to full and appropriate resuscitative attempts. Although these catastrophes are rare, the practitioner is well advised to inject no more than 5 mL of the drug at any one time, to wait 4–5 minutes, then to repeat the procedure until the desired volume has been delivered. The maximum concentration of bupivacaine now allowed by the FDA for obstetric epidural anesthesia is 0.5%. The toxic dose is now considered 1–2 mg/kg for bupivacaine.

## Local Infiltration Analgesia

Local tissue infiltration of dilute solutions of anesthetic drugs generally yields satisfactory results because the target is the fine nerve fibers. Nevertheless, one must recall the dangers of systemic toxicity when large areas are anesthetized or when reinjection is required. It is good practice, therefore, to calculate in advance the milligrams of drug in the volume of solution that may be required to keep the total dosage below the accepted toxic dose.

Infiltration in or near an area of inflammation is contraindicated. Injections into these zones may be followed by rapid systemic absorption of the drug owing to the increased vascularity of the inflamed tissues. Moreover, the injection may introduce or aggravate infection.

## Regional Analgesia

**A. Lumbar Epidural Block:** These analgesic techniques have become more popular recently, because they are well suited to obstetric anesthesia. Either bolus injections or continuous infusion of local anesthetics are used for labor, vaginal delivery, or cesarean surgery (Fig 26–4). Narcotics are often added to supplement the quality of the block.

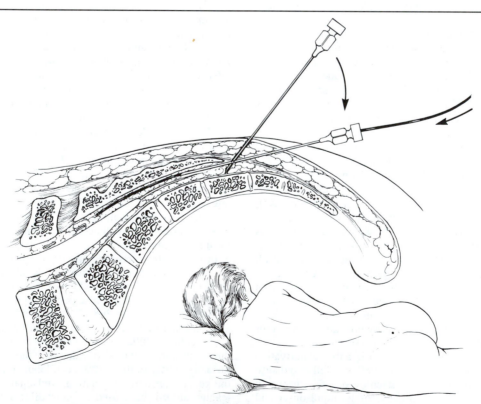

**Figure 26–4.** Caudal catheter in place for continuous caudal anesthesia.

After the patient is evaluated, an epidural block may be placed once labor is established. Drug dosages can be adjusted as circumstances change. The catheter can be used for surgery and postoperative analgesia if necessary. The second stage of labor is prolonged by epidural anesthesia; however, the duration of the first stage is unaffected. The use of outlet forceps is increased, but fetal outcome is not adversely affected by epidural block.

The epidural block technique must be exact, and inadvertent massive (high) spinal anesthesia occasionally occurs. Other undesirable reactions include the rapid absorption syndrome (hypotension, bradycardia, hallucinations, convulsions), postpartum backache, and paresthesias. Epidural block should eradicate pain between T10 and L1 for first stage, and between the T10 and S5 for the second stage of labor.

The procedure is as follows: Inject 3 mL of a 1.5% aqueous solution of lidocaine or similar agent into the catheter as a test dose. If spinal anesthesia does not result after 5–10 minutes, inject an additional 5 mL. Inject 10 mL of the anesthetic solution in total to slowly accomplish an adequate degree and suitable level of anesthesia. Once the block is established, reinjection of 8–10 mL of solution every 60–90 minutes, or a continuous infusion of 8–12 mL/hr will maintain the block for labor. Bupivacaine, 0.125–0.25%, is most often used for an epidural block.

The mother is nursed in a wedged or lateral position to avoid aortocaval compression. The sympathectomy produced by the block predisposes the patient to venous pooling and reduced venous return. Maternal blood pressure must be measured frequently when the epidural is in effect.

**B. Caudal Block:** Caudal anesthesia is an epidural block approached through the caudal space. It can provide selective sacral block for second-stage labor; however, it is rarely used now because of complications specific to the obstetric patient. The descent of the fetal head against the perineum, in addition to the sacral edema at term, obscures the landmarks of the sacral hiatus. This makes the caudal procedure technically challenging, and reports of transfixing the rectum and fetal skull puncture with the epidural needle have led many anesthesiologists away from this technique. Lumbar epidural anesthesia is considered a safer alternative.

**C. Spinal Anesthesia:** Spinal anesthesia is currently used to alleviate the pain of delivery and the third stage of labor. Short-acting agents (5% lidocaine, 50 mg) or long-acting drugs (1% tetracaine, 4 mg) are used. Brief or minimal spinal anesthesia is far safer than prolonged spinal anesthesia, which is not recommended for obstetric use. The advantages of spinal anesthesia are that no fetal hypoxia ensues unless hypotension occurs, blood loss is minimal, the mother remains conscious to witness delivery, no inhalation anesthetics or analgesic drugs are required, the technique is not difficult, and good relaxation of the pelvic floor and lower birth canal is achieved. Prompt anesthesia is achieved within 5–10 minutes, and there are fewer failures than with caudal anesthesia. The dosage of spinal anesthetic is small. Complications are fewer and easier to treat. Hypotension is rare with the doses used. Spinal headache occurs in 1–2% of patients, however, and operative delivery is more often required because voluntary expulsive efforts are eliminated. Drug reactions (eg, hypotension) may occur. Respiratory failure may occur if the anesthetic ascends within the spinal cord owing to rapid injection or straining by the patient.

The procedure is as follows:

1. Inject 50 mg of lidocaine 5% or 4 mg of tetracaine as 1% solution with 10% glucose, or comparable drug, slowly into the third or fourth lumbar interspace between contractions. Have the patient lying on her side or sitting up. Elevate her head on a pillow immediately after the injection. Tilt the table up or down to achieve a level of anesthesia at or near the umbilicus. Anesthesia will be maximal in 3–5 minutes and will last for 1 hour or longer.

2. Obtain and record the blood pressure and respiratory rate every 3 minutes for the first 10 minutes and every 5 minutes thereafter.

3. Give oxygen for respiratory depression and mild hypotension. In addition, administer vasopressors such as ephedrine, 5–10 mg intravenously, if blood pressure decreases more than 20% of baseline or to less than 100 mm Hg systolic and is not responsive to intravenous fluids and lateral tilt.

**D. Paracervical Block:** (Fig 26–5.) Paracervical block is no longer considered a safe technique for the obstetric patient. In the past, paracervical anesthesia was used to relieve the pain of the first stage of labor. Pudendal block was required for pain during the second stage of labor. Sensory nerve fibers from the uterus fuse bilaterally at the 4–6 o'clock and 6–8 o'clock positions around the cervix in the region of the cervical-vaginal junction. Ordinarily, when 5–10 mL of 1% lidocaine or its equivalent is injected into these areas, interruption of the sensory input from the cervix and uterus promptly follows.

Many now consider paracervical block to be contraindicated in obstetrics because of the potential adverse fetal effects. There are many reports in the literature that place the incidence of fetal bradycardia at 8–18%. Recent work with accurate fetal heart rate monitoring associated with continuous uterine contraction patterns, however, suggests that the incidence is closer to 20–25%. Some researchers have attempted to investigate the significance of the bradycardia. One explanation is that an acid-base disturbance in the fetus does not occur unless the bradycardia lasts longer than 10 minutes and that neonatal depression is rare unless associated with delivery during the period of bradycardia. There seems to be little difference in the incidence and severity of fetal bradycardia by paracervical block between compli-

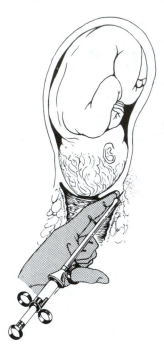

**Figure 26–5.** Paracervical block. This block is considered by many to be contraindicated in pregnancy.

cated and uncomplicated patients. Other disadvantages of paracervical block include maternal trauma and bleeding, fetal trauma and direct injection, inadvertent intravascular injection with convulsions, and short duration of the block.

**E. Pudendal Nerve Block:** Pudendal block has been one of the most popular of all nerve block techniques in obstetrics. The infant is not depressed, and blood loss is minimal. The technique is simplified by the fact that the pudendal nerve approaches the spine of the ischium on its course to innervate the perineum. Injection of 10 mL of 1% lidocaine on each side will achieve analgesia for 30–45 minutes about 50% of the time.

Both the transvaginal and transcutaneous methods are useful for administering a pudendal block. The transvaginal technique has important practical advantages over the transcutaneous technique. The "Iowa trumpet" needle guide may be used, and the operator's finger should be placed at the end of the needle guide to palpate the sacrospinous ligament, which runs in the same direction and is just anterior to the pudendal nerve and artery. It is usually very difficult to appreciate the sensation of the needle puncturing the ligament. This facet of the technique (no definite end point) may make it difficult for the inexperienced person to perform. Aspiration of the syringe for possible inadvertent entry into the pudendal artery should be accomplished, and, if no blood is

returned, 10 mL of local anesthetic solution should be injected in a fan-like fashion on the right and left sides. The successful performance of the pudendal block requires injection of the drug at least 10–12 minutes before episiotomy. Often, in clinical practice, pudendal block is performed within 4–5 minutes of episiotomy. Hence, there may not be adequate time for the local anesthetic to take effect.

**1. Advantages and disadvantages**–Enthusiasm for pudendal nerve block has been due to its safety and ease of administration and the rapidity of onset of effect. Disadvantages include maternal trauma, bleeding, and infection; rare maternal convulsions due to drug sensitivity; occasional complete or partial failure; and regional discomfort during administration.

The pudendal perineal block, like any other nerve block, demands some technical experience and knowledge of the innervation of the lower birth canal. Nevertheless, in spite of a well-placed bilateral block, skip areas of perineal analgesia may be noted. The reason for this may be that although the pudendal nerve of S2–S4 derivation does contribute to the majority of fibers for sensory innervation to the perineum, other sensory fibers are involved also. For example, the inferior hemorrhoidal nerve may have an origin independent from that of the sacral nerve and therefore will not be a component branch of the pudendal nerve. In this case, it must be infiltrated separately. In addition, the posterior femoral cutaneous nerve (S1–S3) origin may contribute an important perineal branch to the anterior fourchette bilaterally. In instances in which this nerve plays a major role in innervation, it must be blocked separately by local skin infiltration.

Two other nerves contribute to the sensory innervation of the perineum: the ilioinguinal nerve, of L1 origin, and the genital branch of the genitofemoral nerve, of L1 and L2 origin. Both of these nerves sweep superficially over the mons pubis to innervate the skin over the symphysis of the mons pubis and the labium majus. Occasionally, these nerves must also be separately infiltrated to provide optimal perineal analgesic effect. It should be apparent, then, that a simple bilateral pudendal nerve block may not be effective in many cases. For maximum analgesic effectiveness, in addition to a bilateral pudendal block, superficial infiltration of the skin from the symphysis medially to a point halfway between the ischial spines may be necessary. Thus, a true perineal block may be regarded as a regional technique.

Either lumbar epidural or caudal epidural block should eradicate pain between the T10 and S5 level for the second stage. All these nerves are denervated, since they all are derived from L1—S5 segments.

**2. Procedure**–(Fig 26–6.)

a. Palpate the ischial spines vaginally. Slowly advance the needle guide toward each spine. After

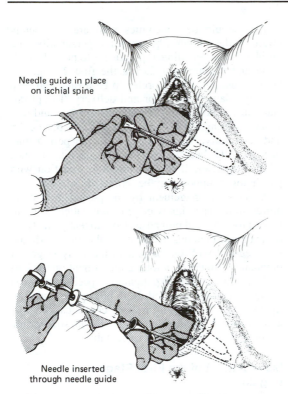

Needle guide in place on ischial spine

Needle inserted through needle guide

**Figure 26–6.** Use of needle guide ("Iowa trumpet") in pudendal anesthetic block. (Reproduced, with permission, from Benson RC: *Handbook of Obstetrics & Gynecology,* 8th ed. Lange, 1983.)

placement is achieved, the needle is advanced through the guide to penetrate approximately 0.5 cm. Aspirate and, if not in a vessel, deposit 5 mL below each spine. This blocks the right and left pudendal nerves. Refill the syringe when necessary, and proceed in a similar manner to anesthetize the other areas specified. Keep the needle moving while injecting and avoid the sensitive vaginal mucosa and periosteum.

b. Withdraw the needle and guide about 2 cm and redirect toward an ischial tuberosity. Inject 3 mL near the center of each tuberosity to anesthetize the inferior hemorrhoidal and lateral femoral cutaneous nerves.

c. Withdraw the needle and guide almost entirely and then slowly advance toward the symphysis pubica almost to the clitoris, keeping about 2 cm lateral to the labial fold and about 1–2 cm beneath the skin. The injection of 5 mL of lidocaine on each side beneath the symphysis will block the ilioinguinal and genitocrural nerves.

If the procedure just explained is not hurried and is skillfully done, there will be slight discomfort during injections only. Prompt flaccid relaxation and good anesthesia for 30–60 minutes can be expected.

## Undesirable Side Effects of Spinal or Epidural Anesthesia

The most serious consequence of spinal or epidural anesthesia has been very rare mortality. However, between 1978 and 1983, maternal deaths associated with the use of 0.75% bupivacaine for cesarean section delivery and labor were reported. These deaths were attributed to venous uptake of the drug and immediate and lasting myocardial depression from the local anesthetic, which did not respond to appropriate cardiac resuscitative efforts. Lower concentrations and doses appear to have solved the problem. Most side effects of spinal or epidural anesthesia are secondary to the block of the sympathetic nerve fibers that accompany the anterior roots of the spinal thoracic and upper lumbar nerves (thoracolumbar outflow). Thus, many physiologic regulating mechanisms are disturbed. The blood lumbarpressure falls as the result of loss of arterial resistance and venous pooling—assuming no compensation by change of the patient's position (eg, Trendelenburg position). If high thoracic dermatomes (T1–T5) are blocked, alteration of the cardiac sympathetic innervation slows the heart rate and reduces cardiac contractility. Epinephrine secretion by the adrenal medulla is depressed. Concomitantly, the unopposed parasympathetic effect of cardiac slowing alters vagal stimulations. As a result of these and related changes, shock follows promptly, especially in hypotensive or hypovolemic patients. Moreover, a precipitous fall in the blood pressure of the arteriosclerotic hypertensive patient is inevitable.

Fluids, oxygen therapy for adequate tissue perfusion, shock position to encourage venous return, and pressor drugs given intravenously are recommended.

Post-dural puncture headache (PDPH) due to leakage of cerebrospinal fluid through the needle hole in the dura in the past has been an early postoperative complication in up to 15% of patients. Small-caliber needles (25F) decrease the incidence of headache to 8–10%. More recently, the introduction of pencil-point Whitacker and Sprotte spinal needles, the incidence of PDPH is now 1–2%. Therapy for PDPH includes recumbent position, hydration, sedation, and, in severe cases, injection of 10–20 mL of the patient's fresh blood to "seal" the defect epidurally.

Rarely, spinal or epidural anesthesia has caused nerve injury and transient or permanent hypesthesia or paresthesia. Excessive drug concentration, sensitivity, or infection may have been responsible for some of these complications. The incidence of serious complications of spinal or epidural anesthesia is considerably less than that of cardiac arrest during general anesthesia.

## Prevention & Treatment of Local Anesthetic Overdosage

The correct dose of any local anesthetic is the smallest quantity of drug in the greatest dilution that will provide adequate analgesia. The pregnant patient is more likely to have an intravascular drug injection because of the venous distention in the epidural space and may be more susceptible to the toxic effects of local anesthetics (Table 26–3). Injection of the drug into a highly vascularized area will result in more rapid systemic absorption than, eg, injection into the skin. To prevent too-rapid absorption, the operator may add epinephrine to produce local vasoconstriction and prolong the anesthetic. A final concentration of 1:200,000 is desirable, especially when a toxic amount is approached. Epinephrine is contraindicated, however, in patients with increased cardiac irritability of medical or drug origin.

The treatment of local anesthetic overdosage manifested by central nervous system toxicity (a convulsion) is generally achieved very effectively and without incident. However, the administrator must be aware of certain basic principles. These consist of the recognition of prodromal signs of a central nervous system toxic reaction and immediate treatment as required. A toxic central nervous system reaction to local anesthetics consists of ringing in the ears, diplopia, perioral numbness, and deep, slurred speech. An adequate airway must be maintained, and the patient should receive 100% oxygen, with respiratory assistance if necessary. Protection of the patient's airway and immediate injection of thiopental, 50 mg, or midazolam, 1–2 mg, usually stop the convulsion immediately. In the past, succinylcholine was recommended. This drug is a potent neuromuscular relaxant, which requires placement of an endotracheal tube with positive pressure ventilation. Studies have indicated that cellular metabolism is greatly increased during convulsive episodes, so that a definite increase in cellular oxygenation occurs—hence the use of a depressant selective for the hypothalamus and thalamus, because these sites are the foci of irritation.

## ANALGESIA FOR INTRAPARTUM OBSTETRICS

For ideal anesthetic management of intrapartum analgesia, the physician who has an established rapport with the patient should be responsible. Any sub-

stitutes should be colleagues who are completely aware of the patient's background, personality, and problems. Current clinical practice is to provide analgesia and not amnesia during the first 2 stages of labor. Most parturients prefer to be awake and help the physician during labor and delivery. The physician must be aware of the patient's attitude and personality during labor. A mother who has been calm and cooperative during the antepartum period may unexpectedly become anxious or distraught once labor progresses. If this occurs, mild sedation with psychologic support may be indicated.

Analgesia management by the physician also requires some basic knowledge of the patient's gestational problems and prognosis. Consequently, the types of analgesic methods available to the patient should be discussed with the patient in the early stages of pregnancy. However, a total commitment on the part of the physician and the patient to a specific analgesia method should be avoided. Both primiparas and multiparas may develop unforeseen complications that could make the method agreed upon undesirable and, in some cases, medically unacceptable.

### Management of the First Stage (Fig 26–7)

The management of labor analgesia can be deter-

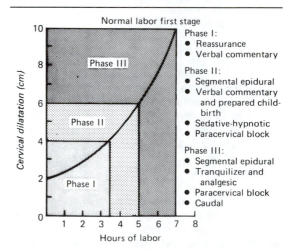

**Figure 26–7.** First-stage management in a primipara may be divided into 3 phases. Phase I (early labor) should be managed by simple reassurance and verbal commentary if the patient has had adequate antepartum education. An epidural may be performed once labor is well established. Phase II may be handled by a segmental epidural block, continued reassurance, a sedative-hypnotic drug, narcotic, or a tranquilizer. The accentuated phase of labor (phase III) may be handled by segmental epidural block, a combination tranquilizer and analgesic, or a caudal epidural block. However, use of reassurance and verbal commentary in conjunction with prepared childbirth methods may be adequate for some patients to tolerate the discomfort of phase III labor.

**Table 26–3.** Toxic doses of local anesthetics commonly used in obstetrics.

| Drug | Toxic Dose |
|---|---|
| Lidocaine | 5 mg/kg, plain<br>7mg/kg, with epinephrine |
| Bupivacaine | 1.5 mg/kg* |
| Chloroprocaine | 10 mg/kg |
| Tetracaine | 1 mg/kg |

*Doses as low as 90 mg have produced cardiac arrest; Albright GA, Anesthesiology (1979).

mined only when the patient experiences the pain and decides on options with the help and reassurance of her physician.

## Management of the Second Stage

**A. Epidural Block:** If an epidural technique is utilized for first-stage pain relief, it may be extended to cover the second stage. Assuming that a lumbar catheter alone is utilized, the segmental block can be extended to include sacral dermatomes with a larger volume of local anesthetic. Sacral block is present in only 3.5% of patients with the initial epidural dose. This increases to 65% of patients with repeated injections. It is therefore important for the anesthesiologist to assess the degree of sacral anesthesia that is present when a "perineal dose" is requested. No further dosing may be needed, or 10–12 mL of local anesthetic will usually produce sacral block if none is present at the time of delivery.

The timing of second-stage analgesia must be managed carefully because 10–12 minutes are required for a good sacral block to develop after the injection described above. If a caudal catheter is used, 10 mL of 2% lidocaine should be injected into the caudal epidural space; within 5–8 minutes, good sacral analgesia should be present. This technique rarely fails to produce bilateral analgesia, and its onset is more rapid. A 2% solution is preferred for the second stage for a more complete motor block of the pudendum.

**B. Subarachnoid Block:** Subarachnoid block may also be utilized for good second-stage analgesia and muscle relaxation of the perineum. The technique may be performed with the patient in either the sitting or lateral recumbent position. The latter is the most common position for subarachnoid block and is infinitely more comfortable for the patient. An important feature is the total amount of drug used. Four milligrams of 1% tetracaine 6–8 mg of 0.75% bupivacaine or 50 mg of 5% lidocaine are adequate for a low spinal block of dermatomes T10–S5. The block will last only 50–70 minutes and therefore should be used only if delivery is imminent.

One of the advantages of subarachnoid block is the rapid onset of both sensory and motor blockade. Careful attention must be paid to changes in the sensory level and blood pressure. The latter must be recorded every 2–3 minutes for the first 10 minutes to be certain that sudden undetected hypotension does not occur. Thereafter, the blood pressure may be recorded every 5 minutes for 30 minutes.

**C. Pudendal Block:** Pudendal block, when performed correctly, will suffice also for second-stage pain relief. As outlined above, performance of the pudendal nerve block is not as simple as many physicians believe. Inadequate perineal analgesia often occurs because of lack of knowledge of the sensory distribution to the perineum. Nonetheless, a good bilateral pudendal block combined with superficial injection of the triangular area between the midportion

of the symphysis pubica and halfway to a line drawn to the spinous process often will effect complete perineal analgesia. In spite of this, more analgesia is usually needed for an indicated forceps delivery. If forceps extraction is necessary, a caudal or subarachnoid block it may be needed to utilize to achieve complete perineal anesthesia.

**D. Special Problems:**

**1. Midforceps delivery**–Since precise timing and specific requirements for rotation of the fetus may be necessary, the obstetrician must carefully choose the best analgesia for midforceps delivery. Each patient's requirements vary and every situation must be evaluated on an individual basis. Midforceps delivery involves both rotation and traction. Therefore, the anesthetic regimen must provide relaxation as well as analgesia for the perineum, lower vagina, and upper birth canal. In order for the obstetrician to perform the procedures necessary for delivery, it is necessary to provide optimal conditions so that maternal and fetal trauma can be minimized. Regional analgesia with a lumbar, caudal epidural, or subarachnoid block is preferred, since these blocks provide analgesia and optimal relaxation.

**2. The trapped head**–On the rare occasion when the breech delivery is complicated by a trapped head, the application of forceps or other manipulations may be required urgently. If an epidural block is in place, no further analgesia will be required; however, if one is not in place, immediate anesthesia and pelvic relaxation will be required to facilitate rapid delivery and minimize trauma. The only acceptable technique for this purpose is general anesthesia with halothane after suitable protection of the patient from the hazards of aspiration. Protection should include use of antacid, 30 mL orally; adequate oxygenation; glycopyrrolate, 0.2 mg intravenously; tubocurarine, 3 mg intravenously; followed by thiopental, 200 mg intravenously; succinylcholine, 80–100 mg intravenously; and rapid intubation with cricoid pressure.

## ANESTHESIA FOR THE FETUS AT RISK

### Premature Labor

**A. Psychoanalgesia:** Familiarize the patient before labor (if possible) with a relaxation technique (Lamaze or Dick-Read) and the use of her delivery powers to reduce tension and pain (psychoprophylaxis). Establish rapport and provide emotional support. Use reassurance and kindly direction. Use suggestion and hypnosis when feasible. Psychoprophylaxis has been most successful, but fewer than 20% of patients can be carried through labor and delivery with hypnosis alone.

**B. Regional Analgesia:** Conduction analgesia is usually more desirable than inhalation or parenteral analgesia. All regional blocking agents are rapidly absorbed. These agents may intoxicate the fetus when overdosage occurs, with resultant apnea and vascular collapse due to medullary depression, bradycardia due to the quinidine-like effect on the myocardium, and convulsions due to cortical excitation. These agents with the amide molecular linkage (lidocaine, mepivacaine, and prilocaine) have a stability that resists enzymatic splitting and rapidly cross the placental barrier intact. In contrast, local anesthetics with an ester bond (procaine, 2-chloroprocaine, and tetracaine) are metabolized in the plasma and placenta with only minor transfer to the fetus.

**1. Pudendal nerve block–**The nerves supplying the lower birth canal are anesthetized by blocking the pudendal nerve at the ischial spines. Transvaginal injection is preferred. A spinal needle with an Iowa trumpet needle guide is used (Fig 26–8), and the procedure can be carried out without assistance.

Identify the ischial spines on each side by digital examination through the elastic vagina. Then note the sacrospinous ligament across the sacrospinous notch above and posterior to the spines.

**2. Lumbar epidural block–**Continuous lumbar epidural block may be a safe method of anesthesia in the delivery of a jeopardized fetus if properly performed by well-trained personnel. It may be selected in maternal complications such as congenital or acquired heart disease, pulmonary disorders, diabetes, preeclampsia-eclampsia, hypertension, and renal or hepatic disease. It may be the best technique for pre-

mature or postmature labor, prolonged labor, or cervical dystocia. The low-dosage technique can be augmented to produce anesthesia for cesarean section delivery.

**3. Caudal block–**Epidural placement of an anesthetic solution in the caudal canal (caudal block), although it involves less risk of dural puncture, requires more medication (with attendant fetal risks), and the procedure blocks a larger nerve distribution, with the hazard of hypotension. The anesthetic may also lead to failure of spontaneous internal rotation.

**4. Spinal block–**Maternal hypotension with decreased uterine blood flow is the greatest risk to the fetus when subarachnoid (spinal) block is used. It is useful only during delivery because it is a "single shot" technique with a duration of action of only 50–70 minutes.

**5. General anesthesia–**General anesthetics may be useful adjuncts in certain high-risk patients. It should be stressed, however, that all general anesthetics cross the placenta and can depress the fetus. General anesthetics may be selected if regional anesthetics are contraindicated, if deep uterine relaxation is necessary, for alleviation of constriction rings, for relief of tetanic uterine contractions, or when prompt deep anesthesia is necessary.

### Multiple Pregnancy

**A. Psychoanalgesia:** The psychoprophylactic technique helps to prepare the patient for the intrapartum experience. When the labor progresses normally, psychoanalgesia can effectively reduce apprehension and enhance the pleasurable aspects. It may also prepare the patient for an understanding of some of the complications of multiple pregnancy (uterine inertia in the first stage of labor, uterine atony in the third stage, and possible need for cesarean section delivery) and reduce the total amount of drugs required for analgesia.

**B. Pudendal Nerve Block:** Pudendal nerve block often is preferred because it allows more spontaneous management during delivery and because the fetus or newborn is not exposed to excess drug (local anesthetic). Many physicians are not aware that regardless of the area of injection of the local anesthetic agent, the drug exposure to the fetus is similar. Nevertheless, it is true that with the exception of local perineal injection or a low caudal (S2–S4), pudendal block does allow for the most spontaneous second-stage management.

**C. Epidural Block:** This technique is useful as a first-stage analgesic method, but only a segmental type should be utilized (T10–L2) to prevent the increased hazard of hypotension secondary to a combined large-segment sympathetic block and vena cava occlusion. Ideal management here entails the use of lumbar epidural block for the first stage and low caudal for the late second stage of labor. Epidural anesthesia does not effect fetal outcome with twin de-

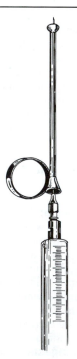

**Figure 26–8.** "Iowa trumpet" needle guide assembled. (Reproduced, with permission, from Benson RC: *Handbook of Obstetrics & Gynecology, 8th ed.* Lange, 1983.)

livery, but has the advantage of enabling the obstetrician to intervene more easily if the second twin presents abnormally. The need for a general anesthetic can be avoided if an epidural is in place and a cesarean section is required urgently for delivery of the second twin.

**D. Spinal Block:** The low subarachnoid block is rarely used during termination of the second stage for crowning, delivery, and episiotomy. A low spinal block does not provide a high enough block for cesarean section, if it is required urgently (eg, in malpresentation or cord prolapse of the second twin). Therefore, an epidural anesthetic is always preferable for the labor and delivery of multiple births.

**E. Inhalation Analgesics:** The only inhalation anesthetic that is analgesic at low concentration is nitrous oxide. Experience is needed to use this drug safely because the pregnant patient is sensitive to its anesthetic effects and can easily become obtunded. Loss of airway reflexes and aspiration are causes of maternal mortality.

General endotracheal anesthesia can be used for cesarean section delivery of twins. Neonatal depression is more likely if the induction-delivery time is long (> 8 minutes), especially if the uterine incision to delivery time is also prolonged (> 3 minutes).

# ANALGESIA FOR ABNORMAL OBSTETRICS

Abnormal obstetrics may include conditions that compromise both the fetus and the mother. Analgesia management in acute and chronic fetal distress and in maternal complications such as preeclampsia-eclampsia, hypertension, heart disease, and diabetes will be discussed. Finally, the analgesic management of obstetric complications such as placenta previa, cord prolapse, abruptio placentae, and breech presentation will be considered.

## Acute Fetal Distress

Acute fetal distress usually occurs intrapartum, without previously suspected fetal compromise. It may be heralded clinically by either the sudden appearance of meconium, the development of bradycardia, or a deceleration pattern detected by fetal monitoring. With continuous heart rate-monitoring equipment, a severe deceleration may be designated as variable or late. In either case, because uterine perfusion presently is correlated with blood pressure, it may be assumed that a maternal pressure fall greater than 20% of the baseline systolic figure will produce a substantial reduction in uterine perfusion. Because this will aggravate any acute intrapartum fetal distress, hypotension should be avoided. Although the incidence and degree of hypotension after sympathetic blockade can be minimized by thorough evaluation, fluid preloading, and patient positioning, it may occur even in the best circumstances. With defi-

nite documentation of severe intrapartum distress, therefore, analgesic techniques should be chosen that are not associated with hypotensive sequelae.

Hypotension is more frequent with spinal anesthesia, and therefore this technique is usually contraindicated when fetal distress exists. A systemic technique may be used, but recall that the systemic administration of narcotics and barbiturates may cause neonatal depression after delivery. The use of a narcotic antagonist such as naloxone (Narcan) may reverse the effect of antepartum narcotics. The anesthetic selection during labor with mild fetal distress is usually either a small dose of intravenous tranquilizer and narcotics or a segmental epidural block. If severe fetal distress requires immediate cesarean delivery, time must not be spent placing a regional block. General endotracheal anesthesia is required in this circumstance to enable the most speedy delivery of the distressed fetus.

## Chronic Fetal Distress

A serious problem in anesthetic management occurs when acute intrapartum distress is superimposed on chronic fetal distress. Underlying chronic distress may be preeclampsia-eclampsia, hypertension, postmaturity, or diabetes. These disorders all reduce fetal reserve. The anesthesiologist must meticulously avoid or manage even mild hypotension, since the primary aim should be maintenance of uterine blood flow. The probable choices are no analgesia, minimal systemic analgesia, or segmental epidural block.

## Maternal Complications

**A. Preeclampsia-Eclampsia:** This syndrome (often called toxemia of pregnancy) is composed of the triad of hypertension, generalized edema, and proteinuria. It accounts for almost 20% of maternal deaths per year in the USA. The primary pathologic characteristic of this disease process is generalized arterial spasm. As gestation lengthens, there is a tendency toward a fluid shift from the vascular to the extravascular compartment with resultant hypovolemia—in spite of an expanded extracellular fluid space. The most significant electrolyte disturbances are those of sodium and chloride. Although both salt and water are retained in the extracellular space, sodium and chloride values in the intravascular compartment are subnormal. This is not reflected by serum electrolyte values because of hypovolemia. Arterial spasm takes its toll via the cardiovascular system.

It is estimated that nearly 50% of eclamptic patients who die have myocardial hemorrhages or areas of focal necrosis. Major disorders of central nervous system function probably are caused by cerebral vasospasm. It is obvious that optimal anesthetic management of these patients during the intrapartum period must include a careful preanesthetic evaluation of the cardiovascular and central nervous systems. If, after searching appraisal, the patient appears to be suffering from a mild form of the disease, one may institute almost any of the aforementioned anesthetic techniques. Nevertheless, the complications of hypotension should be avoided.

The majority of patients with preeclampsia-eclampsia should be medicated with magnesium sulfate so the need for substantial analgesia is reduced. Preference may be given to segmental epidural block with small increments of anesthetic following adequate fluid replacement. Adequate fluid replacement in some of these patients may necessitate the intravenous administration of 1–2 L of lactated Ringer's solution. An alternative method is administration of very small increments of narcotic to produce mild analgesia. Again, use of a narcotic, which will pass the placental barrier and perhaps eventually depress the fetus, is potentially hazardous for these patients, whose infants may be primarily depressed because of the original disease process.

The physiologic changes of severe preeclampsia-eclampsia are exaggerated by regional block due to a restricted intravascular volume, and this may result in considerable depression of blood pressure. A small subgroup of these patients suffer from a reduced cardiac output (compared to normal pregnancy), decreased intravascular fluid space, and marked increases in systemic vascular resistance (SVR). Patients with severe hemodynamic changes may require direct monitoring of pulmonary artery and wedge pressures to manage labor and the effects of epidural anesthesia. Uterine blood flow is increased with epidural block because of the favorable reduction of SVR, as long as central filling pressures and mean arterial pressure are well maintained.

Epidural and spinal block are avoided if coagulopathy exists.

**B. Hemorrhage and Shock:** Intrapartum obstetric emergencies demand immediate diagnosis and therapy for a favorable outcome for the mother and fetus. Placenta previa and abruptio placentae are accompanied by serious maternal hemorrhage. Aggressive obstetric management may be indicated, but superior anesthetic management will play a major role in the reduction of maternal and fetal morbidity and mortality rates. The primary threat to the mother is that of blood loss, which reduces her effective circulating blood volume and her oxygenation potential. Similarly, the chief hazard to the fetus is diminished uteroplacental perfusion secondary to maternal hypovolemia and hypotension. The perinatal mortality rate associated with placenta previa and abruptio placentae ranges from 15–20% in some studies up to 50–100% in others. The overall morbidity and mortality rates for both the fetus and the mother depend on the gestational age and health of the fetus, the extent of the hemorrhage, and the therapy given.

Good anesthetic management demands early consultation. Reliable intravenous lines should be established early. In addition, recommendations for the treatment and control of shock must be formulated. Prompt cesarean section delivery is often indicated. Ketamine can support blood pressure for induction. A modified nitrous oxide-oxygen relaxant method of general anesthesia will provide improved oxygenation for both the mother and the fetus and will have a minimal effect on the maternal blood pressure. As surgery progresses, it may be necessary to administer large volumes of warm blood, intravenous fluids, or even vasopressors when imperative. Vaginal delivery is rarely possible except after fetal death and when maternal risk is minimal. If there has been considerable blood loss, analgesia for such a procedure should not include regional techniques, which may result in substantial maternal sympathetic blockade. This restricts the choices to systemic tranquilizers or sedatives.

**C. Umbilical Cord Prolapse:** Umbilical cord prolapse is an acute obstetric emergency that involves a critical threat to the fetus. Often, because of confusion, irrational behavior by the medical staff may threaten the mother's life. For example, a haphazard rapid induction of anesthesia without attention to many of the essential safety details may be attempted. Naturally, prolapse of the umbilical cord is incompatible with fetal survival unless the fetal presenting part is elevated at once and maintained in that position to avoid compression of the cord. There should then be adequate time for a methodical, safe induction of anesthesia. General anesthesia is induced as soon as the abdomen is prepped and draped. In the rush of the emergency situation, the anesthesiologist must remain meticulous in his assessment and management of the mother's airway. A failed intubation and its consequent cardiorespiratory arrest constitute the leading cause of anesthetic maternal mortality.

**D. Breech Delivery:** Anesthesia for breech delivery may seem to be a simple matter, but hazards to the life of the fetus and mother may develop. It is vital that the anesthesiologist be notified early in labor in order to become familiar with the situation, examine the patient, and prepare equipment for rapid induction when necessary. The anesthetic emergency usually involves rapid induction and intubation of the mother followed by adequate uterine relaxation with halothane. The primary purpose of anesthesia for breech delivery is to allow for a difficult delivery of the aftercoming head. The anesthesiologist who is not consulted until delivery of the breech has occurred cannot be expected to provide immediate safe, adequate uterine relaxation in such a brief period of time.

This problem is compounded by the lack of molding of the head of the fetus, so that the unknown midpelvis may also threaten the safety of delivery. This situation is made worse if an ill-considered attempt is made to relax and dilate the cervix with a uterine relaxant. The lower portion of the cervix is chiefly connective tissue that cannot be relaxed with any anesthetic. Cervical dilatation normally takes 1 hour for each 2 cm of dilatation, and this process cannot be accelerated even by profound myometrial relaxation with a potent inhalation anesthetic. Persistent forceful attempts at dilatation will only produce maternal trauma—possibly rupture of the lower uterine segment, with serious fetal morbidity or even death.

Epidural anesthesia may be used for the labor patient with a breech presentation. The need for breech extraction is not increased by the use of epidural anesthesia, and a functioning epidural may avoid the need for general anesthesia should an emergency arise at delivery.

If an epidural block is not in place at the time of delivery, the anesthesiologist must be prepared to proceed with an immediate endotracheal general anesthesia if the aftercoming fetal head becomes trapped. Drugs, monitors, and anesthetic equipment must be prepared in anticipation of such an event.

Because breech delivery is associated with a high perinatal mortality rate, excellent communication and cooperation between the obstetrician and the anesthesiologist is greatly needed to effect an atraumatic delivery.

**E. Anesthesia for Emergency Cesarean Section:** General anesthesia is the technique most suitable for the urgent cesarean section delivery. It entails placement of an endotracheal tube with an inflated cuff to protect the patient from aspiration of gastric contents into the lung after administration of adequate barbiturate and a muscle relaxant to facilitate endotracheal intubation. Several safety measures must be taken: (1) Give 30 mL of a nonparticulate antacid (sodium citrate) within 15 minutes of induction. (2) Accomplish denitrogenation with 100% oxygen by tight mask fit. (3) Inject thiopental, 2.5 mg/kg intravenously. (4) Apply cricoid pressure. (5) Give succinylcholine, 100–120 mg intravenously. (6) Intubate the trachea and inflate the cuff. (7) Give 6–8 deep breaths of 100% oxygen. (8) Continue to administer nitrous oxide 50% with oxygen 50%, 0.5% halothane, and maintain relaxation with vecuranium or atracurium. (9) Supplement with short-acting narcotics and midazolam after the baby is delivered.

The steps just mentioned should be instituted rapidly and with effective communication between the anesthesiologist and the obstetrician, who should be scrubbed and prepared to make the incision. With this technique, anesthesia can be induced and the fetus delivered within 30 minutes from the time cesarean section is ordered. To avoid vena cava occlusion from the heavy uterus, a wedge should be placed under the patient's right hip or the operating table rotated slightly to the left.

# ANESTHESIA FOR NONOBSTETRIC COMPLICATIONS

Anesthesiologists use the following classification system developed by the American Society of Anes-

thesia. It is used in both emergency and nonemergent situations to record physical status and to ascertain that proper materials are available for the anticipated procedure.

**Class 1.** No organic, physiologic, biochemical, or psychiatric disturbance.

**Class 2.** Mild to moderate systemic disturbance that may or may not be related to the reason for surgery. (Examples: Heart disease that only slightly limits physical activity, essential hypertension, anemia, extremes of age, obesity, chronic bronchitis.)

**Class 3.** Severe systemic disturbance that may or may not be related to the reason for surgery. (Examples: Heart disease that limits activity, poorly controlled hypertension, diabetes mellitus with vascular complications, chronic pulmonary disease that limits activity.)

**Class 4.** Severe systemic disturbance that is life-threatening with or without surgery. (Examples: Congestive heart failure, crescendo angina pectoris, advanced pulmonary, renal, and hepatic dysfunction.)

**Class 5.** Moribund patient who has little chance of survival but is submitted to surgery as a last resort (resuscitative effort). (Examples: Uncontrolled hemorrhage as from a ruptured abdominal aneurysm, cerebral trauma, pulmonary embolus.)

**Emergency operation (E).** Any patient in whom an emergency operation is required. (Example: An otherwise healthy 30-year-old female who requires a dilatation and curettage for moderate but persistent hemorrhage [ASA class 1E].)

## Hypertension

Preexisting hypertensive cardiovascular disease in a pregnant woman should be differentiated from preeclampsia-eclampsia. Unlike the latter, the manifestations of hypertensive disease usually are present before the 24th week of pregnancy and persist after delivery. There is usually a long history of hypertension with superimposed proteinuria and edema. The untreated disease by itself presents a serious challenge to the obstetrician and increases maternal and fetal risk. Chronic hypertension does not specifically contraindicate any of the anesthetic options, but the anesthesiologist must assess and manage abnormalities of volume and vascular resistance to avoid hypotension. Systemic analgesia with sedatives and tranquilizers may be selected for first-stage pain relief, but a hazard still remains. A chronically deprived fetus exposed to a systemic depressant may suffer serious consequences during and after delivery. Second-stage analgesia may be managed using one of the following: true saddle block, sacral caudal block, pudendal nerve block, or inhalation analgesia.

## Heart Disease

Pregnancy superimposed on heart disease presents serious problems in anesthetic management. Patients with functional class I or II rheumatic or congenital heart disease usually fare well throughout pregnancy. Except for patients with fixed cardiac output (moderate to severe aortic stenosis or mitral stenosis), regional analgesia epidural block provides ideal management of first- and second-stage pain relief. This avoids undesirable intrapartum problems such as anxiety, tachycardia, increased cardiac output, and the Valsalva maneuver. The lumbar epidural 4 catheter may be activated for first-stage analgesia with sensory levels of T10 through L2 segments. With the restricted epidural technique, wide variations in blood pressure usually will be avoided and adequate analgesia provided.

An important drug in the treatment of heart disease today is the potent sympathetic blocking drug propranolol. The obstetric anesthesiologist should consider patients taking therapeutic doses of propranolol to be beta-blocked pharmacologically. Both the maternal and fetal cardiovascular systems may be poorly responsive to sympathetic discharges mediating beta$_1$ compensatory reactions to stress. As a result, positive chronotropic and inotropic responses may be sluggish. Additionally, the uterine beta$_2$-adrenergic receptors may also be blocked, rendering the uterus more responsive to exogenous oxytocin. Finally, since propranolol may also antagonize uteroplacental renin and since uteroplacental renin may be vital to regulation of uterine blood flow (ie, increasing flow), one must be cautious about the delicate balance of fetal blood flow in such patients. In one reported incident, fetal distress was perhaps precipitated by such an interaction of propranolol and oxytocin.

Patients with valvular heart disease need to be thoroughly assessed prior to the onset of labor so that the anesthesiologist can determine the risks of regional block, tolerance to volume loading, and sympathectomy and determine the need for invasive monitoring. These patients need thorough physical examination, ECG, echocardiography, and Doppler assessment of valve areas and left ventricular function.

Patients with stenotic lesions may not tolerate fluid loading nor sympathetic block. Epidural narcotic anesthesia does not provide complete analgesia for labor but may be an appropriate choice if the patient does not tolerate the autonomic effects of local anesthetics. Patients with regurgitant valve lesions generally do well with this afterload reduction of epidural local anesthesia. Central monitoring of preload is indicated with severe lesions.

Marfan's syndrome and ischemia heart disease require early and aggressive management of labor pain to avoid hypertension and tachycardia. Early lumbar epidural anesthesia with narcotic/local anesthetic mixtures is recommended.

## Diabetes Mellitus

Diabetes presents unique problems in anesthetic management because of the hazard to the fetus. The patient with diabetes requires a detailed regimen of antepartum care that extends through the intrapartum and the neonatal period. Moreover, hypotension presents an anesthetic hazard in situations of reduced fetal reserve common to diabetes. The latent phase of labor is best managed with psychologic support, mild sedatives, or tranquilizers. The latter part of the first stage may be managed with small intravenous doses of narcotics or epidural block. If labor continues without signs of fetal distress and analgesia for the second stage is desired, either local or pudendal block, epidural or saddle block is appropriate. If a patient is allowed to undergo the stress of labor but fetal decompensation is evident, operative delivery must be performed at once, with emphasis on the avoidance of hypotension. Careful regional block can be used if time permits. If time does not permit placement of a regional block, emergency general endotracheal anesthesia is indicated. Blood glucose levels should be measured intraoperatively because the unconscious patient cannot report hypoglycemia.

## Gastrointestinal Difficulties

Gastrointestinal nonstriated muscle has diminished tone and motility during pregnancy. Some medical gastrointestinal difficulties present special problems in management during the intrapartum period. **Peptic ulcer** often improves during pregnancy, but in some cases the disease worsens in the last trimester and causes serious problems during labor and the immediate postpartum period. Ulcer perforation and hematemesis are rare in labor. Nonetheless, good management of analgesia during delivery is necessary to decrease anxiety and apprehension.

**Ulcerative colitis** may become worse during pregnancy. Perinatal and maternal mortality rates are not increased, because symptomatic management usually is adequate. **Regional ileitis** may also become more severe during pregnancy.

**Chronic pancreatitis** may be reactivated during pregnancy. **Acute pancreatitis** occasionally occurs in the third trimester. The significant laboratory values are elevated serum amylase and reduced serum calcium, along with typical symptoms of epigastric pain and nausea and vomiting.

Sympathetic blocking techniques are not contraindicated for anesthetic management of the first and second stages of labor in these gastrointestinal disorders that may coincide with pregnancy. It is clinically desirable to alleviate anxiety and apprehension in the first stage of labor, since tension may exacerbate the disease process. Therefore, a tranquilizer/narcotic combination early in the first stage of labor should be considered and then lumbar epidural block for first- and second-stage management. Subarachnoid block may be used to manage the second stage of labor successfully, with use of a true saddle block obtunding chiefly the sacral fibers.

## Psychiatric Disorders

Most patients approaching delivery look upon the experience as one of the happiest times of their lives. However, some patients undergo severe emotional stresses during the third trimester and as delivery nears.

The obstetrician and the anesthesiologist should talk openly with a psychiatric patient about problems of labor and delivery management and offer suggestions for management of discomfort so that she will have minimal emotional stress. The ideal technique is the combined use of lumbar epidural block for the first stage and lumbar or caudal epidural block for the second stage. It is best to carefully point out to the patient the reasons for choosing the technique and to review the technical points of the procedure so that she will not be alarmed when the block is attempted. These techniques are preferred because they afford early and continuous analgesia during labor and delivery.

## TREATMENT OF COMPLICATIONS OF ANESTHETICS

### Resuscitation of the Mother

Anesthesia is responsible for 10% of maternal mortality. The most common cause of maternal death is failure to intubate the trachea at induction of general anesthesia. Less frequently, maternal death is due to inadvertent intravascular injection of local anesthetic (toxic reaction) or inadvertent intrathecal injection of anesthetic (total spinal).

When faced with maternal cardiovascular collapse, full cardiopulmonary resuscitation (CPR) is indicated:

1. Establish a patent airway.
2. Aspirate mucus, blood, vomitus, etc, with a tracheal suction apparatus. Use a laryngoscope for direct visualization of air passages and intubate the trachea.
3. Administer oxygen by artificial respiration if respirations are absent or weak. If high spinal anesthesia has occurred, continue to ventilate the patient until paralysis of the diaphragm has dissipated.
4. Give vasopressors intravenously (ephedrine, 10–20 mg). Place the patient in the wedged supine position with the feet elevated and give transfusions of plasma, plasma expanders, and blood for traumatic or hemorrhagic shock.
5. Specifically treat cardiac arrhythmias, as per Advanced Cardiac Life Support (ACLS) recommendations.
6. Provide external cardiac massage in the absence of adequate rhythm and blood pressure.
7. Consider immediate cesarean section delivery to salvage fetus and improve venous return, if patient does not immediately respond to efforts.

Full cardiopulmonary arrest can be averted if the prodromal symptoms are recognized and immediately treated. A total spinal block is recognized by excessive and dense sensory and motor block to a test injection of local anesthesia through the epidural catheter. Further injections are avoided, and the patient's blood pressure is supported with fluid, positioning, and vasopressors.

An intravascular injection of local anesthetic is recognized early by symptoms of drowsiness, agitation, tinnitus, perioral tingling, bradycardia, and mild hypotension. The patient should be immediately given 100% oxygen and a small dose of valium (5 mg), midazolam (1 mg) or pentothal (50 mg). Further treatment may not be needed. The patient must be watched closely and the epidural catheter removed.

## ANESTHESIA FOR CESAREAN SECTION DELIVERY

With few exceptions, all cesarean section deliveries in the USA are performed with spinal, epidural, or general anesthesia. When these techniques are done effectively, maternal and neonatal outcome is good.

### Regional Analgesia

**A. Lumbar Epidural Block:** Lumbar epidural blockade may be utilized for cesarean section analgesia and for providing adequate analgesia for operative delivery. As mentioned, the major hazard of the regional analgesic technique is blockade of sympathetic fibers and a decrease in vascular resistance, venous pooling, and hypotension. However, this can be greatly alleviated by elevation of the patient's right hip to avoid compression of the vena cava by the gravid uterus when the patient is lying on the operating table. In addition, the anesthesiologist may rotate the operating table 15–20 degrees to the left to rotate the uterus away from the vena cava.

An epidural catheter can be placed immediately prior to surgery, or a catheter used to provide pain relief for labor can be reinjected for the surgery. After the catheter is suitably placed and taped in position, the patient should be rotated slightly out of the supine position to remove the hazard of vena cava occlusion when local anesthetic is injected as a test dose. Lidocaine 2% with epinephrine 1:200,000 may be used, or lidocaine 2% without epinephrine if there is cardiovascular instability. Bupivacaine 0.5–0.75% or mepivacaine 1.5% with or without epinephrine, as described for lidocaine, may also be used. The total dosage for the therapeutic test is approximately 3 mL, which is an adequate amount to ascertain whether or not inadvertent subarachnoid injection of the drug has occurred. Incremental injections of 5 mL are then titrated to produce a T4–T6 sensory level. Usually a total volume of 18–20 mL of local anesthetic is required.

The blood pressure is monitored every 5 minutes

and the dermatome levels examined every 5 minutes for the first 20 minutes to ascertain the height and density of the analgesic block. It is usually necessary to wait only 15–20 minutes for an adequate analgesic block for incision. During this time, the patient's abdomen is surgically scrubbed and prepared and the patient draped for cesarean section delivery. If a brief episode of hypotension occurs, the patient is given a rapid infusion of lactated Ringer's solution. In addition, the uterus must be shifted away from the vena cava. If these measures are not sufficient to relieve a brief episode of hypotension, one may utilize 5–10 mg of ephedrine intravenously for a mild vasopressor effect.

**B. Subarachnoid Block:** The subarachnoid block technique provides a regional analgesic method that has certain advantages and disadvantages compared with the lumbar epidural method. The advantages are the immediate onset of analgesia, so that there is no waiting for the block to become effective, and the absence of drug transmission from the maternal to the fetal compartment, because the anesthetic is deposited in the subarachnoid space in such small quantities. In addition, subarachnoid block may be a simpler technique to perform, since the end point is definite—the identification of fluid from the subarachnoid space. The disadvantages are a more profound and rapid onset of hypotension and more frequent nausea and vomiting, due either to unopposed parasympathetic stimulation of the gastrointestinal tract or to hypotension. Subarachnoid block is usually achieved via the paramedian or midline technique, which cannot be detailed here. The agents most commonly used for subarachnoid analgesia include tetracaine 1% (usually 6–8 mg), lidocaine 5% (50–75 mg), or bupivacaine (10–12.5%). As with the lumbar epidural technique, the patient is prehydrated with 500–1000 mL of lactated Ringer's solution.

After the technical aspects of the procedure have been completed, the patient is placed in the supine position with the uterus displaced to the left as just described. If hypotension occurs, the uterus should be pushed farther to the left to improve return of blood from the lower extremities into the circulation and increase right atrial pressure and, therefore, cardiac output, and a bolus of Ringer's lactate is given. If these measures are not successful, the patient should receive ephedrine, 5–10 mg intravenously, to sustain a mild vasopressor effect. During a period of hypotension, the mother should receive oxygen by mask to increase oxygen delivery to the uteroplacental bed. Newer spinal needles are associated with a low incidence (1–2%) of spinal headache (PDPH). As a result, spinal anesthesia is becoming more popular for elective cesarean surgery.

## General & Local Anesthesia

General anesthesia is indicated for cesarean section delivery when regional techniques cannot be used because of coagulopathy, infection, hypovolemia, or urgency. Some patients prefer to be "put to sleep" and refuse regional techniques.

Ideally, general anesthesia for cesarean section delivery should cause the mother to be unconscious, feel no pain, and have no unpleasant memories of the procedure, while the fetus should not be jeopardized, with minimal depression and intact reflex irritability.

General anesthesia for cesarean section delivery is substantially modified from the typical nonobstetric technique. A rapid sequence technique is used with cricoid pressure to prevent aspiration, with recognition that the risks for the term obstetric patient include (1) full stomach (and aspiration), (2) difficulty with laryngoscopy and intubation, (3) rapid desaturation if intubation is unsuccessful.

**A. Patient Preparation:** Preoperative medication is not usually required when the patient is brought to the cesarean section room. Alert the patient preoperatively that she may have a lucid "window" during the operative procedure when she has pain or hears voices. Explain that this is due to the necessity of maintaining a light analgesic state to protect the fetus from large doses of drugs. She should also be prepared with 30 mL of nonparticulate antacid to offset gastric acidity. The patient is then given 100% oxygen with a close-fitting mask for 3 minutes prior to induction.

**B. Procedure:** As the surgeon is ready to make the incision, thiopental, 2.5 mg/kg, should be injected intravenously and cricoid pressure exerted by an assistant. Immediately, succinylcholine, 120–140 mg intravenously, should be administered, and intubation and inflation of the cuff performed. Intubation is confirmed by auscultation and monitoring end-tidal $CO_2$ before the cricoid pressure is released and the incision made. After 6–8 breaths of 100% oxygen, the patient should be given nitrous oxide 50% with oxygen 50% until delivery of the fetus. Low concentrations of halothane (0.5%) will reduce the incidence of awareness. Intermediate-acting muscle relaxants maintain paralysis. An attempt must be made to keep the induction-to-delivery time under 10 minutes. Five minutes are required for redistribution of barbiturate back across the placenta into the maternal compartment. After delivery of the fetus, the nitrous oxide concentration may be increased to 70% if oxygen saturation is more than 8%, and intravenous narcotics and benzodiazepines injected intravenously for supplemental anesthesia.

The patient should be fully awakened and on her side before extubation. Postoperative analgesia can be provided by patient-controlled (PCA) administration of morphine or meperidine.

With this approach, good neonatal outcomes are anticipated if induction-delivery times and uterine invasion to delivery times are kept to a minimum.

# REFERENCES

Bacigalupo G, Riese S, Rosendahl H, Saling E: Quantitative relationships between pain intensities during labor and beta-endorphin and cortisol concentrations in plasma. Decline of the hormone concentrations in the early postpartum period. J Perinat Med 1990;18:289.

Berg TG, Rayburn WF: Effects of analgesia on labor. Clin Obstet Gynecol 1992;35:457.

Bonica JJ: Labour pain. In: *Textbook of Pain,* 2nd ed. Wall PD, Melzack R (editors). Churchill Livingstone, 1989.

Bonica JJ: *Principles and Practice of Obstetric Analgesia and Anesthesia.* FA Davis, 1994.

Brown WU Jr et al: Newborn blood levels of lidocaine and mepivacaine in the first postnatal day following maternal epidural anesthesia. Anesthesiology 1975;42:698.

Browning AJF et al: Maternal and cord plasma concentrations of β-lipotrophin, β-endorphin and Y-lipotrophin at delivery; Effect of analgesia. Br J Obstet Gynaecol 1983;90:1152.

Buchan PC: Emotional stress in childbirth and its modifications by variations in obstetric management. Epidural analgesia and stress in labor. Acta Obstet Gynecol Scand 1980;59(4):319.

Chan EC, Smith R, Lewin T et al: Plasma corticotropin-releasing hormone, beta-endorphin and cortisol interrelationships during human pregnancy. Acta Endocrinol 1993;128:339.

Cheetham RW, Rzadkowolski A: Psychiatric aspects of labour and the puerperium. S Afr Med J 1980;58(20):814.

Clark SL, Cotton DB: Clinical indications for pulmonary artery catheterization in the patient with severe preeclampsia. Am J Obstet Gynecol 1988;158:453.

Cohen SE et al: Epidural fentanyl/bupivacaine mixtures for obstetric analgesia. Anesthesiology 1987;67:403.

Confino E: Extradural analgesia in the management of singleton breech delivery. Br J Anaesth 1985;57:892.

Crawford JS: *Principles and Practices of Obstetric Anaesthesia,* 5th ed. Blackwell Scientific Publications, 1984.

Datta S et al: Neonatal effect of prolonged anesthetic induction for cesarean section. Obstet Gynecol 1981;58:331.

Delke I, Minkoff H, Grunebaum A: Effect of Lamaze childbirth preparation on maternal plasma beta-endorphin immunoreactivity in active labor. Am J Perinatol 1985;2(4):317.

Detrick JM, Pearson JW, Frederickson RCA: Endorphins and parturition. Obstet Gynecol 1985;65:647.

Edward ND, Hartley M, Clyburn P, Harmer M: Epidural pethidine and bupivacaine in labour. Anaesthesia 1992;47:435.

Facchinetti F et al: Fetomaternal opioid levels and parturition. Obstet Gynecol 1983;62:764.

Frahm R, Mundt A: Labor pain from the viewpoint of the modern knowledge of pain physiology. Zentralbl Gynakol 1986;108:203.

Goebelsmann U et al: Beta-endorphin in pregnancy. Eur J Obstet Gynecol Reprod Biol 1984;17:77.

Hoffman DI et al: Plasma β-endorphin concentrations prior to and during pregnancy, in labor, and after delivery. Am J Obstet Gynecol 1984;150(5):492.

Jevremovic M, Terzic M, Kartaljevic G et al: The opioid peptide, beta-endorphin, in spontaneous vaginal delivery and cesarean section. Srp Arh Celok Lek 1991;119:271.

Kanto J: Pharmacokinetics and sedative effect of midazolam in connection with cesarean section performed under epidural anesthesia. Acta Anaesthesiol Scand 1984;28:116.

Ketscher KD, Kindt J, Retzke U: Effect of modified obstetrical neuroleptanalgesia on the duration of labor and uterine contractions. Zentralbl Gynakol 1986;108:1251.

Khan GQ, Lilford RJ: Wound pain may be reduced by prior infiltration of the episiotomy site after delivery under epidural analgesia. Br J Obstet Gynaecol 1987;94:341.

Koehntop DE et al: Pharmacokinetics for fentanyl in neonates. Anesth Analg 1986;65:227.

Kofinas GD, Kofinas AD, Tavakoli FM: Maternal and fetal β-endorphin release in response to the stress of labor and delivery. Am J Obstet Gynecol 1985;152:56.

Lieberman BA: The effects of maternally administered pethidine or epidural bupivacaine on the fetus and newborn. Br J Obstet Gynaecol 1979;86:598.

Lynch C et al: Anesthetic management and monitoring of a parturient with mitral and aortic valvular disease. Anesth Analg 1982;61:788.

McDonald JS: Preanesthetic and intrapartal medications. Clin Obstet Gynecol 1977;20:447.

Melzack R et al: Severity of labour pain: Influence of physical as well as psychologic variables. Can Med Assoc J 1984;130:579.

Mitrani A et al: Use of propranolol in dysfunctional labour. Br J Obstet Gynaecol 1975;82:651.

Moore DC, Batra MS: The components of an effective test dose prior to epidural block. Anesthesiology 1981;55:693.

Neumark J, Hammerle AF, Biegelmayer C: Effects of epidural analgesia on plasma catecholamines and cortisol in parturition. Acta Anaesthesiol Scand 1985;29:555.

Ohno H et al: Maternal plasma concentrations of catecholamines and cyclic nucleotides during labor and following delivery. Res Commun Chem Pathol Pharmacol 1986;51(2):183.

O'Sullivan GM et al: Noninvasive measurement of gastric emptying in obstetric patients. Anesth Analg 1987;66: 505.

Pohjavuori M et al: Stress of delivery and plasma endorphins and catecholamines in the newborn infant. Biol Res Pregnancy Perinatol 1986;7:1.

Rauaisauanen I et al: β-Endorphin in maternal and umbilical cord plasma at elective cesarean section and in spontaneous labor. Obstet Gynecol 1986;67(3):384.

Ramler D, Roberts J: A comparison of cold and warm sitz baths for relief of postpartum perineal pain. J Obstet Gynecol Neonatal Nurs 1986;15:471.

Rees GAD et al: Diabetes, pregnancy and anesthesia. Clin Obstet Gynecol 1982;9:311.

Rochat RW et al: Maternal mortality in the United States: Report from the Maternal Mortality Collaborative. Obstet Gynecol 1988;72:91.

Rosaeg OP, Yarnell RW: The Obstetrical Anesthesia Assessment Clinic: A review of six years experience. Can J Anesth 1003;40:346.

Ross BK et al: Sprotte needle for obstetric anesthesia: Decreased incidence of post dural puncture headache. Reg Anesth 1992;17:29.

Savona-Ventura C, Sammut M, Sammut C: Pethidine blood concentrations at time of birth. Int J Gynaecol Obstet 1991;36:103.

Shnider SM et al: Maternal catecholamines decrease during labor after lumbar epidural anesthesia. Am J Obstet Gynecol 1983;147:13.

Slavazza KL et al: Anesthesia and analgesia for vaginal childbirth: Differences in maternal perceptions. J Obstet Gynecol Neonatal Nurs 1985;14:321.

Swartz J et al: The effects of general anaesthesia on the asphyxiated foetal lamb in utero. Can Anaesth Soc J 1985;32:577.

Thacker SB, Banta HD: Benefits and risks of episiotomy: An interpretative review of the English language literature, 1860–1980. Obstet Gynecol Surv 1983;38(6):322.

Vella LM et al: Epidural fentanyl in labour: An evaluation of the systemic contribution. Anaesthesia 1985;40:741.

Weissberg N, Schwartz G, Shemesh O et al: Serum and mononuclear cell potassium, magnesium, sodium and calcium in pregnancy and labor and their relation to uterine muscle contraction. Manges Res 1992;5:173.

Williamson P, English EC: Stress and coping in first pregnancy: couple-family physicians interaction. J Fam Pract 1981;13(5):629.

Westgren M, Lindahl SGE, Norden NE: Maternal and fetal endocrine stress response at vaginal delivery with and without an epidural block. J Perinat Med 1986;14:235.

Worthington EL Jr: Labor room and laboratory: Clinical validation of the cold pressor as a means of testing preparation for childbirth strategies. J Psychosom Res 1982;26:223.

Yarnell RW et al: Sacralization of epidural block with repeated doses of 0.25% bupivacaine during labor. Reg Anesth 1990;15:275.

# Operative Delivery

# 27

*Ralph W. Hale, MD*

The term "operative delivery" denotes any obstetric procedure in which active measures are taken to accomplish delivery. The procedures, which should be used only upon clear indications, are often major ones whose success depends not only on the skill with which they are used but also on the proper timing of their use.

In former years the ability to perform a difficult vaginal delivery was an essential part of obstetric practice. In current practice one mark of a skilled obstetrician is the ability to avoid difficult vaginal delivery. However, the obstetrician should have sufficient knowledge and experience to be able to intervene vaginally when indicated and to perform the obstetric operation that is safest for mother and baby. This chapter considers the obstetric operations in modern use that should be within the competence of each obstetrician.

## FORCEPS OPERATIONS

The obstetric forceps is an instrument designed to assist the delivery of the baby's head. It is used either to expedite delivery or to overcome or correct certain abnormalities in the cephalopelvic relationship that interfere with advancement of the head in labor.

The primary functions of the forceps are traction (either for assistance in the terminal phase of labor or to deal with arrest of the head) and rotation (in cases in which there is no disproportion but the head presents with an unfavorable diameter).

Forceps delivery may be indicated in the interests of mother or baby, and when properly performed it may be lifesaving.

### THE OBSTETRIC FORCEPS

The obstetric forceps consists of 2 matched parts that articulate, or "lock." Each part is composed of a blade, shank, lock, and handle (Fig 27–1). Each blade is so designed that it possesses 2 curves: the cephalic curve, which permits the instrument to be applied accurately to the sides of the baby's head; and the pelvic curve, which conforms to the curved axis of the maternal pelvis. The tip of each blade is called the toe.

The front of the forceps is the concave side of the pelvic curve. The blades are referred to as left and right according to the side of the mother's pelvis on which they lie after application. According to the rule of the forceps, the handle of the left blade is held in the left hand and the blade is applied to the left side of the mother's pelvis; the handle of the right blade is then held in the right hand and inserted so as to lie on the right side of the mother's pelvis. When the blades are inserted in this order, the right shank comes to lie atop the left so that the forceps articulate, or lock, as the handles are closed.

Physicians have been making modifications in one or more of the 4 basic parts since forceps were first invented. Although more than 600 kinds of forceps have been described, only a few are currently in use.

Obstetric forceps may be divided into 2 groups: classic forceps and special forceps (Fig 27–2). Classic forceps are those with the usual cephalic and pelvic curves and English lock; the Simpson and Elliot forceps are the prototypes. Special forceps are those designed to solve specific problems; those in modern use are the Piper, Kielland, and Barton forceps.

## INDICATIONS & CONDITIONS FOR FORCEPS DELIVERY

In each of the following indications for forceps delivery, it should be emphasized that cesarean section is an alternative procedure that may or may not be appropriate under the prevailing circumstances. Recognizing the inherent risks of both procedures, the obstetrician must decide which operation—vaginal delivery or cesarean section—will be safer for mother and baby. In modern obstetrics there is rarely a place for the difficult forceps delivery that endangers either mother or child. Likewise the obstetrician's training

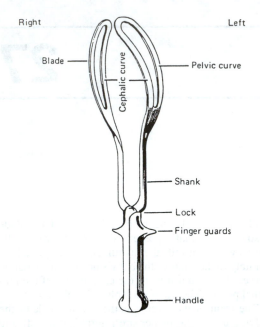

**Figure 27–1.** DeLee modification of Simpson forceps. Reproduced, with permission, from Benson RC: *Handbook of Obstetrics & Gynecology*, 8th ed. Lange, 1983.)

and experience must be a prime consideration in deciding between a forceps delivery and a cesarean section.

### Prophylaxis

The principle of prophylactic forceps was first enunciated by DeLee in 1920. Although it instantly provoked bitter denunciation as "meddlesome midwifery," it was generally accepted that when the perineum and coccyx offered the only resistance to delivery, the use of episiotomy and outlet forceps was indeed prophylactic because the fetal head was spared unpredictable stress—especially compression against the perineum. Rationale for this acceptance included the belief that the second stage of labor was significantly shortened, greatly minimizing the patient's physical discomfort whereas the repair of a cleanly incised wound rather than of a jagged, laceration facilitated healing and recovery of the pelvic floor and perineal structures. Episiotomy is still the most frequently performed obstetric operation although it is becoming far less common than in the past and current trends are to use it even less. Prophylactic forceps has no place in modern routine obstetrics. Any use of a forceps must be predicated on an existing condition for which a forceps is indicated.

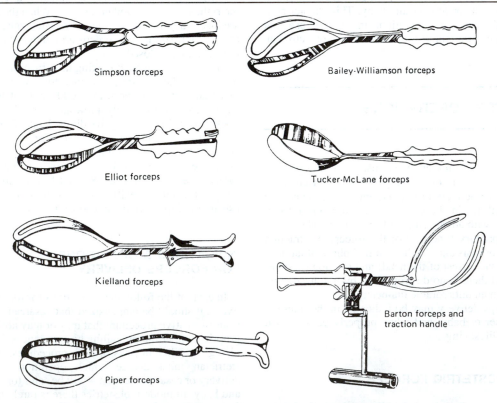

**Figure 27–2.** Commonly used forceps. (Reproduced, with permission, from Benson RC: *Handbook of Obstetrics & Gynecology*, 8th ed. Lange, 1983.)

## Dystocia

During the second stage, when labor fails to progress or a second stage exceeding 2 hours occurs the use of forceps should be considered. However, good judgment is necessary to decide whether continued labor, forceps delivery, or cesarean section is indicated.

**A. Uterine Inertia:** Uterine inertia may account for both failure to progress and prolongation of the second stage of labor. In such cases, oxytocin should be considered initially if disproportion has been excluded. If the conditions for forceps delivery have not been met, cesarean section may be appropriate. Uterine inertia may also be responsible for failure of the head to rotate to the anterior position. In such cases, artificial rotation is usually not difficult, but the obstetrician must decide whether cesarean section would be safer. A critical factor is the station of the fetal head when forceps are considered. No rotations should be used at a station above the bispinous level or 0.

**B. Faulty Cephalopelvic Relationships:** Despite contractions of good quality, arrest may occur in the following circumstances: (1) if an unfavorable diameter of the head presents to the pelvis (eg, occiput anterior [OA] in a flat pelvis); (2) if the position is such that the head cannot negotiate the pelvic curve (eg, certain cases of occiput posterior [OP]); or (3) if cephalopelvic disproportion exists. In the latter case, molding of the head may overcome minor degrees of disproportion and permit the head to advance without injury. After 1–2 hours of voluntary bearing down in the second stage, the physician must determine whether vaginal delivery by forceps is safe and appropriate or whether true disproportion requiring cesarean section for delivery is present.

## Maternal & Fetal Indications for Forceps Delivery

Maternal and fetal indications for forceps delivery include circumstances in which continuation of the second stage of labor would constitute a significant threat to the mother or the baby or those circumstances in which the mother can no longer satisfactorily assist in delivering the infant as with regional anesthesia. Forceps delivery in such cases should impose no additional risk on either or cesarean section is preferable.

**A. Maternal Indications:** The second stage can be shortened in cases of exhaustion, severe cardiac or pulmonary problems accompanied by dyspnea, and intercurrent debilitating illness.

**B. Fetal Indications:** The primary fetal indication for terminating the second stage prematurely is fetal distress, as manifested by fetal heart tones (FHTs) with a rate of less than 100 or more than 160 beats/min, late deceleration patterns, or gross irregularity. In many of these cases, unless delivery is imminent cesarean section is preferable to forceps delivery.

## Conditions for Forceps Delivery

The use of forceps is permissible only when all of the following conditions prevail, regardless of the urgent need for delivery.

(1) **The cervix must be fully dilated.** Extraction of the head through an incompletely dilated cervix invariably produces ragged, bleeding tears that may extend into the broad ligament of the uterus. The uterine support may be damaged also, thus setting the stage for later prolapse.

(2) **The membranes must be ruptured.** Forceps should not be applied before the membranes rupture. If the membranes are intact and forceps are used, they will slip, and traction upon the membranes may detach the edge of the placenta.

(3) **The head must be engaged to a station below + 2.** Engagement means that the biparietal diameter of the fetal head has passed the plane of the inlet. If the head is not molded, the tip of the vertex, at the time of engagement, is at 0 station; in extreme molding with a large caput succedaneum, the scalp may be almost at the introitus when the biparietal diameter is still at the level of the inlet. The higher the station of the head, the greater the likelihood of serious damage to mother or baby. One should not apply forceps if the sinciput can be felt above the symphysis.

(4) **The head must present correctly.** All vertex presentations and all face presentations with chin anterior are suitable. Neither brow presentation nor face presentation with chin posterior is suitable for application of forceps. One may apply forceps to the aftercoming head in breech presentation, provided the head is engaged and is in the OA position.

(5) **There must be no significant cephalopelvic disproportion.** In the case of a "tight fit," one may advance the head, provided that only moderate traction is needed; it is potentially severely damaging to use extreme force to drag the head past significant bony resistance.

(6) **The bladder should be empty.** The bladder should be drained by catheterization before forceps are used. It must be emphasized that merely meeting the foregoing conditions does not justify forceps delivery. A specific indication for the application of forceps must be present, and the timing of the procedure is of vital importance. Countless obstetric disasters have resulted from the inappropriate or too early use of forceps and from the use of forceps when another mode of delivery would have been preferable.

## CLASSIFICATION & DEFINITIONS OF FORCEPS DELIVERIES

Until 1949, low forceps was defined as "forceps extraction when the head rests upon the perineum, or lies well below the line joining the ischial spines." This definition was very misleading because it included some formidable extractions from the midpelvis. In 1949, the authors of 4 major obstetric textbooks (N.J. Eastman, J.P. Greenhill, C.O. McCormick, and Paul Titus) agreed to state in their books the following definition of low forceps: "Low forceps is the application of forceps when the head is visible, the skull is on the pelvic floor, and the sagittal suture is in the anteroposterior diameter of the pelvis."

The classification of forceps deliveries currently approved by The American College of Obstetricians and Gynecologists was adopted in 1988 and uses the leading bony part of the fetal skull and its relationship to the maternal ischial spines in centimeters as the point of reference. Part of this definition is as follows:

(1) **"Outlet forceps** is the application of forceps when a) the scalp is visible at the introitus without separating the labia, b) the fetal skull has reached the pelvic floor, c) the sagittal suture is in the anteriorposterior diameter or in the right or left occiput anterior or posterior position, and d) the fetal head is at or on the perineum." According to this definition, rotation cannot exceed 45 degrees. There is no difference in perinatal outcome when deliveries involving the use of outlet forceps are compared with similar spontaneous deliveries, and there are no data to support the concept that rotating the head on the pelvic floor 45 degrees or less increases morbidity. Forceps delivery under these conditions may be desirable to shorten the second stage of labor—when indicated.

(2) **"Low forceps** is the application of forceps when the leading point of the skull is at a station + 2 cm or more and not on the pelvic floor. Low forceps have 2 subdivisions: a) rotation 45 degrees or less (eg, left occipitoanterior to occiput anterior, left occipitoposterior to occiput posterior), and b) rotation more than 45 degrees."

(3) **"Midforceps** is the application of forceps when the head is engaged but the leading point of the skull is above station + 2 cm. Under unusual circumstances, such as the sudden onset of severe fetal or maternal compromise, application of forceps above station + 2 may be attempted while simultaneously initiating preparations for a cesarean delivery in the event that the forceps maneuver is unsuccessful. Under no circumstances, however, should forceps be applied to an unengaged presenting part or when the cervix is not completely dilated."

(4) **High forceps** is the application of forceps at any time prior to the engagement of the fetal head. This procedure is inappropriate in modern obstetrics and has been replaced by the use of cesarean section.

The foregoing definitions refer only to the station of the head at the time the operation is begun. Two additional definitions apply to special circumstances.

(5) **Failed forceps** denotes an unsuccessful attempt at forceps delivery and abandonment of this effort in favor of cesarean section.

(6) **Trial forceps** is a tentative, cautious traction with forceps with the intent of abandoning attempts at delivery if undue resistance is encountered. Since there is also the intent to deliver with forceps if feasible, the term "trial forceps" is appropriate.

## CHOICE & APPLICATION OF FORCEPS

The results of forceps delivery depend far more on the judgment and skill of the operator than on the selection of any particular instrument. Certain instruments clearly are preferable to others for particular problems, however, and it is important to know exactly what is to be accomplished and which instrument is safest and most effective for the specific difficulty encountered. Some of the forceps used most frequently are shown in Figure 27–2. It is important for obstetricians in training to become familiar with all the standard instruments and to select the ones that will form the basis of their armamentarium. The obstetrician should generally settle on one instrument for outlet forceps; one instrument for traction in the OA position; one instrument for traction and rotation in the occiput transverse (OT) position; and one instrument for application to the aftercoming head.

(1) **For outlet forceps,** in which no significant traction is needed, and there is minimal molding of the fetal head, the Tucker-McLane instrument is preferable. The Tucker-McLane forceps has the advantage of overlapping shanks, which do not spread and extend the perineum as the head is brought through the introitus. The disadvantage is that the blades may not fit the head well, especially if there is extensive molding. If any significant traction is exerted, the fetal cheeks may be marked or cut over the zygoma. Tucker-McLane forceps are most applicable for infants without significant molding (rapid primigravid or multigravid deliveries).

(2) **For traction in the OA** (or in one of the oblique anterior positions or with a fetus with marked molding of the head), the Simpson forceps or one of its modifications (DeLee-Simpson, DeWeiss, or Elliot) is often used. If applied correctly and if traction is made in the proper diameter of the pelvis, considerable force may usually be applied without fetal injury. Moreover, the Simpson and DeLee-Simpson instruments generally cannot be locked or articulated properly except when they are applied accurately— unlike the Tucker-McLane forceps, which usually can be locked regardless of the accuracy of their application.

(3) **For rotation from the OP to the OA,** many obstetricians prefer either the Tucker-McLane or the Luikart forceps. The Kielland forceps is also applicable for rotation from posterior to anterior.

(4) **For transverse arrest,** either the Barton or the Kielland forceps is applicable.

(5) **For application to the aftercoming head,** American obstetricians prefer the Piper forceps. The long-shanked classic forceps is also applicable.

Two methods of application are available:

(1) **Cephalic application** denotes the deliberate and accurate application of the forceps to the sides of the baby's head parallel to a line from the chin to a point between the anterior and posterior fontanelles. The blades should be somewhat closer to the posterior than the anterior. Cephalic application is possible in OA, OT, OP, face presentation with chin anterior, and for the aftercoming head (Fig 27–3).

(2) **Pelvic application** is made by applying the blades and locking the forceps, by force if necessary, without reference to the position of the head. This application is condemned in modern obstetrics because it imposes dangerous (even lethal) stresses that the fetal head can rarely withstand. If a proper cephalic application cannot be made, some other method of management is mandatory.

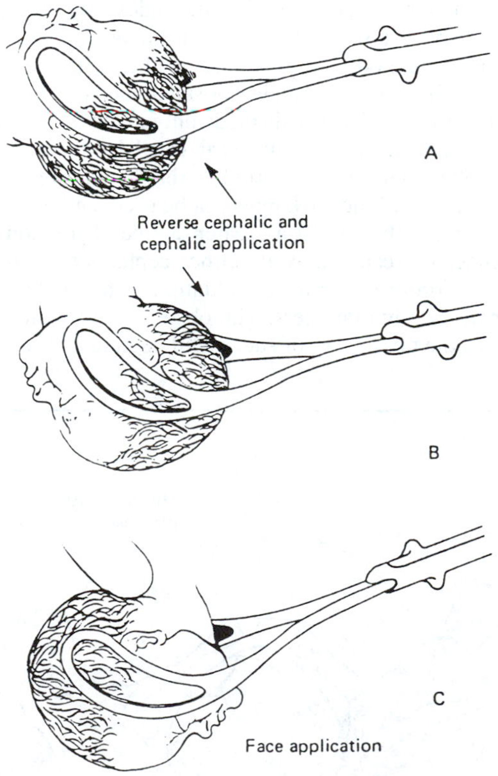

## PREPARATION OF THE PATIENT FOR FORCEPS DELIVERY

The lithotomy position is required, and the patient's buttocks should extend 5 cm beyond the end of the table. The legs should be comfortably placed in stirrups with the hips flexed and abducted. A low position is usually preferable to prevent excessive stretching of the perineum.

If conduction anesthesia is to be used, it must be administered prior to the foregoing steps in delivery. If pudendal block or local infiltration is to be used, it should be administered after the preliminary examination has been made and all is in readiness for delivery. An appropriate and effective anesthetic is essential to the performance of any forceps delivery.

### The Preliminary Examination

Before application of the forceps, a careful examination must be made to determine the following:

(1) **The position of the fetal head,** which is usually easily determined by first locating the lambdoid sutures and then determining the direction of the sagittal suture. The posterior fontanelle is readily evident after the 3 sutures running into it are identified. If the most accessible fontanelle is found to have 4 sutures running into it, it is the anterior fontanelle and the position is usually OP. In the presence of marked edema of the scalp or caput succedaneum, both sutures and fontanelles may be masked, and position can be determined only by feeling an ear and then noting the direction of the pinna.

(2) **The station of the fetal head,** determined by noting the relationship of the presenting bony part to the ischial spines. In labor that proceeds swiftly without complication, such a determination is usually accurate. When the first or, especially, the second stage is prolonged and is further complicated by marked molding and a heavy caput, this relation may suggest a false level of the head in the pelvis. If the head can be felt above the symphysis, forceps should not be used.

(3) **The adequacy of the pelvic diameters** of the midpelvis and outlet, determined by noting the following: (a) the prominence of the spines, the degree to which they shorten the transverse diameter of the midpelvis, and the amount of space between the spine and the side of the fetal head; (b) the contour of the accessible portion of the sacrum and the amount of space posterior to the head usually based on the length of the sacrospinous ligament; and (c) the width of the subpubic arch.

This kind of appraisal is not needed or feasible in

Reverse cephalic and cephalic application

Face application

**Figure 27–3.** Forceps correctly applied along occipitomental diameter of head in various positions of the occiput. **A:** Occiput posterior. **B:** Occiput anterior. **C:** Mentum anterior. (Reproduced, with permission, from Benson RC: *Handbook of Obstetrics & Gynecology*, 8th ed. Lange, 1983.)

outlet forceps, but for indicated low forceps or midforceps it is essential to know whether the anteroposterior (AP) or the transverse diameter is the shorter so that the biparietal diameter can be brought through it.

## FORCEPS DELIVERY: POSITION OCCIPUT ANTERIOR

An episiotomy was formerly considered an essential part of almost all forceps deliveries. It was usually made after the preliminary examination but before the application of forceps. However, current thought is mixed. The trend among many obstetricians is to perform an episiotomy only as the head is being delivered and then only if the perineum appears to be tearing. The individual obstetrician needs to carefully evaluate his or her preference and the current clinical findings before performing "routine episiotomy."

The method of forceps delivery in OA is shown in Figures 27–4 to 27–7. The legends should be given special attention. This technique is applicable to both outlet forceps and midforceps delivery when the head is in the direct OA position or in one of the oblique diameters.

The operator should be seated in front of the patient, and all maneuvers should be made carefully and slowly.

### Application of Forceps

The left handle is held between the thumb and fingers of the left hand, and, by means of 2 or 3 fingers of the right hand, the blade is guided to its correct position on the left side of the fetal head. This is repeated with the right hand and the right blade, using the fingers of the left hand to guide the blade. The handles are depressed slightly before locking in order to place the blades properly along the optimal diameter of the fetal head.

### Articulation of Forceps

The forceps are so designed that if the application is accurate they should lock easily as the handles are closed. If the handles are askew or if any force is needed to achieve precise articulation, the application is faulty and the position must be checked again by noting the relation of each blade to the lambdoid suture. If simple manipulation of the blades does not permit easy articulation, the forceps should be removed, the position verified (by feeling an ear, if necessary), and the blades reapplied correctly.

### Traction

Different obstetricians hold forceps for traction in different ways. One method is to grasp the crossbar of the handle between the index and middle fingers of the left hand from underneath (DeLee-Simpson forceps) and to insert the middle and index finger of the right hand in the crotch of the instrument from above. Another method is to grasp the handles with the fingers on the top of the handles or shanks and the thumbs on the bottom. Traction is made only in the axis of the pelvis along the curve of the birth canal. No more force is applied than can be exerted by the flexed forearms; the muscles of the back must not be used, and the feet must not be braced. If a greater degree of traction is needed, the cause may be either cephalopelvic disproportion or an error in evaluation of the wide and narrow pelvic diameters. The obstetrician should reassess the possibility of successful vaginal delivery.

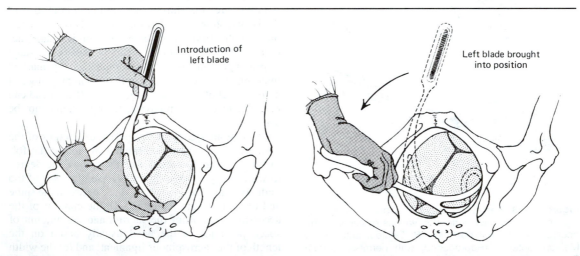

**Figure 27–4.** Introduction of left blade (left blade, left hand, left side of pelvis). The handle is held with the fingers and thumb, not clenched in the hand. The handle is held vertically. The blade is guided with the fingers of the right hand. Placement of blade is completed by swinging the handle down to the horizontal plane.

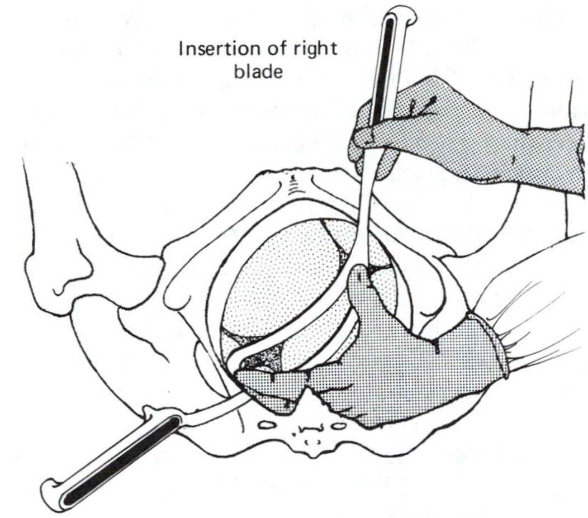

Insertion of right
blade

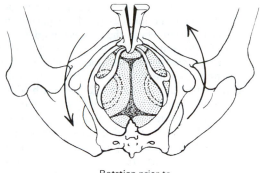

Rotation prior to
traction

**Figure 27–5.** Introduction of right blade (right blade, right hand, right side of pelvis). The left blade is already in place. The handle is grasped with the fingers and thumb, not gripped in the whole hand. The handle is held vertically.

**Figure 27–7.** Traction on forceps. Some operators prefer to place the fingers of their right hand in the crotch of the instrument to facilitate traction. If heavier traction is needed, no more force should be used than can be exerted by flexed forearms.

During normal labor, the head is relieved of pressure between uterine contractions; during a contraction the pressure increases gradually, is sustained at its maximum for 15–30 seconds, and wanes gradually. Similarly, traction on the forceps should also be applied gradually, sustained at its maximum intensity for not more than 30 seconds, and released gradually. When traction ceases, the handles are separated slightly and the head is allowed to recede at will. Traction may be resumed after 15–20 seconds. If time allows, traction is most effectively exerted with contractions.

### Delivery of the Head

As the head begins to distend the perineum, both the amount and the direction of traction must be altered. The farther the head advances, the less the resistance offered both by the pelvis and by the soft parts; hence, only minimal traction should be applied as the head is about to be delivered. Unless traction is controlled carefully, the head will "jump" over the coccyx and cause extension of the episiotomy or tearing of the perineum.

The head negotiates the final portion of the pelvic curve by extension, and the physician should simulate this movement by elevating the handles of the forceps more and more as the head crowns (Fig 27–8). If the

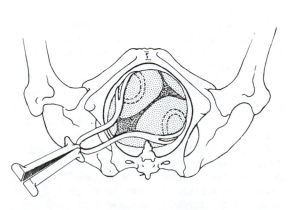

**Figure 27–6.** Both blades introduced. The 2 handles are brought together and locked. If application is correct, the handles lock precisely, without force.

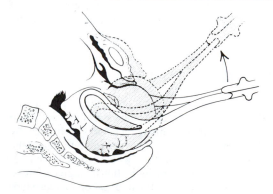

**Figure 27–8.** Upward traction with low forceps. As the head extends, the handles are raised until they pass the vertical. Little force is needed. One hand suffices; the other hand may support the perineum. (Figures 27–5 through 27–8 are reproduced, with permission, from Benson RC: *Handbook of Obstetrics & Gynecology*, 8th ed. Lange, 1983.)

forceps are allowed to remain in place throughout delivery of the head, the handles will have passed the vertical plane as delivery of the head is completed. It is preferable to remove the forceps as the head crowns in the reverse order of their application by first disarticulating the forceps and raising the right handle until the blade is delivered. The left blade is then removed in similar fashion. Early removal of the forceps is less important when a mediolateral episiotomy is used, because minor degrees of extension do not matter. When a median episiotomy or no episiotomy is performed, early removal of the forceps reduces the size of the spheroid that must pass through the introitus and thus reduces the likelihood of tears or extension.

After removal of the forceps, the head may recede; however, if the forceps have not been removed too soon, the head can be delivered readily by use of the Ritgen maneuver during the next contraction.

### The Use of Forceps When Anterior Rotation Is Not Complete

If it is necessary to intervene when the sagittal suture has passed the transverse plane of the pelvis but has not reached the exact anterior position, the physician may obtain a precise cephalic application by "wandering" the appropriate blade of the forceps toward the parietal bone that lies farthest anteriorly and inserting the other blade a little more posteriorly than is done in the direct OA position. For example, if the position is right OA, the left blade is inserted on the left side of the pelvis as if the position were OA; the blade is wandered anteriorly by placing the tips of the right index and middle fingers under the heel of the blade. Using this point as a fulcrum, the physician wings the blade into the correct position on the head by gentle lever motions of the handle. The right blade usually can be inserted directly into its correct position, but if it skips toward the right lateral aspect of the pelvis it can be wandered posteriorly in a similar manner.

## MIDFORCEPS DELIVERY

Several older series of cases indicated increased morbidity, with lowered Apgar ratings and increased neurologic deficits, among newborns delivered by midforceps. Although it is not possible to gauge the skill and experience of those who performed the midforceps operations or the indication or degree of difficulty of each procedure, the implication of such studies is that midforceps should be performed only if cesarean section would not offer a better solution to the problem. Recent reports using the newer definitions have not found the same findings. They indicate that when properly performed, midforceps cause no increase in infant morbidity or mortality. Obstetricians should be able to recognize appropriate mid-

forceps deliveries and perform them safely, and they should also be able to determine when vaginal delivery will be difficult and traumatic. In the context of current definitions, midforceps delivery from a level higher than station + 2 cm is rarely indicated and cesarean section is usually preferable.

### Conduct of the Second Stage

The lower the head at the time delivery begins, the less chance of injury to mother and baby. Also, the deeper the head is in the birth canal, the greater the likelihood of spontaneous rotation of the occiput to the anterior. Accordingly, the conduct of the second stage of labor is of special importance.

**A. Bladder:** Because a full bladder can impede the second stage of labor, it should be emptied whenever it can be felt abdominally.

**B. Dehydration:** Most labors are now conducted with an infusion running, which usually prevents dehydration. If dehydration occurs, it can lead to decelerative patterns in the FHTs, maternal exhaustion, and ineffective voluntary effort.

**C. Voluntary Efforts:** The patient's voluntary efforts may not be crucial if the pelvis is large and the baby is small. In contrast, if there is borderline disproportion (a "tight fit"), strong voluntary effort may be essential for safe delivery. Accordingly, anything that impairs the patient's ability to bear down (eg, heavy systemic analgesia or conduction anesthesia used too early) should be avoided. In cases in which voluntary effort is needed, the delivery table should be equipped with handles the patient may pull on while straining, and the knees should be flexed far back on the abdomen so the axis of uterine force is directly into the inlet.

**D. Uterine Contractions:** Uterine contractions during the second stage normally occur at 2-minute intervals. The contractions are of strong intensity and last 45–50 seconds. A delay in the interval between contractions or in their duration or intensity causes inertia that may be sufficient to delay or even stop progress. The management of second-stage inertia is judicious use of oxytocin. An infusion pump designed to administer exact amounts of oxytocin at a preselected rate is essential (a drip should not be used). In addition, during the second stage the infusion should be started at a rate of 0.5 mU/min. This may be increased by 0.5 mU/min at 5-minute intervals. If the desired result has not been achieved within 60 minutes, the infusion should be abandoned and other steps taken to accomplish delivery.

**E. Length of the Second Stage:** The length of the second stage is determined by the effectiveness of the contractions and the rate of progress. In the past an active second stage was terminated after 1–2 hours because of the increasing danger of uterine rupture or construction ring dystocia. However, most of these studies were based on older literature.

With the use of intrapartum monitoring and a fetus

that is tolerating labor well, the length of the second stage is no longer a critical indication for operative delivery. If satisfactory but slow progress is occurring, 3 or more hours may be acceptable. On the other hand, after 2 hours, a thorough evaluation must be made to rule out an unsuspected delaying factor.

**F. Anesthesia:** Anesthesia that is satisfactory for forceps delivery in most cases is satisfactory for low midforceps delivery also.

**G. Cephalopelvic Relationships:** A knowledge of variations in pelvic architecture and their effect on the mechanism of labor is essential for the proper performance of any midforceps delivery. As a rule, the midpelvis and outlet can be adequately evaluated by digital examination during or before labor. However, if the adequacy of these diameters is questionable or if the head does not readily engage, x-ray pelvimetry may be helpful. The mechanism of labor that is typical of each of the pure pelvic types is diagrammed in Figure 27–9. Because most pelves are of mixed type, combinations of these mechanisms usually are encountered.

Two facts are important in appraising and predicting the mechanism of labor: (1) The biparietal diameter is the shortest diameter of the head; therefore, his diameter should be directed through the narrowest diameter of the pelvis. (2) The occiput tends to rotate to the widest, most ample portion of the pelvis at any given level. Regardless of the position at which arrest

occurs, it is essential that the area of greatest narrowing be determined, either by palpation or by a trial of traction or both, and that the biparietal diameter of the head be brought through it safely.

### Midpelvic Arrest, Position Occiput Anterior

In the presence of uterine contractions of good quality and adequate voluntary effort, arrest in the anterior position most frequently results from the combination of slight transverse narrowing of the midpelvis (caused by either prominent spines or converging side walls) and a slightly forward lower sacrum. Usually, classic forceps are applied to the OA and traction applied as outlined above. If undue resistance is encountered, the head may be elevated slightly, rotated by the forceps to an oblique diameter, and traction repeated. If marked resistance is again encountered, the forceps should be removed and both the position and the pelvic features reevaluated. Cesarean section should be selected in almost all cases of arrest in the anterior or oblique position if heavy resistance is encountered on traction.

### Midpelvic Arrest, Position Occiput Posterior

As shown in Figure 27–9, an anthropoid pelvis predisposes to the posterior mechanism of labor. In about 70% of cases, an effective second stage results in spontaneous rotation of the occiput to the anterior position and an uneventful delivery. In the remaining

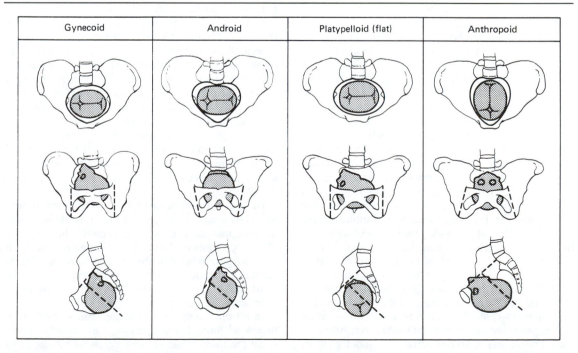

**Figure 27–9.** Diagrammatic representation of 4 maternal pelvic types (Caldwell-Moloy) and the influence of characteristic pelvic variations on mechanism of labor. (Reproduced, with permission, from Danforth DN, Ellis AH: Midforceps delivery: A vanishing art? Am J Obstet Gynecol 1983;86:29.)

cases, the head arrests in the posterior position. In the OP position, the choice of an appropriate method of delivery depends on the configuration of the pelvis.

**A. Delivery in the Occiput Posterior Position, Face to Os Pubis:** In the classic anthropoid pelvis, this is the customary method of delivery. When the sacrum flares widely posteriorly and the head is low in the pelvis, the pelvic floor may offer the only resistance to delivery. In such cases, it is entirely appropriate to make a wide episiotomy, apply classic forceps to the head in the posterior position, and deliver the fetus face to os pubis if there is no significant resistance (see Fig 27–3). On the other hand, if there is resistance the head must be rotated to the anterior position before extraction.

**B. Rotation to the Anterior Position and Midforceps Delivery:** When the head is in the anterior position, it must negotiate the terminal portion of the pelvic curve by extension; when it is in the posterior position, however, the chin is already flexed on the thorax as much as possible and cannot advance unless there is virtually no terminal pelvic curve. If the arrest occurs at or above station + 2 cm, cephalopelvic disproportion is usually the cause, and delivery should be by cesarean section. However, if the head is well molded, advanced as far as possible by the patient's voluntary effort, and deeply engaged, rotation is almost invariably not only feasible but very easily accomplished. It is emphasized that rotation, either manually or by forceps, is an essential skill required of all obstetricians.

Assisted rotation to the anterior is required in 2 circumstances.

(1) In the patient whose sacrum curves slightly forward, ample space for rotation at the level of arrest exists if the side walls are straight or divergent. If uterine force is sufficient, the occiput should rotate spontaneously away from the forward lower sacrum, and the baby will be delivered in the manner described for the anterior position. The cause of this type of arrest is uterine inertia or inadequate voluntary effort. Rotation in this circumstance is rarely difficult and can usually be facilitated by gently inserting the tips of the fingers of one hand onto the posterior fontanelle against the lambdoid suture that is on the same side as the baby's back. Elevating the head slightly and moving the lambdoid suture toward the side of the baby's back generally will move the head to the anterior position. Delivery may then be accomplished by application of classic forceps as in the anterior position or by voluntary expulsion.

(2) In the presence of a slightly forward lower sacrum and transverse narrowing of the midpelvis (due to prominent spines or converging sidewalls), arrest in the posterior position is inevitable, regardless of the effectiveness of uterine forces or voluntary effort, because there is an insufficient transverse diameter to permit the longer AP dimension of the head to rotate through it. Generally, assisted rotation will be

needed, and it usually must be done above the level of arrest. A "spiral extraction" has no place in the management of this problem, since it forces the long diameter of the head to adapt to the narrow diameter of the pelvis. Irreparable damage to mother and baby may result. There are 2 techniques of assisted rotation: manual and forceps. Manual rotation usually is preferred by obstetricians who have relatively small, narrow hands; forceps rotation generally is selected if the hand is large or the fingers short. Both techniques are acceptable and widely used. It is important to master one or the other and use it exclusively unless some unusual problem should require a variant.

**C. Manual Rotation:** The rotation maneuver described by W. C. Danforth (1932) is perhaps most widely used (Fig 27–10). Anesthesia must be sufficient to relax the uterus for this maneuver. The right hand is used regardless of whether the head is to be rotated to the right or to the left. Working on the assumption that the position is ROP, the operator introduces the right hand into the vagina. With the fingers spread widely, the thumb is directed posteriorly in the pelvis and the fingers anteriorly; the head is grasped with the entire hand and turned to the OA position. It is important that the left (external) hand assist in this maneuver by applying pressure on the shoulder through the lower part of the mother's right abdomen. If necessary, the head may be elevated slightly to gain a little more space, but it should not be disengaged. The head is rotated slightly beyond the exact anterior position to allow for the tendency of the presenting part to slip back. The right thumb is now withdrawn from the vagina, leaving the fingers in contact with the side of the infant's face to prevent the head from rotating back to the posterior position. The left blade of the forceps is introduced in the usual manner, using the fingers in the vagina as a guide. The right blade is then introduced, and the delivery proceeds as in the anterior position. If the head lies in the LOP position, the maneuver is reversed, although the right hand is still used. The use of the right hand always makes it possible to introduce the left blade first and obviates the need to readjust the handles for locking, as would be necessary if the right blade were introduced first.

**D. Forceps Rotation:** Forceps rotation is maligned by many on the grounds that it is likely to produce vaginal tears and severely damage the baby, but if it is performed skillfully, deliberately, and with knowledge of what must be accomplished, it safe, effective, and extremely simple. Many experienced obstetricians prefer it to manual rotation because of its simplicity and safety.

In all operations in which the head is rotated by means of forceps, the operator must clearly understand the movements of the forceps within the birth canal. If any classic forceps with the standard pelvic curve is held horizontally and the instrument rotated while keeping the handles in the same axis, the tips of

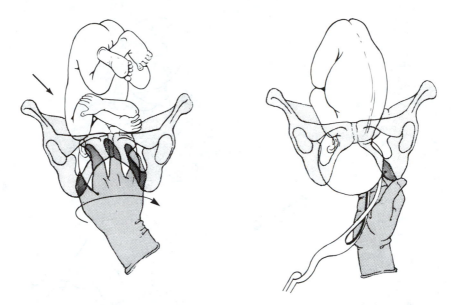

**Figure 27–10.** Manual rotation. *Left:* Head grasped by whole right hand and rotated to anterior position. Left hand (upper arrow) pushes shoulder toward woman's left, aiding rotation. *Right:* Anterior rotation complete. Right hand maintains head in anterior position while left blade of forceps is applied. (Redrawn and reproduced, with permission, from Danforth WC: The treatment of occiput posterior with special reference to manual rotation. Am J Obstet Gynecol 1932;23:360.)

the blades will describe an arc. Causing the handles to describe a wide arc, however, makes it possible to rotate the forceps so that the tips of the blades remain in the same place (Fig 27–11). The operator who performs a forceps rotation must constantly be aware of the position of each portion of the entire forceps blade and must cause the handles to describe a sufficiently wide arc so that the blades will not deviate from the axis of the pelvis or the space available in the birth canal. Most maternal and fetal injuries result from failure to observe this maxim.

Many techniques of forceps rotation have been described, and several are not recommended either because they are awkward or because the chance of injury to mother and baby seems to be excessive. Included in this category are (1) the spiral extraction using a classic forceps followed by reapplication of the forceps; (2) DeLee's key-and-lock maneuver; and (3) Bill's rotation.

The preferred technique is the Stillman maneuver, or the classic Scanzoni maneuver because these 2 procedures are very similar. The steps in the Stillman rotation are as follows (Fig 27–12).

(1) The Tucker-McLane forceps (or equivalent) is placed by an accurate cephalic application with the pelvic curve of the forceps toward the infant's face.

(2) The head is pushed upward gently in the birth canal for a distance of 1–3 cm above the level of arrest, or until an outpouring of amniotic fluid occurs, suggesting that the head has been elevated sufficiently to permit easy rotation.

(3) While the head is held at this slightly higher

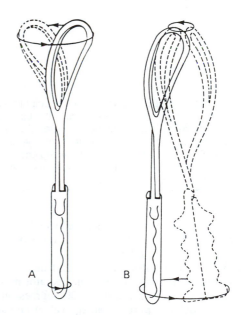

**Figure 27–11.** Action of forceps in rotation of head in occiput posterior position. **A:** Incorrect technique. If handles are merely turned in the same axis, the tips of the blades swing widely, making rotation impossible and damaging soft parts. **B:** Correct technique. The handles are first elevated and then describe a wide arc; the tips of the blades remain at approximately the same point, and the blades remain in the same axis throughout rotation. (Redrawn and reproduced, with permission, from Douglas RG, Stromme WG: *Operative Obstetrics,* 2nd ed. Appleton-Century-Crofts, 1976.)

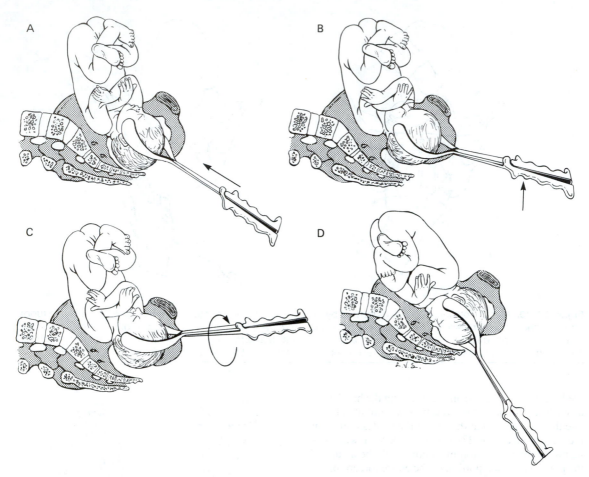

**Figure 27–12.** Forceps rotation of head in occiput posterior position. **A:** Tucker-McLane forceps are applied accurately to the head. The head is elevated in axis of the birth canal. **B** and **C:** The handles are elevated and rotated to the right. According to this technique, the head is rotated only through a short arc (during which it advances slightly), elevated again, and so rotated through short arcs until the anterior position is reached. **D:** Rotation complete, handles pointing downward. Forceps are then removed (leaving one blade in place) and replaced by DeLee-Simpson forceps for delivery. (Redrawn and reproduced, with permission, from Danforth DN: A method of forceps rotation in persistent occiput posterior. Am J Obstet Gynecol 1953;65:120.)

level, the handles of the forceps are elevated so as to center the blades in the birth canal in the axis they will occupy throughout the rotation.

(4) When the handles are raised and the head is held at this slightly higher level, the operator moves the handles through an arc of 15–30 degrees only; this causes the head to rotate an equivalent amount. As the head rotates, it tends to descend slightly, returning to the level of arrest. If the Scanzoni method is used, the operator does not stop at 15–30 degrees, but continues through 180 degrees in a slow but deliberate rotation. If the head does not turn easily, the Stillman maneuver is indicated.

(5) The head is again elevated above the level of arrest from its new position and again rotated through a short arc of 15–30 degrees, during which time it tends to advance again to the former level of arrest.

The operator repeats the maneuver, swinging the handles widely, until the position reaches OA. When the rotation is completed, the handles will point toward the floor. Slight traction is then made to fix the head in its new position.

(6) The left blade of the rotating forceps, now lying on the right side of the mother's pelvis, is removed and replaced by the right blade of the DeLee-Simpson forceps. Next, the right blade of the rotating forceps is removed and replaced by left blade of the DeLee-Simpson (or similar) forceps. (Both blades of the rotating forceps should not be removed at once. If one blade is left in place at all times, the head will be prevented from rotating back to the posterior position.)

(7) Because the right blade of the DeLee-Simpson forceps has been applied first, the handles must be positioned for locking. This done, the extraction is

accomplished by intermittent traction as though the position initially had been OA.

The foregoing steps in the rotation should be carried out slowly, deliberately, and with the utmost gentleness. The procedure should require only about 1 minute. The operator's grip on the handles should be sufficiently delicate so that any resistance, however slight, will be perceived immediately. If resistance occurs at any point in the rotation or if the FHTs indicate fetal distress, the head should be returned immediately to its original posterior position and rotation carried out in the opposite direction. During the various steps in the rotation, an assistant may direct the anterior shoulder across the abdomen as described for manual rotation.

### Midpelvic Arrest, Position Occiput Transverse

Transverse arrest may result either from failure of the uterine forces of contraction or from borderline cephalopelvic disproportion. It occurs most frequently in the following situations:

**A. En Route to the Anterior from a Primary Occiput Posterior Position:** In the presence of an anthropoid inlet, straight or divergent sidewalls, and a slightly forward lower sacrum or heavy pelvic floor, spontaneous rotation to the anterior position will occur if uterine powers are adequate. If uterine inertia occurs or if the voluntary efforts are insufficient, progress may cease when the head has reached the transverse position but has only partially rotated. In this case, rotation to the anterior position usually can be accomplished digitally by placing 2 fingers against the anterior lambdoid suture and turning the head anteriorly beneath the symphysis. If this cannot be achieved and there is sufficient room behind the head in the hollow of the sacrum, classic forceps often can be applied easily to the head in the transverse position. The blade that is to lie anteriorly (the left blade in right OT, the right blade in left OT) is introduced to the proper side of the mother's pelvis and wandered anteriorly; the opposite blade then is introduced posteriorly, the forceps are locked, and the head is rotated to the anterior position and extracted.

A third means of dealing with this problem is to rotate the head (pressure against the lambdoid suture usually suffices) back to the posterior position, which can be done with remarkable ease, and then to use either forceps or manual rotation and delivery as outlined above.

Kielland forceps may be used by those experienced in their use. The "classic" application of Kielland forceps is shown in Figure 27–13. An alternative method of application is to introduce the blade that is to lie anteriorly on the lateral side of the mother's pelvis and to "wander" it anteriorly until it comes into position over the parietal bone.

**B. En Route to the Anterior From a Primary Transverse Position:** In a gynecoid pelvis, the

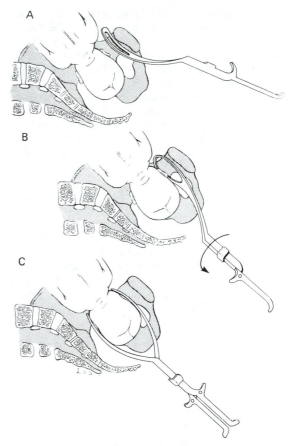

**Figure 27–13.** Classic application of Kielland forceps. **A:** Introduction of first blade (in this case, left blade, since position is ROT). **B:** Concavity of blade looks upward, and the tip of the blade is rotated toward the patient's right (as shown by arrow) through arc of 180 degrees until the blade lies in contact with the head. **C:** Instrument applied, right blade having been introduced posteriorly. Note that the buttons point toward the occiput. (Redrawn and reproduced, with permission, from Danforth WC: In: *Obstetrics and Gynecology.* Curtis AH [editor]. Saunders, 1933.)

customary mechanism of labor is engagement and descent in the transverse position, followed by flexion of the head and rotation to the anterior position as the result of slight transverse narrowing of the midpelvis and the normal tendency of the occiput to rotate away from the pelvic floor. If the AP at the outlet and lower midpelvis is normal, rotation to the anterior position and extraction are indicated. Sometimes this can be accomplished digitally. If not, manual rotation or application of classic or Kielland forceps to the head in the transverse position is appropriate.

**C. Flat Pelvis, Primary Transverse Position:** According to the classic mechanism of labor in the flat pelvis, the head engages in the transverse position and advances through the midpelvis in the transverse position without anterior rotation. If the lower sacrum permits, anterior rotation may occur on the pelvic floor; if the lower sacrum is also forward, the head actually may be born in the transverse position. In this instance, the pelvic curve will be negotiated by lateral flexion of the head.

In the management of transverse arrest of this type, rotation to the anterior and extraction from the anterior position are specifically contraindicated because they would bring the long AP diameter of the head through the shortened AP diameter of the pelvis. The head must be advanced in the transverse position and allowed to rotate to the anterior position only when it has reached a level at which the anteroposterior diameters are favorable. The Barton forceps is preferred for cases of transverse arrest in which the head must be advanced in the transverse position. The Kielland forceps may also be used in this situation, although the application of traction is more difficult and less precise. Application of the Kielland and the Barton forceps is shown in Figures 27–13 and 27–14, respectively. The technique of rotation and delivery with the Barton forceps is shown in Figure 27–15.

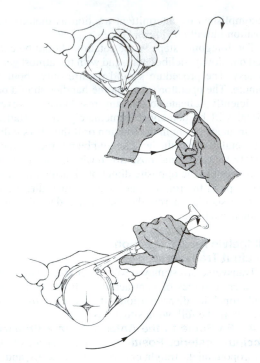

**Figure 27–15.** Completion of rotation using Barton forceps for advancement of the head in the transverse position. (Redrawn and reproduced, with permission, from Bachman C: The Barton obstetric forceps: A review of its use in 55 cases. Surg Gynecol Obstet 1927;45:805.)

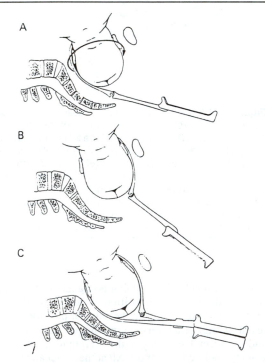

**Figure 27–14.** Application of Barton forceps for advancement of the head in the transverse position. **A:** Introduction of anterior hinged blade posteriorly, behind the head. **B:** Anterior blade has been wandered to position over anterior parietal bone. **C:** Posterior blade introduced, forceps locked. The traction bar, as shown in Fig 27–2, is now affixed to facilitate traction in the proper pelvic diameter. (Redrawn and reproduced, with permission, from Barton LJ, Caldwell WE, Studdiford WE: A new obstetric forceps. Am J Obstet Gynecol 1928;15:16.)

Like the Kielland forceps, the Barton forceps should be used only by operators who have experience in its use and are able to predict with confidence that delivery can be safely and easily accomplished by this means. Also, as with Kielland forceps, the position of Barton forceps in the obstetrician's armamentarium is daily becoming more tenuous: If the choice is offered, most problems for which these forceps are really needed are preferably dealt with by cesarean section. With the Barton forceps, traction is made with the head in the transverse position and is continued until the occiput is felt to rotate to the anterior. When the anterior rotation is achieved, the head has passed the area of major obstruction and little force is needed; the traction bar is removed and, with the handles pointing toward one maternal thigh or the other, the delivery is accomplished by continued slight traction.

## Forceps Delivery in Face Presentation

If the chin is anterior, the same indications, conditions, and stipulations apply for forceps delivery as in the OA position. The classic forceps are applied to the occipitomental diameter of the head (see Fig 27–3); elevating the handles as the head advances causes the chin to come under the symphysis, and the occiput emerges posteriorly.

If the chin is posterior, rotation of the chin to the anterior position sometimes occurs spontaneously as labor progresses. If not, it is virtually impossible to accomplish artificial rotation safely. Extraction with the chin in the posterior position will almost surely damage the infant regardless of how small it is or how large the pelvis is. Forceps delivery is contraindicated, and cesarean section is required.

### Forceps Delivery in Brow Presentation

An average-sized fetal head cannot enter even a large pelvic inlet when the brow presents. Some brow presentations convert to an occiput presentation spontaneously during the first stage of labor or can be converted to either occiput or face presentation, in which case labor should be managed accordingly. If a brow presentation fails to convert to a favorable position (chin anterior or occipital presentation) or cannot be converted readily, the infant must be delivered by cesarean section.

## DANGERS & COMPLICATIONS OF FORCEPS DELIVERIES

A number of injuries to both mother and baby can result from the use of forceps, many of them serious and some fatal. With regard to the mother, injuries range from simple extension of the episiotomy to rupture of the uterus or bladder. The baby may sustain transient facial paralysis, irreparable intracranial damage, among other injuries. Almost all of the serious injuries and many of the minor ones inflicted by obstetric forceps result form errors in judgment rather than from lack of technical skill. Such errors include failure to recognize the essential conditions for forceps delivery and lack of an appropriate indication for the operation, as outlined above; intervention too early, before maximal molding and descent have been achieved by the patient's voluntary efforts; relentless traction in the presence of unrecognized cephalopelvic disproportion; errors in diagnosis of the position of the head, with consequent application of forceps to the wrong diameter; and an incomplete knowledge of the architecture of the particular pelvis in question, with an attempt to advance the head in the wrong diameter.

Fortunately, most physicians who care for obstetric patients quickly develop respect for the operation of forceps delivery and an intuitive knowledge of when and how a patient can be delivered most safely. It is also essential for physicians to be able to admit an error in judgment and resort to cesarean section when confronted with a forceps delivery of unusual difficulty.

## THE VACUUM EXTRACTOR

The vacuum extractor, introduced by Malmström in 1954, is designed to assist delivery by the application of traction to a suction cup attached to the fetal scalp. The instrument has been widely used with good reported results. The vacuum extractor gains its purchase by pulling the scalp into a specially designed cup whose diameter at the rim is smaller than that above the rim; a consequence is distortion of the scalp into the somewhat grotesque caput succedaneum, called a "chignon," which, at least hypothetically, could lead to serious injury to the scalp and to the delicate cranial and intracranial tissues of the fetus. The data from reports in which the instrument is used extensively attest to its safety, provided the instrument is used correctly. The instrument lacks the precision of forceps and disregards the finer details of pelvic architecture as well as the mechanism of labor—all essential and traditional parts of skillful forceps delivery.

The vacuum extractor as designed by Malmström, has the following components: a specially designed suction cup, a hose connecting the suction cup to a suction pump with intervening trap bottle and manometer, and a chain inside the hose that connects the suction cup to a crossbar for traction (Fig 27–16). The design of the cup, smaller at the rim than above the rim, permits the scalp to be anchored in the peripheral reaches of the cup. Three sizes (40 mm, 50 mm, and 60 mm) are available. Two important modifications of the device have simplified its use. Bird's modification of the suction cup permits far more efficient traction and also eliminates the need to thread the chain through the hose (Fig 27–17). Use of a soft Silastic cup in preference to a metal cup reportedly simplifies the procedure. The soft cup is easier to manipulate, and a suitable vacuum is attained more quickly. Hand-held vacuum pumps, as well as mechanical pumps with built-in regulators have added to the safety of the procedure.

The procedure begins with selection of the largest cup that can be easily introduced. This is positioned to cover the posterior fontanelle so that the sagittal and lambdoid sutures are symmetrically palpable at the cup's periphery. Negative pressure is induced until a negative pressure of 0.6 kg/cm$^2$ is attained.

Once the cup has been applied, traction is made intermittently, coincident with uterine contractions and supplemented by the mother's bearing-down efforts as needed. The direction of traction is determined with due attention to the pelvic curve of Carus, depending on the station of the head at the time; it should be perpendicular to the cup to prevent the cup from slipping off the scalp. Traction should be sus-

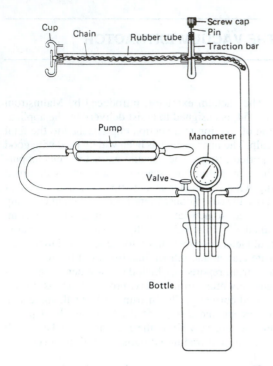

Figure 27–16. Modified Malmström vacuum extractor. (Reproduced, with permission, from Benson RC: *Handbook of Obstetrics & Gynecology*, 8th ed. Lange, 1983.)

tained and even throughout the uterine contraction and should be discontinued between contractions. There is disagreement in reference to the acceptable number of pulls before the procedure is halted. In general, if descent occurs with each episode of trac-

tion, 3 to 5 pulls should be sufficient to accomplish delivery. If no descent occurs or the cup slips off after 2 to 3 pulls, cesarean section is the preferable recourse, since failure of vacuum extraction implies cephalopelvic disproportion. The cup should not be allowed to remain in place for more than 30 minutes, because of the possibility of damage to the scalp.

Anesthesia requirements are usually less than for forceps delivery. Pudendal block usually suffices, and in many cases no anesthesia may be needed or local infiltration of the perineum may be sufficient.

Several studies have compared neonatal results by type of delivery—spontaneous vacuum extraction, forceps, or cesarean section. In the study reported by Greis et al (1981), neither perinatal mortality nor serious traumatic complications were attributable to vacuum extraction if the instrument was used judiciously. Apgar scores were similar in each of the groups. Except for the incidence of "chignon," skin bruises and lacerations were less frequent in the group delivered by vacuum extraction than in the group delivered by forceps. Cephalhematoma can be expected in a high percentage of babies delivered by vacuum extraction, but unlike the customary cephalhematomas, they tend to vanish in 2–5 days.

Complications due to vacuum extraction are usually attributed to improper use, ie, failure to recognize the circumstances in which it is contraindicated, overlong or incorrectly applied traction, use of excessive negative pressure, overlong application of the suction cup to the scalp, and failure to prevent cervical or vaginal tissue from entering the cup.

Use of the vacuum extractor is obviously contraindicated in the presence of cephalopelvic disproportion; in breech, brow, or face presentation; or if the head of a fetus is not engaged in the pelvis. It should

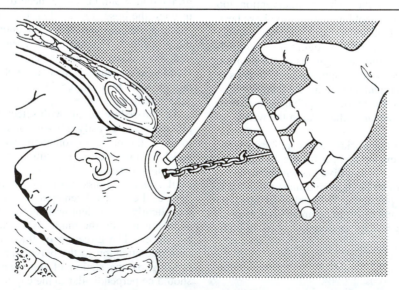

Figure 27–17. Bird's modification of Malmström's vacuum extractor.

not be used if the membranes are intact. The propriety of its use in preterm delivery is unsettled.

Vacuum extraction technique has been used successfully for delivery of a second twin in preference to version and extraction or cesarean section. Those who are experienced in its use find it to be suitable in occiput posterior presentations. If the interspinous diameter is wide, spontaneous rotation to the anterior usually occurs as the head is advanced. Attempts to rotate the head by turning the instrument usually fail, because the cup either detaches or turns only on the scalp. The trend is away from forceps delivery. As more and more cesarean sections are performed in order to avoid forceps delivery, fewer obstetricians will gain the skills that are essential to the performance of forceps delivery. The vacuum extractor has gained acceptance as a means of avoiding both forceps delivery and, in some cases, cesarean section.

# REPAIR OF LACERATIONS

Regardless of the ease or difficulty of labor, it is an essential part of each delivery to make a careful examination for lacerations and, if any are found, to repair them immediately. The following types of lacerations may occur: vestibular, perineal (including 3-degree lacerations), vaginal, cervical, and uterine (rupture).

## Diagnosis
Vestibular and perineal lacerations are immediately evident, and instruments are not needed in diagnosis.

Vaginal lacerations can usually be felt digitally, but extent and accessibility can be determined only by exposing the vagina under strong surgical light, using appropriate retractors held in place by an assistant. This is especially true of vaginal lacerations over very prominent, spike-like ischial spines. If the laceration is high in the vagina or in the cervix, a retractor is held anteriorly to expose the posterior vaginal wall. A retractor placed laterally may also be needed.

To expose the cervix, the retractor may be used posteriorly and anteriorly. The cervix is grasped with 2 ring or sponge forceps (2–3 cm apart); moving them "hand over hand," it is possible to inspect the entire circumference of the cervix. The integrity of the anal sphincter and the anterior rectal wall is tested by a finger in the rectum (after which the glove is discarded).

## Management
Vestibular lacerations usually occur in explosive deliveries. Even if extensive, they tend to heal quickly and neatly. Sutures are rarely required unless there is active bleeding.

First-degree lacerations of the perineum or vagina not involving underlying tissues rarely require sutures. Second-degree lacerations should be repaired. The tissues tend to be frayed and in some cases macerated, making identification more difficult than in episiotomy repair; however, the principles and technique are similar (Fig 27–18). Number 000 or 0000 chromic catgut or polyglycolic suture should be used.

In third-degree laceration of the perineum (involving the anal sphincter), it is usually difficult to identify the severed ends of the sphincter. However, their position is often marked by a dimple that appears on the anal skin a little anterior to the anal orifice. One may secure the ends of the sphincter by an Allis forceps or by probing to the level of the dimple with the suture needle. After this tissue is secured on both sides, the ends are approximated with a figure-of-8 suture or interrupted suturing of the fibrous sheath encasing the sphincter.

In fourth-degree laceration of the perineum, the rectal mucosa is torn. This must be repaired separately from the rest of the tissue. The usual fashion is a mucosal approximating stitch of chromic or polyglycolic suture to bring the edges together and then a second layer overlapping the first. The repair then continues as described for a third-degree laceration. Even the slightest rectal tear requires careful repair to avoid fistula formation.

Cervical lacerations less than ½ inch (1.5 cm) in length usually heal without leaving a defect and require no repair. Those longer than 1.5 cm should be repaired with interrupted sutures of No. 0 or 00 chromic or polyglycolic catgut about ¼ in (.5 cm) apart, so placed as to include about 1 cm of tissue lateral to the edge of the tear. The first suture is placed at the exact apex. If this cannot be seen, a suture is placed at the highest accessible point and used for traction to expose the higher reaches of the tear. The same technique is used for high vaginal lacerations.

Uterine rupture must be treated by laparotomy. In some cases, the tear is such that the edges can be accurately apposed in the same way as one would repair a cesarean section incision, leaving the uterus fit for future childbearing. If the integrity of the uterus cannot be assured, hysterectomy is appropriate.

# CESAREAN SECTION

The term "cesarean section" denotes the delivery of fetus, placenta, and membranes through an incision in the abdominal and uterine walls. This definition excludes the obsolete operation of vaginal cesarean section in which transvaginal access to the fetus is achieved by incising the anterior lip of the cervix and

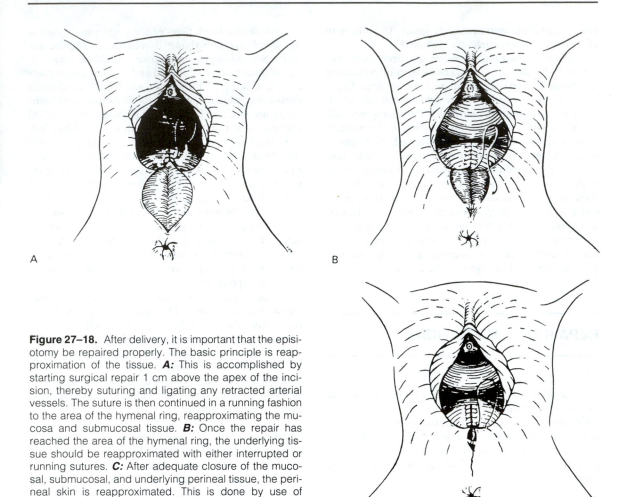

**Figure 27–18.** After delivery, it is important that the episiotomy be repaired properly. The basic principle is reapproximation of the tissue. **A:** This is accomplished by starting surgical repair 1 cm above the apex of the incision, thereby suturing and ligating any retracted arterial vessels. The suture is then continued in a running fashion to the area of the hymenal ring, reapproximating the mucosa and submucosal tissue. **B:** Once the repair has reached the area of the hymenal ring, the underlying tissue should be reapproximated with either interrupted or running sutures. **C:** After adequate closure of the mucosal, submucosal, and underlying perineal tissue, the perineal skin is reapproximated. This is done by use of subcuticular stitches, although interrupted stitches are occasionally used.

lower uterine segment. The term also excludes the operation involving the recovery, through an abdominal incision, of a fetus lying free in the abdominal cavity after secondary implantation or uterine rupture. The correct term for the surgical delivery of a previable infant is **hysterotomy**.

The first cesarean section performed on a patient is known as primary cesarean section; subsequent procedures are referred to as secondary, tertiary, and so on, or simply as repeat cesarean section.

An elective cesarean section is one that is performed before the onset of labor or before the appearance of any complication that might constitute an urgent indication.

## Historical Note

Historians agree that the term "cesarean section" has nothing to do with the birth of Julius Caesar. It has been suggested that the term is derived from the *lex caesarea*, a decree said to have continued under

the rule of the Caesars from the time of Numa Pompilius (715–672 BC) requiring that before burial of any women dying in late pregnancy the child be removed from the uterus. Certain historians also disapprove of this derivation. The term probably derives from the Latin word *caedere*, "to cut" (past participle *caesum*, "cut").

The first documented operation on a living patient (who died on the 25th postoperative day) was done in 1610. The first successful cesarean section in the USA was done in a cabin near Staunton, Virginia, in 1794; both mother and baby survived.

In early cesarean section, no sutures were placed in the uterus, and sepsis was likely in those who survived the initial hemorrhage from the open uterine sinuses. Two reports, in 1876 and 1882, did much to lower the mortality rate, which theretofore had varied from 50–85%. The first, by Porro, concerned a patient in whom the corpus uteri was excised because of uncontrollable hemorrhage from the uterine wound.

He sutured the cervix into the lower angle of the incision for drainage. Although the operation was extremely formidable, it provided a means of controlling hemorrhage; in addition, it prevented the later development of metritis and parametritis that so often led to peritonitis and death.

The second report, by Sçanger, emphasized the desirability of suturing the uterine defect before closing the abdomen. In the latter part of the 19th century, the advent of anesthesia and aseptic surgical techniques resulted in further reduction of the mortality rate. The term "Porro operation" is still used inaccurately (although less frequently) to designate the procedure of cesarean section-hysterectomy; the Sçanger operation is now known as classic cesarean section, in which the uterine incision is made in a longitudinal direction through the corpus uteri.

The lower uterine segment or low cervical cesarean section was designed, performed, and recommended by Osiander in 1805 but gained no recognition until 1906, when Frank recalled Osiander's operation and made the first of many modifications. The place of this operation in modern obstetrics was largely established by DeLee's repeated emphasis on its safety and relative lack of immediate and late sequelae compared with the Sçanger incision. DeLee's enthusiasm was not greeted by universal accord, and criticism arose from high places. In 1919, J. Whitridge Williams, responding to DeLee's thesis, declared that when "the old-fashioned, conservative (classic) operation is properly done, the danger of a weakened scar is very slight, and the probability of rupture remote." Williams' opinions have proved to be in error.

Before the advent of antibiotics, it was recognized that after the membranes had been ruptured for 10–12 hours, the performance of cesarean section imposed a threat of intractable sepsis; with each hour that passed, the hazard increased by almost geometric progression. Accordingly, it soon became an all but inviolable rule that cesarean section was forbidden for any patient in whom the membranes had been ruptured for more than 12 hours and that, regardless of the problem, delivery was to be accomplished vaginally. This policy saved the lives of many women, but in cases of cephalopelvic disproportion it also imposed a need for craniotomy, sometimes on the living baby, or a technique called **extraperitoneal cesarean section**. This was accomplished by entering the uterus without entering the abdominal cavity. A difficult task, it is rarely used in modern obstetrics.

Today, refinements in surgical technique, asepsis, antibiotic therapy, blood transfusion, and anesthesia have reduced but not eliminated the risks associated with cesarean section. The attainment of good results requires appropriate surgical and perinatal conditions and full knowledge of the possible consequences of deviating from the principles on which this major operation is based.

## General Considerations

In the past 20 years, the rate of cesarean section has steadily increased from about 5% to more than 20%. The reasons for this are (1) increasing avoidance of midforceps and vaginal breech deliveries, (2) greater awareness of serious fetal distress with use of fetal monitoring during labor, and (3) the belief that once a woman has had one cesarean delivery, all subsequent pregnancies must be delivered by cesarean section. In order for the percentage of cesarean deliveries to be reduced, it must be recognized that many women who have had a cesarean delivery can be delivered vaginally in subsequent pregnancies, especially when the indication for the initial procedure is no longer present.

Cesarean section is not to be taken lightly, and unless the indications are unmistakable one should pause to consider its risks versus its benefits. The maternal mortality rate associated with cesarean section varies in different series from 4 per 10,000 to 8 per 10,000. In one series, the risk of death from cesarean section was found to be 26 times greater than with vaginal delivery. Ledger (1977) observed that the most seriously ill of all postpartum patients with hospital-acquired infections are those who have been monitored by internal leads before they come to cesarean section. As to the fetal effects, it is clear that cesarean section is far preferable to a difficult vaginal delivery, but there is no conclusive proof that liberal use of cesarean section has done anything to improve the mental performance or reduce the incidence of neurologic deficits of children or adults in our population.

## Indications

Cesarean section is used in cases in which vaginal delivery either is not feasible or would impose undue risks on mother or baby. Some of the indications are clear and absolute (eg, central placenta previa, obvious cephalopelvic disproportion); others are relative. In some cases, fine judgment is needed to determine whether cesarean section or vaginal delivery would be better. It is not possible to prepare a complete list of indications, for there is hardly an obstetric complication that has not been dealt with by cesarean section. The following indications are the most common.

**A. Cephalopelvic Disproportion:** Cases in which the head is too large to come through the pelvis should be managed by cesarean section. The term **contracted pelvis** is sometimes listed as an indication; this is not a precise designation, because a small baby can sometimes negotiate a small pelvis, just as a large pelvis may be inadequate for a very large baby.

Extreme cases of cephalopelvic disproportion can sometimes be identified before the onset of labor, whereas in others a test or trial of labor is required. A **test of labor** is defined as 2 hours of good voluntary effort in the second stage of labor with ruptured membranes. If the baby cannot be safely delivered vaginally by this time, cesarean section is elected. In a **trial of labor,** this conclusion is reached either prior to full dilatation of the cervix or before 2 hours of the second stage have elapsed.

Test of labor is now a rarity. Fetal monitoring is used in cases of possible disproportion, and evidence of fetal distress almost always appears before the test can be completed. If the head fails to descend at an appropriate rate, cesarean section is usually the proper course.

**Inlet disproportion** can often be diagnosed with reasonable accuracy by careful pelvic examination supplemented by x-ray pelvimetry. However, unless the findings are absolute, it is best to await the onset of labor before making the diagnosis. In the primigravida, inlet disproportion should be suspected if the patient begins labor with the fetal head unengaged; in a significant number of such patients, the head fails to engage and cesarean section is indicated.

**Midpelvic disproportion** may be suspected if the AP diameter is short, the ischial spines are very prominent, the sacrospinal ligament is less than 5 cm, and the baby is large. Cesarean section should be selected, usually after a trial of labor, if the head can still be felt above the symphysis or if the vertex fails to advance beyond station + 2 cm. A trial of forceps may or may not be necessary to make this decision.

Outlet disproportion usually requires a trial of forceps before one can decide definitely that safe vaginal delivery is not possible. In general, x-ray pelvimetry and digital examination are unsatisfactory for assessment of the outlet.

**B. Uterine Inertia:** Uterine inertia (either primary or secondary to abnormal fetal position) is a common indication for cesarean section. A labor curve can be extremely helpful in evaluating the course of labor and in bringing instant attention to the appearance of uterine inertia. If the cervix fails to dilate at a rate of 1 cm/h, one should recognize the possibility of dysfunctional labor. As noted elsewhere in this book (see Chapter 25), many of these cases are resolved by oxytocin infusion, but if not, cesarean section is appropriate.

**Failure to progress** is a diagnosis that has become more common in the last 10 years. It is a nebulous term that can include inertia or cephalopelvic disproportion. The patient's labor progress becomes stalled during the course labor and before full dilation. When this has remained unchanged for 2–3 hours, the patient needs a careful reevaluation including the labor pattern, contractions, and evaluation of the pelvis. The diagnosis invariably results in cesarean section; therefore, all possible factors must be considered before the diagnosis is made.

**C. Placenta Previa:** If expectant treatment is not suitable because the pregnancy has proceeded beyond 36 weeks or because bleeding from the uterus is severe, cesarean section should be performed for placenta previa.

**D. Premature Separation of the Placenta:** In all cases of definite abruptio placentae, the membranes should be ruptured at once, regardless of the intended method of delivery, the degree of separation, or the development of shock. In moderate abruption (ie, separation of more than one-fourth but less than two-thirds of the placental surface), cesarean section should be selected (1) if fetal distress occurs; (2) if effective labor does not immediately follow rupture of the membranes; or (3) if vaginal delivery is unlikely to occur within 2 hours. In severe abruption (separation of more than two-thirds of the placental surface), cesarean section should be selected for immediate delivery if (1) if the baby is still alive; (2) if effective labor does not immediately follow rupture of the membranes; or (3) if imminent vaginal delivery cannot be anticipated within 2 hours; or (4) if the baby shows signs of compromise.

**E. Malposition and Malpresentation:** Posterior chin position and transverse lie in labor are in themselves indications for cesarean section; attempts to convert these positions to favorable ones are almost invariably futile and may be damaging. Brow presentation during labor warrants cesarean section unless a cautious attempt at conversion to an occipital or anterior chin position is successful. Shoulder presentation and compound presentation are variants of transverse lie and, with few exceptions, are best managed by cesarean section.

**F. Preeclampsia-Eclampsia:** Medical management is of course an integral part of the treatment of preeclampsia-eclampsia, but the definitive treatment is delivery. Induction of labor should be initiated in most cases; however if this is not feasible, the solution is cesarean section.

**G. Fetal Distress:** Fetal monitoring both before labor (nonstressed and stressed techniques) and during labor may disclose fetal problems that would not otherwise be evident. Consequently, the number of cesarean sections performed for the indication of fetal distress or fetal jeopardy has increased. Cesarean section should only be performed immediately in those with persistent abnormal and ominous patterns.

**H. Cord Prolapse:** This complication must be treated by the most expeditious method. If conditions are such that immediate vaginal delivery would be hazardous to the mother or the baby, the patient should be placed in the Trendelenburg position, with the cord protected by the index and middle fingers inside the cervix between the head and the uterine wall, and cesarean section should be performed without changing this position or altering the digital protection of the cord.

**I. Diabetes, Erythroblastosis, and Other Threatening Conditions:** In such conditions as diabetes, Rh incompatibility, or postterm pregnancy, fetal welfare is usually monitored by nonstress or stress testing (contraction stress test, oxytocin challenge test). If the well-being of the fetus seems compromised, it should be decided, first, when to deliver, and, second, how to deliver the fetus. For the most part, a nonreactive nonstress test followed by a positive oxytocin challenge test (late deceleration of FHTs) is an indication for delivery. If the delay involved in induction of labor cannot be justified or if conditions are unfavorable, immediate cesarean section should be chosen. It is usually fruitless to attempt to induce labor without rupturing the membranes simply to avoid a total commitment. The induction is either appropriate or it is not. If it is appropriate, one should proceed by the most effective means; if it is not, no attempt should be made.

**J. Carcinoma of the Cervix:** Cesarean section followed by definitive treatment is indicated when invasive carcinoma of the cervix is diagnosed after 28 weeks of gestation.

**K. The X Factor:** In addition to the absolute indications for cesarean section, there are also relative indications which, considered separately, might not warrant this mode of delivery but which taken together do constitute a valid indication. Eastman, in referring to postmaturity, termed these "X factors": Cesarean section would not be indicated because of postmaturity alone or because of X alone, but it could be indicated because of postmaturity plus X. X might stand for such factors as elderly primigravida, prior infertility problem, ruptured membranes but patient not in labor, or diabetes.

**L. Cervical Dystocia:** In former years, failure of the cervix to dilate properly was considered to be invariably due to incoordinate uterine action. In fact, most cases do result from uterine inertia, but some are the result of cervical scarring following deep cauterization or conization; some occur following failure of the connective tissue mechanisms normally responsible for effacement of the cervix. Although the presence of an additional X factor is often useful in electing cesarean section in cases of cervical dystocia, cesarean section—in the absence of an X factor—may be appropriate for the patient whose cervix remains rigid and fails to dilate more than 3–4 cm despite strong, frequent, first-stage uterine contractions.

**M. Previous Uterine Incision:** A previous uterine incision such as a myomectomy or a prior cesarean section may weaken the uterine wall or predispose to rupture if labor is permitted. The outmoded but entrenched maxim—"Once a cesarean, always a cesarean"—still has a few supporters. There is now ample evidence, however, that many uterine scars are indeed firm and that many patients who have had a prior uncomplicated cesarean section can be delivered easily and with less hazard vaginally than by repeat cesarean section. In general, postcesarean section patients who are suitable candidates for vaginal delivery are (1) those whose operation was of the low cervical (not classic) type; (2) those who begin labor

at or before the estimated date of confinement; and (3) those with nonrecurring conditions. In such cases it is entirely appropriate to rupture the membranes and await progress. One should be prepared for immediate cesarean section if there is an abnormality of labor or if vaginal bleeding or pain indicates that rupture of the scar is occurring. In general, elective repeat cesarean section is indicated (1) for women whose first cesarean section was done because of cephalopelvic disproportion; (although a significant number will deliver vaginally and a trial of labor is acceptable); (2) for those whose labor is likely to be long and tedious (eg, when the patient enters the hospital with ruptured membranes, a high presenting part, and an uneffaced, rigid cervix); (3) for those who have had a prior classic cesarean section or myomectomy in which the uterine cavity was entered; (4) for those who, after viability is reached, experience persistent pain in the region of the uterine incision. If vaginal delivery is allowed to proceed, alert surveillance is essential, since some cesarean section scars do rupture during labor. In the Merrill and Gibbs series, 3 scars ruptured in labor among 526 such patients.

The major hazard in the performance of elective repeat cesarean section is miscalculation of dates, with consequent delivery of a premature baby. Amniocentesis with estimation of surfactant in amniotic fluid is a definitive method of ascertaining fetal age. Serial ultrasound scans during pregnancy can also be helpful in verifying fetal maturity. Such scans are essential in determining a reasonable date for repeat cesarean section if the menstrual dates are uncertain or if the timing of the pregnancy is uncertain—for example, because of oral contraception or amenorrhea prior to conception.

**N. Other Indications:** Unusual and infrequent indications for cesarean section include a tumor obstructing the birth canal, a prior extensive vaginal plastic operation, active herpes genitalis, and severe heart disease or other debilitating condition in which vaginal delivery would impose a greater threat than cesarean section.

## Contraindications

The major contraindication to cesarean section is absence of an appropriate indication. Pyogenic infections of the abdominal wall, an abnormal fetus, a dead fetus, and lack of appropriate facilities or assistants have been suggested as contraindications. In each instance, the hazard of performing an indicated operation in the face of an alleged contraindication must be weighed against the possible consequence of not performing it.

## Preparation for Cesarean Section

**A. Ultrasound Scan:** If serial scans were not done earlier in pregnancy, a scan is desirable prior to nonemergent operations to determine the position and size of the baby, to rule out gross abnormality or twins, and to determine the location of the placenta.

**B. Timing:** The low cervical technique, which is preferred for almost all cesarean sections, is simpler to perform if the lower uterine segment changes of early labor have developed and the bladder fold of peritoneum has advanced upward; hence, for elective repeat cesarean section, it may be desirable to await the onset of labor. In addition, the patient may progress rapidly and deliver vaginally. The wait also ensures that the baby has attained maximum development before delivery. As to the time of day, no operation should be deliberately undertaken during off hours if it can be safely deferred until full staff and full laboratory facilities are available.

**C. Blood for Transfusion:** At least 2 units of packed cells should be available before surgery in the following situations: active bleeding, preeclampsia, overdistention of the uterus, coagulopathy, and oxytocin stimulation. In the absence of these indications, the need for transfusion is unlikely. Accordingly, except for these indications, most obstetric services now limit the preoperative blood preparation to "type and screen" (ABO/Rh typing, screen for unexpected antibodies) and cross-match only when blood is actually needed.

**D. Preoperative Preparation:** Preoperative sedatives should be avoided. A clear antacid (eg, 15 mL of sodium citrate, 0.3 mol/L, in 20% syrup) should be given 1 hour before operation to minimize the effects of aspiration if it should occur during anesthesia. An intravenous 18-gauge needle should be in place and 5% dextrose in lactated Ringer's or similar solution running before the operation begins. A Foley catheter should be in place. Surgical preparations (shaving, antisepsis, enema) are the same as for other abdominal operations and are used at the surgeon's discretion.

## Procedural Details

**A. Prophylactic Antibiotics:** In patients who are at minimal risk for infection, prophylactic antibiotics are not recommended prior to cesarean section. Such patients include those having repeat cesarean section and those in whom vaginal examination is not done after admission to the hospital. Women known to be at risk for infection include those who have had premature rupture of the membranes or prolonged labor, those who have undergone invasive methods of monitoring, or those who have undergone trial or failed forceps delivery. Other risk factors that may be sufficient to warrant use of prophylactic antibiotics are anemia and obesity.

Infants of women at risk for postoperative infection are also at risk for infection, and cultures of both mother and baby are required. Many pediatricians believe that early administration of prophylactic antibiotics to the mother produces fetal levels high enough to vitiate neonatal cultures, so that more extensive evaluation for sepsis may be necessary. Cunningham

et al (1983) suggest that delaying the first dose until after the cord is clamped is just as effective in preventing maternal infection but does not interfere with laboratory workups of the baby. Both aerobic and anaerobic coverage are needed. Several agents have proved effective, although the least expensive effective agent should be used. The usual schedule is followed intravenously immediately after clamping the cord and repeated doses at 4–6-hour intervals for the next 24 hours.

**B. Anesthesia:** Anesthesia for cesarean section is discussed in Chapter 26.

**C. Position on the Table:** Placing the patient in the Trendelenburg position at an angle of 25–30 degrees may be extremely helpful during dissection of the bladder fold and disengagement of the fetal head. If the head is deeply engaged, upward pressure from below by an assistant or use of forceps may be needed.

Tilting the patient slightly to the left moves the uterus to the left of the midline and minimizes pressure on the inferior vena cava.

**D. Abdominal Incision:** Opinions differ regarding the abdominal incision. An increasing number of obstetricians use the transverse incision with or without transection of the rectus muscles because wound dehiscence and postoperative incisional hernia are rare and because the cosmetic result is usually better. In cases of fetal distress or gross obesity, the midline suprapubic incision is preferred because it is much quicker and the exposure for expeditious delivery and dealing with uterine bleeding (by hysterectomy, if needed) is usually better. In the presence of a prior lower abdominal scar, it is important to enter the peritoneal cavity at the upper end of the incision to avoid entering the bladder, which may have been pulled upward on the abdominal wall at the time of closure of the previous incision.

**E. Uterine Incision:** Before the uterine incision is made, laparotomy pads that have been soaked in warm saline and wrung out may be placed on either side of the uterus to catch the spill of amniotic fluid. The degree of dextrorotation should also be determined by noting the position of the round ligaments so that the uterine incision will be centered. Torsion should not be corrected; instead, access to the midline should be obtained by retraction of the abdominal wall to the patient's right.

**F. Heavy Bleeding:** Heavy bleeding from large sinuses in the uterine incision usually can be controlled with large T clamps, but lesser bleeding points should be left to be controlled when closure sutures are placed. It is unwise to routinely place a palisade of clamps on the uterine wall because, even though this may seal the bleeders temporarily, they may begin to bleed again after the patient is in the recovery room.

**G. Encountering the Placenta:** If the placenta is encountered beneath the uterine incision, the operator must try to avoid perforating it; otherwise serious fetal bleeding may result. A way should be found around the placenta and the membranes then ruptured. If this is impossible, an incision may be made through the placenta. However, the baby must be delivered as quickly as possible and the cord clamped immediately to prevent blood loss.

**H. Delivery:** The operator delivers the baby and then separates and extracts the placenta. After delivery of the placenta, oxytocin should be administered. Oxytocin should be given by intravenous drip (10 to 20 units in 1000 mL of 5% dextrose in water) at a rate sufficient to maintain a firm contraction.

**I. Suture of the Uterine Incision:** Swaged needles cause less bleeding and are useful for placing sutures in the uterine wall. The entire thickness of the myometrium should be closed, and no harm is done if the deep sutures include the edge of the endometrium.

## Types of Cesarean Section

The types of cesarean section in modern use are (1) classic cesarean section, (2) low cervical cesarean section, and (3) extraperitoneal cesarean section.

**A. Classic Cesarean Section:** This is the simplest to perform. However, it is also associated with the greatest loss of blood, and it leaves a scar that may rupture in a subsequent pregnancy. Moreover, a loop of small bowel may adhere to the uterine incision and predispose to intestinal obstruction. The currently accepted indications for classic cesarean section are placenta previa (because the incision in the corpus usually avoids the low-lying placenta); transverse lie (in which better access to the baby is provided by the Sauanger incision); and premature delivery (there is little formation of the lower uterine segment). Some prefer the low cervical operation, if possible, for each of these conditions, however.

Classic cesarean section may also be preferred if there is need for extreme haste, because it offers the quickest means of delivering the baby. Nonetheless, the hazards of this procedure must be weighed against the additional minute or so needed to dissect the bladder away from the lower uterine segment and to make the transverse semilunar low cervical incision.

In performing the classic procedure, a vertical incision is made in the corpus; a scalpel is used to enter the uterine cavity; and the incision is enlarged with bandage scissors. Since the incision is relatively high in the uterus, the head is rarely accessible. Accordingly, the feet are grasped and brought through the incision. The remainder of the delivery is accomplished using the several maneuvers appropriate to breech delivery (see Chapter 21). After removal of the placenta and membranes, the uterine defect may be repaired with 3 layers of chromic catgut or an absorbable synthetic suture. No. 0 is recommended for the 2 deeper layers and 00 for the superficial suture to coapt the serosal edges. In placing the superficial layer, a "baseball stitch" minimizes bleeding from the cut edges: Each suture enters the myometrium on the cut surface, emerging on the serosal surface about 3/16 in (5 mm) from the edge, and is so continued side-to-side for the length of the incision.

**B. Low Cervical Cesarean Section:** (Lower uterine segment cesarean section or cervical cesarean section.) The confused terminology of this procedure is understandable: Before labor, when the cervix is closed, uneffaced, and located at about the level of the ischial spines, a transverse uterine incision (which is made ¾–1 in [2–3 cm] superior to the symphysis pubica) necessarily is made in the lower uterine segment; when the cervix is fully dilated and retracted, the anterior lip is just superior to the symphysis and the incision just superior to the symphysis is through the cervix. When the operation is performed after the onset of labor but before full dilatation, there is no indication whether the incision is made in the cervix proper or in the lower uterine segment—a detail of only academic interest.

The steps in the operation are shown in Figure 27–19. The bladder fold of peritoneum is picked up with tissue forceps and incised transversely. By means of finger dissection through the loose areolar tissue, the bladder is separated from the anterior aspect of the uterus interiorly for a distance of 3–4 cm. The bladder is held away from this denuded area by a specially designed bladder retractor, and a transverse incision about 2 cm long is made through the anterior uterine wall. The membranes are preferably left intact, but no real damage follows if they should be ruptured. Using bandage scissors, the operator enlarges the transverse incision in a crescent-shaped path that extends superiorly at the lateral extremities to avoid the uterine vessels.

If it can be readily accomplished, the baby is delivered by elevation with the hand. If it cannot, the baby's face is rotated into the incision, and the left blade of the DeLee cesarean section forceps or the Simpson forceps is introduced and applied to one side of the head. Using this blade as a vectis and combining it with moderate fundal pressure by the assistant, the operator can usually deliver the baby's head with ease; if not, the second blade may be applied. If the face cannot be easily rotated into the incision, the head should be turned to the OA position and delivered using one or both blades of the forceps, as above. Occasionally, with considerable molding and deep engagement, a vertex delivery may be difficult, in which case the baby's feet must be brought down and delivery must be accomplished as in classic cesarean section.

Most obstetricians prefer the transverse semilunar incision. In former years a longitudinal incision, usually extending into the corpus uteri superiorly, was more popular. However, this incision has many of the same complications and risks as those of a classic incision.

The uterine incision generally is repaired using 2 layers of No. 0 or 00 chromic catgut or absorbable synthetic suture. (It is helpful, in gaining exposure for

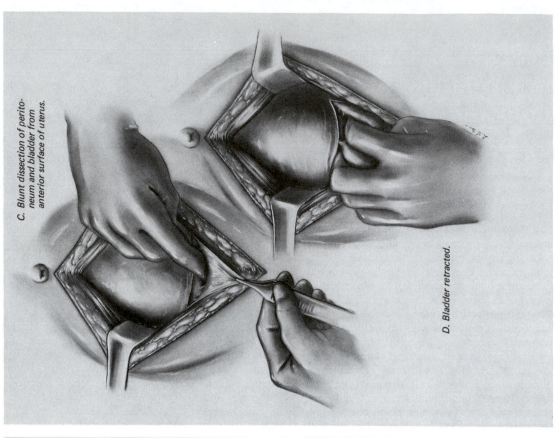

C. Blunt dissection of peritoneum and bladder from
anterior surface of uterus.

D. Bladder retracted.

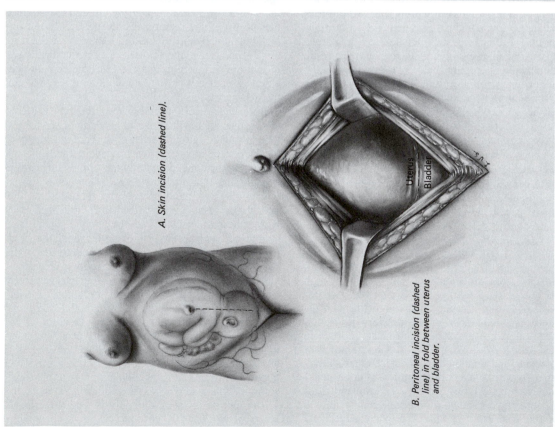

A. Skin incision (dashed line).

Uterus

Bladder

B. Peritoneal incision (dashed
line) in fold between uterus
and bladder.

**Figure 27–19.** Cesarean section. (Reproduced, with permission, from Dunn LG: Cesarean section and other obstetric operations. In: *Obstetrics and Gynecology*, 5th ed. Danforth DN, Scott JR [editors]. Lippincott, 1986.)

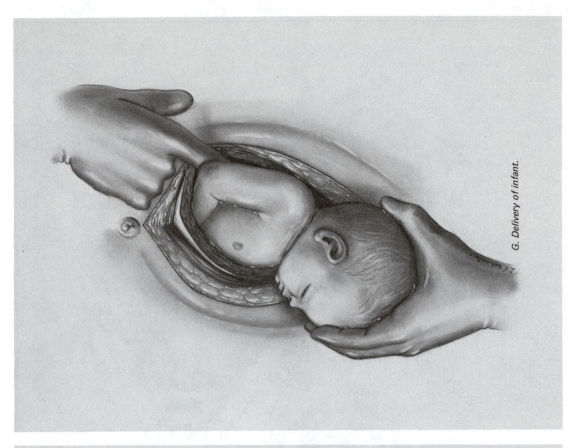

G. Delivery of infant.

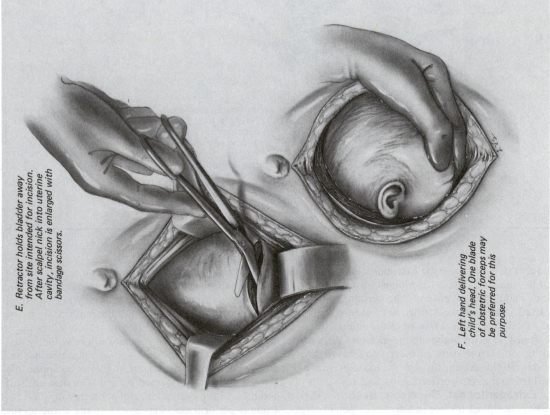

E. Retractor holds bladder away
from site intended for incision.
After scalpel nick into uterine
cavity, incision is enlarged with
bandage scissors.

F. Left hand delivering
child's head. One blade
of obstetric forceps may
be preferred for this
purpose.

**Figure 27–19 (cont'd).** Cesarean section.

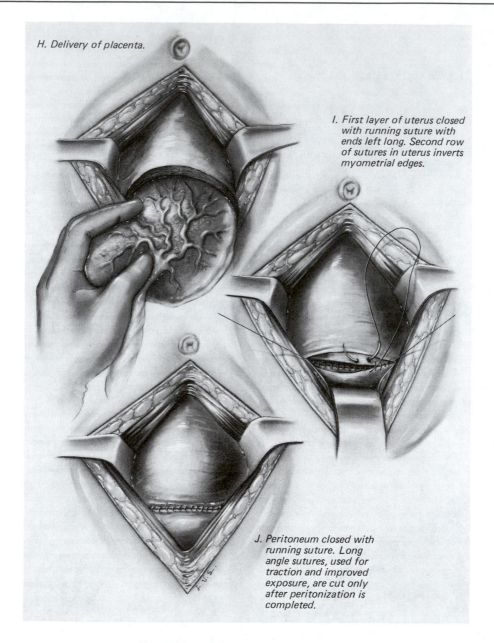

H. Delivery of placenta.

I. First layer of uterus closed with running suture with ends left long. Second row of sutures in uterus inverts myometrial edges.

J. Peritoneum closed with running suture. Long angle sutures, used for traction and improved exposure, are cut only after peritonization is completed.

**Figure 27–19 (cont'd).** Cesarean section.

subsequent steps, to leave the first suture long at each end of the incision. These function as lifting sutures, and they should not be cut until the peritonization is completed.) The peritoneal reflection is sutured either to the superior peritoneal flap or to the anterior uterine wall just superior to the uterine incision. With involution, the uterine incision moves downward into the pelvis. Slight seepage through the incision usually is confined to the retroperitoneal spaces.

**C. Extraperitoneal Cesarean Section:** This procedure, designed for use in infected or potentially infected patients, was introduced before the modern era of antibacterial agents and blood transfusion. The procedure is time-consuming and may not be effective in preventing spillage into the peritoneal cavity, because the peritoneum often is perforated even by the expert. Although the operation was virtually discarded more than 20 years ago, the question has recently been raised whether it might not be applicable for the potentially infected patient. The data are still too meager for evaluation, and at present most obstetricians perform cesarean hysterectomy if the uterus is frankly infected; if it is only potentially infected, they perform low cervical cesarean section with prophylactic antibiotic coverage.

## Complications & Prognosis

The major factors affecting healing of the uterine incision are hemostasis, accuracy of apposition, quality and amount of suture material, and avoidance of infection and tissue strangulation. Unfortunately, little information about the integrity of a particular scar in a subsequent pregnancy is gained by inquiry as to the presence or absence of postoperative infection and the location of the incision.

In a later pregnancy, pain in the area of the scar may suggest dehiscence. About 50% of all ruptures of uterine scars occur before the onset of labor. The incidence of rupture is about 1–2% of classic scars and 0.5–1% in cases of low cervical cesarean section. Rupture of the classic scar is usually catastrophic, occurring suddenly, totally, and with partial or total extrusion of the fetus into the abdominal cavity. Shock due to internal hemorrhage is a prominent sign. Rupture of the low cervical scar is usually more subtle and is characterized principally by pain and occasionally by evidence of slower internal bleeding. Some ruptures are entirely silent, and during repeat cesarean section myometrial fenestrations covered only by visceral peritoneum may be noted.

**A. Maternal Morbidity and Mortality:** Average maternal morbidity and mortality rates after cesarean section suggest that the risk from the operation per se is very small. Some large series with no postoperative deaths have been reported. In other series, incidences of mortality have ranged from 40 to 80 per 100,000 cases. In general, it is reasonable to conclude that the risk of death following cesarean delivery is at least twice the risk following vaginal delivery. Such figures are difficult to interpret, however, because of the great variability of indications and complications. Even in the most favorable cases variable factors exist, including spill of amniotic fluid and blood into the peritoneal cavity; ease or difficulty of delivering the baby through the uterine incision; amount of incisional bleeding; and patient response to anesthesia. Factors contributing heavily to postoperative complications are prior internal monitoring, prolonged rupture of the membranes, unsuccessful prior efforts at vaginal delivery, hemorrhage, uterine rupture, and countless other obstetric problems that may have compromised the patient and for which emergency cesarean section was performed. See Prophylactic Antibiotics, earlier in this chapter, for a discussion of the risk of postoperative infection.

The longer the operative procedure, the greater the likelihood of postoperative complications. As Victor Bonney noted in an early edition of his classic *Gynecological Surgery*, "An operation rapidly yet correctly performed has many advantages over one technically as correct, yet laboriously and tediously accomplished." Most cesarean sections should be completed in less than 1 hour unless significant technical problems are encountered.

Disasters following cesarean section are rare. Some clearly are not preventable. Others are due directly to faulty surgical technique, especially lack of attention to hemostasis, inept or ill-chosen anesthesia, inadequate blood replacement or transfusion of mismatched blood, and mismanagement of infection.

**B. Perinatal Morbidity and Mortality:** Perinatal problems are as difficult to assess as maternal ones. Data suggest that spontaneous vaginal delivery in the uncomplicated multipara is less hazardous for the baby than repeat elective cesarean section and that if elective cesarean section is performed, regional anesthesia appears to be less noxious than general anesthesia.

The first conclusion will be acceptable to most: Spontaneous vaginal delivery is usually the most normal of births, whereas repeat cesarean section may entail time-consuming procedures such as dissection of an adherent bladder, aspiration of amniotic fluid during attempts at delivery, fetal hypoxia if the placenta is encountered beneath the prior incision, and the occasional need for version to accomplish delivery.

It must be emphasized that iatrogenic prematurity is still an important consequence of elective cesarean section. Whenever repeat cesarean section is contemplated or whenever risk factors make it necessary to terminate the pregnancy before term, every effort must be made to establish an accurate term date, preferably by ultrasound scans at 20–21 weeks' gestation and again at 30–31 weeks. If gestational age is still in doubt, the lecithin: sphingomyelin ratio or amniotic fluid phosphatidylglycerol concentration should be determined before operation.

Some evidence suggests that cesarean section per se contributes in some unknown way to increased occurrence of respiratory problems in the newborn, and this underscores the desirability of examination of the infant by a pediatrician as soon as possible after delivery.

## Elective Procedures Coincidental to Cesarean Section

**A. Appendectomy:** Appendectomy should not be performed routinely at the time of cesarean section. An appendectomy may seem to be "innocuous," only to result in obstruction and peritonitis.

**B. Myomectomy:** Myomectomy is permissible at the time of cesarean section only if the tumor is pedunculated. Extracting intramural tumors can provoke intense and uncontrollable bleeding. Also, myomas almost invariably regress after pregnancy; indeed, even large myomas are sometimes not palpable 3 months after delivery.

**C. Tubal Ligation:** This procedure is usually offered to the multiparous patient at the time of the cesarean section. If a Pomeroy sterilization procedure is done, the fimbriated end of the tube must first be identified (the round ligament has been mistaken for the tube) and the operation performed at the junction of the mid and outer thirds of the tube. Caution should be used to avoid excessive pulling on the tube, which could rupture veins in the broad ligament.

## Cesarean Hysterectomy

A major indication for cesarean hysterectomy is inability to stop bleeding from the uterine incision. A second important indication, formerly more common than at present is a frankly infected uterus. Other indications are rupture of the uterus in which repair is impractical, placenta accreta, uterine hemorrhage from uncontrollable atony, and large uterine myomas.

Cesarean hysterectomy should never be done as a means of sterilization. The procedure is too formidable for this purpose alone; postpartum tubal ligation is far less hazardous and is highly effective if done properly.

The superiority of total over subtotal hysterectomy has been amply demonstrated, and it is now accepted that the cervix should be removed in all cases unless doing so would impose undue risk or serious technical problems. At the time of cesarean section, it is also preferable to remove the cervix if the patient's condition is good and if there is no contraindication to prolonging operating time by 10–15 minutes. Supravaginal hysterectomy should be performed only when it is desirable to terminate the operation quickly. A risk of leaving the cervix is postoperative hemorrhage and thus good hemostasis is critical.

The technical aspects of hysterectomy at the time of cesarean section do not differ basically from those of hysterectomy in the nonpregnant patient except that all structures and cleavage planes are highly vascular and the tissues are friable. At least 4 units of matched blood must be at hand. In one study, blood replacement was needed in 98% of the indicated cesarean hysterectomies and in 66% of the elective sterilization group; two-thirds of the patients in the elective group received an average of 1.6 units of blood.

## Postmortem Cesarean Section

Postmortem cesarean section is a difficult problem for the following reasons.

(1) The possibility of litigation is introduced if the operation is done without informed consent of the next of kin (usually an impractical detail in these circumstances) or if it is not done in the interests of the baby.

(2) The definition of legal death is not fully established, but most agree that in the adult, irreversible brain damage results after 5 minutes or more of total anoxia. There is inconclusive evidence that the fetal brain may be more resistant to hypoxia than that of the adult. The prospects for a healthy baby depend to a certain extent on whether the mother's death was instantaneous or whether she was moribund for an extended period.

Regardless of how quickly the operation is done after the mother's death, the outlook for the baby is bleak. Jeffcoate (1976), the preeminent Liverpudlian obstetrician-gynecologist, commented that some "continue to report with misplaced pride the delivery by postmortem caesarean section of babies which have suffered so much cerebral anoxia whilst in utero that they are permanently crippled mentally and physically as well as being motherless."

Arthur (1978) has reviewed the subject and suggests that with modern life-support systems, the outlook for the baby may be immeasurably improved if the operation can be performed when death is imminent but has not yet occurred. According to a news release from the Roanoke (Virginia) Memorial Hospital, a brain-dead woman who had been kept breathing by respirator for 84 days was delivered by cesarean section of a 3-lb 11-oz (1.67-kg) apparently normal baby. Life support was withdrawn after delivery.

## Fetal Injury

While performing a cesarean section, most emphasis is placed on careful dissection of maternal tissues. The obstetrician must be just as careful with the fetus. The incision in the uterus can lacerate the infant if it is too deep. Although this is an unusual occurrence, it does occur in 0.2 to 0.4% of all cesarean sections. The usual site is on the face in the area of the cheek. It may also occur on the buttock, ear, head, or any other body site under the incision. To avoid this injury completely is probably impossible. However, careful incision through the uterine layers will minimize any laceration that may occur.

## VAGINAL DELIVERY FOLLOWING PREVIOUS CESAREAN SECTION (VBAC)

A marked rise in the incidence of cesarean section deliveries has occurred in the USA over the past 15 years, and rates of 25–70% are common in those hospitals that encourage or require a trial of labor following a previous cesarean section. Factors responsible for the increase include the relative safety of the procedure and concern about malpractice litigation. In 1981, the National Institutes of Health consensus Development Task Force on Cesarean Birth undertook a study of the trend toward cesarean section delivery. Vaginal delivery is associated with fewer delivery risks, requires less anesthesia, poses a lower potential for postpartum morbidity, involves a shorter hospital stay, saves money, and encourages earlier and often smoother interaction between mother and infant.

Since 30% of cesarean sections are performed solely because of previous cesarean section, a substantial (and beneficial) decrease in incidence would occur if VBAC were more widely adopted in the absence of contraindications. In recent studies 60–80% of all patients who undergo a trial of labor after previous cesarean section have a successful vaginal delivery when the obstetrician actively promotes VBAC. In the case of cesarean delivery performed for malpresentation and other indications not necessarily recurring in subsequent pregnancies, vaginal delivery should occur in 75–80% subsequent pregnancies. Previous vaginal delivery is an indicator of probable success in future vaginal delivery.

### Indications

Criteria for vaginal delivery following previous cesarean section may include the following. (1) The patient agrees to the procedure. (2) A low transverse uterine incision was used. (3) The original indication for cesarean section was a cause not necessarily recurring in subsequent pregnancies. (4) The postoperative course was benign. (5) The current pregnancy is not complicated by macrosomia, malposition, multiple gestation, or other conditions that would be likely to preclude vaginal delivery.

### Contraindications

Although authorities agree that a previous classic uterine incision is an absolute contraindication to vaginal delivery in later pregnancies, other contraindications are less clear. For example, there appears to be little increased risk in attempting a trial of labor in the presence of mild macrosomia, and many authors now feel that the occurrence of 2 prior cesarean sections is no longer an absolute contraindication.

### Management

**A. Definitions:** *Dehiscence* is the unsuspected and undiagnosed silent separation of a uterine scar from a previous cesarean section; it is usually limited to the immediate area of the scar. *Rupture* is the sudden separation of the scar, usually with hemorrhage; the laceration may be extensive. A rupture is termed *complete* if it communicates with the peritoneal cavity and *incomplete* if the visceral peritoneum is intact. The incidence of uterine dehiscence increases by only 15% if there have been 2 previous cesarean sections but increases by nearly 200% if there have been 3 previous cesareans. Exact information on the safety of vaginal delivery in the presence of low vertical cesarean scars is lacking.

**B. Oxytocin:** Judicious use of oxytocin appears to be safe in vaginal delivery following previous cesarean section. Several reports show no greater incidence of necessary cesarean section, dehiscence or rupture of the scar, uterine atony, hemorrhage, transfusion, hysterectomy, birth trauma, or adverse neonatal outcome with carefully controlled infusion of oxytocin.

**C. Epidural Anesthesia:** The role of epidural anesthesia in vaginal delivery following previous cesarean section remains controversial. Although pain may not be a reliable sign of uterine rupture and epidural anesthesia may not completely block the pain associated with such an event, the concern is that epidural anesthesia could potentially mask the rupture, thereby jeopardizing both mother and infant. On the other hand, epidural anesthesia removes the fear of labor pain and helps the obstetrician encourage VBAC.

**D. Complications:** The most feared complication is uterine rupture, although 44–60% of these ruptures precede the onset of labor and are most frequently associated with a classic incision. Current studies cite a maternal mortality rate of about 1% and a perinatal mortality rate of about 50% in association with uterine rupture, although exact data are unavailable. The institution in which delivery is to occur must therefore be fully capable of managing possible uterine rupture. Equipment for both maternal and electronic fetal monitoring and appropriate obstetric and neonatal facilities must be available. A large-bore intravenous catheter must be used, and type-specific blood for possible maternal transfusion must be at hand. Appropriate anesthesia, a fully equipped operating room, and obstetric and neonatal staff experienced in emergency care all must be immediately available.

## REFERENCES

### FORCEPS DELIVERY

ACOG Committee Opinion No. 59. February 1988: Obstetric Forceps.

ACOG Technical Bulletin No. 152: February 1991: Operative Vaginal Delivery (in press).

Barton LJ, Caldwell WE, Studdiford WE: A new obstetric forceps. Am J Obstet Gynecol 1928;15:16.

Bashore RA, Phillips WH Jr, Brinkman CR: A comparison of the morbidity of midforceps and cesarean delivery. Am J Obstet Gynecol 1990;162(6):1428.

Chiswick ML, James DK: Kielland's forceps: Association with neonatal morbidity and mortality. Br Med J 1979;1:7.

Cibils LA, Ringler GE: Evaluation of midforceps delivery as an alternative. J Perinatol Med 1990;18(1):5.

Danforth DN: A method of forceps rotation in persistent occiput posterior. Am J Obstet Gynecol 1953;65:120.

Danforth WC: The treatment of occiput posterior with special reference to manual rotation. Am J Obstet Gynecol 1932:23:360.

DeLee JB: The prophylactic forceps operation. Am J Obstet Gynecol 1920;1:34.

Dierker LR Jr et al: Midforceps deliveries: Long-term fetal outcome of infants. Am J Obstet Gynecol 1986; 154:764.

Gilstrap LC II et al: Neonatal acidosis and method of delivery. Obstet Gynecol 1984;63:681.

Hagadorn-Freathy AS, Yeomans ER, Hankins GDV. Validation of the 1988 ACOG forceps classification system. Obstet Gynecol 1991;77:356.

Healy DL, Laufe LE. Survey of obstetric forceps training in North America in 1981. Am J Obstet Gynecol 1985;151:54.

Kadar N, Romero R: Prognosis for future childbearing after midcavity instrumental deliveries in primigravidas. Obstet Gynecol 1983;62:166.

Kong AS, Bates SJ, Rizk B: A randomized comparison of assisted vaginal delivery by obstetric forceps and polyethylene vacuum cup. Br J Anaesth 1992; 68(3): 252.

Robertson PA, Laros RK Jr, Zhao RL: Neonatal and maternal outcome in low-pelvic and midpelvic operative deliveries. Am J Obstet Gynecol 1990; 162(6): 1436.

Yancy MK, Harlass FE, Benson W, Brady K: The perioperative morbidity of scheduled cesarean hysterectomy. Obstet Gynecol 1992 Feb;81(2):206.

Zlatnik FJ: Mechanism of normal labor. In: *Danforth's Obstetrics and Gynecology*, 5th ed. Scott JR, et al (editors). Lippincott, 1990.

## VACUUM EXTRACTOR

Berkus MD et al: Cohort study of Silastic obstetric vacuum cup deliveries: Safety of the instrument. Obstet Gynecol 1985;66:503.

Bird GC: Modification of Malmström's vacuum extractor. Br Med J 1969;3:526.

Dell DL, Sightler SE, Plauche WC: Soft cup vacuum extraction: A comparison of outlet delivery. Obstet Gynecol 1985;66:624.

Greis BJ, Bieniarz J, Scommegna A: Comparison of maternal and fetal effects of vacuum extraction with forceps or cesarean deliveries. Obstet Gynecol 1981; 57:571.

Leijon I: Neurology and behavior of newborn infants delivered by vacuum extraction on maternal indication. Acta Paediatr Scand 1980;69:625.

Malmström T: The vacuum extractor, an obstetrical instrument. Acta Obstet Gynecol Scand 1954;4(Suppl): 33.

Pelosi MA, Pelosi MA 3d: A randomized comparison of assisted vaginal delivery by obstetric forceps and polyethylene vacuum cup. Obstet Gynecol 1992; 79(4):638.

Williams MC, Knuppel RA, O'Brien WF et al: A randomized comparison of assisted vaginal delivery in term pregnancies. Obstet Gynecol 1991;78(5 Pt 1):789.

## CESAREAN SECTION

Arthur RK: Postmortem cesarean section. Am J Obstet Gynecol 1978;132:175.

Brocke-Utne JG et al: Advantages of left over right lateral tilt for cesarean section. S Afr Med J 1978;54: 489.

Chang PL, Newton ER: Predictors of antibiotic prophylactic failure in post-cesarean endometritis. Obstet Gynecol 1992;80(1):117.

Cunningham FG et al: Perioperative antimicrobials for cesarean delivery: Before or after cord clamping? Obstet Gynecol 1983;62:151.

Danforth DN: Cesarean section. JAMA 1985;253:811.

Evrard JR, Gold EM: Cesarean section: Risk/benefit. Perinatol Care 1978;2:4.

Faro S, Martens MG, Hammill HA, Riddle G, Tortolero G: Antibiotic prophylaxis: Is there a difference? Am J Obstet Gynecol 1990;162(4):900;discussion:907.

Flaksman FJ, Vollman RH, Benfield DG: Iatrogenic prematurity due to elective termination of the uncomplicated pregnancy: A major perinatal health care problem. Am J Obstet Gynecol 1978;132:885.

Gibbs RS, Blanco JD, St. Clair PJ: A case-control study of wound abscess after cesarean delivery. Obstet Gynecol 1983;62:498.

Gonik B, Shannon RL et al: Why patients fail antibiotic prophylaxis at cesarean delivery: Histologic evidence for incipient infection. Obstet Gynecol 1992;79(2): 179.

Hertz RH et al: Clinical estimation of gestational age:Rules for avoiding preterm delivery. Am J Obstet Gynecol 1978;131:395.

Hjalmarson O et al: The importance of neonatal asphyxia and cesarean section as risk factors for neonatal respiratory disorders in an unselected population. Acta Paediatr Scand 1982;71:403.

Jeffcoate N: Medicine versus nature. J R Coll Surg Edinb 1976;21:263.

Ledger WJ: Hospital-acquired obstetric infections. In: *Infections in the Female*. Lea & Febiger, 1977.

Mann LL, Gallant J: Modern indications for cesarean section. Am J Obstet Gynecol 1979;135:437.

Neuhoff D, Burke MS, Porreco RP: Cesarean birth for failed progress in labor. Obstet Gynecol 1989; 73(6) 915.

Nielsen TF, Hauokeganard KH: Postoperative cesarean section morbidity: A prospective study. Am J Obstet Gynecol 1983;146:911.

NIH Consensus Development Task Force: Statement on cesarean childbirth. Am J Obstet Gynecol 1981;139: 902.

Pastorek JG, Sanders CV Jr: Antibiotic therapy for post-cesarean endomyometritis. Rev Infect Dis 1991;13 (Suppl 9):S752.

Perlo M, Curet LB: The effect of fetal monitoring on cesarean section morbidity. Obstet Gynecol 1979;53: 354.

Rosen MG, Debanne SM, Thompson K: Arrest disorders and infant brain damage. Obstet Gynecol 1989;74(3 Pt 1):321.

Shiono PH, McNellis D, Rhoads GG: Reasons for the rising cesarean delivery rates: 1978–1984. Obstet Gynecol 1987;69(5):696.

Speert H: Cesarean section. In: *Obstetrics and Gynecology in America: A history*, ACOG, 1980, p. 150.

Studd J: Partograms and nomograms of cervical dilatation in management of primigravid labour. Br Med J 1973;4:451.

Yancy MK, Herpolsheimer A, Jordan GD et al: Maternal and neonatal effects of outlet forceps of delivery compared with spontaneous vaginal delivery in term pregnancies. Obstet Gynecol 1991;78(4):646.

## VAGINAL DELIVERY FOLLOWING PREVIOUS CESAREAN SECTION

Brody CZ, Kosasa TS, Nakayama RT: Vaginal birth after cesarean section in Hawaii. Experience at Kapiolani Medical Center for Women and Children. Hawaii Med J 1993 Feb; 52(2):38.

Flamm BL, Newman LA, Thomas SJ et al: Vaginal birth after cesarean delivery:Results of a 5-year multicenter collaborative study. Obstet Gynecol 1990;76(5 Pt 1):750.

Horenstein JM, Phelan JP: Previous cesarean section: The risks and benefits of oxytocin usage in a trial of labor. Am J Obstet Gynecol 1985;151:564.

Phelan JP et al: Vaginal birth after cesarean. Am J Obstet Gynecol 1987;157:1510.

Raynor BD: The experience with vaginal birth after cesarean delivery in a small rural community practice. Am J Obstet Gynecol 1993;168(1 Pt 1):60.

Rosen MG, Dickinson JC, Westhoff CL: Vaginal birth after cesarean: a meta-analysis of morbidity and mortality. Obstet Gynecol 1991;77(3):465.

Stovall TG et al: Trial of labor in previous cesarean section patients, excluding classical cesarean sections. Obstet Gynecol 1987;70:513.

# 28

# Postpartum Hemorrhage & the Abnormal Puerperium

*Sabrina D. Craigo, MD, and Peter S. Kapernick, MD*

## POSTPARTUM HEMORRHAGE

### Definition

Postpartum hemorrhage denotes excessive bleeding (> 500 mL in vaginal delivery) following delivery. Hemorrhage may occur before, during, or after delivery of the placenta. Actual measured blood loss during uncomplicated vaginal deliveries has been shown to average 700 mL, and blood loss may often be underestimated. Nevertheless, the criterion of a loss of 500 mL is acceptable on historical grounds and because 1 unit (U) of blood also contains 500 mL. The parallel has obvious value in estimating the need for transfusion.

Blood lost during the first 24 hours after delivery is early postpartum hemorrhage; blood lost between 24 hours and 6 weeks after delivery is late postpartum hemorrhage.

### Incidence

The incidence of excessive blood loss following vaginal delivery is 5–8%. Postpartum hemorrhage is the most common cause of excessive blood loss in pregnancy, and most transfusions in pregnant women are performed to replace blood lost after delivery. Hemorrhage is the third leading cause of maternal mortality in the USA and is directly responsible for about one-sixth of maternal deaths (Atrash et al, 1990). In less-developed countries, hemorrhage is among the leading obstetric causes of maternal deaths.

### Morbidity & Mortality

Although any woman may suffer excessive blood loss during delivery, women already compromised by anemia or intercurrent illness are more likely to demonstrate serious deterioration of condition, and anemia and excessive blood loss may predispose to subsequent puerperal infection. Major morbidity associated with transfusion therapy (eg, hepatitis, human immunodeficiency virus infection, transfusion reactions) is infrequent but it is not insignificant. Moreover, other types of treatment for anemia may involve some risk.

Postpartum hypotension may lead to partial or total necrosis of the anterior pituitary gland and cause postpartum panhypopituitarism, or Sheehan's syndrome, which is characterized by failure to lactate, amenorrhea, decreased breast size, loss of pubic and axillary hair, hypothyroidism, and adrenal insufficiency. The condition is rare (< 1 in 10,000 deliveries). A woman who has been hypotensive postpartum and who is actively lactating probably does not have Sheehan's syndrome. Hypotension can also lead to acute renal failure and other organ system injury. In extreme hemorrhage, sterility will result from hysterectomy performed to control intractable postpartum hemorrhage.

### Etiology

Causes of postpartum hemorrhage include uterine atony, obstetric lacerations, retained placental tissue, and coagulation defects.

**A. Uterine Atony:** Postpartum bleeding is physiologically controlled by constriction of interlacing myometrial fibers that surround the blood vessels supplying the placental implantation site. Uterine atony exists when the myometrium cannot contract.

Atony is the most common cause of postpartum hemorrhage (50% of cases). Predisposing causes include excessive manipulation of the uterus, general anesthesia (particularly with halogenated compounds), uterine overdistention (twins or polyhydramnios), prolonged labor, grand multiparity, uterine leiomyomas, operative delivery and intrauterine manipulation, oxytocin induction or augmentation of labor, previous hemorrhage in the third stage, uterine infection, extravasation of blood into the myometrium (Couvelaire uterus), and intrinsic myometrial dysfunction.

**B. Obstetric Lacerations:** Excessive bleeding from an episiotomy, lacerations, or both cause about 20% of postpartum hemorrhages. Lacerations can involve the uterus, cervix, vagina, or vulva, and they usually result from precipitate or uncontrolled delivery or operative delivery of a large infant. However, they may occur after any delivery. Laceration of blood vessels underneath the vaginal or vulvar epithelium results in hematomas. Bleeding is concealed and can be particularly dangerous, since it may go unrecognized for several hours and only become apparent when shock occurs.

Episiotomies may cause excessive bleeding if they involve arteries or large varicosities, if the episiotomy is large, if there is a delay between episiotomy and delivery, or if there is a delay between delivery and repair of the episiotomy (Odell and Seski, 1947).

Persistent bleeding (especially bright red) and a well-contracted, firm uterus suggest bleeding from a laceration or from the episiotomy. When cervical or vaginal lacerations are identified as the source of postpartum hemorrhage, repair is best performed with adequate anesthesia.

Spontaneous rupture of the uterus is rare. Risk factors for this complication include grand multiparity, malpresentation, previous uterine surgery, and oxytocin induction of labor. Rupture of a previous cesarean section scar after vaginal delivery may be an increasingly important cause of postpartum hemorrhage.

**C. Retained Placental Tissue:** Retained placental tissue and membranes cause 5–10% of postpartum hemorrhages. Retention of placental tissue in the uterine cavity occurs in placenta accreta, in manual removal of the placenta, in mismanagement of the third stage of labor, and in unrecognized succenturiate placenta.

Lee and coworkers (1981) have used ultrasonography to visualize retained tissue in the endometrial cavity in a few cases of immediate postpartum hemorrhage. The technique is probably better used in cases of hemorrhage occurring a few hours after delivery or in late postpartum hemorrhage. Transvaginal duplex Doppler imaging is also effective in evaluating these patients (Achiron et al, 1993). These noninvasive methods of evaluation can identify retained blood clots or placental tissue. If the endometrial cavity appears empty, unnecessary dilatation and curettage may be avoided.

**D. Coagulation Defects:** Coagulopathies in pregnancy may be acquired coagulation defects seen in association with several obstetric disorders, including abruptio placentae, excess thromboplastin from a retained dead fetus, amniotic fluid embolism, severe preeclampsia, eclampsia, and sepsis (see Chapter 59). These coagulopathies may present as hypofibrinogenemia, thrombocytopenia, and disseminated intravascular coagulation. Transfusion of more than 8 U of blood may in itself induce a dilutional coagulopathy.

Von Willebrand's disease, autoimmune thrombocytopenia, and leukemia may also occur in pregnant women.

## Risk Factors

Prevention of hemorrhage is preferable to even the best treatment. All patients in labor should be evaluated for risk of postpartum hemorrhage. Risk factors include coagulopathy, hemorrhage, or blood transfusion during a previous pregnancy; anemia during labor; grand multiparity; multiple gestation; large infant; polyhydramnios; dysfunctional labor; oxytocin induction or augmentation of labor; rapid or tumultuous labor; severe preeclampsia or eclampsia; vaginal delivery after previous cesarean birth; general anesthesia for delivery; and midforceps delivery.

## Management

**A. Predelivery Preparation:** All obstetric patients should have blood typed and screened on admission. Patients identified as being at risk for postpartum hemorrhage should have their blood typed and cross-matched immediately. The blood should be reserved in the blood bank for 24 hours after delivery. A large-bore intravenous catheter should be securely taped into place after insertion. Delivery room personnel should be alerted to the risk of hemorrhage. Severely anemic patients should be transfused as soon as cross-matched blood is ready.

With increasing concerns associated with blood transfusion, autologous blood donation in obstetric patients at risk for postpartum hemorrhage has been advocated. Despite careful evaluation for risk factors, with the exception of cases of placenta previa, our ability to predict which patients will have hemorrhage and require blood transfusion remains poor; therefore, the cost of such an approach may not be justified (Andres et al, 1990; Combs et al, 1992).

**B. Delivery:** Following delivery of the infant, the uterus is massaged in a circular or back-and-forth motion until the myometrium becomes firm and well contracted. Excessive and vigorous massage of the uterus before, during, or after delivery of the placenta may interfere with normal contraction of the myometrium and instead of hastening contraction may lead to excessive postpartum blood loss.

**C. Third Stage of Labor Normal Placental Separation:** The placenta typically separates from the uterus and is delivered within 5 minutes of delivery of the infant. Attempts to speed separation are of no benefit and may cause harm. Spontaneous placental separation is impending if the uterus becomes round and firm, a sudden gush of blood comes from the vagina, the uterus seems to rise in the abdomen, and the umbilical cord moves down out of the vagina.

The placenta can then be removed from the vagina by gentle traction on the umbilical cord. Prior to placental separation, gentle steady traction on the cord combined with upward pressure on the lower uterine segment (Brandt-Andrews maneuver) ensures that the placenta can be removed as soon as separation occurs and provides a means of monitoring the consistency of the uterus. Adherent membranes can be removed by gentle traction with ring forceps. The placenta is inspected for completeness immediately after delivery.

## Manual Removal of the Placenta

Opinion is divided about the timing of manual removal of the placenta. In the presence of hemorrhage, it is obviously unreasonable to wait for spontaneous separation, and manual removal of the placenta should be undertaken without delay.

Efforts to promote routine manual removal of the placenta were often made in the past. The rationale includes shortening the third stage of labor, decreasing blood loss, developing experience in manual removal as practice for dealing with placenta accreta, and providing a way to simultaneously explore the uterus. These real or potential benefits must be weighed against the discomfort caused to the patient, the risk of infection, and the risk of causing more bleeding by interfering with normal mechanisms of placental separation.

**Technique.** The uterus is stabilized by grasping the fundus with a hand placed over the abdomen. The other hand traces the course of the umbilical cord through the vagina and cervix into the uterus to palpate the edge of the placenta. The membranes at the placental margin are perforated, and the hand is inserted between the placenta and the uterine wall, palmar side toward the placenta. The hand is then gently swept from side to side and up and down to peel the placenta from its attachments to the uterus. When the placenta has been completely separated from the uterus, it is grasped and pulled from the uterus.

The fetal and maternal sides of the placenta should be inspected to ensure that it has been removed in its entirety. On the fetal surface, incomplete placental removal is manifested as interruption of the vessels on the chorionic plate, usually shown by hemorrhage. On the maternal surface, it is possible to see where cotyledons have been detached. If there is evidence of incomplete removal, the uterus must be re-explored and any small pieces of adherent placenta removed. The uterus should be massaged until a firm myometrial tone is achieved.

## Immediate Postpartum Period

Uterotonic agents may be administered as soon as the infant's anterior shoulder is delivered, but this risks entrapment of the placenta or of an undiagnosed second twin inside a tightly contracted uterus. Oxytocin or an ergot alkaloid given later, at the time of placental separation, avoids these dangers without necessarily incurring markedly increased blood loss. Routine administration of oxytocics during the third stage reduces the blood loss of delivery and decreases the chances of postpartum hemorrhage by 40% (Elbourne et al, 1988). Oxytocin, 10–20 U/L of isotonic saline, or other intravenous solution by slow intravenous infusion or 10 U intramuscularly, can be used in every patient after delivery of the infant. Bolus administration should not be used, since large doses (> 5 U) can cause hypotension. Ergot alkaloids (eg, methylergonovine maleate, 0.2 mg intramuscularly) can also be routinely used but they are not more effective than oxytocin and pose more risk, since they may rarely cause marked hypertension. This occurs most commonly in intravenous administration or when regional anesthesia is used. Ergot alkaloids should not be used in hypertensive women or in women with cardiac disease.

## Repair of Lacerations

If bleeding is excessive before placental separation, manual removal of the placenta is indicated. Otherwise, excessive manipulation of the uterus should be avoided.

The vagina and cervix should be carefully inspected immediately after delivery of the placenta, with adequate lighting and assistants available. The episiotomy is quickly repaired after massage has produced a firm, tightly contracted uterus. A pack placed in the vagina above the episiotomy helps to keep the field dry; attaching the free end of the pack to the adjacent drapes reminds the operator to remove it after the repair is completed.

The tendency of bleeding vessels to retract from the laceration site is the reason for one of the cardinal principles of repair. Begin the repair above the highest extent of the laceration. The highest suture is also used to provide gentle traction to bring the laceration site closer to the introitus. Hemostatic ligatures are then placed in the usual manner, and the entire birth canal is carefully inspected to make sure that there are no additional bleeding sites. Extensive inspection also provides time to confirm that prior hemostatic efforts have been effective.

A cervical or vaginal laceration extending into the broad ligament should not be repaired vaginally. Laparotomy with evacuation of the resultant hematoma and hemostatic repair or hysterectomy is required.

Large or expanding hematomas of the vaginal walls require operative management for proper control. The vaginal wall is first exposed by an assistant. If a laceration accompanies the hematoma, the laceration is extended so that the hematoma can be completely evacuated and explored. When the bleeding site is identified, a large hemostatic ligature can be placed well above the site. This ensures hemostasis in the vessel, which is likely to retract when lacerated. The hematoma cavity should be left open to allow drainage of blood and ensure that bleeding will not be concealed if hemostasis cannot be achieved.

If there is no laceration in the vaginal side wall when a hematoma is identified, then an incision must be made over the hematoma to allow treatment to proceed as outlined above.

Following delivery, recovery room attendants should frequently massage the uterus and check for vaginal bleeding.

## Evaluation of Persistent Bleeding

If vaginal bleeding persists after delivery of the placenta, aggressive treatment should be initiated. It is not sufficient to perform perfunctory uterine massage, for instance, without searching for the cause of the bleeding and initiating definitive treatment. The following steps should be undertaken without delay:

(1) Manually compress the uterus.

(2) Obtain assistance.

(3) If not already done, obtain blood for typing and cross-matching.

(4) Observe blood for clotting to rule out coagulopathy.

(5) Begin fluid or blood replacement.

(6) Carefully explore the uterine cavity.

(7) Completely inspect the cervix and vagina.

(8) Insert a second intravenous catheter for administration of blood or fluids.

**D. Measures to Control Bleeding:**

**1. Manual exploration of the uterus**–The uterus should be explored immediately in women with postpartum hemorrhage. Manual exploration should also be considered after delivery of the placenta in the following circumstances: (1) when vaginal delivery follows previous cesarean section; (2) when intrauterine manipulation, eg, version and extraction, has been performed; (3) when malpresentation has occurred during labor and delivery; (4) when a premature infant has been delivered; (5) when an abnormal uterine contour has been noted prior to delivery; and (6) when there is a possibility of undiagnosed multiple pregnancy—to rule out twins.

Ensure that all placental parts have been delivered and that the uterus is intact. This should be done even in the case of a well-contracted uterus. Exploration performed for reasons other than the evaluation of hemorrhage should also confirm that the uterine wall is intact and should attempt to identify any possible intrauterine structural abnormalities. Manual exploration of the uterus does not increase febrile morbidity, blood loss, or the incidence of asymptomatic bacteriuria postpartum (Berger et al, 1981; Blanchette, 1977).

**Technique.** Place a fresh glove over the glove on the exploring hand. Form the hand into a cone and gently introduce it by firm pressure through the cervix while the fundus is stabilized with the other hand. Sweep the backs of the first and second fingers across the entire surface of the uterus, beginning at the fundus. In the lower uterine segment, palpate the walls with the palmar surface of one finger. Uterine lacerations will be felt as an obvious anatomic defect. All exploration should be gentle, since the postpartum uterus is easily perforated.

Uterine rupture detected by manual exploration in the presence of postpartum hemorrhage requires immediate laparotomy. A decision to repair the defect or proceed with hysterectomy is made on the basis of the extent of the rupture, the patient's desire for future childbearing, and the degree of the patient's clinical deterioration.

**2. Bimanual compression and massage**–The most important step in controlling atonic postpartum hemorrhage is immediate bimanual uterine compression, which may have to be continued for 20–30 minutes or more. Fluid replacement should begin as soon as a secure intravenous line is in place. Typed and cross-matched blood is given when it is available. Manual compression of the uterus will control virtually all cases of hemorrhage due to uterine atony, retained products of conception, and coagulopathies, and it may even control bleeding from a lacerated cervix.

**Technique.** Place a hand on the patient's abdomen and grasp the uterine fundus; bring it down over the symphysis pubis. Insert the other hand into the vagina and place the first and second fingers on either side of the cervix and push it cephalad and anteriorly. The pulsating uterine arteries should be felt by the fingertips. Massage the uterus with both hands while compression is maintained. Prolonged compression (20–30 minutes) may be required but is almost always successful in controlling bleeding.

Insert a Foley catheter into the bladder during compression and massage, since vigorous fluid and blood replacement will cause diuresis. A distended bladder will interfere with compression and massage, contribute to the patient's discomfort, and may itself be a major contributor to uterine atony.

**3. Curettage**–Curettage of a large, soft postpartum uterus can be a formidable undertaking, since the risk of perforation is high and the procedure commonly results in increased rather than decreased bleeding. The suction curet, even with a large cannula, covers only a small area of the postpartum uterus, and its size and shape increase the likelihood of perforation. A large blunt curet, the "banjo" curet, is probably the safest instrument for curettage of the postpartum uterus. It may be used when manual exploration fails to remove fragments of adherent placenta.

Curettage should be delayed unless bleeding cannot be controlled by compression and massage alone. Overly vigorous puerperal curettage can result in focal complete removal of the endometrium, particularly if the uterus is infected, with subsequent healing characterized by formation of adhesions and **Asherman's syndrome** (amenorrhea and secondary sterility due to intrauterine adhesions and uterine synechiae). If circumstances permit, ultrasonic evaluation of the postpartum uterus may distinguish those patients who will benefit from curettage from those who should be managed without it.

**4. Uterine packing**–Although once widely used for control of obstetric hemorrhage, uterine packing is no longer favored. The uterus may expand to considerable size after delivery of the placenta, thus accommodating both a large volume of packing material and a large volume of blood. The technique also demands considerable technical expertise.

**5. Uterotonic agents**–Oxytocin 20–40 U/L of crystalloid should be infused, if not already running, at a rate of 10–15 mL/minute. Methylergonovine, 0.2

mg, can be given intramuscularly, but is contraindicated if the patient is hypertensive. Intramyometrial injection of prostaglandin $F_{2\alpha}$ ($PGF_{2\alpha}$) to control bleeding was initially described in 1976 (Corson and Bolognese, 1977). Intravaginal or rectal prostaglandin suppositories, intrauterine irrigation with prostaglandins, and intramyometrial injection of prostaglandins have also been reported to control hemorrhage from uterine atony. Intramuscular administration of 15-methylprostaglandin analog was successful in treating 85% of patients with postpartum hemorrhage due to atony (Buttino and Garite, 1986; Hayashi et al, 1984). Failures in these series occurred in women who had uterine infections or unrecognized placenta accreta. Side effects are usually minimal, but may include transient oxygen desaturation, bronchospasm, and, rarely, significant hypertension (Hankins et al, 1988; Toppozada et al, 1981).

**6. Radiographic embolization of pelvic vessels**–Embolization of pelvic and uterine vessels by angiographic techniques has controlled otherwise intractable hemorrhage in 37 of 38 cases reported (Alvarez et al, 1992). In institutions with trained interventional radiologists, it is certainly worth considering in women of low parity as an alternative to hysterectomy. With the patient under local anesthesia, a catheter is placed in the aorta and fluoroscopy is used to identify the bleeding vessel. Pieces of absorbable gelatin sponge (Gelfoam) are injected into the damaged vessel, or into the internal iliac vessels if no specific site of bleeding can be identified. If bleeding continues, further embolization can be performed. This technique has the advantage of being effective even when the cause of hemorrhage is extrauterine and in the presence or absence of uterine atony. Many authors recommend embolization before internal iliac ligation, because ligation obstructs the access route for angiography. Adequate recanalization occurs to maintain fertility.

**7. Operative management**–The patient's wishes regarding further childbearing should be made clear as soon as laparotomy is contemplated for the management of postpartum hemorrhage. If the patient's wishes cannot be ascertained, the operator should assume that the childbearing function is to be retained. Whenever possible, the spouse or family members should also be consulted prior to laparotomy.

**a. Pressure occlusion of the aorta**–Immediate temporary control of pelvic bleeding may be obtained at laparotomy by pressure occlusion of the aorta, which will provide valuable time to treat hypotension, obtain experienced assistants, identify the source of bleeding, and plan the operative procedure. In the young and otherwise healthy patient, pressure occlusion can be maintained for several minutes without permanent sequelae.

**b. Uterine artery ligation**–During pregnancy, 90% of the blood flow to the uterus is supplied by the uterine arteries. Direct ligation of these easily accessible vessels can successfully control hemorrhage in 75–90% of cases (Fahmy, 1987; O'Leary and O'Leary, 1974), particularly when the bleeding is uterine in origin. Recanalization can occur and subsequent pregnancies have been reported.

**Technique.** The uterus is lifted upward and away from the side to be ligated. Absorbable suture on a large needle is placed around the ascending uterine artery and vein on one side of the uterus, passing through the myometrium 2–4 cm medial to the vessels and through the avascular area of the broad ligament. The suture includes the myometrium to fix the suture and to avoid tearing the vessels. The same procedure is then performed on the opposite side. If the ligation is performed during cesarean section, the sutures can be placed just below the uterine incision under the bladder flap. It is not necessary to mobilize the bladder otherwise. Bilateral ovarian artery ligation can also be performed in an attempt to reduce blood flow to the uterus. This should be performed with absorbable suture near the point of anastomoses between the ovarian artery and the ascending uterine artery at the utero-ovarian ligament (Cruikshank and Stoelk, 1983).

**c. Internal iliac artery ligation**—Bilateral internal iliac (hypogastric) artery ligation is the surgical method most often used to control severe postpartum bleeding (Fig 28–1). Exposure can be difficult, particularly in the presence of a large boggy uterus or hematoma. Failure rates of this technique can range as high as 57% (Evans and McShane, 1985), but may be related to the skill of the operator, the cause of the hemorrhage, and the patient's condition before ligation is attempted.

**Technique.** The peritoneum lateral to the infundibulopelvic ligament is incised parallel with the ligament, or the round ligament is transected. In either case, the peritoneum to which the ureter will adhere is dissected medially, which removes the ureter from the operative field. The pararectal space is then enlarged by blunt dissection. The internal iliac artery on the lateral side of the space is isolated and doubly ligated (but not cut) with silk ligatures at its origin from the common iliac artery. The operator must be careful not to tear the adjacent thin veins. Blood flow distally to the uterus, cervix, and upper vagina is not occluded, but the pulse pressure is sufficiently diminished to allow hemostasis to occur by in situ thrombosis. Fertility is preserved, and subsequent pregnancies are not compromised.

**d. Hysterectomy**—Hysterectomy is the definitive method of controlling postpartum hemorrhage. Simple hemostatic repair of a ruptured uterus with or without tubal ligation in a woman of high parity or in poor condition for more extensive surgery may be preferred unless she has intercurrent uterine disease. The procedure is undoubtedly lifesaving.

**8. Blood replacement**–Blood and fluid replacement are required for successful management of

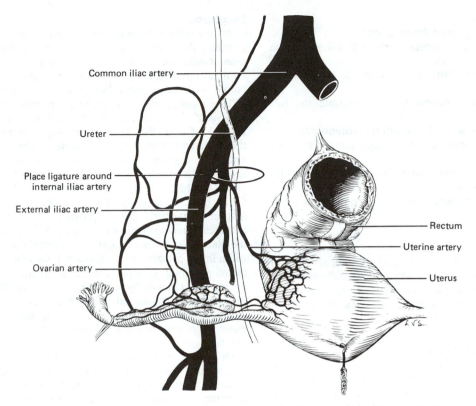

**Figure 28–1.** Location of ligatures for right internal iliac (hypogastric) artery ligation.

postpartum hemorrhage. In patients with severe hemorrhage, massive transfusions may be necessary. Component therapy is advocated, with transfusion of packed cells, platelets, fresh frozen plasma, and cryoprecipitate when indicated. Blood products should be obtained and given without delay when needed, since postponing transfusion may only contribute to the development of disseminated intravascular coagulation. Nolan and Gallup (1991) recently reviewed the approach to and management of massive transfusion in obstetric patients.

**E. Management of Delayed Postpartum Hemorrhage:** Delayed postpartum hemorrhage (bleeding 2 weeks or more after delivery) is almost always due to subinvolution of the placental bed. Involution of the placental site is normally delayed when compared with that of the rest of the endometrium, but for unknown reasons, in subinvolution, the adjacent endometrium and the decidua basalis have not regenerated to cover the placental implantation site. The involutional processes of thrombosis and hyalinization have failed to occur in the underlying blood vessels, so that bleeding may occur with only minimal trauma or other (unknown) stimuli. Although the cause of subinvolution is unknown, faulty placental implantation, implantation in the poorly vascularized lower uterine segment, and persistent in-

fection at the implantation site have been suggested as possible factors. Delayed postpartum hemorrhage is seldom due to retained placental tissue.

Because late postpartum bleeding is due to subinvolution of the implantation site, curettage is not likely to result in decreased uterine bleeding. Uterine compression and bimanual massage, as previously described, controls this type of bleeding, but it may be necessary to continue compression and massage for 30–45 minutes or longer.

Broad-spectrum antibiotics should be started when resuscitation allows. Oxytocin, 10 U intramuscularly every 4 hours or 10–20 u/L intravenous solution by slow continuous infusion, 15-methyl $PGF_{2\alpha}$ (Prostin 15M), 0.25 mg intramuscularly every 2 hours or ergot alkaloids, eg, methylergonovine maleate, 0.2 mg orally every 6 hours, should be administered for at least 48 hours.

## PLACENTA ACCRETA

A layer of decidua normally separates the placental villi and the myometrium at the site of placental implantation. A placenta that directly adheres to the myometrium without an intervening decidual layer is termed placenta accreta.

## Classification

### A. By Degree of Adherence:

**1. Placenta accreta vera**–Villi adhere to the superficial myometrium.

**2. Placenta increta**–Villi invade the myometrium.

**3. Placenta percreta**–Villi penetrate the full thickness of the myometrium.

### B. By Amount of Placental Involvement:

**1. Focal adherence**–A single cotyledon is involved.

**2. Partial adherence**–One or several cotyledons are involved.

**3. Total adherence**–The entire placenta is involved.

## Incidence

Estimates of the incidence of placenta accreta (all forms) vary from 1 in 2000 to 1 in 7000 deliveries. Placenta accreta vera accounts for about 80% of abnormally adherent placentas; placenta increta, 15%; and placenta percreta, 5%.

## Morbidity & Mortality

The immediate morbidity associated with an abnormally adherent placenta is that associated with any type of postpartum hemorrhage. Massive blood loss and hypotension can occur. Intrauterine manipulation necessary to diagnose and treat placenta accreta may result in uterine perforation and infection. Sterility may occur as a result of hysterectomy performed to control bleeding.

Recurrence may be common with lesser degrees of adherence.

## Etiology

Both excessive penetrability of the trophoblast and defective or missing decidua basalis have been suggested as causes of placenta accreta. Histologic examination of the placental implantation site usually demonstrates the absence of the decidua and Nitabuch's layer. Cases of placenta accreta have been seen in the first trimester, suggesting that the process may occur at the time of implantation and not later in gestation.

Although the exact cause is unknown, several clinical situations are associated with placenta accreta, eg, previous cesarean section, placenta previa, grand multiparity, previous uterine curettage, and previously treated Asherman's syndrome.

These conditions share a common possible defect in formation of the decidua basalis. The incidence of placenta accreta in the presence of a placenta previa after 1 previous uterine incision is 24%, after 2 is 48%, and after 4 is 67% (Clark et al, 1985). The incidence of placenta accreta after successful treatment of Asherman's syndrome is 8% (Schenker and Margalioth, 1982).

## Diagnosis

Adverse effects from placenta accreta in pregnancy or during the course of labor and delivery are uncommon. Rarely, intra-abdominal hemorrhage or placental invasion of adjacent organs prior to labor has occurred, with the diagnosis being made at laparotomy.

Tabsh and coworkers (1982) have reported the diagnosis of placenta increta prior to delivery based on the lack of a sonolucent area normally seen beneath the implantation site during ultrasonographic examination. More recently, sonographic antenatal diagnosis of the less invasive placental accreta has been reported (Finberg and Williams, 1992; Guy et al, 1990). Color Doppler imaging appears to be particularly helpful in diagnosis. The diagnosis is more often established when no plane of cleavage is found between the placenta or parts of the placenta and the myometrium in the presence of postpartum hemorrhage. Retained placental parts prevent the myometrium from contracting and thereby achieving hemostasis. Bleeding can be brisk. Inspection of the already separated placenta shows that portions are missing, and manual exploration may produce additional placental fragments.

Delayed spontaneous separation of the placenta is also an indication of an unusually adherent placenta. Focal or partial involvement may be manifested as difficulty in establishing a cleavage plane during manual removal of the placenta. Removal of a totally adherent placenta is very difficult. Persistent efforts to manually remove a totally adherent placenta are futile and waste time, and they result in even more blood loss. Preparation for hysterectomy should begin as soon as the diagnosis is suspected.

## Management

Fluid and blood replacement should begin as soon as excessive blood loss is diagnosed. It may be necessary to insert a second large-bore intravenous catheter. Evaluation of puerperal hemorrhage should be performed as outlined above.

Conservative treatment of placenta accreta in women of low parity has occasionally succeeded. The placenta (or portions of it) is left in situ if bleeding is minimal and will later slough off. Successful subsequent pregnancies have been reported, although the risk of recurrence of placenta accreta may be high. In up to 72% of cases of placenta accreta, particularly those associated with placenta-previa, hysterectomy is required (Clark et al, 1985).

Successful conservative treatment of placenta percreta is rare, but the conservative approach may be a reasonable option if only focal defects are present, blood loss is not excessive, and the patient is interested in preserving fertility (Cox et al, 1988). However, additional resection of adjacent organs, such as partial cystectomy, may be necessary in placenta percreta, and the condition has a high perinatal mortality rate (96%) in the cases reported.

## UTERINE INVERSION

### Definition

Uterine inversion is the prolapse of the fundus to or through the cervix so that the uterus is in effect turned inside out. Almost all cases of uterine inversion occur after delivery and may be worsened by excess traction on the cord before placental separation. Nonpuerperal uterine inversion is very rare and is usually associated with tumors (eg, polypoid leiomyomas).

### Classification

If the uterus is inverted but does not protrude through the cervix, the inversion is incomplete. In complete inversion, the fundus has prolapsed through the cervix. Occasionally, the entire uterus may prolapse out the vagina.

Puerperal inversion has also been classified on the basis of its duration. Acute inversion occurs immediately after delivery and before the cervix constricts. Once the cervix constricts, the inversion is termed subacute. Chronic inversion is noted more than 4 weeks after delivery. Today, nearly all cases of uterine inversion are of the acute variety and are recognized and treated immediately after delivery.

### Incidence

The incidence of uterine inversion has varied in series reported within the past 30 years from 1 in 4000 to 1 in 100,000 deliveries; an incidence of 1 in 20,000 is frequently cited. One worker reported no inversions in over 10,000 personally conducted deliveries. More recent reviews indicate a greater incidence of uterine inversion, approximately 1 in 2000–2500 deliveries (Read et al, 1980; Watson et al, 1980).

### Morbidity & Mortality

The morbidity and mortality associated with uterine inversion correlate with the degree of hemorrhage, the rapidity of diagnosis, and the effectiveness of treatment.

The immediate morbidity is that associated with any postpartum hemorrhage; however, endomyometritis frequently follows uterine inversion. The intestines and uterine appendages may be injured if they are entrapped by the prolapsed uterine fundus. Death has occurred from uterine inversion, although with prompt recognition, definitive treatment, and vigorous resuscitation, the mortality rate in this condition should be quite low.

### Etiology

The exact cause of uterine inversion is unknown, and the condition is not always preventable. The cervix must be dilated and the uterine fundus must be relaxed for inversion to occur. Rapid uterine emptying may contribute to uterine relaxation.

Conditions that may predispose women to uterine inversion include fundal implantation of the placenta, abnormal adherence of the placenta (partial placenta accreta), congenital or acquired weakness of the myometrium, uterine anomalies, protracted labor, previous uterine inversion, intrapartum therapy with magnesium sulfate, strong traction exerted on the umbilical cord, and fundal pressure.

Many cases of uterine inversion result from mismanagement of the third stage of labor in women who are already at risk for developing uterine inversion. The following maneuvers are to be avoided: excessive traction on the umbilical cord, excessive fundal pressure, excessive intra-abdominal pressure, and excessively vigorous manual removal of the placenta.

### Diagnosis

The diagnosis of uterine inversion is usually obvious. Shock and hemorrhage are prominent, as well as considerable pain. A dark red-blue bleeding mass is palpable and often visible at the cervix, in the vagina, or outside the vagina. A depression in the uterine fundus or even an absent fundus is noted on abdominal examination.

### Treatment

Successful management of patients with uterine inversion depends on prompt recognition and treatment. If initial measures fail to relieve the condition, it may progress to the point at which operative treatment or even hysterectomy is necessary. Shock associated with uterine inversion is typically profound. Hemorrhage can be massive, and hypovolemia should be vigorously treated with fluid and blood replacement.

**A. Manual Repositioning of the Uterus:** Treatment should begin as soon as the diagnosis of uterine inversion is made. Assistance is vital. An initial attempt should be made to reposition the fundus. The inverted fundus, along with the placenta if it is still attached, is slowly and steadily pushed upward in the axis of the uterus (Fig 28–2). If the placenta has not separated, do not remove it until an adequate intravenous infusion has been established.

If the initial attempt fails, induce general anesthesia, preferably with a halogenated agent (eg, halothane) to provide uterine relaxation. Tocolytics may be useful in producing uterine relaxation, particularly in subacute cases. Either intravenous magnesium sulfate or Terbutaline, 0.25 mg given as a bolus dose intravenously, has been successfully used to achieve uterine relaxation in subacute inversion and neither has been associated with bleeding (Catanzarite et al, 1986).

**Technique.** The operator's fist is placed on the uterine fundus, and the fundus is gradually pushed back into the pelvis through the dilated cervix. The general anesthetic or uterine relaxant is then discontinued. Infusion of oxytocin or ergot alkaloids is started and fluid and blood replacement continued. Alternatively, prostaglandins may be used to effect

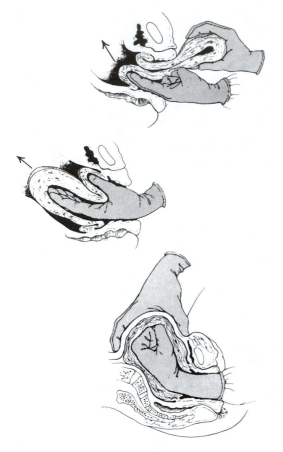

**Figure 28–2.** Replacement of an inverted uterus.

uterine contraction after repositioning. Bimanual uterine compression and massage are maintained until the uterus is well contracted and hemorrhage has ceased. The placenta can then be removed.

Antibiotics should be started as soon is as practical. Oxytocics or ergot alkaloids are continued for at least 24 hours. Frequent determinations of the hematocrit should be made to ascertain the need for further blood replacement. Iron supplements should begin with resumption of oral intake.

**B. Surgical Repositioning of the Uterus:** Surgical repositioning of the uterus is rarely necessary in contemporary medical practice in the USA. However, when all other efforts have failed to reposition the everted uterus, operative intervention may be lifesaving. This is generally accomplished by a vertical incision through the lower uterine segment directly posterior. The uterus is repositioned by either pulling from above or, very rarely, pushing from below (using a sterile glove). The incision is then repaired as would be any uterine incision. Blood replacement, antibiotics, and careful monitoring are necessary for successful perioperative management.

# ABNORMALITIES OF THE PUERPERIUM

When compared with the dramatic and climactic events of delivery, the puerperium may seem uneventful. Nevertheless, significant physiologic changes occur during this interval, and these undoubtedly influence many of the problems that often arise rapidly and without warning. Hypotension and shock demand urgent treatment and careful follow-up. Cardiac monitoring and insertion of Swan-Ganz or central venous pressure catheters may be prudent to permit rapid evaluation of hemodynamic status. Appropriate medical and surgical consultation is also recommended.

## POSTPARTUM & PUERPERAL INFECTIONS

Infections are among the most prominent puerperal complications. An improved understanding of the natural history of female genital infections and the availability of powerful antibiotics may have produced a complacent attitude toward puerperal infections that is as yet unrealistic. Postpartum infections are still costly to both patients and society, and they are associated with an admittedly small but not negligible threat of serious disability and death.

Puerperal morbidity due to infection has occurred if the patient's temperature is higher than 38°C (100.4°F) on 2 separate occasions at least 24 hours apart following the first 24 hours after delivery. Overt infections can and do occur in the absence of these criteria, but fever of some degree remains the hallmark of puerperal infection, and the patient with fever can be assumed to have a genital infection until proved otherwise.

### Incidence

Puerperal infectious morbidity affects 2–8% of pregnant women and is more common in those of low socioeconomic status, those who have undergone operative delivery, those with premature rupture of the membranes, those with long labors, and those with multiple pelvic examinations.

### Morbidity & Mortality

Postpartum infections are responsible for much of the morbidity associated with childbirth, and they either are directly responsible for or contribute to the death of about 8% of all pregnant women who die each year. The costs are also considerable, not only in additional days of hospitalization and medications but also in time lost from work.

Sterility may result from the sequelae of postpartum infections, eg, periadnexal adhesions. Hysterectomy is occasionally required in patients with serious postpartum or postoperative infection.

## Pathogenesis

The flora of the birth canal of pregnant women is essentially the same as that of nonpregnant women, although variations in culture techniques and in the study populations have produced markedly different results. The vaginal flora typically includes aerobic and anaerobic organisms that are commonly considered pathogenic (Table 28–1). Several mechanisms appear to prevent overt infection in the genital tract, eg, the acidity of the normal vagina; thick, tenacious cervical mucus; and maternal antibodies to most vaginal flora.

During labor and particularly after rupture of the membranes, some of these protective mechanisms are no longer present. Examinations and invasive monitoring apparatus probably facilitate the introduction of vaginal bacteria into the uterine cavity. Bacteria can be cultured from the amniotic fluid of most women undergoing intrauterine pressure monitoring, but overt postpartum infection is seen in fewer than 10% of these cases (Listwa et al, 1976). Contractions during labor may spread bacteria present in the amniotic cavity to the adjacent uterine lymphatics and even into the bloodstream.

**Table 28–1.** Percentage of organisms isolated from the vagina or cervix in normal pregnant and nonpregnant women.

| Organism | Percentage Isolated |
|---|---|
| **Aerobic bacteria** | |
| *Lactobacillus* | 17–97 |
| Diphtheroids | 14–83 |
| *Staphylococcus epidermidis* | 7–67 |
| *Staphylococcus aureus* | 0–12 |
| Alpha-hemolytic streptococci | 2–53 |
| Beta-hemolytic streptococci | 0–93 |
| Nonhemolytic streptococci | 4–37 |
| Group D streptococci | 4–44 |
| *Escherichia coli* | 0–28 |
| *Gardnerella vaginalis* | 40–43 |
| *Neisseria gonorrhoeae* | 1–7 |
| *Mycoplasma* | 15–72 |
| *Ureaplasma* | 40–95 |
| **Anaerobic bacteria** | |
| *Lactobacillus* | 11–72 |
| *Bacteroides fragilis* | 0–20 |
| *Bacteroides* species | 0–50 |
| *Fusobacterium* species | 0–18 |
| *Peptococcus* species | 0–71 |
| *Peptostreptococcus* species | 12–40 |
| *Veillonella* species | 0–27 |
| *Clostridium* species | 0–17 |
| *Bifidobacterium* species | 0–32 |
| *Eubacterium* species | 0–36 |

(Reproduced and modified, with permission, from Sweet RL: Perinatal infections: Bacteriology, diagnosis, and management. In: *Principles & Practice of Obstetrics & Perinatology*, 1981. Iffy L, Kaminetzky HA (editors). Copyright © 1981. Reprinted by permission of John Wiley & Sons, Inc.)

The postpartum uterus is initially devoid of mechanisms that keep it sterile, and bacteria may be recovered from the uterus in nearly all women in the postpartum period. Whether or not disease is clinically expressed depends on the presence of predisposing factors, the duration of uterine contamination, and the type and amount of microorganisms involved. The necrosis of decidua and other intrauterine contents (lochia) promotes an increase in the number of anaerobic bacteria, heretofore limited by lack of suitable nutrients and other factors necessary for growth.

Sterility of the endometrial cavity returns by the third or fourth postpartum week. Granulocytes that penetrate the endometrial cavity and the open drainage of lochia are effective in preventing infection in most patients.

## Etiology

Almost all postpartum infections are caused by bacteria normally present in the genitalia of pregnant women. The lochia is an excellent culture medium for organisms ascending from the vagina. In women who have undergone cesarean section, more devitalized tissue and foreign bodies (sutures) are present, providing additional fertile ground for possible contamination and subsequent infection. About 70% of puerperal soft tissue infections are mixed infections consisting of both aerobic and anaerobic organisms; infections occurring in women undergoing cesarean section are more likely to be serious.

## General Evaluation

The source of infection should be identified, the likely cause determined, and the severity assessed. Most women with fever in the postpartum period have endometritis. Urinary tract infection is the next most common infection. Neglected or virulent endomyometritis may progress to more serious infection. Generalized sepsis, septic pelvic thrombophlebitis, or pelvic abscess may be the end result of an initial infection of the endometrial cavity.

## 1. ENDOMETRITIS

### Etiology

All of the following circumstances have led to higher than normal postpartum infection rates: prolonged rupture of the membranes (> 24 hours), chorioamnionitis, excessive number of digital vaginal examinations, prolonged labor (> 12 hours), toxemia, intrauterine pressure catheters (> 8 hours), fetal scalp electrode monitoring, preexisting vaginitis or cervicitis, operative vaginal deliveries, cesarean section, intrapartum and postpartum anemia, poor nutrition, obesity, low socioeconomic status, and coitus near term.

Cesarean section and low socioeconomic class are consistently associated with higher rates of postpartum infection, and cesarean section is easily the most common identifiable risk factor for development of puerperal infection. Some series report an infection rate of 40–80% following cesarean section delivery. Postpartum infection is more likely to be serious after cesarean section than after vaginal delivery.

## Clinical Findings

**A. Symptoms and Signs:** Fever and a soft, tender uterus are the most prominent signs of endometritis. The lochia may or may not have a foul odor. Leukocytosis (white blood cell count > 10,000/μL) is seen. In more severe disease, high fever, malaise, abdominal tenderness, ileus, hypotension, and generalized sepsis may be seen. Movement of the uterus causes increased pain.

**1. Fever–**Although it is true that the puerperium is a period of high metabolic activity, this factor should not raise the temperature above 37.2°C (99°F) and then only briefly in the first 24 hours postpartum. Modest temperature elevations may occur with dehydration. Any woman with a fever over 38°C (100.4°F) at any time in the puerperium should be evaluated.

Endometritis results in temperatures ranging from 38°C to over 40°C (100.4°F to over 104°F), depending on the patient, the causative microorganism, and the extent of infection. The lower range of temperatures is more common. Endometritis usually develops on the second or third postpartum day. Early fever (within hours of delivery) and hypotension are almost pathognomonic for infection with beta-hemolytic streptococci.

**2. Uterine tenderness–**The uterus is soft and exquisitely tender. Motion of the cervix and uterus may cause increased pain.

Abdominal tenderness is generally limited to the lower abdomen and does not lateralize. A carefully performed baseline examination should include an adnexal evaluation. Adnexal masses palpable on abdominal or pelvic examination are not seen in uncomplicated endometritis, but tubo-ovarian abscess may be a later complication of an infection originally confined to the uterus. Bowel sounds may be decreased and the abdomen distended and tympanitic.

Pelvic examination confirms the findings disclosed by abdominal examination.

**B. Laboratory Findings:**

**1. Hematologic findings–**Leukocytosis is a normal finding during labor and the immediate puerperal period. White blood cell counts may be as high as 20,000/μL in the absence of infection; higher counts may thus be anticipated in infection. Bacteremia is present in 5–30% of women with uncomplicated endometritis (Sorrell et al, 1981). *Mycoplasma* is also frequently recovered from the blood of patients with postpartum fever (Eschenbach et al, 1982). Infections with *Bacteroides* as the predominant organism are frequently associated with positive blood cultures.

**2. Urinalysis–**Urinalysis should be routinely performed in patients thought to have endometritis, since urinary tract infections are often associated with a clinical picture similar to that of mild endometritis. If pyuria and bacteria are noted in a properly collected specimen, appropriate antibiotic therapy for urinary tract infections should be started and a portion of the specimen sent for culture.

**3. Lochia cultures–**Bacteria colonizing the cervical canal and ectocervix can almost always be recovered from lochia cultures, but these may not be the same organisms causing endometritis. Accurate cultures can be achieved only if specimens obtained transcervically are free from vaginal contamination. Material should be obtained using a speculum to allow direct visualization of the cervix and a gloved culture device (a swab that is covered while it is passed through a contaminated area, then uncovered to obtain a culture from the desired area). Transabdominal aspiration of uterine contents does secure an uncontaminated specimen, but routine use of this technique is probably not justified, and confirmation of placement within the uterine cavity may be difficult. Unless special means are taken to prevent cervical contamination and to ensure the recovery of anaerobic species, results of lochia cultures must be interpreted with great care.

**4. Bacteriologic findings–**Although the organisms responsible for puerperal infections vary considerably from hospital to hospital, most puerperal infections are due to anaerobic streptococci, gram-negative coliforms, *Bacteroides* species, and aerobic streptococci. *Chlamydia* and *Mycoplasma* are also implicated in many postpartum infections, but clinical isolates are rare because of the difficulty in culturing these organisms. Gonococci are recovered in varying degrees. The percentage of representative microorganisms recovered from women with endometritis is set forth in Table 28–2.

Patterns of bacterial isolates in puerperal infections in the patient's hospital are more important in guiding selection of appropriate antibiotics than are studies from the literature.

**a. Aerobic bacteria–**Group A streptococci are no longer a major cause of postpartum infection, but infection with these organisms still occurs occasionally. If more than an isolated instance of infection due to these streptococci occurs, immediate measures should be taken to halt a potential epidemic. Penicillin is highly effective.

In as many as 30% of women with clinically recognized endometritis, group B streptococci are partly or wholly responsible for the infection. Classic presenting signs are high fever and hypotension shortly after delivery. However, group B streptococci are commonly recovered from the vaginas of pregnant women whether or not they have endometritis. Why some women with positive cultures develop serious illness whereas others do not undoubtedly depends on the

**Table 28–2.** Percentage of organisms recovered from women with postpartum endomyometritis.

| Organism | Percentage Isolated |
|---|---|
| **Aerobic bacteria** | |
| Group A streptococci | 2–6 |
| Group B streptococci | 6–21 |
| Group D streptococci | 3–14 |
| *Enterococcus* | 12–21 |
| Other streptococci | 32 |
| *Staphylococcus epidermidis* | 28 |
| *Staphylococcus aureus* | 10 |
| *Escherichia coli* | 13–36 |
| Gonococci | 1–40 |
| *Gardnerella vaginalis* | 16 |
| **Anaerobic bacteria** | |
| *Bacteroides fragilis* | 19–75 |
| *Bacteroides* species | 17–100 |
| *Peptococcus* | 4–40 |
| *Peptostreptococcus* | 15–54 |
| *Veillonella* species | 10 |
| *Clostridium* species | 4–32 |

presence of predisposing factors as well as other, as yet unknown, elements. It is interesting that positive cultures in women do not correlate well with incidence of streptococcal infection in their newborns. Penicillin is the treatment of choice for patients with endometritis.

Group D streptococci, which include *S faecalis,* are common isolates in endometritis. Ampicillin in high doses is the treatment of choice. Aminoglycosides are also effective against this group.

*Staphylococcus aureus* is not commonly seen in cultures from women with postpartum infections of the uterus. *S epidermidis* is frequently recovered from women with postpartum infections. These organisms are typically not seen in pure culture. When established staphylococcal infections require treatment, nafcillin, cloxacillin, or cephalosporins should be used.

Among the gram-negative aerobic organisms likely to be recovered in postpartum uterine infections, *Escherichia coli* is the most common. In postpartum uterine infections, *E coli* is more likely to be isolated from seriously ill patients, whereas in urinary tract infections, it is the most commonly isolated organism but is not necessarily found in the sickest patients. Hospital-acquired *E coli* is most susceptible to aminoglycosides and cephalosporins.

The incidence of *Neisseria gonorrhoeae* is 2–8% in pregnant women antepartum. Unless repeat screening examinations and treatment of patients with positive cultures are undertaken in women near term, the incidence of asymptomatic endocervical gonorrhea at delivery is probably only slightly less, and it is reasonable to believe that some cases of puerperal endometritis are gonococcal in origin.

*Gardnerella vaginalis,* a cause of vaginitis, is seen in isolates from women with postpartum infections, usually in those with a polymicrobial cause, although pure isolates have been reported.

Other gram-negative bacilli that are commonly encountered on medical and surgical wards (eg, *Klebsiella pneumoniae, Enterobacter, Proteus,* and *Pseudomonas* species) are uncommon causes of endometritis.

**b. Anaerobic bacteria**—Anaerobic bacteria are involved in puerperal infections of the uterus in at least 50% and perhaps as many as 95% of cases. They are much less commonly seen in urinary tract infections. Anaerobic peptostreptococci and peptococci are commonly recovered in specimens from women with postpartum infection, particularly with other anaerobic species. Clindamycin, chloramphenicol, and the newer cephalosporins are active against these organisms.

*Bacteroides* species and in particular *B fragilis* are commonly found in mixed puerperal infections. These are likely to be the more serious infections (eg, puerperal pelvic abscess, cesarean section wound infections, and septic pelvic thrombophlebitis). When infection with this organism is suspected or confirmed, clindamycin, chloramphenicol, or third-generation cephalosporins should be used.

Gram-positive anaerobic organisms are represented only by *Clostridium perfringens,* which is not infrequently isolated from an infected uterus but which is a rare cause of puerperal infection.

**c. Other organisms**—*Mycoplasma* and *Ureaplasma* species are common genital pathogens that have been isolated from the genital tract and blood of postpartum women both with and without overt infection. These pathogens are frequently found in the presence of other bacteria. The role of these organisms in puerperal infections is unknown.

*Chlamydia trachomatis* is now thought to be the leading cause of pelvic inflammatory disease in some populations. Since the population most at risk for pelvic inflammatory disease is the same as that most likely to become pregnant, it is not surprising that *Chlamydia* is in some way involved in puerperal infections, but it is infrequently isolated as a cause of early postpartum endometritis. *Chlamydia* is more frequently associated with mild late-onset endometritis, so cultures for this organism should be obtained from patients with endometritis diagnosed several days after delivery. *Chlamydia* is difficult to culture, and it is possible that as more effective culture techniques become available, the place of this organism in the morbidity associated with postpartum infections may be clarified.

## Differential Diagnosis

In the immediate postpartum period, involuntary chills are common and are not necessarily an indication of overt infection. Lower abdominal pain is also common as the uterus undergoes involution with continuing contractions.

Extragenital infections are much less common than endometritis and urinary tract infections. Most of them can be effectively ruled out by history and examination alone. Patients should be asked, at a minimum, about coughing, chest pain, pain at the insertion site of intravenous catheters, breast tenderness, and leg pain. Examination of the breasts, chest, intravenous catheter insertion site, and leg veins should determine whether these areas might be the source of the postpartum fever. Chest x-rays are rarely of benefit unless signs and symptoms point to a possible pulmonary cause of the fever.

## Treatment

The choice of antibiotics for treatment of endometritis depends on the suspected causative organisms and the severity of the disease. If the illness is serious enough to require antibiotics, initial therapy should use intravenous antibiotics in high doses. Factors reinforcing the need for this approach include the large volume of the uterus, the expanded maternal blood volume, the brisk diuresis associated with the puerperium, and the difficulty of achieving adequate tissue concentrations of the antibiotic distal to the thrombosed myometrial blood vessels. Clindamycin plus an aminoglycoside is a standard first-line regimen. Single-agent therapy with second- or third-generation cephalosporins is an acceptable alternative.

The response to therapy should be carefully monitored for 24–48 hours. Deterioration or failure to respond both clinically and on laboratory test results requires a complete reevaluation. Ampicillin is added when the patient has a less than adequate response to the usual regimen, particularly if *Enterococcus* species are suspected.

Intravenous antibiotics are continued until the patient has been afebrile for 24–48 hours (Duff, 1986; Morales et al, 1989). Randomized and prospective trials have shown that additional treatment with oral antibiotics after intravenous therapy is unnecessary (Dinsmoor et al, 1991). Patients with documented concurrent bacteremia can be treated similarly, unless the patient has persistently positive blood cultures or a staphylococcal species cultured. If the patient remains febrile despite the standard antibiotic regimens, further evaluation should be initiated to look for abscess formation, hematomas, wound infection, and septic pelvic thrombophlebitis.

For patients known to be infected or at extremely high risk for infection at the time of delivery, initial therapy with 2- or 3-drug regimens in which one of the agents is clindamycin is prudent. Single-agent intravenous infusion of broad-spectrum agents such as piperacillin or cefoxitin appear to be equally effective.

## 2. URINARY TRACT INFECTION

About 2–4% of women develop a urinary tract infection postpartum. Following delivery, the bladder and lower urinary tract remain somewhat hypotonic, and residual urine and reflux result. This altered physiologic state, in conjunction with catheterization, birth trauma, conduction anesthesia, frequent pelvic examinations, and nearly continuous contamination of the perineum, is sufficient to explain the high incidence of lower urinary tract infections postpartum. In many women, preexisting asymptomatic bacteria, chronic urinary tract infections, and anatomic disorders of the bladder, urethra, and kidneys contribute to urinary tract infection postpartum.

## Clinical Findings

**A. Symptoms and Signs:** Urinary tract infection usually presents with dysuria, frequency, urgency, and low-grade fever; however, an elevated temperature is occasionally the only symptom. White blood cells and bacteria are seen in a centrifuged sample of catheterized urine. A urine culture should be obtained. The history should be reviewed for evidence of chronic antepartum infections. If a woman has had an antepartum urinary tract infection, it is likely that postpartum infection is caused by the same organism. Repeated urinary tract infections call for careful postpartum evaluation. Urethral diverticulum, kidney stones, and upper urinary tract anomalies should be ruled out.

Urinary retention postpartum in the absence of regional anesthesia or well after its effects have worn off almost always indicates urinary tract infection.

Pyelonephritis may be accompanied by fever, chills, malaise, and nausea and vomiting. Characteristic signs of kidney involvement associated with pyelonephritis include costovertebral angle tenderness, dysuria, pyuria, and, in the case of hemorrhagic cystitis, hematuria.

**B. Laboratory Findings:** *E coli* is easily the most common organism isolated from infected urine in postpartum women (about 75% of cases). Other gram-negative bacilli are much less likely to be recovered. *E coli* is less likely to be the causative organism in women who have had repeated urinary tract infections in the recent past.

## Treatment

Antibiotics with specific activity against the causative organism are the cornerstone of therapy in uncomplicated cystitis. These include sulfonamides, nitrofurantoin, trimethoprim-sulfamethoxazole, oral cephalosporins (cephalexin, cephradine), and ampicillin. Some hospitals report a high incidence of microbial resistance to ampicillin. The oral combination of amoxicillin-clavulanic acid provides a better spectrum of bacterial sensitivity. Sulfa antibiotics can be used safely in women who are breastfeeding if the infants are term without hyperbilirubinemia or suspected glucose-6-phosphate dehydrogenase deficiency. High fluid intake should be encouraged.

Pyelonephritis requires initial therapy with high doses of intravenous antibiotics, eg, ampicillin, 8–12 g/d, or first-generation cephalosporins (cefazolin,

3–6 g/d; cephalothin, 4–8 g/d). An aminoglycoside can be added when resistant organisms are suspected or when the patient has clinical signs of sepsis. A long-acting third-generation cephalosporin such as ceftriaxone, 1–2 g every 12 hours, may also be used. The response to therapy may be rapid, but some women respond with gradual defervescence over 48 hours or longer. Urine cultures should be obtained to guide any necessary modifications in drug therapy if the patient's response is not prompt. Even with prompt resolution of fever, antibiotic therapy should be continued intravenously or orally for a total of 10 days of therapy. Urine for culture should also be obtained at a postpartum visit after therapy has been completed.

## 3. PNEUMONIA

Women with obstructive lung disease, smokers, and those undergoing general anesthesia have an increased risk of developing pneumonia postpartum.

### Clinical Findings

**A. Symptoms and Signs:** Symptoms and signs are the same as those of pneumonia in nonpregnant patients: productive cough, chest pain, fever, chills, rales, and infiltrates on chest x-ray. In some cases, careful differentiation from pulmonary embolus is required.

**B. X-Ray and Laboratory Findings:** Chest x-ray confirms the diagnosis of pneumonia. Gram-stained smears of sputum and material for culture should be obtained.

*Streptococcus pneumoniae* and *Mycoplasma pneumoniae* are the 2 most likely causative organisms. *S pneumoniae* can easily be identified on gram-stained smears. Infection with *M pneumoniae* can be suspected on clinical grounds.

### Treatment

Appropriate antibiotics, oxygen (if the patient is hypoxic), intravenous hydration, and pulmonary toilet are the mainstays of therapy.

## 4. CESAREAN SECTION WOUND INFECTION

### Incidence

Wound infection occurs in 4–12% of patients following cesarean section.

### Etiology

The following risk factors predispose to subsequent wound infection in women undergoing cesarean section: obesity, diabetes, prolonged hospitalization before cesarean section, prolonged rupture of the membranes, chorioamnionitis, endomyometritis, prolonged labor, emergency rather than elective indications for cesarean section, and anemia.

### Clinical Findings

**A. Symptoms and Signs:** Fever with no apparent cause, which persists to the fourth or fifth postoperative day strongly suggests a wound infection. Wound erythema and tenderness may not be evident until several days after surgery. Occasionally, wound infections are manifested by spontaneous drainage, often accompanied by resolution of fever and relief of local tenderness. Rarely, a deep-seated wound infection becomes apparent when the skin overtly separates, usually after some strenuous activity by the patient.

**B. Laboratory Findings:** Gram-stained smears and culture of material from the wound may be helpful in guiding selection of the initial antibiotic. Blood cultures may be positive in the patient with systemic sepsis due to wound infection. The organisms responsible for most wound infections originate on the patient's skin. *S aureus* is the organism most commonly isolated. *Streptococcus* species, *E coli,* and other gram-negative organisms that may originally have colonized the amniotic cavity are also seen. Occasionally, *Bacteroides,* which comes only from the genital tract, is isolated from material taken from serious wound infections.

Rarely, necrotizing fasciitis and the closely related synergistic bacterial gangrene can involve cesarean section incisions. They are recognized by their intense tissue destruction and rapid extension. Radical debridement of necrotic and infected tissue is the cornerstone of treatment.

### Treatment

**A. Initial Evaluation:** The incision should be opened along its entire length and the deeper portion of the wound gently explored to determine whether fascial separation has occurred. If the fascia is not intact, the wound is dissected to the fascial level, debrided, and repaired. Wound dehiscence has a high mortality rate and should be treated aggressively. Dehiscence is uncommon in healthy patients and with Pfannenstiel incisions. The skin may be left open to undergo delayed closure or to heal by primary intention.

If the fascia is intact, the wound infection can be treated by local measures.

**B. Definitive Measures:** Mechanical cleansing of the wound is the mainstay of therapy for cesarean wound infection. Opening the wound encourages drainage of infected material. The wound may be packed with saline-soaked gauze 2–3 times per day, which will remove necrotic debris each time the wound is unpacked. The wound may be left open to heal, or it may be closed secondarily when granulation tissue has begun to form.

### Antibiotic Prophylaxis for Cesarean Section

The high rate of infection (averaging 35–40%) following cesarean section is reason enough to consider prophylactic perioperative antibiotic administration in high-risk patients. If possible, a single drug should be used because of the convenience. The drug should have a wide spectrum of activity, including reasonably good activity against pathogens likely to be present at the incision site. The dosage regimen should be designed to ensure adequate tissue levels at the time the operation begins or shortly thereafter. The drug should not be one that is used to treat serious, established infections. The duration of therapy should be short. (Antibiotics administered for more than 48 hours can hardly be called prophylactic.) The drug should be free of major side effects and should be relatively inexpensive.

One drug commonly used is cefazolin, 1 g intravenously, when the umbilical cord is clamped, followed by 2 similar doses at 6-hour intervals. A single dose has been shown to be as effective as a 3-dose regimen (Duff, 1987). Almost all studies of the use of prophylactic antibiotics in patients with cesarean section deliveries have shown significant reductions in the incidence of infection, regardless of the drugs, doses, and schedules used. No regimen has provided total protection against the incidence of fever and associated morbidity, however, nor has one completely prevented serious postoperative infections. Low-risk women, ie, those undergoing elective cesarean section and are not in active labor, do not benefit to the same degree from prophylactic antibiotics.

## 5. EPISIOTOMY INFECTION

It is surprising that infected episiotomies do not occur more often than they do, since contamination at the time of delivery is universal. Subsequent contamination during the healing phase must also be common, yet infection and disruption of the wound are infrequent—0.5–3% (Thacker and Banta, 1983). The excellent local blood supply is suggested as an explanation for this phenomenon.

### Etiology

In general, the more extensive the laceration or episiotomy, the greater the chances for infection and breakdown of the wound. More tissue is devitalized in a large episiotomy, thereby providing greater opportunity for contamination. Women with infections elsewhere in the genital area are probably at greater risk for infection of the episiotomy.

### Clinical Findings

**A. Symptoms and Signs:** Pain at the episiotomy site is the most common symptom. Spontaneous drainage is frequent, so a mass rarely forms. Incontinence of flatus and stool may be the presenting symptom of an episiotomy that breaks down and heals spontaneously.

Inspection of the episiotomy site shows disruption of the wound and gaping of the incision. A necrotic membrane may cover the wound and should be debrided if possible. A careful rectovaginal examination should be performed to determine whether a rectovaginal fistula has formed. The integrity of the anal sphincter should also be evaluated.

**B. Laboratory Findings:** Infection with mixed aerobic and anaerobic organisms is common. *Staphylococcus* may be recovered from cultures of material from these infections. Culture results are frequently misleading, since the area of the episiotomy is typically contaminated with a wide variety of pathogenic bacteria.

### Treatment

Initial treatment should be directed toward opening and cleaning the wound and promoting the formation of granulation tissue. Warm sitz baths or Hubbard tank treatments help the debridement process. Attempts to close an infected, disrupted episiotomy are likely to fail and may make ultimate closure more difficult. Surgical closure by perineorrhaphy should be undertaken only after granulation tissue has thoroughly covered the wound site, which on average occurs by 6 days postpartum (Hankins et al, 1990).

## 6. MASTITIS

Congestive mastitis, or breast engorgement, is more common in primigravidas than in multiparas. Infectious mastitis and breast abscesses are also more common in women pregnant for the first time and are seen almost exclusively in nursing mothers.

### Etiology

Infectious mastitis and breast abscesses are uncommon complications of breastfeeding. They almost certainly occur as a result of trauma to the nipple and the subsequent introduction of organisms from the infant's nostrils to the mother's breast. *S aureus* contracted by the infant while in the hospital nursery is the usual causative agent.

### Clinical Findings

**A. Symptoms and Signs:** Breast engorgement usually occurs on the second or third postpartum day. The breasts are swollen, tender, tense, and warm. The patient's temperature may be mildly elevated. Axillary adenopathy can be seen.

Mastitis presents 1 week or more after delivery. Usually only 1 breast is affected and often only 1 quadrant or lobule. It is tender, reddened, swollen, and hot. There may be purulent drainage, and aspiration may produce pus. The patient is febrile and appears ill.

**B. Laboratory Findings:** The organism responsible for infectious mastitis and breast abscess is almost always *S aureus*. *Streptococcus* species and

*E coli* are occasionally isolated. Leukocytosis is evident.

## Treatment

**A. Congestive Mastitis:** The form of treatment depends on whether or not the patient plans to breastfeed. If she does not, tight breast binding, ice packs, restriction of breast stimulation, and analgesics help to relieve pain and suppress lactation. Medical suppression of lactation probably does not hasten involution of congested breasts unless it is begun very early after delivery. Bromocriptine (Parlodel), 2.5 mg twice daily orally for 10 days, is an effective regimen. For the woman who is breastfeeding, manually emptying the breasts following infant feeding is all that is necessary to relieve discomfort.

**B. Infectious Mastitis:** Infectious mastitis is treated in the same way as congestive mastitis. Local heat and support of the breasts help to reduce pain. Cloxacillin, dicloxacillin, nafcillin, or a cephalosporin—antibiotics with activity against the commonly encountered causative organisms—should be administered. Infants tolerate the small amount of antibiotics in breast milk without difficulty. It may be prudent to check the infant for possible colonization with the same bacteria present in the mother's breast.

If an abscess is present, incision and drainage are necessary. The cavity should be packed open with gauze, which is then advanced toward the surface in stages daily. Most authorities recommend cessation of breastfeeding when an abscess develops. Antistaphylococcal antibiotics should be prescribed. Inhibition of lactation is also recommended.

## DISORDERS OF LACTATION

### Inhibition & Suppression of Lactation

Anatomic alteration of the breasts during pregnancy prepares them for sustained milk production shortly after delivery. The rapid decrease of serum estrogen and progesterone levels postpartum does not occur in prolactin levels, which decrease much more slowly. The breast is no longer subject to the inhibitory effects of the steroid hormones and now comes under the influence of high prolactin levels to begin sustained milk production.

Colostrum is secreted in late pregnancy and for the first 2–3 days postpartum. It is higher in protein (much of which may be antibodies) and minerals and lower in carbohydrates and fat than is later breast milk. Prior to full milk production, from the second to the fourth postpartum days, the breasts become enlarged, engorged, and tender. The breast lobules enlarge, and alveoli and blood vessels proliferate. Milk production truly begins around the third or fourth postpartum day. Fortuitously, infants may frequently take this long to feel a sensation of hunger and develop the neuromuscular control necessary to successfully empty the breast.

In spite of the manifold benefits of breastfeeding for both infants and mothers, at least a third of all women who give birth today do not wish to nurse, and perhaps an additional 10–20% discontinue attempts within a few weeks of delivery. For these women, inhibition of lactation for relief of breast congestion and tenderness may be necessary.

**A. Physical Methods of Suppression of Lactation:** Inhibition of physical stimuli that encourage milk secretion can prevent lactation. Tight breast binding, avoidance of any tactile breast stimulation, ice packs, and mild analgesics (eg, aspirin or ibuprofen) are effective in inhibiting lactation and relieving the symptoms of breast engorgement in 50% of women. Physical methods successfully inhibit lactation and prevent breast engorgement either before the onset of lactation or after it has been established for some time.

**B. Hormonal Suppression of Lactation:** Large doses of estrogen alone have been used to suppress lactation; they do inhibit milk production, probably by acting directly on the breast. Estrogens are somewhat more successful than physical methods alone. Side effects are tolerable in young women who have had vaginal deliveries, but increased rates of thrombophlebitis and pulmonary embolism are seen in women over age 35, in those who have undergone cesarean section, and in those with difficult deliveries. For these reasons, pure estrogens are no longer used for suppression of lactation as they once were. Furthermore, drug-induced suppression of lactation is not very effective after lactation has been established.

An ergot derivative, bromocriptine (Parlodel), has strong prolactin-inhibiting and thus lactation-inhibiting properties. In the dosage ranges used to suppress lactation, the drug is relatively free of serious side effects. Minor side effects include nausea and nasal congestion. More serious associations with hypertension, cerebral vascular accidents, and myocardial infarction have also been reported. The risks seem to be reported frequently when bromocriptine is used in patients with pregnancy-induced hypertension. Drawbacks of bromocriptine therapy include the necessity for prolonged treatment (10–14 days) and a more rapid resumption of ovulation. A significant number of women have rebound lactation (18–40%). The Food and Drug Administration removed painful breast engorgement as an indication for the use of bromocriptine in 1989. The FDA noted that although there is no clear proof of adverse effects of these medications, there is no proved health benefit, so "even anecdotal safety concerns become important, because of their unfavorable effects on the benefit-risk ratio" (ACOG newsletter, 1990). In women with severe congestive mastitis, bromocriptine may be a reasonable treatment option.

## Inappropriate Lactation

Lactation is physiologic in late pregnancy and for a considerable period of time after delivery. In the woman who has not lactated for 1 year or more or who has never been pregnant, lactation may indicate a significant endocrinopathy (see Chapter 12).

## POSTPARTUM MONITORING

Serious and acute obstetric and postanesthetic complications often occur during the first few hours immediately following delivery. The patient should therefore be transferred to a recovery room where she can be constantly attended to and where observation of bleeding, blood pressure, pulse, and respiratory change can be made every 15 minutes for at least 1–2 hours after delivery or until the effects of general or major regional anesthesia have disappeared. On return to the patient's room or ward, the patient's blood pressure should be taken and the measurement repeated every 12 hours for the first 24 hours and daily thereafter for several days. Preeclampsia-eclampsia, infection, or other medical or surgical complications of pregnancy may require more prolonged and intensive postpartum care.

## POSTPARTUM COMPLICATIONS

### 1. COMPLICATIONS OF ANESTHESIA

The most common respiratory complications that follow general anesthesia and delivery are airway obstruction or laryngospasm and vomiting with aspiration of vomitus. Bronchoscopy, tracheostomy, and other related procedures must be done promptly as indicated. Hypoventilation and hypotension may follow an abnormally high subarachnoid block. Because serum cholinesterase activity is lower during labor and the postpartum period, hypoventilation during the early puerperium may also follow the use of large amounts of succinylcholine during anesthesia for cesarean section. Brief postpartum shivering is commonly seen after completion of the third stage of labor and is no cause for alarm. The cause of the shivering is unknown, but it may be related to loss of heat, or it may be a sympathetic response. Subcutaneous emphysema may make its appearance postpartum after vigorous bearing-down efforts. Most cases resolve spontaneously.

Hypertension in the immediate puerperium is most often due to excessive use of vasopressor or oxytocic drugs. It must be treated promptly with a vasodilator. Hydralazine, 5 mg administrated slowly intravenously, usually reduces the blood pressure.

Postanesthetic complications that manifest themselves later in the puerperium include postsubara-chnoid puncture headache, atelectasis, renal or hepatic dysfunction, and neurologic sequelae.

Postpuncture headache is usually located in the forehead, deep behind the eyes; occasionally, the pain radiates to both temples and to the occipital region. It usually begins on the first or second postpartum day and lasts 1–3 days. Because new mothers frequently develop various types of headache, the correct diagnosis is essential. An important characteristic of post-spinal puncture headache is increased pain in the sitting or standing position and significant improvement when the patient is supine. The mild form is relieved by aspirin or other analgesics. Headache is due to leakage of cerebrospinal fluid through the site of dural puncture into the extradural space. It is advisable to supplement the daily oral intake of fluids with at least 1 L of 5% glucose in saline intravenously. Administration of 7–10 mL of the patient's own blood into the thecal space at the point of previous needle insertion will "patch" the leaking point and relieve the headache in most patients. Subdural hematoma is a rare complication of chronic leakage of cerebrospinal fluid and resultant loss of support to intracranial structures.

A small percentage of women who develop headaches during this time also show symptoms of meningeal irritation. Headache due to aseptic chemical meningitis is not relieved by lying down. Lumbar puncture reveals a slightly elevated pressure and an increase in spinal fluid protein and white blood cells but no bacteria. Symptoms usually disappear 1–3 days later, and the spinal fluid returns to normal within 4 days with no sequelae. Treatment is conservative and includes supportive measures, analgesics, and fluids.

Neurologic problems in the puerperium sometimes follow traumatic childbirth, eg, injury to the femoral nerve caused by forceps when the patient was in the lithotomy position. Such complications are rarely bilateral, which aids in the differential diagnosis of a spinal cord lesion. Evidence of more serious neurologic sequelae following regional or general anesthesia for delivery requires consultation with the anesthesiologist or a neurologist.

### 2. POSTPARTUM CARDIAC PROBLEMS

The puerperium is relatively complicated for the patient with congenital or acquired heart disease. Following delivery, the cardiovascular system responds with sharply increased cardiac output as a result of unimpeded venous return from the lower extremities and pelvis. This produces a relative bradycardia that may persist for several days. For the initial few days after delivery, the intracellular water and sodium retained during pregnancy are mobilized and contribute to increasing cardiac output. A concomitant postpartum diuresis gradually mitigates the bradycardia and increases cardiac output (see Chapter 7).

## Valvular Heart Disease

The management principles underlying treatment of valvular heart disease in the postpartum period are those begun in the intrapartum period: antibiotic prophylaxis of bacterial endocarditis, careful fluid and electrolyte administration, accurate (often continuous invasive) monitoring, and frequent physical examination to detect changes in cardiovascular status. Return to an ambulatory status soon after delivery reduces the possibility of thrombophlebitis. The postpartum period is also a time for the patient to carefully consider further childbearing options in light of the fetal outcome and the possible progression of heart disease during the antecedent pregnancy.

Women whose valvular heart disease required systemic anticoagulation before delivery should continue the treatment postpartum; however, oral anticoagulants may be used instead of heparin. There are no reports of problems in term breastfed infants of women taking warfarin or dicumarol. Other oral anticoagulants are contraindicated if the patient is breastfeeding.

## Postpartum Cardiomyopathy

A cardiomyopathy unique to the latter half of pregnancy and the puerperium has been described by numerous investigators. The incidence is estimated to be 1 in 4000 deliveries. Congestive heart failure, cardiomegaly, and cardiac arrhythmias develop in otherwise healthy young women. A number of causes—viral, immunologic, toxic, genetic—have been suggested, but none has been confirmed. A high incidence of myocarditis (29%) has been reported (O'Connell et al, 1986). The clinical presentation of disease and the appearance of heart muscle on histologic examination do not differ from those of idiopathic cardiomyopathy.

Patients with postpartum cardiomyopathy are generally in their mid 20s to early 30s. The disease is more common in blacks and parous women. Twin pregnancy is reported in 7–10% of patients with this disorder. Patients usually present a few days to several weeks postpartum in florid congestive heart failure. Treatment with digitalis, diuretics, oxygen, bed rest, and salt restriction relieves symptoms in most cases. Cardiac function returns to normal within 6 months in over 50% of women with this disorder. Slow improvement, continued cardiac symptoms, or deterioration characterizes the course of other patients. Recurrence of disease in a subsequent pregnancy has been described but is not inevitable. Cardiac transplantation has been used successfully in a few women with severe progressive disease. Lee and Cotton (1989) have reviewed the literature on this disorder.

## 3. POSTPARTUM PULMONARY PROBLEMS

Return to nonpregnant pulmonary physiology occurs by 6 weeks after delivery. Except for women undergoing general anesthesia, the puerperium is not a time of special concern. The factors placing pregnant women at risk for highly destructive chemical aspiration pneumonitis (gastric pH < 2.5 and fasting gastric contents > 25 mL) persist for at least 48 hours after delivery (James et al, 1984). Thus, women undergoing general anesthesia in the puerperium (eg, for tubal ligation) are at a high risk for aspiration. A nonparticulate antacid should be used preoperatively for women undergoing general anesthesia in the puerperal period as well as other anesthetic techniques (rapid sequence induction of anesthesia, endotracheal intubation, and preanesthetic fasting) designed to prevent aspiration of gastric contents.

Pulmonary hypertension, either primary or secondary to congenital heart disease, is an overt threat to the mother's life in the intrapartum and postpartum periods. The most important management principle is to use invasive monitoring to avoid hypovolemia (see Chapter 59).

## 4. POSTPARTUM THYROIDITIS

Several studies have shown that thyroid abnormalities, probably of immunologic origin, are common in the postpartum period (Jansson et al, 1984: Nikolai et al, 1987). In susceptible populations, 5–11% of women may be affected. Postpartum thyroiditis usually presents with mild transient hyperthyroidism 1–3 months postpartum, followed by mild and transient hypothyroidism. Suppression of hyperthyroid symptoms or temporary thyroid hormone supplementation may be necessary, but most women recover completely and are euthyroid within 6–9 months after delivery. A significant number of women, however, will remain hypothyroid (Lervang et al, 1987). The recurrence risk for postpartum thyroiditis in a subsequent pregnancy is 10–25% (Walfish, 1985).

## 5. POSTPARTUM THROMBOPHLEBITIS & THROMBOEMBOLISM

Historically, the puerperium has been known as the time when severe thrombophlebitic conditions and pulmonary embolism occur, probably as a result of the once-prevalent recommendation of prolonged bed rest following parturition. Even though contemporary postpartum management encourages early ambulation, puerperal thrombophlebitis and thromboembolism remain a serious problem.

Thrombophlebitis requires careful and prolonged medical management. The risk of recurrence in a subsequent pregnancy is substantial, and a history of thrombophlebitis may prohibit the future use of oral contraceptives and replacement estrogens.

The incidence of thrombophlebitic conditions is difficult to estimate since the clinical diagnosis of these disorders is highly unreliable. One study of venographically confirmed deep venous thrombosis reported 1.3 antepartum cases per 10,000 deliveries and 6.1 postpartum cases per 10,000 deliveries (Kierkegaard, 1983). Most studies confirm that the incidence of superficial thrombophlebitis, deep venous thrombosis, and pulmonary embolism, is 2–6 times higher in the postpartum period than in the antepartum period. (Methods of diagnosis and treatment of thromboembolic conditions are discussed in Chapter 43).

## 6. POSTPARTUM NEUROPSYCHIATRIC COMPLICATIONS

### Peripheral Nerve Palsy

Nerve palsies involving pelvic nerves or parts of the lumbosacral plexus result from pressure by the presenting part or trauma by obstetric forceps. Typically, the palsy occurs after prolonged labor in a nullipara, and presents as unilateral footdrop noted when ambulation resumes after delivery. Most cases resolve spontaneously in a matter of days or weeks. A few may have a more protracted course. Electromyography may help in predicting the course of the disorder.

### Seizures

Postpartum seizures immediately raise the possibility of eclampsia, but if the interval since delivery is greater than 48 hours, other etiologies should be considered. In the absence of a prior history of epilepsy or signs of pregnancy-induced hypertension, a thorough evaluation to determine the cause of the seizures must be performed.

### Postpartum Depression

Considering the excitement, anticipation, and tension associated with imminent delivery; the marked hormonal alterations following delivery; and the substantial new burdens and responsibilities that result from childbirth, it is not surprising that some women experience depression after delivery. The incidence of postpartum depression is difficult to estimate, but the disorder is common. The disorder in its usual form is self-limited and benign.

In women who suffered from depression before they became pregnant and in those without effective support mechanisms, the severity of depression may be more profound and the consequences far more serious. An openly psychotic state may develop within a few days after delivery and render the woman incapable of caring for herself or her newborn. In some cases she may harm her infant and herself.

Psychiatric consultation should be obtained for the postpartum woman who shows symptoms of severe depression or overt psychosis. Nursery personnel are often the first to notice that the new mother does not devote the usual amount of attention to her newborn (see Chapter 60).

## REFERENCES

Achiron R et al: Transvaginal duplex Doppler ultrasonography in bleeding patients suspected of having residual trophoblastic tissue. Obstet Gynecol 1993;81:507.

Alvarez M et al: Prophylactic and emergent arterial catheterization for selective embolization in obstetric hemorrhage. Am J Perinatol 1992;9(5/6):441.

American College of Obstetrics and Gynecology Newsletter 1990 April:8.

Andres RL, Piacquadio KM, Resnik R: A reappraisal of the need for autologous blood donation in the obstetric patient. Am J Obstet Gynecol 1990; 163:1551.

Atrash HK et al: Maternal mortality in the United States, 1979–1986. Obstet Gynecol 1990; 76:1055.

Berger E, Gillieson MS, Walters JH: Puerperal febrile complications and cervical flora following elective manual exploration of the uterus. Am J Obstet Gynecol 1981;139:320.

Blanchette H: Elective manual exploration of the uterus after delivery: A study and review. J Reprod Med 1977;19:13.

Buttino L Jr, Garite TJ: The use of 15 methyl $F_{2\alpha}$ prostaglandin (Prostin 15M) for the control of postpartum hemorrhage. Am J Perinatol 1986;3:241.

Catanzarite VA et al: New approaches to the management of acute puerperal uterine inversion. Obstet Gynecol 1986;68:75.

Clark SL, Koonings PP, Phelan JP: Placenta previa/accreta and prior cesarean section. Obstet Gynecol 1985;66:89.

Combs CA, Murphy EL, Laros RK: Cost-benefit analysis of autologous blood donation in obstetrics. Obstet Gynecol 1992;80:621.

Corson SL, Bolognese RJ: Postpartum uterine atony treated with prostaglandins. Am J Obstet Gynecol 1977;129:918.

Cox SM, Carpenter RJ, Cotton DB: Placenta percreta: Ultrasound diagnosis and conservative surgical management. Obstet Gynecol 1988;71:454.

Cruikshank SH, Stoekl EM: Surgical control of pelvic hemorrhage: Ovarian artery ligation. Am J Obstet Gynecol 1983;147:724.

Dinsmoor MJ, Newton ER, Gibbs RS: A randomized, double-blind, placebo-controlled trial of oral antibiotic therapy following intravenous antibiotic therapy for postpartum endometritis. Obstet Gynecol 1991;77:60.

Duff P: Prophylactic antibiotics for cesarean delivery: A simple cost-effective strategy for prevention of postoperative morbidity.

Elbourne D, Prendiville W, Chalmers I: Choice of oxytocic preparation for routine use in the management of the third stage of labour: An overview of the evidence from controlled trials. Br J Obstet Gynecol 1988;95:17.

Eschenbach DA et al: Isolation of mycoplasmas and bacteria from the blood of postpartum women. Am J Obstet Gynecol 1982;143:104.

Evans S, McShane P: The efficacy of internal iliac artery

ligation in obstetric hemorrhage. Surg Gynecol Obstet 1985;160:250.

Fahmy K: Uterine artery ligation to control postpartum hemorrhage. Int J Gynaecol Obstet 1987;25:363.

Finberg HJ, Williams JW: Placenta accreta: Prospective sonographic diagnosis in patient with placenta previa and prior cesarean section. J Ultrasound Med 1992;11:333.

Guy GP, Peisner DB, Timor-Tritsch IE: Ultrasonographic evaluation of uteroplacental blood flow patterns of abnormally located and adherent placentas. Am J Obstet Gynecol 1990;163:723.

Hankins GDV et al: Early repair of episiotomy dehiscence. Obstet Gynecol 1990;75:48.

Hankins GDV et al: Maternal arterial desaturation with 15-methyl prostaglandin $F_2$ alpha for uterine atony. Obstet Gynecol 1988;72:367.

Hayashi RH, Castillo MS, Noah ML: Management of severe postpartum hemorrhage with a prostaglandin $F_2$ alpha analogue. Obstet Gynecol 1984;63:806.

James DF, Gibbs CP, Banner T: Postpartum perioperative risk of aspiration pneumonia. Anesthesiology 1984;61:756.

Jansson R et al: Autoimmune thyroid dysfunction in the postpartum period. J Clin Endocrinol Metab 1984;58:681.

Kierkegaard A: Incidence and diagnosis of deep vein thrombosis associated with pregnancy. Acta Obstet Gynecol Scand 1983;62:239.

Lee W, Cotton DB: Peripartum cardiomyopathy: Current concepts and clinical management. Clin Obstet Gynecol 1989;32(1):54.

Lee CY, Madrazo B, Drukker BH: Ultrasonic evaluation of the postpartum uterus in the management of postpartum bleeding. Obstet Gynecol 1981;58:227.

Lervang HH, Pryds O, Ostergaard Kristensen HP: Thyroid dysfunction after delivery: Incidence and clinical course. Acta Med Scand 1987;222:369.

Listwa HM et al: The predictability of intrauterine infection by analysis of amniotic fluid. Obstet Gynecol 1976;48:31.

Morales WJ et al: Short course of antibiotic therapy in treatment of postpartum endomyometritis. Am J Obstet Gynecol 1989;161:568.

Nikolai TF, Turney SL, Roberts RC: Postpartum lymphocytic thyroiditis: Prevalence, clinical course, and long-term follow-up. Arch Intern Med 1987;147:221.

Nolan TE, Gallup DG: Massive transfusion: A current review. Obstet Gynecol Survey 1991;46(5):289.

O'Connell JB et al: Peripartum cardiomyopathy: Clinical, hemodynamic, histologic, and prognostic characteristics. J Am Coll Cardiol 1986;8:52.

Odell LD, Seski A: Episiotomy blood loss. Am J Obstet Gynecol 1947;54:51.

O'Leary JL, O'Leary JA: Uterine artery ligation for control of post cesarean section hemorrhage. Obstet Gynecol 1974;43:849.

Read JA, Cotton DB, Miller FC: Placenta accreta: Changing clinical aspects and outcome. Obstet Gynecol 1980;56:31.

Schenker JG, Margalioth EJ: Intrauterine adhesions: An updated appraisal. Fertil Steril 1982;37:593.

Sorrell TC et al: Antimicrobial therapy of postpartum endomyometritis. 2. Prospective, randomized trial of mezlocillin versus ampicillin. Am J Obstet Gynecol 1981;141:246.

Tabsh KMA, Brinkham CR III, King W: Ultrasound diagnosis of placenta increta. J Clin Ultrasound 1982;10:288.

Thacker SB, Banta HD: Benefits and risks of episiotomy: An interpretive review of the English language literature, 1860–1980. Obstet Gynecol Surv 1983;38:322.

Toppozada M et al: Control of intractable atonic postpartum hemorrhage by 15-methyl prostaglandin $F_{2\alpha}$. Obstet Gynecol 1981;58:327.

Veille JC: Peripartum cardiomyopathies: A review. Am J Obstet Gynecol 1984;148:805.

Walfish PG, Chan JYC: Postpartum hyperthyroidism. Clin Endocrinol Metab 1985;14:417.

Watson P, Besch N, Bowes WA Jr: Management of acute and subacute puerperal inversion of the uterus. Obstet Gynecol 1980;55:12.

# 29

# Neonatal Resuscitation & Care of the Newborn at Risk

*Emily R. Baker, MD, & Barbara Shephard, MD*

## PERINATAL RESUSCITATION

When a high-risk mother and fetus are identified, plans for appropriate management must be made immediately. These plans should consider not only the best time and method of delivery but also the level of care required by both mother and infant. It may be best to transfer the mother to a tertiary-care perinatal center well before delivery, particularly if she is to be delivered before term. Such planning requires the combined efforts of obstetricians, pediatricians, perinatologists, neonatologists, and skilled nurses. However, not all high-risk mothers can be transferred prior to delivery, and indeed, the delivery of an infant requiring resuscitation cannot always be anticipated. At every delivery, there should be at least one person skilled in complete neonatal resuscitation, and all of the equipment necessary for a complete resuscitation should be present in the delivery room.

## Delivery Room Management

Optimal resuscitation of the high-risk, premature, or depressed neonate requires as much notice as possible, and ready communication between the obstetric and pediatric staffs is critical. When a depressed or premature neonate is expected, the resuscitation team should comprise a two-person team capable of complete resuscitation. The Apgar score, an objective evaluation of the newborn's condition, is generally assigned at 1 and 5 minutes. Assessment of the infant and necessary interventions should begin immediately at birth, the Apgar may then be useful as an assessment of the effectiveness of the resuscitation effort.

Figure 29–1 provides an outline that is recommended by the American Academy of Pediatrics (AAP) and the American Heart Association for the general care of depressed infants in the delivery room.

**A. Initial Steps:** The steps in resuscitation begin with preventing heat loss by immediately drying the infant and providing a warm environment (eg, preheated overhead warmer bed), clearing the airway by positioning and suctioning if needed, and assessing adequacy of the infant's breathing. If an infant is not breathing, tactile stimulation while 100% oxygen is administered by face mask is usually sufficient to stimulate breathing. If breathing does not begin within a few seconds, positive pressure ventilation with a bag and mask should be initiated. The pressure required for initial breaths is 30–40 mm Hg. This will expand the lungs, clear fetal lung fluid, and facilitate the increase in pulmonary perfusion that is required in transition from fetal circulation (Fig 29–2). Ventilation should also be initiated if the infant's heart rate (HR) is < 100 beats/min.

**B. Ventilation:** Either a small anesthesia bag with a manometer or a small self-inflating bag with an oxygen reservoir may be used, as long as the mask is the proper size to create a seal over the mouth and nose but not over the eyes. High oxygen concentration (90–100%) should be used. If the infant is profoundly depressed, intubation and ventilation via endotracheal tube may be elected, if staff well-skilled in intubation is present. A respiratory rate of 40–60 breaths/min should be provided at pressures to cause chest wall expansion. The infant's HR should be checked and should be > 100 beats/min. Most infants will respond to adequate expansion of the lung with spontaneous respirations. If not, adequacy of bag and mask ventilation should be checked, or endotracheal intubation should be considered.

**C. Chest Compressions:** Techniques for infant chest compressions are shown in Figure 29–3. The rate should be 120 beats/min. It is the rare infant that does not respond within 30 seconds of such ventilatory and cardiac resuscitation. If the HR rises, ventilation should continue until regular spontaneous respiration begins. If the infant does not respond, medications should be administered.

**D. Medications:** The use of drugs or volume expansion is rarely needed in the delivery room and should not be given until adequate ventilation and circulation have been established for a minimum of 30 seconds. Table 29–1 lists the medications used with doses and routes of administration when needed for neonatal resuscitation. The preferred route is intravenous (IV) via the umbilical vein, which can be easily

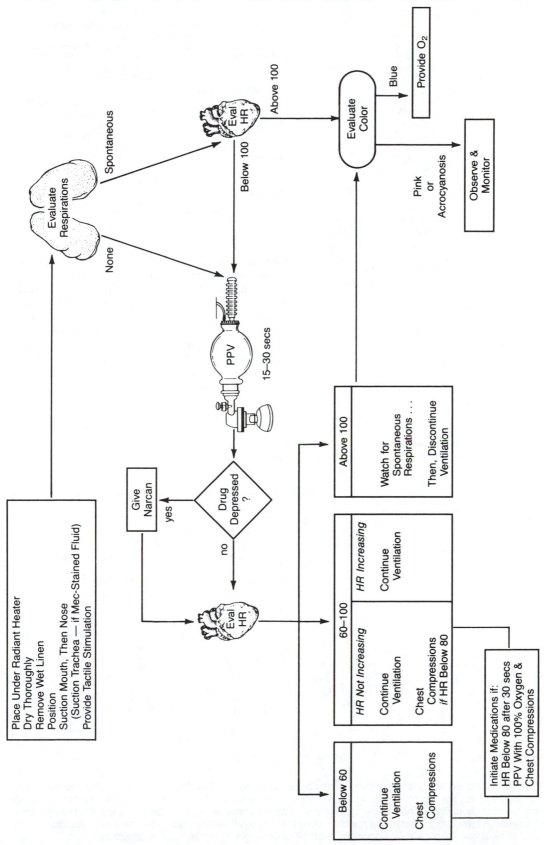

**Figure 29–1.** Flow diagram for neonatal resuscitation. (Reproduced, with permission, from *Textbook of Neonatal Resuscitation*, 1987, 1990. Copyright American Heart Association.)

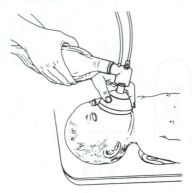

**Figure 29–2.** The technique of bag and mask ventilation of the newborn. The neck should be slightly extended. An anesthesia bag should have a manometer attached; a self-inflating bag should have an oxygen reservoir attached. (Reproduced, with permission, *Textbook of Neonatal Resuscitation,* 1987, 1990. Copyright American Heart Association.)

**Table 29–1.** Neonatal resuscitation and newborn infant drug doses.

| | |
|---|---|
| **Epinephrine** | (1:10,000) 0.2 mL/kg IV or ET. Give rapidly. Dilute 1:1 with saline for ET use. |
| **Volume Expansion** | (whole blood, saline, 5% albumin, ringers lactate) 10 mL/kg. Give over 5–10 minutes. |
| **NaHCO$_3$** | (0.5 mEq/mL) 1–2 mEq/kg IV. Give slowly, only if ventilation adequate. |
| **Naloxone** | (0.4 mg/mL) 0.1 mg/kg = 0.25 mL/kg IV, ET, IM, SQ. Give rapidly. |
| **Glucose** | D$_{10}$W 2 mL/kg IV. Give over 1–2 minutes. |

cannulated. However, dilute epinephrine is often effective when given via endotracheal tube (ET) and naloxone can be given IV or ET and may sometimes be effective if given intramuscularly (IM).

Naloxone, a narcotic antagonist, is the first drug to be administered when respiratory depression due to recent maternal narcotic treatment is suspected. Note, however, that naloxone is contraindicated for the infant of a narcotic-addicted mother, since it may elicit immediate withdrawal and result in severe seizures. Volume expanders are indicated when acute bleeding and signs of hypovolemia, such as pallor, weak pulses, and hypotension, are present. Sodium bicarbonate may be given when metabolic acidosis is documented or assumed due to prolonged asphyxia, after ventilation is established. Atropine and calcium are not currently thought to be helpful in the acute phase of neonatal resuscitation.

**E. Intubation:** The resuscitator must be skilled in intubation, since failed attempts at intubation may greatly jeopardize an already compromised infant. The heart rate should be constantly monitored during this procedure, since reflex bradycardia resulting from the underlying disorder or stimulation of the hy-

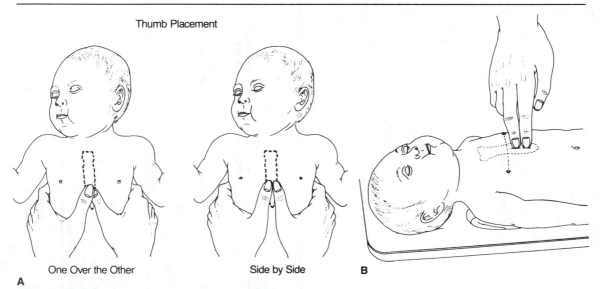

Thumb Placement

One Over the Other                Side by Side                **B**

**A**

**Figure 29–3.** **A:** Thumb technique for performing chest compressions on an infant. The two thumbs, either side by side or one overlapping the other, are used to depress the lower third of the sternum, with the hands encircling the torso and the fingers supporting the back. **B:** Two-finger method for performing chest compressions on the infant. The tips of the middle finger and either the index finger or ring finger of one hand are used to compress the lower third of the sternum. (Reproduced with permission, from *Textbook of Neonatal Resuscitation,* 1987, 1990. Copyright American Heart Association).

popharynx may occur. If intubation is unsuccessful within 20–30 seconds or if it is unclear whether the endotracheal tube is in the trachea or the esophagus, ventilation with a bag and mask should be resumed.

**F. Meconium Aspiration:** Term and postterm infants who are stressed are likely to pass meconium in utero or during delivery and are at risk of developing meconium aspiration syndrome. Meconium passes slowly from the upper to the lower airways, a pattern that explains the clinical presentation of progressive respiratory distress that eventually develops into full-blown pneumonitis. To prevent meconium aspiration, the obstetrician should suction the infant's oropharynx and nasopharynx before the infant takes its first breath. If the meconium is thick or particulate and the infant is depressed, the infant should be intubated for tracheal suction (Fig 29–4). If the infant is vigorous, the need for intubation is less clear, although most agree that in the presence of thick or particulate meconium, tracheal suctioning is advised. Delivery rooms should be equipped with adequate mechanical or wall suction for use by both obstetricians and pediatricians. Mouth suction, such as into the DeLee suction trap, should never be performed, given the risk of infectious agent exposure including hepatitis B virus and HIV.

**G. Pulmonary Hypertension of the Newborn:** Perinatal asphyxia as well as meconium aspiration may result in persistent pulmonary hypertension of the newborn (PPHN) (Fig 29–5). Hypoxia, acidosis, and hypercapnia, probably acting through elevated

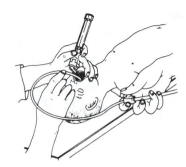

**Figure 29–4.** Resuscitation of an infant born after passage of meconium. The obstetrician aspirates the oropharynx and naxopharynx with mechanical suction before the infant utters its first cry. The infant is then intubated and the upper airway suctioned. (Reproduced with permission, from *Textbook of Neonatal Resuscitation,* 1987, 1990. Copyright American Heart Association).

plasma concentrations of potent vasoconstrictors such as thromboxane, prevent the reduction of pulmonary vascular resistance and establishment of pulmonary blood flow that accompany normal delivery. Persistent pulmonary hypertension of the newborn may also occur in association with sepsis, pulmonary hypoplasia, or congenital diaphragmatic hernia. Treatment consists of vigorous resuscitation and measures to maintain systemic blood pressure with generous use of pressor agents (eg, dopamine and dobutamine) and reduce pulmonary vascular resis-

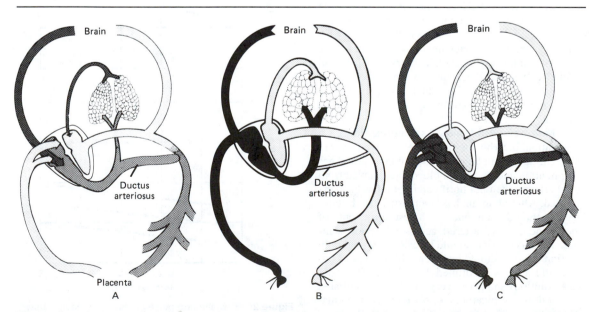

**Figure 29–5.** **A:** The normal fetal circulation, with saturated blood coursing from the umbilical vein to the right side of the heart. Right-to-left shunting of saturated blood occurs across the ductus arteriosus. **B:** Normal transition to extrauterine life. Some transient left-to-right shunting across the ductus arteriosus may occur. **C:** Persistent pulmonary hypertension. Because of persistence of elevated pulmonary vascular resistance into the neonatal period, little blood flow to the lungs is allowed, and excessive right-to-left shunting of unsaturated blood occurs across the ductus arteriosus.

tance. In PPHN, the pulmonary vasculature is very sensitive to hypoxia and acidosis. When possible, $PaO_2$ should be maintained in the 80–100 mm Hg range. Higher $PaO_2$ has not been shown to improve outcome and may be detrimental. Respiratory acidosis should be corrected, but attempts to induce alkalosis by hyperventilation, although controversial, are no longer standard. Rather, administration of alkali to induce *metabolic* alkalosis can effectively lower pulmonary vascular resistance without contributing to barotrauma and worsening lung disease. Vasodilating agents (eg, tolazoline) can be very useful in lowering pulmonary vascular resistance but because of potential severe complications are generally reserved for the most refractory pulmonary hypertension. The use of paralytic agents is controversial, but most infants should be sedated with morphine or fentanyl since they are exquisitely sensitive to external stimuli. Persistent pulmonary hypertension can be idiopathic. In some babies who have died from this, excessive hypertrophied pulmonary arteriolar musculature has been found. These infants are indistinguishable clinically from those with persistent pulmonary hypertension of the newborn due to other causes. This vascular smooth muscle maldevelopment may be a consequence of chronic intrauterine hypoxia or other situations resulting in sustained pulmonary hypertension in utero. The ECMO Registry of the Extracorporeal Life Support Organization reports that nearly 800 neonates have been treated with extracorporeal membrane oxygenation (ECMO) as of early 1993. The indicating diagnosis for many of these infants was PPHN with or without meconium aspiration syndrome, pneumonia, or sepsis. Most criteria for treatment with ECMO include failure of conventional medical management such that an 80% chance of death is anticipated. Yet survival rates with ECMO treatment of these patients now exceed 75%. As of 1990, there were 73 centers using ECMO as routine treatment for severe respiratory failure in newborns.

**H. Metabolic Acidosis:** As mentioned, during a resuscitation, bicarbonate should not be given prior to documenting metabolic acidosis with cord blood gas determination and/or arterial blood gas sampled from the infant, and then not until ventilation has been established. After an infant has been resuscitated, stabilization should continue with establishment of venous and usually arterial access for blood sampling. The base deficit should be calculated, but only a portion (1/4–1/2) should be given initially. Bicarbonate should always be diluted 1:1 with sterile water (4.2% solution) and given very slowly. Concentrated or rapid doses of bicarbonate, particularly in premature infants, increase the risk of intraventricular hemorrhage. It should not be administered via umbilical venous catheter unless the tip is documented in the inferior vena cava, or severe hepatic damage, scarring, and subsequent portal hypertension could result.

Frequent arterial blood gases should be followed after treatment.

## Blood Pressure

Figure 29–6 shows normal blood pressure ranges for full term-infants relative to their birth weight. The normal ranges for small preterm infants are generally lower. Infants who have been asphyxiated may be hypovolemic. Hypovolemia may be diagnosed by measuring arterial blood pressure. However, infants who are acidotic may have falsely high arterial blood pressure readings. Noting that the infant is pale with cool extremities and slow capillary filling (> 3 seconds) can help assess the circulatory status. Correction of blood pressure should be achieved slowly unless the infant is extremely hypotensive, since premature and term infants have limited autoregulatory capabilities in the cerebrum, and rapid shifts in systemic arterial blood pressure and volume will be immediately reflected in the cerebral vasculature. Such fluctuations may increase the risk of intraventricular hemorrhage in a premature infant and brain damage in a term infant. Hypovolemia is best

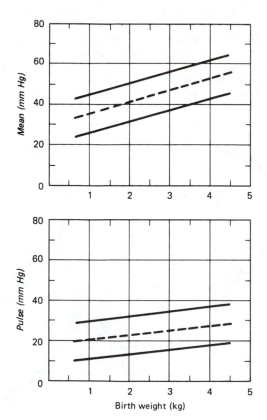

**Figure 29–6.** Mean and pulse pressures of healthy newborn infants relative to birth weight during the first 12 hours of life. (Reproduced, with permission, from Versmold HT et al: Aortic blood pressure during the first 12 hours of life in infants with birth weight 610–4220 grams. Pediatrics 1981;67:607.)

treated with whole blood; however, 5% albumin or normal saline 10 mL/kg intravenously, can also be used. Uncross-matched O-negative whole blood or packed red blood cells may also be used in emergencies when the hematocrit is low.

## Metabolic Considerations

Infants who are stressed in utero are at increased risk of developing hypoglycemia and hypocalcemia as neonates.

**A. Hypoglycemia:** Hypoxia, acidosis, and alterations in blood pressure occurring in utero will stimulate catecholamine release and mobilize fetal hepatic glycogen stores. Premature infants (whether stressed in utero or not) are at great risk of hypoglycemia because of limited glycogen stores. Untreated hypoglycemia can result in myocardial failure and brain damage. Hypoglycemia is best treated with a slow infusion of 10% glucose, 10–15 mL/kg of body weight.

**B. Hypocalcemia:** Hypocalcemia often develops in asphyxiated newborns. Asphyxia initially increases both total and ionized serum calcium concentrations. With correction of acidosis or development of alkalosis with sodium bicarbonate therapy, calcium is cleared from the intravascular space, and hypocalcemia develops. Premature infants may also develop hypocalcemia later in the neonatal period because of their limited body stores. Sustained hypocalcemia may also cause seizures, neuromuscular alterations, and heart failure. Hypocalcemia should be corrected with a slow intravenous infusion of calcium gluconate, 100 mg/kg. Daily maintenance doses of calcium for premature infants should also be provided (100–200 mg/kg/d intravenously).

**C. Heat Loss:** Throughout resuscitation, heat loss must be minimized. Initially, the infant should be dried and placed on a warm, dry mattress. The infant's temperature should be maintained with a servomechanism-controlled overhead radiant heater to maintain thermoneutral status. A hat should be placed on the infant's head, and heat loss due to convection should also be minimized.

## THE PRETERM INFANT

Resuscitation and care of the infant with respiratory distress syndrome are discussed in other sections of this chapter.

## General Fluid Balance

For immediate newborn care, administration of fluids should be based on the degree of prematurity and the severity of illness. Fluid restriction will facilitate closure of the ductus arteriosus and will avoid the numerous problems associated with congestive heart failure due to a patent ductus arteriosus that can complicate the infant's later course. However, enough fluid must be provided for sometimes enormous, insensible water losses by evaporation from the skin and respiratory tract, which can be affected by open radiant warmer beds, phototherapy, and humidified ventilatory support. Careful, ongoing clinical evaluation of hydration and close monitoring of urine output and weight changes are required.

## Nutritional Considerations

**A. Premature Infants:** Small premature infants (< 1500g, < 32 weeks' gestation) and all sick premature infants require intravenous glucose initially, 5–7 mg/kg/min, to maintain glucose homeostasis and plasma glucose concentrations of 40–180 mg/dL. Nutrition should then be provided either parenterally or enterally to meet the infant's caloric needs of 100–150 kcal/kg of body weight per day. When enteral feeds are possible, human milk is considered the preferred nutritional source for premature infants because of its unique composition and the well-established immunologic, nutritional, and psychologic advantages. Although it has been suggested that enteral feedings increase the risk of necrotizing enterocolitis, no studies have confirmed this impression. Indeed, early enteral feedings may reduce the risk of hyperbilirubinemia and enhance the infant's ability to tolerate feeding. Parenteral nutrition should be provided whenever enteral feedings are withheld or insufficient for longer than a few days. Prolonged total parenteral nutrition should be avoided, when possible, since it greatly increases the risk of cholestatic jaundice. Nurseries should follow consistent regimens for providing nutrition, whether enteral or parenteral methods are selected.

**B. Carbohydrates:** The carbohydrate offered to a neonate should provide about 40% of the total calories administered. Any increase in the rate or concentration of intravenous glucose must be implemented slowly, since the premature infant's ability to modulate insulin and glucagon secretion is quite sluggish when compared with that of older children and adults. Glucose offered enterally should not be hyperosmolar.

**C. Amino Acids:** Intravenous amino acids should not exceed 3–3.5 g of protein per kilogram of body weight per day, since doses exceeding this amount can cause metabolic acidosis, hepatic and renal damage, and possibly brain damage. Doses exceeding this amount do not improve weight gain. Some amino acids that are nonessential for term infants and older children (eg, cystine, cysteine, tyrosine, and taurine) are essential for premature infants, since the enzymes necessary for synthesis of these amino acids do not appear until late in gestation. With enteral feedings, it should be remembered that milk from the mother who has delivered prematurely offers a greater caloric density and more favorable amino acid and lipid composition than milk from a mother who has delivered at term. Currently available formulas for premature infants provide proteins and essential amino acids similar to those found in preterm human milk.

**D. Lipids:** Intravenous lipid preparations provide both calories and essential fatty acids with low osmolality. Parenteral lipids should not exceed 40% of the total calories provided in 24 hours. High doses of intravenous lipids have been associated with hypoxia and worsening of the alveolar-arterial oxygen gradient when given over short periods of time. Careful monitoring of respiratory variables is therefore indicated, and lipid emulsions should be administered over prolonged infusion periods. Parenteral lipid solutions are invaluable for the support of very tiny infants who require as many calories as possible with limited fluid administration. Formulas prepared for preterm infants contain up to half of the fat blend as medium chain triglycerides (MCT), which are more readily absorbed from the premature gut.

**E. Calcium and Iron:** Fetal stores of iron and calcium are normally established during the third trimester. Premature infants are therefore at great risk of developing osteopenia, since they have limited calcium stores, a higher rate of bone growth and mineralization, and relatively poor absorption of dietary calcium. With either enteral or parenteral nutrition, every attempt should be made to provide a minimum of 130 mg of calcium per 100 kcal. This does not approach the amount of calcium normally acquired by the fetus during the third trimester, however, and careful observation for the possible development of osteopenia is therefore mandatory in premature infants. The available formulas for premature infants offer more calcium than standard formulas. In addition, the presence of MCT oil is believed to enhance calcium absorption by improving fat absorption and will therefore reduce the risk of osteopenia. If small premature infants are to be provided breast milk, human milk fortifier should be used since prolonged provision of human breast milk alone may not meet the calcium needs of the very premature infant.

Premature infants are born with decreased iron stores because most iron is accumulated toward the end of pregnancy. The exact age at which iron supplementation should be started has not been clearly established. Iron supplementation has been shown to increase the requirements for vitamin E, and thus could increase the risk of hemolysis due to vitamin E deficiency. When erythropoiesis has begun (as evidenced by reticulocytosis), iron supplementation can be provided in some of the preterm formulas or as an additive to human milk-fed babies. Earlier administration of exogenous iron will not stimulate erythropoiesis. The AAP recommends that serum vitamin E levels be closely monitored in preterm infants receiving iron supplementation prior to 2 months of age.

**Heat Conservation**

The decision to use an open radiant heater bed or closed incubator should be based on the routine operations of the nursery. Both systems offer advantages and disadvantages. Radiant heater beds offer caretakers ready access to unstable infants; however, heat losses due to convection and increased insensible water loss due to evaporation are greater than with incubators. Incubators are particularly useful for very premature infants, whose insensible fluid losses can be considerable. In addition, a heat shield can be placed over the infant in an incubator; this will decrease radiant heat losses even further. Double-walled incubators will also accomplish this purpose. They may also shield the infant from some extraneous noise, light, and air currents. Incubators, however, limit access and may obstruct the care of an acutely ill infant. With either system, skin or environmental temperature should be adjusted to maintain a thermoneutral state and minimize caloric expenditure and oxygen consumption.

# DISEASES OF THE PREMATURE NEONATE

## RESPIRATORY DISTRESS SYNDROME (RDS, Hyaline Membrane Disease)

Respiratory distress syndrome is caused by a functional deficiency of the pulmonary surfactant system. Pulmonary surfactant is a surface-active complex of phospholipids and proteins that reduces alveolar surface tension and prevents atelectasis. In addition, inhibitors of surfactant function may limit the surfactant's effectiveness as respiratory distress syndrome progresses. The progressive generalized atelectasis of RDS results in a loss of functional residual capacity and mismatched ventilation and perfusion. Increased alveolar-arterial differences, ventilatory failure with consequent cyanosis, tachypnea, and grunting at end expiration result, the last finding representing the infant's attempt to maintain alveolar distention during exhalation.

### Clinical Findings

**A. Signs:** Tachypnea, retractions, and grunting generally begin soon after birth and become progressively more severe. In babies not treated with surfactant replacement therapy, decreased air exchange and cyanosis worsen for the first 24–48 hours. The very premature infant may present with or develop apnea due to RDS. Since it has little chest wall muscularity or stability, the infant is unable to sustain respiration against the generalized atelectasis.

**B. Laboratory Findings:** Affected infants are hypoxic and often hypercapnic and acidotic. These

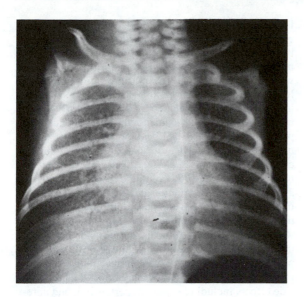

**Figure 29–7.** Chest x-ray of an infant with respiratory distress syndrome. The "ground-glass" appearance results from generalized atelectasis.

stresses may cause hypotension. Chest x-ray shows characteristic low lung volumes and a diffuse ground-glass appearance caused by atelectasis, which develops during the first 6 hours of life (Fig 29–7). Pulmonary function studies demonstrate increased work of breathing and diminished compliance, lung volume, and functional residual capacity.

**C. Associated Disorders:** While all premature infants are at great risk of developing RDS (incidence is approximately 60% at 29 weeks' gestation), other conditions are also associated with this disorder. Maternal diabetes mellitus increases the risk of RDS because the associated fetal hyperinsulinism limits the induction of enzymes necessary for surfactant production. Acidosis during labor and delivery can cause or worsen RDS by limiting surfactant production. Evaluation of fetal lung maturity by testing amniotic fluid for the presence of surfactant (L/S ratio, presence of phosphatidylinositol and phosphatidylglycerol, foam stability test) assists both obstetric and neonatal management. Corticosteroids administered to the mother to encourage maturation of the fetal lungs have been well shown to reduce the incidence and severity of RDS, as well as bronchopulmonary dysplasia in infants born prior to 32 weeks' gestation.

### Differential Diagnosis

The differential diagnosis of RDS includes bacterial and viral pneumonias, transient tachypnea of the newborn (TTN), and aspiration syndromes including meconium and amniotic fluid. TTN is self-limited (by definition resolving within 24 hours of birth) and generally requires minimal oxygen therapy. Viral pneumonias generally manifest streaky infiltrates on x-ray and can thereby be distinguished from RDS. On the other hand, bacterial pneumonias, particularly those caused by group B beta-hemolytic streptococci, often mimic RDS in both their clinical and their radiologic presentation. In fact, they may coexist with RDS, given the higher attack rate of bacterial pathogens in premature infants. For this reason, blood cultures should be obtained, culture of cerebrospinal fluid (CSF) should be considered, and antibiotic therapy should be considered in the initial management of an infant with presumed RDS.

### Treatment

For optimal care, a premature infant at risk for RDS should be delivered in a perinatal center with a pediatric resuscitation team in attendance. Early treatment to establish oxygenation, ventilation, and correction of acidosis and hypotension will moderate the clinical course of RDS. This is important, since acidosis and hypotension can destroy surfactant present in the lungs and impede production of surfactant by type II alveolar cells. In addition, early stabilization of the infant may reduce the risk of numerous other complications of prematurity, eg, intraventricular hemorrhage and necrotizing enterocolitis.

Several approaches exist for providing respiratory support to the premature infant with RDS. In general, infants with mild disease may simply be maintained in an environment with increased oxygen. Physical signs of respiratory distress as well as fractional inspired oxygen ($FIO_2$) and arterial blood gas tensions and pH must be closely monitored so that any worsening of condition—manifested by decreasing arterial oxygen tension ($PaO_2$) and increasing arterial carbon dioxide tension ($PaCO_2$)—can be quickly detected.

Infants with moderate to severe RDS (inability to maintain $PaO_2$ > 50 mm Hg with $FIO_2$ of .50–.80 or inability to maintain $PaCO_2$ < 50 mm Hg) require assisted ventilation. Numerous approaches, including continuous positive airway pressure or intermittent mandatory ventilation with either pressure-or volume-limited ventilators, are possible. Continuous positive airway presssure (CPAP) alone is often sufficient, particularly in larger premature infants. CPAP should be started earlier, ie, when $FIO_2$ reaches 0.5. When intermittent mandatory ventilation is used, positive end-expiratory pressure (4–8 cm water) is necessary in order to limit atelectasis at the end of expiration. Respiratory rate, inspiratory and expiratory time, inspiratory pressure or volume, and end-expiratory pressure can be adjusted to maintain $PaO_2$ between 50 and 70 mm Hg; $PaCO_2$ up to 50–60 mm Hg can be tolerated and may reduce barotrauma, which is thought to contribute to chronic lung disease. Frequent measurement of arterial blood gas tensions and pH or O2 saturation is necessary. If transcutaneous or oxygen saturation monitors are used to measure oxygenation, correlation with arterial blood samples is necessary so that use of ventilatory therapy can be minimized to avoid its toxic effects.

A number of exogenous surfactant preparations have undergone numerous clinical trials. Two are Federal Drug Administration (FDA) approved for general clinical use in the United States: a synthetic surfactant (EXOSURF Neonatal, Burroughs Wellcome Company, Research Triangle Park, NC) and a modified natural bovine surfactant (SURVANTA, Ross Laboratories, Division of Abbott Laboratories, Columbus, Ohio). There is now plentiful evidence that surfactant replacement therapy decreases the severity of RDS, decreases neonatal mortality, and increases survival without bronchopulmonary dysplasia. Dosing variables, including size of dose, method of administration, timing of first dose, and total number of doses, remain active areas of investigation. In addition, there is now evidence that replacement surfactant is even more effective in infants that have been treated prenatally with corticosteroids.

## Complications

**A. Retinopathy of Prematurity:** Retinopathy of prematurity (ROP, previously called retrolental fibroplasia), is a vasoproliferative retinal disorder that primarily affects premature, very low birth weight (VLBW) infants. It has been associated with prolonged exposure to high concentrations of oxygen in blood but can develop even in room air, particularly in the most immature infants. Studies indicate that oxygen therapy alone does not cause ROP and that other factors that have not yet been entirely elucidated are associated with its development. The more immature the infant, the greater is the risk of ROP. The theory of pathogenesis includes retinal vessel spasm, proliferation, hemorrhage, and fibrosis. ROP may regress spontaneously or progress to complete retinal detachment. It is responsible for producing visual loss or blindness in hundreds of children every year in the USA. Cryotherapy appears to be a promising means of treating this condition and may reduce the incidence of retinal detachment by up to 50%. Other treatment and prevention approaches under investigation include laser therapy and supplemental oxygen therapy. All infants born at < 30 weeks' gestation or < 1300 and all infants < 35 weeks or < 1800 who have received oxygen therapy should be screened for ROP by 4–8 weeks' of age.

**B. Bronchopulmonary Dysplasia:** Prolonged exposure of the immature lung to high oxygen concentrations and barotrauma pressure can result in bronchopulmonary dysplasia characterized pathologically by scarring of the airways and lung parenchyma, and clinically by supplemental oxygen requirement, increased airway reactivity, and a tendency toward pulmonary edema. It is not yet clear what part is played by the numerous contributing factors in the development of the disorder. The immature lung may lack sufficient antioxidant enzymes to scavenge damaging oxygen radicals; in addition, the exuberant inflammatory response of the immature lung may cause excessive scarring and fibrosis. Infants with bronchopulmonary dysplasia often require prolonged ventilatory support and environments with increased oxygen. Patience is required during treatment, since overzealous attempts to reduce supportive therapy will fail and possibly worsen the infant's condition. Bronchospasm, which often occurs with this disorder, can be effectively treated with bronchodilators (eg, theophylline and selective B-2 agonists). Fluid restriction and the use of diuretics may reduce interstitial edema and improve lung function. Excessive osteopenia due to urinary calcium wasting and nephrocalcinosis are two side effects of this therapy. Corticosteroid administration can improve lung function in some infants with bronchopulmonary dysplasia (BPD) but can have significant side effects including sepsis, hypertension, and adrenal malfunction. Studies of corticosteroids administered locally (ie, inhaled) are in progress with the hope of providing the pulmonary improvements with fewer adverse systemic effects.

**C. "Air Leaks":** This risk of pulmonary interstitial edema (PIE) pneumothorax, pneumomediastinum, or pneumopericardium exists in any premature infant requiring assisted ventilation. The development of any of these "air leaks" is the result of overdistention and rupture of alveoli and is typically signaled by a decrease in $PaO_2$ and blood pressure and, in the case of pneumothorax, narrowing of the pulse pressure. PIE is a serious complication with significant mortality in small premature infants. Treatment attempts include positioning and altering mechanical ventilation in an attempt to minimize gas trapping. Pneumothorax can be immediately evacuated with needle and syringe aspiration; however, all symptomatic or "tension" pneumothoraces require placement of a chest tube attached to an underwater seal and suction device, since the likelihood of reaccumulation of a gas in the pleural space following needle aspiration is great, especially during positive pressure ventilation. Chest and pericardial tubes should remain in place for at least 24–48 hours so that sufficient healing will occur to prevent recurrence of pneumothorax.

## HEART DISEASE

The incidence of congenital heart disease is the same in premature and term infants and ranges from 3 to 8/1000 live births. The incidence of patent ductus ateriosus is greatly increased in premature infants. Premature delivery does not automatically trigger closure of the ductus; continued hypoxia as a result of severe respiratory distress syndrome may maintain ductal patency, possibly because of the continued local production of vasodilator prostanoids such as prostaglandin E.

Early in RDS, when pulmonary vascular resistance is elevated, blood may shunt from right to left through the patent ductus. With resolution of RDS, pulmonary vascular resistance decreases and left-to-right shunting develops, both of which can complicate the ventilatory management of an infant with RDS, since the development of congestive heart failure will prolong the need for assisted ventilation. Prolonged ductal patency is also implicated in the etiology of bronchopulmonary dysplasia, necrotizing enterocolitis, and intraventricular hemorrhage.

The diagnosis of congestive heart failure due to patent ductus arteriosus is suggested by a systolic murmur over the precordium, rales at the lung bases, wide pulse pressure, and bounding peripheral pulses. The "machinery murmur" characteristic of patent ductus arteriosus in older children is rarely heard in premature infants. Chest x-ray demonstrates cardiac enlargement and fluid in the lung fields. Echocardiography and Doppler flow methods will delineate the patent ductus.

Closure of the ductus can be achieved in premature infants who have RDS by stringent limitation of fluid administration early in the disease. In symptomatic infants, early administration of indomethacin, a potent inhibitor of prostaglandin synthesis, may close the ductus. The drug may also be used later in the clinical course when congestive heart failure develops or if the duct reopens. Known complications of indomethacin therapy include transient renal failure and gastrointestinal bleeding. Indomethacin has been implicated in increasing the incidence of necrotizing enterocolitis and has been used in research trials for prevention of intraventricular hemorrhage. Congestive heart failure in the premature infant is best treated with fluid restriction and diuretics. Surgical ligation of the ductus is indicated in symptomatic infants if two courses of indomethacin therapy are unsuccessful or if indomethacin is contraindicated.

Preserving the patency of the ductus can be lifesaving in a number of different heart defects including those with restriction of pulmonary blood flow, transposition of the great vessels, or severe left ventricular outflow obstruction. Infusion of prostaglandin E will maintain ductal patency in preparation for neonatal transport or cardiac surgery.

## HYPERBILIRUBINEMIA

Most neonates develop some degree of jaundice during the newborn period because of a relatively rapid rate of hemolysis of fetal red blood cells and immature hepatic mechanisms for bilirubin conjugation and excretion. Certain disorders are associated with an increased degree of or prolonged hyperbilirubinemia as a result of altered rates of red cell breakdown, conjugation of bilirubin, and excretion of conjugated bilirubin. It should be noted that in the term infant, the severity of disease (as manifested by the extent of jaundice) correlates reasonably well with plasma bilirubin concentrations. However, this is not the case in premature infants.

### Etiology

**A.** Increased Rate of Hemolysis: These neonates have increased unconjugated bilirubin concentration and an increased reticulocyte count.

   **1.** Newborns with positive Coombs' test (this category includes all patients with isoimmunization, including ABO incompatibility, Rh incompatibility, etc).

   **2.** Neonates with negative Coombs' test.

      a. Abnormal red cell membrane, including spherocytosis, elliptocytosis, pyknocytosis, stomatocytosis.

      b. Red cell enzyme abnormalities: glucose 6-phosphate dehydrogenase deficiency, pyruvate kinase deficiency.

      c. Sepsis (eg, Clostridia).

**B.** Decreased Rate of Conjugation: These newborns have elevated levels of unconjugated bilirubin and a normal reticulocyte count.

   **1.** Immaturity of bilirubin conjugation ("physiologic jaundice").

   **2.** Congenital familial nonhemolytic jaundice (inborn errors of metabolism affecting glucuronyl transferase system and bilirubin transport).

   **3.** Breast milk jaundice.

**C.** Abnormalities of Excretion or Reabsorption: These neonates have elevated levels of conjugated and unconjugated bilirubin, negative Coombs' test, and normal reticulocyte count.

   **1.** Hepatitis.

      a. Infection.

      b. Toxic (eg, parenteral nutrition).

   **2.** Metabolic abnormalities.

      a. Galactosemia.

      b. Glycogen storage diseases.

      c. Maternal diabetes.

      d. Cystic fibrosis.

      e. $\alpha$-1 antitrypsin deficiency.

   **3.** Obstruction to biliary flow.

      a. Extrahepatic biliary atresia.

      b. Choledochal cyst.

      c. Alagille syndrome (paucity of intrahepatic bile ducts).

      d. Inspissated bile syndrome.

   **4.** Sepsis (eg, E. coli).

   **5.** Gastrointestinal obstruction (due to increased enterohepatic circulation of bilirubin).

The serum concentration of unconjugated bilirubin should be checked in all jaundiced infants, because in

**Table 29–2.** Indirect bilirubin concentration (mg/dL).

| BW (kg) | 5–6 | 7–9 | 10–12 | 13–15 | 16–20 | > 20 |
|---|---|---|---|---|---|---|
| < 1.0 | Phototherapy | | Think of exchange | | Exchange transfusion | |
| 1.0–1.5 | | Phototherapy | | Think of exchange | Exchange transfusion | |
| 1.5–2.0 | | | Phototherapy | | Think of exchange | Exchange transfusion |
| 2.0–2.5 | | | | Phototherapy | Think of exchange | Exchange transfusion |
| > 2.5 | | | | | Phototherapy | Think of exchange |

Guidelines for suggested bilirubin levels for phototherapy or exchange transfusion based on birth weight and clinical course of the infant. (Reproduced, with permission, from Harvey-Wilkes K, 1993).

some infants hyperbilirubinemia may cause sensorineural hearing loss or kernicterus.

Bilirubin concentrations that pose a definite risk to premature infants have not been established, although it is generally held that the acidosis, hypoxia, and fluid shifts that frequently complicate a premature infant's clinical course greatly increase the risk of central nervous system damage at relatively low bilirubin concentrations.

**Treatment**

1. Infant approaching phototherapy level (and being fed)

    a. Increase frequency of enteral feedings if possible. DeCarvahlo et al have shown that infants fed every 2 hours had increased frequency of stooling and lower bilirubin levels than those fed every 3 or 4 hours. Intake volume and weight gain/loss were similar between the two groups, thus the difference was not due to hydration, but to the increased frequency of stooling and thus, decreased contribution of the "enterohepatic circulation" of bilirubin.

    b. It is not necessary (or advisable) to discontinue breast milk. If the mother's milk has not "come in" yet, or she cannot nurse every 2–3 hours, or the infant seems thirsty supplement with formula. Water has been shown to *increase* the "enterohepatic circulation" of bilirubin.

2. Phototherapy is an important treatment method that uses radiant energy to isomerize bilirubin to a soluble form that is excreted by both the kidneys and gastrointestinal tract. When phototherapy is used, the infant's eyes must be covered to prevent potential damage to the rods and cones. Phototherapy lessens jaundice, so that skin appearance can no longer be used as a measure of bilirubin concentrations. It also substantially increases insensible fluid loss, so that fluid therapy must be managed accordingly. Use of phototherapy

in infants with conjugated hyperbilirubinemia may result in bronze baby syndrome. The National Institute of Child Health and Human Development determined that phototherapy used to control serum bilirubin is safe and as effective in preventing brain injury as exchange transfusion.

3. A double-volume exchange transfusion through an umbilical arterial or venous catheter is performed when serum bilirubin approaches a level at which neurologic damage can occur. Fresh O-negative, low-antibody-titer whole blood should be used. The risks of exchange transfusion include catheter accidents, infection, and acute blood pressure changes that can increase the risk of hemorrhage or cause or worsen congestive heart failure.

Guidelines for suggested bilirubin levels for phototherapy or exchange transfusion based on birth weight and clinical course of the infant are shown in Table 29–2.

## HEMATOLOGIC DISORDERS

### Isoimmunization

See Chapter 13.

### Hemorrhagic Diseases of the Newborn (Hypoprothrombinemia)

Levels of vitamin K-dependent clotting factors (factors II, VII, IX, and X) are normal at birth but decrease within 2–3 days. In vitamin K-deficient infants, these levels may be very low, resulting in prolonged bleeding times. The reported incidence of classic hemorrhagic disease of the newborn ranges from 1.7% of births to 5.4/100,000 births. Bleeding may occur into the skin or gastrointestinal tract, at the site of injection or circumcision, or at internal sites.

Small amounts of vitamin K are generally sufficient to correct clotting factor defects. All newborns should receive vitamin K, 1 mg intramuscularly, on admission to the nursery.

## Anemia

Placenta previa, abruptio placentae, velamentous cord insertion, a torn cord or placenta, or twin-to-twin transfusion may result in hemorrhage and consequent anemia. Anemia may also result from accelerated red cell hemolysis due to isoimmunization, membrane defects, hemoglobinopathy, enzymopathy or microangiopathic hemolysis. A regenerative anemia is rare. Treatment depends on the severity of anemia. If hypotension or hypo perfusion develops, as characterized by a capillary filling time exceeding 3 seconds, volume expansion is indicated. The asymptomatic term infant with a hematocrit between 20 and 30% may not require transfusion; supplemental iron (3–6 mg/kg/d of elemental iron orally) should be given and the infant followed closely. While transfusions are often required, recombinant human erythropoietin has been used successfully for anemia of prematurity and has been suggested for hyporegenerative anemia following in-utero transfusion for maternal isoimmunization.

## Polycythemia

A venous hematocrit exceeding 65% is considered polycythemia in a neonate and is found in 2–6% of newborns. Blood viscosity increases roughly exponentially with increases in hematocrit. Polycythemia is associated with twin-to-twin transfusion and enhanced placental transfusion due to late cord clamping; it is also noted in infants of diabetic mothers, small for gestational age (SGA) infants, and infants with congenital, adrenal hyperplasia, thyrotoxicosis, or Down's syndrome.

The complications of polycythemia per se are related to volume overload and congestive heart failure. Hyperviscosity, on the other hand, causes sludging in the vascular bed, and complications include infarction of the cerebral, mesenteric, and renal vascular beds. Clinical manifestations include tachypnea, central nervous system disturbances, and hypoglycemia.

Therapy calls for reducing the hematocrit with partial exchange transfusion. The volume of blood to be exchanged for plasma or saline is calculated as follows:

Volume of = blood x (observed – desired
blood to be   volume   hemocrit     hemocrit)
exchanged (mL)
                                   ————————————————
                                   observed hemocrit

Phlebotomy alone should never be performed. Intravenous hydration may be sufficient to reduce the hematocrit. It is likely that early partial exchange transfusion will limit or prevent most of the complications of hyperviscosity, although controversy exists over the value of partial exchange transfusion in asymptomatic polycythemic infants.

## GASTROINTESTINAL DISORDERS

### Necrotizing Enterocolitis

Necrotizing enterocolitis occurs mainly in premature infants and is characterized by necrosis and sloughing of the bowel mucosa from the muscularis. In severe situations, bowel perforation and dissection of gas into the hepatic portal tree can occur. Necrotizing enterocolitis typically develops in the small intestine. Infants will develop feeding intolerance and abdominal distention, pass bloody stools, and demonstrate intramural gas in dilated loops of bowel on x-ray.

The causes of necrotizing enterocolitis are unclear. In relatively large premature infants (about 34 weeks' gestation), the period of greatest risk for the development of necrotizing enterocolitis is the first 2 weeks of life. Smaller and more immature infants have a longer risk period, and the onset is often delayed. Necrotizing enterocolitis is known to occur in both sporadic and epidemic patterns. The etiology of necrotizing enterocolitis is felt to be multifactorial. Hypoxic-ischemic states, bacteria, and enteral feeding all have potential roles in mediating bowel injury.

If necrotizing enterocolitis is suspected or diagnosed, feedings should be discontinued and the bowel decompressed with low-pressure suction applied to a soft feeding tube. Blood and stool cultures should be obtained and antibiotics and parenteral nutrition administered. Careful surveillance should be maintained for acidosis and hypovolemia. Surgical consultation should be obtained early. Frequent abdominal x-rays should be obtained to monitor disease progression. The need for 0 surgical treatment is based on resolution or progression of the disease. The overall survival rate is 70–80%, and approximately 60% will develop sepsis. Of those treated medically, 11–36% will develop strictures.

### Diaphragmatic Hernia

Diaphragmatic hernia is a congenital malformation in which herniation of abdominal organs into a hemithorax occurs because of a defect in the diaphragm. Hernias on the left, due to a defect in the foramen of Bochdalek, account for 70% of diaphragmatic hernias. Infants with diaphragmatic hernias present with cyanosis and severe respiratory distress immediately after birth. Because the abdominal viscera are in the chest, the abdominal contour is scaphoid, and breath sounds are diminished or absent. With assisted ventilation, the gastrointestinal tract fills with gas, further compromising ventilation. Successful management depends on early diagnosis, decompression of the stomach and intestines with continuous suction, appropriate ventilation with an endotracheal tube, and circulatory support. Immediate surgical intervention is indicated.

Prognosis for survival depends on the severity of pulmonary hypoplasia and pulmonary hypertension and on the presence of associated structural or chromosomal abnormalities. Extracorporeal membrane oxygenation has been used successfully for diaphragmatic hernia therapy in selected cases, although the impact on overall survival rates is controversial. While early results of attempts at in-utero repair have been discouraging, active research on fetal surgery techniques continues.

## Omphalocele & Gastroschisis

Both omphalocele and gastroschisis require immediate care in the delivery room. In omphalocele, part or all of the intestines as well as the liver and spleen may be visible in a sac protruding through the abdominal wall. In gastroschisis, abdominal organs protrude through a congenital fissure of the abdominal wall. In both disorders, the externalized viscera should be covered with gauze soaked in warm, sterile saline and covered with a sterile plastic bag. Every effort should be made to avoid trauma to the viscera before corrective surgery.

## Tracheoesophageal Fistula & Esophageal Atresia

Atresia of the esophagus with an associated fistula between the distal segment of the esophagus and the trachea is the most frequently occurring esophageal anomaly. Less common are esophageal atresia without fistula, and the H-type fistula. Esophageal atresia should be suspected in cases of polyhydramnios. The earliest sign of tracheoesophageal fistula is regurgitation of saliva on the first feeding. Aspiration may occur and cause choking and coughing. As inspired air is drawn through the fistula, abdominal distention may occur.

Tracheoesophageal fistula can be diagnosed by passing a catheter through the nose or mouth down into the fistula and obtaining an x-ray of the upper airway. Contrast studies to determine the type of lesion should be performed only by a skilled pediatric radiologist at a tertiary-care hospital.

## RENAL FAILURE

Severe perinatal asphyxia, cardiorespiratory arrest, hemorrhage, or other stresses that acutely limit perfusion of the kidneys may cause cortical or medullary necrosis. This is characterized by anuria or oliguria and is followed by polyuria if the infant survives. Decreased urine output also occurs with indomethacin therapy or with clot formation in the renal arteries occurring as a complication of the use of umbilical catheters.

When renal failure is suspected in an infant with decreased urine output (normal, 1–2 mL/kg of body weight/h), fluid challenge with intravenous fluids, 10–20 mL/kg of body weight, followed by furosemide, 1–2 mg/kg intravenously, should be performed. If urine output increases, fluid administration should be increased. Dopamine, 5 µg/kg/min, may improve renal perfusion and output at this time. If fluid challenge fails to stimulate urine production, fluid administration should be limited to replacement of insensible losses and urine output. Serum electrolyte concentrations should be measured frequently so that metabolic derangements associated with renal failure can be detected. These include hyponatremia, hyperkalemia, hyperphosphatemia, hypocalcemia, and metabolic acidosis. Hypertension may also occur. The characteristic electrocardiographic changes associated with hyperkalemia in adults may not develop in infants. Hyperkalemia may be treated acutely with intravenous sodium bicarbonate, insulin and glucose, or ion exchange resin enemas (eg, sodium polystyrene sulfonate [Kayexalate], 1 g/kg in sorbitol).

In some newborns with acute renal failure, dialysis is considered. Peritoneal dialysis is preferred to hemodialysis in newborns because of less technical difficulty and similar effectiveness. Continuous arteriovenous hemofiltration is an alternative technique for removal of excess fluid without dialysis, and it may also be considered.

Acute oliguric failure in the newborn carries a mortality rate of 50%. Nonoliguric renal failure has a much better prognosis.

## CENTRAL NERVOUS SYSTEM DISORDERS

### Newborn Encephalopathy

Newborn encephalopathy occurs at a rate of 1–6/1000 term births depending on severity. The use of fetal heart rate monitoring does not seem to have had a major impact of the incidence. This condition has been given a variety of names including hypoxic-ischemic encephalopathy and postasphyxial encephalopathy. An undefined proportion of newborn encephalopathy is felt to be due to hypoxia and ischemia, which can occur prior to labor or during labor and delivery. Depending on the timing and severity of the insult, the manifestations include irritability, tremor, stupor, seizures, coma, and death.

Supportive care includes maintenance of nutrition, respiratory support, and anticonvulsants for seizures. CT scan, cranial ultrasound, and EEG are useful in determining the site of brain lesions. The prognosis for infants who have suffered hypoxic ischemic encephalopathy is unpredictable. The risk of long-term impairment of cognitive and psychomotor development to survivors is approximately 25%. The prognostic value of measures of intrapartum asphyxia such as Apgar scores are especially poor. Perinatal asphyxia is felt to account for only 8–15% of cases of cerebral palsy, and most survivors of asphyxia do not have cerebral palsy.

## Seizures

The cause of seizures must be quickly identified. The infant should be evaluated for treatable causes such as hypoglycemia, hypocalcemia, acidosis, and sepsis. Initial management should ensure adequate ventilation, oxygenation, and perfusion Phenobarbital, 15–20 mg/kg IV, is the treatment of choice. If seizures continue, a second and third dose (10 mg/kg) may be given, to a maximum of 30–40 mg/kg. With high doses of phenobarbital, the infant should be observed carefully for respiratory depression. If phenobarbital fails to control seizures, phenytoin, 15–20 mg/kg IV, may be administered. The rate of administration should not exceed 1 mg/kg/min to avoid depression of cardiac rhythm. Diazepam, 0.1 mg/kg intravenously, may be administered, but it acts synergistically with phenobarbital to depress respiration. If plasma levels of 30–45 mg/mL of phenobarbital and 10–20 mg/mL of phenytoin fail to control seizures, paraldehyde (0.1–0.3 mL/kg diluted 1:1 or 1:2 in mineral oil) may be administered rectally.

## Intracranial Hemorrhage in the Premature Infant

Up to 50% of premature infants develop some degree of intracranial hemorrhage. These hemorrhages most commonly initiate in the fragile capillaries of the germinal matrix layer of the subependymal region, the ventricles, and the periventricular white matter. A commonly used grading system defines grade I as germinal matrix hemorrhage, grade II as blood within but not distending the lateral ventricles, grade III as blood distending the ventricles, and grade IV as parenchymal involvement. It is not clear whether low grade hemorrhage has an impact on long-term outcome, while the more severe grades are associated with a higher incidence of adverse neurologic outcome and posthemorrhagic hydrocephalus.

The development of intraventricular hemorrhage is thought to relate to fluctuation in cerebral blood flow and pressure and is associated with hypercapnia, rapid volume expansion, seizures, and pneumothorax. No specific preventative therapy is presently available. Abrupt increase in blood pressure should be avoided. Blood gas values should be monitored frequently, and coagulopathies should be corrected.

All infants with identified hemorrhage should be followed with serial cranial ultrasounds or CT scans to check for extension of bleeding and the development of posthemorrhagic hydrocephalus. If hydrocephalus progresses, serial lumbar puncture or neurosurgery to drain cerebrospinal fluid may be indicated.

## INFECTIONS

Signs of infection in the newborn may be as subtle as slight temperature instability and jaundice or as overt as respiratory distress and shock. Whenever an infection is suspected, samples of blood, urine, and, when appropriate, cerebrospinal fluid should be obtained for examination and culture. A complete blood count, smear for differential, and a platelet count should also be obtained. Thrombocytopenia and both of the extremes of neutrophil count suggest sepsis. Broad spectrum antibiotics to cover both gram-positive and gram-negative organisms should be initiated. When culture results become available, drugs may be changed as necessary.

In infants born more than 24 hours after rupture of the membranes, white blood cell counts and blood cultures should be obtained. The decision to initiate antibiotic therapy should be based on the infant's clinical status.

Group B streptococcus is the most common cause of neonatal sepsis. Although approximately 30% of pregnant women are colonized with these organisms, and there is a 70% rate of vertical transmission of colonization, relatively few infants actually develop sepsis. Those who do often present with respiratory difficulties that mimic RDS. Risk factors for the development of rarely onset group B streptococcal sepsis include premature delivery, rupture of membranes greater than 18 hours, maternal fever in labor, and multiple gestation. Intrapartum chemoprophylactic strategies have been developed to decrease the risk of sepsis. Treatment consists of intravenous penicillin and ampicillin. A sample of cerebrospinal fluid should be examined to check for signs of meningitis. Other bacteria that cause neonatal sepsis and meningitis include *E coli, Listeria monocytogenes,* and staphylococci.

Infants thought to have viral infections acquired in utero require antibody titers and cultures to confirm the diagnosis. Infants who are shedding virus may require isolation. Evaluation for potential long-term difficulties such as impaired hearing and cognitive development should be carried out (brain stem auditory evoked potentials, neurosonograms, etc).

Infants with herpesvirus infections such as herpes simplex and varicella may require acyclovir therapy. Infants born to mothers who develop chicken pox within 5 days of delivery should be given varicella-zoster immune globulin prophylaxis.

Hepatitis immune globulin and hepatitis vaccine should be given to infants born to mothers with hepatitis B surface antigenemia. Hepatitis vaccine has also been added to the schedule of routine pediatric vaccination. The first dose is given prior to hospital discharge.

Infants delivered of mothers with human immunodeficiency virus (HIV) infection should be identified. The risk of vertical transmission is approximately 25–30%. Early initiation of antiviral and antibacterial treatment is of significant benefit to the infant. Breastfeeding is contraindicated when formula feeding is available.

Infection with cytomegalovirus poses a great threat

to the fetus and neonate and may even be fatal in utero. Intrauterine infection occurs in 0.5–3 of all live births and is the most common congenital infection. Although infection in most infants is asymptomatic and goes unrecognized, some infants with cytomegalovirus infection are at risk for severe deficits in cognitive and psychomotor development, and they may demonstrate varying degrees of sensorineural hearing loss. Primary maternal infection carries the greatest risk of transmission and of severe sequelae. Recurrent infection is thought rarely to cause congenital infection with adverse outcome. Cytomegalovirus can be transmitted in breast milk.

*Chlamydia trachomatis* is a gram-negative bacterium acquired by the newborn at delivery that can cause both conjunctivitis and pneumonitis during the later neonatal period. Conjunctivitis develops 5–12 days after birth and can be severe, resulting in conjunctival scarring if untreated. Pneumonitis develops within the first 3 months of life. The infant is typically afebrile and tachypneic and has a short, abrupt cough. Treatment of chlamydial conjunctivitis includes oral erythromycin and topical sulfacetamide ointment for the eyes.

## DRUG & ALCOHOL ADDICTION

There has been a dramatic increase in the past decade in the number of infants born to mothers using legal and illegal substances that can harm the fetus. The most commonly used currently are cocaine and other stimulants. Infants born to these women have an increased incidence of prematurity, low birth weight, and congenital infections. Other problems for which they may be at risk include drug withdrawal, visual dysfunction, vascular accidents resulting in cerebral infarcts, necrotizing enterocolitis, and limb anomalies. They appear to be at greater risk for sudden infant death syndrome (SIDS).

Infants born to narcotic-addicted women are more likely to be born prematurely and intrauterine growth restricted. They may undergo withdrawal and manifest the neonatal abstinence syndrome findings of tremors, irritability, hyperactivity, diarrhea, sweating, sneezing, and possibly seizures. Toxicologic analysis of urine can confirm the in utero exposure to drugs such as cocaine and opiates.

Many passively addicted infants can be treated without medication; holding, rocking, swaddling, and frequent feedings may be sufficient. Infants who fail to respond to symptomatic treatment will require pharmacologic therapy. The AAP recommends drug phenobarbital as the drug of choice, 5–10 mg/kg/d initially IM, then orally after good control has been achieved. If treatment with phenobarbital fails, dilute tincture of opium (DTO), diazepam, and chlorpromazine have also been used.

Maternal alcohol use during early gestation causes a teratogenic syndrome of fetal malformation. The fetal alcohol syndrome includes growth retardation, microcephaly, characteristic facial features, mental retardation, and cardiac and renal abnormalities.

Excessive ingestion of alcohol by the mother during late pregnancy may result in withdrawal symptoms in the infant that generally begin on the first day and may include tremors, hyperactivity, seizures, and hypoglycemia.

Multiple-drug abuse is common among substance-abusing women; simultaneous use of more than one drug should be suspected when fetal exposure to one drug has been identified. Furthermore, IV drug abusers are the second largest risk group for HIV infection. Infants born to a substance abuser should be evaluated for HIV infection.

## THE INFANT WITH DEVELOPMENTAL ABNORMALITIES

Infants born with developmental abnormalities need prompt evaluation by pediatricians, clinical geneticists, perinatologists, and other clinicians with expertise in dysmorphology. Most of these experts will be found in referral centers, which may necessitate transfer of a child born in a community hospital. The purpose of the following discussion is to outline certain principles of dysmorphology, to define commonly used terminology, and to furnish a method of assessment and a method of counseling for parents of dysmorphic offspring.

### Principles of Dysmorphology

(1) Most defects are nonspecific. An isolated defect does not generally allow diagnosis of a specific syndrome. For example, facial clefts occur in trisomy 13 syndrome, but not all infants with facial clefts have trisomy 13 syndrome.

(2) The overall pattern of defects is important for diagnosis. Thus, the presence of minor anomalies may be very useful in diagnosis.

(3) Not every malformation reported in a syndrome is necessary for diagnosis. Rarely does a patient exhibit every malformation reported with any given syndrome; and the same patient may exhibit variability from one side of the body to the other in those defects capable of being bilateral. This variance of expression is common to virtually all syndromes. For example, the characteristics of clefting, polydactyly, and cardiac defects form a basis for the diagnosis of trisomy 13 syndrome. However, only 60–80% of pa-

tients with this syndrome will have each of these specific anomalies.

(4) Similar phenotypes may mask different syndromes. Individuals with Marfan syndrome appear similar to individuals with homocystinuria; however, genetically, biochemically, and medically they are dissimilar.

## Terminology

An anomaly or malformation is a primary structural defect that results from a localized developmental error, eg, cleft lip. A deformation is an alteration in the structure or shape of a previously normally formed part, eg, clubfoot. A syndrome is a recognized pattern of malformations with the same cause and not the result of an isolated morphogenic error. Down's syndrome (trisomy 21 syndrome) is an example. A **sequence** is a pattern of malformations caused by a single developmental abnormality that leads to a cascade of defects, eg, Potter's sequence. Anomalies that occur together more frequently than expected by chance but that do not represent a syndrome are known as an association.

## Assessment of Developmental Defects

**A. Thorough Physical Examination:** Careful definition and recording of the anomalies and their extent is mandatory. This facilitates categorization of the errors, separation of primary and secondary defects, and definition of problems requiring immediate attention. The temptation to make a diagnosis based on preliminary information must be avoided. The information communicated (to families or other health care providers) should be descriptive and should serve to facilitate any further evaluation.

**B. History:** If physical examination alone is insufficient for diagnosis, the taking of a detailed history is imperative. The history should include at least the following information: a thorough history of this pregnancy with emphasis on the first trimester, including potential teratogen exposure and illness during pregnancy; a reproductive history; a 3-generation pedigree; and a complete maternal medical history.

**C. Genetic or Dysmorphic Consultation:** Given the extraordinary emotional impact of most anomalies, it is usually prudent to seek consultation from clinical geneticists, dysmorphologists, or appropriate pediatric subspecialists. With even the most obvious diagnoses it may assist the family in their acceptance of the problem.

**D. Photography:** Photographs permanently document the findings and may later serve to confirm the diagnosis or assist in study and consultation. They may be crucial should a severely malformed infant die before it can be evaluated by a dysmorphologist.

**E. Radiography:** Many syndromes have well-defined radiographic findings, but diagnosis may be difficult in certain cases. Selected radiographs, in-cluding whole-body radiographs of the infant that has died, may facilitate the diagnosis.

**F. Laboratory Evaluation:** The need for laboratory evaluation depends on the nature of the defect. In some cases, no laboratory evaluation is necessary. However, in many it is prudent to obtain cytogenetic studies. In other situations, it may be necessary to obtain microbiologic, immunologic, histologic, and metabolic studies.

**G. Autopsy:** In the event of the infant's death, autopsy may facilitate diagnosis. The type and extent of specific abnormalities must be recorded if the autopsy is to provide meaningful information.

## Counseling for Developmental Disabilities

Counseling for developmental disabilities can be difficult, and it may require a significant amount of time. It may be adequately provided by the primary physician who is sufficiently motivated and prepared, although the assistance of specialists can be helpful. Preparation for counseling includes (1) allocating enough time for a meaningful discussion (2) having adequate information about the abnormality (3) being comfortable dealing with this type of situation and (4) being able to listen carefully and be sensitive to the family's needs. Careful attention to questions will generally uncover misinformation.

While counseling for each family must be individualized, certain basic elements of counseling should be included (Table 29–3). Definitive counseling may require several visits, because factors such as stress may preclude normal assimilation of information.

The parents' adjustment to and acceptance of the situation may well depend upon the physician's initial introduction and explanations. Concerned relatives, friends, and medical staff often give the parents well-meaning but misdirected information. Parents frequently attempt to relate something they did or did not do during the course of the pregnancy to the defect. Careful consideration and factual explanation of the perceived relationship between the defect and the

**Table 29–3.** Elements of counseling
for developmental defects.[1]

Description of the anomalies present
The cause of the condition (if known)
An indication of the prognosis
A discussion of immediate options
Therapeutic means that may be necessary
The potential for recurrence
The mode of inheritance (if known)
Late complications to be expected
In cases of death, the autopsy findings
Thorough answering of questions
Provisions for familial emotional support

[1]Modified and reproduced, with permission, from: Pernoll ML, King CR, Prescott GH: Genetics in Obstetrics and Gynecology. In: *Obstetrics and Gynecology Annual: 1980.* Vol 9, p 31. Wynn RM (editor). Appleton-Century-Crofts, 1980.

time when the event occurred often assist in answering such questions. For example, the mother with a viral illness at 24 weeks' gestation may be reassured that this was not the cause of her infant's cleft palate.

Parents and siblings may experience psychologic trauma, which must be recognized in order to be managed effectively. This trauma may be expressed individually or collectively as shame, guilt, anger, denial, intellectualization, fear, depression, and a sense of failure. The family may consider the infant's condition to be retribution for a real or imagined sin. Blame between the parents will require thoughtful exploration and explanation. Sexual dysfunction often develops after the birth of an anomalous child. The entire family constellation must be considered for counseling to be effective.

## REFERENCES

Abbasi S, Bhutani VK, Gerdes JS: Long-term pulmonary consequences of respiratory distress syndrome in preterm infants treated with exogenous surfactant. J Pediatr 1993;122:446.

Allan WC: The IVH complex of lesions: Cerebrovascular injury in the preterm infant. Pediatr Neurol 1990;8:529.

American Academy of Pediatrics Committee on Bioethics: Treatment of critically ill newborns. Pediatrics 1983; 72:565.

American Academy of Pediatrics Committee on Drugs: Naloxone dosage and route of administration for infants and children: Addendum to emergency drug doses for infants and children. Pediatrics 1990;86:484.

American Academy of Pediatrics Committee on Drugs: Neonatal drug withdrawal. Pediatrics 1983;72:895.

American Academy of Pediatrics Committee on Drugs: Psychotropic drugs in pregnancy and lactation. Pediatrics 1982;69:241.

American Academy of Pediatrics Committee on Fetus and Newborn: Recommendations on extracorporeal membrane oxygenation. Pediatrics 1990;85:618.

American Academy of Pediatrics Committee on Fetus and Newborn: Surfactant replacement therapy for respiratory distress syndrome. Pediatrics 1991;87:946.

American Academy of Pediatrics Committee on Fetus and Newborn: Vitamin E and the prevention of retinopathy of prematurity. Pediatrics 1985;76:315.

American Academy of Pediatrics Committee on Infectious Diseases and Committee on Fetus and Newborn: Guidelines for prevention of group B streptococci (GBS) infection by chemoprophylaxis. Pediatrics 1992; 90:775.

Apgar V: A proposal for a new method of evaluation of the newborn infant. Curr Res Anesth Analg 1953;32:260.

Avery GB et al: Controlled trial of dexamethasone in respiratory-dependent infants with bronchopulmonary dysplasia. Pediatrics 1985;75:106.

Bada HS et al: Asymptomatic syndrome of polycythemic hyperviscosity: Effect of partial plasma exchange transfusion. J Pediatr 1992;120:579.

Barst RJ, Gersony WM: The pharmacological treatment of patent ductus arteriosus. Drugs 1989;38:249.

Bartlett RH: Extracorporeal life support for respiratory failure in children and adults: An introduction to ECLS. University of Michigan Medical Center, Ann Arbor, MI June 19–20, 1993.

Berseth CL: Effect of early feeding on maturation of the infant's small intestine. J Pediatr 1992;120:947.

Bloom RS, Cropley C: *The Textbook of Neonatal Resuscitation.* Chameides L, AHA/AAP Neonatal Resuscitation Steering committee (eds). American Heart Association, 1990.

Boon AW, Milner AD, Hopkin IE: Lung expansion, tidal exchange, and formation of the functional residual capacity during resuscitation of asphyxiated neonates. J Pediatr 1979;95:1031.

Briggs GG, Freeman RK, Yaffee SJ: *Drugs in Pregnancy and Lactation: A Reference Guide to Fetal and Neonatal Risk,* 3rd ed. Williams and Wilkins, 1990.

Brown MS, Berman ER, Luckey DL: Prediction of the need for transfusion during anemia of prematurity. J Pediatr 1990;116:773.

Buck ML: Prostaglandin $E_1$ treatment of congenital heart disease: Use prior to Neonatal transport. DICP Ann Pharmacother 1991;25:408.

Carson BS et al: Combined obstetric and pediatric approach to prevent meconium aspiration syndrome. Am J Obstet Gynecol 1976;126:712.

Canarelli JP et al: Ligation of the patent ductus arteriosus in premature infants—indications and procedures. Eur J Pediatr Surg 1993;3:3.

Caplan MS, MacGregor SN: Perinatal management of congenital diaphragmatic hernia and anterior abdominal wall defects. Clin Perinatol 1989;16:917.

Carmi D et al: Polycythemia of the preterm and full-term newborn infant: Relationship between hematocrit and gestational age, total blood solutes, reticulocyte count, and blood pH. Biol Neonate 1992;61:173.

Crowley P, Chalmers I, Keirse MJNC: The effects of corticosteroid administration before preterm delivery: An overview of the evidence from controlled trials. Br J Ob Gynaecol 1990;97:11.

Cryotherapy for Retinopathy of Prematurity Cooperative Group: Multicenter trial of cryotherapy for retinopathy of prematurity: Preliminary results. Pediatrics 1988;81:697.

Cunningham AS et al: Tracheal suction and meconium: A proposed standard of care. J Pediatr 1990;116:153.

DeCarvahlo M, HollM, Harvey D: Effects of water supplementation of physiological jaundice in breastfed babies. Arch Dis child 1981;56:568.

DeCarvahlo M, Klause MH, Merkatz RB: Frequency of breastfeeding and serum bilirubin concentration. Am J Dis Child 1982;136:737.

Dubowits LMS, Dubowitz V: *Assessment of Gestational Age in the Newborn: A Clinical Manual.* Addison-Wesley, 1977.

Emmerson AJB et al: Double blind trial of recombinant

human erythropoietin in preterm infants. Arch Dis Child 1993;68:291.

Fowler KB et al: The outcome of congenital cytomegalovirus infection in relation to maternal antibody status. N Engl J Med 1992;326:663.

Frank L: Antioxidants, nutrition, and bronchopulmonary dysplasia. Clin Perinatol 1992;19:541.

Fujiwara T et al: Surfactant replacement therapy with a single postventilatory dose of a reconstituted bovine surfactant in preterm neonates with respiratory distress syndrome: Final analysis of a multicenter, double-blind, randomized trial and comparison with similar trials. Pediatrics 1990;86:753.

Gerdes JS: Clinicopathologic approach to the diagnosis of neonatal sepsis. Clin Perinatol 1991;18:361.

Gibson DL et al: Retinopathy of prematurity-induced blindness; birth weight specific survival and the new epidemic. Pediatrics 1990;86:405.

Göbel W, Richard G: Retinopathy of prematurity—current diagnosis and management. Eur J Pediatr 1993;152:286.

Goldfarb J: Breastfeeding: AIDS and other infectious diseases. Clin Perinatol 1993;20:225.

Gross SJ, Slagle TA: Feeding the low birth weight infant. Clin Perinatol 1993;20:193.

*Guidelines of Perinatal Care.* 3rd ed. American Academy of Pediatrics/American College of Obstetricians and Gynecologists, Freeman RK (ed.), 1992.

Halac E et al: Prenatal and postnatal corticosteroid therapy to prevent neonatal necrotizing enterocolitis: A controlled trial. J Pediatr 1990;117:132.

Holtzman RB et al: Perinatal management of meconium staining of the amniotic fluid. Clin Perinatol 1989;16:825.

Howard CR, Weitzman M: Breast or bottle: Practical aspects of infant nutrition in the first 6 months. Pediatr Ann 1992;21:619.

Hudak BB, egan EA: Impact of lung surfactant therapy on chronic lung diseases in premature infants. Clin Perinatol 1992;19:591.

Hull J, Dodd K: What is birth asphyxia? Br J Obstet Gynaecol 1991;98:953.

Jacobs MM, Phibbs RH: Prevention, recognition, and treatment of perinatal asphyxia. Clin Perinatol 1989;16:785.

Javitt J, Cas RD, Chiang Y: Cost-effectiveness of screening and cryotherapy for threshold retinopathy of prematurity. Pediatrics 1993;91:859.

Johnson L et al: Effect of sustained pharmacologic vitamin E levels on the incidence and severity of retinopathy of prematurity: A controlled trial. J Pediatr 1989;114:827.

Jones KL: *Smith's Recognizable Patterns of Human Malformation,* 4th ed. Saunders, 1988.

Karlowicz MG, Adelman RD: Acute renal failure in the neonate. Clin Pediatr 1992;19:139.

Klebanoff MA et al: The risk of childhood cancer after neonatal exposure to vitamin K. N Engl J Med 1993;329:905.

Kliegman RM: Models of the pathogenesis of necrotizing enterocolitis. J Pediatr 1990;117:52.

Knight DB: Patent ductus arteriosus: How important to which babies? Early Hum Dev 1992;29:287.

Kosloske AM: A unifying hypothesis for pathogenesis and prevention of necrotizing enterocolitis. J Pediatr 1990;117:568.

Kwong MS, Holm BA, Egan EA: Use of surfactant in the delivery room. Clin Perinatol 1989;16:853.

Lamp KC, Reynolds MS: Indomethacin for prevention of neonatal intraventricular hemorrhage. DICP 1991;25:1344.

Levine RL, Fredericks WR, Rapoport SI: Entry of bilirubin into the brain due to opening of the blood-brain barrier. Pediatrics 1982;69:255.

Leviton A, Nelson KB: Problems with definitions and classifications of newborn encephalopathy. Pediatr Neurol 1992;8:85.

Linderkamp O et al: The effect of early and late cord-clamping on blood viscosity and other hemorheological parameters in full-term neonates. Acta Pediatr 1992;81:745.

Low JA: The relationhhip of asphyxia in the mature fetus to long-term neurologic outcome. Clin Obstet Gynecol 1993;36:82.

Mammel MC et al: Controlled trial of dexamethasone therapy in infants with bronchopulmonary dysplasia. Lancet 1983;1:1356.

Martin GI, Sindel BD: Neonatal management of the very low birth weight infant: The use of surfactant. Clin Perinatol 1992;19:461.

Ment LR: Intraventricular hemorrhage of the preterm infant. Pages 315–318, in: *Principles and Practice of Pediatrics.* DeAngelis CD, Feigin RD, Warshaw JB (eds) Lippincott, 1990.

Molenaar JC et al: Congenital diaphragmatic hernia, what defect? J Pediatr Surg 1991;26:248.

Nelson KB, Ellenberg JH: Antecedents of cerebral palsy. N Engl J Med 1986;315:81.

Northway WH: An introduction to bronchopulmonary dysplasia. Clin Perinatol 1992;19:489.

Ogata ES: Perinatal carbohydrate metabolism in the fetus and neonate and altered neonatal glucoregulation. Pediatr Clin North Am 1986;33:25.

Ogata ES: Problems of the infant of the diabetic mother. In: *Pediatrics.* Rudolph A (ed.). Appleton-Century-Crofts, 1982.

Ogata ES et al: Pneumothorax in the respiratory distress syndrome: Incidence and effect on vital signs, blood gases, and pH. Pediatrics 1976;58:177.

Papile LA et al: Posthemorrhagic hydrocephalus in low-birth-weight infants: Treatment by serial lumbar punctures. J Pediatr 1980;97:273.

Pearson HA: Anemia in the newborn: A diagnostic approach. Semin Perinatol 1991;15:2.

Pearlman JM et al: Reduction in intraventricular hemorrhage by elimination of fluctuating cerebral blood-flow velocity in preterm infants with respiratory distress syndrome. N Engl J Med 1985;312:1353.

Pinckert TL, Golbus MS: Fetal surgery. Clin Perinatol 1988;15:943.

Pitt J: Perinatal human immunodeficiency virus infection. Clin Perinatol 1991;18:227.

Polin RA: Management of neonatal hyperbilirubinemia: Rational use of phototherapy. Biol Neonate 1990;58(Suppl 1):32.

Polin RA, Yoder MC, Burg FD: *Workbook in Practical Neonatalogy.* 2nd ed. Sunders, 1993.

Reller MD et al: Ductal patency in neonates with respiratory distress syndrome. A randomized surfactant trial. Am J Dis Child 1991;145:1017.

Reller MD et al: The timing of spontaneous closure of the ductus arteriosus in infants with respiratory distress syndrome. Am J Cardiol 1990;66:75.

Remington JS, Klein JO (eds): *Infectious Diseases of the Fetus and Newborn Infant,* 3rd ed. Saunders, 1990.

Samanek M et al: Prevalence, treatment and outcome of heart disease in live-born children: A prospective analysis of 91,832 live-born children. Pediatr Cardiol 1989; 10:205.

Scheidt PC et al: Phototherapy for neonatal hyperbilirubinemia: Six-year follow up of the National Institute of Child Health and Human Development clinical trial. Pediatrics 1990;85:455.

Schulman JL: Coping with major disease: Child, family pediatrician. J Pediatr 1983;102:988.

Schumacher RE et al: Follow-up of infants treated with extracorporeal membrane oxygenation for newborn respiratory failure. Pediatrics 1991;87:451.

Shaffer SG, Weismann DN: Fluid requirements in the preterm infant. Clin Perinatol 1992;19:233.

Shannon KM: Anemia of prematurity: Progess and prospects. Am J Pediatr Hematol Oncol 1990;12:14.

Singer L, Arendt R, Minnes S: Neurodevelopmental effects of cocaine. Clin Perinatol 1993;20:245.

Stolar CJ, Snedecor SM, Bartlett RH: Extracorporeal membrane oxygenation and neonatal respiratory failure: Experience from the extracorporeal life support organization. J Pediatr Surg 1991;26:563.

Taeusch HW, Ballard RA, Avery ME: *Diseases of the Newborn.* Saunders, 1991.

Tammela OK, Koivisto ME: Fluid restriction for preventing bronchopulmonary dysplasia? Reduced fluid intake during the first weeks of life improves the outcome of low-birth-weight infants. Acta Pediatr 1992;81:207.

Thorp JA et al: Hyporegenerative anemia associated with intrauterine transfusion in rhesus hemolytic disease. Am J Obstet Gynecol 1991;165:79.

Van Marter LJ et al: Maternal glucocorticoid therapy and reduced risk of bronchopulomary dysplasia. Pediatrics 1990;86:331.

Vannucci RC: Current and potentially new management strategies for perinatal hypoxicischemic encephalopathy. Pediatrics 1990;85:961.

Volpe JJ: Intraventricular hemorrhage in the premature infant—current concepts. Part II. Ann Neurol 1989;25:109.

Volpe JJ: Neonatal seizures: Current concepts and revised classification. Pediatrics 1989;84:422.

Von Kries R, Hanawa Y: Neonatal vitamin K prophylaxis. Report of scientific and standardization subcommittee on perinatal haemostasis. Thromb Haemost 1993;69:293.

Ward SLD, Keens TG: Prenatal substance abuse. Clin Perinatol 1992;19:849.

Weakley DR, Spencer R: Current concepts in retinopathy of prematurity. Early Hum Dev 1992;30:121.

Wiswell TE, Henley MA: Intratracheal suctioning, systemic infection, and the meconium aspiration syndrome. Pediatrics 1992;89:203.

# Gynecologic History, Examination, & Diagnostic Procedures

# 30

*Charles Kawada, MD*

A good gynecologist regards each patient at every visit as a whole person and pays careful attention to emotional as well as physical needs. The initial approach to the gynecologic patient and the general diagnostic procedures available for the investigation of gynecologic complaints are presented here. Although other aspects of the general medical examination are left to other texts, concern for the patient's total health and well-being is mandatory.

## THE PERIODIC HEALTH SCREENING EXAMINATION

It is now a generally accepted part of the physician's responsibility to advise patients to have periodic medical evaluations. The frequency of visits varies according to the patient's problem.

The periodic health screening examination helps detect the following ailments of women that are especially amenable to early diagnosis and treatment: diabetes mellitus; urinary tract infection or tumor; hypertension; malnutrition or obesity; thyroid dysfunction or tumor; and breast, abdominal, or pelvic tumor. These conditions can be detected by a review of systems, with specific questions regarding recent abnormalities or any variation in function. Determination of weight, blood pressure, and urinalysis, which can be done in minutes, may reveal variations from the previous examination. An examination of the thyroid gland, breasts, abdomen, and pelvis, including a Papanicolaou (Pap) smear, should then be performed. A rectal examination is also advisable, and a conveniently packaged test for occult blood (Hemoccult) is now available and recommended for patients over 40 years of age.

The physician should also be concerned about conditions other than purely somatic ones. Unless a patient's problems require the services of a psychiatrist or some other specialist, the doctor should be prepared to act as a counselor and work with the patient during a mutually agreeable time when it is possible to listen to her problems without being hurried and to give support, counsel, and other kinds of help as required.

## HISTORY

To adequately evaluate the gynecologic patient, it is important to establish a rapport during the history taking. The patient must be allowed to tell her story to an interested listener, who does not allow body language or facial expressions to imply disinterest or boredom. One should avoid cutting off the patient's story, since doing so may obscure important clues or other problems that may have contributed to the reasons for the visit.

The following outline varies from the routine medical history because, in evaluating the gynecologic patient, the problem can often be clarified if it is obtained in the following order.

### Identifying Information

**A. Age:** Knowledge of the patient's age sets the tone for the complaint and the approach to the patient. Obviously, the problems and the approach to them vary at different stages in a woman's life (pubescence, adolescence, childbearing years, and pre- and postmenopausal years).

**B. Last Normal Menstrual Period:** The date of onset of the last normal menstrual period (LNMP) is important to define. A missed period, irregularity of periods, erratic bleeding, or other abnormalities may all imply certain events that are more easily diagnosed when the date of onset of the LNMP is established.

**C. Gravidity and Parity:** The process of taking the patient's obstetric history is detailed in Chapter 9, but the reproductive history should be recorded as part of the gynecologic evaluation. A convenient symbol for recording the reproductive history is a 4-digit code denoting the number of term pregnancies, premature deliveries, abortions, and living children (TPAL); eg, 2-1-1-3 means 2 term pregnancies, 1 premature delivery, 1 abortion, and 3 living children.

## Chief Complaint

The chief complaint is usually best elicited by asking "What kind of problem are you having?" or "How can I help you?" It is important to listen carefully to the way in which the patient responds to this question and to allow her to fully explain her complaint. The patient should be interrupted only to clarify certain points that may be unclear.

## Present Illness

Each of the problems the patient describes must be obtained in detail by questioning regarding what exactly is the problem, where exactly the problem is occurring, the date and time of onset, whether the symptoms are abating or getting worse, the duration of the symptoms when they do occur, and how these symptoms are related to or influence other events in her life. For example, the site, duration, and intensity of pain must be accurately described. Often helpful in evaluating the intensity of pain is getting a sense of how the pain affects her life: "Does the pain prevent you from standing or walking?"

It is important to maintain eye contact with the patient and to listen to every word. Do not rely on a patient's sophistication as a measure of her knowledge of anatomy and medical terminology. It is important for the physician to judiciously adjust the level of terminology according to the patient's knowledge and vocabulary. Communicating with the patient in this manner may help the physician obtain an accurate history and establish rapport.

In addition to physiologic events and the life cycle, symptoms described could be related to the beginning of a new job, the beginning of a new relationship or difficulties in the current relationship, an exercise regimen, new medication, and any emotional changes in the patient's life.

## Past History

After the physician is satisfied that all possible information concerning the present illness and the important corollaries has been obtained, the past history should be elicited.

**A. Contraception:** Continuing with the history, it is important to elicit whether the patient is using or needs some form of contraception. If she is using contraception, her level of satisfaction with her chosen method should be determined. In patients taking oral contraceptives, the history should reflect the agent and dose, whether there is a great variation in the time of day she takes her pill, and any impact the pill has had on other physiologic functions. It is also extremely important to ask questions during the remainder of the history and to key the physical examination to ascertain whether there are any contraindications to the patient's current form of contraception.

**B. Medications and Habits:** Any medications, prescribed or otherwise, that are being taken or that were being taken when symptoms first occurred

should be described. Particular attention must be directed to use of hormones, steroids, and other compounds likely to influence the reproductive tract. In addition to medications the patient should be questioned concerning her use of recreational drugs. It must be ascertained whether the patient smokes and, if so, how much and for how long. It is also important to ascertain the amount of alcohol ingested, if any. This questioning provides an ideal time to indicate the health risks of various habits.

**C. Medical:** It is important to discover any history of prior serious medical and psychiatric illnesses and whether hospitalization was required. Particularly important are illnesses in the major organ systems. It is also important to know whether there is a major endocrinopathy in the patient's history. Notable weight gain or loss prior to the onset of the patient's current symptoms should be detailed. Other important details include when she had her last physical examination including pelvic examination and Pap smear.

**D. Surgical:** The surgical history includes all operations, the dates performed, and associated postoperative or anesthetic complications.

**E. Allergies:** Questioning should continue relating any possible allergic reactions to drugs or specific foods. The reaction produced (eg, rash, gastrointestinal upset) must be elicited and the approximate time when it occurred ascertained. Any testing to confirm or deny the observation must be noted.

**F. Bleeding Diatheses:** Determining whether or not the patient bleeds excessively in relation to prior surgery or small trauma is important. A history of easy bruising or of bleeding from the gums while brushing teeth may be useful in this judgment. Suspicion of a bleeding problem indicates the need for further laboratory evaluation.

**G. Obstetrics:** The obstetric history includes each of the patient's pregnancies listed in chronologic order. The date of birth; sex and weight of the offspring; duration of pregnancy; length of labor; type of delivery; type of anesthesia; and any complications should be included.

**H. Gynecologic:** The first item in the gynecologic past history is the menstrual history: age at menarche, interval between periods, duration of flow, amount and character of flow, degree of discomfort, and age at menopause. The menstrual history is often an important clue in the diagnosis.

A prior history of sexually transmitted disease (STD) needs to be detailed. Although in the past it was more common to note only gonorrhea and syphilis, it is important to also document exposure to HIV, herpesvirus, *Chlamydia,* and papillomavirus. Any treatment or admissions to the hospital for treatment of salpingitis, endometritis, or tubo-ovarian abscess must be carefully documented. Attempts to assess the impact of these processes in relation to ectopic pregnancy, infertility, and the type of contraception must be elicited.

Although its significance is less than that of the

prior stated diseases, the occurrence of episodes of vaginitis should not be dismissed. Their frequency and the medications used to treat them should be discussed. In the case of such infections, it is important to detail whether or not it was a pathologic situation or merely a misinterpreted physiologic circumstance.

**I. Sexual:** The sexual history should be an integral part of any general gynecologic history. In taking a sexual history, the physician must be nonjudgmental and not embarrassed or critical.

Questions that may be covered include the following. Is she currently sexually active? Is the relationship satisfactory to her and, if not, why not? A question regarding whether the patient is heterosexual or gay is important but often difficult to ask because the question may be offensive to some patients. It is important, however, not to assume that a relationship is heterosexual because a gay woman will lose all rapport with the physician when the physician is insensitive to such issues.

**J. Social:** A social history can be an extension of earlier questions pertaining to the marital and sexual history. Knowing the type of work the patient does (including the amount of physical exercise entailed), something of her education, and her community activities may assist in ascertaining the patient's relationship to her entire environment.

The patient's involvement with her own health care should be carefully elicited, including her attention and knowledge concerning diet, health screening examinations, exercise, and recreation.

## Family History

The patient's family history must include the state of health of immediate relatives (parents, siblings, grandparents, and offspring). In addition to listing these relatives, it is useful in cases where genetic illnesses may be apparent to record a 3-generation pedigree.

The incidence of familial heart disease, hypertensive renal or vascular disease, diabetes mellitus (insulin-dependent or non-insulin-dependent), vascular accidents, and hematologic abnormalities should be ascertained. If the patient has a problem with hirsutism or if she perceives an excessive hair growth, it is important to elicit whether anyone in her family has the same distribution of hair growth. Familial history of breast and ovarian cancers are important to elicit since a close familial history may require additional testing and close follow-up. It is important to relate the time of menopause in the mother or grandmother and to ascertain a history of osteoporosis.

## PHYSICAL EXAMINATION

The physical examination is most useful if it is conducted in an environment that is aesthetically pleasing to the patient. Adequate gowning and draping assist in the prevention of embarrassment. Often a physician's assistant conducts the patient to the dressing area and gives explicit instructions about what to take off and how to put on her gown and then may assist in draping the patient.

A physician may have a female assistant remain in the examining room to assist when necessary, but whether or not she remains solely as a chaperone depends on local custom, legal requirements, and the preference of the patient and the physician. A chaperone is not customarily or legally required, but the physician must be selective in this matter and have an assistant present during the examination of an overly fearful or potentially seductive patient. If the patient wants her husband, relative, or a female friend to be present, the request should be honored unless, in the physician's judgment, some impropriety might result or such an arrangement would interfere with the examination or with obtaining an accurate history.

### General Examination

If the gynecologist is the primary care physician for the patient, a general physical examination should be performed yearly or whenever the situation warrants. A complete examination obviously provides more information, demonstrates the physician's thoroughness, and establishes rapport with the patient.

### General Evaluation

**A. Vital Signs:** As part of every examination—whether for a specific problem, routine annual examination, or a return visit for a previously diagnosed problem—the patient should be weighed and her blood pressure taken. Postmenopausal patients should have their height measured to document whether there is loss of height from osteoporosis and vertebral fractures. Before she empties her bladder for the examination, it should be determined whether the urine will need to be sent for urinalysis, culture, or pregnancy testing.

The examination of the chest should include visual examination for any skin lesions and symmetry of movement. Auscultation and percussion of the lungs are important for excluding primary pulmonary problems such as asthma and pneumonia. The examination of the heart includes percussion for size and auscultation for arrhythmias and significant murmurs.

### Breast Examination
### (See also Chapter 62.)

Breast examination should be a routine part of the physical examination. Breast cancer will occur in 1 in 11 women in the USA. Physicians who treat women should educate patients in the technique of self-examination, since the well-prepared patient is one of the most accurate screening methods for breast disease.

The physical examination provides an ideal time to ascertain the frequency and methodology of breast self-examination. It also is an ideal time to teach the patient how to perform breast self-examination. The patient should be advised to examine herself in the mirror, looking for skin changes or dimpling, and then carefully palpate all quadrants of the breast. Most women prefer to do this with soapy hands while showering or bathing. The examination should be repeated at the same time each month, preferably 1 week after the initiation of the menses, when the breasts are least nodular; postmenopausal women should perform self-examination on the same day each month.

Baseline mammography is recommended for every woman at age 35. The frequency of subsequent mammography or the earlier use of mammography depends on both the individual women and her family history. Patients with a positive family history of breast cancer should have a mammogram at an earlier age, particularly those whose mother or sister developed premenopausal breast cancer. In general, after the baseline mammography, a mammogram should be repeated every 2 years from ages 40 to 50 and annually thereafter. Ultrasonography will now reliably differentiate solid from cystic lesions; this technique complements but does not supplant mammography. Indeed, breast self-examination, physician examination, mammography, and ultrasonography are complementary and all should be employed in the early detection of breast cancer.

The correct technique for breast examination is demonstrated in Figure 30–1. If abnormalities are en-

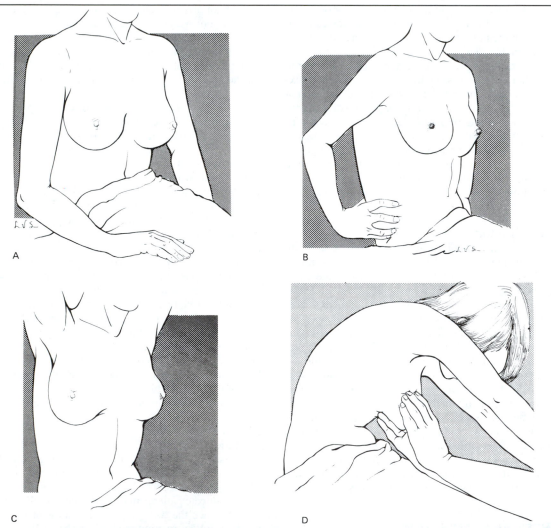

**Figure 30–1.** Breast examination by the physician. **A:** Patient is sitting, arms at sides. Perform visual inspection in good light, looking for lumps or for dimpling or wrinkling of skin. **B:** Patient is sitting, hands pressing on hips so that pectoralis muscles are tensed. Repeat visual inspection. **C:** Patient is sitting, arms above head. Repeat visual inspection of breasts and also perform visual inspection of axillae. **D:** Patient is sitting and leaning forward, hands on examiner's shoulders, the stirrups, or her own knees. Perform bimanual palpation, paying particular attention to the base of the glandular portion of the breast.

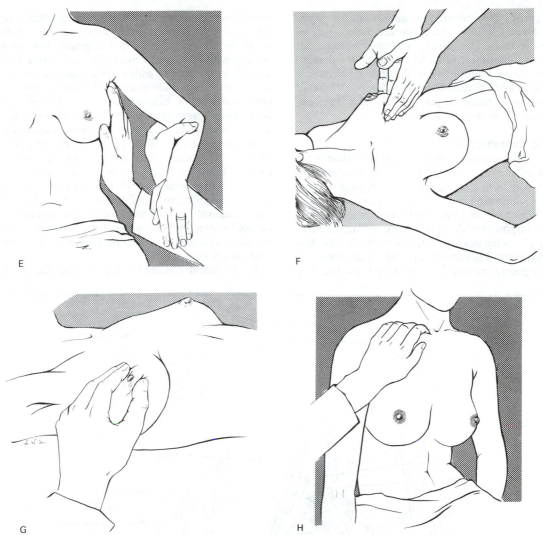

**Figure 30–1 (cont'd).** **E:** Patient is sitting, arms extended 60–90 degrees. Palpate axillae. **F:** Patient is supine, arms relaxed at sides. Perform bimanual palpation of each portion of breast (usually each quadrant, but smaller sections for unusually large breasts). Repeat examinations **C, E,** and **F** with patient supine, arms above head. **G:** Patient is supine, arms relaxed at sides. Palpate under the areola and nipple with the thumb and forefinger to detect a mass or test for expression of fluid from the nipple. **H:** Patient is either sitting or supine. Palpate supraclavicular areas.

countered, a decision should be reached concerning the need for mammography (or other imaging methods) or direct referral to a breast surgeon unless the gynecologist is trained in performing breast biopsies. Skin lesions, particularly eczematous lesions in the area of the nipple, should be closely observed; if they are not easily cured by simple measures, they should be biopsied. An eczematous lesion on the nipple or areola may represent Paget's carcinoma.

## Abdominal Examination

The patient should be lying completely supine and relaxed; the knees may be slightly flexed and supported as an aid to relaxation of the abdominal mus-

cles. Inspection should detect irregularity of contour or color. Auscultation should follow inspection but precede palpation because the latter may change the character of intestinal activity. Palpation of the entire abdomen—gently at first, then more firmly as indicated—should detect rigidity, voluntary guarding, masses, and tenderness. If the patient complains of abdominal pain or if unexpected tenderness is elicited, the examiner should ask her to indicate the point of maximal pain or tenderness with one finger. Suprapubic palpation is designed to detect uterine, ovarian, or urinary bladder enlargements. A painful area should be left until last for deep palpation; otherwise, the entire abdomen may be guarded voluntarily. As a final part of the abdominal examination, the physician should carefully check for any abnormality of the abdominal organs: liver, gallbladder, spleen, kidneys, and intestines. In some instances, the demonstration of an abnormality of the abdominal muscle reflexes may be diagnostically helpful. Percussion of the abdomen should be performed to identify organ enlargement, tumor, or ascites.

## Pelvic Examination

The pelvic examination is a feared procedure in the minds of many women and must be conducted in such a way as to allay her anxieties. A patient's first pelvic examination may be especially disturbing, so it is important for the physician to attempt to allay fear and to inspire confidence and cooperation. The empathic physician usually finds that by the time the history has been obtained and a painless and nonembarrassing general examination performed, a satisfactory gynecologic examination is not a problem. Relaxing surroundings; a nurse or attendant chaperone if indicated; warm instruments; and a gentle, unhurried manner with continued explanation and reassurance are helpful in securing patient relaxation and cooperation. This is especially true with the woman who has never had a pelvic examination before. In these patients a one-finger examination and a narrow speculum often are necessary. In some cases, vaginal examination is not possible; palpation of the pelvic structures by rectal examination is then the only recourse. Occasionally an ultrasound examination may be helpful in ascertaining whether the pelvic organs are normal in size and configuration in patients from whom adequate relaxation of the abdominal muscles cannot be obtained. If a more definitive pelvic examination is essential, it can be performed with the patient anesthetized.

**A. External Genitalia (Fig 30–2):** The pubic

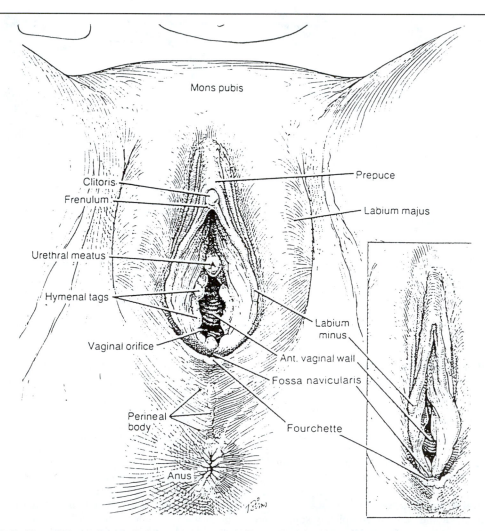

**Figure 30–2.** Normal external genitalia in a mature woman. (Reproduced, with permission, from Benson RC: *Handbook of Obstetrics & Gynecology*, 8th ed. Lange, 1983.)

hair should be inspected for its pattern (masculine or feminine), for the nits of pubic lice, for infected hair follicles, or for any other abnormality. The skin of the vulva, mons pubis, and perineal area should be examined for evidence of dermatitis or discoloration. The glans clitoridis can be exposed by gently retracting the surrounding skin folds. The clitoris is at the ventral confluence of the 2 labia; it should be no more than 2.5 cm in length, most of which is subcutaneous. The major and minor labia are usually the same size on both sides, but a moderate difference in size is not abnormal. Small protuberances or subcutaneous nodules may be either sebaceous cysts or tumors. External condylomata are often found in this area. The urethra, just below the clitoris, should be the same color as the surrounding tissue and without protuberances. Normally, vestibular (Bartholin's) glands can be neither seen nor felt; enlargement, therefore, may indicate an abnormality of this gland system. The area of vestibular glands should be palpated by placing the index finger in the vagina and the thumb outside and gently feeling for enlargement or tenderness (Fig 30–3). The perineal skin may be reddened as a result of vulvar or vaginal infection. Scars may indicate obstetric lacerations or surgery. The anus should also be inspected at this time for the presence of hemorrhoids, fissures, irritation, or perianal infections (eg, condylomata or herpesvirus).

**B. Hymen:** An unruptured hymen may present in many forms, but only a completely imperforate hymen is pathologic (Fig 30–4). After rupture, it also may be seen in various forms (Fig 30–5). After the

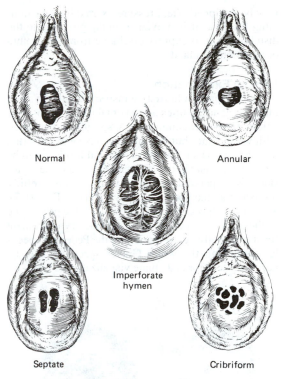

Normal

Annular

Imperforate hymen

Septate

Cribriform

**Figure 30–4.** Unruptured hymen.

birth of several children, the hymen may almost disappear.

**C. Perineal Support:** To determine the presence of pelvic relaxation, the physician spreads the labia with 2 fingers and tells the patient to "bear down." This will demonstrate urethrocele, cystocele, rectocele, or uterine prolapse, although sometimes an upright position may be necessary to demonstrate a complete prolapse of the uterus (see Chapter 41).

**D. Urethra:** Redness of the urethra may indicate infection or a urethral caruncle or carcinoma. The paraurethral glands are situated below the urethra and empty into the urethra just inside the meatus. With the labia spread adequately for better vision, the urethra

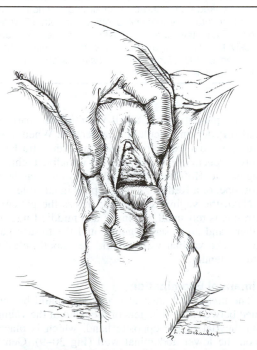

**Figure 30–3.** Palpation of vestibular glands.

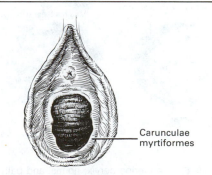

Carunculae myrtiformes

**Figure 30–5.** Ruptured hymen (parous introitus.)

may be "stripped" (ie, pressure exerted by the examining finger as it is moved from the proximal to the distal urethra) to express discharge from the urethra or paraurethral glands.

## Vaginal Examination

The vagina should first be inspected with the speculum for abnormalities and to obtain a Pap cytosmear before further examination. A speculum dampened with warm water but not lubricated is gently inserted into the vagina so that the cervix and fornices can be thoroughly visualized (Fig 30–6). After the cytosmear is prepared, the vaginal wall is again carefully inspected as the speculum is withdrawn (Fig 30–7). The type of speculum used depends on the preference of the physician, but the most satisfactory instrument for the sexually active patient is the Pederson speculum, although the wider Graves speculum may be necessary to afford adequate visualization (Fig 30–8).

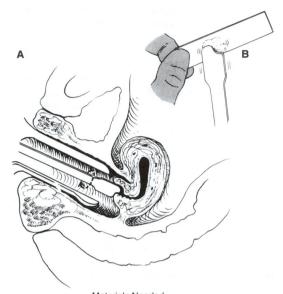

**Materials Needed**

One cervical spatula, cut tongue depressor, cotton swab, or small brush made especially for obtaining endocervical cells.

One glass slide (one end frosted). Identify by writing the patient's name on the frosted end with a lead pencil.

One speculum (without lubricant).

One bottle of fixative (75% ethyl alcohol) or spray-on fixative, eg, Aqua-Net or Cyto-Spray.

**Figure 30–7.** Preparation of a Papanicolaou smear **A:** Obtain cervical scraping from complete squamocolumnar junction by rotating 360 degrees around the external os. **B:** Place the material an inch from the end of the slide and smear along the slide to obtain a thin preparation. Use a saline soaked cotton swab or small endocervical brush and place into the endocervical canal and rotate 360 degrees. Place this specimen onto the same slide and quickly fix with fixative. (Reproduced, with permission, from Benson RC: *Handbook of Obstetrics and Gynecology*, 8th edition, Lange, 1983.)

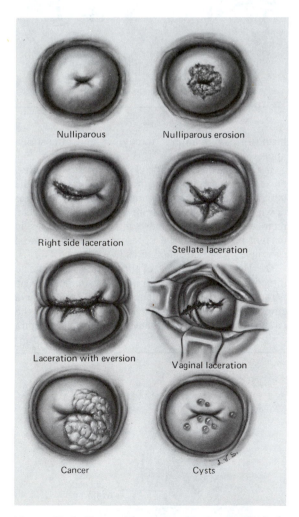

**Figure 30–6.** The uterine cervix: normal and pathologic appearance.

For the patient with a small introitus, the narrow-bladed Pederson speculum is preferable. When more than the usual exposure is necessary, an extra large Graves speculum is available. To visualize a child's vagina, a Huffman or nasal speculum, a large otoscope, or a Kelly air cystoscope is invaluable.

Next, the vagina is palpated; unless the patient's introitus is too small, the index and middle finger of either hand are inserted gently and the tissues palpated. The vaginal walls should be smooth, elastic, and nontender.

## Bimanual Examination

The uterus and adnexal structures should be outlined between the 2 fingers of the hand in the vagina and the flat of the opposite hand, which is placed upon the lower abdominal wall (Fig 30–9). Gentle palpation and manipulation of the structures will de-

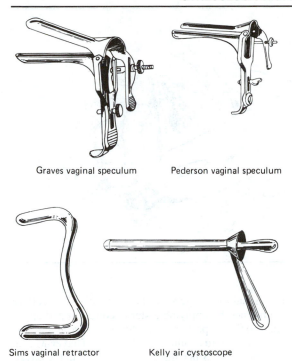

Graves vaginal speculum      Pederson vaginal speculum

Sims vaginal retractor      Kelly air cystoscope

**Figure 30–8.** Specula. (Reproduced, with permission, from Benson RC: *Handbook of Obstetrics & Gynecology,* 8th ed. Lange, 1983.)

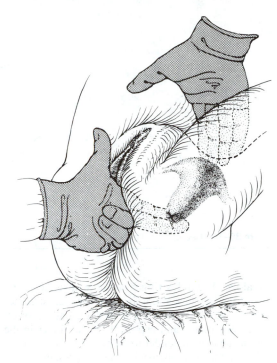

**Figure 30–9.** Bimanual pelvic examination.

lineate position, size, shape, mobility, consistency, and tenderness of the pelvic structures—except in the obese or uncooperative patient or in a patient whose abdominal muscles are taut as a result of fear or tenderness. Tenderness can be elicited either on direct palpation or on movement or stretching of the pelvic structures.

**A. Cervix:** The cervix is a firm structure traditionally described as having the consistency of the tip of the nose. Normally it is round and approximately 3–4 cm in diameter. Various appearances of the cervix are shown in Figure 30–6. The external os is also round and virtually closed. Multiparous women may have an os that has been lacerated. An irregularity in shape or nodularity may be due to one or more nabothian cysts. If the cervix is extremely firm, it may contain a tumor, even cancer. The cervix (along with the body of the uterus) normally is moderately mobile, so that it can be moved 2–4 cm in any direction without causing undue discomfort. (When examining a patient, it is helpful to warn her that she will feel the movement of the uterus but that ordinarily this maneuver is not painful.) Restriction of mobility of the cervix or corpus often follows inflammation, neoplasia, or surgery.

**B. Corpus of the Uterus:** The corpus of the uterus is approximately half the size of the patient's fist and weighs approximately 70–90 g. It is regular in outline and not tender to pressure or moderate motion. In most women, the uterus is anteverted; in about one-third of women, it is retroverted (see Chap-

ter 41). A retroverted uterus is usually not a pathologic finding. In certain cases of endometriosis or previous salpingitis, it may be that the "tipped" uterus is a result of adhesions caused by the disease process. The uterus is usually described in terms of its size, shape, position, consistency, and mobility.

**C. Adnexa:** Adnexal structures (uterine tubes and ovaries) cannot be palpated in many overweight women, because the normal tube is only about 7 mm in diameter and the ovary no more than 3 cm in its greatest diameter. In very slender women, however, the ovaries nearly always are palpable and, in some instances, the oviducts as well. In the postmenopausal woman usually no adnexal structures can be palpated. Unusual tenderness or enlargement of any adnexal structure indicates the need for further diagnostic procedures; an adnexal mass in any woman is an indication for investigation.

## Rectovaginal Examination

At the completion of the bimanual pelvic examination, a rectovaginal examination should always be performed. The well-lubricated middle finger of the examining hand should be inserted gently into the rectum to feel for tenderness, masses, or irregularities. When the examining finger has been inserted a short distance, the index finger can then be inserted into the vagina until the depth of the vagina is reached (Fig 30–10). It is much easier to examine some aspects of the posterior portion of the pelvis by rectovaginal examination than by vaginal examina-

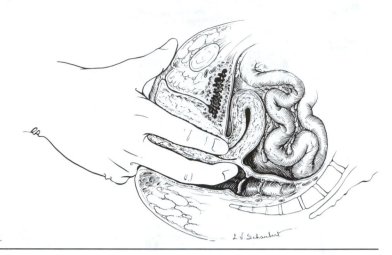

**Figure 30–10.** Rectovaginal examination.

tion alone. The index finger can now raise the cervix toward the anterior abdominal wall, which stretches the uterosacral ligaments. This is not usually painful; if it causes pain—and especially if the finger in the rectum can palpate tender nodules along the uterosacral ligaments—endometriosis may be present.

### Occult Bleeding Due to Gastrointestinal Cancer

Cancer of the gastrointestinal tract is the fourth most common cancer in women, after cancer of the breast, lung, and reproductive organs. The physician should check for occult bleeding from the gastrointestinal tract by performing a guaiac test on feces adhering to the examination glove following the rectovaginal examination. Several commercial test kits are now available.

An early gastrointestinal tract lesion may not bleed continuously and may be associated with a false-negative result. Therefore, testing should be done at each routine health screening visit. If the patient has recently eaten a large amount of meat, a false-positive reaction may result. Therefore, patients with a positive guaiac test should be placed on a meat-free diet for 3 days, and the test should then be repeated. Patients can be given a test kit to take home and mail back to the physician.

### DIAGNOSTIC OFFICE PROCEDURES

Certain diagnostic procedures may be performed in the office because complicated equipment and general anesthesia are not required. Other office diagnostic procedures useful in specific situations (eg, tests used in infertility evaluation) will be found in appropriate chapters elsewhere in this book.

### Tests for Vaginal Infection

If abnormal vaginal discharge is present, a sample of vaginal discharge should be scrutinized. A culture is obtained by applying a sterile cotton-tipped applicator to the suspect area and then transferring the suspect material to a culture medium, eg, Thayer-Martin or Transgrow. Since this is inconvenient in the physician's office, most laboratories supply a prepackaged kit that allows the physician to put the cotton-tipped applicator into a sterile container, which is then sent to the laboratory. A *Chlamydia* swab should be obtained from the endocervix and sent for identification. The vaginal discharge can also be tested for the vaginal pH. An acidic pH of 4–5 is consistent with fungal infection, whereas an alkaline pH of 5.5–7 suggests infections such as bacterial vaginosis and *Trichomonas*.

**A. Saline (Plain Slide):** To demonstrate *Trichomonas vaginalis* organisms, the physician mixes on a slide 1 drop of vaginal discharge with 1 drop of normal saline warmed to approximately body temperature. The slide should have a coverslip. If the smear is examined while it is still warm, actively motile trichomonads can usually be seen.

The saline slide can also be used to look for the mycelia of the fungus, *Candida albicans*, which appear as segmented and branching filaments. The slide can be useful in looking for bacterial vaginosis by looking for "clue cells," epithelial cells covered from edge to edge by short coccobacilli-type of bacteria.

**B. Potassium Hydroxide:** One drop of an aqueous 10% potassium hydroxide solution is mixed with 1 drop of vaginal discharge on a clean slide and covered with a coverslip. The potassium hydroxide dissolves epithelial cells and debris and facilitates visualization of the mycelia of a fungus causing vaginal infection. The slide can be brought near the nose to see if the discharge has a "fishy" odor. This odor is strongly suggestive of bacterial vaginosis, a common vaginal infection associated with a mixed anaerobic bacterial flora. In addition, this same slide with a coverslip can be magnified with a microscope to visualize mycelia that may have been hidden away by debris with just the saline smear.

**C. Bacterial Infection:** Bacterial infection may be present, especially if there is an ischemic lesion such as after radiation therapy for cervical carcinoma, or if a patient is suspected of having *bacterial vaginosis, gonorrhea,* or a *Chlamydia trachomatis* infection. Material from the cervix, urethra, or vaginal lesion may be smeared, stained, and examined microscopically, or the material may be cultured.

### Fern Test for Ovulation

The Fern test can determine the presence or absence of ovulation or the time of ovulation. When cervical mucus is spread upon a clean dry slide and allowed to dry in air, it may or may not assume a frond-like pattern under the microscope (sometimes seen grossly). The fern frond pattern indicates an estrogenic effect on the mucus without the influence of progesterone; thus, a non-frond-like pattern can be interpreted as showing that ovulation has occurred (Fig 30–11).

### Schiller Test for Neoplasia

Although colposcopy is more accurate, the Schiller test can be performed when cancer or precancerous changes of the cervix or vaginal mucosa is suspected. The suspect area is painted with Lugol's (strong io-

dine) solution; any portion of the epithelium that does not accept the dye is abnormal because of the presence of scar tissue, neoplasia and precursors, and columnar epithelium. Biopsy should be performed in this area if there is any suspicion of cancer.

### Biopsy

**A. Vulva and Vagina:** For biopsy of the vulva or vagina, a 1–2% aqueous solution of a standard local anesthetic solution can be injected around a small suspicious area and a sample obtained with a skin punch or sharp scalpel. Bleeding can usually be controlled by pressure or by Monsel's solution, but occasionally a clip or suture is necessary.

**B. Cervix:** Colposcopically directed biopsy is the method of choice for the diagnosis of cervical lesions, either suspected on visualization or indicated after an abnormal Pap smear. Colposcopy should reveal the full columnar-squamous "transformation zone" (TZ) at the juncture of the exocervix and endocervix. In addition, it may be advisable to sample the endocervix by curettage. Specific instruments have been devised for cervical biopsy (Fig 30–12). The cervix is less sensitive to cutting procedures than the vagina, so that one or more small biopsies of the cervix can be taken with little discomfort to the patient. Bleeding usually is minimal and controlled with light pressure for a few minutes or by the use of Monsel's solution when colposcopy is not available. A "4-quadrant" biopsy of the squamocolumnar junction may be taken at 12, 3, 6, and 9 o'clock. A Schiller test may often more quickly direct the physician to the area that should be biopsied.

**C. Endometrium:** Endometrial biopsy can be helpful in the diagnosis of ovarian dysfunction (eg, infertility) and as a screening test for carcinoma of the uterine corpus. The endometrial biopsy may be performed with a Duncan curet (see Fig 30–12) or by passing any of several available hollow endometrial biopsy curets into the uterine cavity and using suction to aspirate fragments of endometrium into the curet (Fig 30–13). Since either procedure usually causes a cramp, the patient should be warned, and the examiner should take as few strokes of the curet as possible. Newer flexible suction cannulas such as the Pipelle have increased the yield of endometrial tissue obtained and decreased the discomfort level for the patient.

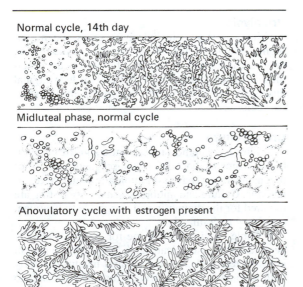

Normal cycle, 14th day

Midluteal phase, normal cycle

Anovulatory cycle with estrogen present

**Figure 30–11.** Patterns formed when cervical mucus is smeared on a slide, permitted to dry, and examined under a microscope. Progesterone makes the mucus thick and cellular. In the smear from a patient who failed to ovulate (bottom), there is no progesterone to inhibit the estrogen-induced fern pattern. (Reproduced, with permission, from Ganong WF: *Review of Medical Physiology*, 12th ed. Lange, 1985.)

## DIAGNOSTIC LABORATORY PROCEDURES

Routine procedures that are not discussed here but should be considered with periodic primary care visits include a complete blood count (including differential white cell count), glucose screening, a lipid profile, and thyroid function tests. The frequency with which these tests are given should be at the dis-

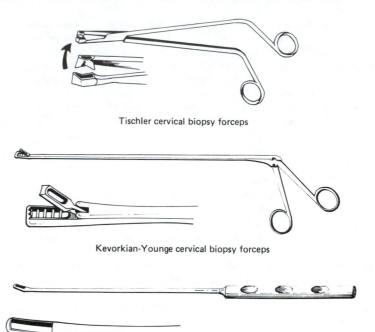

Tischler cervical biopsy forceps

Kevorkian-Younge cervical biopsy forceps

**Figure 30–12.** Biopsy instruments.

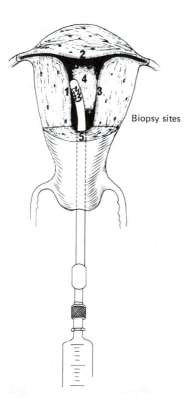

Biopsy sites

**Figure 30–13.** Sites of endometrial biopsy. (Reproduced, with permission, from Benson RC: *Handbook of Obstetrics & Gynecology*, 8th ed. Lange, 1983.)

cretion of the physician based on risk factors and presenting complaints.

### Urinalysis

Urinalysis should include both gross and microscopic examinations. A microscopic examination may reveal crystals or bacteria, but unless the specimen is collected in a manner that will exclude vaginal discharge, the presence of bacteria is meaningless (see below).

### Urine Culture

Studies have demonstrated that a significant number of women (about 3% of nonpregnant and 7% of pregnant women) have asymptomatic urinary tract infections. Culture and antibiotic sensitivity testing are required for the diagnosis and as a guide to treatment of urinary tract infections.

Reliable specimens of urine for culture often can be obtained by the "clean catch" method: the patient is instructed to cleanse the urethral meatus carefully with soap and water, to urinate for a few seconds to dispose of urethral contaminants, and then to catch a "midstream" portion of the urine. It is essential that the urine not dribble over the labia, but this may be difficult for some patients to accomplish.

A more reliable method of collecting urine for culture is by sterile catheterization performed by the physician or nurse. However, care must be exercised in catheterization to guarantee that infection is not introduced by faulty technique. When correctly performed, catheterization rarely causes infection of the urinary tract.

## Other Cultures

**A. Urethral:** Urethral cultures are indicated if a sexually transmitted disease is suspected.

**B. Vaginal:** Determining the cause of vaginal infection is usually simple, and a culture is usually unnecessary, since visual inspection or microscopic examination will usually enable the physician to make a diagnosis, eg, curd-like vaginal material that reveals mycelia (candidiasis). However, in questionable cases, a culture should be obtained.

**C. Cervical:** As in the case of the urethra, the usual indication for a culture of cervical discharge is the suspected presence of a sexually transmitted disease.

## Specific Tests

**A. Herpesvirus hominis:** Herpesvirus hominis (herpes genitalis, usually type 2) is a frequently seen vulvar lesion (see Chapter 38). It is most easily diagnosed by the cytopathologist, who finds typical cellular changes. The virus can be demonstrated by culturing, but the process is expensive and slow.

**B. Chlamydial Infections:** These sexually transmitted infections are now considered to be more prevalent than gonorrhea. Positive serologic tests may show only that the patient had an infection years ago. Culturing is slow, expensive, and frequently unavailable. Fluorescent antibody testing is the most commonly done method of diagnosis with a sensitivity of greater than 90%.

**C. Human Immunodeficiency Virus:** Acquired immunodeficiency syndrome (AIDS) has become one of the most difficult issues to be confronted with. The need for screening for human immunodeficiency virus (HIV) for the general population has become more pressing since the largest increase in incidence is in the young heterosexually active female with no other risk factors. An accurate blood test is available for diagnosis. Prior to having the blood drawn, the physician must discuss with the patient about the accuracy of the blood test for diagnosing the presence of the HIV virus. She must also be made aware that there are infrequent false-positive tests. At the present time, a written consent must be signed by the patient prior to having the blood drawn.

## Other Specific Tests

Specific diagnostic laboratory procedures may be indicated for some of the less common venereal diseases, eg, lymphogranuloma venereum and hepatitis B. These will be indicated in the discussions of the specific diseases in other chapters in this book.

## Pregnancy Testing

Pregnancy testing is discussed in Chapter 9.

## Papanicolaou Smear of Cervix

The Pap smear is an important part of the gynecologic examination. The frequency of the need for this test is in dispute at this time; epidemiologic statistics have led some physicians to state that for the average woman, a smear test every 2 or 3 years is adequate. This recommendation is based on the observation that most cervical cancers are slow-growing. However, because rapidly growing cervical cancers are occasionally reported and because there is always a possibility of false-negative laboratory reports, the American College of Obstetricians and Gynecologists at this time continues to advocate annual smears. Even those who advocate less frequent smears generally agree that patients at risk should have annual smear tests. Those at risk include women with multiple sexual partners, a history of sexually transmitted disease, genital condylomata, and prior abnormal Pap smears.

Aside from premalignant and malignant changes, other local conditions can often be suspected by the cytologist. Viral infections such as herpes simplex and condylomata acuminata can be seen as mucosal changes. Actinomycosis and *Trichomonas* infections can be detected on a Pap smear.

The Pap smear is a screening test only; positive tests are an indication for further diagnostic procedures such as colposcopy, cervical biopsy or conizations, endometrial biopsy, or D&C. The properly collected Pap smear can accurately lead to the diagnosis of carcinoma of the cervix in about 95% of cases. The Pap smear is also helpful in the detection of endometrial abnormalities such as endometrial polyps, hyperplasia, and cancers, but it picks up less than 50% of cases.

The techniques of collection of a Pap smear may vary, but the following is a common procedure.

The patient should not have douched within no less than 24 hours before the examination and should not be menstruating. The speculum is placed in the vagina after being lubricated with water only. With the cervix exposed, either a cotton-tipped applicator slightly dampened with saline solution or a specially designed plastic or wooden spatula is applied to abrade the surface slightly and to pick up cells from the squamocolumnar area of the cervical os. Care should be taken to ascertain that endocervical cells are also obtained. If this is not accomplished with the spatula, a cotton-tipped applicator or small brush is now available for this purpose; it can be inserted into the cervical canal of most women and rotated, picking up endocervical cells more efficiently. These 2 specimens may be mixed or put on the slide separately according to the preference of the examiner. A preservative is applied immediately to prevent air drying, which will compromise the interpretation. The slide is sent to the laboratory with an identification sheet containing pertinent history and findings (see Fig 30–7).

A vaginal smear from the lateral vaginal wall may be obtained for hormonal evaluation, which is a

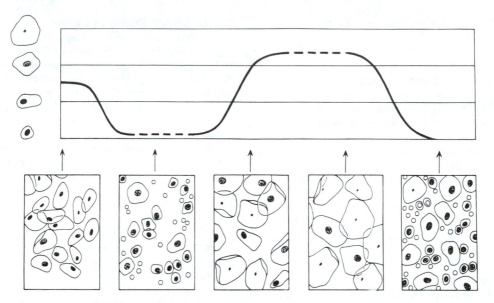

**Figure 30–14.** Vaginal cytologic picture in various stages of life. ***Top:*** Graphic representation of the maturation of vaginal epithelium. ***Bottom:*** Left to right: Epithelial maturation at birth; atrophic cell picture in childhood; beginning of estrogenic influence in puberty; complete maturation in the reproductive period; regression in old age. (Reproduced, with permission, from Beller FK et al: *Gynecology: A Textbook for Students.* Springer-Verlag, 1974.)

rough indicator of the amount of estrogen stimulation present in a given patient. A vaginal smear is also important in detecting diethylstilbestrol (DES)-related changes on the vagina and also for detecting vaginal malignancies. Figure 30–14 shows vaginal cytology during different stages of life.

The laboratory reports the Pap smear using the Bethesda System as developed by the 1988 National Cancer Institute Workshop, which has advocated a standardized reporting system for cytologic reports. An adaptation of the Bethesda System is shown on Table 30–1.

**Table 30–1.** Adapted from Bethesda System of Cytologic Results.

1. Adequacy of Sample
   a) Satisfactory for evaluation
   b) Satisfactory for evaluation but limited by (specific reason)
   c) Unsatisfactory
2. Descriptive Diagnosis
   a) Normal
   b) Benign cellular changes:
      1. Infection (trichomonas, candida, etc)
      2. Reactive changes (inflammation, atrophy, etc)
   c) Epithelial cell abnormalities:
      1. Atypical squamous cells of undetermined significance.
      2. Low grade squamous intraepithelial lesion including human papilloma virus and mild dysplasia (CIN I)
      3. High grade squamous intraepithelial lesions including moderate/severe dysplasia/carcinoma-in-situ (CIN II and III and CIS)
   d) Glandular cell abnormalities (adenocarcinoma, atypical glandular cells, etc.)

## Colposcopy

The colposcope is a binocular microscope used for direct visualization of the cervix (Fig 30–15). Magnification as high as 60 is available, but the most popular instrument in clinical use has a 13.5 magnification that effectively bridges the gap between what can be seen by the naked eye and by the microscope. Some colposcopes are equipped with a camera for single or serial photographic recording of pathologic conditions.

Colposcopy does not replace other methods of diagnosing abnormalities of the cervix but is instead an additional and important tool. The 2 most important groups of patients who can benefit by its use are (1) patients with an abnormal Pap smear test and (2) "DES babies," who may have dysplasia of the vagina or cervix (see Chapter 35).

The colposcope is able to see areas of cellular dysplasia and vascular or tissue abnormalities not visible otherwise, which makes it possible to select areas most propitious for biopsy. Stains and other chemical agents are also used to improve visualization. The colposcope has reduced the need for doing blind cervical biopsies where the rate of finding abnormalities was low. In addition, the necessity for doing cone biopsies, a procedure with a high morbidity rate, has been greatly reduced. Therefore, the experienced colposcopist is able to find focal cervical lesions, obtain directed biopsy at the most appropriate sites, and make decisions about the most appropriate therapy largely based on what is seen through the colposcope (Fig 30–16).

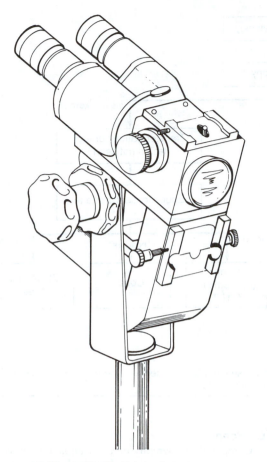

**Figure 30–15.** Zeiss colposcope.

## Hysteroscopy

Hysteroscopy is the visual examination of the uterine cavity through a fiberoptic instrument, the hysteroscope. In order to inspect the interior of the uterus with the hysteroscope, the uterine cavity is inflated with a solution such as saline or dextran or by carbon dioxide insufflation. Intravenous sedation and paracervical block are oftentimes adequate for hysteroscopy so long as prolonged manipulation is not required.

Hysteroscopic applications include evaluation for abnormal uterine bleeding, resection of uterine synechiae and septa, removal of polyps and IUDs, resection of submucous myomas, and endometrial ablation. Most of these therapeutic maneuvers require extensive manipulation so that regional or general anesthesia is required.

Hysteroscopy should be performed only by physicians with proper training. The tip of the instrument should be inserted just beyond the internal cervical os and then advanced slowly, with adequate distention under direct vision.

Hysteroscopy is often used in conjunction with an-

other operative procedure such as curettage or laparoscopy.

Failure of hysteroscopy may be due to cervical stenosis, inadequate distention of the uterine cavity, bleeding, or excessive mucus secretion. The most common complications include perforation, bleeding, and infection. Perforation of the uterus usually occurs at the fundus. Unless there is damage to a viscus or internal bleeding develops, surgical repair may not be required. Bleeding generally subsides, but fulguration following attempts to remove polyps or myomas may be required to stop bleeding in some cases. Parametritis or salpingitis, rarely noted, usually necessitates antibiotic therapy.

## Culdocentesis

The passage of a needle into the cul-de-sac—culdocentesis—in order to obtain fluid from the pouch of Douglas is a simple diagnostic procedure that can be performed in the office or in a hospital treatment room (Fig 30–17). The type of fluid obtained indicates the type of intraperitoneal lesion, eg, bloody with a ruptured ectopic pregnancy; pus with acute salpingitis; ascitic fluid with malignant cells in cancer.

## Radiographic Diagnostic Procedures

There are many common radiologic procedures that may be helpful in the diagnosis of pelvic conditions. The "flat film" will show calcified lesions, teeth, or a ring of a dermoid cyst and will indicate other pelvic masses by shadows or displaced intestinal loops. The use of contrast media is indicated frequently to help delineate pelvic masses or to rule out metastatic lesions. Barium enema, upper gastrointestinal series, intravenous urogram, and cystogram may be helpful.

## Hysterography & Hysterosalpingography

The uterine cavity and the lumens of the oviducts can be outlined by instillation of contrast medium through the cervix, followed by fluoroscopic observations or film. The technique was first widely used for the diagnosis of tubal disease as part of the investigation of infertile women; its use is now being extended to the investigation of uterine disease.

To diagnose tubal patency or occlusion, the medium is instilled through a cervical cannula; the filling of the uterine cavity and the spreading of the medium through the tubes is watched via a fluoroscope, with the radiologist taking "spot" films at intervals for subsequent, more definitive, scrutiny. If there is no occlusion, the medium will reach the fimbriated end of the tube and spill into the pelvis—evidence of tubal patency. This procedure will also reveal an abnormality of the uterus, eg, congenital malformation, submucous myomas, endometrial polyps.

## Angiography

Angiography is the radiographic demonstration of contrast medium in the blood vascular system. By

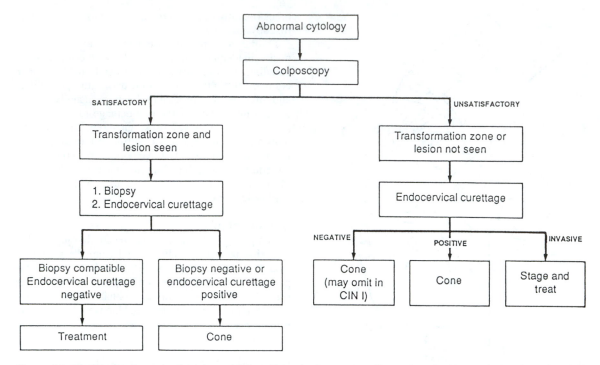

**Figure 30–16.** Diagnostic evaluation of a suspicious Papanicolaou smear. (Reproduced, with permission, from Gant NF, Cunningham FG: *Basic Gynecology and Obstetrics*. Appleton & Lange, 1993:223).

demonstrating the vascular pattern of an area, tumors or other abnormalities can be delineated. It is also used in delineating continued bleeding from pelvic vessels postoperatively or bleeding from infiltration by cancer in cancer patients. These vessels can then be embolized with synthetic fabrics to stop the bleeding and therapy avoiding the necessity of a major abdominal operation in a very compromised patient.

## CT Scan

Computed tomography or CT scan is a diagnostic imaging technique that provides high-resolution 2-dimensional images. The CT scan takes cross-sectional images through the body at very close intervals so that multiple "slices" of the body are obtained. The beam transmission is measured and calculated through an array of sensors that are about

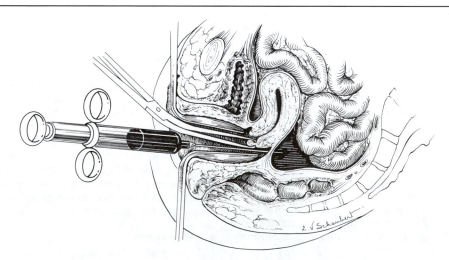

**Figure 30–17.** Culdocentesis.

100 times more sensitive than conventional x-rays. The computer is able to translate the densities of different types of tissues into gray-scale pictures that can be read on an x-ray film or on a television monitor.

Contrast media can be given orally, intravenously, or rectally to outline the gastrointestinal and urinary systems to help differentiate these organ systems from the pelvic reproductive organs. In gynecology, the CT scan is most useful in accurately diagnosing retroperitoneal lymphadenopathy associated with malignancies. It has also been used to determine depth of myometrial invasion in endometrial carcinoma as well as extrauterine spread. It is an accurate tool for locating pelvic abscesses that cannot be located by ultrasonography. Often a needle can be placed into an abscess pocket to both drain the abscess and find out what organism may be involved. Pelvic thrombophlebitis can often be diagnosed by CT scan as an adjunct to clinical suspicion. Common abnormalities such as ovarian cysts and myomas are also easily diagnosed (Fig 30–18).

## Magnetic Resonance Imaging (MRI)

Magnetic resonance imaging (MRI) is a diagnostic imaging technique creating a high-resolution, cross-sectional image of the body like a CT scan. The technique is based on the body absorbing radiowaves from the machine. A small amount of this energy is absorbed by the nuclei in the various tissues. These nuclei act like small bar magnets and are influenced by the magnetic field created by the machine. These nuclei then emit some of the radiowaves back out of the body and are picked up by sensitive and sophisticated receivers that are then translated into images by computer technology.

The advantages of MRI include the fact that it uses nonionized radiation that have show no adverse or harmful effects on the body. It is superior to the CT scan in its ability to differentiate different types of tissue, including inflammatory masses, cancers, and abnormal tissue metabolism. Its disadvantages are mainly its high cost and the fact that calcifications are poorly demonstrated. Its main use in gynecology appears to be for staging and following up pelvic cancers. MRI's use in obstetrics is mainly experimental

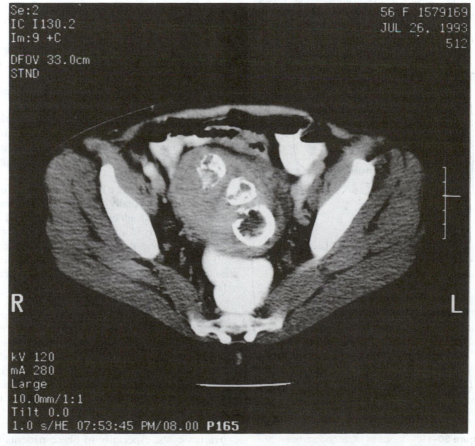

**Figure 30–18.** CT scan of the pelvis showing a large fibroid uterus with three calcified fibroids in the body of the uterus. (Picture courtesy of Dr. Barbara Carter, New England Medical Center, Boston.)

and may be limited because of fetal movement making it unsuitable for most studies.

Potentially, evaluation of placenta blood flow may be obtained by MRI as well as being an accurate method of doing pelvimetry.

## Ultrasonography

Ultrasonography records high-frequency sound waves as they are reflected from anatomic structures. As the sound wave passes through tissues, it encounters variable acoustic densities; each of these tissues returns a different echo, depending on the energy reflected. This echo signal, which can be measured, can be converted into a 2-dimensional picture of the area under examination with the relative densities being translated into gray-scale images.

Ultrasonography is a simple and painless procedure that has the added advantage of avoiding any radiation hazard. It is especially helpful in patients in whom an adequate pelvic examination may be difficult such as in children, virginal women, and those who cannot cooperate.

The pelvis and lower abdomen are scanned and recorded at regular intervals of distance, using a sector scanner that provides a better 2-dimensional picture than the linear array scanner (Fig 30–19). Generally, the scan is performed with the bladder full; this elevates the uterus out of the pelvis, displaces air-filled loops of bowel, and provides the operator with an index of density—a sonographic "window" differentiating the pelvic organs.

Ultrasonography can be helpful in the diagnosis of almost any pelvic abnormality, since all structures, normal and abnormal, can usually be demonstrated. In most instances, a clinical picture has been developed—by history, physical examination, or both—before ultrasonograms are obtained. The scan thus often will corroborate the clinical impression, but it may also uncover an unexpected condition that the clinician should recognize.

There are many indications for ultrasonography. Normal early pregnancy can be diagnosed as can pathologic pregnancies such as incomplete and missed abortions and hydatidiform moles. Ultrasonography can also be extremely helpful in avoiding the placenta and fetus with midtrimester amniocentesis. The uses for ultrasound examination in obstetrics are discussed elsewhere in this book.

Ultrasonography may be used to locate a lost intrauterine device or a foreign body in the vagina of a child. Congenital malformations such as a bicornate uterus or a vaginal agenesis can be detected. Ultrasound examination is useful in the placement of uterine tandems for radiation therapy for endometrial cancer and for guidance during second-trimester abortion procedures.

The more common uses for ultrasonography include the diagnoses of pelvic masses. Often because of their location, attachment, and density, myomas can be diagnosed without too much difficulty (Fig 30–20A).

Adnexal masses can also be found with relative ease by ultrasonography, although an accurate diagnosis is more difficult because of the various types of adnexal masses that can be found (Fig 30–20B and C.)

Ovarian cysts can be described as being unilocular or multilocular, totally fluid-filled or partially solid. A very common adnexal mass, a dermoid cyst, can have characteristic ultrasound findings because of fat tissue and bone densities seen in these cysts (Fig 30–20D). Pelvic abscesses can be diagnosed by ultrasonography, especially if there is a well-encapsulated large abscess pocket.

In addition to the traditional abdominal scan, the vaginal probe scan has become a useful modality. The vaginal probe is used for determining early gestations and can diagnose a pregnancy as early as 5 weeks from the last normal menstrual period. Ectopic pregnancies can sometimes be seen on vaginal ultrasonography, but it is more useful for excluding an intrauterine gestation when there is a suspicion of an ectopic pregnancy.

Ultrasonography is commonly used to diagnose ovarian cysts, especially in obese patients in whom

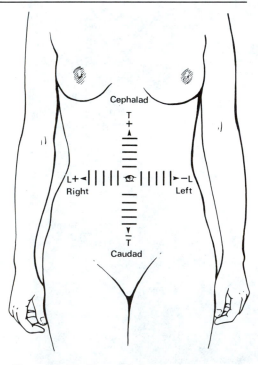

**Figure 30–19.** Planes of ultrasonograms.

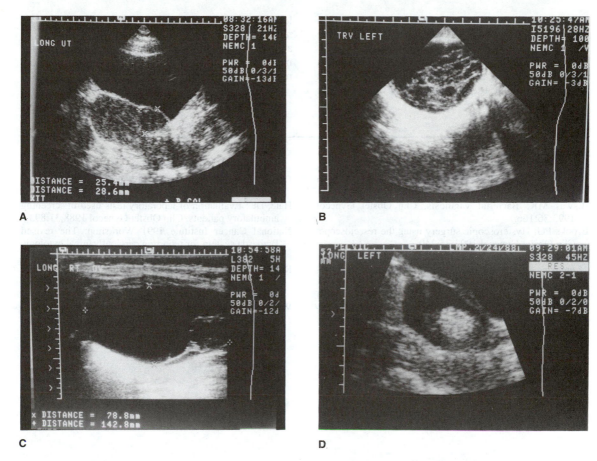

**Figure 30–20. A:** Longitudinal view of the uterus with anterior fibroid outlined by the x's; bladder anterior. **B:** Transverse section through an endometrioma with multiple loculations and debris. **C:** Longitudinal view of large ovarian cyst outlined by the +'s and x's with a focal multicystic area. **D:** Longitudinal view of a dermoid cyst showing areas of fat within the cyst. (Pictures courtesy of Dr. Frederick Doherty, New England Medical Center, Boston.)

abdominal scans are of limited use. The vaginal scan is used very often in in vitro fertilization to determine follicular size and to predict the best time for ovum retrieval.

### Carbon Dioxide Laser

Controlled tissue vaporization by laser is a modality for the treatment of cervical, vaginal, or perineal condylomata and dysplasia. It also can be used for conization of the cervix for diagnosis of dysplasia or carcinoma within the cervical canal.

The vaporization procedure is not difficult, but training is essential, especially in the physics of laser and the potential risks of laser therapy not only to the patient but to the operator and others in the immediate vicinity. Antiseptic preparation of the vagina should be gentle, to avoid trauma to the tissue that is to be examined histologically. Local anesthesia, with or without preliminary intravenous sedation, is usually adequate.

Advantages of the laser method of cervical conization are the following: little or no pain; a low incidence of infection, because the beam sterilizes the tissues; decreased blood loss, since the laser instrument—at a decreased energy level—is a hemostatic agent; less tissue necrosis than occurs with electrocautery (but probably the same as with excision by a sharp knife); and a decreased incidence of postoperative cervical stenosis (see also Chapter 58).

### Loop Electrosurgical Excision Procedure

Loop electrosurgical excision procedure (LEEP) is a new modality of therapy for vulvar and cervical lesions. LEEP uses a low-voltage, high-frequency alternating current that limits thermal damage at the same time having good hemostatic properties. It is most commonly used for excision of vulvar condylomata and cervical dysplasias and for cone biopsies of the cervix.

The technique requires the use of local anesthesia and then the use of a wire loop cautery unit that will cauterize and cut the desired tissue. Various size loops are used for different size specimens. The major advantages of LEEP include its usefulness in an office setting with a lower equipment cost, minimal damage to the surrounding tissue, and the low morbidity associated with it.

## REFERENCES

Bachmann GA, Leiblum SR, Grill J: Brief sexual inquiry in gynecologic practice. Obstet Gynecol 1989;73:425.

Biswas MK: Bacterial vaginosis. Clin Obstet Gynecol 1993;36:166.

Brooks PG: Hysteroscopic surgery using the resectoscope. Clin Obstet Gynecol 1992;35:249.

*Cervical cytology: Evaluation and management of abnormalities.* American College of Obstetricians and Gynecologists Technical Bulletin 1993:184.

Coppleson M, Pixley EC, Reid BC: Colposcopic features of papillomavirus infection and premalignancy in the female lower genital tract. Obstet Gynecol Clin North Am 1987;14:451.

Dodd G: American Cancer Society guidelines on screening for breast cancer: An overview. CA 1992;42:177.

Hale, DC: Evaluation of laboratory tests used in screening ambulatory patients. Clin Obstet Gynecol 1988;31:893.

National Cancer Institute 1991 Workshop: The revised Bethesda system for reporting cervical/vaginal cytologic diagnoses. J Reprod Med 1992;37:383.

Riccio TJ et al: Magnetic resonance imaging as an adjunct to sonography in the evaluation of the female pelvis. Magn Reson Imaging 1990;8:699.

Wright TC et al: Treatment of cervical intraepithelial neoplasia using the loop electrosurgical excision procedure. Obstet Gynecol 1992;79:173.

# Pediatric & Adolescent Gynecology

# 31

*David Muram, MD*

Until recently, even physicians did not fully appreciate that female infants, children, and adolescents might develop the same gynecologic disorders as adult women. Inspection of the external genitalia has now become an integral step of the routine well child examination, permitting early detection of infections, labial adhesions, congenital anomalies, and even genital tumors. A complete gynecologic examination is mandatory whenever a child has symptoms or signs of a genital disorder.

The reproductive tract in children and adolescents differs in both structure and function from that of adult females. Physicians involved in the care of children and adolescents must be aware of the differences, so that diagnosis and management are accurate and appropriate. Specially designed equipment must be used (eg, vaginoscope, virginal vaginal speculum) to prevent undue discomfort and consequent anxiety about future examinations.

## ANATOMIC & PHYSIOLOGIC CONSIDERATIONS

### Newborn Infants

During the first few weeks of life, the newborn female responds physiologically to stimulation by placentally acquired maternal sex hormones. The effects may be seen for about 1 month, rarely longer. The most obvious manifestation, breast budding, occurs in nearly all female infants born at term. Sometimes, breast enlargement is marked, and, occasionally, there may be small amounts of fluid discharged from the nipples. No treatment is required or desirable. Repeated examinations may lead to bruising of the breast tissue or infection.

The external genitalia are also hormonally affected. The labia majora are bulbous, and the labia minora are thick and protruding (Fig 31–1). The clitoris is relatively large but has a normal index of 0.6 cm$^2$ or less.* The effects of maternal estrogens are particularly evident in the hymen, which initially is turgid and purple-red, covers the external urethral orifice, and projects from the slightly gaping vulva. Vaginal discharge is common, since the cervical glands secrete a considerable amount of mucus, which mixes with exfoliated vaginal cells.

The internal genital organs are also stimulated by maternal estrogens. The vagina is 4 cm in length, and vaginal secretions are acidic in nature. Lactobacilli are present in the vagina. The uterus is enlarged (4 cm in length) and has no axial flexion; the ratio between the cervix and the corpus is 3:1. The columnar epithelium protrudes through the external cervical os, producing a reddened zone of "physiologic eversion." The ovaries, which are embryologically derived from near the T10 level, are abdominal organs in early childhood and are not palpable on pelvic or rectal examination. Occasionally, as estrogen levels decline following birth, the stimulated endometrial lining is shed, and vaginal bleeding occurs. Such bleeding usually stops within 7–10 days after birth.

### Young Children

In early childhood, the female genital organs receive little estrogen stimulation. This causes the labia majora to be flat and the labia minora and hymen to be extremely thin (Fig 31–2). The smooth skin of the labia minora has the same appearance as hairless skin elsewhere on the body. The clitoral prepuce is hidden in the small cleft of the vulva. The mucous membrane of the introitus is pink and somewhat moist. The clitoris is relatively small, but the clitoral index is unchanged. The vagina, although slightly longer (~ 5 cm), has a thin pink atrophic mucosa with relatively few rugae and very little resistance to trauma and infection. The vaginal barrel contains neutral or slightly alkaline secretions and mixed bacterial flora. The cervix in childhood is flush with the vaginal vault, since the vaginal fornices do not develop until puberty. The cervix is not palpable—even visualization is sometimes difficult—and the cervical opening appears as a small slit. The uterus regresses in size; not until age 6 years does it regain the size present at birth. The ovaries contain small follicles during infancy. As the

---

*Clitoral index (cm$^2$) = length (cm) width (cm), ie, a clitoris 1 cm long 0.5 cm wide = 0.5 cm$^2$.

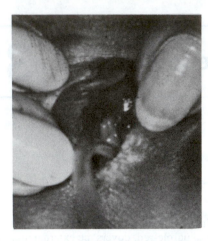

**Figure 31–1.** External genitalia of a newborn female. Note the hypertrophy and turgor of the vulvar tissues. A small catheter is inserted into the vagina to demonstrate patency. (Reproduced [as are a number of other illustrations in this chapter] from Huffman JW: The Gynecology of Childhood and Adolescence. Saunders, 1968.)

child approaches menarche, a significant increase in the number and size of ovarian follicles can be observed.

These anatomic differences are particularly important when a laparotomy is performed. The operator cannot rely on inspection alone to determine the size and shape of the uterus. The uterus may be merely a strip of dense tissue in the anteromedial area of the broad ligaments. Palpation may aid in delineating the

uterine outline. As the child matures, the ovaries become larger and descend into the true pelvis. The number of larger follicles increases, and these may attain a significant size prior to their regression. Because of this follicular development, the ovary may appear cystic. However, a biopsy is not required. Removal of an ovary must be done carefully, because injury to adjacent structures may easily occur.

## Older Children

During late childhood (age 7–10 years), the external genitalia again show signs of estrogen stimulation: the mons pubis thickens, the labia majora fill out, and the labia minora become rounded. The hymen becomes thicker (Fig 31–3), losing its thin, almost transparent character. Hymenal orifice diameters vary as a function of hymenal shape, estrogen status, advancing age, position during the examination and degree of relaxation. The vagina elongates to 8 cm, the mucosa becomes thicker, the corpus uteri enlarges, and the ratio of cervix to corpus becomes 1:1. The cervix is still flush with the vault. However, some estrogen stimulation exists, and a maturation index performed at this time will show, in addition to

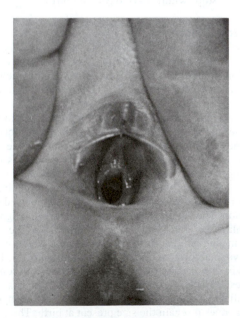

**Figure 31–2.** External genitalia of a child 3 years of age.

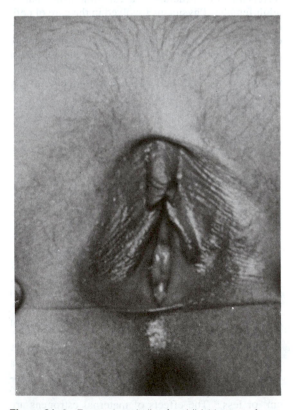

**Figure 31–3.** External genitalia of a child 11 years of age. Early estrogen response is evidenced by the fuller labia, wrinkling of the vulvar mucosa, and thickening of the hymen.

basal cells, parabasal cells and occasional superficial cells (ie, the maturation index is beginning to shift to the right, and a typical report may show 75/25/0 or 70/25/5).

When the girl is age 9–10 years, uterine growth occurs and the shape of the uterus is altered, primarily as a result of myometrial proliferation rather than endometrial development. It is not until menarche is imminent that rapid endometrial proliferation occurs. Until then, there is gradual thickening of the endometrium and a modest increase in the depth and complexity of the endometrial glands. The ovaries, formerly spindle-shaped and elongated, become larger and descend farther into the pelvis as menarche approaches. The number of large ovarian follicles increases, and although they are in various stages of development, none results in ovulation. Some may grow to a considerable size and then regress.

### Young Adolescents

During early puberty (age 10–13 years), the external genitalia take on the adult appearance. The major vestibular glands (Bartholin's glands), which apparently have no secretory function during the neonatal period and early childhood, begin to produce mucus just prior to menarche. The vagina reaches its adult length (10–12 cm). It is more distensible; the mucosa becomes thick and moist; the vaginal secretions are acidic; and lactobacilli reappear. With the development of the vaginal fornices, the cervix becomes separated from the vaginal vault, and the differential growth of the corpus and cervix is more pronounced. The corpus becomes twice as large as the cervix, yet there is no flexion of the axis. The ovaries descend into the true pelvic cavity.

Secondary sexual characteristics develop, often rapidly, during the late premenarcheal period. The body habitus, which during early childhood differs little from that of a boy's, becomes rounded, especially the shoulders and hips. Accelerated somatic growth velocity (the adolescent growth spurt) occurs, and at the same time, breast buds appear and gradually increase in size to form small mounds. Physiologic leukorrhea is noted.

**Table 31–1.** Tanner classification of female adolescent development.

| Stage | Breast Development | Pubic Hair Development |
|---|---|---|
| I | Papillae elevated (pre-adolescent), no breast buds | None |
| II | Breast buds and papillae slightly elevated | Sparse, long, slightly pigmented |
| III | Breasts and areolae confluent, elevated | Darker, coarser, curly |
| IV | Areolae and papillae project above breast | Adult-type pubis only |
| V | Papillae projected, mature | Lateral distribution |

Pubic hair growth appears to be under the hormonal control of adrenal androgens. Initially, one may observe sparse, long, slightly curly, and pigmented hair over the pubic area. With time, there is increased quantity of coarse, pigmented curled hair. The pubic hair pattern assumes the characteristic triangle with the base above the mons pubis. Hair growth in the axilla appears later, also as a result of adrenocorticosteroid hormone stimulation. The development of secondary sexual features has been described by Marshall and Tanner and is summarized in Table 31–1 (see also Fig 6–3). This descriptive method should be used to document progress through puberty.

## GYNECOLOGIC EXAMINATION OF INFANTS, CHILDREN, & YOUNG ADOLESCENTS

An infant girl should have her first gynecologic examination in the delivery room or the nursery as part of the routine newborn evaluation. It is unnecessary, in most cases, to perform an internal examination. Most gynecologic abnormalities that should be recognized at this stage are limited to the external genitalia. Some defects require immediate correction and may suggest the presence of other abnormalities (eg, congenital adrenal hyperplasia) for which immediate medical therapy is required if potentially lethal complications are to be prevented. Even if management of the anomaly can be safely delayed until early adulthood, early diagnosis allows for better planning of treatment and gives the physician the opportunity to provide emotional support for patients for whom treatment is unavailable.

Inspection of the external genitalia should be incorporated into every well child examination. In the absence of gynecologic symptoms, a comprehensive internal gynecologic examination is usually not warranted until sexual activity is contemplated or initiated. In asymptomatic patients who are not sexually active, the American College of Obstetricians and Gynecologists recommends that a gynecologic examination be done at age 18 years. Finally, adolescents who were exposed in utero to diethystilbestrol should be examined immediately following menarche or at age 13 years, whichever comes first.

### Examination of the Newborn Infant

**A. General Examination:** As in adults, the first step in a genital evaluation of the newborn is a careful general examination, which may reveal abnormalities suggesting genital anomaly (eg, webbed neck, abdominal mass, edema of the hands and legs, coarctation of the aorta). Then, the external genitalia are inspected and palpated. Each structure is evaluated: Does it appear normal? Is it in its proper location? Will it function normally later in life?

**B. Clitoris:** The clitoris deserves particular attention, because enlargement in the newborn is almost always associated with congenital adrenal hyperplasia. Other causes must also be considered (eg, true hermaphroditism, male pseudohermaphroditism).

**C. Vagina:** The vaginal orifice should be evident when the labia are separated or retracted. If it is not, it can be found by gently inserting a small, well-lubricated pediatric feeding tube (Fig 31–1). When an opening cannot be found, the infant most likely has an imperforate hymen or vaginal agenesis. Infrequently, associated inguinal hernias suggest the possibility that the child is a genetic male, particularly when there is a mass in the hernial sac. If the vaginal orifice cannot be located, further investigation is warranted.

**D. Rectoabdominal Examination:** To complete the primary evaluation, a rectoabdominal examination is performed. Usually, the uterus and adnexa in the newborn cannot be palpated on rectal examination. Occasionally, a small central mass representing the uterine cervix can be felt on examination. When an ovary is palpable, it denotes a marked enlargement and warrants further investigation (eg, ultrasonography) to rule out the presence of an ovarian tumor. Negative findings are valuable because they generally exclude a pelvic tumor. Rectal examination also confirms patency of the anorectal canal.

## Examination of the Premenarcheal Child

Children of all ages are very sensitive to a physician's attitude. They tend to withdraw from a doctor or nurse who is hurried, brusque, or indifferent but react positively to someone who is kind, warm, interested, and patient. Parents may be helpful in the examination of a young child because they provide a sense of security and may also distract the patient. Children up to 5 years of age become apprehensive when placed on the examination table. Placing them on the parent's lap affords a better opportunity to perform an adequate examination (Fig 31–4). Older children may be placed on the examination table, but the use of stirrups is not generally necessary if the patient is asked to flex her knees and abduct her legs.

Studies have shown that young patients, adolescents in particular, prefer a physician who wears a white coat. Similarly, parents of young children would like the physician who cares for their children to be dressed in professional attire such as a white coat and tie. In addition, sexual abuse of children is not uncommon in today's society, and many prevention programs for children emphasize that private parts should not be touched or seen by strangers. The physician is a stranger to the child. As a uniform, the white coat identifies the physician and his or her role, which may involve inspection and occasional palpation of private areas. Uniforms and the presence of the mother at the time of examination may create a distinctive atmosphere that would not contradict the teaching given in education programs aimed at abuse prevention. Explaining procedures to the older child and asking her to help with the examination are of definite value. The child's being involved and help-

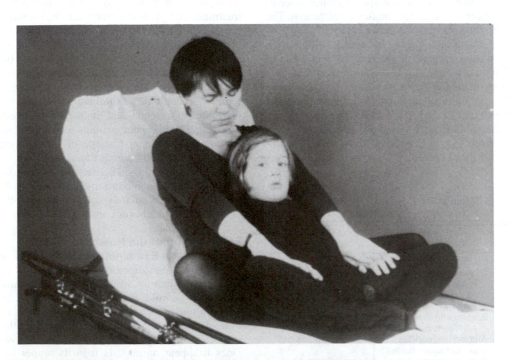

**Figure 31–4.** Child is positioned on mother's lap. Child feels secure in mother's arms. Mother can assist by supporting child's legs, providing excellent view of the genital area (Photo courtesy of Dr. T. Anglin.)

ing the physician decrease her apprehension by providing a sense of control.

**A. Physical Examination:**

**1. General inspection—**The examination begins with an evaluation of the general appearance, nutritional status, body habitus, and any gross congenital anomalies. General uncleanliness suggests bad perineal hygiene, which may contribute to vulvovaginitis in young girls.

**2. Breasts—**The breasts should be inspected and palpated. Breast budding usually does not begin until age 8–9 years. It is common and normal for a small, firm, flat "button" to form beneath the nipple at the start of breast growth. Prominence of the nipple and breast development at an earlier age may be early signs of sexual precocity.

**3. Abdomen—**Inspection and palpation of the abdomen should precede examination of the genitalia. If the child is ticklish, having her place one hand on or under the examiner's hand usually will overcome that difficulty. Light palpation and slow movement from one area to the other will elicit most information.

The ovary of a premenarcheal child is situated high in the pelvis. This location and the small size of the pelvic cavity tend to force ovarian tumors toward the midabdomen above the true pelvic brim. Thus, large neoplasms of the ovary are likely to be mistaken for other abdominal masses (eg, polycystic kidney). Inguinal hernia is less common in females than in males (about 1:10) but does occur, usually with no discomfort. An excellent method of demonstrating an inguinal hernia is to have the child stand up and increase the intra-abdominal pressure by blowing up a rubber balloon.

**4. Genitalia—**The vulva and vestibule may be exposed by light lateral and downward pressure on each side of the perineum. When exposure of the vaginal walls is necessary, the labia may be grasped between the examiner's thumb and forefinger and pulled forward, downward, and sideways. Particular note should be made as to whether the mother has properly cleansed the child's anogenital region or if the perineal hygiene practiced by an older girl is adequate. The examiner should also look for skin lesions, perineal excoriations, ulcers, and tumors. A zone of inflammation below the urethral meatus may explain dysuria in a child. Signs of hormonal stimulation in early childhood and absence of such signs later in childhood are important signs of many endocrine disorders associated with precocious or delayed puberty. Attention should be paid to vulvar inflammation and vulvar and vaginal discharge.

Enlargement of the clitoris is of diagnostic significance. Preputial adhesions may be important when an accumulation of smegma beneath the prepuce becomes an irritant. The vestibule may not be visible because of labial adhesions or congenital anomalies. The former condition is frequently mistaken for vagi-

nal agenesis or imperforate hymen. The patency of the hymenal orifice must be ensured. This can be easily accomplished with a small well-lubricated feeding tube.

It is impossible to perform a digital vaginal examination in a child whose vagina is normal-sized for her age. Gentle rectal digital examination can be accomplished and should not cause pain, but the small size of the uterus and ovaries, the firmness of the abdominal wall, and the resistance most children offer to the examination render accurate intrapelvic evaluation difficult. It can be assumed that if the uterus and ovaries are not palpable, the child has no genital tumor. If the presence of a pelvic tumor is suspected, and the neoplasm cannot be palpated on rectal examination, other diagnostic procedures (eg, sonography, laparoscopy) should be performed.

**B. Vaginoscopy:** Instrumentation is often required when it is necessary to carefully visualize the upper third of the vagina, eg, searching for a source of abnormal vaginal bleeding. Instrumentation is also required in some patients to confirm patency of the genital tract, to detect and remove foreign bodies, and to exclude penetrating injuries. In the latter case, the examination is often performed under general anesthesia. Figure 31–5 demonstrates the office vaginoscope, which is essentially a hollow cylinder with a removable obturator. Additionally, a cystoscope (air or water), urethroscope, or laparoscope may be used. The water cystoscope allows some distention of the vagina and thus better visualization of the vaginal mucosa. At the same time, the water irrigates secretions, blood, and debris (Fig 31–6).

When a vaginoscope is inserted, a progressive stepwise approach decreases apprehension. First, the child should be allowed to touch the lubricated instrument with her index finger, and it is pointed out to her

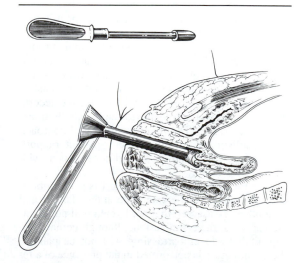

**Figure 31–5.** Huffman vaginoscope being used for examination of a premenarcheal child.

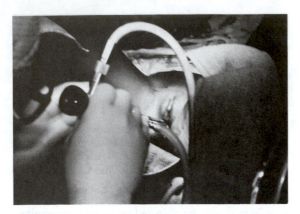

**Figure 31–6.** Performing vaginoscopy under anesthesia using a water cystoscope.

that it feels slippery, cool, and perhaps strange. Then, the instrument is placed against the inner thigh and the labia majora, and it is repeated that this feels cool, slippery, and unusual. Only then is the instrument passed through the hymenal orifice.

In infancy and childhood, the hymenal orifice normally will admit a 0.5-cm vaginoscope. An instrument 0.8 cm in diameter can be used to examine most older premenarcheal girls. If the aperture is too small for an instrument to be passed without discomfort, vaginoscopy should not be further attempted without general anesthesia. Persistent manipulation of sensitive tissues without anesthesia will be traumatic and counterproductive.

## Examination of the Young Adolescent

The adolescent girl's first trip to the gynecologist is often laden with fear and apprehension. Girlfriends may have told her harrowing stories they have heard about vaginal examinations. Thus, time spent in putting the patient at ease and winning her confidence will save time and frustration in the examining room. The physician should make it clear that the adolescent is the patient, not her mother, who usually accompanies her. The girl, not her mother, is asked for routine information that will go on the record. Questions about sexual behavior and sexually transmitted diseases (STDs) require delicacy of approach and establishment of good doctor-patient rapport. Obviously, such questions should not be asked with the mother present.

After the history is taken, the girl is given a brief description of what the examination entails. She and her mother are assured that her hymen will not be injured and that the examination, although perhaps uncomfortable and embarrassing, will not be painful. The examination is performed in the presence of a female assistant, who must constantly reassure the young patient.

Examination of the breasts is an integral part of the physical examination of every female patient. The technique of self-examination should be described, and information should be given to the patient at this time.

Explanations of what is being done are given throughout the examination, particularly when the genitalia are examined. The examination is also used to provide the patient with health maintenance instructions and explanations about her body and its various functions. The physician is at a disadvantage when he or she attempts to show the genitalia to the patient. Many adolescents are not familiar with the appearance of their own genitalia, and explanations about anatomic details and function may seem abstract to these young patients. Some physicians use mirrors during the examination to show normal anatomic details, demonstrate abnormalities, to explain treatment plans, and to provide explanations regarding health maintenance. The use of mirrors is often cumbersome, and many physicians and patients find it less than satisfactory. The mirrored image is generally small and placement of the mirror at the foot of the bed forces the patient to strain in order to view the mirrored image.

Lastly, the physician who is demonstrating the genitalia is never certain what image is actually viewed by the patient. Recently, many physicians have begun using a colposcope for the genital examination of young children. The colposcope may be attached to a video camera and a TV monitor. With the monitor placed behind the physician, the patient is able to view the same findings with the physician. This provides an enlarged image seen simultaneously by the examiner and the patient, and permits direct communication, particularly in difficult cases. Although this equipment is desirable, cost may be prohibitive.

Following inspection of the genitalia, a speculum is inserted into the vagina. The introitus of most adolescents is about 1 cm in diameter and will admit a narrow speculum without difficulty. The Huffman-Graves long-bladed instrument is preferable to the short-bladed Graves speculum, because the Huffman speculum is designed to allow for easy inspection of the cervix in adolescents, in whom the vagina is 10–12 cm long (Fig 31–7). In a patient with a large hymenal opening, bimanual examination is performed by inserting a finger into the vagina. If the hymenal orifice is too small for digital examination, rectal examination may be performed.

Following the examination, the girl is given an opportunity to talk to the examiner alone. She needs to believe that she can relay her concerns to the physician, who will respect her confidence. Problems may be discussed with both the girl and her mother, but only after the physician and the patient have completed their discussion and agreed what will be held in confidence. Under no circumstances should the

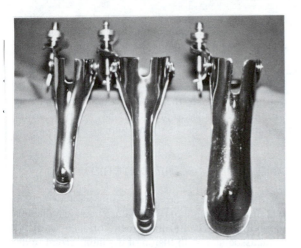

**Figure 31–7.** The Huffman-Graves speculum (*middle*) is as long as the adult Graves speculum (*right*) and as narrow as the short pediatric Graves speculum (*left*).

physician violate the patient's request for secrecy. If the physician believes the parents should be aware of all details, the patient must be so advised and convinced that it would be for her own benefit.

### Examination of a Child Victim of Sexual Abuse

Many children who are possible victims of sexual abuse are brought into a hospital emergency room or to their physician's office for a comprehensive medical evaluation. After a child has been identified as a victim of sexual abuse, the examining physician must obtain special informed consent from the child's legal guardian, properly signed and witnessed. In addition to permission for examination and treatment, this consent should include permission to collect evidenciary materials, take photographs, and release the information to the proper authorities.

**A. History:** It is important to obtain a detailed history from the child. When obtained from a young child, an account of the incident is extremely valuable. It can later be used in court as evidence, or it may reveal an unusual area of injury and, thus, uncommon sites for collection of evidence. The examiner should note the child's composure, behavior, and mental state, as well as how she interacts with her parents and other persons. It is also important to know how and by whom the child sustained the injury. Victims of physical or sexual abuse must be removed immediately from an unsafe environment.

The information should be recorded carefully in the child's own words. Although a detailed history is desirable, the patient should not be made to repeat the account of the incident over and over. When it is impossible to obtain a history from a very young child, the physician is then compelled to accept an account

of the incident from relatives, police officers, neighbors, or other sources, including other children.

**B. Physical Examination:** The physical examination has two purposes–to detect injuries and to collect samples that can later be used as evidence.

**1. Detection of injuries**–Colposcopy has been used to complement the examination of child victims of sexual abuse. The genitalia are inspected under regular illumination and through a green filter, which better demonstrates vascular patterns. The colposcope can be used to obtain photographs, which may be added to the medical record, introduced as evidence, and reviewed to refresh the examiner's memory. No solutions or dyes need to be applied to the genitalia during the examination, although some investigators have reported that the use of toluidine blue dye accentuated minor mucosal injuries. The use of a colposcope may enhance the physical findings; however, the experience of most physicians in the use of the colposcope for this purpose is limited. Therefore, colposcopic findings should be interpreted with caution. Vulvar irritation is fairly common in small children as a result of poor local hygiene, maceration of the skin due to wetness from diapers, or excoriations caused by local infection. Such nonspecific findings, enhanced by the colposcope, should not be regarded as diagnostic of sexual abuse.

**2. Collection of evidence**–During the general inspection, all foreign material such as sand and grass should be removed and placed in clearly labeled envelopes. Scrapings from underneath the fingernails and loose hairs on the skin are collected. A Wood's lamp can be used to detect the presence of seminal fluid on the patient's body, since the ultraviolet light causes semen to fluoresce. The stain may be lifted off the skin with moistened cotton swabs for further analysis. Semen can be detected on the skin many hours after the assault.

If vaginal penetration is suspected, vaginal fluid is collected and sent for the appropriate cultures, wet mount preparation, cytology, acid phosphatase determination, and enzyme p30.

An immediate wet mount preparation done by the examining physician may detect motile sperm. Culture swabs are obtained from the rectum, vagina, urethra, and pharynx, even if the patient denies orogenital contact. All specimens must be clearly labeled and the containers and envelopes sealed and signed by the examiner. The kit is then given to the police investigator who signs for it in the record and on the routing slip. All persons handling the materials must sign for it. Such a system is necessary to maintain the chain of evidence; otherwise, these specimens may not be admissible in court. If the kit needs to be stored in the physician's office, it must be placed in an inaccessible area, preferably locked, until it can be given to the police investigator, or to the forensic laboratory. (See also Chapter 61.)

# CONGENITAL ANOMALIES OF THE FEMALE GENITAL TRACT

Congenital anomalies of the genitalia may be divided into those that suggest sexual ambiguity (intersex problems) and those that do not. Intersex individuals have significant ambiguity of the external genitalia, so that the true gender cannot be immediately determined. This category includes genetic males and is discussed in detail in Chapter 5.

## ANOMALIES OF THE VULVA & LABIA

As in any other part of the body, minor differences in the contour or size of vulvar structures are not unusual. Often there is considerable variation in the distance between the posterior fourchette and the anus or between the urethra and the clitoris, giving the vulva different appearances. Sometimes, the vulva is situated deep between the bulging sides of the perineum, forming a "vulva retrousse." This is more common in muscular adolescent girls in whom the perineal body is exceptionally thick and wide. Rare anomalies of the vulva include bifid clitoris, which occurs in conjunction with bladder exstrophy; a caudal appendage resembling a tail; congenital prolapse of the vagina; variations in the insertion of the bulbocavernosus muscle, which may alter the appearance of the labia majora, and at times, obliterate the fossa navicularis. Duplication of the vulva is an extremely rare anomaly, which may be associated with duplication of the urinary and intestinal tracts.

Frequently, there is a considerable variation in the size and shape of the labia minora. One labium minor may be considerably larger than the other, or both labia may be unusually large. These changes have been wrongly assumed by some to be the result of masturbation. The child and her parents need reassurance that these variations are inherited and thus are simple congenital anomalies, which usually require no treatment (Fig 31–8). If the asymmetry is significant or if the large labia are pulled into the vagina during intercourse, the hypertrophied labia may be trimmed surgically to provide a more symmetric appearance and to relieve dyspareunia.

## ANOMALIES OF THE CLITORIS

Clitoral enlargement almost invariably suggests that the infant was exposed in utero to elevated levels of androgens. Such enlargement of the clitoris is often associated with fusion of the labioscrotal folds; this is discussed in Chapter 5. Enlargement of the clitoris caused by a benign neoplasm has been observed in a few infants. Von Reklinghausen's neurofibromatosis, lymphangiomas, and fibromas may involve the clitoris and cause enlargement. When an isolated neoplasm causes enlargement of the clitoris, therapy consists of excision of the neoplasm and thereby reduction of the clitoris to normal size.

Clitoral agenesis is a very rare condition. Splitting or duplication of the clitoris represents longitudinal splitting of the clitoris caused by failure of the corpora to fuse in the midline. Bifid clitoris usually occurs in conjunction with bladder exstrophy, epispadias, and absence or cleavage of the symphysis pubis. The labia majora are widely separated, and the labia minora are separated anteriorly but can be traced posteriorly around the vaginal orifice. The uterus often shows a fusion deformity, and the vaginal orifice is narrow. The vagina is shortened and rotated anteriorly. The pelvic floor is incomplete, and uterine prolapse is often observed in these patients. Other congenital anomalies may be present, eg, spina bifida. At puberty, pubic hair growth is absent over the midline.

## ANOMALIES OF THE HYMEN

The hymen has more apparent variations in structure than any other part of the female genitalia: the orifice may vary in diameter; there may be one or more small orifices; instead of a thin membrane, the hymenal diaphragm may be thickened and fibrous, forming a firm partition. A thick median ridge separating 2 lateral hymenal orifices may suggest a septate vagina. Occasionally, what appears to be an imperforate hymen is found to have one or more tiny openings and is called a microperforate hymen.

Although most of these variants are of no clinical significance, hymenal anomalies require surgical correction if they block the escape of vaginal secretions or menstrual fluid, interfere with intercourse, or pre-

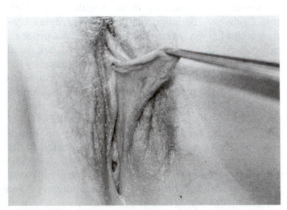

**Figure 31–8.** Labial asymmetry resulting from enlargement of the left labium minor.

vent the performance of vaginoscopy or treatment of a vaginal disorder.

## Imperforate Hymen

The hymen may be a solid membrane without an aperture (imperforate hymen). An imperforate hymen is believed to represent a persistent portion of the urogenital membrane and occurs when the mesoderm of the primitive streak abnormally invades the urogenital portion of the cloacal membrane. The solid membrane causes obstruction of the vagina, and accumulation of secretions may cause vaginal distention. When a mucocolpos develops, the membrane is seen as a bulging, shiny, thin protuberance (Fig 31–9), and the distended vagina forms a large mass that may interfere with urination, and at times may be mistaken for an abdominal tumor.

Imperforate hymen without a mucocolpos forms a fibrous, smooth surface between the labia minora and is difficult to differentiate from an absent vagina. Sonographic evaluation of the pelvis can identify the uterus, cervix, and vagina and thus distinguish between these 2 conditions.

Imperforate hymen often is not diagnosed until an adolescent girl presents with complaints of primary amenorrhea and recurrent pelvic pain. Occasionally, the first symptom may be urinary retention caused by pressure from a large hematocolpos on the bladder and urethra. Inspection of the vulva generally reveals a dome-shaped, purplish-red hymenal membrane bulging outward as a result of the accumulation of blood above it. On rectal examination, the distended vagina is palpable as a large cystic mass. The blood fills the vagina (hematocolpos) and then the uterus (hematometra) and may spill through the uterine tubes into the peritoneal cavity. Endometriosis and vaginal adenosis are known but not inevitable complications.

Imperforate hymen must be corrected. In infants, the central portion of the membrane is lifted up and snipped away with scissors; sutures usually are not

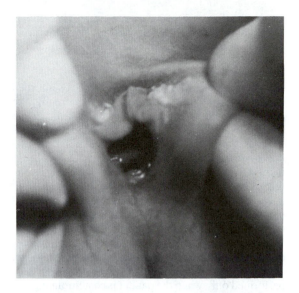

**Figure 31–10.** Newborn infant following excision of an imperforate hymen. Forward traction on the labia majora provides unimpaired view of the hymenal ring. Note the large opening created. No bleeding was noted and no sutures were required.

necessary (Fig 31–10). In postmenarcheal girls, a large central portion of the membrane should be removed; if an incision alone is performed, the edges tend to coalesce. As these edges adhere, the obstructing membrane may reform. Follow-up evaluation of the vagina and pelvis should be deferred for 4–6 weeks to reduce the risk of introducing infection.

## ANOMALIES OF THE VAGINA

### 1. TRANSVERSE VAGINAL SEPTUM

Transverse vaginal septa are the result of faulty canalization of the embryonic vagina and therefore are present at birth. They are usually found in the midvagina but may occur at any level. When the septum is located in the upper vagina, it is likely to be patent, whereas those located in the lower part of the vagina are more often complete. An undiscovered imperforate transverse septum may lead to the formation of a large mucocolpos in infancy or to obstruction of menstrual flow in adolescence.

An incomplete septum is usually asymptomatic, and therefore does not require correction during childhood or early adolescence. The central aperture allows for vaginal secretions and menstrual flow to egress from the vagina. However, an incomplete septum may cause dyspareunia, and the septum should be excised in symptomatic patients.

A complete septum results in signs and symptoms similar to those of an imperforate hymen. Unfortu-

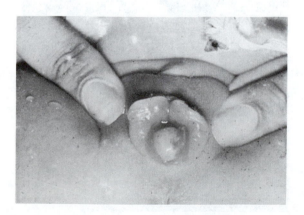

**Figure 31–9.** Mucocolpos in newborn infant.

nately, the diagnosis of a transverse vaginal septum is often delayed until after menarche when menstrual blood is trapped behind an obstructing membrane.

## Treatment

If the diagnosis of a complete septum is established prior to menarche, it should be incised, creating an aperture to allow drainage. Incision of a complete septum should be done only when the upper vagina is distended and the membrane is bulging. The distention confirms the presence of an upper vaginal segment and facilitates the procedure and reduces the risk of injury to adjacent structures.

Occasionally, there is some narrowing of the vaginal canal at the site of the septum. Because of the technical difficulties in performing intravaginal surgery on immature structures, it is best to limit the procedure only to the establishment of vaginal drainage. Surgical correction of vaginal narrowing should be performed only when the patient is contemplating initiation of sexual activity, at which time the membrane should be excised along with the ring of dense subepithelial connective tissue surrounding the vagina at the level of partition. The mucosa of the upper vagina should then be sutured to the mucosa of the lower vagina. In instances in which the length of the obstructing membrane is such that reanastomosis is not possible, the operator may leave an indwelling Lucite form in the vagina. The form allows for egress of menstrual flow and maintains vaginal patency and width. With time, re-epithelialization occurs, and the form may be removed in 4–6 months.

## 2. LONGITUDINAL VAGINAL SEPTUM

Duplication of the vagina is an extremely rare condition, often associated with duplication of the vulva, bladder, and uterus. Each part of the vagina is encircled with a separate muscular layer. A more common anomaly occurs when the distal ends of the Müllerian ducts fail to fuse properly, forming a longitudinal vaginal septum. Both parts of the vagina are encircled by one muscular layer, and a fibrous septum lined with epithelium divides the vagina. The uterus may be bicornuate, with 1 or 2 cervices (Fig 31–11).

Asymptomatic longitudinal septa require no treatment. Division of the septum is indicated when dyspareunia is present, when obstruction of drainage from one half of the vagina is noted or when it appears that the septum will interfere with vaginal delivery.

## 3. VAGINAL AGENESIS

The external genitalia of patients with vaginal agenesis (**Rokitansky syndrome**) are normal. A ruffled ridge of tissue represents the hymen (Fig 31–12). Inside this circle of tissue is an indentation marking

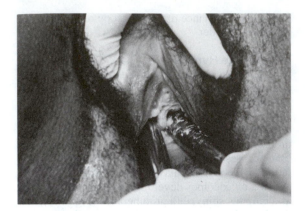

**Figure 31–11**. Longitudal septum dividing the vagina.

the spot where the introitus would normally be found. In most patients, the uterus and tubes are absent, or present as rudimentary vestiges. Other developmental defects are often present as well, affecting the urinary tract (45–50%), the spine (10%), and, less frequently, the middle ear and other mesodermal structures. Therefore, at some time during childhood, an evaluation of the urinary tract and spine and a hearing test should be given.

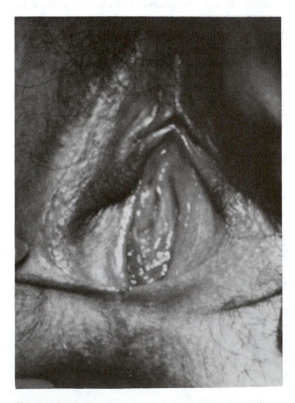

**Figure 31–12.** Vaginal agenesis in a girl 16 years of age.

Persons with Rokitansky syndrome are genetic females; they develop normally in adolescence and have all the typical feminine attributes, except that they suffer from primary amenorrhea and infertility. However, serum testosterone or a karyotype should be obtained from all patients with vaginal agenesis to identify the rare instances in which müllerian agenesis represents the effects of testicular activity, indicating male pseudohermaphroditism.

## Treatment

Creation of a satisfactory vagina is the objective in the treatment of patients with vaginal agenesis. Exploratory laparotomy, or laparoscopy, is not indicated in these patients, and the creation of a vagina should be deferred until the girl is contemplating an active sexual life. Nonoperative creation of a vagina using the method described by Frank, and later modified by Ingram (1981), is relatively risk-free, but requires motivation and patient cooperation. The region that the vagina would occupy is a potential space filled with comparatively loose connective tissue, which is capable of considerable indentation. The patient is given a series of dilators of graduated sizes and lengths and is taught how to place them against the vaginal dimple and apply constant pressure. This maneuver is repeated daily for 20–30 minutes with wider, longer dilators. The procedure takes a few months to complete and requires persistence and patience. If it fails, the next step is usually the McIndoe procedure, which involves the creation of a cavity by surgical dissection between the urethra and bladder anteriorly and the perineal body and rectum posteriorly. The cavity is then lined by a split-thickness skin graft overlying a plastic or soft silicone mold. Although the use of an amnion graft in lieu of skin had been described, the risk of transferring the AIDS virus made the use of this membrane a less desirable alternative.

An alternative procedure is the Williams vulvovaginoplasty, which utilizes the labia majora to construct a coital pouch. The procedure is relatively simple. The labia are placed under tension. A U-shaped incision is carried from the level of the urethra along the margins of the labia majora to the midpoint between the posterior fourchette and the anus. The vulvar skin is dissected from the subcutaneous fat to allow approximation without tension. Closure is in 3 layers. First, layer closure of the incision begins posteriorly and proceeds anteriorly, approximating the inner layer of skin. Interrupted sutures are then used to approximate the subcutaneous tissues; then, the outer layer of skin is closed over the midline.

## 4. PARTIAL VAGINAL AGENESIS

Partial vaginal agenesis occurs when a large portion of the vaginal plate, usually the distal part, fails to canalize. The affected vaginal segment of the vagina is replaced by a soft mass of tissue. The cause of this uncommon anomaly is unknown. Absence of the distal vagina may be identified when the infant is examined at birth, and sonographic visualization of the upper vagina, cervix, and uterus serves to distinguish it from Rokitansky syndrome.

If the uterus has developed normally, the upper part of the vagina fills with blood when menstruation begins. The symptoms are similar to those associated with imperforate hymen after the menarche. Vulvar inspection reveals findings identical with those of vaginal agenesis, but rectoabdominal palpation reveals a large, boggy pelvic mass. Diagnostic imaging using sonography, computed tomography, or magnetic resonance imaging, will confirm the diagnosis.

## Treatment

Although it is impossible to specify a standard procedure for the management of patients with partial vaginal agenesis, obstruction to menstrual flow must be corrected. In some, drainage of the uterus can be achieved through a reconstructed vagina. In others, particularly when the uterus is rudimentary, consideration may be given to performing a hysterectomy.

## ANOMALIES OF THE UTERUS

Most uterine anomalies are asymptomatic and therefore are not detected during childhood or early adolescence. Symptoms during adolescence caused by retention of menstrual flow are likely to occur in only 2 types of anomalies: rudimentary uterine horn and unicornuate uterus with paramesonephric vaginal cyst. Pain may suggest the existence of these anomalies. Asymptomatic abnormalities often escape detection until they interfere with reproduction.

## 1. RUDIMENTARY UTERINE HORN

Failure of fusion of the müllerian duct may result in 2 separate uterine bodies. Maldevelopment of one body creates a small rudimentary uterine horn. Sometimes, this rudimentary horn is separated from the remainder of the uterus and does not communicate with the other uterine cavity or the vagina. When menstruation occurs, the blood cannot escape and is trapped in the rudimentary cavity, resulting in severe dysmenorrhea, hematometra, or pyometra. If pregnancy occurs in a rudimentary horn, it may result in rupture, a complication that is potentially fatal for both mother and fetus (Fig 31–13).

Diagnostic imaging may aid in the early recogni-

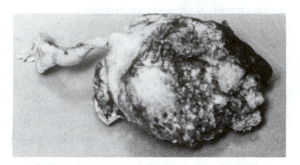

**Figure 31–13.** Pregnancy in a noncommunicating rudimentary uterine horn that has resulted in rupture.

tion of such an abnormality. Ideally, a rudimentary horn should be resected before the woman conceives a child. The tube and ovary on the affected side can be preserved, provided that the blood supply is not impaired. If the endometrial cavity of the remaining horn is entered during the operation, cesarean section is a reasonable mode of delivery for any subsequent pregnancies.

## 2. UNICORNUATE UTERUS WITH PARAMESONEPHRIC CYST

A unicornuate uterus is occasionally accompanied by an anomaly of the opposite paramesonephric duct,

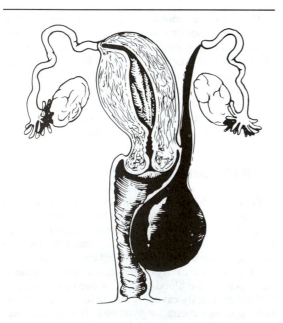

**Figure 31–14.** Unicornuate uterus with paramesonephric vaginal cyst. The endometrium lining the upper part of the cyst bleeds at menarche, and the blood, filling the lower part of the cyst, forms a mass protruding into the vagina.

creating a lateral vaginal wall cyst with an endometrial lining. As a result, the cyst fills with blood following menarche and produces a vaginal mass (Fig 31–14). Excision of a small segment of the wall between the cyst and the vagina often provides adequate drainage. Attempts to remove the cyst may involve extensive dissection, with potential damage to the urethra, bladder, or ureter.

## ANOMALIES OF THE OVARIES

At about the fifth week of gestation, the midportion of the urogenital ridge, close to the mesonephric duct, thickens to form the gonadal ridge. Located along the urogenital ridge, an additional ovary is infrequently found, separated from the normal ovaries (supernumerary ovary). Similarly, excess ovarian tissue may be observed near a normally placed ovary and connected to it (accessory ovary).

During development, the testes are drawn into the scrotum by the gubernaculum testis. Similarly, an ovary, particularly if it contains testicular elements, may be drawn by the round ligament into the inguinal canal or the labium majus. A firm inguinal mass should alert the examiner to the possible presence of an aberrant gonad, possibly containing testicular elements, even though the external genitalia are female. A karyotype should be obtained when a girl presents with an inguinal gonad. At the time of hernia repair, the gonad should be biopsied. If it proves to be an ovary, it should be returned to the peritoneal cavity and the hernia repaired. If a testis is identified, the gonad should be removed.

The infant with gonadal dysgenesis may demonstrate other signs of the typical syndrome (eg, cutis laxa and edema of the dorsal surfaces of the hands and feet). The diagnosis is difficult in premenarcheal girls who have none of the obvious signs. It is important to search for the following signs: height and weight below the third percentile, broad chest and small nipples, webbed neck, coarctation of the aorta, prominent epicanthal folds, nevi, and other somatic anomalies (eg, short fourth metacarpal).

The loss or deletion of an X chromosome usually causes rapid atresia of germ cells, so at the time of birth or soon afterward, only nonfunctioning streak gonads remain. In most adults with gonadal dysgenesis, the normal gonad is replaced by a white fibrous streak, 2 to 3 cm long and about 0.5 cm wide, located in the gonadal ridge. Histologically, the streak gonad is characterized by interlacing waves of dense fibrous stroma, indistinguishable from normal ovarian stroma.

Although oocytes are present in children and sometimes in adolescents, they are usually absent in 45,X adults. Lack of oocytes is caused by increased atresia and failure of germ cell formation. The process of atresia is sometimes incomplete, and in such patients, pubertal changes, spontaneous menstruation, and even pregnancies have been reported. Incomplete depletion of germ cells is more common in patients with mosaicism. The parents need to know what is likely in the child's medical future. They must understand that their baby has normal female organs except for impaired ovarian development; that she will need hormonal replacement therapy later; and that she may be able to have children by in vitro fertilization (donor egg), ovum transfer, or embryo transfer, or she may adopt children.

Most patients, however, are identified during adolescence, when they present with delayed pubertal development. Gonadal dysgenesis is discussed in further detail later in this chapter.

## ANOMALIES OF THE URETHRA & ANUS

Failure of a newborn infant to pass meconium or urine demands investigation. Passage of feces or urine through the vagina suggests a fistulous communication, and usually either the urethra or the anus is imperforate. Anal and rectal anomalies are classified according to Ladd and Gross (Table 31–2). In general, anomalies are divided into 2 major groups: those that form complete obstruction of the intestinal tract and those that are associated with some type of abnormal opening or fistula.

Only broad generalizations can be offered regarding the management of urogenital anomalies of this type, because the findings are so dissimilar. The following general principles may serve as guidelines. (1) Obstruction of the intestinal tract must be corrected.

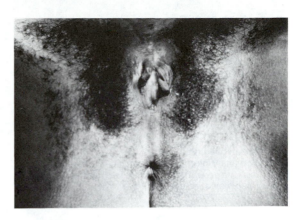

**Figure 31–15.** An adolescent girl following repair of bladder exstrophy. Note the bifid clitoris and anterior displacement of the vagina.

(2) Obstruction of the urinary tract must be relieved (this may require an initial ureterostomy or cystostomy). (3) If the urogenital sinus cannot be used later as a urethra, a permanent diversion (eg, ileal conduit) must be created. (4) If fecal contamination of the urinary tract is present, it is essential that it be corrected, usually with a temporary colostomy.

### Epispadias & Bladder Exstrophy

Epispadias denotes the failure of normal fusion of the anterior wall of the urogenital sinus, resulting in a urethra that opens cephalad to a bifid clitoris under the symphysis pubis (Fig 31–15). Occasionally, the defect is more extensive, involving the bladder and the anterior abdominal wall, causing exstrophy of the bladder. Both conditions may be associated with defects involving the anterior pelvic girdle, resulting in diminished pelvic support. Uterine and vaginal vault prolapse as well as anterior displacement of the vagina are common gynecologic complications. Rarely, vaginal and uterine prolapse may occur in the absence of other malformations. Major urologic reconstruction is required immediately, although the gynecologic defects can be repaired at a later date, usually during adolescence.

## GYNECOLOGIC DISORDERS IN PREMENARCHEAL CHILDREN

### VULVOVAGINITIS

Vulvovaginitis is probably the most common gynecologic disorder in children. The child is susceptible to infections for the following reasons: (1) lack of

**Table 31–2.** Malformations of the anus and rectum.

| | Female | Male |
|---|---|---|
| Anal stenosis | | |
| Imperforate anal membrane | | |
| Anal agenesis | With fistula<br>Anoperineal (ectopic perineal anus, anovulvar)<br>Without fistula | With fistula<br>Anoperineal (ectopic perineal anus, anocutaneous [covered anus]) or anourethral (bulbar or membranous)<br>Without fistula |
| Rectal agenesis | With fistula<br>Rectovestibular, rectovaginal, rectocloacal (urogenital sinus)<br>Without fistula | With fistula<br>Rectourethral, rectovesical<br>Without fistula |
| Rectal atresia | | |

Reproduced, with permission, from Ladd WE, Gross RE: Congenital malformations of the anus and rectum: Report of 162 cases. Am J Surg 1934;23:167.

**Table 31–3.** Classification of vulvovaginitis according to cause.

**Nonspecific vulvovaginitis**
Polymicrobial infection associated with disturbed homeostasis: secondary to poor perineal hygiene or a foreign body

**Vulvovaginitis due to secondary inoculation**
Infection resulting from inoculation of the vagina with pathogens affecting other areas of the body by contact or bloodborne transmission: secondary to upper respiratory tract infection or urinary tract infection

**Specific vulvovaginitis**
Specific primary infection, most commonly sexually transmitted: *Neisseria gonorrhoeae, Gardnerella vaginalis,* herpesvirus, *Treponema pallidum,* others

estrogen (which makes the vaginal mucosa thin and atrophic); (2) contamination by stool and other debris (in young children, perineal hygiene is often less than adequate); and (3) possibly impaired immune mechanisms of the vagina. See Table 31–3 for classification according to cause.

## Clinical Findings

Acute vulvovaginitis may denude the thin vulvar or vaginal mucosa, but bleeding is usually minimal. As a rule, mucopurulent or purulent discharge is present. Vaginal discharge may vary from minimal to copious, and at times it is bloodstained. Symptoms vary from minor discomfort to relatively intense perineal pruritus. The irritating discharge inflames the vulva and often causes the child to scratch the area to the point of bleeding. The child often complains of a burning sensation accompanied by a foul-smelling discharge. Many patients experience a burning sensation particularly during urination, when urine flows over the inflamed tissues. An erroneous diagnosis of lower urinary tract infaction may be made, especially when leukocytes are found in a voided urine specimen. Therefore, it is advisable to rule out vulvovaginitis before treatment is instituted for urinary tract infection. Inspection of the vagina reveals an area of redness and soreness that may be minimal or may extend laterally to the thighs and backward to the anus.

Evaluation of the vaginal secretions should include the following:

1. Smears for Gram's stain
2. Bacterial cultures
3. Cultures for mycotic organisms
4. Wet prep for:
   a. Mycotic organisms
   b. White and red blood cells
   c. Vaginal epithelium (estrogen effect)
   d. *Trichomonas*
   e. Parasitic ova

The diagnosis is suspected by the typical appearance of the inflamed tissue. A wet mount preparation reveals numerous leukocytes and occasional red blood cells. Culture of vaginal secretions will identify the offending organism.

Improvement of perineal hygiene is important to relieve the symptoms and to prevent recurrences. The child is instructed to sit in the tub, open her thighs, and wash the vulvar area with warm water and soap. There is no need to put soap in the vagina. Following the bath, the child is told to pat dry the vulvar area. Bubble baths and detergent washing of underpants should be avoided. Loose-fitting, white cotton undergarments are worn. Antimicrobial therapy would be expected to contribute to clinical improvement. Amoxicillin (20–40 mg/kg/day in 3 divided doses) is effective against a variety of potentially pathogenic organisms in nonspecific vulvovaginitis. When the infection is severe and extensive mucosal damage is seen, a short course of topical estrogen cream is given to promote healing of vulval and vaginal tissues. When irritation is intense, hydrocortisone cream may be necessary to alleviate the itch. In children with a first-time documented infection, vaginoscopy can be delayed. In recurrent infections refractory to treatment or associated with a foul-smelling, bloody discharge, vaginoscopy is necessary to exclude a foreign body or tumor.

## FOREIGN BODIES

Vaginal foreign bodies induce an intense inflammatory reaction and result in a bloodstained, foul-smelling discharge. Usually, the child does not recall inserting the foreign object or will not admit to it. The most commonly found foreign bodies are rolled pieces of toilet paper, which appear as amorphous conglomerates of grayish material, in which white and red blood cells are embedded. Radiographs cannot be depended on to reveal a foreign body, because many objects are not radiopaque. Vaginoscopy is essential to discover and remove objects and to exclude other causes of bleeding. Foreign bodies in the lower third of the vagina can be flushed out with a warm saline irrigation. Even after removal, if the vagina cannot be adequately inspected in the office, vaginoscopy is indicated to confirm that no other foreign bodies are present in the upper vagina. Recurrences are common, and proper instructions regarding perineal hygiene should be given to the mother and the child.

## URETHRAL PROLAPSE

Occasionally, vulvar bleeding is the result of urethral prolapse. The urethral mucosa protrudes through the meatus and forms a hemorrhagic, sensitive vulvar mass (Fig 31–16). Prolapse of the urethra is diagnosed when the urethral orifice is identified in the center of the mass and the mass is separated from

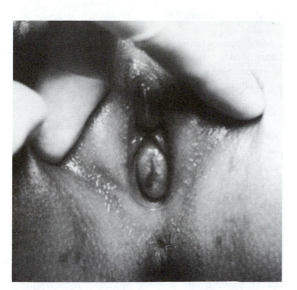

**Figure 31–16.** Urethral prolapse in a child aged 6 years.

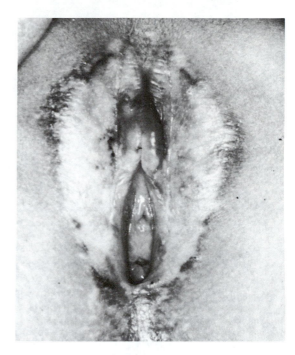

**Figure 31–17.** Lichen sclerosus of vulva of 6-year-old child.

the vagina. When the lesion is small and urination is unimpaired, a short course of therapy using estrogen cream is beneficial. When urinary retention is present, if the lesion is large and necrotic, if medical therapy fails, or if the child is being examined under anesthesia, resection of the prolapsed tissue should be performed and an indwelling catheter inserted for 24 hours.

## LICHEN SCLEROSUS

Lichen sclerosus of the vulva is a hypotrophic dystrophy. Although it usually affects women in the postmenopausal age group, it is occasionally seen in young children. Histologically, the findings in the postmenopausal age group and in young children are similar, mainly flattening of the rete pegs, hyalinization of the subdermal tissues, and keratinization. The lesion in children has no known malignant potential if only hypoplastic dystrophy is present.

The clinical presentation is that of flat ivory papules which may coalesce into plaques or, in extreme cases, involve the entire vulva (Fig 31–17). Usually, the lesion does not extend laterally beyond the middle of the labia majora nor does it encroach into the vagina. The clitoris is frequently involved as well as the posterior fourchette and the anorectal area. Occasionally, there are skin lesions affecting extragenital areas. Although most lesions are predominantly white, some have pronounced vascular markings. They tend to bruise easily, forming bloody blisters, and they are susceptible to secondary infections. The symptoms consist of vulvar irritation, dysuria, and pruritus. Scratching is common and occasionally may provoke bleeding or lead to secondary infection.

Although histologic confirmation is necessary in postmenopausal women, it is not always indicated in children. If the lesions appear to be lichen sclerosus to the experienced observer, histologic confirmation is not required.

Treatment usually consists of improved local hygiene, reduction of trauma, and short-term use of hydrocortisone cream to alleviate the pruritus. Treatment may be repeated when exacerbation occurs. Marked improvement in symptoms and in the appearance of the skin lesions is described following puberty. Review of the literature suggests more than 50% of children improve significantly or recover during puberty.

## LABIAL ADHESION

Labial adhesion is common in prepubertal children. It may be asymptomatic and therefore undiagnosed in many youngsters. The cause is not known but is probably related to the low levels of estrogens in prepubertal children. The skin covering the labia is extremely thin, and local irritation induces scratching, which may denude the labia. The labia then adhere in the midline, stick to each other, and reepithelialization occurs on both sides, with the labia remaining fused in the midline (Fig 31–18). It is important to differentiate this condition from congenital absence of the vagina.

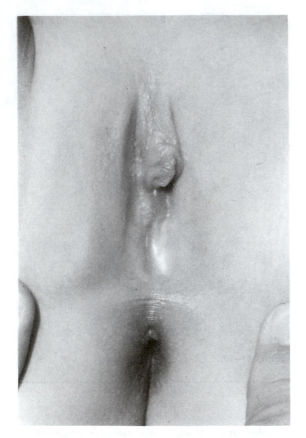

**Figure 31–18.** Labial adhesion in a young girl. Note the translucent vertical line in the center where the labia are fused together.

Most children with small areas of labial adhesions are completely asymptomatic. When symptoms occur, they usually relate to interference with urination or accumulation of urine behind the membrane. Thus, dysuria, burning pain at urination, and recurrent vulvar and vaginal infections are the cardinal symptoms. On rare occasions, urinary retention may occur.

Asymptomatic minimal-to-moderate labial fusion need not be treated. Symptomatic fusion may be treated with a short course of Premarin cream applied twice daily for 7–10 days; this may separate the labia. When medical treatment fails or if severe urinary symptoms exist, separation of the labia is indicated. This can be done as an office procedure using 1–2% topical xylocaine gel.

Because of low levels of estrogen, recurrences of labial adhesion are common until puberty. Following puberty, the condition resolves spontaneously, not to recur until after the menopause. Improved perineal hygiene and removal of any vulvar irritants may prevent recurrences. Proper instructions to mother and child should be given at that time.

## GENITAL INJURIES

Most injuries to the genitalia during childhood are accidental. Many are of minor significance, but a few are life-threatening and require surgical intervention. The physician must determine how the child sustained the injury, bearing in mind that the child requires protection if she is the victim of physical or sexual abuse.

### 1. VULVAR INJURIES

Contusion of the vulva usually does not require treatment. A hematoma manifests itself as a round, tense, ecchymotic, tender mass (Fig 31–19). A small vulvar hematoma can usually be controlled by pressure with an ice pack. The vulva should be kept clean and dry. A large hematoma, or one that continues to increase in size, may need to be incised, the clotted blood removed, and the bleeding points ligated. If the source of bleeding cannot be found, the cavity should be packed with gauze and a firm pressure dressing applied. The pack is removed in 24 hours. Prophylactic broad-spectrum antibiotics may be advisable.

When a large hematoma obstructs the urethra, it is necessary to insert a catheter, usually by a suprapubic approach. X-ray of the pelvis may be necessary to rule out pelvic fracture. In very young patients and in those with severe trauma, it may be necessary to perform the examination under general anesthesia.

### 2. VAGINAL INJURIES

Usually, there is only a small amount of bleeding from a hymenal injury. However, when the hymen is lacerated or when there is other evidence that an object has entered the vagina or penetrated the perineum, a detailed examination must be carried out to exclude injuries to the upper vagina or intrapelvic

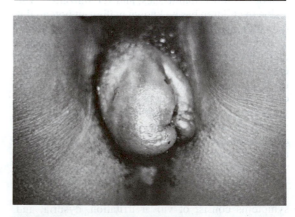

**Figure 31–19.** A large vulvar hematoma secondary to bicycle injury.

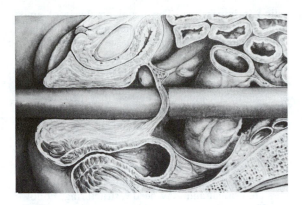

**Figure 31–20.** Transvaginal perforation of cul-de-sac and penetration of peritoneal cavity by a fall on a mop handle. Scanty bleeding from a hymenal tear was the only symptom on admission.

viscera (Fig 31–20). An intravaginal examination is required, even though the child is not in pain and there is little bleeding. Most injuries are not serious, but there could be an extensive tear, even with peritoneal perforation, without notable symptoms for several hours after the accident.

Most vaginal injuries involve the lateral walls. Generally, there is relatively little blood loss, and the child does not have much pain if only the mucosa is damaged. If the laceration extends to the vaginal vault, exploration of the pelvic cavity is necessary to rule out extension into the broad ligament or peritoneal cavity. Bladder and bowel integrity must be confirmed by catheterization and rectal palpation. Because of the small caliber of the organs involved, special instruments, as well as proper exposure and assistance, may be required for repair of vaginal injuries in young girls. Many vaginal lacerations are limited to the mucosal and submucosal tissues and are repaired with fine suture material after complete hemostasis is secured.

A vaginal wall hematoma from a small vessel may stop bleeding spontaneously. Larger vessels may form large, tense hematomas that distend the vagina and require evacuation and ligation of the bleeding vessel. When a vessel is torn above the pelvic floor, a retroperitoneal hematoma may develop. If the hematoma is enlarging, a laparotomy must be performed, the clot removed, and the bleeding vessel ligated. Alternatively, the bleeding may be controlled by angiographic embolization of the bleeding vessel.

## 3. ANOGENITAL INJURIES CAUSED BY ABUSE

Many children who are victims of sexual abuse do not sustain physical injuries, and an examination is not expected to detect signs of abuse. Even when injured, many of these children may not be seen for weeks, months, or even years after the incident occurred. The delay allows for semen and debris to wash away and for most, if not all, injuries to heal.

Injuries to the vulva may be caused by manipulation of the vulva or introitus, without vaginal penetration, or by friction of the penis against the child's vulva ("dry intercourse"). Erythema, swelling, skin bruising, and excoriations are found on the labia and vestibule. These injuries are superficial and often limited to the vulvar skin; they should resolve within a few days and require no special treatment.

Meticulous perineal hygiene is important in the prevention of secondary infections. Sitz baths should be used to remove secretions and contaminants. In some patients with extensive skin abrasions, broad-spectrum antibiotics should be given as prophylaxis. Large vulvar tears require suturing, which is best done under general anesthesia, using fine absorbable sutures. Bite wounds on the genitalia should be irrigated copiously and necrotic tissue cautiously debrided. A noninfected fresh wound can often be closed primarily, but most bite wounds should be left open. Closure is completed when granulation tissue is formed. After 3–5 days, secondary debridement may be required to remove necrotic tissues. Antitetanus immunization should be given if the child is not already immunized. Broad-spectrum antibiotics should be used for therapy rather than prophylaxis.

Most vaginal injuries occur when an object penetrates the vagina through the hymenal opening. Such penetration may result in a laceration or a tear of the hymenal ring as well as associated vaginal injuries. A detailed examination is necessary to exclude injuries to the upper vagina. The management of vaginal lacerations had been described earlier in this chapter.

Examination of the anus and rectum is easier than examination of the vagina, and most children tolerate it well. Since the anal sphincter and anal canal allow for some dilatation, a tear of the anal mucosa or sphincter rarely occurs following a digital assault. However, penetration by a larger object almost always results in some degree of injury, which varies from swelling of the anal verge to gross tearing of the sphincter. In the period immediately following penetration, the main findings are sphincter laxity and swelling and small tears of the anal verge. If the sphincter is not severed, it may be seen in spasm and will not permit a digital examination. Within days, the swelling subsides and the mucosal tears heal, occasionally forming skin tags. If not severed, the anal sphincter regains function. Repeated anal penetration over a prolonged period may cause the anal sphincter to become loose, forming an enlarged opening that can easily admit 2 or more fingers. The anal mucosa thickens and loses its normal folds.

Occasionally, child victims of abuse have contracted an STD. If the child is asymptomatic, prophylactic antibiotic therapy is not necessary. Instead, treatment should be deferred until the results of cultures and the serologic tests for syphilis (VDRL) become available so that optimal therapy may be instituted. If vulvovaginitis is clinically suspected on the initial visit, appropriate antibiotic therapy is given. If the infection is severe, a short course of topical estrogen cream is given to promote healing of vulval and vaginal tissues. When irritation is intense, hydrocortisone cream may be necessary to alleviate itching. A repeat VDRL to detect seroconversion is required 6 weeks later.

Although the likelihood of a child becoming infected with HIV as a result of sexual abuse is relatively low, many victims and their families are concerned about this possibility. Unfortunately, HIV infection in children can result in a prolonged clinical latency and can masquerade as other pathologic conditions. One study reported that 41 HIV-infected children were identified by HIV antibody tests conducted during sex abuse assessments on 5622 children. Thirteen children had alternative risk factors, but 28 children lacked any alternative transmission route to that of sexual abuse. Eighteen of these 28 victims were female and 20 were African-American. The mean age was 9 years. Coinfection with another STD occurred in 9 (33%) cases.

It has been shown that siblings and close friends of sexual abuse victims are likely to have been abused as well. Thus, HIV testing may be required in siblings of children with documented HIV infections. A recent report evaluated the prevalence of sexual abuse among siblings and other children cohabiting with sexually abused HIV-positive children. The study group consisted of 22 siblings or other children who lived in the homes of 14 previously described HIV-infected sexually abused children. Eleven of the 22 cohabiting children were confirmed to have been sexually abused and 4 (18%) were suspected of having been sexually abused. Seven (32%) of the cohabiting children could not be examined, and it was not known whether they had been sexually abused. Obviously, all these children were exposed to HIV and should be properly counseled.

### Protective Services & Counseling

It is imperative to ensure that the child is being discharged to a safe environment. Sometimes it is advisable to admit the child to the hospital or utilize temporary placement. All patients who are suspected of being victims of child sexual abuse should be referred to Child Protective Services for further evaluation.

In the period immediately following sexual assault or disclosure of sexual abuse, the child and her family often require intensive day-to-day emotional support, counseling, and guidance. Child victims often show signs of depression and have feelings of guilt, fear, and low self-esteem. Appropriate referral for coun-

seling is imperative. The major emphasis of emotional support involves strengthening the child's ego, improving her self-image, and helping her to learn to trust others and feel secure again. To begin the strengthening process, the child needs to realize that she was a victim. She must be encouraged to express her feelings of anger and hurt so that these feelings may be later expressed without experiencing further guilt. Often, the child has both positive and negative feelings toward the perpetrator and may need help in sorting out these feelings. Sometimes the child blames her parents for not protecting her. The child's relationships with her parents and other family members are critical and may need restructuring. Following this crisis intervention phase, a treatment program using individual and peer-group therapy is initiated. The patient and her family should be offered treatment for as long as they need it.

## GENITAL NEOPLASMS

Genital tumors, although uncommon, must be considered whenever a girl is found to have a chronic genital ulcer, nontraumatic swelling of the external genitalia, tissue protruding from the vagina, a fetid or bloody discharge, abdominal pain or enlargement, or premature sexual maturation. Despite their rarity, virtually every type of genital neoplasm reported in adults has also been found in girls under 14 years of age. About 50% of the genital tumors in children are premalignant or malignant.

### 1. BENIGN TUMORS OF THE VULVA & VAGINA

Teratomas, hemangiomas, simple cysts of the hymen, retention cysts of the paraurethral ducts, benign granulomas of the perineum, and condylomata acuminata are some of the benign vulvar neoplasms observed in children and adolescents.

Obstruction of a paraurethral duct may form a relatively large cyst distorting the urethral orifice. The recommended treatment is incision and drainage, marsupialization or excision.

Teratomas usually present as cystic masses arising from the midline of the perineum. Although a teratoma in this area may be benign, local recurrence is likely. To prevent recurrences, a generous margin of healthy tissue is excised about the periphery of the mass.

Capillary hemangiomas usually disappear as the child grows older and thus require no therapy except for reassurance to the mother. Cavernous hemangiomas, in contrast, are composed of vessels of considerable size, and injury to them may cause serious hemorrhage. They are best treated surgically.

Most benign tumors of the vagina in children are unilocular cystic remnants of the mesonephric duct

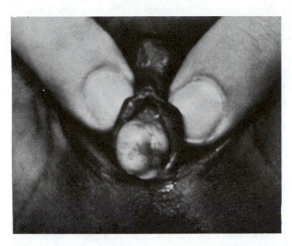

**Figure 31–21.** Simple vulvar or hymeneal cyst arising posterior to the urethra of newborn infant. (Courtesy of H Cohen et al and Am J Dis Child.)

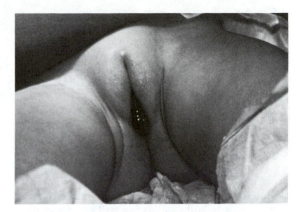

**Figure 31–22.** Botryoid sarcoma presenting as a hemorrhagic growth extruding from the vagina.

(Fig 31–21). Small cysts of the mesonephric duct (Gartner's duct) do not require surgery when they are asymptomatic. Large cysts (eg, those that block the vagina) must be treated surgically. The technical difficulties associated with excision of a large mesonephric cyst from the wall of the vagina in an infant may be considerable. Removal of a large portion of the cyst wall and marsupialization of the edges, which prevents reaccumulation of fluid, is usually sufficient.

## 2. MALIGNANT TUMORS OF THE VAGINA & CERVIX

Embryonal Carcinoma of the Vagina (Botryoid Sarcoma) Embryonal vaginal carcinomas are most commonly seen in very young girls (< 3 years old). The tumor usually involves the vagina, but the cervix may be affected as well, particularly in an older child. The tumors arise in the submucosal tissues and spread rapidly beneath an intact vaginal epithelium. The vaginal mucosa then bulges into a series of polypoid growths (thus, the term botryoid sarcoma; Fig 31–22). The diagnosis is made on the basis of histologic evaluation of a biopsy specimen, but routine microscopic evaluation may lead to an erroneous diagnosis of these lesions as benign. Striated muscle fibers are not always seen, and most of the tumor demonstrates myxomatous changes. Electron microscopy may be required to confirm the diagnosis of embryonal rhabdomyosarcoma.

In recent years, there has been marked progress in the treatment of embryonal carcinoma. Combination chemotherapy regimens—often, vincristine, dactinomycin (Actinomycin D), and cyclophosphamide—

have been used with success. Following a course of chemotherapy lasting for at least 6 months, the tumor is reexamined and rebiopsied. If following chemotherapy no residual tumor is found, surgical extirpation may not be required. If tumor is present and is amenable to surgical removal, radical hysterectomy and vaginectomy may be performed. The ovaries are preserved, and exenteration is not recommended. If the tumor is unresectable, radiation therapy is used to further shrink and control tumor growth. Following surgery, chemotherapy should be continued for another 6–12 months.

### Other Malignant Tumors of the Vagina

Three types of vaginal carcinoma may appear during childhood and the early teens. Endodermal carcinoma occurs most often in young children. Carcinoma arising in a remnant of a mesonephric duct (mesonephric carcinoma) occurs more often in girls 3 years of age or older. Clear cell adenocarcinoma of müllerian origin, often associated with a history of antenatal exposure to diethylstilbestrol (DES), is encountered most frequently in postmenarcheal teenaged girls. The clinical features and treatment of malignant lesions of the vagina and cervix are similar to those in adult women (see Chapters 45 and 46).

### 3. OVARIAN TUMORS

Even though ovarian tumors are the most common genital neoplasm encountered in children and adolescents, they represent only 1% of all neoplasms in premenarcheal children. Ovarian tumors of all varieties (except Brenner tumors) have been reported in premenarcheal children, with benign cystic teratomas accounting for at least 30%. The incidence of malignant degeneration of neoplasms is higher in children than in adolescents or adult women. Clinical signs often differ from those in adults. The 2 most common symptoms are abdominal pain and an abdominal mass. The small pelvic cavity of a child causes most ovarian tumors to rise above the pelvic inlet and present abdominally. Acute symptoms of severe pain, peritoneal irritation, or intra-abdominal hemorrhage resulting from a tumor accident (torsion, rupture, perforation) may lead to an erroneous diagnosis of appendicitis, intussusception, or volvulus. At least 25% of all childhood ovarian tumors elude diagnosis until exploratory laparotomy is performed. Tumors of the ovary should be considered in the differential diagnosis of most disorders causing abdominal pain or mass in a child. Pelvic (rectal) examination may be helpful if the tumor is in the pelvis but will not detect most abdominal tumors.

Clinical features, diagnosis, and treatment of specific ovarian tumors in mature teenagers and adults are described in Chapter 37. The management of ovarian neoplasms in premenarcheal children varies from that in older patients because continued ovarian function is necessary to complete sexual and somatic maturation in children. Therefore, greater attempts should be made to preserve ovarian function.

Conservative surgery (unilateral salpingo-oophorectomy) is justified for most premenarcheal patients with stage I cancer of the ovary, provided that it can be shown that the tumor is limited to the ovary. It should be documented that the tumor is unilateral, that there are no diaphragmatic or omental metastases, and that there is no extension to the para-aortic or pelvic lymph nodes; peritoneal washings should not contain tumor cells. Obviously, if a tumor has extended beyond the ovary, more radical surgery (bilateral salpingo-oophorectomy with hysterectomy) is indicated.

## DISORDERS OF SEXUAL MATURATION

### ACCELERATED SEXUAL MATURATION

Puberty is the process by which sexually immature persons become capable of reproduction. These changes occur largely as the result of maturation of the hypothalamic-pituitary-gonadal axis. As a rule, breast development, cornification of the vaginal mucosa, and growth of genital hair precede uterine bleeding by about 2 years. The normal sequence of events in sexual development is outlined in Figure 31–23. Usually, initial growth acceleration occurs first. Breast budding occurs between ages 9 and 11 years and is followed by pubarche and a marked increase in growth rate, often referred to as the adolescent growth spurt. The first menstrual period occurs at an average age of 12.8 years in girls in the USA. Regular ovulatory cycles, 20 months later, mark the end of the pubertal changes.

Sexual precocity is the onset of sexual maturation at any age that is 2.5 SD earlier than the normal age. At present, the appearance of any secondary sexual characteristics before 8 years of age or onset of men-

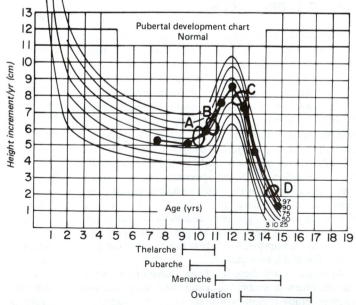

**Figure 31–23.** A pubertal development chart for a normally developing female adolescent. Growth data are converted to growth velocity and plotted. The growth velocity curve shows initial acceleration in growth followed by the growth spurt and subsequent deceleration. Superimposed on this curve are the following pubertal events: A, thelarche; B, pubarche; C, menarche; D, onset of ovulation. (From Reindollar RH, Mcdonough PG: Delayed sexual development: Common causes and basic clinical approach. Pediatr Ann 1981;10:178.)

**Table 31–4.** Classification of patients with accelerated sexual maturation.

**Complete Forms**

**GnRH Dependent**
Idiopathic Precocious Puberty
CNS Lesions
   Congenital malformations
   Neoplasms
   Space occupying lesions
   Hydrocephalus
   Injuries

**GnRH Independent (Peripheral)**
Exogenous sex steroids
Endogenous production of sex steroids
   Ovarian cysts
   Ovarian neoplasms
   Feminizing adrenal tumors
McCune Albright Syndrome
Thyroid dysfunction

**Incomplete Forms**
Premature Thelarche
Premature Adrenarche
Premature menarche

arche prior to age 10 is considered precocious. Sexual precocity may be classified as (1) gonadotropin-releasing hormone (GnRH)-dependent precocious puberty, (2) GnRH-independent precocious puberty; or (3) precocious pseudopuberty, also called isolated partial development or incomplete precocious puberty (Table 31–4).

## GnRH-Dependent Precocious Puberty

GnRH-dependent precocious puberty is a normal pubertal development that occurs at an earlier age. Premature reactivation of the hypothalamic-pituitary axis occurs. It is followed by gonadotropin secretion, which in turn stimulates the gonads to produce steroid hormones, and subsequently, pubertal changes. GnRH-dependent precocious puberty is seen more frequently in girls than in boys. The cause of such early development often remains unclear and has been labeled as idiopathic. A familial form does exist, but is more commonly seen in boys.

Occasionally, precocious puberty is associated with central nervous system (CNS) abnormalities, including hypothalamic hamartomas. With improved imaging techniques, it is now apparent that many cases of what was once considered to be idiopathic precocious puberty are in fact associated with hypothalamic hamartomas. Other CNS neoplasms are associated with precocious puberty, including optic gliomas, neurofibromas, as well as other CNS neoplasms. Cranial irradiation and CNS injuries may also be associated with precocious puberty. Finally, prolonged excessive therapy with exogenous sex steroids may accelerate hypothalamic-pituitary axis maturation resulting in precocious puberty.

## GnRH-Independent Precocious Puberty

**A. Endogenous Estrogens:** The ovary in the newborn female contains 1–2 million primordial follicles, most of which undergo atresia during childhood without producing significant quantities of estrogen. However, large follicular cysts capable of estrogen production occur occasionally and may cause early feminization. Benign tumors of the ovary (eg, teratoma, cystadenoma) may produce estrogen or may induce surrounding ovarian tissue to produce steroids. Granulosa cell tumors capable of estrogen production are a rare cause of prepubertal feminization. Other tumors of extragonadal origin may produce estrogens, including adrenal adenomas and hepatomas, but these are extremely rare.

**B. Exogenous Estrogens:** Accidental ingestion of estrogens or prolonged use of creams containing estrogens is a possible, though uncommon cause of early feminization. If exposure to estrogens is documented, prompt discontinuation is the proper treatment.

**C. McCune-Albright Syndrome:** Polyosthotic fibrous dysplasia, irregular cutaneous pigmentation, and precocious puberty occurring together are the cardinal signs of McCune-Albright syndrome (Fig 31–24). Affected children usually present at a younger age than those with idiopathic precocious puberty. Vaginal bleeding occurs early and in most is the first sign of puberty. The diagnosis is made on the basis of skin pigmentation and demonstration of bone lesions or pathologic fractures. The exact cause is unknown; a primary ovarian abnormality with premature estrogen production has been suggested.

The prognosis for children with McCune-Albright syndrome is unfavorable. Adult height is significantly reduced not only because of early epiphyseal closure but also because of pathologic bone fractures. As adults, most patients have menstrual abnormalities and many are infertile.

**D. Precocious Pseudopuberty:** Occasionally, for reasons that remain unclear, only one sign of pubertal development is present (breast development, pubic hair, or menstruation). This is possibly the result of transient elevations of the levels of circulating steroid hormones or, possibly, to extreme sensitivity of the end organ, eg, breast tissue, to the low, prepubertal levels of sex hormones. Such isolated development, however, may represent the initial sign of precocious puberty, and these patients should be reevaluated at regular intervals.

**E. Premature Thelarche:** Premature thelarche is the isolated development of breast tissue prior to age 8, most commonly occurring between 1 and 3 years of age. It may affect one or both breasts (Fig 31–25). On examination, the somatic growth pattern is not accelerated, bone age is not advanced, and smear of vaginal secretions fails to show estrogen effect. The diagnosis is made by exclusion of other disorders. Surgical biopsy of the breast is

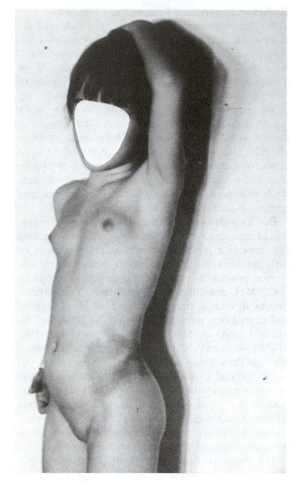

**Figure 31–24.** Six-and-a-half-year-old child with McCuneAlbright syndrome. (Reproduced, with permission, from Huffman JW: Gynauakologie des Kindes. Urban & Schwarzenberg, 1975.)

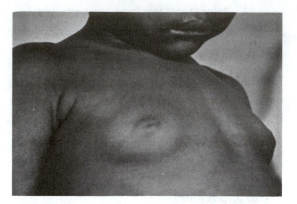

**Figure 31–25.** Premature thelarche in a child 5 years of age.

contraindicated, because too extensive excision of tissue may cause permanent damage to the breast.

**F. Premature Pubarche:** Premature pubarche is the isolated development of pubic or axillary hair prior to age 8 years without other signs of precocious puberty (Fig 31–26). Such hair growth may be idiopathic and of no clinical significance. In some studies, these children tended to be slightly taller, had marginally advanced bone age, and had slightly elevated serum DHEA levels.

Early pubarche may be a sign of excess androgen production due to enzyme deficiency (congenital adrenal hyperplasia) or tumor (Leydig cell tumor). Thorough evaluation of adrenal and gonadal function and assessment of androgen production are necessary to exclude such abnormalities. The diagnosis of idiopathic premature pubarche is made

only after such an evaluation fails to detect an abnormality.

**G. Premature Menarche:** Premature menarche denotes the appearance of cyclic vaginal bleeding in children in the absence of other signs of secondary sexual development. The cause is unknown but may be related to increased end organ sensitivity of the endometrium to low prepubertal levels of estrogens. Alternatively, bleeding may be related to transient elevation of estrogens due to premature follicular development. These patients have estradiol levels in the prepubertal range, and cytologic smears of vaginal secretions indicate lack of estrogenic stimulation. When patients are given GnRH, the response of the pituitary gland is similar to that seen in prepubertal children.

The diagnosis of premature menarche is formulated by exclusion following investigation of other causes of vaginal bleeding and is confirmed when the cyclic nature of the bleeding becomes apparent. The prognosis is excellent. Adult height is uncompromised; the menstrual pattern is normal; and fertility potential remains unimpaired.

## EVALUATION OF THE PATIENT WITH VAGINAL BLEEDING

Vaginal bleeding in children requires a thorough evaluation and accurate diagnosis. In general, 2 sources of bleeding should be suspected: (1) the endometrium (bleeding is usually a manifestation of precocious puberty; see following text) and (2) a local vulvar or vaginal lesion (eg, vulvovaginitis, foreign bodies, urethral prolapse, trauma, botryoid sarcoma, adenocarcinoma of cervix or vagina, and vulvar skin disorders).

Vaginal bleeding during childhood should always alert the physician to the possibility of a genital

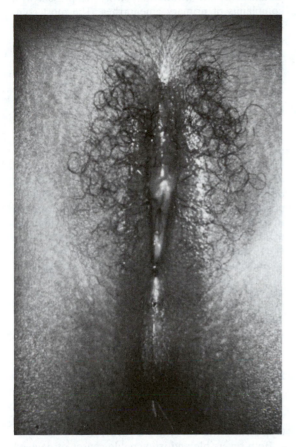

**Figure 31–26.** Premature pubarche in a child 4 years of age.

tumor. Vaginoscopy and examination under anesthesia are the mainstays of evaluation to exclude the presence of tumors, foreign bodies, and other local lesions. Benign tumors of the vulva and vagina are rare in childhood, and those that do occur seldom cause bleeding. Malignant neoplasms usually bleed from necrotic or ulcerative areas that appear early in their development. Thorough examination, including vaginoscopy, is mandatory, and all suspicious lesions require biopsy for diagnosis. Genital tract neoplasms are discussed elsewhere in this chapter.

### Evaluation of the Patient with Precocious Puberty

When evaluating the patient with sexual precocity, the age at onset, duration, and progression of signs and symptoms constitute important historical information. Family history and review of systems may add important facts. Detailed examination shows the typical changes which include the following:

**General changes:** Enhancement of general growth

is coincident with the onset of estrogen-stimulated change. The child often exhibits accelerated growth velocity, tall stature for age, and advanced skeletal maturation.

**Skin:** Additional androgen-dependent findings include acne and adult-type body odor.

**Breast development:** Breast development is at least at Tanner stage II, with the areolae having a broadened, darkened, "stimulated" appearance.

**Genitalia:** Genital changes include fullness of the labia and pink dulling of the vaginal mucosa, reflecting estrogen-induced thickening of the genital tissues. Increased vaginal secretions may result in leukorrhea. Dark, coarse pubic hair may be present.

### Diagnosis

The diagnosis of GnRH-dependent precocity requires demonstration of pubertal gonadotropin secretion. The diagnostic evaluation required to document early pubertal development and differentiate central from peripheral causes includes the determination of serum luteinizing hormone (LH), follicle-stimulating hormone (FSH), estradiol levels, and a GnRH stimulation test. In patients with GnRH-dependent precocious puberty, the results of these tests will be in the normal pubertal range. In addition, these patients will require diagnostic imaging to document skeletal age, and the absence of gonadal or CNS lesions.

### Treatment of GnRH-Dependent Precocious Puberty

The treatment of choice for GnRH-dependent precocious puberty is a GnRH analog (GnRHa). Analogs of GnRH are modifications of the native hormone, which have greater resistance to degradation and increased affinity for the pituitary GnRH receptors. This treatment induces down-regulation of receptor function, resulting in temporary, reversible inhibition of the H-P-O axis, as reflected by minimal or no response to GnRH stimulation, and regression of the manifestations of puberty.

Treatment with GnRHa decreases gonadotropins and sex steroids to prepubertal levels, which is followed by regression of secondary sexual features. Treatment also causes a deceleration in the skeletal maturation rate. Treatment with GnRHa preserves, or even improves predicted height, unless bone age is so advanced that further growth is precluded. Treatment is continued until puberty is appropriate based on age, emotional maturity, height, and height potential. Resumption of puberty occurs promptly after discontinuation of GnRHa therapy.

### DELAYED SEXUAL MATURATION

Delayed sexual development has been defined as the absence of normal pubertal events at an age 2.5 SD from the mean. The absence of thelarche by age

13 years or the absence of menarche by age 15 is an indication for investigation. However, evaluation need not always be delayed until such strict criteria are met. The concern of the patient, her family, or the referring physician is reason enough for initiating an evaluation. Some degree of sexual maturation occurs in over 30% of patients with gonadal dysgenesis; therefore, a patient who presents following the larche with a delay in the orderly progression of pubertal development should also undergo investigation. Delayed sexual development may be classified according to gonadal function (Table 31–5).

## 1. DELAYED MENARCHE WITH ADEQUATE SECONDARY SEXUAL DEVELOPMENT

Patients with functioning gonads and delayed sexual maturation usually consult a physician in their midteens because of amenorrhea. Most have well-formed female configuration with adequately developed breasts. Many of these patients suffer from inappropriate hypothalamic-pituitary-ovarian feedback mechanism leading to anovulation and androgen excess. Primary amenorrhea may persist until a progestin challenge is given. Patients should be monitored for continued menstrual shedding. Persisting amenorrhea is treated with progestins administered every other month to prevent endometrial hyperplasia. A sexually active girl should be given oral contraceptives rather than cyclic progestins. Further evaluation is required in patients with persistent menstrual abnormalities, since similar clinical manifestations are also encountered in adolescents with adult-onset congenital adrenal hyperplasia and those with polycystic ovarian disease.

**Table 31–5.** Classification of patients with delayed sexual maturation.

**Delayed Menarche with Adequate Secondary Sexual Development**
Anatomic genital abnormalities
Inappropriate positive feedback
Androgen insensitivity syndromes (complete forms)

**Delayed Puberty with Inadequate or Absent Secondary Sexual Development**
Hypothalamic-pituitary dysfunction (low FSH)
  Reversible: Constitutional delay, weight loss due to extreme dieting, protein deficiency, fat loss without muscle loss, drug abuse
  Irreversible: Kallmann's syndrome, pituitary destruction
Gonadal failure (high FSH)
  Abnormal chromosomal complement (e.g. Turner's syndrome)
  Normal chromosomal complement: chemotherapy, irradiation, infection, infiltrative or autoimmune disease, resistant ovary syndrome

**Delayed Puberty with Heterosexual Secondary Sexual Development (Virilization)**
Enzyme deficiency (eg, 21α-hydroxylase deficiency), neoplasm, male pseudohermaphroditism

Most patients with congenital anomalies of the paramesonephric (Müllerian) structures present with complaints of primary amenorrhea. The most common defect is congenital absence of the uterus and vagina; other causes are imperforate hymen, transverse vaginal septa, and agenesis of the cervix. Gynecologic examination supplemented by ultrasonography establishes the diagnosis of these congenital anomalies, which are discussed in detail earlier in this chapter.

The complete forms of androgen insensitivity (Fig 31–27) are also associated with amenorrhea and normal breast development. Affected persons have normal testicular function but are not responsive to male concentrations of testosterone, and the development of breasts is secondary to the small amounts of unopposed estrogens produced by the testis. Pubic and axillary hair is scant or often absent. A short blind vaginal pouch is present. Once pubertal development has been completed, surgical extirpation of the gonads and reconstruction of the vagina are necessary.

The possibility of pregnancy in an adolescent who has not begun to menstruate is highly unlikely but must be borne in mind when considering causes of delayed menarche in patients with normal pubertal development.

## 2. DELAYED PUBERTY WITH INADEQUATE OR ABSENT SECONDARY SEXUAL DEVELOPMENT

### Hypothalamic-Pituitary Dysfunction

Both reversible and irreversible causes of delayed puberty secondary to lack of maturation or function of the hypothalamus and pituitary have been described.

The onset of puberty depends on an ill-defined stage of maturity that is reflected in skeletal age. Maturation is partly genetically determined but also depends on multiple environmental factors; thus, the chronologic age of puberty varies considerably. Statistical limits of normal variation in a defined population group indicate that by definition, 2.5% of all normal adolescents will develop later than the age defined as "normal." This group has been labeled "late bloomers," or having a constitutional delay in the maturation process. Although these patients are normal, absence of signs of puberty (including the growth spurt) often concerns the patient when her adolescent friends have developed secondary sexual features and gained the characteristic increase in height.

The diagnosis of hypothalamic-pituitary dysfunction is made by exclusion of other causes of delayed sexual maturation. The GnRH challenge test differentiates constitutional delay from similar conditions associated with a deficiency of GnRH. Reassurance is the only treatment necessary, but the patient must be kept under observation until regular menstrual cycles are established. Occasionally, an adolescent requires hormonal replacement therapy because of emotional distress over her condition.

Isolated deficiency of GnRH, often associated with intracranial anomalies and anosmia (**Kallmann's syndrome**), is uncommon. Patients suspected of having the syndrome should be carefully tested for anosmia, although many have only a minor impairment. These patients fail to develop secondary sexual features, and blood levels of gonadotropins are very low. Following GnRH challenge, a rise in gonadotropin levels is noted. Estrogen replacement therapy is used to initiate and sustain sexual development. Induction of ovulation with human menopausal gonadotropins or GnRH is necessary when pregnancy is desired.

A pituitary or parasellar tumor, particularly craniopharyngioma or pituitary adenoma, must be considered in the evaluation of a patient with delayed sexual maturation. Craniopharyngiomas are rapidly growing tumors that often develop in late childhood. Pituitary adenomas are slow-growing, may become symptomatic during puberty, and may interfere with sexual maturation. An occult pituitary prolactinoma in adolescents with unexplained delayed sexual maturation must also be ruled out. Serum prolactin levels should be measured yearly in patients with unexplained delayed sexual maturation.

Weight loss due to extreme dieting, marked protein deficiency, and fat loss without notable loss of muscle (often seen in athletes) may also delay or suppress hypothalamic pituitary maturation. Heroin addiction may cause amenorrhea, but its effects on sexual maturation have not been documented.

## Gonadal Failure

Most patients with gonadal dysgenesis present during adolescence with delayed puberty and primary amenorrhea. If untreated, estrogen and androgen levels are decreased and FSH and LH levels are increased. Estrogen-dependent organs show the predictable effects of hormonal deficiency. Breasts contain little parenchymal tissue, and the areolar tissue is only slightly darker than the surrounding skin; the well-differentiated external genitalia, vagina, and müllerian derivatives remain small. Pubic and axillary hair fail to develop in normal quantity.

However, normal pubertal development, menstruation, and even pregnancies have been reported in adults with gonadal dysgenesis. It is possible that a few of these persons maintain some germ cells to adulthood. Spontaneous development is more commonly observed in patients with mosaicism with a 46,XX line. The rare offspring of these women probably do not have an increased risk for chromosomal abnormalities.

Some patients may have ovarian failure even though they have a normal chromosome complement and 2 intact sex chromosomes (46,XX). An autosomal recessive form of ovarian failure has been demonstrated in some families. Other causes of follicular depletion include chemotherapy, irradiation, infections (eg, mumps), infiltrative disease processes of the ovary (eg, tuberculosis), autoimmune diseases, and unknown environmental agents.

A karyotype is necessary to rule out the presence of Y chromosome material. DNA probes and H-Y antigen assays have also been used to identify Y chromosome material. A high incidence of neoplastic changes in the gonadal ridge has been reported in the presence of a Y chromosome; thus, prophylactic gonadectomy is recommended (Fig 31–28). Replacement hormonal therapy is then given in a cyclic manner.

The resistant ovary syndrome is characterized by delayed menarche or primary amenorrhea, a 46,XX chromosome complement, high FSH levels, and ovaries with apparently normal follicular apparatus that do not respond to endogenous gonadotropins. It is assumed that absence of follicular receptors for gonadotropins is responsible for ovarian dysfunction in these patients. These individuals may have normally developed secondary sexual characteristics. Estrogen replacement therapy is required to prevent long-term complications of estrogen deficiency (eg, vaginal dryness, osteoporosis). Pregnancies have been reported in some patients treated with Pergonal or following discontinuation of estrogen therapy.

## 3. DELAYED PUBERTY WITH HETEROSEXUAL SECONDARY SEXUAL DEVELOPMENT

Virilization at puberty is the result of elevated androgens from adrenal or gonadal sources. These may be the result of an enzyme deficiency (eg, late-onset congenital adrenal hyperplasia) or a neoplasm (eg, Leydig cell tumor).

A small group of patients are male pseudohermaphrodites. These are adolescents who are being reared as girls and have female external genitalia, intra-abdominal or ectopic malfunctioning testes, and a normal 46,XY chromosomal complement. The diagnosis and treatment of intersex disorders are discussed in Chapter 5.

## Evaluation of the Patient with Delayed Sexual Development

Determination of gonadal function can be accomplished by obtaining a medical history and performing a detailed physical examination, supplemented by selected laboratory studies. Historical information should center around previous growth and pubertal development. Linear and velocity growth charts as well as a pubertal development chart clarify previous growth patterns and are useful in subsequent follow-up. Knowledge of previ-

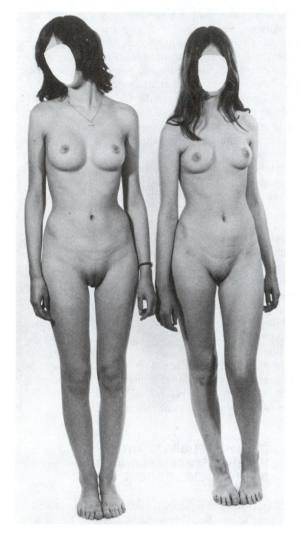

**Figure 31–27.** XY sisters with androgen insensitivity syndrome. (Courtesy of CJ Dewhurst.)

pelvic sonogram to confirm uterine absence and ovarian presence.

Absence of pubic hair is suggestive of the androgen insensitivity syndrome. Karyotype will identify the 46,XY cell line in patients with testicular feminization syndrome (Fig. 31–28). Patients with complete pubertal development, evidence of continued estrogen production, and normal müllerian systems probably have inappropriate positive feedback and thus chronic anovulation. Progesterone challenge in such patients is helpful. A withdrawal bleed signifies a normal müllerian system and continued estrogen production.

When breast development is minimal, the usual diagnosis is lack of gonadal function. Serum gonadotropin assays are performed for further elucidation. Elevated FSH levels suggest gonadal failure. Other endocrine profiles should be obtained if hypothyroidism, congenital adrenal hyperplasia, or Cushing's syndrome is suspected. Karyotype is necessary in all patients with gonadal failure and will identify both normal and abnormal chromosome complements. The presence of a Y chromosome in either group dictates gonadal removal.

Low FSH levels suggest an interference with hypothalamic-pituitary maturation and gonadotropin release. Skull films and prolactin assays must be obtained for all patients to rule out the presence of pituitary or hypothalamic tumors. Appropriate endocrine evaluation identifies the occasional patient with hypothyroidism or congenital adrenal hyperplasia and the rare patient with Cushing's syndrome. Diagnosis of Kallmann's syndrome is suspected in hypogonadotrophic patients who have an associated anosmia, and it is confirmed when GnRH challenge tests are performed. The presumed diagnosis of constitutional delay is made by exclusion of all other causes and by the typical GnRH release patterns after GnRH challenge.

ous medical disorders may immediately identify the cause of aberrant puberty.

Physical examination must include height and weight assessments and a careful search for somatic anomalies. Staging of pubertal development by Tanner criteria is most important in the determination of gonadal function. Presence of breast development signifies prior gonadal function. A vaginal smear for cytohormonal evaluation can determine whether the gonad is continuing to produce estrogen. Pelvic and rectal examination will identify patients with an obstructed outflow tract, as well as patients with congenital absence of the vagina and uterus. Further confirmation of patients with Rokitansky sequence is dependent on a karyotype to identify normal 46,XX complement, and a

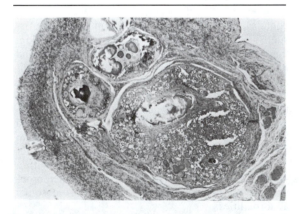

**Figure 31–28.** Gonadoblastoma developing in a gonadal ridge in a patient with gonadal dysgenesis and 45,XO/46,XY karyotype.

# PREGNANCY IN CHILDREN & ADOLESCENTS

## PRECOCIOUS (JUVENILE) PREGNANCY

Precocious, or juvenile, pregnancy is rare. The youngest known patient was a Peruvian girl aged 5 years, 8 months, who was delivered at term by cesarean section in 1939 of a healthy male infant weighing 2950 g (6 lb, 8 oz). Both mother and infant survived. In every reported instance, the underage mothers were sexually precocious, most having menstruated for several years before becoming pregnant. Juvenile pregnancy per se does not increase the chance of congenital anomalies in the offspring, but in many cases the mother is a victim of sexual abuse, and if the pregnancy is the result of incest, there is a greater likelihood of genetic malformations carried by recessive genes.

Most precocious mothers and their babies have not done well; there is an increased incidence of spontaneous abortion, pregnancy-induced hypertension, and premature labor and delivery. In patients under 9 years of age, less than 50% have normal labor, and there is a 35% likelihood of neonatal loss.

The underage mother and her family may need psychiatric counseling, both during pregnancy and following delivery. Lessening the emotional, social, and medical trauma associated with such a gestation is an important task for all who assist in the care of the pregnant child.

## ADOLESCENT PREGNANCY

The USA endures the highest teenage pregnancy rate (9.5%) of any Western nation, thereby taxing both the economic resources of society and the adjustment capacities of single mothers, since few adolescents are opting to marry early. In one decade, from 1972 to 1982, the estimated percentage of teenage girls who were sexually active rose from 28% to 42%. Similar increase was noted in the young teenagers' birth rate (ages 15–17), which have risen to 37.5% in 1990—the highest rate since 1977. Yet conventional sex education programs have shown little impact on lowering the risks of contagion or conception. [Moreover, a clearly negative relationship between completed fertility and intelligence seems to be emerging from recent, large-sample research. Despite these distressing trends, the mass media purvey and exploit the excitement of sex without giving comparable attention to its dangers or to means for preventing pregnancy and disease. For instance, a typical family will observe over 9000 sexual encounters and references yearly during prime-time television view-ing, but will see many fewer depictions of ways to avert health hazards, let alone to engage in contraception.] The rate of teenage pregnancy in the USA is twice that of Canada, England, or France and 7 times that of the Netherlands. The rate of teenage abortion is also higher in the USA than in other Western countries for which data are available, and teenagers in the USA use contraceptives less frequently and use less effective methods of contraception. Problems of cost and fears of lack of confidentiality appear to inhibit young women from obtaining contraceptives. The result is an increase in teenage pregnancy rates.

For years it has been accepted that adolescent pregnancy is a high-risk pregnancy. Many studies have shown that the outcome of adolescent pregnancy is less satisfactory than that of a pregnancy in the general population. The lifestyle of an adolescent girl may be detrimental to the pregnancy. Many adolescents come from low socioeconomic backgrounds, having poor education and perhaps poor general health due to inadequate nutrition, cigarette smoking, drug abuse, or STDs. Nutrition is an important problem. Bone mineral content, iron stores, and caloric intake are often reduced among adolescent girls, and iron deficiency anemia is frequently found. Proper education and dietary counseling may improve nutritional status and prevent anemia.

Optimal care should be given to teenage mothers not only to improve the pregnancy outcome but also to enhance their social, educational, and emotional adjustment. The young mother's program established in 1965 by the Yale New Haven Center is an example of a comprehensive care program. There are indications that such a program reduces significantly the hazards in this high-risk group. Other studies have concluded that complications of labor and delivery are highly dependent on the quality of prenatal care.

Preeclampsia-eclampsia, which is more common in a first pregnancy, occurs more frequently among adolescents than among adult women, perhaps because of high-risk factors just mentioned. There seems to be no intrinsic predisposition to preeclampsia-eclampsia in adolescents, and when proper prenatal care is provided, the incidence is greatly reduced.

Prematurity and small-for-dates infants are a major problem in adolescent pregnancies. Predisposing factors are high-risk factors such as low prepregnancy weight, poor weight gain, adverse socioeconomic conditions, cigarette smoking, anemia, first pregnancy, and deficient prenatal care, all of which occur more commonly in adolescents. Nutritional deficit is extremely important. If the teenage mother is more than 10% below her ideal weight, she is more likely to produce an underweight baby. If the teenager gains less than 20 lbs during her pregnancy, she is at risk of having a low birth weight baby. If she is more than 10% under ideal weight and gains less than 20 pounds during the pregnancy, she is in double jeopardy.

Thus, to minimize prenatal complications and improve maternal and fetal outcome, the young patient should be enrolled in an aggressive prenatal care program that addresses the unique problems of the adolescent patient.

## REFERENCES

Bays J, Chadwick D: Medical diagnosis of the sexually abused child. Child Abuse Negl 1993;17:91.

Berenson AB: Appearance of the hymen at birth and one year of age: A longitudinal study. Pediatrics 1993;91:820.

Berenson AB, Heger AH, Andrews S: Appearance of the hymen in newborns. Pediatrics 1991;87:458.

Berenson AB, Heger AH, Hayes JM et al: Appearance of the hymen in prepubertal girls. Pediatrics 1992;89:387.

Bourguignon JP, Franchimont P, Ernould C, Geubelle F: Delayed puberty: From pathophysiology to therapy. In: *Adolescence in Females.* pp. 389–404. Venturoli S, Flanigni G, Givens JR (editors). YearBook Medical Publishers, 1985.

Cutler GB Jr, Laue L: Congenital adrenal hyperplasia due to 21-hydroxylase deficiency. N Eng J Med 1990;323:1806.

Daugaard G, Hansen HH, Rorth M: Treatment of malignant germ cell tumors. Ann Oncol 1990;1:195.

Dewhurst CJ: *Practical Pediatric & Adolescent Gynecology.* Marcel Dekker, 1980.

Dewhurst J: *Female Puberty and Its Abnormalities.* Churchill Livingstone, 1984.

Dewhurst J: Lichen sclerosus of the vulva in childhood. Pediatr Adolesc Gynecol 1983;1:149.

Emans SJH, Goldstein DP: *Pediatric and Adolescent Gynecology,* 3rd ed., pp. 1–45. Little, Brown & Co., 1990.

Finkelhor D, Hotaling G, Lewis IA, Smith C: Sexual abuse in a national survey of adult men and women: Prevalence, characteristics, and risk factors. Child Abuse Negl 1990;14:19.

Frank R: Formation of artificial vagina without operation. Am J Obstet Gynecol, 1938;35:1053.

Friedrich EG Jr: *Vulvar Disease.* 2nd ed., WB Saunders, 1983.

Gale CL, Muram D, Adamec TA: The effects of estrogen on wound healing. Adolesc Pediatr Gynecol 1993;6:160.

Gardner JJ: Descriptive study of genital variation in healthy, nonabused premenarchal girls. J Pediatr 1992;120:251.

Gellert GA, Durfee MJ, Berkowitz CD et al: Situational and sociodemographic characteristics of children infected with human immunodeficiency virus from pediatric sexual abuse. Pediatrics 1993;91:39.

Grant DB, Muram D, Dewhurst J: Precocious puberty: Implications on adult reproductive function, pp. 335–340. In: *Adolescence in Females.* Venturoli S, Flanigni C, Givens JR (editors). YearBook Medical Publishers, 1985.

Griffin JE, Edwards C, Madden JD et al: Congenital absence of the vagina. The Mayer-Rokitansky-Kuster-Hauser syndrome. Ann Intern Med 1976;85:224.

Grumbach MM, Conte FA: Disorders of sexual differentiation. In: *Williams Textbook of Endocrinology,* 7th ed., pp. 312–401. Wilson JD, Foster DW (editors). WB Saunders, 1985.

Gutman LT, St. Claire KK, Weedy C et al: Sexual abuse of human immunodeficiency virus-positive children. Outcomes for perpetrators and evaluation of other household children. Am J Dis Child 1992;146:1185.

Heger A, Emans JE: *Evaluation of the Sexually Abused Child.* Oxford University Press, 1992.

Heller ME, Dewhurst J, Grant DB: Premature menarche without other evidence of precocious puberty. Arch Dis Child 1979;54:472.

Hintz RL: New approaches to growth failure in Turner syndrome. Adolesc Pediatr Gynecol 1989;2:172.

Hobbs CJ, Wynne JM. Child abuse: Buggery in childhood—A common syndrome of child abuse. Lancet 1986;2:792.

Hobbs CJ, Wynne JM. Sexual abuse of English boys and girls: The importance of anal examination. Child Abuse Negl 1989;13:195.

Huffman JW, Dewhurst CJ, Capraro VJ: *The Gynecology of Childhood and Adolescence,* 2nd ed., pp. 76–100. WB Saunders, 1981.

Imperato-McGinley J, Gautier T, Pichardo M, Shackleton C: The diagnosis of 5 alpha-reductase deficiency in infancy. J Clin Endocrinol Metab 1986;63:1313.

Ingram JM: The bicycle seat stool in the treatment of vaginal agenesis and stenosis: A preliminary report. Am J Obstet Gynecol 1981;140:867.

Jones HW Jr, Rock JA: *Reparative and Constructive Surgery of the Female Genital Tract.* Williams & Wilkins, 1983.

Kaneti J, Lieberman E, Moshe P, Carmie R: A case of ambiguous genitalia owing to neurofibromatosis: Review of the literature. J Urol 1988;140:584.

Lavery JP et al: Pregnancy outcome in a comprehensive teenage parent program. Adolesc Pediatr Gynecol 1988;1:34.

Lavery JP, Sanfilippo JS: *Pediatric and Adolescent Obstetrics and Gynecology.* Springer-Verlag, 1985.

Lowy G: Sexually transmitted diseases in children. Pediatr Dermatol 1992;9:329.

Marshall WA, Tanner JM: Variation in the pattern of pubertal changes in girls. Arch Dis Child 1969;44:291.

McCann J, Voris J: Perianal injuries resulting from sexual abuse: A longitudinal study. Pediatrics 1993;91:390.

McCann J, Voris J, Simon M: Genital injuries resulting from sexual abuse: A longitudinal study. Pediatrics 1992;89:307.

McCann J, Voris J, Simon M, Wells R: Comparison of genital examination techniques in prepubertal girls. Pediatrics 1990;85:182.

McCann J, Voris J, Simon M, Wells R: Perianal findings in prepubertal children selected for nonabuse: A descriptive study. Child Abuse Negl 1989;13:179.

McCann J, Wells R, Simon M, Voris J: Genital findings in prepubertal girls selected for nonabuse: A descriptive study. Pediatrics 1990;86:428.

McCauley J, Gorman RL, Guzinski G: Toluidine blue in the detection of perineal lacerations in pediatric and adolescent sexual abuse victims. Pediatrics 1986;78:1039.

McDonough PG, Tho PT: The spectrum of 45,X/46,XY gonadal dysgenesis and its implications (a study of 19 patients). Pediatr Adolesc Gynecol 1983;1:1.

Meneses MF, Ostrowski ML: Female splenic-gonadal fusion of the discontinuous type. Hum Pathol 1989;20;486.

Muram D, Dewhurst J: The inheritance of intersexuality. Can Med Assoc J 1984;130:121.

Muram D, Dewhurst J, Grant DB: Premature menarche: A follow-up study. Arch Dis Child 1983;58:142.

Muram D, Dorko B, Brown JG, Tolley EE: Sexual abuse in Shelby County, Tennessee: A new epidemic? Child Abuse Negl 1991;15:523.

Muram D, Elias S: Child sexual abuse—Genital findings in prepubertal girls. II. Comparison of colposcopic and unaided examination. Am J Obstet Gynecol 1989;160:333.

Muram D, Elias S: The treatment of labial adhesions in prepubertal girls. Surg Forum 1988;34:464.

Muram D, Gale CL, Thompson E, Marina N: Ovarian cancer in children and adolescents. Adolesc Pediatr Gynecol 1992;5:21.

Muram D, Gold JJ: Physicians' dress style and the examination of young children. Adolesc Pediatr Gynecol 1990;3:158.

Muram D, Grant DB, Dewhurst J: Precocious puberty: A follow-up study. Arch Dis Child 1984;59:77.

Muram D, Jones CE: The use of video-colposcopy in the gynecologic examination of children and adolescents. Adolesc Pediatr Gynecol 1993;6:154.

Muram D, McAlister MS, Winer-Muram HT, Smith WC: Asymptomatic rupture of a rudimentary uterine horn. Obstet Gynecol 1987;69:486.

Muram D, Rau F: Anatomic variations of the bulbocavernosus muscle. Adolesc Pediatr Gynecol 1991;4:85.

Muram D, Rosenthal TL, Tolley EA et al: Teenage pregnancy: Dating and sexual attitudes. J Sex Education Ther 1993;18:264.

Muram D, Speck PM, Gold SS: genital abnormalities in female siblings and friends of child victims of sexual abuse. Child Abuse Negl 1991;15:105.

Muram D, Spence JEH: Rupture of a rudimentary uterine horn in an adolescent girl, followed by a successful pregnancy. Pediatr Adolesc Gynecol 1993;1:53.

Muram D: Anal and perianal abnormalities seen in prepubertal victims of abuse. Am J Obstet Gynecol 1989;161:278.

Muram D: Child sexual abuse—Genital findings in prepubertal girls. I. The unaided medical examination. Am J Obstet Gynecol 1989;160:328.

Muram D: Child sexual abuse: Correlation between genital findings and sexual acts. Child Abuse Negl 1989;13:211.

Muram D: Congenital malformations. In: *Textbook of Gynecology. Copeland LJ (editor). WB Saunders, 1993.*

Muram D: Genital tract trauma in pre-pubertal children. Pediatr Ann 1986;15:616.

Muram D: Vaginal bleeding in children and adolescents. Obstet Gynecol Clin North Am 1990;17:389.

Persaud D, Chandwani S, Rigaud M et al: Delayed recognition of human immunodeficiency virus infection in preadolescent children. Pediatrics 1992;90:688.

Pinsky L, Kaufman M: Genetics of steroid receptors and their disorders. Adv Hum Genet 1987;16:299.

Pinsky L, Kaufman M, Levitsky LL: Partial androgen resistance due to a distinctive qualitative defect of the androgen receptor. Am J Med Genet 1987;27:459.

Pokorny S: Anatomic detail of the prepubertal hymen. Am J Obstet Gynecol 1987;157:950.

Reindollar RH, McDonough PG: Delayed sexual development: Common causes and basic clinical approach. Pediatr Ann 1981;10:30.

Reindollar RH, Tho SPT, McFonough PG: Abnormalities of sexual differentiation. Clin Obstet Gynecol 1987;30:697.

Rock JA, Azziz R: Genital anomalies in childhood. Clin Obstet Gynecol 1987;30:682.

Rogol AD, Rosen SW: LH and FSH responses to LHRH in patients with congenital anosmia and hypogonadotropic hypogonadism. In: *The LH Releasing Hormone.* Beling CG, Wentz AC (editors). Masson, 1980.

Rosenthal TL, Muram D, Tolley EA et al: Teenage pregnancy: Predicting the adolescent at risk. J Sex Education Ther 1993;18:277.

Sanfilippo J, Muram D, Lee P, Dewhurst JC (eds): *Pediatric and Adolescent Gynecology. Pediatric and Adolescent Gynecology.* WB Saunders Co, 1994.

Shulman L, Wachtel S, Wachtel G et al: Marker chromosomes in gonadal dysgenesis: Avoiding unnecessary surgery. Adolesc Pediatr Gynecol 1992;5:39.

Siegel SF, Finegold DN, Murray PJ, Lee PA: Assessment of Clinical hyperandrogenism in adolescent girls. Adolesc Pediatr Gynecol 1992;5:13.

Siegel SF, Finegold DN, Urban MD et al: Premature pubarche: Etiological heterogeneity. J Clin Endocrinol Metab 1992;74:239.

Simpson JL: *Disorders of Sexual Differentiation: Etiology and Clinical Delineation.* Academic Press, 1976.

Simpson JL: Phenotypic-karyotypic correlations of gonadal determinants: Current status and relationship to molecular studies. In: *Proceedings 7th International Congress Human Genetics* (Berlin, 1986), pp. 224–232). Sperling K, Vogel F (eds). Springer-Verlag, 1987.

Slaughter L, Brown C: Colposcopic findings in victims of sexual assault. Am J Obstet Gynecol 1992;166:83.

Ulloa-Aguirre A, Carranza-Lira S, Mendez JP et al: Incomplete regression of müllerian ducts in androgen insensitivity syndrome. Fertil Steril 1990;53:1024.

Verp M S, Simpson J L: Abnormal sexual differentiation and neoplasia. Cancer Genet Cytogenet 1987;25:191.

Winer-Muram HT, Muram D, Emerson D, Boulden T: The sonographic features of the peripubertal ovaries. Adolesc Pediatr Gynecol 1989;2:158.

Wu PC, Huang RL, Lang JH et al: Treatment of malignant ovarian germ cell tumors with preservation of fertility: A report of 28 cases. Gynecol Oncol 1991;40:2.

Wynne JM: Injuries to the genitalia in female children. South African Med J 1980;57:47.

Zacharias L, Rand WM, Wurtman RJ: A prospective study of sexual development and growth in American girls: The statistics of menarche. Obstet Gynecol Surv 1976;31:325.

# Complications of Menstruation; Abnormal Uterine Bleeding

*Melvin V. Gerbie, MD*

---

## COMPLICATIONS OF MENSTRUATION

### PREMENSTRUAL SYNDROME

#### Essentials of Diagnosis

- Symptoms include edema, weight gain, restlessness, irritability, and increased tension.
- Symptoms must occur in the second half of the menstrual cycle.
- There must be a symptom-free period of at least 7 days in the first half of the cycle.
- Symptoms must occur in each of 3 consecutive cycles.
- Symptoms must be severe enough to require medical advice or treatment.

#### General Considerations

Premenstrual syndrome (PMS) is a psychoneuroendocrine disorder with biologic, psychologic, and social parameters. It is both difficult to define adequately and quite controversial. Some authorities consider it one of the world's most common diseases; yet others consider it a nonissue. Indeed, one major difficulty in detailing whether PMS is a disease or a description of physiologic changes is its extraordinary prevalence. Up to 90% of women suffer some recurrent PMS symptoms; 20–40% are mentally or physically incapacitated to some degree, and 5% experience severe distress. The highest incidence is in the women in their late 20s to early 30s. PMS is rarely encountered in adolescents.

According to Dalton (1984), PMS sufferers exhibit (at the minimum) edema, weight gain, feelings of restlessness, irritability, and increased tension. The classic criteria for PMS require that the patient have symptoms in the second half of the menstrual cycle and a symptom-free period of at least 7 days in the first half of the cycle. The symptoms must occur in each of 3 consecutive cycles and must be severe enough to require medical advice or treatment.

Unfortunately, authorities disagree concerning both symptoms and criteria. Other symptoms commonly included in PMS are abdominal discomfort, breast tenderness, headaches, bloating, clumsiness, accident proneness, sleep changes, and mood swings. Behavioral changes include social withdrawal, altered daily activities, increased crying, and changes in sexual desire. In all, more than 150 symptoms have been related to PMS. Thus, the symptom complex of PMS has not been totally defined.

The potential relationship between PMS and antisocial behavior has resulted in successful courtroom defenses of female offenders in England. US courts have not been as accepting of PMS as a defense, but legal argument was incorporated into statute with the Insanity Defense Reform Act of 1985 [18 U.S.C.A. 20 (Supp. 1985)], which provides that PMS may be argued as a mitigating factor in criminal behavior if it is connected with a psychosis. Arguments for and against such defenses have been the subject of a number of publications. Although such controversy is interesting, discussion of it exceeds the limitations of this medical text.

#### Pathogenesis

The etiology of the symptom complex of PMS is not known, although several theories have been proposed, including estrogen-progesterone imbalance, excess aldosterone, hypoglycemia, hyperprolactinemia, and psychogenic factors. Excess or abnormal prostaglandin activity may also be a cause; this is presumed because nonsteroidal antiinflammatory agents often relieve symptoms. A popular theory is that the premenstrual fall in endogenous endorphins precipitates the symptoms of PMS. Eliminating cyclic fluctuations without adding steroid hormones might therefore provide rational treatment. Gonadotropin-releasing hormone (GnRh) analog treatment has been successful in some short-term trials for patients with debilitating symptoms. However, long-term studies of the effectiveness and safety of this treatment are needed.

#### Clinical Findings

A careful history and physical examination are

most important to exclude organic causes of PMS localized to the reproductive, urinary, or gastrointestinal tracts. Most patients readily describe their symptoms, but careful questioning may be needed with some patients who may be reluctant to do so. Although it is important not to lead a patient to exaggerate her concerns, it is equally important not to minimize them.

Symptoms of PMS may be specific, well-localized, and recurrent. They may be exacerbated by emotional stress. Migraine-like headaches may also occur, often preceded by visual scotomas and vomiting. Symptomatology varies from patient to patient but is often consistent in the same patient.

A psychiatric history should be obtained, with special attention paid to a personal history of psychiatric problems or a family history of affective disorders. A mental status evaluation of affect, thinking, and behavior should be performed and recorded. A prospective diary correlating symptoms, daily activities, and menstrual flow can be very useful to document changes and to encourage patients' participation in their care.

General measures advocated by some authorities (but of undocumented efficacy) include the daily diary of symptoms and regular exercise, restriction of salt, sugar, caffeine, and alcohol intake, and cessation of smoking. Relaxation techniques (including biofeedback), behavioral techniques, and group support may be of assistance. Vitamin $B_6$ (50–100 mg/d) has reportedly been helpful but remains unproved.

If underlying psychiatric illness is suspected, a psychiatric evaluation is indicated. The most common associated psychiatric illness is depression, which generally responds to antidepressant drugs and psychotherapy. It should also be recalled that psychiatric illnesses have premenstrual exacerbations and medications should be altered accordingly.

### Treatment

With both definition and etiology unclear, therapy is extremely controversial. Therapeutic recommendations have included vitamins and minerals; natural substances for sedation, diuresis, and laxations; and progesterone. Definitive therapy or programs have not emerged. Progesterone (400 mg/d as a vaginal suppository) in the second half of the menstrual cycle has been recommended, but this has not been confirmed as being effective in double-blind studies. Oral micronized progesterone has been used in a double-blind crossover study (Dennerstein et al, 1985), with significant improvement in those patients receiving the medication. Other progesterone derivatives such as megestrol acetate or medroxyprogesterone acetate have also been used with mixed success; these substances are much less expensive and easier to use. Spironolactone is the most frequently chosen diuretic for symptoms related to cyclic edema, but chlorothiazides may be as effective.

The dose of diuretic should be kept to a minimum. Bromocriptine may be useful for the patient with hyperprolactinemia, mastodynia, and breast engorgement. As noted, antiprostaglandins may be helpful. Use of oral contraceptives may produce symptoms similar to those of PMS, but paradoxically, in many patients, symptoms of premenstrual discomfort are relieved by their use. Placebo effects may occur with any of the therapeutic regimens, including danocrine or GnRh analogs. The addition of estrogen and progestin to a GnRh regimen may obviate the long-term problems of osteoporosis and lipid metabolism caused by the use of GnRh alone.

The physician should be prepared to spend as much time as necessary with patients with this disturbing syndrome. There is no "quick-fix" that works for all patients, and support is as essential to management as are most medications. If a physician cannot take enough time, the patient with PMS may be better served by referral to a special clinic.

## MASTODYNIA

Pain and, usually, swelling of the breasts caused by edema and engorgement of the vascular and ductal systems is termed mastodynia, or **mastalgia.** It is common in women with PMS and may be the only symptom of this syndrome in some. Although most women have varying degrees of breast tenderness in the second half of the menstrual cycle, the term mastodynia is reserved for severe symptoms associated with no palpable abnormality on breast examination except obvious tenderness and perhaps generalized thickening of tissue. Examination is always necessary to rule out neoplasm, although most malignant tumors are painless. In postpartum patients, mastitis must be considered.

The presence of solitary or multiple cystic areas suggests **mammary dysplasia (fibrocystic disease, fibrodysplasia).** The diagnosis can usually be confirmed by aspiration, but excisional biopsy is occasionally necessary. Serial mammograms or ultrasound examinations can be used to help monitor these patients. (See also Chapter 62.)

### Treatment

Management of painful breasts due to fibrocystic changes consists of support of the breasts, avoidance of methylxanthenes (coffee, tea, chocolate, cola drinks), and occasional use of a mild diuretic. In the absence of cystic changes and other contraindications, mastodynia can be treated with low-dose testosterone (5 mg on alternate days when symptoms occur). If any signs of virilization occur, the drug must be discontinued. Danazol (Danocrine), 100–400 mg/d for up to 6 months, may produce long-term resolution of symptoms. Use of vitamin E, 1200–1800 U/d, has had mixed results.

## DYSMENORRHEA

Dysmenorrhea, or **painful menstruation,** is the most common complaint of gynecologic patients. Many women experience mild discomfort during menstruation, but the term "dysmenorrhea" is reserved for those women whose pain prevents normal activity and requires medication, whether over-the-counter or by prescription.

There are 3 types of dysmenorrhea: (1) primary (no organic cause), (2) secondary (pathologic cause), and (3) membranous (cast of endometrial cavity shed as a single entity). This discussion will focus mainly on primary dysmenorrhea. Secondary dysmenorrhea is discussed elsewhere in this book in association with specific diseases and disorders (eg, endometriosis, adenomyosis, pelvic inflammatory disease [particularly in patients with residuals of pelvic infection], cervical stenosis, fibroid polyps, and, possibly, uterine displacement with fixation).

Membranous dysmenorrhea is rare; it causes intense cramping pain due to passage of a cast of the endometrium through an undilated cervix. Another cause of dysmenorrhea that should be considered is cramping due to the presence of an intrauterine device (IUD).

### Pathogenesis

It has long been known that pain during menstruation is associated with ovulatory cycles. The mechanism of pain has only recently been attributed to prostaglandin activity. Prostaglandins are present in much higher concentrations in women with dysmenorrhea than in those with mild or no pain.

Psychologic factors may be involved, including attitudes passed from mother to daughter. Girls should receive accurate information about menstruation before menarche; this can be provided by parents, teachers, physicians, or counselors. Emotional anxiety due to academic or social demands may also be a cofactor.

### Clinical Findings

Reactions to pain are subjective, and questioning by the physician should not lead the patient to exaggerate or minimize her discomfort. History taking is most important and should include the following questions: When does the pain occur? What does the patient do about the pain? Are there other symptoms? Do oral contraceptives relieve or intensify the pain? Is the pain becoming more severe over time?

Because dysmenorrhea is almost always associated with ovulatory cycles, it does not usually occur at menarche but rather later in adolescence. Typically, pain occurs on the first day of the menses, usually about the time the flow begins, but it may not be present until the second day. Nausea and vomiting, diarrhea, and headache may occur. The specific symptoms associated with endometriosis are not present.

The physical examination does not reveal any significant pelvic disease. When the patient is symptomatic, she has generalized pelvic tenderness, perhaps more so in the area of the uterus than of the adnexa. Occasionally, ultrasonography or laparoscopy is necessary to rule out pelvic abnormalities such as endometriosis, pelvic inflammatory disease, or an accident in an ovarian cyst.

### Differential Diagnosis

The most common misdiagnosis of primary dysmenorrhea is secondary dysmenorrhea due to endometriosis. With endometriosis, the pain usually begins 1–2 weeks before the menses, reaches a peak 1–2 days before, and is relieved at the onset of flow or shortly thereafter. Severe pain during sexual intercourse or findings of adnexal tenderness or mass or cul-de-sac modularity, particularly in the premenstrual interval, help to confirm the diagnosis. (See also Chapter 40.) A similar pain pattern occurs with adenomyosis, although in an older age group and in the absence of extrauterine clinical findings.

### Treatment

Aspirin or acetaminophen may relieve mild discomfort. For severe pain, codeine or other stronger analgesics may be needed and bed rest may be desirable. Occasionally, emergency treatment with parenteral medication may be necessary. Analgesics may cause drowsiness at the dosages required.

**A. Antiprostaglandins:** Antiprostaglandins are now used for the treatment of dysmenorrhea. The newer, stronger, faster-acting drugs appear to be more useful than aspirin. Aspirin intolerance and gastrointestinal problems are the main contraindications to their use. Ibuprofen has been extremely effective. Over-the-counter formulations of ibuprofen are available; dosages must be adjusted to compare with prescription products. The drug must be used at the earliest onset of symptoms, usually at the onset of bleeding or cramping.

Antiprostaglandins work by blocking prostaglandin synthesis and metabolism; once the pain has been established, antiprostaglandins are not nearly as effective as with early use.

**B. Oral Contraceptives:** Cyclic administration of oral contraceptives, usually in the lowest dosage but occasionally with increased estrogen, prevent pain in most patients who do not obtain relief from antiprostaglandins or cannot tolerate them. The mechanism of pain relief may be related to absence of ovulation or to altered endometrium resulting in decreased prostaglandin production. In women who do not require contraception, oral contraceptives are given for 6–12 months. Many women continue to be free of pain after treatment has been discontinued.

**C. Surgical Treatment:** In a few women, no medication will control dysmenorrhea. Cervical dilatation is of little use. Uterosacral ligament division and presacral neurectomy are infrequently performed, although some physicians consider these to be important adjuncts to conservative operation for endometriosis. Newer laparoscopic techniques have reopened the question of the value of this procedure either in patients with no pathology or those with endometriosis.

Adenomyosis, endometriosis or residual pelvic infection unresponsive to medical therapy or conservative surgical therapy may eventually require hysterectomy with or without ovarian removal in extreme cases. Very rarely a patient with no organic source of pain may eventually require hysterectomy to relieve symptoms.

## ABNORMAL UTERINE BLEEDING

Abnormal uterine bleeding includes abnormal menstrual bleeding and bleeding due to other causes such as pregnancy, systemic disease, or cancer. The diagnosis and management of abnormal uterine bleeding present some of the most difficult problems in gynecology. Patients may not be able to localize the source of the bleeding from the vagina, urethra, or rectum. In childbearing women, a complication of pregnancy must always be considered, and one must always remember that more than 1 diagnosis may be present, eg, uterine myomas and cervical cancer.

### Patterns of Abnormal Uterine Bleeding

The standard classification for patterns of abnormal bleeding recognizes 7 different patterns.

(1) **Menorrhagia (hypermenorrhea)** is heavy or prolonged menstrual flow. The presence of clots may not be abnormal but may signify excessive bleeding. "Gushing" or "open-faucet" bleeding is always abnormal. Submucous myomas, complications of pregnancy, adenomyosis, endometrial hyperplasias, malignant tumors, and dysfunctional bleeding are causes of menorrhagia.

(2) **Hypomenorrhea (cryptomenorrhea)** is unusually light menstrual flow, sometimes only "spotting." An obstruction such as hymenal or cervical stenosis may be the cause. Uterine synechiae (Asherman's syndrome) can be causative and are diagnosed by hysterogram or hysteroscopy. Patients receiving oral contraceptives occasionally complain of light flow and can be reassured that this is not significant.

(3) **Metrorrhagia (intermenstrual bleeding)** is bleeding occurring at any time between menstrual periods. Ovulatory bleeding occurs at midcycle as spotting and can be documented with basal body temperatures. Endometrial polyps and endometrial and cervical carcinomas are pathologic causes. In recent years, exogenous estrogen administration has become a common cause of this type of bleeding.

(4) **Polymenorrhea** describes periods that occur too frequently. This is usually associated with anovu-lation and rarely with a shortened luteal phase in the menstrual cycle.

(5) **Menometrorrhagia** is bleeding that occurs at irregular intervals. The amount and duration of bleeding also vary. Any condition that causes intermenstrual bleeding can eventually lead to menometrorrhagia. Sudden onset of irregular bleeding episodes is an indication of malignant tumors or complications of pregnancy.

(6) **Oligomenorrhea** describes menstrual periods that occur more than 35 days apart. Amenorrhea is diagnosed if there is no menstrual period in more than 6 months. Bleeding is usually decreased in amount and associated with anovulation, either from endocrine causes (eg, pregnancy, pituitary-hypothalamic causes, menopause) or systemic causes (eg, excessive weight loss). Estrogen-secreting tumors produce oligomenorrhea prior to other patterns of abnormal bleeding.

(7) **Contact bleeding (postcoital bleeding)** is self-explanatory but must be considered a sign of cervical cancer until proved otherwise. Other causes of contact bleeding are much more common, including cervical eversion, cervical polyps, and cervical or vaginal infection (eg, due to *Trichomonas*). A negative cytologic smear does not rule out invasive cervical cancer, and colposcopy or biopsy or both may be necessary.

## EVALUATION OF ABNORMAL UTERINE BLEEDING

The time-honored method for the evaluation of abnormal bleeding is dilatation and curettage (D&C) performed under general anesthesia. Although D&C is still essential in some cases, hysteroscopy provides a more precise diagnosis by allowing visualization and directed biopsy. With either modality, most patients can be properly evaluated either in the office or, occasionally, in the outpatient department with local anesthesia.

**A. History:** Many causes of bleeding are strongly suggested by the history alone. Note the amount of menstrual flow, the length of the menstrual cycle and menstrual period, the length and amount of episodes of intermenstrual bleeding, and any episodes of contact bleeding. Note also the last menstrual period, the last normal menstrual period, age at menarche and menopause, and any changes in general health. The patient must keep a record of bleeding patterns to determine whether bleeding is abnormal or only a variation of normal. However, most women have an occasional menstrual cycle that is not in their usual pattern. Depending on the patient's age and the pattern of the bleeding, observation may be all that is necessary.

**B. Physical Examination:** Abdominal masses and an enlarged, irregular uterus suggest myoma. A symmetrically enlarged uterus is more typical of adenomyosis or endometrial carcinoma. Atrophic and inflammatory vulvar and vaginal lesions can be visualized, and cervical polyps and invasive lesions of cervical carcinoma can be seen. Rectovaginal examination is especially important to identify lateral and posterior spread or the presence of a barrel-shaped cervix. In pregnancy, a decidual reaction of the cervix may be the source of bleeding. The appearance is a velvety, friable erythematous lesion on the ectocervix.

**C. Cytologic Examination:** Although most useful in diagnosing asymptomatic intraepithelial lesions of the cervix, cytologic smears can help screen for invasive cervical (particularly endocervical) lesions. Although cytology is not reliable for the diagnosis of endometrial abnormalities, the presence of endometrial cells in a postmenopausal woman is abnormal unless she is receiving exogenous estrogens. Likewise, women in the secretory phase of the menstrual cycle should not shed endometrial cells. Of course, a cytologic examination that is positive or suspicious for endometrial cancer demands further evaluation.

Tubal or ovarian cancer also can be suspected on a cervical smear. The technique of obtaining a smear is important, since a tumor may be present only in the endocervical canal and may not shed cells to the ectocervix or vagina. Laboratories should report the presence or absence of endocervical cells. The current use of a spatula and endocervical brush in nonpregnant patients has significantly increased the adequacy of the cytologic smears from the cervix. Soon most laboratories will be using the Bethesda system. Histologic prediction is preferred to the older numerical classification. Any abnormal smear requires further evaluation. (See also Chapter 47.)

Instruments used in collection of endometrial cells include the endometrial brush and Isaacs' endometrial aspiration instrument. Cytologic changes in the endometrium do not correlate well with histologic changes, and these techniques are not widely used.

**D. Endometrial Biopsy:** Traditional methods of endometrial biopsy include use of the Novak suction curet, the Duncan curet, or the Kevorkian curet. Cervical dilatation is not necessary with these instruments. Small areas of the endometrial lining are sampled. These techniques are useful in evaluation of infertility as well as in patients being considered for or receiving exogenous estrogens.

**E. Histologic Examination:** The Vabra aspirator is used to obtain tissue for histologic examination. A narrow (3–4 mm) suction curet with a vacuum pump is used to perform curettage of an adequate endometrial sample, which allows histologic diagnosis of hyperplasias and endometrial carcinoma. The endometrial Pipelle or Z-Sampler has further simplified endometrial sampling. These flexible polypropylene suction cannulas have an outer diameter of 3.1 mm and their use is almost painless in most situations,

with particular ease of use in the postmenopausal woman. The histologic specimens compare favorably with Vabra aspirations (Kaunitz, 1988). These techniques have almost replaced D&C as the method of choice in the diagnosis of abnormal uterine bleeding. For full evaluation of bleeding, endocervical curettage should also be done to localize the source of bleeding. If no cause of bleeding can be found or if the tissue obtained is inadequate for diagnosis, D&C must be performed.

**F. Hysterosalpingography:** X-ray following injection of contrast medium into the cervix has been proposed as an adjuvant means of diagnosis in endometrial carcinoma. A theoretic objection is that the procedure may cause cells to spread through the uterine tubes.

**G. Hysteroscopy:** Direct visualization by endoscopy is receiving more attention as an aid in the diagnosis of abnormal bleeding. With improving technology, this is being done more frequently as an office procedure.

**H. Dilatation and Curettage:** D&C is the "gold standard" for the diagnosis of abnormal uterine bleeding. It can be done under local or general anesthesia, almost always in an outpatient or ambulatory setting. With general anesthesia, relaxation of the abdominal musculature is greater, allowing for a more thorough pelvic examination, more precise evaluation of pelvic masses, and more complete curettage. Curettage of the endocervix should be performed before sounding of the endometrial cavity or dilatation of the cervix is done.

**I. Other Diagnostic Procedures:** Assay of the beta-subunit of human chorionic gonadotropin (hCG) may be used for complications of pregnancy and trophoblastic disease. Pelvic ultrasonography and laparoscopy may help to evaluate uterine and adnexal masses.

## General Principles of Management

In making the diagnosis, it is important not to assume the obvious. A careful history and pelvic examination are vital. The possibility of pregnancy must be considered as well as use of oral contraceptives, IUDs, and hormones. Adequate sampling of the endometrium is essential for a definitive diagnosis.

Improved diagnostic techniques and treatment have resulted in decreased use of hysterectomy to treat abnormal bleeding patterns. If pathologic causes (eg, submucous myomas, adenomyosis) can be excluded, if there is no significant risk of cancer developing (as from atypical endometrial hyperplasia), and if there is no acute life-threatening hemorrhage, most patients can be treated with hormone preparations. Myomectomy can be suggested for myoma if the patient wishes to retain her potential for childbearing.

## ABNORMAL UTERINE BLEEDING DUE TO GYNECOLOGIC DISEASES & DISORDERS

Genital conditions that cause abnormal bleeding can be classified by location as follows:

**(1) Vulva and vagina:** Atrophic vulvitis or vaginitis, traumatic lacerations (eg, hymenal tears, ulcerations due to use of tampons), infection (vulvovaginitis), cancer (eg, sarcoma botryoides in the very young, vaginal carcinoma in older women).

**(2) Cervix:** Eversion (ectropion), cervical polyps, cancer, pedunculated myomas.

**(3) Uterus:** Endometritis, hyperplasias, cancer, endometrial polyps, adenomyosis, submucous myomas, use of oral contraceptives, perforation due to use of IUDs.

**(4) Uterine tubes:** Salpingitis, tumors, tubal pregnancy.

**(5) Ovaries:** Estrogen-producing tumors, other cancers, functional ovarian cysts.

Many cases of bleeding are iatrogenic (eg, due to use of IUDs or oral contraceptives). The IUD should be removed or the oral contraceptives modified or discontinued; any subsequent episodes of bleeding should be reported and then evaluated. Younger patients with rare episodes of irregular bleeding should also record the bleeding episodes for a few months to determine a pattern. Basal body temperature graphs will aid in determining the presence of ovulatory or anovulatory cycles.

The site of bleeding must be determined. Multiple sites may be present (eg, vaginal spotting due to infection with *Trichomonas* and endometrial bleeding due to endometrial carcinoma). Persistent or recurrent bleeding following resolution of infection indicates that another cause exists.

## ABNORMAL UTERINE BLEEDING DURING PREGNANCY

See Chapter 20.

## ABNORMAL BLEEDING DUE TO NONGYNECOLOGIC DISEASES & DISORDERS

In the differential diagnosis of abnormal bleeding, nongynecologic causes of bleeding (eg, rectal or urologic disorders) must be ruled out, because patients may have difficulty differentiating the source of bleeding. Gynecologic and nongynecologic causes of bleeding may coexist. Systemic disease may cause abnormal uterine bleeding. For example, myxedema usually causes amenorrhea, but less severe hypothyroidism is associated with increased uterine bleeding. Liver disease interferes with estrogen metabolism and may cause variable degrees of bleeding. Both of these conditions are usually clinically apparent before gynecologic symptoms appear. Blood dyscrasias and coagulation abnormalities can also produce gynecologic bleeding. Patients receiving anticoagulants or adrenal steroids may expect abnormalities. Extreme weight loss due to eating disorders, exercise, or dieting may be associated with anovulation and amenorrhea.

## DYSFUNCTIONAL UTERINE BLEEDING

Exclusion of pathologic causes of abnormal bleeding establishes the diagnosis of dysfunctional uterine bleeding. Although a persistent corpus luteum cyst or short luteal phase can produce abnormal bleeding associated with ovulation, most patients are anovulatory. The exact cause of anovulation is not truly understood but probably represents dysfunction of the hypothalamic-pituitary-ovarian axis, resulting in continued estrogenic stimulation of the endometrium. The endometrium outgrows its blood supply, partially breaks down, and is sloughed in an irregular manner. Conversion from proliferative to secretory endometrium corrects most acute and chronic bleeding problems. Organic causes of anovulation must be excluded (eg, thyroid or adrenal abnormalities).

Dysfunctional bleeding occurs most commonly at the extremes of reproductive age (20% of cases occur in adolescence and 40% in patients over age 40). Management depends on the age of the patient (adolescent, young woman, or premenopausal woman). The diagnosis is made by history, absence of ovulatory temperature changes, low serum progesterone and results of endometrial sampling in the older woman.

### Treatment

**A. Adolescents:** Because the first menstrual cycles are frequently anovulatory, it is not unusual for menses to be irregular, and explanation of the reason is all that is necessary for treatment. Heavy bleeding—even hemorrhage—may occur. Diagnostic procedures are usually not necessary in young patients, but pelvic examination must be performed to exclude pregnancy or pathologic conditions. Although high-dose parenteral estrogens were used previously, estrogens given orally should be adequate for all patients except those requiring curettage to control hemorrhage. Numerous regimens are available, including estrogens followed by progesterone, progesterone alone, or combination oral contraceptives. The dose of conjugated estrogens is 2.5 mg 4 times a day; bleeding is usually controlled within 2–3 days. Estrogens must be continued for 20–25 days at a lower dose (1.25 mg) and medroxyprogesterone acetate, 10 mg/d, added for the last 5 days. Increased dosages of estrogen may be needed if bleeding persists for more than 2–3 days.

Oral contraceptives, 3–4 times the usual dose, are just as effective and may be simpler to use than sequential hormones. Again, the dose is lowered after a few days and the lower dose is continued for the next few cycles, particularly to raise the hemoglobin levels in an anemic patient. Medroxyprogesterone acetate, 10 mg/d for 10 days, can be used in patients who have proliferative endometrium on biopsy. In patients receiving cyclic therapy, 3–6 courses are usually administered, after which treatment is discontinued and further evaluation is performed if necessary.

**B. Young Women:** In patients age 20–30 years old, pathologic causes are more common and diagnostic procedures are more often necessary, particularly endometrial biopsy or aspiration. Hormonal management is the same as for adolescents.

**C. Premenopausal Women:** In the later reproductive years, even more care must be given to excluding pathologic causes because of the possibility of endometrial cancer. Aspiration, curettage, or both should clearly establish anovulatory or dyssynchronous cycles as the cause before hormonal therapy is started. Recurrences of abnormal bleeding demand further evaluation.

**D. Surgical Measures:** For patients whose bleeding cannot be controlled with hormones, who are symptomatically anemic, and whose lifestyle is compromised by persistence of irregular bleeding, abdominal or vaginal hysterectomy may be necessary. Endometrial ablation techniques using a laser, roller ball, or resectoscope preceded by GnRh analogs are useful in patients who have personal or medical contraindications to hysterectomy. Definitive surgery may also be needed for coexistent endometriosis, myoma, and disorders of pelvic relaxation.

## POSTMENOPAUSAL BLEEDING

Postmenopausal bleeding may be defined as bleeding that occurs after 12 months of amenorrhea in a middle-aged women. When amenorrhea occurs in a younger person for 1 year and premature ovarian failure or menopause has been diagnosed, episodes of bleeding may be classified as postmenopausal, although resumption of ovulatory cycles can occur. Follicle-stimulating hormone (FSH) levels are particularly helpful in the differential diagnoses of menopausal versus hypothalamic amenorrhea. An FSH level greater than 30/mL is highly suggestive of menopause.

Postmenopausal bleeding is more likely to be caused by pathologic disease than is bleeding in younger women, and it must always be investigated. Nongynecologic causes must be excluded; these are also more likely to be caused by pathologic disease in older women, and the patient may be unable to determine the site of bleeding. The source of bleeding should not be assumed as nongynecologic unless there is good evidence or proper evaluation has excluded gynecologic causes.

Neither normal ("functional") bleeding nor dysfunctional bleeding should occur after menopause. Although pathologic disorders are more likely, other causes may also occur. Atrophic or anovulatory endometrium is not unusual. Secretory patterns should not occur unless the patient has resumed ovulation or has received progesterone therapy.

After nongynecologic causes of bleeding are excluded, gynecologic causes must be considered.

**A. Exogenous Hormones:** The most common cause of postmenopausal uterine bleeding is the use of exogenous hormones. In the past, face creams and cosmetics contained homeopathic amounts of estrogens, but this is highly unlikely today. Careful history taking becomes vital, since patients may not follow specific instructions on the use of estrogen and progesterone therapy.

Recent recommendations for long-term estrogen/progesterone administration for prevention of osteoporosis has improved lipid levels, and improved quality of life have caused resumption of regular menstrual bleeding in many patients. Use of hormones for the treatment of endometrial hyperplasia is discussed in Chapter 35. However, when abnormal bleeding occurs (while taking hormones, with intercourse) or when bleeding is particularly heavy, it must be evaluated. In the past, hormones were discontinued for a period of time to see whether bleeding would stop, but current thought holds that the patient should be examined and the cause of bleeding identified, if possible. If endometrial hyperplasia is found, specific attention must be paid to the presence of atypia and treatment by increasing the progesterone component or by hysterectomy should be considered.

**B. Vaginal Atrophy and Vaginal and Vulvar Lesions:** Bleeding from the lower reproductive tract is almost always related to vaginal atrophy, with or without trauma. Examination reveals thin tissue with ecchymosis. Rarely, there will be a tear at the introitus or deep in the vagina requiring suturing. With vulvar dystrophies, there may be a white area and cracking of the skin of the vulva. Cytologic study of material obtained from the cervix and vagina will reveal immature epithelial cells with or without inflammation. After excluding coexisting upper tract lesions, treatment can include local or systemic estrogen therapy for vaginal lesions. Vulvar lesions need further diagnostic evaluation to determine the proper treatment.

**C. Tumors of the Reproductive Tract:** The differential diagnosis of organic causes of postmenopausal uterine bleeding includes endometrial hyperplasias (simple, complex, and atypical), endometrial polyps, endometrial carcinoma or other more rare tumors such as cervical or endocervical carcinoma, uterine sarcomas (including mixed mesodermal and myosarcomas), and, even more rarely, uterine tube and ovarian cancer. Estrogen-secreting ovarian tumors should also be considered.

Uterine sampling must be done and tissue must be obtained. Endocervical curettage should be done along with any endometrial sampling technique. If a diagnosis cannot be established or is questionable with office procedures, D&C must be done. Hysteroscopy done in the office or operating room may prove helpful in locating endometrial polyps or fibroid pol-yps that could be missed even by fractional curettage. Pelvic ultrasonography may be extremely helpful in the diagnosis of ovarian tumors and in evaluation of the thickness of the endometrium, as well as in the discerning between uterine myomas and adnexal tumors. Recurring episodes of postmenopausal bleeding may rarely require hysterectomy, even when a diagnosis cannot be established by endometrial sampling.

## REFERENCES

Budoff PW: Use of prostaglandin inhibitors in the treatment of PMS. Clin Obstet Gynecol 1987;30:453.

Carter J et al: Transvaginal ultrasound in gynecologic oncology. Obstet Gynecol Surv 1991;46:687.

Dalton K: *The Premenstrual Syndrome and Progesterone Therapy*, 2nd ed. Year Book, 1984.

Dawood MY: Dysmenorrhea. J Reprod Med 1985;30:154.

Dennerstein L et al: Progesterone and the premenstrual syndrome: A double blind crossover trial. Br Med J 1985; 290:1617.

Freeman EW et al: Evaluating premenstrual symptoms in medical practice. Obstet Gynecol 1985;65:500.

Ghadirian AM, Kamaraju LS: Premenstrual mood changes in affective disorders. Can Med Assoc J 1987;136:1027.

Kaunitz AM et al: Comparison of endometrial biopsy with the endometrial Pipelle and Vabra aspirator. J Reprod Med 1988;33:427.

Loffer K et al: Hysteroscopy, combined with selective endometrial sampling, compared with D and C for abnormal uterine bleeding: The value of a negative hysteroscopic view. Obstet Gynecol 1989;73:16.

Mortola JF et al: Successful treatment of severe premenstrual syndrome by combined use of gonadotropin-releasing hormone agonist and estrogen/progestin. J Clin Endocrinol Metab 1991;71;252.

Muse K et al: Clinical experience with the use of GnRH agonists in the treatment of premenstrual syndrome. Obstet Gynecol Surv 1989;44;317.

Pitkin RM, Scott JR (editors): *Clinical Obstetrics and Gynecology*. vol. 30, No. 2. Lippincott, 1987.

Tjaden B et al: The efficacy of presacral neurectomy for the relief of midline dysmenorrhea. Obstet Oncol 1990; 76:1989.

# 33

# Contraception & Family Planning

*Ronald T. Burkman, MD\**

## I. CONTRACEPTION

One of the most sensitive and intimate decisions made by an individual or by a couple is that of fertility control. This decision is often based on deeply held religious or philosophical convictions. Thus, the clinician must approach the patient's fertility needs with particular sensitivity, empathy, maturity, and nonjudgmental behavior.

However, it must be recognized that there is a considerable need for contraception. For example, in 1987, of the 6.3 million pregnancies that occurred in the USA, an estimated 57% were unintended. Furthermore, it is important to recognize that some socioeconomic changes are occurring in the USA that affect contraceptive practice. Adolescents are experiencing higher rates of pregnancy; in 1989, the birth rate for women 15–17 years old was 8% higher than that in 1988. Women in the later stages of the reproductive lifespan are now tending to delay childbearing until they are in their 30s and 40s. In 1990, the US census documented for the first time that there were more women aged 30–44 years than those aged 15–29 years—a demographic shift that will continue into the next century. Thus, health care professionals who provide contraception need to meet the needs of women with divergent social or economic circumstances.

### Individual Indications for Birth Control

Contraception is practiced by most couples for personal reasons. Many couples wish not to have children at a particular time (spacers) or to have no children or no more children (limiters). Others desire to avoid childbearing because of the effects of preexisting illness on the pregnancy, eg, severe diabetes, or because pregnancy may be life-threatening to the mother as in the case of severe aortic stenosis. For all of these types of decisions, clinicians must provide accurate information about the benefits and risks of both pregnancy and contraception. However, medical conditions that may substantially increase the risk of using some form of birth control usually increase the risks associated with pregnancy to an even greater extent. Finally, as a matter of policy, some countries, especially those that are less developed, promote contraception in an effort to curb undesired population growth.

### Legal Aspects of Contraception

Contraceptives are prescribed, demonstrated, and sold in most states of the USA without restriction.

Despite high rates of unprotected intercourse and unintended pregnancy, the pros and cons of providing contraceptive information and materials to teenagers have been vigorously debated. A regulation proposed in 1982 for federally funded family planning programs in the USA would have required personnel at family planning facilities to notify the parent or guardian of any person under the age of 18 years at least 10 working days before the clinic would be able to provide a prescription contraceptive to the teenager. This proposal was declared unconstitutional by the courts. Furthermore, in 1977, the United States Supreme Court provided a ruling that minors have a constitutional right of access to contraceptives. Most states either have legislation that permits access to contraception for persons under 18 or have not addressed the issue legislatively. Most physicians agree that teenagers should be given contraceptive advice and prescriptions within the confines of appropriate legal restraints. However, they must be careful to avoid imposing their own religious or moral views on their patients.

Health care providers must provide all persons requesting contraception with detailed information about the use of the method or methods, benefits, risks, and side effects so that an informed choice can be made relative to a particular method. Not only is the provision of this information of ethical and legal importance, but also such counseling is likely to ensure that the method will be used appropriately with overall improved compliance. Documentation of the discussion with the patient and her understanding of what has been said is of legal importance.

In particular, when using methods that require in-

*The author would like to acknowledge the contributions of Dr. Tatum to this chapter over the years.

strumentation or some type of surgical approach and that also may require intervention by a health care professional for discontinuation (eg, IUD, injectable or implantable progestin, or sterilization), use of signed consent forms that outline the information discussed and the patient's understanding is important. Such a form serves as evidence, if needed, that counseling about use of a particular birth control method was given; that the patient appeared competent to understand what was said to her; and that she consented to receive contraceptive management in the manner specified.

# METHODS OF CONTRACEPTION

The available methods of contraception may be classified in many ways. For the sake of this discussion, traditional or folk methods are coitus interruptus, postcoital douche, lactational amenorrhea, and periodic abstinence (rhythm, natural family planning). Barrier methods include condoms (male and female), diaphragm, cervical cap, vaginal sponge, and spermicides. Hormonal methods encompass oral contraceptives and injectable or implantable long-acting progestins. In addition, the intrauterine contraceptive device (IUD) and sterilization (tubal ligation, vasectomy) are also part of the contraceptive armamentarium. However, sterilization is discussed elsewhere in this book.

## COITUS INTERRUPTUS

One of the oldest contraceptive methods is withdrawal of the penis before ejaculation. This results in deposition of the semen outside the female genital tract. It has the disadvantage of demanding sufficient self-control by the man so that withdrawal can precede ejaculation. Although the failure rate is probably higher than that of most methods, reliable statistics are not available. Failure may result from escape of semen before orgasm or the deposition of semen on the external female genitalia near the vagina.

## POSTCOITAL DOUCHE

Plain water, vinegar, and a number of "feminine hygiene" products are widely used as postcoital douches. Theoretically, the douche serves to flush the semen out of the vagina, and the additives to the water may possess some spermicidal properties. Nevertheless, sperm have been found within the cervical mucus within 90 seconds after ejaculation. Hence, the method is ineffective and unreliable.

## LACTATIONAL AMENORRHEA

Women are less fertile when nursing than after weaning, and deliberate continuation of nursing after it is no longer necessary for infant nutrition has long been a widespread contraceptive method. The delay in recurrence of ovulation after delivery is due in part to hypophyseal or hypothalamic stimuli from nursing during amenorrhea. Nonetheless, the duration of suppression of ovulation is variable. Recent studies have indicated that lactational amenorrhea can be reasonably effective as a method of contraception if certain principles are followed. First, when using lactation as a method of birth control, the mother must provide breastfeeding as the only form of infant nutrition. Supplemental feedings may alter both the pattern of lactation and the intensity of infant suckling, which secondarily may affect suppression of ovulation. Second, amenorrhea must be maintained. Finally, the method should be practiced as the only form of birth control for a maximum of 6 months after birth. When these principles are followed, most studies have shown a failure rate of only 2%.

## MALE CONDOM

The latex rubber or animal intestine condom, or contraceptive sheath, serves as a cover for the penis during coitus and prevents the deposition of semen in the vagina. The advantages of the condom are that it provides highly effective inexpensive contraception, protection against sexually transmitted diseases (STDs) and is convenient to use. Some condoms now contain a spermicide, which may offer further protection against failure particularly if the condom breaks. Furthermore, spermicides also offer protection against STDs, and further benefit is gained with the addition of such agents. Given the concern about both STDs and the HIV epidemic, condom use should be a significant consideration for persons who are at risk for contracting such infections.

The condom probably is the most widely used mechanical contraceptive in the world today. Most condoms are made of latex that is 0.3–0.8 mm thick; a membrane that is impervious to both sperm and most bacterial and viral organisms that cause STDs or HIV infection. However, the less commonly used lamb's intestine condom is not impermeable to such organisms. The failure of all condoms are due to imperfections of manufacture (about 3 per 1000); errors of technique such as applying the condom after some semen has escaped into the vagina; and escape of semen from the condom as a result of failure to withdraw before detumescence. Adding a small quantity of spermicide nonoxynol 9 within the condom may reduce the failure rate if the condom breaks during coitus. In overall use, failure rates with condoms range from 2–15% in the first year of use.

When greater contraceptive effectiveness is desired, a second method such as contraceptive vaginal jelly or foam should be used in conjunction with the condom. This significantly reduces the chances for condom failure due to mechanical or technical deficiencies. No association has been established between the use of vaginal contraceptives (spermicides) and the occurrence of congenital malformations, if a pregnancy occurs.

## FEMALE CONDOM

Female condoms (Reality Vaginal Pouch) are now being introduced in the USA. The design is that of a pouch made of thin polyurethane material with 2 flexible rings at each end. One ring fits into the depth of the vagina, and the other ring sits outside the vagina near the introitus. Although initial studies suggest that the failure rate is somewhat higher than that of male condoms (an estimated 26% for the first year), these studies were of relatively short duration so that estimated failure rates may not reflect what may be achieved with longer-term use. Female condoms have the advantage of being in the control of the female partner and of offering some protection against STDs. Significant disadvantages may be their cost and overall bulkiness. However, in initial clinical trials, the overall acceptability rate for women users was 65–70%, whereas 75–80% of their partners liked the device.

## VAGINAL DIAPHRAGM

The diaphragm is a mechanical barrier between the vagina and the cervical canal. Diaphragms are circular rings ranging from 50–105 mm in diameter, which are designed to fit in the vaginal cul-de-sac and cover the cervix. Although the designs vary, the arcing spring version is probably the easiest to use for most women. A contraceptive jelly or cream should be placed on the cervical side of the diaphragm before insertion, since the device is ineffective without it. This medicament serves also as a lubricant for the insertion. Additional jelly should be introduced into the vagina on and around the diaphragm after it is securely in place. When the diaphragm is of proper size (as determined by pelvic examination and trial with fitting rings) and is used according to directions, its failure rate is 2–20 pregnancies per 100 women per year of exposure. The diaphragm has the disadvantages of requiring fitting by a physician or a trained paramedical person and the necessity for anticipating the need for protection. Failures may result from im-

proper fitting or placement and dislodgement of the diaphragm during intercourse. As with condoms, diaphragms also offer some protection against STDs, an effect that may be due primarily to the concomitant use of a spermicide. The only side effects are vaginal wall irritation, usually with initial use or if the device is too tightly fit, and an increased risk of urinary tract infections.

## CERVICAL CAP

Cervical caps are small cup-like diaphragms placed over the cervix. They are supposed to be held in place by "suction." To provide a successful barrier against sperm, they must fit tightly over the cervix. Because of variability in cervical size, individualization is almost essential. This greatly limits the practical usefulness of the method. Tailoring the cap to fit each cervix is difficult. In addition, many women are unable to feel their own cervix and thus have great difficulty in placing the cap correctly over the cervix. Because of these problems, the cervical cap has few advantages over the traditional vaginal diaphragm. Although some advocates of the cervical cap recommend that it remain in place for 1 or 2 days at a time, a foul discharge often develops after about 1 day's use. With proper use, the efficacy of the cervical cap is similar to that of the diaphragm, with dislodgement being the most frequently cited cause of failure in most reports. In any event, due to the difficulty associated with proper fitting and routine insertion, it is doubtful that the cap in its present state of development will play an important role in contraception.

## CONTRACEPTIVE SPONGE

A contraceptive vaginal sponge (Today) is available for over-the-counter sales in the USA. Overall rates of conception with this product are similar to those with the diaphragm. However, parous women tend to have higher pregnancy rates perhaps secondary to dislodgement during intercourse. The sponge is made of polyurethane and contains the spermicide nonoxynol 9, which is released by wetting of the sponge and by the action of intercourse. The spermicide is effective for 24 hours. A built-in loop facilitates removal of the sponge.

Although there have been concerns about the risk of toxic shock syndrome associated with use of the sponge, the highest rates in reported series have been only about 10 cases per 100,000 users annually. Most reports suggest that prolonged use is a risk factor for the development of this syndrome.

## SPERMICIDAL PREPARATIONS

Spermicidal vaginal jellies, creams, gels, suppositories, and foams, in addition to their killing effect on sperm, also act as a mechanical barrier to entry of sperm into the cervical canal. The majority of spermicides marketed in the USA contain nonoxynol 9, which is a long-chain surfactant that is toxic to spermatozoa. Spermicides may be used alone or in conjunction with a diaphragm or condom. Some of the foam tablets and suppositories require a few minutes for adequate dispersion throughout the vagina, and failures may result if dispersion is not allowed to occur. In general, when used alone, spermicides have a failure rate of about 15% per year. Infrequently, these chemical agents may irritate the vaginal mucosa and external genitalia. Spermicides that contain nonoxynol 9 also exert significant prophylactic effects against the common sexually transmitted organisms *Neisseria gonorrhoeae, Treponema pallidum, Candida albicans, Trichomonas vaginalis* as well as HIV virus.

Although concern was raised by a few uncontrolled reports in the past, the possible risk of congenital disorders in babies born to mothers who used vaginal spermicides is not supported by well-controlled data.

## PERIODIC ABSTINENCE

It has long been known that women are fertile for only a few days of the menstrual cycle. The periodic abstinence or rhythm method of contraception requires that coitus be avoided during the time of the cycle when a fertilizable ovum and motile sperm could meet in the oviduct. Fertilization takes place within the tube, and the ovum remains in the tube for about 3 days after ovulation; hence, the fertile period is from the time of ovulation to 2–3 days thereafter.

Accurate prediction or indication of ovulation is essential to the success of the rhythm method. Accordingly, the types of periodic abstinence vary in their approaches to determining the fertile period.

(1) The **calendar method,** predicts the day of ovulation by means of a formula based on the menstrual pattern recorded over a period of several months. Ovulation ordinarily occurs 14 days before the first day of the next menstrual period. The fertile interval should be assumed to extend from at least 2 days before ovulation to no less than 2 days after ovulation. An interval of 1–2 days of abstinence either way increases the likelihood of success. Successful use of this approach is based on the knowledge that the luteal phase of a menstrual cycle is relatively constant at 14 days for normal women. Furthermore, for this approach to be successful as the only form of contraception requires regular menstrual cycles so that the various timing schedules retain validity. Although this is the most commonly used method of period abstinence, it is also the least reliable with failure rates as high as 35% in 1 year's use.

(2) A somewhat more efficacious approach to periodic abstinence is the temperature method, since more reliable evidence of ovulation may be obtained by recording the basal body temperature (BBT). The vaginal or rectal temperature must be recorded upon awakening in the morning before any physical activity is undertaken. Although it is often missed, there is a slight drop in temperature 24–36 hours after ovulation. The temperature then rises abruptly about 0.3–0.4°C (0.5–0.7°F) and continues on this plateau for the remainder of the cycle. The third day after the onset of elevated temperature is considered to be the end of the fertile period. For reliability, care must be taken by the woman to ensure that true basal temperatures are recorded, ie, that hyperthermia due to other causes does not provide misleading information.

(3) The **combined temperature and calendar method** uses features of both the previously mentioned methods to more accurately predict the time of ovulation. Failure rates of only 5 pregnancies per 100 couples per year have been reported in studies of well-motivated couples.

(4) The **cervical mucus (Billings) method** uses changes in cervical mucus secretions as affected by menstrual cycle hormonal alterations to predict ovulation. Starting several days before and until just after ovulation, the mucus becomes thin and watery, whereas at other times the mucus is thick and opaque. Women using this approach are trained to evaluate their mucus on a daily basis. Success rates are similar to those described for the combined temperature and calendar method. Advantages of this approach include relative simplicity and lack of a requirement for charting; disadvantages include difficulty in evaluating mucus in the presence of vaginal infection and the reluctance of some women to evaluate such secretions.

(5) The **symptothermal method,** if used properly, is probably the most effective of all the periodic abstinence approaches. It combines features of both the cervical mucus and the temperature methods. In addition, symptoms that may occur just prior to ovulation such as bloating and vulvar swelling are used as adjuncts to predict the likely occurrence of ovulation.

The most accurate method of determining ovulation time is to demonstrate the luteinizing hormone (LH) peak in serum specimens. Because of the cost and the time required for the serial measurements of LH that are essential to indicate the abrupt increment, this method is impractical as a method of birth control. It is valuable in the treatment of infertility, however, when the optimal time for coitus or artificial insemination is of great importance.

Figure 33–1 shows the relationships among ovulation, BBT, serum levels of LH and follicle-stimulating hormone (FSH), and menses. At least 20% of fertile women have enough variation in their cycles that reliable prediction of the fertile period is impossible.

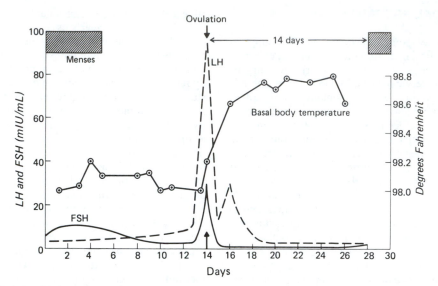

**Figure 33–1.** Relationship between ovulation and basal body temperature and luteinizing hormone (LH) and follicle-stimulating hormone (FSH) surges in the normal menstrual cycle.

Epidemiologic studies of women using the rhythm method have suggested an increased incidence of congenital anomalies such as anencephaly and Down's syndrome among children resulting from unplanned pregnancies. Delayed fertilization has been shown in animal experiments to result in an increased incidence of aneuploidy and polyploidy in offspring, thus suggesting a possible explanation for similar human fetal anomalies. However, despite a theoretical explanation for the occurrence of such birth defects, it is important to recognize that much of the data are subject to bias so that it would be inappropriate to conclude that such associations have been conclusively proved.

## ORAL HORMONAL CONTRACEPTIVES

The oral contraceptives in general use are synthetic steroids similar to the natural female sex hormones— the estrogens and progestins. These steroids are used in doses and in combinations that provide contraception by inhibiting ovulation.

The 2 principal regimens of oral contraception, when first developed were combined and sequential. In the combined method, pills containing estrogen and progestin are taken each day for 20–21 days. The sequential method, in which an estrogen pill was taken each day for 15–16 days followed by an estrogen-progestin pill each day for 5 days, has been abandoned in the USA because several studies showed a higher than normal incidence of endometrial cancer in women using this method of contraception.

The combined regimen is begun either with the onset of the menstrual cycle or on the Sunday closest to the start of menses. Since most oral contraceptive preparations are packaged in 28-day regimens (the last 7 days being placebos), the Sunday start approach may be easier to follow for most women. However, a good practice is to recommend use of an additional form of contraception during the first cycle to maximize efficacy. Withdrawal bleeding can be expected within 3–5 days after completion of the 20- or 21-day regimen.

The serum levels of FSH and LH throughout the normal menstrual cycle are shown in Figure 33–2A. During a typical cycle under the combined oral contraceptive regimen (Fig 33–2B), there is no rise during the first half of the cycle; thus, follicle growth is either not initiated or, if initiated, recruitment does not occur, ovulation does not occur, and consequently there is no FSH and LH surge. During the sequential oral contraceptive regimen (Fig 33–2C), the estrogen stimulates LH secretion in an irregular manner. There is no concomitant early rise in FSH when progestin is added, and another LH surge usually is produced. When a progestin-only regimen (Fig 33–2D) is followed (eg, with the minipill; see section "Minipill"), there are multiple LH surges but no significant changes in FSH levels. For the reasons given, these oral contraceptive regimens significantly alter the physiologic hormonal balance. The minipill regimen causes the least derangement, but its efficacy as a contraceptive is less than that of combined oral contraception. Moreover, occasional amenorrhea may occur.

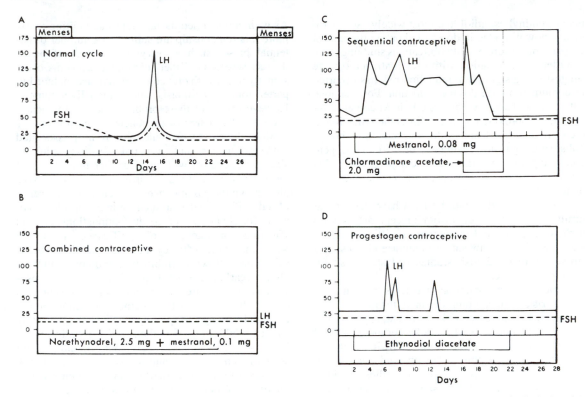

**Figure 33–2.** Serum levels (in mIU/mL) of follicle-stimulating hormone (FSH) and luteinizing hormone (LH) during the menstrual cycle, with and without oral contraception. **A:** During a normal cycle without medication. **B:** During atypical cycle with combined medication (see text). **C:** During a typical cycle with sequential medication (see text). **D:** During progestin-only medication. (Reproduced, with permission, from Odell WD, Moyer DL: Physiology of Reproduction. Mosby, 1971.)

## Advantages

Major noncontraceptive advantages derived from use of oral contraceptives in the USA alone include approximately 50,000 hospitalizations averted annually for conditions that include benign breast disease, retention cysts of the ovaries, iron deficiency anemia and pelvic inflammatory disease. Recent studies in the USA and Great Britain have shown that users of oral contraceptives have almost complete protection against ectopic pregnancies. Oral contraceptive use is estimated to prevent about 10,000 hospitalizations for this life-threatening complication annually in the USA alone.

Although there were initial concerns about oral contraceptives and carcinogenicity, recent studies have suggested that users of the combined oral contraceptives have only 50% of the risk of developing endometrial cancer than do nonusers. This protection appears after 1 year of use of oral contraceptives; after 5 years the risk is further reduced to 34%. Protection may persist for 10 or more years after discontinuation of pill use.

Recent ongoing studies at the Centers for Disease Control and several other smaller studies confirm that pill users experience a rate of ovarian cancer that is 60% that of non-pill users. In these studies, the protective effect persists for as long as 10 years after oral contraceptives are discontinued. This protective effect appears to be greater for nulliparas than for parous women.

Other health benefits include a decrease in menstrual blood loss; a reduction in incidence of dysmenorrhea; protection against salpingitis; and protection against osteoporosis.

## Disadvantages & Side Effects

Much attention has been paid to a possible relationship between the use of oral contraceptives and the incidence of thromboembolic disease, including pulmonary embolism and cerebral thrombosis. Between 1967 and 1969, reports of retrospective studies in the Great Britain and the USA provided statistically valid data indicating that deep vein thrombosis, pulmonary embolism, and cerebral thrombosis occur 3–6 times more frequently in users of oral contraceptives than in nonusers. However, since those earlier reports were published, the dosages of steroids contained in oral contraceptives have been reduced 3 to 4 times. In particular, ethinyl estradiol, the most widely used estrogen, is now provided in doses of about 35 μg in most preparations. More recent publications studying these disorders in association with oral contraceptive use suggest that a significant reduction risk has occurred in conjunction with dosage reduction. For example, data from a pharmacy-based study in Michigan demonstrated approximately a 2½ times the reduction in the estimated incidence of deep venous thromboembolism among women using less than 50 μg estrogen-containing oral contraceptives compared with that found in women using preparations containing more than 50 μg.

Studies in Sweden and the USA have had similar results. Furthermore, data from 2 recent large studies in the USA failed to demonstrate a statistically significant association between oral contraceptive use and stroke, although British studies still show risk for thrombotic stroke.

Some users of oral contraceptives may have a greater risk of developing coronary thrombosis than nonusers. The increased risk, if present, appears to be confined to older users who smoke 1 or more packs of cigarettes per day. Furthermore, following oral contraceptive use, the Nurses Health Study has shown that past oral contraceptive use, regardless of duration, does not increase the risk of subsequent cardiovascular disease including myocardial infarction. Although the progestins contained in oral contraceptives may change the lipid/lipoprotein profile in an adverse direction, the advent of new progestins and dosage reductions have led to a reduction in the magnitude of such changes. In addition, estrogen affects such profiles in a favorable direction and also has direct effects on vessel walls that reduce risk of atherosclerosis. Thus, the interaction of the 2 steroids combined with recent dosage and formulation changes has led to preparations that are essentially neutral relative to their effects on the cardiovascular system.

Although epithelial abnormalities of the uterine cervix among users of oral contraceptives were at one time a matter of concern, the preponderance of evidence cannot demonstrate that the use of oral contraceptives neither causes nor predisposes to the development of cancer of the cervix. A major problem with studies attempting to examine this relationship is the confounding that occurs with risk factors such as multiple sexual partners, age at first intercourse, and frequency of sexual activity.

The association between oral contraceptive use and breast cancer has been extensively studied during the past decade. At this time, it is unclear whether any positive association exists. The data in some studies suggest that long-term oral contraceptive use before childbearing may increase the risk of premenopausal breast cancer. However, some data also suggest that use may also offer modest protection against the more common postmenopausal form of this cancer.

As with cervical neoplasia, studies attempting to explore this relationship are subject to a number of potential biases such as varying practices of breast disease screening. Other infrequent problems occasionally noted with oral contraceptive use include hypertension, cholelithiasis, and benign liver tumors. However, none of these problems occurs frequently enough to be of significant concern to most users.

Since the current formulations are now associated with significant reductions in risk of serious sequelae, side effect control will be of greater importance to most users in the future. Furthermore, studies have also shown that compliance is affected by occurrence of side effects and that such "minor" problems account for about 40% of the discontinuations. Factors affecting compliance are of significance particularly when one studies efficacy. For example, the theoretical failure rate with combination oral contraceptives after 1 year's use is less than 1%. However, the use-effectiveness failure rate in some studies is as high as 4–6%. Intermenstrual bleeding including breakthrough bleeding and spotting may be experienced by about 10–20% of users in the first few months of use. With today's formulations, at about 6 months of use such problems stabilize and are seen in only about 5% of users. Missed menstrual periods or amenorrhea is relatively infrequent and of little clinical significance except that it can raise concern as to whether a contraceptive failure has occurred. Nausea may be seen in up to 10% of users; as with intermenstrual bleeding, this is a duration effect that declines rapidly after several months of use. With current formulations, acne tends to improve or show little change. Furthermore, significant headache disturbances and weight gain are far less frequent than reported with higher-dose preparations.

Since compliance and a good understanding of how to take oral contraceptives are important to their successful use, health care providers should take the time at the initial visit to explain the packaging of the brand being prescribed, discuss the side effects, review how to start the first cycle, and discuss what to do when pills are missed. It should be emphasized that the patient package insert provides useful information on these topics. In addition, users should be encouraged to contact their provider or someone in the office or clinic who is familiar with oral contraceptive health care if problems occur. Finally, users should be advised to use alternate forms of contraception if oral contraceptive use is interrupted because of forgotten pills or the occurrence of side effects.

Table 33–1 lists the currently available oral contraceptives and their contents.

## The "Minipill" or Progestin-Only Pill

The idea of administering small daily amounts of a progestin arose when clinical experience with some of the low-dose combination pills indicated that con-

**Table 33–1.** Oral contraceptive agents in use. The estrogen-containing compounds are arranged in order of increasing content of estrogen (ethinyl estradiol and mestranol have similar potencies).

| | Estrogen (mg) | Progestin (mg) | |
|---|---|---|---|
| **Combination tablets** | | | |
| Loestrin 1/20 | Ethinyl estradiol 0.02 | Norethindrone acetate | 1 |
| Loestrin 1.5/30 | Ethinyl estradiol 0.03 | Norethindrone acetate | 1.5 |
| Ovcon-35 | Ethinyl estradiol 0.035 | Norethindrone | 0.4 |
| Brevicon | Ethinyl estradiol 0.035 | Norethindrone | 0.5 |
| Modicon | | | |
| Nordette | Ethinyl estradiol 0.03 | L-Norgestrel | 0.15 |
| Ortho-Cept, Desogen | Ethinyl estradiol 0.30 | Desogestrel | 0.15 |
| Marvelon | Ethinyl estradiol 0.30 | Gestodene | 0.075 |
| Ortho-Cyclen | Ethinyl estradiol 0.35 | Norgestimate | 0.25 |
| Lo/Ovral | Ethinyl estradiol 0.03 | DL-Norgestrel | 0.3 |
| Ovral | Ethinyl estradiol 0.05 | DL-Norgestrel | 0.5 |
| Norlestrin 1/50 | Ethinyl estradiol 0.05 | Norethindrone acetate | 1 |
| Norlestrin 2.5/50 | Ethinyl estradiol 0.05 | Norethindrone acetate | 2.5 |
| Demulen | Ethinyl estradiol 0.05 | Ethynodiol diacetate | 1 |
| Ovcon-50 | Ethinyl estradiol 0.05 | Norethindrone | 1 |
| Norinyl 1/50 | Mestranol 0.05 | Norethindrone | 1 |
| Ortho-Novum 1/50 | | | |
| **Combination tablets—multidose** | | | |
| **Biphasic** | | | |
| Ortho-Novum 10/11 | | | |
| Day 1–10 | Ethinyl estradiol 0.035 | Norethindrone | 0.5 |
| Day 11–21 | Ethinyl estradiol 0.035 | Norethindrone | 1 |
| **Triphasic** | | | |
| Tri-Norinyl | | | |
| Day 1–7 | Ethinyl estradiol 0.035 | Norethindrone | 0.5 |
| Day 8–16 | Ethinyl estradiol 0.035 | Norethindrone | 1 |
| Day 17–21 | Ethinyl estradiol 0.035 | Norethindrone | 0.5 |
| Day 22–28 | | Placebo | |
| Triphasil, Trilevlen | | | |
| Day 1–6 | Ethinyl estradiol 0.030 | Levonorgestrel | 0.05 |
| Day 7–11 | Ethinyl estradiol 0.040 | Levonorgestrel | 0.075 |
| Day 12–21 | Ethinyl estradiol 0.030 | Levonorgestrel | 0.125 |
| Day 22–28 | | Placebo | |
| Ortho-Novum 7/7/7 | | | |
| Day 1–7 | Ethinyl estradiol 0.035 | Norethindrone | 0.5 |
| Day 8–14 | Ethinyl estradiol 0.035 | Norethindrone | 0.75 |
| Day 15–21 | Ethinyl estradiol 0.035 | Norethindrone | 1 |
| Day 22–28 | | Placebo | |
| Ortho-Tricept, Tri-Desogen | | | |
| Day 1–7 | Ethinyl estradiol 0.35 | Desogestrel | 0.05 |
| Day 8–14 | Ethinyl estradiol 0.30 | Desogestrel | 0.10 |
| Day 15–21 | Ethinyl estradiol 0.30 | Desogestrel | 0.15 |
| Day 22–28 | | Placebo | |
| Tri-Marvelon | | | |
| Day 1–6 | Ethinyl estradiol 0.30 | Gestodene | 0.05 |
| Day 7–11 | Ethinyl estradiol 0.40 | Gestodene | 0.07 |
| Day 12–21 | Ethinyl estradiol 0.30 | Gestodene | 0.10 |
| Day 22–28 | | Placebo | |
| Ortho-Tri-Cyclen | | | |
| Day 1–7 | Ethinyl estradiol 0.35 | Norgestimate | 0.180 |
| Day 8–14 | Ethinyl estradiol 0.35 | Norgestimate | 0.215 |
| Day 15–21 | Ethinyl estradiol 0.35 | Norgestimate | 0.250 |
| **Daily progestin tablets** | | | |
| Micronor | . . . | Norethindrone | 0.35 |
| Nor-QD | . . . | Norethindrone | 0.35 |
| Ovrette | . . . | DL-Norgestrel | 0.075 |

Some of the above oral contraceptives are available as generic formulations.

traception was being provided even though ovulation was not always inhibited. Subsequent studies demonstrated that a small daily quantity of a progestin alone would provide reasonably good protection against pregnancy without suppressing ovulation. The method has the following advantages: (1) Because no estrogen is given, the side effects attributable to the estrogen component of conventional oral contraceptives are eliminated; (2) the minipill is taken every day; ie, no special sequence of pill-taking is necessary. The mechanism of contraceptive action of the microdose nonstop progestins is not known. It has been suggested that the cervical mucus becomes less permeable to sperm and that endometrial activity goes out of phase, so that nidation is thwarted even if fertilization does occur. In clinical tests, the use of microdoses of progestins has resulted in a pregnancy rate of about 2–7 per 100 woman years.

Progestin is associated with some side effects, mainly irregularity of the ovulatory cycle and ectopic pregnancies, and these significantly reduce its contraceptive acceptability. Its overall effectiveness is less than that of combination pills. Currently, the minipill is thought to be useful in only a few patients, ie, in those having a documented hypersensitivity to estrogens and perhaps for the lactating woman.

### Postcoital or "Morning-After" Pill

Actually, there is no "morning-after" pill as such. Large doses of diethylstilbestrol (25–50 mg/d for 5 days) after unprotected intercourse, around the time of ovulation was first shown to be effective in preventing pregnancy; however, if the uptake of estrogen coincides with ovulation or entrance of the ovum into the tube, transport of the ovum through the tube may be markedly accelerated. Under these conditions, fertilization may not take place; or, if fertilization has already occurred, the ovum may reach the endometrial cavity prematurely and may not achieve nidation. If coitus takes place 2–6 days before ovulation, the high doses of estrogen effectively suppress ovulation. If coitus takes place 4 or more days after ovulation, fertilization would not take place anyway. Obviously, the use of high doses of estrogen probably will protect against pregnancy, provided that the estrogen is given coincident to the transport of the egg through the uterine tube or long enough before ovulation to effect suppression of ovulation.

The incrimination of nonsteroidal estrogens such as diethylstilbestrol (DES) in the etiology of clear cell vaginal carcinoma of female progeny has suggested that the use of this drug as a morning-after contraceptive may be unwise. Other estrogens such as ethinyl estradiol, conjugated equine estrogens, and stilbestrol diphosphate have been used with varying degrees of success. The potential carcinogenic effect of estrogen on female progeny in later life is not relevant to the morning-after use of estrogens because of the very limited duration of use and the presumed resistance to the preimplanted

blastocyst to drugs that may modify organogenesis. The principal side effects associated with the use of estrogens for this purpose are bloating and the distressing nausea and vomiting that occur during the drug regimen. The reported failure rates range from 0–2.4%. The use of estrogens as morning-after contraceptives should not be advised unless it is understood that congenital malformation is possible if pregnancy occurs.

More recent studies have shown that the provision of 2 tablets of an oral contraceptive containing 50 μg of ethinyl estradiol and 0.5 mg of norgestrel (Ovral) followed by 2 more tablets in 12 hours is also highly effective as a form of postcoital contraception. It has been estimated that the failure rate with this approach is only 1–1.5%. Furthermore, nuisance side effects such as nausea are less common because of reduced dosages of the steroids. Regardless of the approach chosen, women using the morning-after pill should be followed up within 3–4 weeks to assess efficacy as well as to initiate another contraceptive method, if needed.

## HORMONAL CONTRACEPTION BY INJECTION OR IMPLANTATION

Steroid sex hormones may be injected intramuscularly to provide a depot that, depending on the drug, dosage, and formulation, may provide contraception for 1 month, 6 months, or even 1 year. A pure progestin may be used, or the injection may consist of a combination of a progestin with an estrogen. Most of these regimens prevent ovulation by suppression of anterior pituitary function.

The compound that has been most widely used worldwide for contraception is medroxyprogesterone acetate (Depo-Provera). The most extensively evaluated regimen consists of 150 mg every 90 days. This results in marked interference with the midcycle production of LH. Ovulation is suppressed, although small amounts of FSH may be produced and some ovarian follicle development may occur. Because of the marked imbalance of estrogen and progesterone produced as a consequence of pituitary suppression, the endometrium usually is atrophic, and uterine bleeding is either irregular or absent for months. For example, in sharp contrast to Norplant (an implantable contraceptive that releases levonorgestrel), about 60% of users of the injection method of progestin administration experience amenorrhea after 1 year of use. Nonetheless, contraceptive effectiveness is very high. Published failure rates of 0.3% in the first year of use indicate that this injectable form of birth control is one of the most effective available. After the injections are discontinued, there may be considerable delay in reestablishment of regular ovulation and corresponding true menstrual bleeding. However, fertility rates are essentially normal at about 18 months after discontinuation.

Approximately a 2-fold increased risk of premenopausal breast cancer among women under 35 years using medroxyprogesterone was reported in one study, although the overall risk of breast cancer in older postmenopausal users was not elevated. Whether or not this constitutes a significant risk requires confirmation in other studies.

Bone mineral density may be reduced among those who receive injections of medroxyprogesterone. However, like breast cancer, this potential problem is based on data from only one study. Side effects other than irregular bleeding that may be encountered are weight gain, headache, nervousness, abdominal discomfort, dizziness, and fatigue. An advantage of the drug is that its use is independent of coitus or a daily activity like pill taking; a disadvantage is the need for injections every 3 months.

Norplant, which is a system that contains 36 mg of levonorgestrel in each of 6 Silastic rods, is another form of progestin contraception. The Silastic rods, which are placed subdermally in the inside upper arm, provide contraceptive protection for up to 5 years. Efficacy is high and first-year pregnancy rates are only 0.2% with cumulative 5-year rates of 3.9%. As with most progestins, pregnancy protection is likely for many women because of ovulation inhibition. However, since a significant number of women may ovulate while using the Norplant system, other mechanisms such as thickening of the cervical mucus are also of importance.

Major potential health sequelae have not been identified in association with use of Norplant, but side effects are fairly common. Some degree of menstrual irregularity such as increased flow or spotting has been reported in up to 60% of Norplant users in the first year. However, the occurrence of such side effects is time-dependent, with the rate declining by about 50% after 1 year. Headache is cited as the reason for discontinuation of Norplant in about 20% of women. Weight change and mastalgia are also reported with varying frequency among users. Like medroxyprogesterone, a significant advantage of the system is long-term effectiveness in a method that is independent of coitus or a daily activity, eg, taking a pill. The disadvantage is the requirement that a health care provider remove the rods via a minor surgical procedure.

After discontinuation of Norplant, there appears to be no significant delay in restoration of fertility, in contrast to that which occurs with injected medroxyprogesterone.

## INTRAUTERINE CONTRACEPTIVE DEVICES

The intrauterine device (IUD or IUCD) is made of plastic or metal or a combination of these materials. It is introduced into the endometrial cavity through the cervical canal. A large variety of shapes and sizes have been tried, with varying degrees of contraceptive effectiveness.

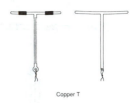

Copper T

**Figure 33–3.** Currently available intrauterine contraceptive devices in the USA.

At the present time, only 2 IUDs are available for use in the USA—the Progestasert and the Copper TCu 380A—the Paragard (Fig 33–3). The Progestasert-T is made of a special polymer that includes a reservoir containing 38 mg progesterone, which is released at a rate of 65 μg per day. However, due to this design, the useful lifespan of this device is only 1 year. The Paragard is wound with copper wire resulting in a surface area of copper of 300 mm$^2$ on the vertical arms and 40 mm$^2$ on each of the transverse arms. The lifespan of this device is at least 8 years.

Just how IUDs act to prevent conception is not known. The most widely observed phenomenon is mobilization of leukocytes in response to the presence of the foreign body. The leukocytes aggregate around the IUD in the endometrial fluids and mucosa and, to a lesser extent, in the stroma and underlying myometrium. It is hypothesized that the leukocytes produce an environment hostile to the fertilized ovum. In laboratory animals, this leukocytic infiltration apparently is not dependent on microbial invasion. In human beings, the uterine cavity sterilizes itself, usually within 2–4 weeks after the device is inserted. Other theories regarding the mechanism of action are spermicidal activity with copper devices, disruption of endometrial maturation with the progesterone-releasing device, alteration of normal tubal cilial action, and even disruption of normal oocyte maturation. In short, the mechanism of action is not established. Furthermore, there are no data to suggest that a major mechanism of action may be that of an abortifacient.

Efficacy with the Paragard device is high with a failure rate of less than 1% per year with prolonged use. In contrast, the Progestasert-T has a failure rate of about 1–1.5% with 25% of the pregnancies being ectopic. These data suggest that the latter device, unlike many contraceptive choices, offers no protection against extrauterine pregnancy.

It is felt by many practitioners that it is best to insert an IUD during a menstrual period because the cervical canal is fully patent then and the patient is least likely to be pregnant (Fig 33–4). Furthermore, the endometrial cavity may be more distensible at this time in the cycle, and uterine cramps, if they occur as a result of insertion, will be less noticeable. However,

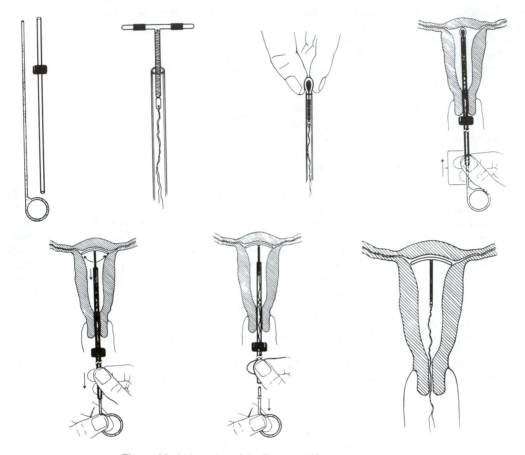

**Figure 33–4.** Insertion of the Paragard (Copper Tcu 380A).

insertion can be accomplished at any other time if this is desired or is more convenient for the patient.

After a pelvic examination has shown that the external and internal genitalia are normal, an antiseptic is used to cleanse the cervix. A single-toothed tenaculum is then placed on the anterior lip of the cervix and gentle traction is applied. This traction tends to reduce the angle between the cervix and the fundus and facilitates introduction of the uterine sound.

After the direction and depth of the uterine cavity have been determined by means of the sound, the device is inserted with the aid of the appropriate insertion tube. Most inserters are equipped with a guide that indicates the direction and the plane in which the device will lie when it emerges from the insertion tube into the cavity. Currently available devices are freed within the uterine cavity by withdrawal of the insertion tube over the plunger rather than by being pushed out of the inserted tube and into the uterine cavity by the plunger. This withdrawal technique reduces the chances for perforation of the uterine wall.

Most IUDs have a monofilament plastic tail or strand that extends through the cervix so that the patient can feel the thread and thus be certain the device is staying in place. Moreover, the tail facilitates removal when desired.

**Complications of Insertion**

There may be moderate discomfort or pain when the uterus is sounded or when the IUD is inserted. In general, the larger the IUD, the more likely it is to cause pain. The pain and occasional syncopal reactions are due to dilatation of the cervical canal and distention of the endometrial cavity. Paracervical anesthesia is desirable, since both pain and syncope are significantly reduced. Mild analgesics may be helpful for several hours following IUD insertion.

Partial or complete perforation of the uterus is a rare complication of IUD insertion. It can be avoided by meticulous care in ascertaining the position and size of the uterus and by strict adherence to the recommended insertion procedure.

The presence of the IUD may elicit uterine cramps (an attempt by the uterus to rid itself of the device) for hours or days after insertion. With larger devices, the intensity of the cramps may require removal of the IUD.

## Disadvantages & Side Effects

**A. Pregnancy:** If pregnancy occurs and the patient wishes it to continue, the IUD may be removed by traction on the plastic tail. If gentle traction does not effect prompt and easy removal, it is probably best to leave the device in place. However, the incidence of spontaneous abortion with a device in situ is about 50%, whereas the normal incidence is 12% or higher. Removal of the IUD reduces the risk of spontaneous abortion to about 20–25% and virtually eliminates the risk of septic abortion. Relative to extrauterine pregnancy, IUDs, except for the Progestasert-T, reduce the risk of ectopic pregnancy 2-fold or greater compared with noncontraceptors. Although about 5% of the pregnancies that occur with an IUD in situ are ectopic, the overall contraceptive action of IUDs reduces the risk of all pregnancies and the absolute risk of an ectopic pregnancy. Data involving the Progestasert-T suggests that ectopic pregnancy protection does not occur with that device; there is even some data that indicate that the risk may be 50% or more greater in comparison with that of noncontraceptors. There is no increased incidence of congenital abnormalities in babies who are conceived with the IUD in utero.

**B. Expulsion:** Most spontaneous expulsions of IUDs occur in the first few months after their insertion—most frequently during menstruation. The incidence of expulsion varies with the stiffness, size, and shape of the device. In general, the expulsion rate is roughly proportional to the degree of distortion of the endometrial cavity brought about by the presence of the IUD. The patient should examine herself periodically, and routinely after her menses, to be assured that the tail of the device is still present, ie, that the device is in place. If the tail cannot be felt and the patient is unaware of having expelled the device, she should see her physician. Until her appointment, alternate contraception should be used. Expulsion may have gone unnoticed, the plastic filament may have been drawn back into the cervix or endometrial cavity, the device may have perforated the uterine wall at insertion and passed into the peritoneal cavity (< 1 out of 1000 insertions), or the tail may have separated from the device and been expelled unnoticed.

The correct explanation can be found by careful inspection or by exploration of the endometrial cavity with an ultrasound examination or, if necessary, by an x-ray examination that includes an anterior-posterior as well as a lateral film and using a sound to localize the uterine cavity. (All IUDs available in the USA are radiopaque because of their metallic components or because they have been impregnated with barium sulfate.)

**C. Bleeding or Pain:** Either bleeding or pain or both are common reasons for removal of an IUD and discontinuation of this method of contraception. As is the case with expulsions, the incidence of pain or bleeding is more or less proportional to the degree of endometrial compression and myometrial distention brought about by the IUD. Thus, an IUD that conforms to the natural size and shape of the endometrial cavity is likely to cause less pain or bleeding than one that distorts the cavity and the uterine wall.

**D. Pelvic Infection:** A number of epidemiologic studies have documented the association between IUD use and pelvic inflammatory disease or salpingitis. However, more recent studies that have controlled for risk factors associated with salpingitis have better clarified the extent of risk. It appears that the highest risk (3- to 4-fold increase) occurs around the time of insertion, suggesting that endometrial cavity contamination in the presence of a foreign body (the IUD) is the major mechanism. No evidence of an increased risk of salpingitis is found 3–4 months after insertion or thereafter in women who don't have risk factors for STDs or salpingitis. In addition, it appears that women at risk for STDs, ie, those with multiple sexual partners or prior STDs, have a significantly higher risk of infection than other women.

Two studies conducted in the USA have also shown a modest increased risk of primary tubal infertility with IUD use. However, at the time of the data collection, copper-bearing IUDs were not in widespread use. Whether or not the risk of tubal infertility would be modified significantly with such devices is unclear. However, subgroup analyses in the 2 data sets suggest a trend that the risk of tubal infertility for low-risk women, eg, parous, married women, would be lower with copper IUD's than with plastic, inert devices.

*Actinomyces israelii* infection has been reported in association with IUD use. Most diagnoses have been made using the appearance of colonies on cervicovaginal Papanicolaou (Pap) smears due to the difficulty of culturing the organism. However, when evaluated, the accuracy of such diagnoses is highly variable. Although one study suggested an increased risk of salpingitis among IUD users when *A israelii* was detected on Pap smear, other investigators have not attempted to verify the association. It is also possible that the detection on Pap smear may represent colonization of the organism on the appendage (string), since *A israelii* has been shown to grow better on surfaces. Furthermore, *A israelii* was detected in presumably normal vaginal flora in about 20% of asymptomatic women in 1 study.

## Contraindications to the Use of IUDs

Absolute contraindications to IUD use are current pregnancy; undiagnosed abnormal vaginal bleeding; acute cervical, uterine, or salpingeal infection; past salpingitis; and suspected gynecologic malignancy. Relative contraindications include nulliparity or high priority attached to future childbearing; prior ectopic pregnancy; history of STDs; multiple sexual partners; moderate or severe dysmenorrhea; congenital anomalies of the uterus or other abnormalities such as leiomyomas; chronic menometrorrhagia; iron deficiency anemia; valvular heart disease; frequent expulsions or problems with prior IUD use; age younger than 25 years (due to higher prevalence of *Chlamydia* infections); and Wilson's disease (if a copper IUD is contemplated).

## Suitable Candidates for an IUD

The most suitable candidates for IUD use are parous women in a mutually monogamous relationship, who do not have a current or prior history of STDs or salpingitis. Other potential candidates include women desiring a method of high efficacy that is free of daily or coitally related activity and women who cannot use hormonal contraception due to side effects or medical conditions. Studies among diabetic IUD users have shown that use is highly effective with no increase in rate of pelvic infection.

Finally, it should be noted that several recent surveys of contracepting women indicate that IUD users are highly satisfied with their method.

## Indications for Removal of an IUD

The major reason for IUD removal is desire for pregnancy. Medical reasons for removal are partial expulsion, usually occurring in the first few months of use; persistent cramping, bleeding, or anemia, accounting for about 20% of removals during the first 3 months; acute salpingitis or *Actinomyces* infection on Pap smear; pregnancy (for the reasons previously cited); intra-abdominal placement/perforation; and significant postinsertion pain, which may indicate improper placement or partial perforation.

# II. INDUCED ABORTION

Induced abortion is the deliberate termination of pregnancy in a manner that ensures that the embryo or fetus will not survive. Attitudes of society toward elective abortion have undergone marked changes in the past few decades. In some situations the need for abortion is accepted by most people, but political and medical attitudes regarding induced abortion have continued to lag behind changing philosophies. Some religious concepts remain unchanged, resulting in personal, medical, and political conflicts.

About one-third of the world's population lives in nations with nonrestrictive laws governing abortion. Another third live in countries with moderately restrictive abortion laws, ie, where unwanted pregnancies may not be terminated as a matter of right or personal decision but only on broadly interpreted medical, psychologic, and sociologic indications. The remainder live in countries where abortion is illegal without qualification or is allowed only when the woman's life or health would be severely threatened if the pregnancy were allowed to continue.

An estimated 1 out of every 4 pregnancies in the world is terminated by induced abortion, making it perhaps the most common method of reproduction limitation. In the USA, estimates of the number of criminal abortions performed prior to legalization of the procedure ranged from 0.25–1.25 million per year. The number of legal abortions now being performed in this country approximates 1 abortion per 4 live births. In 1985, there were more than 1 million legal abortions in the USA, or 353.8 per 1000 live births.

The procedures being used in the USA for legally induced abortions during the first trimester are relatively safe. Table 33–2 shows that first-trimester legal abortions are consistently safer for the woman than if she used no birth control method and gave birth. Note also in Table 33–2 that whereas the number of maternal deaths related to births steadily increased from 5.6 to 22.6 per 100,000 women as age increased, age-related increase in number of deaths per 100,000 women per year from legal abortions was insignificant.

In general, the risk of death from legal abortion is lowest when it is performed at 8 menstrual weeks or sooner. Table 33–3 shows the relationship between death due to legal abortion and the gestational age at the time of the procedure.

Paracervical anesthesia has replaced general anesthesia in many health settings, resulting in fewer complications relevant to anesthesia. Midtrimester abortion techniques are still problematic and are asso-

**Table 33–2.** Pregnancy-related deaths per 100,000 women per year in developed countries compared with deaths resulting from legal abortion as a means of contraception.

| Type of Birth Control | Age Groups (Years) | | | | | |
|---|---|---|---|---|---|---|
| | 15–19 | 20–24 | 25–29 | 30–34 | 35–39 | 40–44 |
| No birth control; birth related | 5.6 | 6.1 | 7.4 | 13.9 | 20.8 | 22.6 |
| First trimester abortion only; method related | 1.2 | 1.6 | 1.8 | 1.7 | 1.9 | 1.2 |

(Adapted from Tietze C: Induced abortion: 1977 supplement, Table 11. *Rep Popul Fam Plann* 1977;14[2nd ed. Suppl]: 16.)

**Table 33–3.** Death-to-case for legal abortions by weeks of gestation (USA, 1972–1975).

| Weeks of Gestation | Deaths per 100,000 Procedures |
|---|---|
| 8 or less | 0.7 |
| 9–10 | 1.9 |
| 11–12 | 4.1 |
| 13–15 | 7.5 |
| 16–20 | 19.6 |
| 21 or more | 22.9 |

(Adapted from Tyler CW Jr: In: *Abortion Surveillance, 1975.* Center for Disease Control, United States Department of Health, Education, and Welfare Annual Summary 1975, April 1977, p. 36.)

ciated with a higher mortality rate. Hysterectomy carries a far greater risk than induction of labor by amnio-infusion or dilatation and evacuation.

## Legal Aspects of Induced Abortion in the United States

The United States Supreme Court ruled in 1973 (1) that the restrictive abortion laws in the USA were invalid, largely because these laws invaded the individual's right to privacy, and (2) that an abortion could not be denied to a woman in the first 3 months of pregnancy. The Court indicated that after 3 months a state may "regulate the abortion procedure in ways that are reasonably related to maternal health" and that after the fetus reaches the stage of viability (about 24 weeks) the states may refuse the right to terminate the pregnancy except when necessary for the preservation of the life or health of the mother. Still, much opposition is raised by various "right-to-life" groups and religious groups. In spite of this opposition, over 1 million procedures are still performed annually in the USA, with about one-third being performed on teenaged women. This emphasizes dramatically the inadequacy of sex education and the need for greater availability of adequate contraceptive methods in order to avoid such pregnancy wastage.

The patient must be informed regarding the nature of the procedure and its risks, including possible infertility or even continuation of pregnancy. The rights of the spouse, parents, or guardian must also be considered and permission obtained when indicated (until the individual woman's rights are clearly established).

State laws must be obeyed with special reference to residence, duration of pregnancy, indications for abortion, consent, and consultations required.

## Evaluation of Patients Requesting Induced Abortion

Patients give varied reasons for requesting abortion. Since in some cases the request is made at the urging of the woman's parents or in-laws, husband, or peers, every effort should be made to ascertain that the patient herself desires abortion for her own reasons. In addition, one should be certain that she knows she is free to choose among other methods of solving the problem of unplanned pregnancy, eg, adoption or single-parent rearing.

Although the majority of abortions are performed as elective procedures, ie, because of social or economic reasons as opposed to medical reasons, some women still request such services for medical or surgical indications. For example, for women with certain medical conditions, such as Eisenmenger's complex and cystic fibrosis, continuation of pregnancy may pose a threat to the life of the mother. Other indications are pregnancy resulting from a rape or pregnancy with a fetus affected with a major disorder, eg, trisomy 13. In any event, the ultimate decision rests with the pregnant woman.

Help from social agencies should be made available as necessary. A complete social history, medical history, and physical examination are required. Particular attention must be given to uterine size and position; the importance of accurate calculation of the duration of pregnancy (within 2 weeks but preferably within 1 week) cannot be overstated. With uncertainty, pelvic sonography should be used liberally. Routine laboratory tests should include pregnancy tests, urinalysis, hematocrit, Rh typing, serologic tests for syphilis, culture for gonorrhea, and Pap smear.

## Methods of Induced Abortion

Numerous methods are used to induce an abortion: suction or surgical curettage; induction of labor by means of intra- or extraovular injection of a hypertonic solution or other oxytocic agent; dilatation and evacuation; extraovular placement of devices such as catheters, bougies, or bags; hysterotomy—abdominal or vaginal; hysterectomy—abdominal or vaginal; and menstrual regulation.

The method of abortion used is determined primarily by the duration of pregnancy, with consideration for the patient's health, the experience of the physician, and the available physical facilities.

Suction curettage on an outpatient basis under local or light general anesthesia can be accomplished with a high degree of safety. The safety of outpatient abortion and the shortage of hospital beds have led to the development of single-function, "free-standing" abortion clinics. In addition to providing more efficient counseling and social services, these clinics have effectively reduced the cost of abortion. Many hospitals have "short-stay units," matching the efficiency of the outpatient clinics but also offering the back-up facilities of the general hospital.

**A. Suction Curettage:** Suction curettage is the safest and most effective method to terminate pregnancies of 12 weeks' duration or less. This technique has gained rapid worldwide acceptance, and over

90% of induced abortions in the USA are now performed by this method. The procedure involves dilatation of the cervix by instruments or by hydrophilic *Laminaria* tent (see following text), followed by the insertion of a suction cannula of the appropriate diameter into the uterine cavity (Fig 33–5). Standard negative pressures used are in the range of 30–50 mm Hg. Many physicians follow aspiration with light instrumental curettage of the uterine cavity.

The advantages of suction over surgical curettage are that the former empties the uterus more rapidly, minimizes blood loss, and reduces the likelihood of perforation of the uterus. However, failure to recognize perforation of the uterus with a cannula may result in serious damage to other organs. Knowledge of the size and position of the uterus and the volume of the contents is mandatory for safe suction curettage. Moreover, extreme care and slow minimal dilatation of the cervix, with special consideration for the integrity of the internal os, should prevent injury to the cervix or uterus. Attention to the decrease in uterine size that occurs with rapid evacuation helps to avoid uterine injury.

When performed in early pregnancy by properly trained physicians, suction curettage should be associated with a very low failure rate; the complication rate should be under 1% for infection, about 2% for excessive bleeding, and under 1% for uterine perforation. The risk of major complications such as persistent fever, hemorrhage requiring transfusion, and unintended major surgery ranges between 0.2 and 0.6% and is proportional to pregnancy duration. The incidence of mortality for suction curettage is about 1 in 100,000 patients.

**B. Surgical Curettage:** Surgical ("sharp") curettage has been used for first-trimester abortion in the absence of suction curettage equipment. This procedure is performed as a standard D&C, such as for the diagnosis of abnormal uterine bleeding or for the removal of endometrial polyps. The blood loss, duration of surgery, and likelihood of damage to the cervix or uterus are greatly increased when surgical curettage is used. In addition, the risk of uterine synechiae or Asherman's syndrome is also increased with this approach. Accordingly, suction curettage is generally much preferred for carrying out first-trimester termination procedures than is sharp curettage.

**C. Induction of Labor by Intra-amniotic Instillation:** The Japanese developed this technique for induced abortion after the first trimester. Currently, it is used almost exclusively for initiating midtrimester abortion. The original procedure was to perform amniocentesis, aspirate as much fluid as possible, and then instill into the amniotic sac 200 mL of hypertonic (20%) sodium chloride solution. In most (80–90%) cases, spontaneous labor and expulsion of the fetus and placenta would occur within 48 hours. Modifications of this technique have developed, primarily to reduce the injection-abortion interval—and as a result of the development of other agents that, instilled intra-amniotically, will initiate labor.

Because of the problems associated with hypertonic sodium chloride, many clinicians have used intra-amniotic hyperosmolar (59.7%) urea, usually with oxytocin or prostaglandin or intra-amniotic prostaglandin alone. These approaches result in injection-abortion intervals of 16–17 hours for urea and 19–22 hours for prostaglandin. The urea is instilled in a fashion similar to that described for hypertonic sodium chloride; the prostaglandin, most frequently $PGF_{2\alpha}$, is usually instilled as a single dose of 40–50 mg or as 2 doses of 25 mg instilled 6 hours apart. When using oxytocin to augment these agents, note

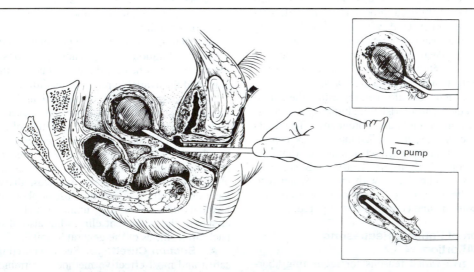

**Figure 33–5.** Suction method for induced abortion.

that because of the relative insensitivity of the myometrium to oxytocin at this stage of pregnancy, doses as high as 332 mU/minute are required to produce uterine contractions. To avoid water intoxication, the oxytocin is made up in highly concentrated solutions and given at slow rates.

It is advantageous to soften the "unripe" cervix with *Laminaria* tents placed in the cervix a few hours before amniocentesis is performed. Such an approach markedly reduces the risk of cervical injury.

Midtrimester induced abortion by this method must be done with scrupulous aseptic surgical technique, and the patient must be monitored until the fetus and placenta are delivered and postabortion bleeding is under control. The complication rate is high—up to 20% in some institutions—and the mortality rate is comparable to that of term parturition. Fortunately, because first-trimester abortion is now more readily available, more women are consulting their physicians early and thus availing themselves of the much safer suction curettage.

Several types of complications are associated with the use of instillation agents. Retained placenta is the most common problem; rates ranging from 13–46% have been reported. The placenta can usually be removed with ring forceps and large curets without difficulty with the patient under local anesthesia. Hemorrhage may be caused by retained products or atony; coagulopathy is seen in up to 1% of patients in whom hypertonic sodium chloride is used. Infection can also be encountered, but is reduced significantly by the use of prophylactic antibiotics in high-risk situations, eg, in patients with early ruptured membranes and during injection-abortion intervals greater than 24 hours. Cervical laceration can also occur; a complication that is reduced by the use of *Laminaria* tents. Hypernatremia can occur with the use of hypertonic sodium chloride if the drug is absorbed rapidly by the placental bed or if it is given by error intravascularly.

Failure of labor to expel the products of conception necessitates either a repetition of the procedure if the membranes are still intact or oxytocin stimulation, usually by intravenous injection or use of the dilatation and evacuation technique.

Emotional stress is an important factor for many women, since they are awake at the time of the expulsion of the fetus and the fetus is well formed. (The emotional stress is also a factor for hospital personnel—a problem impossible to avoid.)

**D. Induction of Labor with Vaginal Prostaglandins:** Prostaglandin $E_2$ given intravaginally can also be used to induce midtrimester abortion. Vaginal suppositories containing 20 mg are used every 3–4 hours until abortion occurs; the presence or absence of labor determines whether to stop the prostaglandin $E_2$. Treatment-abortion intervals, rates of incomplete abortion, and complications are similar to those described for instillation agents. The major disadvan-

tages are significant gastrointestinal side effects, a higher incidence of live abortion, and a more frequent occurrence of fever.

**E. Dilatation and Evacuation:** This technique for inducing midtrimester abortion is essentially a modification of suction curettage. Because fetal parts are larger at this stage of pregnancy, serial placement of *Laminaria* tents is used by most operators to effect cervical dilatation with less likelihood of injury. Larger suction cannulas and specially designed forceps are used to extract tissue. In most instances, the operation can be performed in the outpatient setting using paracervical block anesthesia and intravenous sedation on patients with pregnancies of up to 18 weeks' gestation. Complications include hemorrhage (usually due to atony or laceration), perforation, and, rarely, infection. Retained tissue is uncommon, especially when careful inspection of tissue for completion is carried out at the end of each procedure. Compared with instillation techniques or vaginal prostaglandin, the overall incidence of complications (in pregnancies up to 18 weeks' gestation) is less with dilatation and evacuation. In addition, the technique is preferred by most patients because it is an outpatient procedure and the woman does not undergo labor.

**F. Hysterotomy and Hysterectomy:** The use of hysterotomy and hysterectomy is currently reserved for special circumstances such as in failure to complete a midtrimester abortion due to cervical stenosis or in the management of other complications. Both approaches, compared with other techniques discussed, have unacceptably high rates of morbidity and mortality and neither should be used as a primary method.

**G. Menstrual Regulation:** Menstrual regulation consists of aspiration of the endometrium within 14 days after a missed menstrual cycle or within 42 days after the beginning of the last menstrual period by means of a small cannula attached to a source of low-pressure suction such as a syringe or other suction machine. This is a simple and safe procedure that can be readily performed in the office or outpatient clinic, usually without any anesthetic, although paracervical block can be used if necessary. Menstrual regulation was used extensively in the 1970s and 1980s before reliable, inexpensive, and sensitive urine pregnancy tests were available. It offered a safe early approach to pregnancy termination; however, about 40% of women were not pregnant at the time of the procedure. With the advent of urine pregnancy tests that have the ability to document pregnancy even before a missed menstrual period, standard first-trimester suction curettage is probably more widely used. Complications are similar to that described for suction curettage except that persistent pregnancy is more common, particularly when very early menstrual regulation procedures are performed.

**H. RU-486:** RU-486 (mifepristone) is a synthetic drug developed by French pharmacologists, which acts at least partially as an antiprogestational agent. When given orally in conjunction with a prostaglandin, it effects first-trimester abortion. Complications include failure to terminate a pregnancy, incomplete abortion, and significant uterine cramping. At this time the drug is not available for use in the USA.

### Follow-up of Patients After Induced Abortion

Follow-up care after all procedures must be ensured. After abortion by all methods, human $RH_o$ (D) immune globulin ($Rh_o$GAM) should be administered promptly if the patient is Rh-negative, unless it is known that the male partner was Rh-negative. The patient should take her temperature several times daily and report fever or unusual bleeding at once. She should avoid intercourse or the use of tampons or douches for at least 2 weeks. The physician should discuss with the patient the possibility that emotional depression, similar to that following term pregnancy and delivery, may occur after induced abortion. Follow-up care should include pelvic examination to rule out endo- and parametritis, salpingitis, failure of involution, or continued uterine growth. Finally, effective contraception should be made available according to the patient's needs and desires.

### Long-term Sequelae of Induced Abortion

A large number of studies have been conducted during the past 2 decades to examine the possible long-term sequelae of elective induced abortion. Most of the attention has focused on subsequent reproductive function; unfortunately, many of the studies have had inherent biases and serious methodologic flaws. Despite these problems, enough information is available to provide relative estimates of potential risks. Data from some studies suggest that midtrimester pregnancy loss is more common in women who have undergone 2 or more induced or spontaneous abortions. However, women who have undergone one procedure have essentially the same risk as women who have experienced a single term pregnancy. Relative to low birth weight, only women who have undergone a first-trimester procedure by sharp curettage under general anesthesia appear to have increased risks. The reason for this association might be related to the method of dilatation used. Finally, studies that have examined both ectopic pregnancy and infertility have failed to show any consistent association between these adverse events and prior induced abortion.

## REFERENCES

### GENERAL

Burkman RT: *Handbook of Contraception and Abortion.* Little, Brown, 1989.

Comp PC, Zacur HA: Contraceptive choices in women with coagulation disorders. Am J Obstet Gynecol 1993;168:1990.

Corson SL, Derman R, Tyrer LB: *Fertility Control.* Little, Brown, 1985.

Hankoff LD, Darney PD: Contraceptive choices for behaviorally disordered women. Am J Obstet Gynecol 1993;168:1986.

Harlap S, Kost K, Forrest JD: Preventing pregnancy, protecting health: A new look at birth control choices in the United States. Alan Guttmacher Institute, 1991.

Knopp RH, LaRosa JC, Burkman RT: Contraception and dyslipidemia. Am J Obstet Gynecol 1993;168:1994.

Loriaux DL, Wild RA: Contraceptive choices for women with endocrine complications. Am J Obstet Gynecol 1993;168:2021.

Mattson RH, Rebar RW: Contraceptive methods for women with neurologic disorders. Am J Obstet Gynecol 1993;168:2027.

McGregor JA, Hammill HA: Contraception and sexually transmitted diseases: Interactions and opportunities. Am J Obstet Gynecol 1993;168:2033.

Mestman JH, Schmidt-Sarosi C: Diabetes mellitus and fertility control: Contraception management issues. Am J Obstet Gynecol 1993;168:2012.

Mishell DR: Contraception. N Engl J Med 1989;320(12):777.

Ory HW et al: Making choices: Evaluating the health risks and benefits of birth control methods. Alan Guttmacher Institute, 1983.

Speroff L, Darney PD: *A Clinical Guide for Contraception.* Williams & Wilkins, 1992.

Sullivan JM, Lobo RA: Considerations for contraception in women with cardiovascular disorders. Am J Obstet Gynecol 1993;168:2006.

### CONTRACEPTION IN THE ADOLESCENT

Greydanus DE, McAnarney E: Contraception in the adolescent: Current concepts for the pediatrician. Pediatrics 1980;65:1.

Ory HW et al: The pill at 20: An assessment. Fam Plann Perspect 1980;12:278.

Sulak PJ, Haney AF: Unwanted pregnancies: Understanding contraceptive use and benefits in adolescents and older women. Am J Obstet Gynecol 1993;168: 2042.

### LACTATIONAL AMENORRHEA

Kennedy KI, Visness CM: Contraceptive efficacy of lactational amenorrhoea. Lancet 1992;339:227.

Population Information Program, The Johns Hopkins University Family Planning Programs: Breastfeeding, fertility, and family planning. Population Report Series J, No. 24, Nov–Dec 1981.

## CONDOM

Connell EB, Tatum HJ: Barrier methods of contraception. Creative Infomatics, 1985.

## DIAPHRAGMS

Davidson AJ, Chen JH, Judson FN et al: Barrier contraceptives and sexually transmitted diseases in women: A comparison of female-dependent methods and condoms. Am J Public Health 1992;82(5):669.

Hooton TM, Hiller S, Johnson C et al: *Escherichia coli* bacteriuria and contraceptive method. JAMA 1991; 265(1): 64.

Population Information Program, The Johns Hopkins University Family Planning Programs: New development in vaginal contraception. Population Report, Series H, No. 7, Jan–Feb 1984.

## SPERMICIDAL PREPARATIONS

Abrutyn D, McKenzie BE, Nadaskay N: Teratology study of intravaginally administered nonoxynol 9-containing contraceptive cream in rats. Fertil Steril 1982;37:113.

Cutler JC et al: Vaginal contraceptives as prophylaxis against gonorrhea and other sexually transmitted diseases. Adv Planned Parenthood 1977;12:45.

Jick H et al: Vaginal spermicides and congenital disorders. JAMA 1981;245:1329.

Kreiss J, Ngugi E, Holmes K et al: Efficacy of nonoxynol 9 contraceptive sponge use in preventing heterosexual acquisition of HIV in Nairobi prostitutes. JAMA 1992; 268:477.

## HORMONAL CONTRACEPTIVES

Baird DT, Glasier AF: Drug therapy: Hormonal contraception. N Engl J Med 1993;328:1543.

Bottiger LE, Boman G, Eklund G et al: Oral contraceptives and thromboembolic disease: Effects of lowering estrogen content. Lancet 1980;i:1097.

Brinton LA et al: Risk factors for benign breast disease. Am J Epidemiol 1981;113:203.

Burkman RT: Lipid and lipoprotein changes in relation to oral contraception and hormonal replacement therapy. Fertil Steril 1988;49(5):39s.

Clarkson TB, Shively CA, Morgan TM et al: Oral contraceptives and coronary artery atherosclerosis of cynomolgus monkeys. Obstet Gynecol 1990;75(2):217.

Corson SI: Contraceptive efficacy of a monophasic oral contraceptive containing desogestrel. Am J Obstet Gynecol 1993;168:1017.

Croft P, Hannaford PC: Risk factors for acute myocardial infarction in women: Evidence from the Royal College of General Practitioners' Oral Contraception Study. Br Med J 1989;298(3):165.

Gerstman BB, Piper JM, Tomita DK et al: Oral contraceptive estrogen dose and the risk of deep venous thromboembolic disease. Am J Epidemiol 1991; 133(1):32.

Huggins GR, Zucker PK: Oral contraceptives and neoplasia: 1987 update. Fertil Steril 1987;47(5):733.

Institute of Medicine: *Oral Contraceptives and Breast Cancer.* Washington, DC: National Academy Press, 1991.

Kaufman DW et al: Decreased risk of endometrial cancer among oral contraceptive users. N Engl J Med 1980; 303: 1045.

Kaunitz AM: Combined oral contraception with desogestrel/ethinyl estradiol: Tolerability profile. Am J Obstet Gynecol 1993;168:1028.

Kleerekoper M, Brienza RS, Schultz LR et al: Oral contraceptive use may protect against low bone mass. Arch Intern Med 1991;151:1971.

Kritz-Silverstein D, Barrett-Connor E: Bone mineral density in postmenopausal women as determined by prior oral contraceptive use. Am J Public Health 1993; 83:100.

London RS: The new era in oral contraception: Pills containing gestodene, norgestimate, and desogestrel. Obstet Gynecol Surv 1992;47:777.

Ory H: The noncontraceptive health benefits for moral contraceptive use. Fam Plann Perspect 1982;14:182.

Patsch W, Brown SA, Gotto AM et al: The effect of triphasic oral contraceptives on plasma lipids and lipoproteins. Am J Obstet Gynecol 1989;161(5):1396.

Plummer FA, Simonsen JN, Cameron DW et al: Cofactors in male-female sexual transmission of human immunodeficiency virus type 1. J Infect Dis 1991;163: 233.

Porter JB, Hunter JR, Danielson DA et al: Oral contraceptives and nonfatal vascular disease-recent experience. Obstet Gynecol 1982;59:299.

Porter JB, Hunter JR, Jick H et al: Oral contraceptives and nonfatal vascular disease. Obstet Gynecol 1985; 66:1.

Rosenberg L, Kaufmann DW, Helmrich SP et al: Myocardial infarction and cigarette smoking in women younger than 50 years of age. JAMA 1985;253:2965.

Rosenberg L, Palmer JR, Clarke EA et al: A case-control study of the risk of breast cancer in relation to oral contraceptive use. Am J Epidemiol 1992;136:1437.

Rosenberg L, Palmer JR, Lesko SM et al: Oral contraceptive use and the risk of myocardial infarction. Am J Epidemiol 1990;131(6):1009.

Shoupe D, Mishell DR, Bopp BL et al: The significance of bleeding patterns in Norplant implant users. Obstet Gynecol 1991;77(2):256.

Sivin I: International experience with Norplant and Norplant-2 contraceptives. Stud Fam Plann 1988;19: 81.

Sivin I, Stern J, Diaz S et al: Rates and outcomes of planned pregnancy after use of Norplant capsules, Norplant II rods, or levonorgestrel-releasing of copper TCu 380 Ag intrauterine contraceptive devices. Am J Obstet Gynecol 1992;166(4):1208.

Stadel BV: Oral contraceptives and premenopausal breast cancer in nulliparous women. Contraception 1988;38(3): 287.

Stampfer MJ, Willett WC, Colditz GA et al: A prospective study of past use of oral contraceptive agents and risk of cardiovascular diseases. N Engl J Med 1988;319(20): 1313.

Stampfer MJ, Willett WC, Colditz GA et al: Past use of oral contraceptives and cardiovascular disease: A meta-analysis in the context of the Nurses' Health Study. Am J Obstet Gynecol 1990;163(1):285.

Thomas DB: Oral contraceptives and breast cancer: Review of the epidemiologic literature. Contraception 1991; 43(6):597.

Thorogood M, Mann J, Murphy M et al: Fatal stroke and use of oral contraceptives: Findings from a case-control study. Am J Epidemiol 1992;136:35.

The Walnut Creek Contraceptive Drug Study: A Prospective Study of the Side-Effects of Oral Contraceptives. Vol. 3. US Government Printing Office, 1981.

Wingo PA, Lee NC, Ory HW et al: Age-specific differences in the relationship between oral contraceptive use and breast cancer. Obstet Gynecol 1991;78(2): 161.

Yuzpe AA, Lancee WI: Ethinyl estradiol and dl-norgestrel as a postcoital contraceptive. Fertil Steril 1977;28:932.

## INTRAUTERINE CONTRACEPTIVE DEVICES

Alvarez F, Brache V, Fernandez E et al: New insights on the mode of action of intrauterine contraceptive devices in women. Fertil Steril 1988;49(5):768.

Burkman RT, Damewood MT: *Actinomyces* and the intrauterine contraceptive device. In: Zatuchni GI, Goldsmith A, Sciarra JJ (editors): PARFR Series on Fertility Regulation: Intrauterine Contraception-Advances and Future Prospects. Philadelphia: Harper & Row, 1985, p 427.

Burkman RT, Schlesselman S, McCaffrey L et al: The relationship of genital tract *Actinomycetes* and the development of pelvic inflammatory disease. Am J Obstet Gynecol 1982;143(6):585.

Burkman RT and the Women's Health Study: Association between intrauterine device and pelvic inflammatory disease. Obstet Gynecol 1981;57(3):269.

Cramer DW et al: Tubal infertility and the intrauterine device. N Engl J Med 1985;312:941.

Daling JR, Weiss NS, Voigt LF et al: The intrauterine device and primary tubal infertility. N Engl J Med 1992;326(3):203.

Daling JR et al: Primary tubal infertility in relation to the use of an intrauterine device. N Engl J Med 1985; 312:937.

Eschenbach DA, Harnisch JP, Holmes KK: Pathogenesis of acute pelvic inflammatory disease: Role of contraception and other risk factors. Am J Obstet Gynecol 1977;128:838.

Grimes DA: Intrauterine devices and pelvic inflammatory disease: Recent developments. Contraception 1987;36(1):97.

IUDs: An appropriate contraceptive for many women. Popul Rep Series B, No. 4, July 1982.

Keebler C, Chatwani A, Schwartz R: Actinomycosis infection associated with intrauterine contraceptive devices. Am J Obstet Gynecol 1983;145:596.

Lee NC, Rubin GL, Borucki R: The intrauterine device and pelvic inflammatory disease revisited: New results from the Women's Health Study. Obstet Gynecol 1988;72:1.

Lee NC et al: Type of intrauterine device and the risk of pelvic inflammatory disease. Obstet Gynecol 1983; 62:1.

Sivin I, Diaz J, Alvarez F et al: Four-year experience in a randomized study of the Gyne T 380 Slimline and the standard Gyne T 380 intrauterine contraceptive devices. Contraception 1993;47:37.

Sivin I, Schmidt F: Effectiveness of IUD's: A review. Contraception 1987;36(1):55.

Sivin I, Tatum HJ: Four years' experience with the TCU 380A intrauterine contraceptive device. Fertil Steril 1981;36:159.

Tatum HJ, Connell EB: A decade of intrauterine contraception: 1976–1986. Fertil Steril 1986;46:173.

Vessey MP, Lawless M, McPherson K et al: Fertility after stopping use of intrauterine contraceptive device. Br Med J 1983;286:106.

## INDUCED ABORTION

Baulieu EE: RU-486 as an antiprogesterone steroid: From receptor to contragestion and beyond. JAMA 1989;262:1808.

Burkman RT, Atienza MF, King TM et al: Hyperosmolar urea for elective midtrimester abortion: Experience in 1913 cases. Am J Obstet Gynecol 1978; 131(1):10.

Castadot RG: Pregnancy termination: Techniques, risks, and complications and their management. Fertil Steril 1986;45(1):5.

Cates W Jr, Smith JC: Mortality from legal abortion in the United States, 1972–1976. In: The Safety of Fertility Control. Keith LG, Kent DK, Brittain JR (editors). Springer, 1980.

Centers for Disease Control: Mortality Vital Statistics. Vol. 37, No. 6 (Suppl). Sept 30, 1988, p 42. US Dept of Health and Human Services.

Couzinet B, Strat NL, Ulmann A et al: Termination of early pregnancy by the progesterone antagonist RU 486 (mifepristone). N Engl J Med 1986;315:1565.

Grimes DA, Cates W Jr: The comparative efficacy and safety of intraamniotic prostaglandin $F_{2\alpha}$a and hypertonic saline for second-trimester abortion: A review and critique. J Reprod Med 1979;22:248.

Grimes DA, Cates W Jr: Complications from legally-induced abortion: A review. Obstet Gynecol Surv 1979;34:177.

Grimes DA, Schulz KF, Cates W et al: Midtrimester abortion by dilatation and evacuation: A safe and practical alternative. N Engl J Med 1977;296:1141.

Grimes DA et al: Local versus general anesthesia: Which is safer for performing suction curettage abortions? Am J Obstet Gynecol 1979;135:1030.

Grimes DA et al: Maternal death at term as a late sequela of failed attempted abortion. Adv Planned Parenthood 1979;14:77.

Hogue CJW, Cates W, Tietze C: The effects of induced abortion on subsequent reproduction. Epidemiol Rev 1982;4:66.

Peyron R, Aubeny E, Targosz V et al: Early termination of pregnancy with mifepristone (RU 486) and the orally active prostaglandin misoprostol. N Engl J Med 1993;328:1509.

Segal SJ: Mifepristone (RU 486). N Engl J Med 1990; 322(10):691.

# Benign Disorders of the Vulva & Vagina

# 34

*Stephen L. Curry, MD, & David L. Barclay, MD*

Benign vulvar and vaginal disorders are common in the practice of gynecology. A thorough understanding of the physiology and pathology of these areas is of importance in diagnosing and treating these disorders. It is also very important for the care givers to teach their patients the normal and the abnormal. For example, young girls often receive little or no instruction in perineal hygiene, and teenage girls are often misinformed about the presumed necessity for douching or the use of feminine hygiene products, which may do more harm than good.

In prepubertal girls, the absence of endogenous estrogen results in a thin vaginal epithelium deficient in glycogen. This predisposes to bacterial infection, the most common gynecologic disorder in this age group.

During the reproductive years, the vaginal epithelium matures. However, coitus, contraceptive agents, feminine hygiene practices, and the wearing of tight, nonabsorbent, heat-retaining clothing (panty hose, etc) predispose to the development of vulvovaginal inflammation.

In postmenopausal patients, the level of endogenous estrogen decreases. The cells of the vaginal mucosa and vulvar skin lose glycogen, and vaginal acidity declines, resulting in fragile atrophic tissues that are susceptible to trauma and infection.

The anatomy of the vulva is described on page 11. The vulvar skin is responsive to hormonal stimulation and provides a warm, moist environment that is exposed to urinary and fecal soiling. The first symptom of vaginal irritation is often vulvar pruritus, which commonly results from contact with the vaginal discharge, often compounded by overlying garments made of synthetic fabrics that are heat- and moisture-retaining.

Evaluation of a patient with vulvar symptoms requires a detailed history and physical examination, including inspection of other mucosal and skin surfaces. Feminine hygiene products and contraceptives should be identified, as well as antibiotics that may alter the vaginal flora, resulting in overgrowth of *Candida albicans*. A family history of diabetes mellitus or an obstetric history of excessively large infants strongly suggests the possibility of diabetes, which also predisposes to candidiasis.

## LEUKORRHEA

Although the term *leukorrhea* literally means a white discharge, the color may vary depending on the cause. The most common cause of leukorrhea is a vaginal infection. Other causes range from the normal milky vaginal discharge seen in the premenarcheal girl to blood-tinged discharge caused by cancer of the vagina or cervix. Before the menarche, there may be a scant vaginal discharge that ordinarily does not cause irritation and is not considered abnormal. Inspection of the vagina in an adolescent girl may reveal a small amount of white mucoid material in the vaginal vault that is the result of normal desquamation and accumulation of vaginal epithelial cells. Vaginal discharge in the sexually mature woman is considered abnormal if soiling of the clothing occurs, if the odor is offensive, or if irritation interferes with function.

### Pathologic Physiology

The pathophysiology of leukorrhea due to vaginitis must be considered by age groups because of the influence of endogenous and exogenous estrogen and sexual activity. Under the influence of estrogens, the vaginal epithelium thickens and large quantities of glycogen are present in the epithelial cells. The collection of intraepithelial glycogen results in the production of lactic acid. This acid environment (pH 3.5–4.0) fosters the growth of a normal vaginal flora, chiefly lactobacilli (Döderlein's bacilli) and acidogenic corynebacteria. *Candida* organisms may be present but in small numbers because of the preponderance of bacteria. Normally, no trichomonads are present.

Relative lack of estrogen in the premenarcheal child results in a thin vaginal mucosa that is poorly resistant to infection. Estrogen depletion due to aging, ovariectomy, or pelvic irradiation causes atrophy of the vaginal mucosa, a reduction in glycogen content, and a decrease in the acidity of the vaginal fluid. A thin vaginal mucosa is susceptible to trauma. The bacterial population of the vagina changes from predominantly lactobacilli to a mixed flora consisting chiefly of pathogenic cocci.

Other factors that tend to make the vagina more alkaline are infected cervical mucus, menstrual fluid, and the vaginal transudate that occurs with sexual excitement. In addition, the male ejaculate is alkaline.

Although *C albicans* may be a normal inhabitant of the vagina, other types of vaginitis, eg, *Gardnerella (Haemophilus) vaginalis* vaginitis, are related to sexual activity and should be considered sexually transmitted diseases. In resistant cases, therefore, the male partner should wear a condom or undergo treatment concurrently.

## Etiology

**A. Foreign Bodies:** Foreign bodies commonly cause vaginal discharge and infection in preadolescent girls. Paper, cotton, or other materials may be placed in the vagina and cause secondary infection. Children may require vaginoscopic examination under anesthesia to identify or rule out foreign body or tumor high in the vaginal vault. In adults, a forgotten menstrual tampon or contraceptive device may cause malodorous leukorrhea. The diagnosis can usually be made by pelvic examination.

**B. Bacterial Infection:** In the premenarcheal and postmenopausal hypoestrogenic vagina, a mixed bacterial flora may be expected, particularly in the presence of trauma or a foreign body. A specific diagnosis can be made only by preparation of stained smears and cultures, although culture reports may be misleading because of identification of mixed flora.

*G vaginalis* may be the most common cause of symptomatic bacterial vaginal infection. Other significant bacteria are *Neisseria gonorrhoeae, Chlamydia, Mycoplasma hominis,* and *Ureaplasma urealyticum.* Each bacterial agent is associated with characteristic symptoms.

**C. Viral Infections:** The DNA viruses that affect the vulva and vagina are of the herpesvirus, poxvirus, and papovavirus types. The herpesviruses that affect the lower genitalia are herpes simplex, varicella, herpes zoster, and cytomegalovirus.

**D. Candidiasis:** *Candida* species belong to the family Cryptococcaceae. Of the *Candida* species, *Candida albicans* most frequently causes human disease, and it has the ability to form both spores and pseudohyphae. *C albicans* is frequently a normal inhabitant of the mouth, throat, large intestine, and vagina. Clinical infection is occasionally associated with a systemic disorder (eg, diabetes mellitus), pregnancy, nondiabetic glycosuria, a diet consisting of large amounts of fruit or sugar, debilitation, corticosteroids, antibiotics, and possibly oral contraceptives.

**E. Trichomoniasis:** *Trichomonas vaginalis* is a unicellular flagellate protozoan. Humans are host to 3 *Trichomonas* species, but *T vaginalis*, which is found in the vagina, may be the only species that causes disease. *T vaginalis* organisms are larger than polymorphonuclear leukocytes but smaller than mature epithelial cells. Trichomoniasis is an infestation not only of the vagina but also of the lower urinary tract in both men and women. It is a sexually transmitted disease; other forms of transmission are infrequent, because large numbers of organisms are required to cause symptoms.

**F. Cervicitis:** Chronic cervicitis associated with hypertrophy or eversion of the endocervical mucosa may produce a copious mucopurulent discharge. A variety of aerobic and anaerobic organisms can be cultured from cervical mucus. The alkaline cervical mucus may cause a sufficient change in vaginal pH to alter the bacterial flora, enhancing the environment for other pathogenic organisms. Herpesvirus often causes a necrotic exophytic cervical lesion that may be confused with cancer. Other causes of cervicitis are *N gonorrhoeae, Chlamydia trachomatis,* and *T vaginalis.* Benign cervical polyps and cancer of the cervix are other causes of mucopurulent discharge and bleeding.

**G. Atrophic Vaginitis:** Prepubertal, lactating, and postmenopausal women lack the vaginal stimulation of endogenous estrogen production. The pH of the vagina is abnormally high, and the normally acidogenic flora of the vagina may be replaced by mixed flora. The vaginal mucosa is thinned, and the epithelium is thus more susceptible to both infection and trauma. Although most patients are asymptomatic, many postmenopausal women report vaginal dryness and dyspareunia. Some of the symptoms of irritation are caused by secondary infection.

**H. Other Causes:**

**1. Cervical mucorrhea or vaginal epithelial discharge**–An unusually large cervical ectropion may cause an excessive discharge of cervical mucus from normal endocervical cells. Vaginal adenosis may cause the same type of vaginal discharge. The discharge is mucoid and clear or slightly cloudy, but there is no itching, burning, or odor. Patients may equate the discharge with vaginal infection and seek treatment. One must always consider the possibility of adenocarcinoma of the endocervix or clear cell carcinoma of the cervix or vagina.

A gray-white, pasty discharge, which causes no irritation or odor and occasionally is quite profuse, may be caused by excessive **desquamation** of normal vaginal epithelial cells. Excessive but normal vaginal secretions may appear in the speculum blade as a clump or curd and be confused with a *Candida* infection. Here, the vaginal pH is normal. Microscopically, the secretions show normal bacterial flora, a heavy spread of mature vaginal squamae, and no increase in leukocytes.

**2. Pinworms (Enterobius vermicularis)**–Vaginal infestation by this organism may cause vaginitis, usually in children. The source of infection is fecal soiling of the introitus, and the result is an extremely pruritic perineal area. The parasite may be detected by pressing a strip of adhesive cellulose tape to the perineum and then adhering the tape to a slide. Microscopic examination may reveal the characteristic double-walled ova.

**3. Entamoeba histolytica**–*E histolytica* infection of the vagina and cervix is quite common in developing countries but rare in the USA. Severe infection may resemble cervical cancer, but symptoms are chiefly due to involvement of the vulvar skin. Trophozoites of *E histolytica* may be demonstrated in wet mount preparations from the vagina or, occasionally, on a Papanicolaou smear. Because the intestinal tract is infected also, appropriate stool studies should be conducted.

**4. Desquamative inflammatory vaginitis**–This disorder demonstrates clinical and microscopic features of postmenopausal atrophic vaginitis but may develop in premenopausal women with normal estrogen levels. The cause is unknown. The primary complaint is discharge, vaginal soreness, and occasional spotting. The process is patchy and usually localized to the upper half of the vagina. The discharge contains many immature epithelial and pus cells not due to any identifiable cause. Synechiae may develop in the upper vagina, causing partial occlusion, and response to treatment is poor.

**5. Vaginal ulcers**–Most vaginal ulcers are caused by the improper use of menstrual tampons. Other causes listed previously must be excluded.

**6. Vaginitis emphysematosa**–This disorder is characterized by multiple gas-filled cystic structures on the vaginal and cervical mucosa. There is usually a concomitant infection by *G vaginalis, T vaginalis,* or both. The process is probably a rare manifestation of one or both infections, and the blebs disappear on eradication of these organisms.

**7. Nonspecific vaginitis**–Nonspecific vaginitis was defined in the past as a vaginal infection in which *C albicans, T vaginalis,* or *N gonorrhoeae* organisms were not identified. In recent years, *G vaginalis* has been considered to be the cause in many cases. Other possible causes of leukorrhea or vulvovaginitis without obvious cause are allergic states; chemical irritants; cunnilingus; and, possibly, excessive sexual activity.

### Clinical Findings

A vaginal discharge is considered abnormal by the patient if there is an increase in volume (especially if there is soiling of the clothing), an objectionable odor, or a change in consistency or color (Table 34–1). Characteristics depend on the cause. Secondary irritation of the vulvar skin may be minimal or extensive, causing pruritus or dyspareunia.

The patient should be examined as soon as possible

**Table 34–1.** Diagnosis of major causes of vaginitis.

| | Symptom | pH | Discharge | Wet Smear |
|---|---|---|---|---|
| *Candida* | Pruritus | 4.0–5.0 | Thick, curdy | Hyphae |
| *Tricho-monas* | Discharge | 5.0–7.0 | Thin, copious | Motile protozoa |
| *Gardnerella* | Odor | 4.0–6.0 | Scant, nonirritating | Clue cells |

after the onset of symptoms if not actively menstruating. She should be instructed not to douche. After a clinical history is obtained, the vulva, vagina, and cervix should be thoroughly inspected (Table 34–2). A history of previous vaginal infections may be important. The pH of secretions in the blade of the vaginal speculum should be determined, and a small amount of secretion should be placed on each of 2 glass slides. One slide should be treated with 10% warm potassium hydroxide and the other diluted with warm normal saline. A transient "fishy odor" after application of 10% potassium hydroxide is characteristic of *Gardnerella* infection; this is the so-called sniff or whiff test. White blood cells and epithelial cells will be digested, enhancing detection of the candidal pseudohyphae and spores. Motile trichomonads may be detected under low power on the saline-diluted slide. The bacteria-covered "clue cells" of *G vaginalis* should also be sought on this slide. These are epithelial cells whose cytoplasmic membrane cannot be seen because of the attached bacteria. Next, the relative number of leukocytes should be noted and the maturity of the epithelial cells determined. Secretions from the normal vagina have few leukocytes, and the epithelial cells are mature. Patients with vaginitis or cervicitis show many white blood cells, and the presence of intermediate or basal cells indicates inflammation of the vaginal epithelium. Selective cultures may be performed for trichomoniasis, bacteria, and rarely candidiasis (Figs 34–1 to 34–4).

**A. Foreign Bodies:** (See earlier) Changes in the vagina caused by improper use of vaginal tampons have been described. Symptoms of abnormal vaginal discharge and intermenstrual spotting may be secondary to drying of the vaginal mucosa, and microulceration may be detected by colposcopy. Ulcerative lesions are typically located in the vaginal fornices, and they have rolled, irregular edges with a red granulation tissue base. Regenerating epithelium at the ulcer edge may shed cells that may be interpreted as

**Table 34–2.** Diagnosis of vaginitis.

Obtain history, symptoms.
Examine vulva, vaginal walls, and cervix.
Check pH of discharge.
Prepare wet smear with saline.
Prepare potassium hydroxide smear ("sniff test").

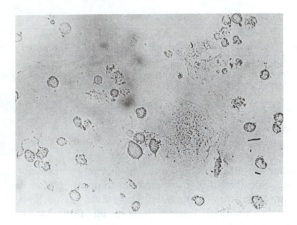

**Figure 34–1.** Saline wet mount with motile trichomonads in the center.

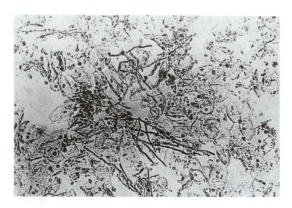

**Figure 34–3.** Saline wet mount demonstrating Candida albicans.

atypical, suggesting dysplasia. The lesions heal spontaneously after use of vaginal tampons is discontinued (Fig 34–5).

**Toxic shock syndrome** (see also Chapter 38) is the most serious complication of improper use of vaginal tampons. Symptoms consist of a high fever ≥ 38.9°C 102°F and may be accompanied by severe headache, sore throat, vomiting, and diarrhea. The disease may resemble viremia or meningitis. Progressive hypotension may occur and proceed to shock levels within 48 hours. Palmar erythema and a diffuse sunburnlike rash have also been described. Superficial desquamation of the palms and soles often follows within 2–3 weeks. Elevated blood urea nitrogen or oliguria may herald renal involvement. Cardiac dysfunction and central nervous system symptoms have also been reported. The syndrome has been linked to staphylococcal vaginal infection in healthy young women having an otherwise normal menstrual period. The skin rash usually disappears in 24–48 hours, but on occasion a patient will have a recurrent maculopapular, morbilliform eruption between the sixth and tenth days. Although it has been estimated that 70–80% of women in the USA use tampons, the incidence of toxic shock syndrome is only 6.2 per 100,000 menstruating women per year. Women who have had toxic shock syndrome are at considerable risk for recurrence and should not use tampons until it has been demonstrated that *S aureus* is eradicated from the vagina. This disease entity was not identified before 1974, and it appears to occur in women who wear a tampon continuously throughout the menstrual period.

**B. Bacterial Infections:** In the premenopausal and postmenopausal patient, the hypoestrogenic vagina is susceptible to bacterial infection characterized by discharge and spotting. Inspection of the vagina will rule out a foreign body. Microscopic examination of vaginal secretions is necessary for detection of the more common causes of vaginitis and will demonstrate intermediate and parabasal epithelial cells.

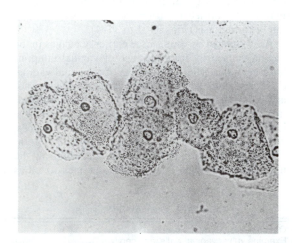

**Figure 34–2.** Saline wet mount of clue cells from Gardnerella vaginalis infection. Note the absence of inflammatory cells.

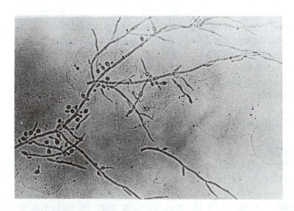

**Figure 34–4.** KOH preparation showing branched and budding Candida albicans.

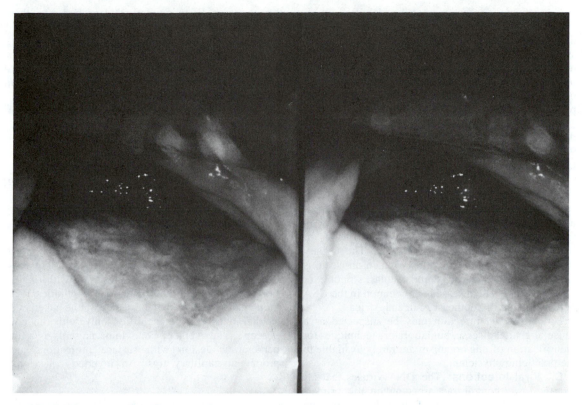

**Figure 34–5.** Colposcopic view of ulcer anterior to cervix caused by prolonged use of a vaginal tampon.

Bacterial cultures are usually not helpful because of the mixed flora without predominant organisms.

*G vaginalis* is the most common cause of bacterial vaginitis in the sexually active mature patient. The patient complains of a malodorous, nonirritating discharge, and examination reveals homogeneous, gray-white secretions with a pH of 5.0–5.5. A transient "fishy odor" may be released upon application of 10% potassium hydroxide to the vaginal secretions on a glass slide. A wet mount preparation of physiologic saline mixed with vaginal secretions should be examined under low-power and high-power objectives. There are few white blood cells and lactobacilli. The characteristic "clue cells" are identified as numerous stippled or granulated epithelial cells (see Fig 34–2). This appearance is caused by the adherence of almost uniformly spaced *G vaginalis* organisms on their surfaces. The cells may be completely or only partially covered. Clumps of *G vaginalis* organisms may also be noted attached to the edges of epithelial cells or floating free in the preparation. A gram-stained smear reveals large numbers of small gram-negative bacilli and a relative absence of lactobacilli. Cultures are seldom necessary to establish a diagnosis.

Symptoms of infection by *N gonorrhoeae* may be quite severe, but up to 85% of infected female patients have no symptoms. The incidence of the disease has risen steadily, and a prevalence of 10%, detected by cervical cultures, has been reported from family planning clinics. A 2–3% prevalence has been reported in patients served by private practitioners. The gonococcus affects primarily the glandular structures of the cervix, vulva, perineum, and anus. The cervical canal, urethra, paraurethral glands, and anus are the most commonly affected sites. Although clinically evident infection of the vagina is only transitory, it is the second most common site of a positive culture in infected patients who have had a hysterectomy. It is also a cause of vaginitis in premenarchial and postmenarchial females. In acute disease, the gram-stained smear will identify the gram-negative diplococci within leukocytes, but the diagnosis must be confirmed by culture.

A nonlubricated speculum should be inserted into the vagina and the cervix inspected. A sterile moistened swab should be inserted into the endocervix and rotated. If there is excessive cervical mucus, it should be removed before the sample is taken. A slide for gram stain is made, and the appropriate culture tube is inoculated. Other sites for culture, in order of preference, are the urethra, rectum and mouth. It is estimated that approximately 15–20% of patients with lower genital tract infection will develop an infection of the upper genital tract.

*C trachomatis* infections can be identified by recently developed tests for office use. Chlamydiazyme detects live and dead organisms from an endocervical swab, and the results are available in less than 4 hours. A similar test for gonorrhea (Gonozyme) may be prepared from the same endocervical swab. A fluorescein-labeled monoclonal antibody test is also prepared from an endocervical swab, and the result is available within 1 hour. Both types of tests reportedly demonstrate sensitivity and specificity of at least 95%. Complement fixation tests for lymphogranuloma venereum are more accurate than the Frei skin test, which is no longer used. A titer greater than 1:28 should be expected in most infected females. The disease affects primarily the vulvar tissues. Retroperitoneal lymphadenopathy may be present. The initial lesion is a transient, painless vesicular lesion or shallow ulcer at the inoculation site. The tertiary stage of the disease, when most women are seen, is characterized by anal or genital fistulas, stricture, or rectal stenosis. The disease is uncommon in the USA but is endemic in Southeast Asia and Africa.

*U urealyticum* infection may be suspected as a cause of genital disease, but laboratory techniques for identification of this organism are rarely available to the practicing physician.

**C. Viral Infections:** The DNA viruses that affect the lower genital tract are symptomatic, primarily because of involvement of the vulvar skin. Two exceptions are herpesvirus hominis and the human papillomavirus. The latter causes condylomas of the vaginal mucosa that can be confused with or related to epithelial dysplasia. The herpesvirus may cause superficial ulcerations or an exophytic necrotic mass involving the cervix, which, in turn, causes profuse vaginal discharge. The cervix may be quite tender to manipulation and may bleed easily. The primary lesion lasts 2–6 weeks and heals without scarring. Recurrent infections may also cause cervical lesions. The virus may be isolated by culture from ulcers or ruptured vesicles. Cervical cytologic examination may reveal multinucleated giant cells with intranuclear inclusions.Approximately 83% of patients will develop antibodies to herpesvirus type 2 in a minimum of 21 days following a primary infection. (See Viral Infections later.)

Herpesvirus hominis (herpes simplex) has 2 immunologic variants, type 1 and type 2, distinguished by certain biologic differences and neutralization titrations, despite the presence of across-reactive antigen. In general, type 1 virus is isolated "above the waist" and type 2 "below the waist." Approximately 10–15% of genital herpes infections are caused by type 1 virus.

Human papillomaviruses not only cause condylomatous warts of the genitalia but have also been implicated as a cause of cancer. The virus is very small and contains all its genetic information on a single molecule of DNA, but it has not been possible to culture the virus. By using viral DNA probes, more than 50 types of human papillomavirus have been identified, some of which appear to have oncogenic potential, particularly types 16 and 18.

The human papillomavirus causes condylomata acuminata of the cervix, vagina, skin of the vulva, perineum, and perianal areas. The viruses are sexually transmitted, affect the same age group as other venereal diseases, and infect both partners. The exophytic or papillomatous condyloma is the typical lesion and the only one recognized before 1976. Since that time, other varieties have been identified in the vagina, particularly by colposcopic examination (Fig 34–6). These are the flat, the "spiked," and the inverted condyloma. The flat condyloma appears as a white lesion with a somewhat granular surface; a mosaic pattern and punctation may also be present, suggesting vaginal intraepithelial neoplasia, which must be excluded by biopsy. The florid, papillomatous condyloma shows a raised white lesion with finger-like projections often containing capillaries. Although large lesions may be seen with the naked eye, smaller ones can be identified only with the colposcope. The "spiked" condyloma presents as a hyperkeratotic lesion with surface projections and prominent capillary tips. An inverted condyloma

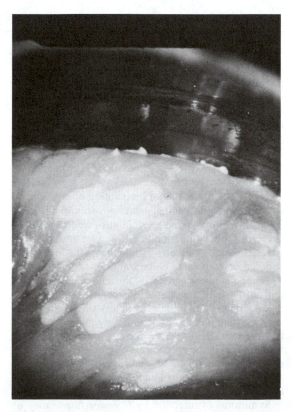

**Figure 34–6.** Vaginal condylomata acuminata as seen with a colposcope (× 13).

grows into the glands of the cervix but has not been identified on the vaginal mucosa. Condylomatous vaginitis causes a rather rough vaginal surface, demonstrating white projections from the pink vaginal mucosa.

Koilocytes are superficial or intermediate cells characterized by a large perinuclear cavity that stains only faintly. They are said to be pathognomonic of human papillomavirus infection. Careful, colposcopically directed biopsies must be taken to exclude intraepithelial neoplasia. The chief histologic difference between dysplasia and condyloma is the direction of progression of cellular atypia. In dysplasia, the dysplastic cells move toward the surface, whereas changes from condyloma progress from the epithelial surface inward toward the basal membrane.

Vaginal discharge and pruritus are the most common symptoms of florid condylomas. In addition, there may be occasional postcoital bleeding. No specific symptoms are associated with other types of condylomas. The entire lower genital tract is usually involved by subclincal or florid lesions whenever lesions are found on the vulva. Cellular immunity is lowered during pregnancy or in the diabetic or renal transplant patient, so that massive proliferation of condylomas may occur, and these are difficult to treat. Laryngeal papilloma and vulvar condylomas in infants delivered through an infected vaginal canal have been reported.

**D. Candidiasis:** Intense vulvar pruritus is the principal symptom of vaginal candidiasis and may interfere with normal activity. The symptoms correlate positively with the extent of vulvar erythema. A burning sensation may follow urination, particularly if there is maceration or excoriation of the skin from scratching. Widespread involvement of the skin adjacent to the labia may suggest an underlying metabolic problem, eg, diabetes. The labia minora may be erythematous, edematous, and excoriated. Typical thrush patches are uncommon in nonpregnant patients. Clinical manifestations tend to be more severe just prior to menstruation, and infections become refractory during pregnancy. The ubiquitous nature of the organism allows repeated infections that may be interpreted as a chronic resistant infection.

Diagnosis is based on the clinical features of the disease as well as the demonstration of candidal mycelia. Identification of *C albicans* depends on the finding of filamentous forms (pseudohyphae) of the organism (see Fig 34–4). Vaginal wall exudate is mixed in 10–20% potassium hydroxide, placed on a coverslip, and examined microscopically. The organism may be grown on Sabouraud's or Nickerson's medium in an incubator or, less well, at room temperature.

**E. Trichomonas Vaginalis Vaginitis:** Trichomoniasis tends to be worse just after menstruation or during pregnancy. Persistent leukorrhea is the principal symptom of trichomoniasis with or without sec-

ondary vulvar pruritus. Leukorrhea is characteristically profuse, extremely frothy, greenish, and, in severe cases, foul-smelling. The characteristics and volume of the discharge may be altered by douching, prior medications, or duration of disease. In chronic infections, the quantity of discharge may be decreased and the color may be gray or even light green to yellow. The pH of the vagina usually exceeds 5.0. Involvement of the vulva may be limited to the vestibule and labia minora, although a profuse discharge often causes inflammation of the labia majora, perineum, and adjacent skin surfaces. The labia minora may become edematous and tender. Urinary symptoms may occur; however, burning with urination is most often associated with severe vulvitis, particularly if there has been excoriation of the skin from scratching. Gentle inspection of the vaginal mucosa with a speculum may reveal generalized vaginal erythema with multiple small petechiae, so-called strawberry spots, which may be confused with epithelial punctation. The diagnosis is confirmed by finding characteristic motile flagellates in a wet mount preparation using physiologic saline and a drop of vaginal fluid on a slide covered with a coverslip (see Fig 34–1).

**Complications**

A solid foreign body retained in the vagina of a child over a prolonged period may erode into the bladder or rectum. Similarly, a retained vaginal pessary in an elderly patient not only causes infection but may become encrusted and erode the wall of the vagina. A spectrum of illness associated with menstrual tampon use has been described, the most severe manifestation being toxic shock syndrome.

*G vaginalis* vaginitis is accompanied by acute symptoms, but there may be no systemic manifestations or chronic complications. Two exceptions are puerperal morbidity and infection and septicemia after abdominal hysterectomy, with gaseous crepitation in the abdominal incision.

Gonorrheal infections cause acute lower tract symptoms, and the newborn may develop conjunctivitis by contamination during vaginal delivery. Ascending infection, with salpingitis, tubo-ovarian abscess, and peritonitis, may follow vaginal infection.

*C trachomatis* causes a purulent cervicitis that can be symptomatic. Recent reports, particularly from Scandinavian countries, have suggested that 50% or more of upper tract infections (salpingitis) may be due to *C trachomatis*. The infection tends to have a milder clinical course than gonococcal salpingitis but may be a significant cause of tubal occlusion and infertility. It has been suggested that atypical cytologic findings are more common in patients who have a culture-proved chlamydial cervicitis. The organism is transmitted to the male urethra, causing nongonococcal urethritis. It is also responsible for inclusion conjunctivitis of the newborn.

Lymphogranuloma venereum is characterized by

chronic lymphadenitis, rectal stricture, vulvar elephantiasis, and chronic hypertrophic changes of the vulvar skin. *Mycoplasma* infections may cause infertility, spontaneous abortion, postpartum fever, nongonococcal urethritis in men, and possibly salpingitis and pelvic abscess.

Herpesvirus infection is a major clinical problem causing the following problems: recurrent and disabling symptomatic disease, venereal transmission or infection of the newborn. The immunosuppressed patient is particularly susceptible to refractory local infection and viremia. The acquired immunodeficiency syndrome should be considered in patients with recurrent herpesvirus infections.

Cytomegalovirus infection ordinarily causes no symptoms in the maternal host, but it may be the most common cause of congenital infection; it affects the central nervous system primarily.

The various manifestations of papillomavirus infection in humans have only recently been recognized. Multifocal acute, commonly recurrent disease is often difficult to treat, particularly in the pregnant or immunosuppressed patient. Some varieties of papillomavirus are associated with dysplasia and cancer of the lower genital tract and perianal skin. Laryngeal papillomas and vulvar condylomas in infants are caused by infection contracted during vaginal delivery.

*Candida* infections tend to recur and are often interpreted as chronic refractory vulvovaginitis. The organisms are particularly difficult to eradicate during pregnancy or in the immuno-suppressed or diabetic patient. Chronic vaginal candidiasis occurs in women with human immunodeficiency virus infection.

Severe trichomonal vaginitis can lead to sufficient change in the epithelial surface of the cervix and vagina so that cytologic preparations may be interpreted as dysplastic. The infection must be treated and the cytologic study repeated.

## Prevention

Prevention is largely a matter of patient education. The adolescent girl should be instructed in feminine hygiene and the role of douches and feminine hygiene sprays explained. Immediate and long-term consequences of exposure to sexually transmitted diseases should be part of the educational curriculum for all adolescents. Care must be taken in selection of a sexual partner, and barrier-type contraception may be helpful.

## Treatment

**A. General Measures:** Coitus should be avoided until cure has been achieved—or a condom should be used, especially if there are frequent recurrences of infection. The sexual partner also should be treated if infection is repeated. Associated vulvar pruritus may be treated with local applications of corticosteroid lotion or nonoily cream. Cornstarch or talcum powder may prevent or alleviate chafing.

**B. Local Nonspecific Measures:** During a period of specific treatment, the external genitalia should be kept clean by gentle sponging. Dryness must be encouraged and may be accomplished with a hair dryer. Tight-fitting or synthetic fiber clothing should not be worn. Occasional douching with a dilute vinegar solution (60 mL of white vinegar to 1 L of warm water) may improve the patient's sense of well-being. This rarely causes irritation. Excessive douching often increases secretion of mucus and compounds the problem.

**C. Surgical Measures:** Cauterization incision of Skene's glands, or marsupialization of a Bartholin duct cyst may be required to eradicate a focus of infection. Cancer must first be ruled out.

**D. Specific Measures:*** Treat infections with specific drugs, including those listed below. If sensitivity develops, discontinue medication and substitute another drug as soon as practicable. When necessary, continue treating the patient during menstruation. Refractory patients may respond to vaginal acidification using Aci-jel.

**1. Foreign bodies–**Treatment consists of complete removal of the foreign body. Rarely, specific systemic antibiotics may be administered for ulceration or cellulitis of the vagina or vulva.

Dryness or ulceration of the vagina secondary to use of menstrual tampons is transient and heals spontaneously. Ulcers have been observed also in women who have worn tampons between menstrual periods for excessive vaginal discharge. **Toxic shock syndrome** should be suspected in any menstruating woman with a sudden onset of febrile illness. The tampon should be removed, cultures prepared, and the vagina thoroughly cleansed to decrease the inoculum of responsible organisms. Appropriate supportive measures should be instituted and a β-lactamaseresistant penicillin administered to those not allergic to the drug. Recovered patients are prone to recurrence and should discontinue use of tampons.

**2. Atrophic vaginitis–**In most women, an atrophic vagina is asymptomatic. Symptoms may be due to secondary bacterial infection or dyspareunia. Treatment includes intravaginal application of an estrogen cream. Because approximately one-third of the estrogen will be absorbed into the systemic circulation, such treatment may be contraindicated in patients who have had cancer of the breast or endometrium. Insertion of one-half to 1 applicatorful of cream each night for 1 week may cause breast tenderness. Maturation of the vaginal mucosa ordinarily eradicates a bacterial infection but may predispose the patient to a secondary trichomonal or candidal vaginitis. Instillation approximately twice weekly thereafter should maintain the vaginal mucosa. If

---

*Gonorrhea is discussed in Chapter 38.

there are no contraindications, systemic estrogens therapy should be considered.

### 3. Bacterial infections–

**a. G vaginalis–**The treatment of choice for *G vaginalis* is oral metronidazole, 500 mg twice daily for 6 days. A single dose of 2 g has proved effective in treatment of adolescent patients, but in general a 5- to 7-day course of treatment is more effective. Although it is recommended that sexual partners be treated simultaneously, it is unclear whether this significantly decreases the incidence of recurrent disease. Contraindications to metronidazole include certain blood dyscrasias and central nervous system diseases. An important side effect is intolerance to alcohol. The drug is contraindicated during early pregnancy and lactation.

Cephradine, 500 mg by mouth 4 times daily for 6 days, will eliminate *G vaginalis* from the vagina and relieve symptoms but has little effect on the anaerobic flora of the vagina. Other oral and vaginal preparations have been prescribed but have not proved useful. Douching removes malodorous secretions temporarily but does not cure the infection.

**b. C trachomatis–**If a purulent cervicitis suggests *C trachomatis* endocervicitis, the diagnosis can be confirmed by one of the office tests. A concurrent gonococcal infection should be considered. If the patient is not pregnant, tetracycline, 500 mg 4 times daily; minocycline, 50 mg 2 times daily; or doxycycline, 100 mg 2 times daily, should be administered by mouth for 7–10 days. If the patient is allergic to tetracycline or is pregnant, then erythromycin, 500 mg 4 times daily for 10 days, is acceptable. The cervix should be recultured after treatment. It should be remembered that *C trachomatis* has been implicated as a causative agent in salpingitis.

If treatment of mycoplasmal infection is indicated, the tetracyclines are the most useful drugs. Demeclocycline and doxycycline are recommended. Therapeutic doses should be administered to the patient and her sexual partner for 10 days.

### 4. Viral infections–

**a. Herpesvirus hominis–**The symptoms of herpesvirus hominis infection are due to lesions of the vaginal introitus or skin of the vulva and perineum. Rarely, a necrotizing cervicitis that may ascend into the uterine cavity causes leukorrhea. Disseminated disease is unusual except in a newborn or an immunosuppressed patient. Therapy is discussed later under Viral Infections of the Vulva & Vagina.

**b. Condylomata acuminata–**Condylomata acuminata are manifestations of infection of the lower genital tract with a human papillomavirus. One should anticipate infection of cells of the entire tract from the cervix to the vulvar and perianal skin. Before treatment, the entire area should be inspected with a colposcope. Lesions may ascend into the anal canal or urethral meatus. The virus is present in normal cells as well as those involved in condylomatous growths. For that reason, recurrence after treatment is common. Cure of clinically identifiable disease probably depends on the responsiveness of the patient's immune system. On gross examination, condylomas cannot always be distinguished from dysplastic warts. Therefore, biopsy of one or more lesions may be useful. Condylomas of the cervix should always undergo colposcopically directed biopsy. Treatment is the same as that for cervical dysplasia.

Prior to treatment, other causes of vaginitis should be sought and treated. The genital area should be kept clean and dry. Diabetes, if present, should be well controlled. Prevention of recurrence is difficult in patients who are immunosuppressed or receiving long-term corticosteroid treatment.

Condylomas of the vagina are usually multifocal, and colposcopic examination is essential to determine the extent of disease. The mucosa readily absorbs drugs instilled into the vagina, and the rectum and bladder may be adversely affected by vigorous treatment. Bichloracetic acid or trichloracetic acid is the treatment of choice. A 50% solution can be used in the vagina and on the cervix. If an 80% solution is used on the vulva, one must be careful not to use excessive amounts, which might burn the normal skin.

Fluorouracil cream 5% is effective in treating dysplasia and carcinoma in situ of the vagina and in eradicating condylomatous warts, particularly early lesions. The warts are sensitive to this medication, and one course of treatment is usually sufficient. The patient is reexamined several days after the first course, and a second course may be instituted if necessary. Before application of the intravaginal cream, the vaginal introitus should be liberally lubricated with petroletum. This therapy should not be employed in pregnancy because of the known fetotoxic effects.

Cryosurgery, electrosurgery, simple surgical excision, and laser vaporization may be used in the vagina for a localized lesion. The advantages of this approach are immediate reduction in size of the antigenic mass and removal of contagious material.

Florid growth of vaginal condylomas during pregnancy may necessitate cesarean section to avoid bleeding and soft tissue dystocia. In addition, laryngeal papillomas and vulvar condylomas of the offspring may follow vaginal delivery. Acetic acid treatment, as described earlier, should be utilized in the last 4 weeks to avoid cesarean section if possible. Electrocoagulation, cryotherapy, or laser therapy should be used before 32 weeks' gestation to avoid posttreatment necrosis lasting as long as 4–6 weeks.

The long-term course of untreated vaginal condylomas is unknown. In any event, spontaneous resolution occasionally occurs within 12–24 months. In some clinics, treatment is not prescribed unless there are symptoms or evidence (from a biopsy specimen) of atypia for which treatment would be the same as that for vaginal intraepithelial neoplasia. Use of a condom should assist in the prevention of viral transmission to sexual partners.

**5. Candida albicans vaginitis**–Treatment is limited to patients with symptoms who have *Candida* organisms present. Short-term or irregular and erratic treatment is often unsuccessful. Infection in a postmenopausal or breast-feeding woman or premenarcheal child may be an indicator of diabetes. The blood glucose in diabetics should be controlled, and complicating medications, eg, systemic antibiotics, should be discontinued. Nonabsorbent undergarments must not be worn, and self-medication and feminine hygiene products should be discontinued. The sexual partner should be examined in all instances of poor response to treatment, and intercourse should be discontinued unless a condom is used. Therapy for acute symptomatic vulvovaginitis should be modified in chronic or resistant cases (Fig 34–7).

Anti-*Candida* preparations must be applied topically to be effective. The following drugs are useful in treatment of acute vaginal candidiasis.

**a.** Clotrimazole, 1% cream (Gyne-Lotrimin or Mycelex-G), 1 applicatorful (about 5 g) inserted high in the vaginal canal at bedtime for 7 nights. Treatment may be extended to 14 or more days in chronic, refractory cases. The cream should also be applied to the vulvar skin 3 or 4 times daily for pruritus. One vaginal tablet (100 mg) may be substituted for the cream; it is less messy but may be less effective. Two tablets inserted nightly 3 times may be as effective as 7 days of treatment with 1 tablet. Recently, a one-night treatment consisting of a 500-mg clotrimazole tablet has been recommended. The tablet's lactic acid component produces a high level of acidity that increases the degree and duration of fungicidal activity. The drug dissolves in the vagina and remains active in secretions for 3–4 days. Treatment, if given for more than 1 day, is continued without interruption during menstruation. Medication is contraindicated in women who have shown hypersensitivity to any component of the preparation.

**b.** Miconazole nitrate, 2% (Monistat 7 Vaginal Cream), 1 applicatorful placed high in the vagina each night for 7 applications. A 100-mg miconazole suppository may be substituted for the cream. A 200-mg suppository inserted intravaginally, once daily at bedtime for 3 consecutive nights, is reportedly as effective as longer treatment.

**c.** Butoconazole nitrate, 2% (Femstat Vaginal Cream), 1 applicatorful placed high in the vagina at bedtime for 3–5 nights.

**d.** Terconazole, 0.4% (Terazol 7 Vaginal Cream), 1 applicatorful vaginally at bedtime for 7 nights. Terconazole, 80 mg (Terazol 3 Vaginal Suppositories), may also be used, 1 suppository vaginally at bedtime for 3 nights.

Clotrimazole, miconazole, butoconazole, and terconazole have not been studied during the first trimester of pregnancy. Nystatin, 100,000 unit (Mycostatin Vaginal Tablets), 1 tablet vaginally at bedtime for 2 weeks, may be used during the first trimester. Patients who have demonstrated sensitivity to clotrimazole or miconazole products may be treated with boric acid powder, 600 mg in a gelatin capsule. One capsule is placed high in the vagina each night for 2 weeks or nightly for 1 week followed by twice weekly for 3 weeks.

*Candida* vulvitis usually responds to topical applications of clotrimazole cream. If this is not successful, a topical corticosteroid cream (Mycolog, Lotrisone) reduces the inflammatory reaction and relieves itching. Lotrisone contains a potent corticosteroid and

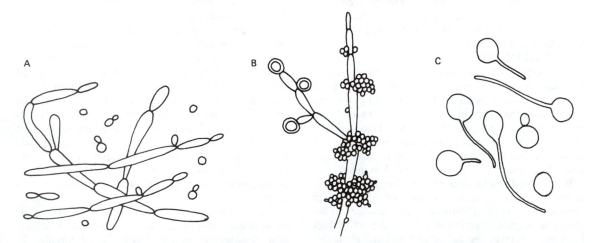

**Figure 34–7.** *Candida albicans.* **A:** Blastospores and pseudohyphae in exudate. **B:** Blastospores, pseudohyphae, and conidia in culture at 20°C. **C:** Young culture forms germ tubes when placed in serum for 3 hours at 37°C. (Reproduced with permission, from Brooks GF, Butel JS, Ornston LN: *Jawetz, Melinick, & Adelberg's Medical Microbiology,* 19th ed. Appleton & Lange, 1991.)

should not be used extensively on pregnant patients, in large amounts, or for prolonged periods of time. Adverse reactions to topical anesthetics outweigh the possible benefits of use for relief of symptoms. Gentian violet, while effective treatment for *Candida*, causes such discoloration of tissues and clothing that it is generally poorly accepted by patients.

Chronic and recurring infections may be a result of decreased host immunity or reinfection. There is no uniformly successful treatment plan. It has been suggested that treatment of *C albicans* in the digestive tract would decrease the incidence of recurrence; however, controlled studies have not confirmed that suggestion. Estrogen treatment of postmenopausal patients may precipitate or aggravate recurrent candidiasis. Some studies have implicated oral contraceptives as a predisposing factor. Systemic antibiotics, particularly tetracycline, increase the number of candidal organisms in the lower bowel and vagina. Organisms in the preputial folds of the clitoris and the partner's foreskin may be a source of reinfection. Therapeutic alternatives are (1) prolonged treatment beyond the usual 7- to 14-day regimen, (2) self-medication for 3–5 days at the first evidence of symptoms, or (3) prophylactic treatment for several days before each menstrual period or during antibiotic therapy. Periodic examination is necessary to demonstrate that recurrent infections are in fact due to *Candida*. A recent report suggests that recurrent symptomatic infections may, in some instances, be due to *Candida tropicalis*, an organism resistant to imidazole drugs. Ketoconazole, an oral antimycotic, is under investigation. Acidification of the vagina is a valuable option for chronic or recurrent infections.

**6. Trichomonas vaginalis vaginitis**–Because there are inaccessible foci of trichomonads in the urinary tracts of both sexes, a systemic agent is indicated. Most men with affected sexual partners also harbor the organism but are asymptomatic. For this reason, both partners should be treated simultaneously. Meanwhile, intercourse should be avoided unless a condom is used. Douching may temporarily remove odorous secretions and relieve symptoms. Metronidazole is the only systemic agent approved for use in the USA (Fig 34–8).

**a. Metronidazole (Flagyl, Protostat)**–Both partners should be treated simultaneously with metronidazole, one 250-mg tablet orally 3 times daily for 7 days. A 1-day treatment regimen that may be as effective consists of administration of 2 g in a single dose. In resistant cases, which most likely are reinfection, oral courses of metronidazole may be repeated after 4–6 weeks if the presence of trichomonads has been confirmed and the white blood cell and differential counts are normal. An undesirable side effect is nausea or emesis with alcohol consumption. Moreover, approximately 2% of patients report the onset of nausea several hours after administration of metronidazole alone. Contraindications to metronidazole

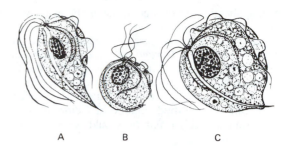

**Figure 34–8.** *Trichomonas vaginalis* as found in vaginal and prostatic secretions. **A:** Normal trophozoite. **B:** Round form after division. **C:** Common form seen in stained preparation. Cysts not found. (Reproduced with permission, from Brooks GF, Butel JS, Ornston LN: *Jawetz, Melinick, & Adelberg's Medical Microbiology,* 19th ed. Appleton & Lange, 1991.)

include certain blood dyscrasias and central nervous system diseases. Administration is contraindicated during early pregnancy and lactation. An oncogenic effect has been demonstrated in animals but not in human beings.

**b. Other drugs**–Patients who develop side effects from metronidazole may be treated with antitrichomonal suppositories (eg, Vagisec Plus [polyoxyethylene nonyl phenol, aminacrine, sodium edetate, and docusate sodium]), one inserted deep into the vagina twice daily for 2 weeks and then for at least 1 week after no organisms are identified on a vaginal smear. Although temporary relief of symptoms may be achieved, complete cure is seldom attained.

**7. Cervicitis**–Treatment depends on the etiologic agent. If an organism is identified, it should be treated specifically. Purulent cervicitis without an identifiable cause may be secondary to *C trachomatis* infection and can be treated with tetracycline or erythromycin. An occasional patient may require cryosurgery, cautery, or carbon dioxide laser vaporization after a premalignant or malignant lesion has been excluded by cytologic examination and coloscopy and has indicated biopsies including an endocervical curettage.

**8. Mucorrhea and epithelial discharge**–Excessive but normal vaginal discharge from severe cervical ectropion, vaginal adenosis, or vaginal epithelial surface should be treated by reassurance. Continuous use of a vagina tampon could be dangerous. Occasional douching may help control the discharge and relieve symptoms. Cryosurgery or carbon dioxide laser treatment of the cervix is occasionally beneficial.

**9. Other causes**–Pinworm and *Entamoeba histolytica* infestations of the vagina are treated specifically.

Desquamative inflammatory vaginitis in a patient with normal ovarian activity is a diagnosis of exclusion. Treatment has not been defined but has included local applications of estrogenic, antibiotic, and corticosteroid preparations.

Vaginitis emphysematosa is a manifestation of vaginitis caused by *G vaginalis* or *T vaginalis* and should be treated specifically with metronidazole.

The diagnosis of nonspecific vaginitis is seldom justified, but in an occasional patient no specific cause can be identified. Emotional factors causing psychosomatic vulvovaginitis should be considered in the history.

**E. Treatment Failure:** Persistent leukorrhea in spite of apparently adequate therapy requires complete reevaluation to detect recurrent or persistent disease or to establish a new diagnosis. Factors that compromise host defenses or modify the normal physiology of the vagina must be assessed and the sexual partners examined.

## Prognosis

An orderly approach to the diagnosis of the bacterial, candidal, or protozoal causes of leukorrhea and appropriate specific treatment, when available, should lead to cure. Viral infections, on the other hand, cannot be treated specifically, and the long-term serious consequences to the patient and her offspring pose significant clinical problems that cannot be resolved at this time. Improvement in laboratory technology and availability of diagnostic studies will prove or disprove the suggested roles of some currently recognized organisms and will identify others.

## PRINCIPLES OF DIAGNOSIS OF VULVAR DISEASES

A complete history of potential causes of vulvar irritation such as creams, powders, soaps, type of underware, and cleansing techniques should be noted. Careful inspection, palpation, and liberal use of colposcopy or magnifying glass is followed by biopsy of any suspicious areas, lesions, or discolorations.

## Pruritus

Pruritus is the most common symptom of vulvar disease. The term pruritus vulvae denotes intense itching of the vulvar skin and mucous membranes due to any cause. Specific diagnosis depends on a thorough history, a physical examination that includes inspection of all body surfaces, and, in most instances, an adequate biopsy.

## Ulceration, Tumor, Dystrophy

Ulcerative lesions suggest a granulomatous sexually transmitted disease or cancer. Therefore, appropriate tests for sexually transmitted disease should be conducted along with biopsy to rule out primary or coexisting cancer. Well-circumscribed solid tumors should be excised widely and submitted for micro-

scopic examination. Diffuse, dystrophic white lesions may demonstrate great histologic variability. A colposcope should be used to select the most suitable biopsy sites. A satisfactory full-thickness biopsy of the skin and tumor can be obtained with a dermatologic punch biopsy instrument under local anesthesia.

## Abnormalities of Pigmentation

The color of vulvar skin or lesions depends principally upon the vascularity of the dermis, the thickness of the overlying epidermis, and the amount of intervening pigment, either melanin or blood pigments. A dystrophic lesion of the vulva may have a white appearance due primarily to a decrease in vascularity **(lichen sclerosus et atrophicus)** or an increase in the keratin layer **(lichen simplex chronicus)** that has undergone maceration from the increased moisture in the vulvar area. During the acute phase of lichen sclerosus, the vulvar skin is moderately erythematous. As the lesion matures, it becomes hyperkeratotic and develops a typical white appearance resembling cigarette paper. The epidermal thickening of neoplasia obscures the underlying vasculature and, in conjunction with the macerating effect of the moist environment, usually produces a hyperplastic white lesion. A diffuse white lesion of the vulva is also produced by loss or absence of melanin pigmentation, eg, **vitiligo**, a heredity disorder. **Leukoderma** is a localized white lesion resulting from transient loss of pigment in a residual scar after healing of an ulcer.

A red lesion results from thinning or ulceration of the epidermis, the vasodilatation of inflammation or an immune response, or the neovascularization of neoplasia. With ulceration of the epithelium, there is loss of areas of epidermis, and the vascular dermis is apparent. Acute candidal vulvovaginitis, as seen in diabetic patients, is a typical example of vulvar erythema secondary to inflammation and the local immune response. One variety of invasive epidermoid cancer is characterized by a velvety red lesion that spreads over the vulvar skin. **Psoriasis and Paget's disease** are other examples of diseases that produce basically red lesions.

Dark lesions are due to an increased amount or concentration of melanin or blood pigments. These may occur after trauma. A persistent dark lesion on the vulvar skin or mucosa is usually either a nevus or a melanoma. **Melanosis**, or lentigo, is a benign, darkly pigmented, flat lesion that may be confused with a melanoma. In the occasional case of carcinoma in situ of the vulvar skin, atypical squamous cells are unable to contain the melanin pigment. As a consequence, it is concentrated in local macrophages, causing dark coloration of the tumor. Vulvar skin may darken following the use of estrogen cream applied to the vulva and vagina for the treatment of vaginitis or after oral contraceptive use.

## VASCULAR & LYMPHATIC DISEASES OF THE VULVA & VAGINA

The vulva and vagina have a rich vascular and lymphatic supply. These channels may undergo obstruction, dilatation, rupture, or infection or may develop tumorous lesions, which are usually malformations rather than true neoplasms.

### Varicosities

Varicosities of the vulva involve one or more veins. Severe varicosities of the legs and vulva may be aggravated during pregnancy. Symptomatic vulvar varices in a patient who is not pregnant are uncommon and may indicate vascular disease in the pelvis, either primary or secondary to tumor masses. Regardless of the cause, varicosities may cause considerable discomfort, consisting of pain and a sense of heaviness, and a large mass of veins may be apparent. Rupture of a vulvar varicosity during pregnancy may cause profuse hemorrhage. Acute thrombosis or phlebitis usually causes acute pain and tenderness. An examination should be performed with the patient in the standing position, which distends the veins; otherwise, the correct diagnosis may not be considered.

Treatment of vulvar and vaginal varicosities is seldom necessary, although symptoms might be quite severe during pregnancy. Support clothing such as panty hose or leotards usually provides effective support, even in pregnant patients. Operation is usually necessary only for rupture and hemorrhage, which are rare. Swelling tends to decrease considerably after the 36th week of pregnancy. Management of the pregnancy should be guided by ordinary obstetric principles. Vaginal delivery is usually advisable.

### Edema

The loose integument of the vulva predisposes to edema from a variety of causes. Vascular or lymphatic obstruction may be the result of neoplasm or infection such as lymphogranuloma venereum, which can cause extensive lymphatic obstruction and gross deformity of the vulvar tissues. If resolution does not occur after specific antibiotic treatment, vulvectomy may be indicated.

Accidental trauma from a bicycle accident in a young girl or a blow or kick to the pudendum may cause painful swelling. An ice pack applied to the perineum after acute trauma tends to retard the development of edema; 1–2 days later, warm packs or sitz baths assist in resolution of the associated inflammation or hematoma.

Severe vulvar edema may be associated with systemic disorders that cause generalized edema, eg, congestive heart failure, nephrotic syndrome, or pre-eclampsia-eclampsia. Acute edema may be a manifestation of a systemic allergic reaction or local contact dermatitis. Dependent edema is occasionally seen in neurologic patients confined to bed.

### Hematoma

The vulva has a rich blood supply, and the unusually distensible tissues often do not limit hemorrhage when a vessel is ruptured. Blunt trauma to the vulva, particularly in the pregnant patient, results in rapid development of hematoma and associated edema. An ice pack should be applied to the perineum after acute trauma. However, if a hematoma is not self-limiting and continues to expand, the area should be incised, specific bleeders ligated, and the wound packed but left unsutured. There are usually multiple bleeding sites, and ligation of individual bleeding points is ordinarily not curative. Antibiotics should be administered on an individual basis depending on the amount of tissue trauma and contamination from the original traumatic event.

### Granuloma Pyogenicum

Pyogenic granuloma is considered to be a varient of capillary hemangioma. It is usually single, raised, and dull red and seldom exceeds 2 cm in size (Fig 34–9). It is important because it tends to bleed easily when traumatized. Wide excision biopsy is indicated

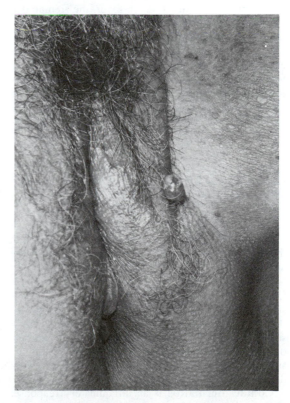

**Figure 34–9.** Pyogenic granuloma.

to alleviate symptoms and to rule out malignant melanoma.

## Senile Hemangioma

Senile hemangiomas are usually multiple small, dark blue, asymptomatic papules discovered incidentally during examination of an older patient. Excision biopsy is indicated only if they bleed repeatedly.

## Hemangiomas in Children

Childhood hemangiomas, usually diagnosed in the first few months of life, may vary in size from small strawberry hemangiomas to large cavernous ones. They tend to be elevated and bright red or dark, depending on their size and the thickness of the overlying skin. Those that tend to increase in size during the first few months of life are most likely to become static or regress without therapy after about age 1½.

Although most of these tumors can be observed without treatment, larger ones require dermatologic consultation regarding therapy.

## Lymphangioma

Lymphangiomas are tumors of lymphatic vessels and may be difficult to differentiate microscopically from hemangiomas unless blood cells are present within the vessels. **Lymphangioma cavernosum** may cause a diffuse enlargement of one side of the vulva and extend down over the remainder of the vulva and perineum. If the tumor is sufficiently large, it should be surgically excised. **Lymphangioma simplex** tumors (circumscription tumors) are usually small, soft, white or purple nodules or small wartlike lesions most frequently seen on the labia majora. Lymphangiomas are usually asymptomatic, but on occasion an associated pruritus or formication may be intense and the involved skin must be excised.

## DISORDERS OF OTHER SYSTEMS WITH VULVAR MANIFESTATIONS

## Leukemia

Nodular infiltration and ulceration of the vulva and the rectovaginal septum occasionally occur with acute leukemia.

## Dermatologic Disorders

Recurrent ulcerations of the mucous membranes of the mouth and vagina may be a manifestation of **disseminated lupus erythematosus**. Bullous eruptions of apparently normal skin and mucous membrane surfaces of the vulva may be one of the first evidences of **pemphigus vulgaris**.

**Contact dermatitis** is an inflammatory response of the vulvar tissues to agents that may either be locally irritating or induce sensitivity upon contact. The local reaction to a systematically administered drug is termed **dermatitis medicamentosa**.

**Psoriasis** is a chronic relapsing dermatosis that may also affect the scalp, the extensor surfaces of the extremities, the trunk, and the vulva. The vulvar skin may be the only body surface affected, and the lesions appear typically erythematous, resembling fungal infection, but without the silver scaly crusts that occur on the other parts of the body (Fig 34–10).

An underlying adenocarcinoma may occasionally be associated with **acanthosis nigricans**, a benign hyperpigmented lesion characterized by papillomatous hypertrophy. Pseudoacanthosis nigricans is a benign process that may appear on the skin of the vulva and inner thighs in obese and darkly pigmented women.

**Intergrigo** is an inflammatory reaction involving the genitocrural folds or the skin under the abdominal panniculus. It is common in obese patients and results from persistent moistness of the skin surfaces. An associated superficial fungal or bacterial infection may be present. The area appears either erythematous or white from maceration. Measures that promote dryness, eg, absorbent cotton undergarments and dusting with cornstarch powder, may be helpful.

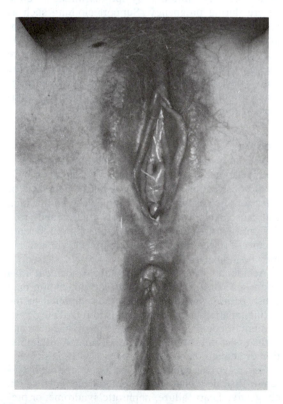

**Figure 34–10.** Typical lesions of psoriasis with a sharp outline and bright red surface.

## Diabetes Mellitus

Diabetes mellitus is the systemic disease most commonly associated with chronic pruritus vulvae. It has been suggested that half of diabetic women develop chronic vulvitis sufficiently characteristic to be designated **diabetic vulvitis**. The cause is a chronic vulvovaginal candidiasis. Thus, diabetes mellitus must be considered in any patient who responds poorly to treatment of vulvovaginal candidiasis. Glycosuria is apparently not necessary to produce diabetic vulvitis. A 2-hour postprandial blood sugar or glucose tolerance test may be necessary to detect otherwise asymptomatic diabetes. If the condition persists without control of the systemic disorder, the skin will often undergo lichenification and secondary bacterial infection. Chronic dermatitis may develop that is compatible with lichen simplex chronicus (neurodermatitis). On occasion, bacterial infection may result in acute vulvar abscesses, chronic subcutaneous abscesses, and draining sinuses. These may be unresponsive to therapy if the diabetes is not controlled. Management of the acute phase consists of control of the metabolic disorder and specific therapy for candidiasis.

## Behçet's Syndrome

Behçet's syndrome is a rare disorder of unknown cause characterized by recurrent oral and genital ulcerations. The ulcers are preceded by small vesicles or papules and last for a variable period of time. Ocular lesions begin as superficial inflammation and may proceed to iridocyclitis and even blindness. Monarticular arthritis and central nervous system symptoms are manifestations of severe disease. The syndrome may be an expression of vasculitis or perhaps of collagen disease rather than of viral infection—an earlier theory. Behçet's syndrome, together with disseminated lupus erythematosus and pemphigus, is included in the differential diagnosis of recurrent aphthous ulcers of the oral or vaginal mucosa. There is no specific therapy—only palliative treatment. Systemic corticosteroids have provided the most consistent relief. Patients with Behçet's syndrome require consultation and long-term management by a dermatologist.

## VIRAL INFECTIONS OF THE VULVA & VAGINA

Systemic viral infections in children, eg, varicella and rubeola, may involve the skin and mucosa of the vulva. The principal viruses that affect the vulva and vagina are DNA viruses, primarily of the herpesvirus, poxvirus, and papovavirus types. In adults, the principal viral infections of the lower genital tract are herpes genitalis, herpes zoster, molluscum contagiosum, condyloma acuminatum.

## 1. HERPES GENITALIS

Herpesvirus hominis infection of the lower genital tract (herpes genitalis) may be the most common sexually transmitted disease. It has been reported that about 10% of women seen in private practice demonstrate serologic evidence of prior exposure to the virus. The infection is acquired in early adult life with the onset of sexual activity. Approximately 85% of primary infections are secondary to herpesvirus hominis type 2, and the remainder are caused by type 1. Despite the presence of adequate humoral and cell-mediated immunity, the DNA viruses of the herpes group reactivate periodically. Between recurrent infections, the virus persists in a latent phase in sensory sacral ganglia. Type 2 virus has been recovered from the cervices of asymptomatic women and from the urethras and prostates of asymptomatic men. Transmission to a sexual partner or newborn can occur in the absence of symptoms. The virus frequently is associated with other sexually transmitted diseases.

Herpetic genital infection is either primary or secondary. The incubation period of primary infection is 2–7 days. Prodomal symptoms of tingling or itching occur shortly before vesicular eruptions appear. The vesicles erode rapidly, resulting in painful ulcers distributed in small patches, or they may involve most of the vulvar surfaces (Fig 34–11). Urinary symptoms develop, eg, dysuria or even urinary retention that requires catheter drainage of the bladder. Bilateral inguinal adenopathy, fever, and malaise accompany severe infections. Herpetic cervicitis causes a profuse watery discharge. Rarely, disseminated infection follows a primary herpesvirus type 2 genital infection. Considering the number of women who have positive herpes antibody titers, the initial infection in some must be asymptomatic. Lesions may persist for 2–6 weeks, after which healing occurs without scarring. Virus can be removed from vesicle fluid during the acute phase, but organisms usually cannot be recovered by 2 weeks after healing of the primary lesions. Approximately 85% of patients develop antibodies to type 2 virus within 21 days of primary infection.

Type 2 virus is much more likely to cause recurrent genital disease than is type 1. Recurrent symptomatic disease is more frequent in men than in women, although clinical recurrence may not be as easily detectable in women. Approximately 50% of patients will have a recurrence within 6 months of primary infection; the median time to recurrence in women is approximately 40–45 days. Virus is usually not recoverable within 7 days after healing of recurrent lesions.

In recurrent disease, ulcers tend to be smaller, fewer in number, and confined to one area of the vulva, vagina, or cervix. Extragenital sites, such as fingers, buttocks, and trunk (**eczema herpeticum**), have been described. Prodromal symptoms of itching and burning at the site of future lesions and occasion-

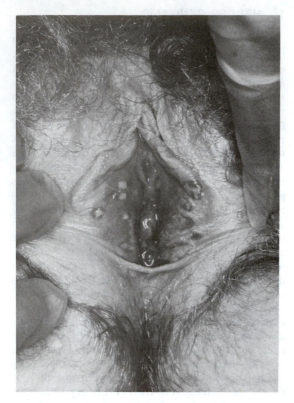

**Figure 34–11.** Ulcerating vesicles of herpes genitalis.

ally pain radiating to the back and down the legs have been reported. Inguinal adenopathy and systemic symptoms ordinarily do not recur. Healing is usually complete in 1–3 weeks. Why periodic active viral replication causes shedding of infectious virus and recurrent or reactivated clinical disease is unknown. Exogenous factors known to contribute to reactivation of herpesvirus include fever, emotional stress, and menstruation. Immunosuppressed patients are prone to develop extensive local disease and systemic dissemination. Whether frequent coitus promotes recurrent disease is unknown.

Primary infection can usually be distinguished from recurrent disease on the basis of history and clinical findings. Virus is easily recoverable from the acute lesion—if facilities for virus culture are available. Otherwise, a scraping taken from the ulcer and stained as a Papanicolaou smear often will demonstrate characteristic giant cells indicative of viral infection. Nonetheless, these may be confused with malignant cells even by a pathologist. Other cells demonstrate a homogeneous "ground-glass" appearance of cellular nuclei with numerous small intracellular, scattered basophilic particles and acidophilic inclusion bodies. Unsuspected disease is occasionally detected incidentally on a cervical or vaginal smear. The sensitivity of such smears is about 50%.

Several immunologic assays for detecting herpesvirus antigen have been developed. Viral particles in vesicular lesions can be identified with electron microscopy. Serologic tests are best utilized to determine whether the patient has been infected in the past. A 4-fold or higher increase in neutralizing or complement fixation antibody titers between acute and convalescent sera may be useful to document a primary infection. Only 5% of patients with recurrent infection demonstrate a 4-fold or higher rise in antibody titer.

It is estimated that the incidence of neonatal herpes simplex virus infection ranges from 1 in 5000 to 1 in 20,000 live births. Infection in the newborn is associated with a mortality rate of 60% and at least one-half of the survivors have significant neurologic or ocular sequelae, or both. The risk of infection for an infant born vaginally to a mother with a primary genital infection is 40–50%, and the risk in the presence of a recurrent infection is estimated to be 5%. However, most infants who develop a herpetic infection are born to women with no history or clinical evidence of active infection during pregnancy. Therefore, it is difficult to identify women whose infants are in jeopardy. It is recommended that, at the initial prenatal interview, all patients be asked whether or not they or their sexual contacts are known to have had genital herpetic lesions. Recommendations for management of potentially infected patients are in the process of change; therefore, consultation should be sought for current opinion concerning this problem.

The lesions of herpesvirus infection are self-limiting, and they heal spontaneously unless they become secondarily infected. Symptomatic treatment includes good genital hygiene, loose-fitting undergarments, cool compresses or sitz baths, and oral analgesics. Local analgesics are contraindicated because they may cause severe contact dermatitis. Indications for hospitalization for management of a severe primary infection are urinary retention, severe headache or other systemic symptoms, temperature greater than 101°F (38.3°C), or possibly a large number of lesions. Immunosuppressed patients are prone to systemic dissemination and should be managed carefully. In the hospitalized patient, acyclovir may be given intravenously. Reportedly, these patients become virus-free, heal, and are pain-free sooner than untreated patients. Patients not requiring hospitalization may be treated with oral or topical acyclovir. Treatment has not been shown to prevent recurrent episodes of genital herpes. Acyclovir has not been approved for use in pregnancy.

Recurrent herpes can be treated with either topical or oral acyclovir. Oral acyclovir prevents or reduces the frequency and severity of recurrence in the majority of patients studied.

Avoidance of direct contact with active lesions is one sure way to prevent spread of the disease. However, contact with an individual with subclinical disease must result in some primary infections. The general rules for prevention of dissemination are as follows: (1) Precautions are unnecessary in the absence of active lesions. (2) Small lesions situated away from the oral or vaginal orifices may be covered with adhesive or paper tape during coitus. (3) In the presence of active lesions, whether or not the partner contracts the disease depends on previous exposure to herpes. A nonimmune partner usually will be infected. If a regular partner has had genital herpes or has not been infected after prolonged exposure, no precautions will be necessary. If a casual partner has had a history of genital herpes, a contraceptive cream or foam should be used, followed by genital cleansing with soap and water. If a partner has no past history of genital herpes, a condom should be used but may be of limited value.

## 2. HERPES ZOSTER
### (Shingles)

Zoster is an inflammatory disorder in which a painful eruption of groups of vesicles is distributed over an area of skin corresponding to the course of one or more peripheral sensory nerves.The causative agent is varicella zoster virus. The lesion is commonly unilateral and not infrequently attacks one buttock or thigh or the vulva on one side. The vesicles may rupture and crust over, although they usually dry, forming a scab that ultimately separates. The primary purposes of treatment are alleviation of pain, resolution of vesicles, and prevention of secondary infection and ulceration.

## 3. MOLLUSCUM CONTAGIOSUM

These benign epithelial virus-induced tumors are dome-shaped, often umbilicated, and vary in size up to 1 cm. The lesions are often multiple and are mildly contagious. The microscopic appearance is characterized by numerous inclusion bodies (molluscum bodies) in the cytoplasm of the cells. Each lesion may be treated by desiccation, freezing, or curettage and chemical cauterization of the base.

## 4. CONDYLOMA ACUMINATUM

Condylomata acuminata (sexually transmitted genital warts) are caused by a virus of the papovavirus group. Papillary growths, small at first, tend to coalesce and form large cauliflowerlike masses that proliferate profusely during pregnancy.

Before treatment is undertaken, the entire lower genital tract from the cervix to perianal skin should be examined with the colposcope, and a cytologic smear taken from the cervix. Considering the frequent coex-

istence of other sexually transmitted diseases, appropriate studies are indicated. There is considerable variation in oncogenic potential of human papovaviruses; a biopsy may be indicated. The incubation period for appearance of clinical disease after exposure is 3 months or longer. Apparent clinical disease may represent only a small area of the infected surface. Prompt recurrence after treatment may represent reinfection or clinical manifestation of latent disease. During treatment, the patient should keep the area as clean as possible and abstain from sexual intercourse or have her partner use a condom. If clinical disease recurs, the sexual partner should be examined and treated as necessary. Penile, urethral, and perianal warts in the male may be overlooked.

Standard treatment is to cover the wart with bichloracetic or trichloracetic acid every week until the wart is gone. Alternative forms of therapy are cryosurgery, electrosurgical destruction, excision, and laser vaporization. Some authors recommend laser vaporization of all visible lesions plus a margin of normal adjacent skin under colposcopic guidance. Intralesional interferon has been shown to be effective in refractory cases.

Condylomatous warts may grow rapidly during pregnancy. Warts at the vaginal introitus may bleed during delivery and predispose the newborn to genital warts or laryngeal papillomatosis. Condylomata recognized early in pregnancy should be treated early enough to allow healing prior to delivery. If treatment is not successful, delivery by cesarean section should be considered.

## INFESTATIONS OF THE VULVA & VAGINA*

## 1. PEDICULOSIS PUBIS

The crab louse *(Pthirus pubis)* is transmitted through sexual contact or from shared infected bedding or clothing. The louse eggs are laid at the base of a hair shaft near the skin. The eggs hatch in 7–9 days, and the louse must attach to the skin of the host to survive. Intense pubic and anogenital itching results. Minute pale-brown insects and their ova may be seen attached to terminal hair shafts. Treatment is with gamma benzene hexa-chloride (Kwell) cream, 1%, left on for 12–24 hours and then removed by washing. The treatment may be repeated in 4 days if necessary. Treat all contacts and sterilize clothing that has been in contact with the infested area.

## 2. SCABIES

*Sarcoptes scabiei* causes intractable itching and excoriation of the skin surface in the vicinity of min-

---

*Trichomoniasis is discussed on p 624.

ute skin burrows where parasites have deposited ova. The itch mite is transmitted, often directly, from infected persons. The patient should take a hot soapy bath, scrubbing the burrows and encrusted areas thoroughly. Gamma benzene hexachloride (Kwell) cream or lotion (1%) should be applied to the entire body from the neck down, with particular attention to the hands and wrists, axillas, breasts, and anogenital region. The treatment should be repeated in 24 hours but without a bath. Twenty-four hours after the second application of cream, a bath should be taken and all potentially infected clothing or bedding washed or dry-cleaned. All contacts or persons in the family must be treated in the same way to prevent reinfection. Therapy should be repeated in 10–14 days if new lesions develop.

### 3. ENTEROBIASIS
### (Pinworm, Seatworm)

*Enterobius vermicularis* infection is common in children. Nocturnal perineal itching is described by the patient, and perianal excoriation may be observed. Apply adhesive cellulose tape to the anal region, stick the tape to a glass slide, and examine under the microscope for ova. Insist that patients wash hands and scrub their nails after each defecation. Underclothes must be boiled.

Apply ammoniated mercury ointment to the perineal region twice daily for relief of itching. Pinworms succumb to systemic treatment with pyrantel pamoate, mebendazole, or pyrvinium pamoate.

## MYCOTIC INFECTIONS
## OF THE FEMALE GENITAL TRACT*

### 1. FUNGAL DERMATITIS
### (Dermatophytoses)

**Tinea cruris** is a superficial fungal infection of the genitocrural area that is more common in men than in women. The most common organisms are *Trichophyton mentagrophytes* and *T rubrum*. The initial lesions usually are on the upper inner thighs and are well circumscribed, erythematous, dry scaly areas that coalesce. Scratching causes lichenification and a gross appearance similar to neurodermatitis. The diagnosis depends upon microscopic examination (as for *Candida*); culture on Sabouraud's medium is final proof. Treatment with 1% haloprogin or tolnaftate (Tinactin) is effective.

*Tinea versicolor* usually involves the skin of the trunk, although occasionally the vulvar skin is in-

volved. The lesions are usually multiple and may have a red, brown, or yellowish appearance. The diagnostic studies are as outlined for other fungal infections. Treatment with selenium sulfide suspension (Selsun) daily for 5–7 days is usually curative.

### 2. DEEP CELLULITIS CAUSED BY FUNGI

**Blastomycosis and actinomycosis** are examples of deep mycoses that usually affect internal organs but may also involve the skin. Involvement of the vulvar skin in these diseases is very rare in the USA. The diagnosis is usually made by laboratory exclusion of the granulomatous sexually transmitted diseases, tuberculosis, and other causes of chronic infection.

Treatment of blastomycosis with amphotericin B or hydroxystilbamidine is not very satisfactory. Actinomycosis can usually be treated successfully with penicillin.

## OTHER INFECTIONS
## OF THE VULVA & VAGINA

### 1. IMPETIGO

Impetigo is caused by hemolytic *Staphylococcus aureus* or streptococci. The disease is autoinoculable and spreads rapidly to various parts of the body, including the vulva. Thin-walled vesicles and bullae develop that display reddened edges and crusted surfaces after rupture. The disease is common in children, particularly on the face, hands, and vulva.

The patient must be isolated and the blebs incised or crusts removed aseptically. Neomycin or bacitracin should be applied twice a day for 1 week. Bathing with an antibacterial soap is recommended.

### 2. FURUNCULOSIS

Vulvar folliculitis is due to a staphylococcal infection of hair follicles. Furunculosis occurs if the infection spreads into the perifollicular tissues to produce a localized cellulitis. Some follicular lesions are palpable as tender subcutaneous nodules that resolve without suppuration. A furuncle begins as a hard, tender subcutaneous nodule that ruptures through the skin, discharging blood and purulent material. After expulsion of a core of necrotic tissue, the lesion heals. New furuncles may appear sporadically over a period of years.

Minor infections may be treated by applications of topical antibiotic lotions. Deeper infections may be brought to a head with hot soaks, after which the pustule should be incised and drained. Appropriate sys-

---

*Candidiasis is discussed on p 620.

temic antibiotics are warranted when extensive furunculosis is noted.

## 3. ERYSIPELAS

Erysipelas is a rapidly spreading erythematous lesion of the skin caused by invasion of the superficial lymphatics by β-hemolytic streptococci. Erysipelas of the vulva is exceedingly rare and is most commonly seen after trauma to the vulva or a surgical procedure. Systemic symptoms of chills, fever, and malaise associated with an erythematous vulvitis suggest the diagnosis. Vesicles and bullae may appear, and erythematous streaks leading to the regional lymph nodes are typical.

The patient should be placed at bed rest and given systemic (preferably parenteral) penicillin or tetracycline orally in large doses.

## 4. HIDRADENITIS

Hidradenitis suppurativa is a refractory infection of the aprocrine sweat glands, usually caused by staphylococci or streptococci. The apocrine sweat glands of the vulva become active after puberty. Inspissation of secretory material and secondary infection may be related to occlusion of the ducts. Initially, multiple pruritic subcutaneous nodules appear that eventually develop into abscesses and rupture. The process tends to involve the skin of the entire vulva, resulting in multiple abscesses and chronic draining sinuses. Treatment early in the disease consists of drainage and administration of antibiotics based on organism sensitivity tests. Severe chronic infections may not respond to medical therapy, and the involved skin and subcutaneous tissues must be removed down to the deep fascia. This may necessitate a filet and curettage or a complete vulvectomy. The area will not heal after primary closure; therefore, the wound must be left open and allowed to heal by secondary intention.

## 5. TUBERCULOSIS
### (Usually Vulvovaginal Lupus Vulgaris)

Pudendal tuberculosis is manifested by chronic, minimally painful, exudative "sores" that are tender, reddish, raised, moderately firm and nodular, with central "apple jelly"-like contents. Ulcerative, undermined, necrotic discharging lesions develop later. There is some tendency toward healing with heavy scarring. Induration and sinus formation are common in the scrofulous type of infection. Cancer and sexually transmitted disease must be ruled out and tuberculosis sought elsewhere.

Wet compresses of aluminum acetate (Burow's) solution are helpful. Systemic antituberculosis chemotherapy should be given.

## VULVAR DYSTROPHIES

Vulvar dystrophies represent a spectrum of atrophic and hypertrophic lesions caused by a diverse number of stimuli that result in circumscribed or diffuse white lesions of the vulva. The lesions do not necessarily have a uniform microscopic appearance throughout, and there may be areas of dysplasia merging with frank cancer. Multiple biopsies are therefore necessary, and the toluidine blue test and colposcopy may be of assistance in delineating areas of maximum epithelial hyperactivity most suitable for biopsy. These lesions have been classified as shown in Table 34–3.

### Clinical Findings

**A. Hypertrophic Dystrophies:** Benign epithelial thickening and hyperkeratosis may be the result of chronic vulvovaginal infections or other causes of chronic irritation. During the acute phase, as in diabetic vulvitis, the lesions may be red and moist and demonstrate evidence of secondary infection. The condition is exacerbated by the accompanying pruritus, which leads to rubbing and scratching. This becomes involuntary over time. As epithelial thickening develops, the environment of the vulva causes maceration and a raised white lesion that may be circumscribed or diffuse and may involve any portion of the vulva, adjacent thighs, perineum, or perianal skin. These lesions have been designated **lichen simplex chronicus or neurodermatitis**.

Either intraepithelial or invasive malignant tumors may appear as a circumscribed, raised white lesion of the vulvar skin or as multifocal areas of cancer in a diffuse hypertrophic lesion. Differentiation can only be achieved by evaluating multiple biopsies. Whether or not a hypertrophic white lesion is a premalignant

**Table 34–3.** Classification of vulvar dystrophies adopted by the International Society for the Study of Vulvar Disease.

| | Clinical Features | Histologic Features |
|---|---|---|
| Lichen sclerosus | Pruritic, thin, parchmentlike "atrophic area"; introital stenosis. | Thin, loss of rete, homogenization, inflammatory infiltrate. |
| Hyperplastic[1] | Pruritic, thick, gray or white plaques on skin or mucosa. | Acanthosis, hyperkeratosis, inflammatory infiltrate. |
| Mixed[1] | Areas compatible with both forms may be present at the same time. | (See above.) |

[1]Atypia may accompany hyperplastic dystrophy and is graded as mild, moderate, or severe.

disorder is debatable. Patients must be reexamined periodically, and one should not hesitate to take additional biopsy specimens. Extended observation of lesser degrees of dysplasia is warranted, but excision of the more advanced lesion is indicated.

**B. Atrophic Dystrophies:** With aging, there is a decrease in endogenous estrogen, and atrophic changes in the vulvar skin and subdermal tissues usually occur some years after advanced atrophy of the vaginal mucous membrane. There will be contracture of the vaginal introitus, and the skin becomes thin, fragile, and easily traumatized. The chief symptoms are dysuria, pruritus, and dyspareunia.

**Lichen sclerosus et atrophicus** is a dermatologic disorder of unknown origin and the most common cause of an atrophic dystrophy. The vulva is the skin surface most frequently affected and may be the only one, although the skin of the back, the axillas, beneath the breasts, the neck, and the arms may be affected also. The cause is unknown. White women over age 65 are most often affected, although the disease does occur in younger women. During the acute phase, the lesion may have a reddish or purple appearance and classically involves the vulva, perineum, and perianal area in an hourglass pattern (Fig 34–12). The skin is thin, wrinkled, and has a cigarette-paper appearance. As the disease progresses, the vulvar structures contract and the labia minora blend into the labia majora. Although the process is primarily one of atrophy of the skin, areas of dysplasia and invasive cancer may develop, and suspicious areas must be biopsied (Fig 34–13). The chief symptom is intense pruritus. This leads to rubbing and scratching, which may lead to areas of hypertrophy and, thus, mixed dystrophy.

### Diagnosis of Dystrophic Lesions

Initial evaluation of the patient with a white lesion of the vulva includes inspection of other body surfaces and a complete gynecologic examination. One or more biopsies may be taken using the toluidine blue test or colposcope to assist in determining the most appropriate sites. All these conditions are chronic; therefore, periodic reexamination is indicated, and additional biopsies can be taken of areas that appear to have changed in appearance and become particularly hypertrophic.

### Pathology

Definitive diagnosis depends on histologic examination of biopsy specimens. Characteristic microscopic findings in hypertrophic dystrophies (lichen simplex chronicus) are hyperkeratosis and acanthosis, producing thickening of the epithelium and elon-

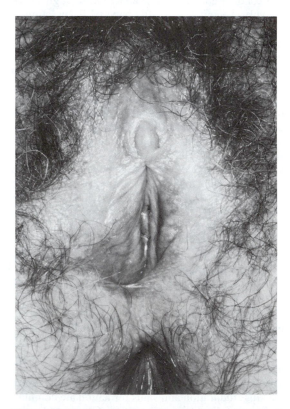

**Figure 34–13.** Advanced lesion of lichen sclerosus et atrophicus. The labia minora and prepuce of the clitoris have blended into the labial skin. Focal dysplasia was present in the posterior third of the right labium majus.

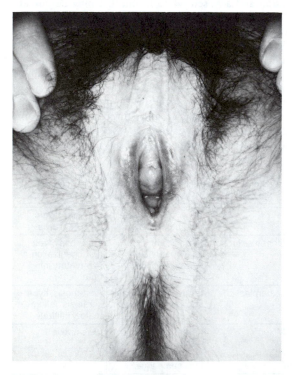

**Figure 34–12.** Early lesion of lichen sclerosus tatrophicus—typical hourglass configuration.

gation of the rete pegs. Atypical hyperplasia, or carcinoma in situ, is characterized by a pronounced degree of pleomorphism and loss of cellular polarity in the epithelium.

The microscopic appearance of lichen sclerosus et atrophicus is typical. In the well-developed lesion, there is hyperkeratosis, epithelial atrophy, and flattening of the rete pegs. Beneath the epidermis is a zone of homogenized collagenous tissue that is acellular and pink in appearance (Fig 34–14). Neoplastic changes are similar to those described in hypertrophic lesions.

### Treatment

Treatment is based on the histologic diagnosis. Assume that all patients are scratching. For the hypotrophic lesions, stopping the pruritus and building up the epithelium is accomplished by using a mild hydrocortisone cream in the morning and 2% testosterone cream at night. An oral antihistamine is given at bedtime to decrease pruritus. Hypertrophic lesions are treated twice a day with hydrocortisone cream to decrease the pruritus and inflammation. Vulvar epithelium takes at least 6 weeks to heal.

Patient should be encouraged to carefully follow the vulvar drying regimen. They should avoid tight slacks and synthetic underwear. They should not rub their vulva with towels or toilet paper. They should cleanse daily with a mild soap and use a hair dryer regularly to keep the vulvar skin dry.

Refractory patients may respond to more potent steroid creams, alcohol injections, steroid injections, or surgical removal. Surgery should be avoided if at all possible because of the high recurrence rate.

### Prognosis

In the absence of malignant epithelial changes, the principal goal is to relieve symptoms, mainly pruritus. Symptoms are usually relieved, but a significant change in histopathologic appearance of the skin seldom is achieved. Periodic reexamination is necessary to detect any malignant changes.

## VULVAR VESTIBULITIS

This recently recognized condition is characterized by postcoital vulvar burning that eventually becomes constant. It is localized to the posterior fourchette and can be so severe as to create abstinence. The condition either resolves spontaneously in 6–12 months or becomes chronic and persistent. Other inflammatory conditions and dystrophic changes must be ruled out. Colposcopically the minor vestibular glands are erythematous, and the pain can be elicited by touching these area by the blunt end of a Q-tip.

### Pathology

On biopsy of the area one finds nonspecific inflammation of the minor gland ducts. This area becomes intensely white when painted with acetic acid, however, to date no evidence of papilloma virus has been detected.

### Treatment

Initial treatment is with biweekly bichloracetic acid 4 times followed by 6 weeks' observation. If the condition is not cleared, then vestibulectomy is recommended. It is important to remove the posterior hymenal ring and mobilized the posterior vagina to bring it out to the perineal skin. Deep dissection and fine suture material insure the best possible results. The patient should be cautioned that surgery is only 80% effective.

## VULVODYNIA

Diffuse vulvar burning or pain without visible evidence of any abnormality of the epithelium has been called essential vulvodynia. Similar findings can follow surgery to the vulva, laser therapy, or chronic inflammation. This condition appears to be a peripheral neuralgia and in many cases responds to a short course of tricyclic antidepressants.

## BENIGN CYSTIC TUMORS

### Clinical Findings

**A. Cysts of Epidermal Origin:** Cysts of epidermal origin are lined with squamous epithelium and filled with oily material and desquamated epithelial cells. Epidermal inclusion cysts may result from traumatic suturing of skin fragments during closure of the vulvar mucosa and skin after trauma or episiotomy. However, most epidermal cysts arise from occlusion of pilosebaceous ducts. These cysts are usually small, solitary, and asymptomatic.

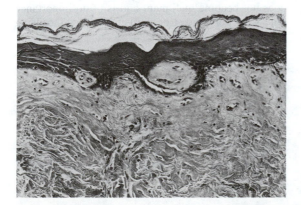

**Figure 34–14.** Microscopic appearance of lichen sclerosus et atrophicus, characterized by hyperkeratosis, flattened epidermis, and hyalinization of the dermis.

### B. Sebaceous and Sweat Gland Cysts:

**1. Sebaceous cysts**–The occlusion of a duct to a sebaceous gland results in accumulation of sebaceous material and develops into a sebaceous cyst. These cysts are frequently multiple and almost always involve the labia majora. They are generally asymptomatic; however, acutely infected cysts may require incision and drainage.

**2. Apocrine sweat gland cysts**–Aprocrine sweat glands are numerous in the skin of the labia majora and mons pubis. They become functional after puberty. Occlusion of the ducts results in an extremely pruritic microcystic disease called **Fox-Fordyce disease**. Chronic infection in the apocrine glands, usually with streptococci or staphylococci, results in multiple subcutaneous abscesses and draining sinuses. The condition is called **hidradenitis suppurativa**.

A diverse group of benign cystic or solid tumors of apocrine sweat gland origin present as small subcutaneous, often asymptomatic tumors. **Hidradenoma and syringoma** are examples of these tumors.

**C. Less Common Cysts:** A variety of other infrequent cystic vulvar tumors must be considered in differential diagnosis. Anteriorly, a Skene duct cyst or urethral diverticulum may be visible, suggesting a vulvar tumor. An inguinal hernia may extend into the labium majus, causing a large cystic dilatation. Occlusion of a persistent processus vaginalis (canal of Nuck) may cause a cystic tumor or hydrocele. Dilatation of paramesonephric duct vestiges usually produces cystic vaginal tumors; rarely, the vaginal introitus is involved. Supernumerary mammary tissue that persists in the labia majora may form a cystic or solid tumor or even an adenocarcinoma; engorgement of such tissue in the pregnant patient can be symptomatic.

### Diagnosis & Treatment

The diagnosis of small cystic structures on the vulva is ordinarily made by clinical examination or by excision biopsy, which also serves as treatment.

## BARTHOLIN'S DUCT CYST & ABSCESS

Obstruction of the main duct of Bartholin's gland results in retention of secretions and cystic dilatation. Infection is an important cause of obstruction. However, inspissated mucus and congenital narrowing of the duct may also be causes. Secondary infection may result in recurrent abscess formation.

A gland and duct are located deep in the posterior third of each labium majus. Enlargement in the postmenopausal patient should arouse a suspicion of cancer, and biopsy is indicated.

### Clinical Findings

Acute symptoms are ordinarily the result of infec-tion, which results in pain, tenderness, and dyspareunia. The surrounding tissues become edematous and inflamed, and a fluctuant mass usually is palpable.

Small, noninflamed cysts are asymptomatic and of little consequence unless progressive enlargement compromises the vaginal introitus or acute infection intervenes. Unless there is an extensive inflammatory process, few systemic symptoms or signs of infection are likely.

### Treatment

Primary treatment consists of drainage of the infected cyst or abscess, preferably by marsupialization or insertion of a Ward catheter (Fig 34–15). Simple incision and drainage may provide temporary relief. However, the opening tends to become obstructed, and recurrent cystic dilatation and infection may result. Appropriate antibiotics should be given if considerable surrounding inflammation develops.

### Prognosis

Recurrent infection resulting in cystic dilatation of the duct is the rule unless a permanent opening for drainage is established.

## BENIGN SOLID TUMORS

A benign solid tumor may be an incidental finding at the time of pelvic examination, or it may be of sufficient size to interfere with function or produce symptoms due to irritation and bleeding. The diagnosis should be established by excision or biopsy. The clinical features of a representative sample of solid vulvar tumors will be described.

### Acrochordon

An acrochordon is a flesh-colored, soft polypoid tumor of the vulvar skin that has been called a fibroepithelial polyp or simply a skin tag. The tumor does not become malignant and is of no importance unless the polypoid structure is traumatized, causing

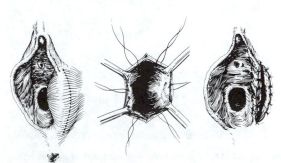

**Figure 34–15.** Marsupialization of a vestibular duct (Bartholin's) cyst.

bleeding. Simple excision biopsy in the office is ordinarily adequate therapy.

## Pigmented Nevi

Pigmented lesions of the vulva or vagina suggestive of nevi should be removed by wide excision, or a representative portion of the tumor biopsied to diagnose or exclude melanoma. A nevus on the vulvar skin may be flat, slightly elevated, papillomatous, dome-shaped, or pedunculated. Melanomas of the vulva are uncommon neoplasms constituting only 1–3% of vulvar cancers. They are extremely aggressive malignant lesions and may rise from pigmented nevi of the vulva. **Melanosis** of the vaginal mucosa or vulvar skin is a benign, flat, darkly pigmented lesion that can usually be differentiated from a nevus without histologic examination.

## Leiomyoma, Fibroma, Lipoma

Tumors of mesodermal origin occur infrequently on the vulva, but they can become very large. A **leiomyoma** arises from muscle in the round ligament and appears as a firm, symmetric, freely movable tumor deep in the substance of the labium majus.

**Fibromas** arise from proliferation of fibroblasts and vary in size from small subcutaneous nodules found incidentally to large polypoid tumors. Large tumors often undergo myxomatous degeneration and are very soft and cystic to palpation.

**Lipomas**, consisting of a combination of mature fat cells and connective tissue, cannot be differentiated from degenerated fibromas except by histopathologic examination.

Small tumors can be removed under local anesthesia in the office; large ones require general anesthesia and operating room facilities. The diagnosis of sarcoma depends on histologic examination.

## Neurofibromas

Neurofibromas are fleshy polypoid lesions and may be solitary, solid tumors of the vulva or associated with generalized neurofibromatosis (Recklinghausen's disease). They arise from the neural sheath and are usually small lesions of no consequence. Multiple disfiguring tumors of the vulva may interfere with sexual function and thus require vulvectomy.

## Granular Cell Myoblastoma (Schwannoma)

Granular cell myoblastoma is usually a solitary, painless, slow-growing, infiltrating but benign tumor of neural sheath origin, most commonly found in the tongue or integument, although about 7% involve the vulva. The usual picture is of small subcutaneous nodules 1–4 cm in diameter. With increasing size, they erode through the surface and result in an ulcerative lesion that may be confused with cancer. The margins of the tumor are indistinct, and wide local excision is necessary to resect completely cells extending into contiguous tissues. The area of resection must then be periodically reexamined and secondary excision performed promptly if recurrence is suspected.

## REFERENCES

### GENERAL

Advances in Candida management: A symposium. The Female Patient 1896;1:5. [Entire issue.]

Bacterial vaginosis: A symposium. Am J Obstet Gynecol 1993;441. [Entire issue.]

Current Considerations in the Obstetric and Gynecologic Management of Herpes Simplex Virus Infection. J Reprod Med 1986;31(Suppl):357. [Entire issue.]

Horowitz BJ, Mardh PA: *Vaginitis And Vaginosis.* Wiley-Liss, 1991.

Kaufman RH, Friedrich EG, Gardner HL: *Benign Diseases of the Vulva and Vagina*, 3rd Ed. Year Book Medical Publishers, 1989.

Proceedings of the 11th International Congress of the International Society for the Study of Vulvar Disease. J Reprod Med 1993;38:1.

Reid R (ed.): Human papillomavirus. Obstet Gynecol Clin North Am 1987;14. [Entire issue.]

Ridley CM: *The Vulva.* Churchill Livingstone, 1988.

Vulvovaginal candidiasis: A symposium. J Reprod Med 1986;31:(Suppl)639. [Entire issue.]

Vulvovaginitis: Causes and therapies: A symposium. Am J Obstet Gynecol. 1991;165(Suppl):1163. [Entire issue.]

### SPECIFIC

Abd-Rabbo MS, Atta MA: Aspiration and tetracycline sclerotherapy: A novel method for management of vaginal and vulval gartner cysts. Int J Gynecol Obstet 1991;35:235.

Andersch B, et al: Bacterial vaginosis and the effects of intermittent prophylactic treatment with an acid lactate gel. Gynecol Obstet Invest 1990;30:114.

Andersen PG, et al: Treatment of Bartholin's Abscess: Marsupialization versus incision, curretege and suture under antibiotic cover. A randomized study with 6 months followup. Acta Obstet Gynecol Scand 1992; 71:59.

Bauer HM, et al: Genital human Papillomavirus infection in female university students as determined by a PCR-based method. JAMA 1991;265:472.

Bergerdn C, et al: Multicentric human Papillomavirus infections of the female genital tract: Correlation of viral types with abnormal mitotic figures, colposcopic presentation and location. Obstet Gynecol 1987;69: 736.

Brown 2A, et al: Effects on infants of a first episode of genital herpes during pregnancy. N Engl J Med 1987; 69:1246.

Dalziel KL, Wojnarowska F, Millard P: The treatment of vulval lichen sclerosus with a very potent topical steroid (Clobetasol Propionate 0.05%). Br J Dermatol 1991;124:461.

DeVilliers EM, et al: Human papillomavirus DNA in women without and with cytologic abnormalities: Results of a 5-year follow-up study. Gynecol Oncol 1992;44:33.

Follen MM, et al: Colposcopic correlates of cervical papillomavirus infection. Am J Obstet Gynecol 1987; 157:809.

Friedrich EG: Vulvar vestibulitis syndrome. J Reprod Med 1987;32:110.

Furlonge B, et al: Vulvar vestibulitis syndrome: A clinicopathological study. Br J Obstet Gynecol 1991;93: 703.

Grossman JH, Galask RP: Persistent vaginitis caused by metronidazole-resistant trichomonas. Obstet Gynecol 1990;76:521.

Horowitz BJ: Interferon therapy for condylomatous vulvitis. Obstet Gynecol 1989;73:446.

Horowitz BJ: Mycotic vulvovaginitis: A broad overview. Am J Obstet Gynecol 1991;165:1188.

Horsburg CR, et al: Preventive strategies in sexually transmitted diseases for the primary care physician. JAMA 1987;258:815.

Hughes VL, Hillier SL: Microbiologic characteristics of lactobacillus products used for colonization of the vagina. Obstet Gynecol 1990;75:244.

Kaplowitz LG, et al: Prolonged continuous Acyclovir treatment of normal adults with frequently recurring genital herpes simplex virus infection. JAMA 1991; 265:747.

Kent HL: Epidemiology of vaginitis. Am J Obstet Gynecol 1991;165:1168.

Krebs HB: Treatment of vaginal condylomata acuminata by weekly topical application of 5-fluorouracil. Obstet Gynecol 1987;70:68.

Lafferty WE, et al: Recurrences after oral and genital herpes simplex virus infection: Influence of site of infection and viral type. N Engl J Med 1987;316:1444.

Larsson PG, Platz-Christensen JJ: Enumeration of clue cells in rehydrated air-dried vaginal wet smears for the diagnosis of bacterial vaginosis. Obstet Gynecol 1990;76:727.

McKay M, et al: Vulvar vestibulitis and vestibular papillomatosis: Report of the ISSVD Committee on Vulvodynia. J Reprod Med 1991;36:413.

McKay M: Vulvodynia: Diagnostic patterns. Dermatol Clin 1992;28:123.

Mann MS, et al: Vulvar vestibulitis: Significant clinical variables and treatment outcome. Obstet Gynecol 1992;79:122.

Marinof SC, Turner ML: Vulvar vestibulitis syndrome: An overview. Am J Obstet Gynecol 1991;165:1228.

Markowicz LE, et al: Toxic shock syndrome: Evaluation of national surveillance data using a hospital discharge survey. JAMA 1987;258:75.

Michlewitz H, et al: Vulvar vestibulitis-subgroup with Bartholin gland duct inflammation. Obstet Gynecol 1989;73:410.

Nash JD, et al: Biologic course of cervical human papillomavirus infection. Obstet Gynecol 1987;69:160.

Neri A, Peled Y, Braslavski D: Vulvar leiomyoma. Acta Obstet Gynecol Scand 1993;72:221.

Prober CG, et al: Low risk of herpes simplex virus infections in neonates exposed to the virus at the time of vaginal delivery to mothers with recurrent genital herpes simplex virus infections. N Engl J Med 1987;316: 240.

Quinn TC, et al: Detection of Chlamydia trachomatis cervical infection: A comparison of Papanicolaou and immunofluorescent staining with cell culture. Am J Obstet Gynecol 1987;157:394.

Redondo-Lopez V, Cook RL, Sohel JD: Emerging role of lactobacilli in the control and maintenance of the vaginal bacterial microflora. Rev Infect Dis 1990; 12:856.

Reed BD: Risk factors for candida vulvovaginitis. Obstet Gynecol 1992;47:551.

Reid R, et al: Sexually transmitted papillomaviral infections. 1. The anatomic distribution and pathologic grade of neoplastic lesions associated with different viral types. Am J Obstet Gynecol 1987;156:212.

Rhoads JL, et al: Chronic vaginal candidiasis in women with human immunodeficiency virus infection. JAMA 1987;257:3105.

Ridley CM: Genital lichen sclerosis (lichen sclerosis et Atrophicus) in childhood and adolescence. J Roy Soc Med 1993;86:69.

Schover LR, Youngs DD, Cannata R: Psychosexual aspects of the evaluation and management of vulvar vestibulitis. Am J Obstet Gynecol 1992;167:630.

Sweet RL, et al: Chlamydia trachomatis infection and pregnancy outcome. Am J Obstet Gynecol 1987;156: 824.

Thomason JL, Gelbart SM, Scaglione NJ: Bacterial vaginosis: Current review with indications for asymptomatic therapy. Am J Obstet Gynecol 1991;165: 1210.

Turner ML, Marinoff SC: Pudendal neuralgia. Am J Obstet Gynecol 1991;165:1233.

Van Heusden AM, et al: Single-dose oral fluconazole versus single-dose topical miconazole for the treatment of acute vulvovaginal candidiasis. Acta Obstet Gynecol Scand 1990;60:417.

# Benign Disorders of the Uterine Cervix

# 35

*Edward C. Hill, MD, & Martin L. Pernoll, MD*

## CONGENITAL ANOMALIES OF THE CERVIX

The cervix, as the lowermost portion of the uterus, develops embryologically by fusion of the two müllerian ducts with subsequent resorption of the midline septum resulting from the fusion (Fig 35–1). Anomalous development of the cervix results from (1) aplasia of all, or portions of, the müllerian ducts, (2) failure of fusion of all, or portions or, the müllerian ducts, (3) failure of resorption of all, or portions of, the midline septum.

### Aplasia

If only one müllerian duct develops, the result is a unicornuate uterus with its own cervix and vagina (Fig 35–2). Rudimentary horns, communicating and noncommunicating, functioning and nonfunctioning, all without cervices, are the result of incomplete development of one müllerian duct. Both the cervix and vagina are absent in congenital absence of the vagina, the Mayer-Rokitansky-Küster-Hauser syndrome, in which the müllerian ducts develop normally in a karyotypic female (XX) only to the point where both fallopian tubes are formed. Often a tiny, midline nubbin of a vestigial nonfunctioning uterus is present, but no functioning corpus, cervix, or vagina exists (Fig 35–3). Ovarian development is normal. The condition often is not recognized until adolescence when primary amenorrhea prompts clinical investigation. Karyotyping distinguishes it from the androgen insensitivity syndrome (XY), in which the testes are intra-abdominal or located in the inguinal canal.

Treatment options include (1) the development of a neovagina by dilatation (the Ingram bicycle seat method), (2) surgical construction of a neovagina using split-thickness skin grafts (MacIndoe method) or the Williams technique using the labia to form a tube. Most authorities recommend an initial trial of the nonsurgical approach, but it takes several months to accomplish and requires a well-motivated patient.

Cervical and vaginal aplasia may occur in spite of normal development of the uterine corpus and fallopian tubes. This is rare but is seen in the young patient with primary amenorrhea, cyclic lower abdominal pain, absence of a vagina, and with a midline uterine mass distended by a hematometra (Fig 35–4). Cervical aplasia carries a high risk of extensive pelvic endometriosis due to retrograde menstruation. To preserve childbearing function, attempts have been made to correct this condition surgically, and a few pregnancies have been recorded; however, the risks of serious morbidity and even mortality are high and the success rates are extremely low, prompting some authorities to recommend hysterectomy.

Magnetic resonance imaging usually is definitive in defining the various forms of müllerian duct aplasia.

### Failure of Fusion

Uterus didelphys with two separate uterine horns, each with its own cervix separated by a longitudinal vaginal septum, occurs as a result of complete failure of the müllerian ducts to fuse. The diagnosis is easily missed because one side usually predominates, and insertion of the vaginal speculum into this side obscures the opposite vagina and cervix. A variant of this is the uterus didelphys in which there is no introitus for the second vagina, it failing to communicate with the urogenital sinus. This vagina ends blindly; therefore, with puberty and the onset of menstrual function, blood is trapped in the blind vagina. As the menses continue, not only does hematocolpos develop but it may progress to involve the ipsilateral corpus and fallopian tube in a hematometra and hematocolpos (Fig 35–5). Again, there is increased risk of pelvic endometriosis due to retrograde menstruation.

Fusion of the müllerian ducts usually begins at the caudal end and proceeds in a cephalic direction. Partial failure of fusion, then, is responsible for varying degrees of bicornuate uteri, the complete form leaving a vascular, fibromuscular septum, the lowermost portion of which is located at the level of the internal cervical os (Fig 35–6). The partial form divides the two horns at varying levels above the cervix. An arcu-

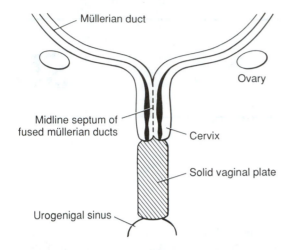

**Figure 35–1.** Fusion of müllerian ducts to form cervix and corpus uteri.

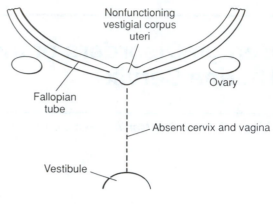

**Figure 35–3.** Congenital absence of vagina.

ate uterus is the minimal manifestation of fusion failure and may not be clinically significant.

## Failure of Resorption

Resorption of the midline septum resulting from fusion of the two müllerian ducts normally begins at the level of the internal cervical os and progresses in both a caudad and cephalad direction. If there is complete failure of resorption, the cervix and corpus are divided by a longitudinal midline septum, the completely septate uterus (Fig 35–7). The septum in this case consists primarily of relatively avascular fibrous connective tissue rather than the vascular fibromuscular septum found in the bicornuate uterus. Moreover, the uterine corpus is unified and not bicornuate. Arrest in the resorptive process in a cepahalic direction produces varying degrees of septation of the cor-

pus above the level of the internal os ranging from complete division of the endometrial cavity to minimal septation at the fundus only.

Müllerian duct fusion and septal resorption failures usually are discovered as a result of a complicated pregnancy (during abortion, cesarean section delivery, or manual removal of the placenta) or during infertility investigation (hysterosalpingography, sonography, laparoscopy, hysteroscopy). All these anomalies carry varying degrees of risk of pregnancy wastage due to spontaneous abortion, intrauterine fetal growth retardation, and prematurity. Uterine anomalies are implicated in approximately 15% of couples experiencing repeated pregnancy loss. It is surprising that some of the more spectacular anomalies such as uterus didelphys carry a smaller risk (43%) than those that are more subtle, such as the septate uterus (70–88%). Magnetic resonance imaging is very helpful in defining the various müllerian duct anomalies resulting from failure of fusion or septal resorption. When pregnancy wastage does become a problem, treatment varies from hysteroscopic resection of the

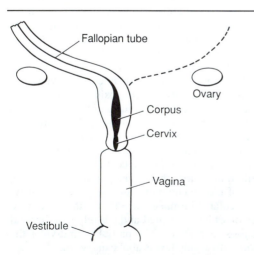

**Figure 35–2.** Unicornuate uterus.

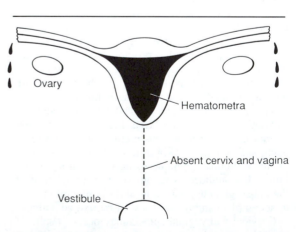

**Figure 35–4.** Cervical aplasia with hematometra and retrograde menstruation.

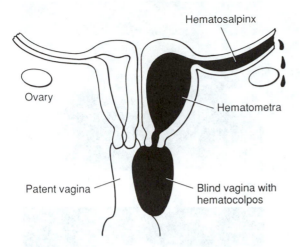

**Figure 35–5.** Uterus didelphys with blind vagina hematocolpos, hematometra, hematosalpinx, and retrograde menstruation.

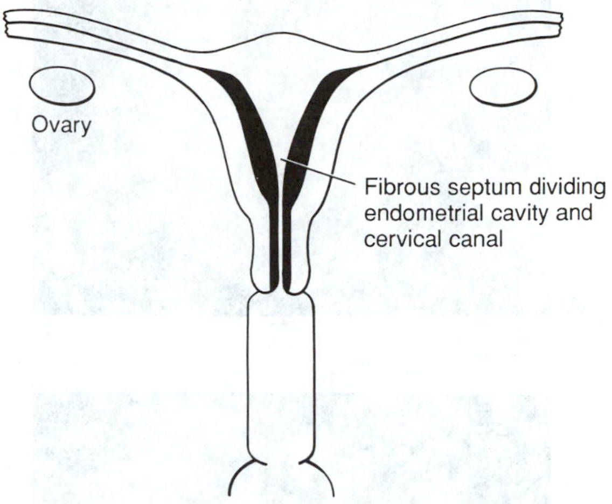

**Figure 35–7.** Complete septate uterus.

relatively avascular septum of the septate uterus to the Strassman unification procedure for the bicornuate uterus.

## CERVICAL CHANGES RELATED TO DIETHYLSTILBESTROL EXPOSURE IN UTERO

Congenital anomalies of the cervix related to intrauterine exposure to diethylstilbestrol (DES) deserve special consideration, because they are encountered

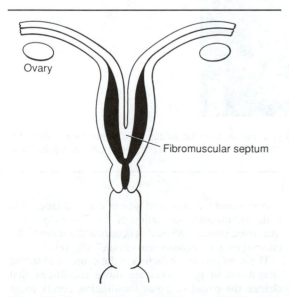

**Figure 35–6.** Complete bicornuate uterus with fibromuscular septum at level of internal cervical os.

in about two-thirds of exposed female offspring and an estimated 1 million such young women are in the USA alone. Although unusual cervical configurations are common in these individuals, the risk of clear cell cancer is thought to be 0.14–1.4 per 1000.

The cervical changes due to DES exposure have been classified as follows (Sandberg, 1976; Fig 35–8): (1) circular sulcus, complete or incomplete; (2) recessed area surrounding the external os; (3) portio vaginalis completely covered by columnar epithelium; (4) pseudopolyp formation due to localized, eccentric hypertrophy of endocervical tissue (not shown in illustration); and (5) and (6) anterior cervical lip protuberances, rough or smooth. These changes are often associated with certain anomalies of the vagina such as incomplete septa, fibrous bands, narrowing of the vaginal apex, and vaginal adenosis.

Some of the cervical changes associated with DES exposure predispose to cervical incompetence in pregnancy, and an increased incidence of spontaneous abortion premature delivery and ectopic pregnancies has been reported.

## CERVICAL INJURIES

### Lacerations

Cervical lacerations are common in both normal and abnormal deliveries. Unless the cervix is routinely inspected following the completion of the third stage of labor, injury may go undetected until after it heals with one or more lacerations. Most obstetric lacerations occur on either side of the cervix at about 6 or 9 o'clock positions. They may vary in length from small notches less than 1 cm deep to extensive tears extending upward into the lower uterine seg-

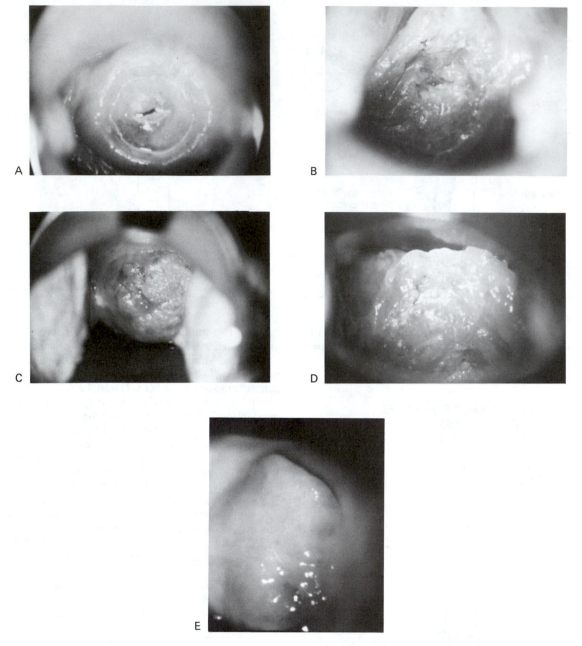

**Figure 35–8.** Cervical changes in women exposed to DES in utero. *A:* Circular sulcus. *B:* Central depression and ectopy. *C:* Portio vaginalis covered by columnar epithelium (ectopy). *D:* Anterior cervical protuberance (rough). *E:* Anterior cervical protuberance (smooth).

ment. Bleeding from deep lacerations may be brisk, requiring immediate repair to control hemorrhage. Thus, cervical examination is mandatory in every case of immediate (or delayed) postpartum hemorrhage. Examination must include not only inspection but careful palpation of the upper angle of the laceration because the visible portion may represent only the lower margin of a wound that may extend into the uterus.

A less easily recognized type of cervical laceration is the submucosal separation of the fibrous connective tissue stroma. When this occurs at the level of the internal os, an "incompetent cervix" may result.

The most important factors in the cause of obstetric lacerations of the cervix are those conditions that change the ovoid shape of the dilating cervix to an ellipsoid with resulting increased regional tension on the cervical tissues. This may occur during the delivery of unusually large babies or when the presentation is an occiput posterior or breech. Lacerations also occur when delivery is attempted before the cervix is completely dilated or effaced.

Nonobstetric lacerations of the cervix may occur during instrumental procedures, eg, dilatation and curettage (D&C) or placement of radioactive sources. Postmenopausal atrophy, chronic inflammation, or malignant cervical disease predisposes to such iatrogenic lacerations.

## Perforations

Perforation of the cervix may occur during self-induced abortion with sharp objects, eg, wires or darning or knitting needles, or inadvertently during sounding of the uterus, cervical dilatation, insertion of radioactive sources, or conization of the cervix. The urinary bladder may be injured also because of its close proximity to the anterior aspect of the cervix.

## Ulcerations

Ulceration of the cervix may result from pressure necrosis due to a vaginal pessary in the vagina or a cervical stem pessary. Cervical ulceration may also develop with uterine prolapse when the cervix protrudes through the vaginal introitus.

## Annular Detachment

Annular detachment of the cervix is a rare complication resulting from compression necrosis of the cervix during labor. It occurs when the external os fails to dilate and the blood supply is compromised by pressure of the fetal head. The diagnosis is made when the detached ring or portion of cervix is expelled prior to delivery of the presenting part of the fetus.

## Complications of Cervical Injuries

Hemorrhage is the most immediate and serious complication of cervical laceration. Although external bleeding is usually present, intra- or extraperitoneal hemorrhage may occur when the cervical tear extends into the uterus. The clinical picture then is that of hypovolemic shock out of proportion to visible blood loss.

Cervical incompetence results from unrecognized or improperly repaired lacerations through the internal os. Repeated or habitual abortion, often occurring during the second trimester of pregnancy, may be due to cervical incompetence.

## CERVICAL INFECTIONS

### Essentials of Diagnosis

- Leukorrhea—purulent or mucopurulent discharge with disagreeable odor.
- Vulvovaginal irritation (itching or burning) if associated with vaginitis.
- Red, edematous cervix.
- Tenderness on cervical motion.
- Often asymptomatic.
- Colposcopic changes (possibly the only clinical manifestation).
- Atypical epithelial cells and inflammatory cells on cytologic examination.
- Positive laboratory studies for pathogens.

### General Considerations

Acute or chronic infectious cervicitis probably is the most common gynecologic disorder, affecting more than 50% of all women at some time during their adult life. The squamous epithelium of the cervix, being in direct continuity with that of the vagina, is subject to all of the vaginal infections whether viral, spirochetal, fungal, bacterial, or parasitic in origin. In addition, the cervix may be the site of specific infections in the absence of vaginal disease. *Chlamydia trachomatis, Neisseria gonorrhoeae,* and the herpes simplex virus, all sexually transmitted, are the major causes of infectious cervicitis. Although not producing a cervicitis per se, the human papillomavirus (HPV), the etiologic agent of condylomata accuminata of the vulva, perianal skin and vagina, also frequently infects the cervix and plays a significant role in the development of cervical cancer.

Syphilis, tuberculosis, granuloma inguinale, lymphogranuloma venereum, chancroid, actinomyocosis, and schistosomiasis may also involve the cervix, but rarely. Enterococci, staphylococci, and streptococci, organisms often found in the normal vagina, may establish a foothold in obstetric lacerations of the cervix as well as cause postpartum endometritis and parametritis. These infections may become chronic in old, healed cervical lacerations. Cervical hypertrophy and elongation, producing a "pseudoprolapse," may follow. Acute and chronic infectious cervicitis therefore represents a problem of considerable complexity requiring accurate assessment, appropriate treatment, and careful follow-up.

### Etiology and Pathogenesis

*C trachomatis,* the agent responsible for so-called **nongonorrheal urethritis** in the male, is sexually transmitted, invading the columnar epithelium of the cervix. Being the most prevalent of the organisms infecting the cervix primarily, it causes an estimated 4 million cases per year in the USA. With the cervix as a reservoir, the organism may be carried by hand to the eye where it causes trachoma and inclusion conjunctivitis. It may infect the fetus in its passage through the birth canal. Or, it may ascend via the endometrial cavity to the fallopian tubes to cause salpingitis as well as pelvic and perihepatic peritonitis. It has been implicated as the agent responsible for the Fitzhugh-Curtis syndrome (violin-string adhesions between the liver and the parietal peritoneum). *C trachomatis* and *N gonorrhoeae* often are coagents in the etiology of acute and chronic cervicitis and salpingitis. An estimated 20% of men and 40% of women harboring *N gonorrhoeae* in their genital tracts also have *C trachomatis* infection.

*N gonorrhoeae* is a common cause of cervicitis, also infecting the columnar epithelium of the endocervix, the mature squamous epithelium of the adult cervix and vagina being resistant to the invading organism. As in the case of *Chlamydia* infections, the cervix acts as a nidus for ascending infection of the endometrium and the fallopian tubes, the upward invasion often occurring after a menstrual period and the loss of the protective mucous plug.

Herpes simplex virus (HSV, herpes genitalis) infection produces cervical lesions similar to those found on the vulva. Vesicular at first, the lesion becomes ulcerative. Primary infections may be extensive and severe, producing constitutional symptoms of low-grade fever, myalgia, and malaise lasting about 2 weeks. The ulcers eventually heal, but recurrences of lesser severity and duration are common. Herpes simplex type 2 (HSV-2) is the etiologic agent in more than 90% of genital herpes infections, the remainder being due to herpes simplex type 1 (HSV-1), the cause of the common labial cold sore or fever blister. Orogenital contact is thought to be responsible. After the initial infection has healed, the virus continues to reside in the epithelial cells of the cervix, and viral shedding occurs in asymptomatic patients. Infection of infants in their passage through the birth canal has led to the practice of cesarean section in women who have evidence of active infection at term. HSV infections also have been associated with cervical cancer. Women with antibodies to HSV-2 have a higher incidence of intraepithelial neoplasia as well as invasive malignancy, although a direct etiologic link has not been established.

The cervical lesions of human papillomavirus (HPV), also sexually transmitted, are flatter and moister than the typical genital warts (condylomata accuminata) seen on the vulva and perianal skin. In fact, often they are invisible to the naked eye, becoming visible only after the application of a dilute solution of acetic acid (aceto-white epithelium) or by colposcopic examination (white epithelium, mosaicism, and coarse punctation). More than 65 types of HPV have been identified. Benign lesions of the cervix are associated with types 6 and 11 whereas types 16, 18, 45, and 56 are more often found in association with cervical intraepithelial neoplasia and invasive cancers. Approximately one-third of women with HPV infection have a coexistent cervicitis caused by other organisms. The presence of cervicitis does not significantly affect the clinical course of the HPV lesions.

## Cytopathology

The Papanicolaou smear often reflects the pathologic changes of cervical infections. A few inflammatory cells are seen normally in the smear, particularly immediately before, during, and immediately after the menses. However, large numbers of polymorphonuclear leukocytes and histiocytes indicate an acute cervicitis. At times the inflammatory exudate may be so dense that it obscures the epithelial cells, in which case the smear test should be repeated after the inflammatory process has been treated and cleared. Epithelial cell changes commonly are associated with cervical inflammation and must be distinguished from those related to neoplastic disease. Nuclear enlargement, clumping of chromatin, hyperchromatism, and nucleoli as well as cytoplasmic eosinophilia and poorly defined cell membranes often are seen. These are the findings of "cytologic atypia" and are nonspecific. Frequently, however, a specific diagnosis can be made either by directly identifying the offending organism or organisms or by noting typical changes in the epithelial cells characteristic of a specific type of infection. For example, the organisms of trichomoniasis and moniliasis can be identified directly on the Pap smear. HPV, of course, cannot be seen but the infection is characterized by squamous epithelial cell enlargement, multinucleation and the perinuclear "halo" effect of koilocytosis. The so-called "balloon-cell" is almost pathognomonic of this condition. Cellular changes of mild dysplasia (low-grade squamous intraepithelial lesion [SIL]), moderate or severe dysplasia (carcinoma-in-situ [CIS], high-grade SIL) and even invasive cancer may be associated findings.

Greatly enlarged, multinucleated cells with ground-glass cytoplasm and nuclei containing characteristic inclusion bodies are indicative of infection by HSV.

## Histopathology of Cervical Infections

The histopathologic findings of cervical infection also are both nonspecific and specific. Characteristically, both *N gonorrhoeae* and *C trachomatis* infections produce a nonspecific acute inflammatory reaction. Because of edema and increased vascularity, the cervix becomes swollen and reddened. Stromal edema and infiltration by polymorphonuclear leukocytes are seen microscopically, and there may be focal loss of overlying mucous membrane.

As the acute process subsides, the swelling and redness disappear, and the polymorphonuclear leukocytes are replaced by lymphocytes, plasma cells, and macrophages—the histologic picture of chronic cervicitis. Irritation due to infection causes the glandular epithelium to hyperfunction, and mucus mixed with inflammatory cells produces a copious purulent or mucopurulent exudate, which may be clinically apparent only by introducing a cotton swab into the cervical canal. Because the infected clefts and crypts drain poorly, they become dilated and often obstructed, leading to microabscess formation. With long-continued inflammation, proliferation of fibrous connective tissue in the cervical stroma occurs. This results in hypertrophy and elongation of the cervix, and, if this process is extreme, the portio vaginalis may actually protrude beyond the vaginal introitus, giving the impression of a prolapse of the uterus.

On numerous occasions a histopathologic diagnosis of chronic cervicitis is made based on the finding of small collections of lymphocytes in the cervical stroma. This is a characteristic of the cervix of almost all parous women, and, unless there is some clinical manifestation of cervicitis, it is probably not a significant finding.

The gross appearance of acute cervicitis must be distinguished clinically and at times histologically from the red, granular inflamed-appearing cervix of cervical ectopy in which variable portions of the cervical portio vaginalis are covered by endocervical, mucus-secreting epithelium or by a thin layer of immature metaplastic epithelium. Particularly in younger women, the squamocolumnar junction, instead of being located at or near the external os, is found on the surface of the portio. Being covered only by a single layer of columnar cells, the underlying vascular stroma is clearly visible, producing a red, granular appearance. In the past this has been called a cervical "erosion." "Erosion" is not a proper term for cervical redness except as an acute, limited denudation of mucous membrane as might be seen with an especially virulent acute cervicitis or following punch biopsy, cauterization, cryotherapy, laser treatment, loop excision, cone biopsy, or radiation therapy.

The location of the squamocolumnar function of the cervix is not static throughout life but undergoes continuous change. Through the process of squamous metaplasia, columnar epithelium on the portio vaginalis is gradually converted to stratified squamous epithelium. Initially the stratified metaplastic epithelium is thin and immature, but, with the passage of time, becomes thicker and more mature, eventually taking on the appearance of "original squamous epithelium." Microscopically, the squamocolumnar junction rarely demonstrates an abrupt transition from squamous to columnar epithelium but instead is marked by a zone of immature squamous metaplasia (Fig 35–9 and 35–10). This change from a mucous membrane covered by a single layer of columnar epithelium to one of stratified squamous epithelium not only is a continuously ongoing process but is accelerated during 3 periods of a woman's life: fetal existence, adolescence, and the first pregnancy.

By the time a woman reaches the fifth decade, the squamocolumnar junction has receded into the endocervical canal, and the portio vaginalis is completely covered by squamous epithelium. In the process, however, the deeper crypts and clefts of columnar epithelium are bridged over and occluded by metaplastic epithelium, obstructing the egress of mucus, producing the common, typical nabothian cysts of the cervix. To the naked eye, the presence of nabothian

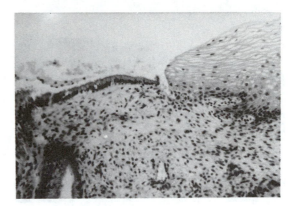

**Figure 35–9.** Abrupt transition, squamocolumnar junction.

cysts indicates that this area at one time was occupied by columnar epithelium which has undergone transformation. Therefore, the nabothian cyst is the hallmark of the "transformation zone," the area in which epithelial neoplasia first appears.

Certain pathologic findings are specific in that they may implicate specific organisms. For example, microscopic examination of a cervical biopsy obtained from a vesicular lesion may demonstrate intraepithelial, multinucleated giant cells containing nuclear inclusions surrounded by a clear halo typical of HSV infection. Colposcopically directed biopsy of an area of white epithelium, coarse punctation, or mosaicism may show a flat, thickened, squamous epithelium whose superficial layers are occupied by cells demonstrating large cytoplasmic vacuoles, devoid of glycogen, surrounding shrunken, hyperchromatic nuclei and cell membranes that are thickened and eosinophilic. These are the typical histologic findings of HPV infection (Fig 35–11). They may be associated with the findings of intraepithelial neoplasia. (See Chapter 47.)

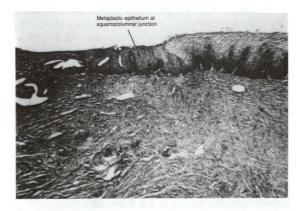

**Figure 35–10.** Metaplastic epithelium at the squamocolumnar junction.

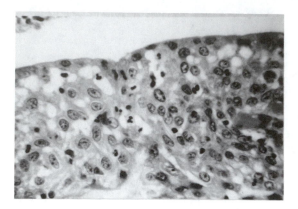

**Figure 35–11.** Squamous epithelium showing histologic changes of HPV infection.

## Clinical Findings

### A. Symptoms and Signs:

**1. Acute cervicitis**–The primary symptom of acute cervicitis is a purulent vaginal discharge. The appearance of the discharge is variable—often thick and creamy as in gonorrheal infection; foamy and greenish-white as in trichomonal infection; white and curd-like in candidiasis; and thin and gray in *Gardnerella vaginalis* infection. Chlamydial infections often produce a purulent discharge from an angry, reddened, congested cervix. The discharge is often indistinguishable from that due to gonorrheal cervicitis and has been characterized as mucopurulent. If yellow mucopus is seen on a cotton-tipped applicator placed in the cervical canal in the presence or absence of *N gonorrhoeae,* chlamydial infection should be suspected.

**a. Leukorrhea**—In leukorrhea caused by endocervical inflammation, the characteristics vary with the menstrual cycle. In the absence of infection, the cervical mucus is thin, clear, and acellular at the time of ovulation or after moderate estrogen stimulation. Normally, in the late secretory phase, the mucus is slightly mucopurulent, and it is tenacious and viscid.

**b. Infertility**—A thick, glutinous, acidic, pus-laden cervical mucus is noxious to sperm and prevents fertilization.

**c. Pelvic discomfort**—Vulvar burning and itching may be prominent symptoms. Gonorrheal cervicitis may be accompanied by urethritis with frequency, urgency, and dysuria. If associated with acute salpingitis, the symptoms and signs will be those of pelvic peritonitis.

**d. Sexual dysfunction**—Constitutional symptoms do not usually occur as a result of acute cervicitis alone, but an associated parametritis may cause dyspareunia or discomfort in the lower abdomen.

**e. Physical signs**—Inspection of the cervix initially infected by *N gonorrhoeae* generally reveals an acutely inflamed, edematous cervix with a purulent discharge escaping from the external os. In trichomonal infection, the telltale strawberry petechiae may be visible on the squamous epithelial surface of the portio vaginalis as well as the adjacent vaginal mucosa. As noted previously, mucopurulent endocervical exudate is the hallmark of *C trachomatis infection.* In candidiasis, there is likely to be a white cheesy exudate that is difficult to wipe away and that, if scraped off, usually leaves punctate hemorrhagic areas. Colposcopic findings of acute cervicitis are those primarily of an altered microangioarchitecture with marked increase in the surface capillaries, which, viewed end-on, may show a pattern of diffuse "punctation." Trichomoniasis is typified by characteristic double-hairpin capillaries. The capillary pattern of inflammation should not be confused with that of neoplasia. In an inflammatory process, the colposcopic picture is diffuse with ill-defined margins as contrasted with the localized and sharply demarcated vascular changes associated with intraepithelial neoplasia. It should be emphasized that invasive cancers often are secondarily infected so that, in addition to the colposcopic changes associated with frank malignancy, those related to inflammation are also present. Colposcopy also readily identifies the fine villiform pattern of cervical ectopy (Fig 35–12).

**f. Metrorrhagia**—Hyperemia of the infected cervix may be associated with freely bleeding areas. Cervical ooze may account for intermenstrual (often postcoital) spotting.

**g. Abortion**—Cervicitis may be followed by endometritis with subsequent abortion.

**2. Chronic cervicitis**–In chronic cervicitis, leukorrhea may be the chief symptom. Although it may not be as profuse as in acute cervicitis, this discharge may also cause vulvar irritation. The discharge may be frankly purulent, varying in color, or it may present simply as thick, tenacious, turbid mucus. Intermenstrual bleeding may occur.

Associated eversion may present as a velvety to granular perioral redness or as patchy erythema due to scattered squamous metaplasia (epithelialization or

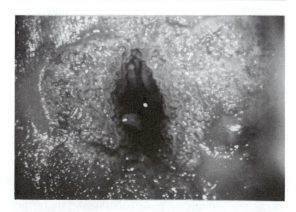

**Figure 35–12.** Colposcopic view of villiform pattern of cervical ectopy.

epidermization). Nabothian cysts in the area of the so-called transformation zone often occur. The Schiller test may show poorly staining or nonstaining areas. There is often some tenderness and thickening in the region of the uterosacral ligaments on pelvic examination, and motion of the cervix may be painful.

Lower abdominal pain, lumbosacral backache, dysmenorrhea, or dyspareunia may occur occasionally related to an associated parametritis. Infertility may be due to the inflammatory changes resulting in a tacky cervical mucus that is acidic and otherwise "hostile" (toxic) to sperm. Urinary frequency, urgency, and dysuria may be seen in association with chronic cervicitis. These symptoms are related to an associated subvesical lymphangitis, not to cystitis.

Inspection of the chronically infected cervix often reveals only abnormal discharge.

**a. Cervical dystocia**—Fibrosis and stenosis of the cervix may follow chronic cervical infection. Delayed or incomplete dilatation of the cervix may result.

**b. Laceration, eversion, and hypertrophy of the cervix**—Laceration, eversion, and hypertrophy of the cervix may be apparent, together with nabothian cysts. Patulousness of the deeply lacerated external os often exposes the endocervical canal, which may bleed when wiped with a cotton applicator. The portio and the upper vagina usually appear normal in cervicitis.

**B. Laboratory Findings:**

**1. Smears**—Wet smear preparations of the exudate diluted with isotonic saline solution usually demonstrate the motile flagellated *T vaginalis* organisms when present. A similar suspension in 10% potassium hydroxide may disclose the spores and mycelia of *Candida albicans*. Yeast organisms should be cultured on Nickerson's or comparable medium. The speckled-appearing "clue cell" of *G vaginalis* is suggestive of this type of cervicitis-vaginitis. Ten or more polymorphonuclear leukocytes per high-power field (magnification × 1000) in a gram-stained endocervical smear or a frankly mucopurulent exudate obtained from the endocervix on a cotton swab are indicative of acute cervicitis.

In acute gonorrheal cervicitis, a gram-stained smear of cervical exudate may show the typical coffee-bean-shaped, paired, gram-negative, intracellular diplococci of *N gonorrhoeae*. This finding is adequate for the initiation of definitive therapy. However, one must not confuse this organism with nonpathogenic diplococci that may be found in the lower reproductive tract.

In chronic infections, the cervical mucus is thick and tenacious and contains clumps of pus cells and cervical debris.

In chronic gonococcal infections, the gram-stained smear usually fails to reveal specific pathogens. Culture on Thayer-Martin medium may be diagnostic.

**2. Cultures**—Culture of the material obtained from the cervix on Thayer-Martin or blood agar medium provides a positive diagnosis. Culture is essential for a definite diagnosis of gonorrhea despite a finding of intracellular diplococci. A single culture from the cervix on Thayer-Martin medium will detect *N gonorrhoeae* in 90–93% of infected women. The addition of a culture obtained from the anal canal increases the sensitivity of diagnosis by 6–10%. Chlamydiae are obligate intracellular organisms and cannot be cultured on artificial media, requiring tissue culture for definitive diagnosis. Most clinical laboratories are not equipped for this; therefore, although culture is the most sensitive test, the clinician must rely primarily on a direct fluorescent antibody (DFA) or an enzyme immunoassay (EIA) test. Both are 75–85% sensitive and 97–98% specific, so false-positive results are a problem.

**3. Cytology**–(See section on cytopathology.)

**4. Blood studies**–In uncomplicated cervicitis not accompanied by salpingitis, the white count may be normal or only a slight leukocytosis and sedimentation rate elevation may be present. In any patient with gonorrhea, syphilis must be ruled out by appropriate serologic tests.

**5. Mucus studies**–In patients under investigation for the cause of infertility, a postcoital examination of the cervical mucus (Sims-Huhner test) usually shows a paucity of spermatozoa, and those that are present may demonstrate poor motility and short survival times. The dried mucus smear never shows a normal "fern" pattern in cervicitis.

**6. Urine studies**–A clean-catch or catheterized urine specimen in patients with cervicitis usually contains only occasional white cells, rare or absent erythrocytes, and no casts. Culture of the urine is generally negative in urethritis and trigonitis secondary to cervicitis.

**C. X-Ray Findings:** In the presence of an acute cervicitis, hysterography is contraindicated. In chronic cervicitis, the introduction of a radiopaque dye (eg, Salpix) into the canal may demonstrate the hypertrophied endocervical rugae.

**Differential Diagnosis**

The leukorrhea of cervicitis can be distinguished from that of tension states and the physiologic outpouring of mucus at the time of ovulation by the fact that in the latter condition the mucus is clear and shows only rare leukocytes on microscopic examination.

Rectovaginal examination should be done to distinguish the signs and symptoms of pelvic tenderness, induration, and mass formation above the cervix when discharge is noted from the cervix.

Cervicitis must be distinguished from early neoplastic processes. This may not be easy, because inflammatory conditions may alter the epithelial cells to produce atypia on cytologic examination. Colposcopy is useful (see sections on cervical dysplasia and cervical cancer). Cytologic examination of cervical scrapings as well as mucosa from endocervical aspiration and histologic examination of biopsy specimens from any suspect areas should help to distinguish chronic cervicitis from a developing cancer of the cervix. Consider also the lesions of syphilis and chancroid as well as the chronic granulomatous ulcerations of tuberculosis and granuloma inguinale.

## Complications

Leukorrhea, cervical stenosis, and infertility are sequelae of chronic cervicitis. Salpingitis is common with gonorrhea and acute postabortal cervicitis. Chronic infection of the lower and subsequently the upper urinary tract may follow persistent cervicitis. Salpingitis is a common complication of gonorrheal, chlamydial, and postabortion cervicitis.

Carcinoma of the cervix usually occurs in sexually active, parous women. Examination often reveals neglected cervical lacerations and chronic infection; however, these cannot be implicated as causes of cervical cancer.

## Prevention

Gonorrheal herpetic and chlamydial cervicitis can be prevented by the avoidance of sexual contact with infected persons or the use of a condom for protection during coitus. The condom also protects against HPV infection.

The avoidance of surgical or obstetric trauma and the prompt recognition and proper repair of cervical lacerations help to prevent the subsequent development of a chronically infected cervix.

When surgical removal of the corpus of the uterus is indicated, the cervix should be removed also if this is feasible.

## Treatment

Selection of the most appropriate treatment depends on the age of the patient and her desire for pregnancy; the severity of the cervical involvement; the presence of complicating factors (eg, salpingitis); and previous treatment.

Instrumentation and vigorous topical therapy should be avoided during the acute phase of cervicitis and before the menses, when ascending infection may occur.

**A. Acute Cervicitis:** When acute cervicitis is associated with vaginitis due to a specific organism, treatment must be directed accordingly.

Metronidazole (Flagyl) is specific for the treatment of *T vaginalis* infection. The dosage (for men and women) is 2 g orally, once only. Metronidazole is contraindicated during the first trimester of pregnancy because of possible teratogenicity.

Candidiasis may be treated topically with fungicidal preparations such as Nystatin vaginal suppositories (100 mg) inserted twice daily for 10 days.

*Gardnerella* infection usually responds to oral metronidazole, 500 mg twice daily for 7 days (~10% more effective than 2 g orally, once only). Resistant or recurrent cases may respond to ampicillin or amoxicillin with clavulanic acid (Augmentin).

See Chapter 38 for treatment of *N gonorrhoeae* infection. Chlamydial cervicitis is best treated with doxycycline, 100 mg twice daily for 1 week. Erythromycin should be substituted in pregnant women.

**B. Chronic Cervicitis:** Chronic cervicitis in an asymptomatic patient, as manifested by a purulent or mucopurulent exudate, found either grossly on a cotton swab from the endocervix or microscopically as 10 or more polymorphonuclear leukocytes per high-power field, should be treated. In the absence of evidence of *N gonorrhoeae,* treatment for *C trachomatis* in the form of doxycycline, 100 mg twice daily for 1 week is recommended.

Because of the frequent coexistence of gonorrheal and chlamydial infections and because *C trachomatis* is not responsive to antibiotics that are used to treat gonorrhea, the addition of doxycycline, 100 mg twice daily for 1 week, to the therapeutic regimen for gonorrhea is recommended.

Chronically infected, old, healed obstetric lacerations should also be treated.

**1. Medical treatment**–A chronic purulent discharge from the cervical canal of an otherwise normal-appearing cervix should be cultured and sensitivity tests should be ordered. Antibiotic treatment should be given systemically (orally or parenterally) rather than topically because there is little justification for treating deep-seated endocervical infections, which often are unresponsive to vaginal chemotherapy.

Medical treatment should be used initially for patients during and after the childbearing period. If the patient is unimproved after 2–3 months, minor surgical therapy is indicated.

**2. Surgical treatment**–Before treating cervicitis surgically, consider the results desired; the likelihood of postoperative bleeding, infection, stricture formation, and infertility; and the implications for vaginal delivery in future pregnancies. Cervical cauterization or office dilatation of the cervix must not be done in the premenstrual period because of the danger of ascending infection and postoperative infection, but puncture biopsy of nabothian cysts may be done at any time during the cycle.

Other surgical procedures may be used if the canal is widely exposed by lacerations or for severe chronic cervicitis. These procedures include light electrocauterization with low-frequency current using a nasal tip or small Post electrode, or mild electrocoagulation with a high-frequency monopolar electrode.

With electrocoagulation (and electrosurgery), both incision and coagulation are possible, and the penetration of heat and destruction of diseased gland tissue are uniform and controllable. For these reasons, most physicians prefer coagulation to cauterization, although both methods, if used with skill and restraint, give satisfactory results. Coagulation should be done radially.

When chronic cervicitis is accompanied by ectropion (ectopy, eversion), the most successful treatment is destruction of the involved tissues by electrocauterization, cryosurgery, or laser beam.

Electrocauterization is best performed in a radial strip fashion with either a thermal or a spark-type electrocautery within a few days following the completion of a menstrual period. Because of the paucity of nerve endings carrying pain sensation from the cervix, this can be done in the office without anesthesia. It should not be performed in an acutely inflamed cervix, since this may produce a spread of infection into the parametrial tissues. In addition, it should not be done before the possibility of an early cervical cancer has been eliminated by cytologic and biopsy examinations.

Cryosurgery destroys tissue by freezing. The refrigerants (carbon dioxide, Freon, nitrous oxide, or nitrogen—all in liquid state) are passed through a hollow probe placed in the cervical canal and against the external os. The advantages are the ease of administration and lack of discomfort when compared with thermal or electrocauterization. Moreover, postoperative bleeding and cervical stenosis are uncommon after cryosurgery. This treatment method has some disadvantages. The depth of tissue destruction is no more than 3–4 mm, and the profuse vaginal discharge that occurs for 2–3 weeks following its application is annoying.

In laser therapy, a high-energy beam of light in the infrared spectrum is directed to the cervix, resulting in complete vaporization of cells. As a result, there is no necrotic tissue slough and no resulting leukorrhea. The degree of cellular destruction is easily controlled, and the cervix heals with less scarring than with other methods. Disadvantages are the relatively large size and high cost of the equipment as well as the special training required.

The aim of the above-mentioned treatment methods is destruction of infected tissues with subsequent healing by fibroblastic proliferation and reepithelialization. Anesthesia is usually unnecessary for minor surgical treatment. Complete healing may take up to 6 weeks. The cervix should be inspected again at the end of this time to be certain that healing is satisfactory. It is rarely necessary to cauterize a second time. If cauterization must be repeated, however, it should be done 1–2 months after the initial treatment to encourage healing.

Many complications of cauterization result from injudicious or overly vigorous use of these methods. Reactivation of salpingitis may occur if treatment is given in the presence of acute cervicitis. Cervical ste-

nosis may follow deep cauterization or cryotherapy carried high into the endocervical canal. Cauterization or freezing of a cervix that contains an unrecognized malignant tumor will mask the neoplastic process, resulting in further delay in its recognition and perhaps serious consequences.

On rare occasions, it may be necessary to repair the lacerated cervix or remove a considerable portion of the cervix to eradicate a deep-seated infection. The latter requires loop excision, conization (Fig 35–13), or cervical amputation in the patient in whom it is important to preserve childbearing function. In patients with extensive chronic cervicitis who are beyond the childbearing years or who do not want more children, total hysterectomy may be the best method of management. This is particularly true when there is a second indication such as cervical dysplasia, symptomatic pelvic floor relaxation, or a need for sterilization.

## Treatment of Complications

**A. Cervical Hemorrhage:** This may follow electrocauterization, loop excision, cryosurgery, laser vaporization, trachelorrhaphy, or cervical amputation and may require suture and ligation of the bleeding vessels. Usually, point coagulation of bleeding areas is successful. Styptics such as Monsel's solution applied topically with snug vaginal packing may be helpful.

**B. Salpingitis:** Inflammation of the uterine tubes usually necessitates the administration of a broad-spectrum antibiotic.

**C. Leukorrhea:** Discharge is usually due to persistent cervicitis caused by pyogenic organisms. In acute cases the endocervix should be cultured and suitable antibiotic treatment given. In chronic cases, retreatment of cervicitis is indicated.

**D. Cervical Stenosis:** The gentle passage of graduated sounds through the cervical canal at weekly intervals during the intermenstrual phase for 2–3 months following treatment will prevent or correct stenosis.

**E. Infertility:** The absence of cervical mucus necessary for sperm migration often causes infertility and may be due to too extensive destruction (cauterization, freezing, or vaporization) or removal (conization, trachelorrhaphy, amputation of the cervix) of the endocervical glandular cells. Conjugated estrogenic substances (Premarin) or equivalent, 0.3 mg daily by mouth for 3–4 days prior to and on the day of ovulation may stimulate the remaining endocervical cells to produce more mucus. Assisted reproductive techniques may be required.

**F. Chronic Urinary Tract Infection:** The type of antiinfective therapy depends on the organism and the results of sensitivity tests.

## Prognosis

With conservative, systemic, and persistent ther-

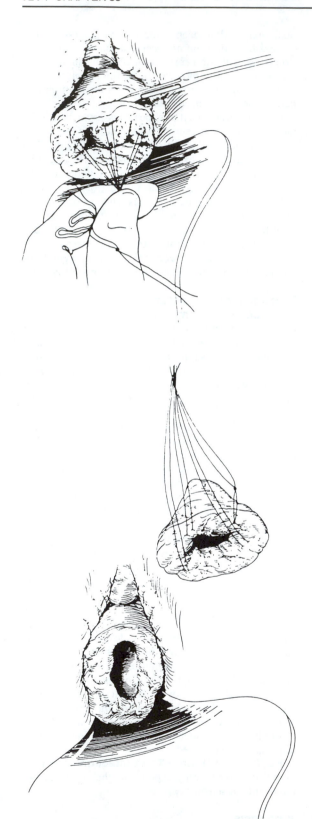

**Figrue 35–13.** Conization of the cervix.

apy, cervicitis can almost always be cured. With neglect or overtreatment, the prognosis is poor. Mild chronic cervicitis usually responds to therapy in 4–8 weeks; more severe chronic cervicitis may require 2–3 months of treatment.

## GRANULOMATOUS INFECTIONS OF THE CERVIX*

Tuberculosis, tertiary syphilis, and granuloma inguinale may on rare occasions be manifested by chronic cervical lesions. These lesions usually take the form of nodules, ulcerations, or granulation tissue. They produce a chronic inflammatory exudate characterized histologically by lymphocytes, giant cells, and histiocytes. They may simulate carcinoma of the cervix and must be distinguished from this and other neoplastic diseases.

### Tuberculosis

In 1986, the steadily decreasing incidence of tuberculosis in the USA over the previous several decades was reversed. Since then the risk has increased, particularly for Blacks, Hispanics, and Asians. Some of this increase has been attributed to the epidemic spread of the human immunodeficiency virus (HIV). Genitourinary tuberculosis is almost always secondary to infection elsewhere in the body, usually pulmonary, but active pulmonary disease can be documented in only one-third of patients. Vascular dissemination is responsible for infection of the fallopian tubes in almost all patients with genital tuberculosis, and involvement of the endometrium follows in 90%. Cervical disease is thought to be secondary to involvement of the endometrium but is rare, occurring in only 1%. In the past, genital tuberculosis has accounted for only 1% of patients with pelvic inflammatory disease; however, in European and Asian countries, the occurrence ranges from 2% to 10%. With increasing numbers of immigrants to the USA and with the rise in incidence of AIDS in US women, an increase in the incidence of pelvic tuberculosis can be expected.

The chief clinical manifestations of cervical involvement are a foul-smelling discharge and contact bleeding. The cervix may be hypertrophied and nodular, without any visible lesion on the portio vaginalis, or speculum examination may demonstrate either an ulcerative or a papillary lesion, thus resembling neoplastic disease.

The diagnosis of tuberculosis of the cervix must be made by biopsy. Histologically, the disease is characterized by tubercles undergoing central caseation. Because such lesions may be caused by other organisms,

*Syphilis and granuloma inguinale are discussed in Chapter 38.

it is necessary to demonstrate the tubercle bacillus by acid-fast stains or by culture.

The reader is referred to other texts for the details of medical therapy of genital tuberculosis. Most patients are cured by medical management alone; patients who respond poorly or who have other problems (eg, tumors, fistulas) may require total hysterectomy and bilateral salpingo-oophorectomy after a trial of chemotherapy.

## RARE INFECTIOUS DISEASES OF THE CERVIX

**Lymphogranuloma venereum,** a chlamydial infection, and *chancroid*, caused by *Haemophilus ducreyi*, may attack the cervix along with other areas of the reproductive tract.

**Cervical actinomycosis** may occur as a result of contamination by instruments and by intrauterine devices. The cervical lesion may be a nodular tumor, ulcer, or fistula. Prolonged penicillin or sulfonamide therapy is recommended.

**Schistosomiasis of the cervix** is usually secondary to involvement of the pelvic and uterine veins by the blood fluke *Schistosoma haematobium*. Cervical schistosomiasis may produce a large papillary growth that ulcerates and bleeds on contact, simulating cervical cancer. In other instances, it may be found in endocervical polyps, causing intermenstrual and postcoital bleeding. An ovum can occasionally be identified in a biopsy specimen taken from the granulomatous cervical lesion. The diagnosis is usually made, however, by recovering the parasite from the urine or feces. Chemical, serologic, and intradermal tests for schistosomiasis are also available.

**Echinococcal cysts** may involve the cervix. Treatment consists of surgical excision.

## CYSTIC ABNORMALITIES OF THE CERVIX

### Nabothian Cysts

When a tunnel or cleft of tall columnar endocervical epithelium becomes sealed off, either through an inflammatory process or as a result of epidermidization (squamous metaplasia), mucous secretions become entrapped, producing a cyst of microscopic to macroscopic size. These nabothian cysts develop frequently, but they reach clinical significance only when they are so numerous that they produce marked enlargement of the cervix due to the retention of mucus. On the portio vaginalis of the cervix their presence serves as an indication that the portio was at one time the site of ectopic endocervical epithelium that has been replaced by squamous epithelium. The nabothian cyst farthest away from the external cervical os on the portio indicates the extent of the "transformation zone."

### Mesonephric Cysts

Microscopic remnants of the mesonephric (wolffian) duct are often seen deep in the stroma externally in the normal cervix. Occasionally they become cystic, forming structures up to 2.5 mm in diameter lined by ragged cuboid epithelium. They may be confused with deeply situated nabothian cysts, but their location and the wolffian-type cells lining the cysts serve as useful distinguishing features.

### Endometriosis

Endometriosis occasionally produces small reddish or purplish cystic structures on the portio vaginalis of the cervix. These usually measure several millimeters in diameter, but cysts larger than 1 cm have occasionally been reported. Endometriosis involves the cervix primarily by implantation during delivery or surgery or by direct extension from the cul-de-sac, in which case the adjacent vagina also is usually involved. Biopsy showing typical endometrial glands and stroma is diagnostic. These areas of ectopic endometrium usually respond to hormonal stimuli during the menstrual cycle. Intermenstrual and postcoital bleeding, dysmenorrhea, and dyspareunia may be associated symptoms. Rarely, the lesions may resemble cervical cancer; hence, the diagnosis of endometriosis depends on biopsy. Small lesions may be destroyed by cauterization, but larger ones must be excised.

## CERVICAL STENOSIS

Cervical stenosis—of congenital, inflammatory, neoplastic, or surgical origin—may be partially or even completely occlusive. Most cases of cervical stenosis follow extensive surgical manipulation of the cervix (eg, electrocoagulation, cryotherapy, laser vaporization, conization, or cervical amputation) or radiation therapy. Marked to complete obstruction to menstrual drainage will result in hematometra, typified by cryptomenorrhea or amenorrhea; abdominal discomfort; and a soft, slightly tender midpelvic mass. Pyometra may develop in the postmenopausal woman with cervical stenosis and always raises the suspicion of an associated endometrial carcinoma. Both hematometra and pyometra are readily confirmed by pelvic ultrasonography.

Cautious dilatation of the cervix is recommended, with drainage of the entrapped fluid. Cultures and sensitivity tests should be done and, with appropriate antibiotic coverage, cervical or endometrial tissue or both should be obtained to rule out cancer. The endocervical canal should receive minimal caustic therapy or electrotherapy for chronic cervicitis to avoid cervical stenosis. Removal of the cicatrix by laser vaporization has been effective in cases of postconization stenosis.

## BENIGN NEOPLASMS OF THE CERVIX

### 1. MICROGLANDULAR HYPERPLASIA OF THE ENDOCERVICAL MUCOSA

Microglandular (adenomatous) hyperplasia of the endocervix, an abnormal response to the hormonal stimulus of oral contraceptive medication, may occur in occasional patients. It may also result from inflammation. Grossly, adenomatous hyperplasia appears as exuberant granular tissue within the cervical canal, often extruding beyond the cervical os. The disorder may be mistaken for cancer, but biopsy should make the distinction. Microscopically, it presents as a collection of closely packed cystic spaces lined by nonneoplastic columnar epithelium and filled with mucus.

### 2. CERVICAL POLYPS

#### Essentials of Diagnosis

- Intermenstrual or postcoital bleeding.
- A soft, red pedunculated protrusion from the cervical canal at the external os.
- Microscopic examination confirms the diagnosis of benign polyp.

#### General Considerations

Cervical polyps are small pedunculated, often sessile neoplasms of the cervix. Most originate from the endocervix; a few arise from the portio (Fig 35–14). They are composed of a vascular connective tissue stroma and covered by columnar, squamocolumnar, or squamous epithelium. Polyps are relatively common, especially in multigravidas over 20 years of age. They are rare before the menarche, but an occasional polyp may develop after menopause. Asymptomatic polyps often are discovered on routine pelvic examination. Most are benign, but all should be removed and submitted for pathologic examination because malignant change may occur. Moreover, some cervical cancers present as a polypoid mass.

Polyps arise as a result of focal hyperplasia of the endocervix. It is not known whether this is due to chronic inflammation, an abnormal local responsiveness to hormonal stimulation, or a localized vascular congestion of cervical blood vessels. They are often found in association with endometrial hyperplasia, suggesting that hyperestrinism plays a significant etiologic role.

Endocervical polyps are usually red, flame-shaped, fragile growths and may vary in size from a few millimeters in length and diameter to larger tumors 2–3 cm in diameter and several centimeters long. These polyps are usually attached to the endocervical mucosa near the external os by a narrow pedicle, but occasionally the base is broad. On microscopic examination, the stroma of a polyp is composed of fibrous connective tissue containing numerous small blood vessels in the center. There is often an extravasation of blood and a marked infiltration of the stroma by inflammatory cells (polymorphonuclear neutrophils, lymphocytes, and plasma cells). The surface epithelium resembles that of the endocervix, varying from typical picket fence columnar cells to areas that show squamous metaplasia and mature stratified squamous epithelium. The surface often is thrown into folds much as is the normal endocervical mucosa.

Ectocervical polyps are pale, flesh-colored, smooth, and rounded or elongated, often with a broad pedicle. They arise from the portio and are less likely to bleed than endocervical polyps. Microscopically, they are more fibrous than endocervical polyps, having few or no mucous glands. They are covered by stratified squamous epithelium.

Metaplastic alteration is common. Inflammation, often with necrosis at the tip (or more extensively), is typical of both polyp types.

The incidence of malignant change in a cervical polyp is estimated to be less than 1%. Squamous cell carcinoma is the most common type, although adenocarcinomas have been reported. Endometrial cancer may involve the polyp secondarily. Sarcoma rarely develops within a polyp.

Botryoid sarcoma, an embryonal tumor of the cervix (or vaginal wall) resembling small pink or yellow grapes, contains striated muscle and other mesenchymal elements. It is extremely malignant.

Most polypoid structures are vascular and often infected and are subject to displacement or torsion. Discharge commonly results, and bleeding, often metrorrhagia of the postcoital type, follows.

Chronic irritation and bleeding are annoying and cause cervicitis, endometritis, and parametritis; salpingitis may develop if these are not treated successfully.

Because polyps are a potential focus of cancer, they must be examined routinely for malignant characteristics on removal.

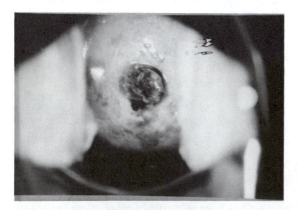

**Figure 35–14.** Cervical polyp.

## Clinical Findings

**A. Symptoms and Signs:** Intermenstrual or postcoital bleeding is the most common symptom of the presence of cervical polyps. Leukorrhea and hypermenorrhea have also been associated with cervical polyps.

Abnormal vaginal bleeding is often reported. Postmenopausal bleeding is frequently described by older women. Infertility may be traceable to cervical polyps and cervicitis.

Cervical polyps appear as smooth, red, finger-like projections from the cervical canal and are usually about 1–2 cm in length and 0.5–1 cm in diameter. Generally they are too soft to be felt by the examining finger.

**B. X-Ray Findings:** Polyps high in the endocervical canal may be demonstrated by hysterography and often are a significant finding in hitherto unexplained infertility.

**C. Laboratory Findings:** Vaginal cytology will reveal signs of infection and often mildly atypical cells. Blood and urine studies are not helpful.

**D. Special Examination:** A polyp high in the endocervical canal may occasionally be seen with the aid of a special endocervical speculum or by hysteroscopy. Some polyps are found only at the time of diagnostic D&C in the investigation of abnormal bleeding.

## Differential Diagnosis

Masses projecting from the cervix may be polypoid but not polyps. Adenocarcinoma of the endometrium or endometrial sarcoma may present at the external os or even beyond. Discharge and bleeding usually occur.

Typical polyps are not difficult to diagnose by gross inspection, but ulcerated and atypical growths must be distinguished from small submucous pedunculated myomas or endometrial polyps arising low in the uterus. These often result in dilatation of the cervix, presenting just within the os and resembling cervical polyps. The products of conception, usually decidua, may push through the cervix and resemble a polypoid tissue mass, but other signs and symptoms of recent pregnancy generally are absent. Condylomata, submucous myomas, and polypoid carcinomas are diagnosed by microscopic examination.

## Complications

All cervical polyps are infected, some by virulent staphylococci, streptococci, or other pathogens. Serious infections occasionally follow instrumentation for the identification or removal of polyps. A broad-spectrum antibiotic should be administered at the first sign or symptom of spreading infection.

Acute salpingitis may be initiated or exacerbated by polypectomy.

It is unwise to remove a large polyp and then do a hysterectomy several days thereafter. Pelvic peritonitis may complicate the latter procedure. A delay of several weeks or a month between polypectomy and hysterectomy is recommended.

## Prevention

Because of the possible role of chronic inflammation in polyp formation, cervicitis must always be treated promptly.

## Treatment

**A. Medical Measures:** Culture and sensitivity tests of cervical discharge and appropriate therapy are indicated if infection is present.

**B. Specific Measures:** Most polyps can be removed in the physician's office. This is done with little bleeding by grasping the pedicle with a hemostat or uterine packing forceps and twisting it until the growth is avulsed. Large polyps and those with sessile attachments may require electrosurgical excision and suturing. It may be wise in some cases to perform these procedures in the hospital because of the risk of hemorrhage.

If the cervix is soft, patulous, or definitely dilated and the polyp is large, surgical D&C should be done, especially if the pedicle is not readily visible. Exploration of the cervical and uterine cavities with the polyp forceps and curet may disclose multiple polyps or other important lesions.

All tissue must be sent to a pathologist to be examined for cancer.

**C. Local Measures:** Warm acetic acid douches after polypectomy usually suffice to control an inflammatory reaction. Prophylactic antibiotic therapy is not usually necessary.

## Prognosis

Simple removal of cervical polyps is usually curative.

## 3. PAPILLOMAS OF THE CERVIX

### Essentials of Diagnosis

- Asymptomatic.
- Papillary projection from the exocervix.
- The presence of koilocytes with or without cytologic atypia.
- Colposcopic identification.

### General Considerations

Cervical papillomas are benign neoplasms found on the portio vaginalis of the cervix. They are of 2 types: (1) The typical solitary papillary projection from the exocervix, composed of a central core of fibrous connective tissue covered by stratified squamous epithelium. This is a true benign neoplasm, and the cause is unknown. (2) Condylomata of the cervix, which may be present in various forms ranging from a slightly raised area on the exocervix that appears white after acetic acid application (on colposcopy) to the typical condyloma acuminatum. These are usually multiple and are caused by HPV infection, a sexually transmitted disease. Similar lesions of the vagina and vulva are often, but not always, present. Evidence of HPV infection can be found in 1–2% of cytologically screened women. The incidence is much higher in women attending sexually transmitted disease clinics.

## Clinical Findings

**A. Symptoms and Signs:** There are no characteristic symptoms of cervical papillomas; they are often discovered on routine pelvic examination or colposcopic examination for dysplasia revealed by Papanicolaou smear.

**B. Laboratory Findings:** Cytologic findings of koilocytes—squamous cells with perinuclear clear halos—are strongly suggestive of HPV infection. Dysplastic squamous cells are frequently found in association with koilocytes. Biopsy of involved epithelium reveals papillomatosis and acanthosis. Mitoses may be frequent, but in the absence of neoplastic change, the cells are orderly with regular nuclear features. Koilocytes predominate in the superficial cells.

## Complications

Intraepithelial neoplasia is associated with certain types of HPV infection (see Dysplasia of the Cervix, Chapter 47). The presence of condylomata of the portio vaginalis substantially increases the risk of squamous cell carcinoma of the cervix.

## Prevention

Contraception with condoms and possibly other barrier methods may prevent primary infection and reinfection.

## Treatment

Solitary papillomas should be surgically excised and submitted for pathologic examination. Likewise, biopsies of flat condylomata should be submitted for histopathologic examination. Flat condylomata may be completely removed with the punch biopsy forceps if they are small. More extensive lesions may require electrodesiccation, cryotherapy, loop excision, or laser vaporization. Topical 5-fluorouracil cream (Efudex) has also been used successfully, but patient compliance is low because of discomfort. Dysplasia associated with HPV infection should be managed according to the severity and extent of the dysplastic process (see Dysplasia of the Cervix, Chapter 47).

## Prognosis

Because the entire lower genital tract is a target area for HPV infection, long-term follow-up with attention to the cervix, vagina, and vulva is necessary. Excision of solitary, non-HPV-related papillomas is curative.

## 4. LEIOMYOMAS OF THE CERVIX

The paucity of smooth muscle elements in the cervical stroma makes leiomyomas arising primarily in the cervix uncommon. The ratio of corpus leiomyomas to cervical leiomyomas is in the range of 12:1.

Although myomas are usually multiple in the corpus, cervical myomas are most often solitary and may be large enough to fill the entire pelvic cavity, compressing the bladder, rectum, and ureters (Fig 35–15). Grossly and microscopically, they are identical with leiomyomas arising elsewhere in the uterus.

## Clinical Findings

**A. Symptoms and Signs:** Cervical leiomyomas are often silent, producing no symptoms unless they become very large. Symptoms are those due to pressure on surrounding organs such as the bladder, rectum, or soft tissues of the parametrium or obstruction of the cervical canal. Frequency and urgency of urination are the result of bladder compression. Urinary retention occasionally occurs as a result of pressure against the urethra. Hematometra may develop with obstruction of the cervix.

If the direction of growth is lateral, there may be ureteral obstruction with hydronephrosis. Rectal en-

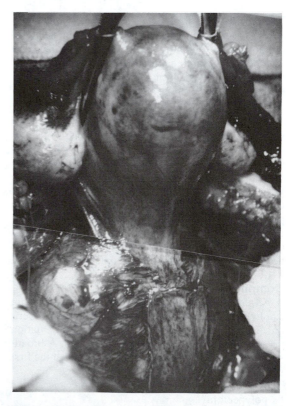

**Figure 35–15.** Large cervical leiomyoma filling true pelvis.

croachment causes constipation. Dyspareunia may occur if the tumor occupies the vagina. In pregnancy, because of their location, large cervical leiomyomas, unlike those involving the corpus, are apt to cause soft tissue dystocia, preventing descent of the presenting part in the pelvis.

Cervical leiomyomas of significant size can be readily palpated on bimanual examination.

**B. Imaging:** A plain film may demonstrate the typical mottled calcific pattern associated with cervical leiomyomas. Hysterography may define distortion of the endocervical canal. Intravenous urography may demonstrate ureteral displacement or obstruction. MRI is diagnostic.

## Treatment

Small, asymptomatic cervical leiomyomas should be observed for rate of growth. If they become larger,

they should be removed, and it may be possible to enucleate a single, small tumor via the vaginal route. However, because cervical tumors are often associated with multiple leiomyomas of the corpus, the surgical approach is usually an abdominal one and the treatment is either a multiple myomectomy or total hysterectomy, depending on the clinical circumstances and the need to preserve the uterus for childbearing.

Because of the proximity of the pelvic ureter to the cervix, this structure may be in jeopardy in any operation involving a cervical leiomyoma, and precautions should be taken to prevent its injury.

## Prognosis

Recurrence of cervical leiomyomas after surgical removal is rare.

## REFERENCES

### ANOMALIES OF THE CERVIX

Buttram VC Jr, Gibbons WE: Müllerian anomalies: A proposed classification (an analysis of 144 cases). Fertil Steril 1979;32:40.

Carrington BM et al: Müllerian duct anomalies: MR imaging. Radiology 1990;176:715.

Kalstone C: Cervical stenosis in pregnancy: A complication of cryotherapy in diethylstilbestrol-exposed women. Am J Obstet Gynecol 1992;166:502.

Sandberg EC: Benign cervical and vaginal changes associated with exposure to stilbestrol in utero. Am J Obstet Gynecol 1976;125:777.

### CERVICAL INFECTIONS

Addess DG et al: *Chlamydia trachomatis* infection in women attending urban midwestern family planning and community health clinics: Risk factors, selective screening, and evaluation of non-culture techniques. Sex Transm Dis 1990;17:138.

Brown ZA et al: Neonatal herpes simplex infection in relation to asymptomatic maternal infection at the time of labor. N Engl J Med 1991;324:1247.

Carlson JA Jr et al: Clinical and pathologic correlation of endometrial cavity fluid detected by ultrasound in the postmenopausal patient. Obstet Gynecol 1991;77:119.

Centers for Disease Control: 1989 Sexually transmitted disease guidelines. MMWR 1989;38(Suppl 8).

Frisch LE, Buckley LD, Chalem SA: Inflammatory epithelial changes and nonviral cervicovaginal pathogens. Acta Cytol 1990;34:129.

Handsfield HH: Old enemies: Combating syphilis and gonorrhea in the 1990s. JAMA 1990;264:1451.

Horn JE et al: Genital human papillomavirus infections in patients attending an inner-city STD clinic. Sex Transm Dis 1991;18:183.

Judson FN et al: Multicenter study of a single 500 mg dose of cefotaxime for treatment of uncomplicated gonorrhea. Sex Transm Dis 1991;18:41.

Karchmer AW: Sexually transmitted diseases, Chapter 7. *Infectious Diseases.* Sci Am Med 1989.

Kataja V et al: Prognostic factors in human papillomavirus infections. Sex Transm Dis 1992;19:154.

Katz BP et al: A randomized trial to compare 7- and 21-day tetracycline regimens in the prevention of recurrence of infection with *Chlamydia trachomatis*. Sex Transm Dis 1991;18:36.

Knud-Hansen et al: Surrogate methods to diagnose gonococcal and chlamydial cervicitis: Comparison of leukocyte esterase dipstick, endocervical gram stain, and culture. Sex Transm Dis 1991;18:211.

Krettek JE et al: *Chlamydia trachomatis* in patients who used oral contraceptives and had intermenstrual spotting. Obstet Gynecol 1993;81:728.

Lorincz AT et al: Human papillomavirus infection of the cervix: Relative risk associations of 15 common anogenital types. Obstet Gynecol 1992;79:328.

Magat AH et al: Double-blind randomized study comparing amoxicillin and erythromycin for the treatment of *Chlamydia trachomatis* in pregnancy. Obstet Gynecol 1993;81:745.

Nieminen P et al: Cervical human papillomavirus deoxyribonucleic acid and cytologic evaluations in gynecologic outpatients. Am J Obstet Gynecol 1991;164:1265.

Paavonen J et al: Etiology of cervical inflammation. Am J Obstet Gynecol 1986;154:556.

Paavonen J et al: Randomized treatment of mucopurulent cervicitis with doxycycline or amoxicillin. Am J Obstet Gynecol 1989;161:128.

Portilla I et al: Oral cefixime versus intramuscular ceftriaxone in patients with uncomplicated gonococcal infections. Sex Transm Dis 1992;19:94.

Rieder HL et al: Tuberculosis in the United States. JAMA 1989;262:385.

Schachter J et al: Experience with the routine use of

erythromycin for chlamydial infections in pregnancy. N Engl J Med 1986;314:276.

Schachter J: Why we need a program for the control of *Chlamydia trachomatis*. (Editorial.) N Engl J Med 1989;320:802.

Schachter J: Chlamydial infections. West J Med 1990; 153:523.

Smith JR et al: Prevalence of *Chlamydia trachomatis* infection in women having cervical smear tests. BMJ 1991;302:413.

Stenberg K, Per-Anders M: Genital infection with *Chlamydia trachomatis* in patients with chlamydial conjunctivitis: Unexplained results. Sex Transm Dis 1991;18:1.

Sutherland AM: Postmenopausal tuberculosis of the female genital tract. Obstet Gynecol 1982;59:545.

Sutherland AM: Gynaecological tuberculosis: Analysis of a personal series of 710 cases. Aust NZ J Obstet Gynecol 1985;25:203.

Yliskoski M et al: Clinical course of cervical human papillomavirus lesions in relation to coexistent cervical infections. Sex Transm Dis 1992;19:137.

## CERVICAL POLYPS

Kerner H, Lichtig: Müllerian adenosarcoma presenting as cervical polyps: A report of seven cases and review of the literature. Obstet Gynecol 1993;18:655.

# Benign Disorders of the Uterine Corpus

# 36

*Alvin S. Wexler, MD, & Martin L. Pernoll, MD*

## LEIOMYOMA OF THE UTERUS (Fibromyoma, Fibroid, Myoma)

### Essentials of Diagnosis

- Mass: irregular enlargement of the uterus.
- Bleeding: hypermenorrhea, metrorrhagia, dysmenorrhea.
- Pain: torsion or degeneration.
- Pressure: symptoms from neighboring organs.

### General Considerations

Uterine leiomyomas are benign, uterine neoplasms composed primarily of smooth muscle. Leiomyomas are present in 20–25% of reproductive-age women, but for an unknown reason, leiomyoma are 3–9 times more frequent in black than white women. Indeed, by the fifth decade as many as 50% of black women will have leiomyomata.

The etiology of this common tumor is not known. Leiomyomas are not detectable before puberty and, being hormonally responsive, normally grow only during the reproductive years. While they can occur as isolated microscopic growths, they are more commonly multiple. They are usually less than 15 cm in size but rarely may reach enormous proportions, weighing more than 45 kg (100 lb).

While usually asymptomatic, leiomyomata can produce a wide spectrum of problems including metrorrhagia and menorrhagia, pain, and even infertility. Indeed, excessive uterine bleeding from leiomyomas is one of the most common indications for hysterectomy in the USA.

Perhaps the most consequential aspect of asymptomatic leiomyomas is their ability to mask other simultaneous and potentially lethal pelvic tumors. The physician should not be deceived into following "asymptomatic myomas" without unequivocal substantiation that an underlying uterine tube, ovarian, or bowel carcinoma does not also exist. Occasionally it is necessary to differentiate leiomyomata from leiomyosarcoma. The latter occurs infrequently (see p. 733) and is malignant.

### Pathogenesis

The cause of uterine leiomyomata is not known. There is evidence that each individual leiomyoma is unicellular in origin (monoclonal) from glucose-6-phosphate dehydrogenase studies. While there is no evidence to suggest that estrogens cause leiomyomas, they are certainly implicated in their growth. Leiomyomas contain estrogen receptors in higher concentrations than in the surrounding myometrium but in lower concentrations than in the endometrium. Data concerning progesterone receptors in leiomyomata are inconsistent. Leiomyomas generally increase in size with estrogen therapy and during pregnancy but decrease in size and even disappear following menopause.

The hypothesis that human growth hormone (HGH) is related to the development of leiomyomas has been largely dispelled by radioimmunoassay studies of HGH in pregnant patients and in patients taking estrogens, but there is speculation that leiomyoma growth in pregnancy is related to synergistic activity of estradiol and human placental lactogen (HPL).

### Pathology

Leiomyomas are usually multiple, discrete, and spherical, or irregularly lobulated. Although leiomyomas have a false capsular covering, they are clearly demarcated from the surrounding myometrium and can be easily and cleanly enucleated from the surrounding tissue. On gross examination in transverse section, they are buff-colored, rounded, smooth, and usually firm. Generally they are lighter in color than the myometrium (Fig 36–1). When a fresh specimen is sectioned, the tumor surface projects above the surface of the surrounding musculature, revealing the pseudocapsule.

**A. Classification:** Uterine leiomyomas originate in the myometrium and are classified by anatomic location (Fig 36–2). Submucous leiomyomas lie just beneath the endometrium and tend to compress it as they grow toward the uterine lumen. Their impact on the endometrium and its blood supply most often leads to irregular uterine bleeding. Leiomyo-

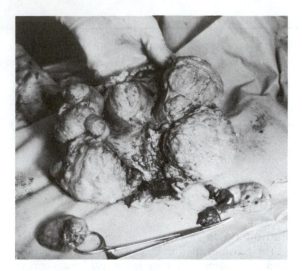

**Figure 36–1.** Multiple leiomyomas. Cervix is opened at the bottom.

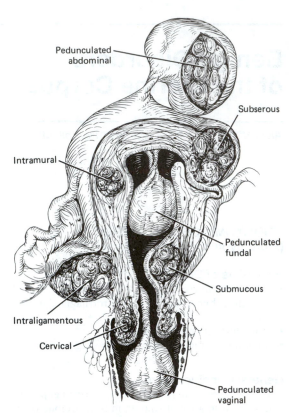

**Figure 36–2.** Myomas of the uterus.

mata may also develop pedicles and protrude fully into the uterine cavity. Occasionally they may even pass through the cervical canal while still attached within the corpus by a long stalk. When this occurs leiomyomata are subject to torsion or infection, conditions that must be taken into consideration before treatment.

Intramural or interstitial leiomyomas lie within the uterine wall, giving it a variable consistency. Subserous or subperitoneal leiomyomata may lie just at the serosal surface of the uterus or may bulge outward from the myometrium. The subserous leiomyomata may also become pedunculated. If such a tumor acquires an extrauterine blood supply from omental vessels, its pedicle may atrophy and resorb; the tumor is then said to be parasitic. Subserous tumors arising laterally may extend between the 2 peritoneal layers of the broad ligament to become intraligamentary leiomyomas. This may lead to compromise of the ureter and/or pelvic blood supply.

**B. Microscopic Structure:** Nonstriated muscle fibers are arranged in interlacing bundles of varying size running in different directions (whorled appearance). Individual cells are spindle-shaped, have elongated nuclei, and are quite uniform in size. Characteristically, varying amounts of connective tissue are intermixed with the smooth muscle bundles. Leiomyomata are sharply demarcated from surrounding normal musculature by a pseudocapsule of areolar tissue and compressed myometrium. The arterial density of a leiomyoma is less than that of the surrounding myometrium, and the small arteries that supply the tumor are less tortuous than the adjacent radial arteries. The arteries penetrate the myoma randomly on its surface and are oriented in the direction of the muscle bundles; thus, they present no regular

pattern. One or 2 major vessels are found in the base or pedicle. The venous pattern appears to be even more sparse, but this may be in part artifactual because of the difficulty encountered in filling the venous circulation under artificial conditions.

**C. Secondary Changes:** There may be areas of hyalinization, liquefaction (cystic degeneration), calcification, hemorrhage, fat, or inflammation within leiomyomata. While these secondary alterations are histologically interesting, they usually have little clinical significance. Whether or not leiomyosarcomas are a malignant alteration within a mature leiomyoma, as is commonly stated, or arise de novo remains an unsettled issue. Extraordinarily cellular myomas have often been misinterpreted as sarcomas because the criteria used to differentiate leiomyoma from sarcoma are imprecise and often subjective. Ultrastructural studies suggest that leiomyoma and leiomyosarcoma are distinct entities and that the cellular leiomyoma is merely a variety of the common leiomyoma.

**1. Benign degeneration**–Benign degeneration is of the following types:

**a. Atrophic**–Signs and symptoms regress or disappear as the tumor size decreases at menopause or after pregnancy.

**b. Hyaline**–Mature or "old" leiomyomas are white but contain yellow, soft, and often gelatinous areas of hyaline change. These tumors are usually asymptomatic.

**c. Cystic**–Liquefaction follows extreme hyalinization, and physical stress may cause sudden evacuation of fluid contents into the uterus, the peritoneal cavity, or the retroperitoneal space.

**d. Calcific (calcareous)**–Subserous leiomyomata are most commonly affected by circulatory deprivation, which causes precipitation of calcium carbonate and phosphate within the tumor.

**e. Septic**–Circulatory inadequacy may cause necrosis of the central portion of the tumor followed by infection. Acute pain, tenderness, and fever result.

**f. Carneous (red)**–Venous thrombosis and congestion with interstitial hemorrhage are responsible for the color of a leiomyoma undergoing red degeneration (Fig 36–3). During pregnancy, when carneous degeneration is most common, edema and hypertrophy of the myometrium occur. The physiologic changes in the leiomyoma are not the same as in the myometrium; the resultant anatomic discrepancy impedes the blood supply, resulting in aseptic degeneration and infarction. The process is usually accompanied by pain but is self-limited. Potential complications of degeneration in pregnancy include preterm labor and, albeit rarely, initiation of disseminated intravascular coagulation.

**g. Myxomatous (fatty)**–This uncommon and asymptomatic degeneration follows hyaline and cystic degeneration.

**2. Malignant transformation**–Malignant transformation (leiomyosarcomas) are reported to develop with a frequency of 0.1–0.5% that of diagnosed leiomyomata.

### Clinical Findings

**A. Symptoms:** Symptoms are present in only

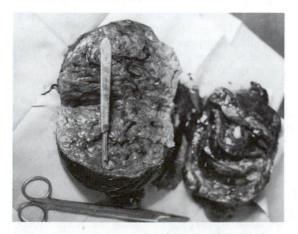

**Figure 36–3.** Carneous (red) degeneration. Note the congested, dark appearance as compared with Figure 36–1.

35–50% of patients with leiomyomas. Thus, most leiomyomata do not produce symptoms, and even very large ones may remain undetected, particularly by the obese patient. Symptoms from leiomyomas depend on their location, size, state of preservation and whether or not the patient is pregnant.

**1. Abnormal uterine bleeding**–Abnormal uterine bleeding is by far and away the most common and most important clinical manifestation of leiomyomas, being present in up to 30% of patients. The abnormal bleeding commonly produces iron deficiency anemia, which may become uncontrollable with iron therapy if the bleeding is heavy and protracted.

Bleeding from a submucous leiomyoma may occur from interruption of the blood supply to the endometrium, distortion and congestion of the surrounding vessels, particularly the veins, or ulceration of the overlying endometrium. Most commonly, the patient has prolonged, heavy menses (menorrhagia), premenstrual spotting, or prolonged light staining following menses; however, any type of abnormal bleeding is possible.

Minor degrees of metrorrhagia (intermenstrual bleeding) may be associated with a tumor that has areas of endometrial venous thrombosis and necrosis on its surface, particularly if it is pedunculated and partially extruded through the cervical canal.

**2. Pain**–Leiomyomata are rarely painful unless vascular compromise occurs. Thus, pain may result from degeneration associated with vascular occlusion, infection, torsion of a pedunculated tumor, or myometrial contractions to expel a subserous myoma from the uterine cavity. The pain associated with infarction from torsion or red degeneration can be excruciating and produce a clinical picture consistent with acute abdomen.

Large tumors may produce a sensation of heaviness in the pelvic area or perhaps a discomfort described as a "bearing-down" feeling. Tumors that become impacted within the bony pelvis may press on nerves and create pain radiating to the back or lower extremities. Backache is such a common general complaint that it is usually difficult to ascribe it specifically to myomas.

**3. Pressure effects**–Pressure effects are unusual and difficult to directly relate to leiomyomata, except in certain circumstances. Intramural or intraligamentous leiomyomata may distort or obstruct other organs. Parasitic tumors may cause intestinal obstruction if they are large or involve omentum or bowel. Cervical tumors may cause serosanguineous vaginal discharge, vaginal bleeding, dyspareunia, and infertility. Large cervical tumors may fill the true pelvis and displace or compress the ureters, bladder, or rectum.

Compression of surrounding structures may result in urinary symptoms or hydroureter. Large tumors may cause pelvic venous congestion and lower extremity edema or constipation. Rarely, an impacted tumor may lead to urinary retention because of pressure on the urethra. A posterior fundal leiomyoma may carry the uterus into extreme retroflexion, distorting the bladder base and causing urinary retention. This may present as intermittent overflow incontinence produced by elongation of the urethra with loss of sphincter control—a situation identical to sacculation of the uterus during early pregnancy. The condition is relieved by dislodging the uterus from the true pelvis with the patient in the knee-chest position.

**4. Infertility**–Inability to conceive may be the presenting complaint, but leiomyomata are the sole cause of infertility in only 2–10% of patients. The association of infertility and leiomyomata may signal a pedunculated endometrial tumor; but, infertility secondary to leiomyoma may also be related to abnormal uterine bleeding (or blood flow), abnormal uterine or tubal motility or interference with sperm transport.

**5. Spontaneous abortion**–The incidence of spontaneous abortion secondary to leiomyoma is unknown but is possibly 2 times the incidence in normal pregnant women. For example, the incidence of spontaneous abortion prior to myomectomy is approximately 40% and following myomectomy is approximately 20%.

**B. Examination:** Myomas are easily discovered by routine bimanual examination of the uterus or sometimes by palpation of the lower abdomen. Uterine retroflexion and retroversion may obscure the physical examination diagnosis of even moderately large leiomyomata. When the cervix is pulled up behind the symphysis, large fibroids are usually implicated. The diagnosis is obvious when the normal uterine contour is distorted by one or more smooth, spherical, firm masses, but often it is difficult to be absolutely certain that such masses are part of the uterus. A pelvic ultrasound generally assists in establishing the diagnosis, as well as excluding pregnancy as a cause of the uterine enlargement.

**C. Laboratory Findings:** As noted earlier, anemia is a most common consequence of leiomyomata. This is due to the excessive uterine bleeding and depletion of iron reserves. However, occasional patients display erythrocytosis. The hematocrit returns to normal levels following removal of the uterus, and elevated erythropoietin levels have been reported in such cases. Moreover, the recognized association of polycythemia and renal disease has led to speculation that leiomyomas may compress the ureters to cause ureteral back pressure and thus induce renal erythropoietin production.

Leukocytosis, fever, and an elevated sedimentation rate may be present with acute degeneration or infection.

**D. Imaging:** Pelvic ultrasound examinations have reached a level of technical sophistication to be of usefulness in these cases. While ultrasound should never be a substitute for a thorough pelvic examination, it can be extremely helpful in identifying leiomyomata, detailing the cause of other pelvic masses and in the identification of pregnancy. Moreover, ultrasonography is of particular usefulness in the obese individual.

Large leiomyomata typically appear as soft tissue masses on x-rays of the lower abdomen and pelvis; however, attention is sometimes drawn to the tumors by calcifications. Hysterosalpingography may be useful in detailing an intrauterine leiomyoma in the infertile patient.

Intravenous urography is indispensable in the workup of any pelvic mass, because it frequently reveals ureteral deviation or compression and identifies urinary anomalies. It is essential at operation to know the anatomic position and number of ureters and kidneys.

Magnetic resonance imaging (MRI) is highly accurate in depicting the number, size, and location of leiomyomata, but it is rarely necessary.

**E. Special Examinations:** Hysteroscopy may assist in identification, as well as be used for removal, of a submucous leiomyomata. Laparoscopy is often definitive in establishing the precise origin of the leiomyomata and is increasingly being used for myomectomy (see later).

**Differential Diagnosis**

The diagnosis of uterine myoma is not usually difficult, although any pelvic mass, including pregnancy, may be mistaken for leiomyomata. Indeed, leiomyoma is a common preoperative diagnosis for ovarian carcinoma, endolymphatic stromal meiosis, tubo-ovarian abscess, and endometriosis. Modern imaging techniques may clarify the diagnosis, particularly in obese women or when palpation is difficult for other reasons, eg, when the abdominal muscles are tense.

Ovarian cysts or neoplasia must be considered in the differential diagnosis of uterine leiomyomata. Other adnexal considerations include tubo-ovarian inflammatory or neoplastic masses. Uterine enlargement simulating leiomyomata may be due to pregnancy (including subinvolution), endometrial cancer, adenomyosis, myometrial hypertrophy, or congenital anomalies. Adnexa, omentum, or bowel adherent to the uterus also may be erroneously diagnosed as leiomyomata. Because a fetus may exist within an obviously myomatous uterus, a pregnancy test should be obtained in all women of childbearing age.

The most common symptom of leiomyomata, recurrent abnormal bleeding, may be caused by any of the numerous conditions that affect the uterus. Adenocarcinoma of the endometrium or uterine tube, uterine sarcomas, and ovarian carcinomas are the most lethal and therefore the most important to be excluded. Hyperplasia, polyps, irregular shedding, dysfunctional (nonorganic) bleeding, tubal carcinoma, ovarian neoplasms, endometriosis, adenomyosis, and exogenous estrogens or steroid hormones may all cause abnormal bleeding.

The definitive diagnosis can be established by endometrial biopsy or fractional dilation and curettage (D&C). The latter procedure should be considered essential in the workup of any patient with abnormal bleeding or a pelvic mass who has not recently had an evaluation of her endocervical canal and endometrial cavity by curettage. Even in the presence of uterine leiomyomas, other conditions can coexist and must be ruled out before definitive therapy.

## Complications

**A. Myomas and Pregnancy:** The literature is replete with indications that myomectomy does improve the chance of conception in some women even after other causes of infertility have been excluded. The reported incidence of pregnancy following myomectomy is about 40% in previously infertile women.

During the second and third trimesters of pregnancy, myomas may rapidly increase in size and undergo vascular depravation and subsequent degenerative changes. Clinically this most commonly leads to pain and localized tenderness (see carneous degeneration, earlier) but may also initiate preterm labor. Expectant management with bed rest and narcotics is virtually always successful in alleviation of the pain, but tocolytics may be necessary to control the uterine contractions. Once the acute episode is over, most patients can be carried to term without further complication.

During labor, leiomyomas may produce uterine inertia, fetal malpresentation, or obstruction of the birth canal. In general, leiomyomas tend to rise out of the pelvis as pregnancy progresses, and vaginal delivery may be accomplished. Nevertheless, a large cervical or isthmic myoma may be rather immobile and may necessitate cesarean delivery. Leiomyomas may interfere with effective uterine contraction immediately after delivery; therefore, the possibility of postpartum hemorrhage should be anticipated.

**B. Complications in Nonpregnant Women:** As noted previously, heavy bleeding with anemia is the most common complication of myomas. Urinary or bowel obstruction from large or parasitic myomas is much less common, and malignant transformation is rare. Ureteral injury or ligation is a well-recognized complication of surgery for leiomyomas, particularly cervical.

## Precautions

Estrogens must be used with caution in post menopausal patients with leiomyomas. The dose should be the lowest necessary to control symptoms, and the size of the tumors should be closely followed with pelvic examinations (every 6 months) and imaging studies as necessary. Oral contraceptives should be used with caution in all premenopausal patients with leiomyomas.

## Treatment

Choice of treatment depends on the patient's age, parity, pregnancy status, desire for future pregnancies, general health, and symptoms, as well as the size, location, and state of preservation of the leiomyomas.

**A. Emergency Measures:** Blood transfusions may be necessary to correct anemia. Packed red blood cells given over several days should be used for the patient with chronic anemia, eventhough profound, because the patient may have abnormal blood volume and rapid transfusion of whole blood could precipitate acute heart failure. Surgery is usually indicated for these cases when they become hemodynamically stable. Emergency surgery is indicated for infected leiomyomata, acute torsion, or intestinal obstruction caused by a pedunculated or parasitic myoma. Myomectomy is generally contraindicated during pregnancy, except for a very occasional symptomatic torsion.

**B. Specific Measures**

**1. Nonpregnant women–**In most instances, myomas do not require treatment, particularly if there are no symptoms or if the patient is postmenopausal. However, other causes of pelvic masses (see earlier) must be ruled out. The clinical diagnosis of myoma must be unequivocal, and the patient should be examined every 6 months.

Although no definitive medical therapy is currently available for leiomyomata, the gonadotropin-releasing hormone (GnRH) anagonists have proven very useful for limiting the growth or to cause a decrease in tumor size. Examples of the clinical situations where GnRH anagonists may be useful include control of bleeding from leiomyomata (except the polypoid submucous, which may actually be worsened), the unstable or unsuitable surgical candidate, the shrinkage of size sufficient to allow laparoscopically assisted vaginal hysterectomy, or vaginal hysterectomy and in certain cases for myomectomy. In the latter case several authorities have noted that use for more than 3 months makes myomectomy more difficult. Unfortunately, in all circumstances GnRH anagonists may be used only temporarily, because they create an artificial menopause.

It is impossible to precisely define the size to which a myomatous uterus may be safely allowed to grow, and each case must be individualized. However, many gynecologists urge removal when the mass becomes larger than a pregnant uterus of 12–14 weeks' gestation. Such a size precludes ovarian evaluation on pelvic examination. Large tumors pose difficult surgical problems of exposure and vascular control, particularly if the mass is cervical or intraligamentary and has displaced the ureter. Intramural and subserous myomas rarely require operation unless they are larger than a 12- to 14-week pregnancy or may be associated with other pathology. Growing cervical myomas larger than 3–4 cm in diameter should be removed to avoid a more difficult operative procedure in the future.

Depending on the size, and location of such myomas and the presence of other pelvic disease (such as pelvic inflammatory disease or endometriosis), surgical extirpation may be difficult and challenging.

**2. Puerperal**–Surgical indications during pregnancy (for leiomyomata) are discussed earlier. If removal of leiomyomata is required following pregnancy, it should be deferred as much as 12 weeks following delivery, when uterine vascular supply has returned to prepregnant levels, involution of the uterus has occurred, and regression of the tumor is complete.

**C. Supportive Measures:** All patients should have a cervical Papanicolaou smear. Before definitive surgery, necessary blood volume should be replenished, and other measures such as the administration of prophylactic antibiotics or heparin should be considered. Mechanical and antibiotic bowel preparation should be routinely employed when difficult pelvic surgery is anticipated!

**D. Surgical Measures:**

**1. Evaluation for other neoplasia**–Imaging most often must be accompanied by endometrial evaluation to rule out other pelvic neoplastic processes. The endometrial evaluation may be accomplished by endometrial biopsy in the uncomplicated patient but may necessitate hysteroscopy in the more complicated case. Fractional curettage should be performed if there is any possibility of endometrial cancer. Occasionally examination under anesthesia is necessary but has largely been replaced by the measures noted earlier to rule out coexisting problems, especially cancer.

**2. Myomectomy**–Myomectomy should be planned for the symptomatic patient who wishes to preserve fertility, but one can never be certain, before operation, that myomectomy can be accomplished easily. Myomectomy is quite successful for control of chronic bleeding associated with leiomyomata. Increasingly myomectomy is being performed through the hysteroscope in cases of submucous leiomyomata and through the laparoscope for those that are subserous. Indeed, these less invasive procedures are liberalizing the surgical indications for myomectomy.

A pedunculated submucous myoma protruding into the vagina can sometimes be removed vaginally with a looped wire snare or by hysteroscopy. This is most useful if other tumors do not obviously require removal. If the pedunculated myoma cannot be removed vaginally, careful biopsy should be performed to rule out leiomyosarcoma or a mixed mesodermal sarcoma. Both of these tumors are known to protrude through the cervix in older women and may be clinically indistinguishable from an infarcted prolapsed myoma (Fig 36–4). Since infection is usual in this setting, prophylactic antibiotics should be utilized.

**3. Hysterectomy**–Uteri with small myomas may be removed by total vaginal hysterectomy, particularly if vaginal relaxation demands repair of cystocele, rectocele, or enterocele.

When numerous large tumors (especially intraligamentary myomas) are found, total abdominal hysterectomy is indicated. If the ovaries are diseased

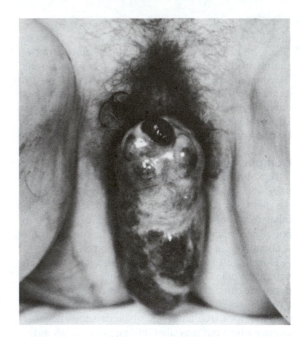

**Figure 36–4.** Prolapsed and partially infarcted myoma.

or if their blood supply has been destroyed, oophorectomy is necessary; otherwise, the ovaries should be preserved in young women. Ovaries generally are preserved in premenopausal women and removed in women after the age of 45, although there is no consensus about the virtue of conserving or removing them during this transitional period.

**E. Surgical Treatment of Complications From Myomas During Pregnancy:** Patients who have undergone previous multiple myomectomy, particularly if the endometrial cavity was entered, have less risk of uterine rupture if delivered by cesarean section. In some cases, cesarean hysterectomy is a sensible solution to the problem of myomas in a pregnant woman who wants no more children.

On the other hand, although rather small myomas may increase appreciably during pregnancy, they usually regress after delivery. Furthermore, one must not overlook the hazards—blood loss and possible urinary tract damage—associated with removal of a huge puerperal uterus. The mere presence of myomas that were not clinically of much significance before pregnancy should not be cited as an indication for cesarean hysterectomy in the absence of compelling reasons for abdominal delivery or for removal of the uterus.

**Prognosis**

Hysterectomy with removal of all leiomyomas is curative. Myomectomy, when it is extensive and significantly involves the myometrium or penetrates the endometrium, may necessitate cesarean delivery of subsequent pregnancies. Recurrence of myomas following myomectomy occurs in 15–40% of patients, and two-thirds of these require further surgical treatment.

## ADENOMYOSIS

### Essentials of Diagnosis

- Premenstrual and comenstrual dysmenorrhea.
- Diffuse globular uterine enlargement.
- Hypermenorrhea.
- Softening of areas of adenomyosis just prior to or during the early phases of menstruation.

### General Considerations

Adenomyosis is defined by the presence of endometrial glands and stroma within the myometrium, ie, the endometrium is growing beneath the basement membrane, marking its separation from the myometrium. Although histologic sections often show direct continuity of ectopic endometrial islands with the mucosal surface, many foci of adenomyosis appear isolated, perhaps because their connections with the surface have been interrupted by fibrosis and areas of musculature. As adenomyosis becomes more advanced, the uterus is diffusely enlarged and globular because of hypertrophy of the smooth muscle elements adjacent to the ectopic glands.

Occasionally the glandular elements are encased in smooth muscle tumors grossly similar to leiomyomata. The latter condition has been termed an adenomyoma, which implies an isolated, distinct regional abnormality. However, a scattered, diffuse type also occurs. Neither type characteristically has the sharp limitation or pseudocapsule found in leiomyomata.

The cause of adenomyosis is unknown, but it occurs infrequently in nulliparas. It is primarily a disorder of parous women over age 30 and often is associated with menorrhagia and increasingly severe secondary dysmenorrhea. The reported incidence of adenomyosis varies widely (8–40%) in routine sampling of surgically removed uteri.

It causes symptoms in approximately 70% of proved cases; about 30% of cases are asymptomatic and are discovered accidentally. The condition regresses after the menopause. The pathologic diagnosis depends, obviously, on the diligence with which the specimens are assessed and on whether or not examples of minimal muscular invasion (adenomyosis subbasalis) are included.

### Pathology

The myometrial thickening produced by adenomyosis is usually diffuse and of uniform consistency rather than irregularly nodular (as with myomas). The fundus generally is the site of adenomyosis. It may involve either or both walls of the uterus, to create a globular enlargement (usually 10–12 cm in diameter, Fig 36–5a). The consistency of the uterus is irregularly firm, and it has enhanced vascularity. The cut surface appears convex (bulging) and exudes serum. The cut surface may have a whorl-like or granular trabecular pattern, and there may be coarse stippling or granular trabeculation with small yellow or brown cystic spaces containing fluid or blood (Fig 36–5b). Small hemorrhagic areas represent endometrial islands in which menstrual bleeding has occurred. The endometrial-myometrial juncture is often indiscernible. Leiomyomas and adenomyosis may coexist in the same specimen.

The microscopic pattern is one of endometrial islands scattered through myometrium. Depth of penetration can be graded, and opinion varies concerning what constitutes true adenomyosis rather than superficial extension of basal endometrium. Degrees of involvement have been described on the basis of the numbers of endometrial glands observed within one

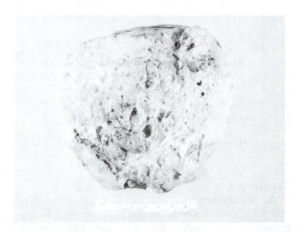
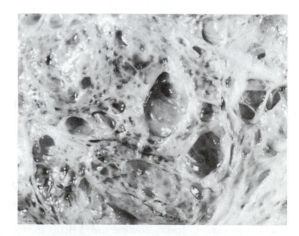

**Figure 36–5.** Adenomyosis. **A:** Gross view showing globular mass. **B:** Close-up view showing stippled trabeculation with small cystic spaces containing fluid or blood.

low-power field, but this is somewhat impractical because of variations in the distribution of glandular elements from one area to another.

Myometrial hypertrophy and hyperplasia are almost invariably apparent around the endometrial islets, and phagocytosed hemosiderin occasionally may be seen in the muscularis. If the degree of involvement is marked, the ectopic endometrium may show cyclic changes identical to those of normal endometrium, but in most instances the aberrant tissue appears to respond fairly well to estrogen though not to progesterone. When endometrial hyperplasia involves the mucosal layer, the same histologic pattern may be seen in the ectopic islands. The ectopic endometrium may also participate in the decidual changes characteristic of pregnancy.

## Clinical Findings

**A. Symptoms and Signs:** Significant degrees of adenomyosis are associated with hypermenorrhea in fully 50% of patients, and about 30% have an acquired, increasingly severe form of dysmenorrhea. However, only about 20% of women with adenomyosis are likely to have both of these classic complaints.

Despite widespread knowledge of the major symptoms of adenomyosis, the correct preoperative diagnosis is made in somewhat less than one-third of all instances. Failure to make the diagnosis preoperatively is largely the consequence of failure to think of it, although coexisting lesions such as myomas, endometrial polyps, endometrial hyperplasia, endometrial carcinoma, or endometriosis may disguise the symptomatology.

**1. Hypermenorrhea**–It is claimed that even adenomyosis subbasalis may produce hypermenorrhea in a high proportion of cases. This would seem to invalidate the contention that increased menstrual flow results from interference with normal myometrial contraction when large areas of musculature are disrupted by numerous endometrial islands. Nevertheless, there is clearly a positive correlation between the degree of involvement (as opposed to depth of penetration), vascularity, and the occurrence of menorrhagia, whatever the precise explanation for the increased bleeding may be.

**2. Dysmenorrhea**–Dysmenorrhea is directly related to the depth of penetration and degree of involvement, and probably results from myometrial contractions invoked by premenstrual swelling and menstrual bleeding in endometrial islands. The uterus is usually tender and slightly softened by bimanual examination done premenstrually (Halban's sign).

**B. Imaging:** The often diffuse nature of adenomyosis makes pelvic ultrasound less useful for diagnosis than it is in other conditions. Contrast hysterography may be diagnostic in some cases, but the yield is too low to justify routine use. MRI is useful for the diagnosis of adenomyosis, but the cost of the procedure precludes its routine use.

## Differential Diagnosis

1. Pregnancy may be ruled out with a pregnancy test.

2. Submucous leiomyomas may be present in 50–60% of cases of adenomyosis and the two bear differentiation. Leiomyomas may cause excessive and progressive menorrhagia and pain. The uterus is firm and nontender, even during menstruation, and discomfort occurs if the leiomyoma is pedunculated and in the process of extrusion. Diagnosis is confirmed by D&C.

3. Endometrial cancer is diagnosed by D&C.

4. Idiopathic hypertrophy of the Uterus must be considered if menorrhagia occurs without dysmenorrhea or uterine tenderness.

5. Pelvic congestion syndrome (Taylor's syndrome) is characterized by the chronic complaints of continuous pelvic pain and menometrorrhagia and is characteristically described in patients of hysterical personality type. In some instances, the uterus is enlarged, symmetric, and minimally softened; the cervix may be cyanotic and somewhat patulous.

6. Pelvic endometriosis is marked by premenstrual and intramenstrual dysmenorrhea, adherent adnexal masses, and "shotty" cul-de-sac or uterosacral ligament nodulations. The disorder is associated with adenomyosis in about 15% of patients.

## Complications

Chronic severe anemia may result from persistent menorrhagia.

Primary adenocarcinoma has rarely been observed in islands of aberrant endometrium within myometrium provided the surface endometrium is normal. On the other hand, endometrial adenocarcinoma is often associated with islands of malignant glands in the muscularis, but it may be impossible to determine whether there has been myometrial metastasis from the primary surface tumor or development of carcinoma within a focus of adenomyosis. However, if the surface tumor is markedly anaplastic and the myometrial islets exhibit well-differentiated glands, it seems reasonable to conclude that the latter are not metastases.

When the stromal component of endometrium, without glands, invades the myometrium, the resulting "tumor" is referred to as endolymphatic stromal myosis, or stromatosis. This entity is not dependent on ovarian hormonal production and therefore is not truly comparable to adenomyosis.

## Prevention

Adenomyosis cannot be prevented.

## Treatment

**A. Hysterectomy:** Although focal adenomyomas may occasionally be successfully removed, hysterectomy is the only other definitive treatment for adenomyosis. Hysterectomy is also the only way to establish the diagnosis with certainty. Whether the ovaries should be removed depends, as in many other situations, on the patient's age and the presence of obvious ovarian lesions or generalized pelvic endometriosis.

**B. Chemotherapy:** Various sex hormone regimens have been unsuccessful in control of adenomyosis caused by symptomatology. Oral contraceptives usually accentuate pain or bleeding. Women near the menopause may be managed for an appreciable time with an analgesic alone, anticipating resolution of symptoms following cessation of menses. (See also Chapter 50.)

## Prognosis

Hysterectomy is curative.

## ENDOMETRIAL POLYPS

### Essentials of Diagnosis

- Menometrorrhagia or postmenopausal bleeding.
- Direct visualization and biopsy (hysteroscopy).

### General Considerations

"Polyp" is a general descriptive term for any mass of tissue that projects outward or away from the surface of surrounding tissues. A polyp is grossly visible as a spheroidal or cylindric structure that may be either pedunculated (attached by a slender stalk) or sessile (relatively broad-based) (Fig 36–6).

Benign endometrial polyps are common in the endometrial cavity at all ages but particularly at age 29–59; with their greatest incidence after age 50. They consist of stromal cores with mucosal surfaces projecting above the level of the adjacent endometrium.

Endometrial polyps must be differentiated from submucous myomas, malignant neoplasms (especially mixed sarcomas), and even retained fragments of placental tissue (which may grossly assume a polypoid architecture).

Polyps may be single or multiple and may range in size from 1 to 2 mm in diameter to masses that fill or even distend the uterine cavity. Most polyps arise in the fundal region and extend downward. Occasionally, an endometrial polyp may project through the external cervical os and may even extend to the vaginal introitus (Fig 36–7). Postmortem examinations have shown that about 10% of uteri contain presumably asymptomatic polyps.

Polyps may undergo malignant change, and isolated endometrial carcinomas and sarcomas have been identified in solitary polyps. When this occurs, the prognosis is more favorable than for uterine carcinoma or sarcoma in general, providing there is no evidence of spread beyond the polyp on analysis of the hysterectomy specimen.

The histogenesis of endometrial polyps is not clear. Unresponsive areas of endometrium often remain in situ, along with the basalis, during menstrual shedding, and such an area may serve as the nidus of a polyp. However, not even the smallest polyps studied by histologic sectioning have given a wholly

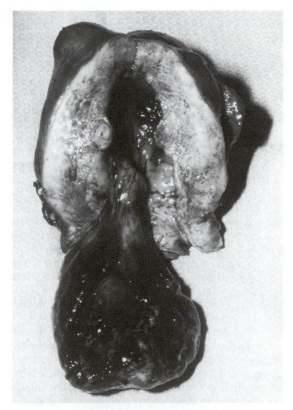

**Figure 36–7.** Large, partially infarcted endometrial polyp prolapsed through the cervical os.

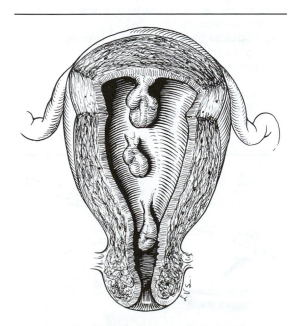

**Figure 36–6.** Endometrial polyps.

acceptable clue as to the precise mechanism of formation. Polyps are considered to be estrogen-sensitive; their response to estrogen is similar to that of the surrounding endometrium, and their association with other proliferative endometrial lesions (such as hyperplasia and endometrial carcinoma) is well recognized.

## Pathology

Grossly, an endometrial polyp is a smooth, red or brown, ovoid body with a velvety texture ranging from a few millimeters to several centimeters in widest diameter. A large polyp usually tapers to an obvious pedicle; a small polyp, when cut longitudinally, often presents a rather cylindric silhouette, with rounding at the distal end. Uterine polyps are of the same color as the surrounding endometrium unless they are infarcted, in which case they are dark red. A sectioned polyp may have a spongy appearance if it contains many dilated glandular spaces.

The microscopic pattern of an endometrial polyp is a mixture of (1) generally dense fibrous tissue—the stroma; (2) impressively large and thick-walled vascular channels; and (3) glandlike spaces, of variable size and shape, lined with endometrial epithelium. The relative amounts of these 3 components vary considerably. The surface of an intact polyp in a functioning uterus usually is covered by a layer of endometrium resembling that of the remainder of the endometrial surface, but beneath this exterior there are glandular components that are seemingly much older, and these apparently do not participate in menstrual shedding.

Squamous metaplasia of the surface epithelium is not uncommon. The subsurface epithelial spaces are often compared with basal endometrial glands unresponsive to progesterone, but they tend to form bizarre shapes and become quite dilated. Hence, a fragment of polyp may be mistaken for the cystic variety of endometrial hyperplasia ("Swiss cheese" endometrium). The distal or dependent portion of a polyp may show marked engorgement of blood vessels, hemorrhage into the stroma, inflammatory cells, and perhaps ulceration at the surface.

Adenocarcinoma may develop within an otherwise benign polyp, usually at some distance from its base or pedicle. On the other hand, a benign polyp may exist in an area of endometrial carcinoma. Thus, when a harmless-appearing polyp is recovered from the bleeding uterus of a post menopausal woman, there is no guarantee that a more serious lesion does not exist elsewhere in the cavity.

Polyps that contain interlacing bands of smooth muscle are called pedunculated adenomyomas. Generally, these have broad bases and are associated with adenomyosis of the uterus. In the same uterine cavity, endometrial polyps may coexist with pedunculated leiomyomas. In cases of hyperplasia of the endometrium, the abundant overgrowth of tissue may produce a gross pattern called multiple polyposis. Curet-

tage of such lesions may suggest the presence of adenocarcinoma because of the unexpected volume of tissue obtained.

## Clinical Findings

**A. Symptoms and Signs:** In a uterus of normal size, a history of regularly recurring menorrhagia suggests the possibility of endometrial polyps. Presumably, a large polyp, with its central vascular component, may participate in menstrual bleeding and add greatly to the total blood loss. Polyps may be the source of minor premenstrual and postmenstrual bleeding, allegedly because the polyp's dependent tip is the first endometrial area to degenerate and the last to obtain a new epithelial covering and cease bleeding after the menstrual slough.

The sudden occurrence of considerable bleeding in a postmenopausal woman, often accompanied by crampy uterine pain, may result from an infarcting large polyp. Such bleeding episodes usually are of limited duration and are not life-threatening.

These explanations are highly speculative, but it is true that duration and volume of menstruation often are lessened and the end points of the bleeding phase become more clear-cut by the removal of one or more endometrial polyps. In the postmenopausal woman, bleeding from polyps is usually light and is often described as "staining" or "spotting." A polyp should be suspected when bleeding continues following a D&C that has produced only benign normal tissue.

**B. Imaging:** Pelvic ultrasound often does not reveal endometrial polyps, while MRI is diagnostic but rarely employed because of cost. Polyps may be evident on a hysterosalpingogram as irregularities in the outline of the uterine cavity or as filling defects. However, this technique has largely been replaced by office hysteroscopy.

**C. Special Examinations:** Hysteroscopy is an excellent technique for evaluating and treating endometrial polyps.

## Treatment

**A. Surgical Excision:** Direct visualization of polyps by hysteroscopy has greatly aided in their

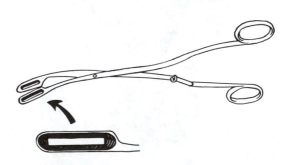

**Figure 36–8.** Overstreet polyp forceps.

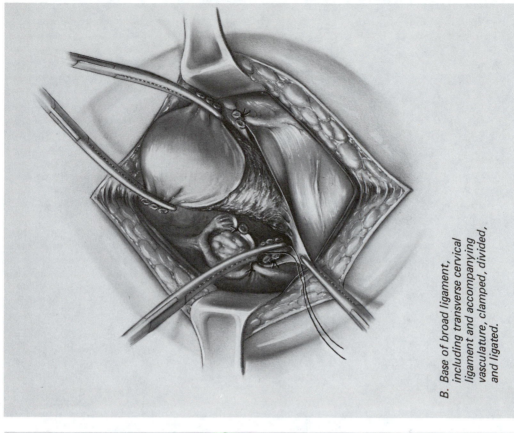

B. Base of broad ligament, including transverse cervical ligament and accompanying vasculature, clamped, divided, and ligated.

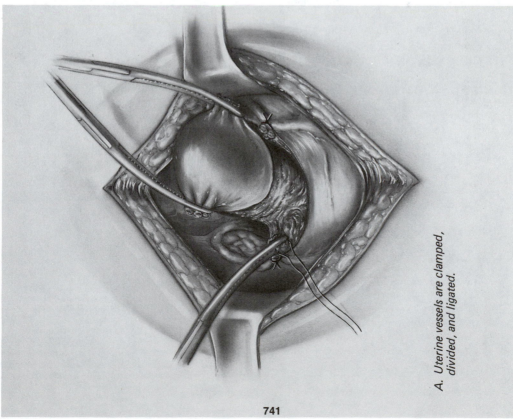

A. Uterine vessels are clamped, divided, and ligated.

**Figure 36–9.** Richardson technique for conservative hysterectomy. (continued)

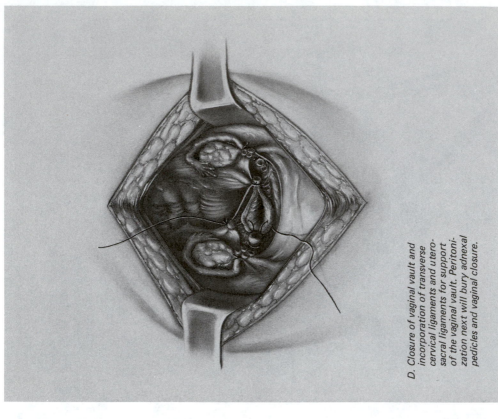

*D. Closure of vaginal vault and incorporation of transverse cervical ligaments and utero-sacral ligaments for support of the vaginal vault. Peritonization next will bury adnexal pedicles and vaginal closure.*

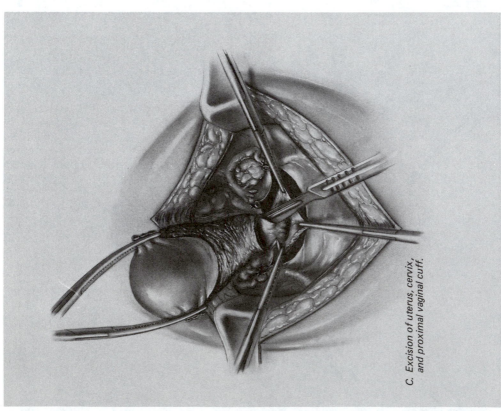

*C. Excision of uterus, cervix, and proximal vaginal cuff.*

**Figure 36–9 (cont'd).** Richardson technique for conservative hysterectomy.

identification and removal. The stalk may be identified, and, under direct visualization, hysteroscopic instruments used to remove the polyp. With larger polyps it may be necessary to section the tumor to portions that may be removed through the cervix. Many authorities recommend curettage of the point of insertion of the stalk into the endometrium-myometrium. Additionally, the direct visualization of the endometrium and selected biopsies can rule out endometrial atypias or dysplasias.

To avoid overlooking a polyp during curettage of the uterus (D&C), the endometrial cavity must be explored separately with a grasping forceps (such as an Overstreet polyp forceps (Fig 36–8) or a Randall stone clamp), preferably at the beginning of the curettage procedure.

Despite this precaution, all too frequently polyps are missed and remain in the uterus after curettage, only to be discovered later when menorrhagia persists and a hysterectomy is performed. At other times, only a portion of a polyp may be removed by curettage, and rather brisk bleeding will continue postoperatively from the residual basal portion of the lesion. A very large polyp may have to be severed at its base with a wire snare or scissors. In all cases, a fractional curettage should follow any nonvisualizing attempt at polyp removal, whether it was successful or not, in order to rule out endometrial carcinoma.

The imprecision of the nonvisualizing techniques have led to the emergence of hysteroscopy as the "gold standard" for both diagnosis and treatment of endometrial polyps.

A polyp should be labeled as such, preserved separately in fixative solution, and sent to the pathology laboratory as a separate specimen, because it may prove to be the most significant portion of the total tissue sample. If it is intermingled with other curettings or biopsies, there is no assurance that it will become a part of the material chosen for histologic sectioning.

**B. Chemotherapy:** There is no specific hormonal therapy for endometrial polyps.

**C. Hysterectomy:** Simple excision is adequate for a benign polyp, but if areas of carcinoma or sarcoma are discovered, hysterectomy should be performed. In a premenopausal patient, persistence of abnormal uterine bleeding after removal of an apparently benign polyp (or some portion of it) may be an indication for hysterectomy (Fig 36–9). Uteri removed for this reason occasionally contain additional polyps, submucous leiomyomata, or (rarely) a small area of carcinoma in a relatively inaccessible location.

### Prognosis

Removal is curative for that polyp, but recurrence is frequent. Hysterectomy is definitive but usually unnecessary if cancer has been ruled out.

## REFERENCES

**UTERINE LEIOMYOMATA**

Berkeley AS, De Cherney AH, Polan ML: Abdominal myomectomy and subsequent fertility. SurgGynecol Obstet 1983;156:319.

Bezjian AA: Pelvic masses in pregnancy. Clin Obstet Gynecol 1984;27:402.

Carlson KJ, Nichols, DH, Schiff I: Indications for hysterectomy. N Eng J Med 1993;328:856.

Davis JL et al: Uterine leiomyoma in pregnancy—a prospective study. Obstet Gynecol 1989;86:127.

Fedele L et al: Treatment with GnRH agonist before myomectomy and the risk of short-term myoma recurrence. Br J Obstet Gynaecol 1990;5:393.

Gross BH, Silver TM, Jaffe MH: Sonographic features of uterine leiomyomas: Analysis of 41 proven cases. J Ultrasound Med 1983;2:401.

Jonas HS, Masterson BJ: Giant uterine tumors: Case report and review of the literature. Obstet Gynecol 1977;50(Suppl 1):2s.

Moghissi KS: Hormonal therapy before surgical treatment for uterine leiomyomas. Surg Gynecol Obstet 1991;172:497.

Marugo M et al: Estrogen and progesterone receptors in uterine leiomyoma. Acta Obstet Gynecol Scand 1989;8:731.

Neuwirth RS, Amin HK: Excision of submucous fibroids with hysteroscopic control. Am J Obstet Gynecol 1976;126:95.

Valle RF: Hysteroscopy. Curr Opio Obstet Gynecol 1991;3:422.

**ADENOMYOSIS**

Azziz R: Adenomyosis: Current perspectives. Obstet Gynecol Clin North Am 1989;16:221.

Hernandez E, Woodruff DJ: Endometrial adenocarcinoma arising in adenomyosis. Am J Obstet Gy 1980;138:827.

Kilkku P, Erkkola R, Grauonroos M: Non-specificity of symptoms related to adenomyosis: A prospective comparative study. Acta Obstet Gynecol Scand 1984;63:229.

Luciano AA, Pitkin RM: Endometriosis: Approaches to diagnosis and treatment. Surg Annu 1984;16:297.

Thomas JS Jr, Clark JF: Adenomyosis: a retrospective view. J Natl Med Assoc 1989:81:969.

**ENDOMETRIAL POLYPS**

Holst J, Koskela O, von Schoultz B: Endometrial findings following curettage in 2018 women according to age and indications. Ann Chir Gynae col 1983;72:274.

Siegler AM: Panoramic CO2 hysteroscopy. Clin Obstet Gynaecol 1983;26:242.

# 37

# Benign Disorders of the Ovaries & Oviducts

*James E. Wheeler, MD, & J.Donald Woodruff, MD*

Benign disorders of the adnexa may be divided into nonneoplastic lesions and neoplastic lesions. The nonneoplastic lesions are frequently a cause of infertility. Most of these are of inflammatory origin and are discussed fully in Chapter 38. Noninflammatory and physiologic cysts and benign ovarian and tubal neoplasms are discussed in this chapter (Table 37–1). Malignant epithelial tumors and nonepithelial tumors are covered in Chapter 49.

## DEVELOPMENT OF BENIGN ADNEXAL DISORDERS

Benign adnexal disorders develop almost exclusively during the years between menarche and the menopause. They may produce local discomfort, menstrual dysfunction, impairment of fertility, or, rarely, debility and death due to local problems such as intestinal or ureteral obstruction.

One exception to the usual age distribution is precocious puberty. Most precocious puberty is isosexual, in which a premature release of gonadotropins from the pituitary stimulates sexual development. Pseudoprecocity occurs when a functioning ovarian tumor (granulosa cell tumor or thecoma) produces sufficient estrogens that breast development, pubic and axillary hair, and genital organ growth take place in the absence of ovulation. Gonadal stromal lesions in premenarcheal girls are generally benign, which is not true of the childhood germ cell lesions. Thus, precocious puberty as well as any palpable ovarian enlargement in infancy or childhood must be considered abnormal and must be further investigated.

## PHYSIOLOGIC ENLARGEMENT

### FUNCTIONAL CYSTS

A cyst is a sac containing fluid or semisolid material. Ovarian cysts may develop at any time but are most common from puberty to the menopause.

Many are small and clinically unimportant; however, each potentially represents an early manifestation of a benign or malignant neoplasm. Physical examination may disclose a 5- to 6-cm enlarged ovary in which ultrasonography demonstrates the presence of a 2- to 3-cm cyst. Although such "cysts" in the premenopausal female are common, the patient must be followed up carefully and true neoplasia ruled out. If cysts persist (eg, > 60 days) with normal menstrual cycles, the enlargement should be considered neoplastic. Conversely, if the tumor disappears during this time, it is most likely a functional cyst. Functional cysts—eg, **follicle cysts** or **corpus luteum cysts**—are normal transient structures usually related to aberrations of ovulation. They may be symptomatic and usually are unilateral. Bleeding from a hemorrhagic corpus luteum may produce acute pelvic pain, rectal tenesmus, and, on rare occasions, shock, thus simulating the picture of ruptured extrauterine pregnancy. Inflammatory ovarian disorders generally are related to salpingitis, appendicitis, or peritonitis, although even viral or parasitic infections may occur.

### Follicle Cysts

Follicle cysts are common (Fig 37–1). They are usually larger than the typical preovulatory follicle and vary in size from 3 to 8 cm or more in diameter. These cysts represent the failure of the fluid in an incompletely developed follicle to be reabsorbed; they are classically asymptomatic. Bleeding and torsion are rare. Occasionally, such cysts are associated with an isolated menstrual abnormality such as a prolonged intermenstrual interval or short cycle. Large

**Table 37–1.** Classification of ovarian tumors based on pathophysiology and embryology.

I. **Nonneoplastic lesions:**
  A. Inflammatory diseases of the ovary: Adhesive disease due to subacute or chronic infections; endometriosis or peritoneal inclusions.
  B. Nonneoplastic cysts of the ovary: Granulosa and theca lutein cysts; Stein-Leventhal ovary; diffuse or focal proliferations, eg, thecosis, cortical granulomas, luteoma of pregnancy.

II. **Ovarian neoplasia (mesothelial [stromoepithelial] tumors** with or without functioning stroma):
  A. Mesothelial tumors (primarily epithelial): Serous mucinous, endometrioid, "mesonephroid" tumors, true mesotheliomas.
  B. Mesothelial tumors (primarily stromal): Fibroadenoma, cystadenofibroma, Brenner tumor:
    1. Low functional potential.
    2. High functional potential: Granulosa-theca cell and Sertoli-Leydig cell tumors; gonadal stromal tumors with varying degrees of differentiation.
  C. Stromal (mesenchymal) tumors (of variable functional potential): Fibroma, fibromyoma, fibrothecoma, thecoma (luteoma), gonadal stromal tumors, sarcoma.
  D. Metastatic tumors and secondary malignant tumors.

III. **Germ cell tumors and associated gonadal aberrations:**
  A. Dysgerminoma
  B. Teratomas
    1. Embryonal
      a. Immature-embryoid: Poorly differentiated elements of one or all germ cell layers.
      b. Mature: Monoplastic (eg, struma ovarii); polyplastic (common benign teratoma).
    2. Extraembryonal
      a. Endodermal sinus.
      b. Polyvesicular vitelline (yolk sac).
      c. Choriocarcinoma.
  C. Dysgenetic gonad: Gonadoblastoma.

IV. **Functioning ovarian tumors:**
  See groups IIB2, IIC, IIIB1b, and VE. In addition to the classic "functioning tumors" noted in these groups, primarily granulosa-theca cell and theca cell lesions, any lesion with gonadal stroma, particularly the mucinous tumors (benign or malignant), may demonstrate hormonal activity. It is important to note that the histology of the lesion *does not* identify the type of functional activity, eg, a number of histologically classic granulosa cell tumors have been associated with masculinization of the host.
  In many classifications, these "functioning tumors" are classified as "sex cord stromal" lesions. However, there are no sex cords in the female gonad at any time, during embryogenesis or later. Lesions of this type are composed of more or less gonadal stroma, usually with a definitive epithelial component.

V. **Parovarian lesions:**
  A. Cysts, hydatids.
  B. "Mesonephroma" (ie, metamesonephroma).
  C. Hilar cell tumor.
  D. Adrenal rest tumor.
  E. "Arrhenoblastoma."

VI. **Other tumors (rarely in ovary): Hemangiopericytoma,** myoma, angioma, argentaffin tumor; hypernephroma.

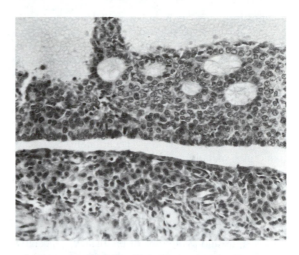

**Figure 37–1.** The wall of a "follicle" cyst showing the proliferating granulosa cells with tiny cystic Call-Exner bodies in the superior portion of the figure. They have artifactually pulled away from the underlying theca cells.

cysts may cause aching pelvic pain, dyspareunia, and, occasionally, abnormal uterine bleeding associated with a disturbance of the ovulatory pattern. Salpingitis, endometriosis, lutein cysts, and neoplastic cysts must be considered in the differential diagnosis.

Most follicle cysts disappear spontaneously within 60 days without treatment. Use of oral contraceptives may help establish a normal rhythm. Such medication is contraindicated if there is a possibility of pregnancy. Although fetal abnormalities are rare in association with such therapy, one should be alert to the medicolegal aspects involved. Any cyst that enlarges or persists longer than 60 days, particularly if a normal menstrual period intervenes, probably is not a functioning cyst. Laparoscopy is indicated. Puncture of such cysts under ultrasonographic direction is a controversial procedure. If the cyst is neoplastic, tumor cells may escape into the abdominal cavity. Laparoscopic cystectomy may be possible but is not recommended because of the controversial pathologic possibilities.

## Lutein Cysts

Two types of lutein cysts are recognized: granulosa lutein and theca lutein cysts.

**A. Corpus Luteum (Granulosa Lutein) Cysts:** These are functional, nonneoplastic enlargements of the ovary. Following ovulation, the granulosa cells lining the follicle become luteinized. In the stage of vascularization, blood accumulates in the central cavity, the corpus hemorrhagicum. Resorption of the blood results in a corpus luteum cyst. A persistent corpus luteum cyst may cause local pain and tenderness and either amenorrhea or delayed menstruation, thus simulating the clinical picture associated with ectopic pregnancy. If symptoms are present, prompt diagnostic studies are in order to rule out eccyesis. A corpus luteum cyst may encourage torsion of the ovary, causing severe pain; or it may rupture and bleed, in which case laparoscopy or laparotomy is usually required to control hemorrhage into the peritoneal cavity. Unless acute complications develop, symptomatic therapy is indicated.

**B. Theca Lutein Cysts:** These cysts are rarely large; they are usually bilateral and are filled with clear, straw-colored fluid. Theca lutein cysts are found in association with polycystic ovarian disease, hydatidiform mole, choriocarcinoma, and chorionic gonadotropin or clomiphene therapy.

Abdominal symptoms are minimal. A sense of pelvic weight or aching may be described. Rupture of the cyst may result in intraperitoneal bleeding. Continued signs and symptoms of pregnancy, especially hyperemesis and breast paresthesias, are also reported.

Laboratory studies may disclose startlingly high titers of chorionic gonadotropin. Dilation and curettage should be done if there is any question of retained products of conception, mole, or choriocarcinoma. Extrauterine pregnancy should be considered. If normal menses resume, the possibility of bilateral ovarian neoplasm (eg, dermoid cyst) must be ruled out.

Surgery is rarely required. The cysts disappear spontaneously following termination of the molar pregnancy, treatment of the choriocarcinoma, or discontinuation of gonadotropin therapy. However, such resolution may take months to occur.

If the patient is postmenopausal, ovarian enlargement should be investigated promptly regardless of its size.

## HYPERTHECOSIS

Hyperthecosis, or thecomatosis, commonly produces no gross enlargement of the ovary (Fig 37–2). Thus, the lesions are demonstrable only by histologic examination of the excised gonad. They are characterized by nests of stromal cells demonstrating increased cytoplasm, simulating the changes seen in the normal theca after stimulation by pituitary gonadotropin. In the premenopausal woman, hyperthecosis is associated with virilization and clinical findings similar to those seen in polycystic ovarian disease (see following text). These alterations also may be associated with postmenopausal bleeding and endometrial hyperplasia.

## POLYCYSTIC OVARIAN DISEASE
## (Stein-Leventhal Syndrome)

Polycystic ovarian disease is characterized by bilaterally enlarged polycystic ovaries, secondary amen-

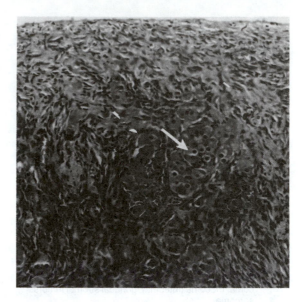

**Figure 37–2.** In hyperthecosis, nests of rounded eosinophilic luteinized stroma cells are found in the ovarian cortex.

orrhea or oligomenorrhea, and infertility. About 50% of patients are hirsute, and many are obese. The syndrome affects females between the ages of 15 and 30 years. Many cases of female infertility secondary to failure of ovulation are due to polycystic ovarian disease. The disorder is presumably related to hypothalamic pituitary dysfunction. However, the primary ovarian contribution to the problem has not been clearly defined.

The enlarged, "sclerocystic" ovaries with smooth, pearl-white surfaces but without surface indentations have been called "oyster ovaries." Many small, fluid-filled follicle cysts lie beneath the thickened fibrous surface cortex (Fig 37–3). Luteinization of the theca interna is usually observed, and occasionally there is focal stromal luteinization.

An interesting corollary to the polycystic ovary syndrome is the large edematous ovary syndrome initially reported by Sternberg. This unilaterally enlarged ovary is characterized by edematous stroma with nests of luteinized stromal cells. The classic patient is masculinized. Unilateral oophorectomy is associated with reversion of symptomatology.

### Diagnosis

A presumptive diagnosis of polycystic ovarian disease often can be made from the history and initial examination. A normal puberty and early adolescence with menses are followed by episodes of amenorrhea that become progressively longer. The enlarged ovaries are identifiable on pelvic examination in about 50% of patients.

Urinary 17-ketosteroids are minimally elevated,

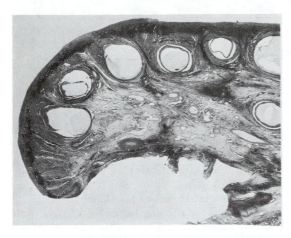

**Figure 37–3.** Polycystic ovary with a thickened capsule and prominent subcapsular cysts. Note lack of corpora lutea or corpora albicantia due to anovulation.

but estrogen and follicle-stimulating hormone (FSH) excretion are normal. Luteinizing hormone (LH) levels are elevated, and the LH surge is absent. Some patients have an increased $\Delta^4$-androstenedione output; others excrete considerable amounts of dehydroepiandrosterone. Adrenocorticosteroid hormone titers are normal. Basal body temperature records and endometrial biopsies confirm anovulation.

Currently, the accepted diagnostic techniques are ultrasonography and laparoscopy. Adrenocortical hyperplasia or tumor is ruled out, since signs of defeminization are absent and adrenal function is normal. Dexamethasone suppression test results are negative with an adrenal tumor unless the tumor is pelvic in origin. A virilizing ovarian tumor is an unlikely diagnosis because the ovarian enlargement is bilateral and rarely do voice changes or clitoral hypertrophy occur.

### Treatment

For polycystic ovarian disease, clomiphene citrate (Clomid), 50–100 mg/day for 5–7 days cyclically, will be successful in inducing ovulation in most cases. In the recalcitrant case, the experienced clinician may add human menopausal gonadotropin to produce the desired ovulation. Rarely is wedge resection necessary; however, the results of such surgery have been eminently successful in restoring ovulation and fertility. Periovarian adhesions may result from this procedure.

Since patients with polycystic ovarian disease are chronically anovulatory, the endometrium is stimulated by estrogen alone; endometrial hyperplasia, both typical and atypical, is thus more frequent in patients with polycystic ovarian disease and long-term anovulation. Well-differentiated endometrial cancer has been reported in patients with prolonged anovula-

tion and the associated persistent estrogen stimulation. Many of these markedly atypical endometrial features can be reversed by large doses of progestational agents such as megestrol acetate (Megace), 40–60 mg/day for 3–4 months. Follow-up endometrial biopsy is mandatory to determine endometrial response and subsequent recurrence.

## LUTEOMA OF PREGNANCY

Tumor-like nodules of lutein cells may form in the ovaries during pregnancy, often both multifocal and bilateral. The nodules range up to 20 cm in diameter, but most often are in the 5–10 cm range. On section they form well-delineated, soft brown masses with focal hemorrhage. Microscopically they are formed of sheets of large luteinized cells with abundant cytoplasm and relatively uniform nuclei with occasional mitoses. Clinically they appear ominous to the obstetrician who becomes aware of them only when the abdomen is open at the time of cesarean section delivery. Unilateral salpingo-oophorectomy may be done for frozen section in the belief that the large masses must be malignant. A confirmatory biopsy is adequate, and follow-up will reveal total regression a few months later.

## DIAGNOSIS OF OVARIAN NEOPLASMS

The ovarian tumor represents the greatest contemporary challenge to the gynecologic diagnostician, therapist, and investigator. Study of the patient with an adnexal mass should include examinations that have the following goals:

1. To evaluate the patient's general physical condition and to inspire confidence and assure the patient of her physician's concern.
2. To identify the presence or absence of urinary tract or intestinal disease.
3. To correlate the lesion with any physiologic or endocrinologic abnormalities, eg, amenorrhea, hirsutism, or endometrial proliferation.
4. To determine associated karyotypic abnormalities with or without other clinical evidence of sex ambiguity.
5. To diagnose the presence of neoplasia at other pelvic or extrapelvic sites, eg, metastatic disease.

Routine use of CT and MRI scans are not advocated as initial studies. Nevertheless, radiologic scans and even laparoscopy may be necessary, particularly in obese patients, if less costly means of investigation (eg, ultrasonography) are not diagnostic in the presence of ambiguous pelvic findings.

Prompt, accurate diagnosis and appropriate treatment must be the physician's goals when an ovarian enlargement is identified. The following factors must always be considered: (1) the age of the patient, (2) the size and persistence of the enlargement, (3) the involvement of one or both ovaries, (4) adherence of adnexal structures, (5) hormone production, (6) other pelvic abnormalities, and (7) ascites.

## Treatment of Ovarian Tumors

Severe pain, internal bleeding, or sepsis associated with ovarian enlargement requires prompt operation. Conversely, observation to confirm the persistence and to establish the character of an ovarian enlargement is the best policy when the lesion is cystic and associated with menstrual irregularities or when evidence of pelvic inflammatory disease as a cause of the adnexal mass is present. Conversely, if the tumor is solid or if the cystic mass is asymptomatic and persistent through at least one menstrual cycle, prompt and thorough investigation is imperative. After a diagnosis of ovarian neoplasia, cystic or solid, is established, definitive surgery and adjunctive therapy are mandatory if survival rates are to be improved. The surgeon must be prepared to carry out a full staging procedure and any ancillary surgery (such as bowel resection) that may be required.

Peritoneal fluid (free or from washings) should be obtained at the time of laparotomy for evaluation of cell content. Addition of heparin to the fluid will prevent coagulation if blood is present. The cell content must be evaluated accurately to prevent an overdiagnosis of cancer due to the proliferation of atypical reactive mesothelial cells.

Excision of some ovarian enlargements—eg, endometriosis or dermoid cysts—with preservation of the remainder of the ovary is feasible and desirable. Other benign lesions in young women, especially large cystic tumors such as cystadenomas, may require unilateral oophorectomy, depending on the histopathologic features. Bisection of a grossly normal ovary should be avoided, since postincision adhesions may interfere with fertility.

Prophylactic oophorectomy in women under the age of 40 years who are undergoing hysterectomy for benign disease is of questionable value and must be a decision reached by careful discussion with the patient and her family. Nevertheless, the surgeon should never "tie his hands," since unexpected pathologic findings may necessitate bilateral salpingo-oophorectomy. Conversely, if after the menopause pelvic surgery is indicated for other reasons, removal of the ovaries should be considered, since approximately 6% of ovarian neoplasms develop in retained ovaries.

The role of the gynecologist is that of primary diagnostician and physician in charge of therapy to whom the patient may turn both for care and for comfort, regardless of the outcome of therapy or how discouraging the prognosis.

# NEOPLASTIC LESIONS

## EPITHELIAL TUMORS

Epithelial tumors account for approximately 60–80% of all true ovarian neoplasms and includes the common serous, mucinous, endometrioid, clear cell and transitional cell (Brenner) tumors, and the stromal tumors with an epithelial element. The epithelium of these tumors arises from a common anlage, ie, the mesothelium lining the coelomic cavity and ovarian surfaces (Fig 37–4). This basic thesis explains the similarity of the epithelia of the upper genital canal—endocervix, endometrium, and endosalpinx—to those found in the ovarian tumors. Most tumors presumably arise from invaginated surface epithelium (Fig 37–4) and proliferation or malignant degeneration in the epithelial lining of the resulting surface inclusion cyst (Fig 37–5). The epithelial tumors are classified on the basis of their histologic appearance.

## 1. SEROUS TUMORS

Serous tumors are, by definition, characterized by a proliferation of epithelium resembling that which lines the fallopian tube. They are virtually all cystic and may attain a size large enough to fill the abdominal cavity, but they are usually smaller than their mucinous counterparts. Benign lesions are commonly unilocular, have a smooth lining surface, and contain thin, clear yellow fluid. Focal proliferation of the underlying stroma may produce firm papillary projections into the cyst, forming a serous cystadenofibroma (Fig 37–6). It is important to study these papillary projections thoroughly to rule out atypical proliferation. Some serous tumors consist of benign stromal proliferation interspersed with tiny serous cysts, **serous adenofibromas.** The histopathology of benign serous tumors remains remarkably uniform, section after section. Conservative therapy is in order.

### Pathology

The simple serous cystadenoma may attain tremendous size. If multiloculated, all cyst cavities must be examined grossly to rule out a focus of potentially malignant solid or papillary growth. The cells lining the cyst are a mixed population of ciliated and secretory cells similar to those of the endosalpinx.

### Clinical Findings

Serous tumors have been reported in all age groups. The low-grade neoplasms generally are found in patients in their 20s and 30s, whereas the an-

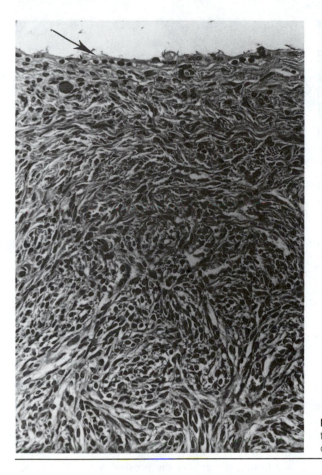

**Figure 37–4.** The surface epithelium (mesothelium) of the ovary forms an inconspicuous, usually flat, layer of cells over the underlying ovarian cortex.

aplastic counterpart occurs more commonly in peri- and postmenopausal women.

As occurs with most epithelial ovarian tumors, patients with serous tumors show no classic symptoms. Most of these tumors are found on routine pelvic examination. In other cases, the presenting symptoms include nonspecific pelvic discomfort, a palpable abdominal swelling, or ascites. Extra-abdominal disease is rarely found in any "ovarian malignancy" except in the terminal stage. As with all ovarian enlargements, the tumors must be differentiated from intestinal and urinary tract lesions. In addition to differentiating the latter from a true pelvic neoplasm, it is important to appreciate the possibility that the intestine may be involved in the neoplastic process. "Uterine myoma" is the primary physician diagnosis in about one-third of all ovarian tumors. Thus, laparotomy should be performed if, because of the distortion of the pelvic architecture, ovarian neoplasms cannot be ruled out after ultrasonography or appropriate radiologic studies.

**Treatment**

The preferred treatment for all ovarian tumors is surgical excision with careful exploration of the abdominal contents. A midline incision should be made for adequate exploration. Frozen section is helpful in identifying the type and neoplastic potential of the tumor. However, since it is impossible to sample adequately a tumor of the size of the usual ovarian neoplasm, final opinion and prognosis *must* be based on analysis of permanent, rather than frozen, sections. Therefore, in the patient desirous of retaining fertility, the surgeon must err on the side of retention of the uterus and contralateral ovary if there is the slightest doubt as to malignancy on the part of the pathologist.

## 2. MUCINOUS TUMORS

Mucinous tumors account for approximately 10–20% of all epithelial ovarian neoplasms; about 85% of them are benign. The benign tumors are typically found in women in the third through the fifth decades.

**Pathology**

Mucinous cysts are usually smooth-walled; true papillae are rare (compared with the serous variety). The tumors generally are multilocular, and the mucus-containing locules appear blue through the tense capsule (Fig 37–7). Bilateral tumor develop-

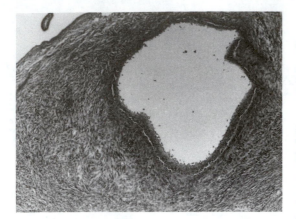

**Figure 37–5.** Most surface (germinal) inclusion cyst, such as the one shown here, undergo a serous (tubal) metaplasia. If larger than 1 cm in diameter by definition they are termed cystadenoma.

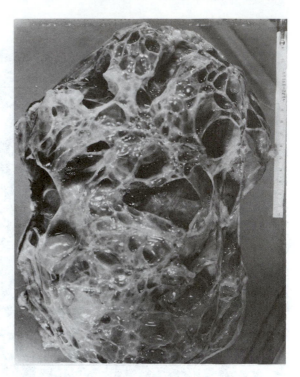

**Figure 37–7.** Multilocular mucinous cystadenoma of ovary.

ment occurs in 8–10% of all cases, whether the tumors are benign or malignant. The internal surface is lined by tall columnar cells with dark, basally situated nuclei and mucinous cytoplasm as shown in Figure 37–8.

The epithelium of mucinous cysts resembles that of the endocervix in about 50% of the cases; in the other 50%, mucin-containing goblet cells are present resembling colonic epithelial cells. Careful study of mucinous neoplasms has shown that there may be great variation in histologic appearance from area to area, with some areas appearing benign whereas others are of low malignant potential or frankly malignant. Hence, sampling must be more extensive than in the typical serous tumor.

## Clinical Findings

Mucinous tumors are the largest tumors found in

the human body; 15 reported tumors have weighed over 70 kg (154 lb). Consequently, the more massive the tumor, the greater the possibility that it may be mucinous. They generally are asymptomatic, and the patient is seen because of either an abdominal mass or nonspecific abdominal discomfort. Uncommonly in postmenopausal patients, luteinization of the stroma

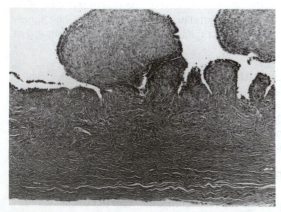

**Figure 37–6.** Serous cystadenofibromas usually form unilocular cysts with firm white papillations protruding into the cyst, seen here microscopically.

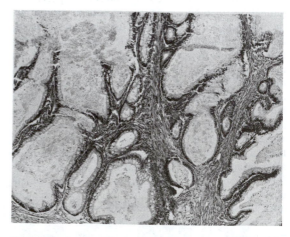

**Figure 37–8.** Mucinous cystadenoma. The lining cells are tall and columnar with basally situated nuclei. Generous sampling of these tumors is necessary to rule out a higher grade lesion.

may result in hormone production (usually estrogen) and associated hyperplasia of the endometrium with vaginal bleeding. During pregnancy, hormonal stimulation may result in virilization.

**Pseudomyxoma peritonei,** the accumulation of thick intraperitoneal mucin, may result from dissemination of mucin from a mucinous tumor through the ovarian stroma with spillage into the peritoneal cavity. Usually, however, an appendiceal mucinous cystadenoma is also present and is believed to be the source of mucin. Cytologically bland but mucin-producing tumor cells are commonly present in the mucin, and the clinical course of most patients is multiple reaccumulations of mucin over the years with eventual bowel obstruction.

### Treatment

If the tumor is encapsulated, a unilateral salpingo-oophorectomy is acceptable in patients with pseudomyxoma peritonei; 5–10% dextrose should be injected into the abdominal cavity to liquefy the mucin so that it may be evacuated.

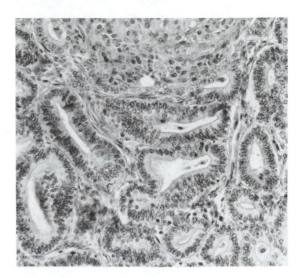

**Figure 37–9.** Endometrioid cystadenomas contain a proliferation of bland endometrial-like glands without the stroma of endometriosis.

### 3. ENDOMETRIOID LESIONS

Endometrioid lesions include benign tumors, tumors of low malignant potential, and malignant variants. Endometriosis of the ovary (see Chapter 40) represents a benign "tumor-like" condition rather than a true neoplasm. The only clearly recognizable benign endometrioid tumors are the **endometrioid adenofibroma** and the **proliferative endometrioid adenofibroma.**

### Pathology

Endometrioid tumors are characterized by proliferation of benign nonspecific stroma in which bland endometrial-type glands may be found. If the epithelial growth is exuberant but cytologically benign, it is termed a proliferative rather than a low malignant potential tumor, since the prognosis appears to be invariably excellent (Fig 37–9).

Clinically affected patients present with symptoms related to the mass, or it is found incidentally on pelvic examination.

### 4. CLEAR CELL (MESONEPHROID) TUMORS

Like the endometrioid tumors, clear cell tumors in their benign form are virtually limited to clear cell adenofibromas in which a solid proliferation of nonspecific stroma contains small cytologically bland glands formed by columnar cells with clear cytoplasm. Clinically they appear like any other benign ovarian mass and are diagnosed only on histologic examination. The prognosis is excellent.

### 5. TRANSITIONAL CELL (BRENNER) TUMORS

Transitional cell tumors, over 98% of which are benign, represent adenofibromas in which the proliferating epithelial element has a transitional cell appearance. This represents metaplasia as is seen in the cervix so frequently. Brenner tumors represent 1–2% of primary ovarian tumors and are unilateral in nearly 95% of cases. They are frequently so small as to be incidental findings at operation. However, the tumor may reach 5–8 cm in diameter and present as an adnexal mass at pelvic examination. On section they are firm and pale yellow or white (Fig 37–10). The epithelium is composed of nests of cells with ovoid nuclei with a prominent longitudinal groove ("coffee-bean nuclei"; Fig 37–11). Occasionally there is a mucinous metaplasia of the cells in the center of one or more of these nests, which may account for the 10% incidence of mucinous cystadenomas found associated with Brenner tumors. The Walthard rest found as a 1-mm cyst beneath the serosa of the fallopian tube appears to represent an inclusion cyst in which the mesothelium has undergone a similar transitional cell metaplasia.

### Clinical Findings

Solid adenofibromatous neoplasms are commonly mistaken for uterine myomas. Consequently, if a solid pelvic neoplasm is situated so that it prevents careful evaluation of the adnexa, operative removal is indicated, regardless of its origin.

### Treatment

Treatment for Brenner tumors is primarily surgical

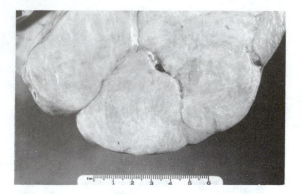

**Figure 37–10.** The cut surface of a Brenner tumor is a firm, solid, and yellowish-white, and resembles a fibrothecoma.

and is done to establish the diagnosis and remove the tumor.

# BENIGN TUMORS OF THE OVIDUCT

Since benign lesions of the uterine tube are routinely asymptomatic and rarely large enough to be palpable—with the exception of the paratubal or parovarian cyst—the diagnosis is made incidentally at the operating table or in the pathology laboratory.

## CYSTIC TUMORS

Cystic tumors of the uterine tube are extremely common at or near the fimbriated end, the so-called

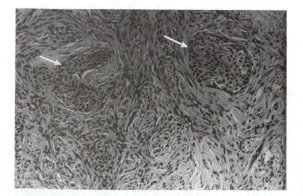

**Figure 37–11.** In a transitional cell (Brenner) tumor, islands of bland transitional cells proliferate, accompanied by a prominent proliferation of benign spindley fibroblast-like cells.

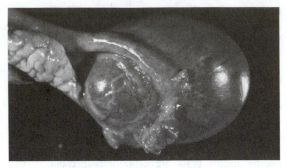

**Figure 37–12.** Parovarian cyst. Note the orientation of the cyst to the fimbriated end of the oviduct.

hydatid of Morgagni. These clear fluid-filled cysts are usually about 1 cm in diameter and are lined by tubal-type epithelium. Rarely do these cysts cause symptoms, and they are most often found inadvertently during a pelvic operative procedure. On rare occasions, torsion may produce an acute surgical emergency. Occasionally, a larger paratubal or parovarian cyst may develop, especially in the broad ligament (Fig 37–12). These cysts are almost always serous tumors of low malignant potential with a benign clinical outcome. Cysts arising from the mesonephric remnants normally found adjacent to the tube are extremely uncommon.

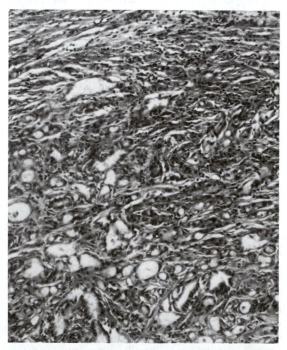

**Figure 37–13.** Adenomatoid tumor (Benign mesothelioma) with tiny slit-like spaces and glands invading the muscular wall of the tube.

The epithelium is low, flat, and nonsecretory and the surrounding muscle prominent; consequently, dilatation is unusual.

## EPITHELIAL TUMORS

Benign epithelial tumors of the uterine tube are extremely rare. The polyps that occur in the cornual portion appear to be of endometrial rather than tubal origin.

## ADENOMATOID TUMORS

The adenomatoid tumor is probably the most common benign tumor found in the uterine tube. It actually represents a benign mesothelioma, but the compact nature of the adenomatous pattern may be mistaken for malignancy (Fig 37–13). Adenomatoid lesions rarely measure more than 1–1.5 cm. They are always incidental findings when the adnexa are removed for other purposes. Similar lesions, usually cystic, may involve the myometrium or ovary. The so-called "metaplastic tumor" of the fallopian tube is not a tumor. It may represent a variant of the "Arias-Stella reaction" and is seen in the postpartum period.

## OTHER BENIGN TUBAL AND PARATUBAL TUMORS

Other benign tubal tumors, such as leiomyomas and teratomas are rare, as are benign adnexal tumors of probable wolffian origin. Adrenal cortical nests, however, are common incidental findings in the broad ligament as yellowish ovoid nodules 3–4 mm in diameter.

## REFERENCES

Bell DA, Scully RE: Benign and borderline clear cell adenofibromas of the ovary. Cancer 1985;56:2922.

Blaustein A: Peritoneal mesothelium and ovarian surface cells-shared characteristics. Int J Gynecol Pathol 1984; 3:361.

Blaustein A et al: Inclusions in ovaries of females aged day 1–30 years. Int J Gynecol Pathol 1982;1:145.

Gramlich T, Austin RM, Lutz M: Histologic sampling requirements in ovarian carcinoma: A review of 51 tumors. Gynecol Oncol 1990;32:249.

Russell P, Bannatyne P: *Surgical Pathology of the Ovaries.* Churchill Livingstone, 1989.

Santini D et al: Brenner tumor of the ovary: A correlative histologic, histochemical, immunohistochemical, and ultrastructural investigation. Hum Pathol 1989;20:787.

Scully RE: Tumors of the ovary and maldeveloped gonads. In: *Atlas of Tumor Pathology.* Washington, DC, Armed Forces Institute of Pathology, Fascicle 16, series 2, 1979.

Shevchuk MM, Fenoglio CM, Richart RM: Histogenesis of Brenner tumors. I. Histology and ultrastructure. Cancer 1980;46:2607.

Snyder RR, Norris HJ, Tavassoli, F: Endometrioid proliferative and low malignant potential tumors of the ovary: A clinicopathologic study of 46 cases. Am J Surg Pathol 1988;12:661.

Wheeler JE: Diseases of the fallopian tube. In: *Blaustein's Pathology of the Female Genital Tract,* 4th ed. Kurman RJ (editor). Springer-Verlag, 1994.

Young RH, Gilks CB, Scully RE: Mucinous tumors of the appendix associated with mucinous tumors of the ovary and pseudomyxoma peritonei: A clinicopathological analysis of 22 cases supporting an origin in the appendix. Am J Surg Pathol 1991;15:415.

# 38 Sexually Transmitted Diseases & Pelvic Infections

*Susan M. Ramin, MD, George D. Wendel, Jr., MD, & David L. Hemsell, MD*

## SEXUALLY TRANSMITTED DISEASES

The term "sexually transmitted diseases" is used to denote disorders spread principally by intimate contact. Although this usually means sexual intercourse, it also includes close body contact, kissing, cunnilingus, anilingus, fellatio, mouth-breast contact, and anal intercourse. Many sexually transmitted diseases can be acquired by transplacental spread or perinatally. The organisms involved are peculiarly adapted to growth in the genital tract and are present in body secretions or blood.

The list of organisms traditionally thought of as causing sexually transmitted diseases has been extended to include cytomegalovirus, herpes simplex virus types I and II, *Chlamydia*, group B *Streptococcus*, molluscum contagiosum virus, *Sarcoptes scabiei*, hepatitis viruses, and human immunodeficiency virus (HIV). Some diseases spread by body contact but not necessarily by coitus—eg, pediculosis pubis and molluscum contagiosum—are discussed with the dermatitides rather than here; herpes genitalis is discussed in Chapter 34.

## 1. GONORRHEA

### Essentials of Diagnosis

- Most affected women are asymptomatic carriers.
- Purulent vaginal discharge.
- Frequency and dysuria.
- Recovery of organism in selective media.
- May progress to pelvic infection or disseminated infection.

### General Considerations

*Neisseria gonorrhoeae* is a gram-negative diplococcus that forms oxidase-positive colonies and ferments glucose. The organism may be recovered from the urethra, cervix, anal canal, or pharynx. Optimal recovery of the organism is with use of Thayer-Martin or Martin-Lester (Transgrow) medium. *N gonorrhoeae* is killed rapidly by drying, sunlight, heat, and most disinfectants.

The columnar and transitional epithelium of the genitourinary tract is the principal site of invasion. The organism may enter the upper reproductive tract (Fig 38–1), causing salpingitis with its attendant complications. It has been estimated that after exposure to an infected partner, 20–50% of men and 60–90% of women become infected. Without therapy, 10–17% of women with gonorrhea develop pelvic infection. Depending on the geographic location and population involved, *N gonorrhoeae* is often present with other sexually transmitted diseases. Traditionally, women with gonorrhea are considered to be at risk for incubating syphilis. Recently, it has been shown that 20–40% also have *Chlamydia* infection.

### Clinical Findings

#### A. Symptoms and Signs:

**1. Early symptoms**–Most women with gonorrhea are asymptomatic. When symptoms occur, they are localized to the lower genitourinary tract and include vaginal discharge, urinary frequency or dysuria, and rectal discomfort. The incubation period is only 3–5 days.

**2. Discharge**–The vulva, vagina, cervix, and urethra may be inflamed and may itch or burn. Specimens of discharge from the cervix, urethra, and anus should be taken for culture in the symptomatic patient. A stain of purulent urethral exudate may demonstrate gram-negative diplococci in leukocytes. Similar findings in a purulent cervical discharge are less conclusively diagnostic of *N gonorrhoeae*.

**3. Bartholinitis**–Unilateral swelling in the inferior lateral portion of the introitus suggests involvement of Bartholin's duct and gland. In early gonococcal infections, the organism may be recovered by gently squeezing the gland and expressing pus from the duct. Enlargement, tenderness, and fluctuation may develop, signifying abscess formation. *N gonorrhoeae* is then less frequently recovered; however, the prevalence of infection with other bacteria

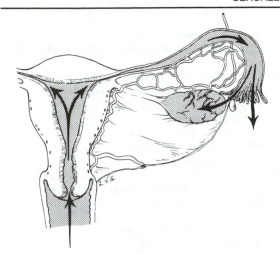

**Figure 38–1.** Intra-abdominal spread of gonorrhea and other pathogenic bacteria.

merits a search for these pathogens. Spontaneous evacuation of pus often occurs if drainage by incision is not done. The infection may result in asymptomatic cyst formation.

**4. Anorectal inflammation**–Anal itching, pain, discharge, or bleeding occurs rarely. Most women are asymptomatic and acquire infection by perineal spread of vaginal secretions rather than by anal intercourse.

**5. Pharyngitis**–Acute pharyngitis and tonsillitis rarely occur; most infections are asymptomatic.

**6. Disseminated infection**–For unknown reasons, asymptomatic carriers can develop systemic infection. Commonly, a triad of polyarthralgia, tenosynovitis, and dermatitis is seen, or purulent arthritis without dermatitis. Septicemia is more common in the first clinical setting and *N gonorrhoeae* cultured from joint aspirates in the latter. Endocarditis and meningitis have been described.

**7. Conjunctivitis**–In adults, ophthalmic infection is usually due to autoinoculation. Ophthalmia neonatorum may result from delivery through an infected birth canal.

**8. Vulvovaginitis in children**–Gonococcal invasion of nonkeratinized membranes in prepubertal girls produces severe vulvovaginitis. The typical sign is a purulent vaginal discharge with dysuria. The genital mucous membranes are red and swollen. Infection is commonly introduced by adults, and in such cases the physician must consider the possibility of child abuse.

**B. Laboratory Findings:** A presumptive diagnosis of gonorrhea can be made based on examination of the stained smear; however, confirmation requires positive identification on selective media. Secretions are examined under oil immersion for presumptive identification. Gram-negative diplococci that are oxi-

dase-positive and obtained from selective media (Thayer-Martin or Transgrow) usually signify *N gonorrhoeae*. Carbohydrate fermentation tests may be performed, but, in addition to being time-consuming and expensive, they occasionally yield other species of *Neisseria*. Cultures therefore are reported as "presumptive for *N gonorrhoeae*." Chlamydial cultures or direct smear testing (ELISA or immunofluorescent staining) of the cervix and a serologic test for syphilis should also be obtained.

## Complications

The major complication in the female is salpingitis and the complications that may arise from salpingitis (see p 770). *N gonorrhoeae* can be recovered from the cervix in about 50% of women with salpingitis. Resistant strains of *N gonorrhoeae* have emerged in some geographic areas owing to their capacity to produce penicillinase or owing to chromosome-mediated resistance. Some strains are also resistant to spectinomycin and tetracycline. Follow-up cultures are essential in these settings, at least by 7 days after completion of therapy.

## Differential Diagnosis

See Chapter 34.

## Prevention

Gonorrhea is a reportable disease that can be controlled only by detecting the asymptomatic carrier and treating her and her sexual partners. All high-risk populations should be screened by routine cultures. Reexamination is mandatory to rule out re-infection or failure of therapy. The use of condoms will protect against gonorrhea.

## Treatment

*Note:* Any patient with gonorrhea must be suspected of also having other sexually transmitted diseases, eg, syphilis and chlamydial infection, and managed accordingly. Treatment should cover *N gonorrhoeae, Chlamydia trachomatis*, and incubating syphilis.

**A. Uncomplicated Infections:** Guidelines issued by the Centers for Disease Control (CDC) for therapy of uncomplicated infection in adults are as follows: (1) Recommended regimens: (a) Ceftriaxone, 125 mg intramuscularly once, plus doxycycline, 100 mg orally twice daily for 7 days; (b) cefixime 0.4 g orally once, plus doxycycline as above; (c) ofloxacin 0.4 g, or ciprofloxacin 0.5 g, orally once in nonpregnant patients over 17 years, plus doxycycline as above. (2) Alternative regimens: (a) spectinomycin, 2 g intramuscularly once, followed by doxycycline, as above, for patients who cannot take cephalosporins or quinolones; not reliable for pharyngeal infection; (b) ceftizoxime, 0.5 g, cefotaxime 0.5 g, cefotetan 1 g, or cefoxitin 1 g, intramuscularly once, plus doxycycline as above; (c) enoxacin, 0.4 g or norfloxacin 0.8 g, orally once, in nonpregnant patients over 17, plus doxycycline as above.

For patients in whom tetracyclines are contraindicated or not tolerated, erythromycin base or stearate, 500 mg, or erythromycin ethylsuccinate, 800 mg, may be taken orally 4 times daily for 7 days. Follow-up cultures are not essential for patients treated with any of the above regimens. Patients should return for examination if symptoms persist after treatment.

The incidence of penicillinase-producing strains of *N gonorrhoeae* (PPNG) is increasing and is spreading from coastal areas to the center of the USA. It is unresponsive to previously recommended conventional therapy such as penicillin, ampicillin, or amoxicillin, so the production of penicillinase should be tested for. Currently recommended cephalosporins and quinolones and regimens with β-lactamase inhibitors are effective therapy against PPNG strains.

**B. Acute Salpingitis:** See p 769.

**C. Disseminated Infections:** Disseminated gonococcal infection should be treated in the hospital initially. Evidence for endocarditis or meningitis should be sought. Recommended regimens include ceftriaxone, 1 g intramuscularly or intravenously every 24 hours, or cefotaxime or ceftizoxime, 1 g intravenously every 8 hours. For patients with β-lactamase allergy, spectinomycin, 2 g intramuscularly every 12 hours can be used. Testing for Chlamydia should be performed or therapy given. Therapy should be given for a total of 1 week; oral medications include cefixime, 0.4 g every 12 hours or ciprofloxacin, 0.5 g every 12 hours if not pregnant.

**D. Neonates and Children:** Infants born to women with untreated gonorrhea should be treated with ceftriaxone, 25–50 mg/kg intravenously or intramuscularly, not to exceed 125 mg. It should be given cautiously to premature or hyperbilirubinemic infants.

## Prognosis

The prognosis for patients with gonorrhea with prompt treatment is excellent. Infertility may result from even a single episode. Fewer cases are reported to the CDC yearly over the past 10 years.

## 2. SYPHILIS

## Essentials of Diagnosis

*Primary syphilis:*
- Painless genital sore (chancre) on labia, vulva, vagina, cervix, anus, lips, or nipples.
- Painless, rubbery, regional lymphadenopathy followed by generalized lymphadenopathy in third to sixth weeks.
- Darkfield microscopic findings positive.
- Positive serologic test in 70% of cases.

*Secondary syphilis:*
- Bilaterally symmetric extragenital papulosquamous eruption.
- Condyloma latum, mucous patches.
- Darkfield findings positive in moist lesions.
- Positive serologic test for syphilis.
- Lymphadenopathy

*Congenital syphilis:*
- History of maternal syphilis.
- Positive serologic test for syphilis.
- Stigmata of congenital syphilis (eg, x-ray changes of bone, hepatosplenomegaly, jaundice, anemia).
- Normal examination or signs of intrauterine infection.
- Often stillborn or premature.
- Enlarged, waxy placenta.

*Latent syphilis:*
- History or serologic evidence of previous infection.
- Absence of lesions.
- Serologic test usually reactive; titer may be low.

## General Considerations

The rates of syphilis in women during their reproductive years are the highest that have been observed since the 1940s. Syphilis is caused by *Treponema pallidum*, transmitted by direct contact with an infectious moist lesion. Treponemes pass through intact mucous membranes or abraded skin. Ten to 90 days after the treponemes enter, a primary lesion (chancre) develops. The chancre persists for 1–5 weeks and then heals spontaneously but may persist with signs of secondary disease. Serologic tests for syphilis are usually nonreactive when the chancre first appears but become reactive 1–4 weeks later. Two weeks to 6 months (average, 6 weeks) after the primary lesion appears, the generalized cutaneous eruption of secondary syphilis may appear. The skin lesions heal spontaneously in 2–6 weeks. Serologic tests are almost always positive during the secondary phase. Latent syphilis may follow the secondary stage and may last a lifetime, or tertiary syphilis may develop. The latter usually becomes manifest 4–20 or more years after the disappearance of the primary lesion.

In one-third of untreated cases, the destructive lesions of late (tertiary) syphilis develop. These involve skin or bone (gummas), the cardiovascular system (aortic aneurysm or insufficiency), and the nervous system (meningitis, tabes dorsalis, paresis). The complications of tertiary syphilis are fatal in almost one-fourth of cases, but one-fourth never show any ill effects.

## Clinical Findings

**A. Symptoms and Signs:**

**1. Primary syphilis**–The chancre (Fig 38–2) is an indurated, firm, painless papule or ulcer with raised borders. Groin lymph nodes may be enlarged, firm, and painless. Genital lesions are not usually

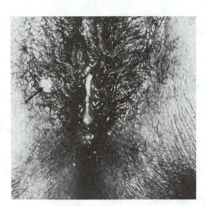

**Figure 38–2.** Chancre of primary syphilis (**arrow**).

seen in women unless they occur on the external genitalia; however, careful examination may reveal a typical cervical or vaginal lesion. Primary lesions may occur on any mucous membrane or skin area of the body (nose, breast, perineum), and darkfield examination is required for all suspect lesions. Serologic tests should be done every week for 6 weeks or until positive.

**2. Secondary syphilis–**Signs of diffuse systemic infection become evident as the spirochetes spread hematogenously. A "viral syndrome" presentation often with diffuse lymphadenopathy is not uncommon. The characteristic dermatitis appears as diffuse, bilateral, symmetric, papulosquamous lesions that often involve the palms and soles. Lesions may also cover the trunk and be macular, maculopapular, papular, or pustular. Other systemic manifestations include patchy alopecia, hepatitis, and nephritis. Moist papules can be seen in the perineal area (condyloma latum). Mucous patches may also be seen; like condyloma latum, they are darkfield-positive, infectious lesions. Serologic tests for syphilis are invariably reactive in this stage.

**3. Latent syphilis–**With resolution of the lesions of primary and secondary infection or the finding of a reactive serologic test without a history of therapy, a patient passes into latency. Persons are infectious in the first 1–2 years of latency, with clinical relapses resembling the secondary stage occurring in about 25% of cases in the first year. The United States Public Health Service defines early latent syphilis as disease of less than 1 years' duration and includes it in the category of "early or infectious syphilis, with primary and secondary lues." Late latent syphilis is infection of indeterminate or greater than 1 year's duration; consideration must be given to possible asymptomatic neurosyphilis in this setting.

**4. Syphilis during pregnancy–**The course of syphilis is unaltered by pregnancy, but misdiagnoses are common. The chancre is often unnoticed or internal and not brought to medical attention. Chancres,

mucous patches, and condyloma latum are often thought to be herpes genitalis. The dermatoses can resolve prior to diagnosis, or they may be misdiagnosed.

The effect of syphilis on pregnancy outcome can be profound. The risk of fetal infection depends on the degree of maternal spirochetemia (greater in the secondary stage than in the primary or latent stages) and the gestational age of the fetus. Treponemes may cross the placenta at all stages of pregnancy, but fetal involvement is rare before 18 weeks because of fetal immunoincompetence. After 18 weeks, the fetus is able to mount an immunologic response, and tissue damage may result. The earlier in pregnancy the fetus is exposed, the more severe the fetal infection and the greater the risk of premature delivery or stillbirth. Antepartum infection in late pregnancy does not necessarily result in congenital infection, since only 40–50% of such infants will have definite congenital infection. Placental infection can occur with resultant endarteritis, stromal hyperplasia, and immature villi. Grossly, the placenta looks hydropic (pale yellow, waxy, and enlarged). Hydramnios is frequently noted in association with symptomatic congenital infection.

**5. Congenital syphilis–**Most infants with congenital syphilis are born to women of low socioeconomic status with inadequate or no prenatal care. Either these neonates may be affected at birth from intrauterine infection (hepatosplenomegaly, osteochondritis, jaundice, anemia, skin lesions, rhinitis, lymphadenopathy, nervous system involvement), or symptoms may develop weeks or months later. The clinical spectrum of congenital infection is analogous to adult secondary disease, since the disease is systemic from onset due to transplacental hematogenous inoculation.

Since the antibodies from the maternal compartment are of the IgG class, they freely cross the placenta, giving most neonates a reactive serologic test if the mother's test was reactive. With symptomatic neonatal infection, often the cord blood serologic test will be higher in titer than the maternal test. There is no clinically reliable neonatal IgM serologic test. Other diagnostic aids include long-bone survey and lumbar puncture, which may help diagnose asymptomatic systemic infection requiring more intense therapy.

The newborn may have lymphadenitis and an enlarged liver and spleen. The bones usually reveal signs of osteochondritis and an irregular epiphyseal juncture (Guaaerin's line) on x-ray. The eyes, central nervous system structures, and other organs may reveal abnormalities at birth, or defects may develop later in untreated cases.

Any infant with the stigmata of syphilis should be placed in isolation until a definite diagnosis can be made and treatment administered.

Newborns with congenital syphilis may appear healthy at birth but often develop symptoms weeks or months later. Examine the body for stigmata of syphilis at intervals of 3 weeks to 4 months. If the mother's serologic test is positive at delivery, the baby's test will also be positive. Obtain serial quantitative serologic tests of the infant's blood for 4 months. A rising titer indicates congenital syphilis, and treatment is indicated.

**B. Laboratory Findings:**

**1. Identification of organism**–*T pallidum* can usually be identified by darkfield examination of specimens from cutaneous lesions, but the recovery period of the treponeme is very brief; in most cases, diagnosis depends on the history and serologic tests. An immunofluorescent technique is now available for dried smears. Silver staining for *T pallidum* of biopsy specimens, placental sections, or autopsy material may confirm the diagnosis in difficult cases. Motile spirochetes can be identified in amniotic fluid obtained transabdominally in women with syphilis and fetal death. Polymerase chain reaction is extremely specific for detection of *T pallidum* in amniotic fluid and neonatal serum and spinal fluid.

**2. Serologic tests**–Diagnostic tests after the primary or secondary moist lesion has disappeared are confined largely to serologic testing. Serologic tests become positive several weeks after the primary lesion appears.

**a. Nontreponemal tests**–These measure reaginic antibody detected by highly purified cardiolipin-lecithin antigen. They can be performed rapidly, relatively easily, and inexpensively. Nontreponemal tests are used principally for syphilis screening, but they are relatively specific, so they are not absolute for syphilis and false-positive reactions may occur. Nontreponemal tests currently in use are flocculation procedures that include the VDRL slide test, rapid reagin test, and automated reagin test for screening procedures in the field. The latter tests are more sensitive but less specific than the VDRL. If they are positive, the activity should be verified, and the degree of reactivity should be checked by the VDRL test. Complement fixation tests, eg, Kolmer, are no longer used in the USA.

The VDRL test (the nontreponemal test in widest use) generally becomes positive 3–6 weeks after infection, or 2–3 weeks after the appearance of the primary lesion; it is almost invariably positive in the secondary stage. The VDRL titer is usually high in secondary syphilis and tends to be lower or even nil in late forms of syphilis, although this is highly variable. A 4-fold falling titer in treated early syphilis or a falling or stable titer in latent or late syphilis indicates satisfactory therapeutic progress. False-positive serologic reactions are frequently encountered in a wide variety of situations, including collagen diseases, infectious mononucleosis, malaria, many febrile diseases, leprosy, vaccination, drug addiction, old age, and possibly pregnancy. False-positive reac-

tions are usually of low titer and transient and may be distinguished from true positives by specific treponemal antibody tests.

**b. Treponemal antibody tests**—The fluorescent treponemal antibody absorption (FTA-ABS) test and microhemagglutination assay for *T pallidum* (MHA-TP) detect antibody against *Treponema* spirochetes. Both tests are more sensitive and specific than nontreponemal tests (except the MHA-TP test with primary disease; Table 38–1). These tests remain positive despite therapy, and so are not given titers or used to follow serologic response to treatment.

## Differential Diagnosis

Primary syphilis must be differentiated from chancroid, granuloma inguinale, lymphogranuloma venereum, herpes genitalis, carcinoma, scabies, trauma, lichen planus, psoriasis, drug eruption, aphthosis, mycotic infections, Reiter's syndrome, and Bowen's disease.

Secondary syphilis must be differentiated from pityriasis rosea, psoriasis, lichen planus, tinea versicolor, drug eruption, "id" eruptions, perleche, parasitic infections, iritis, neuroretinitis, condyloma acuminatum, acute exanthems, infectious mononucleosis, alopecia, and sarcoidosis.

## Prevention

If the patient is known to have been exposed to syphilis, do not wait for the disease to develop to the clinical or reactive serologic stage before giving preventive treatment. Even so, every effort should be made to reach a diagnosis, including a complete physical examination, before administering preventive treatment.

Prenatal care is often underutilized or unavailable in geographic areas where congenital syphilis occurs. Education concerning the preventive value of prenatal care in these high-risk, generally low socioeconomic groups is essential. All pregnant women should undergo a routine serologic test for syphilis at the first visit. The test should be repeated between 28 and 32 weeks' of gestation. If the test is positive, attention must be given to the patient's prior serologic test and therapy (if any) for syphilis. If doubt exists as to whether or not the patient has active syphilis, repeat therapy is far better than the risk of congenital syphilis in the neonate.

**Table 38–1.** Percent sensitivity of serologic tests in untreated syphilis.

| Type of Test | Stage of Disease | | | |
|---|---|---|---|---|
| | Primary | Secondary | Latent | Late |
| VDRL | 59–87 | 100 | 73–91 | 37–94 |
| FTA-ABS | 86–100 | 99–100 | 96–99 | 96–100 |
| MHA-TP | 64–87 | 96–100 | 96–100 | 94–100 |

Reproduced, with permission, from Holmes KK et al (editors): *Sexually Transmitted Diseases.* McGraw-Hill, 1984.

Syphilis is still a serious public health problem. Teaching young people about the disease and its consequences is still the best method of control. Use of a condom, together with soap and water decontamination after coitus, would prevent most cases. If a lesion develops, a physician should be notified at once. All exposed persons must be sought and treated and the case reported to the communicable disease service in the city or state.

## Treatment

**A. Early Syphilis and Contacts:** (Primary, secondary, and latent syphilis of less than 1 year's duration.)

1. Benzathine penicillin G, 2.4 million units intramuscularly once.

2. Tetracycline hydrochloride, 500 mg orally 4 times daily or 100 mg doxycycline twice daily for 14 days, for nonpregnant penicillin-allergic patients.

3. Erythromycin (stearate, ethylsuccinate, or base), 500 mg orally 4 times daily for 15 days (30 g total), if the patient is penicillin-allergic and tetracycline is not tolerated or is contraindicated. Erythromycin estolate should not be administered to pregnant women because of potential drug-related hepatotoxicity.

**B. Late Syphilis:** (Includes latent syphilis of indeterminate duration or more than 1 year's duration, except neurosyphilis.)

1. Benzathine penicillin G, 2.4 million units intramuscularly for 3 successive weeks (7.2 million units total).

2. Tetracycline hydrochloride, 500 mg orally 4 times daily or 100 mg doxycycline twice daily for 14 days, for penicillin-allergic patients.

**C. Syphilis in Pregnancy:** Treat as indicated above, except that tetracycline is not recommended. If serologic tests are equivocal (eg, possible biologic false-positive), it is better to err on the side of early treatment. Penicillin-allergic patients may be given oral desensitization therapy using gradually larger doses of phenoxymethyl penicillin suspension to achieve a temporary tolerant state that allows parenteral penicillin therapy. This is particularly useful in circumventing compliance problems due to hyperemesis or drug-induced gastric upset.

**D. Congenital Syphilis:** Adequate maternal treatment before 16–18 weeks' gestation prevents congenital syphilis. Treatment thereafter may arrest fetal syphilitic infection, but some stigmata may remain.

1. Benzathine penicillin G, 50,000 U/kg intramuscularly as a single injection, for asymptomatic infants without neurosyphilis.

2. Aqueous crystalline penicillin G, 50,000 U/kg intravenously every 8–12 hours, or procaine penicillin G, 50,000 U/kg intramuscularly once daily for 10–14 days, for symptomatic infants or those with neurosyphilis.

**E. Jarisch-Herxheimer Reaction:** A febrile reaction may occur in 50–75% of patients with early syphilis treated with penicillin. This occurs 4–12 hours after injection and is completed by 24 hours. Its cause is uncertain but may involve a release of treponemal toxic products upon organism lysis. The reaction is generally benign but may trigger labor in pregnant women. Prophylaxis with antipyretics or corticosteroids is of unknown value.

**F. Coexisting Infection With HIV:** No specific changes in treatment are currently necessary, but close follow-up is necessary to ensure adequate treatment.

## 3. HERPES SIMPLEX

Vulvovaginal infections with herpes simplex virus have assumed a primary role in sexually transmitted diseases because of frequent incapacitation from pain as well as prohibitive risks of death or morbidity to the newborn exposed to maternal lesions. These infections are discussed in Chapter 34.

## 4. TRICHOMONAS VAGINITIS

See Chapter 34.

## 5. CHLAMYDIAL INFECTIONS

### Essentials of Diagnosis

- Mucopurulent cervicitis.
- Salpingitis.
- Urethral syndrome.
- Nongonococcal urethritis in male consort.
- Neonatal infections.
- Lymphogranuloma venereum.

### General Considerations

The spectrum of genital infections caused by serotypes of *Chlamydia trachomatis* has only become recently appreciated. Over 4 million cases of chlamydial infection occur yearly. Genital infection with this organism is the most common sexually transmitted bacterial disease in women. There has been a dramatic increase in the number of women with this infection reported to the CDC over the past 10 years. Chlamydiae are obligate intracellular microorganisms that have a cell wall similar to that of gram-negative bacteria. They are classified as bacteria and contain both DNA and RNA; they divide by binary fission, but like viruses, they grow intracellularly. They can be grown only by tissue culture. With the exception of the L serotypes, chlamydiae attach only to columnar epithelial cells without deep tissue invasion. As a result of this characteristic, clinical infection may not be apparent. For example, infections of the eye, respiratory tract, or genital tract are accompanied by discharge, swelling, erythema, and pain localized in these areas only. *C trachomatis* infections are associated with many adverse sequelae due to chronic inflammatory changes as well as fibrosis (eg, tubal infertility and ectopic pregnancy). The hypothesis for the pathogenesis of chlamydial disease has been an immune-mediated response, which has been supported by the observations of *C trachomatis* vaccine studies in humans and monkeys as well as other animal model studies. There is recent evidence that a 57-kDa chlamydial protein, which is a member of 60 kDa heat-shock proteins, plays a role in the immunopathogenesis of chlamydial disease.

Certain factors may be predictive of women with a greater likelihood of having *C trachomatis*. Sexually active women younger than 20 years of age have chlamydial infection rates 2–3 times higher than older women. The number of sexual partners and, in some studies, lower socioeconomic status are associated with higher chlamydial infection rates. Persons who use barrier contraception are less frequently infected by *C trachomatis* than those who use no contraception, and women who use oral contraceptives may have a higher incidence of cervical infection than women not using oral contraceptives. Cervical infection in pregnant women varies from 2 to 24% and is most prevalent in young, unmarried women of lower socioeconomic status in inner-city environments. The CDC recommends screening sexually active adolescent girls at their routine yearly gynecologic examination as well as women aged 20–24 years, and especially those who have new or multiple partners and who inconsistently use barrier contraceptives.

## Clinical Findings

**A. Symptoms and Signs:** It is not uncommon for women with chlamydial infection to be asymptomatic. Women with cervical infection generally have a mucopurulent discharge with hypertrophic cervical inflammation. Salpingitis may be unassociated with symptoms.

**B. Laboratory Findings:** The diagnosis of chlamydial infection is based solely on laboratory tests. Diagnosis of *C trachomatis* using cell culture isolation has a sensitivity of 70–90%; however, this specialized modality is not yet widely available. Cell culture is the detection method of greatest specificity (almost 100%), but the cost can be prohibitive, and a 3- to 7-day delay in diagnosis is required. Despite its disadvantages, cell culture is presently the standard for quality assurance of nonculture chlamydia tests. The CDC recommends cell culture for specimens from the urethra, rectum, and vagina of prepubertal girls and the nasopharynx of infants. In infants with inclusion conjunctivitis, Giemsa stain of purulent discharge from the eye is used to identify chlamydial inclusions, but similar stained slides of exudates in adults with genital infections are only about 40% ac-

curate in the diagnosis of these infections. Serologic methods, either the complement fixation or microimmunofluorescent test, are not totally accurate, because 20–40% of sexually active women have positive antibody titers. In fact, most women with microimmunofluorescent antibody do not have a current infection.

Moss and colleagues (1993) examined antibody responses to chlamydia species in patients who attended a genitourinary clinic and found that up to 50% of all chlamydia–IgG-positive cases were due to nongenital chlamydiae (*C pneumoniae* and *C psittaci*). The low specificity of the chlamydia serology tests is attributed to these antibodies as well as to the presence of group-specific antibodies. It is therefore of utmost importance to use serologic tests capable of distinguishing antibodies to *C trachomatis* from antibodies to *C pneumoniae* and *C psittaci* (nongenital chlamydial pathogens). Direct-smear fluorescent antibody testing requires a fluorescence microscope, and processing time is only 30–40 minutes. Sensitivity is 90% or higher, with a specificity of 98% or higher if an experienced microscopist and a satisfactory specimen are available. This appears to be the most promising test, and when tissue samples (endometrial or uterine tube) are being evaluated, it has been reported to be more accurate. Polymerase chain reaction (PCR), ligase chain reaction, and current DNA probes used in the detection of *C trachomatis* may be more rapid and less expensive. Nucleic acid hybridization methods (DNA probe) require only 2–3 hours for processing time. The DNA probe assay is specific for *C trachomatis*; cross-reactivity with *C pneumoniae* and *C psittaci* has not been reported. To ensure high specificity, a competitive probe assay has been produced and is currently undergoing evaluation in clinical trials. Recent reports indicate PCR positivity with negative culture. PCR may be the most sensitive and specific test method for chlamydia.

## Differential Diagnosis

Mucopurulent cervicitis is frequently caused by *N gonorrhoeae*, and selective cultures for this organism should be performed. As discussed above, *C trachomatis* alone may be associated with as many as 20–35% of cases of acute salpingitis in the USA. In both cervicitis and salpingitis, cultures may frequently be positive for both organisms.

## Complications

Adverse sequelae of salpingitis, specifically infertility due to tubal obstruction and ectopic pregnancy, are the most dire complications of these infections. Pregnant women with cervical chlamydial infection can transmit infections to their newborns; there is evidence that up to 50% of infants born to such mothers will have inclusion conjunctivitis. In perhaps 10%, an indolent chlamydial pneumonitis develops at 2–3 months of age. This pathogen may also cause otitis media in the neonate. Whether or not maternal cervical infection with *Chlamydia* causes significantly increased fetal and perinatal wastage by abortion, premature delivery, or stillbirth remains uncertain.

Increasing evidence exists that chlamydial infection in pregnancy is a risk marker for premature delivery and postpartum infections. Women at greatest risk are those with recent chlamydial infection detected by antichlamydial IgM. Those with chronic or recurrent infection do not have increased risks of preterm delivery. It is hypothesized that asymptomatic cervicitis predisposes to mild amnionitis. This event activates phospholipase $A_2$ to release prostaglandins, which cause uterine contractions that may lead to premature labor. Chlamydial infection is associated with higher rates of early postpartum endometritis as well as a delayed infection from *Chlamydia* that often presents several weeks postpartum.

## Treatment

In most cases, *Chlamydia* can be eradicated from the cervix by tetracycline, 500 mg orally 4 times daily, or doxycycline, 100 mg orally twice daily, for a minimum of 7 days. Compliance with treatment may play a major role in controlling chlamydial infections. Katz and associates (1992) evaluated the compliance with antichlamydial and antigonorrheal therapy and found that 63% of patients being treated with the standard 7-day regimen of tetracycline or erythromycin were compliant. When tetracyclines are contraindicated or not tolerated, erythromycin base, 500 mg, or erythromycin ethylsuccinate, 800 mg, orally 4 times daily should be given for a minimum of 7 days. An alternative regimen for patients who cannot tolerate erythromycin is amoxicillin, 500 mg orally 3 times daily for 7–10 days. Martin and colleagues (1992) have shown that a single 1-g oral dose of azithromycin, a new azalide antibiotic, is also effective in the treatment of uncomplicated genital chlamydial infections. Ofloxacin, 300 mg orally twice daily for 7 days, is the only quinolone effective against chlamydial infection. Its use is contraindicated during pregnancy or in patients under 18 years of age. Another regimen with less efficacy is sulfisoxazole, 500 mg orally 4 times daily for 10 days. Giving high doses of ampicillin has resulted in the elimination of *C trachomatis* from the cervices of women with acute salpingitis. Addition of the irreversible β-lactamase enzyme inhibitor sulbactam increases in vitro antichlamydial activity.

Current studies indicate that 3–5% of pregnant women and as many as 15% of sexually active nonpregnant women have an asymptomatic chlamydial cervical colonization. It is not known whether attempts to eradicate asymptomatic colonization will prevent chlamydial cervicitis, salpingitis, or neonatal infections. Posttreatment cultures are not usually advised if doxycycline, azithromycin, or ofloxacin is taken as above; cure rates should be higher than 95%. Retesting may be considered 3 weeks after completing treatment with erythromycin, sulfisoxazole, or amoxicillin. A positive posttreatment culture is more likely to represent noncompliance by the patient or sexual partner or reinfection rather than antibiotic resistance. It is important that the sexual partner be treated.

## 6. LYMPHOGRANULOMA VENEREUM

### Essentials of Diagnosis

- Rectal ulceration, inguinal lymphadenopathy, or rectal stricture.
- Positive complement fixation test.

### General Considerations

The causative agent of lymphogranuloma venereum is one of the aggressive L serotypes (L1, L2, or L3) of *C trachomatis*. It is encountered more frequently in the tropical and subtropical nations of Africa and Asia but is also seen in the southeastern USA. Transmission is sexual; men are affected more frequently than women (6:1). The incubation period is 7–21 days.

### Clinical Findings

**A. Symptoms and Signs:** (Fig 38–3)

1. Early in the course of the disease, a vesicopustular eruption may go undetected; with inguinal (and vulvar) ulceration, lymphedema, and secondary bilateral invasion, an excruciating condition arises. Sitting or walking may cause pain. During the inguinal bubo phase, the groin is exquisitely tender. A hard cutaneous induration (red to purplish-blue) is a notable feature. This usually occurs within 10–30 days after exposure and may be bilateral. Anorectal lymphedema occurs early; defecation is painful, and the stool may be blood-streaked.

2. Later, as the lymphedema and ulceration undergo cicatrization, rectal stricture makes defecation difficult or impossible. Vaginal narrowing and distor-

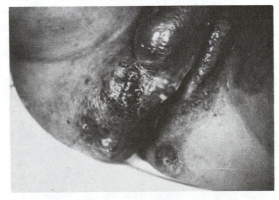

**Figure 38–3.** Lymphogranuloma venereum. Note involvement of perineum and spread over buttocks.

tion may end in severe dyspareunia. In the late phase, systemic symptoms—fever, headache, arthralgia, chills, and abdominal cramps—may develop.

**B. Laboratory Findings:** The diagnosis can be proved only by isolating *C trachomatis* from appropriate specimens and confirming the immunotype. These procedures are seldom available, so less specific tests are used.

A complement fixation test using a heat-stable antigen that is group-specific for all *Chlamydia* species is available. This test is positive at a titer of $\geq 1:16$ in more than 80% of cases of lymphogranuloma venereum. If acute or convalescent sera are available, a rise in titer is particularly helpful in making the diagnosis. Application of the microimmunofluorescent test may be useful also.

## Differential Diagnosis

As with any disseminated disease, the systemic symptoms of lymphogranuloma venereum may resemble meningitis, arthritis, pleurisy, or peritonitis. The cutaneous lesions must be differentiated from those of granuloma inguinale, tuberculosis, early syphilis, and chancroid. In case of colonic lesions, proctoscopic examination and mucosal biopsy are needed to rule out carcinoma, schistosomiasis, and granuloma inguinale.

## Complications

Perianal scarring and rectal strictures—late complications—can involve the entire sigmoid, but the urogenital diaphragm is rarely involved. Vulvar elephantiasis (esthiomene) produces marked distortion of the external genitalia.

## Prevention

Lymphogranuloma venereum is reportable. Avoiding infectious contact with a carrier is achieved by use of a condom or by refraining from coitus. Definite exposure can be treated with sulfonamides or tetracyclines.

## Treatment

**A. Chemotherapy:** Doxycycline, 100 mg twice daily orally, should be given for 21 days according to tolerance. If disease persists, the course should be repeated. Alternative regimens include tetracycline, erythromycin, or sulfisoxazole, 500 mg orally 4 times daily for 21 days.

**B. Local and Surgical Treatment:** Anal strictures should be dilated manually at weekly intervals. Severe stricture may require diversionary colostomy. If the disease is arrested, complete vulvectomy may be done for cosmetic reasons. Abscesses should be aspirated, not excised.

## 7. BACTERIAL VAGINOSIS (*Corynebacterium vaginale* Vaginitis; *Gardnerella vaginalis* Vaginitis)

Although bacterial vaginosis is the most prevalent vaginal infection, almost 50% of affected women are asymptomatic. The term bacterial vaginosis refers to the intricate changes of vaginal bacterial flora with a loss of lactobacilli, an increase in vaginal pH (pH > 4.5), and an increase in multiple anaerobic and aerobic bacteria. *Gardnerella vaginalis* (formerly designated *C vaginale* and *Haemophilus vaginalis*) is a small, nonmotile, nonencapsulated, pleomorphic rod that stains variably with Gram's stain. It is spread by sexual contact and, though of low virulence, causes vaginitis. The disorder may be atypical and even more troublesome when *G vaginalis* coexists with more virulent organisms. *G vaginalis* is not the only cause of bacterial vaginosis. The characteristic fishy odor of bacterial vaginosis is due to anaerobic bacteria, such as *Bacteroides*, *Prevotella*, *Peptostreptococcus*, and *Mobiluncus* sp, and genital mycoplasmas.

*G vaginalis* infection is often overlooked. It may be suspected on the basis of the microscopic appearance of unstained exfoliated vaginal cells in a wet preparation that appears to be dusted with many small dark particles, actually *G vaginalis* organisms. These "clue cells" are presumptive evidence of the presence of this organism. In case of mixed infection (eg, with *Candida albicans*), it may not be possible to make the diagnosis except by culture. Gram stain is another method useful in making the diagnosis of bacterial vaginosis.

## Treatment

Specific therapy for vaginal infection caused by *G vaginalis* and *C vaginale* has been neglected, owing in part to the rather innocuous symptoms reported. Standard teaching held that vaginally applied sulfonamide cream was adequate, but now this seems doubtful. Another regimen of questionable benefit is oral ampicillin, 500 mg 4 times daily for 1 week. Guidelines issued by the CDC for therapy are as follows: (1) recommended regimen: oral metronidazole, 500 mg twice daily for 7 days. (2) alternative regimens: (a) oral metronidazole 2 g, in a single dose; (b) oral clindamycin 300 mg twice daily for 7 days; (c) clindamycin cream, 2%, one applicatorful (5 g) intravaginally at night for 7 days; (d) metronidazole gel, 0.75%, one applicatorful (5 g), intravaginally, twice daily for 5 days. Four randomized controlled trials have demonstrated overall cure rates of 95% for the 7-day metronidazole regimen and 84% for the single 2 g regimen.

## 8. CHANCROID
### (Soft Chancre)

### Essentials of Diagnosis
- Painful, tender genital ulcer.
- Culture positive for *Haemophilus ducreyi*.
- Inguinal adenitis with erythema or fluctuance.

### General Considerations
Chancroid is a sexually transmitted disease characterized by a painful genital ulcer. It is endemic in many areas of the USA, although it occurs more frequently in Africa, the West Indies, and Southeast Asia. The causative organism is the gram-negative rod *H ducreyi*. Exposure is usually through coitus, but accidentally acquired lesions of the hands have occurred. The incubation period is short: the lesion usually appears in 3–5 days or sooner. An increased rate of HIV infection has been reported among patients with this genital ulcer disease; chancroid is a cofactor for HIV transmission. Moreover, 10% of patients with genital chancroid may have coinfection with herpes or syphilis.

### Clinical Findings
**A. Symptoms and Signs:** The early chancroid lesion is a vesicopustule on the pudendum, vagina, or cervix. Later, it degenerates into a saucer-shaped ragged ulcer circumscribed by an inflammatory wheal. Typically, the lesion is very tender and produces a heavy, foul discharge that is contagious. A cluster of ulcers may develop.

Painful inguinal adenitis is noted in over 50% of cases. The buboes may become necrotic and drain spontaneously.

**B. Laboratory Findings:** Syphilis must first be ruled out. Clinical diagnosis is more reliable than smears or cultures because of the difficulty of isolating this organism. Isolation of *H ducreyi* is diagnostic, but isolation occurs in less than one-third of cases. Aspirated pus from a bubo is the best material for culture.

### Differential Diagnosis
Syphilis, granuloma inguinale, lymphogranuloma venereum, and herpes simplex may coexist with chancroid and need to be ruled out.

### Prevention
Chancroid is a reportable disease. Routine antibiotic prophylaxis is not warranted. Condoms can give protection. Soap and water liberally used are relatively effective. Education is essential.

### Treatment
**A. Local Treatment:** Good personal hygiene is important. The early lesions should be cleansed with mild soap solution. Sitz baths are beneficial.

**B. Antibiotic Treatment:** The susceptibility of *H ducreyi* to antimicrobial agents varies by locality. Consultation with the nearest STD clinic may reveal information about current susceptibilities and effective treatment regimens. Guidelines issued by the CDC for genital chancroid are as follows: (1) Recommended regimens are (a) azithromycin 1 g orally once; (b) ceftriaxone 250 mg intramuscularly as a single dose; (c) erythromycin base 500 mg orally 4 times daily for 7 days. (2) Alternative regimens are (a) amoxicillin 500 mg with clavulanic acid 125 mg orally 3 times daily for 7 days; (b) ciprofloxacin 500 mg orally twice daily for 3 days in nonpregnant patients over 17. The course may have to be repeated. Fluctuant lymph nodes may need to be aspirated through normal adjacent skin. Incision and drainage of the nodes is not recommended, since it will delay healing.

### Prognosis
Untreated or poorly managed cases of chancroid may persist, and secondary infection may develop. Frequently, the ulcers heal spontaneously. If not treated, they may cause deep scarring with sequelae in men.

## 9. GRANULOMA INGUINALE
### (Donovanosis)

### Essentials of Diagnosis
- Ulcerative vulvitis, chronic or recurrent.
- Donovan bodies revealed by Wright's or Giemsa's stain.

### General Considerations
Granuloma inguinale is a chronic ulcerative granulomatous disease that usually develops in the vulva, perineum, and inguinal regions (Fig 38–4). The disease is almost nonexistent in the USA. It is most common in India, Brazil, the West Indies, some South Pacific islands, and parts of Australia, China, and Africa. The causative organism is *Calymmatobacterium granulomatis* (Donovan body). Donovan bodies are bacteria encapsulated in mononuclear leukocytes. Transmission is via coitus, and the incubation period is 8–12 weeks.

### Clinical Findings
**A. Symptoms and Signs:** Although granuloma inguinale most often involves the skin and subcutaneous tissues of the vulva and inguinal regions, cervical, uterine, orolabial, and ovarian sites have been reported. A malodorous discharge is characteristic. The disorder often begins as a papule, which then ulcerates, with the development of a beefy-red granular zone with clean, sharp edges. The ulcer shows little tendency to heal, and there are usually no local or systemic symptoms. Healing is very slow, and satellite ulcers may unite to form a large lesion. Lymphatic

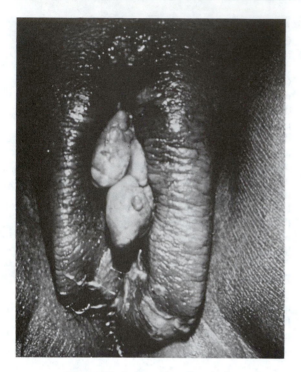

**Figure 38–4.** Granuloma inguinale.

permeation is rare, but lymphadenitis may result when the cutaneous lesion becomes superimposed on lymphatic channels. Inguinal swelling is common, with late formation of abscesses (buboes). Rarely, granuloma inguinale may be manifested by chronic cervical lesions. These lesions usually take the form of redness or ulceration, or they form granulation tissue. They produce a chronic inflammatory exudate characterized histologically by lymphocytes, giant cells, and histiocytes. They may mimic carcinoma of the cervix and must be distinguished from this as well as other neoplastic diseases.

The chronic ulcerative process may involve the urethra and the anal area, causing marked discomfort. Introital contraction may make coitus difficult or impossible; walking or sitting may become painful. The possibility of the coexistence of another venereal disease must be considered. Spread to other areas occurs in about 7% of patients.

**B. Laboratory Findings:** Direct smear from beneath the surface of an ulcer may reveal gram-negative bipolar rods within mononuclear leukocytes. These are seen best in Wright-stained smears. When smears are negative, a biopsy specimen should be taken. Biopsy of the lesion generally shows granulation tissue infiltrated by plasma cells and scattered large macrophages with rod-shaped cytoplasmic inclusion bodies (Mikulicz cells). Pseudoepitheliomatous hyperplasia often is seen at the margin of the ulcer.

The diagnosis of granuloma inguinale is made by demonstrating, in biopsy or smear material stained with Wright's, Giemsa's, or silver stain, large mononuclear cells having one or more cystic inclusions containing the so-called Donovan bodies—small round or rod-shaped particles that stain purple in traditional hematoxylin and eosin preparations.

### Prevention

Personal hygiene is the best method of prevention. Therapy immediately after exposure may abort the infection.

### Treatment

Tetracycline is the drug of first choice. The recommended dose is 500 mg orally 4 times daily for at least 3 weeks. Occasionally, doses of 40–60 g may be used. Erythromycin, 500 mg 4 times daily for 2–3 weeks, is also effective. Doxycycline, 100 mg orally, or sulfamethoxazole, 1 g orally, twice daily for at least 3 weeks may be used. Penicillin is not effective, but chloramphenicol, 500 mg orally 3 times daily, is often effective.

## 10. CONDYLOMATA ACUMINATA (Venereal Warts)

See Chapter 34.

## 11. HUMAN IMMUNODEFICIENCY VIRUS (HIV) INFECTION

### Essentials of Diagnosis

*Asymptomatic Infection*
- HIV antibody, antigen, or culture.
- High-risk group member.
- HIV antibody, antigen, or culture.
- Mononucleosis-like syndrome with weight loss, fever, night sweats.
- Neurologic involvement.
- Lymphadenopathy.
- Pharyngitis.
- Erythematous maculopapular rash.
- Extragenital lymphadenopathy.

*Acquired Immunodeficiency Syndrome (AIDS)*
- HIV antibody, antigen, or culture.
- Any of the above signs or symptoms.
- Opportunistic infections.
- Cognitive difficulties or depression.
- Kaposi's sarcoma.
- CD4+ counts below 200 CD4 lymphocytes/mm$^3$.

### General Considerations

Since 1981 there have been over 200,000 cases of acquired immunodeficiency syndrome (AIDS) reported in the USA. The CDC estimated in 1991 that between 1 and 1.5 million people in the USA were infected with HIV. Unfortunately, no reliable sero-prevalence studies are available for the general population. The best estimates of the incidence of HIV infection in the USA are likely to come from ongoing serologic surveillance studies in sentinel areas and hospitals. In the general population, HIV infection is most prevalent in gay or bisexual men, intravenous drug abusers, and hemophiliacs. Approximately 11% of the cases of AIDS in the USA in 1989 occurred in women, most clustered in the large metropolitan areas of New York City, New Jersey, and Miami. The high-risk groups for women, in decreasing order of frequency, are intravenous drug abusers, those with heterosexual contacts with men in high-risk groups, recipients of unscreened transfusions, and prostitutes.

Over 80% of the cases of AIDS in women occur in women of reproductive age, making heterosexual and perinatal transmission important concerns. Minorities are overly represented in the reported AIDS cases: more blacks than Hispanics and more Hispanics than whites have been reported to the CDC. Most HIV infections in the United States are due to HIV-1. The prevalence of HIV-2 in this country is very low. HIV-2 is endemic in parts of West Africa and has been reported increasingly in Angola, Mozambique, Portugal, and France.

## Modes of Transmission

Although many speculations exist about the modes of HIV transmission, HIV infection may be acquired in only 3 ways.

First, HIV infection may be acquired by sexual contact. Transmission has been reported from male to male, male to female, female to male, and, recently, female to female. The risk appears to be greatest for the female sexual partners of men with AIDS, followed in decreasing order by intravenous drug abusers, bisexual men, transfusion recipients, and hemophiliacs. Other factors that increase the risk for heterosexual acquisition of HIV infection are the number of exposures to high-risk sexual partners; anal-receptive intercourse; and infection with other sexually transmitted diseases such as syphilis, genital herpes, chancroid, and condylomata acuminata.

The second means by which HIV transmission can occur is by parenteral exposure to blood or bodily fluids such as with intravenous drug use or occupational exposure.

The third means by which HIV infection can occur is by transmission from an infected woman to her fetus or infant.

## Course of Infection

The chance of acquiring HIV infection through sexual contact is unknown. Approximately 5% of the cases reported to the CDC appear to be acquired through heterosexual contact; some of the cases without risk factors may be heterosexually acquired. The percentage of cases arising from heterosexual contact is larger in women than in men, probably because transmission can occur more easily from male to female. This is due to 2 reasons: (1) the concentration of HIV in semen is high and (2) coitus causes more breaks in the introital mucosa than in the penile skin. It is hypothesized that these breaks in the mucosa, similar to those that occur with anal-receptive intercourse, increase the chances for acquiring HIV through sexual contact. The presence of a genital ulcerative disease also increases the risk of infection in a similar fashion.

The natural course of HIV infection is becoming better understood. HIV is a single-stranded RNA-enveloped retrovirus that attaches to the CD4 receptor of the target cell and integrates into the host genome. If they become infected, most patients develop anti-HIV antibody within 12 weeks after exposure. As many as 45–90% of patients develop an acute HIV-induced retroviral infection in the first few months after infection. This is similar to mononucleosis, with symptoms of weight loss, fever, night sweats, pharyngitis, lymphadenopathy, erythematous maculopapular rash, and extragenital lymphadenopathy. This syndrome usually resolves within several weeks, and the patient becomes asymptomatic. HIV-infected individuals ultimately show evidence of progressive immune dysfunction and the condition progresses to AIDS as immunosuppression continues and systemic involvement becomes more severe and diffuse. The CDC case definition of AIDS is an HIV-infected person with a specific opportunistic infection (eg, *Pneumocystis carinii* pneumonia, central nervous system toxoplasmosis), neoplasia (eg, Kaposi's sarcoma), dementia encephalopathy, wasting syndrome, or a CD4 lymphocyte count less than $200/mm^3$. A patient without laboratory evidence of infection may also be diagnosed with AIDS if one of the indicator diseases is present and there is no explanation for the immune dysfunction. The chance of becoming symptomatic after HIV-seropositive conversion is approximately 54% within 10 years (data from the San Francisco Gay Men's Cohort Study).

Unfortunately, the mortality rate for patients with AIDS is greater than 90% and at present does not appear to be altered by antiviral agents such as zidovudine (AZT). Further research in the development of antivirals and vaccines is in progress.

## Prevention of HIV Infection

To decrease the risk of acquiring HIV infection through sexual contact, "safer sex" guidelines have been established. These include a reduction in the number of sexual partners, especially those who are in high-risk groups, and use of condoms for all coital activity. Latex condoms lubricated with Nonoxynol 9, a spermicide that inactivates HIV in vitro, are the most effective.

Education and counseling for detection of HIV-infected patients and prevention of HIV infection are difficult tasks. HIV infection in women appears to be a disease of drug users and sexual partners of high-risk men. Groups to whom information must be targeted are intravenous drug users and ethnic minorities groups, particularly blacks and Hispanics. Counseling must not only stress behavior modification but also reinforce those behavioral changes through culturally significant and sensitive messages. In general, reduction of high-risk behavior and use of safer sex guidelines have been the 2 main areas of education and counseling.

The general preventive guidelines for seropositive women include the following:

(1) Refraining from donating blood, plasma, organs, or tissue.

(2) Being in a mutually monogamous sexual relationship.

(3) Using condoms with spermicide.

(4) Avoiding pregnancy.

## HIV Infection During Pregnancy

Maternal transmission of HIV can occur transplacentally before birth, peripartum by exposure to blood and bodily fluids at delivery, or postpartum through breastfeeding. The risks of perinatal transmission are not clearly elucidated, because they are based on small prospective studies and sibling studies. The range of perinatal infection rate has been 20–50%, with an average of about 30%. However, a recent report by the European Collaborative Study found a 13% maternal-fetal transmission rate. The risk appears to be higher in subsequent pregnancies if a patient has delivered one infected infant; in this setting the risk may be 37–65%. Unfortunately, no known factors modify the risk of perinatal transmission. The mode of delivery does not play a role in increasing or decreasing the risks of developing pediatric AIDS.

Many of the concerns about the effect of pregnancy on HIV infection are unanswered. Does the altered immune status of pregnancy accelerate the progression of HIV infection? Clinically, progression from asymptomatic infection to AIDS is uncommon in pregnancy. However, 45–75% of women will develop symptomatic HIV infection within 2–3 years postpartum if their child was infected. Whether this represents an accelerated progression of HIV infection or demonstrates more effective perinatal transmission in women with longstanding infection is unknown. Delays in the diagnosis of acute HIV infection may occur, since some of the symptoms of early HIV infection may mimic those of the first trimester of pregnancy. Additionally, pregnant women may not receive treatment, since many of the drugs used to treat HIV infection and opportunistic infections are potentially teratogenic. Finally, the effect of a therapeutic termination of pregnancy on the ultimate progress of HIV infection is unknown.

Prenatal care must be individualized, with referral to support systems ideally occurring during the pregnancy rather than postpartum. Screening for other sexually transmitted diseases (eg, syphilis, gonorrhea, and herpes simplex virus infection) is important. Other specific HIV-related infections must be sought, including *Pneumocystis carinii* pneumonia, *Mycobacterium* tuberculosis, cytomegaloviral infection, toxoplasmosis, and candidiasis. As a minimum, HIV-infected patients should receive a shielded chest x-ray, a tuberculin skin test with controls, and cytomegalovirus and toxoplasmosis baseline serologic tests. Susceptible patients should receive hepatitis B virus, pneumococcal, and influenza vaccines. CD4+ lymphocyte cell counts should be monitored each trimester. A CD4+ count of less than $200/mm^3$ is an indication for prophylaxis against *Pneumocystis carinii* pneumonia and antiviral treatment after the first trimester.

Peripartum care should include universal application of infection control guidelines to avoid exposure to blood and bodily fluids. These include water-repellant gowns, double gloves, hand-washing between patient contacts, goggles for significant splash exposures, and wall or bulb suction. Needles should not be recapped. A 1:10 sodium hypochlorite solution should be used to clean instruments. Fetal scalp sampling and scalp electrodes should be avoided because they could become portals of entry for infection.

Postpartum care should entail a continuance of blood and bodily fluids precautions with proscription of breast-feeding. Family planning and safer sex counseling can be continued in the postpartum period with strong consideration given to tubal ligation. Medical and support system referrals should be initiated prior to discharge from the hospital, if possible.

## Pediatric HIV Infection

Over 1000 cases of pediatric AIDS have been reported in the USA, accounting for 1–2% of the total reported cases. Eighty percent of these are perinatally acquired, occurring in infants born to women in high-risk groups: intravenous drug users, partners of high-risk men, or women with AIDS. The progression to infection appears to be faster than in adults, and pediatric AIDS carries a mortality rate similar to that found in adults.

Identification of infected neonates is difficult, because maternal anti-HIV IgG crosses the placenta. Thus, most infants are born with HIV seropositivity, which may persist up to 15 months by the enzyme immunoassay (EIA) technique. An HIV IgM has been described that may help identify fetal HIV infection, but it is not yet approved for general use. An HIV embryopathy similar to the fetal alcohol syndrome has been described. Since many of the high-risk mothers have multifactorial perinatal problems, assigning the cause of the syndrome to HIV is uncertain.

Infant care involves many of the same guidelines as maternal peripartum care. Blood and bodily fluid precautions, as well as immunosuppression care guidelines, should be exercised. Consultation with a pediatric immunologist to plan neonatal and follow-up care should begin prior to discharge from the hospital. Circumcision should be discouraged. Prior to discharge, detailed home-care instruction should be given regarding avoidance of bodily secretions.

## Guidelines for HIV Testing

HIV serologic testing should include pretest and posttest counseling about interpretation of the test results. After obtaining informed consent from the patient, confidentiality must be maintained concerning the test results. Situations in which HIV testing should be offered include the following:

(1) Women who have used intravenous drugs.
(2) Women who have engaged in prostitution.
(3) Women with sex partners who are HIV-infected or are at risk for HIV infection.
(4) Women who have sexually transmitted diseases.
(5) Women who have lived in communities or were born in countries where the prevalence of HIV infection (especially heterosexually acquired HIV infection) among women is high.
(6) Women who received blood transfusions between 1978 and 1985.
(7) Women undergoing medical evaluation or treatment for clinical signs and symptoms of HIV infection.
(8) Women who have been inmates in correctional systems.
(9) Women who consider themselves at risk.

## HIV Antibody Testing

The diagnosis of HIV infection is usually by HIV-1 antibody tests. Routine testing for HIV-2, other than at blood banks, is currently not recommended unless a patient is at risk for HIV-2 infection or has clinical findings of HIV disease and has had a negative HIV-1 antibody test. Refer to recent reviews cited in the references for details of the criteria for HIV antibody detection. In general, the enzyme-linked immunosorbent assay (ELISA) functions as a screening test for exposure to HIV. Most patients exposed to HIV develop detectable levels of antibody against the virus by 12 weeks after exposure. The presence of antibody indicates current infection, although the patient may be asymptomatic for years. The sensitivity and specificity of the ELISA test is 99% when it is repeatedly reactive. Thus, the test for HIV antibody is considered negative if the ELISA is nonreactive, and indicates a lack of HIV infection unless it is too early to detect antibody production.

The probability of a false-negative test in an uninfected woman is remote unless she is in the "window" before antibody is produced. A positive test result occurs when an ELISA is repeatedly reactive followed by a positive Western blot assay. The Western blot assay is reactive when a critical pattern of specific antibodies are detected against the 3 main gene products of HIV. The probability that an abnormal testing sequence will falsely identify a patient as HIV-infected is from less than 1 to 5 in 100,000 persons. Individuals in high-risk groups should be retested in 3 months; they are likely to become positive. The status of those without associated risk factors is likely to remain indeterminate, but persistent indeterminate status is not diagnostic of HIV infection.

## PELVIC INFECTIONS

Because of their common occurrence and often serious consequences, infections are among the most important problems encountered in the practice of gynecology. A wide variety of pelvic infections, ranging from uncomplicated gonococcal salpingo-oophoritis to septicemic shock following rupture of a pelvic abscess, confront the general physician as well as the gynecologist.

The following is a general classification of pelvic infections by frequency of occurrence:

(1) Pelvic inflammatory disease
  (a) Acute salpingitis
    (i) Gonococcal
    (ii) Nongonococcal
  (b) IUD-related pelvic cellulitis
  (c) Tubo-ovarian abscess
  (d) Pelvic abscess
(2) Puerperal infections
  (a) Cesarean section (common)
  (b) Vaginal delivery (uncommon)
(3) Postoperative gynecologic surgery
  (a) Cuff cellulitis and parametritis
  (b) Vaginal cuff abscess
  (c) Tubo-ovarian abscess
(4) Abortion-associated infections
  (a) Postabortal cellulitis
  (b) Incomplete septic abortion
(5) Secondary to other infections
  (a) Appendicitis
  (b) Diverticulitis
  (c) Tuberculosis

"Pelvic inflammatory disease" (PID) is a general term for acute, subacute, recurrent, or chronic infection of the oviducts and ovaries, often with involvement of adjacent tissues. Most infections seen in clinical practice are bacterial, but viral, fungal, and parasitic infections may occur. The term PID is vague at best and should be discarded in favor of more specific terminology. This should include identification of the affected organs, the stage of the infection, and, if possible, the causative agent. This specificity is especially important in view of the rising incidence of venereal disease and its complications.

The three proposed pathways of dissemination of microorganisms in pelvic infections are depicted in Figures 38–1, 38–5, and 38–6. Lymphatic dissemination (Fig 38–5), typified by postpartum, postabortal, and some IUD-related infections, results in extraperitoneal parametrial cellulitis. In Fig 38–1, the endometrial-endosalpingeal-peritoneal spread of microorganisms is depicted; this represents more common forms of nonpuerperal PID, in which pathogenic bacteria gain access to the lining of the uterine tubes, with resultant purulent inflammation and egress of pus through tubal ostia into the peritoneal cavity. These infections are represented by endometritis, adnexal infection, and peritonitis. In rare instances, certain diseases (eg, tuberculosis) may gain access to pelvic structures by hematogenous routes (Fig 38–6).

Early recognition and treatment of the various entities that make up PID are mandatory so that specific therapy can be instituted to prevent damage to the reproductive system. Repeated sexual contacts with multiple partners predispose to subsequent reinfection or superinfection, spreading the disease throughout the reproductive system and resulting in sterility and an increased risk for tubal pregnancy.

The initial gonococcal infection (more common in young single women of low parity) may be relatively asymptomatic, and the patient may not be seen until recurrent infection with irreversible pathologic changes has taken place. Gonorrhea involving only the lower genital tract and urethra is often asymptomatic; severe symptomatic gonorrhea implies tubal and peritoneal involvement. If the initial infection is limited to the lower tract, proper therapy may prevent further sequelae. The presence of endosalpingitis or ovarian infection carries a graver prognosis in regard to future fertility.

Originally, it was thought that the gonococcus was the only organism responsible for nonpuerperal acute

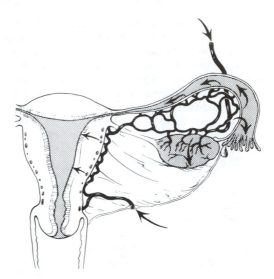

**Figure 38–6.** Hematogenous spread of bacterial infection (eg, tuberculosis).

pelvic inflammation. More recent data indicate that *N gonorrhoeae* is isolated in only 40–60% of women with acute salpingitis. In Sweden, *C trachomatis* was estimated to cause 60% of cases of salpingitis. Although direct evidence of such infection, eg, recovery from tubal culture, is lacking in most studies done in the USA, authorities believe that this pathogen may be responsible for 20–35% of such pelvic infections. It is unclear how frequently salpingitis is caused by chlamydiae alone or by chlamydiae in association with other invasive microorganisms. Regardless of the initiating factors, nongonococcal pathogens that comprise the normal vagina flora may become involved in many cases of acute salpingitis-peritonitis.

*N gonorrhoeae* was present alone or with other pathogens in 65% of the specimens. Chow et al (1975) reported positive cul-de-sac fluid cultures in 18 (90%) of 20 patients with acute salpingitis compared with 8 normal patients with negative results.

If the infectious process continues, pelvic adhesions become more pronounced, and tissue planes are lost. It becomes difficult to identify the tubes and ovaries in the inflammatory mass, which may include omental and intestinal attachments. Further progression causes tissue necrosis with abscess formation. Containment of the purulent exudate under pressure becomes impossible at certain sites, and pus is released into the peritoneal cavity. This is usually at the site of an adhesion to a nearby organ, and the point of rupture can often be identified at operation. Abscess formation may be localized in either or both of the tubes and ovaries without leakage or rupture. Another possibility is accumulation of purulent material walled off in the cul-de-sac.

Recent observations have shown these pelvic in-

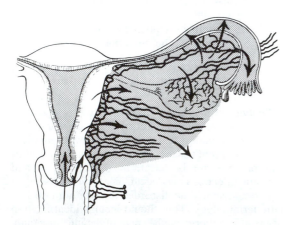

**Figure 38–5.** Lymphatic spread of bacterial infection.

fections to be polymicrobial with mixed anaerobic and aerobic bacteria. Anaerobes predominate and frequently coexist with aerobes. In some cases, aerobes alone are isolated. With further advanced disease, such as abscess formation, anaerobic organisms seem to predominate. All these bacteria are members of the normal vaginal and endocervical flora and include *Bacteroides*, *Escherichia coli*, aerobic streptococci, and anaerobic cocci (*Peptostreptococcus* and *Peptococcus*). Virtually any organism indigenous to the normal vaginal or gastrointestinal flora may be isolated if specific techniques are used. Direct immunofluorescent antibody testing of cervical smears of 500 asymptomatic women showed *C trachomatis* in 10%. Of women recently treated as outpatients for acute salpingitis, 16% had *C trachomatis* in endocervical specimens and 8% had the organism in the endometrial cavity (obtained with a double-lumen catheter-protected brush). From the same sites, *N gonorrhoeae* was identified in 68% and 65%, respectively. Great numbers of both aerobes and anaerobes were recovered from endometrial cultures; 10% had group B *Streptococcus*, 10% had *Bacteroides fragilis* sp, 55% had *Streptococcus faecalis*, 65% had *Staphylococcus epidermidis*, 75% had anaerobic *Streptococcus* sp, and 65% had *Prevotella bivius* in that location. Whether this is a result of infection or is flora from the lower tract and endometrium is under evaluation.

Many factors may account for adverse sequelae of these pelvic infections, eg, infertility and pain. Delay in initiation of treatment is associated with later symptomatology. Likewise, inadequate therapy due to improper antimicrobial selection, insufficient dosage, or inadequate duration of therapy may be responsible for subsequent problems. An inflammatory process that is allowed to continue—for whatever reason—results in anatomic derangements with adhesive attachments to nearby organs. An ovulation site in an ovary may serve as a portal of entry for extension of the infection into the ovarian stroma, and this sets the stage for formation of tubo-ovarian abscesses.

The most important factor in the diagnosis in women with pelvic infections is clinical awareness by the physician. For patients with high-risk factors, eg, postoperative pelvic surgery, postpartum, or postabortal, fever is usually the first clue. For women without these factors, a high index of suspicion is important. If gonorrhea is suspected, a Gram-stained smear of endocervical purulent material or fluid obtained by culdocentesis may be helpful. The Gram-stained smear may be lifesaving in the woman now only infrequently seen with serious infection due to *Clostridium perfringens*. Except for isolation of *N gonorrhoeae* with specialized media, cultures taken from women with pelvic infections currently are not useful for clinical management. Since these infections are usually polymicrobial, sophisticated techniques are necessary for microbiologic identification.

These are time-consuming, and by the time the results become available to the clinician, the woman has usually been cured with empiric antimicrobial drug therapy.

Ultrasonography has become a useful means of diagnosis of adnexal and pelvic masses. When ultrasound diagnosis is compared with laparoscopic diagnosis, it is about 90% accurate. Thickening is noted in the pelvic areas during the inflammatory process. Ultrasonography is most valuable in following the progression or regression of an abscess after it has been diagnosed. The borders of an abscess conform to the surrounding pelvic structures and as such do not give a well-defined border as noted in ovarian cyst. Unfortunately, x-ray films (kidney, ureter, bladder [KUB]) are of little help in pelvic infections because they seldom identify pelvic masses. X-rays often identify adynamic ileus, which frequently accompanies pelvic peritonitis. Chest films are necessary if pneumonia is suspected and to detect the presence of free air under the diaphragms.

Complete reliance cannot be placed on the white blood count because it may be elevated, normal, or decreased in patients with moderate to severe infections.

Culdocentesis (cul-de-sac tap) may be helpful in the diagnosis of suspected pelvic infection. Other conditions that may simulate infection can be ruled out by means of this simple procedure. The rectouterine pouch (of Douglas) is punctured with a long spinal needle to obtain a sample of the contents of the peritoneal cavity after vaginal membrane prep with povidone-iodine or similar agents. Culdocentesis is easy to perform and may be done with or without local anesthesia in the hospital or in the office. One milliliter of sterile saline anesthetizes the vaginal membrane and peritoneum. Culdocentesis is indicated whenever peritoneal material is needed for diagnosis. Cultures for aerobic and anaerobic organisms may also be obtained. Contraindications include a cul-de-sac mass or a fixed retroflexed uterus. For differential evaluation of fluid obtained by culdocentesis, see Table 38–2.

## PELVIC INFLAMMATORY DISEASE

### 1. ACUTE SALPINGITIS-PERITONITIS

**Essentials of Diagnosis**

- Onset of lower abdominal and pelvic pain, usually following onset or cessation of menses and associated with vaginal discharge, abdominal, uterine, adnexal, and cervical motion tenderness, plus one or more of the following:
  (a) Temperature above 38°C (100.4°F).
  (b) Leukocyte count greater than 10,000/μL.
  (c) Inflammatory mass (examination or sonography).

**Table 38–2.** Differential evaluation of fluid obtained by culdocentesis.

| Finding | Implications for Diagnosis |
|---------|----------------------------|
| Blood | Ruptured ectopic pregnancy. Hemorrhage from corpus luteum cyst. Retrograde menstruation. Rupture of spleen or liver. Gastrointestinal bleeding. Acute salpingitis. |
| Pus | Ruptured tubo-ovarian abscess. Ruptured appendix or viscus. Rupture of diverticular abscess. Uterine abscess with myoma. |
| Cloudy | Pelvic peritonitis (such as is seen with acute gonococcal salpingitis). Twisted adnexal cyst. Other causes of peritonitis: appendicitis, pancreatitis, cholecystitis, perforated ulcer, carcinomatosis, echinococcosis. |

(d) Gram-negative intracellular diplococci in cervical secretions.

(e) Purulent material (WBC) from peritoneal cavity (culdocentesis or laparoscopy).

## General Considerations

There is generally an acute onset of pelvic infection, often associated with invasion by *N gonorrhoeae* and involving the uterus, tubes, and ovaries, with varying degrees of pelvic peritonitis. In the acute stage, there is redness and edema of the tubes and ovaries with a purulent discharge oozing from the ostium of the tube.

## Clinical Findings

**A. Symptoms and Signs:** The insidious or acute onset of lower abdominal and pelvic pain usually is bilateral and only occasionally unilateral. There may be a sensation of pelvic pressure, with back pain radiating down one or both legs. In most cases, symptoms appear shortly after the onset or cessation of menses. There is often an associated purulent vaginal discharge.

Nausea may occur, with or without vomiting, but these symptoms may be indicative of a more serious problem (eg, acute appendicitis). Headache and general lassitude are common complaints.

Fever is not necessary for the diagnosis of acute salpingitis, although its absence may indicate other disorders, specifically ectopic pregnancy. In one study (Westrom et al, 1979), only 30% of women with laparoscopically confirmed acute salpingitis had fever. Although standardization of criteria for diagnosis of acute salpingitis to include fever greater than 38°C (100.4°F) may greatly aid clinical research, such a distinction may result in many women with acute pelvic infection being erroneously diagnosed and inadequately treated.

Abdominal tenderness is often encountered, usually in both lower quadrants. The abdomen may be somewhat distended, and bowel sounds may be hypoactive or absent. Pelvic examination may demonstrate inflammation of the periurethral (Skene) or Bartholin glands as well as a purulent cervical discharge. Bimanual examination typically elicits extreme tenderness on movement of the cervix and uterus and palpation of the parametria.

**B. Laboratory Findings:** Leukocytosis with a shift to the left is usually present; however, the white count may be normal. A smear of purulent cervical material may demonstrate Gram-negative kidney-shaped diplococci in polymorphonuclear leukocytes. These organisms may be gonococci, but definitive cultures on selective media are advised. Penicillinase production should also be confirmed.

Culdocentesis generally is productive of "reaction fluid" (cloudy peritoneal fluid) which, when stained, reveals leukocytes with or without gonococci or other organisms. Culture and sensitivity testing of organisms from culdocentesis samples may be done.

**C. X-Ray Findings:** X-ray examination of the abdomen may show signs of ileus, but this finding is nonspecific. Air may be seen under the diaphragm with a ruptured tubo-ovarian or pelvic abscess and demands immediate laparotomy in addition to combination antimicrobial therapy.

## Differential Diagnosis

Acute salpingitis must be differentiated from acute appendicitis, ectopic pregnancy, ruptured corpus luteum cyst with hemorrhage, diverticulitis, infected septic abortion, torsion of an adnexal mass, degeneration of a leiomyoma, endometriosis, acute urinary tract infection, regional enteritis, and ulcerative colitis.

## Complications

Complications of acute salpingitis include pelvic peritonitis or generalized peritonitis, prolonged adynamic ileus, severe pelvic cellulitis with thrombophlebitis, abscess formation (pyosalpinx, tubo-ovarian abscess, cul-de-sac abscess) with adnexal destruction and subsequent infertility, and intestinal adhesions and obstruction. More rarely, dermatitis, gonococcal arthritis, or bacteremia with septic shock may occur.

## Prevention

Approximately 15% of women with asymptomatic gonococcal cervical infection develop acute salpingitis. Detection and treatment of these women and their sexual partners should therefore prevent a substantial number of cases of gonococcal pelvic infection. Early diagnosis and eradication of minimally symptomatic disease (cervicitis, urethritis) also usually prevent salpingitis.

## Treatment

As with most female pelvic infections, the microbial etiologic agents are not readily apparent when clinical infection is diagnosed, and because of the myriad of pathogens described above, empiric therapy is given. The majority of women who present with acute salpingitis-peritonitis have clinical disease of mild-to-moderate severity that usually responds well to outpatient antibiotic therapy. Hospitalization usually is warranted for women who are more severely ill as well as for women in whom the exact diagnosis is uncertain. Prepubertal children and pregnant women with this diagnosis should be hospitalized for therapy, as should women with a suspected abscess, women unable to tolerate outpatient oral therapy, and women who have not responded to outpatient therapy. Although it has not been clinically proved that inpatient therapy is associated with improved future fertility, those women who desire future fertility may benefit from inpatient therapy if only by reason of compliance. Some authors believe that all women with this infection should receive inpatient therapy.

**A. Outpatient Therapy:** Outpatient therapy for women with acute salpingitis may be undertaken if the temperature is less than 39°C (102.2°F), lower abdominal findings are minimal, and the patient is not "toxic" and can take oral medication. These women may be treated with antibiotics, IUD removal, analgesics, and bed rest. Regimens recommended by the CDC (September, 1993) include (1) cefoxitin, 2 g intramuscularly, plus probenecid, 1 g orally, followed by 14 days of doxycycline, 100 mg orally twice daily, or tetracycline, 500 mg orally 4 times daily; (2) ceftriaxone, 250 mg intramuscularly, or equivalent cephalosporin (eg, ceftizoxime or cefotaxime) intramuscularly with probenecid, 1 g orally, followed by 14 days of doxycycline, 100 mg orally twice daily, or tetracycline, 500 mg orally 4 times daily; (3) ofloxacin 400 mg orally twice daily for 14 days plus clindamycin 450 mg orally 4 times daily or metronidazole 500 mg orally twice daily for 14 days. Patient compliance may be better with doxycycline, which is also more active against certain anaerobes; it is also more expensive. Tetracycline, 500 mg orally 4 times daily for 10 days, has proved effective in clinical studies. Erythromycin base or stearate, at a dosage of 500 mg orally 4 times a day for 7 days, may be substituted in patients who are allergic or have contraindications to tetracycline. Refer the patient to the city or county health department or STD clinic for contact surveillance. All male sexual partners of women treated for this acute infection should be examined for sexually transmitted diseases and promptly treated with a regimen effective against uncomplicated gonococcal and chlamydial infections.

**B. Inpatient Therapy:** Inpatient therapy is prudent for patients with a temperature over 39°C (102.2°F), for those with guarding and rebound tenderness in lower quadrants, or for patients who look "toxic." Hospitalization of these patients is necessary for therapy and for watching for signs of complications or deterioration. The following measures should be taken.

1. Maintain bed rest.
2. Restrict oral feeding.
3. Administer intravenous fluids to correct dehydration and acidosis.
4. Use nasogastric suction in the presence of abdominal distention or ileus.
5. No standardization of inpatient antimicrobial therapy for women with acute salpingitis has yet been established. Symptomatic response and adverse sequelae are related to the severity of tubal inflammatory disease and the development of adnexal abscesses. The CDC recommends one of the following regimens: (1) doxycycline, 100 mg intravenously or orally twice daily, plus cefoxitin, 2 g intravenously 4 times daily or cefotetan 2 g intravenously twice daily, for at least 48 hours after the patient shows clinical improvement, followed by doxycycline, 100 mg orally twice a day to complete 14 days of therapy; (2) clindamycin, 900 mg intravenously 3 times daily, plus gentamicin 2 mg/kg intravenously and then 1.5 mg/kg intravenously every 8 hours, given as above in women with normal renal function, followed by doxycycline, 100 mg twice daily or clindamycin, 450 mg orally 4 times daily for 14 days. The incidence of infertility after the first episode of salpingitis is about 12%. Because infertility increases with the degree of inflammatory response,

intensive broad-spectrum therapy should reduce complications.

6. Exploratory laparotomy should be performed if there is clinical suspicion of abscess rupture. More gynecologists are successfully performing just a linear salpingostomy, as might be done for ectopic pregnancy, when pyosalpinx is identified. Percutaneous drainage may avoid operation.

7. Continual evaluation by the same experienced clinician is of paramount importance to maintain accuracy and continuity of clinical observation.

## Prognosis

A favorable outcome is directly related to the promptness with which adequate therapy is begun. For example, the incidence of infertility is directly related to the severity of tubal inflammation judged by laparoscopic examination. A single episode of salpingitis has been shown to cause infertility in 12–18% of women (Westrom et al, 1979). Tubal occlusion was demonstrated in only about 10% of these patients regardless of whether or not there had been a gonococcal or nongonococcal infection. Nongonococcal infection predisposed more commonly to ectopic pregnancy, and thus carried a worse prognosis for subsequent viable pregnancy. The ability and willingness of the patient to cooperate with her physician are important to the outcome of patients with the milder cases who are adequately treated on an outpatient basis. Follow-up care and education are necessary to prevent reinfection and complications.

## 2. RECURRENT OR CHRONIC PELVIC INFECTION

### Essentials of Diagnosis

- History of acute salpingitis, pelvic infection, or postpartum or postabortal infection.
- Recurrent episodes of acute reinfection or recurrence of symptoms and physical findings less than 6 weeks after treatment for acute salpingitis.
- Chronic infection may be relatively asymptomatic or may provoke complaints of chronic pelvic pain and dyspareunia.
- Generalized pelvic tenderness on examination; usually less severe than with acute infection.
- Thickening of adnexal tissues, with or without hydrosalpinx (often).
- Infertility (commonly).

### General Considerations

Recurrent pelvic inflammatory disease begins as does primary disease, but preexisting tubal tissue damage may result in more severe infection. Chronic pelvic infection implies the presence of tissue changes in the parametria, tubes, and ovaries. Adhesions of the peritoneal surfaces to the adnexa as well as fibrotic changes in the tubal lumen are usually present. Hydrosalpinx or tubo-ovarian "complexes" may be present. Chronic inflammatory lesions usually are secondary to changes induced by previous acute salpingitis but may represent an acute reinfection.

The diagnosis of chronic pelvic infection generally is difficult to make clinically. It has been erroneously applied to almost any cause of chronic pelvic pain. However, it may be the cause of pain in less than 50% of such women (Cunanan et al, 1983).

### Clinical Findings

**A. Symptoms and Signs:** Recurrent infection usually has the same manifestations as acute salpingitis (see previous text), and a history of pelvic infection can usually be obtained. Pain may be unilateral or bilateral, and dyspareunia and infertility are often reported. The patient may be febrile, with tachycardia; however, unless an acute reinfection is present, the fever is minimal. There is tenderness upon movement of the cervix, uterus, or adnexa. Adnexal masses may be present, as well as thickening of the parametria.

**B. Laboratory Findings:** Cultures from the cervix usually do not show gonococci unless reinfection is present. Leukocytosis may be demonstrated if active infection is superimposed on chronic changes.

### Differential Diagnosis

Any patient with suspected chronic pelvic infection who presents with pelvic tenderness but without fever must be suspected of having an ectopic pregnancy. Other conditions to be considered include endometriosis, symptomatic uterine relaxation, appendicitis, diverticulitis, regional enteritis, ulcerative colitis, ovarian cyst or neoplasm, and acute or chronic cystourethritis.

### Complications

The complications of chronic or recurrent pelvic infection include hydrosalpinx, pyosalpinx, and tubo-ovarian abscess; infertility or ectopic pregnancy; and chronic pelvic pain of varying degrees.

### Prevention

Prompt and adequate treatment of acute pelvic infections is the essential preventive measure. Education about avoidance of venereal infection is also important.

### Treatment

**A. Recurrent Cases:** Treat for acute salpingitis (see previous text). If an IUD is in place, treatment may be started, and the IUD should be removed.

**B. Chronic Cases:** Long-term antimicrobial administration is of questionable benefit but is worthy of trial in young women of low parity. Therapy with a tetracycline, ampicillin, or a cephalosporin, 500 mg 4 times daily for 3 weeks, may occasionally be beneficial, but changes responsible for symptoms are usually not due to active infection. Symptomatic relief can be achieved by use of analgesics such as aspirin or acetaminophen with or without codeine. Careful follow-up, preferably by the same physician, may detect serious sequelae, eg, tubo-ovarian abscess.

If the patient remains symptomatic after 3 weeks of antibiotic therapy, other causes must be considered. Consider laparoscopy or exploratory laparotomy to rule out other causes, eg, endometriosis.

If infertility is a problem, verify tubal patency by means of hysterosalpingography or laparoscopy and retrograde injection of methylene blue solution. It is important to prescribe antibiotics prior to and following either procedure because acute reinfection is common.

Total abdominal hysterectomy with bilateral adnexectomy may be indicated if the disease is far advanced and the woman is symptomatic or if an adnexal mass is demonstrated. Consideration may be given to resection or drainage of the abscess if preservation of fertility is desired. In many instances, CT-directed percutaneous drainage may avoid laparotomy.

### Prognosis

With each succeeding episode of recurrent pelvic infection, the prognosis for fertility dramatically decreases. Likewise, the chances of an ectopic gestation increase with ensuing episodes of acute infection. These sequelae are undoubtedly due to chronic infection, which is the postinflammatory end result of one or multiple infections. Superimposition of acute infection on chronic disease is also associated with a higher incidence of tubo-ovarian and other pelvic abscesses.

## 3. PELVIC (CUL-DE-SAC) ABSCESS

Pelvic abscess is an uncommon complication of chronic or recurrent pelvic inflammation. It may occur as a sequela to acute pelvic or postabortal infection. Abscess formation is frequently associated with organisms other than the gonococcus, commonly anaerobic species, especially *Bacteroides*.

Any of the symptoms of acute or chronic pelvic inflammation may be present together with a fluctuant mass filling the cul-de-sac and dissecting into the rectovaginal septum. These patients usually have more severe symptoms. They may complain of painful defecation and severe back pain, rectal pain, or both. The severity of symptoms is often directly proportionate to the size of the abscess, but occasionally even a large pelvic abscess may be totally asymptomatic. One woman who was admitted to the obstetric service with "fetal heart tones" was ultimately drained of 3000 mL of pus through a colpotomy incision.

### Differential Diagnosis

The following conditions must be considered: tubo-ovarian abscess, periappendiceal abscess, ectopic pregnancy, ovarian neoplasm, uterine leiomyoma, retroflexed and incarcerated uterus, endometriosis, carcinomatosis, and diverticulitis with perforation.

### Treatment

In addition to the measures outlined in the previous section, the following are required:

(1) Antibiotics to include anaerobic as well as aerobic microorganisms: (a) penicillin G, 20–30 million units intravenously per 24 hours, and chloramphenicol, 4–6 g intravenously per 24 hours; (b) penicillin G, 20–30 million units or ampicillin 8 g intravenously per 24 hours; clindamycin, 900 mg intravenously 3 times daily; and gentamicin, 5 mg/kg intravenously per 24 hours. Metronidazole may be substituted for clindamycin at a dose of 15 mg/kg loading dose then 7.5 mg/kg 4 times daily; (c) cefoxitin, 8–12 g intravenously per 24 hours, and gentamicin or tobramycin, 5 mg/kg intravenously per 24 hours; (d) cefotaxime, 6–8 g intravenously per 24 hours. **Caution:** Rare idiosyncratic reactions in the form of blood dyscrasias have been reported with chloramphenicol. With almost any effective therapeutic regimen, antibiotic-associated enterocolitis (diarrhea) is a complication that demands immediate evaluation, including testing for the presence of *Clostridium difficile* toxin. Pseudomembranous colitis is rare.

(2) Reevaluate abdominal findings frequently to detect peritoneal involvement.

(3) If the abscess is dissecting the rectovaginal septum and is fixed to the vaginal membrane, colpotomy drainage with dissection of sacculations is indicated. This space should be actively drained with a large catheter, such as a Cook catheter, and preferably irrigated with sterile saline solution every 4 hours until the space is obliterated.

(4) If fever persists in the face of altered antimicrobial therapy but there is no evidence of abscess rupture or dissection of the rectovaginal septum, percutaneous drainage and irrigation may obviate laparotomy (Figs 38–7 to 38–9).

(5) If the patient's condition deteriorates despite aggressive management, perform exploratory laparotomy. In patients with recurrent infections and loss of reproductive function, total abdominal hysterectomy with bilateral salpingo-oophorectomy and lysis of adhesions offers the only cure. The patient's age and parity and the degree of involvement of the tubes and ovaries determine the extent of surgery when there is some likelihood of preservation of reproductive function. Clinical judgment is difficult and tends to favor surgery. Conservative surgery for women desiring future fertility is appropriate in many cases.

### Prognosis

With early treatment, the prognosis for the woman with a well-localized abscess is good. Antibiotic treatment is essential; drainage may be necessary. Rupture into the peritoneum is a serious complication and demands immediate abdominal exploration. The prognosis for fertility is very poor following this type of abscess.

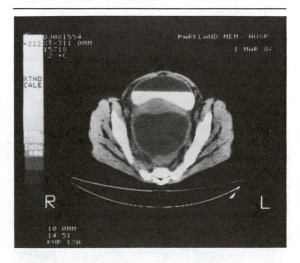

**Figure 38–7.** Pelvic CT scan, with bladder and contrast medium on top, uterus and thickened broad ligaments centrally, and the posterior pelvis filled with abscess.

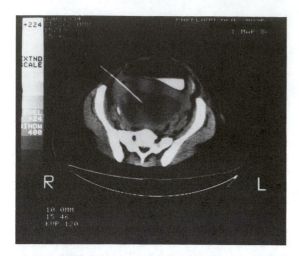

**Figure 38–8.** Pelvic CT scan with percutaneous drainage in process.

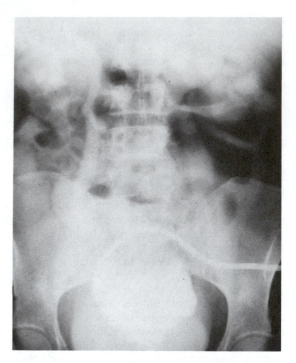

**Figure 38–9.** Cook catheter is in abscess cavity. Note the mild bilateral hydroureter caused by abscess compression at the pelvic brim.

## 4. TUBO-OVARIAN ABSCESS

### Essentials of Diagnosis

- History of pelvic infection. Tubo-ovarian abscess may present as a complication of acute salpingitis, including the initial episode.
- Lower abdominal and pelvic pain of varying degrees.
- Nausea and vomiting.
- Adnexal mass, usually extremely tender.
- Fever, tachycardia.
- Rebound tenderness in lower quadrants.
- Adynamic ileus.
- Culdocentesis productive of gross pus in case of rupture. (Contraindicated in cases of posterior pelvic abscess.)

### General Considerations

Tubo-ovarian abscess formation may occur following an initial episode of acute salpingitis but is usually seen with recurrent infection superimposed on chronically damaged adnexal tissue. Initially there is salpingitis with or without ovarian involvement. The inflammatory process may subside spontaneously or in response to therapy; however, the result may be anatomic derangement, with fibrinous attachments to nearby organs (Figs 38–10 and 38–11). Involvement of the adjacent ovary, usually at an ovulation site, may serve as the portal of entry for extension of infection and abscess formation. Pressure of the purulent exudate may cause rupture of the abscess with resultant fulminating peritonitis, necessitating emergency laparotomy.

Slow leakage of the abscess may cause formation of a cul-de-sac abscess (see previous text). Culdocentesis into an abscess of this type will yield exudate like that of a ruptured tubo-ovarian abscess. Clinical appraisal usually will differentiate the two conditions, but if any doubt exists, treatment should be as specified for ruptured tubo-ovarian abscess.

These abscesses may occur in association with use of an IUD or in the presence of granulomatous infection (eg, tuberculosis, actinomycosis). Disease is usually bilateral, although unilateral disease is more common than previously observed and may account for 20–40% of such abscesses even in the absence of IUD usage. Abscesses are usually polymicrobial.

*Actinomyces israelii*, a normal anaerobic commensal of the gastrointestinal tract, has been identified in 8–20% of women who have an IUD. Most patients are asymptomatic, but up to 25% are reported to develop symptoms of pelvic infection. Controversy exists as to whether an IUD should be removed from an asymptomatic woman with evidence of *Actinomyces* on Papanicolaou smear or culture. If the IUD is removed, a new IUD should not be inserted until the organism is no longer present; this rarely takes longer than one menstrual cycle. Antimicrobial therapy with penicillin should be reserved for symptomatic patients. Surgical drainage is usually required for actinomycotic abscesses, which are almost always the result of intestinal infections such as appendicitis but may be associated with use of an IUD.

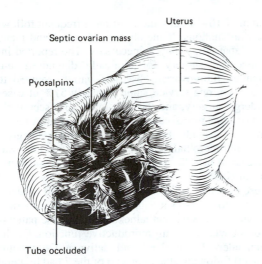

**Figure 38–10.** Tubo-ovarian abscess. (Reproduced, with permission, from Benson RC: *Handbook of Obstetrics & Gynecology*, 8th ed. Lange, 1983.)

## Clinical Findings

**A. Symptoms and Signs:** The clinical spectrum varies greatly and may range from total absence of symptoms in a woman who, on routine pelvic examination, is found to have an adnexal mass, to a moribund patient presenting with acute abdomen and septicemic shock.

The typical patient with tubo-ovarian abscess is usually young and of low parity, with a history of previous pelvic infection. No age group, however, is exempt. The duration of symptoms for these women is usually about 1 week, and the onset is usually about 2 weeks or more after a menstrual period, in contrast to that which occurs in uncomplicated acute salpingitis, in which symptoms usually appear shortly after the onset or cessation of menses. The typical symptoms are pelvic and abdominal pain, fever, nausea and

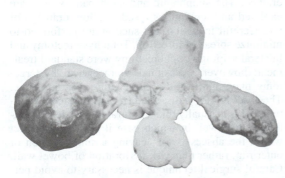

**Figure 38–11.** Uterus with myoma, unruptured right tubo-ovarian abscess, and chronic inflammatory left tubo-ovarian cyst.

vomiting, and tachycardia. Four-quadrant abdominal tenderness and guarding may be present. Adequate pelvic examination is often impossible because of tenderness, but an adnexal mass may be palpated. Culdocentesis may lacerate (rupture) a pelvic abscess, so this procedure must be performed with extreme caution, if at all.

Signs and symptoms of ruptured tubo-ovarian abscess may resemble those of any acute surgical abdomen, and a careful history and an alert clinician are essential to ensure an accurate diagnosis. Signs of actual or impending septic shock frequently accompany a ruptured abscess and include fever (occasionally hypothermia), chills, tachycardia, disorientation, hypotension, tachypnea, and oliguria.

**B. Laboratory Findings:** Laboratory findings are generally of little value. The white count may vary from leukopenia to marked leukocytosis. Urinalysis may demonstrate pyuria without bacteriuria.

**C. X-Ray Findings:** Plain films of the abdomen (KUB) usually demonstrate findings of a dynamic ileus and may arouse suspicion of adnexal mass. Free air may be seen under the diaphragm with ruptured tubo-ovarian abscess.

**D. Ultrasonography:** Ultrasonography may be helpful and can be used with fewer complications to the patient. It can be of great help in following the patient and detecting changes that may take place such as progression, regression, formation of pus pockets, rupture, and so on.

**E. Special Examinations:** Culdocentesis fluid obtained in a woman with an unruptured tubo-ovarian abscess may demonstrate the same cloudy "reaction fluid" seen in acute salpingitis. With a leaking or ruptured tubo-ovarian abscess, however, grossly purulent material may be obtained.

## Differential Diagnosis

An unruptured tubo-ovarian abscess must be differentiated from an ovarian cyst or tumor, unruptured ectopic pregnancy, periappendiceal abscess, uterine leiomyoma, hydrosalpinx, perforation of the appendix, perforation of a diverticulum or diverticular abscess, perforation of peptic ulcer, and any systemic disease that causes acute abdominal distress (eg, diabetic ketoacidosis, porphyria). If an abscess does not respond to medical therapy and colpotomy is not possible, CT or MRI scanning may disclose the cause (Fig 38–12).

## Complications

Unruptured tubo-ovarian abscess may be complicated by rupture with sepsis, reinfection at a later date, bowel obstruction, infertility, and ectopic pregnancy.

Ruptured tubo-ovarian abscess is a surgical emergency and is frequently complicated by septic shock,

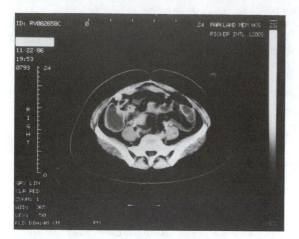

**Figure 38–12.** CT scan showing thickened appendix with intraluminal purulence. The source of this woman's pelvic abscess was a ruptured appendix.

intra-abdominal abscess (eg, subphrenic abscess), and septic emboli with renal, lung, or brain abscess.

## Treatment

**A. Unruptured Asymptomatic Tubo-ovarian Abscess:** Treatment is similar to that of chronic salpingitis: long-term antibacterial therapy and close follow-up. If the mass does not begin to subside within 15–21 days or becomes larger, drainage is indicated. At exploration, total hysterectomy and bilateral adnexectomy were usually performed; however, in selected cases, unilateral salpingo-oophorectomy or linear salpingostomy with copious irrigation and suction drainage may be considered (see Recurrent or Chronic Pelvic Infection, in previous text).

**B. Unruptured Symptomatic Tubo-ovarian Abscess:** Treatment consists of immediate hospitalization, bed rest in the semi-Fowler position, close monitoring of vital signs and urinary output, frequent gentle abdominal examination, nasogastric suction if necessary, and intravenous sodium-containing fluids. Intensive antimicrobial therapy should be instituted and should include either clindamycin, metronidazole, or chloramphenicol because of their specific activity against anaerobes. The following combinations, given in appropriate intravenous doses, are recommended for these severely ill patients: (1) penicillin G and chloramphenicol; (2) penicillin G, ampicillin, or gentamicin plus metronidazole or clindamycin.

Laparotomy is mandatory in all cases of suspected leakage or rupture as well as in all cases that do not respond to medical management and percutaneous drainage is not possible.

If initial therapy is successful, the patient is kept on antibiotics (eg, oral tetracycline, 500 mg 4 times daily, or doxycycline, 100 mg twice daily) for a min-imum of 10–14 days and must have frequent follow-up examinations. If the abscess persists—and many do—laparotomy may be necessary. The reported incidence of surgery for clinically diagnosed, unruptured tubo-ovarian abscesses varies from 30 to 100%. On one service, approximately 57% of cases undergo surgery, and the remaining 43% seemingly respond to aggressive medical management. A recent prospective study (Hemsell, 1985) found that aggressive antimicrobial treatment with cefotaxime was successful in 95% of 40 women with abscesses ranging in size from 4 × 4 to 13 × 15 cm. Only 12% of these patients underwent hysterectomy and bilateral adnexectomy 1–33 months following initial therapy because of a persistent adnexal mass. These patients did not wish to retain reproductive function. Of the remainder, 7 conceived and delivered 26 months (mean) following study entry; 6 of the 7 had bilateral abscesses at sonography. These data support the theory that conservative therapy can be successful.

**C. Ruptured Tubo-ovarian Abscess:** This is an acute life-threatening catastrophe requiring immediate medical therapy associated with operation. In addition to the procedures described above, the following may be necessary:

1. Monitoring of the hourly urinary output with an indwelling catheter in place.

2. Monitoring of central venous pressure.

3. Administration of oxygen by mask.

4. Rapid replacement of fluid and perhaps blood to maintain blood pressure and ensure urine output of > 30 mL/h.

5. Rapid evaluation and preparation for immediate operation. The patient's systemic deficiencies should first be corrected by intravenous fluids and blood if needed.

6. Surgical measures—The anesthesiologist must be completely informed of the patient's condition. A low midline incision is made to allow for cephalad extension. When the abdomen is opened, pus is obtained for aerobic and anaerobic cultures. The bowel is inspected and all loculated abscesses identified and drained. The subphrenic and subhepatic spaces are explored and loculations lysed to allow drainage of pus. Careful irrigation and suction are performed to minimize spread of infection. Total hysterectomy and bilateral salpingo-oophorectomy were standard treatment; however, occasional supracervical hysterectomy may significantly shorten the operating time. The abscess wall is dissected from the adjacent structures. This is usually thick, indurated, and densely adherent to bowel, in which case it is best to dissect within the abscess wall, leaving a small portion of outer rim, rather than risk perforation of bowel wall. Careful surgical technique is necessary to avoid perforation of the bowel or ligation and transection of the ureters. The vaginal cuff is left open after a hemostatic interlocking continuous suture has been applied around the edge of the cuff.

Active drainage of the pelvis is done routinely. Active suction through the abdominal wall provides the best result with the least contamination. The drains are left in place as long as purulent material is recovered. The fascia is closed with wide monofilament synthetic or wire sutures. Retention sutures may be used. The subcutaneous space is left open. In some cases, only drainage may be possible.

## Prognosis

**A. Unruptured Abscess:** Generally the patient with an unruptured abscess has an excellent prognosis. Medical therapy, followed by judicious surgical treatment, yields good results in the usual case. Unruptured localized abscesses that do not respond to aggressive medical management by improvement in signs and symptoms and decreasing size are best drained or removed surgically if inaccessible to percutaneous or transvaginal drainage. Many clinically diagnosed unruptured tubo-ovarian abscesses may represent only acute salpingitis with omental and intestinal adhesions, which respond promptly to adequate antibiotic therapy. Serial ultrasonography may help to identify the true unruptured tubo-ovarian abscesses. The outlook for fertility, however, is greatly reduced. The risk of reinfection must be considered if definitive surgical treatment has not been performed, but the incidence of reinfection in our prospectively studied patient population is less than 10%.

**B. Ruptured Abscess:** Before effective means of treating overwhelming septicemia became available and the need for immediate surgical intervention was recognized, the mortality rate from ruptured tubo-ovarian abscess was 80–90%. With modern therapeutic resources, both medical and surgical, the mortality rate should be less than 5%.

## POSTOPERATIVE PELVIC INFECTIONS

### Essentials of Diagnosis

- Recent pelvic surgery.
- Pelvic or low abdominal pain or pressure.
- Fever and tachycardia.
- Purulent, foul discharge.
- Constitutional symptoms: malaise, chills, etc.
- Vaginal cuff tenderness with cellulitis or abscess.

### General Considerations

Patients who have had gynecologic surgery, especially hysterectomy, may develop postoperative infections of the remaining pelvic structures. These infections include simple cuff induration (cellulitis), infected cuff hematoma (cuff abscess), salpingitis, pelvic cellulitis, suppurative pelvic thrombophlebitis, and tubo-ovarian abscess with or without rupture. The incidence of such infections has been significantly reduced, from 32% after abdominal hysterectomy and 57% after vaginal hysterectomy in women given placebo to about 5% in women given a single dose of antimicrobial prophylaxis.

The pathogenesis of posthysterectomy infection is simple and straightforward; the apex of the vaginal vault consists of crushed, devitalized tissue, and the loose areolar tissue in the parametrial areas usually oozes postoperatively. These conditions provide an ideal medium for the myriads of pathogens that normally inhabit the vagina and are inoculated into the operative site during surgery.

The term "pelvic cellulitis" implies that the soft tissue of the vaginal apex and adjacent parametrial tissues have been invaded by bacteria. In addition, the serum and blood at the cuff apex may become infected, resulting in an infected hematoma, which is, in essence, a cuff abscess. The infection is treated at this point by establishing adequate drainage combined with antibiotic therapy. Infection may extend via lymphatic channels to the adnexa, resulting in salpingitis. Pelvic veins may become involved in the infectious process, particularly if *Bacteroides* or anaerobic streptococci are predominant pathogens. Rarely, septic emboli to the lungs, brain, spleen, and elsewhere may occur.

The incidence of posthysterectomy infection varies considerably with the population studied. Among private patients, it is about 5–30%; among clinic patients, the rate approaches 50% without prophylaxis.

### Clinical Findings

The diagnosis of postoperative pelvic infection is made clinically; laboratory studies may be useful in establishing the specific etiologic diagnosis and determining the sensitivity of the recovered bacteria to various antibiotics.

**A. Symptoms and Signs:** Any postoperative gynecologic patient who develops fever may have atelectasis, phlebitis, upper urinary tract infection, or pelvic infection; these conditions may or may not require antimicrobial therapy. Although some investigators have stated that fever due to postoperative pelvic infection usually does not occur before the third or fourth postoperative day, up to 50% of patients develop temperatures of 38.3–39.4°C (101–103°F) by the 24th—36th postoperative hour. Recurrent temperature elevation without symptoms occurs a mean of 50 hours after hysterectomy in our patient population and disappears without therapy. Temperature elevations associated with symptoms and physical findings of infection occur later. The mean time of this diagnosis in our patients is about 80 hours. The patients fall into 2 distinct groups; those who ultimately require parenteral antimicrobial therapy do not experience early asymptomatic temperature elevation.

Within 2 days following hysterectomy, the surgical margin of the vagina (vaginal cuff) appears hyperemic and edematous, and there is almost always a purulent or seropurulent exudate, regardless of the clinical condition of the patient and whether or not fever is present. When palpated, this site is usually indurated and tender—findings common to most healing wounds and not indicative of a need for antimicrobial therapy. When natural defense mechanisms of the host are inadequate for the inoculum, lymphatic extension of the infection to adjacent tissues results in pelvic cellulitis, demonstrable on pelvic examination as tender induration in the parametrial areas. The infection may involve the tubes and ovaries, with resultant abscess formation in unresponsive patients. At this point, the patient will begin to complain of lower abdominal, pelvic, or back pressure or pain. Abdominal distention due to ileus may develop, as may urinary symptoms due to perivesical irritation.

The diagnosis of suppurative pelvic thrombophlebitis is rare and usually is not apparent until after the sixth postoperative day, at which time the patient continues to have hectic spiking fever of 39–40.5°C (102.2–105°F) with a diurnal variation. The pelvic findings are usually unrevealing except for mild pelvic tenderness. Surprisingly, the woman's general health often is good unless septic embolization has occurred.

An infected pelvic hematoma is impossible to palpate early, but it can be diagnosed by sonography. Recurring temperature elevation is the principal indicator of this type of infection. Rarely do these patients have symptoms, and their examination is usually unremarkable. This problem can be suspected when the hematocrit is lower than anticipated. Onset is frequently at the same time other pelvic infections begin.

**B. Laboratory Findings:** Unfortunately, as previously outlined, the polymicrobial nature of these infections prohibits accurate identification of the offending microorganisms in a reasonable time period. For this reason, broad-spectrum empirical antimicrobial administration is necessary.

Serial complete blood counts usually demonstrate leukocytosis but occasionally enable the physician to detect concealed hemorrhage, which may harbor a large pelvic abscess. Urinalysis is rarely helpful.

**C. X-Ray Findings:** Chest films are unrevealing in most cases but can be useful if pulmonary complications are suspected.

**D. Ultrasonography:** Pelvic sonograms may prove helpful in detecting either retroperitoneal or tubo-ovarian abscesses that develop as a complication of cuff infection.

### Differential Diagnosis

Pulmonary atelectasis may become manifest within 12–36 hours after operation. This can usually be detected by auscultation and confirmed by chest x-ray. Aspiration pneumonitis must always be considered if pulmonary problems develop.

Deep vein thrombophlebitis of the lower extremities is rarely detected clinically and, when present, is seldom accompanied by significant fever. Superficial phlebitis of the upper extremity due to an indwelling venous catheter may cause significant pyrexia. Long-term (48–72 hours) infusion of intravenous antimicrobials increases the likelihood of phlebitis. Although the routine of changing the intravenous site every 48 hours may prevent this complication, it will respond to warm soaks and antiinflammatory agents, such as aspirin, if it does develop.

Upper urinary tract infection may also account for the fever. Because of the liberal use of indwelling catheters in gynecologic surgery, significant bacteriuria commonly develops; however, this rarely causes fever unless pyelonephritis develops.

Fever from abdominal wound infection usually becomes manifest on or after the fourth postoperative day. Examination of the abdominal wound is mandatory in all febrile patients. It may be necessary to probe the abdominal incision carefully, regardless of its appearance, especially if the pelvic examination is unrevealing.

### Complications

Complications of postoperative pelvic infection include extensive pelvic or intra-abdominal abscesses, tubo-ovarian abscess with or without rupture, intestinal adhesions and obstruction, septic pelvic thrombophlebitis with metastatic abscesses, and septicemia.

### Prevention

Many attempts have been made to decrease infectious morbidity following gynecologic surgical procedures. None have been uniformly successful, but the following measures may be of some help:

(1) Preoperative cleansing of the vagina for several days with douches containing bactericidal or bacteriostatic agents (eg, hexachlorophene, povidone-iodine).

(2) Preoperative insertion of antibacterial vaginal creams or suppositories, especially if cervicitis, bacterial vaginosis, or vulvovaginitis is present.

(3) Preparation of the vagina with hexachlorophene or povidone-iodine solution just prior to surgery.

(4) Meticulous attention to hemostasis at operation and gentle handling of tissues. The use of large, strangulating hemostatic sutures should be avoided; nonreactive suture material should be used.

(5) If hemostasis is less than desirable but maximal under given circumstances, suction drainage of that area should be accomplished. This may be done with the vaginal surgical margin left open or closed at hysterectomy.

(6) Antimicrobial prophylaxis beginning preoperatively has been shown by many to significantly reduce pelvic infectious morbidity following vaginal and abdominal hysterectomy. Some controversy regarding this treatment still exists, however. Before

using prophylaxis, one should consider the guidelines proposed by Ledger (1975): (a) Morbidity on a specific service should be significant enough to warrant attempts to decrease it. (b) Antimicrobials of relatively insignificant toxicity but proved value should be used. (c) The first dose should be given preoperatively to ensure adequate tissue concentrations at the time of surgery. Increasingly, studies show that a single preoperative dose is as effective as multiple doses in preventing major infection. Use of many different antimicrobials has been associated with dramatic lowering of pelvic infection morbidity rates. Recent comparative studies indicate that the newer, more expensive semisynthetic cephalosporins and penicillins are more effective than the older agents. In otherwise uncomplicated cases, pelvic infections developing despite prophylaxis generally are mild in nature, although severe infections and resultant complications are not always prevented.

(7) Severe, more advanced infections may be prevented by early diagnosis, drainage (including an open vaginal cuff), and prompt treatment of mild infections.

## Treatment

If a cuff hematoma or abscess is found, adequate drainage may be established by separating the apposed vaginal edges with ring forceps or some other suitable instrument. Care must be taken not to disrupt the intact peritoneum. The usual supportive measures are instituted, and antibiotic therapy is begun. Many of the newer semisynthetic cephalosporins and expanded spectrum penicillins have proved valuable as single-agent therapy for these infections. Rarely, the addition of metronidazole to these regimens may be necessary to effect a cure.

In most cases, the patient with postoperative pelvic infection becomes afebrile within 48–72 hours. If a large, infected pelvic hematoma has developed, more prolonged treatment will be necessary. Large hematomas may be drained and irrigated from below by means of a Foley catheter or Penrose drain introduced into the abscess cavity. Suction drains should be used whenever possible.

A postoperative tubo-ovarian abscess is treated expectantly as outlined above in the section on unruptured tubo-ovarian abscess. If intra-abdominal rupture of a pelvic abscess or tubo-ovarian abscess is suspected, immediate laparotomy is indicated.

Persistent fever and clinical signs of unresponsiveness to therapy may indicate septic pelvic thrombophlebitis, which is generally a diagnosis of exclusion after a 7- to 10-day course of antibiotics. Intermittent intravenous heparin therapy, 5000 U every 4 hours, should be given. Persistence of fever in spite of heparin therapy suggests abscess formation. Abscesses—as well as septic thrombophlebitis—are usually associated with an aerobic bacteria, and antimicrobial therapy should include clindamycin, chloramphenicol, or metronidazole in addition to other agents effective against aerobic microorganisms.

## PELVIC TUBERCULOSIS

### Essentials of Diagnosis

- Infertility.
- Active or healed pulmonary tuberculosis.
- Findings by hysterosalpingography or laparoscopy.
- Recovery of *Mycobacterium tuberculosis* from either menstrual fluid or biopsy specimen.

### General Considerations

In the USA, pelvic tuberculosis is becoming a rare entity. When it does occur, it usually represents secondary invasion from a primary lung infection via the lymphohematogenous route (Fig 38–6). The overall incidence of pelvic tuberculosis in patients with pulmonary tuberculosis is approximately 5%. Prepubertal tuberculosis rarely results in genital tract infection.

After the pelvic organs become affected (Fig 38–13), direct extension to adjacent organs may occur. Older studies in the USA indicated that the oviducts were most frequently involved (90%) and the endometrium next most frequently (70%). More recent studies in Scotland, where the disease is still prevalent, showed endometrial involvement in more than 90% of cases and tubal involvement in only 5%.

### Clinical Findings

**A. Symptoms and Signs:** The only complaint may be infertility, although dysmenorrhea, pelvic pain, and evidence of tuberculous peritonitis may also

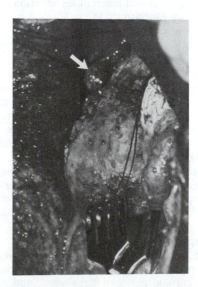

**Figure 38–13.** Miliary tuberculosis involving the uterus and peritoneum.

be present. Endometrial involvement may result in amenorrhea or some other disturbance of the cycle. Abdominal or pelvic pain from this infection is commonly associated with low-grade fever, asthenia, and weight loss. The diagnosis can usually be established on the basis of a complete history and physical examination, chest x-ray and lung scan, and appropriate tests such as a tuberculin (Mantoux) test, sputum smears, and sputum cultures. Tuberculosis of the female genital tract is usually secondary to hematogenous spread involving the endometrium, tubes, and ovaries. The manifestations are usually those of chronic pelvic disease and sterility. Gross ascites with fluid containing more than 3 g of protein per 100 mL of peritoneal fluid is characteristic of tuberculous peritonitis.

Pelvic tuberculosis is usually encountered in the course of a gynecologic operation done for other reasons. Although it may be mistaken for chronic pelvic inflammation, some distinguishing features usually can be found: extremely dense adhesions without planes of cleavage, segmental dilatation of the tubes, and lack of occlusion of the tubes at the ostia. If the internal genitalia are involved, with disseminated granulomatous disease of the serosal surfaces, ascites usually is present. Clinical diagnosis is difficult.

**B. Laboratory Findings:** The best direct method of diagnosis in suspected genital tuberculosis is detection of acid-fast bacteria by means of the Ziehl-Neelsen stain followed by culture on Lowenstein-Jensen medium. The specimen may be from menstrual discharge, from curettage or biopsy, or from peritoneal biopsy in cases where ascites is present. A rapid sedimentation rate, peripheral blood eosinophilia, and a strongly positive Mantoux test are additional evidence of tuberculous infection.

**C. X-Ray Findings:**

**1. Chest x-ray**–A chest x-ray should be taken in any patient with proved or suspected tuberculosis of other organs or tissues.

**2. Hysterosalpingography**–The tubal lining may be irregular, and areas of dilatation may be present. Saccular diverticula extending from the ampulla and giving the impression of a cluster of currants are characteristic of granulomatous salpingitis. Other findings that should arouse suspicion are calcifications of the periaortic or iliac lymph nodes.

**D. Special Examinations:** Visual inspection (laparoscopy) as well as aspiration of fluid for culture and biopsy of affected areas is possible and often diagnostic.

## Differential Diagnosis

Pelvic tuberculosis should be differentiated from schistosomiasis, enterobiasis, lipoid salpingitis, carcinoma, chronic pelvic inflammation, and mycotic infections.

## Complications

Sterility and tuberculous peritonitis are possible sequelae of pelvic tuberculosis.

## Treatment

**A. Medical Measures:** To prevent the emergence of drug-resistant strains, the initial therapy of tuberculous infection should include four drugs. The drug regimen for the first 2 months of treatment should include isoniazid, rifampin, pyrazinamide, and streptomycin or ethambutal. Once drug susceptibility results are available, the drug regimen can be appropriately changed. Treatment should be continued for 24–36 months, since extrapulmonary tuberculosis is more difficult to eradicate. Culture and sensitivity studies are necessary to detect variants that may be resistant to the usual combination of tuberculostatic drugs.

**B. Surgical Measures:** Although the primary treatment is medical, surgery plays a role in some cases of pelvic tuberculosis. If the diagnosis of pelvic tuberculosis is made prior to operation, medical therapy is given for 12–18 months. The ultimate indications for surgery include (1) masses not resolving with medical therapy, (2) resistant or reactivated disease, (3) persistent menstrual irregularities, and (4) fistula formation.

## Prognosis

The prognosis for life and health is excellent if chemotherapy is instituted promptly, although the prognosis for fertility is poor.

## TOXIC SHOCK SYNDROME

### Essentials of Diagnosis

- Fever of 38.9°C (102°F) or higher.
- Diffuse macular rash.
- Desquamation (1–2 weeks after onset of illness; affects particularly palms and soles).
- Hypotension (systolic > 90 mm Hg for adults, or orthostatic syncope).
- Involvement of 3 or more of the following organ systems: gastrointestinal, muscular, mucous membrane, renal, hepatic, hematologic, central nervous system.

### General Considerations

Toxic shock syndrome was first described in children in 1978 but was very quickly identified as an illness occurring primarily in menstruating women 12–24 years of age. An association with use of superabsorbent tampons was made by the CDC. The majority of cases have occurred in California, Minnesota, Wisconsin, Utah, and Iowa. Peak incidence was reported in August, 1980. It is not known whether the abrupt decline in incidence has been due to changes in tampon use, improvements in manufacture, or reduction in disease severity due to early recognition. Of the approximately 30 million menstruating women in the USA, it is estimated that 70% use tampons and over 50% of those use superabsorbent types. Almost 1,000,000 women are at theoretic risk. The incidence in menstruating women is now 6–7:100,000 annually. Toxic shock syndrome has also been reported in women after delivery and in those using a diaphragm, in men and women following surgical procedures, or associated with soft tissue abscesses or osteomyelitis. The incidence of nonmenstrual disease has shown only a slight increase in the past 10 years.

The cause of toxic shock syndrome is preformed toxins produced by *Staphylococcus aureus*, so that colonization or infection by this microorganism must occur. A pyrogenic toxin has been identified in persons with this syndrome. As implied, this toxin induces high fever and may enhance susceptibility to endotoxins that cause shock as well as liver, kidney, and myocardial damage. Other unrecognized toxins may play a role. How toxins gain access to the circulatory system is unknown. Tampon use has been associated with this syndrome, but evidence for the mechanism of toxin entry remains obscure. Insertion could cause mucosal damage. Vaginal ulcerations due to pressure changes usually are not observed, although vaginal erythema commonly is present. Superabsorbent tampons may obstruct the vagina, resulting in retrograde menstruation and peritoneal absorption of bacteria or toxin. Tampons may be associated with increased numbers of aerobic bacteria due to oxygen trapped in interfibrous spaces. The longer a tampon is left in place, the greater the risk for development of this syndrome.

### Clinical Findings

**A. Symptoms and Signs:** Onset is usually sudden, with high fever, watery diarrhea, and vomiting—the triad often seen with viral gastroenteritis. Myalgia, headache, and sometimes sore throat may be present as well as erythroderma and conjunctivitis, as frequently seen with viral infections. Unlike most viral infections, however, this disorder may progress to hypotensive shock within several hours (usually < 48 hours). Timely diagnosis is critical, and the key is the fact that the woman is menstruating or using tampons. The patient will appear obviously acutely ill, with a fever of 39°C (102.2°F) or higher. An erythematous, sunburn-like rash is seen over the face, proximal extremities, and trunk. Dehydration is evident, and the patient will have tachycardia and perhaps hypotension. The conjunctiva will be erythematous as will the pharynx, and there usually will be muscle and abdominal tenderness. A vaginal examination must be performed; if a tampon is present, it must be removed. Mucosal lesions should be sought, and a culture for *S aureus* performed. If nu-

chal rigidity, headache, or disorientation unexplained by hypotension or fever is present, a lumbar puncture must be performed to rule out meningitis. During convalescence, desquamation can be striking.

**B. Laboratory Findings:** Since this is a multisystem syndrome, a battery of tests should be performed. These tests should initially include a complete blood count with differential, electrolyte measurements, urinalysis, urea nitrogen measurement, creatinine measurement, and hepatic function tests. Other tests are performed as indicated by clinical symptoms and signs. Cultures should be made of blood, throat secretions, and probably cerebrospinal fluid. A vaginal culture will yield penicillinase-producing *S aureus*.

### Differential Diagnosis

Other systemic diseases characterized by rash, fever, and systemic complications should be considered. Most patients will not have an obvious source of infection such as a recent incision, soft tissue abscess, or osteomyelitis, but these should be sought. Kawasaki's disease of young children is similar but not as severe, since hypotension, renal failure, and thrombocytopenia do not occur and the incidence of myalgia, diarrhea, and hepatic damage is greatly decreased. Scarlet fever must be excluded. Rocky Mountain spotted fever, leptospirosis, and measles may be excluded by appropriate serologic tests. Gram-negative sepsis must be excluded by both blood and cerebrospinal fluid cultures.

### Complications

Approximately 30% of women who develop toxic shock syndrome have recurrences. The greatest risk for recurrence is during the first 3 menstrual periods following treatment, and the recurrent episode may be less or more severe than the initial one. The incidence is reduced to less than 5% if antistaphylococcal antibiotic therapy is given during therapy of the initial occurrence. Half of the women who developed this disease in Wisconsin during the infancy of its recognition each have had 3 recurrences. Cervicovaginal and nasal cultures for *A aureus* should be negative twice, 4 weeks apart, prior to resumption of tampon use. Women can almost entirely eliminate the risk of this illness by not using tampons and may substantially reduce the risk by intermittent use of tampons during menstruation.

### Treatment

Aggressive supportive therapy is imperative for a successful outcome. Appropriate initial management begins with fluid and electrolyte resuscitation—up to 12 L/d. Packed red blood cells and coagulation factors may be necessary. Central venous or pulmonary wedge pressures and urine output must be monitored to guide therapy. Laboratory studies and appropriate cultures must be obtained early. Dopamine infusion at 2–5 µg/kg/min may be necessary if fluid volume alone does not correct hypotension. Mechanical ventilation may be necessary if adult respiratory syndrome develops, and hemodialysis may be necessary if renal failure develops. Corticosteroid therapy (methylprednisolone, 30 mg/kg, or dexamethasone, 3 mg/kg as a bolus and repeated every 4 hours as necessary), if instituted early, may reduce the severity of illness and duration of fever. Naloxone has resulted in reversal of hypotension in seriously compromised patients by antiendorphin activity. Although *S aureus* is not present in the blood, treatment with a β-lactamase-resistant antibiotic such as nafcillin, oxacillin, or methicillin (1 g intravenously every 4 hours) should be given. If penicillin allergy is present, vancomycin, 500 mg every 6 hours, should be given. Dose reduction is necessary with renal impairment. Until gram-negative sepsis has been excluded, an aminoglycoside should be included with caution, since there will be altered renal function. The mortality rate associated with toxic shock syndrome is 3–6%. The 3 major causes of death are adult respiratory distress syndrome, intractable hypotension, and hemorrhage secondary to disseminated intravascular coagulopathy.

# REFERENCES

## GENERAL

Centers for Disease Control: 1993 Sexually Transmitted Disease Treatment Guidelines. MMWR 1993;(In Press):1.

King KK et al (editors): *Sexually Transmitted Diseases,* 2nd ed. McGraw-Hill, 1990.

## GONORRHEA

Britigan BE, Cohen MS, Sparling PF: Gonococcal infection: A model of molecular pathogenesis. N Engl J Med 1985;312:1683.

Centers for Disease Control: Plasmid-mediated antimicrobial resistance in *Neisseria gonorrhoeae*—United States, 1988 and 1989. MMWR 1990;39:284.

Centers for Disease Control: Guide for the diagnosis of gonorrhea. USPHS, 1985.

Dallabetta G, Hook EW: Gonococcal infections. Infect Dis Clin North Am 1987;1:25.

Thin RN, Shaw EJ: Diagnosis of gonorrhea in women. Br J Vener Dis 1979;55:10.

## SYPHILIS

Berman SM et al: Low birth weight, prematurity, and postpartum endometritis. Association with prenatal cervical *Mycoplasma hominis* and *Chlamydia trachomatis* infections. JAMA 1987;257:1189.

Centers for Disease Control: Recommendations for diagnosing and treating syphilis in HIV-infected patients. MMWR 1988;37:600.

Centers for Disease Control: Congenital syphilis—New York City, 1986–1988. MMWR 1989; 38:826.

Centers for Disease Control: Regional and temporal trends in the surveillance of syphilis, United States, 1986–1990. MMWR 1992a;40:29.

Cohen I, Veille J-C, Calkins BM: Improved pregnancy outcome following successful treatment of chlamydial infection. JAMA 1990; 263:3160.

Crombleholme WR et al: Amoxicillin therapy for *Chlamydia trachomatis* in pregnancy. Obstet Gynecol 1990; 75:752.

Katz BP et al: Compliance with antibiotic therapy for *Chlamydia trachomatis* and *Neisseria gonorrhoeae.* Sex Transm Dis 1992;19:351.

Musher DM: Syphilis. Infect Dis Clin North Am 1987; 1:83.

Wendel GD: Gestational and congenital syphilis. Clin Perinatol 1988;15:287.

Wendel GD et al: Penicillin allergy and desensitization in serious infections during pregnancy. N Engl J Med 1985;312:1229.

Wendel GD et al: Examination of amniotic fluid in diagnosing congenital syphilis with fetal death. Obstet Gynecol 1989;74:967.

Wendel GD et al: Identification of *Treponema pallidum* in amniotic fluid and fetal blood from pregnancies complicated by congenital syphilis. Obstet Gynecol 1991;78:890.

## CHLAMYDIAL INFECTIONS

Centers for Disease Control: Chlamydia trachomatis infections. Policy guidelines for prevention and control. MMWR 1985;34:53.

Gravett MG et al: Independent associations of bacterial vaginosis and Chlamydia trachomatis infection with adverse pregnancy outcome. JAMA 1986;256:1899.

Hammerschlag MR et al: Efficacy of neonatal ocular prophylaxis for the prevention of chlamydial and gonococcal conjunctivitis. N Engl J Med 1989; 320: 769.

Hoyme UB, Kiviat N, Eschenbach DA: Microbiology and treatment of late postpartum endometritis. Obstet Gynecol 1986;68:226.

Martin DH et al: A controlled trial of a single dose of azithromycin for the treatment of chlamydial urethritis and cervicitis. N Engl J Med 1992;327:921.

Martin DH, Vaginal Infections and Prematurity Study Group: Erythromycin treatment of *Chlamydia trachomatis* infections during pregnancy. Abstract No.683, 30th Interscience Conference on Antimicrobial Agents and Chemotherapy, Atlanta GA, October 1990.

McGregor JA, French JI: *Chlamydia trachomatis* infection during pregnancy. Am J Obstet Gynecol 1991; 164:1782.

Morrison RP: Chlamydial hsp 60 and the immunopathogenesis of chlamydial disease. Semin Immunol 1991; 3:25.

Morrison RP et al: Chlamydial disease pathogenesis. The 57-kD Chlamydial hypersensitivity antigen is a stress response protein. J Exp Med 1989;170:1271.

Moss TR et al: Antibodies to chlamydia species in patients attending a genitourinary clinic and the impact of antibodies to *C pneumoniae* and *C psittaci* on the sensitivity and specificity of *C. trachomatis* serology tests. Sex Transm Dis 1993;20:61.

Nettleman MD, Bell TA: Cost-effectiveness of prenatal testing for *Chlamydia trachomatis*. Am J Obstet Gynecol 1991;164:1289.

Rettig PJ: Perinatal infections with *Chlamydia trachomatis*. Clin Perinatol 1988;15:321.

Ryan GM et al: *Chlamydia trachomatis* infection in pregnancy and effect of treatment on outcome. Am J Obstet Gynecol 1990;162:34.

Sanders LL, Harrison R, Washington AE: Treatment of sexually transmitted chlamydial infections. JAMA 1986;255:1750.

Schacter J: Breaking the chain of chlamydial infection. Contemporary Obstet Gynecol 1987;30(1):146.

Schacter J et al: Experience with the routine use of erythromycin for chlamydial infections in pregnancy. N Engl J Med 1986;314:276.

Schacter J et al: Prospective study of perinatal transmission of *Chlamydia trachomatis*. JAMA 1986;255:3374.

Schacter J: Why we need a program for the control of chlamydia trachomatis. N Engl J Med 1989;320:803.

Sweet RL et al: *Chlamydia trachomatis* infection and pregnancy outcome. Am J Obstet Gynecol 1987;156:824.

Wagar EA et al: Differential human serologic response to two 60,000 molecular weight *Chlamydia trachomatis* antigens. *J Infect Dis 1990;162:922.*

Wendel GD, Cunningham FG: Sexually transmitted diseases in pregnancy. Williams Obstetrics, 18th ed (Suppl 13). Norwalk CT, Appleton & Lange, August/September 1991.

Witkin SS et al: Cell-mediated immune response to recombinant 57-kDa heat-shock protein of *Chlamydia trachomatis* in women with salpingitis. J infect Dis 1993;167:1379.

Yuan Y et al: Monoclonal antibodies define genus-specific, species-specific, and cross-reactive epitopes of the chlamydial 60-kilodalton heat shock protein (hsp60): Specific immunodetection and purification of chlamydial hsp60. Infect Immunol 1992;60:2288.

## BACTERIAL VAGINOSIS

Eschenbach DA et al: Prevalence of hydrogen peroxide-producing *Lactobacillus* species in normal women and women with bacterial vaginosis. J Clin Microbiol 1989;27:251.

Eschenbach DA et al: Diagnosis and Clinical manifestations of bacterial vaginosis. Am J Obstet Gynecol 1988;158:819.

Spiegel CA: Bacterial vaginosis. Clin Microbiol Rev 1991;4:485.

Thomason JL, Gelbart SM, Scaglione NJ: Bacterial vaginosis: Current review with indications for asymptomatic therapy. Am J Obstet Gynecol 1991;165:1210.

## CHANCROID

Bodhidatta L et al: Evaluation of 500 and 1,000 mg doses of ciprofloxacin for the treatment of chancroid. Antimicrob Agents Chemother 1988;32:723.

Dylewski J et al: Single-dose therapy with trimethoprim-sulfamethoxazole for chancroid in females. Sex Transm Dis 1986;13:166.

Naamara W et al: Treatment of chancroid with ciprofloxacin. Am J Med 1987;82:317.

Naamara W et al: Treating chancroid with Enoxacin. Genitourin Med 1988;64:189.

Schmid GP et al: Chancroid in the United States: Reestablishment of an old disease. JAMA 1987;258:3265.

## GRANULOMA INGUINALE

Latif A, Mason P, Paraiwa E: Treatment of donovanosis. Sex Transm Dis 1988;15:27.

## HUMAN IMMUNODEFICIENCY VIRUS

Centers for Disease Control: Additional recommendations to reduce sexual and drug abuse-related transmission of HTLV-III/LAV. MMWR 1986;35:152.

Centers for Disease Control: Human immunodeficiency virus infection in the United States: A review of current knowledge. MMWR 1987;36(Suppl 6):1.

Centers for Disease Control: Public Health Service guidelines for counseling and antibody testing to prevent HIV infection and AIDS. MMWR 1987;36:509.

Centers for Disease Control: Recommendations for assisting in the prevention of perinatal transmission of HTLV-III/LAV and AIDS. MMWR 1985;34:721.

Centers for Disease Control: Update: Universal precautions for prevention of transmission of human immunodeficiency virus, hepatitis B virus, and other bloodborne pathogens in health-care setting. MMWR 1988;37:377.

Centers for Disease Control: The second 100,000 cases of acquired immunodeficiency syndrome—United States, June 1981–December 1991. MMWR 1992; 41:28.

Centers for Disease Control: Update: Barrier protection against HIV infection and other sexually transmitted diseases. MMWR 1993;42:589.

Curran JW et al: Epidemiology of HIV infection and AIDS in the United States. Science 1988;239:610.

Ellerbrock TV et al: Epidemiology of women with AIDS in the United States, 1981 through 1990. JAMA 1991; 265:2971.

European Collaborative Study: Children born to women with HIV-1 infection: Natural history and risk of transmission. Lancet 1991;337:253.

Friedland G, Klein R: Transmission of the human immunodeficiency virus. N Engl J Med 1987;317:1125.

Glatt AE, Chirgwin K, Sheldon HL: Treatment of infections associated with human immunodeficiency virus. N Engl J Med 1988;22:1439.

Gloeb DJ, O'Sullivan MJ, Efantis J: Human immunodeficiency virus infection in women. Am J Obstet Gynecol 1988;159:756.

Guinan ME, Hardy A: Epidemiology of AIDS in women in the United States, 1981 through 1986. JAMA 1987;257:2039.

Ho D, Romerantz R, Kaplan J: Pathogenesis of infection with human immunodeficiency virus. N Engl J Med 1987;317:278.

Landesman S et al: Serosurvey of human immunodeficiency virus infection in parturients: Implications for human immunodeficiency virus testing programs of pregnant women. JAMA 1987;258:2701.

Minkoff HL: Care of pregnant women infected with human immunodeficiency virus. JAMA 1987;258:2714.

Minkoff H et al: Pregnancies resulting in infants with acquired immunodeficiency syndrome or AIDS-related complex. Obstet Gynecol 1987;69:285.

O'Brien TR, George JR, Holmberg SD: Human immunodeficiency virus type 2 infection in the United States: Epidemiology, diagnosis, and public health implications. JAMA 1992;267:2775.

Peterman TA, Curran JW: Sexual transmission of human immunodeficiency virus. JAMA 1986;256:2222.

Pyun K et al: Perinatal infection with human immunodeficiency virus: Specific antibody responses by the neonate. N Engl J Med 1987;317:611.

Qazi QH et al: Lack of evidence for craniofacial dysmorphism in perinatal human immunodeficiency virus infection. J Pediatr 1988;112:7.

Sperling RS, Stratton P,and the Members of the Obstetric-Gynecologic Working Group of the AIDS Clinical Trials Group of the National Institute of Allergy and Infectious Diseases: Treatment options for human immunodeficiency virus-infected pregnant women. Obstet Gynecol 1992;79:443.

## PELVIC INFLAMMATORY DISEASE

Centers for Disease Control: *Chlamydia trachomatis* Infections: Policy Guidelines for Prevention and Control. Publication 00-4770. August, 1985.

Chow AW et al: The bacteriology of acute pelvic inflammatory disease: Value of cul-de-sac cultures and relative importance of gonococci and other aerobic or anaerobic bacteria. Am J Obstet Gynecol 1975;122:876.

Cunanan RG Jr et al: Laparoscopic findings in patients with pelvic pain. Am J Obstet Gynecol 1983;146:589.

Hager WD et al: Criteria for diagnosis and grading of salpingitis. Obstet Gynecol 1983;61:113.

Holmes KK: The *Chlamydia* epidemic. JAMA 1981;245:1718.

Sweet RL: Diagnosis and treatment of pelvic inflammatory disease in the emergency room. Sex Transm Dis 1981;8(Suppl):156.

Sweet RL et al: Use of laparoscopy to determine microbiologic etiology of acute salpingitis. Am J Obstet Gynecol 1979;134:68.

Treharne JD et al: Antibodies to *Chlamydia trachomatis* in acute salpingitis. Br J Vener Dis 1979;55:28.

Westrom L et al: Infertility after acute salpingitis: Results of treatment with different antibiotics. Curr Ther Res 1979;26(Suppl):752.

## TUBO-OVARIAN ABSCESS

Bhagavan BS, Gupta PK: Genital actinomycosis and intrauterine contraceptive devices: Cytopathologic diagnosis and clinical significance. Hum Pathol 1978;9:567.

Cunningham FG, Hemsell DL: Management of ruptured pelvic abscesses. Contemp Obstet Gynecol 1981;18:107.

Hemsell DL et al: Cefotaxime treatment for women with community-acquired pelvic abscesses. Am J Obstet Gynecol 1985;151:771.

Jones MC et al: The prevalence of actinomycetes-like organisms found in cervicovaginal smears of 300 IUD wearers. Acta Cytol 1979;23:282.

Rivlin ME: Conservative surgery for adnexal abscess. J Reprod Med 1985;30:726.

## POSTOPERATIVE PELVIC INFECTIONS

Hemsell DL et al: Cefoxitin for prophylaxis in premenopausal women undergoing vaginal hysterectomy. Obstet Gynecol 1980;56:629.

Hemsell DL et al: Prevention of major infection following elective abdominal hysterectomy: Individual determination required. Am J Obstet Gynecol 1983;147:520.

Ledger WJ, Gee C, Lewis WP: Guidelines for antibiotic prophylaxis in gynecology. Am J Obstet Gynecol 1975;121:1038.

## PELVIC TUBERCULOSIS

Centers for Disease Control: Initial therapy for tuberculosis in the era of multidrug resistance. Recommendations of the advisory council for the elimination of tuberculosis. MMWR 1993;42:1.

Hutchins C: Tuberculosis of the genital tract: A changing picture. Br J Obstet Gynaecol 1977;84:534.

## TOXIC SHOCK SYNDROME

Centers for Disease Control: Toxic-shock syndrome: United States. MMWR 1980;29:229.

Garbe PL et al: *Staphylococcus aureus* isolates from patients with nonmenstrual toxic shock syndrome: Evidence for additional toxins. JAMA 1985;253:2538.

Todd JK et al: Corticosteroid therapy for patients with toxic shock syndrome. JAMA 1984;252:3399.

# Antimicrobial Chemotherapy

# 39

*Ronald S. Gibbs, MD*

## ANTIMICROBIAL CHEMOTHERAPY

Although microbial infection has always been a threat to obstetric or gynecologic patients, gratifying developments in antimicrobial therapy have led to marked improvements in outcome and have contributed mightily to decreases in puerperal and postoperative mortality.

However, antimicrobial drugs are effective adjuncts, not panaceas. On occasion, improper application of antimicrobials not only fails to cure the patient but may contribute significantly to morbidity and mortality. Widespread improper administration of antimicrobials may also favor the emergence of drug-resistant organisms, enhance the risk of hospital infections, dangerously sensitize the population, and carry the risk of serious direct toxic effects. Accordingly, we must all guard against a casual, cavalier attitude toward use of the life-improving drugs and use them wisely.

## PRINCIPLES OF SELECTION OF ANTIMICROBIAL DRUGS

Several special conditions pertain to most infections encountered in obstetric and gynecologic practice. First, infections are common. Second, our patients (with the exception of some elderly and some oncology patients) are generally healthy and free of debilitating illness. Third, many infections, especially postpartum, postoperative infection and pelvic inflammatory disease, are polymicrobial in origin, involving an array of aerobes, anaerobes, genital mycoplasmas, and often *Chlamydia trachomatis*. Fourth, when a clinical diagnosis of infection is made, empiric antibiotic therapy is usually indicated before culture results are available. Fifth, because of limitations in laboratory technique, culture results may not be available in a timely fashion or may not even be

performed at all. Thus, although general principles of good antimicrobial selection should generally be applied, knowledge of these special conditions is also essential.

To serve as a guide to wise selection, two helpful tables are provided. Table 39–1 shows drugs of choice, by organism. Since the clinician is usually not able to predict the infecting organism or combination of organisms with any degree of confidence, Table 39–2 shows appropriate selections, by clinical diagnosis.

Proper use of antimicrobial drugs gives striking therapeutic results, but these drugs can create serious complications and should therefore be administered only upon proper indication.

The following steps merit consideration in each patient.

**A. Etiologic Diagnosis:** Formulate an etiologic diagnosis based on clinical observations. Microbial infections are best treated early. Therefore, the physician must attempt to decide on clinical grounds (1) whether the patient has a microbial infection that can probably be influenced by antimicrobial drugs, and (2) the most probable infectious agent causing the disorder ("best guess").

**B. "Best Guess":** Based on a best guess about the probable cause of the patient's infection, the physician should choose a drug (or drug combination) that is likely to be effective against the suspected microorganism.

**C. Laboratory Control:** Before beginning antimicrobial drug treatment, obtain meaningful specimens, if available, for laboratory examination to determine the causative infectious organism and, if desirable, its susceptibility to antimicrobial drugs.

**D. Clinical Response:** Based on the clinical response of the patient, evaluate the laboratory reports and consider the desirability of changing the antimicrobial drug regimen. Laboratory results should not automatically overrule clinical judgment. The isolation of an organism that reinforces the initial clinical impression is a useful confirmation. Conversely, laboratory results may contradict the initial clinical impression and may force its reconsideration. If the

**Table 39–1.** Drug selection for commonly encountered organisms in obstetric-gynecologic practice ($\pm$ = alone or combined with)

| Suspected or Proved Etiologic Agent | Drug(s) of First Choice | Alternative Drug(s) |
|---|---|---|
| **Gram-negative cocci** | | |
| Gonococcus | Ceftriaxone | Spectinomycin, cefoxitin, ciprofloxacin, norfloxacin; amoxicillin, only if proved *not* to be resistant. |
| **Gran-positive cocci** | | |
| Pneumococcus (*Streptococcus pneumoniae*) | Penicillin[1] | Erythromycin,[3] cephalosporin[4] |
| *Streptococcus*, hemolytic, groups A, C, G | Penicillin[1] | Erythromycin,[3] cephalosporin[4] |
| group b | Penicillin, ampicillin | Erythromycin, clindamycin, vancomycin |
| *Streptococcus viridans* | Penicillin,[1] $\pm$ aminoglycosides[5] | Cephalosporin,[4] vancomycin |
| *Staphylococcus*, non-penicillinase-producing | Penicillin[1] | Cephalosporin,[4] vancomycin |
| *Staphylococcus*, penicillinase-producing | Penicillinase-resistant penicillin[5] | Vancomycin, cephalosporin[4] |
| *Streptococcus faecalis* | Ampicillin + aminoglycoside[5] | Vancomycin |
| **Gram-negative rods** | | |
| *Acinetobacter* (*Mima-Herellea*) | Aminoglycoside[5] $\pm$ imipenem | Minocycline, TMP-SMX[7] |
| *Bacteroides*, oropharyngeal strains | Penicillin,[1] clindamycin | Metronidazole, cephalosporin[4,8] |
| *Bacteroides*, gastrointestinal and pelvic strains | Metronidazole, clindamycin | Cefoxitin, chloramphenicol |
| *Enterobacter* | Newer cephalosporins[8] | Aminoglycoside,[5] TMP-SMX[7] |
| *Escherichia coli* (sepsis) | Aminoglycoside[5] $\pm$ ampicillin | Newer cephalosporins,[8] TMP-SMX[7] |
| *Escherichia coli* (first urinary tract infection) | Sulfonamide,[10] TMP-SMX[7] | Ampicillin, cephalosporin[4] |
| *Klebsiella* | Newer cephalosporins,[8] aminoglycoside[5] | Chloramphenicol, TMP-SMX[7] |
| *Proteus mirabilis* | Ampicillin | Newer cephalosporins,[8] aminoglycoside[5] |
| *Proteus vulgaris* and other species | Newer cephalosporins[8] | Aminoglycosides[5] |
| *Pseudomonas aeruginosa* | Aminoglycoside[5] + ticarcillin | Newer cephalosporins[8] $\pm$ aminoglycoside |
| *Serratia, Providencia* | Newer cephalosporins,[8] aminoglycoside[5] | TMP-SMX[7] |
| **Gram-positive rods** | | |
| *Actinomyces* | Penicillin[1] | Tetracycline[9] |
| *Bacillus* (eg, anthrax) | Penicillin[1] | Erythromycin[3] |
| *Clostridium,* (eg, gas gangrene, tetanus) | Penicillin,[1] clindamycin | Metronidazole |
| *Corynebacterium* | Erythromycin[3] | Penicillin,[1] cephalosporin[4] |
| *Listeria* | Ampicillin $\pm$ aminoglycoside[5] | TMP-SMX[7] |
| **Spirochetes** | | |
| *Borrelia* (Lyme disease, relapsing fever) | Tetracycline[9] | Penicillin[1] |
| *Treponema* (syphilis, yaws, etc) | Penicillin[1] | Erythromycin,[3] tetracycline[9] |
| **Mycoplasma** | Tetracycline[9] | Erythromycin (for *U. urealyticum*); Clindamycin (for *M. hominis*) |
| **Chlamydiae** (*C trachomatis, C psittaci*) | Tetracycline[9]; Azithromycin | Erythromycin[3] or clindamycin |

[1]Penicillin G is preferred for parenteral injection; penicillin V for oral administration—to be used only in treating infections due to highly sensitive organisms.

[2]Oral sulfisoxazole and trisulfapyrimidines are highly soluble in urine; parenteral sodium sulfadiazine can be injected intravenously in treating severely ill patients.

[3]Erythromycin estolate is best absorbed orally but carries the highest risk of hepatitis; especially in pregnancy; erythromycin stearate and erythromycin ethylsuccinate are also available.

[4]Older cephalosporins are cephalothin, cefazolin, cephapirin, and cefoxitin for parenteral injection; cephalexin and cephradine can be given orally.

[5]Aminoglycosides—gentamicin, tobramycin, amikacin, netilmicin—should be chosen on the basis of local patterns of susceptibility.

[6]Parenteral nafcillin or oxacillin; oral dicloxacillin, cloxacillin, or oxacillin.

[7]TMP-SMX is a mixture of 1 part trimethoprim and 5 parts sulfamethoxazole.

[8]Newer cephalosporins (1968) include cefotaxime, cefoperazone, cefuroxime, ceftriaxone, ceftazidime, ceftizoxime, and others.

[9]All tetracyclines have similar activity against microorganisms. Dosage is determined by rates of absorption and excretion of various preparations. Tetracyclines should not be used in pregnancy.

[10]First choice for previously untreated urinary tract infection is a highly soluble sulfonamide (see Note 2). TMP-SMX[7] is acceptable.

**Table 39–2.** Drug selection for commonly encountered infections in obstetric/gynecologic practice.

| Suspected or Proved Infection | Drug(s) of First Choice | Alternate Drug(s) |
|---|---|---|
| **Sexually Transmitted Infections** | | |
| Syphilis | Benzathine penicillin | A tetracycline |
| Genital herpes | Acyclovir | — |
| Gonorrhea | Ceftriaxone | Spectinomycin, cefoxitin, cipro- or norfloxacin; amoxicillin only if source proved *not* to be resistant |
| *C trachomatis* | Tetracycline, azithromycin | Erythromycin, amoxicillin or clindamycin in pregnancy |
| Pelvic inflammatory disease | Cefoxitin (or alternate) plus doxycycline; clindamycin plus gentamicin | Norfloxacin |
| **Vaginitis** | | |
| Trichomonas vaginalis | Metronidazole | |
| Candidiasis | See text for selection, many choices | |
| Bacterial vaginosis | Metronidazole | Clindamycin |
| **Obstetric Infection** | | |
| Puerperal endometritis | Clindamycin plus gentamicin | Several including cefoxitin or cefotetan; ampicillin plus sulbactam |
| Clinical chorioamnionitis | Ampicillin plus gentamicin, plus clindamycin if cesarean delivery | As for endometritis |
| Sepsis | Clindamycin plus gentamicin, plus ampicillin | Metronidazole plus gentamicin, plus ampicillin |
| Pyelonephritis—1st episode | First-generation cephalosporin | Third-generation cephalosporin |
| Recurrent | Ampicillin plus gentamicin | Same |
| **Gynecologic Infection** | | |
| Posthysterectomy cuff infection | As for endometritis | As for endometritis |
| Abdominal wound infection | Drainage ± antibiotics as for endometritis | |

specimen was obtained from a site normally devoid of bacterial flora and not exposed to the external environment (eg, blood, amniotic fluid), the recovery of a microorganism is a significant finding even if the organism recovered is different from the clinically suspected etiologic agent and may force a change in antimicrobial treatment. On the other hand, the isolation of unexpected microorganisms from genital tract, gut, or surface lesions (sites that have a complex flora) must be critically evaluated before drugs are abandoned that were judiciously selected on the basis of an initial best guess for empiric treatment.

**E. Drug Susceptibility Tests:** Some microorganisms are fairly uniformly susceptible to certain drugs; if such organisms are isolated from the patient, they need not be tested for drug susceptibility. For example, group A and B streptococci, and clostridia respond predictably to penicillin. On the other hand, enteric gram-negative rods are sufficiently variable in their response to warrant drug susceptibility testing when they are isolated from a significant specimen.

Antimicrobial drug susceptibility tests may be done on solid media as "disk tests," in broth tubes, or in wells of microdilution plates. The latter method yields results usually expressed as MIC (minimal inhibitory concentration). In some infections, the MIC permits a better estimate of the amount of drug required for therapeutic effect in vivo. Disk tests usually indicate whether an isolate is susceptible or resistant to drug concentrations achieved in vivo with conventional dosage regimens, thus providing valuable guidance in selecting therapy.

When there appear to be marked discrepancies between test results and clinical response of the patient, the following possibilities must be considered:

1. Failure to drain a collection of pus or to remove a foreign body.

2. Choice of inappropriate drug, dose, or route of administration.

3. Failure of a poorly diffusing drug to reach the site of infection (eg, central nervous system) or to reach intracellular phagocytosed bacteria.

4. Superinfection in the course of prolonged chemotherapy. After suppression of the original infection or of normal flora, a second type of microorganism may establish itself against which the originally selected drug is ineffective.

5. Emergence of drug-resistant or tolerant organisms.

6. Participation of 2 or more microorganisms in the infectious process, of which only one was originally detected and used for drug selection.

**F. Adequate Dosage:** To determine whether the proper drug is being used in adequate dosage, a serum assay may be performed. However, in obstetric-gynecologic practice, performing antibiotic levels is usually unnecessary except in selected cases of aminoglycoside use, such as in obese women, in women with renal insufficiency (here, another class of drugs would generally be preferable), in patients with longer courses (> 7 days), and in patients not responding to therapy.

**G. Route of Administration:** The absorption of oral penicillins, tetracyclines, erythromycin, etc, is impaired by food. Therefore, these oral drugs must be given between meals.

When an antibiotic is administered intravenously, the following cautions should be observed:

1. Give in neutral solution (pH 7.0–7.2) of sodium chloride (0.9%) or dextrose (5%) in water.

2. Administer by intermittent (every 2–6 hours) addition to the intravenous infusion ("bolus injection") to avoid inactivation (by temperature, changing pH, etc) and prolonged vein irritation from high drug concentration, which favors thrombophlebitis.

3. Change the infusion site every 48 hours to reduce the chance of superinfection.

**H. Duration of Antimicrobial Therapy:** Generally speaking, effective antimicrobial treatment results in reversal of the clinical and laboratory parameters of active infection and marked clinical improvement within a very few days. Treatment may, however, have to be continued for varying periods to effect cure. For instance, acute cystitis in women may respond in just 1–3 days.

To minimize untoward reactions from drugs and the likelihood of superinfection, treatment should be continued only as long as necessary to eradicate the infectious agent.

For most postoperative and postpartum infections, intravenous antibiotics may be discontinued after the patient has been afebrile for 48–72 hours. Furthermore, in most patients who respond promptly to such intravenous treatment, oral antibiotic therapy is unnecessary.

**I. Adverse Reactions:** The administration of antimicrobial drugs is commonly associated with untoward reactions. These fall into several groups.

**1. Hypersensitivity–**The most common reactions are fever and skin rashes. Hematologic or hepatic disorders and anaphylaxis are rare.

**2. Direct toxicity–**Most common are nausea and vomiting and diarrhea. More serious toxic reactions are impairment of renal, hepatic, or hematopoietic functions or damage to the eighth nerve.

**3. Suppression–**Suppression of normal microbial flora and "superinfection" by drug-resistant microorganisms, or continued infection with the initial pathogen through the emergence of drug-resistant variants.

## Oliguria, Impaired Renal Function, & Uremia

Oliguria, impaired renal function, and uremia have an important influence on antimicrobial drug dosage, since most of these drugs are excreted—to a greater or lesser extent—by the kidneys. Only minor adjustment in dosage or frequency of administration is necessary with relatively nontoxic drugs (eg, penicillins) or with drugs that are detoxified or excreted mainly by the liver (eg, erythromycins or chloramphenicol). On the other hand, aminoglycosides (gentamicin, tobramycin, amikacin, etc), tetracyclines, and vancomycin must be drastically reduced in dosage or frequency of administration if toxicity is to be avoided in the presence of nitrogen retention. The administration of such drugs during renal failure should be guided by intermittent direct assay of drug concentration in serum.

---

# ANTIMICROBIAL DRUGS

---

## PENICILLINS

The penicillins are a large group of antimicrobial substances, all of which share a common chemical nucleus (6-aminopenicillanic acid) that contains a $\beta$-lactam ring essential to their biologic activity. All $\beta$-lactam antibiotics inhibit formation of microbial cell walls. In particular, they block the final transpeptidation reaction in the synthesis of cell wall mucopeptide (peptidoglycan), and they activate autolytic enzymes in the cell wall. These reactions result in bacterial cell death.

### Antimicrobial Activity

The initial step in penicillin action is the binding of the drug to cell receptors and penicillin-binding proteins (PBPs). The PBPs of different organisms differ in number and affinity for a given drug. After penicillins have attached to receptors, peptidoglycan synthesis is inhibited because the activity of transpeptidation enzymes is blocked. The final bactericidal action is the activation of autolytic enzymes in the cell wall, which results in cell lysis. Organisms that are defective in autolysin function are inhibited but not killed (**tolerant organisms**) by $\beta$-lactam antibiotics. Organisms that produce $\beta$-lactamases are resistant to some penicillins because the $\beta$-lactam ring is broken and the drug inactivated. Only organisms that are actively synthesizing peptidoglycan (in the process of multiplication) are susceptible to $\beta$-lactam antibiotics. Nonmultiplying organisms or those lacking cell walls (L forms) are not susceptible but may act as **persisters.**

One million units of penicillin G equal 0.6 g. Other penicillins are prescribed in grams. A blood level of 0.01–1 µg/mL of penicillin G or ampicillin is lethal for most susceptible gram-positive microorganisms. Most β-lactamase–resistant penicillins are 5–50 times less active against penicillin G-susceptible organisms.

Penicillins can be arranged into groups:

1. Highest activity against gram-positive organisms but susceptible to hydrolysis by β-lactamases, eg, penicillin G, benzathine penicillin.

2. Relatively resistant to β-lactamases but of lower activity against gram-positive organisms and inactive against gram-negative ones, eg, nafcillin.

3. Relatively high activity against both gram-positive and gram-negative organisms but destroyed by β-lactamases (penicillinases), eg, ampicillin, amoxicillin, ticarcillin, piperacillin.

4. Stable to gastric acid and suitable for oral administration, eg, penicillin V, cloxacillin, ampicillin, amoxicillin.

5. Combinations of penicillins with β-lactamase inhibitors, eg, ampicillin plus sulbactam, carbenicillin plus clavulanic acid.

## Resistance

Resistance to penicillins falls into several categories:

1. Production of β-lactamases, eg, by staphylococci, gonococci, *Haemophilus*, coliform organisms.

2. Lack of penicillin-binding proteins; impermeability of cell envelope to penicillins so that they cannot reach receptors.

3. Failure of activation of autolytic enzymes in the cell wall; "tolerance," eg, in staphylococci, group B streptococci.

4. Cell wall-deficient (L) forms or mycoplasmas, which do not synthesize peptidoglycans.

## Absorption, Distribution, & Excretion

After parenteral administration, absorption of most penicillins is complete and rapid. After oral administration, only a portion of the dose is absorbed (from $1/20$ to $1/3$, depending on acid stability, binding to foods, and the presence of buffers). To minimize binding to foods, oral penicillins should not be preceded or followed by food for at least 1 hour.

After absorption, penicillins are widely distributed in body fluids and tissues. With parenteral doses of 3–6 g (5–10 million units) per 24 hours of any penicillin injected by continuous infusion or divided intramuscular injections, average serum levels of the drug reach 1–10 units (0.6–6 μg) per mL.

In many tissues, penicillin concentrations are equal to those in serum. Lower levels are found in central nervous system. However, with active inflammation of the meninges, as in bacterial meningitis, penicillin levels in the cerebrospinal fluid exceed 0.2 μg/mL with a daily parenteral dose of 12 g.

Most of the absorbed penicillin is rapidly excreted by the kidneys into the urine—90% by tubular secretion. Tubular secretion can be partially blocked by probenecid (Benemid), 0.5 g every 6 hours by mouth, to achieve higher systemic levels.

Renal excretion of penicillin results in very high levels in the urine. Thus, systemic daily doses of 6 g of penicillin may yield urine levels of 500–3000 μg/mL—enough to suppress not only gram-positive but also many gram-negative bacteria in the urine (provided they produce little β-lactamase).

## Indications, Dosages, & Routes of Administration

The penicillins have been among the most effective and the most widely used antimicrobial drugs. All oral penicillins must be given 1 hour away from mealtimes to reduce binding and acid inactivation. Blood levels of all penicillins can be raised by simultaneous administration of probenecid, 0.5 g every 6 hours orally (10 mg/kg every 6 hours).

**A. Penicillin G:** In obstetric-gynecologic practice, this is the drug of choice for infections caused by group A and B streptococci, *Treponema pallidum*, aerobic gram-positive rods, clostridia, *Actinomyces*, and some *Bacteroides* species.

Penicillin G is no longer the drug of choice for gonococci because of widespread resistance. Enterococci are unusual streptococci because they are not susceptible to penicillin G alone, but to a synergistic combination of penicillin G plus an aminoglycoside or, in milder infections, to ampicillin alone. Penicillin remains the drug of choice for other bacteria occasionally encountered such as pneumococci and meningococci.

**1. Intramuscular or intravenous**–Although most of the above-mentioned infections respond to aqueous penicillin G in daily doses of 0.6–5 million units administered by intermittent intramuscular injection, larger amounts (6–50 g daily) given by intermittent intravenous infusion are usually used. Sites for such intravenous administration are subject to thrombophlebitis and superinfection and must be rotated every 2–3 days. In enterococcal infections, an aminoglycoside is given simultaneously with large doses of a penicillin.

**2. Oral**–Penicillin V is indicated only in minor infections (eg, of the respiratory tract or its associated structures) in daily doses of 1–4 g (1.6–6.4 million units). Oral administration is subject to too many variables to be relied on in seriously ill patients.

**B. Benzathine Penicillin G:** This penicillin is a salt of very low water solubility. It is injected intramuscularly to establish a depot that yields low but prolonged drug levels. An injection of 2.4 million units intramuscularly once a week for 1–3 weeks is satisfactory for treatment of syphilis. An injection of 1.2–2.4 million units intramuscularly every 3–4 weeks provides satisfactory prophylaxis for rheumatics against reinfection with group A streptococci. There is no indication for using this drug by mouth.

**C. Ampicillin, Amoxicillin, Carbenicillin, Ticarcillin, Piperacillin, Meziocillin, Aziocillin:** These drugs have greater activity against gram-negative aerobes than penicillin G but are destroyed by penicillinases (β-lactamases).

Ampicillin can be given orally in divided doses, 2–3 g daily, to treat urinary tract infections with coliform bacteria, enterococci, or *Proteus mirabilis*. It is ineffective against *Enterobacter* and *Pseudomonas*. Amoxicillin, 500 mg every 8 hours, is similar to ampicillin but is better absorbed. A single dose of amoxicillin, plus probenecid, is no longer recommended for gonorrhea.

Carbenicillin is more active against *Pseudomonas* and *Proteus*, but resistance emerges rapidly. Ticarcillin resembles carbenicillin but gives higher tissue levels. In susceptible populations of *Pseudomonas* sp, resistance to these drugs may emerge rapidly. Because carbenicillin and ticarcillin also possess moderate activity against the wide array of bacteria involved in pelvic infections, they have been used with fairly good success as single-agent therapy. Carbenicillin indanyl sodium can be given orally for some urinary tract infections. Piperacillin and similar (listed) drugs all resemble ticarcillin but are somewhat more active against some gram-negative aerobes, especially *Pseudomonas*. Mixtures of clavulanic acid with amoxicillin or ticarcillin are somewhat protected against destruction by β-lactamases and have been used for treatment of some lactamase producers, eg, *Haemophilus influenzae*.

**D. β-Lactamase–Resistant Penicillins:** Cloxacillin, nafcillin, and others are relatively resistant to destruction by β-lactamase. The only indication for the use of these drugs is infection by β-lactamase–producing staphylococci.

**1. Oral–**Oxacillin, cloxacillin, dicloxacillin, or nafcillin may be given in doses of 0.25–0.5 g every 4–6 hours in mild or localized staphylococcal infections. Food markedly interferes with absorption.

**2. Intravenous–**For serious systemic staphylococcal infections, nafcillin, 6–12 g, is given intravenously, by adding 1–2 g every 2 hours to a continuous infusion of 5% dextrose in water.

**E. Combinations of Penicillins plus β-Lactamase Inhibitors:** Because of their wide spectrum of activity against bacteria involved in pelvic infections, these combinations have been successful in many circumstances. Ampicillin plus sulbactam (Unasyn), 3 g every 6 hours, or carbenicillin plus clavulanic acid (Timentin), 3.1 g every 6 hours, may be given as the regimen in such polymicrobial infections.

**Adverse Effects**

The penicillins undoubtedly possess less direct toxicity than any other antibiotics. Most of the serious side effects are due to hypersensitivity.

**A. Allergy:** All penicillins are cross-sensitizing and cross-reacting. Any preparation containing penicillin may induce sensitization, including foods or cosmetics. In general, sensitization occurs in direct proportion to the duration and total dose of penicillin received in the past. Skin tests with penicilloyl-polylysine, with alkaline hydrolysis products (minor antigen determinants), and with undegraded penicillin can identify many hypersensitive individuals. Among positive reactors to skin tests, the incidence of subsequent immediate (IgE-mediated) penicillin reactions is high. Although many persons develop IgG antibodies to antigenic determinants of penicillin, the presence of such antibodies is not correlated with allergic reactivity (except rare hemolytic anemia). A history of a penicillin reaction in the past is not reliable; however, in such cases the drug should be administered with caution; ie, have available an artificial airway, 1% epinephrine in a syringe, running intravenous fluids, and competent personnel standing by, or a substitute drug should be given.

Allergic reactions may occur as typical anaphylactic shock, typical serum sickness type reactions (urticaria, fever, joint swelling, angioneurotic edema, intense pruritus, and respiratory embarrassment occurring 7–12 days after exposure), a variety of skin rashes, oral lesions, fever, nephritis, eosinophilia, hemolytic anemia and other hematologic disturbances, and vasculitis. The incidence of hypersensitivity to penicillin is estimated to be 3–5% among adults in the USA. Acute anaphylactic life-threatening reactions are fortunately very rare (0.05%). Ampicillin produces skin rashes (mononucleosis-like) 3–5 times more frequently than other penicillins, but some ampicillin rashes are not allergic. Methicillin and other penicillins can induce interstitial nephritis; nafcillin is less nephrotoxic than methicillin.

**B. Toxicity:** Since the action of penicillin is directed against a unique bacterial structure, the cell wall, it is virtually without effect on animal cells. The toxic effects of penicillin G are due to the direct irritation caused by intramuscular or intravenous injection of exceedingly high concentrations (eg, 1 g/mL). A rare patient receiving more than 50 g of penicillin G daily parenterally has exhibited signs of cerebrocortical irritation as a result of the passage of large amounts of penicillin into the central nervous system. With doses of this magnitude, direct cation toxicity ($Na^+$, $K^+$) can also occur. Potassium penicillin G contains 1.7 meq of $K^+$ per million units (2.7 meq/g), and potassium may accumulate in the presence of renal failure. Carbenicillin contains 4.7 meq of $Na^+$ per gram—a risk in heart failure.

Large doses of penicillins given orally may lead to gastrointestinal upset, particularly nausea and diarrhea. These symptoms are most marked with oral ampicillin or amoxicillin. Oral therapy may also be accompanied by luxuriant overgrowth of staphylococci, *Pseudomonas*, *Proteus*, or yeasts, which may occasionally cause enteritis. Superinfections in other organ systems may occur. Carbenicillin and ticarcillin may damage platelet function, cause bleeding, or result in hypokalemic alkalosis.

## CEPHALOSPORINS

The cephalosporins are structurally related to the penicillins. They consist of a β-lactam ring attached to a dihydrothiazoline ring. Substitutions of chemical groups at various positions on the basic structure have resulted in a proliferation of drugs with varying pharmacologic properties and antimicrobial activities.

The mechanism of action of cephalosporins is analogous to that of the penicillins: (1) binding to specific penicillin-binding proteins that serve as drug receptors on bacteria, (2) inhibition of cell wall synthesis, and (3) activation of autolytic enzymes in the cell wall that result in bacterial death. Resistance to cephalosporins may be due to poor permeability of the drug into bacteria, lack of penicillin-binding proteins, or degradation by β-lactamases.

Cephalosporins have been divided into 3 major groups or "generations," based mainly on their antibacterial activity: First-generation cephalosporins have good activity against aerobic gram-positive organisms and many community-acquired gram-negative organisms; second-generation drugs have a slightly extended spectrum against gram-negative bacteria, and some are active against anaerobes; and third-generation cephalosporins have less activity against gram-positives but are extremely active against most gram-negative bacteria. Not all cephalosporins fit neatly into this grouping, and there are exceptions to the general characterization of the drugs in the individual classes; however, the generational classification of cephalosporins is useful for discussion purposes.

## 1. FIRST-GENERATION CEPHALOSPORINS

### Antimicrobial Activity

These drugs are very active against gram-positive cocci, including pneumococci, viridans streptococci, group A and B streptococci, and *Staphylococcus aureus*. Like all cephalosporins, they are inactive against enterococci and methicillin-resistant staphylococci. Among gram-negative bacteria, *Escherichia coli*, *Klebsiella pneumoniae*, and *Proteus mirabilis* are usually sensitive except for some hospital-acquired strains. There is very little activity against such gram-negatives as *Pseudomonas aeruginosa*, indole-positive *Proteus* sp, *Enterobacter* spp, *Serratia marcescens*, *Citrobacter* spp, and *Acinetobacter* spp.

Anaerobic cocci are usually sensitive, but most *Bacteroides* species are not.

### Pharmacokinetics & Administration

**A. Oral:** Cephalexin, cephradine, and cefadroxil are absorbed from the gut to a variable extent. After a 500-mg oral dose, serum levels range from 15 to 20 µg/mL. Urine concentrations are usually very high, but in other tissues the levels are variable and usually lower than in the serum. Cephalexin and cephradine are given orally in doses of 0.25–0.5 g 4 times daily (15–30 mg/kg/d). Cefadroxil can be given in doses of 0.5–1 g twice daily.

Dosage should be reduced in renal insufficiency: for $Cl_{cr}$ 20–50 mL/min, give half the normal dose; for $Cl_{cr} < 20$ mL/min, give one-fourth the normal dose.

**B. Intravenous:** Cefazolin has a longer half-life than cephalothin or cephapirin. After an intravenous infusion of 1 g, the peak serum level of cefazolin is 90–120 µg/mL, whereas cephalothin and cephapirin reach levels of 40–60 µg/mL. The usual doses of cefazolin for adults are 1–2 g intravenously every 8 hours (50–100 mg/kg/d) and for cephalothin and cephapirin 1–2 g every 4–6 hours (50-200 mg/kg/d). In patients with impaired renal function, dosage adjustment somewhat as for oral dosage is needed.

**C. Intramuscular:** Both cephapirin and cefazolin can be given intramuscularly, but pain on injection is less with cefazolin.

### Clinical Uses

Although the first-generation cephalosporins have a broad spectrum of activity and are relatively nontoxic, they are rarely the drugs of choice. Oral drugs are indicated for treatment of urinary infections in patients who are allergic to sulfonamides or penicillins, and they can be used for minor staphylococcal infections in penicillin-allergic patients. Oral cephalosporins may also be preferred for minor polymicrobial infections (eg, cellulitis, soft tissue abscess). Oral cephalosporins should not be relied on in serious systemic infections.

Intravenous first-generation cephalosporins penetrate most tissues well and are among the drugs of choice for gynecologic and cesarean section prophylaxis. More expensive second- and third-generation cephalosporins offer no advantage over the first-generation drugs for surgical prophylaxis and should not be used for that purpose.

Other major uses of intravenous first-generation cephalosporins include infections for which they are the least toxic drugs (eg, *Klebsiella* infections) and infections in persons with a history of mild penicillin allergy (not anaphylaxis).

First-generation cephalosporins do not penetrate into the cerebrospinal fluid and cannot be used to treat meningitis.

## 2. SECOND-GENERATION CEPHALOSPORINS

Second-generation cephalosporins are a heterogeneous group with marked individual differences in activity, pharmacokinetics, and toxicity. In general, all of them are active against organisms also covered by first-generation drugs, but they have an extended gram-negative coverage. Indole-positive *Proteus* and *Klebsiella* spp (including cephalothin-resistant strains) are usually sensitive. In addition, cefoxitin and cefotetan are active against *Bacteroides fragilis* and some strains of *Serratia* but have poor activity against *Enterobacter* and *H influenzae*. Against gram-positive organisms, these drugs are less active than the first-generation cephalosporins. Like the latter, second-generation drugs have no activity against *P aeruginosa* or enterococci.

### Pharmacokinetics & Administration

After an intravenous infusion of 1 g, serum levels range from 75–125 µg/mL. Because of differences in drug half-life and protein binding, intervals between doses vary greatly. For cefoxitin (short half-lives), the interval is 4–6 hours; cefoxitin, 50–200 mg/kg/d.

Drugs with longer half-lives can be injected less frequently: cefotetan, 1–2 mg every 8–12 hours; and cefonicid or ceforanide, 1–2 g (15–30 mg/kg/d) once or twice daily. In renal failure, dosage adjustments are required.

### Clinical Uses

Because of their activity against *B fragilis*, cefoxitin and cefotetan are widely used to treat polymicrobial obstetric and gynecologic infections. There is no evidence that they are more effective than first-generation cephalosporins, and they are more expensive.

## 3. THIRD-GENERATION CEPHALOSPORINS

### Antimicrobial Activity

These drugs are active against staphylococci (not methicillin-resistant strains) but less so than first-generation cephalosporins. They have no activity against enterococci but may inhibit nonenterococcal streptococci. A major advantage of the new cephalosporins is their expanded gram-negative coverage. In addition to organisms inhibited by other cephalosporins, they are consistently active against *Enterobacter* spp, *Citrobacter freundii*, *S marcescens*, *Providencia* spp, *Haemophilus* spp, and *Neisseria* spp, including β-lactamase—producing strains. Two drugs—ceftazidime and cefoperazone—have good activity against *P aeruginosa*, whereas the others inhibit only 40–60% of strains. *Listeria* spp, *Acinetobacter* spp, and non-*aeruginosa* strains of *Pseudomonas* are variably sensitive to third-generation cephalosporins. Only ceftizoxime and moxalactam have good activity against *B fragilis*.

### Pharmacokinetics & Administration

After an intravenous infusion of 1 g, serum levels of these drugs range from 60 to 140 µg/mL. They penetrate well into body fluids and tissues. The half-life of these drugs is variable: ceftriaxone, 7–8 hours; cefoperazone, 2 hours; the others, 1–1.7 hours. Consequently, ceftriaxone can be injected every 12–24 hours in a dose of 15–30 mg/kg/d (or 30–50 mg/kg every 12 hours in adult meningitis and 50 mg/kg every 12 hours in infants). Cefoperazone can be given every 8–12 hours in a dose of 25–100 mg/kg/d, and the other drugs of the group every 6–8 hours in doses ranging from 2 to 12 g/d depending on the severity of the infection. Cefoperazone and ceftriaxone are eliminated primarily by biliary excretion, and no dosage adjustment is required in renal insufficiency. The other drugs are eliminated by the kidney and thus require dosage adjustments in renal insufficiency.

### Clinical Uses

Ceftriaxone 250 mg intramuscularly is now the drug of choice for treating uncomplicated gonorrhea. It is combined with doxycycline for cotreatment of chlamydia.

In obstetric-gynecologic practice, these agents generally have been used sparingly. Some members such as cefoperazone have been moderately successful as single-agent therapy in treating postoperative infections, but there are other choices with more favorable spectra.

## ADVERSE EFFECTS OF CEPHALOSPORINS

### Allergy

Cephalosporins are sensitizing, and a variety of hypersensitivity reactions occur, including anaphylaxis, fever, skin rashes, nephritis, granulocytopenia, and hemolytic anemia. The incidence of cross-allergy between cephalosporins and penicillins is not certainly known but is estimated to be about 6–10%. Persons with a history of anaphylaxis to penicillins should not receive cephalosporins.

### Toxicity

Local pain can occur after intramuscular injection, or thrombophlebitis after intravenous injection. Hypoprothrombinemia is a potential adverse effect of cephalosporins that have a methylthiotetrazole group (eg, cefamandole, moxalactam, cefoperazone). Administration of vitamin K, 10 mg twice weekly, can prevent this complication. Moxalactam interferes with platelet function and has been associated with severe bleeding. Drugs containing the methylthiotetrazole ring can also cause severe disulfiram-like reactions, and use of alcohol or medications containing alcohol (eg, theophylline) must be avoided.

### Superinfection

Many newer cephalosporins have little activity against gram-positive organisms, particularly staphylococci and enterococci. Superinfection with these organisms—as well as with fungi—may occur.

## NEW BETA-LACTAM DRUGS

### Monobactams

Monobactams are drugs with a monocyclic β-lactam ring, which are resistant to β-lactamases and are active against gram-negative organisms (including *Pseudomonas*) but not against gram-positive organisms or anaerobes. Aztreonam resembles aminoglycosides in activity. The usual dose is 1–2 g intravenously every 6–8 hours. Clinical uses of aztreonam alone are limited because of the availability of third-generation cephalosporins with a broader spectrum of activity and minimal toxicity. However, in combination with a drug such as clindamycin, aztreonam provides a regimen with a broad activity and appears equivalent to clindamycin-gentamicin in efficacy. Although aztreonam has potentially less toxicity than gentamicin, gentamicin is much less expensive, and the majority of obstetric-gynecologic patients are at low risk for gentamicin toxicity. The place of aztreonam remains to be established.

### Carbapenems

This new class of drugs is structurally related to β-lactam antibiotics. Imipenem, the first drug of this type, has a wide spectrum with good activity against many gram-negative rods, gram-positive organisms, and anaerobes. It is resistant to β-lactamases but is inactivated by dipeptidases in renal tubules. Consequently, it must be combined with cilastatin, a dipeptidase inhibitor, for clinical use.

The half-life of imipenem is 1 hour. Penetration into body tissues and fluids, including the cerebrospinal fluid, is good. The usual dose is 0.5–1 g intravenously every 6 hours. Dosage adjustment is required in renal insufficiency. Because imipenem has an unusual spectrum, it should be reserved for special cases such as treatment of highly resistant organisms. It should be used as a first-line treatment for pelvic infections.

The most common adverse effects of imipenem are nausea, vomiting, diarrhea, reactions at the infusion site, and skin rashes. Seizures can occur in patients with renal failure. Patients allergic to penicillins may be allergic to imipenem as well.

## ERYTHROMYCIN GROUP (Macrolides)

The erythromycins inhibit protein synthesis and are bacteriostatic or bactericidal against gram-positive organisms in concentrations of 0.02–2 μg/mL. *Chlamydia*, *Ureaplasma urealyticum*, *Legionella*, and *Campylobacter* are also susceptible. Activity is enhanced at alkaline pH.

Erythromycins are the drugs of choice in chlamydial infections, or in pneumonia caused by mycoplasmas or *Legionella*. They are useful as substitutes for penicillin in persons who are allergic to penicillin and for tetracyclines in pregnancy in the treatment of *Chlamydia* and *Ureaplasma*.

### Dosages

**A. Oral:** Erythromycin base, stearate or estolate, 0.25–0.5 g every 6 hours (for children, 40 mg/kg/d), or erythromycin ethylsuccinate, 0.4–0.6 g every 6 hours. The estolate derivative should not be used during pregnancy since it causes hepatic enzyme elevations.

**B. Intravenous:** Erythromycin lactobionate or gluceptate, 0.5 g every 12 hours.

### Adverse Effects

Nausea and vomiting and diarrhea may occur after oral intake. Erythromycin estolate probably more than the other salts can produce acute cholestatic hepatitis (fever, jaundice, impaired liver function) because of hypersensitivity. Most patients recover completely.

## TETRACYCLINE GROUP

The tetracyclines have common basic chemical structures, antimicrobial activity, and pharmacologic properties. Microorganisms resistant to one tetracycline show cross-resistance to all tetracyclines.

### Antimicrobial Activity

Tetracyclines are inhibitors of protein synthesis and are bacteriostatic for many gram-positive and gram-negative bacteria. They are strongly inhibitory for the growth of mycoplasmas, rickettsiae, chlamydiae, and some protozoa (eg, amebas). Equal concentrations of all tetracyclines in blood or tissue have approximately equal antimicrobial activity. However, there are great differences in the susceptibility of different strains of a given species of microorganism, and laboratory tests are therefore important. Because of the emergence of resistant strains, tetracyclines have lost some of their former usefulness against gram-negative and gram-positive bacteria, but they have new usefulness in treating sexually transmitted organisms. Tetracyclines alone are no longer considered adequate therapy for gonorrhea, but the drug of choice for chlamydia.

## Absorption, Distribution, & Excretion

Tetracyclines are absorbed somewhat irregularly from the gut. Absorption is limited by the low solubility of the drugs and by chelation with divalent cations, eg, $Ca^{2+}$ or $Fe^{2+}$. A large proportion (80%) of orally administered tetracycline remains in the gut lumen, modifies intestinal flora, and is excreted in feces. With full systemic doses (2 g/d), levels of active drug in serum reach 2–10 μg/mL. Tetracyclines are specifically deposited in growing bones and teeth, bound to calcium.

Absorbed tetracyclines are excreted mainly in bile and urine. Up to 20% of oral doses may appear in the urine after glomerular filtration. Urine levels may be 5–50 μg/mL or more. With renal failure, doses of tetracyclines must be reduced or intervals between doses increased.

Minocycline and doxycycline are well absorbed from the gut but are excreted more slowly than others, leading to accumulation and prolonged blood levels. Renal clearance ranges from 9 mL/min for minocycline to 90 mL/min for oxytetracycline. Doxycycline does not accumulate greatly in renal failure and can be used in uremia.

## Indications, Dosages, & Routes of Administration

Tetracyclines are the drugs of choice in chlamydial and genital mycoplasmal infections.

**A. Oral:** Tetracycline hydrochloride and oxytetracycline are dispensed in 250 mg capsules. Give 0.25–0.5 g orally every 6 hours. Doxycycline, 100 mg twice daily, is equally as effective as tetracycline hydrochloride, 2 g/d.

Doxycycline and minocycline are available in capsules containing 50 or 100 mg or as powder for oral suspension. Give doxycycline, 100 mg every 12 hours on the first day and 100 mg/d for maintenance.

**B. Intravenous:** Several tetracyclines are formulated for parenteral administration in individuals unable to take oral medication. The dose is generally similar to the oral dose (see manufacturers' instructions).

## Adverse Effects

**A. Allergy:** Hypersensitivity reactions with fever or skin rashes are uncommon.

**B. Gastrointestinal Side Effects:** Gastrointestinal side effects—especially diarrhea, nausea, and anorexia—are common. These can be diminished by reducing the dose or by administering tetracyclines with food or carboxymethylcellulose, but sometimes they force discontinuance of the drug. After a few days of oral use, the gut flora is modified so that drug-resistant bacteria and yeasts become prominent. This may cause functional gut disturbances, anal pruritus, and even enterocolitis with shock and death.

**C. Bones and Teeth:** Tetracyclines are bound to calcium deposited in growing bones and teeth, causing fluorescence, discoloration, enamel dysplasia, deformity, or growth inhibition. This risk must be considered if tetracyclines are given to pregnant women.

**D. Liver Damage:** Tetracyclines can impair hepatic function or even cause liver necrosis, particularly during pregnancy, in the presence of preexisting liver damage, or with doses of more than 3 g intravenously.

**E. Kidney Damage:** Outdated tetracycline preparations have been implicated in renal tubular acidosis and other renal damage. Tetracyclines may increase blood urea nitrogen when diuretics are administered.

**F. Other:** Tetracyclines, principally demeclocycline, may induce photosensitization, especially in blonds. Intravenous injection may cause thrombophlebitis, and intramuscular injection may induce local inflammation with pain. Minocycline causes vestibular reactions (dizziness, vertigo, nausea) in 30–60% of cases after doses of 200 mg daily.

## AMINOGLYCOSIDES

The aminoglycosides are a group of bactericidal drugs sharing chemical, antimicrobial, pharmacologic, and toxic characteristics. The group includes widely used drugs such as gentamicin and tobramycin. All these agents inhibit protein synthesis in bacteria by attaching to and inhibiting the function of the 30S subunit of the bacterial ribosome. Resistance is based on (1) a deficiency of the ribosomal receptor (chromosomal mutant); (2) the enzymatic destruction of the drug (plasmid-mediated transmissible resistance of clinical importance) by acetylation, phosphorylation, or adenylation; or (3) a lack of permeability to the drug molecule or failure of active transport across cell membranes. The last-named form of resistance can be chromosomal (eg, streptococci are relatively impermeable to aminoglycosides), or it may be plasmid-mediated (clinically significant resistance among gram-negative enteric bacteria). Anaerobic bacteria are often resistant to aminoglycosides because transport across the cell membrane is an oxygen-dependent energy-requiring process.

All aminoglycosides are more active at alkaline than at acid pH. All are potentially ototoxic and nephrotoxic, although to different degrees. All can accumulate in renal failure; therefore, dosage adjustments must be made in uremia.

Aminoglycosides are used most widely against gram-negative enteric bacteria or when there is a suspicion of sepsis. In the treatment of bacteremia or endocarditis caused by fecal streptococci or by some gram-negative bacteria, the aminoglycoside is given together with a penicillin to enhance permeability and facilitate the entry of the aminoglycoside.

## General Properties of Aminoglycosides

Because of the similarities of the aminoglycosides, a summary of properties is presented briefly before each drug is taken up individually for a discussion of its main clinical uses.

**A. Physical Properties:** Aminoglycosides are water-soluble and stable in solution. If they are mixed in solution with β-lactam antibiotics, they may form complexes and lose some activity.

**B. Absorption, Distribution, Metabolism, and Excretion:** Aminoglycosides are well absorbed after intramuscular or intravenous injection but are not absorbed from the gut. They are distributed widely in tissues and penetrate pleural, peritoneal, or joint fluid in the presence of inflammation. They enter the central nervous system to only a slight extent after parenteral administration. There is no significant metabolic breakdown of aminoglycosides. The serum half-life is 2–3 hours; excretion is mainly by glomerular filtration. Urine levels are 10–50 times higher than serum levels. Aminoglycosides are removed fairly effectively by hemodialysis but irregularly by peritoneal dialysis.

**C. Dose and Effect in Cases of Impaired Renal Function:** In persons with normal renal function, the dose of gentamicin is 3–7 mg/kg/d, usually injected in 3 equal amounts every 8 hours. In pregnancy, even higher doses of gentamicin may be necessary as the increases in glomerular filtration often lead to more rapid antibiotic excretion.

In persons with impaired renal function, excretion is diminished and there is a danger of drug accumulation with increased side effects. Therefore, if the interval is kept constant, the dose has to be reduced, or the interval must be increased if the dose is kept constant. Nomograms have been constructed relating serum creatinine levels to adjustments of treatment regimens. One widely used formula uses a multiplication factor (gentamicin = 8, tobramycin = 6) times the serum creatinine value (mg/dL) to give the interval between doses in hours. However, there is considerable variation in aminoglycoside levels in different patients with similar creatinine values. Therefore, it is highly desirable to choose an alternate drug or monitor drug levels in blood whenever possible to avoid severe toxicity when renal functional capacity is rapidly changing.

**D. Adverse Effects:** All aminoglycosides can cause varying degrees of ototoxicity and nephrotoxicity. Ototoxicity can present either as hearing loss (cochlear damage) that is noted first with high-frequency tones, or as vestibular damage, evident by vertigo, ataxia, and loss of balance. Nephrotoxicity is evident with rising serum creatinine levels or reduced creatinine clearance.

In very high doses, aminoglycosides can be neurotoxic, producing a curare-like effect with neuromuscular blockage that results in respiratory paralysis. This has been most common in gynecologic surgery when solutions containing aminoglycosides have been used for peritoneal irrigation. Calcium gluconate or neostigmine can serve as antidote. Rarely, aminoglycosides cause hypersensitivity and local reactions.

## 1. GENTAMICIN

Gentamicin is the most widely used aminoglycoside antibiotic on obstetric-gynecologic services. In concentrations of 0.5–5 μg/mL, gentamicin is bactericidal not only for staphylococci and coliform organisms but also for many strains of *Pseudomonas*, *Proteus*, and *Serratia*. Enterococci are resistant. With doses of 3–7 mg/kg/d, serum levels reach 3–8 μg/mL. Gentamicin may be synergistic with ticarcillin against *Pseudomonas*. However, the 2 drugs should not be mixed in vitro.

## Indications, Dosages, & Routes of Administration

Gentamicin is used in severe infections caused by gram-negative bacteria. *Klebsiella-Enterobacter*, *Proteus*, *Pseudomonas*, and *Serratia*. The dosage is 3–7 mg/kg/d intramuscularly (or intravenously) in 3 equal doses for 7–10 days. In urinary tract infections caused by these organisms, 0.8–1.2 mg/kg/d is given intramuscularly for 5–10 days. It is necessary to monitor renal function by checking serum creatinine every few days and to reduce the dosage or lengthen the interval between doses if renal function declines. About 2–3% of patients develop vestibular dysfunction and loss of hearing when peak serum levels exceed 10 μg/mL. Serum concentrations should be monitored by laboratory assay in selected circumstances (see previous text).

## 2. TOBRAMYCIN

Tobramycin is an aminoglycoside that closely resembles gentamicin in antibacterial activity and pharmacologic properties and exhibits partial cross-resistance. Tobramycin may be effective against some gentamicin-resistant gram-negative bacteria, especially *Pseudomonas*. A daily dose of 3–5 mg/kg is given in 3 equal amounts intramuscularly or intravenously at intervals of 8 hours. In uremia, the suggested dose is 1 mg/kg intramuscularly every 6 (serum creatinine value [in mg/dL]) hours. However, blood levels should be monitored. Tobramycin may be less nephrotoxic than gentamicin; their ototoxicity is similar.

## SPECTINOMYCIN

Spectinomycin is an aminocyclitol antibiotic, related to the aminoglycosides. Its sole indication is for the treatment of β-lactamase—producing gonococci or gonorrhea in a penicillin-hypersensitive person. One injection of 2 g (40 mg/kg) is given. About 5–10% of gonococci are resistant. There usually is pain at the injection site, and there may be nausea and fever.

## SULFONAMIDES

Since 1935, more than 150 different sulfonamides have been marketed. The increasing emergence of sulfonamide resistance (eg, among streptococci, meningococci, and shigellae) and the higher efficacy of other antimicrobial drugs have drastically curtailed the number of specific indications for sulfonamides as drugs of choice. The present indications for the use of these drugs can be summarized as follows:

**(1) First (previously untreated) infection of the urinary tract:** Many coliform organisms, which are the most common causes of urinary infections, are still susceptible to sulfonamides or to trimethoprim-sulfamethoxazole.

**(2) Parasitic diseases:** The combination of trimethoprim with sulfamethoxazole is often effective for prophylaxis or for treatment of *Pneumocystis carinii* pneumonia in immunocompromised individuals. Similar combinations (eg, Fansidar) are sometimes effective in falciparum malaria. The combination of a sulfonamide with pyrimethamine is used in the treatment of toxoplasmosis.

### Dosages & Routes of Administration

For systemic disease, the soluble, rapidly excreted sulfonamides (eg, sulfadiazine, sulfisoxazole) are given orally in an initial dose of 2–4 g (40 mg/kg) followed by 0.5–1 g (10 mg/kg) every 4–6 hours. Trisulfapyrimidines USP may be given in the same total doses. Urine must be kept alkaline.

For urinary tract infections (first attack, not previously treated), trisulfapyrimidines or sulfisoxazole is given in a dose of 2–4 g daily. Following one course of sulfonamides, resistant organisms usually prevail. Simultaneous administration of a sulfonamide, 2 g/d orally, and trimethoprim, 400 mg/d orally, may be more effective than either one alone.

Long-acting sulfonamides (eg, sulfamethoxypyridazine) have a significantly higher rate of toxic effects than the short-acting sulfonamides.

### Adverse Effects

Sulfonamides produce a wide variety of side effects—due partly to hypersensitivity, partly to direct toxicity—which must be considered whenever unexplained symptoms or signs occur in a patient who may have received these drugs. Except in the mildest reactions, fluids should be forced and, if symptoms and signs progressively increase, the drugs should be discontinued. Precautions to prevent complications (see text that follows) are important.

**A. Systemic Side Effects:** Fever, skin rashes, urticaria; nausea and vomiting or diarrhea; stomatitis, conjunctivitis, arthritis, exfoliative dermatitis; hematopoietic disturbances, including thrombocytopenia, hemolytic (in G6PD deficiency) or aplastic anemia, granulocytopenia, leukemoid reactions; hepatitis, polyarteritis nodosa, vasculitis, Stevens-Johnson syndrome; psychosis; and many others.

**B. Urinary Tract Disturbances:** Sulfonamides may precipitate in urine, especially at neutral or acid pH, producing hematuria, crystalluria, or even obstruction. They have also been implicated in various types of nephritis and nephrosis. Sulfonamides and methenamine salts should not be given together.

### Precautions in the Use of Sulfonamides

(1) There is cross-allergenicity among all sulfonamides. Obtain a history of past administration or reaction. Observe for possible allergic responses.

(2) Keep the urine volume above 1500 mL/d by forcing fluids. Check urine pH—it should be 7.5 or higher. Give alkali by mouth (sodium bicarbonate or equivalent, 5–15 g/d). Examine fresh urine for crystals and red cells every 5–7 days.

(3) Check hemoglobin, white blood cell count, and differential count once weekly to detect possible disturbances early in high-risk patients.

## TRIMETHOPRIM

This folate antagonist can act together with sulfonamides or alone. Trimethoprim, 100 mg orally every 12 hours, is effective in urinary tract infections. Trimethoprim-sulfamethoxazole mixtures are a choice in *P carinii* pneumonia (see Sulfonamides), *Shigella* enteritis, *Serratia* sepsis, and other diseases. Such mixtures (trimethoprim, 80 mg, and sulfamethoxazole, 400 mg) can also be effective chemoprophylaxis for recurrent urinary tract infections; give ½ tablet daily or 1 tablet 3 times weekly. The side effects of trimethoprim resemble those of the sulfonamides.

## SPECIALIZED DRUGS AGAINST GRAM-POSITIVE BACTERIA

### 1. CLINDAMYCIN

Clindamycin resembles erythromycin and is active against gram-positive organisms (except enterococci). Clindamycin, 0.15–0.3 g orally every 6 hours yields serum concentrations of 2–5 μg/mL. The drug is widely distributed in tissues. Excretion is through the bile and urine. It is an alternative to erythromycin as substitutes for penicillin. Clindamycin is effective against most strains of *Bacteroides* and is a drug of choice in polymicrobial aerobic-anaerobic infections, when used in combination with an aminoglycoside. Seriously ill patients are given clindamycin, 600 mg (20–30 mg/kg/d) intravenously during a 1-hour period every 6 hours or 900 mg every 8 hours. A new preparation, 2% vaginal clindamycin cream, when used nightly (5–7 mL) is highly effective in treating bacterial vaginosis.

Common side effects are diarrhea, nausea, and skin rashes. Impaired liver function and neutropenia have been noted. If 3–4 g are given rapidly intravenously, cardiorespiratory arrest may occur. Bloody diarrhea with pseudomembranous colitis has been associated with clindamycin administration and has caused some fatalities. This is due to necrotizing toxin produced by *Clostridium difficile*, which is clindamycin-resistant and increases in the gut with the selection pressure exerted by administration of this drug. The organism is sensitive to vancomycin, and the colitis rapidly regresses during oral treatment with vancomycin (see below).

## 2. AZITHROMYCIN

Azithromycin is the first of the azalide antibiotics that are chemically similar to the macrolides such as clindamycin and erythromycin. With excellent in vitro activity against *C trachomatis* and with favorable kinetics including sustained high concentration in tissue (even though serum concentrations are low), azithromycin (1 g orally once) has been as effective as doxycycline (100 mg twice daily for 7 days), 97% versus 95%, respectively in treating chlamydia urethritis and cervicitis. Side-effects were similar, mainly gastrointestinal, and were mild to moderate. Because this 1 g dose of azithromycin is not adequate for treating gonorrhea, cotreatment with single-dose ceftriaxone (250 mg intramuscularly) is necessary. Because this drug has not been widely used in pregnancy, alternate treatment is preferable.

## 3. METRONIDAZOLE

Metronidazole is an antiprotozoal drug that also is strikingly active against most anaerobes, including *Bacteroides* species. Metronidazole is well absorbed after oral administration and is widely distributed. The drug is metabolized in the liver, and dosage reduction is required in the presence of hepatic insufficiency. Metronidazole can also be given intravenously or by rectal suppository, with serum levels

equivalent for both routes. Metronidazole is used to treat amebiasis and also the following:

(1) *Trichomonas* vaginitis responds to either a single dose (2 g) or to 250 mg orally 3 times daily for 7–10 days. Both sexual partners should be treated.

(2) Bacterial vaginosis (formerly nonspecific vaginitis) responds to 500 mg orally 3 times daily for 5 days or to vaginal cream, 5–7 mL, applied nightly for 5 nights. Single-dose treatment is less effective, and treatment of sexual partners is not recommended since this does not decrease recurrences in the female.

(3) In anaerobic or mixed infections, metronidazole can be given orally or intravenously 500 mg 3 times daily (30 mg/kg/d).

(4) As an alternative to oral vancomycin for antibiotic-associated colitis, give 500 mg 3 times daily orally.

Adverse effects of metronidazole include stomatitis, nausea, diarrhea, and disulfiram-like reactions. With prolonged use, peripheral neuropathy may develop.

## 4. VANCOMYCIN

Vancomycin is bactericidal for most gram-positive organisms, particularly staphylococci. Resistant mutants are very rare, and there is no cross-resistance with other antimicrobial drugs. Vancomycin is not absorbed from the gut. It is given orally (2 g/d) only for the treatment of antibiotic-associated enterocolitis. For systemic effect, the drug must be administered intravenously. After intravenous injection of 0.5 g over a period of 20 minutes, blood levels of 10 μg/mL are maintained for 1–2 hours. Vancomycin is excreted mainly through the kidneys but may accumulate in the kidneys in the event of liver failure. In renal insufficiency, the half-life may be up to 8 days. Thus, only 1 dose of 0.5–1 g may be given every 4–8 days to a uremic individual undergoing hemodialysis.

The only indications for parenteral vancomycin are serious staphylococcal infection or enterococcal endocarditis (in combination with an aminoglycoside). Vancomycin, 0.5 g, is injected intravenously over a 20-minute period every 6–8 hours (for children, 20–40 mg/kg/d).

Vancomycin is irritating to tissues; chills, fever, and thrombophlebitis sometimes follow intravenous injection. Rapid infusion may result in diffuse hyperemia (**red man syndrome**); this can be avoided by giving infusions over 1 hour. Vancomycin is sometimes ototoxic and (perhaps) nephrotoxic.

## 5. QUINOLONES

Quinolones are synthetic analogs of nalidixic acid and are active against many gram-positive and gram-negative bacteria. All quinolones inhibit bacterial

DNA synthesis by blocking the enzyme DNA gyrase. The earlier quinolones (nalidixic acid, oxolinic acid, cinoxacin) did not achieve systemic antibacterial levels and thus were useful only as urinary antiseptics. The newer fluoroquinolones (eg, norfloxacin, ciprofloxacin, enoxacin, oxofloxacin, pefloxacin) have greater antibacterial activity, achieve clinically useful levels in blood and tissues, and have low toxicity. They are active against a wide variety of aerobic bacteria but not against clinically important anaerobes. After oral administration, these newer fluoroquinolones are well absorbed and widely distributed, with a serum half-life of 3–8 hours. They are excreted mainly by tubular renal secretion or glomerular filtration. Up to 20% of the dose is metabolized by the liver.

The proper indications for individual fluoroquinolones are now being defined. Most of them are effective in urinary tract infections, even when caused by multiresistant bacteria, eg *Pseudomonas aeruginosa*. Norfloxacin, 400 mg, or ciprofloxacin, 500 mg (orally twice daily) is effective for this purpose. However, less expensive antimicrobials are usually preferable. Some of these preparations are effective in treating *C trachomatis*. These same quinolones are likely to offer an alternative in the treatment of pelvic inflammatory disease. Intravenous as well as oral preparations are available.

Because they inhibit DNA gyrase, they should not be used in pregnancy.

The most pronounced adverse effects are nausea, vomiting, diarrhea, headache, dizziness, insomnia, occasional skin rashes, and impairment of liver function.

## URINARY ANTISEPTICS

Urinary antiseptics exert antimicrobial activity in the urine but have little or no systemic antibacterial effect. Their usefulness is limited to urinary tract infections.

## 1. NITROFURANTOIN

Nitrofurantoin is bacteriostatic and bactericidal for both gram-positive and gram-negative bacteria in urine. The drug has no systemic antimicrobial activity. Its activity in urine is enhanced at pH 5.5 or below. Microbial resistance does not emerge rapidly.

The average daily dose in urinary tract infections is 100 mg orally 4 times daily (for children, 5–10 mg/kg/d), taken with food.

Oral nitrofurantoin often causes nausea and vomiting. Hemolytic anemia occurs in G6PD deficiency. Hypersensitivity may produce skin rashes and pulmonary infiltration. In uremia, there is virtually no excretion of nitrofurantoin into the urine and no therapeutic effect.

## 2. NALIDIXIC ACID & OXOLINIC ACID

Nalidixic acid and oxolinic acid are older quinolones with no systemic effect. Resistant mutants tend to emerge fairly rapidly in susceptible bacterial populations. In urinary tract infections, the adult dosage is 1 g orally 4–6 times daily. Adverse reactions are those of the quinolones (see previous text).

## ANTIFUNGAL DRUGS

Most antibacterial drugs have no effect on yeasts and fungi. Others (eg, amphotericin B) are relatively effective in some systemic mycotic infections but are difficult to administer because of toxicity. New imidazoles are fairly effective and relatively nontoxic. Topical preparations such as 2% miconazole, 1% clotrimazole, 2% butoconazole, or 0.4% terconazole have all been used effectively in vaginal candidiasis. Ketoconazole can be given orally, 200–600 mg once daily, preferably with food. It is well absorbed, reaches serum levels of 2–4 μg/mL, and is degraded in tissues, thus requiring no renal or biliary excretion. It has a dramatic therapeutic effect on chronic vaginal candidiasis. Ketoconazole blocks the synthesis of adrenal steroids and can cause gynecomastia. Adverse effects are mild, with nausea, headache, skin rashes, and occasional elevations in transaminase levels. If evidence of liver dysfunction persists, the drug should be discontinued.

Fluconazole also appears to be effective in recurrent or refractory vaginal candidiasis and is less hepatotoxic.

## ANTIMICROBIAL DRUGS USED IN COMBINATION

### Indications

Possible reasons for using 2 or more antimicrobials simultaneously instead of a single drug are as follows:

(1) To treat presumably mixed infections. Each drug is aimed at an important pathogenic microorganism.

(2) To institute prompt presumptive treatment in desperately ill patients suspected of having a serious microbial infection. A good guess about the most probable 2 or 3 pathogens is made, and drugs are aimed at those organisms. Before such treatment is started, it is essential that adequate specimens be obtained for identifying the etiologic agent in the laboratory. Gram-negative sepsis and peritonitis of uncer-

tain cause are important diseases in this category at present.

(3) To achieve bactericidal synergism. In a few infections, eg, enterococcal sepsis, a combination of drugs is more likely to eradicate the infection than either drug used alone.

## Disadvantages

The following disadvantages of using antimicrobial drugs in combinations must always be considered:

(1) The physician may feel that since several drugs are already being given, everything possible has been done for the patient. This attitude leads to relaxation of the effort to establish a specific diagnosis. It may also give the physician a false sense of security.

(2) The more drugs that are administered, the greater the chance for drug reactions to occur or for the patient to become sensitized to drugs.

(3) The cost may be unnecessarily high.

(4) Antimicrobial combinations often accomplish no more than an effective single drug.

## ANTIMICROBIAL CHEMOPROPHYLAXIS IN SURGERY

A major portion of all antimicrobial drugs used in hospitals is used on surgical services with the stated intent of "prophylaxis."

Several general features of "surgical prophylaxis" are applicable.

(1) Prophylactic administration of antibiotics should generally be considered only if the expected rate of infectious complications is high or where a possible infection would have a catastrophic effect.

(2) If prophylactic antimicrobials are to be effective, a sufficient concentration of drug must be present at the operative site to inhibit or kill bacteria that might settle there. Thus, it is essential that drug administration begin immediately before (or in cesarean section) just after operation begins.

(3) Prolonged administration of antimicrobial drugs tends to alter the normal flora of organ systems, suppressing the susceptible microorganisms and favoring the implantation of drug-resistant ones. Thus, antimicrobial prophylaxis should last only 1–3 doses.

(4) Systemic antimicrobial levels usually do not prevent wound infection, pneumonia, or urinary tract infection if physiologic abnormalities or foreign bodies are present.

In hysterectomy and nonelective cesarean section, the administration of a broad-spectrum bactericidal drug from just before until 1 day after the procedure has been found effective. Thus, cefazolin, eg 1 g intravenously given before pelvic operations and again for 1–2 doses after the end of the operation, results in a demonstrable lowering of the risk of deep infections at the operative site.

Other forms of surgical prophylaxis attempt to reduce normal flora or existing bacterial contamination at the site. Thus, the colon is routinely prepared not only by mechanical cleansing through cathartics and enemas but also by the oral administration of poorly absorbed drugs (eg, neomycin, 1 g, plus erythromycin base, 0.5 g, every 6 hours) for 1–2 days before operation.

In all situations in which antimicrobials are administered with the hope that they may have a prophylactic effect, the risk from these same drugs (allergy, toxicity, selection of superinfecting microorganisms) must be evaluated daily, and the course of prophylaxis must be kept as brief as possible.

## ANTIVIRAL CHEMOPROPHYLAXIS & THERAPY

Several compounds can suppress development of viral diseases. Of these, acyclovir is important in gynecologic practice.

Acyclovir (acycloguanosine [Zovirax]) inhibits replication of herpesviruses in infected cells. When given intravenously (15 mg/kg/d), acyclovir is effective in controlling disseminating herpesvirus infections in immunocompromised patients; it can also markedly reduce pain and extent of lesions in primary genital herpes infections of women. In herpetic encephalitis and in neonatal herpetic dissemination, acyclovir is more effective than vidarabine. There is no effect on cytomegalovirus or Epstein-Barr virus infections, but acyclovir can arrest the progression of varicella and herpes zoster, especially in immunocompromised patients.

Oral acyclovir, 200 mg 5 times daily for adults, has therapeutic effects similar to those of intravenous acyclovir, particularly in primary genital herpes simplex infections. When taken prophylactically in patients with frequent (> 6/y) episodes, it can reduce the frequency of recurrent lesions for up to 3 years. However, no regimen of acyclovir can block the establishment of latency or permanently eliminate recurrences.

Topical acyclovir ointment (5% in polyethylene glycol) (Zovirax) applied several times daily can limit pain and virus shedding and reduce healing time in primary genital herpes infections. In recurrent herpetic lesions, the effect is minimal or questionable. Topical acyclovir has no effect on the incidence or severity of herpetic recurrences. Topical acyclovir produces few and mild side effects. In most instances, however, oral acyclovir is preferable. Although its use in pregnancy has not been extensive, data so far are reassuring in that there have been no side-effects peculiar to the pregnant woman or the fetus.

# REFERENCES

## GENERAL

Daffos F et al: Prenatal management of 746 pregnancies at risk for congenital toxoplasmosis. N Engl J Med 1988;318:271.

Sweet RL, Gibbs RS: *Infectious Diseases of the Female Genital Tract,* 2nd ed. Williams & Wilkins, 1990.

Walker CK, Landers DV: Anti-infective drugs in obstetrics and gynecology. Current Opinion Obstet Gynecol 1991;3:698.

## PENICILLINS & CEPHALOSPORINS

Mercer LJ: Use of expanded spectrum cephalosporins for the treatment of obstetrical and gynecological infections. Obstet Gynecol Survey 1988;43(9):569.

Donowitz GR, Mandell GL: Beta-lactam antibiotics (2 parts). N Engl J Med 1988;318:419, 490.

Wendel GD et al: Penicillin allergy and desensitization in serious infections during pregnancy. N Engl J Med 1985;312:1229.

## SEXUALLY TRANSMITTED DISEASES

1989 Sexually Transmitted Diseases Treatment Guidelines. Morbidity and Mortality Weekly Report 1989; 38:S–8.

Martin DH et al: A controlled trial of a single dose of azithromycin for the treatment of chlamydial urethritis and cervicitis. N Engl J Med 1992;327:921.

## ANAEROBIC INFECTIONS

Sanders CV, Aldridge KE: Antimicrobial therapy of anaerboic infections, 1991. Pharmacotherapy 1991; 11(2Pt 2):72S.

Rosenblatt JE, Edson RS: Metronidazole. Mayo Clin Proc 1987;62:1013.

## QUINOLONES

Hooper DC, Wolfson JS: Fluoroquinolone antimicrobial agents. N Engl J Med 1991;324(6):384.

## ANTIMICROBIAL CHEMOPROPHYLACTIC

Hemsell DL: Prophylactic antibiotics in gynecologic and obstetric surgery. Rev Infect Dis 1991;13(Suppl 10):821.

## ANTIVIRAL AGENTS

Kaplowitz LG et al: Prolonged continuous acyclovir treatment of normal adults with frequently recurring genital herpes simplex virus infection. JAMA 1991;265(Suppl 6):747.

Andrews EB et al: Acyclovir in pregnancy registry: six years' experience. Obstet Gynecol 1992;79(1):7.

Baker DA: Herpes simplex virus infections. Obstet Gyencol 1992;4:676.

# Endometriosis

# 40

*Kenneth N. Muse, Jr., MD, & Michael D. Fox, MD*

Endometriosis is a disorder in which abnormal growths of tissue, histologically resembling the endometrium, are present in locations other than the uterine lining. Although endometriosis can occur very rarely in postmenopausal women, it is found almost exclusively in women of reproductive age. All other manifestations of endometriosis exhibit a wide spectrum of expression. The lesions are usually found on the peritoneal surfaces of the reproductive organs and adjacent structures of the pelvis, but they can occur anywhere in the body (Fig 40–1). The size of the individual lesions varies from microscopic to large invasive masses that erode into underlying organs and cause extensive adhesion formation. Similarly, women with endometriosis can be completely asymptomatic or may be crippled by pelvic pain and infertility.

Endometriosis is a common and important health problem of women. Its exact prevalence is unknown because surgery is required for its diagnosis, but it is estimated to be present in 10% of all reproductive-age women. It is seen in 1–2% of women undergoing sterilizations or sterilization reversal, in 10% of hysterectomy surgeries, in 16–31% of laparoscopies, and in 53% of adolescents with pelvic pain severe enough to warrant surgical evaluation. Endometriosis is the commonest single gynecologic diagnosis responsible for hospitalization of women aged 15–44, being found in over 6% of patients.

Adenomyosis, also called endometriosis interna, is the presence of endometrial glands and stroma within the myometrium; it is generally thought to be unrelated to endometriosis. Adenomyosis is discussed in Chapter 36.

## Pathogenesis

The cause of endometriosis is unknown. Several theories have been offered to explain its occurrence, but none have satisfactorily explained all of the features of the disease. The theories fall into groups, and are not mutually exclusive.

A theory of retrograde menstruation was proposed during the 1920s. It was postulated that endometriosis occurred because viable fragments of endometrium were shed at the time of menstruation and passed through the uterine tubes. Once in the pelvic cavity, the tissue became implanted on peritoneal surfaces and grew into endometriotic lesions. Subsequent observations have confirmed that some degree of retrograde menstruation normally occurs in women with patent tubes, that outflow tract obstructions (cervical stenosis, transverse vaginal septa) increase the incidence of endometriosis, and that intentional deposition of endometrium onto peritoneum can initiate endometriosis. Also, the risk of developing the disease is higher in women with prolonged menstrual flow and in those with short menstrual cycle lengths (more menses per year). This theory is simple, attractive, and easily explains why endometriosis is most commonly found on the peritoneal surfaces of the ovaries, cul-de-sac, and bladder and why lesions may develop in episiotomies and other incisions. However, it does not explain why all women do not develop endometriosis nor does it explain the rare cases of endometriosis in the lung, brain, or other soft tissues or in nonmenstruating subjects (women with Turner's syndrome or with absent uteri).

Other workers proposed that endometrial tissue could be transported by lymphatic or hematogenous routes, and a theory of coelomic metaplasia was postulated. In the latter, peritoneum is induced to undergo metaplasia into endometrial tissue by some stimulus (menstrual fluid or other irritants, cyclic ovarian hormones, etc).

A role for the immune system in the origin of endometriosis was suggested by workers studying monkeys with spontaneous endometriosis that mounted a lesser immune response to endometrial antigens than control animals. Also, the peritoneal fluid of women with endometriosis has been noted to have increased immunosuppressive properties and lymphocytes with decreased natural killer cell activity. Endometriosis may occur when a deficiency in cellular immunity allows menstrual tissue to implant and grow on the peritoneum.

Genetic influences in the development of endometriosis have been described. Studies have found that 7–9% of endometriosis patients' first-degree female relatives are diagnosed with the disease—signifi-

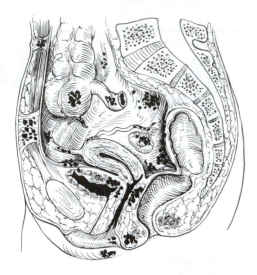

**Figure 40–1.** Common sites of endometrial implants (endometriosis). (Reproduced, with permission, from Way LW [editor]: Current Surgical Diagnosis & Treatment, 7th ed. Lange, 1985.)

cantly greater than the control rate of 1–2%. Further investigation failed to link endometriosis with the presence of particular HLA antigens.

## Pathology

The gross appearance of endometriosis at operation is usually quite characteristic and, to an experienced surgeon, is sufficient for diagnosis. The smallest (and presumably earliest) implants are red, petechial lesions on the peritoneal surface. With further growth, menstrual-like detritus accumulates within the lesion, giving it a cystic, dark brown, dark blue, or black appearance. The surrounding peritoneal surface becomes thickened and scarred. These "powder burn" implants typically attain a size of 5–10 mm in diameter. With progression of disease, the number and size of lesions increase, and extensive adhesions may develop. When present on the ovary, cysts may enlarge to several centimeters in size and are called "endometriomas" or "chocolate cysts." Severe disease can erode into underlying tissues and distort the remaining organs with extensive adhesions. In addition to these traditional presentations, endometriosis lesions can have a variety of nonclassical appearances: clear vesicles, white or yellow spots or nodules, circular folds of peritoneum ("pockets"), and visually normal peritoneum (lesions so small they can only be detected microscopically).

The distribution of lesions also exhibits a characteristic pattern. Solitary lesions are possible, but multiple implantations are the rule. The most common site of disease is the ovary (approximately half of all cases), follwed by the uterine cul-de-sac, uterosacral ligaments, the posterior surfaces of the uterus and broad ligament, and the remaining pelvic peritoneum. Implants may occur over the bowel, bladder, and ureters; rarely, they may erode into underlying tissue and cause blood in the stool or urine, or their associated adhesions may result in stricture and obstruction of these organs. Implants can occur deep in tissue, especially on the cervix, posterior vaginal formix, or within wounds contaminated by endometrial tissue. Very rarely, endometriosis is found distant from the pelvis, in such sites as the lung, brain, and kidney. Pleural implantations are associated with recurrent right pneumothoraces at the time of menses, termed "catamenial pneumothorax." Similarly, lesions in the central nervous system can cause catamenial seizures.

The microscopic finding that these lesions are composed of tissue histologically resembling endometrial glands and stroma gives endometriosis its name (Fig 40–2). The normal endometrial appearance is best seen in small, early lesions; with advanced disease, cyst formation, and fibrosis, the wall of the implant is lined by a monolayer of cells, if at all. Blood is present inside the cyst, and hemosiderin-laden macrophages are found in the cyst wall.

Although endometriosis resembles the uterine endometrium histologically, further assumptions about similarities between the tissues must be made with great caution. Simultaneous biopsies of implants and endometrium have found the implants often to be histologically out of phase with the uterine tissue. Also, the characteristic changes of estrogen and progesterone receptors present in endometrium across the menstrual cycle are absent in endometriosis implants. Endometriosis implants, unlike endometrium, do not respond to progesterone in vitro by the induction of 17β-hydroxysteroid dehydrogenase activity, the enzyme that in the luteal phase converts estradiol to the less potent estrone.

## Pathologic Physiology

The mechanisms by which endometriosis causes pelvic pain and infertility are only partially understood. It is generally agreed that pelvic pain occurs premenstrually in endometriosis patients. Because of this, pain from endometriosis is thought to be due to stimulation from estrogen and progesterone during the menstrual cycle; the tissue of the implant is stimulated to grow in much the same way as is the endometrium. The implants enlarge and may undergo secretory change and bleeding; however, the fibrotic tissues surrounding the implants prevent the expansion and escape of hemorrhagic fluid that occurs in the uterus. With subsequent cycles, this process repeats itself. Pain is produced by pressure and inflammation within and around the lesion, by traction on adhesions associated with the lesions, by the number of implants and their proximity to nerves and other sensitive structures, and by the mass effect of large lesions. Although this sequence of events explains

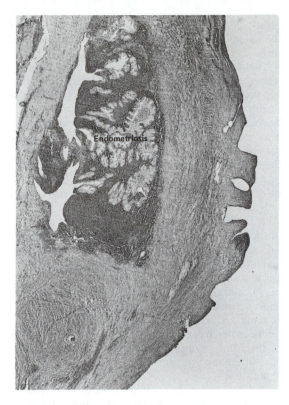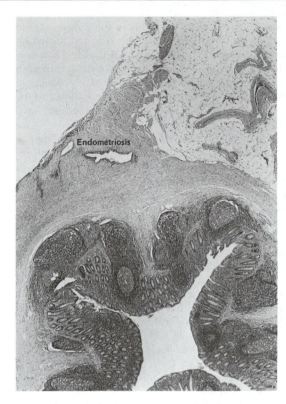

**Figure 40–2.** Histologic appearance of endometriosis. A: Endometriosis of ovary. B: Endometriosis of cervix. (Courtesy of Eugene H. Ruffolo, MD.)

why premenstrual pelvic pain can occur in endometriosis, it is incomplete, because many patients with extensive endometriosis have no pain. It is a common observation that the occurrence and severity of pain from endometriosis bear little relationship to the amount and distribution of the disease.

The relationship between endometriosis and infertility has been more extensively investigated. Moderate and severe endometriosis is associated with pelvic adhesions that distort pelvic anatomy, prevent normal tubo-ovarian apposition, and encase the ovary. Implants can destroy ovarian and tubal tissue, although occlusion of uterine tubes is rare.

It is not difficult to understand how advanced disease can result in infertility, but minimal or mild endometriosis, in which pelvic anatomy is entirely normal except for a few peritoneal surface lesions, can also cause infertility. The mechanism by which this occurs is unknown. Various theories have been proposed to explain this phenomenon.

Several investigators have examined peritoneal fluid abnormalities. The peritoneal fluid is an ultrafiltrate of plasma, with less than 5 mL normally present in the pelvis. After ovulation, a transient rise to approximately 20 mL occurs. The volume of peritoneal fluid and the concentrations of various hormones and other substances in it affect the processes of ovulation, ovum pickup, tubal function, and so on. The normal role of the peritoneal fluid and its constituents in these processes, and how it is altered by endometriosis, are largely unknown. Peritoneal fluid volume has been reported to be altered in endometriosis patients, but studies have led to inconsistent results.

Similarly, reports are contradictory as to whether endometriosis patients have elevations in peritoneal fluid prostaglandins F2 alpha and E2. Prostaglandins are normally secreted by the endometrium and by endometriosis lesions; an increase in peritoneal fluid prostaglandin levels could theoretically decrease fertility by altering ovulation, tubal motility, nidation, and luteal phase adequacy. The conflicting reports may result from fluctuations that normally occur across the cycle in prostanoid production, as well as variations in the lesions' synthesis of prostaglandins; small red petechial implants have been found to secrete more prostaglandins than larger, powder burn ones.

Several disorders of menstrual cyclicity and ovulation have been suggested as a basis for the infertility caused by mild endometriosis. The rate of anovulation among endometriosis patients is 11–27%. Nearly half become pregnant when this problem is also treated. More subtle problems in folliculogenesis in endometriosis patients have been reported, including lower serum estradiol levels, smaller follicle size during follicular growth, and lower oocyte fertilization rates and pregnancy rates in assisted reproduction. Problems with ovum pickup by the Fallopian tube and embryo implantation in the endometrium have also been suggested.

An increased incidence of luteal phase deficiency in infertile women with endometriosis has been reported by many authors, based on steroid levels in pooled midluteal serum samples, basal temperature graphs, or endometrial biopsies. More recent reports, using more stringent criteria, have been unable to confirm this association.

In the luteinized unruptured follicle syndrome (LUFS), the menstrual cycle is ovulatory by all standard criteria (temperature, serum progesterone, endometrial biopsy), but ovulation does not actually occur, and the ovum remains within the ovary. The incidence of LUFS has been reported to be significantly increased in infertile women with endometriosis. Subsequent studies in women have confirmed that LUFS does occur but is not more common in endometriosis patients. Current research indicates that LUFS is an occasional, nonrecurring event in 5–10% of normal cycles.

Immunologic phenomena have been incriminated as a cause of infertility in mild endometriosis. Serum complement levels were reported to be low, with complement present in the endometrium of endometriosis patients. Serum antibodies to endometriosis lesions and the endometrium were also noted. The immune system was postulated to attack the implants and, subsequently, normal endometrium, thus interfering with gamete transport or nidation. However, subsequent studies were unable to confirm these findings.

As noted previously, deficient cellular immunity to endometrium has been reported in endometriosis. This may also adversely effect normal nidation and other reproductive processes. Other studies have shown that the number or activity of peritoneal macrophages may be increased in endometriosis, possibly causing excessive prostaglandins to be released locally by the macrophages, sperm transport, or function to be attacked by the cells, and cytokines (inflammatory mediators including interleukin-1) to be released from pelvic lymphocytes.

Endometriosis was linked in the past to an increased incidence of spontaneous abortions; however, further studies have not supported this association.

## Clinical Findings

Endometriosis is common among women of reproductive age. Its prevalence increases to 30–40% among infertile women. Clinical findings vary greatly depending on the number, size, and extent of the lesions and on the patient population being examined.

The diagnosis of endometriosis is often strongly suspected from a patient's initial history. Infertility and pelvic pain are the cardinal symptoms. Most patients complain of constant pelvic pain or a low sacral backache that occurs premenstrually and subsides after menses begins. Dyspareunia is often present, particularly with deep penetration. Lesions involving the urinary tract or bowel may result in bloody urine or stool in the perimenstrual interval. Implantations on or near the external surfaces of the cervix, vagina, vulva, rectum, or urethra may cause pain or bleeding with defecation, urination, or intercourse at any time of the menstrual cycle. Adhesions from endometriosis may cause discomfort at any time of the cycle, and a sensation of pelvic pressure may result if large masses are present. Premenstrual spotting may occur and is more likely to be associated with endometriosis than with luteal-phase inadequacy. It must be emphasized, however, that many patients either have no symptoms or have infertility as their only symptom and that the extent of disease often has little correlation with the severity of symptoms.

The physical examination may also be helpful in discerning whether endometriosis is present. Classically, pelvic examination reveals tender nodules in the posterior vaginal fornix and pain upon uterine motion. The uterus may be fixed and retroverted due to cul-de-sac adhesions, and tender adnexal masses may be felt because of the presence of endometriomas. Careful inspection may reveal implants in healed wounds, especially episiotomy and cesarean section incisions, in the vaginal fornix, or on the cervix. Biopsy may be required to prove that the lesions are due to endometriosis. However, many patients have no abnormal findings on physical examination.

For the vast majority of patients, endometriosis is included in the differential diagnosis of infertility or pelvic pain. Endometriosis should be suspected in any patient of reproductive age complaining of pain or infertility. Medical treatment can be given for pelvic pain thought to be due to endometriosis, but the specific diagnosis of endometriosis should not be made unless documented by direct visualization. The final diagnosis of endometriosis can only be made at laparoscopy or laparotomy, by direct observation of the implants. Occasionally, an isolated endometrioma is removed, and the diagnosis must be made histologically by the demonstration of "endometrial" glands and stroma or of hemosiderin-laden macrophages in the cyst wall.

Except for special circumstances, such as urography or sigmoidoscopy for suspected bowel or urinary involvement, ancillary diagnostic studies (ultrasound, x-rays, CT scans) are of little help in diagnosis.

## Complications

True complications of endometriosis are few. Implants over the bowel or ureters may cause obstruction and silent impairment of renal function. The erosive nature of the lesions in advanced aggressive disease can cause a myriad of symptoms, depending on the tissue damaged. Endometriomas can cause ovarian torsion or can rupture and spill their irritating contents into the peritoneal cavity, resulting in a chemical peritonitis. Excision of endometriosis causing catamenial seizures or pneumothorax may be necessary.

## Differential Diagnosis

The varied presentations of endometriosis mandate that it be considered in the differential diagnosis of virtually all pelvic disease. In particular, the pain, infertility, and adhesions associated with endometriosis must be distinguished from similar symptoms accompanying pelvic inflammatory disease, pelvic tumors, and dysmenorrhea. Usually this will require operative evaluation. A patient with a persistent adnexal mass greater than 5 cm should never be presumed to have an endometrioma even if endometriosis has been diagnosed previously. Such masses require surgical diagnosis.

## Prevention

Prevention of endometriosis is not currently possible. Traditionally, women with relatives affected by endometriosis—or in whom the diagnosis has recently been made—are advised not to postpone childbearing. The merits of this advice have not been proved. Similarly, whether or not multiple maneuvers aimed at preventing menstrual reflux or soiling of the peritoneal cavity with endometrial fragments (hysterosalpingograms during menses, cervical dilatations, etc) actually decrease the risk of endometriosis is unknown. Tubal ligations close to the uterine cornua may form fistulas, and endometriosis may subsequently develop at that site; more distal ligation would prevent this complication.

The use of tampons or diaphragms has not been shown to prevent or cause endometriosis. Previously, oral contraceptives were thought to prevent further spread of endometriosis by limiting endometrial growth and diminishing the endometrium available for retrograde reflux through the uterine tubes. However, the presence of endometriosis maybe was associated with high previous estrogen exposure, such as diethylstilbestrol (DES) administration and the use of oral contraceptives containing estrogen doses greater than 50 µg. Low-dose oral contraceptives are not related to an increase in endometriosis.

## Classification

Several classification schemes to assist in describing the anatomic location and severity of endometriosis at operation have been created. Although none is entirely satisfactory, the scoring systems are useful for reporting operative findings and for comparing the results of various treatment protocols. The revised American Fertility Society classification is given in Table 40–1.

## Treatment

Treatment options are dictated by the patient's desire for future fertility, her symptoms, the stage of her disease, and to some extent her age. It must be emphasized that therapy for endometriosis requires operative inspection of the lesions for correct diagnosis and staging and to be sure that the patient's symptoms are attributable to endometriosis only.

**A: Observation:** In asymptomatic patients, those with mild discomfort, or infertile women with minimal or mild endometriosis, expectant management may be appropriate. Although endometriosis is generally felt to be a progressive disease, there is no evidence that treating an asymptomatic patient will prevent or ameliorate the onset of symptoms later. Many reports have found expectant management of infertile women with minimal or mild endometriosis to be as successful as medical or surgical therapies.

**B. Analgesic Therapy:** Analgesic treatments include nonsteroidal antiinflammatory agents and prostaglandin synthetase-inhibiting drugs. These drugs are appropriate sole therapy for endometriosis when the patient has mild premenstrual pain from minimal endometriosis, no abnormalities on pelvic examination, and no desire for immediate fertility.

**C. Pseudopregnancy:** Endometriosis is similar to the endometrium in its response to changing levels of gonadal steroids. Because the lesions of endometriosis seem to regress during pregnancy, "pseudopregnancy" hormonal therapies were developed, using either constant daily administration of a progestin or oral contraceptives. The aim of therapy is to create constant high levels of progestins, as seen in pregnancy, to thin the endometrium and cause its regression with pseudodecidual changes. Medroxyprogesterone acetate, 10–30 mg daily, is commonly given, as are continuous oral contraceptive pills (no hormone-free interval at the end of each cycle). Pseudopregnancy relieves pelvic pain in most patients, but the pregnancy rates of 20–40% associated with it are clearly inferior to other regimens. Depression, bloating, weight gain, and significant breakthrough bleeding are found with these treatments, limiting their usefulness. Currently, pseudopregnancy is best reserved for patients with milder forms of endometriosis who do not desire immediate fertility and are unable to take other treatments.

**D. Pseudomenopause:** Endometriosis is uni-

**Table 40–1.** Revised American Fertility Society classification of endometriosis, 1985[1,2]

| Endometriosis | Less Than 1 cm | 1–3 cm | More Than 3 cm |
|---|---|---|---|
| Peritoneum | | | |
| Superficial | 1 | 2 | 4 |
| Deep | 2 | 4 | 6 |
| Ovary[3] | | | |
| Superficial | 1 | 2 | 4 |
| Deep | 4 | 16 | 20 |

| | Partial | Complete |
|---|---|---|
| **Posterior cul-de-sac obliteration** | 4 | 40 |

| Adhesions | Less Than 1/3 Enclosure | 1/3–2/3 Enclosure | More Than 2/3 Enclosure |
|---|---|---|---|
| Ovary[3] | | | |
| Filmy | 1 | 2 | 4 |
| Dense | 4 | 8 | 16 |
| Uterine tube[3] | | | |
| Filmy | 1 | 2 | 4 |
| Dense | 4[4] | 8[4] | 16 |

[1]Data reproduced, with permission, from American Fertility Society: Revised classification of endometriosis: 1985. *Fertil Steril* 1985;43:351.
[2]Scoring: Stage 1 disease (minimal) = 1–5, stage 2 (mild) = 6–15, stage 3 (moderate) = 16–40, stage 4 (severe) = more than 40.
[3]Each ovary and uterine tube is scored separately.
[4]If the fimbriated end of the tube is completely enclosed, the score is 16.

versally noted to regress after bilateral oophorectomy or menopause; this forms the basis for "pseudomenopause" therapy, in which a medication attempts to reduce endogeneous estrogen and progesterone production to constant low levels. This therapy is the medical treatment of choice for endometriosis.

**1. Danazol**–The original pseudomenopause treatment is danazol, a weak androgen that is the isoxazole derivative of 17α-ethinyl testosterone (ethisterone). Danazol acts via several mechanisms to treat endometriosis. It acts at the hypothalamic level to inhibit gonadotropin release, which in turn lowers ovarian production of sex steroids and prevents ovulation. Danazol binds to androgen receptors in the endometriotic implants, directly inhibiting implant growth. In addition, danazol binds strongly to sex hormone-binding globulin and corticosteroid-binding globulin, thus displacing native testosterone and allowing it to act against the implants as well. The increased androgenic environment acts on the liver to decrease sex hormone binding globulin concentrations, freeing more androgens to be active (as well as estrogens; free estrogen levels may approach normal during danazol therapy). Danazol inhibits the steroidogenic enzymes in the ovary that synthesize estrogen. Together, these actions decrease estrogen receptor stimulation within the lesions, thus inhibiting their growth.

The dosage of danazol is 800 mg/d in divided doses for 6 months. Because of its high cost, attempts have been made to reduce this daily dosage. How-

ever, if pregnancy does not result after therapy with a lower dosage, the question remains whether the larger dosage would have been successful. Furthermore, danazol is an effective contraceptive when taken in doses of 800 mg/d; this alleviates the concern that it has been associated with virilization of a female fetus in pregnant women. Some androgen-related, anabolic side effects of danazol may be beneficial (such as preservation of bone mass), but adverse effects are common and include acne, oily skin, deepening of the voice, weight gain, edema, and adverse plasma lipoprotein changes. Most changes are reversible upon cessation of therapy, but some (such as deepening of the voice) may not be.

Interpretation of various studies using danazol to treat endometriosis is difficult; as a rule, danazol treatment seems to be superior to pseudopregnancy. Pain relief is usually impressive. In infertile patients, pregnancy rates vary with the stage of disease. In mild endometriosis, danazol treatment is probably no better than expectant management, and patients with severe disease will not see resolution of their adhesions or endometriomas from this therapy. Endometriosis symptoms usually recur several months after treatment.

**2. GnRH agonists**–Gonadotropin-releasing hormone (GnRH) agonists are congeners of the 10-amino-acid peptide hormone GnRH.

**Other hormonal therapies**–Gestrinone is an antiestrogen, antiprogesterone steroid with effects similar to those of danazol. It is not currrrently available in the USA. In the past, methyltestosterone, 5–10 mg/d, was used to decrease pain. Although this regimen was effective, androgenic side effects were prominent, and ovulation was not inhibited. If the patient became pregnant, a female fetus could become virilized.

**E. Surgical Treatment:** In women with complaints of infertility who have severe disease or adhesions or are older, conservative surgical therapy is the treatment of choice. This surgery attempts to excise or destroy all endometriotic tissue, remove all adhesions, and restore pelvic anatomy to the best possible condition. Presacral neurectomy or uterosacral ligament ablation to relieve pain and a uterine suspension procedure may be performed as required, although the efficacies of these treatments are controversial. Conservative surgery has traditionally been performed at laparotomy, but a laparoscopic approach is associated with a shorter hospital stay and less morbidity, and it may be more cost-effective. This is particularly true in contemporary practice, where this therapy is usually performed at the time of the initial, diagnostic laparoscopy. Reported pregnancy rates following conservative surgery are inversely proportionate to the severity of the disease and vary greatly. In counseling patients, approximate pregnancy rates of 75% for mild disease, 50–60% for moderate disease, and 30–40% for severe disease should be quoted; however, individualization of therapy is stressed.

If the patient does not desire future childbearing and has severe disease or symptoms, definitive surgery is appropriate and often curative. This entails total abdominal hysterectomy, bilateral salpingo-oophorectomy, and excision of remaining adhesions or implantations. If endometriosis remains after excision, postoperative medical therapy may be indicated. After this or after complete excision, hormone replacement therapy is indicated. Estrogen-progestin therapy may be used without reactivating the endometriosis, but individualization of therapy is required.

**F. Assisted Reproduction:** Infertile women with endometriosis who are older, or who have failed other therapies for infertility, can undergo assisted reproduction (in vitro fertilization, gamete intra-fallopian transfer, etc) with success rates similar to those seen in women with other diagnoses. The relatively short time required with this option may make it the mose efficacious of all infertility therapies for endometriosis. Women with more severe disease have decreased success.

**Prognosis**

Proper counseling of patients with endometriosis requires attention to several aspects of the disorder. Of primary importance is the initial operative staging of the disease to obtain adequate information on which to base future decisions about therapy. The patient's symptoms and desire for childbearing dictate appropriate therapy. Most patients can be told that they will be able to obtain significant relief from pelvic pain and that treatment will assist them in achieving pregnancy.

Long-term concerns must be more guarded in that all current therapies offer relief but not cure. Even after definitive surgery, endometriosis may recur, but the risk is very low (about 3%). The risk of recurrence is not significantly increased by estrogen replacement therapy. After conservative surgery, reported recurrence rates vary greatly but usually exceed 10% in 3 years and 35% in 5 years. Pregnancy delays but does not preclude recurrence. Recurrence rates after medical treatment also vary and are similar to or higher than those reported following surgical treatment.

Although many patients are concerned that endometriosis will progress inexorably, experience has been that conservative surgery avoids the necessity for hysterectomy in the great majority of cases. The course of endometriosis in any individual is impossible to predict at present, and future treatment options should greatly improve what can now be offered.

## REFERENCES

### EPIDEMIOLOGY

Cramer DW et al: The relation of endometriosis to menstrual characteristics, smoking, and exercise. JAMA 1985;225:1904.

Wheeler JM: Epidemiology and prevalence of endometriosis. Infertil Reprod Med Clin N Amer 1992;3:545.

### PATHOGENESIS

Coxhead D, Thomas EJ: Familial inheritance of endometriosis in a British population: A case control study. J Obstet Gynaecol 1993;13:42.

Oosterlynck DJ et al: Immunosuppressive activity of peritoneal fluid in women with endometriosis. Obstet Gynecol 1993;82:206.

Ramey JW, Archer DF: Peritoneal fluid: Its relevance to the development of endometriosis. Fertil Steril 1993; 60:1.

### PATHOLOGY

Bergqvist A, Ferno M: Estrogen and progesterone receptors in endometriotic tissue and edometrium: Comparison according to localization and recurrence. Fertil Steril 1993;60:63.

Murphy AA et al: Unsuspected endometriosis documented by scanning electron microscopy in visually normal peritoneum. Fertil Steril 1986;46:52.

## PATHOLOGIC PHYSIOLOGY

Pittaway DE, Ellington CP, Klimek M: Preclinical abortions and endometriosis. Fertil Steril 1988;49:221.

Rodrigues-Escudero FJ et al: Does minimal endometriosis reduce fecundity? Fertil Steril 1988;50:522.

Steele RW, Dmowski WP, Marmer DJ: Deficient cellular immunity in endometriosis. Am J Reprod Immunol 1984;6:33.

Switchenko AC, Kauffman RS, Becker A: Are there endometrial antibodies in sera of women with endometriosis? Fertil Steril 1991;56:235.

Syrop CH, Halme J: Peritoneal fluid environment and infertility. Fertil Steril 1987;48:1.

## CLINICAL FINDINGS

Fedele L et al: Pain symptoms associated with endometriosis. Obstet Gynecol 1992;79:767.

## COMPLICATIONS

Schorlemmer GR, Battaglini JW: Pneumothorax in menstruating females. Contemp Furg 1982;20:53.

Zwas FR, Lyon DT: Endometriosis: An important condition in clinical gastroenterology. Dig Dis Sci 1991;36:353.

## CLASSIFICATION

American Fertility Society: Revised classification of endometriosis: 1985/ Fertil Steril 1985;43:351.

## TREATMENT

Barbieri RL: Hormonal treatment of endometriosis: The estrogen threshold hypothesis. Am J Obstet Gynecol 1992;166:740.

Barbieri RL, Ryan KJ: Danazol: Endocrine pharmacology and therapeutic applications. Am J Obstet Gynecol 1981;141:453.

Cook AS, Rock JA: The role of laparoscopy in the treatment of endometriosis. Fertil Steril 1991;55:663.

Coronado C et al: Surgical treatment of symptomatic colorectal endometriosis. Fertil Steril 1990;53:411.

Dlugi AM, Miller JD, Knittle J: Lupron depot (leuprolide acetate for depot suspension) in the treatment of endometriosis: A randomized placebo-controlled, double blind study. Fertil Steril 1990;54:419.

Henzl MR et al: Administration of nasal nafarelin as compared with oral danazol for endometriosis: A multicenter double-blind comparative trial. N Engl J Med 19888;318:485.

Krasnow JS, Berga SL: Endometriosis and gamete intrafallopian transfer. Assisted Reprod Rev 1993;3:121.

Luciano AA, Turksoy RN, Carleo J: Evaluation of oral medroxyprogesterone acetate in the treatment of endometriosis. Obstet Gynecol 1988;72:323.

Maouris P: Asymptomatic mild endometriosis in infertile women: The case for expectant management. Obstet Hynecol Surv 1991;46:548.

Surrey ES et al: The effects of combining norethindrone with a gonadotropin-releasing hormone agonist in the treatment of symptomatic endometriosis. Fertil Steril 1990;53:620.

# Relaxation of Pelvic Supports

# 41

*Clyde H. Dorr, II, MD*

## CYSTOCELE & URETHROCELE

### Essentials of Diagnosis

- Sensation of vaginal fullness, pressure, "falling out."
- Feeling of incomplete emptying of the bladder, often stress incontinence, urinary frequency; perhaps a need to push the bladder up in order to void.
- Presence of a soft, reducible mass bulging into the anterior vagina and distending the vaginal introitus.
- With straining or coughing, increased bulging and descent of the anterior vaginal wall and urethra.

### General Considerations

Defects in the pelvic supporting structures result in a variety of clinically evident pelvic relaxation abnormalities. Pelvic supportive defects may be classified according to their anatomic location.

**Sheath defects**
Midline defects
Precervical superior vesicovaginal fascial avulsions
Postcervical superior colporectovaginal fascial avulsions
Midurethral transverse fascial defects
**Paravaginal defects**
Paraurethral defects
Paravesical defects
Pararectal defects
**Lateral vaginal defects**
Lateral vesicovaginal defects
Lateral rectovaginal defects (both corrected by using paravaginal repair as are the paravaginal defects)
**Perineal defects**
Midline defects
Sulcal defects (repair affected primarily by musculofascial reapproximation for both)

Better understanding of the pathophysiology of the pelvic supportive defects, their causes, and clinical presentations allows the individualization of the therapy most likely to successfully affect long-term therapy for each patient.

Cystocele, descent of a portion of the posterior bladder wall and trigone into the vagina, is usually due to the trauma of parturition. The stretching, attenuation, or actual laceration of the so-called pubovesicocervical fascia produced by the birth of a large baby, multiple or operative deliveries, and prolonged labors increase the possibility and degree of cystocele (Figs 41–1 and 41–2). Urethrocele (sagging of the urethra) is commonly associated with cystocele, often in women who have urinary stress incontinence. However, urethrocele is not a cause of urinary incontinence (see Chapter 42, "Gynecologic Urology"). Sagging of the urethra is the result of the shearing effect of the fetal head on the urethra and its attachments beneath the symphysis pubica—an occurrence that appears to be more common in women with wide gynecoid subpubic arches. A narrow android subpubic arch displaces the fetal head posteriorly, providing a measure of protection to the anterior vaginal wall and the urethra.

Cystourethrocele (simultaneous occurrence of cystocele and urethrocele) may occur in nulliparous women, apparently as a result of congenital inadequacy of the endopelvic connective tissues or fascia and of the musculature of the pelvic floor.

Although a degree of cystourethrocele is demonstrable in virtually all parous women during childbearing years, the condition may not progress and may cause no symptoms. Treatment in such cases is not usually required until after the menopause, when the pelvic fascial and muscular supports become attenuated by slowly progressive involutional changes.

### Clinical Findings

**A. Symptoms:** A small cystocele causes no significant symptoms, and in many cases fairly large ones cause no noteworthy complaints. A cystocele may be large enough to bulge out of the vaginal introitus, and the patient may complain of vaginal pressure or a protruding mass that gives her the feeling that she is "sitting on a ball." Symptoms are aggravated by vigorous activity, prolonged standing, coughing, sneezing, or straining. Relief can be obtained by rest and by assuming a recumbent or prone position.

Although urinary incontinence is the most com-

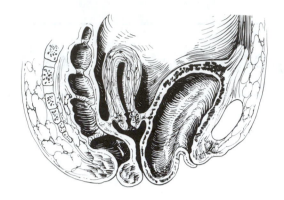

**Figure 41–1.** Cystocele.

mon and most important symptom associated with cystocele, this disorder as such does not cause incontinence, and its repair does not correct stress incontinence. Stress incontinence is the result of relaxation of the musculofascial supporting tissues of the urethra. Unless special attention is directed to the urethral supports, operative correction of a large cystocele may cause rather than correct stress incontinence.

The vaginal pressure of a cystocele may be interpreted as incomplete bladder emptying and thus may lead to frequent efforts to empty the bladder. This has given rise to the popular misconception that cystocele is commonly responsible for large volumes of residual urine with accompanying problems of cystitis, trigonitis, urethritis, urinary urgency and frequency, and dysuria. It is true that a large cystocele projecting well outside the introitus is responsible for significant residual urine. This could lead to bladder infection and symptoms of inflammation. However, many patients in this category have learned through experi-

ence that complete bladder emptying can be achieved either by voiding again after several minutes ("double voiding") or by manually reducing the cystocele into the vagina prior to voiding. Unless the patient has significant volumes of residual urine, as demonstrated by catheterization, cystocele operations performed primarily to relieve symptoms of chronic inflammation of the urinary tract (ie, urgency, frequency, dysuria, chronic cystitis) will be unsuccessful.

**B. Signs:** Examination of the patient with cystocele (preferably with a full bladder) reveals a relaxed vaginal outlet with a thin-walled, rather smooth, bulging mass involving the anterior vaginal wall below the cervix. When the perineum is depressed and the patient is asked to strain, the mass descends and, depending on the degree of relaxation, distends or projects through the vaginal introitus. When there is an associated urethrocele, a downward and forward rotational "sliding" of the urethra and its external meatus is noted; asking the patient with a partially filled bladder to cough while straining may demonstrate stress incontinence of urine.

**C. Laboratory Findings:** (See also Chapter 42.) Examination of a catheterized urine specimen may reveal evidence of infection. The volume of residual urine should be determined by catheterization after voiding. Unless the patient has a significant volume of residual urine, the cystocele probably is not responsible for urinary tract infection. Any urinary tract infection requires complete investigation prior to correction of the cystocele.

**D. X-Ray Findings:** If the cystocele is associated with urethrocele, stress incontinence, or symptoms suggestive of chronic urinary tract infection, x-ray study can be helpful. Cystoscopy and urethroscopy, especially when the bladder has been filled with $CO_2$, can be helpful in diagnosis. With contrast medium in the bladder and perhaps a metal bead chain in the urethra, anteroposterior and especially lateral views may demonstrate the cystocele (descent of the bladder base and trigone) and loss of the normal posterior urethrovesical angle.

Cinefluorography (without the bead chain) while voiding may reveal a patulous (funneled) proximal urethra, perhaps an occult diverticulum of the urethra or bladder, or other anomaly as a cause of urinary tract infection.

Ceptometrics should be performed in all patients with urinary incontinence. Video urethroscopy and urinary dynamics studies should be performed when appropriate (See Chapter 42, "Gynecologic Urology").

### Differential Diagnosis

Tumors of the urethra and bladder are much more indurated and fixed than cystoceles.

A large urethral diverticulum may look and feel like a cystocele but usually is more lateral, sensitive,

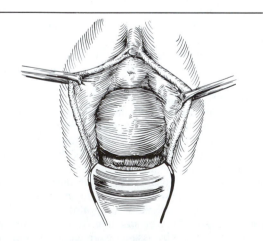

**Figure 41–2.** Cystocele.

and painful; compression, as a rule, will express some purulent material from the urethral meatus.

A true bladder diverticulum is rare in the trigonal portion of the bladder. The diverticulum may appear somewhat asymmetric. Without cystoscopic or cinefluorographic study, it may go undetected.

Enterocele of the anterior vaginal wall (see later in chapter), although rare, may occur in patients who have had a hysterectomy. It can be distinguished from a cystocele by identifying the loops of intestine contained in the hernial sac. Enterocele can be demonstrated by inserting a probe into the bladder; by vaginal palpation over the tip of the probe, one can detect the unusually thick anterior vaginal wall and perhaps note intestinal crepitation. This maneuver may also be helpful in differentiating the anterior vaginal mass produced by a previous interposition operation that interposed the uterine fundus (or just the uterine isthmus) between the bladder and the vaginal wall.

## Complications

A large cystocele, perhaps in association with uterine prolapse, may lead to acute urinary retention. Recurrent urinary tract infection may occur in patients in whom bladder emptying is incomplete.

## Prevention

Intrapartum and postpartum exercises, especially those designed to strengthen the levator and perineal muscle groups (Kegel), often help improve or maintain pelvic support. Obesity, chronic cough, straining, and traumatic deliveries must be corrected or avoided. Estrogen therapy following the menopause helps to maintain the tone of pelvic musculofascial tissues and thereby prevent or postpone the appearance of cystocele and other forms of relaxation.

## Treatment

**A. Medical Measures:** The patient with a small or moderate-sized cystocele requires reassurance that the pressure symptoms are not the result of a serious condition and that, even though the relaxation may progress slowly over several years, no serious illness will result. With this conservative approach, surgical correction of a cystocele is rarely indicated in a woman in her childbearing years who may still wish to have children. If the young woman does present with significant symptoms related to the cystocele—or with a disturbing degree of urinary incontinence—temporary medical measures may provide adequate relief until she has had all the babies she wants, whereupon a definitive operative procedure can be accomplished.

**1. Pessary–**A vaginal pessary (Smith-Hodge, ball, bee cell), or even a tampon in the lower part of the vagina, may provide adequate temporary support of the bladder and urethra and good urinary control. For the elderly patient with complicating medical factors who is therefore a poor operative risk, the temporary use of a vaginal pessary may provide relief of symptoms until her general condition has improved.

Prolonged use of pessaries, despite the utmost care, eventually leads to pressure necrosis and vaginal ulceration.

**2. Exercises–**In younger patients, some improvement of pressure symptoms and of urinary control may be obtained by using Kegel isometric exercises for 6–12 months to tighten and strengthen the pubococcygeus muscles. Objective evidence of improved support of the pelvic floor may be noted. Kegel exercises can be of greatest benefit when used prophylactically, beginning in pregnancy and continuing during and after the puerperium. In older patients, Kegel exercises rarely provide more than partial relief.

**3. Estrogens–**In postmenopausal women, estrogen replacement therapy (conjugated estrogens) for a number of months may greatly improve the tone, quality, and vascularity of the musculofascial supports. Nevertheless, one cannot expect that severe anatomic injury (large cystocele with associated stress incontinence) will be corrected by medical measures.

**B. Surgical Measures:** Cystocele alone (without concomitant uterine prolapse, rectocele, or enterocele) rarely becomes large enough or causes symptoms that require operative correction. It is only when the cystocele is large, when it is responsible for urine retention and recurrent bladder infections, or when it is associated with bladder and urethral changes responsible for stress incontinence that operative repair is required.

Anterior vaginal colporrhaphy is the most effective surgical treatment for cystocele (Fig 41–3). This is often combined with vaginal hysterectomy and posterior colpoperineorrhaphy because, ordinarily, the cystocele represents only one component of a generalized relaxation of urogenital musculofascial supporting tissues. In preventing further pregnancies, hysterectomy also averts the problem of vaginal delivery, which would destroy the bladder support provided by the anterior colporrhaphy.

Obliterative vaginal operations (vaginectomy, Le Fort's operation) may effectively correct a cystocele (Fig 41–4). Unfortunately, operations of this type may not correct associated stress incontinence; in fact, traction produced by the obliterating scar tissue under the bladder neck and the urethra may actually cause or aggravate stress incontinence.

Similarly, transabdominal repair of the cystocele (along with total abdominal hysterectomy) may be elected to correct the cystocele. When an abdominal approach is essential for other pelvic conditions, however, a retropubic urethrovesical suspension (Burch/Marshall-Marchetti-Krantz) can be combined with abdominal cystocele repair to correct or prevent the development of stress incontinence.

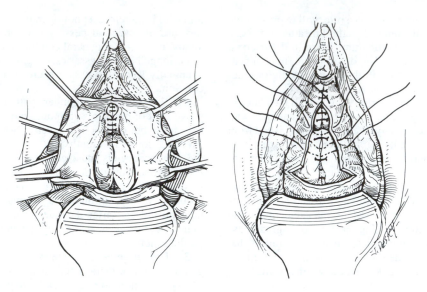

**Figure 41–3.** Repair of cystocele and plication of urethra for correction of stress incontinence of urine.

## Prognosis

The prognosis after anterior colporrhaphy is excellent in the absence of a subsequent pregnancy or comparable factors (eg, constipation, obesity, large pelvic tumors, bronchitis, bronchiectasis, heavy manual labor) that increase intra-abdominal pressure. Recurrence of the cystocele after anterior colporrhaphy is rather common when a generalized relaxation of pelvic supports has been overlooked or ignored; in such cases, subsequent progression of uterine prolapse, enterocele, and rectocele leads to disruption of the cystocele repair.

## Vaginal Defects & Cystocele

It was previously stated that colporrhaphy is the most effective surgical treatment for cystocele. For decades, anterior colporrhaphy (midline plication) has remained the traditional method of cystocele repair. Rediscovery of paravaginal defects has led to work during the past 2 decades that has greatly increased our understanding of pelvic relaxation, including cystocele.

Cystocele may be associated with midline, lateral, and superior (vesicovaginal) fascial or supportive defects (Fig 41–5). These defects may occur alone or in combination. The reason anterior colporrhaphy has been reasonably successful is because midline defects are so common. Other defects, if present, must be identified and repaired. Lateral (paravaginal) defects are also common, occur in combination with midline defects, and are frequently associated with superior vesicovaginal fascial defects. Cystoceles caused by paravaginal defects may need to be repaired transabdominally (paravaginal repair). Those

with a combination of defects require a combined surgical approach. To repair only a midline defect and leave paravaginal and/or superior vesicovaginal defects unrepaired does not restore normal anatomy and may lead to recurrence of cystocele.

Cystoceles are classified as either anterior or posterior, according to their position in relation to the interureteric ridge. Descent anterior to the interureteric ridge is called an **anterior cystocele**; descent posterior to the ridge is called a **posterior cystocele.** Anterior cystoceles are usually associated with rotational descent of the bladder neck and are often associated with stress urinary incontinence. Posterior cystocele may be of the **distention type** (intrinsic damage to the vaginal wall), the **displacement type** (damage to lateral fascial and muscular supports outside the vagina), or a combination of the 2 types. Appropriate understanding of all defects involved is clearly necessary to plan the proper corrective surgical approach.

## RECTOCELE

### Essentials of Diagnosis

- Difficult evacuation of feces.
- Sensation of vaginal fullness ("falling out" pressure).
- Presence of a soft, reducible mass bulging into the lower half of the posterior vaginal wall; frequently a flat, lacerated perineal body.

### General Considerations

Rectocele is a rectovaginal hernia caused by dis-

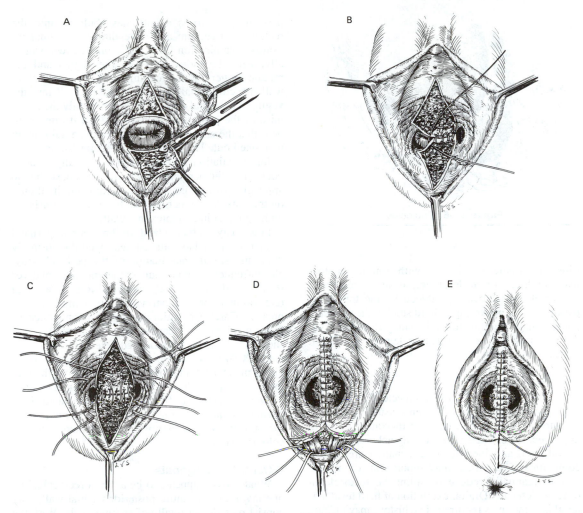

**Figure 41–4.** Goodall-Power modification of Le Fort's operation.

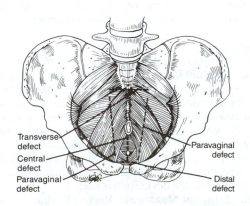

**Figure 41–5.** Four areas in which pubocervical fascia can break or separate—the four defects.

ruption, during childbirth, of the fibrous connective tissue (rectovaginal fascia) between the rectum and the vagina (Figs 41–6 and 41–7). Some degree of damage always occurs during delivery—particularly of a large fetus or one presenting by the breech—and during multiple delivery. Early and adequate episiotomy reduces the amount of damage done to rectovaginal fascia and to perineal muscles by the presenting part.

Even though all multiparas have some degree of rectocele, the condition may not become manifest until the woman has passed the childbearing years and frequently not until several years after the menopause. This manifestation is due to the slowly progressive involutional changes in the pelvic musculofascial supporting tissues.

In addition to parturition and the inherent tone and quality of the patient's tissues, bowel habits may be an important factor in the development of rectocele.

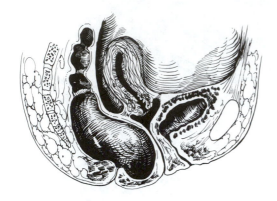

**Figure 41–6.** Rectocele.

Lifelong chronic constipation with straining at stool may produce—or at least aggravate—a rectocele; conversely, a rectocele produced by the trauma of parturition, by pocketing of hard stool in the rectocele pouch, may "aggravate" mismanaged bowel syndrome. Thus, the cause of rectocele may be difficult to distinguish from the effect of rectocele.

## Clinical Findings

**A. Symptoms:** A small rectocele, demonstrable in virtually all multiparous patients, usually causes no symptoms. With more extensive relaxation (ie, with larger rectoceles), sensations of vaginal pressure, rectal fullness, and incomplete evacuation are typical complaints. The patient may report that it is necessary to manually reduce or splint the rectocele in order to defecate. Digital extraction of hard fecal material is sometimes required. The history may include prolonged, excessive use of laxatives or frequent enemas.

**B. Signs:** Inspection of the area, with the patient straining and perhaps with slight depression of the

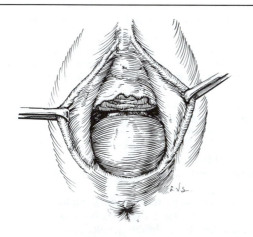

**Figure 41–7.** Rectocele.

perineum, discloses a soft mass bulging into the rectovaginal septum and distending the vaginal introitus. Examination (best accomplished rectovaginally, with the index finger in the vagina and the middle finger in the rectum) reveals a soft, thin-walled rectovaginal septum projecting well into the vagina. The septal defect may involve only the lower third of the posterior vaginal wall, but it often happens that the entire length of the rectovaginal septum is thinned out. The finger in the rectum confirms anterior sacculation into the vagina. Actually, a deep pocket into the perineal body may be noted, so that on apposition of the finger in the rectum and the thumb on the outside, the perineal body seems to consist of nothing but skin and intestinal wall.

Previously unrecognized or unrepaired perineal lacerations may have almost destroyed the normally thick and strong musculature of the perineal body. Not infrequently, this traumatic attenuation involves some or all of the anal sphincter. Rarely, a small rectovaginal (or rectoperineal) fistula may also be present. Careful questioning about incontinence of feces or flatus and careful inspection of the area should disclose these associated defects.

**C. X-Ray Findings:** Although lateral x-ray views made after a barium enema will show the rectocele, this procedure is not essential for diagnosis. However, rectocele frequently is associated with "hemorrhoidal bleeding"; when this occurs, proctoscopic study is necessary to exclude a concomitant colonic lesion.

## Differential Diagnosis

What grossly appears to be a "high rectocele," ie, one involving the entire posterior vaginal wall, may consist partially or totally of an enterocele. With the patient standing, straining, and squatting slightly, rectovaginal examination will confirm the presence of abdominal contents sliding into the enterocele sac, and bowel crepitation may be noted.

Digital examination will also disclose tumors of the rectovaginal septum (lipomas, fibromas, sarcomas) that may produce a classic rectocele appearance.

## Treatment

Fecal impaction may require digital extraction.

**A. Medical Measures:** Medical management of a symptomatic rectocele is usually advisable until the patient has completed her family. Increased fluid intake and correction of faulty diet and bowel habits may be beneficial. Laxatives and rectal suppositories may be required. As a temporary measure, a large vaginal pessary of the round ball or inflatable doughnut type may provide relief if the perineum is adequate to retain the device in the vagina.

**B. Surgical Measures:** Rectocele alone (without associated enterocele, uterine prolapse, and cystocele) seldom requires surgical management. However, when the rectocele becomes so large that fecal evacuation is difficult, or the patient finds it necessary to manually reduce the rectocele into the vagina to expedite expulsion of feces, or the rectocele protrudes enough to cause discomfort or tissue breakdown, surgical repair is indicated (Fig 41–8).

Posterior colpoperineorrhaphy is usually curative. The posterior midline incision includes the perineum and the posterior vaginal wall, and it must be extended high enough to enable the surgeon to rule out the presence of an enterocele. For the latter purpose, it is frequently necessary to extend the dissection of the rectovaginal septum up to the level of the posterior vaginal fornix and to open the cul-de-sac of the peritoneum. Adequate repair includes plication of the rectovaginal fascia, excision of the redundancy of the posterior vaginal wall, and midline approximation of the levator and perineal muscles. However, over-zealous perineorrhaphy should be avoided if preservation of sexual function is desirable.

Postoperative avoidance of straining, coughing, and strenuous activity is advisable. Careful instruction about diet to avoid constipation, about intake of fluids, and about the use of stool-softening laxatives and lubricating suppositories is necessary to ensure permanent integrity of the rectocele repair.

### Prognosis

Recurrence of rectocele after adequate colpoperineorrhaphy is uncommon if chronic constipation has been corrected, subsequent vaginal delivery is

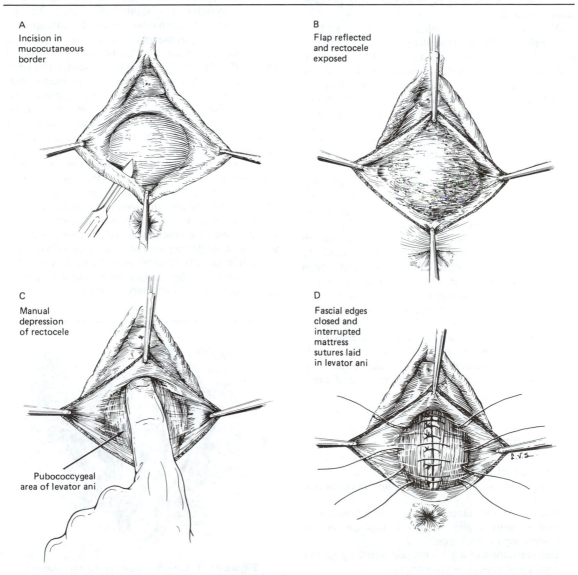

**Figure 41–8.** Repair of rectocele.

avoided, and a concomitant enterocele and uterine prolapse have not been overlooked.

## Vaginal Defects & Rectocele

As with the anterior vaginal wall, defects may occur in the posterior vaginal wall and its supports. Three basic types of damage have been described:

1. Damage to the vaginal wall itself, probably secondary to overdistention at childbirth.

2. Stretching of the lateral attachments of the vagina to the pelvic side wall, probably secondary to increased intra-abdominal pressure or as a result of certain forces during labor and birth.

3. Tearing, as well as stretching, of the lateral attachments of the vagina to the pelvic side wall.

Each of these types of damage may exist alone or in combination and may be associated with perineal defects as well.

Rectoceles may be further categorized as **low, midvaginal,** or **high,** depending on where the defect occurs in the posterior vaginal wall. Defects in the perineum, which may be associated with posterior vaginal wall defects, must also be recognized and repaired appropriately, since this adds considerable support to the lower anterior vaginal wall and urethra.

Additionally, levator ani defects leading to the **perineal descent syndrome** have been described. These defects are felt by some to constitute a major problem in disorders of the pelvic floor.

Clinically, perineal descent is associated with difficulty with defecation, rectal discharge and bleeding, deep perineal pain, and sometimes, rectal prolapse. Patients may complain that they feel as if they are "sitting on a ball." Eventually this defect may lead to neuropathy and anal incontinence. A levatorplasty has been devised for repair of this defect. It has been used as an adjunct to pelvic floor reconstruction with good results. The procedure has also been used for patients with anal incontinence with some success.

Although perineal descent is not present in every patient who has a rectocele, when it is present, it must be recognized and repaired if normal anatomy is to be restored. It should not be assumed that all difficulty with defecation is due to the presence of a rectocele.

## ENTEROCELE

### Essentials of Diagnosis

• Uncomfortable pressure and a falling-out sensation in the vagina.

• Associated with uterine prolapse or subsequent to hysterectomy in any age group; most common in postmenopausal women.

• Demonstration of a mass bulging into the posterior fornix and upper posterior vaginal wall.

## General Considerations

Enterocele is a herniation of the rectouterine pouch (pouch of Douglas) into the rectovaginal septum (Fig 41–9). This presents as a bulging mass in the posterior fornix and upper posterior vaginal wall. A similar hernial sac through the cul-de-sac, but extending posteriorly, may present through the anal canal as a rectal prolapse. Extremely large cul-de-sac hernias may present in both directions—anteriorly as an enterocele extending out through the vaginal introitus and posteriorly as a rectal prolapse out through the anal canal, creating a "saddle hernia" on both sides of the perineal body.

Enterocele may be congenital or acquired; the latter is much more common. The congenital form rarely causes symptoms. Enterocele does not appear to progress in size, and its discovery is usually incidental to hysterectomy or other procedures. The acquired form of enterocele occurs in multiparous menopausal or postmenopausal women and almost invariably is associated with other manifestations of musculofascial weakness such as uterine prolapse, cystocele, and rectocele. The trauma of many pregnancies and vaginal deliveries (perhaps breech extractions, forceps rotations), large pelvic tumors, marked obesity, ascites, chronic bronchitis, and other factors that increase intra-abdominal pressure are of etiologic importance.

Uterine prolapse is almost always accompanied by some degree of enterocele, and, as the degree of uterine descent progresses, the size of the hernial sac increases. Similarly, posthysterectomy prolapse of the vaginal vault (in a sense, an incisional hernia) usually is the result of a potential or actual enterocele that was overlooked (not repaired) at the time of hysterectomy. Rarely, after hysterectomy, the enterocele is located anterior to the vaginal vault, where it may be easily confused with ordinary cystocele.

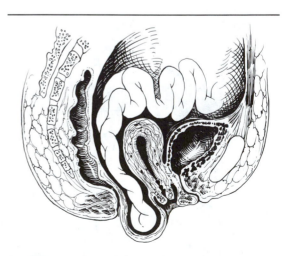

**Figure 41–9.** Enterocele and prolapsed uterus.

## Clinical Findings

**A. Symptoms:** The pelvic and abdominal symptoms produced by an enterocele are nonspecific and perhaps are actually the result of downward traction of the lower abdominal viscera. Aching discomfort frequently is described, along with the sensation of vaginal pressure and fullness commonly noted with other forms of prolapse. Gastrointestinal symptoms can rarely, if ever, be attributed to an enterocele. Peculiarly, the small bowel almost never becomes adherent to or incarcerated in the enterocele—not even in the tight-necked hernial sac that is characteristic of the congenital type of enterocele. This effect does not apply to the thin-walled posthysterectomy enteroceles (vaginal vault prolapse), many of which contain adherent small intestine and some of which produce obstructive symptoms and even (rarely) rupture spontaneously to eviscerate through the vagina.

**B. Signs:** Rectovaginal examination, especially with the patient standing, reveals a reducible thickness or bulging of the upper rectovaginal septum. After exposing the entire posterior vaginal wall (by elevating the anterior vaginal wall and cervix with a Sims retractor or a single blade of a vaginal speculum) and inserting a finger in the rectum to delineate the extent of the rectocele, one frequently can observe gradual filling and distention of the enterocele sac as the patient "strains down." With similar exposure of the posterior vaginal wall, failure of a proctoscopic light source to transilluminate the upper rectovaginal septum may suggest the presence of an enterocele. In the case of a large, thin-walled enterocele, small bowel peristalsis will be visible. Occasionally, to obtain filling of the hernial sac, it is essential to examine the patient in a standing-straining position.

**C. X-Ray Findings:** Lateral pelvic x-ray views obtained during barium studies of the small bowel may reveal prolapse of the ileum into the enterocele.

## Differential Diagnosis

High rectocele and cystocele (when an anterior enterocele is suspected) are the most common causes of difficulty in differential diagnosis. Careful examination and palpation of the region (previously described) will delineate these conditions.

Soft tumors (lipoma, leiomyoma, sarcoma) of the upper rectovaginal septum are more fixed and are nonreducible.

In obese women, a downward sliding of rectosigmoid and perirectal fatty tissues may occur. This may almost exactly mimic an enterocele and may be distinguished only at operation, when the cul-de-sac of the peritoneum is found to be in a normal position, without herniation.

## Prevention

Neglected, obstructed labor and traumatic delivery, which weaken uterovaginal supports, should be avoided. Factors that increase intra-abdominal pressure (obesity, chronic cough, straining, ascites, large pelvic tumors) should be corrected promptly. At hysterectomy (abdominal or vaginal), a diligent effort must be made to detect and repair any potential or actual enterocele. (See Chapter 44.)

## Treatment

**A. Emergency Measures:** With complete eversion of the vagina by the enterocele, trophic ulceration, edema, and fibrosis of the vaginal walls may occur to such a degree that the prolapsing mass cannot be reduced. Rest in bed (with the foot of the bed elevated) and wet packs applied to the vagina will reduce edema and allow replacement of the vagina, and vaginal packing can be used to maintain reduction until local conditions permit operative correction.

Rupture of the enterocele, with evisceration of the small intestine, is managed best by prompt reduction of the prolapsing loops of small intestine followed by simple closure of the tear in the vaginal wall. Rest in bed, prophylactic broad-spectrum antibiotics, and a supporting vaginal pack (or pessary, if it can be retained) should be instituted postoperatively. Definitive repair of the ruptured enterocele can be accomplished immediately if the patient's general condition warrants. If the prolapsing bowel has become gangrenous, operation should be limited to resection of the involved segment of the bowel—in other words, definitive repair of the enterocele should be deferred until the patient's condition is less precarious.

**B. Medical Measures:** Many patients with large enteroceles are elderly; others are grossly obese. While the patient's general health is being improved, the prolapsing vaginal hernia can be reduced with a pessary if it can be retained. Occasionally, packing the reduced vagina with cotton tampons or gauze impregnated with medicaments (bacteriostatic, estrogenic) is more effective than using a pessary. If immediate operative correction is not essential, a rigorous program of weight reduction for several months may be extremely beneficial for the very obese patient and may increase her chances of eventually obtaining a successful repair.

**C. Surgical Measures:** Enterocele repair may be accomplished transabdominally or transvaginally. In the abdominal operation, the enterocele sac is obliterated and the uterosacral ligaments and endopelvic fascia are approximated with concentric purse-string sutures as described by Moschowitz (Fig 41–10). However, inasmuch as symptomatic enterocele almost invariably is associated with other forms of musculofascial weakness (uterine prolapse, cystocele, rectocele), a transvaginal operation may provide the best route of repair and offer the greatest likelihood of permanent correction of the enterocele. This procedure includes excision and high ligation of the enterocele sac (a cardinal principle of any hernia repair) and approximation of the uterosacral ligaments and endopelvic fascia anterior to the rectum

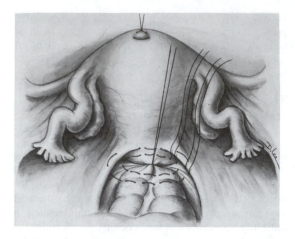

**Figure 41–10.** Transabdominal correction of enterocele (Reproduced with permission, from Moschowitz AV: The pathogenesis, anatomy, and cure of prolapse of the rectum. Surg Gynecol Obstet 1992;15:7

**Table 41–1.** Results after 197 operations for posthysterectomy enterocele and vaginal vault prolapse.

| Operation | No. of Patients | Result | | | Follow-up | |
| | | Good | Fair | Poor | Lost | > 5 Yr |
|---|---|---|---|---|---|---|
| Abdominal (presacral suspension) | 11 | 9 | 0 | 1 | 1 | 7 |
| Combined vaginal and abdominal | 6 | 6 | 0 | 0 | 0 | 4 |
| Vaginal | 180* | 142 | 9 | 9* | 20 | 128 |
| Total | 197 | 157† | 9 | 10 | 21 | 139 |

Reproduced, with permission, from Symmonds RE et al: Posthysterectomy enterocele and vaginal vault prolapse. Am J Obstet Gynecol 1981;140:852.
*A second operation was successful in 7 patients.
†Operation was successful in 89% of those with follow-up.

(floor of cul-de-sac). Concomitant vaginal hysterectomy, anterior (cystocele) and posterior (rectocele) colporrhaphy, and perineorrhaphy greatly augment the support.

Posthysterectomy enterocele with prolapse of the vaginal vault is also best managed by the transvaginal route (Table 41–1). This procedure makes use of the same supporting tissue commonly used in ordinary vaginal hysterectomy and anteroposterior colporrhaphy (Figs 41–11 and 41–12).

Sometimes—not often—it is necessary to accomplish suspension of the prolapsing vaginal vault. This may be accomplished transvaginally or transabdominally. Because the normal vaginal axis is directed some distance posteriorly (almost horizontally when the patient is in an erect position), operative correction by any means, whether by the vaginal or the abdominal route, should restore a normal vaginal axis. This is accomplished by suspension of the vaginal apex far back on the uterosacral ligaments, the presacral fascia, or the sacrospinous ligaments. The suspension can be provided by use of nonabsorbable sutures, autogenous fascia, or prosthetic material (eg, Dacron, Teflon, or Marlex mesh). Techniques that suspend the vaginal vault from the anterior abdomi-

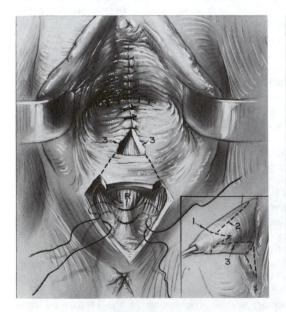

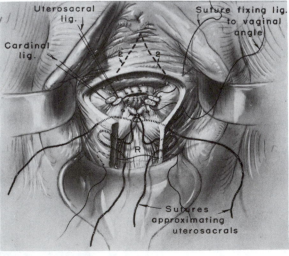

**Figure 41–11.** Correction of vaginal prolapse after hysterectomy. *R,* rectum.

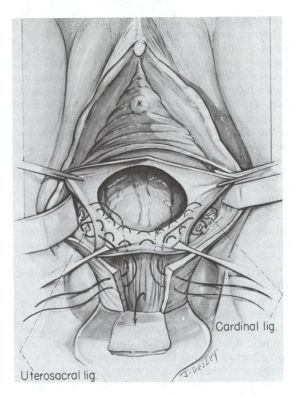

**Figure 41–12.** Symmonds' modification of the McCall enterocele repair (after vaginal hysterectomy and repair).

nal wall should be avoided because they bring the axis of the vagina too far forward and leave a hiatus posteriorly, which promotes recurrence of the enterocele.

A popular method of vaginal vault suspension is that of unilateral fixation to the sacrospinous ligament. In this technique the vaginal mucosa is separated from the rectovaginal tissues, and the associated enterocoele is identified and repaired (as previously described). Perforation through the right or left rectal pillar is usually easily accomplished by directing blunt dissection toward the ischial spine through the loose areolar tissue. After an appropriate location on the sacrospinous ligament is identified (usually 2–3 cm medial to the ischial spine), one of several techniques may be used to safely pass 2 or more permanent (or delayed absorbable) ligatures through the ligament to the submucosal apex of the vagina. Tying the sutures brings the vaginal apex to that sacrospinous ligament and a posterior colporrhaphy is then performed (as noted previously). Closing the dead space by intermittently suturing the vaginal mucosa to the underlying reconstituted rectovaginal septum may be useful. Necessary correction of urinary system abnormalities may precede or follow this procedure.

The vaginal positioning to the right or left seemingly is minimal after healing occurs and has not con-

stituted a problem. Indeed, vaginal connection to both sacrospinous ligaments is not recommended because it causes excessive lateral stretching of the vaginal apex. Vaginal vault suspension to one or both sacrospinous ligaments has the potential of injury to the pudendal nerve or pudendal vessels and is often technically difficult. Thus, it requires a skilled surgeon and should be undertaken only by those familiar with the technique (see Nichols, 1985).

Vaginal obliterative procedures (Le Fort's operation, vaginectomy) may be used in patients who do not require preservation of vaginal function. Unless the hernial sac is obliterated or removed, however, the enterocele may recur, perhaps in the form of a hernia of the perineum or of the ischiorectal fossa.

**D. Supportive Measures:** As with hernias of other types, obesity, chronic cough, and constipation should be corrected. Strenuous lifting, straining, and vigorous activity (calisthenics, bowling, etc) should be avoided for at least 6 months postoperatively.

### Prognosis

The outlook after proper enterocele repair is excellent. Techniques that repair only the enterocele (neglecting the associated cystocele, rectocele, and uterine prolapse) and those that suspend the vaginal vault (or the intact uterus) without obliterating the hernial sac are associated with a high incidence of recurrence.

### Vaginal Defects & Enterocele

Enteroceles are related to superior vaginal defects and may occur with or without associated uterine or vaginal vault prolapse. They may be classified as **anterior, posterior,** or **lateral** to the vagina, with or without vaginal vault prolapse. Additionally, they may be classified as **central, right,** or **left** in relation to the uterosacral ligaments or as **complete** (involving both the cul-de-sac and the uterosacral ligaments). Although some enteroceles may be **congenital** and some **iatrogenic,** most are of the **pulsion** or **traction** type. Enterocele may be associated with uterine prolapse or with posthysterectomy vaginal prolapse. Rarely a pudendal enterocele or a "saddle enterocele" (concomitant anterior and posterior enterocele) may occur.

Although surgical repair of an enterocele always involves excision of the sac and ligation of the sac orifice as high as possible, because of its association with other vaginal defects, those defects must also be understood, identified, and repaired. Unrecognized and unrepaired defects can lead to recurrence or to the later development of enterocele, if one is not already present. Failure to repair such defects as cystocele, rectocele, early vaginal prolapse or any supravaginal, or even lateral vaginal support defects, increases the risk of enterocele or recurrence. Not only should these defects be repaired at the time of enterocele repair, prophylactic corrections should be carried out when an enterocele is not present, ie, shortening and plication of elongated, strong uterosacral ligaments; excision and high ligation of excessive posterior cul-de-sac peritoneum; wedging and closure of a wide vaginal cuff.

The surgical techniques used must be directed at the enterocele and all associated specific defects. A combination of procedures is most frequently necessary. No single procedure can be standardized to correct all defects.

## Vaginal Defects & Vaginal Prolapse

Vaginal prolapse may occur in association with uterine prolapse or in a posthysterectomy patient and is one of the most troubling types of pelvic relaxation defects that a patient may experience. Although frequently associated with cystocele, rectocele, and enterocele, vaginal prolapse may or may not coexist with these conditions. Identification of each of these defects is mandatory, since each should be repaired to restore normal function. Vaginal prolapse, particularly massive posthysterectomy vaginal prolapse, is related to the adequacy of vaginal vault support and is a complex problem. To achieve the goals of restoration of normal anatomy and function and prevention of recurrence, the surgeon must appreciate the cause of each type of defect present and be able to tailor the surgical approach to the individual patient.

Correction of vaginal prolapse requires: consideration of hysterectomy, if the uterus is present; repair and prevention of enterocele; repair of cystocele and rectocele; correction and prevention of stress urinary incontinence; vaginal vault suspension (colopexy); restoration of normal vaginal caliber, length, and angle; correction of levator defects; and repair of a defective perineum. Transvaginal, transabdominal, or a combination of both approaches may be necessary. Failure to repair any of the specific defects present may well lead to new difficulties or to recurrence. There is no single surgical procedure that is always curative for this condition, and cure is effected by tailoring the operation to the patient. Possibly more than with any other pelvic support relaxation disorder, correct surgical treatment of complete vaginal prolapse requires a thorough understanding of all the vaginal defects present.

## UTERINE PROLAPSE

### Essentials of Diagnosis

- Firm mass in the lower vagina; cervix projecting through the vaginal introitus; vaginal inversion, with the cervix and uterus projecting between the legs.
- Sensation of vaginal fullness or pressure; lower abdominal pulling or aching; low backache.

## General Considerations

Uterine prolapse (pelvic floor hernia, pudendal hernia; is abnormal protrusion of the uterus through the pelvic floor aperture or genital hiatus (Fig 41–13). Like cystocele, rectocele, and enterocele—conditions with which it is usually associated—uterine prolapse occurs most commonly in multiparous white women as a gradually progressive result of childbirth injuries to the endopelvic fascia (and its condensations, the uterosacral and cardinal ligaments) and lacerations of muscle, especially the levator muscles and those of the perineal body. Uterine prolapse may also be the result of pelvic tumor; sacral nerve disorders, especially injury to S1–S4 (as in spina bifida); diabetic neuropathy; caudal anesthesia accidents; and presacral tumor. Additional factors promoting uterine prolapse are (1) systemic conditions, including obesity, asthma, chronic bronchitis, and bronchiectasis; and (2) local conditions such as ascites and large uterine and ovarian tumors.

A congenital type of uterine prolapse is seen rarely in newborn infants during vigorous crying or vomiting. It is also seen occasionally in nulliparous, even virginal, females with intact, strong levator muscles and a narrow genital hiatus; apparently, prolapse in these cases is the result of an inherent weakness of the endopelvic fascial supports of the uterus and vagina. In uterine prolapse of the common type, symptoms may not occur until many years after the causative event (eg, traumatic delivery). This finding suggests that aging and involutional attenuation of the supporting structures play an important role.

A uterus that is in a retroverted position is especially subject to prolapse; with the corpus aligned

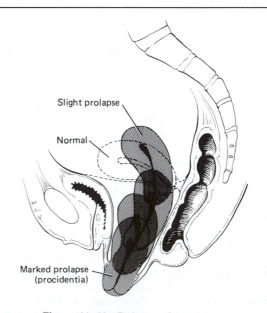

**Figure 41–13.** Prolapse of the uterus.

with the axis of the vagina, anything increasing intra-abdominal pressure exerts a piston-like action on the uterus, driving it down into the vagina.

Prolapse of a cervical stump (after subtotal abdominal hysterectomy) does not differ in any significant way from prolapse of an intact uterus. Admittedly, the oviducts and the utero-ovarian and round ligaments have been divided, but these structures do not contribute to the support of the cervical stump (or the uterus).

The degree of uterine prolapse parallels the extent of separation or attenuation of its supporting structures. In slight intravaginal or incomplete prolapse, the uterus descends only partway down the vagina; in moderate prolapse, it descends to the introitus, and the cervix protrudes slightly beyond; and in marked or complete prolapse (procidentia), the entire cervix and uterus protrude beyond the introitus and the vagina is inverted.

The principal components of the basin-like pelvic floor are the pelvic bones (including the coccyx), the endopelvic fascia, and the levator and perineal muscles. These structures normally support and maintain the position of the pelvic viscera despite great increments of intra-abdominal pressure that occur with straining, coughing, and heavy lifting when the patient is in the erect position. The urogenital hiatus ("anterior levator muscle gap"), which permits the urethra, vagina, and anus to emerge from the pelvis, is a site of potential weakness. Attenuation of the pubococcygeal and puborectal portions of the levator muscles, whether as the result of a traumatic delivery or of involutional changes, widens the levator gap and converts this potential weakness to an actual defect. If there has been a concomitant injury or attenuation of the endopelvic fascia (uterosacral and cardinal ligaments, rectovaginal and pubocervical fascia), heightened intra-abdominal pressure gradually leads to uterine prolapse along with cystocele, rectocele, and enterocele. If the integrity of the endopelvic fascia and its condensations has been maintained, the incompetency of the genital hiatus and levator muscles may be associated only with elongation of the cervix.

Anterior and posterior vaginal relaxation, as well as incompetency of the perineum, often accompanies prolapse of the uterus. Large cystocele is more common than rectocele in prolapse because the bladder is more easily carried downward than is the rectum. Prior to the menopause, the prolapsed uterus hypertrophies and is engorged and flabby. After the menopause, the uterus atrophies. In procidentia, the vaginal mucosa thickens and cornifies, coming to resemble skin.

## Clinical Findings

**A. Symptoms and Signs:** With mild prolapse (1st degree; cervix palpable as a firm mass in the lower third of the vagina), few symptoms can be at-tributed to the relaxation. With moderate prolapse (2nd degree; cervix visible and projecting into or through the vaginal introitus), the patient may experience a falling-out sensation or may report that she is sitting on a ball; of less significance may be a sensation of heaviness in the pelvis, low backache, and lower abdominal and inguinal pulling discomfort. In cases of severe prolapse (procidentia; 3rd degree), the cervix and entire uterus project through the introitus and the vagina is totally inverted. Frequently, this large mass has one or more areas of easily bleeding atrophic ulceration.

In premenopausal women with prolapse, leukorrhea or menometrorrhagia frequently develops as a result of uterine engorgement. Infertility is often related to excessive discharge. Once well established, however, pregnancy usually continues to term. After the menopause, excessive vaginal mucus and bleeding may be due to atrophic ulceration and infection of the prolapse.

Compression, distortion, or herniation of the bladder by the displaced uterus and cervix may be responsible for accumulation of residual urine, which leads to urinary tract infection, frequency and urgency, and overflow voiding. Incontinence is rare, but does occur. Constipation and painful defecation occur with prolapse because of pressure and rectocele. Ease and completeness of voiding and defecation may follow manual reduction of the prolapse by the patient. Cramping and obstipation may follow intestinal constriction within a large enterocele.

**B. Pelvic Examination:** With the patient bearing down or straining (perhaps in a standing position), pelvic examination reveals descent of the cervix to the lower third of the vagina (mild prolapse), descent past the introitus (moderate prolapse), or descent of the entire uterus through the introitus (severe prolapse). As the uterus progressively descends, some degree of cystocele and enterocele must develop concomitantly as a result of anatomic fixation of the bladder base and of the cul-de-sac to anterior and posterior uterocervical surfaces. In fact, a supposed uterine prolapse unaccompanied by cystocele and enterocele is almost invariably the result of cervical elongation (see following section).

The uterine tubes, ovaries, bladder, and distal ureters are drawn downward by the prolapsing uterus. Uterine or adnexal neoplasms and ascites associated with uterine prolapse should be noted.

Rectovaginal examination may reveal a rectocele. An enterocele may be behind and perhaps below the cervix, but in front of a rectocele. Placement of a metal sound or firm catheter within the bladder may determine the extent of concomitant cystocele.

## Differential Diagnosis

Cervical elongation presents the most troublesome problem in differential diagnosis. The distinction is important because vaginal hysterectomy (the customary operative treatment for uterine prolapse) may be difficult when performed for cervical elongation. With cervical elongation, vaginal examination discloses that the anterior, posterior, and lateral vaginal fornices are at their customary high level and descend minimally with straining; the anterior and upper posterior vaginal walls are well supported (little or no cystocele or enterocele); and the uterine corpus remains in a relatively high and posterior position.

Cervical tumors—as well as endometrial tumors (pedunculated myoma or endometrial polyps)—if prolapsed through a dilated cervix and presenting in the lower third of the vagina may be confused with mild or moderate uterine prolapse. Prolapse of the uterus must also be distinguished from cystocele, rectocele, uterine inversion, fecal impaction, or a large bladder stone. Myomas or polyps may coexist with prolapse of the uterus and cause unusual symptoms.

Despite the variety of possibilities, the history and physical findings in uterine prolapse are so characteristic that diagnosis is usually not a problem.

## Complications

Leukorrhea, abnormal uterine bleeding, and abortion may result from infection or from disordered uterine or ovarian circulation in prolapse. Chronic decubitus ulceration may develop in procidentia, but whether or not the ulcers predispose to cancer is uncertain. Urinary tract infection may occur with prolapse because of cystocele; and partial ureteral obstruction, with hydronephrosis, may occur in procidentia. Hemorrhoids result from straining to overcome constipation. Small bowel obstruction may occur within a deep enterocele.

## Prevention

Prenatal and postpartum Kegel exercises to strengthen the levator muscles, early and adequate episiotomy, and avoidance of traumatic delivery tend to prevent or at least to minimize prolapse. Prolonged estrogen therapy for menopausal and postmenopausal women tends to maintain the tone and integrity of the endopelvic fascia and pelvic floor musculature.

## Treatment

**A. Emergency Measures:** Infrequently, a patient with moderate to severe prolapse becomes pregnant. The rapidly enlarging uterus may become incarcerated within the true pelvis or, in procidentia, even outside the pelvis. It is imperative that the uterus be replaced and that the patient remain in bed until the uterus is large enough to prevent recurrence of the prolapse. An incarcerated, edematous procidentia may lead to urethral (even ureteral) obstruction, anuria, and uremia; therefore, prompt reduction of the prolapse is essential.

**B. Medical Measures:** A vaginal pessary (inflatable doughnut, Menge, Gellhorn, bee cell) may be used either as palliative therapy if surgical treatment is contraindicated or as a temporary measure in mild to moderate prolapse. The use of a pessary may assist in determining whether or not the rather ambiguous symptoms reported by the patient are actually produced by the uterine prolapse. In procidentia, reduction of the uterus followed by packing of the vagina to maintain uterine position may be necessary in the preoperative management of an ulcerated, infected prolapse.

In postmenopausal patients, the administration of estrogen (systemically or vaginally) will improve the tissue tone and facilitate correction of an atrophic, perhaps ulcerative, vaginitis. Biopsies should be taken of ulcerated areas; D&C may be necessary to investigate bleeding and to rule out cancer. Prescribe vaginal creams (eg, Aci-Jel), acetic acid douches, medicated tampons, or chemotherapy for ulceration. Treat urinary tract infection, diabetes mellitus, or cardiovascular complications appropriately. Prescribe laxatives or enemas for constipation.

**C. Surgical Measures:** Uterine prolapse may remain constant for many years or may progress very slowly, depending somewhat on the patient's age and activity. Even though one can be certain that the condition will not regress and that operation will eventually be required, its correction is not urgent, and surgical treatment should be deferred until the prolapse gives rise to significant symptoms.

Selection of a surgical approach for uterine prolapse depends on a number of variables: the patient's age, her desire for pregnancy or preservation of vaginal function, the degree of prolapse, and the presence of associated conditions (cystocele, stress incontinence, enterocele, rectocele). In general, symptoms associated with mild to moderate uterine prolapse are not severe. Thus, in the younger patient whose subsequent pregnancy may well nullify any benefits derived from an operative repair, it is customary to defer operative treatment until the childbearing years have passed or the patient has had all the babies she wants. Operations of the Manchester type were at one time recommended for the young patient with prolapse; but this procedure, which includes amputation of the cervix, has fallen into disfavor because it is associated with a high incidence of infertility and premature labor. The pelvic floor should be restored. Otherwise, vaginal hysterectomy with correction of hernial defects may be elected.

Most patients with uterovaginal prolapse have a composite lesion, ie, symptoms related to a moderate degree of uterine prolapse plus a moderate degree of cystocele, stress incontinence, enterocele, rectocele, and perineal relaxation. To provide good support for the vaginal vault and vaginal wall, the best surgical management consists of a composite operation. In addition to vaginal hysterectomy, the operation must include repair of actual or potential enterocele, careful anterior colporrhaphy to correct the cystocele and stress incontinence, and posterior colpoperineorrhaphy extending well up the posterior vaginal wall (Fig 41–14). If preservation of vaginal function is not important, narrowing and shortening the vagina by the removal of much of the anterior and posterior vaginal walls with the colporrhaphy, when combined with a high approximation of the levator muscles and with perineorrhaphy, will ensure the success of the operative repair. Vaginal obliterative operations (Le Fort's operation or vaginectomy) are rarely indicated or necessary; they may induce urinary incontinence, and they seldom correct an existing incontinence.

Uterine prolapse can be managed by an abdominal approach that includes total abdominal hysterectomy and the obliteration of any associated enterocele. However, this method is rather cumbersome and time-consuming; furthermore, it is permanently successful only when combined with transvaginal repair of cystocele and rectocele. Uterine suspensions—even ventrofixation of the corpus to the abdominal wall—are not effective in the treatment of prolapse.

In postmenopausal women who are sexually active, vaginal hysterectomy and repair are preferable to interposition procedures. In elderly patients, colpocleisis or colpectomy is infrequently chosen.

**D. Supportive Measures:** If the patient is obese, she should be encouraged to lose weight. Tight girdles and garments that increase intra-abdominal pressure and other factors (occupational or physical) that have a similar effect should be avoided or corrected.

**E. Treatment of Complications:** Infection of the operative area or of the urinary tract may require antibiotic therapy. Prescribe a pessary or reoperate for recurrence.

### Prognosis

Vaginal hysterectomy with anteroposterior colpoperineorrhaphy provides excellent and permanent vaginal support and, if good healing occurs, preservation of vaginal function as well. Recurrent vaginal prolapse may result from generalized relaxation (unrepaired cystocele, rectocele, or enterocele) or from occupational factors such as heavy lifting or straining.

### Vaginal Defects & Uterine Prolapse

Uterine prolapse is the result of genital prolapse and not the cause. It may or may not be associated with cystocele, rectocele, or enterocele. The defects causing uterine prolapse are defects in the supravaginal supports, primarily the uterosacral and paracervical ligaments. Three sites of damage have been suggested:

1. Upper steadying apparatus damage (round and broad ligaments).

2. Middle holding group damage (cardinal-uterosacral ligament complex).

3. Lower supporting group damage (pelvic and urogenital diaphragms, perineum and its associated muscles).

These defects may occur singly or in combination. Depending on the exact defect or combination of defects present, abnormalities ranging from uterine retrodisplacement to procidentia associated with cystocele, rectocele, and enterocele may occur. Since these defects are usually progressive, failure to repair all defects present may lead to new difficulties or recurrence. For example, to perform a vaginal hysterectomy for early uterine descensus, but not address the weaknesses in support at the vaginal cuff can lead to later development of an enterocele and/or vaginal vault prolapse. Additionally, failure to correct asymptomatic cystocele and rectocele at the time of hysterectomy not only increases the risk of vaginal vault prolapse, but also leaves the vagina with an abnormal depth and angle.

The importance of understanding the etiology of the various defects before attempting surgical correction of a prolapsed uterus cannot be overstated. Simply performing hysterectomy is insufficient.

## MALPOSITIONS OF THE UTERUS ("Tipped Uterus")

Significant displacement of the uterus may cause signs or symptoms such as pelvic pain, backache, menstrual aberrations, and infertility. Displacement may be lateral, anterior, or posterior. Virtually all women with symptoms that may be due to displacements are premenopausal. Almost all postpartum patients have a temporarily retroposed (tipped) uterus. Some retrodisplacements are secondary to defects in the supravaginal supports either congenital or acquired. Women with such defects may be at greater risk of developing other pelvic support problems later, ie, uterine descensus, vaginal prolapse, cystocele, and rectocele.

The uterus is not a fixed organ, and the position may vary transiently as a result of pelvic inclination or prolonged sitting, standing, or lying. The body of the uterus is directed forward in 80% of women; in the remainder, it is directed backward, but fewer than 5% of these women have a bona fide complaint referable to posterior version of the uterus. Normally, the cervix is directed posteriorly in the vaginal vault in nulliparas. After parturition, the cervix is often in the vaginal axis, an attitude caused by retrodisplacement of the corpus. The cervix and uterus often are aligned following relaxation of the pelvic floor. Laxity of the transverse cervical and round ligaments accounts for a posterior deviation in uterine position. Moderate uterine prolapse is usually associated with a retroposed uterus.

**Retroversion** implies that the axis of the body of the uterus is directed to the hollow of the sacrum, al-

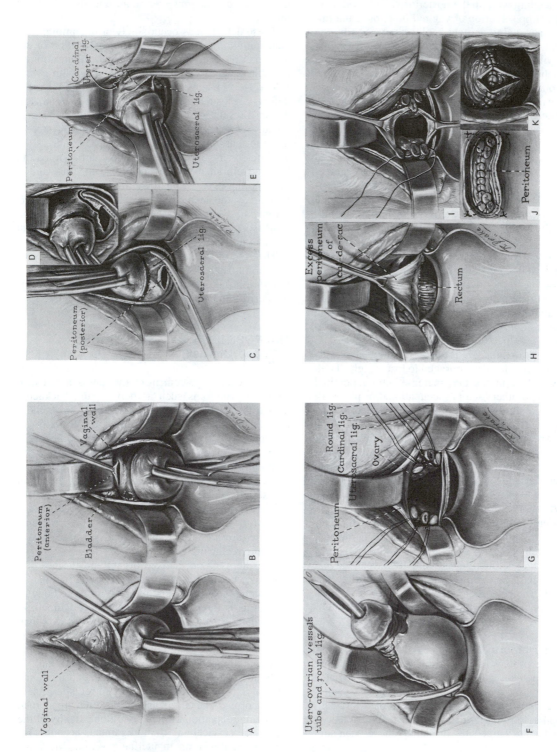

**Figure 41–14.** Vaginal hysterectomy for uterine prolapse.

though the cervix remains in its normal axis. If angulation of the corpus on the cervix is extreme, the term **retroflexion** is preferred. **Retrocession** implies that both the cervix and the uterus have gravitated backward toward the sacrum. Acute **anteversion** probably does not cause either obstruction to uterine discharge or circulatory alteration or dysmenorrhea—a reversal of opinion of a generation or more ago. Free **dextroversion** or levoversion is of little clinical importance unless tumors, shortened supports, or other disorders are present.

Adherent lateral deviation of the uterus may indicate primary pelvic disease (eg, salpingitis). Enlargement of the uterus, whether by pregnancy or tumor, may alter the relative position of that organ. Pelvic infections or endometriosis may obliterate the cul-de-sac. A pyosalpinx or hydrosalpinx may drag the corpus backward and downward by its weight, whereupon adhesions add restriction to cause immobility (Figs 41–15 to 41–18).

The patient's complaints are not often due solely to free retroposition. Nevertheless, dysmenorrhea and menometrorrhagia may be due to utero-ovarian congestion; backache is frequently caused by similar turgescence or taut uterosacral ligaments. Prolapse of the ovaries may cause dyspareunia in uterine retroposition.

Constipation due to displacement of the bowel or pressure by the uterine fundus on the rectum is possible but unlikely. Bladder dysfunction secondary to malposition of the uterus rarely occurs.

Early in pregnancy, a retroposed uterus may become incarcerated, often because of adhesions; the anteriorly displaced cervix may exert pressure on the urethrovesical juncture, causing urinary retention. In addition, because adherence may interfere with uterine blood flow, abortion may result.

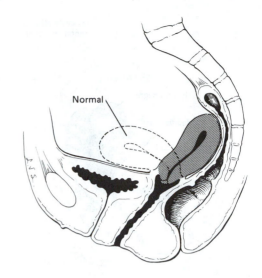

**Figure 41–16.** Retrocession of uterus.

## Clinical Findings

**A. Symptoms and Signs:** Pelvic pain, backache, abnormal menstrual bleeding, and infertility are commonly, but uncritically, related to malposition of the uterus. A combined abdominal and rectovaginal examination should be done to determine uterine position and to estimate the degree of misalignment of the uterus and cervix as well as the degree of adherence and tumefaction.

**B. X-Ray Findings:** Hysterography will reveal malposition of the uterus, especially when both anteroposterior and lateral films are obtained. Pneumoperitoneum or contrast medium within the rectum and bladder will enhance hysterography, especially when malposition is related to pelvic tumors.

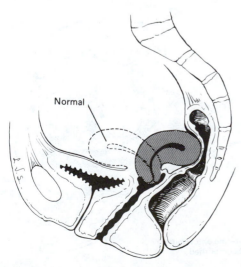

**Figure 41–15.** Retroflexion in an anteverted uterus.

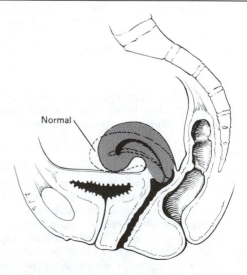

**Figure 41–17.** Acute anteflexion of uterus.

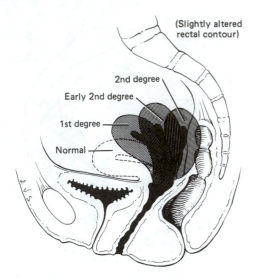

**Figure 41–18.** Degrees of retroversion of uterus without retroflexion.

**C. Special Examinations:** In examining a non-pregnant patient, gently insert a sterile curved uterine sound into the uterine cavity after applying a topical antiseptic to the external cervical os and distal canal. The direction of the instrument will indicate the position of the corpus.

## Differential Diagnosis

A fundal myoma or ovarian tumor resting in the cul-de-sac may be mistaken for a retroposed fundus and vice versa.

Adherent retroposition of the uterus may cause the same symptoms as uterine malposition. Basically, however, the disorder may be salpingitis, endometriosis, or neoplasia. Uterine retroposition does not inevitably cause backache, which is frequently due to orthopedic disorders. Abnormal posture, fatigue, myositis, arthritis, and herniation of an intervertebral disk should be considered as possible causes of backache.

## Prevention

Avoidance of the causes of pelvic infection and early, specific therapy when infection occurs will reduce the incidence of adherent malposition of the uterus.

## Treatment

Retroposition of the uterus is now regarded as important clinically when replacement and support by a vaginal pessary relieve the symptoms. *Note:* Knee-chest exercises alone are of questionable value.

**A. Emergency Measures:** An incarcerated, non-adherent uterus must be surgically elevated, especially in the case of a pregnant patient who develops acute urinary retention or seems likely to abort. Rectovaginal manipulation of the corpus with the pa-

tient in the knee-chest position may facilitate restoration of uterine anteposition.

**B. Specific Local Measures:** In the nonpregnant patient, neither an asymptomatic retroposition nor a normally involuting retroposed puerperal uterus requires treatment. For the gynecologic patient with pelvic pain or abnormal bleeding and for the recently delivered woman with subinvolution and persistent lochia or bleeding, the uterus should be repositioned and a properly fitted vaginal pessary inserted (see following text). Unless discomfort develops, permit the pessary to remain in place for 6–8 weeks and record the result. If anteversion and relief follow pessary support, no further therapy will be necessary. Reinsert the pessary after 2 months if symptoms recur.

Bimanual replacement of retrodisplaced uterus is performed as follows: With the patient in the lithotomy position, insert 1 or 2 gloved fingers into the vagina, elevate the fundus, and press against the cervix. With the other hand, bring the corpus forward (Fig 41–19). Fit a vaginal pessary of the Hodge type to support the uterus in anteposition.

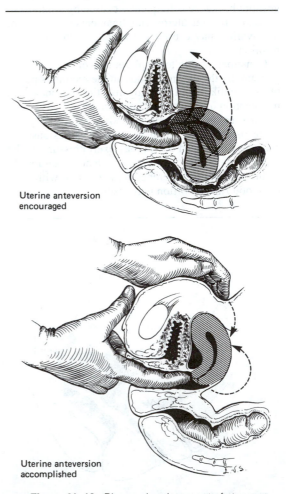

Uterine anteversion encouraged

Uterine anteversion accomplished

**Figure 41–19.** Bimanual replacement of uterus.

If this procedure is not successful, insert a pessary of the Hodge type into the posterior vaginal fornix (Fig 41–20). Have the patient sit up and then assume the knee-chest position. Apply pressure on the lateral bars of the pessary and displace the cervix backward while the patient coughs; the nonadherent uterus usually falls forward. Require the patient to slip slowly into the prone position and then into the lithotomy position. Seat the pessary so as to maintain the uterus in anteposition.

**C. Surgical Measures:** Suspend the uterus as a primary procedure if repeated replacement of the corpus by the use of a pessary has alleviated symptoms and signs or if adherence of the uterus and prolapse of the adnexa are probable causes of disability.

Suspend the uterus as the concluding step in an operation performed to eliminate specific pelvic disease (eg, tubal plastic procedures).

**D. Treatment of Complications:** Occasional warm acetic acid douches or the use of vaginal creams (eg, Aci-Jel) may relieve irritation and prevent discharge caused by a vaginal pessary. (Even a well-fitted one may cause irritation.)

## Prognosis

If correction of the uterine malposition follows an accurate diagnosis of symptomatic displacement, the outlook is good. It is poor if uterine suspension is done without a convincing indication.

## VAGINAL PESSARIES

The vaginal pessary is a prosthesis of ancient lineage, now made of rubber or plastic material, often with a metal band or spring frame. A great many types have been devised, but fewer than a dozen are basically unique and specifically helpful.

Pessaries are principally used to support the uterus, cervical stump, or hernias of the pelvic floor. They are effective because they reduce vaginal relaxation and increase the tautness of the pelvic floor structures. Little or no leverage is involved. The retrodisplaced uterus remains forward after it is repositioned and a pessary inserted because the tension produced on the uterosacral ligaments draws the cervix backward. In most cases, adequate support anteriorly and a reasonably good perineal body are required; otherwise, the pessary may slip from behind the symphysis and extrude from the vagina.

## Indications & Uses
### A. Obstetric:

1. To avert threatened abortion presumed to be due to marked uterine retroposition and chronic passive congestion.

2. To promote healing of atrophic cervical ulceration associated with prolapse during pregnancy.

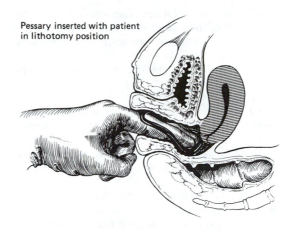

Pessary inserted with patient in lithotomy position

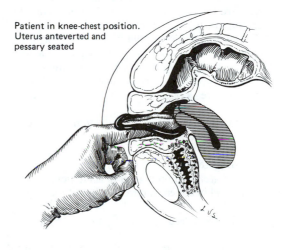

Patient in knee-chest position. Uterus anteverted and pessary seated

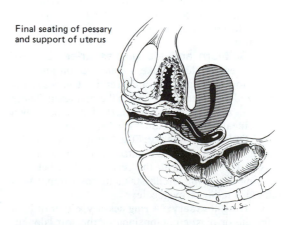

Final seating of pessary and support of uterus

**Figure 41–20.** Insertion of Hodge pessary if bimanual replacement of uterus is not successful.

3. To relieve acute urinary retention or pain due to retroposition of the uterus in midpregnancy.

4. To prevent or relieve postpartum subinvolution or retroversion.

5. To protect against abortion in cervical incompetence.

**B. Gynecologic:**

1. To treat poor-risk patients or those who refuse operation for uterine prolapse or other genitourinary hernias.

2. To serve as a preoperative aid in the healing of cervical stasis ulcerations associated with uterine prolapse.

3. To reduce cystocele or retrocele.

4. To alleviate menorrhagia, dysmenorrhea, or dyspareunia related to free uterine retroposition and adnexal prolapse.

5. To determine whether hysteropexy will relieve backache due to retroversion.

6. To control urinary stress incontinence by exerting pressure beneath the urethra or by improving the posterior urethrovesical angle.

7. To aid conception in the management of infertility, because the cervix may be displaced anteriorly, away from the posterior fornix seminal pool, or because there may be angulation of tubes or chronic passive congestion secondary to retroposition.

8. To facilitate hysteropexy by holding the uterus in position for operation.

## Contraindications

Pessaries are contraindicated in acute genital tract infections and in adherent retroposition of the uterus.

## Types of Pessaries
## (Fig 41–21)

**A. Hodge Pessary:** (Smith-Hodge, or Smith and other variations.) This is an elongated, curved ovoid. One end is placed behind the symphysis and the other in the posterior vaginal fornix. The anterior bow is curved to avoid the urethra; the cervix rests within the larger, posterior bow. This type of pessary is used to hold the uterus in place after it has been repositioned.

**B. Gellhorn and Menge Pessaries:** Both of these types are shaped like a collar button and provide a ring-like platform for the cervix. The pessary is stabilized by a stem that rests on the perineum. These pessaries are used to correct marked prolapse when the perineal body is reasonably adequate.

**C. Gehrung Pessary:** The Gehrung pessary resembles 2 firm letter U's attached by crossbars. It rests in the vagina with the cervix cradled between the long arms; this arches the anterior vaginal wall and helps reduce a cystocele.

**D. Ring Pessary:** A ring pessary, either of hard vulcanite or plastic composition or the soft "doughnut" type, distends the vagina and elevates the cervix.

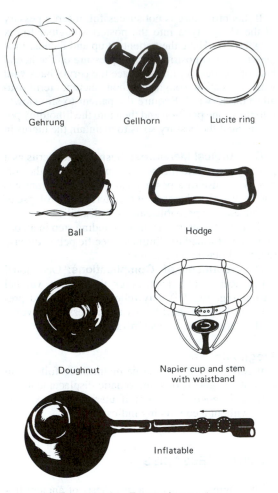

**Figure 41–21.** Types of pessaries.

Cystocele and rectocele are reduced considerably by a ring pessary.

**E. Ball or Bee Cell Pessary:** (Fig 41–22) A hollow plastic ball or sponge rubber (bee cell) pessary functions much like a ring pessary and is used for similar purposes. A moderate intact perineum is necessary for retention.

**F. Napier Pessary:** A uterine supporter (Napier pessary) is a cup-and-stem arrangement supported by a belt. This device elevates the cervix and uterus and holds them in place. It is used in cases of marked prolapse when the perineum is incompetent, especially in a patient who cannot withstand an operation.

**G. Inflatable Pessary:** The inflatable pessary (Milex) functions much like a doughnut pessary. The ball valve is moved "up" and "down." When the ball is in the down position, air inflates the pessary; when in the up position, the air is sealed in and inflation is maintained.

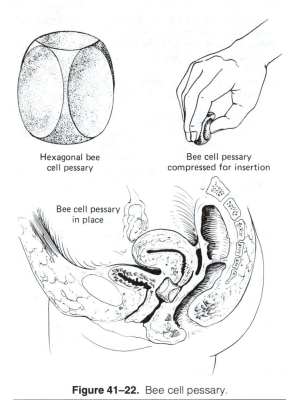

Hexagonal bee
cell pessary

Bee cell pessary
compressed for insertion

Bee cell pessary
in place

**Figure 41–22.** Bee cell pessary.

## FITTING OF PESSARIES

Pessaries that are too large cause irritation and ulceration. Those that are too small may not stay in place and may protrude. Bee cell and inflatable pessaries should be removed nightly to cleanse and to preserve the vaginal mucosa.

To determine the proper length of a pessary, pass a pair of uterine dressing forceps, using the finger as a guide, into the vagina to the top of the posterior vaginal vault. Mark the shank of the forceps at the introitus with a finger or piece of tape. Withdraw the forceps and measure the distance from the marked point to the tip of the blades. This dimension minus 1 cm is the appropriate length of the pessary. To obtain the width (assuming that an ovoid rather than a round pessary is required), introduce the forceps to about the level of the cervix and separate the handles until the blades touch the walls of the vagina. Note the distance between the handles; then close the instrument and withdraw it. Separate the handles to the distance noted and measure between the tips of the blades. This measurement represents the greatest diameter of the pessary.

The pessary should be lubricated and inserted with its widest dimension in the oblique diameter of the vagina to avoid painful distention at the introitus. With a finger of the opposite hand, depress the perineum to widen the introitus.

The Hodge pessary should be rotated slightly after it is in the vagina; then, using the forefinger of one hand, slip the posterior bar behind the cervix. The anterior bar should then be brought upward so that the pessary will be wholly within the vagina (ie, no portion of it visible).

The forefinger should pass easily between the sides of the frame and the vaginal wall at any point; otherwise, the pessary is too large. A solid vulcanite pessary can be molded in hot water and reshaped for a better fit.

After the pessary has been fitted, the patient should be asked to stand, walk, and squat to determine whether pain occurs, whether the pessary becomes displaced, and whether the uterus remains in position. She should be shown how to withdraw the pessary if it becomes displaced or is uncomfortable, and cautioned that a contraceptive vaginal diaphragm cannot be used while a vaginal pessary is in place.

Frequent low-pressure acetic acid douches or acidic vaginal creams are helpful while vaginal pessaries are being worn. Pessaries should be removed and cleaned once every month; or a pessary of slightly different size and shape can be substituted. During pregnancy—and as a preoperative trial in gynecologic patients—a pessary should be worn for approximately 3 months. In many causes during pregnancy, if uterine retroposition is corrected with a pessary, the uterus will remain forward after the pessary is removed.

Vaginal pessaries are not curative of prolapse, but they may be used for months or years for palliation with proper supervision.

A neglected pessary may cause fistulas or favor genital infections, but it is doubtful that cancer ever occurs as a result of wearing a modern pessary.

## REFERENCES

### CYSTOCELE

Baden WF, Walker T: *Surgical Repair of Vaginal Defects.* JB Lippincott, 1992:237.

Beecham CT: Classification of vaginal relaxation. Am J Obstet Gynecol 1980;136:957.

Macer GA: Transabdominal repair of cystocele: A 20 year experience, compared with the traditional vaginal approach. Am J Obstet Gynecol 1978;131:203.

Nichols DH: Effects of pelvic relaxation on gynecologic urologic problems. Clin Obstet Gynecol 1978; 21:759.

Nichols, DH: *Gynecologic and Obstetric Surgery.* CV Mosby, 1993:339.

White GR: Cystocele: A radical cure by suturing lateral sulci of vagina to white line of pelvic fascia. JAMA 1909;53:1707.

Word BH, Montgomery HA: "Vaginal Approach to Anterior Paravaginal repair: Alternative Techniques," In: *Surgical Repair of Vaginal Defects.* Baden W, Walker T, (eds). JB Lippincott, 1992:195.

## RECTOCELE

Benson JT: Vaginal approach to posterior vaginal defects: The perineal site. In: *Surgical Repair of Vaginal Defects.* Baden W, Walker T, (eds). JB Lippincott, 1992:226, 232.

Kuhn RJ, Hollyock VE: Observations on the anatomy of the rectovaginal pouch and septum. Obstet Gynecol 1982;59:445.

Nichols DH: *Gynecologic and Obstetrics Surgery,* CV Mosby, 1993:365.

Parks AG, Porter NH, Hardcastle J: The syndrome of the descending perineum. Proc R Soc Med 1966;59:477.

## ENTEROCELE

Beecham CT, Beecham JB: Correction of prolapsed vagina or enterocele with fascia lata. Obstet Gynecol 1973;42:542.

Birnbaum SJ: Rational therapy of the prolapsed vagina. Am J Obstet Gynecol 1973;115:411.

Desai VB: Marlex mesh prosthesis for massive vaginal prolapse. Int Surg 1987;72:160.

Drutz HP, Cha LS: Massive genital and vaginal vault prolapse treated by abdominal-vaginal sacropexy with use of Marlex mesh: Review of the literature. Am J Obstet Gynecol 1987;156:387.

Feldman GB, Birnbaum SJ: Sacral colpopexy for vaginal vault prolapse. Obstet Gynecol 1979;53:399.

Fox PF, Kowalczyk, AC: Ruptured enterocele. Am J Obstet Gynecol 1971;111:592.

Hendee AE, Berry CM: Abdominal sacropexy for vaginal vault prolapse. Clin Obstet Gynecol 1981;24: 1217.

Langmade CF, Oliver JA, White JS: Cooper ligament repair of vaginal vault prolapse twenty-eight years later. Am J Obstet Gynecol 1978;131:134.

Miyazaki FS: Miya hook ligature carrier for sacrospinous ligament suspension. Obstet Gynecol 1987;70: 286.

Moschcowitz AV: The pathogenesis, anatomy and cure of the prolapse of the rectum. Surg Gynecol Obstet 1992;15:7.

Nichols DH: *Gynecologic and Obstetric Surgery.* CV Mosby, 1993:427.

Nichols DH: Relaxed vaginal outlet, rectocele and enterocele. Chap 24, pp 569–595. In: *TeLinde's Operative Gynecology,* 6th ed. Mattingly RF, Thompson JD (editors). JB Lippincott, 1985.

Pelosi MA et al: Use of dermal graft in the surgical repair of vaginal vault prolapse. Obstet Gynecol 1980;55: 385.

Ranney B: Enterocele, vaginal prolapse, pelvic hernia: Recognition and treatment. Am J Obstet Gynecol 1981; 140:53.

Richter K, Albrich W: Long-term results following fixation of the vagina on the sacrospinal ligament by the vaginal route (vaginae fixatio sacrospinalis vaginalis). Am J Obstet Gynecol 1981;141:811.

Symmonds RE et al: Posthysterectomy enterocele and vaginal vault prolapse. Am J Obstet Gynecol 1981; 140: 852.

Tancer JL, Fleischer M, Berkowitz BS: Simultaneous colpo-recto-sacropexy. Obstet Gynecol 1987;70:951.

Wilensky AV, Kaufman PA: Vaginal hernia. Am J Surg 1940;49:31.

Yates MJ: An abdominal approach to the repair of posthysterectomy vaginal inversion. Br J Obstet Gynecol 1975;82:817.

Zacharin RF: *Pelvic Floor Anatomy and the Surgery of Pulsion Enterocele.* Springer-Verlag, 1985.

Zacharin RF: Pulsion enterocele: Review of functional anatomy of the pelvic floor. Obstet Gynecol 1980;55: 135.

## UTERINE PROLAPSE

Ardekany MS, Rafee R: A new modification of colpocleisis for treatment of total procidentia in old age. Int J Gynaecol Obstet 1978;15:358.

Azpuru CE: Total rectal prolapse and total genital prolapse: A series of 17 cases. Dis Colon Rectum 1974; 17:528.

Baden WF, Walker T: *Surgical Repair of Vaginal Defects.* JB Lippincott, 1992:248.

Bonney V: The principles that should underlie all operations for prolapse. J Obstet Gynaecol Br Emp 1934; 41:669.

Bonney V: The sustentacular apparatus of the female genital canal: The displacements that result from the yielding of its several components, and their appropriate treatment. J Obstet Gynaecol Br Commonw 1914; 45:328.

Chambers CB: Uterine prolapse with incarceration. Am J Obstet Gynecol 1975;122:459.

Elkin M et al: Ureteral obstruction in patients with uterine prolapse. Radiology 1974;110:289.

Feroze RM: Vaginal hysterectomy and repair. Clin Obstet Gynaecol 1978;5:545.

Lavery JP, Boey CS: Uterine prolapse with pregnancy. Obstet Gynecol 1973;42:681.

Pratt JH: Vaginal hysterectomy. In: *Complications in Obstetrics and Gynecology.* Harper & Row, 1981.

Wheeless CR Jr: Total vaginal hysterectomy. In: *Atlas of Pelvic Surgery. Lea & Febiger, 1981.*

# Gynecologic Urology

# 42

*Jack R. Robertson, MD, & David B. Hebert, MD*

The female reproductive tract and lower urinary tract are closely related embryologically and anatomically. A distinction between pathologic gynecologic and urologic conditions is often difficult to make in women, and disease processes in one tract often result in symptoms referable to the other.

## ANATOMY & PHYSIOLOGY

Although the bladder is composed of 3 layers of smooth muscle, these layers are so densely interwoven that they cannot be distinctly dissected from one another. Two of these layers extend into the urethra in well-defined longitudinal and circular or spiral layers. In some anatomic specimens, decussations of striated muscle from the pubococcygeus muscle attach to the urethra, but this cannot be demonstrated in all instances, and anatomists have long argued whether or not a true striated muscle urethral sphincter exists. Functionally, however, the pubococcygeus muscle acts as the striated muscle sphincter of the urethra.

The autonomic and somatic nervous systems control the storage and expulsion of urine (Fig 42–1). Parasympathetic nerves originating from S2–4 stimulate bladder contractions through the release of acetylcholine (cholinergic nerve fibers). Preganglionic sympathetic fibers arising from T10–L2 are also cholinergic, but the postganglionic fibers innervating both the bladder and the urethra act through the release of norepinephrine (adrenergic nerve fibers). Beta-adrenergic fibers terminate mainly in the bladder and alpha-adrenergic fibers mostly in the urethra. The alpha-adrenergic component of the sympathetic nervous system contracts the smooth muscle of the urethra, while the beta-adrenergic component relaxes both the bladder and the urethra. The somatic nervous system innervates the striated muscle of the urethra through the pudendal nerve. The parasympathetic, sympathetic, and somatic nervous systems control micturition through complex reflex interactions and by their direct actions on the bladder and urethra.

The detrusor muscle has the intrinsic ability to relax in response to increasing bladder volume, so that the bladder can fill without concomitant increase in intraluminal pressure. Disease processes that alter this intrinsic ability, whether they be local (eg, scarring from birth trauma) or systemic, may affect bladder function and sensation. The detrusor muscle is unique in that it is under voluntary control even though it is smooth muscle; it contracts to empty the bladder when called upon to do so in socially acceptable situations but remains relaxed when micturition is inappropriate.

## HISTORY & PHYSICAL EXAMINATION

### Common Symptoms of Urinary Tract Disorders

**A. Dysuria:** Painful urination is usually described as a burning sensation that occurs when urine passes through the urethra. The most common causes are urethritis or cystitis. Dysuria may also result from trauma, chemical irritation, or atrophy due to estrogen deficiency. Dysuria should be differentiated from burning due to contact of urine with inflamed vulvar or vaginal epithelium.

**B. Frequency:** A patient with urinary frequency urinates more often than usual. An individual typically urinates 2–7 times a day during waking hours. Frequency has many causes, including infection, excessive diuresis, and social or emotional problems. Frequency must be assessed based on changes in the usual voiding intervals for a given patient.

**C. Enuresis:** Bed wetting is common in young children but usually resolves after maturation of the nervous system and development of subconscious cortical control over micturition. Enuresis in an adult almost always indicates a neurologic or psychogenic disorder.

**D. Nocturia:** Waking to void more than once per night is often associated with sleep disorders, but it may also be due to infection or neurologic abnormalities. In the elderly, nocturia is common and does not necessarily indicate a pathologic condition. Any assessment of nocturia should consider voided vol-

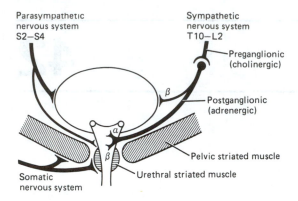

**Figure 42–1.** Innervation of the lower urinary tract.

umes, since diuresis on assuming the recumbent position is common in individuals with peripheral edema or congestive heart failure.

**E. Urgency:** The strong or sudden desire to void occurs in over 80% of patients evaluated for lower urinary tract symptoms, and it is the most common urinary complaint.

**F. Hesitancy:** The inability to readily start and maintain the urinary stream suggests either poor urethral relaxation or poor detrusor contraction, but it may also result from partial urethral obstruction due to severe relaxation of pelvic supports.

**G. Postvoiding Fullness:** The patient feels that the bladder is not completely empty after voiding. Postvoiding fullness in most patients is associated with disorders causing irritation (eg, infection, inflammation, foreign bodies, trauma) and low residual urine volumes. Elevated residual urine due to dennervation is not usually associated with postvoiding fullness, since the patient typically has both sensory and motor dennervation. Postvoiding fullness is common in irritative lesions, relaxation of pelvic supports, and vaginal atrophy.

**H. Stress Incontinence:** Involuntary loss of urine occurs during activities that increase intra-abdominal pressure, eg, coughing, sneezing, or exercise. The amount of leakage, frequency of leakage, and degree of social embarrassment should be noted.

**I. Urge Incontinence:** Leakage of urine that is associated with a strong desire to void constitutes urge incontinence. The urge may be sudden or gradual in onset. Urge incontinence and stress incontinence may occur simultaneously.

## History

The medical and surgical history is important in the assessment of lower urinary tract symptoms. Attention should be directed particularly to medications, obstetric deliveries, pelvic or back surgery, neurologic disorders, and systemic diseases. The chronologic development of symptoms should be de-

termined. The degree of social dysfunction associated with incontinence is a crucial consideration, since a life-threatening condition is rarely responsible for this annoying symptom.

## Physical Examination

A general physical examination should precede the genitourinary examination. A basic neurologic assessment must also be included to rule out neurologic causes of urinary tract disorders.

**A. Pelvic Examination:** The pelvic examination should assess the effect of pelvic masses (eg, neoplasm, abscess, nonneoplastic cyst, hydrosalpinx) on the bladder and urethra. The presence and degree of relaxation of pelvic support are evaluated. A Sims speculum, or the posterior blade of a Graves speculum, may be used to depress the posterior wall or elevate the anterior wall of the vagina to visualize the amount of descent of the opposite wall and vaginal side walls (Fig 42–2). Suburethral masses, scarring, and fistulas may be visualized.

The vagina is inspected for discharge or other evidence of a localized abnormality that may involve the urethra. Inspection of the urethral meatus may reveal a caruncle, neoplasia, stenosis, or paraurethral (Skene's) duct abnormalities. Evidence of vaginal atrophy should be noted, since the response of the vagina and urethra to estrogen stimulation is similar. Atrophic urethral changes are one of the most common causes of lower urinary tract symptoms.

**1. Cotton-tipped applicator (Q-tip) test—**An accurate assessment of bladder or urethral descent during straining requires objective measurement by means of the cotton-tipped applicator test or radiographic techniques (Fig 42–3). The cotton-tipped applicator test is performed by placing a lubricated

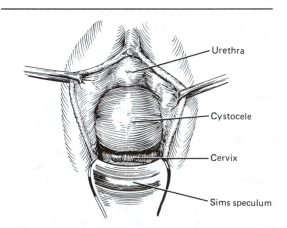

**Figure 42–2.** Sims speculum used to inspect the anterior vaginal wall. The anterior blade of a bivalved speculum does not allow adequate visualization and may support the vaginal wall, leading to errors in judgment of the degree of relaxation.

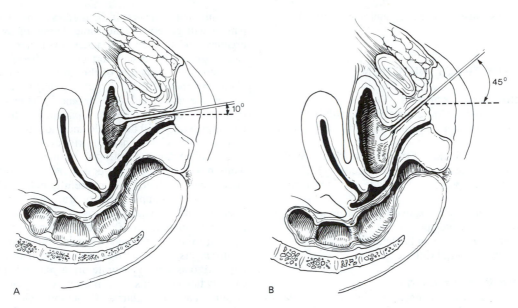

**Figure 42–3.** The cotton-tipped applicator (Q-tip) test for the assessment of urethral and bladder support. **A:** The resting angle of the cotton-tipped applicator is normal. **B:** With straining, the urethrovesical junction descends, causing the end of the stick to rotate upward.

cotton-tipped applicator in the urethra with the cotton tip at the urethrovesical junction. The patient lies in the supine position. The angle formed by the applicator stick and an imaginary line drawn parallel to the floor is measured while the patient is resting and while she performs the Valsalva maneuver (forced exhalation against a closed glottis). An angle of less than 15 degrees both during rest and during the Valsalva maneuver constitutes a good result and demonstrates good anatomic support. An angle of more than 30 degrees during the Valsalva maneuver indicates poor anatomic support. An angle of 15–30 degrees is considered inconclusive.

**2. Palpation–**Palpation of the bladder or urethra may reveal a suburethral mass or tenderness. Stripping the urethra with a fingertip from the urethrovesical junction to the meatus often reveals urethral discharge when a diverticulum is present.

**3. Urinary stress test–**The urinary stress test is an important part of the examination. A known volume of fluid (300 mL is a good standard) is instilled in the bladder. The patient may feel that the bladder is relatively full but should not be uncomfortable. The patient then performs the Valsalva maneuver or coughs forcefully 8–10 times while she is standing with feet spread as wide as her shoulders. The perineum is inspected for leakage of urine. Incontinence occurring with stress and ending shortly thereafter suggests poor anatomic support as a likely cause. Delayed or continued leakage suggests disorders of detrusor muscle control, eg, unstable bladder. This test is only suggestive and is not diagnostic of any

specific type of incontinence. It does not permit quantitation of the degree of incontinence, since voluntary compensatory mechanisms often result in less leakage in a laboratory setting than that reported in a more natural setting. A negative test (no leakage) does not rule out incontinence but suggests a mild degree of the disorder, and verification of incontinence by other methods is necessary before institution of surgical or medical therapy.

Another form of the urinary stress test has been encouraged by many authors. Known as the Bonney test, Read test, or Marshall test, this test purports to predict the effectiveness of surgery on the basis of the patient's response to elevation of the anterior vaginal wall or urethrovesical junction during the stress test (if pressure and elevation inhibit incontinence, the patient is thought to be a good candidate for surgery). This test has been proved invalid, since its effect is achieved by mechanical obstruction of the urethra in a manner contrary to the physiologic effect achieved by standard incontinence surgery. The urinary stress test described above is a valuable adjunct to the physical examination, but the effect of elevation of the vaginal wall should not be used to determine the appropriateness of surgical repair for incontinence.

**B. Neurologic Examination:** The neurologic examination focuses on the pelvic floor and lower extremities. Reflexes, sensation, and strength are tested in the lower extremities. Sensation on the perineum, the resting tone of the pubococcygeus muscles and anal sphincter, and voluntary contraction of the pubococcygeus muscles and anal sphincter should be assessed.

## URINARY TRACT INFECTION

### Essentials of Diagnosis

- Urethral discomfort during urination (dysuria).
- A sensation that immediate voiding cannot be delayed (urgency).
- A persistent feeling of the need to void, even after the bladder has been emptied (frequency).
- Inability to prevent immediate voiding (incontinence).
- Fever, chills, and costovertebral angle pain if pyelonephritis develops.
- Pyuria, bacteriuria, or hematuria.
- Positive Bacterial Culture.

### General Considerations

The urinary tract is considered infected if the bacterial count in 2 successive clean-catch urine specimens or in a single catheterized specimen exceeds 105/mL. Urinary tract infection is more common in women than men, and the incidence increases with age. Sexual intercourse and estrogen deficiency are contributing factors. Vaginitis is the most common differential diagnosis and often occurs simultaneously.

### Etiology

Urinary tract infection may ascend from the urethra (urethritis), to the bladder (cystitis), to the kidney (pyelonephritis). Bacteria causing urinary tract infection generally originate in the vagina or the rectum. Sexual intercourse forces bacteria up the urethra and traumatizes the bladder and urethral mucosa, lending them more to infection. Other vaginal factors include contraceptive diaphragms, spermicides, bubble baths, and vaginitis. Vaginal factors occasionally contributing to colonization with pathogenic organisms include poor rectal and perineal hygiene due to conditions such as hemorrhoids, fecal incontinence, and anal fissures may trigger urinary tract infections or increased vaginal pH after menopause and associated changes of decreased lubrication and vascularity increase bacterial colonization of the urethra and bladder. A short urethra or a urethral meatus that opens into the vagina appears to increase the risk of urinary tract infection. The risk of urinary tract infection is also increased in diabetics, the chronically dehydrated patient, infrequent voiders, and patients with persistent residual urine after voiding. Anomalies such as urinary tract obstruction, reflux, congenital abnormalities, diverticula, or calculi also increase the risk of urinary tract infection.

### Clinical Findings

**A. Symptoms and Signs:** Symptoms range from minimal to severe. If the urethra is infected, the patient will generally note some degree of dysuria, urgency, and frequency. Bladder involvement often causes suprapubic discomfort but may be relatively asymptomatic. Palpation of the urethra and bladder elicit tenderness. Bladder irritability may result in incontinence associated with urgency. Patients with cystitis are generally afebrile. A patient with pyelonephritis generally will be febrile and anorexic and may complain of back pain near the kidney.

**B. Laboratory Findings:** If more than 6–8 white blood cells per high-power field are noted on microscopic evaluation of a carefully collected centrifuged urine sample, urinary tract infection is a likely diagnosis. The diagnosis is confirmed by the growth of more than $10^5$ bacteria per milliliter of urine. If excessive vaginal epithelial cells are present on urinalysis, a catheterized urine specimen may be required to assure an accurate urinalysis and culture. Chlamydial urethritis may present with pyuria but negative bacterial cultures. In hemorrhagic cystitis, inflammation causes a disturbing amount of blood in the urine. Epithelial cells are generally not abundant unless the sample has been contaminated by vaginal secretions. White blood cell casts form in the renal tubules of patients with pyelonephritis and may be evident on urinalysis. An elevated white blood cell count in the CBC may support a diagnosis of pyelonephritis in a patient with suggestive symptoms; in a patient with cystitis or urethritis, however, the CBC is usually normal.

### Differential Diagnosis

White blood cells in a urine sample may actually reflect contamination of a urine sample by vaginal secretions, possibly in association with vaginitis. Patients with *Trichomonas* or other forms of vaginitis may complain of dysuria and pelvic pain. It may be difficult for the patient with vulvovaginitis to differentiate between dysuria and vulvar burning from contact with urine during micturition. Pelvic pressure from a mass may be confused with the bladder discomfort associated with cystitis. Normal symptoms of early pregnancy are often confused with cystitis. Urethritis and vulvitis due to herpes infection classically produce dysuria and vulvar burning on urination. A routine pelvic examination should be performed in all women who complain of symptoms that suggest urinary tract infection.

### Treatment

Antibiotics commonly used to treat urinary tract infections include ampicillin, trimethoprim-sulfamethoxazole, cephalosporins, nitrofurantoin, and, in resistant cases, aminoglycosides (Table 42–1). In an uncomplicated first episode of urinary tract infection, trimethroprim-sulfamethoxazole, ampicillin, or nitrofurantoin is effective against **Escherichia coli**, the most likely pathogen. Organisms found in chronic

**Table 42–1.** Antibiotic dosage regimens for the treatment of urinary tract infection.[1]

|  | Oral | Intravenous |
|---|---|---|
| Ampicillin | 250–500 mg 4 times daily | 1–2 g 4 times daily |
| Trimethoprim-sulfamethoxazole | One double-strength tablet (trimethoprim, 160 mg; sulfamethoxazole, 800 mg) 2 times a day | No |
| Cephalosporins | Cephalexin, 250–500 mg 4 times daily | Cefazolin, 1 g 3 times daily |
| Nitrofurantoin | 50–100 mg 4 times daily | No |
| Aminoglycosides | No | Gentamicin, 3 mg/kg/d in 3 divided doses |

[1]Oral regimens are for uncomplicated urethritis and cystitis; Intravenous regimens should be used in pyelonephritis.

or recurrent urinary tract infections are often resistant to commonly used antibiotics. It is always wise to submit a urine sample for culture and sensitivity testing. Patients with cystitis may be started empirically on an antibiotic, which may be changed as needed after the results of sensitivity testing are available. Urinary tract analgesics may be indicated for the first 24–48 hours of antibiotic therapy. Single-dose antibiotic therapy is often effective for mild, uncomplicated cystitis. Septic, anorexic patients with pyelonephritis respond more rapidly to intravenous administration of appropriate antibiotics.

The physician must seek contributing factors in any patient with recurrent urinary tract infection. Thorough evaluation includes vaginal examination to detect cystocele or urethral disorders such as diverticulum, fistula, caruncle, or skene duct abscess. Patients with recurrent infection caused by contamination of the urethra during sexual intercourse may be able to prevent recurrences by voiding immediately after coitus. In some patients, prophylactic doses of a urinary antibiotic taken after intercourse or nightly may be necessary to prevent recurrent cystitis. A sexual history should be taken to include frequency of oral or anal sex and the use of mechanical and chemical contraceptives.

Bacterial persistence after a full course of an appropriate antibiotic chosen according to sensitivity testing indicates the need for cystoscopy and intravenous pyelography to rule out structural abnormalities.

## Complications

Many patients complaining of (often recurrent) dysuria and urinary frequency (particularly if recurrent) do not meet the standard criteria for urinary tract infection. Urinalysis may demonstrate many white blood cells, but no organisms or low colony counts grow on routine cultures. A diagnosis of urethral syndrome is appropriate in these special cases.

Routine culture techniques may fail to demonstrate significant bacterial growth in 30–40% of women complaining of symptoms of urethritis. Effective treatment against all organisms recovered from standard culture should be started even if the count is under $10^5$/mL. Organisms such as *Chlamydia*, anaerobic bacteria, *Mycoplasma*, *Ureaplasma*, and herpes simplex may be responsible in patients with recurrent urethral syndrome. The male partner may require treatment if the organism found can be sexually transmitted. Patients with recurrent urethral syndrome should be examined for anomalies of the urinary tract, eg, urethral stenosis, chemical or mechanical irritation of the urethra, urethral diverticulum, or urethral meatus opening into the vagina.

## URINARY INCONTINENCE

### Etiology

When the urinary tract is intact, continence is maintained as long as the pressure closing the urethra is greater than the intravesical pressure. When the pressure gradient is reversed and the intravesical pressure is greater than the intraurethral pressure, urine is expelled through the urethra. This occurs in voluntary micturition as a result of urethral relaxation and detrusor muscle contraction. Urinary incontinence is leakage of urine due to involuntary reversal of the gradient. Urinary incontinence may be due to any of the following events, alone or in combination: (1) lowered urethral pressure (momentary or continuous), (2) detrusor contractions, (3) greater transmission of intra-abdominal pressure to the bladder than to the urethra, (4) passive increases in intravesical pressure due to distention beyond the elastic limits of the bladder, or (5) bypassing of the continence mechanism due to fistula or ectopic ureter (despite the presence of a normal pressure gradient).

### Classification

Urinary incontinence may be classified into 6 types on the basis of clinical findings: (1) genuine stress incontinence, (2) motor urge incontinence (unstable bladder), (3) sensory urge incontinence, (4) overflow incontinence, (5) bypass incontinence, and (6) psychogenic incontinence.

### Incidence

Several studies indicate that about 50% of all women experience at least occasional incontinence, and 10% experience incontinence regularly. The incidence increases with increased parity and with advancing age (independent of each other). As many as 20% of women over age 75 are affected daily.

Urinary incontinence occurs in over 30% of nursing home residents and is often a major reason for placing individuals in nursing homes. Incontinence prevents many women from fully enjoying their careers, social relationships, and sexual lives. Although severe physical effects are rare, minor discomforts such as vaginal discharge, perineal eruptions, dyspareunia, and unpleasant odors are common.

## 1. GENUINE STRESS INCONTINENCE

Genuine stress incontinence (anatomic stress incontinence, true stress incontinence, urinary stress incontinence) is the involuntary loss of urine through the urethra occurring simultaneously with an increase in intra-abdominal pressure but in the absence of detrusor muscle contraction.

The patient who is continent at rest has an intraurethral pressure that is greater than the intravesical pressure. The pressure difference, or urethral closure pressure (total urethral pressure minus intravesical pressure), represents the margin of continence (Fig 42–4). Because the bladder is an intra-abdominal organ, activities that increase intra-abdominal pressure also increase intravesical pressure by an equal amount. An increase in intra-abdominal pressure is also transmitted to the proximal urethra, though perhaps only partially, so that intraurethral pressure may not increase by the same amount as intravesical pressure. During coughing or exercise, therefore, a deterioration in the margin of continence (urethral closure pressure) may be noted. If the resting intravesical pressure plus any increase in pressure generated during stressful activities exceeds the intraurethral pressure at rest plus any increase in urethral pressure generated during stressful activities, the urethral closure pressure will decrease

to zero, and genuine stress incontinence will result (Fig 42–5).

## Etiology

No hypothesis for the cause of genuine stress incontinence is universally accepted, but proposed mechanisms include the following:

(1) Anatomic descent of the proximal urethra below its normal intra-abdominal position during stressful activities. Increased intra-abdominal pres-

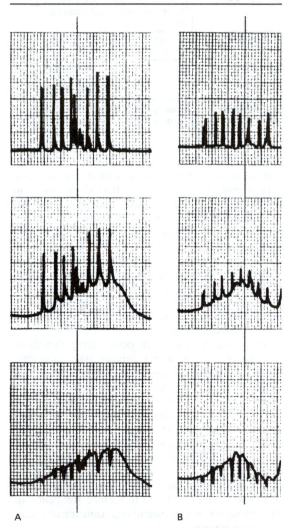

A          B

**Figure 42–5.** The patient coughs repeatedly as tracings are recorded of bladder pressure (top), urethral pressure (middle), and urethral closure pressure (bottom). **A:** Stress continence. Although the spikes recorded during coughing are higher in the bladder than in the urethra, a positive urethral closure pressure is maintained along the length of the urethra. **B:** Stress incontinence. Pressure recorded during coughing is transmitted poorly to the urethra. By electronic subtraction, a zero or negative urethral closure pressure is demonstrated along the entire length of the urethra.

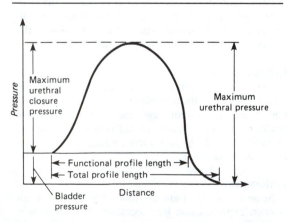

**Figure 42–4.** The urethral pressure profile (at rest) is recorded by measuring the intraluminal pressure along the length of the urethra. The pressure in the urethra is greater than the pressure in the bladder, resulting in urethral closure pressure.

sure is not fully transmitted to the urethra, and the subsequent rise in intraurethral pressure is not as great as the increase in intravesical pressure.

(2) Altered anatomic relationships between the urethra and bladder, so that increases in intra-abdominal pressure result in vector forces directed from the bladder along the axis of the urethra.

(3) Failure of neuromuscular components that reflexly increase intraurethral pressure in response to increases in intra-abdominal pressure in continent patients.

The primary defect in genuine stress incontinence is a greater differential pressure increase in the bladder than in the urethra during stressful activities. However, the urethral closure pressure at rest plays an important role in that the higher the urethral closure pressure prior to stressful activity, the greater the pressure gradient that can be tolerated during stress, and the longer that continence is maintained. Factors that weaken the urethral closing mechanism, eg, estrogen deficiency, scarring, denervation, or medications, may predispose to or exacerbate genuine stress incontinence.

## Diagnosis

No single test is diagnostic of genuine stress incontinence (Table 42–2). Unstable bladder, overflow incontinence, and infection must be ruled out. Objective demonstration of stress incontinence and demonstration of a defect in the anatomic support of the proximal urethra are necessary before a diagnosis can be made and treatment can be started.

## Clinical Findings

**A. Symptoms and Signs:** Almost any lower urinary tract symptom and many vaginal symptoms may be associated with genuine stress incontinence. Stress incontinence is the classic symptom, but frequency, urgency, urge incontinence, and a postvoiding sensation of fullness are common. Dysuria and hematuria are rare in the absence of unrelated gynecologic or urinary tract lesions.

Physical findings are supportive of the diagnosis but not pathognomonic. Cystocele or urethrocele is noted in 75% of patients with genuine stress incontinence, but only half of women with moderate to severe cystocele or urethrocele have genuine stress in-

**Table 42–2.** Criteria for diagnosis of genuine stress incontinence.

Normal urinalysis, negative urine culture
Normal neurologic examination
Poor anatomic support (cotton-tipped applicator test, x-ray, or urethroscopy)
Demonstrable leakage with stress (stress test or pad test)
Normal cystometrogram or urethrocystometry (normal residual urine volumes, bladder capacity, and sensation; no involuntary detrusor contractions)

continence. Efforts to objectively demonstrate poor support of the urethra (cotton-tipped applicator test, x-rays, ultrasonography) are necessary before surgical correction is undertaken, since the goal of almost all standard incontinence procedures is correction of such anatomic defects.

**B. Cotton-tipped Applicator (Q-tip) Test:** The cotton-tipped applicator test is abnormal in 95% of patients with genuine stress incontinence. In about 5%, the test is normal, and incontinence is due to (1) funneling of the proximal urethra, (2) atony of the urethral sphincteric mechanism, or (3) severe scarring of the urethra. A normal test in a patient thought to have genuine stress incontinence is an indication for ultrasonography or radiographic techniques such as a straining cystogram or videocystourethrography to demonstrate urethral funneling or poor urethral support. Poor support may be masked by scarring, which prevents the cotton-tipped applicator from rotating during the test.

**C. Radiographic Studies:** Many physicians feel that radiographic studies are desirable in all patients with urinary incontinence, but the associated cost, discomfort, time, and side effects argue against their routine use. Several authors have found radiographic landmarks and interpretation of cystograms to be inconsistent. Radiographic studies are most useful in the evaluation of patients with recurrent stress incontinence and in those with no abnormality on the cotton-tipped applicator test or pelvic examination.

**D. Urinary Stress Test:** Stress incontinence may be demonstrated by the urinary stress test, which provides gross quantitation of the degree of incontinence, but even under ideal conditions (patient is standing, has a full bladder, and coughs several times), 20% of persons with genuine stress incontinence will not demonstrate incontinence.

**E. Pad Test:** When the stress test is negative (no urine leakage), a pad test may be performed in order to demonstrate incontinence. The patient wears a preweighed sanitary napkin and is requested to exercise, climb stairs, or participate in whatever activities usually result in incontinence. The pad is then reweighed to determine how much urine has been lost. Pad tests are frequently used to assess the degree of incontinence. Any patient who complains of severe incontinence that occurs with minimal stress but who demonstrates only minimal or no leakage on the stress test or pad test must be evaluated for some additional cause of incontinence besides an anatomic abnormality. An alternative method of performing the pad test is to instill colored fluid into the bladder and then check for staining of the sanitary napkin after physical activity.

**F. Laboratory Tests:** Urinalysis and urine culture should be performed in order to detect possible infection.

**G. Cystometry:** A cystometrogram is necessary to rule out unstable bladder, overflow incontinence, reduced bladder capacity, or abnormalities of bladder sensation. Bladder capacities under 300 mL or over 800 mL contraindicate surgery for genuine stress incontinence.

**H. Endoscopy:** Urethroscopy and cystoscopy are useful adjuncts in the assessment of genuine stress incontinence. Diverticula, fistulas, neoplasia, calculi, and inflammatory conditions may be detected. Dynamic urethroscopy affords a functional assessment of the urethrovesical junction during bladder filling as well as during coughing or straining. If anatomic support is adequate during a cough or Valsalva maneuver, the urethrovesical junction closes above the tip of a urethroscope placed in the proximal urethra. Poor anatomic support results in descent of the urethrovesical junction over the tip of the urethroscope when the patient coughs or strains.

**I. Urethral Pressure Profile:** Urethral pressure profiles frequently demonstrate weakness of the urethral sphincteric mechanism at rest in patients with genuine stress incontinence. Urethral weakness at rest occurs in many conditions and is not pathognomonic of genuine stress incontinence. The greatest value of urethral pressure profiles is that the results indicate which patients are not likely to be cured by standard surgical procedures for stress incontinence, since the success rate of surgery in patients with very low resting urethral closure pressure is poor.

## Treatment

**A. Surgical Measures:** Surgical procedures for genuine stress incontinence are divided into those with vaginal approaches and those that use the abdominal route. The goal of most standard incontinence operations is elevation and support of the urethrovesical junction to improve pressure transmission to the urethra during stressful activities.

Assessment of the cure rate of any surgical treatment for genuine stress incontinence must take into account the selection of patients, skill of the surgeon, accuracy of the preoperative diagnosis, length of postoperative follow-up, and criteria for cure.

Reported cure rates for abdominal procedures range from 60 to 100%, with 85–90% being the generally accepted rate. Most failures are due to incorrect preoperative diagnosis, poor surgical technique (failure to correct the anatomic defect), healing failures, secondary causes of incontinence, or a low urethral closing pressure at rest.

Vaginal procedures for incontinence yield reported cure rates ranging from 30 to nearly 100%. The overall long-term success rate for the standard anterior colporrhaphy appears to be no more than 60%. Several authors have reported higher cure rates of 75–85% in carefully selected patients with mild incontinence and minor descent of the urethrovesical junction. Modifications of the anterior colporrhaphy have yielded cure rates approaching or equaling those of abdominal procedures.

No matter which surgical technique is used, the recurrence rate will increase in the later years of long-term follow-up studies. This is in part due to the effects of aging and to the emergence of new pathologic conditions affecting the continence mechanism.

**1. Abdominal procedures**–Abdominal incontinence operations include the Marshall-Marchetti-Krantz procedure, Burch procedure, and many modifications (Fig 42–6). All these procedures follow 2 basic principles and vary only in their implementation: (1) Sutures are placed in the periurethral, vaginal, or paravaginal tissue to elevate the urethrovesical junction, and (2) the elevating sutures are attached to relatively strong and permanent structures. The periosteum of the pubic symphysis (Marshall-Marchetti-Krantz) or Cooper's ligaments (Burch) are most often used, but many other structures may be employed, including the obturator fascia, arcus tendineus of the pelvic fascia, insertion of the rectus fascia, and periosteum of the pubic ramus.

**2. Vaginal procedures**–Vaginal incontinence surgery has evolved from the anterior colporrhaphy described by Kelly (Kelly plication). Anterior colporrhaphy is based on the assumption that weakening or damage of the endopelvic fascia between the bladder and vagina is responsible for poor support of the bladder and urethra. This tissue is plicated in the midline through a vaginal incision. Because the anatomic result and subsequent clinical response are frequently poor and delayed recurrences are common, many variations have been described. Many of those variations use more defined and more permanent anatomic structures than the endopelvic fascia, eg, the pubourethral ligaments, periosteum of the pubic ramus, or the pubococcygeus muscles.

**3. Combined vaginoabdominal technique**– Often referred to as needle procedures, the Pereyra technique and its modifications use a vaginal incision and specially designed ligature carriers to pass sutures through a small abdominal incision to support the paraurethral tissue to the rectus muscles and fascia, thereby incorporating the principles of both vaginal and abdominal techniques. Although short-term results are very good, the incidence of long-term recurrences has been high. The initial procedure has stimulated the development of many modifications that most resemble retropubic procedures performed mainly through the vagina. With these modifications, the cure rates are nearly identical to those of standard abdominal procedures.

**4. Sling procedures and artificial urethral sphincters**–Sling procedures and artificial urethral sphincters may correct incontinence when standard surgical procedures are not likely to succeed. They are primarily used in patients with low urethral closure pressure due to denervation or scarring. Sling procedures use autogenous fascia (rectus fascia, fascia lata, round ligaments) or synthetic material that is passed under the urethra to provide support at the ure-

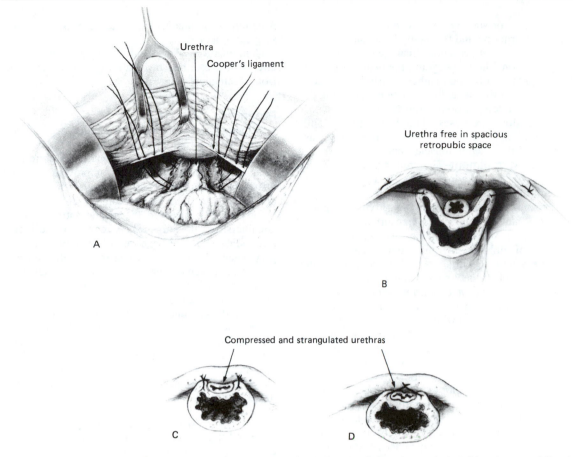

**Figure 42–6.** Abdominal surgical procedure to correct stress incontinence. **A:** Anterior vaginal wall has been mobilized. Two sutures have been placed on either side and far lateral from the midline. Distal sutures are opposite the mid urethra. Proximal sutures are at the end of the vesicourethral junction. Sutures are attached to Coopers ligament. **B:** Cross section shows urethra free in retropubic space with anterior vaginal wall lifting and suppporting it. **C** and **D:** Urethra is compressed and strangulated against pubic bone when vaginal sutures are applied close to the urethra and then fixed to the pubic symphysis. (Reproduced, with permission, from Tanagho EA: Colpocystourethropexy. J Urol 1976;116:751. Copyright 1976 by The Williams & Wilkins Co.)

throvesical junction and partial obstruction of the urethra. A loosely applied sling may not totally prevent incontinence. A tightly applied sling may obstruct the urethra enough to prevent micturition and requires intermittent self-catheterization or micturition by the Credaae maneuver (external abdominal pressure on the bladder).

The artificial urethral sphincter is an effective option for patients with incontinence not amenable to standard surgical treatment because of urethral scarring or atony. The sphincter obstructs the urethra, but an internal pumping system empties the sphincter and relieves the obstruction when the patient desires to void.

**B. Medical Measures:**

**1. Kegel exercises–**Since weakness of the urethral musculature contributes to the severity of incontinence, strengthening of weak pelvic floor muscles may lessen and (in some mild cases) prevent incontinence. Kegel found that repeated contractions of the pubococcygeus muscles were often beneficial. To perform the exercises, the patient squeezes the vaginal muscles or tightens the muscles she normally uses to stop urination. The ability of the patient to isolate and contract the pubococcygeus muscles can be determined by placing two fingertips in the vagina while she attempts to contract the muscles. Lateral pressure on the fingertips indicates muscle contraction. When Kegel exercises are done 150–200 times per day, satisfactory improvement occurs in 15–30% of women with stress incontinence, and another 30–40% report at least some improvement in symptoms. Performing fewer repetitions lowers the effectiveness of the exercises. Women with severe incontinence rarely experience marked improvement. The results of Kegel exercises are directly related to the proficiency at which the exercises are performed. Many patients have difficulty learning to contract the correct muscles or staying on an exercise program. Intensive instruction and follow-up by medical personnel yield results much better than merely instructing the patient on a home program. Perineometers, vaginal weights, and balloon catheters may be placed in the vagina to provide tactile sensation, improving the efficiency of pelvic floor exercises.

Pelvic floor exercises should incorporate both short and long contractions to exercise both fast twitch and slow twitch muscle fibers.

**2. Drug treatment**–The urethra is mainly innervated by the alpha-adrenergic sympathetic nervous system. Elimination of medications that exert ganglionic or alpha-adrenergic blocking activity (eg, guanethidine, methyldopa, and prazosin) may improve urethral tone and result in improved continence. A regimen of alpha-adrenergic agonists may improve genuine stress incontinence; phenylpropanolamine and pseudoephedrine are most commonly prescribed.

Specific therapy of concurrent problems such as infection or inflammatory lesions may be beneficial. Nonspecific treatment with urinary tract analgesics or antispasmodics may lessen the severity of incontinence by reducing irritative symptoms (eg, frequency, urgency, dysuria, postvoiding fullness) that contribute to the patient's overall discomfort.

**3. Estrogen replacement**–Estrogen replacement is vital in those women with localized effects of estrogen deficiency. Estrogen replacement alone relieves stress incontinence in 10–30% of postmenopausal patients, and in many others, symptoms are improved and the response to other forms of therapy is enhanced. Vaginal estrogen therapy appears to provide symptomatic improvement more rapidly than oral replacement, but once symptoms improve, oral and vaginal preparations are equally effective in maintaining the improved status.

**4. Other methods**–Electrical stimulation of the pelvic floor, periurethral injections of Teflon, and other nonsurgical methods are sometimes successful in the treatment of genuine stress incontinence. Electrical stimulation improves continence by increasing urethral closure pressure. Periurethral injections of Teflon or collagen compress the urethral mucosa, providing mild obstruction.

## Complications

Genuine stress incontinence has few and mild physical sequelae but major social and psychologic effects. The surgeon must weigh the social benefits of successful surgery against the risk of a major operative procedure. Urinary tract infection, delayed postoperative voiding, dyspareunia, frequency-urgency syndrome, and surgically induced unstable bladder have been reported even in patients who have undergone successful operation for relief of genuine stress incontinence. Iatrogenic damage to the urinary tract, postoperative fistula, and bladder calculi from sutures penetrating the bladder lumen are rare but potential surgical sequelae.

Complications of medical therapy are chiefly side effects of prescribed medications or local irritation from mechanical devices.

## Prognosis

Although many patients with genuine stress incontinence improve when they are placed on medical regimens, few experience complete resolution of symptoms. Usually, symptomatic improvement rather than outright cure occurs, and cessation of treatment often results in return of symptoms.

Surgery is considered the standard treatment of genuine stress incontinence. A review of the literature indicates a correction rate of 75–85% with surgery when it is well performed in carefully selected patients. An even higher success rate can be achieved if surgery is withheld from those who are better managed medically and if surgical techniques are altered if standard techniques are not likely to be successful. Patients with a poorer prognosis include those with previous surgical failures, poor urethral closing pressure at rest, concomitant local disease, combined urinary incontinence (genuine stress incontinence plus motor urge incontinence), and systemic diseases that make healing or technical performance of surgery more difficult (obesity, diabetes).

A failed surgical procedure increases the likelihood of failure or postoperative complications in subsequent procedures. The operator must avoid the philosophy that a simple, easy procedure may be done first and a preferred procedure reserved for failures or recurrences. The procedure of choice for the first operation should be the one that will yield the best result.

## 2. MOTOR URGE INCONTINENCE (Detrusor Instability, Unstable Bladder)

Motor urge incontinence (unstable bladder, detrusor instability) is the result of involuntary uninhibited detrusor muscle contractions. A hyperreflexic bladder is a bladder that is unstable because of a neurologic cause. Most cases of motor urge incontinence are classified as idiopathic, but infection and obstruction have been cited as possible causes.

Unstable bladder is the second most common cause of urinary incontinence, affecting 1–2% of the adult female population. Because of the large volumes of urine that are lost and the unpredictability of urine loss, this condition usually has a greater detrimental effect on patients than does genuine stress incontinence. Instability of the detrusor muscle is more common in old age and contributes greatly to the costs of health care for the geriatric population.

## Pathophysiology

The initiating event of normal micturition is relaxation of the urethral sphincteric mechanism, followed in 1–3 seconds by contraction of the detrusor muscle. In an unstable bladder, the identical sequence of events occurs despite the efforts of the patient to inhibit them. Typically, involuntary contractions occur at bladder volumes below normal cystometric capacity (the bladder volume that can be tolerated in the awake, unanesthetized state), but they may occur at virtually any volume.

The unstable bladder may contract spontaneously or upon provocation. Reports suggest that 25–50% of patients with unstable bladders are incontinent only in response to provocative stimuli, which may be physical or psychologic, tactile or auditory. Coughing, exercise, running water, or cold may be triggering events. Patients who experience involuntary contractions of the detrusor during stressful activities often present with stress incontinence. On the basis of clinical findings, it may be difficult to determine whether such patients have genuine stress incontinence or bladder instability. Diagnosis is further complicated by the fact that about one-third of all patients with unstable bladder also have genuine stress incontinence. Many patients with combined incontinence have 2 independent conditions. It is apparent that in at least some patients, the conditions are causally related, since medical treatment of the unstable bladder often resolves the genuine stress incontinence. Surgery that corrects genuine stress incontinence also occasionally eliminates concomitant detrusor instability. The exact relationship between these 2 conditions is unknown, but either physiologic or anatomic funneling of the proximal urethra may be responsible.

There is usually an intense urge to urinate shortly before the incontinent episode. Occasionally, particularly when neurologic disease is responsible, leakage of urine may occur without warning, and the patient is only aware of incontinence when she feels herself urinating.

## Clinical Findings

**A. Symptoms and Signs:** The symptoms of unstable bladder are usually multiple, including frequency, urgency, urge incontinence, and stress incontinence.

The physical examination may be normal and rarely provides strong supportive evidence of detrusor instability. Anatomic support of the bladder and urethra may be good or poor. Neurologic signs are typically absent but may be present in cases of detrusor hyperreflexia.

**B. Urologic Studies:** A diagnosis of unstable bladder is suggested when urinary leakage during the urinary stress test is delayed several seconds after stressful activity or when heavy flow continues for several seconds despite the patient's efforts to stop it.

The diagnosis of unstable bladder is confirmed by cystometric demonstration of involuntary detrusor contractions at rest, during bladder filling, or following provocative maneuvers such as coughing, hand washing, or bouncing on the heels while standing. Typically, a smooth rise in pressure occurs simultaneously with visible leakage of urine (Fig 42–7). Simultaneous urethrocystometry measures the intraurethral pressure and intravesical pressure simultaneously. Involuntary contractions are preceded by a fall in urethral pressure just as in normal voiding.

Urethroscopy and cystoscopy often reveal bladder trabeculation due to hypertrophy of the detrusor muscle fascicles. During dynamic urethroscopy, detrusor contractions and urethral relaxation may be visualized simultaneously with either leakage of the filling medium or a measured rise in detrusor pressure. A rigid endoscope placed into the bladder exerts an unphysiologic effect, however, so that results must be verified by standard cystometric techniques.

## Differential Diagnosis

The most common diagnostic problem is the differentiation between unstable bladder and genuine stress incontinence. Provocative cystometry or simultaneous urethrocystometry can usually make the distinction. A more difficult distinction is that between unstable bladder and sensory urge incontinence. In sensory urge incontinence, the patient can usually prevent the leakage of urine with adequate encouragement, whereas with unstable bladder, the patient is unable to inhibit leakage despite strong encouragement and her concerted effort to do so.

## Treatment

The mainstays of treatment for unstable bladder include medication, behavior modification, surgery, or insertion of an indwelling catheter.

**A. Medications:** Anticholinergic agents are the most effective, but bladder analgesics, smooth muscle antispasmodics, calcium channel blockers, and

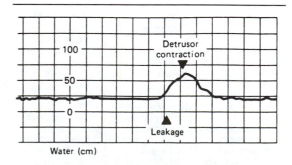

**Figure 42–7.** Unstable bladder. The cystometrogram reveals a detrusor contraction and associated leakage, both involuntary.

prostaglandin synthetase inhibitors are often prescribed alone or in combination (Table 42–3). Fifty to 80% of patients will respond to medication.

**B. Behavior Modification:** Bladder retraining drills, hypnosis, biofeedback, and psychotherapy have been advocated for therapy of unstable bladder. Bladder retraining educates the patient about her bladder problem and may provide a cure without side effects or the morbidity associated with other methods. Bladder retraining yields an initial response rate of over 80% but requires a well-motivated, intelligent patient. The patient is instructed to void according to a schedule that gradually lengthens the interval between voidings. The patient gradually develops the cortical control over the voiding reflex that she has lost. Behavioral techniques are not useful when neurologic disease is responsible for unstable bladder.

**C. Surgery:** Denervation, cystoplasty, and urinary diversion are the surgical procedures advocated for treatment of unstable bladder, but they should be used as a last resort when all other treatments fail. Surgical management is usually reserved for severe permanent bladder instability due to neurologic disease.

**D. Catheterization:** Indwelling catheterization rather than urinary diversion is occasionally used for severely incapacitated patients.

## Prognosis

Although response rates to bladder retraining techniques are good, many patients are not suitable candidates, and the procedure is time-consuming for both physician and patient. Recurrence rates are high, but patients who respond initially usually respond again when retraining techniques are reinstituted.

Response to medications is poorer than to bladder retraining. Side effects of anticholinergic medica-

**Table 42–3.** Drug regimens for treatment of unstable bladder.

| Drug | Trade Name | Dosage |
|------|-----------|--------|
| Oxbutynin | Ditropan | 2.5 mg twice daily to 5 mg 4 times a day |
| Propantheline | Norpanth, Pro-Banthine | 7.5 mg twice daily to 15 mg 4 times a day |
| Imipramine | Tofranil | 25 mg 2–3 times daily |
| Flavoxate | Urispas | 100 mg twice daily to 200 mg 4 times a day |
| Hyoscyamine | Cystospaz, Levsin, many others | 0.125–0.25 mg 3–4 times daily |
| Prostaglandin synthetase inhibitors (nonsteroidal anti-inflammatory agents, eg, ibuprofen, fenoprofen, sulindac) | Advil, Clinoril, Naprosyn, many others | See manufacturer's package insert. |

tions are common at effective dosages. The most common side effect is dry mouth. While less common, dry eyes and blurred vision are usually bothersome enough that the patient will discontinue the medication. Combinations of medications may lower the total dosage of each and decrease the incidence of side effects. When combinations of pharmacologic agents are used, patient compliance becomes difficult to achieve.

## 3. SENSORY URGE INCONTINENCE

Patients with irritative conditions of the lower urinary tract may lose urine either when they perform stressful activities or when bladder volume increases. A diagnosis of sensory urge incontinence is made when this leakage (in association with great urgency) occurs in a stable bladder and is not due to excessive descent of the urethra and bladder. Infection, diverticula, neoplasia, and foreign bodies are common causes of urge incontinence, as are psychologic and neurologic factors.

### Pathophysiology

Sensory urge incontinence is caused by either of 2 physiologic mechanisms: urethral relaxation or voluntary detrusor activity. As the bladder fills, reflex stimulation of the micturition reflex makes the patient aware of an initial urge to urinate; this urge is usually subconsciously inhibited in normal patients. Any condition that irritates the urethra or bladder (eg, infection, trauma) may overstimulate the afferent reflex arc. Urethral relaxation occurs intermittently, allowing small amounts of urine to dribble out and further stimulate the bladder. This urethral relaxation may be purely reflexive or may be voluntary, albeit subconscious, in order to relieve the discomfort the patient feels. During daily activities, when the patient is distracted and cannot concentrate on inhibiting the detrusor reflex, the bladder may contract after the urethra relaxes. The patient, however, maintains the ability to inhibit detrusor contraction and does so when instructed, demonstrating that her bladder is stable.

### Clinical Findings

Sensory urge incontinence is usually associated with a small cystometric capacity, but a normal capacity may be present, and bladder capacity under anesthesia is almost always normal except when there is extensive scarring from radiation or trauma. Urethral relaxation or marked variations in urethral pressure may be found on urethral pressure profiles or simultaneous urethrocystometry. Repeated cystometrograms reveal absence of detrusor activity as long as the patient is encouraged to inhibit her desire to void.

Urethroscopy and cystoscopy are of the utmost importance in the diagnosis of sensory urge incontinence, since most specific therapies are based on endoscopic findings.

Sensory urge incontinence is usually associated with multiple urinary complaints, including dysuria, which is not a common symptom of genuine stress incontinence or unstable bladder.

When there is little or no anatomic defect present in a patient complaining of stress incontinence, sensory urge incontinence may be the correct diagnosis.

### Treatment

Specific therapy is started if it is available. Acute infections respond rapidly to antibiotics, but chronic infection may be associated with residual inflammatory changes (eg, erythema, edema, exudate) that cause symptoms long after treatment has eliminated active infection. Suppressive therapy and symptomatic therapy for chronic urethritis and trigonitis may allow gradual resolution of chronic changes. Mechanical treatments such as urethral dilation or instillation of antiinflammatory agents into the bladder may be beneficial. Surgery is the treatment of choice for diverticula, calculi, and neoplasia. Estrogen deficiency and vaginal diseases (eg, infection, neoplasm, trauma) may cause for sensory urge incontinence, and specific therapy for the underlying disorder usually relieves the urinary symptoms as well as the vaginal symptoms.

### Prognosis

Acute causes of sensory urge incontinence are likely to respond fully to appropriate therapy. Chronic causes often recur or result in partial response.

### 4. OVERFLOW INCONTINENCE

### Etiology

Urinary retention and subsequent overflow incontinence may result from several types of causes.

**A. Neurogenic:** Overflow incontinence due to neurogenic causes may originate in the detrusor secondary to diminished or absent detrusor contractions (denervated bladder) or may start in the urethra as a result of failure of the urethra to relax with voiding attempts (detrusor-sphincter dyssynergia). Diabetes and lower motor neuropathies are common causes.

**B. Obstructive:** Postoperative obstruction, massive relaxation of pelvic supports with urethral kinking, and pelvic masses are the most common obstructive causes.

**C. Pharmacologic:** Ganglionic blocking agents, anticholinergic drugs, alpha-adrenergic agonists, and epidural or spinal anesthesia may cause overflow incontinence.

**D. Overdistention of the Bladder:** Urinary retention is the initiating event and may be idiopathic. Mismanagement of acute or chronic distention results in myogenic decompensation and subsequent overflow incontinence.

**E. Psychogenic:** Chronic psychogenic retention may cause overflow incontinence and is an indication of significant psychiatric illness, usually psychosis or severe depression.

### Clinical Findings

Cystometry reveals a large bladder capacity (often > 1200 mL), usually with decreased sensation. Poor or absent detrusor contractility is noted on pressure-flow micturition studies. Normal detrusor contractility may be present initially when retention is due to obstruction, but contractility gradually lessens.

### Treatment

In acute urinary retention, adequate drainage is important to prevent myogenic decompensation, which may otherwise cause chronic retention, infection, and obstructive uropathy. Medical management is usually directed toward reducing urethral closure pressure and increasing detrusor contractility. Alpha-adrenolytic agents (prazosin, terazosin, phenoxybenzamine) and striated muscle relaxants (diazepam, dantrolene) help reduce bladder outlet resistance. Cholinergic agents (bethanechol) are used to stimulate detrusor tone and contractility.

Intermittent self-catheterization is useful in acute or chronic retention.

### 5. BYPASS INCONTINENCE

Fistulas, ectopic ureters, and urethral diverticula may bypass the normal urethral sphincteric mechanism and result in urinary leakage.

Fistulas usually have an obvious inciting cause, such as surgery, child birth, or trauma. Although leakage due to fistulas is generally continuous, it may be exacerbated by stressful activities and therefore mimic genuine stress incontinence or motor urge incontinence.

A diverticulum may damage the urethra, resulting in incontinence due to low urethral closure pressure. Scarring and inflammation from urethral diverticula often cause sensory urge incontinence. A large diverticulum may also retain urine during micturition and expel it as the patient walks, coughs, and strains. The patient rarely describes a gush of urine, however, as she might in genuine stress incontinence.

Treatment is usually surgical. The prognosis is generally good. Urethral diverticulectomy may cause incontinence if the urethral sphincteric mechanism is damaged.

### 6. PSYCHOGENIC INCONTINENCE

Psychogenic urinary incontinence occurs more frequently in women than in men. Stress incontinence, sensory urge incontinence, motor urge incontinence, urinary retention with overflow, and enuresis may be due to psychogenic causes. Although the diagnosis of psychogenic incontinence is most commonly made in patients with significant psychologic or psychiatric disorders, a psychiatric condition may not be obvious. Since most cases of unstable bladder are idiopathic and since behavioral therapies are successful in this disorder, many authorities believe that unstable bladder is mainly a disease of psychogenic origin.

Although medical treatment may be successful, success is usually short-lived unless the patient's underlying psychologic conflicts are resolved. Patients with psychogenic incontinence frequently undergo multiple surgical operations that stand no realistic chance of curing the problem.

## REFERENCES

### URINARY TRACT INFECTION

Fowler JE, Pulaski ET: Excretory urography, cystography and cystoscopy in the evaluation of women with urinary tract infections: A prospective study. N Engl J Med 1981;304:462.

Lomberg H et al: Correlation of blood group, vesicoureteral reflux and bacterial attachment in patients with recurrent pyelonephritis. N Engl J Med 1983; 309:1189.

McDonald MI et al: Ureaplasma urealyticum in patients with acute symptoms of urinary tract infection. J Urol 1982;128:517.

Neu HC, Parry M: Urinary tract infections—1982: Use of new concepts to guide therapy. Bull NY Acad Med 1983;59:288.

Winick RN et al: Urine culture after treatment of uncomplicated cystitis in women. South Med J 1981;74:166.

### URINARY INCONTINENCE

Andersson KE: Current concepts in the treatment of disorders XXX of micturation. Drugs 1988;35:477.

Bergman A, Ballard CA, Koonings PP: Comparison of three different surgical procedures for genuine stress incontinence: Prospective randomized study. Am J Obstet Gynecol 1989;160:1102.

Blaivas JG: Pathophysiology of lower urinary tract dysfunction. Uro Clin North Am 1985;12:215.

Bradley WE et al: Neurology of micturition. J Urol 1976;115:481.

Brink CA: Absorbent pads, garments, and management strategies. J Geriatr Soc 1990;38:368.

Cantor TJ, Bates CP: A comparative study of symptoms and objective urodynamic findings in 214 incontinent women. Br J Obstet Gynaecol 1980;87:889.

Cardozo LD, Standon SL: Genuine stress incontinence and detrusor instability: A review of 200 patients. Br J Obstet Gynaecol 1980;87:184.

Eaton N: Urinary incontinence in adults. Na Inst Health Concensus Dev Con Consensus Statement 1988;7:1.

Elder DD, Stephenson TP: An assessment of the Frewen regimen in the treatment of detrusor dysfunction in females. Br J Urol 1980;52:467.

Enhorning G: Simultaneous recording of intravesical pressure: A study of urethral closure pressure in normal and stress incontinent women. Acta Chir Scand [Suppl] 1961;No.17 276:9. [Entire issue.]

Fantl JA: Urinary incontinence due to detrusor instability. Clin Obstet Gynecol 1984;27:474.

Fernie GR et al: Urodynamic characterization of incontinence in the elderly by bladder volume. J Urol 1983;129:772.

Fossberg E, Beisland HO: Incompetent urethral closure mechanism in females: Experimental and clinical studies with special reference to diagnosis and classification. Urol Int 1982;37:34.

Fossberg E, Beisland HO, Lundgren RA: Stress incontinence in females: Treatment with phenylpropanolamine. A urodynamic and pharmacological evaluation. Urol Int 1983;38:293.

Hebert DB, Francis LN, Ostergard DR: Significance of urethral vascular pulsations in genuine stress urinary incontinence. Am J Obstet Gynecol 1982;144:828.

Hebert DB, Ostergard DR: Vesical instability: Urodynamic parameters by microtip transducer catheters. Obstet Gynecol 1982;60:331.

Hilton P, Stanton SL: A clinical and urodynamic assessment of the Burch colposuspension for genuine stress incontinence. Br J Obstet Gynaecol 1983;90:934.

Hilton P, Stanton SL: Urethral pressure measurements by microtransducer: The results of symptom free women and those with genuine stress incontinence. Br J Obstet Gynaecol 1983;90:919.

Hilton P, Stanton SL: Use of intravaginal oestrogen cream in genuine stress incontinence. Br J Obstet Gynaecol 1983;90:940.

International Continence Society: First report on standardisation of terminology of lower urinary tract function. Br J Urol 1976;48:39.

Kiesswetter H, Hennrich F, Enclisch M: Clinical and urodynamic assessment of pharmacologic therapy of stress incontinence. Urol Int 1983;38:58.

Kujanauu E: Urodynamic analysis of successful and failed incontinence surgery. Int J Gynaecol Obstet 1983;21:353.

Marchant DJ: Clinical evaluation of urinary incontinence and abnormal anatomy and pathophysiology. Clin Obstet Gynecol 1984;27:434.

Miller RJ, Oldenburg BF: The symptomatic urodynamic and psychodynamic results of bladder reeducation programs. J Urol 1983;130:715.

Montz FJ, Stanton SL: Q-tip test in female urinary incontinence. Obstet Gynecol 1986;67:258.

Olah KS, Bridges N, Denning J, Farrar DJ: The conservative management of patients with symptoms of stress incontinence: A randomized, prospective study comparing weighted vaginal cones and interferential therapy. Am J Obst Gynecol 1990;162:87.

Richardson DA, Ostergard DR: Evolution of surgery for

SUI (stress urinary incontinence). Contemp Obstet Gynecol (March) 1983;21(Special Issue):52.

Stanton SL, Ozsoy C, Hilton P: Voiding difficulties in the female: Prevalence, clinical and urodynamic review. Obstet Gynecol 1983;61:144.

Staskin DR, Zimmern PE, Hadley HR, Raz S: The pathophysiology of stress incontinence. Uro Clin North Am 1985;12:271.

Stower MJ, Massey JA, Fenley RC: Urethral closure in management of urinary incontinence. Urology 1989; 34:246.

Ulmsten U, Henriksson L, Iosif S: The unstable female urethra. Am J Obstet Gynecol 1982;144:93.

Walter S, Kjaergaard B, Lose G, et al: Stress urinary incontinence in postmenopausal women treated with oral estrogen (estriol) and an alpha-adrenoceptor-stimulating agent (phenylproanolamine): A randomized double blind placebo-controlled study. Int Urogynecol J 1990;1:74.

Wein AJ: Pharmacologic treatment of incontinence: National Institute of Health Consensus Development Conference on Urinary Incontinence in Adults., Bethesda, MD, USA, October 3–5, 1988. J Am Geriatr Soc 1990;38:317.

# 43

# Perioperative Considerations in Gynecology

*Michael P. Aronson, MD, Brendan P. Garry, MD, & Paul Summers, MD*

The central focus of the gynecologist is on the normal and pathologic anatomy and function of the female reproductive system. However, since no organ system functions independently, the gynecologist must also be familiar with many pathologic conditions not directly related to the reproductive system but which might affect diagnosis and treatment. At no time is this more crucial than during the perioperative period, ie, just before, during, and immediately after gynecologic surgery.

The differential diagnosis of abdominopelvic pain and dysfunction not directly related to the reproductive system must be fully understood by the gynecologist because many of these entities can present with symptoms suggestive of uterine or adnexal origin. Conversely, the first evidence of nongynecologic disease may be an alteration in the function of the female reproductive system.

This chapter covers the perioperative period: the decision to operate, emergently or electively, and the pre- and postoperative management of those patients. Selected medical and surgical disorders of importance to the gynecologist are reviewed as they relate to management of the surgical patient.

# ACUTE ABDOMEN

## Essentials of Diagnosis (Table 43–1)
Essential Elements:
- Acute onset of severe abdominal pain.
- Signs of peritoneal irritation with guarding and rebound tenderness.
  Frequently Seen:
- Anemia or hypovolemic shock if intraperitoneal hemorrhage exists.
- Varying degrees of gastrointestinal irritation, nausea, and vomiting.
- Elevated white blood cell count (if cause is inflammatory).

- Fever (occasionally).
- Possible complication of pregnancy.

## General Considerations
The diagnosis of acute abdomen has traditionally been based on signs and symptoms of peritonitis, which can be caused by a tremendous array of disease processes. Although the acute abdomen always requires an immediate surgical or medical decision, some patients suffer from a major intra-abdominal pathologic process not associated with peritonitis and should not be considered to have an acute abdomen. An example is of a patient with acute gastrointestinal bleeding who requires emergency care but does not have an acute abdomen in the strictest sense. Although the acute abdomen is not precisely defined, a number of signs and symptoms generally accompany this diagnosis (see Table 43–1.)

It is important to note that although many perceive the acute abdomen as a problem always requiring surgical intervention, in many instances medical management is more appropriate. The presence of an acute abdomen does not dictate the type of management, only the need to come to a rapid decision and implement appropriate therapy as expeditiously as possible.

Finally, it should be stated that an abdomen with generalized peritonitis in all 4 quadrants is commonly termed a "surgical abdomen." If the patient has a rigid abdomen with guarding and rebound tenderness in all 4 quadrants, a clear diagnosis usually cannot be achieved except in the operating room. Ultrasonography, culdocentesis, and other routine tests can often establish whether the process is hemorrhagic or inflammatory, but the specific diagnosis can typically be determined only during laparotomy or laparoscopy.

The patient with a surgical abdomen should never be delayed. The operating room should be notified, large-bore intravenous access obtained, and blood work including a CBC and blood for cross-matching should be sent as the patient is being moved toward the operating room. This is the exceptional case that demands the gynecologic surgeon's total attention and skills. For most patients with localized peritoni-

**Table 43–1.** Differential diagnosis of acute gynecologic intra-abdominal disease.

| Disease | Clinical and Laboratory Findings | | | | | | |
|---|---|---|---|---|---|---|---|
| | CBC | Urinalysis | Pregnancy Test | Ultrasound | Culdocentesis | Fever | Nausea and Vomiting |
| Ruptured ectopic pregnancy | Hematocrit low after treatment of hypovolemia. | Red blood cells rare. | Positive. β-hCG low for gestational age. | Possible adnexal mass. Possible sac-like decidual reaction in uterus. Possible increased free fluid in cul-de-sac. | High hematocrit. Defibrinated, nonclotting sample with no platelets. Crenated red blood cells. | No. | Unusual. |
| Salpingitis | Rising white blood cell count. | White blood cells occasionally present. | Generally negative. | Negative unless pyosalpinx or tubo-ovarian abscess present. | Yellow, turbid fluid with many white blood cells and some bacteria. | Progressively worsening. Spiking. | Gradual onset with ileus. |
| Ruptured ovarian cyst (hemorrhagic) | Hematocrit may be low after treatment of hypovolemia. | Normal. | Usually negative. | No masses. Increase free fluid in cul-de-sac. | Hematocrit generally less than 10%. | No. | Rare. |
| Ruptured ovarian cyst (nonhemorrhagic) | Normal. | Normal. | Generally negative. | No masses. Increased free fluid in cul-de-sac. | Increased clear fluid. | No. | Rare. |
| Torsion of adnexa | Normal. | Normal. | Generally negative. | Adnexal mass common. Decreased flow on doppler study. | Minimal clear fluid if obtained early. | No. | Rare. |
| Degenerating leiomyoma | Normal or elevated white blood cell count. | Normal. | Generally negative. | Pedunculated or uterine mass often with central fluid areas. | Normal clear fluid. | Possibly. | Rare. |

tis, however, a diagnosis can be made outside the operating room, allowing more time for consideration of therapeutic options.

## Etiology and Pathogenesis

The acute abdomen can be caused by a wide variety of problems. Their similar clinical presentation reflects the stimulation of pain receptors in the peritoneum by leakage of purulent matter into the peritoneal cavity, intraperitoneal bleeding, necrosis of an intra-abdominal structure, or inflammation due to infection. Stomach acid, bile, and pancreatic secretions cause intense peritoneal irritation when released into the peritoneal cavity, but urine and ascitic fluid generally do not.

## Clinical Findings

**A. Symptoms and Signs:** The most common symptom of a patient with acute abdomen is pain. It can be generalized or have a maximum intensity in a specific area. The presence of guarding, rebound tenderness, or referred tenderness on abdominal examination can be helpful in localizing the area of greatest peritoneal irritation. On pelvic examination, the patient may exhibit uterine motion tenderness. Although commonly associated with pelvic inflammatory disease, this sign is nonspecific and is likely to be present with a number of irritative pelvic processes.

The irritated peritoneum is most sensitive to stretching and movement, so patients often minimize motion to reduce these stimuli. The patient's position may provide a useful clue to the site of greatest irritation. Patients with pelvic peritonitis are frequently most comfortable with one or both hips flexed, depending on the site and extent of the peritonitis.

The quality of the patient's pain is important. Patients with an intermittent torsion of the adnexa or ruptured ovarian cyst may have had such a pain before. The temporal relationship of the onset of pain to the patient's last menstrual period may give valuable clues, especially regarding possible complications of early pregnancy.

Gastrointestinal symptoms that often accompany the acute abdomen are anorexia, nausea, vomiting, or diarrhea. The extent of bowel involvement depends on the severity of the peritonitis. Patients with mild bowel irritation note decreased appetite. Nausea and vomiting may develop as the bowel becomes more directly involved in the inflammatory process. Further progression leads to inhibition of peristalsis with associated abdominal distention secondary to gas- and fluid-filled loops of bowel. As peristalsis decreases, bowel sounds may be decreased or, eventually, absent. High-pitched bowel sounds and rushes may be heard if obstruction is present.

If the peritoneum covering the bladder or rectosigmoid is irritated first, the patient's initial complaint may be of painful bladder or bowel function. It can be a mistake to assume that a patient complaining of painful bladder filling and emptying merely has cystitis. For example, it is not unusual for a patient to note an episode of urinary or bowel urgency at the time of initial rupture of an ectopic pregnancy or an ovarian cyst.

While taking the history, keep in mind the progression and timing of the appearance of the patient's symptoms. While performing the physical examination, it is necessary to realize that the patient has an evolving process going on. A single examination only assesses a stage of that process. Several serial examinations may be necessary to guide clinical decision making.

**B. Laboratory Findings:** The accurate diagnosis of acute abdomen cannot be based on history and physical examination alone. Routine laboratory studies for all women with pelvic peritonitis should include complete blood count (CBC), urinalysis, and rapid pregnancy test. The CBC may demonstrate either acute blood loss or, if the white blood cell count is elevated, an infectious process.

Urinalysis may demonstrate urinary tract infection, but pyuria may also result from an abscess adjacent to the ureter, as occurs in ruptured retrocecal appendicitis. Gross or microscopic hematuria can reflect the passage of a stone or perhaps exacerbation of an underlying pathologic process such as interstitial cystitis.

Patients with diabetic ketoacidosis may present with severe acute abdominal pain; therefore, testing the blood and urine for glucose and ketones is essential. It is also possible for the stress of an acute abdomen from other causes to initiate or aggravate ketoacidosis in a normally well-controlled diabetic patient. Prior to operating on such patients every effort must be made to fully correct their fluid, glucose, electrolyte, and acidotic status.

A rapid, reliable pregnancy test should always be performed immediately in the female patient with pelvic pain. A patient whose history suggests salpingitis may actually have a ruptured ectopic pregnancy.

In addition, a pregnancy may coexist with an independent pathologic process, in which case the pregnancy may influence management. For example, elective surgery for a degenerating leiomyoma in a pregnant patient would be deferred to the second trimester if possible.

Cervical cultures for *Neisseria gonorrhoeae* and *Chlamydia trachomatis* should also be obtained. Although not useful for immediate management decisions, they may aid in guiding antibiotic therapy if the patient is determined to have a pelvic infection. The erythrocyte sedimentation rate is a nonspecific test for the presence of inflammation and is not very useful in the initial evaluation of the acute abdomen.

**A. Special Examinations:**

**1. Culdocentesis–**Culdocentesis (discussed in Chapters 14 and 30) is an easily performed and important diagnostic procedure that is often overlooked in the current era of high-resolution imaging studies. The contents of the peritoneal cavity can be evaluated by means of culdocentesis in any patient with pelvic peritonitis or pain during uterine and adnexal movement.

Clear, straw-colored peritoneal fluid represents a negative culdocentesis, indicating no intraperitoneal bleeding. An unruptured ectopic gestation could still be present. Large amounts of fluid of this type can indicate a ruptured, nonhemorrhagic ovarian cyst or ascites. Turbid peritoneal fluid containing white blood cells on Gram-stained smear suggests an intrapelvic inflammatory process.

A bloody, nonclotting peritoneal fluid sample with a hematocrit in the range of 15–40% reflects recent hemorrhage into the peritoneal cavity, possibly from ruptured ectopic pregnancy or a bleeding ovarian cyst. In this case, prior clotting of blood in the peritoneal cavity results in crenated red blood cells, defibrination, absence of platelets, and lack of clotting factors in the hemorrhagic fluid aspirated from the cul-de-sac. A bloody aspirate that forms a clot may represent blood inadvertently drawn from vaginal or uterine vessels. An attempted culdocentesis that returns no fluid at all is termed "nondiagnostic."

**2. Radiology–**Transvaginal or transabdominal ultrasound studies have become extremely useful over the past decade in the diagnosis of the acute abdomen. In the pelvis, ultrasonography is useful for characterizing the location and gestational age of early pregnancies, identifying adnexal or uterine masses, and determining the presence or absence of pelvic abscesses or excessive free fluid in the cul-de-sac. Outside the pelvis, ultrasonography is often the initial diagnostic modality used to investigate possible cholecystitis, choledocholithiasis, and appendicitis. In patients too uncomfortable to allow adequate abdominal or bimanual pelvic examination, ultrasound examination plays an even more important role.

Plain x-ray films of the abdomen are less helpful in diagnosing gynecologic causes of acute abdomen but may be helpful in detecting bowel obstruction or paralytic ileus if dilated loops of bowel with air-fluid levels are seen. Free air under the diaphragm on an upright film indicates perforation of a viscous organ and requires immediate intervention. An upright film that does not show the diaphragms should be considered inadequate in the work-up of the acute abdomen. Occasionally, loss of the psoas shadow on the right side is seen, supporting a diagnosis of appendicitis. In addition, renal calculi may be seen on plain films.

**3. Microbiology**–In the acute patient, Gram stains and cultures assume a role of lesser importance. Cervical cultures for *N gonorrhoeae* should be done; however, since this organism may be found on the cervix of asymptomatic as well as symptomatic patients, Gram-stained smears of cervical secretions to detect gram-negative diplococci may be unreliable. Finding *N gonorrhoeae* on the cervix does not prove that peritonitis is due to salpingitis. Conversely, many patients with laparoscopically proven pelvic infections have negative cervical cultures. In the patient who proves to have salpingitis, cervical cultures or cultures of washings done at laparoscopy may help to sharpen the focus of subsequent antibiotic therapy. Cervical material should be submitted for culture in all patients suspected of having gonococcal salpingitis, if only to determine the need for treatment of the sexual partner. *Chlamydia* culture or enzymatic assay are frequently done as well.

# GYNECOLOGIC CAUSES OF ACUTE ABDOMEN

Ruptured ectopic pregnancy (Chapter 14), salpingitis (Chapter 38), and hemorrhagic ovarian cyst (Chapter 37) are the 3 most commonly diagnosed gynecologic conditions presenting as acute abdomen in the emergency room. Degenerating leiomyomas (Chapter 36) and torsion of the adnexa occur less frequently. Typical clinical and laboratory findings for these conditions are shown in Table 43–1. These gynecologic entities are discussed fully in their respective chapters.

The challenge of the acute abdomen is expeditious arrival at an accurate diagnosis and the rapid implementation of a treatment plan. The gynecologist may be the only physician to evaluate the patient and must be capable of entertaining all possible diagnoses in the differential—both gynecologic and nongynecologic. The next section, and Table 43–2, review the most common mongynecologic entities that need to be considered by the gynecologist evaluating the patient with an acute abdomen.

# NONGYNECOLOGIC CAUSES OF ACUTE ABDOMEN

## 1. APPENDICITIS

More than 10% of the general population will develop appendicitis at some time in their lives. Appendicitis is widely recognized as a disease of childhood and is the most common reason for laparotomy in infants and children. In the older patient, however, appendicitis can manifest later and in a more subtle fashion. This can be of great clinical significance in these patients who often have other significant underlying diseases. It is wise to consider the possibility of appendicitis in every patient—regardless of age—who presents in the emergency room with an acute abdomen.

In pregnancy the need to consider appendicitis is of paramount importance. (McGee 378) showed in a 10-year experience at a large teaching hospital a perinatal mortality rate of less than 3% for uncomplicated appendicitis as well as for negative laparotomy. When perforation occurred before surgery, the perinatal mortality rate rose to 20%. As McGee stated, "the maxim regarding acute appendicitis—if in doubt, take it out—is never more true than in pregnancy."

### Clinical Findings

**A. Symptoms and Signs:** It is prudent for the gynecologist to remember that the patient may not present with the "classic" symptoms of appendicitis but may present with many variations that closely mimic other diagnostic entities.

The patient's first symptom may be nausea and loss of appetite. Pain typically begins in the periumbilical area and then gradually shifts to the right lower quadrant. Fever is usually not significant unless the appendix has ruptured. Bowel sounds are reduced, and often no bowel movement will have occurred since the onset of pain. After the patient's pain migrates to the right lower quadrant, tenderness to palpation is most severe at McBurney's point, approximately five centimeters medial to the right anterior superior iliac spine on a line between the anterior superior iliac spine and the umbilicus. As inflammation increases, guarding and rebound tenderness appear at this location. Palpation in the left lower quadrant may produce referred pain in the right lower quadrant.

Some patients note marked discomfort with uterine motion as well as right adnexal tenderness on pelvic examination. These symptoms develop because the inflamed appendix irritates the peritoneum adjacent to the uterus and oviduct and may be improperly interpreted as signs of salpingitis. The patient is generally most comfortable in the supine position with the right hip flexed to minimize tension on the peritoneum adjacent to the appendix.

**B. Laboratory Findings:** The CBC may be normal, but an elevated white blood cell count may develop, especially after rupture of the appendix. Urinalysis results are usually normal unless the inflamed appendix rests adjacent to the ureter, or unless an abscess has formed near the ureter, producing pyuria. If the pregnancy test is positive, the presentation of appendicitis may be significantly altered (see Chapter 24).

**C. Radiologic Findings:** X-ray films of the abdomen may demonstrate an oval calcified fecalith up to 1–2 cm in diameter in the right lower quadrant. A dilated, gas-filled "sentinel loop" of the bowel may also be seen as a result of localized inflammation near the cecum on plain films.

High-resolution ultrasonography with graded compression is proving useful in the diagnosis of acute appendicitis. Abu-Yousef et al (1989) claim a diagnostic sensitivity that varies from 80–95%, a specificity of 95–100%, and an accuracy rate of 91–95%. Ultrasonography also allows some differentiation between the acute appendix and the gangrenous and perforated appendix.

**D. Special Examinations:** Culdocentesis may demonstrate straw-colored, turbid peritoneal fluid containing numerous white blood cells. This finding is not diagnostic for appendicitis but merely reflects the existence of an intraperitoneal inflammatory process; similar findings may be seen in salpingitis and acute regional enteritis.

Laparoscopy may be appropriate in equivocal cases. Considerable technical skill may be required to establish or rule out a diagnosis of appendicitis, depending on the location of the appendix and other intra-abdominal conditions. Removal of the appendix through the laparoscope is then possible as well.

### Differential Diagnosis

On the basis of physical examination alone, it may be difficult to distinguish acute salpingitis from appendicitis. The irritation associated with pelvic inflammatory disease usually extends to both lower quadrants unless unilateral salpingitis (possibly associated with an intrauterine device) is suspected. In contrast to the patient with appendicitis, the patient with salpingitis is more likely to have a fever with an elevated white blood cell count at an earlier stage of her disease. The woman with salpingitis usually develops gastrointestinal symptoms later, since pelvic inflammation spreads from the oviducts to secondarily involve the bowel in the pelvic cavity.

A history of early gastrointestinal symptoms, decreased appetite, and nausea and vomiting is often the most reliable single factor in establishing a diagnosis of appendicitis rather than early pelvic inflammatory disease. The possibility of a ruptured right ovarian cyst must be entertained as well.

In the emergency setting, it is occasionally impossible to differentiate appendicitis from acute regional enteritis (Crohn's disease) with involvement of the terminal ileum. At laparotomy for suspected appendicitis in the patient with regional enteritis, the appendix is normal but the terminal ileum is inflamed. In contrast to the patient with appendicitis, a patient with regional enteritis usually has a history of recent diarrhea (Table 43–2).

Ruptured retrocecal appendicitis may be misdiagnosed as pyelonephritis. The fever, nausea, right-sided back pain, and pyuria from a retrocecal abscess may be mistakenly assumed to be of renal origin.

In the pregnant patient, the enlarging uterus displaces the appendix upward, thereby changing the site of the pain of appendicitis (see Fig 24–1). Pregnant patients with appendicitis also demonstrate less dramatic gastrointestinal symptoms and may even continue to have an appetite. Because of the above, the diagnosis of appendicitis in the pregnant patient is much more likely than in the nonpregnant patient to be made after appendiceal rupture and abscess formation have occurred. This most often leads to premature labor. The risk of early surgical intervention in the gravid patient must be weighed against the considerable risk of premature delivery if appendicitis is indeed present and rupture occurs.

### Treatment

The diagnosis of acute appendicitis requires immediate surgical removal of the appendix either by laparotomy or laparoscopy.

### Complications

Early diagnosis and surgery are essential to prevent rupture of the appendix and the possible complications of recurrent pelvic abscess, wound infection, pelvic adhesions, and, occasionally, infertility.

### 2. ACUTE BOWEL OBSTRUCTION

Bowel obstruction may result from an intrinsic or extrinsic expanding neoplasm, compression of a segment of bowel by a hernia, constriction of the lumen by extrinsic bowel adhesions, or volvulus or intussusception of a segment of bowel. Because of the wide range of causes, all age groups or populations should be considered at risk for development of bowel obstruction. The cause is often not clear until laparotomy is performed. Obstruction due to adhesions is always a possibility if the patient has undergone previous abdominal surgery, especially if the previous surgery was complicated by peritonitis.

### Clinical Findings

**A. Symptoms and Signs:** Nausea and vomiting associated with abdominal distention and severe abdominal pain are the hallmarks of bowel obstruction. Bowel sounds may be absent if obstruction is

**Table 43–2.** Differential diagnosis of acute nongynecologic intra-abdominal disease.

| Disease | Clinical and Laboratory Findings | | | | | |
|---------|------|-----------|------------------|--------------|-------|---------------------|
| | CBC | Urinalysis | Pregnancy Test | Culdocentesis | Fever | Nausea and Vomiting |
| Appendicitis | Normal early; high white blood cell count later. | Normal. | If patient is pregnant, presentation of disease is atypical. | Yellow, turbid fluid with many white blood cells and no bacteria. | Not early in course. | Yes. |
| Retrocecal appendicitis | Normal early; high white blood cell count later. | Many white blood cells if abscess forms. | Not helpful. | May be normal. | Yes in advanced disease. | Variable. |
| Regional enteritis (Crohn's disease) | High white blood cell count. | Normal | Not helpful. | Yellow, turbid fluid with many white blood cells. | Yes if severe. | Yes if severe. Recent history of diarrhea. |
| Colonic diverticulitis | High white blood cell count. | Normal. | Not helpful. | Yellow, turbid fluid with many white blood cells and no bacteria. | Yes if severe. | Variable. |
| Bowel obstruction | High if ischemic bowel damage is present. | Normal. | Not helpful. | Increased amount of fluid with many white blood cells if bowel is ischemic. | Only if bowel is ischemic. | Yes. |

total, or high-pitched if it is partial. The patient may complain of constipation and usually ceases to have bowel movements. A hernia or abdominal mass may be evident on physical examination. Abdominal palpation produces guarding and rebound tenderness.

**B. Laboratory Findings:** Loss of hydrochloric acid through protracted vomiting results in alkalosis with respiratory compensation. Serum bicarbonate levels may be high. Serum potassium levels may be low, indicating general depletion of electrolytes.

**C. X-Ray Findings:** A supine x-ray view of the abdomen demonstrates one or more loops of gas-filled bowel. Air-fluid levels are evident in these loops in upright films (Fig 43–1).

## Differential Diagnosis

Peritonitis with secondary inhibition of peristalsis, generally termed **paralytic ileus,** must be distinguished from bowel obstruction. The patient with paralytic ileus usually experiences constant abdominal pain rather than the cramping abdominal pain associated with bowel obstruction. Treatment of the condition causing peritonitis also results in gradual resolution of paralytic ileus.

## Complications

Marked distention of a segment of bowel may result in vascular compromise, strangulation, and, eventually, bowel perforation with spillage of toxic bowel contents into the abdominal cavity. Dehydra-

tion and loss of electrolytes are associated with accumulation of fluid within the bowel lumen. Hypokalemia may produce electrocardiographic abnormalities if the serum potassium level is lower than 3 meq/L.

## Treatment

Nasogastric suction may be effective in decompressing the distended bowel and may relieve the persistent vomiting and cramping pain associated with bowel obstruction. Surgical correction of the structural abnormality responsible for obstruction is the only definitive treatment. Partial bowel obstruction due to adhesions occasionally subsides while the patient is undergoing nasogastric or long-tube suction. Fluid or electrolyte imbalance must also be corrected, and losses must be compensated for during prolonged suction drainage. Evidence of a perforated viscous organ requires immediate surgical intervention.

## 3. INFLAMMATORY BOWEL DISEASE (ULCERATIVE COLITIS & REGIONAL ENTERITIS [CROHN'S DISEASE])

Ulcerative colitis and regional enteritis represent two distinct forms of inflammatory bowel disease. Inflammation restricted to the colon is termed ulcerative colitis. Regional enteritis (Crohn's disease, terminal ileitis) is characterized by multiple sites of small bowel or colonic inflammation, especially in

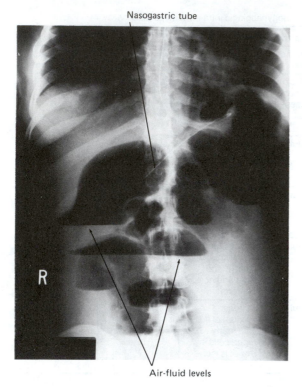

Nasogastric tube

R

Air-fluid levels

**Figure 43–1.** Upright abdominal film demonstrating air-fluid levels in a patient subsequently found to have small bowel obstruction.

the terminal ileum. Women are twice as likely to develop regional enteritis but carry the same risk as men for ulcerative colitis. Inflammatory bowel disease is most likely to develop during the reproductive years.

## Clinical Findings

**A. Symptoms and Signs:** Patients suffering from inflammatory bowel disease generally complain of episodic bloody diarrhea and abdominal pain. Abdominal guarding and rebound tenderness are noted on palpation of the localized area of peritonitis associated with the inflamed segment of bowel. The severity of recurrent episodes of abdominal pain and diarrhea varies widely. Acute regional enteritis with terminal ileitis may mimic appendicitis, although the patient with acute regional enteritis is far more likely to give a history of recent diarrhea.

**B. Laboratory Findings:** The CBC generally shows an elevated white blood cell count with an increased number of polymorphonuclear leukocytes. Culdocentesis should be avoided if inflammatory bowel disease is suspected. If done, however, it would yield turbid fluid containing numerous white cells—largely a result of inflammatory transudate from the inflamed bowel.

**C. X-Ray Findings:** Barium enema and an upper gastrointestinal study with small bowel follow-through may demonstrate either mucosal changes of the bowel consistent with acute inflammation or induration and narrowing of bowel segments, suggesting chronic disease. Involvement of only 1 segment of colon suggests a diagnosis of ulcerative colitis; multiple sites of involvement, often including the terminal ileum, suggest regional enteritis. X-ray studies may be normal in patients with early or inactive inflammatory bowel disease.

**D. Special Examinations:** Endoscopic evaluation with biopsy of areas of inflamed bowel mucosa is the most direct method of diagnosis.

## Differential Diagnosis

Appendicitis, diverticulitis, torsion of the adnexa, and salpingitis may produce physical findings similar to those of acute terminal ileitis. Because of the great difference in appropriate therapy for each of these conditions and because of the serious results of inappropriate treatment, each disease must be ruled out whenever the diagnosis of acute inflammatory bowel disease is suspected.

## Complications

Perforation of the colon and small bowel fistulas are serious inflammatory complications. Appendectomy in a patient with terminal ileitis carries an additional risk of poor healing, abscess formation, and fistula development, especially if the cecum and base of the appendix are involved in the inflammatory process.

## Treatment

Acute inflammatory bowel disease generally responds to administration of corticosteroids. Intravenous metronidazole has been effective in some patients with acute illness. Recurrence may be prevented by long-term administration of sulfasalazine. Therapy is complicated, however, and should be directed by a gastroenterologist. Surgical excision of segments of inflamed bowel may be appropriate in cases of stricture with obstruction, perforation, or massive hemorrhage or in severe cases unresponsive to corticosteroids. Re-anastomosis of bowel after resection for inflammatory bowel disease is often unsuccessful, and resection fails to prevent recurrence, which often occurs just proximal to the anastomotic site. Supportive care, including intravenous fluids, electrolytes, transfusion, antibiotics if sepsis is present, and nutritional replacement for patients with malabsorption, are essential general measures.

## 4. COLONIC DIVERTICULITIS

Diverticula of the distal colon are uncommon in women during the reproductive years, but as many as one-third of postmenopausal women have colonic diverticula demonstrable by barium enema or colonoscopy. Colonic diverticula appear to result from herniation of the bowel mucosa at a site of weakness of the colonic muscularis. The mucosa may be disrupted as the diverticulum enlarges, with resulting bleeding or localized infection. Bleeding may require partial colonic resection. Superficial infection may be self-limiting and associated with mild left lower quadrant pain, which spontaneously subsides as the bowel mucosa heals over a period of 2 or 3 days. Broad-spectrum antibiotics may be necessary if the patient with diverticulitis develops severe left lower quadrant pain, guarding, rebound tenderness, fever, and leukocytosis. Patients not responding to antibiotics or patients with associated pelvic abscess formation require surgical management, including drainage of the pelvic abscess, temporary colostomy, and possible resection of the segment of inflamed or obstructed colon. The surgeon must also rule out carcinoma of the colon, especially in the case of bowel obstruction.

## 5. MECKEL'S DIVERTICULITIS

Meckel's diverticulum, a remnant of the vitelline duct, is found in 2–3% of the general population but is 3 times more common in men than in women. The diverticulum is generally found on the antimesenteric surface of the small bowel, about 80 cm from the ileocecal valve, although the exact distance from the cecum varies greatly. Ectopic secretory gastric mucosa may be found in 20% of patients with Meckel's diverticulum.

If secretory gastric mucosa is present in the diverticulum, ulceration of adjacent bowel mucosa may result in bleeding. Bleeding is an indication for laparotomy in 50% of patients subjected to surgery for complications arising from Meckel's diverticulum. Intestinal obstruction from intussusception of Meckel's diverticulum or obstruction due to volvulus around a vestigial band from the diverticulum to the umbilicus is the reason for an additional 25% of surgical procedures, and Meckel's diverticulitis is the reason for the remaining 25% of surgical cases.

Meckel's diverticulitis is associated with symptoms similar to those of appendicitis, except that abdominal pain is located more medially. Inflamed Meckel's diverticulum may rupture earlier than an inflamed appendix. If the cause of inflammatory peritonitis is unclear at the time of laparotomy, it is important to inspect the entire length of the small bowel for possible inflamed Meckel's diverticulum. An inflamed Meckel's diverticulum should be resected. The base of the diverticulum may be broader than the base of the appendix, so simple ligation may not be possible.

## 6. NEPHROLITHIASIS

Various metabolic factors, in combination with dehydration, may frequently produce supersaturated solutions of relatively insoluble substances that subsequently crystallize in the urine. Men are 2–3 times more likely than women to develop calcium renal stone disease. The less frequently detected struvite (magnesium-ammonium-phosphate), uric acid, and cystine stones are associated with chronic *Proteus* infection of the urinary tract, gout, and cystinuria, respectively.

### Clinical Findings

**A. Symptoms and Signs:** Renal stones may be discovered in any portion of the urinary tract but are most likely to be symptomatic in the ureter. A renal stone passing from the ureteropelvic junction to the bladder usually causes severe ureteral spasm. Ureteral colic generally radiates from the flank on the affected side to the labia or bladder and may occur episodically over several hours or days until the stone passes into the bladder. Although the pain is usually prostrating, the patient experiences no peritonitis and may sometimes be able to remain mobile during the attack. A renal stone may remain lodged at the ureterovesical junction for a long time. In a patient with partial ureteral obstruction, symptoms caused by a renal stone at the ureterovesical junction may mimic the urinary frequency, urgency, bladder discomfort, and hematuria of hemorrhagic cystitis.

Abdominal and pelvic examinations remain normal during an acute attack of ureteral colic, but gentle flank percussion worsens ureteral pain.

**B. Laboratory Findings:** The most helpful initial laboratory test is evaluation for hematuria; blood is found in the urine sample of every patient with renal stone unless total ureteral obstruction exists. Abdominal x-rays are helpful in locating calcium- and magnesium-containing stones. An intravenous pyelogram is useful in assessing ureteral obstruction and secondary renal structural damage. Intravenous pyelogram may also be necessary to locate stones not containing calcium or magnesium (< 10% of all stones), since these are not visible on x-rays. Renal ultrasonography will reveal hydronephrosis or hydroureter if distal obstruction is present.

**C. Special Examinations:** After acute pain has subsided, efforts should be directed toward establishing the cause of renal stone disease. All urine should be filtered to collect stones for analysis of their mineral content. Appropriate metabolic studies to detect hyperuricosuria, hypercalciuria, hyperoxaluria, etc, are dictated by the composition of the stones.

### Treatment

Treatment to prevent recurrent stone formation includes correction of any metabolic abnormalities in the minority of patients who demonstrate such disorders. The most helpful therapy for most patients appears to be conscientious efforts to maintain adequate hydration; consumption of more than 2 L of water daily is advised. Efforts to maintain hydration are especially important after meals and during the night. The pain caused by passage of a stone can be excruciating; adequate pain control is very important.

Obstructing stones lodged in the ureter must occasionally be removed surgically, either by laparotomy or through a cystoscope with the aid of a wire snare attached to a ureteral catheter. Large stones in the renal pelvis or proximal ureter may be pulverized by high-energy shock-wave therapy (extracorporeal shock-wave lithotripsy) to facilitate passage through the ureter.

## 7. OTHER NONGYNECOLOGIC CAUSES

Other causes of acute onset of abdominopelvic pain in the female must also be entertained. Perforation of a peptic ulcer will allow entry of gastric secretions into the peritoneal cavity with resultant severe peritonitis. Acute cholecystitis is most often associated with right upper quadrant pain subsequent to a fatty ingestion. Always keep in mind the remote possibility of a nongynecologic intra-abdominal hemorrhage–either spontaneous or secondary to trauma. Trauma to the left upper quadrant can lead to intraperitoneal splenic hemorrhage that is delayed significantly from the event secondary to capsular containment. Sickle cell crisis can present with severe abdominal pain as can, occasionally, interstitial cystitis.

## THE DECISION TO OPERATE: SCHEDULED GYNECOLOGIC SURGERY

Emergent operations represent a small fraction of all the gynecologic surgical procedures performed. Most operations are planned in an elective fashion with varying degrees of urgency. The patient with a gynecologic malignancy does not have to be rushed to the operating room in the middle of the night, but she wants to plan her procedure within a reasonable period of time. On the other hand, the patient who is having a uterovaginal prolapse repaired has much more leeway to fit her operation into her life rather than having to fit her life around her operation.

Scheduled surgery allows a patient time to get mentally set for the procedure. Patients should be encouraged to assemble support for the postoperative period to help with their recovery or to help cover their responsibilities at work or with child care. The date for an elective gynecologic procedure should always be selected by the patient for the time that is most convenient in her life.

Patients should be encouraged to optimize their physical and emotional conditions prior to scheduled surgery. There is time to attempt to stop smoking, to donate autologous blood for surgery, to lose weight, to take preoperative estrogen or iron, and to take care of any concurrent medical problems before their surgery. In addition, the option exists to postpone a patient's surgery if a respiratory infection or other medical problem develops as the date for surgery approaches.

The indications, workups, and operations for benign and malignant gynecologic conditions are well documented elsewhere in this text. Hysterectomy, laparoscopy, hysteroscopy, and dilatation and curettage (Chapter 45); surgery for pelvic floor relaxation (Chapter 41); infertility surgery (Chapter 58); and surgery for urinary incontinence (Chapter 42) make up a large portion of procedures done for benign disease or dysfunction. Surgeries for gynecologic malignancies are well covered in Chapters 45 through 49.

# PREOPERATIVE CARE

## GENERAL CONSIDERATIONS IN PREOPERATIVE EVALUATION

Preoperative evaluation should include a general medical and surgical history, a complete physical examination, and laboratory tests. An anesthesiologist routinely sees patients preoperatively; however, a patient's medical status may warrant earlier consultation with an anesthesiologist and possibly with physicians in other specialties as well. The medical evaluation must be carried out in such a way as to identify all disorders that might complicate the operative procedure or convalescence. Although "diagnostic overkill" should be avoided, the responsibility of the operating gynecologist is to adequately assess—and take steps to minimize—a given patient's operative risk.

All records of prior hospitalizations should be obtained. Past records may be essential to the interpretation of present findings and may significantly influence the management plan. Patients' ability to recall illnesses and the details of previous surgeries is notoriously inaccurate.

### Laboratory Studies

It has been estimated by Roizen (1989) that by the late 1980s over 40 billion dollars a year was being spent in the United States on preoperative testing. He opined that 60% was wastefully spent on "routine" preoperative laboratory and evaluative studies. Although the efficacy of various preoperative testing regimens has not been established in a prospective, randomized fashion, most gynecologists would agree that preoperative laboratory studies should include at a minimum a CBC, a blood typing and antibody screen, and a urinalysis and culture. Further laboratory tests should be performed only when indicated by the patient's medical condition or by the type of surgery to be performed. A Papanicolaou smear should also be obtained.

A routine chest x-ray and electrocardiogram for all preoperative patients should be discouraged. Sommerville and Murray (1992) showed in their series an overall positive yield for routine chest x-ray of 6%: 17% in those older than 60 years, and 2% in those under 60. Routine electrocardiograms showed an overall positive yield of 7%: 7.4% in those over 40 and 4.5% in those under 40. Finally, they found that investigations prompted by history or physical findings yielded a high positive rate (34% for chest x-ray and 31% for electrocardiograms) and included most of the younger patients who would be missed by an age-only criterion for preoperative testing. It seems reasonable to obtain a preoperative chest x-ray and electrocardiogram on all patients over 45 years old as well as all patients whose medical history or physical findings are matters of concern, regardless of their age.

Blood should be drawn for typing and cross-matching if a need for transfusion is anticipated, especially in patients with abnormal antibodies, which would make intraoperative cross-matching time-consuming (see Chapter 30). If the patient's preoperative hematocrit and physical status permit and if there is an appropriate interval before the anticipated surgery, the possibility of autologous blood donation should be discussed. Directed donor programs can be discussed as well.

Patients scheduled for surgery for menorrhagia with low hematocrit can often be allowed the time to build up their own blood supply through the use of a gonadotropin-releasing hormone (GnRH) agonist and iron supplementation. This can significantly lower the patient's risk for requiring transfusion by starting with a larger red blood cell mass. A GnRH agonist-induced reduction in the size of fibroids, if present, may also help reduce intraoperative blood loss.

More extensive testing tailored to the individual patient's needs can improve the safety of surgical procedures. Fasting and 2-hour postprandial plasma glucose determinations are helpful to exclude diabetes. Platelet count, bleeding time, prothrombin time, and partial thromboplastin time evaluate the adequacy of the clotting system. Liver, renal, and endocrine function testing should be obtained as indicated. A patient with poor pulmonary function might benefit from a baseline arterial blood gas determination. If prolonged parenteral dependency is anticipated, a preoperative laboratory assessment of the patient's nutritional status would be useful. Liver function tests and tumor markers are often obtained in the gynecologic cancer patient (see Chapters 45–49). Finally, testing for HIV antibodies and hepatitis B surface antigen and a serologic test for syphilis, although controversial, may also be appropriate.

Further imaging studies should be obtained only as indicated. Ultrasonography is useful for characterization of pelvic masses. Computed tomography (CT) performs that function as well as giving information regarding the course of the ureters and an assessment of retroperitoneal adenopathy. Intravenous pyelogram demonstrates renal function and architecture while providing information on the course of the ureters and ruling out a dual collecting system. Magnetic resonance imaging, with its superb soft tissue differentiation, can give much information regarding uterine, adnexal, and retroperitoneal architecture. Its clinical usefulness as a preoperative study has not been established. Double contrast barium enema can be useful in identifying bowel lesions or colonic involvement with pelvic masses.

Imaging studies as well as functional studies (eg, pulmonary function tests, stress electrocardiograms, multichannel urodynamics, or anal manometry), are informative but costly. They should be obtained on an individualized basis when the information they give would decrease the patient's perioperative risk, influence the choice of the surgical procedure to be performed, or increase the chances for a successful surgical outcome for the patient. See following section on Assessment and Minimization of Surgical Risk for further discussion of the extended preoperative evaluation.

## Consultations

Because of the increasing tendency to admit patients after surgery, patients should be seen well in advance of their surgical date by the anesthesiologist. This allows for the optimal selection of the type of anesthesia by considering the patient's physical status, prior anesthesia history, proposed surgery, and the personal preferences. Consultation also gives the anesthesiologist an opportunity to allay the patient's anxieties.

Consultations with other physicians should be requested if the surgeon desires advice or assistance with a particularly high-risk surgical candidate or if the proposed procedure involves high risk. Medical preoperative consultation is of particular importance for the older surgery patient as well as the younger patient with known cardiovascular, pulmonary, renal, hematologic, or endocrinologic problems.

Pre-operative urogynecologic consultation, individualized as noted in Chapter 42, can be considered in many cases requiring surgery for urinary incontinence. Consultation with a gynecologic oncologist should be considered pre-operatively when the index of suspicion for malignancy is high.

## Patient-Physician Communication

**A. Informed Consent:** It is imperative for every patient to have a complete understanding of exactly what her procedure will involve, why it is proposed, what alternatives are available, what the chances are for success, and what all the possible complications of the proposed procedure might mean to her in terms of further surgery, disability, or even death. It is important that this dialogue be carried out in layman's terms in the patient's native language and that the patient have ample opportunity to ask any questions that she may have.

To document that this important interaction took place to the satisfaction of the patient, she or her legal guardian should sign a consent form or note. All major points covered in the preoperative discussion should be written on the consent form or within the consent note before it is signed by the patient and the physician. If an interpreter was used, the interpreter should sign this document as well. Permission should be considered as being granted only for the procedures discussed in the preoperative conversation and designated in the consent form or note. This includes optional procedures such as appendectomy.

**B. Patient Education:** In view of the increasing complexity of operative procedures and the associated short- and long-term risks, audiovisual aids may be helpful in the patient counseling process. These aids can supplement, but never replace, the actual communication between the gynecologic surgeon and the patient as outlined above.

A well-prepared video tape with simple diagrams can provide a consistent, in-depth presentation. Patient education pamphlets can serve a similar function. The patient should have an opportunity to ask questions about the film or pamphlet, and any modifications pertinent to her particular case should be explained. As documentation that this patient education was accomplished, it is appropriate to have the patient sign a form indicating that she has viewed the film, discussed it with the physician, and understands its content. If necessary, the film and signed form may serve as evidence that adequate preoperative counseling has been provided.

**C. Documentation:** All details of the history, physical examination, and diagnostic and therapeutic formulations and conclusions of all preoperative consultations must be entered in the patient's chart. This history and physical, or preoperative note, must include a problem-oriented assessment and a clearly delineated plan to address each problem. A note, or consent form as just described, documenting the scope of preoperative counseling must also be entered in the admission record. A carefully completed record is important for health care team communica-

tion and continuity of the patient's care as well as for hospital quality assurance.

## ASSESSMENT AND MINIMIZATION OF SURGICAL RISK

### 1. CARDIOVASCULAR SYSTEM

#### Cardiac Disease

The perioperative period is associated with significant cardiovascular stress. Any patient with heart disease should be considered a high-risk surgical candidate and must be fully evaluated preoperatively. Patients with symptoms of previously undiagnosed heart disease (eg, chest pain, dyspnea on exertion, pretibial edema or orthopnea), new ECG changes, a recent history of congestive heart failure, recent myocardial infarction, or severe hypertension should be evaluated with the assistance of medical or cardiology consultation. Many factors may adversely affect cardiovascular function during and after surgery; for example, fluid shifts, hypotension, electrolyte imbalance, infection, severe pain, apprehension and tachycardia. Perioperative monitoring, anesthesia induction, maintenance techniques, and postoperative care can be tailored to the specific cardiovascular disease, thus improving the patient's chances for a good surgical outcome.

#### Special Studies

**A. Electrocardiography:** An ECG should be obtained on all patients over 45 years of age as well as on younger patients with a history of symptoms of cardiovascular disease. The ECG is of value in identifying the patient with coronary artery disease, ventricular hypertrophy, electrolyte disturbance, arrhythmia, and digitalis or other drug effect. Of prime interest are changes that might indicate coronary artery insufficiency such as ST- and T-wave changes; signs of infarct such as the appearance of Q waves or poor progression of R waves in the anterior chest leads; rhythm changes, particularly atrial fibrillation or flutter and atrioventricular or intraventricular block or ventricular ectopy; and others that might show the effect of systemic disease such as chronic hypertension, left ventricular hypertrophy, and electrolyte imbalance. The age of ECG changes is important since patients with more recent infarcts, for example, have poorer postoperative outcomes than patients with older infarcts. Comparison with older ECGs is important when significant changes do exist. The preoperative ECG should serve as a baseline for subsequent studies if postoperative complications develop.

**B. Echocardiography:** If symptoms of cardiac disease are present, and particularly if an ECG demonstrates potential pathology, a consultation with a cardiologist should be obtained. Generally, an echocardiogram is performed, which will demonstrate any valvular or ventricular wall motion abnormalities resulting from coronary artery insufficiencies or cardiomyopathy. Left ventricular ejection fraction can also be estimated from an echocardiogram.

**C. Dipyrimadole (Persantine)/Thallium Stress Test:** Patients with a significant cardiac history or an abnormal ECG should have a preoperative stress ECG under the direction of the patient's cardiologist. Dipyrimadole or thallium stress tolerance scanning demonstrates older, fibrosed, fixed lesions or areas subject to ischemia and potential infarct. This test identifies ischemia under stress before the patient is subjected to the stress of surgery. The result will guide the gynecologist and anesthesiologist in their invasive monitoring and surgical anesthesia maintenance decisions.

**D. Intraoperative Central Monitoring:** Invasive catheter measurements of intracardiac pressures can often provide useful information regarding cardiovascular dynamics. In most cases, this information can be discerned simply by careful attention to aspects of the physical examination such as blood pressure, pulse, pulse pressure, heart rate, status of neck veins when supine, auscultation and percussion of the chest, presence or absence of edema, and size of the liver. If the preoperative evaluation raises a significant question, direct central venous pressure monitoring should be considered. A Swan-Ganz pulmonary artery catheter is particularly useful when surgery is likely to be prolonged with the history, physical examination, and cardiology testing indicate depressed myocardial function or pulmonary artery hypertension. Specific references to the implementation of monitoring and management of these parameters are found in Chapter 59.

## Varicose Veins and History of Deep Vein Thrombosis

Patients with large, extensive varicosities or a history of thrombophlebitis or thromboembolic events are at risk for developing lower extremity thrombophlebitis or thromboembolic phenomena. This risk may be minimized by prevention of dehydration, early ambulation, and prompt and adequate treatment of cardiac disorders. Except in the patient in whom the risk of pregnancy is high, discontinuance of oral contraceptives 3–4 weeks preoperatively should be considered.

Before the operation, the patient should wear support stockings from toe to thigh. After surgery, these stockings should be worn continuously and discarded only after full ambulation is restored. Pressure on the calf or thigh should be avoided during a long operative procedure. Postoperative leg exercises should be initiated as soon as possible to prevent phlebitis. These may be begun even before ambulation by having the patient press against a footboard whenever supine. When discharged the patient should be advised to avoid prolonged sitting, eg, auto, train, or air travel, during the first month after surgery.

Prophylactic administration of heparin, 5000 U subcutaneously 2 hours before surgery and every 8–12 hours thereafter until full ambulatory status is achieved, may be given to prevent thromboembolization in high-risk cases. No laboratory control is required. Similarly, the use of sequential compression boots intraoperatively and postoperatively until the patient is fully ambulatory helps to prevent thrombosis in high-risk patients. Marshall (1991) reviewed 2 meta-analyses of more than 70 published trials of deep venous thrombosis prophylaxis in general surgical patients. Both studies concluded that prophylaxis significantly reduced the rates of deep venous thrombosis and fatal pulmonary embolism and resulted in improved overall survival. Physical methods such as compression stockings and intermittent pneumatic compression were shown to be as effective as pharmacologic prophylaxis with heparin.

## Valvular Heart Disease

Patients with a history of valvular heart disease or a heart murmur should have echocardiography done if they have not already been evaluated for this. Antibiotic prophylaxis should be administered according to the American Heart Association guidelines.

## 2. PULMONARY SYSTEM

Elective surgery should be postponed if acute upper or lower respiratory tract infection is present. Even mild upper airway infection is associated with an irritable airway, which predisposes to laryngospasm or severe coughing on induction or emergence from anesthesia. Pulmonary infection causes poor ciliary motility, which predisposes to postoperative bronchitis and pneumonia. If emergency surgery is necessary in the presence of a respiratory tract infection, regional anesthesia should be used if possible and aggressive measures should be taken to avoid postoperative atelectasis or pneumonia. If the infection is severe, appropriate antibiotic therapy should be initiated promptly and modified as necessary when the results of cultures become available. The patient should be free from respiratory infection for 1–2 weeks before elective surgery.

Chronic obstructive pulmonary disease, which includes chronic bronchitis, emphysema, and asthma, puts the patient at increased risk in the perioperative period. Optimizing the patient's pulmonary status with chest physical therapy, breathing exercises, and appropriate antibiotics preoperatively decreases the potential for prolonged postoperative ventilation and suture line strain from coughing. Bronchiectasis, relatively uncommon at present, requires the patient to have rigorous chest physiotherapy and antibiotics before surgery. Preoperative pulmonary function tests should be performed to assess the severity and type of disease and to have as a baseline for reference in the postoperative period.

Asthmatic patients and those who smoke are at risk of developing pulmonary complications during or after surgery. Special care must be exercised in the management of such patients. Patients who smoke and for whom general anesthesia by endotracheal intubation is planned should be encouraged to stop smoking for as long as possible before their surgery. Prolonged operations involving general anesthesia or hypoventilation increase the risk of postoperative hypoventilation and other pulmonary problems. Careful evaluation, including chest x-rays and pulmonary function tests, enable the surgeon and his or her consultant to decide when the operation may be safely undertaken and may influence the mode of anesthesia selected.

## 3. RENAL SYSTEM

Renal function should be appraised if there is a history of kidney disease, diabetes mellitus, or hypertension; if the patient is over 60 years of age; or if the routine urinalysis reveals proteinuria, casts, or red cells.

It may be necessary to further evaluate renal function by measuring creatinine clearance, blood urea nitrogen, and plasma electrolyte determinations. An intravenous pyelogram or CT scan may sometimes be indicated for functional as well as anatomic reasons.

## 4. HEMATOLOGIC SYSTEM

### Anemia

Anemia diagnosed in the preoperative obstetric or gynecologic patient usually is of the iron deficiency type caused by inadequate diet, chronic blood loss, or chronic disease. Care must be taken to differentiate iron deficiency anemia from other anemias, eg, sickle cell anemia. Iron deficiency anemia is the only type of anemia in which stained iron deposits cannot be identified in the bone marrow. Megaloblastic, hemolytic, and aplastic anemias usually are easily differentiated from iron deficiency anemia on the basis of the history and simple laboratory examinations. The diagnosis of obscure anemias may require the help of a hematologic consultation.

Patients with iron deficiency anemia respond to oral or parenteral iron therapy. Before elective surgery for menorrhagia, the patient's blood loss may be able to be stopped with a GnRH agonist long enough to allow reversal of the anemia. In emergencies or urgent cases, preoperative blood transfusions, preferably with packed red cells, may be given.

### Von Willebrand's Disease

Von Willebrand's disease is a congenital bleeding disorder characterized by altered factor VIII activity and deficient platelet function. Inheritance is generally autosomal dominant, although a rare autosomal recessive form has been recognized. Clinical manifestations include epistaxis, easy bruisability, hypermenorrhea, and postpartum hemorrhage. Von Willebrand's disease is considered the most common congenital cause of hypermenorrhea. Vaginal bleeding between menses may also occur. Menstrual abnormalities are generally persistent and severe but may be intermittent or moderate, so that milder cases are less likely to be diagnosed. Hypermenorrhea either may develop in affected persons at menarche and persist until the menopause or may not develop until after the second or third decade of life. Von Willebrand's disease is diagnosed in 10 persons per 100,000, but the true incidence is probably somewhat higher. It is possible that the true cause of menstrual abnormalities is undetected in some women with undiagnosed von Willebrand's disease who undergo hysterectomy for hypermenorrhea.

The diagnosis of von Willebrand's disease is confirmed by a prolonged bleeding time, decreased factor VIII activity, and abnormal platelet function. The platelet count is normal. All patients should avoid aspirin and nonsteroidal antiinflammatory medications preoperatively, but this is especially true of the patient with von Willebrand's disease. Treatment with DDAVP 0.3 µg/kg intravenously immediately before surgery may help to improve platelet function. Patients should be given factor VIII and whole blood intraoperatively if needed.

### Thrombocytopenia

The normal platelet count ranges from 150,000 to 350,000/µL. In the patient with thrombocytopenia but normal capillary function, platelet deficiency begins to manifest itself clinically as the count falls below 100,000/µL. Typical manifestations include petechiae on easily traumatized areas of the body, epistaxis, and menorrhagia. Epistaxis and hypermenorrhea may be severe enough to require transfusion. Bleeding into deep muscle and hemarthroses usually do not result spontaneously from thrombocytopenia, but intracranial hemorrhage is a serious risk if the platelet count is very low. The thrombocytopenic patient may require transfusion of platelets before surgery if the platelet count falls too low.

If thrombocytopenia is severe, the deficiency of platelet-produced factors involved in the coagulation cascade may result in some prolongation of clotting time. The most sensitive early clinical measure of platelet deficiency has been thought to be the bleeding time. More recent literature suggests that bleeding time may not be a reliable indicator of platelet function and no study has established that a bleeding time will predict the risk of hemorrhage in individual patients. Spontaneous hemostasis is not expected if the platelet count falls to 10,000/μL or less, and the patient may begin to bleed from all old puncture wounds as the platelet count approaches this threshold.

Bone marrow suppression, autoimmune disease, and platelet consumption are the chief causes of thrombocytopenia. Treatment revolves around treating the underlying cause and support with platelet transfusion and clotting factors as necessary. See also Chapter 22.

## 5. ENDOCRINE SYSTEM

### Diabetes Mellitus

Diabetes is a common disease of disordered metabolism arising largely from altered pancreatic islet cell function. The incidence is higher with age, ranging from 0.1% in children to 2–3% in the general population. Diabetes in nonpregnant patients is defined by the American Diabetes Association as a fasting plasma glucose above 140 mg/dL on more than one occasion. Results on oral glucose tolerance testing are abnormal if fasting blood glucose is over 115 mg/dL, if the 2-hour value is over 140 mg/dL, and if the value in any sample exceeds 200 mg/dL.

Control of diabetes is made especially difficult by the stress of operation, acute infection, anesthesia, and electrolyte imbalance. The operative diabetic patient must be carefully observed and promptly treated before fluid and electrolyte abnormalities, ketosis, hyperglycemia, and infection develop. Diabetics whose disease is out of control are especially susceptible to postoperative sepsis. Preoperative consultation with an internist may be considered to ensure control of diabetes before, during, and after surgery.

Type II diabetes accounts for about ninety percent of cases and is seen in the older, usually more obese, patient population. Insulin production is close to or at normal values, but not appropriate for the blood sugar level. There is also peripheral insulin resistance. These patients develop neither ketoacidoses nor hyperosmolar states. The blood sugar is controlled by diet or oral medication. The oral medications most commonly used are the sulfonylurea derivatives, glyburide (Micronase) or glipizide (Glucotrol). Their duration of action can be greater than 24 hours, and chlorpropamide (Diabinese) may be effective for up to 50 hours. Therefore, it is important to avoid hypoglycemia by closely monitoring blood sugar on the day of surgery and possibly by not using the longer-acting agents for up to 2 days preoperatively.

Type I diabetics tend to be younger and nonobese and have little or no insulin production. They require insulin to avoid development of ketoacidoses, nonketotic hyperosmolar states, and hyperglycemia. In-

sulin-dependent diabetics with good control should be given half of their total morning insulin dose as regular insulin on the morning of surgery. This is preceded or immediately followed by the initiation of a 5% dextrose solution intravenously to prevent hypoglycemia in a fasting patient. Regular insulin should then be given every 6 hours in amounts dictated by plasma glucose, or fingerstick, determinations.

If the diabetes is severe, it may be necessary to admit the patient to the hospital before the operation for glycemic control. Regular insulin may be substituted for long-acting insulin to achieve tighter control. Serum electrolyte determinations should be recorded as points of reference for postoperative management. Fasting plasma glucose should be determined prior to surgery.

Some controversy exists regarding how tightly the blood sugar should be controlled perioperatively. It is generally accepted that keeping the blood sugar in the 100- to 250-mg/dL range in the perioperative period is adequate for most types of surgery. Cardiopulmonary bypass surgery, procedures in pregnancy or after a cerebral ischemic episode, and neurosurgical operations in which maintenance of cerebral autoregulation is important have better results if the blood sugar is more tightly controlled at about 80–130 mg/dL. Tight control is achieved by using an intravenous insulin infusion based on frequent blood sugar estimations.

Occasionally surgery is required emergently in a patient who presents in a hyperglycemic ketoacidotic state. It is important to first correct the fluid and electrolyte status, particularly the potassium levels, but it is not necessary to hold off surgery until complete resolution has occurred. The surgical condition may be the precipitating factor, and final correction may not be possible until surgery is completed. The hyperglycemic ketoacidotic state is treated by giving 10 U of regular insulin intravenously followed by an infusion of insulin based on the formula of the blood sugar divided by 150 U/h. Normal saline solution is given to correct dehydration. Potassium must be supplemented as the insulin drives it into the cells. Total body potassium, despite its initial elevated serum level, may be very depleted. Because there are a fixed number of insulin receptors there is nothing to gain by using higher doses of insulin. Blood glucose levels usually fall at a maximum rate of 100 mg/dL/h, except during the initial rehydration period when the fall is more precipitous.

Chronic medical conditions associated with diabetes may also complicate the perioperative period, eg, hypertension and coronary artery disease. Myocardial ischemia may often be silent in the diabetic with autonomic neuropathy. Autonomic neuropathy is also associated with gastric paresis and increased risk of aspiration. These patients should have an extended cardiac work up and receive metoclopramide as well as a nonparticulate antacid before surgery. Intubation in some patients may be difficult because the atlanto-occipital joint may be involved with the diabetic process.

## Thyroid Disease

Elective surgery should be postponed when thyroid function is suspected of being either excessive or inadequate. Hyperthyroidism is suspected clinically when the patient has a history of weight loss, muscle weakness, a persistently rapid pulse, agitation, tremor, heat intolerance, nervousness or warm skin. The gland either may be diffusely enlarged, as in Graves' disease, or may have only an unobtrusive adenoma. Exophthalmos may be evident. Cardiac signs may be the only clue in the elderly patient (apathetic hyperthyroidism) and may include an unexplained atrial fibrillation or other tachyrhythmia or dysrhythmia. A varying level of ventricular dysfunction is present in all patients with hyperthyroidism.

The patient should be rendered euthyroid before surgery if possible. This may take up to 2 months if antithyroid medications are used in combination with potassium iodine (Lugol's solution). The combination of a beta blocker, usually propranolol (Inderal), and potassium iodide allows surgery in about 14 days. Propranolol blocks the peripheral effects of hyperthyroidism (ie, nervousness, sweating, tachycardia) and may slow the response to atrial fibrillation. It also impairs the conversion of $T_4$ to $T_3$ peripherally. Care must be exercised in the use of propranolol in patients with asthma or congestive heart failure. If surgery is immediately required, propranolol is titrated slowly intravenously in 0.5-mg aliquots until the peripheral signs of thyrotoxicosis have been brought under control. Regional or local anesthesia is preferable. If general anesthesia is required, the airway should be adequately assessed clinically and by x-ray or CT scan for severe tracheal compression or deviation that may interfere with placement of an intratracheal airway.

Severe stress such as that provided by surgery and anesthesia may precipitate a thyroid storm in a person with hyperthyroidism. **Thyroid storm** is a life-threatening event that manifests itself as hyperpyrexia, tachycardia, and cardiovascular instability, and it may be mistaken for malignant hyperthermia.

Hypothyroidism is relatively common in the elderly. It is usually of insidious onset; 95% of cases are due to primary failure of the thyroid to produce adequate $T_4$ and $T_3$. Goiter may be present, and a history of surgery or radioactive iodine treatment may be elicited. There is a slowing down of the metabolism affecting both mental and physical abilities, including a slowing of the heart rate and diminished ventricular contractility in response to catecholamines. Patients are very sensitive to respiratory depressant medications. There is blunting of the stress response, and corticosteroid supplementation may be needed.

In mild to moderate hypothyroidism surgery and anesthesia need not be delayed before treatment is started. If the disease is severe, treatment should be started before surgery, if possible. In all cases, treatment must be started with a very low dose of thyroid replacement therapy to avoid sudden large demands on the myocardium, which may not yet be able to respond appropriately. The usual tests of thyroid function include total $T_4$ and $T_3$ levels, free $T_4$, $T_3$ resin uptake and TSH levels. Preoperative consultation regarding the management of patients with thyroid dysfunction should be sought before major surgery.

## Recent or Current Corticosteroid Use

Patients who are taking corticosteroids, or who have recently stopped them, are under the influence of the adrenal suppressive effects of their medication and are not able to respond to the stress of surgery appropriately. These patients must be provided with intravenous stress dose corticosteroids before, during, and after their surgery.

## 6. OTHER CONDITIONS AFFECTING OPERATIVE RISK

### Pregnancy

The diagnosis of early pregnancy must be considered in the decision to do elective major surgery in the female. Elective surgery generally should be postponed until after delivery. Scheduled surgery that cannot be delayed, such as exploration for an adnexal mass, is best performed in the second trimester whenever possible.

Diagnostic or evaluative procedures necessary in the proper workup for urgently needed surgery override theoretical fetal hazards in the pregnant patient. Appropriate protective measures should be taken to minimize these dangers, such as shielding the uterus from radiation during x-ray studies, using tocolytic agents to prevent premature labor, and considering possible fetal effects when pharmacologic and anesthetic agents are to be used. Hypotension and hypoxia must be meticulously avoided during anesthetic administration or surgical manipulation. Surgery should be performed in the left lateral decubitus position to optimize uterine perfusion. If the surgery is being performed after fetal viability, intraoperative fetal heart rate monitoring should be performed.

The new and more sensitive radioreceptor assay and radioimmunoassay for pregnancy are positive within 10 days of conception, ie, before the anticipated menstrual period. This capability may be important in scheduling elective surgery, especially in gynecologic procedures such as tubal ligation and hysterectomy.

### Age

The 65-year-old and older segment of the population is currently undergoing the most rapid expansion of any demographic group in the USA. This expansion is projected to continue and accelerate well into the next century. The majority of individuals in this age group are women. It has been estimated that over 50% of this older population will, at some point, undergo some surgical intervention. It is clear that the gynecologic surgeon will be caring increasingly for older patients requiring or desiring surgical procedures.

Care of the older patient can present a significant challenge. These persons often have multiple medical problems against a background of a general decline of their physiologic reserve. If care is taken, however, with preoperative evaluation and perioperative management, these patients can do quite well. Age itself is not an independent predictor of surgical risk. The healthy elderly patient, or the carefully evaluated and managed elderly patient with medical problems, should not be discouraged from a beneficial elective procedure.

A careful history and review of systems must be taken and may require the assistance of family members or caretakers. A review of past medical records is crucial. A thorough physical examination must be performed. Appropriate preoperative consultation and extended preoperative evaluation as previously described should be obtained. The results should be reviewed with, and the patient seen by, the anesthesiologist well before the operative date so that an intraoperative management plan can be developed. Finally, meticulous and expeditious technique must be used during surgery to limit the patient's blood loss, operative time, and fluid shifts.

The principles and general considerations of good surgical practice become critically important when the elderly patient is being operated on. Serum electrolytes must be determined preoperatively and any imbalances corrected by appropriate parenteral solutions. Care should be taken not to overload the elderly patient's circulation when administering intravenous fluids, since cardiac, pulmonary, and renal reserves are often diminished. Nutritional deficiencies should be corrected before elective surgery is undertaken if possible. In older patients who are found to be significantly nutritionally deprived, total parenteral nutrition (TPN) may be required before and after surgery.

Fluid intake and urinary output should be monitored carefully and the patient's weight recorded daily. Early ambulation of the patient is very important. The older patient, or one who has been bedridden, requires frequent change of position to prevent the development of a decubitus ulcer. Early ambulation, or aggressive active and passive physical therapy, may prevent many vascular and pulmonary complications.

The elderly patient often requires smaller dosages of medications such as narcotics and anesthetic agents. Barbiturates should especially be prescribed with caution, since mental confusion often results even from small doses.

## Obesity

Obesity puts the patient and every member of the hospital team at a disadvantage in trying to avoid the increased perioperative morbidity associated with it. Every system in the body is affected by this disease.

The anesthesiologist is challenged by difficult intravenous access. These patients have markedly decreased functional residual capacity, making hypoxia a major concern, particularly in a supine or Trendelenburg position. Increased volume and acidity of gastric secretions, along with poor gastroesophageal sphincter tone, increases the risk of pulmonary aspiration. Poor neck extension makes intubation more difficult. The increased work of breathing and tendency to hypoxia occasionally necessitates later extubation and ambulation. In addition, obese patients have an increased potential for hypertension, coronary artery disease, and possibly diabetes.

The surgeon must struggle for exposure. Because of this, there is an increased risk of trauma to adjacent organs. Wound healing is inhibited, and there is an increased risk of postoperative wound seroma and infection. The gynecologic surgeon must plan ahead to make sure extra assistants are available as well as long instruments. The incision should be planned with the patient's body habitus in mind to provide maximal exposure. A mass closure technique with a delayed absorbable or permanent suture should be considered.

Postoperatively, nursing personnel are also at a serious disadvantage. Attempts to achieve ambulation and to prevent respiratory and thromboembolic complications are much more difficult because of the patient's size. These complications are far more likely to occur in patients with obesity than in patients of normal weight. Again, planning beforehand and extra personnel may be the key to a successful postoperative course.

## Drug Allergies & Sensitivities

The obstetric or gynecologic patient who is being evaluated and prepared for a major operation may receive a variety of medications. Drug allergies, sensitivities, incompatibilities, and other adverse effects must be anticipated and prevented if possible. A history of serious reaction or sickness after injection, oral administration, or other use of any of the following substances should be noted and the medication avoided: (1) antibiotic medications, (2) narcotics, (3) anesthetics, (4) analgesics, (5) sedatives, (6) antitoxins or antisera, and (7) antiseptics. Untoward reactions to other medications, foods (eg, milk, chocolate), adhesive tape, and antiseptic solutions, especially iodine, should also be noted.

## Immunologic Compromise

A patient may be considered an immunologically compromised or altered host if her capacity to respond normally to infection or trauma has been significantly impaired by disease or therapy. Obviously, preoperative recognition and special evaluation of these patients are important.

**A. Increased Susceptibility to Infection:** Certain drugs may reduce a patient's resistance to infection by interfering with host defense mechanisms. Corticosteroids, immunosuppressive agents, cytotoxic drugs, and prolonged antibiotic therapy are associated with an increased incidence of superinfection by fungi or other resistant organisms. It is possible that the synergistic combination of radiation, corticosteroids, and serious underlying disease may set the stage for clinical fungal infection.

A high rate of wound, pulmonary, and other infections is seen in renal failure, presumably as a result of decreased host resistance. Granulocytopenia and diseases associated with immunologic deficiency (eg, lymphomas, leukemias, and hypogammaglobulinemia) are frequently complicated by sepsis. The uncontrolled diabetic is also observed clinically to be more susceptible to infection. The acquired immunodeficiency syndrome (AIDS) is associated with increased susceptibility to infection. For a full discussion of HIV infection and AIDS, see Chapter 38.

**B. Delayed Wound Healing:** This problem can be anticipated in certain categories of patients whose tissue repair process may be compromised. Many systemic factors have been alleged to influence wound healing; however, only a few are of clinical significance: protein depletion, ascorbic acid deficiency, marked dehydration or edema, and severe anemia. It has been shown experimentally that hypovolemia, vasoconstriction, increased blood viscosity, and increased intravascular aggregation and erythrostasis due to remote trauma interfere with wound healing, probably by reducing oxygen tension and diffusion within the wound.

Large doses of corticosteroids depress wound healing. This effect apparently is increased by starvation and protein depletion. Wounds of patients who have received large doses of corticosteroids preoperatively should be closed with special care to prevent disruption, inasmuch as healing may be delayed.

Patients who have received anticancer chemotherapeutic agents are just as apt to require surgery as any other population group. Cytotoxic drugs may interfere with cell proliferation and may decrease the tensile strength of the surgical wound. It is wise to assume that healing may be retarded in patients receiving antitumor drugs.

Poor control of blood sugar in diabetic patients is associated with slow healing, poor scar formation, and increased rate of wound infection. Slow healing sometimes is observed in debilitated patients, ie, those with advanced cancer, renal failure, gastrointestinal fistulas, or chronic infection. Protein and other nutritional deficiencies may be major causes of poor wound repair. Decreased vascularity and other local changes occur after a few weeks or months in

tissues that have been heavily irradiated. These are potential deterrents to wound healing as well,(see Chapter 51).

## PREOPERATIVE ORDERS

Presently most patients are admitted to the hospital on the day of their surgery, or they have their surgery as outpatients. Much of the preoperative preparation of the patient that was formerly done in the hospital is now done at home by the patient and her family, since only a small percentage of gynecologic surgical patients are admitted before their surgical date. The following discussion reviews several areas of surgical concern that were formerly addressed in a patient's in-patient, night-before-surgery, preoperative orders.

**A. Skin Preparation:** Many gynecologic surgeons choose to have patients wash the skin over the operative site with povidone-iodine or hexachlorophene the night before the procedure is to be performed and follow with a povidone-iodine preparation just before surgery. It has been shown that wound infection incidence is decreased by shaving the operative site in surgery rather than the night before the procedure. The wound infection rate is lower still with the use of clippers in the operating room or with no hair removal at all.

**B. Diet:** The patient should receive nothing by mouth for at least 8 hours before the operation so that the stomach will be empty at the time of anesthesia.

**C. Preparation of the Gastrointestinal Tract:** Many gynecologic surgeons recommend that a patient use a cleansing enema the night before surgery to make certain that the examination under anesthesia will be accurate and to reduce the need for straining with a bowel movement during the early postoperative period. Mechanical (eg, enemas until clear or an oralosmotic and concentrated electrolyte agent such as and GoLytely) and antibiotic bowel preparation (eg, a combination of oral neomycin and erythromycin) are necessary when the nature of the disease makes the possibility of bowel injury, resection, or purposeful entry likely. Some patients can comfortably complete a GoLytely, or a GoLytely and antibiotic, bowel preparation at home the night before surgery whereas others may require admission the day before to accomplish this.

**D. Sedation:** A sedative-hypnotic may be prescribed to ensure restful sleep the night before the operation.

**E. Preanesthetic Medication:** Preanesthesia medication is not administered until after an intravenous line has been started on the day of surgery. It generally consists of a sedative, such as midazolam, titrated to effect. See also Chapter 26.

**F. Other Medications:** The patient is generally advised to take all of her regular medications on the morning of surgery with sips of water sufficient to swallow them unless there are specific contraindications. Special preoperative orders sometimes must be given for modification of regularly required medications in diabetic patients and patients on anticoagulants or corticosteroids.

**G. Antibiotics:** Preoperative or prophylactic antibiotics are of value especially in cases of expected bowel surgery, abdominal hysterectomy, all major vaginal surgery, and certain cesarean section deliveries. The first-generation cephalosporins have been particularly effective in decreasing postoperative febrile morbidity. Recent experience indicates that single-dose prophylaxis may be as effective as multiple doses.

**H. Blood Transfusions:** In circumstances in which transfusions are not usually required, a type and screen is satisfactory and cost-effective. If major blood loss is anticipated, a full cross-match should be performed. Keep in mind that more blood can be prepared as you are transfusing the units you have already ordered.

Because of current concerns about the risk of transmitting AIDS via transfusion, elective gynecologic surgery patients should be offered the option of autologous blood donation preoperatively. In addition, acute intraoperative autotransfusion should be considered if excessive intraperitoneal blood loss occurs either preoperatively, as in the case of ruptured ectopic pregnancy, or intraoperatively, as in the case of certain radical surgical procedures. Use of a cell saver device, which processes blood aspirated from the surgical field and allows return of the patient's own red blood cells, which have been washed in normal saline, is useful in these large blood loss situations and significantly cuts down on blood bank demand. The device is contraindicated in certain patients, such as those with infection near the operative site or those undergoing cesarean section or cesarean hysterectomy, because thromboplastins from decidual or amniotic fluid may become mixed with the blood.

**I. Bladder Preparations:** For minor procedures, the patient voids prior to being moved to the operating room. If major pelvic surgery is planned, an in-dwelling Foley catheter should be placed when the vaginal preparation is done in the operating room. For prolonged bladder drainage, a suprapubic catheter provides a lower urinary tract infection rate along with the ability to allow voiding trials without multiple urethral catheterizations. Intermittent, clean self-catheterization is another bladder drainage modality that can be taught preoperatively and offers a low postoperative infection rate.

**J. Douches:** An antiseptic douche, eg, with povidone-iodine, is sometimes prescribed prior to gynecologic operations in an attempt to decrease the population of vaginal flora. Its value is not proved, and recent experience suggests that saline douches are as effective.

# POSTOPERATIVE CARE

## IMMEDIATE POSTOPERATIVE CARE

During the immediate postoperative period, maintenance of normal pulmonary and circulatory function should be emphasized. Vital signs and fluid balance should be monitored frequently to facilitate the early diagnosis of shock or pulmonary problems. Bleeding from the surgical site and persisting pulmonary or cardiovascular effects from anesthesia are risks that mandate careful surveillance of all patients in the immediate postoperative period.

### Postoperative Orders

The postsurgical patient is removed to the recovery room, accompanied by the anesthesiologist and the surgeon or other qualified attendant, as soon as she responds. Patients with medical problems may require postoperative admission to an intensive care unit for prolonged ventilation or central monitoring. The nurse receiving the patient should be given a verbal report of her condition in addition to an operative summary and postoperative orders. These should include the following:

**A. Vital Signs:** Record the blood pressure, pulse, and respiratory rate every 15–30 minutes until the patient is stable and hourly thereafter for at least 4–6 hours. Any significant change must be reported immediately. These measurements, including the oral temperature, should then be recorded 4 times daily for the remainder of the postoperative course.

Postoperative fever is a common complication. The cause may be as simple as dehydration or as complex as infection in an obscure location. A search for the cause is mandatory before appropriate treatment can be initiated. Pulmonary, urinary, and pelvic examinations are of primary importance in this evaluation. Thrombophlebitis should also be considered as a possible cause of fever.

**B. Wound Care:** Watch for excessive bleeding (notice abdominal dressing or perineal pads). Determine the hematocrit the day after major surgery and, if there is a question of continued bleeding, repeat as indicated. An abdominal wound should be inspected daily. Skin sutures or clips generally are removed 3–5 days postoperatively and replaced with Steri-Strips.

**C. Medications:** Following major surgery, give narcotic analgesics as needed (eg, meperidine, 75–100 mg intramuscularly every 4 hours, or morphine, 10 mg intramuscularly every 4 hours), to control pain. Recently, injectable nonsteroidal antiinflammatory drugs have become available for postoperative pain control as well. Antiemetics such as promethazine or hydroxyzine may be helpful to suppress nausea as well as to potentiate analgesics.

Patient-controlled analgesia (PCA) is now widely available. With PCA, patients are able to give themselves intravenous pain medication as they need it within the parameters set by the physician. Many patients prefer PCA because it allows them to avoid the "peak and valley" effect of scheduled pain injections.

Many centers are now using intrathecal or epidural opiate injection for relief of postoperative pain. This technique is particularly appropriate for patients who have been given regional anesthesia. A minimal dosage of less than 5 mg of morphine may allow several hours of complete pain relief without compromise of motor activity (ambulation, coughing). Respiratory depression is a hazard, however, and close monitoring of the patient is necessary. Following minor surgery, give mild analgesics as needed. Other medications required by the patient taken prior to surgery (insulin, digitalis, cortisone, or others) should be resumed as required.

**D. Position in Bed:** The patient is usually placed on her side to reduce the risk of inhalation of vomitus or mucus. Other positions desired by the surgeon should be clearly stated, eg, flat with foot of bed elevated.

**E. Drainage Tubes:** Connect the bladder catheter to the gravity drainage system. Written orders for other postoperative drainage and suction catheters should be specific and clear, setting forth the degree of negative pressure desired and the intervals for measurement of drainage volume.

**F. Intake and Output:** Record intake and output of all fluids as well as daily weight.

**G. Fluid Replacement:** Administer fluids orally or intravenously as needed. When deciding how to replace a patient's particular fluid needs, always take into account factors such as intraoperative blood loss and urine output, operating time, intraoperative fluid replacement, and the amount of fluid received in the recovery area. Although each patient and operation are different, an average healthy young patient who has been appropriately replaced intraoperatively will do well with 2400 mL to 3 L of a balanced crystalloid and glucose solution such as 5% dextrose in half-normal saline over the first 24 hours. The rate of intravenous hydration must always be individualized, since many patients require less volume and may become fluid-overloaded at a faster rate. In the patient with normal renal function, adequate fluid replacement should result in a urine output of at least 30 mL/h.

**H. Diet:** Following minor surgery, offer food as desired and tolerated, when the patient is fully awake. After major surgery, disagreement exists on how fast to advance a patient's diet. This again must be individualized to the patient and depends on many factors.

A possible regimen is to allow the patient only sips of tap water on the day of surgery. Do not give ice water, because it may decrease bowel motility significantly. Give clear liquids on the first postoperative day if good bowel sounds are noted and until intestinal gas is passed. Change the diet thereafter to full regular. The time needed to progress to a full diet depends on the extent of the procedure, the duration of anesthesia, and individual variation among patients.

**I. Respiratory Care:** Encourage deep breathing every hour for the first 12 hours and every 2–3 hours for the next 12 hours. Incentive spirometry and the assistance of a respiratory therapist may be of great value, particularly in elderly, obese, or otherwise compromised or immobilized patients.

**J. Ambulation:** Encourage early ambulation and bathroom privileges. If possible, require ambulation on the day of the operation after major surgery.

## RECOVERY FROM MAJOR SURGERY

Even with the trend toward decreasing hospital stays, the patient generally remains hospitalized until recovery of all bodily functions. Normal pulmonary function usually returns after resolution of inhalation anesthesia but may be influenced to some extent by surgical pain during the early postoperative period. Two or three days may pass before return of normal bowel function after laparotomy. The patient with febrile complications generally will not be discharged until she has remained asymptomatic and afebrile for 24 hours.

## OUTPATIENT SURGERY

With the current trend favoring outpatient surgery, the observation period following minor surgery becomes more critical. Following outpatient surgery, patients generally remain hospitalized until mental status, pulmonary, and bladder functions return to normal. Occasionally, admission to the hospital becomes necessary for overnight observation or for further therapy. Although "ambulatory surgery" is designed for the healthy patient who is scheduled for less extensive surgery, to become casual in preparation is to court disaster.

Because these patients play a more active role in the preparation and management of their surgery, the following additional elements must be considered. (1) Preoperative counseling should encompass the same information given the inpatient, but another responsible adult who will provide transportation and postoperative care for the patient should also be present at the session. (2) Emphasis should be placed on the importance of the "nothing by mouth" requirement and on the avoidance of any medications that the surgeon has not prescribed or approved. (3) A hospital must be available for backup if the facility is not hospital-based, and the patient must know where to report if problems arise; this entails establishing 24-hour telephone service for access to medical advice and care. (4) A follow-up call from the physician within 24 hours is often beneficial for picking up early postoperative problems as well as for emotional support for the patient. (5) All postoperative instructions should be reviewed with the patient before her surgery.

## POSTOPERATIVE COUNSELING & RELEASE FROM THE HOSPITAL

Following operation, the patient should receive a careful explanation (both oral and written) of the sur-

gical procedure performed, the findings at surgery, and any postoperative procedures or findings. The postoperative course may be negatively influenced by the patient's anxiety regarding lack of information or unanswered questions. It may be helpful for the physician to refer to preoperative audiovisual aids during the postoperative counseling session.

Every postoperative patient should have a complete physical examination (including a pelvic assessment) before release from the hospital. Findings can be used as a baseline for subsequent follow-up examinations.

The patient should receive oral and written instructions regarding postoperative care at home, including which physical activities she may perform. Appointments should be made for outpatient or office follow-up examinations.

## REFERENCES

### ACUTE ABDOMEN

Beal J: How to diagnose the acute abdomen. Contemp Obstet Gynecol 1983;21(Special issue):13.

Bender JS: Approach to the acute abdomen. Med Clin North Am 1989;73(6):1413.

Laing FC: Ultrasonography of the acute abdomen. Radiol Clin North Am 1992;30(2):389.

MacFayden BV Jr, Wolfe BM, McKernan JB: Laparoscopic management of the acute abdomen, appendix, and small and large bowel. Surg Clin North Am 1992;72(5):1169.

McGee TM: Acute appendicitis in pregnancy. Australian and New Zealand Journal of OB/GYN 1989;29(4):378.

Silen W: *Cope's Early Diagnosis of the Acute Abdomen,* 18th ed. Oxford University Press, 1991.

### APPENDICITIS

Abu-Yousef MM et al: Sonography of acute appendicitis: A critical review. Crit Rev Diagn Imaging 1989;29(4):381.

Buchman TG, Zuidema GD: Reasons for delay of the diagnosis of acute appendicitis. Surg Gynecol Obstet 1984;158:260.

Doherty GM, Lewis FR Jr. Appendicitis: Continuing diagnostic challenge. Emerg Med Clin North Am 1989;7(3):537.

Sreide O: Appendicitis: A study of incidence, death rates, and consumption of hospital resources. Postgrad Med J 1984;60:341.

### DIVERTICULITIS & INFLAMMATORY BOWEL DISEASE

Elfrink RJ, Miedema BW: Colonic diverticula: When

complications require surgery and when they don't. Postgrad Med 1992;92(6):97.

Ertan A: Colonic diverticulitis: Recognizing and managing its presentations and complications. Postgrad Med 1990;88(3):67.

Mowat NAG: Inflammatory bowel disease. Practitioner 1984;228:803.

Oren R, Rachmilewitz D: Preoperative clues to Crohn's disease in suspected, acute appendicitis: Report of 12 cases and review of the literature. J Clin Gastroenterol 1992;15(4):306.

### PERIOPERATIVE EVALUATION AND CARE

Burgos LG et al: Increased intraoperative cardiovascular morbidity in diabetes with autonomic neuropathy. Anesthesiology 1989;70:591.

Celli BR: What is the value of preoperative pulmonary testing? Med Clin North Am 1993;77(2):309.

Croughwell GH et al: Diabetic patients have abnormal cerebral autoregulation during cardiopulmonary bypass. Circulation 1990;82(Suppl IV):407.

Dunnet JM et al: Diabetes mellitus and anesthesia: A survey of the perioperative management of the patient with diabetes mellitus. Anesthesia 1988;43:538.

Ergine PL, Gold SL, Meakins JL: Perioperative care of the elderly patient. World J Surg 1993;17(2):192.

Fleischer LA, Barash PG: Preoperative cardiac evaluation for noncardiac surgery: A functional approach. Anesth Analgesia 1992;74(4):586.

George JN, Shattil SJ: The clinical importance of acquired abnormalities of platelet function. N Engl J Med 1991;324:27.

Gerson MC: Cardiac risk evaluation and management in noncardiac surgery. Clin Chest Med 1993;14(2):263.

Graebe RA: Preoperative and postoperative treatment of

the gynecologic patient. Curr Opin Obstet Gynecol 1991:3(3):362.

Graf G, Rosenbaum S: Anesthesia and the endocrine system. In: *Clinical Anesthesia,* 2nd ed. Barash PG, Cullen BF, Stoelting RK. JB Lippincott, 1992.

Halpern SH: Anesthesia for cesarean section in patients with uncontrolled hyperthyroidism. Can J Anaesth 1989;36:454.

Macpherson DS: Preoperative laboratory testing: Should any tests be "routine" before surgery? Med Clin North Am 1993:77(2):289.

Mishriki YY: Perioperative risk assessment: Common misconceptions. Postgrad Med 1989;85(5):52,59.

Morgensen T, Hjortso NC: Acute hypothyroidism in a severely ill surgical patient. Can J Anaesth 1988; 35:74.

Roizen M: Preoperative patient evaluation. Can J Anaesth 1989;36(3 Pt 2):S13.

Roizen MF: Anesthetic implications of concurrent diseases. In: *Anesthesia,* 3rd ed, vol 1. Miller RD (editor). Churchill Livingstone, 1990.

Sommerville TE, Murray WB: Information yield from routine pre-operative chest radiography and electrocardiography. S Afr Med J 1992:81(4):190.

Watters JM: Preventive measures in the elderly surgical patient. Can J Surg 1991:34(6):561.

Wright RA, Clemente R, Wathen R: Diabetic gastroparesis: an abnormality of gastric emptying of solids. Am J Med Sci 1985;289:240.

## ANTIBIOTIC PROPHYLAXIS

Antimicrobial prophylaxis in surgery. Med Lett 1992; 34:5.

Antimicrobial treatment for gynecologic infections. ACOG Technical Bulletin #153, 1991.

Mittendorf RM, Aronson MP, Berry RL et al: Avoiding serious infection associated with abdominal hysterectomy: A meta analysis of antibiotic prophylaxis. Am J Obstet Gynecol 1993;169:1119.

Stein GE: Patient costs for prophylaxis and treatment of obstetric and gynecologic surgical infections. Am J Obstet Gynecol 1991:164(5 Pt 2):1377.

Walker CK, Landers DV: Anti-infective drugs in obstetrics and gynecology. Curr Opin Obstet Gynecol 1991:3(5):698.

## THROMBOPROPHYLAXIS

Fareed J, Walenga JM, Cornelli U: Antithrombotic drugs in pelvic surgery. Semin Thromb Hemost 1989;15(2): 230.

Husted SE: Principles of thromboprophylaxis in surgical patients. Semin Thromb Hemost 1991;17(Suppl 3): 254.

Marshall JC: Prophylaxis of deep venous thrombosis and pulmonary embolism. Can J Surg 1991;34(6):551.

# Intraoperative and Postoperative Complications of Gynecologic Surgery

# 44

Michael P. Aronson, MD, David Chelmow, MD, & Jack W. Pearson, MD

## INTRAOPERATIVE COMPLICATIONS

There are two truisms concerning intraoperative complications of gynecologic surgery. The first is that if one performs enough gynecologic surgery, one will have complications. The second is that it is a venial sin to cause an intraoperative complication, but a mortal sin not to recognize that one has done so. In this chapter, we will review the keys to avoiding surgical misadventure and to recognizing it when it has occurred: understanding pelvic anatomy, using meticulous and methodical surgical technique, handling tissues gently, and maintaining a constant high index of suspicion. A detailed description of the management of each possible complication of gynecologic surgery is beyond the scope of this text. For this, the reader is referred to the many excellent references at the end of this chapter.

## URINARY TRACT INJURY

### Ureteral Damage

Ureteral injury has occurred in association with most major gynecologic surgical procedures, particularly pelvic cancer surgery, hysterectomy for benign indications, oophorectomy, and suspension of the bladder neck. The reported incidence of ureteral injury during gynecologic procedures ranges from about 0.5% in simple hysterectomies for benign disease to as high as 30% for some older series of Wertheim radical hysterectomies. Isolated statistics such as these, however, have little clinical significance; it is the knowledge, skill, and diligence of the surgeon as well as the difficulty of the surgical procedure that determine the incidence of ureteral injury.

The ureter may be accidentally ligated, kinked, transected, crushed, burned, or devascularized. In gynecologic surgery, injury to the ureter is most likely to occur at the level of the infundibulopelvic ligament, the uterine artery, or the uterosacral ligament. Early recognition of ureteral injury can be crucial for preservation of function of the associated kidney. Repair is most likely to be successful if performed at the time of injury.

The best defense against injury to the ureter is knowledge of its anatomic relations and use of the avascular spaces of the pelvis to identify it intraoperatively (see Chapter 1). This can only be accomplished with good exposure through an adequate incision. On occasion, despite this careful attention, the question of ureteral integrity may arise.

A cystoscope, or other endoscope, can easily be used to prove bilateral ureteral patency at the end of a difficult operation. While the patient is being given 5 mL of indigo carmine intravenously, the bladder should be filled with 300 mL of normal saline. If vaginal surgery is being done, a 70-degree endoscope without its sheath can be gently introduced transurethrally. The ureteral orifices are visualized and a definite blue effluent can easily be seen emanating from the orifices if the ureters are patent. The rest of the bladder should also be examined for gross abnormality or evidence of operative trauma.

If an abdominal procedure is being performed and the entire course of the ureter cannot be visualized, patency can be demonstrated by introducing an endoscope through a cystotomy (Timmons, 1990). The extraperitoneal dome of the bladder is dissected away from the symphysis pubis. Then a purse string suture is placed and a cystotomy made within it. A 0-degree or 30-degree endoscope is placed in the bladder and the pursestring suture cinched tightly. Again, the ureteral orifices can be identified along with the blue effluent of indigo carmine if there is ureteral patency. After the endoscope is removed, the purse string suture is tied and imbricated. Postoperative catheter management is unchanged. If ureteral patency cannot be demonstrated by this technique, further steps can be initiated while the patient is still under anesthesia and the injury is fresh.

In the immediate postoperative period, a high index of suspicion should be maintained regarding the patient who develops flank pain. Urinary tract injury can be detected postoperatively by intravenous pyelogram (IVP) or retrograde x-ray studies. Renal ultrasonography may reveal hydronephrosis or hydroureter. A continuous postoperative watery vaginal discharge is suggestive of vesicovaginal or ureterovaginal fistula. A urinary fistula should also be suspected if laboratory analysis of the fluid draining from a surgical wound or drain demonstrates much higher levels of creatinine than found in the patient's blood sample.

As with all operative complications, the key to a good outcome is early recognition. Different types of ureteral injuries have different presenting symptoms and different management considerations.

**A. Ureteral Ligation:** Accidental ureteral ligation must be discovered within a few weeks if there is to be any hope of restoring renal function. Postoperative signs of ureteral ligation may include flank or pelvic pain, pyelonephritis and sepsis, abdominal swelling secondary to collection of urine (urinoma), and development of a ureterocutaneous fistula. In some patients, kidney failure occurs with no associated warning signs. Graham (1954) reported on 8 patients subjected to intentional ureteral ligation during colon cancer surgery. Only 2 patients experienced asymptomatic loss of renal function on the ligated side, 2 developed pelvic urinomas, and 3 developed ureterocutaneous fistula; 1 patient died of pyelonephritis and septicemia.

**B. Transection:** Continuous leakage of urine into the operative site following ureteral transection increases the likelihood that the injury will be discovered during the operation. Hematuria may occur after transection but cannot be considered a reliable sign of ureteral damage. Transection of the ureter may result in either a pelvic urinoma or ureterocutaneous fistula.

**C. Crush Injury:** There is a significant risk of segmental ureteral necrosis following a surgical clamp crush injury to the ureter. Resection of the crushed ureteral segment and reanastomosis, or performance of ureteroneocystostomy depending on the site of injury, should be considered unless (1) the ureter was clamped for only a brief time, (2) there is no visible damage, and (3) peristalsis persists at the site of injury. In such a case, a double-J ureteral stent should be placed and removed after 4–6 weeks with outpatient cystoscopy.

**D. Devascularization:** Extensive retroperitoneal dissection of the ureter may injure its adventitial vascular supply with subsequent necrosis of the devitalized segment. This risk is greatest in cancer surgery. In the 1950s, Dr. A.H. Palmrich of Vienna anatomically defined this complex of vessels and nerves that supply the ureter. Later series of radical hysterectomies that preserved this complex, by avoiding skeletonization of the ureter, resulted in a dramatic decline in ureteral complications.

### Bladder Injury

Laceration of the bladder can be confirmed by filling the bladder with sterile milk or methylene blue through a urethral catheter and observing leakage of fluid. Use of milk has the advantage of not staining the operative field. All edges of the cystotomy must be visualized and mobilized if necessary. The bladder defect usually is then repaired with 2 layers of absorbable suture after which the bladder is again filled with milk to test for leakage. Uncomplicated recovery is generally the rule. Five to 10 days of catheter drainage, depending on the site and extent of injury, helps to promote healing by preventing bladder distention.

## GASTROINTESTINAL TRACT INJURY

Bowel is highly susceptible to injury during laparotomy. The moment of entry into the peritoneal cavity is a crucial step and should be approached cautiously. Patients with adhesions due to previous surgery, endometriosis, or salpingitis are at high risk for intraoperative bowel injury when adherent bowel is dissected away from the operative site. The risk of bowel laceration is even greater during the acute phase of pelvic infection because of the increased friability of the secondarily inflamed bowel.

Tight abdominal packing, exposure of the bowel serosa with subsequent dehydration, indiscriminate use of unipolar electrocautery, and superficial abrasions from manipulation may be associated with apparently minimal trauma yet ultimately result in postoperative bowel adhesions. Bowel exposure and manipulation must therefore be kept to a minimum during laparotomy.

Complications associated with accidental penetration of bowel during laparotomy arise from bacterial and chemical peritonitis from spillage of bowel contents into the peritoneal cavity. The risk of bacterial peritonitis is clearly greater if the colon is the site of injury. Small bowel injury may produce chemical peritonitis from leakage of secretions from the stomach, gallbladder, and pancreas. Postoperative fever, abdominal distention with evidence of paralytic ileus, and diffuse peritonitis develop within 24 hours after unrecognized overt bowel injury.

Perhaps even more dangerous is the unrecognized, covert injury such as thermal bowel injury from electrocoagulation. A patient with such an injury may appear well in the immediate postoperative period. The delayed onset of symptoms of perforation may be misinterpreted or even overlooked. Such unrecognized injuries can prove lethal. Whether operating transvaginally, by laparotomy or laparoscopically, keep in mind the possibility of unrecognized overt or covert intraoperative bowel injury as the patient moves through the postoperative period.

Injury to the small bowel or stomach can be successfully repaired with 2 layers of interrupted suture. It may be necessary to convert a longitudinal small bowel laceration into a transverse repair to avoid constriction of the bowel lumen. Larger injuries and thermal injuries may require segmental resection using suture techniques or stapling devices.

Most gynecologic surgery patients have not undergone preoperative bowel preparation. Fecal contamination from colonic injury can prevent successful primary repair. If unprepared colon is entered or if injury is extensive, a temporary diverting colostomy proximal to the site of the injury may be necessary to allow healing. Copious irrigation of the abdomen, followed by placement of a closed drainage system at the repair site, decreases the risk of generalized postoperative peritonitis. Abdominal abscess formation, wound infection, enterocutaneous fistula, and extensive bowel adhesions may follow fecal contamination of the abdominal cavity.

## NEUROLOGIC INJURY

### Damage from Patient's Position During Surgery

Unnatural positioning of the patient while under anesthesia may cause significant sensory and motor defects in the extremities. Hyperextension or hyperabduction of an extremity may stretch the corresponding major nerve trunk as it exits the thorax or pelvis. The upper roots of the brachial plexus are especially vulnerable to injury, and transient shoulder pain may occur postoperatively if the shoulder has remained hyperextended during surgery. Femoral neuropathy may occasionally follow procedures carried out in the lithotomy position when the hip has been hyperabducted.

Nerves in the extremities are also vulnerable to injury where they cross over a skeletal prominence. External pressure on these sites during surgery may produce prolonged sensory and motor defects. The most common nerve injury during gynecologic surgery results from compression of the common peroneal nerve at the head of the fibula when the lateral aspect of the leg below the knee rests against a hard leg brace when the patient is in the lithotomy position. The result is loss of sensation in the dorsum of the ankle that is associated with footdrop due to loss of motor function of the peroneus longus and brevis muscles.

Prolonged pressure transmitted through the gluteal muscles may injure the sciatic nerves. Compression of the ulnar nerve against the medial epicondyle of the humerus occurs if the elbow is extended with the wrist pronated and results in nerve injury if the patient's arm remains in this position for prolonged periods.

### Damage During Surgery

The tips of the blades of an improperly placed self-retaining retractor may rest on the psoas muscles. Prolonged pressure may be transmitted to the femoral, ilioinguinal, iliohypogastric, or genitofemoral nerve with resulting painful neuropathy, sensory loss, and muscle weakness. The risk is especially great in the thin patient. Often the external part of the retractor can be bolstered with folded sterile towels to relieve this pressure.

The sciatic or obturator nerves may be at significant risk during radical pelvic cancer surgery, and the long thoracic nerve can be easily damaged during surgery for breast cancer. Careful dissection and a strong anatomic background are the best defenses against these injuries.

## VASCULAR INJURY

### Major Vessel Injury

Incidental injury of major pelvic blood vessels is a rare but potentially catastrophic complication of pelvic surgery. The arterial circulation, with its thick, muscular walls is less often damaged than the thin-walled venous circulation. The inferior vena cava and iliac veins are delicate and are easily injured during lymphadenectomy and other procedures for invasive disease, whereas injury during procedures for benign disease is much less common.

Bleeding from even small injuries to these major vessels can be extremely heavy. If injury occurs, direct pressure should be applied to the injured vessel or the blood supply should be tamponaded by applying pressure proximal to the site of injury. This allows the surgeon time to obtain adequate exposure for repair, to carefully assess the nature and extent of the injury, to summon consultation if necessary, and to have blood products delivered to the operating room while limiting the patient's blood loss. Keeping up with replacement of blood volume with packed red blood cells and blood products is essential.

Small injuries can often be repaired after adequate exposure is obtained and the patient is stabilized with very fine sutures carefully placed in a controlled fashion. Larger injuries may require emergent consultation with a vascular surgeon and may need vessel grafts. In the pregnant patient, many vessels are engorged and may behave as major vessels. The uterine vessels carry 500 mL of blood per minute at term. Laceration of these vessels during cesarean delivery or cesarean hysterectomy can cause massive bleeding.

## Hemorrhage

Even if major vessels are not injured, unexpected and difficult to control bleeding from other sources can occur during any gynecologic surgery. The gynecologic surgeon should be comfortable with the technique of hypogastric artery ligation, which will frequently control such bleeding (see Fig 28–1). This technique involves dissection of the hypogastric artery distal to the bifurcation of the common iliac artery. Two silk ties are then passed under the internal iliac artery and tied approximately 1 cm apart. The artery itself should not be cut. Great care must be taken not to damage the delicate internal iliac vein located immediately posterior and lateral to the hypogastric artery. This ligation acts by decreasing the pulse pressure at the distal bleeding site sufficiently to allow clot formation. Rich collateral circulation exists distal to the ligation, especially from the lumbar and middle sacral circulations. Enough perfusion to the pelvis remains that not only will the pelvic organs remain viable, but the potential for future pregnancy is preserved.

Angiographically guided arterial embolization is another technique that is gaining acceptance for control of massive pelvic hemorrhage (Greenwood, 1987). This technique can be used either intraoperatively or postoperatively in an attempt to avoid a subsequent return to the operating room. Arterial catheters are placed under fluoroscopic guidance, the bleeding sites identified, and embolization done by a variety of techniques. If hypogastric ligation has already been performed, angiographic catheters may not be able to reach the bleeding site, and angiographic embolization may not be possible.

## ANESTHETIC COMPLICATIONS

### Malignant Hyperthermia

One surgical patient in 14,000 has a congenital defect of calcium metabolism that presents as life-threatening hyperthermia during general anesthesia. The administration of succinylcholine or the volatile anesthetic agents can prevent the reuptake of calcium by the sarcoplasmic reticulum in skeletal muscle cells. Massive calcium levels stimulate a dramatic increase in cell metabolism, causing the characteristic symptoms of elevated body temperature, generalized skeletal muscle rigidity, and metabolic acidosis. Fatal cardiac arrhythmias may occur as hyperkalemia develops in association with acidosis.

If malignant hyperthermia develops, all anesthetic agents should be immediately discontinued and dantrolene, given promptly intravenously. Dantrolene exerts its effects by interfering with the release of calcium from the sarcoplasmic reticulum. The dose should be repeated until symptoms subside or until up to a maximum of 10 mg/kg has been given. Dantrolene should be continued postoperatively. Treatment should also be directed toward stabilization of the patient through correction of cardiac arrhythmias, metabolic acidosis, hyperkalemia, and hyperthermia.

### Bronchospasm

Bronchospasm is caused by increased airway reactivity and is detected by wheezing and increased difficulty in ventilating the patient. Patients with known asthma and cardiopulmonary disease are at increased risk for bronchospasm with general anesthesia. However, bronchospasm can also occur in patients without a known history of pulmonary disease. In patients with known disease, consideration is often given to performing procedures under regional anesthesia wherever possible. When bronchospasm does occur intraoperatively, pharmocologic measures such as inhaled beta-mimetics and intravenous corticosteroids should be instituted immediately.

### Hypothermia

Prolonged exposure of the lightly clothed, anesthetized patient with an open abdomen to the relatively cool operating room environment can result in a drop in the core body temperature of several degrees. Severe hypothermia is unusual, but there are important implications for even minor hypothermia. The return to normal body temperature, which often involves shivering, can cause a large increase in oxygen requirements which, in turn, can cause cardiovascular stress, particularly for patients with underlying cardiac or pulmonary disease. Careful attention to patient temperature, including covering the patient and using warmed intravenous fluids and warmed, humidified ventilation can reduce these problems.

### Regional Anesthesia

Regional anesthetic techniques are being used more frequently both for primary anesthesia as well as for relief of postoperative pain. Both epidural and spinal anesthetics are being used with increasing frequency in gynecologic surgery. The most common worrisome problem is respiratory depression. This occurs when the anesthetic level reaches to C3–C5, the level of innervation of the diaphragm. Whenever regional anesthesia is planned, equipment for intubation and mechanical ventilation must be readily available in the event of respiratory depression. These patients must be closely observed both during the procedure and afterward, until the anesthetic agents have been completely metabolized and the anesthetic block resolved as delayed respiratory depression can occur.

The most common and aggravating postoperative problem with regional anesthesia is spinal headache, caused by persistent leakage of cerebrospinal fluid through the hole made by a spinal or epidural needle.

In most instances, headache can be avoided by the use of very small-caliber needles and adequate hydration before, during, and after the procedure. Use of an epidural blood patch technique often gives immediate relief.

### Other Complications

Teeth can be broken or chipped during intubation. Careful technique with the laryngoscope is always required. Some patients, particularly obese patients or patients with short necks, can be very difficult to intubate resulting in laryngeal damage, laryngospasm, or abandonment of the procedure because of inability to intubate the patient. Esophogeal intubation can be catastrophic if unrecognized, but can be avoided by careful attention to laryngeal visualization, $CO_2$ monitoring of exhalation, and careful auscultation. Pneumothorax and aspiration pneumonia, 2 other common complications, will be discussed at length in the section on pulmonary complications. It is thought that death due to anesthetic complication occurs in approximately 1 in 1500–2000 surgical procedures.

## COMPLICATIONS OF ENDOSCOPIC PROCEDURES

Over the past decade, laparoscopy and hysteroscopy have become some of the most frequently performed gynecologic procedures. These procedures are perceived as less invasive, with faster recovery times, and are frequently performed in an outpatient setting. As with many medical and surgical procedures, endoscopic procedures have become accepted faster than the data on their efficacy, safety, and morbidities have been generated. Much of the current data on endoscopic complications is based on case reports and small series. It is becoming clear that despite being considered "minimally invasive," major complications occur with endoscopic surgery. Recognized complications include bowel, bladder, and ureteral injuries, hernias at the trochar sites, catastrophic major vessel injury at the time of trochar insertion, and $CO_2$ embolism. In addition to complications specific to endoscopy, any of the complications associated with traditional gynecologic surgery may still occur.

Great care is necessary to minimize complications from endoscopic procedures. In particular, many of the most serious complications occur at the time of trochar insertion. When inserting the Veress needle, careful attention should be paid to keeping the tip in the midline. The needle should be directed downward at approximately 45 degrees to attempt to avoid the bifurcations of the aorta and inferior vena cava, usually located 1–3 cm below the umbilicus. In patients with a high risk of bowel adhesions to the anterior abdominal wall, some surgeons advocate using an open trochar placement technique, although no objective evidence exists to support this. All other trochars should be placed under direct visualization, with careful attention to avoid the inferior epigastric vessels. When performing operative procedures under laparoscopic guidance, the same attention must be paid to identification of the ureters and other anatomy as in open procedures. Bowel, bladder, and ureter, as well as major vessels, can be injured just as easily and seriously during endoscopic procedures as during laparotomy.

Hysteroscopy has some unique complications. In addition to the risks of uterine perforation, visceral damage, and hemorrhage, life-threatening problems can be caused by the uterine distention media. High molecular weigh dextran can in rare instance cause anaphylaxis or, if used in large amounts, fluid overload secondary to the high osmotic load. Other distending media, including sorbitol and glycine, are sodium-free and may cause hyponatremia or volume overload. When using these media, careful attention must be paid to volume status and electrolytes with correction of abnormalities or discontinuance of the procedure if necessary.

## POSTOPERATIVE COMPLICATIONS

## CARDIOVASCULAR COMPLICATIONS

### 1. SHOCK

The postoperative efficiency of the circulation depends on many factors. Some of the more important of these are blood volume, cardiac function, neurovascular tone, and adrenal secretions (eg, epinephrine, norepinephrine, and adrenocorticosteroids).

Shock, or failure of the circulation, may follow excessive blood loss, escape of vascular fluid into the extravascular compartment ("third spacing"), marked peripheral vasodilatation, cardiac decompensation, sepsis, adrenocortical failure, and pain or emotional distress. A combination of causes may be responsible for shock. Ideally, correct diagnosis of the circulatory problem should be undertaken before proper treatment can be instituted. However, because this complication can be life-threatening, it may be necessary to institute treatment with a presumptive rather than a definitive diagnosis.

Blood loss (hypovolemia) is the most common cause of postoperative shock. The rapid loss of up to 20% of blood volume is classified as mild shock. A healthy patient normally compensates well for a loss of less than 10–20% of their blood volume and is typically asymptomatic, with minimal changes in heart

**Table 44–1.** Some characteristics of different types of shock.

| Type of Shock | History | Physical Findings | Laboratory Findings |
|---|---|---|---|
| Hemorrhagic | Trauma, pregnancy complication. | Acute abdomen, trauma, obvious site of bleeding. | Low hemoglobin/hematocrit, possible clotting deficiency. |
| Cardiogenic | Heart disease. | Pulmonary edema, hepatosplenomegaly, anasarca. | Abnormal blood gases, cardiomegaly or pulmonary edema on chest x-ray. |
| Septic | Infection, illness, abortion. | Febrile, evidence of infection | High white blood cell count, urine white blood cell casts if pyelonephritis. |
| Anaphylactic (allergy) | Bee sting, acute medication administration. | Negative except for shock. | Negative. |

rate, blood pressure, or urine output. A loss of 20–40% usually yields moderate shock, with maximal use of the body's compensatory mechanisms including tachycardia, dropping of urine output, and vasoconstriction yielding cold, clammy, pallid skin. The affected patient's sensorium is usually altered. With unreplaced loss of more than 40% of the blood volume, the body's compensatory mechanisms are overwhelmed, and severe shock occurs. Large blood loss, unless promptly corrected, leads to a drop in cardiac output, a decrease in tissue perfusion, and eventual anoxia and permanent end organ damage.

## General Treatment for All Types of Shock

Shock is an acute emergency that takes precedence over all other problems except acute hemorrhage, cardiac arrest, and respiratory failure. Immediate correction of the underlying disorder is essential.

Treatment should be organized to stop hemorrhage, restore fluid and electrolyte balance, correct cardiac dysfunction, establish adequate ventilation, maintain vital organ perfusion, and avert adrenocortical failure.

Because multiple pathologic mechanisms may be involved, no simple and reliable pattern is seen in a patient going into shock or in her response to treatment. Survival depends on early diagnosis, correct appraisal of physiologic abnormalities, monitoring of essential parameters, and a flexible plan of therapy based on vital signs and laboratory data.

The primary cause of shock must be determined promptly. The history and gross physical findings often permit the differentiation of hemorrhagic, cardiogenic, septic, and allergic types of shock (Table 44–1). Pelvic examination, ultrasound examination, culdocentesis, or paracentesis may be of inestimable value in immediately establishing the presence or absence of postoperative hemoperitoneum. Except in neurogenic shock due to fainting, a self-limiting condition that is treated by placing the patient in the recumbent position and administering stimulants, antishock measures using additional therapy as required for specific problems should be instituted (Table 44–2).

The accurate determination of parenteral fluid requirements depends on continuous clinical observation of blood pressure, temperature, pulse and respiratory rate, mental acuity, skin (color, temperature, and moisture), venous collapse, fluid intake, and urinary output. Frequent monitoring of central venous pressure and urine output with a transurethral catheter and serial determination of serum electrolytes, blood pH, $PO_2$, $PCO_2$, and lactate are essential. Pulmonary artery pressures, left ventricular function, and cardiac output can be assessed with a Swan-Ganz catheter. A peripheral arterial line is helpful for blood gas monitoring and blood drawing. Hemoglobin and hematocrit determinations are not dependable guides to blood replacement in the shock patient because they will not reflect the loss of whole blood until fluid replacement has been given.

Blood should be obtained promptly for crossmatching, hematocrit, coagulation studies, complete blood count, and blood chemistry determinations prior to starting an infusion. If superficial veins have collapsed and peripheral venous access is not possible, a central line should be placed in the subclavian, internal jugular, or femoral vein for intravenous access and central monitoring.

Adequate blood volume must be restored as rapidly as possible. Replacement should be carried out with packed red blood cells (PRBCs) and blood com-

**Table 44–2.** General antishock measures.

1. Place the patient in a recumbent position with foot of bed slightly elevated. Disturb the patient as little as possible. (The extreme Trendelenburg position is no longer recommended, because it may interfere with breathing.)
2. Establish an adequate airway and make certain that pulmonary ventilation is unobstructed. Administer oxygen by nasal catheter, mask, or endotracheal tube as required, especially if dyspnea or cyanosis is present.
3. Keep the patient comfortably warm with blankets. Do not apply external heat, since this will cause peripheral vasodilatation.
4. Control pain and relieve apprehension. Shock patients often have very little discomfort, probably as a result of the physiologic endorphin response to trauma. When required, give a minimum effective parenteral dose of a sedative or, if absolutely necessary, morphine sulfate, 10–15 mg intravenously. Narcotics are contraindicated for patients in coma and those with head injuries or respiratory depression unless mechanical ventilation is immediately available. Avoid overdose of sedative and narcotic drugs.

ponents as necessary for coagulation factors. In general, 1 unit (U) of fresh frozen plasma should be administered with each 5 U of PRBCs to replace clotting factors. Acid-base deficits and electrolyte disturbances may require individual correction. In particular, if large blood volumes are being replaced, calcium should be monitored and replaced as necessary because the citrate in the replacement blood units decreases serum calcium.

Intravenous crystalloid solutions (normal saline or Ringer's lactate) should be infused while awaiting blood components from the blood bank. If the patient has not responded promptly to these measures or if her condition again deteriorates, further intensive monitoring and management will be necessary. (See Chapter 59 for further discussion of management of shock.)

## 2. CARDIAC ARREST

Cardiac arrest occurs most frequently during the induction of anesthesia, but it can also occur during the course of the operation or even in the postoperative period. Predisposing conditions include preexisting heart disease, previous myocardial infarction, shock, hypoventilation, airway (tracheal or pulmonary) obstruction, or drug reaction.

### Clinical Findings

The signs of impending cardiac arrest are rapid fall in blood pressure and irregularity of pulse. This frequently occurs during the administration of anesthesia. The diagnosis should be verified by confirming the absence of pulse and heart sounds by auscultation, and cardiopulmonary resuscitation must be initiated immediately.

### Prevention

A number of measures are helpful in preventing cardiac arrest. Careful monitoring of blood pressure, with prevention of hypotension is essential. If hypotension does occur, immediate treatment is mandatory. Adequate ventilation with oxygen as necessary must be maintained throughout the operative procedure. Pulse oximetry is readily available and is very useful. Most important, patients with cardiac risk factors require a multidisciplinary approach with preoperative consultation with anesthesiologists, cardiologists, and the surgeon. Frequently, a Swan-Ganz catheter and peripheral arterial line is placed before induction of anesthesia to allow intensive monitoring.

### Treatment

Pulmonary ventilation may be accomplished by bag and face mask, until oxygen under pressure can be given. An endotracheal tube should be inserted. Closed chest cardiac massage (Fig 44–1) is the procedure of choice in the attempt to correct the arrest;

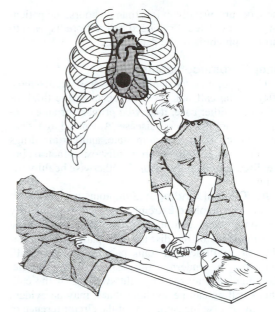

**Figure 44–1.** Technique of closed-chest cardiac massage. Heavy circle in heart drawing shows area of application of force. Circles on supine figure show points of application of electrodes for defibrillation. (Reproduced with permission, from Benson RC: *Handbook of Obstetrics & Gynecology,* 8th ed. Lange, 1983.)

open chest massage is rarely indicated. Electrical stimulation, if available, may be helpful. The gynecologist should be trained in Red Cross Basic Life Support and is usually required to provide emergency treatment only. The subsequent care of the patient should be the responsibility of an expert in critical care medicine.

## 3. THROMBOPHLEBITIS

### Superficial Thrombophlebitis

Superficial thrombophlebitis occurring postoperatively is most common in women with extensive varicosities of the legs. The lithotomy position, with localized pressure on the leg from supports, can contribute. It is usually recognized within the first few days after operation. Additionally, patients may experience superficial thrombosis of veins at intravenous access sites. In many cases, a segment of the superficial saphenous vein becomes inflamed, manifested by redness, localized heat, swelling, and tenderness. This disorder is generally limited to the superficial veins and, in such cases, pulmonary embolism would be unusual. When superficial thrombophlebitis is diagnosed, treatment includes warm, moist packs, elevation of the extremity, and analgesics. Anticoagulants are rarely indicated when only the superficial vessels are involved. As soon as clinical improvement occurs, usually in less than 48 hours, the patient may be ambulated. Prolonged bed rest predisposes to thrombophlebitis of the deep veins.

## Deep Thrombophlebitis

Thrombophlebitis of the deep veins occurs most often in the calf but may also occur in the thigh or pelvis. In either case, it may be primary or an extension of more peripheral disease. Advanced age, obesity, cancer, the postpartum state, and certain drugs (eg, oral contraceptives) are predisposing factors, but the disease frequently occurs in otherwise healthy patients.

**A. Clinical Findings:** Symptoms may be localized to the involved extremity, or the thrombus may be asymptomatic. Pulmonary embolism may be the first evidence of the disease. The patient may complain of a dull ache or frank pain in the leg or calf. There may be tenderness or spasm in the calf muscle. Examination may reveal slight swelling of the calf. This swelling can be so slight that it may be evident only by precise measurement of the circumference of both calves at the same level. Dorsiflexion of the foot may elicit pain in the calf (Homans' sign). Although a positive Homans' sign is specific, the test is not very sensitive (about 25%). A slight elevation of the temperature and pulse is frequently noted. If the disease process is in the femoral vein or in the pelvis, swelling of the extremity may be more evident and severe. Compression ultrasonography, Doppler assessment of the veins proximal to the suspected site of thrombosis, or impedance plethysmography may afford a definite diagnosis. Of the three, compression ultrasonography (when available) is the most simple, sensitive, and specific test. If significant doubt exists after these tests or if anticoagulation would be difficult (eg, because of pregnancy), venography is indicated.

The major complication of deep thrombophlebitis is pulmonary embolism. Chronic venous insufficiency may develop as a long-term consequence of the process.

**B. Treatment:**

**1. Medical treatment–**Once the diagnosis of deep thrombophlebitis has been made, anticoagulants should be started immediately. Heparin, which promptly prolongs clotting time, is the drug of choice; it may be given either intravenously or subcutaneously. However, since it is often difficult to achieve adequate steady-state anticoagulation with subcutaneous administrations, intravenous administration is the accepted initial therapy. Coagulation studies, including a prothrombin time (PT) and partial thromboplastin time (PTT), should be determined before anticoagulant therapy is started; these tests then provide a basis for interpreting the degree of anticoagulation achieved. The PTT should be kept to 2–3 times the control value. Intravenous administration of 1% protamine sulfate counteracts the effect of

heparin quickly on a milligram-for-milligram basis, but it should only be used in an emergency. Heparin should be continued at least 3–5 days after the disappearance of all signs and symptoms and effective oral therapy has been established.

Oral anticoagulants such as dicumarol and warfarin are contraindicated in pregnant patients but are often started at the same time as heparin in other patients. These agents act on different components of the clotting cascade than heparin, and their therapeutic effect is measured by the PT. Whereas heparin prolongs the clotting time almost immediately, the oral anticoagulants do not exert their full effect for 48–72 hours. It is common practice to give heparin for its immediate short-term effect and to replace the heparin with oral anticoagulants for long-term treatment. The PT should be determined before therapy is begun and daily thereafter until equilibrium levels are reached. The objective of therapy is the maintenance of prothrombin activity of 10–30% above control. Emergency reversal can be achieved with 2 U of fresh frozen plasma. Oral anticoagulation is often continued empirically for 6 weeks to 3 months.

Anticoagulation presents significant risks to patients with deep thrombophlebitis, and they must be thoroughly counseled to recognize possible complications of therapy, including hematuria, hemoptysis, hematemesis, melena, and easy bruisability. The patients should be provided with an identification bracelet, identification tag around the neck, or card for their wallet indicating that they are receiving anticoagulant therapy, in case of an accident in which they become unconscious. Patients should also be given a list of over-the-counter medications to avoid including nonsteroidal antiinflammatory drugs, aspirin, and antibiotics, which may affect their anticoagulation.

**2. Local measures–**Local measures in the treatment of deep thrombophlebitis include elevation of the legs to provide good venous drainage and the application of full leg gradient-pressure elastic hose. When inflammation has subsided, usually within 1–2 weeks of starting therapy, full activities may be permitted. The patient should be encouraged to continue to elevate her legs whenever she can. Prolonged sitting and the use of constrictive garments, especially knee high support stockings or hosiery are to be avoided.

**3. Surgical treatment–**Thrombectomy occasionally may be considered for persistent severe swelling of the extremity. An inferior vena cava filter or vena cava ligation may be considered for repeated episodes of pulmonary embolism occurring in spite of adequate anticoagulation or when anticoagulation is absolutely contraindicated.

## Septic Pelvic Thrombophlebitis

Septic pelvic thrombophlebitis is a complication almost unique to pelvic surgery. It is discussed in detail in Chapter 22. The diagnosis of septic pelvic thrombophlebitis is established and effectively managed by clinical trial with heparin in conjunction with antibiotic therapy that affects both aerobic and anaerobic organisms.

## 4. PULMONARY EMBOLISM

Pulmonary embolism is a critical complication of pelvic surgery. This diagnosis should be suspected if cardiac or pulmonary symptoms occur abruptly. Sepsis, obesity, malignancy, and history of pulmonary embolism or deep vein thrombosis are predisposing factors. It is a complication of pelvic or lower extremity thrombophlebitis; nonetheless, pulmonary embolism may precede the diagnosis of peripheral vascular disease. Indeed, in some patients no evidence of thrombophlebitis can be found. Pulmonary embolism may occur at any time, but usually occurs around the seventh to tenth postoperative days. The differential diagnosis includes atelectasis, pneumonia, myocardial infarction, and pneumothorax.

### Clinical Findings

**A. Symptoms and Signs:** Patients with large emboli have chest pain, severe dyspnea, cyanosis, tachycardia, hypotension or shock, restlessness, and anxiety. If the embolus is massive, sudden death may result from acute cor pulmonale. In patients with smaller emboli, the diagnosis is suggested by the sudden onset of pleuritic pain, sometimes in association with blood-streaked sputum. A dry cough may develop. Physical examination may reveal a pleural friction rub. In many cases, no classic diagnostic signs can be elicited.

**B. Laboratory Findings:** A low arterial $PO_2$ is a key finding and should immediately raise suspicion for pulmonary embolus. Moderate leukocytosis (up to 15,000/μL) occurs in 70% of cases. Serum bilirubin is often elevated and is related to heart failure rather than hemorrhage in the lung. Elevated serum lactate dehydrogenase or serum glutamic-oxaloacetic transaminase is seen in about 50% of patients; both enzymes are elevated in about 25% of patients, and both are within the normal range in the remainder.

**C. X-Ray Findings:** Chest x-ray may show no abnormality, or changes may be delayed 24–48 hours. In about 15% of patients, a pulmonary density is present, which is in the periphery of the lung and roughly in the shape of a triangle with its base at the lung surface. Other possible findings are enlargement of the main pulmonary artery, small pleural effusion, and elevated diaphragm. Embolism involves the lower lobes in 75% of cases, more often on the right than the left.

**D. Electrocardiography:** The ECG may show characteristic changes of pulmonary embolism in about one-third of cases. The ECG is principally of interest in differentiating pulmonary embolism from myocardial infarction, which can appear clinically similar.

**E. Lung Scan:** Imaging the lung fields after intravenous injection of radioiodinated, macroaggregated human albumin is a simple and valuable diagnostic procedure that characteristically reveals perfusion defects in the lung areas distal to pulmonary artery obstruction. A negative scan is of great value, because it essentially rules out embolism. However, changes similar to those that occur with pulmonary embolism can be produced by atelectasis, pneumonia, and neoplasm. The ventilation- perfusion comparative scan (V/Q scan) is used to differentiate these entities. It should be noted that a negative scan is reassuring but not totally reliable since there is a 15% false-negative rate. In patients in whom there is a very high clinical suspicion but a low probability V/Q scan, angiography is frequently performed.

**F. Angiography:** Pulmonary angiography should be done if the clinical situation is suggestive and the V/Q scan is indeterminate. It should always be done before an embolectomy is undertaken. It is the most reliable procedure for confirming the diagnosis and determining the location and extent of large emboli. Embolectomy is performed only on selected patients, and a definitive diagnosis is essential. Pressures measured in the right heart and pulmonary artery in conjunction with catheterization for angiography aid in evaluating the degree of right heart failure secondary to pulmonary artery obstruction. Angiography should be preceded by a pulmonary scan; if the scan is negative, massive pulmonary embolus can be virtually ruled out.

In the patient suspected of having a pulmonary embolus, an arterial blood gas, a 12-lead electrocardiogram and chest x-ray should be obtained. If the patient has a low $PO_2$ with no other explanation, a V/Q scan and angiography should be obtained.

### Treatment

Cardiopulmonary resuscitation measures should be instituted as necessary. Close monitoring is essential, as is treatment of acid-base abnormalities and shock. Immediate treatment with heparin is indicated. Because of the high mortality rate associated with pulmonary embolism, it is better to begin heparin therapy even in the absence of a definitive diagnosis if pulmonary embolism is likely. For specific monitoring and management of pulmonary embolus and its complications, see Chapter 59.

## PULMONARY COMPLICATIONS

Pulmonary complications remain one of the major hazards of the postoperative period. About 30% of deaths that occur within 6 weeks after operation are due to pulmonary complications. Postoperative problems vary with the preoperative status of the patient. Chronic bronchitis, emphysema and increased bronchial secretions, which are commonly present in smokers, make these patients particularly susceptible to postoperative respiratory problems. Atelectasis, pneumonia, pulmonary embolism, and respiratory distress syndrome from aspiration, left ventricular failure, fluid overload, or infection are the most common complications.

## 1. ATELECTASIS

Atelectasis is a complication of the very early postoperative period. It consists of areas of airway collapse and is most likely to be seen in patients who already have chronic lung disease. Factors that tend to increase atelectasis in the postoperative period include the diminished functional residual capacity seen in the supine position and "splinting," frequently seen after abdominal surgery. The blood that traverses the capillaries of the areas with atelectasis are not oxygenated, resulting in shunting and hypoxia. Massive atelectasis may occur when a mucous plug or aspirated vomitus occludes a large bronchus, leading to collapse of an entire lobe. Predisposing factors include chronic bronchitis, asthma, smoking, and respiratory infection. Inadequate immediate postoperative attention to deep breathing and delayed ambulation also increase the risk of subsequent pulmonary complications.

### Clinical Findings

The clinical findings vary with the extent of atelectasis. Mild atelectasis is the most common cause of fever in the immediate postoperative period. Usually this is related to underexpansion of the lungs during and after the surgery and is transient. As the patient begins ambulating and mobilizing her secretions, mild atelectasis resolves. The undrained secretions in the segment with atelectasis act as good culture media for bacteria, and if atelectasis is not treated, superimposed pneumonia can develop. Early ambulation, deep breathing exercises, and incentive spirometry can help speed the resolution of atelectasis.

With massive atelectasis, the temperature, pulse rate, and respiratory rate increase sharply. Segments of lung, sometimes entire lobes, may be dull to percussion, with absent breath sounds. Cyanosis may be present. With massive atelectasis, the patient often exhibits shortness of breath. A lateral shift of the mediastinum (ie, displacement of the trachea and heart toward the atelectatic side) may occur. The x-ray findings include patchy opacities and evidence of laterally displaced organs. Multiple small areas of atelectasis and bronchopneumonia, which often have a similar clinical picture, may combine to present as a single disease process. Elevation of temperature and

respiratory rate is the first sign. The patient may complain of an excess of bronchial secretions, with bhonchi and cough. Examination of the chest will detect areas of dullness to percussion, together with bronchial breathing and inspiratory rales. If untreated, atelectasis will progressively worsen.

### Prevention

The prevention of atelectasis requires attention to many details and begins in the preoperative period. Patients should be encouraged to stop smoking. Patients with chronic lung disease should be given antibiotics and chest physical therapy if an acute or chronic infection is suspected. If an element of bronchospasm is present, bronchodilators may be advisable. If upper respiratory infection is present, elective surgery should be postponed until mucociliary function returns to normal. This recovery may take 2–3 weeks.

Intraoperatively, the patient should be ventilated with adequate tidal volumes with the addition of positive end expiratory pressure (PEEP) if signs of atelectasis such as decreasing oxygen saturation become apparent. Intraoperative atelectasis or small airway collapse is more commonly seen in patients with chronic lung disease or obesity and can be aggravated by the Trendelenburg position. Intraoperative humidification and suctioning of secretions are helpful.

Postoperatively, atelectasis is best avoided by minimizing pain, having patients in the sitting position, and encouraging deep breathing and early ambulation. Incentive spirometry devices help patients to perform deep inspiration exercises. Patient-controlled analgesia or use of an epidural catheter for postoperative pain management can help by reducing respiratory depression.

### Treatment

Treatment consists of intensive chest physical therapy and supplemental oxygen. Pain should be controlled, since it is an obstacle to deep breathing. If fever persists and pneumonia develops, antibiotics will be necessary. If the situation deteriorates to the point where there is not adequate tissue oxygenation, intubation and mechanical ventilation will be necessary.

## 2. PNEUMONIA

Pneumonia may follow atelectasis or aspiration of vomitus or other fluid. Abundant tracheobronchial secretions from preexisting bronchitis also predispose to this complication. Fever in the first few postoperative days is usually from atelectasis. If this is followed by higher temperatures, systemic toxicity, and respiratory difficulty, a presumptive diagnosis of pneumonia is justified.

If pneumonia develops, secretions become progressively more abundant and the cough becomes productive. Physical examination may reveal evidence of pulmonary consolidation, and numerous coarse rales often are present. Although the chest x-ray may go on to show diffuse patchy infiltrates or lobar consolidation, this appearance may lag behind the clinical picture by as much as 24 hours.

The treatment of pneumonia includes deep breathing and coughing. The patient should be encouraged to change position frequently. Nasotracheal suction may be used to stimulate the cough reflex. Specific broad-spectrum antibiotic therapy should be instituted and revised as indicated by subsequent sputum culture and sensitivity tests. Induced sputum is more reliable since oral contamination of expectorated specimens can be a problem. Gram's stain of a properly collected sputum can be very helpful.

In desperately weak or debilitated patients with a poor cough reflex, tracheostomy may occasionally be necessary to permit adequate ventilation, suctioning, and bronchoscopy. Positive pressure ventilation may improve the depth of respiration and eliminate the work of breathing in extremely ill patients.

## 3. ASPIRATION PNEUMONITIS

Aspiration of gastric contents into the trachea is associated with many factors such as neurologic disease affecting the gag reflex and vomiting in debilitated patients who do not have the strength to adequately cough. Aspiration of gastric contents into the trachea during induction of anesthesia is the best-known cause, although it is by no means the most common. Aspiration during induction occurs secondary to passive regurgitation of gastric contents, which may be due to a full stomach or poor gastroesophageal sphincter tone (as in hiatal hernia and inflation of the stomach with oxygen), or it may occur in the paralyzed patient in whom some difficulty with intubation is being experienced. The pregnant patient, particularly one having an emergency cesarean delivery, is especially at risk because of slow gastric emptying time and poor gastroesophageal sphincter tone. However, all patients who experience physical trauma have very slow gastric emptying times.

The chances for pulmonary aspiration of acid gastric contents can be minimized by:

1. Doing an awake fiberoptic intubation on patients with predictably difficult airways.

2. Speeding the process of gastric emptying by administering metoclopramide, 10 mg intravenously.

3. Increasing the pH of gastric contents by means of a nonparticulate antacid and use of $H_2$ blockers decreases the pulmonary damage if aspiration does occur.

4. Using a rapid sequence induction with pentothal and cricoid pressure. Cricoid pressure closes off the esophagous to prevent passive regurgitation from reaching the larynx. This pressure is kept on until the position of the tube is verified in the trachea.

If aspiration of gastric contents occurs, an endotracheal tube should be placed immediately and the trachea and bronchi aggressively suctioned and lavaged with saline solution. The outcome depends on the patient's general health and the quantity and acidity of the aspirate. Generally, a small aspiration may be associated with mild atelectasis and cause temporary hypoxia. More severe aspiration may lead to serious hypoxia requiring ventilation. The role of corticosteroids in the management of aspiration remains controversial. Air bronchograms may appear on chest x-ray 12–24 hours after the event. Development of full-blown adult respiratory distress syndrome (ARDS) must be watched for. Treatment of ARDS is considered in Chapter 59.

## 4. TENSION PNEUMOTHORAX

Tension pneumothorax is an uncommon complication and is most likely to occur during the first 24–48 hours after surgery. Pneumothorax can occur during positive pressure ventilation and may not be apparent until the positive pressure is stopped. Pneumothorax presents as acute respiratory distress with distant breath sounds on the affected side and frequently a marked mediastinal shift away from the affected side. The diagnosis is made by chest x-ray. Immediate improvement can be obtained by inserting 1 or more large-bore angiocatheters through the intercostal space at approximately T6–8 with the patient under local anesthesia to allow escape of air until a chest tube can be inserted to reinflate the lung. Chest tube drainage is usually continued for several days, until the air leak has healed.

## 5. ADULT RESPIRATORY DISTRESS SYNDROME (ARDS)

ARDS, a frequently catastrophic postoperative complication, is considered in Chapter 59.

## GASTROINTESTINAL TRACT COMPLICATIONS

### 1. PARALYTIC ILEUS

Some degree of postoperative paralytic ileus must be expected whenever the peritoneal cavity is entered. Gastrointestinal function in the postoperative period must be observed carefully so that the ileus can be minimized. Postoperative ileus may be aggravated by food given too early. The proper rate for advancement of diet remains a matter of style and is done differently by different physicians. Many surgeons encourage their patients to sip tap water (not ice water) on the first day after uncomplicated gynecologic surgery. On the following day, clear fluids are given if bowel sounds are normal. Thereafter, fluids may be taken ad lib, but solid food usually is withheld until the patient passes intestinal gas. At this point, the patient can usually tolerate a regular diet.

## Clinical Findings

Nausea occurring in the immediate postoperative period may be troublesome and is usually anesthesia-related. It may be suppressed with prochlorperazine (Compazine), 5–10 mg intramuscularly or in a 25-mg rectal suppository, promethazine (Phenergan), 25 mg intramuscularly, or trimethobenzamide (Tigan), 200 mg intramuscularly. Nausea or vomiting later in the postoperative period demands diagnostic attention, because the symptom may be due either to adynamic ileus or to partial bowel obstruction.

Ileus is characterized classically by abdominal distention, absence of bowel sounds, and generalized abdominal tympany on percussion. The complication is noted usually within the first 48–72 hours after surgery. On x-ray, there is generalized dilatation and gaseous distention of both small and large bowel, although the small bowel component may be more prominent. Obstipation is also characteristic of postoperative ileus. If ileus is persistent, especially if accompanied by a febrile course, a retained foreign body must be considered. Such an object usually can be ruled out by the same radiologic study. Urologic trauma with resultant extravasation of urine may be an unusual cause of persistent ileus. An intravenous urogram may aid in the diagnosis of urinary extravasation.

## Treatment

If nausea, vomiting, or abdominal distention becomes severe, it may be necessary to insert a nasogastric tube into the stomach. Gastric aspiration usually reveals green to yellow fluids. The distention should lessen with this treatment; if no benefit is noted, bowel obstruction should be suspected.

Some surgeons give a mild laxative such as milk of magnesia or a stool softener such as dioctyl sodium sulfosuccinate (Colace) on the first to third days after operation. A tap water enema for the relief of distention probably should be deferred until the patient has passed gas or has had some bowel movement, evidence that bowel function is returning to normal. Enemas and suppositories are frequently used, but can obscure the diagnosis of a small bowel obstruction by placing air and fluid in the rectum.

Some physicians attempt to minimize postoperative paralytic ileus by giving the patient a pharmacologically inert wetting agent such as simethicone to reduce the surface tension of the intestinal mucus and thereby liberate entrapped gas. Use of sedation and a rectal tube is a time-honored effective measure.

Gastrointestinal complications are most apt to occur after transabdominal operations, but they may complicate vaginal surgery as well. In fact, any serious illness or surgical procedure may cause malfunction of the gastrointestinal tract.

## 2. POSTOPERATIVE INTESTINAL OBSTRUCTION

Bowel obstruction may occur as a complication of any intraperitoneal operation. It is most apt to occur as a consequence of peritonitis or generalized irritation of the peritoneal surface, resulting in varying degrees of adhesions between loops of bowel. Obstruction results when these adhesions trap or kink a segment of intestine.

The resultant partial or complete bowel obstruction due to early adhesions is usually noted between the fifth and sixth postoperative days. However, obstruction can occur sooner. Dense, fibrous adhesions develop after 8–12 weeks and can entrap bowel and cause delayed obstruction with a high incidence of bowel strangulation. Obstruction is associated with significant and even protracted vomiting, accompanied by cramping abdominal pain. On percussion, there may be a localized or focal tympanitic area noted. Bowel rushes heard on auscultation are noted to be synchronous with cramping pain. A flat film of the abdomen usually reveals distention of a portion of small bowel, with air-fluid levels apparent. In general, the colon is free of air.

Small bowel obstruction, with its high incidence of resultant bowel ischemia and infarction, is a life-threatening complication requiring immediate intervention. It is possible to treat postoperative bowel obstruction conservatively by bowel decompression with a nasogastric or long intestinal tube. Long intestinal tubes do not offer any advantage over nasogastric tubes unless properly placed, which generally requires fluoroscopic guidance. Tube decompression often results in realignment of the bowel and relief of the obstruction, or adhesions may relax or be released sufficiently to allow spontaneous decompression. When conservative management is elected, an arbitrary period of decompression should be decided on in advance; if the obstruction does not respond within that period—usually 48–72 hours—reoperation is necessary. Obstruction is associated with large fluid shifts into the bowel lumen, and vigorous hydration and careful electrolyte monitoring are required.

## 3. ACUTE GASTRIC DISTENTION

Acute gastric distention is one of the most common postoperative complications. It is caused by accumulation of air and, to a lesser extent, by gastric juices in the stomach. Most patients with nausea or paralytic ileus swallow air. If intestinal peristalsis is depressed, the swallowed gas accumulates in the stomach. In unusual cases, as gastric distention increases, the movement of the diaphragm may be inhibited. If the patient develops hyperpnea and appears to be splinting her diaphragm and acute gastric distention is the suspected cause, a nasogastric tube should be passed immediately and gastric aspiration continued as long as the ileus persists.

## 4. GASTRIC DILATATION

Gastric dilatation, as opposed to gastric distention, is a grave postoperative complication that has been associated with a mortality rate as high as 50%. In patients with gastric dilatation, the stomach is distended with fluid to such a degree that secondary hemorrhage occurs. The gastric fluid becomes brown or black from the contained hemoglobin. Gastric dilatation may follow untreated gastric distention, but it often is a complication of very serious illnesses associated with low cardiac output. The cause may be outside of the abdomen, eg, with open heart surgery.

Vomiting of brown or black material suggests gastric dilatation or intestinal obstruction. A nasogastric tube should be passed immediately. Decompression of the stomach reverses the gastric distention and secondary bleeding and prevents aspiration. Large quantities of fluid and electrolytes usually have been lost. Shock is often present, and correction of hypovolemia is an essential part of therapy.

## 5. CONSTIPATION, DIARRHEA, AND FECAL IMPACTION

A reduction in the number of bowel movements is to be expected in the early postoperative period because of low food intake and ileus. After gas has been passed rectally, a mild laxative (milk of magnesia, 30 mL orally) may be prescribed. A clear water enema or rectal bisacodyl suppository is also effective.

Fecal impaction is a common cause of diarrhea in the postoperative patient. Whenever the patient develops diarrhea, digital rectal examination should be done immediately. If hard stool is encountered in the ampulla, the diagnosis of fecal impaction is verified. The condition is caused by limitation of oral fluids and is especially common in elderly patients and others confined to bed. It may be aggravated by previous gastrointestinal series or barium enema with accumulation of barium in the colon. The treatment of fecal impaction is digital disimpaction of the firm fecal masses after an oil retention enema.

**Pseudomembranous enterocolitis** may occur as a complication of antibiotic administration. Any antibiotic can alter the bacterial flora of the gastrointestinal tract, occasionally resulting in overgrowth of *Clostridium difficile,* the etiologic organism. Penicillins and cephalosporins are the most frequently implicated agents. The patient typically develops severe diarrhea, and pseudomembranous changes are seen by colonoscopy. The laboratory finding of *C. difficile* toxin in the stool is the usual way of making the diagnosis, with colonoscopy used less frequently. This disease may be particularly devastating and even fatal for the geriatric or debilitated patient. Standard therapy is oral vancomycin, 125 mg every 6 hours for 10 days. Oral metronidazole, 500 mg twice a day for 10 days, is also very effective and somewhat less costly. Careful attention must be paid to replacing fluid and electrolytes in these patients.

## URINARY TRACT COMPLICATIONS

## 1. URINARY RETENTION

Periodic measurement of urine volume provides the most useful method of evaluating the patient's postoperative fluid balance. Except when shock or dehydration intervenes, postoperative fluid needs can be accurately gauged by an hourly, then daily, charting of urinary output.

After a minor procedure, measurement of urinary output can await natural voiding. If fluid therapy has been adequate, the patient should void by the evening of the day of surgery; if she has not voided by then, bladder distention should be suspected. The patient should be encouraged to get out of bed to void. If the normal capacity of the bladder is exceeded (500 mL), serious bladder dysfunction may result. The patient may have to be catheterized if she is unable to void. Sterile technique must be used. Overdistention of the bladder can occur in the patient with a kinked or clotted suprapubic tube or transurethral catheter.

Inability of the patient to void or difficulty in voiding often is due to pain caused by using the voluntary muscles to start the urinary stream. With vaginal plastic procedures or with suprapubic procedures performed to treat urinary incontinence like the Marshall-Marchetti-Krantz operation, sutures near the urethra or urethral edema may make voiding difficult or impossible. Continuous drainage of the bladder probably poses fewer problems than frequent intermittent catheterization when the patient is unable to void.

## Treatment

**A. Postoperative Bladder Drainage:** After a major procedure in which postoperative bleeding or operative damage to the urinary tract is a possibility, bladder drainage by means of a urethral catheter or suprapubic cystotomy tube drainage should be instituted despite the small risk of bladder infection. The catheter usually can be removed within 24–48 hours except after a vaginal plastic procedure bladder neck suspension, or extended operation, which usually requires drainage for a longer time.

If prolonged drainage is required, suprapubic drainage is preferred over urethral catheter drainage by many operators because of patient comfort, ease of care, and a reduced incidence of infection. A suprapubic catheter is also useful in facilitating postoperative voiding trials after urogynecologic procedures. If a patient is facing a prolonged return to normal voiding function and has adequate visual acuity and manual dexterity, intermittent clean self-catheterization can be a very useful bladder drainage modality.

Anxiety can play a significant role in patients with difficulty voiding after surgery. Diazepam may be helpful in management for both its anxiolytic and skeletal muscle relaxant effects.

## 2. OLIGURIA AND ANURIA

Oliguria usually results from volume depletion, which often can be demonstrated by diuresis following the rapid intravenous administration of 500 mL of 5% dextrose in normal saline. Disturbances of electrolyte balance (eg. "water intoxication syndrome") or diminished renal blood flow (cardiac failure, shock) may also cause oliguria as can volume overload with congestive heart failure and pulmonary edema. After these possible causes of oliguria have been eliminated, an underlying serious disorder of the urinary tract should be suspected.

Anuria must be identified promptly. It rarely may be due to bilateral ureteral obstruction, a complication that must be considered when there is no urinary output on the operating table or during the immediate postoperative period. If an IVP fails to reveal the cause of this serious postoperative complication, underlying kidney disease (acute tubular necrosis) should be suspected.

## Treatment

Major surgery often will upset the patient's fluid and electrolyte balance. Prohibition of fluids for at least 12 hours before operation, large insensible water losses during the operation, and inability to tolerate food or fluids postoperatively require major adjustments.

The amount and type of fluid replacement should take into account the fact that preoperative dehydra-

tion may have occurred. In addition, loss of fluid into the bowel and insensible losses from the skin, peritoneal cavity, and lungs may have been substantial. Blood loss must be accurately estimated in the operating room, since excessive blood loss may have depleted the vascular and extracellular fluids. It must be kept in mind that all these losses are generally increased as operating time is prolonged.

In gynecologic surgery, the patients vary in their postoperative fluid replacement needs. The healthy 28-year-old myomectomy patient may require a volume of intravenous fluid that would prove fatal to the frail 68-year-old patient with cardiopulmonary disease who just underwent reconstructive vaginal surgery. Postoperative fluid replacement must be individualized.

On average, the urinary output is above 60 mL/h (1500 mL/d) and ordinarily should not fall below 30 mL/h. The urine specific gravity should range between 1.010 and 1.015. Although there is no "ideal" fluid replacement regimen, a healthy young patient generally should tolerate approximately 3000 mL of intravenous fluid on the first postoperative day. The composition of these fluids should address electrolyte as well as glucose needs. Subsequent fluid requirements should be based on replacement of an average of 1000 mL of daily insensible water loss (higher in febrile patients) plus urinary output. A clinical estimate of the state of hydration can be made by noting the urinary output, moisture of the mucous membranes, and skin turgor. If the patient is unable to take fluids orally in adequate amounts after 48 hours, potassium may need to be added to the intravenous fluids after careful scrutiny of the serum electrolytes. If a complicated major procedure with substantial blood loss has been performed, albumin, plasma, or whole blood may be necessary to adjust the fluid and electrolyte balance.

## 3. URINARY TRACT INFECTION

Urinary tract infection (UTI) may develop in the immediate postoperative period in a patient with preexisting contamination of the urinary tract. This is due to the urinary retention that follows surgery, anesthesia, or immobilization. The bladder usually is uncontaminated before surgery and remains so unless bacteria are introduced by instrumentation or catheterization. Catheter-associated urinary tract infection is the most common nosocomial infection.

The systemic manifestations of UTI usually develop within 24–48 hours after removal of the urinary catheter. Fever from UTI can be high. UTI may be suspected when, despite high fever, the patient does not appear to have the toxic systemic reaction that would be expected with most other conditions that cause high fever. Flank tenderness can be present, suggesting pyelonephritis. Pus or bacteria are seen in the urine sediment. Postvoid residual urine, which may be present, tends to perpetuate the infection and predisposes to ascending infection and pyelonephritis.

Hydration should be increased and activity encouraged to facilitate complete emptying of the bladder. After urine specimens are obtained for culture, appropriate antibiotic therapy should be instituted. Antibiotic coverage may have to be adjusted based on culture and sensitivity results. Reinstitution of catheter drainage may be necessary in patients with a postvoid residual urine of 100 mL or more.

## OTHER INFECTIOUS COMPLICATIONS

### 1. HEMATOMA AND PELVIC ABSCESS

Small hematomas or seromas often resolve spontaneously, but some become infected. Closed-suction drainage is frequently used to prevent intra-abdominal hematoma. Gravity or Penrose drains have a limited role in gynecologic surgery.

Insidious accumulations may occur either in the pelvis or under the fascia of the abdominal rectus muscle. They may be first suspected because of a falling hematocrit in association with a low-grade fever. Ultrasonography is an excellent adjunct to physical examination for diagnosis. The subrectus collection, seen most frequently after a Pfannenstiel or Maylard incision or in conjunction with a retropubic urethropexy, may be difficult to outline clinically but is clearly delineated by ultrasound.

Pelvic hematomas are usually not drained unless they are infected and antibiotic therapy has failed. Drainage of an infected hematoma should be accomplished extraperitoneally. This is simple if it is located in the anterior abdominal wall. However, if it is in the pelvis and easy access is not available at the vaginal vault, an inguinal extraperitoneal approach would be necessary. Consideration should be given to percutaneous drainage (Fabiszewski, 1993). The site and extent of the cavity can be identified by pelvic and abdominal examinations as well as by ultrasonography. If the cavity is not readily accessible for operative drainage by either the abdominal or vaginal route, insertion of a large-caliber "pigtail" catheter with ultrasound or CT scan guidance should be considered.

### 2. WOUND INFECTION

The frequency and degree of postoperative wound infection depend on many factors, such as the patient's age, health, nutritional status, and personal hygiene habits, as well as the presence of malignancy, the use of cortocosteroid medications, history of radiation therapy, and surgical technique. The method of skin preparation prior to surgery is also important. Shaving the operative site may cause folliculitis, resulting in a superficial wound infection. If a shave prep is to be done, it should be done in the operating room just before surgery. Using clippers or omitting shaving entirely yields a lower wound infection rate.

The use of antibiotic prophylaxis has long been known to reduce infection at the incision of uncomplicated vaginal and radical abdominal procedures. Antibiotic prophylaxis has recently been shown by meta-analysis to be effective for routine abdominal hysterectomy as well (Mittendorf et al, 1993). Active infection at the operative site (eg, pelvic abscess, ruptured appendix) or at a distant site will increase the risk of wound infection by direct contamination or hematogenous spread.

The diagnosis of wound infection usually is made during investigation of an unexplained postoperative fever, often on about the fourth or fifth day. This diagnosis is based on the physical findings of redness or induration at the operative site. Facultative and anaerobic gram-negative rods, beta-hemolytic streptococci, and staphylococci are the pathogens most commonly cultured from infected wounds. The wound should be explored and cultured. Ample drainage should be established and appropriate antibiotics ordered to treat adjacent cellulitis. If cellulitis is not present, wound opening and local care are adequate therapy. Damp to dry dressings should be changed 3 times daily and the wound debrided daily until definite improvement is noted. Hydrogen peroxide, iodine compounds, antibiotics, or other chemicals in the wound irrigating solution are sometimes used but have not been proved beneficial and may even be toxic or impede healing. A drain or gauze packing may be required to keep the skin from prematurely sealing the wound.

Open wounds may be treated with irrigation, dressing changes, and periodic debridement until healing by secondary intention is complete. This often takes weeks or even months. Recent literature (Walters et al, 1990) supports a role for early secondary closure of these wounds after all infection is resolved and healing has begun. Healing times can be dramatically shortened. Delayed primary closure should be considered during cases with obvious contamination or infection.

### 3. WOUND DEHISCENCE AND EVISCERATION

The transverse lower abdominal incision used by many gynecologists rarely ruptures. Vertical incisions may carry a somewhat greater risk of breakdown, although fascial integrity and surgical technique of fascial closure are also important risk factors.

Evisceration is disruption of all layers of the abdominal wall with protrusion of the intestines through the incision; it is a critical postoperative complication. The dreaded hallmark of this complication is a profuse serosanguinous discharge exuding from the abdominal incision. It must be emphasized that proper exploration and resolution of this problem should take place in the operating room and not on the ward or in the examining room. When the diagnosis of fascial dehiscence or evisceration is made, secondary closure must be performed immediately with the patient under general anesthesia. Interrupted nonabsorbable sutures through all layers of the abdominal wall are preferred. Broad-spectrum antibiotics should be initiated following wound culture. Consideration should be given to a mass closure technique when risk factors for dehiscence are present to help prevent this complication.

## 4. NECROTIC PHENOMENA

Necrotizing fasciitis, typically a synergistic mixed facultative and anaerobic infection that mainly involves the fascia, has been described in both abdominal and perineal sites and is extremely destructive and rapidly progressive. Early recognition is crucial, and expeditious wide debridement of the necrotic fascia and overlying tissues in the operating room is necessary. A second necrotic complication can result from poor incisional planning. When a new incision is made near and parallel with an existing scar, slough of tissue can result secondary to ischemia. The skin starting at the incision and spreading peripherally is cool, gray, and boggy. Wide debridement in the operating room is usually required. Healing with both phenomena is by secondary intention with skin grafts often being necessary. Both conditions are potentially lethal complications that require timely intervention and should always be considered in the differential diagnosis when wound problems occur.

## REFERENCES

### INTRAOPERATIVE COMPLICATIONS

Burchell RC: Internal iliac artery ligation: Hemodynamics. Obstet Gynecol 1964;24:737.

Burchell RC: Arterial physiology of the human female pelvis. (Editorial.) Obstet Gynecol 1968;31(6):855.

Entrup MH, Davis FG. Perioperative complications of anesthesia. Surg Clin North Am 1991;71:1151.

Gitsch E, Palmrich AH: *Gynecologic Operative Anatomy: The Simple and Radical Hysterectomy.* Walter de Gruyter, 1977.

Graham JW, Goligher JC: The management of accidental injuries and deliberate resection of the ureter during excision of the rectum. Br J Surg 1954;42:151.

Greenwood LH et al: Obstetric and non-malignant gynecologic bleeding: Control with angiographic embolization. Radiology 1987;164:155.

Newton M, Newton ER (editors): *Complications of Gynecologic and Obstetric Management.* WB Saunders, 1988.

Nichols DH (editor): *Clinical Problems, Injuries and Complications of Gynecologic Surgery,* 2nd ed. Williams & Wilkins, 1988.

Nichols DH (editor): *Gynecologic and Obstetric Surgery.* Mosby, 1993.

Thompson JD, Rock JA (editors): *TeLinde's Operative Gynecology,* 7th ed. JB Lippincott, 1992.

Timmons MC, Addison WA: Suprapubic teloscopy: Extraperitoneal intraoperative technique to demonstrate ureteral patency. Obstet Gynecol 1990; 75:137.

### POSTOPERATIVE COMPLICATIONS

AORN Practices Subcommittee: Recommended practices: preoperative skin preparation. AORN J 1988; 48:950.

Boyd ME: Postoperative gynecologic infections. Can J Surg 1987;30:7.

Fabiszewski NL, Sumkin JH, Johns CM: Contemporary radiologic percutaneous abscess drainage in the pelvis. Clin Obstet Gynecol 1993;36:445.

Fabri PJ, Rosemurgy A: Reoperation for small intestinal obstruction. Surg Clin North Am 1991;71(1):131.

Holcroft JW, Blaisdell FW: Shock: Causes and management of circulatory collapse. In: *Textbook of Surgery: The Biological Basis of Modern Surgical Practice.* Sabiston DC (editor). WB Saunders, 1991:34.

Livingston EH, Passaro EP Jr: Postoperative ileus. Dig Dis Sci 1990;35(1):121.

Mittendorf RM, Aronson MP, Berry RL et al: Avoiding serious infection associated with abdominal hysterectomy: A meta analysis of antibiotic prophylaxis. Am J Obstet Gynecol 1993;169:1119.

O'Donohue WJ Jr: Postoperative pulmonary complications. When are preventive and therapeutic measures necessary? Postgrad Med 1992;91(3):167,173.

Persson AV, Davis RJ, Villavincencio JL: Deep venous thrombosis and pulmonary embolism. Surg Clin North Am1991;71(6):1195.

Stamm WE: Catheter associated urinary tract infections: Epidemiology, pathogenesis, and prevention. Am J Med 1991;91(3B):65S.

Sweet RL, Gibbs RS: Wound and episiotomy infection. In: *Infectious Diseases of the Female Genital Tract.* Williams & Wilkins, 1990:374.

Walters MD, Dombroski RA, Davidson SA et al: Reclosure of disrupted abdominal incisions. Obstet Gynecol 1990;76:597.

## LAPAROSCOPIC AND HYSTEROSCOPIC COMPLICATIONS

Baadsgaard SE, Bille S, Egeblad K: Major vascular injury during gynecologic laparoscopy: Report of a case and review of published cases. Acta Obstet Gynecol Scand 1989;68:283.

Brooks PG: Complications of operative hysteroscopy: How safe is it? Clin Obstet Gynecol 1992;35:256.

Grainger DA, Soderstrom RM, Schiff SF et al: Ureteral injuries at laparoscopy: Insights into diagnosis, management, and prevention. Obstet Gynecol 1990; 75:839.

Kadar N, Reich H, Liu CY et al: Incisional hernias after major laparoscopic gynecologic procedures. Am J Obstet Gynecol 1993;168:1493.

L. Russell Malinak, MD, Carol A. Wheeler, MD, & James M. Wheeler, MD

Four of the 10 most commonly performed operations in the USA are dilation and curettage (D&C), tubal sterilization, abdominal hysterectomy, and vaginal hysterectomy. This chapter will review these procedures, as well as other therapeutic operations. Indications, contraindications, technique, and complications will be discussed for each procedure.

## DILATION & CURETTAGE (D&C)

### Indications

The procedure of cervical dilation and uterine curettage is usually performed for one of the following indications: diagnosis and treatment of abnormal uterine bleeding, management of abortion (incomplete, missed, or induced), stenosis, or cancer of the uterus. The diagnosis of abnormal bleeding is discussed in Chapters 32 and 36; D&C as a method of induced abortion is discussed in Chapter 33. This section will discuss the remaining therapeutic uses of D&C.

### Technique

**A. Cervical Dilation:** Dilation of the cervix may be conducted under paracervical, epidural, spinal, or general anesthesia, depending largely on the indication for the procedure. Cervical dilation usually precedes uterine curettage but may be performed as a therapeutic maneuver for acquired or congenital cervical stenosis, dysmenorrhea, or insertion of an intrauterine contraceptive device (IUD) or radium device for treatment of cancer. Dilation may also precede hysterography or hysteroscopy.

The patient is placed in the dorsal lithotomy position, with the back and shoulders supported and the extremities padded. The inner thighs, perineum, and vagina are prepared as for any vaginal operation; the surgeon and assistant should adhere to surgical principles of asepsis. A thorough pelvic examination under anesthesia is mandatory prior to performing cervical dilation, in order to determine the size and

position of the cervix, uterus, and adnexa and the presence of any abnormalities. The patient voids normally before the operation if possible; urinary catheterization is used only if significant residual urine is suspected.

A right-angle retractor is placed anteriorly to gently retract the bladder. A weighted speculum is placed posteriorly to reveal the cervix; this should be removed as soon as possible, certainly within 30 minutes, to avoid undue pressure on the perineal tissues. Under direct vision, the anterior lip of the cervix is grasped with a tenaculum, avoiding the vascular supply at 3 and 9 o'clock. The cervix is grasped firmly but with care taken not to compromise, or especially perforate the endocervical canal. With gentle traction, the cervix can be brought down toward the introitus. Before proceeding further, a complete visual examination should be made of the cervix and the 4 vaginal fornices, because the latter areas (especially posteriorly) are otherwise difficult to examine. Areas that appear abnormal (even benign inclusion cysts) should be noted and followed as appropriate. Areas that are clearly abnormal should be biopsied. After the cervix and vagina are evaluated, the uterine cavity is examined. A uterine sound is gently inserted into the endocervix and then advanced into the uterine cavity in the plane of least resistance and most compatible with the position of the uterus as revealed by pelvic examination. Perforation of the uterus during D&C is most likely to occur at the time of uterine sounding or cervical dilation. Perforation is more likely to occur if the woman has retroversion or anteversion of the uterus or cervical stenosis, is pregnant or has recently given birth, or is postmenopausal; or if the surgeon uses excessive force or faulty technique. If severe cervical stenosis is suspected from the preoperative office examination, cervical softening agents such as prostaglandin $E_2$ gel or *Laminaria* tents may be inserted the day before the planned D&C. The depth of the uterine cavity is recorded as well as any abnormalities such as leiomyomas or septa.

The 2 most common dilators used are the Hegar

and Hank's dilators. Hegar dilators are relatively blunt, gently curved, and numbered sequentially according to width (ie, a No. 7 dilator is 7 mm wide). For most purposes, particularly preceding curettage, dilation to a No. 9 dilator suffices; if dilation is being performed for dysmenorrhea, infertility, or stenosis, dilation should proceed to a No. 11 dilator.

Hank's dilators differ from Hegar dilators in being more gradually tapered ("sharper"); they may have a solid core or a hollow center allowing egress of trapped blood and air. Hank's dilators are measured in French sizes (a No. 20F Hank's dilator is approximately the same diameter as a No. 9 Hegar dilator). The choice of dilator is largely based on surgical training; many prefer not to use the more pointed Hank's dilators in a small postmenopausal uterus.

**B. Endocervical Curettage:** Fractional curettage should be used for abnormal uterine bleeding or if genital tract neoplasia is suspected. The cervical canal should be curetted prior to dilation of the cervix and curettage of the endometrial cavity, in order to preserve the histologic characteristics of the endocervix and prevent contamination of the endometrial sample with endocervical cells. If cervical conization is planned for diagnosis or treatment of cervical intraepithelial neoplasia, uterine sounding precedes conization, but cervical dilation and fractional curettage follow in order to minimize denuding of the endocervical epithelium. The Gusberg curet is a small, slightly curved instrument particularly well suited for endocervical curettage. The curet is placed in the endocervical canal to the level of the internal os; with a firm touch, each of the 4 walls is curetted with a single stroke, with the specimen delivered onto a coated cellulose sponge with a twirling motion of the curet. (The coated cellulose sponge is preferred over ordinary surgical sponges because tissue is less likely to adhere to it.) The cervix is then dilated as described earlier and curettage of the endometrium performed. The endocervical and endometrial specimens are immersed in fixative in separate containers and submitted to the pathologist.

Complications from endocervical curettage are rare in nongravid patients. Because of obvious risks to the fetus and membranes, endocervical curettage is contraindicated in pregnant women. Healing of the curetted endocervix may take 3 weeks or more; the cervical epithelium commonly takes 2 weeks to heal following a routine Papanicolaou smear. Tissue should be allowed to heal before follow-up Papanicolaou smears are taken, because regenerating cells are often mistaken for dysplastic cells.

**C. Endometrial Polypectomy:** The uterine cavity is explored with polyp forceps prior to diagnostic or therapeutic endometrial curettage. It is easier to remove polyps prior to curettage, preserving the histologic integrity necessary to differentiate benign uterine polyps from neoplasia. In a large series advocating routine exploration of the endometrial cavity preceding curettage, 64% of 130 diagnosed endometrial polyps were removed by ureteral stone forceps. Pedunculated or submucous leiomyomas, intrauterine and intracervical synechias, and uterine anomalies may be first suspected at passage of the polyp forceps.

The technique of polypectomy includes gentle insertion of the forceps in the plane most compatible with the position of the uterus (as for uterine sounding). The forceps are opened slightly, rotated 90 degrees, and removed. Many clinicians repeat this procedure through 360 degrees, completely exploring the uterine cavity.

Skillful use of hysteroscopy for diagnosis and treatment of synechias, septa, leiomyomas, and polyps is preferred to blind polypectomy and curettage. With the new, narrow hysteroscope, the procedure may become an office procedure similar to colposcopy for biopsy or laser conization. Recently, second-look hysteroscopy (SLH) has been defined as an important adjunct to uterine surgery for septa or intrauterine adhesions. However, SLH awaits clinical validation of its efficacy.

**D. Endometrial Curettage:** Endometrial curettage is indicated for treatment of complications of pregnancy, including incomplete or missed abortion, postpartum retention of products of conception, placental polyps, and, perhaps, endomyometritis. The procedure is also used in treatment of abnormal uterine bleeding due to pedunculated leiomyomas or polyps or in the occasional case of dysfunctional uterine bleeding that is refractory to medical therapy or life-threatening. The D&C is often both diagnostic and therapeutic.

The technique of endometrial curettage is tailored to the individual patient. In determining the hormone responsiveness of the endometrium, a small but representative sample may be obtained from the anterior and posterior walls. When curettage is being performed therapeutically, a systematic, thorough approach is indicated. The largest sharp curet that can comfortably fit through the dilated cervix is chosen. A serrated curet may cause injury to the underlying basalis layer of the endometrium and myometrium. The anterior, lateral, and posterior walls are scraped with firm pressure in a clockwise or counterclockwise fashion from the top of the uterine fundus down to the internal os. The top of the cavity is curetted with a side-to-side motion. The curettings are retrieved onto the waiting gauze and immersed in fixative as soon as possible. If endometrial curettage is being used for diagnosis of infection (eg, tuberculous endometritis, salpingitis), a portion of the curettings should be placed in containers appropriate for culture (without fixative).

A single curettage will not remove the entire endometrium. Thorough curettage by an experienced gynecologist often removes 50–60% of the endometrium, as determined by immediate post curettage hysterectomy. Gross inspection of curettings is inaccurate in predicting carcinoma. Frozen section gives false results in 25% of patients with suspected cancer. If risk factors for endometrial cancer are present and clinical suspicion for neoplasia persists despite a histologic diagnosis of benign endometrium, further evaluation with hysteroscopic-guided biopsy or hysterectomy is indicated.

Perforation of the uterus occurred in 0.63% of a large series of D&Cs. Perforation is suspected when the sound or curet meets no resistance at the point expected by uterine size, consistency, and position determined by preoperative bimanual examination. Curettage may be continued if the area of suspected perforation is avoided. Should suction curettage be associated with perforation, laparoscopy must be used to continue the procedure to avoid aspiration of bowel into the uterine cavity. In the case of suspected perforation, the patient should be observed for at least 24 hours in the hospital for possible infection or hemorrhage. In a series of 70 uterine perforations, 55 were treated expectantly, and only one patient developed complications (pelvic abscess drained via colpotomy). In 7 patients, hysterectomy was elected but not indicated by operative findings. Today, laparoscopy is the method of choice in evaluating perforations in the hemodynamically stable patient.

**E. Endometrial Biopsy:** Outpatient curettage, or endometrial biopsy, should always be a diagnostic and not a therapeutic technique. The many techniques available, all compared to D&C under adequate anesthesia, are discussed in Chapter 36.

## HYSTEROSCOPY

This section will discuss therapeutic uses of hysteroscopy.

### Indications & Contraindications
See Table 45–1.

### Technique
The hysteroscope is a rigid endoscope similar in design to an operating laparoscope or a urologic resectoscope. Typically 6–10 mm in external diameter, the outer sleeve encloses a fiberoptic light source, a channel used to introduce a medium to distend the uterus, and a channel through which probes, forceps, and electrocautery or laser instruments may be visually directed in the uterine cavity. Viewing angles vary from 10 to 45 degrees.

The uterine cavity, which is normally collapsed, must be distended by a medium: high-molecular-weight dextran mixed 50%–50% with normal saline, sorbitol, glycine, or 5% dextrose in water. $CO_2$, may also be used. Gentle manual pressure is exerted on a syringe containing dextran (usually 50–150 mL). Uterine pressure does not exceed 150 mm Hg under normal conditions, although particular care is exercised in patients with bilateral tubal occlusion that prohibits egress of the dextran. The disadvantage of using dextran is its sticky consistency. Anaphylactic reaction is a rare response to the use of dextran; supportive measures must be instantly available, and an intravenous line should be established in all patients undergoing hysteroscopy.

$CO_2$ gas insufflation is favored by some gyneco-

**Table 45–1.** Indications and contraindications for hysteroscopy.

| Indications | Contraindications |
|---|---|
| **Evaluation and treatment of abnormal uterine bleeding**<br>Perimenopausal bleeding with negative D&C.<br>Directed biopsy in patient with atypical adenomatous hyperplasia but at high risk for hysterectomy.<br>Evaluation of endocervix versus endometrium as origin of biopsy-proved adenocarcinoma.<br>Suspicion (on history or hysterography) of uterine polyp or submucous leiomyoma amenable to hysteroscopic resection.<br>**Evaluation and treatment of infertility**<br>Habitual abortion.<br>Known uterine septum on previous hysterography or curettage.<br>Suspected foreign body (eg, broken or imbedded IUD).<br>Suspected submucous leiomyoma on history, pelvic examination, or laparoscopy.<br>Suspected cornual occlusion on hysterography.<br>Suspected intracervical, intrauterine, or intracornual adhesions.<br>Suspected congenital anomaly (eg, with known urologic anomaly).<br>Possible intrauterine infection (eg, tuberculosis).<br>Intrauterine insemination or embryo transfer in selected patients with known uterine fusion anomaly.<br>Suspected endometrial polyp. | **Absolute contraindications**<br>Pelvic inflammatory disease, especially tubo-ovarian complex.<br>Uterine perforation.<br>Sensitivity to anesthetic or distention medium.<br>Lack of proper equipment, specifically, low-pressure insufflator for $CO_2$ distention.<br>Operator inexperience.<br><br>**Relative contraindications**<br>Heavy bleeding limiting visual field.<br>Known gynecologic cancer, especially endometrial, cervical, tubal, and ovarian, because of theoretic risk of flushing cancer cells into the peritoneal cavity. |

logic surgeons. The addition of a cervical suction cup maintains intrauterine pressure at less than 200 mm Hg. The flow rate must not exceed 100 mL/min to avoid uterine injury or gas embolism; thus, laparoscopic insufflators must never be connected to a hysteroscope. The advantages of $CO_2$ gas over dextran are easier cleansing of instruments and improved comfort for the surgeon. A disadvantage is more difficult visualization due to mixing with blood or debris. This problem is usually surmountable with experience.

A 5% dextrose in water solution requires pressures of 80–120 mm Hg for adequate visualization. This solution is safe and readily available, but visualization is poor because of mixing with blood. This medium is best used for diagnosis when little bleeding is expected; it is rarely the medium of choice in therapeutic hysteroscopy.

More and more instruments are available for use in hysteroscopic procedures, including blunt probes, microscissors, alligator clamps with electrocautery attachment, and a wire loop for excision and coagulation (resectoscope). The argon laser is useful lysing septa, and the neodynium: YAG (yttrium, aluminum, garnet) laser is available for endometrial ablation. (see Table 45–2.)

Local or general anesthetics are chosen on the basis of expected hysteroscopic findings or procedures, concomitant operations planned, and the desires and cooperation of the patient. Most hysteroscopic examinations and virtually all therapeutic procedures are performed under general anesthesia. Following administration of anesthesia, the urinary bladder is drained, and the anterior lip of the cervix is grasped with a tenaculum. The cervix should then be gradually dilated to the same diameter as the external sleeve of the hysteroscope in order to provide a firm fit. Although the lower aspect of the uterine cavity will undoubtedly be entered during cervical dilation, the endometrial cavity should be left as intact as possible in order to optimize hysteroscopic visualization. Concomitant laparoscopy is mandated in any patient in whom a hysteroscopic therapeutic procedure is planned. Uterine perforation may be observed through the laparoscope, and excess dextran may be aspirated from the posterior cul-de-sac after a prolonged procedure.

An assistant must be constantly present during hysteroscopy to monitor uterine insufflation so that the pressure never exceeds 200 mm Hg, and the flow rate of the distending medium never exceeds 100 mL/min. The surgeon must be sitting comfortably, with all instruments available to perform the hysteroscopic procedure safely and expeditiously. Following the procedure, intrauterine instruments should be inspected for their integrity. The microscissors in particular are delicate and could break within the uterus. If dextran is used, it must be immediately flushed from the hysteroscope before it is allowed to dry.

## Complications

Hysteroscopic surgery is generally safe in experienced hands. With laparoscopic observation, the serious complication of uterine perforation can almost always be prevented. If overt bleeding occurs during resection of a septum, polyp, or leiomyoma, the laparoscopic probe can be held against the uterine vessels to slow the blood flow. A Foley catheter may be inserted into the uterine cavity and inflated to provide a tamponade for heavy endometrial bleeding. Infection is an unusual complication following hysteroscopy, although many surgeons administer prophylactic antibiotics (doxycycline, 100 mg twice daily for 7 days). Complications of distending media include ascites and pleural effusion if an excessive amount results in vascular intervasation.

## Prognosis

With proper selection of patients, hysteroscopic surgery has high success rates. Small pedunculated leiomyomas and polyps are usually retrieved by an experienced, patient surgeon. Submucous leiomyomas may be destroyed if they are not too vascular. In a series of 105 septal incisions, 77% were successfully divided; division of the rest was postponed because of bleeding and technical difficulties. In the treatment of intrauterine adhesions, the chance for success and restoration of a normal endometrial cavity depends on the density and extent of the adhesions and the area of normal endometrium remaining after dissection.

Following hysteroscopic surgery in which the endometrium is denuded, postoperative estrogen therapy is prescribed by many physicians to promote rapid endometrial growth.

## LAPAROSCOPY

Laparoscopy (peritoneoscopy) is a transperitoneal endoscopic technique that provides excellent visualization of the pelvic structures and often permits the diagnosis of gynecologic disorders and pelvic surgery without laparotomy.

Most basic laparoscopes are 10 mm in diameter and have a 180-degree viewing angle. The instrument

**Table 45–2.** Comparison of lasers used in treatment of endometriosis.

|  | $CO_2$ | Argon | Nd:YAG |
|---|---|---|---|
| Laser wavelength | 10.6 μm | 0.5 μm | 1.06 μm |
| Depth of tissue destruction | 0.1 mm | 0.5 mm | 4 mm |
| Beam scattering | None | Slight | Significant |
| Effect dependent on tissue color | None | Yes | Yes |
| Delivery by fiberoptic systems | Experimental | Yes | Yes |

has an effective length of over 25 cm and can be utilized with a fiberoptic light box. In order to facilitate visualization, $CO_2$ must be instilled into the peritoneal cavity to distend the abdominal wall.

Use of a pneumatic insufflator permits continuous monitoring of the rate, pressure, and volume of the gas used for inflation. In addition to the equipment used for observation, a variety of other instruments for biopsy, coagulation, aspiration, and manipulation can be passed through separate cannulas or inserted through the same cannula as the laparoscope. A laser ($CO_2$ or Nd:YAG) may be used with the laparoscope. A suitable modification of design provides a true operating laparoscope.

Laparoscopy has been widely used for interval sterilization. When properly performed, fulguration effectively destroys a portion of oviduct, with an extremely low failure rate. An alternative technique is occlusion of the uterine tubes with Silastic bands, Silastic rings, or metal clips. Another frequent use of laparoscopy is for diagnosis of infertility or endometriosis. Some gastroenterologists occasionally use laparoscopy to assess liver disease.

The laparoscope has become an invaluable tool in both diagnostic and operative gynecologic procedures. However, its use requires considerable expertise, and it should always be used by a surgeon familiar with the management of complications. Laparoscopic procedures are *major* intra-abdominal operations performed through small incisions. This technique is rapidly performed; has a low morbidity rate; a short convalescence period; and is less demanding in terms of medical facilities, supplies, and personnel. In many cases, laparoscopy may replace conventional laparotomy for diagnosis and treatment of gynecologic problems. It is a cost-effective outpatient procedure.

## Indications

The indications will increase with the clinician's experience and as technical innovations permit even more complicated procedures.

### A. Diagnosis:

1. Differentiation between ovarian, tubal, and uterine masses, eg, ectopic pregnancy, ovarian cyst, salpingitis, myomas, endometriosis, tuberculosis.

2. Pelvic pain, eg, possible adhesions, endometriosis, ectopic pregnancy, twisted or bleeding ovarian cyst, salpingitis, appendicitis, psychogenic pelvic pain.

3. Disorders of the liver, eg, neoplasia, hepatic cirrhosis, splenomegaly.

4. Genital anomalies, eg, ovarian dysgenesis, uterine maldevelopment.

5. Ascites, eg, ovarian diseases versus cirrhosis.

6. Secondary amenorrhea of possible ovarian origin, eg, polycystic ovarian disease, arrhenoblastoma.

7. Pelvic injuries after penetrating or nonpenetrating abdominal trauma.

8. Staging of Hodgkin's disease and lymphomas.

9. Diagnosis of occult cancer.

### B. Evaluation:

1. Infertility, eg, tubal patency, ovarian biopsy.

2. "Second look" after tubal surgery or treatment of endometriosis.

3. Assessment of pelvic and abdominal trauma.

4. Appraisal of bowel for viability after surgery, for mesenteric thrombosis.

5. Study of pelvic nodes after lymphography.

6. Peritoneal washings for cytology study.

7. Peritoneal culture.

8. Evaluation of uterine perforation.

9. Evaluation of pelvic viscera to determine the feasibility of vaginal hysterectomy.

### C. Therapy:

1. Tubal sterilization:
   a. Electrical: Unipolar or bipolar technique.
   b. Mechanical: Silastic bands, Silastic rings, or metal clips.

2. Lysis of adhesions, with or without laser.

3. Fulguration of endometriosis by laser or thermal cautery.

4. Aspiration of small unilocular ovarian cyst or of fluid for culture.

5. Removal of extruded intrauterine device.

6. Uterosacral ligament division (denervation).

7. Treatment of ectopic pregnancy.

8. Myomectomy.

9. Salpingostomy for phimotic fimbriae.

10. Removal of tuboplastic hoods or splints.

11. Ova collection for in vitro fertilization.

12. GIFT (gamete intrafallopian transfer for fertilization).

13. Mini-wedge resection of ovary.

14. Biopsy of tumor, liver, ovary, spleen, omentum, etc.

15. Placement of intraperitoneal clips as marked for radiotherapy.

16. Oopherectomy.

17. Ovarian cystectomy.

18. Lysis of adhesions or adnexal surgery to allow vaginal hysterectomy ("laporoscopic assisted vaginal hysterectomy").

## Contraindications

Note: Previous intra-abdominal surgery will have been done in 15–18% of patients in large series and usually is not a contraindication to laparoscopy.

**A. Absolute:** Intestinal obstruction, generalized peritonitis.

**B. Relative:** Severe cardiac or pulmonary disease, previous periumbilical surgery, shock, cancer involving anterior abdominal wall.

## Preparation for Laparoscopy

Careful explanation of the contemplated procedure must be given to each patient prior to surgery. Unless the individual is a poor operative risk, laparoscopy is usually an outpatient operation. Preparation includes no solid food for at least 8 hours prior to surgery, no liquids for more than 6 hours preoperatively, a history and physical examination, and routine blood studies. No abdominal or perineal shaving is necessary, but skin preparation with an antiseptic is routine.

## Anesthesia

Local anesthesia, local anesthesia with systemic analgesia, spinal or epidural block techniques, or general anesthesia with or without endotracheal intubation may be used. Acupuncture anesthesia may be effective also. Special hazards of anesthesia exist, eg, reduced diaphragmatic excursion because of the pneumoperitoneum and because the patient may be operated on in the Trendelenburg position. Because of these factors, most procedures in the USA are performed with the patient under general anesthesia with endotracheal intubation. With adequate understanding of the physiology involved, effective anesthesia and laparoscopy can be accomplished safely.

An alternative to general anesthesia is local anesthesia with intravenous sedation. The patient may experience transient discomfort during manipulation of the uterine tubes, but in selected patients this discomfort is easily tolerated. By utilizing local anesthesia, the patient may be discharged 1 hour after the operation.

## Surgical Technique

The patient should be placed in the dorsal lithotomy position and draped after induction of anesthesia and preparation of the abdomen and pelvic area (Fig 45–1). The bladder must be emptied by catheterization to decrease the risk of injury during subsequent introduction and use of other instruments. After careful bimanual examination, a tenaculum is attached to the cervix, and a tubal insufflation cannula is inserted into the cervical canal and finally fixed to the tenaculum so that it can be used as a "handle" to maneuver the uterus. A 1-cm incision is made within or immediately below the umbilicus; a veffes needle is inserted through this incision into the peritoneal cavity. Carbon dioxide should then be introduced and monitored by the pneumatic insufflator. The amount of gas insufflated will vary with the patient's size, the laxity of the abdominal wall, and the planned procedure. In most patients, 2–3 L of gas will be needed to obtain adequate visualization. The maximum insufflation pressure should not exceed 20 mm Hg. The needle is withdrawn and the laparoscopic trocar and cannula inserted. After proper abdominal entry, the trocar may be withdrawn and replaced with the fiberoptic laparoscope. The examiner manipulates the intrauterine cannula so that the pelvic organs can be observed. To test for tubal patency, methylene blue or indigo carmine solution can be injected through the intra-

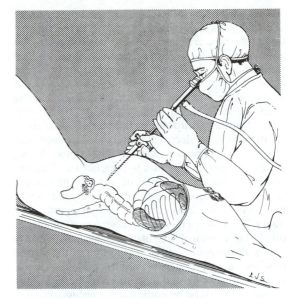

**Figure 45–1.** Pelvic laparoscopy with patient in Trendelenburg position.

uterine cannula. Direct observation of dye leakage attests to tubal patency. A second trocar with a cannula may be inserted under direct laparoscopic vision through a 5-mm transverse midline incision at the pubic hairline. Electrical cutting forceps or an aspiration probe may be used through the second cannula. The use of an operating laparoscope also permits passage of ancillary surgical instruments. Additional punctures are utilized as necessary for the placement of other instruments. Surgical knots may be tied and sutures placed using specially made equipment. The upper abdomen and appendix may be easily visualized.

The operation is terminated by evacuating the insufflated gas through the cannula, followed by removal of all instruments and placement of a 3–0 subcuticular suture for wound closure. A small dressing is applied to the wound. In uncomplicated cases involving diagnosis only, operating time is about 10 minutes. In massively obese patients (> 250 lb) or in patients with previous periumbilical surgery, an open technique may be utilized. A small incision is dissected to the fascia, and the peritoneum is entered under direct visualization. The trocar sleeve is placed in the peritoneal cavity, and Allis forceps or a pursestring suture is used to create an airtight seal. Insufflation is then effected through the sleeve to create the pneumoperitoneum.

**A. Sterilization:** Electrical cautery, Silastic rings or bands, and metal spring clips achieve sterilization by occluding the uterine tubes. About 3% of patients who elect to use these methods of contraception later regret the procedure. Therefore, for women under age

35 and of low parity, techniques resulting in lesser amounts of tissue destruction limited to the midportion of the tube are preferred. The advantages or disadvantages of the different techniques are of less significance than the skill with which a physician can perform any one technique; therefore, choice of method should depend on which technique is most comfortable for the physician.

**1. Cautery (unipolar or bipolar)**–Laparoscopic sterilization with electrical cautery is associated with a very low pregnancy rate (1–4/1000 procedures). Excessive tubal destruction is associated with an unacceptably high incidence of ectopic pregnancy, since it may create a tiny fistula from the uterus into the peritoneal cavity through which sperm may travel. Therefore, when using either form (unipolar or bipolar) of electrical coagulation, one should destroy only a short section of the midportion of the uterine tube, avoiding the uterine cornu if possible. Generally, the tube is burned at 2 different locations, and division of the tube by cutting is not necessary.

**2. Silastic bands**–Tubal occlusion with Silastic bands or rings results in a slightly higher pregnancy rate (6/1000 procedures) but fewer ectopic pregnancies. Mechanical problems in placement of the bands and bleeding from the tubes during the procedure are more common.

**3. Clips**–Tubal occlusion with clips of several types is less frequently employed. Failure rates are higher (20/1000 procedures) than with other techniques and are probably related to poor clip placement.

**B. Infertility:** No study of the infertile patient is complete without laparoscopic study. In procedures of sterilization reversal, laparoscopic visualization may be needed prior to reanastamosis, particularly if the ligation procedure involved electrocautery. Peritubal adhesions may be lysed with electric scissors, and salpingostomy may be accomplished. The minimal trauma of these procedures using laparoscopy and the saving of a major operative procedure are obvious benefits. Laparoscopy should be considered for women with complaints of abnormal bleeding and unexplained pelvic pain. More liberal use of the laparoscope has led to the diagnosis of many unsuspected cases of endometriosis. Hormonal treatment of endometriosis should be withheld until visual or histologic confirmation of the disease is available.

Electrical fulguration of areas of endometriosis or laser destruction of these diseased areas by laparoscopy is a safe, effective, and rapid treatment. The use of laser obviously allows implants on structures such as bowel, bladder, and the fallopian tubes to be treated with a fairly wide margin of safety. Relief may be immediate and striking, whether the woman has complained of dysmenorrhea, dyspareunia, or generalized pelvic pain. Among infertile patients with lesser stages of endometriosis, pregnancy rates

are similar to those in other published studies of treatment with danazol.

In infertility, the laparoscope has been important for ova collection for in vitro fertilization. The newer technique, GIFT (gamete intrafallopian transfer), is effective in couples with nonmechanical causes of infertility and normal fallopian tubes.

**C. Abdominal and pelvic pain:** Laparoscopy has proved invaluable in differentiating various causes of acute and chronic pain. The technique may save the patient the necessity of a major exploratory operation. Fluid aspiration and tissue biopsy are possible through laparoscopy. Also, pelvic and intestinal disease can be differentiated. The appendix may be visualized and acute appendicitis may be diagnosed. Numerous cases of pain caused by intra-abdominal adhesions also have been diagnosed by laparoscopy, and relief has been obtained following laparoscopic adhesion resection.

**D. Trauma**–In cases of intra-abdominal trauma, laparoscopy can be utilized to exclude the need for a major abdominal operation.

**E. Miscellaneous:** "Missing" IUDs have been removed from the intra-abdominal cavity. Mulligan plastic hoods from tuboplasty procedures, "lost" drains, and other foreign material have been removed from the abdomen by operative laparoscopy.

## Postsurgical Care

Patients may be sent home following full recovery from anesthesia, usually in 1–2 hours. Postoperative pain is usually minimal, and patients are discharged with a prescription for a simple oral analgesic. The most common complaint is shoulder pain secondary to subdiaphragmatic accumulation of gas. Patients are encouraged to resume full activity, except for sexual relations, the day following surgery. Sexual relations may be resumed several days postoperatively after a simple procedure, eg, tubal ligation. Following extensive operative laparoscopy or other gynecologic procedures, coitus should be delayed for an appropriate interval, ie, until it is unlikely to cause discomfort or damage to the operative site. Patients should routinely be seen in the office 1–2 weeks postoperatively.

## Complications

When misidentification and luteal phase pregnancies are excluded, the true failure rate for laparoscopic sterilization varies between 0.9 and 6 per 1000 sterilizations, depending in part on the technique used. This rate is similar to that of nonlaparoscopic techniques. A survey conducted by the American Association of Gynecologic Laparoscopists disclosed a complication rate (procedures requiring laparotomy) of 1.6:1000 with sterilization laparoscopy and 3.1:1000 with diagnostic laparoscopy. The higher incidence of complications when the instrument is used for investigation of disease is probably related to the fact that the patients often have had prior laparotomies. As laparoscopists become more experienced, the incidence of complications tends to fall. Complications are infrequent when meticulous care is exercised throughout the procedure.

Large studies of the various sterilization procedures used with laparoscopy do not show any significant change in menstrual patterns following the different procedures, and there is no evidence that sterilization itself alters menstrual patterns.

**A. Pain:** Pain may be referred from the diaphragm to the shoulder or chest due to pressure from unabsorbed gas. Use of smaller volumes of gas will minimize pain. Gas is usually absorbed within hours. Mild analgesics and rest in the recumbent position should alleviate discomfort.

**B. Bleeding:** Insertion of a needle and trocar through the abdominal wall has inherent risks. Proper positioning of the penetrating instrument is essential.

1. Small arterial or venous bleeding usually responds to electrocoagulation or pressure with biopsy forceps. Tubal damage resulting in significant bleeding requiring laparotomy is rare.

2. Ecchymotic areas in the anterior abdominal wall or omentum need no treatment if no active bleeding is visualized.

3. Laceration or puncture injuries of the iliac arteries or veins or of the aorta have been reported. If this is likely to have happened, immediate emergency blood replacement and laparotomy for vascular repair must be instituted.

**C. Puncture injury:** Injury from a trocar requires laparotomy and repair. Puncture injury to the stomach or bowel by the needle during insufflation of gas usually requires no treatment. In selected cases, injuries to the bowel may be repaired via laparoscopy.

**D. Misplacement of gas:** The risk of misplacement of gas into the anterior rectus sheath is minimized by the pneumatic insufflator monitoring equipment, but on occasion it is uncertain whether or not gas has been introduced into the abdominal cavity. Gas disperses rapidly and is absorbed through body tissues, and these qualities provide a safety factor.

**E. Thermal burns:** It was hoped that bipolar sterilization would reduce the number of thermal injuries occurring during laparoscopy, but some still occur. With increased operator experience, the number of serious injuries with unipolar cautery has been reduced drastically. Burn injuries are fewer with improved equipment and operator experience.

**F. Vague unexplained lower abdominal discomfort:** Abdominal discomfort in the days following the procedure must be assessed with the possibility of salpingitis in mind. This is uncommon in patients undergoing tubal ligation but is occasionally seen in patients with preexisting tubal disease and chronic pelvic inflammatory disease. Infections of the surgical wound are rare.

### Mortality Rates Associated With Laparoscopic Sterilization

The Centers for Disease Control studied deaths attributable to tubal sterilization in the USA from 1977 to 1981. Of the 17 deaths associated with laparoscopic sterilization, 6 followed complications of general anesthesia; 5 were due to sepsis (in 3 of these, sepsis was caused by thermal injury to the bowel during electrical sterilization); 3 were due to hemorrhage; and 1 each was due to myocardial infarction, pulmonary embolism, and complete heart block. Obesity was the commonest preexisting condition in patients who died. Some deaths might have been prevented by the use of endotracheal intubation during general anesthesia. Local anesthesia is safe and effective but, regrettably, is not well accepted by patients or physicians in the USA.

## OPERATIONS FOR STERILIZATION OF WOMEN & MEN

Sterilization is a permanent method of contraception that is being chosen by increasing numbers of women and men. Sterilization is the most frequent indication for laparoscopy in the USA (> 1 million women per year). A similar number of men choose partial vasectomy for sterilization.

### TUBAL STERILIZATION

Tubal sterilization was first performed in 1823 to prevent pregnancy in women who would need repeated cesarean sections. Since the first tubal sterilization was performed, over 200 different techniques have been described. In Table 45–3, the most common methods used with conventional laparotomy are listed. In Table 45–4, techniques used with the more popular minilaparotomy are listed. Table 45–5 describes laparoscopic methods.

Rates of tubal sterilization for women of reproductive age increased 164% in the USA between 1970 and 1980. There is an increasing incidence of tubal sterilization in women age 20–24, whereas rates in other age groups appear to be stable. Sterilization rates have increased for both currently and previously married women but remain low for never-married women. Rates for black women are consistently greater than those for Caucasian women. In the USA,

**Table 45–3.** Transabdominal ligation or transection and ligation.[1]

| Method | Failure Rate/1000 (Range) | Morbidity Rate (Incidence) | Procedure Accomplished | |
|---|---|---|---|---|
| | | | Hospital | Outpatient |
| Uchida (Fig 47–1) | Nil | Low | + | + |
| Pomeroy (Fig 47–3) | 0–0.4 | Low | + | + |
| Madlener (same as Pomeroy *except* no tubal resection) | 0.3–2 | Low | + | + |
| Fimbriectomy (Fig 47–4) | Nil | Low | + | + |
| Irving (Fig 47–2) | Nil | Low | + | + |
| Salpingectomy | 0–1.9 | Moderate | + | – |
| Cornual resection | 2.8–3.2 | Moderate | + | – |
| Simple ligation | 20 | Low | + | + |

[1]Modified and reproduced, with permission, from Department of Medical and Public Affairs, George Washington University Medical Center: *Popul Rep*, Series C, No. 7, May 1976.

rates are highest in the South and lowest in the Northeast. Withdrawal of some contraceptives (eg, IUDs) and continued economic and social pressures to limit family size will cause rates of tubal sterilization to increase over the next decade.

## Preoperative Counseling

Clear, comprehensive counseling is essential for women who are considering tubal sterilization. Possible medical and psychologic complications must be carefully outlined (see Complications, later); women are more likely to regret having had the operation if they do not know what to expect.

The physician should be alert to signs that the patient is undecided about having the operation or is being pressured by her husband or others. Regret or dissatisfaction is more common if the procedure is done postpartum than at another time, and these women are more than twice as likely to feel that preoperative counseling was inadequate. Temporary stress associated with the pregnancy may have influenced a premature decision for sterilization in these women. In one study of postpartum and other sterilizations, only 4 of 138 women requested reversal 1 year after sterilization.

Patients should be told that tubal sterilization is usually not reversible. Some methods are sometimes reversible (see Chapter 58). One article estimates that about 1% of women who undergo tubal sterilization request reversal. In general, success is directly related to the amount of normal tube preserved. Less destructive methods such as clips and bands have reversal rates of 84% and 72%, respectively. The reversal rate following the most commonly performed procedure (Pomeroy method) approaches 50% and, following electrocoagulation, 41%. Ectopic pregnancy rates vary from 1.7 to 6.5% following reversal; this incidence may increase to 15% when concomitant tubal disorders (eg, pelvic adhesions) exist at the time of anastomosis or develop subsequent to anastomosis.

It is also important for legal reasons that patients be fully informed of the risks, effectiveness, and chances of reversibility of this operation and of alternative procedures. According to the American College of Obstetricians and Gynecologists, there is no need for a hospital committee to approve or disapprove a request for sterilization if the patient is of legal age and sound mind, irrespective of parity. The United States Supreme Court has ruled that the

**Table 45–4.** Tubal occlusion by minilaparotomy.[1]

| Method | Failure Rate/1000 (Range) | Morbidity Rate (Incidence) | Procedure Accomplished | |
|---|---|---|---|---|
| | | | Hospital | Outpatient |
| Uchida | Nil | Low | + | + |
| Fimbriectomy | Nil | Low | + | + |
| Irving | Nil | Low | + | + |
| Pomeroy | 0–0.4 | Low | + | + |
| Salpingectomy | 0–1.9 | Low | + | + |
| Madlener | 0.3–2 | Low | + | + |
| Simple ligation | 20 | Low | + | + |

[1]Modified and reproduced, with permission, from Department of Medical and Public Affairs, George Washington University Medical Center: *Popul Rep*, Series C, No. 7, May 1976.

**Table 45–5.** Tubal occlusion by laparoscopy.[1]

| | Skill Required | Special Equipment | Failure Rate/1000 (Range) | Morbidity Rate (Incidence) | Procedure Accomplished | |
|---|---|---|---|---|---|---|
| | | | | | Hospital | Outpatient |
| Pomeroy | High | + | ? | Low | + | + |
| Fulguration | | | | | | |
|   Coagulate and excise | High | + | 0–0.6 | Moderate | + | + |
|   Coagulate and divide | High | + | 0.1–2 | High | + | + |
|   Coagulate only | High | + | 1–2 | Low | + | + |
| Clips | | | | | | |
|   Spring-loaded | High | + | 0.2–0.6 | Low | + | + |
|   Tantalum hemoclips | High | + | 5–18 | Low | + | + |
| Bands | | | | | | |
|   Falope ring | High | + | 0.23 | Low | + | + |

[1]Modified and reproduced, with permission, from Department of Medical and Public Affairs, George Washington University Medical Center: *Popul Rep*, Series C, No. 7, May 1976.

husband's signature is not required for regulation of a woman's fertility. Guidelines have been established by the FDA Bureau of Medical Devices to ensure that safe, efficient endoscopes and other devices are used in sterilization procedures.

## Complications

Pain and menstrual disturbances (postbilateral tubal ligation syndrome) have been reported following tubal sterilization. However, prospective controlled studies show that these problems are no more common than in women who have not undergone sterilization. Menstrual changes seem to be related to use of contraceptives—before sterilization. Oral contraceptives are associated with decreased menstrual flow and relief of dysmenorrhea; once they are discontinued, heavier flow and pain may recur. Complaints of menstrual changes are much less frequent in the second half of the first postoperative year.

Patients who have undergone tubal sterilization require hysterectomy more frequently than patients who have not undergone this procedure. This is probably because most women who have tubal sterilizations have had children and are therefore more likely to have disorders typically treated with hysterectomy (eg, symptomatic pelvic relaxation, adenomyosis). Patients should be told that pelvic pain or menstrual disturbances may develop after tubal sterilization but are no more common than in other women of similar age and parity.

Postoperative psychologic problems correlate well with preoperative problems. Even in patients sterilized in the postpartum period, adverse psychologic effects are rare, and psychiatric disturbance is no more common than in the general population.

## Technique

See Figures 45–2 to 45–5.

## OTHER METHODS OF FEMALE STERILIZATION

Because of relatively high morbidity and mortality rates in comparison with tubal occlusion procedures, hysterectomy is justified for sterilization only if there is another unequivocal indication for hysterectomy. Transvaginal tubal ligation via culdotomy or culdoscopy is technically more difficult than transabdominal sterilization and has a higher infection rate. However, there may be less discomfort postoperatively. Experimental methods of transuterine tubal occlusion include electrocoagulation, silicone plugs, clips, and sclerosing liquids. All are investigational at this time.

## VASECTOMY

Partial vasectomy is usually done under local anesthesia via a small incision in the upper outer aspect of the scrotum (Fig 45–6). Sutures or clips are placed tightly around the vas, demarcating a 1- to 1.5-cm segment, which is then excised. The ligated and fulgurated ends are tucked back into the scrotal sac, and the incision is closed. The same procedure is performed on the opposite side. Microscopic examination confirms excision of vasal tissue.

The failure rate with this technique is estimated to be less than 2 in 1000. Sterility is assumed only after ejaculates are completely free of sperm after 3 months and after periodic microscopic analysis.

Complications are infrequent, usually involving slight bleeding, skin infection, and reactions to sutures or local anesthetics. The only reported deaths have been due to tetanus in regions of the world where routine tetanus immunization is not done. Prophylactic tetanus immunization should precede vasectomy.

When vasal anastomosis is attempted (vasovasos-

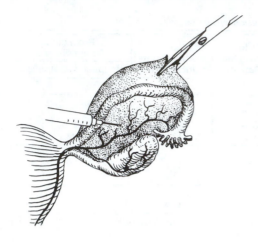

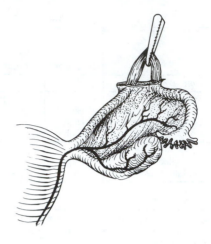

*Saline with epinephrine injected below serosa, which becomes inflated locally. Muscular tube, and even blood vessels, can be separated from serosa, which is then cut open.*

*Muscular tube emerges through opening or is pulled out to form a U shape.*

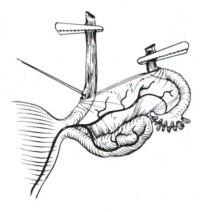

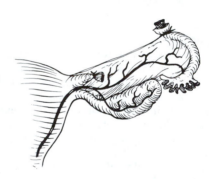

*Fimbriated end is untouched, while the end leading to the uterus is stripped of serosa. This can usually be done without damaging blood vessels.*

*About 5 cm of muscular tube is cut away; the end is buried automatically in serosa. Fimbriated end and serosa opening are closed and tied together.*

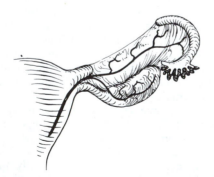

*Blood supply continues normally between ovary and uterus. Hydrosalpinx or adhesion has not been noticed.*

**Figure 45–2.** Uchida method of sterilization. (Reproduced, with permission, from Benson RC: *Handbook of Obstetrics & Gynecology*, 8th ed. Lange, 1983.)

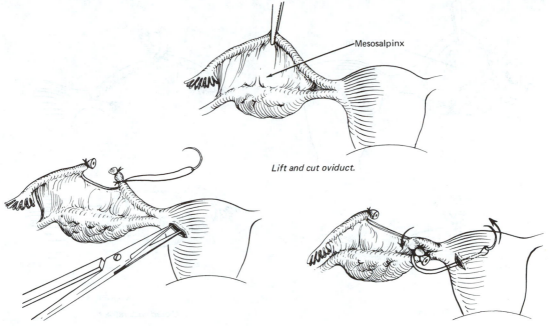

Lift and cut oviduct.

Mesosalpinx

*Double ligation with gut; one tie is left long for traction (special traction suture); mesosalpinx stripped back.*

*Special traction suture inserted in tunnel in anterior uterine wall.*

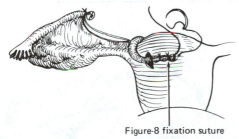

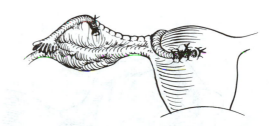

Figure-8 fixation suture

*Traction suture tied and proximal tube sutured in tunnel.*

*Implantation of the proximal tubal limb into a tunnel in the anterior uterine wall.*

**Figure 45–3.** Irving method of sterilization. (Reproduced, with permission, from Benson RC: *Handbook of Obstetrics & Gynecology,* 8th ed. Lange, 1983).

tomy), patency is achieved in approximately 70% of patients. Pregnancy rates are lower (18–60%). Skillful microsurgery performed by an experienced urologist will optimize the chances of pregnancy.

# HYSTERECTOMY

Hysterectomy is complete removal of the uterus, including the cervix. It is the third or fourth most common operation in the USA. With advancements in medical and conservative surgical therapy of gyne-

cologic conditions, the need for hysterectomy has declined. More women now wish to avoid major surgery if equally efficacious alternatives exist. Regulatory boards of gynecologists now support the use of hysterectomy as treatment for conditions refractory to more conservative management.

## Indications

The indications for hysterectomy can be practically divided into those for the treatment of gynecologic cancer and less serious disorders and obstetric complications. Hysterectomy for cancer of the uterus, ovary, and cervix is discussed in Chapters 26 and 47–49. Hysterectomy for obstetric complications, including excessive bleeding and molar pregnancy, is becoming less common (see Chapter 28).

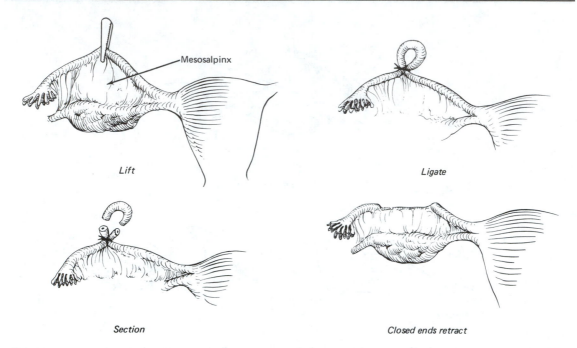

**Figure 45–4.** Pomeroy method of sterilization. (Reproduced, with permission, from Benson RC: *Handbook of Obstetrics & Gynecology,* 8th ed. Lange, 1983.)

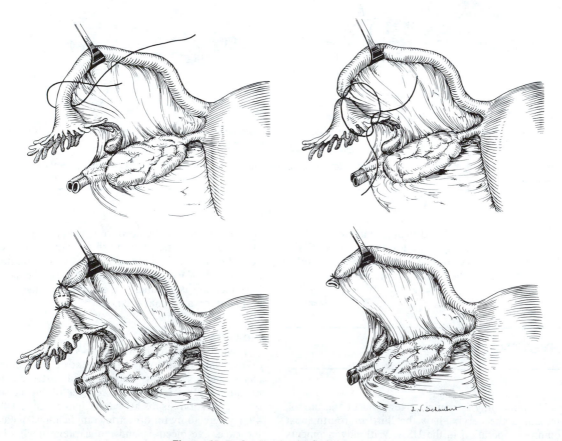

**Figure 45–5.** Sterilization by fimbriectomy.

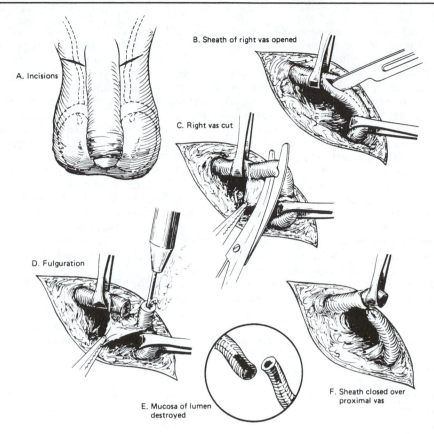

A. Incisions

B. Sheath of right vas opened

C. Right vas cut

D. Fulguration

E. Mucosa of lumen destroyed

F. Sheath closed over proximal vas

**Figure 45–6.** Steps in vasectomy. (Modified from a drawing by S. Taft. Reproduced, with permission, from Schmidt S: Vasectomy should not fail. Contemp Surg 1974;4:13.)

The most common benign diseases and disorders that warrant hysterectomy are shown in Table 45–6.

## Preoperative Evaluation

### A. Diagnostic Tests to Detect Occult Cancer:

All patients anticipating hysterectomy should have a baseline evaluation to detect occult cancer. A Papanicolaou smear should be performed within 3 months before operation, and abnormalities should be followed with colposcopic examination and biopsy before surgery. Cervical conization is indicated prior to hysterectomy if (1) colposcopy fails to demonstrate the entire squamocolumnar junction, where cervical cancers typically arise; (2) colposcopically guided biopsies reveal dysplasia that is more severe by 2 or more grades than that shown on the Papanicolaou smear (eg, carcinoma in situ on smear but mild dysplasia on biopsy); or (3) endocervical curettage demonstrates atypical endocervical cells.

Cervical conization for the previous indications is performed to ensure that occult invasive cancer is not present within the endocervical canal. Frozen-section

**Table 45–6.** Benign diseases and disorders for which hysterectomy may be performed.

Uterine leiomyomas
  Symptomatic (abnormal bleeding or pelvic pressure)
  Asymptomatic (presenting as a large uterus obscuring palpation of the adnexa)
  Rapid growth of the uterus
  Failed conservative management of bleeding (eg, cyclic progestin, D&C) or uterine pain (eg, nonsteroidal anti-inflammatory
    medications)
Symptomatic adenomyosis
Symptomatic endometriosis refractory to conservative surgical or medical therapy
Symptomatic pelvic relaxation syndromes
Chronic incapacitating central pelvic refractory to conservative treatment (eg, hormonal suppression and nonsteroidal anti-
  inflammatory drugs) in a woman with a normal urologic and gastrointestinal evaluation.
Definitive treatment of severe pelvic inflammatory disease or any pelvic abscess involving the genitalia if conservative therapy is
  not possible or desired by the patient

analysis of cervical conization tissue correlates well enough with "permanent" (hematoxylin and eosin) slide analysis that if intraepithelial neoplasia with clear margins is found, the surgeon may, with reasonable certainty, perform a hysterectomy, that will totally include the tumor.

Biospy for endometrial neoplasia must also be considered. Generally any woman over age 35 who present with abnormal uterine bleeding should have endometrial evaluation (D&C, directed biopsies) before hysterectomy. However, certain clinical situations that produce an unopposed estrogen effect on the endometrium warrant preoperative endometrial evaluation at any age: chronic anovulation and secondary oligomenorrhea, unopposed estrogen therapy for menopause, and known ovarian disorders associated with endometrial neoplasia (eg, polycystic ovary syndrome, granulosa cell tumors). Unfortunately, frozen-section analysis of endometrial curettings is neither practical nor accurate, so hysterectomy must wait for permanent section.

Occult cancer may also be present outside the genital tract. All patients should have their stool checked for occult blood preoperatively. In women 35 years or older, xeromammography is standard and is best not postponed until after surgery. With newer monoclonal antibody techniques, patients may one day have a battery of tumor markers screened for ovarian carcinoma before surgery.

**B. Preoperative Evaluation of the Pelvis:** In the woman with a small, mobile uterus with mobile adnexa, little diagnostic evaluation beyond bimanual examination is indicated. However, pelvic disease may have caused disturbance of normal tissue planes imperiling the urologic and gastrointestinal tracts. The following conditions most commonly indicate the need for more extensive evaluation of the pelvis prior to hysterectomy: (1) pelvic inflammatory disease, especially if repeated, chronic or associated with a tubo-ovarian complex (2) endometriosis (3) pelvic adhesions due to other causes of pelvic inflammation (eg, appendicitis, cholecystis, previous pelvic surgery) (4) chronic pelvic pain (5) questionable origin of a palpable pelvic mass (6) clinical suspicion of cancer (eg, palpable adnexa in a postmenopausal woman).

The most commonly utilized preoperative adjunctive diagnostic evaluation is pelvic ultrasound, which has advantages over computed tomography (CT) scan. Magnetic resonance imaging (MRI) holds promise for adnexal evaluation. Ultrasound is helpful in detecting masses in the difficult to examine patient (eg, obese) and in confirming a pelvic mass detected on bimanual examination. However, experienced gynecologic surgeons who palpate a pelvic mass on serial examination, particularly after the bowel is cleansed, rarely need to perform ultrasound examination to confirm the need for exploratory surgery.

Intravenous pyelography (IVP) is helpful in delineating the course of the ureters through the pelvic. A preoperative intravenous pyelogram is especially useful for inflammatory conditions that could distort or obstruct the ureters. Also patients with genital developmental anomalies should have a preoperative intravenous pyelogram to look for concomitant urologic anomalies.

Prehysterectomy evaluation of the colon (beyond screening for occult blood in the stool) is indicated in any patient with symptoms for rectal disease. In most cases, proctoscopy or flexible proctosigmoidoscopy is sufficient. In cases of severe pelvic inflammation, chronic pelvic pain, or suspected cancer, complete colonoscopy or barium enema is indicated. Preoperative diagnosis of bowel disease will aid in the selection of the incision. If necessary, a consultant gastrointestinal surgeon can be present during the operation.

**C. Preoperative Bowel Preparation:** See Chapter 43.

**D. Prophylactic Antibiotics:** Significant infection occurs in about 20% of patients undergoing vaginal or abdominal hysterectomy. Certain risk factors are associated with a higher likelihood of operative site infection. These factors include long operation (> 2¾ hours), no preoperative antibiotic prophylaxis, younger age (premenopausal), clinic patient as compared to private patient, and abdominal incision (Shapiro et al). Patients at highest risk for infection were helped most by use of prophylactic antibiotics. Other studies have confirmed the efficacy of prophylactic antibiotics in reducing operative infection in both abdominal and vaginal hysterectomy.

A broad-spectrum antibiotic should be chosen that will be effective against common (but not necessarily *all*) pathogens causing pelvic infection. The agent should have a low incidence of toxicity and side effects and should be easily administered and cost-effective. Therapeutic levels must be achieved in tissue at the surgical site. It should *not* be an antibiotic reserved for serious infection. Ampicillin, cefazolin, cefoxitin, cephaloradine, cephalothin, cephradine, doxycycline, metronidazole, and penicillin plus streptomycin are all effective. Intravenous or intramuscular administration is usually used, but intraperitoneal irrigation with antibiotic solution is also effective in reducing cuff infections after abdominal hysterectomy. The ideal antibiotic for prophylaxis would be administered once at the time of surgery.

Certain procedures may be used as an alternative to antibiotic prophylaxis, including preoperative hot cervical conization and postoperative suction drainage of the vaginal cuff.

**E. Prophylactic Heparin:** The efficacy of low-dose heparin in preventing thromboembolic complications after surgery is generally accepted but is used in only 25% of hysterectomy patients. Low-dose heparin has been shown to increase blood loss during abdominal hysterectomy, and this risk must be compared to the risk of thromboembolism in individual patients.

A combination of ergotamine derivative and heparin is becoming increasingly popular as a thromboembolic prophylactic agent. The addition of dihydroergotamine is thought to decrease venous stasis and pooling and complement the antithrombin potentiation of heparin.

**F. Blood Products:** Cross-matching of blood is routine in hysterectomy patients. Two to 4 units of blood should be available. It may not be necessary to preoperatively cross-match all patients undergoing hysterectomy. Women who are not at particular risk of needing a transfusion during hysterectomy should at least have blood typing and antibody screening prior to surgery. Patients undergoing peripartum hysterectomy or hysterectomy for gynecologic cancer are more likely to need blood transfusion. Patients undergoing elective hysterectomy are more likely to need a transfusion if the hematocrit is low (30%), if they have pelvic inflammatory disease or pelvic abscess or adhesions, or if colporrhaphy is performed at the time of vaginal hysterectomy.

**G. Informed Consent:** Many women desire, and most insurance companies require, a second opinion prior to scheduling an elective hysterectomy. The patient must understand the diagnosis and be aware of alternative therapies and the risks and benefits of the operation. Common risks of surgery such as cuff cellulitis and blood loss are usually explained during preoperative counseling. The current medicolegal climate mandates the discussion of unusual complications, including the possibility of completing a vaginal operation via an abdominal route and the risks of viral illness following transfusion, severe postoperative infection (including adnexal abscess), ectopic pregnancy, and vaginal vault prolapse. (see also Chapter 63.)

## TECHNIQUE

### Vaginal Versus Abdominal Hysterectomy

The route of hysterectomy is chosen according to the following guidelines:

**A. Pelvic Anatomy:** The ideal candidate for vaginal hysterectomy has a gynecoid pelvis with a pubic arch radius greater than 100 degrees, divergent side walls with widely spread pubic rami, and flat buttocks. Some descent of the uterus is helpful but not mandatory; procidentia makes for a more complicated vaginal hysterectomy because of the greater vulnerability of the prolapsed ureters.

**B. Uterine Size:** Most gynecologists will perform vaginal hysterectomy on a uterus equivalent in size to a uterus at 12 weeks' gestation or smaller. More experienced surgeons will perform what has been termed "heroic" removal of a uterus equivalent in size to that at 20 weeks' gestation.

**C. Adnexa:** In patients with symptoms or pelvic findings suggesting adnexal disease that may indicate adnexectomy, the abdominal route for hysterectomy is preferred.

**D. Gastrointestinal Tract:** Especially in older patients or those with significant history of gastrointestinal complaints, the abdominal approach offers an opportunity for complete examination of the bowel. An exception to this rule is the patient planning concomitant cholecystectomy and hysterectomy; some surgeons feel a vaginal hysterectomy and subcostal incision are preferable to a single midline xiphoid to symphysis incision in terms of wound complications and recuperation time.

**E. Urologic Disorders:** If a retropubic urethropexy is planned, an abdominal route for hysterectomy is preferable. If anterior vaginal colporrhaphy only is planned, vaginal hysterectomy is preferred. Advanced degrees of cystocele, with marked prolapse of the urethrovesical angle, may be best treated with a combined vaginal and abdominal approach (see Chapter 41).

**F. Pelvic Relaxation:** In the case of isolated rectocele, a vaginal approach is preferred. Culdoplasty for enterocele may be performed by either route.

**G. Plastic Procedures:** As more women choose to undergo procedures such as abdominoplasty or suction-assisted lipectomy, an abdominal approach is indicated. Perineorrhaphy and vaginal repairs usually accompany vaginal hysterectomies but can also be done after abdominal hysterectomy.

**H. Medical Disorders:** In patients with significant heart or lung disease, the vaginal approach is preferable when possible because of a lower incidence of postoperative pulmonary complications and earlier ambulation.

**I. Previous Surgery:** Most surgeons are willing to perform a vaginal hysterectomy in patients with previous tubal ligation or cesarean section. The surgery would be more problematic in patients with a history of multiple cesarean births or complications (eg, postpartum endomyoparametritis) or with probable abdominal adhesions from previous laparotomy.

The preceding guidelines may certainly be adjusted to the individual patient based on the surgeon's experience and abilities. An examination performed under anesthesia where the physician is first seeing the patient may help to decide on the approach. Laparoscopic evaluation of the adnexa will further aid in the decision. All patients anticipating vaginal hysterectomy should be told that the operation may have to be completed abdominally if difficulties arise.

### Abdominal Hysterectomy

The technique of abdominal hysterectomy varies according to the indication for the operation, the size and placement of vital structures including the ureters (which may be distorted), and the pelvic anatomy. A standard, well-organized approach to abdominal hysterectomy is essential to avoid incidental injury. Modifications are made as necessary, always within an organized plan of operation.

The anesthetic of choice typically includes general endotracheal intubation, an inhalation agent, and an analgesic. Hysterectomies are of such duration and risk that using a mask alone is unwise. In patients with pulmonary compromise, spinal or epidural anesthesia may be used.

A sterile scrub of the abdomen and vagina is done, and a urinary catheter is placed so that the anesthesiologist can monitor urine output intraoperatively. The choice of incision is based on the suspected disease or disorder; in general, a midline incision extending from 2 fingerbreadths above the pubic symphysis to the umbilicus offers the greatest exposure. One modification of the low transverse incision to improve exposure is the Maylard muscle-splitting procedure or the Cherney detachment of the rectus muscles from their insertion on the pubic symphysis; despite modification, transverse incisions severely limit access to the upper half of the abdomen.

The surgeon and assistants should rinse excessive talcum powder from their gloves before making the incision to prevent granulomatous tissue reaction in the wound. Once the incision is complete, peritoneal fluid may be aspirated if the possibility of gynecologic cancer exists. The pelvic organs are then inspected and the upper abdomen palpated in a systematic fashion: right gutter, right hemidiaphragm, liver, gallbladder, pancreas, stomach (assessing the position of the indwelling gastric decompression tube), and spleen and right hemidiaphragm (gently, because of the risk of trauma to the spleen), left gutter, para-aortic lymph nodes, and omentum. Excessive bowel manipulation should be avoided to decrease the severity of postoperative adynamic ileus; at the least, the appendix and cecum should be inspected as well as the terminal meter of ileum. Older patients and those with gastrointestinal complaints would benefit from careful palpation and inspection of the bowel from rectum to ligament of Treitz. If desired, the wound may be protected with moist towels, a self-retaining retractor placed, and the bowel packed into the upper abdomen.

The classic extrafascial hysterectomy performed by Richardson (1929) remains the mainstay of surgical technique in abdominal hysterectomy (see Fig 36–9). Choice of suture and needle is made according to surgeon experience and preference; 2-0, 0, or 1 absorbable sutures on half-curved taper needles are standard choices. The uterus is grasped either by the fundus with a Massachusetts double-toothed clamp or at the cornu with Ochsner or Kocher clamps. The round ligament is clamped proximal to the uterus; at its midportion, it is ligated by suture, and the suture is tagged with a small hemostat. The round ligament is divided about 0.5 cm proximal to the suture, thus opening the broad ligament at its apex. The anterior

uterine peritoneum may be incised at the vesicouterine junction in preparation for advancement of the bladder. The peritoneum only should be incised; the potentially vascular areolar tissue should be avoided. When this procedure is repeated on the contralateral side, the anterior leaves of the broad ligament are opened, the uterine vessels first become apparent, and attention is then directed to the posterior leaf of the broad ligament.

The posterior leaf of the broad ligament is incised beginning at the ligated round ligament. The extent of the incision is determined by the decision to preserve or remove the adnexa. If the adnexa are to be removed, the peritoneum is incised parallel to the infundibulopelvic ligament to the pelvic sidewall; the loose areolar tissue is dissected medial to the internal iliac (hypogastric) artery, which is typically 0.5 cm thick with a visually appreciable (and certainly palpable) pulse. The dissection will reveal a clear area of peritoneum under the infundibulopelvic ligament; below this area at a variable distance lies the ureter on this medial flap of peritoneum.

The intimate proximity of the ureters to the uterus makes ureteral dissection important. Whereas the ureter is usually 4–6 cm deep to the infundibulopelvic ligament at the lateral margin of the uterus, it is only 0.5–2 cm below this vascular bundle at the level of the pelvic brim. Observing the ureter through the peritoneum or palpating the characteristic "snap" of the ureter should serve only to guide dissection and should not be a substitute for identification of the entire ureter through its pelvic course. The ureter tolerates careful dissection well as long as its blood-carrying adventitia is not stripped away. The ureter can always be found and dissection begun at the pelvic brim, where the ureter passes over the bifurcation of the iliac artery. The most serious ureteral injury is the unrecognized insult. The most common ureteral injuries during hysterectomy occur during ligation of the infundibulopelvic ligament, clamping and suture ligation of the uterosacral-cardinal ligament complex, placement of vaginal angle sutures, ligation of the vesicouterine ligament, ligation of the hypogastric artery as an adjunctive measure to lessen operative blood loss, and reperitonealization of the pelvic floor.

Once the course of the ureters is well established, the adnexal component of the operation is completed. If the adnexa are to be removed, a ligating suture may be passed beneath the infundibulopelvic ligament and above the ureter; this step is repeated for a double ligature as a precaution. Traditionally, the infundibulopelvic ligament is clamped, divided, and ligated; the direct suture technique may avoid undue crushing of tissue. The ligament is ligated again adjacent to the uterus to avoid back bleeding; the infundibulopelvic ligament is divided and the peritoneum incised to the back of the uterine fundus, always cognizant of the proximity of the ureter. If the adnexa are to be preserved, a hole is made in the avascular portion of the posterior leaf of the broad ligament superior to the ureter. The utero-ovarian ligament and fallopian tube are doubly clamped, divided, and ligated, with care taken to avoid incorporation of ovarian tissue into the ligature.

The final step is extending the peritoneal incision posteriorly around the uterus between the medial portions of the uterosacral ligaments. If the incision of the posterior leaf of the broad ligament is extended over the uterosacral ligaments, there is typically significant bleeding just lateral to the insertion of the ligament at the uterus. The advantages of making an incision between the uterosacrals include clear identification of the rectum and its separation from the uterus, ease of suturing the vaginal cuff, and improved mobility of the peritoneum to allow reperitonealization under less tension.

The bladder is advanced down off of the lower uterine segment prior to clamping the uterine vessels. Surgeons-in-training have more difficulty with advancement of the bladder than with other aspects of abdominal hysterectomy. The principal difficulty in mobilization of the bladder is failure to identify the proper cleavage plane between the bladder and the uterus. At the attachment of the bladder to the lower uterine segment, a medianraphe is variably present; it is typically a 1-cm long longitudinal band of thick connective tissue. The raphe is attenuated in pregnant or postmenopausal patients. The raphe is divided at midportion, and loose avascular fibroareolar tissue is seen immediately between the cervix and bladder. The uterus is retracted posteriorly and superiorly, roughly at an angle of 30 degrees to the long axis of the vagina. The midpoint of the peritoneal incision of the bladder flap is gently lifted with forceps; the avascular plane of the vesicovaginal and vesicocervical areolar spaces is continuous once the median raphe is divided. Metzenbaum scissors are pointed to the uterus, and sharp dissection reveals the shiny white pubocervical fascia overlying the cervix. Properly done, the dissection is bloodless, and the plane is recognized by the ease with which the bladder falls away from the cervix. The vesicouterine space is developed 2 cm beyond the anterior vaginal fornix. Care must be exercised in any dissection laterally, because the vesicouterine ligaments ("bladder pillars") may bleed because of the paracervical and paravaginal veins present laterally.

The uterine vessels may be skeletonized by separating the loose avascular areolar connective tissue from the vessels. The intraligamentous course of the ureter is again checked; it is typically 2–3 cm inferolateral to the insertion of the uterine vessels into the uterus. The uterine vessels are clamped with a curved crushing clamp (eg, Heaney, Pfannen, or curved Ballantine clamp). Double-clamping is used for larger vessels. It is not necessary to place another clamp on the uterine side of the pedicle to prevent back bleeding if the uterine arteries on both sides of the uterus are clamped before either pedicle is incised. The clamp is applied at the level of the internal os, with the tip of the clamp at a right angle to the long axis of the cervix; the temptation to clamp the entire cervix and "slide off" dragging paracervical tissue into the pedicle should be avoided in order to minimize the risk of the pedicle slipping out of the clamp. The uterine vessels are then ligated by suture at the tip of the clamp. Occasionally, a second application of the curved clamp is necessary to complete ligation of the uterine vessels.

Next, the cardinal ligament is assessed. Ordinarily, a single application of a straight clamp (Ochsner, Kocher, Ballantine clamp) will include the cardinal ligament to the level of its attachment at the lateral edge of the cervix and upper vagina. A deep knife is often useful in dividing the cardinal ligament adjacent to the uterus, leaving a larger pedicle, which is less likely to slip out of the suture than one remaining after cutting with scissors flush to the clamp. The suture ligature of the cardinal ligament is often tagged to aid in manipulation of the vaginal cuff.

The uterosacral ligaments are clamped at their insertion into the lower cervix, divided at their insertion, and ligated. Alternatively, they may be transected with large Mayo scissors while the vagina is entered posterolaterally. If division and suture ligation of either pedicle of the cardinal-uterosacral ligament complex fails to enter the vagina, the safest approach is to enter the vagina with the knife in the midline, either anteriorly or posteriorly, at the confluence of the vagina with cervix. Once entered, the cervix is circumferentially incised, with long Ochsner clamps used to control point bleeders and elevate the vaginal cuff. The cervix is inspected to ensure complete excision.

Sutures are placed at each lateral vaginal angle to ligate small paravaginal vessels coursing upward through the paravaginal tissues and to provide vaginal vault support. The suture is begun inside the vagina 1 cm from the upper border, then incorporates the cardinal and uterosacral ligaments, and finally transverses the vagina again to end up within the vagina. This suture is tagged, and the procedure is repeated on the contralateral side.

Surgical management of the cuff is individualized. In the case of marked pelvic inflammation and persistent oozing, the cuff may be left open to afford retroperitoneal drainage or allow egress of a closed drain system. In most cases, closing the cuff may reduce granulation tissue and possibly minimize ascension of bacteria from the vagina. The cuff may be closed with either interrupted figure-of-eight sutures or a double running suture; the key points with either closure are inversion of the cut edges into the vagina and hemostasis.

The pelvis is irrigated and hemostasis checked in a systematic fashion from one lateral pedicle to the ipsilateral round ligament pedicle to the cuff and on to the other side. Small bleeding vessels must be ligated to minimize the risk of retroperitoneal hematoma formation, which may expand or become infected. For diffuse oozing, hemostatic agents such as thrombin powder or thrombostatic absorbable sponges may be useful. There is no advantage to closing the parietal peritoneum.

Retained ovaries may be suspended to minimize the risk of torsion and adherence to the vaginal cuff. The utero-ovarian ligament can be conveniently attached to the round ligament stump to suspend the ovaries above the pelvis without placing the infundibulopelvic ligament under tension.

Elective appendectomy at the time of abdominal hysterectomy is losing favor because of lack of demonstrable benefit and increased risk of infection. The abnormal appendix should be removed; in cases of hysterectomy for endometriosis, appendectomy will reveal microscopic endometriotic foci in some 3% of cases.

## Supracervical Hysterectomy

Subtotal hysterectomy is performed less commonly today than in past years because of the availability of antibiotics and better management of anesthesia in the fragile patient and because risk of disease of the uterine cervix remains—most notably, carcinoma. The most common indication now is technical inability to dissect around the cervix due to obliteration of tissue planes by cancer, endometriosis, or pelvic inflammatory disease. For these same indications, intrafascial hysterectomy is associated with less risk to the bladder and rectum because dissection in the distorted planes between the organs is avoided.

Following ligation of the uterine vessels, the uterine fundus may be amputated from the cervix; the level of amputation should be below the internal cervical os to avoid postoperative uterine bleeding from endometrial remnants. The cervical stump is closed with figure-of-eight sutures.

## Vaginal Hysterectomy

Most vaginal hysterectomies are performed under general anesthesia. In the patient with medical complications, particularly pulmonary problems, spinal anesthesia may be elected. Following administration of the anesthetic, a bimanual examination is mandatory before beginning surgery. The perineum is shaved or trimmed as necessary and a sterile wash performed. The patient is placed in a modified dorsal lithotomy position and draped; the surgeon should participate in proper positioning of the patient, because excessive flexion of the hips can stretch the obturator nerves, and excessive extension of the knee can jeopardize the peroneal nerves. All bony prominences and soft tissues in contact with the leg stirrups should be carefully padded.

The urinary bladder may be drained by catheter, but this step is optional. The cervix is grasped with a tenaculum (see Fig 41–13). Passage of a uterine sound will aid in determining the size and position of the uterus; some advocate performing a D&C at this point to rule out pyometra or endometrial neoplasia.

As the surgeon exerts gentle traction downward on the cervix, 2 assistants maintain exposure with lateral vaginal retractors and protect the bladder with an anterior Heaney retractor. If desired, the junction of the vagina and cervix can be injected with a 1% 1:1000 epinephrine solution to minimize blood loss during incision of the cervix. Beginning posteriorly to minimize obscuring the field with blood, the surgeon circumferentially incises the cervix down to the level of the pubovesicocervical fascia. Gentle traction with the bladder retractor and downward traction of the cervix will allow exposure of the fibers of fascia between bladder and cervix, which are incised. When the bladder has been advanced up off of the cervix, attention is given to the posterior attachment of the cervix. While the assistant pulls the uterus upward, the posterior vaginal mucosa is tented away from the cervix. With the patient in the Trendelenburg position to allow as much emptying of the posterior cul-de-sac as possible, the posterior cul-de-sac is incised with a single stroke of the scissors. A retractor is placed within the opening, exposing the uterosacral ligaments. The uterosacral ligaments are grasped with Heaney clamps, making certain that the peritoneum posterior to the ligament is within the clamp. The ligament is cut and ligated with 2–0 or 0 absorbable suture and tagged with a hemostat for later manipulation of the cuff.

The cardinal ligament may next be clamped if the bladder is safely advanced; likewise, the uterine vessels are included in the next application of the Heaney clamps. The anterior cul-de-sac is entered by blunt and sharp dissection to the anterior vesicouterine fold of peritoneum. The anterior retractor is placed within this opening and the bladder is gently lifted upward. The surgeon now clamps, incises, and ligates in pedicles the remaining portions of the broad ligaments bilaterally, incorporating the tissue between the anterior and posterior leaves of the broad ligament. The round ligament, utero-ovarian ligament, and fallopian tube are excised from the uterus and incorporated into these pedicles, and the uterus is removed from the field. A larger uterus may require special manipulation for delivery through the vaginal introitus (eg, bivalving the uterus in the midline, morcellation of the uterus into multiple extractable segments, or myomectomy).

The final suture on the utero-ovarian ligament is tagged to allow careful inspection of the tubes and ovaries. If ovarian disease is suspected or if prophylactic oopherectomy is planned, a clamp is placed above the ovary and uterine tube on the infundibulopelvic ligament for suture ligature, while traction is placed on the last stay suture. The entire ovary must be removed, because an ovarian remnant may become cystic and produce pain many years after the hysterectomy.

Once all pedicles are inspected and found to be hemostatic, the peritoneum is closed with a running 2–0 absorbable suture, incorporating the cardinal and uterosacral ligament pedicles for support of the vaginal vault. Lateral vaginal angle sutures are placed from the vaginal mucosa at 2 o'clock, inside the cuff and including the uterosacral pedicle, then out through the cuff to the 4 o'clock position. If anterior or posterior colporrhaphy is planned, that operation is completed prior to complete closure of the cuff. The cuff may be closed by an interrupted absorbable 0 suture, a running simple suture, or a running vertical mattress technique. The goals of closure are obliteration of the cuff's dead space back to the peritoneum and approximation of the cut edges of the vagina to afford healing and minimize postoperative granulation tissue. Modifications of the just described technique are made by virtually every gynecologic surgeon based on operative findings and experience. Many surgeons will close the posterior cul-de-sac to prevent development of an enterocele or will shorten the uterosacral ligaments to suspend the vaginal vault. As in abdominal hysterectomy, the cuff can be left open to promote drainage with a running locked absorbable 0 suture. Another technique to drain the closure is insertion of a T tube above the cuff, which is associated with a demonstrable reduction in postoperative febrile morbidity.

After the operation is completed, the vagina and perineum are gently cleansed. An indwelling bladder catheter is inserted, although recent studies challenge the need for postoperative indwelling urinary catheters in uncomplicated patients who have vaginal hysterectomy. The patient is returned slowly to the dorsal supine position. A vaginal pack is usually not necessary; it may obscure vaginal cuff bleeding.

## Postoperative Care of the Hysterectomy Patient

The details of postoperative care are dictated by the indications for surgery and the individual patient's overall medical condition. General guidelines include the following:

(1) A Foley catheter is left indwelling for 24 hours; if left longer, urine should be sent for culture at the time of catheter removal.

(2) Prophylactic antibiotics are given only within the first 24 hours postoperatively.

(3) Hydration, 2–3 L/d of balanced electrolyte solution, is given intravenously, depending on blood loss and intraoperative replacement.

(4) Sips of water are given the first night, followed by clear liquids on the next postoperative day or 2.

The diet is advanced based on return of bowel sounds and appetite and the passage of flatus.

(5) Prophylactic heparin therapy or antiembolic stockings are used in patients at risk for thromboembolic complications.

(6) Ambulation is begun on the first postoperative day.

(7) Adequate analgesia is given parenterally.

## Complications

Perioperative deaths may be due to cardiac arrest, coronary occlusion, or respiratory paralysis. Postoperative deaths are usually the result of hemorrhage, infection, pulmonary embolus, or intercurrent disease. A recent study of factors contributing to the risk of death found that abdominal hysterectomies performed for complications of pregnancy or cancer (8% of all hysterectomies) account for 61% of deaths due to hysterectomy. Overall mortality rates for abdominal or vaginal hysterectomy are 0.1–0.2%. Mortality rates increase with age and medical complications for both vaginal and abdominal hysterectomies.

The bladder may be injured in 1–2% of all hysterectomies. Consequences are slight if the injury is to the dome of the bladder—which is usually the case—away from the trigone. The essential point is to recognize urologic injuries and correct them intraoperatively, avoiding the serious postoperative complications that occur from urinary extravasation.

Damage to the bowel is quite uncommon, particularly with vaginal hysterectomy. In preparation for abdominal hysterectomy for suspected extensive or inflammatory pathologic process (eg, ovarian cancer, endometriosis, pelvic inflammatory disease), preoperative bowel preparation will allow incidental colon surgery without the necessity of colostomy. Small bowel injuries, assuming no obstruction, are closed in layers perpendicular to the long axis of the bowel; a running layer of 3–0 sutures in the mucosa is supported by interrupted 2–0 silk sutures in the serosa. If a transmural large bowel injury occurs and no preoperative bowel preparation was given, a temporary diverting colostomy may be indicated to protect the suture line and lower the risk of peritonitis and sepsis.

The most serious postoperative complication is hemorrhage (0.2–2% of patients). Bleeding usually originates at the lateral vaginal angles and is amenable to vaginal resuturing in most cases. Blood products are replaced as needed.

Infection remains the most common complication following hysterectomy. Even with immaculate technique and careful patient selection, the gynecologic surgeon can still expect a 10% rate of postoperative febrile morbidity. A postoperative temperature of 38°C (100.4°F) or higher on 2 consecutive determinations 6 hours apart must be investigated by (1) careful interview of the patient for localizing symptoms (eg, productive cough, intravenous line pain), (2) thorough physical examination (including pelvic examination for inspection and palpation of the cuff), and (3) appropriate laboratory studies (eg, urinalysis, gram-stained smear of sputum, or complete blood count).

Antibiotics are begun only if a focus of infection is identified or highly suspected. Broad-spectrum antibiotics covering anticipated pathogens are prescribed; single-agent semisynthetic penicillins (eg, piperacillin) and cephalosporins (eg, cefoxitin) offer sufficient coverage. In the presence of sepsis, multiagent comprehensive coverage (eg, a penicillin, an aminoglycoside, and an anaerobic agent such as clindamycin or metronidazole) must be prescribed.

Granulation of the vaginal vault is part of the normal healing process and is evident on speculum examination in over half of cases. The granulation is rarely troublesome; light cauterization with silver nitrate sticks or electrocautery eliminates the granulation tissue promptly in most cases. Many suggestions have been made on ways to minimize granulation, including management of the cuff (open versus closed), choice of suture (plain gut versus chromic versus newer synthetics), and drainage techniques. The most important common denominator is close apposition of the cut vaginal edges, which can be accomplished with any of the techniques.

## REFERENCES

Ackerman CFS, MacIsaac SG, Schual R: Vasectomy: Benefits and risks. Int J Gynaecol Obstet 1979;16:493.

Badenoch DF et al: Early repair of accidental injury to the ureter or bladder following gynecological surgery. Br J Urol 1987;59:516.

Bhiwandiwala PP, Mumford SD, Feldblum PJ: A comparison of different laparoscopic sterilization occlusion techniques in 24,439 procedures. Am J Obstet Gynecol 1982; 144:319.

Bhiwandiwala PP, Mumford SD, Feldblum PJ: Menstrual pattern changes following laparoscopic sterilization: A comparative study of electrocoagulation and the tubal ring in 1,025 cases. J Reprod Med 1982;27:249.

Bordahl PE: The social and gynecological long-term consequences of tubal sterilization: A personal six-year follow-up investigation. Acta Obstet Gynecol Scand 1984; 63:487.

Brenner WE: Evaluation of contemporary female sterilization methods. J Reprod Med 1981;26:439.

Chi IC et al: An epidemiologic study of risk factors associated with pregnancy following female sterilization. Am J Obstet Gynecol 1980;136:738.

Cook CL, Benninger TW, Masterson BJ: Teaching laparoscopic sterilization. J Reprod Med 1984;29:693.

Cooper JE et al: Effects of female sterilization: One year follow-up in a prospective controlled study of psychological and psychiatric outcome. J Psychosom Res 1985;29:13.

Corson SL: Major vessel injury during laparoscopy. Am J Obstet Gynecol 1980;138:589.

Daniell J: Operative laparoscopy for endometriosis. Semin Reprod Endocrinol 1985;3:353.

Ellis H, Heddle R: Does the peritoneum need to be closed at lapaortomy? Br J Surg 1977;64:733.

Fedele L et al: Second-look hysteroscopy after conservative surgery of the uterus. Acta Eur Fertil 1986;17:341.

Filmar S, Gomel V. McComb DF: Operative lararoscopy vs. open abdominal surgery: a comparative study on postoperation adhesion formation in the rat model. Fertil Steril 1987;48:486.

Gimpelson RJ: Panoramic hysteroscopy with directed biopsies vs dilatation and curettage for accurate diagnosis. J Reprod Med 1984;29:575.

Goldrath MH, Sherman AI: Office hysteroscopy and suction curettage: Can we eliminate the hospital diagnostic dilatation and curettage? Am J Obstet Gynecol 1985; 152:220.

Grubb GS et al: Regret after decision to have a tubal sterilization. Fertil Steril 1985;44:248.

Hemsell DL et al: Prevention of major infection after elective abdominal hysterectomy: Individual determination required. Am J Obstet Gynecol 1983;147:520.

Hirsch HA, Neeser E: Uncommon indications for laparoscopy. J Reprod Med 1985;30:651.

Holtz G: Laparoscopy in the massively obese female. Obstet Gynecol 1987;69:423.

Hugh TB et al: World J Surg 1990;14:231.

Hulka JF et al: American Association of Gynecologic Laparoscopists' 1985 member survey. J Reprod Med 1987; 32:732.

Krebs HB: Intestinal injury in gynecologic injury: A 10 year experience. Am J Obstet Gynecol 1987;156:264.

Levinson JM: The introduction of laparoscopy in the People's Republic of China. Del Med J 1980;50:147.

Levinson JM: The role of laparoscopy in intra-abdominal diagnosis. Del Med J 1978;50:5.

Lomano JM: Photocoagulation of early pelvic endometriosis with the Nd:YAG laser through the laparoscope. J Reprod Med 1985;30:77.

Millard PR: Laparoscopy in a small community free-standing surgicenter. Am J Obstet Gynecol 1987;156:1480.

Mintz PD, Sullivan MF: Preoperative crossmatch ordering and blood use in elective hysterectomy. Obstet Gynecol 1985;65:389.

Mumford SD et al: Tubal ring sterilization: Experience with 10,086 cases. Obstet Gynecol 1981;57:150.

Palmer RH et al: Cost and quality in the use of bloodbank services for normal deliveries, cesarean sections, and hysterectomies. JAMA 1986;256:219.

Peterson HB et al: Death following puncture of the aorta during laparoscopic sterilization. Obstet Gynecol 1982; 59:133.

Phillips JM et al: The 1979 AAGL Membership Survey Presented at the Annual Meeting of the AAGL. (Nov) 1980.

Phillips JM et al: Endoscopy in Gynecology. American Association of Gynecologic Laparoscopists, 1978.

Rogers SF, Lotze EC, Grunert GM: Endometriosis then and now: Evolution of surgical techniques and treatment. J Reprod Med 1984;29:613.

Shapiro M et al: Benefit-cost analysis of antimicrobial prophylaxis in abdominal and vaginal hysterectomy. JAMA 1983;249:1290.

Shapiro M et al: Risk factors for infection at the operative site after abdominal or vaginal hysterectomy. N Engl J Med 1982;307:1661.

Siegler AM, Hulka J, Peretz A: Reversibility of female sterilization. Fertil Steril 1985;43:499.

Smith GL, Taylor GP, Smith KF: Comparative risks and costs of male and female sterilization. Am J Public Health 1985;75:370.

Tadir Y et al: Actual effective CO2 laser power on tissue in endoscopic surgery. Fertil Steril 1986;45:492.

Wadstrow J, Gerdin B: Closure of the abdominal wall: How and why? Acta Clin Scand 1990;156:75.

Wingo PA et al: The mortality risk associated with hysterectomy. Am J Obstet Gynecol 1985;152:803.

# 46 Premalignant & Malignant Disorders of the Vulva & Vagina

*Donna M. Smith, MD, & David L. Barclay, MD*

## PREINVASIVE DISEASE OF THE VULVA

### General Considerations

The vulvar skin is one component of the anogenital epithelium, extending from the cervix to the perineum and perianal skin. The lower genital tract epithelium is of common cloacogenic origin. Neoplasia of the vulvar skin is often associated with multiple foci of dysplasia in the lower genital tract. The inciting agent has not been identified, but a sexually transmitted agent such as the human papillomavirus is highly suspect (see Chapter 35).

Premalignant lesions of the vulva occur mostly in postmenopausal women in their 50s and 60s. Vulvar dysplasia has been occurring in younger women more frequently in recent years, particularly in those with cervical intraepithelial neoplasia. The disease process is asymptomatic in 50% of women. The most common presenting symptom is pruritus. The diagnosis is made by careful inspection of the vulvar area followed by biopsy of suspicious lesions.

### Pathology

In 1989, the International Congress of the International Society for the Study of Vulvar Disease (ISSVD) adopted a standard of reporting vulvar dysplastic lesions as vulvar intraepithelial neoplasia (VIN) I, II, and III, depending on the degree of epithelial cellular maturation. This terminology has replaced the old and more confusing terms used to describe this disease process such as Bowen's disease, erythroplasia of Queyrat, and bowenoid papulosis. The degree of loss of epithelial cellular maturation in a given lesion defines the grade of VIN. Complete loss of cellular maturation in the full thickness of epithelium is defined as VIN III, which is also synonymous with carcinoma in situ of the vulva.

In contrast to intraepithelial carcinoma of the cervix, which seems to arise from a single point of origin, dysplasia of the vulva is often multicentric. These lesions may be discrete or diffuse, single or multiple, flat or raised. They even form papules and vary in color from the white appearance of hyperkeratotic tumors to a velvety red or black.

The microscopic appearance of dysplastic vulvar lesions is characterized by cellular disorganization and loss of stratification that involves essentially the full thickness of the epithelium. Cellular density is increased, and individual cells vary greatly in size, with giant and multinucleated cells, numerous mitotic figures, and hyperchromatism (Fig 46–1).

### Diagnosis

Possibly 1–2% of young women with cervical dysplasia will be found to have multifocal disease that tends to involve the upper third of the vagina and the vulva, perineum, and perianal areas—these surfaces arising from a common cloacogenic origin. A spectrum of disease may be found ranging from mild dysplasia to carcinoma in situ. Involvement may not be appreciated without careful inspection with and without the green colposcopy filter. The vascular pattern is often much less apparent on the vulva, and the lesions tend to be more hyperkeratotic. An abnormal vascular pattern is most frequently associated with a severe degree of dysplasia, carcinoma in situ, or early invasive disease. Early invasive disease in a rather extensive lesion of carcinoma in situ may be detected by identification of an area of abnormal vasculature. If dysplasia of the vulva is detected in a young woman, colposcopic examination should include thorough evaluation of the cervix and upper vagina. Many times these lesions are associated with condylomata of the genital tract.

### Treatment

It must be assumed that carcinoma in situ of the vulva will progress to invasive cancer if not treated. Although carcinoma in situ of the vulva is being diagnosed more frequently in young women and the true biologic significance of this lesion has not been established, we are obliged to eradicate the disease if possible, using the most conservative treatment available.

The extent of involvement of the vulva, perineum, and perianal skin is defined by colposcopy. Particular attention is given to examination of the perianal skin. The cervix and upper vagina have previously been

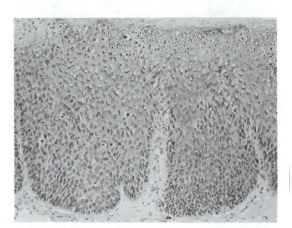

**Figure 46–1.** Carcinoma in situ demonstrating hyperkeratosis, acanthosis, and parakeratosis. The rete ridges are elongated and thickened, and individual cells are atypical.

evaluated by cytologic examination and colposcopy. Circumscribed lesions may be removed by wide local excision. Extensive disease should be treated by total vulvectomy. In younger women, superficial multifocal disease can be treated by a "skinning" procedure in which the excised vulvar skin is replaced with a split-thickness skin graft (Figs 46–2 and 46–3). After either procedure, sexual function can be maintained. Nevertheless, the skinning operation results in a better cosmetic effect and preservation of the clitoris.

Young women exhibiting multifocal small-volume disease varying from mild dysplasia to carcinoma in situ may be treated by laser vaporization. This procedure is particularly valuable in the treatment of lesions around the clitoris and extensive perianal disease. The latter usually involves the perianal skin and does not extend onto the mucosa of the anal canal. The incidence of recurrent disease can be minimized by vaporizing a generous margin of normal skin adjacent to lesions. A lesion of intraepithelial neoplasia can be vaporized without significant destruction of the underlying dermis, resulting in healing with little or no residual scar tissue. The healing phase is quite uncomfortable for the patient.

Topical application of fluorouracil (5-FU) has to be proved useful in the treatment of some lesions, but hyperkeratotic lesions do not respond well. For that reason, the medication is infrequently used.

### Follow-up

Intraepithelial carcinoma of the vulva is often one manifestation of multifocal disease. For this reason, affected patients must be examined periodically for a number of years. Recommended follow-up includes thorough pelvic examinations with colposcopy every 3 to 4 months until the patient is disease-free for 2

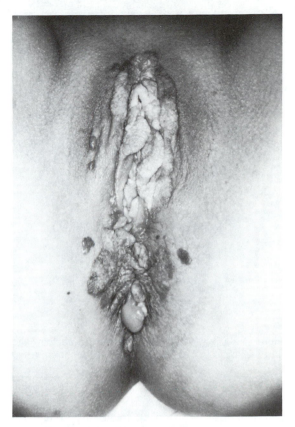

**Figure 46–2.** Diffuse, hypertrophic carcinoma in situ of the vulva and perianal skin. A skinning vulvectomy was performed.

years. If the patient is disease-free for a 2-year period, examinations can be spaced to every 6 months. This is particularly true of patients demonstrating condylomatous dysplasia.

## EXTRAMAMMARY PAGET'S DISEASE

### General Considerations

Paget's disease of the skin is an intraepithelial neoplasia. Reports of long-term survivals suggest that the in situ stage of the disease persists for a long time or that invasive disease is a different clinicopathologic entity. It appears that there are 2 separate lesions: intraepithelial extramammary Paget's disease and pagetoid changes in the skin associated with an underlying adenocarcinoma. Experts believe that an adenocarcinoma associated with Paget's disease arises as a primary adenocarcinoma of the underlying apocrine gland and represents 2 separate diseases and not a spectrum. Approximately 20% of patients with Paget's disease are reported to have an underlying adenocarcinoma. Paget's disease with an underlying ad-

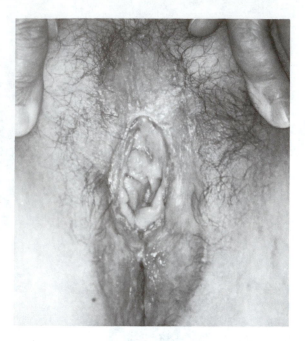

**Figure 46–3.** Appearance after skinning vulvectomy and split-thickness skin grafting of the lesion shown in Fig 46–2.

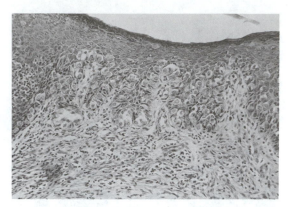

**Figure 46–4.** Paget's disease with typical cells in the basal layer of the epidermis.

enocarcinoma metastasizes frequently to regional lymph nodes and distally. Paget's disease without an underlying adenocarcinoma behaves like an intraepithelial neoplasia and can be treated as such.

## Pathology

The initial lesion may be confused with a number of benign forms of chronic vulvar pruritus. It is a pruritic, slowly spreading, velvety-red discoloration of the skin that eventually becomes eczematoid in appearance with secondary maceration and development of white plaques; it may spread to involve the skin of the perineum, the perianal area, and the adjacent skin of the thigh. Grossly the lesion gives the impression of "cake icing." Because of the serpiginous growth pattern of Paget cells in the basal layer of the epidermis, the true extent of disease is difficult to assess.

Paget's disease of the vulvar skin is an intraepithelial disease. The typical Paget cell, pathognomonic of the disease process, apparently arises from abnormal differentiation of the cells of the basal layer of the epithelium (Fig 46–4). The appearance of malignant cells varies from that of the clear cell of the apocrine gland epithelium to a totally undifferentiated basal cell. It has been suggested that there may be both an intraepithelial and an invasive variety of the disease. The intraepithelial stage of the disease persists for years without evidence of an underlying adenocarcinoma.

## Diagnosis

Paget's disease occurs in women in the seventh decade of life but can be seen in younger patients. Pruritus and tenderness were the most frequent complaints in women with a vulvar lesion. These symptoms may persist for years before the patient seeks medical attention. The lesion may be localized to one labium or involve the entire vulvar area. It is not unusual for the disease process to extend beyond the vulva to involve the perirectal area, buttocks, thighs, inguinal area, and mons. Intraepithelial extramammary Paget's disease presents as a lesion with hyperemic areas associated with superficial white coating to give the impression of "cake icing." Although these lesions can be very extensive, most are confined to the epithelial layer. The diagnosis is made by vulvar biopsy. It is important to palpate the lesion in its entirety. A generous biopsy should be taken of any area that appears to be thickened to rule out an underlying adenocarcinoma.

## Treatment

Since extramammary Paget's disease is an intraepithelial neoplasia it can be treated as such. Wide local excision is the primary treatment modality for this disease process. The lesion needs to be excised in its entirety; however, wide margins need to be removed around the primary lesion since disease often extends beyond the clinically visible erythematous area. Often such a resection involves a complete vulvectomy. Careful histologic examination of the entire operative specimen is necessary to delineate the true extensive disease, ensure free surgical margins, and detect the remote possibility of underlying adenocarcinoma. Patients who have Paget's disease with underlying adenocarcinoma should be treated with a radical vulvectomy and bilateral inguinal lymph node dissection as they would for any other invasive tumor involving the vulvar area.

## Prognosis

Paget's disease of the vulva has a great propensity for local recurrence, which may represent persistence of the disease or development of new disease in the remaining vulvar skin. Extramammary Paget's disease characteristically requires repeated local excisions of recurrent disease after treatment of the primary disease by total vulvectomy. Invasive disease without evidence of lymph node metastases has a favorable prognosis; however, with nodal metastases, the disease is almost invariably fatal.

## CANCER OF THE VULVA

### Essentials of Diagnosis

- Occurs in postmenopausal women.
- Long history of vulvar irritation with pruritus, local discomfort, and bloody discharge.
- Appearance of early lesions like that of chronic vulvar dermatitis.
- Appearance of late lesions like that of a large cauliflower, or a hard ulcerated area in the vulva.
- Biopsy necessary for diagnosis.

### General Considerations

Cancer of the vulva may arise from the skin, subcutaneous tissues, glandular elements of the vulva, or the mucosa of the lower third of the vagina. Approximately 85–90% of these tumors are epidermoid cancers. Less common tumors are extramammary Paget's disease, with underlying adenocarcinoma, carcinoma of Bartholin's gland, basal cell carcinoma, melanoma, sarcoma, and metastatic cancers from other sites.

Cancer of the vulva is responsible for approximately 5% of gynecologic cancers. Vulvar cancer is common in the poor and elderly in most parts of the world, and no race or culture is spared. Vulvar cancer is primarily a disease of postmenopausal women, with a peak incidence in the 60s. In general, the mean age of patients with carcinoma in situ is approximately 10 years less than that for patients with invasive cancer. Intraepithelial cancer of the vulva in women in their 20s and 30s has increased remarkably in recent years coincidentally with an increase in the incidence of diagnosis of dysplasia and carcinoma in situ of the cervix. Occasionally, a vulvar cancer—usually sarcoma botryoides of the vagina or vulva—is diagnosed in a young girl.

The coincidence of carcinoma of the vulva and pregnancy is rare. Treatment can be administered during pregnancy without jeopardizing the fetus.

Considering that cancer of the vulva is a disease of a body surface readily accessible to diagnostic procedures, early diagnosis should be the rule. This is not the case, however, and a 6- to 12-month delay in reporting symptoms of discovery of a tumor is common. Despite the advanced age of many of these pa-

tients and the frequent finding of a moderately large tumor, the disease is usually amenable to surgical therapy. In stage I and II disease, the corrected 5-year survival rate is greater than 90%. A 75% corrected 5-year survival rate for all stages of vulvar cancer is reported by most institutions.

Associated disorders found most frequently with carcinoma of the vulva are obesity, hypertension, and chronic vulvar irritation secondary to diabetes mellitus, granulomatous venereal disease, or vulvar dystrophy.

### Pathology

The gross appearance of vulvar cancer depends on the origin and histologic type. These tumors progress by local extension and involvement of adjacent organs and, with few exceptions, by lymphatic permeation or embolism. The primary route of lymphatic spread is by way of the superficial inguinal, deep femoral, and external iliac lymph nodes (Fig 46–5). Contralateral spread may occur as a result of the rich intercommunicating lymphatic system of the vulvar skin. Direct extension to the deep pelvic lymph nodes, primarily the obturator nodes, occurs in about 3% of patients and seems to be related to midline involvement around the clitoris, urethra, or rectum or to cancer of a vestibular (Bartholin's) gland. Extension of the tumor to the lower and middle thirds of the vagina may also allow access of tumor cells to lymph channels leading to the deep pelvic lymph nodes.

The gross and histologic appearance of the various types of vulvar cancers is as follows.

**A. Epidermoid Cancer:** Epidermoid cancer is by far the most common type of tumor and most fre-

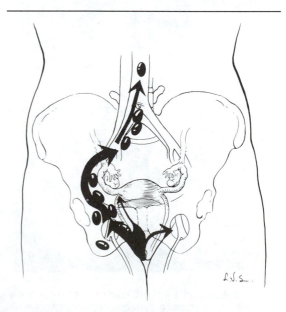

**Figure 46–5.** Lymphatic spread of cancer of the vulva.

quently involves the anterior half of the vulva. In approximately 65% of patients, the tumor arises in the labia majora and minora; and in 25% the clitoris is involved. Over one-third of tumors involve the vulva bilaterally or are midline tumors. These tumors are most frequently associated with nodal spread and in particular bilateral nodal metastases. Midline tumors that involve the perineum do not worsen the outlook unless they extend into the vagina or to the anus and rectum.

Epidermoid cancer of the vulva varies in appearance from a large, exophytic cauliflower-like lesion to a small ulcer crater superimposed on a dystrophic lesion of the vulvar skin (Figs 46–6 and 46–7). Ulcerative lesions may begin as a raised, flat, white area of hypertrophic skin that subsequently undergoes ulceration. Exophytic lesions may become extremely large, undergo necrosis, and become secondarily infected and malodorous. A third variety arises as a slightly elevated, red velvety tumor that gradually spreads over the vulvar skin. There does not appear to be a positive correlation between the gross appearance of the tumor and either histologic grade or frequency of nodal metastases. The primary determinant of nodal metastases is tumor size.

Epidermoid cancers may be graded histologically from I to III. Grade I tumors are well differentiated, often forming keratin pearls; grade II tumors are moderately well differentiated; and grade III tumors

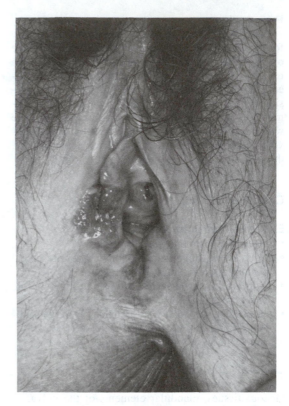

**Figure 46–7.** Ulcerative epidermoid cancer of the vulva.

are composed of poorly differentiated cells. The extent of underlying inflammatory cell infiltration into the stroma surrounding the invasive tumor is variable. The histologic grade of the tumor may be of some significance in small tumors less than 2 cm in diameter. However, the gross size of the tumor is the most significant factor in prognosis.

A variant of epidermoid cancer, **verrucous carcinoma,** is a locally invasive tumor that seldom metastasizes to regional lymph nodes. Grossly, the tumor looks like a mature condylomatous growth. Invading fronds of tumor tend to push the dermal tissue aside, causing diagnostic confusion. Local recurrence is common if a wide vulvectomy is not performed; lymphadenectomy is usually not recommended.

In recent years, an attempt has been made to define a group of early vulvar cancers that might be described as microinvasive cancer and that exhibit little tendency for local recurrence or nodal metastases. Depth of stromal penetration has proved to be the key factor in determining invasive potential of the tumor. Early authors accepted 5 mm or less of dermal invasion as the definition of microinvasion, but this has not been universally accepted. A task force by the International Society for the Study of Vulvar Diseases (1984) suggested that the term "microinvasive cancer of the vulva" be discarded. They defined stage IA

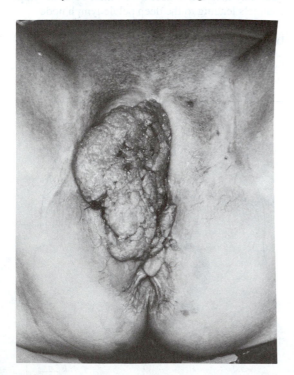

**Figure 46–6.** Large, exophytic epidermoid cancer of the vulva, which was treated by radical vulvectomy and regional lymphadenectomy.

carcinoma of the vulva as a single lesion measuring 2 cm or less in diameter and exhibiting one focus of invasion to a depth of 1 mm or less. The depth of invasion was measured from the epidermal-stromal junction of the most superficial dermal papilla to the deepest point of tumor invasion. Early invasive vulvar carcinoma meeting the above-mentioned histologic criteria can be treated with less radical surgery such as a modified hemivulvectomy with unilateral superficial inguinal lymphadenectomy.

**B. Carcinoma of Bartholin's Gland:** Carcinoma of Bartholin's gland accounts for about 1% of vulvar cancers. Approximately 50% of the tumors are squamous cell. Other types of tumors arising in the Bartholin glands are adenomatous, adenoid cystic (an adenocarcinoma with specific histologic and clinical characteristics), adenosquamous, and transitional cell.

It may be difficult to differentiate by clinical examination a tumor of Bartholin's gland or duct from a benign Bartholin's cyst. Because of its location deep in the substance of the labium, a tumor may impinge upon the rectum and directly spread into the ischiorectal fossa. Therefore, these tumors have access to lymphatic channels draining directly to the deep pelvic lymph nodes as well as the superficial channels draining to the inguinal lymph nodes.

**C. Basal Cell Carcinoma:** Basal cell carcinomas account for 1–2% of vulvar cancers. Most tumors are small papillomatous or elevated lesions. Some are described as pigmented tumors, moles, or simply pruritic maculopapular eruptions. These tumors arise almost exclusively in the skin of the labia majora, although occasionally a tumor can be found elsewhere in the vulva. The tumor is derived from primordial basal cells in the epidermis or hair follicles and is characterized by slow growth, local infiltration, and a tendency to recur if not totally excised. Most basal cell carcinomas of the vulva are of the primordial histologic type. Other histologic varieties that may be found are the pilar, morphea-like, superficially spreading, adenoid, and pigmented cell tumors.

On microscopic examination the typical tumor consists of nodular masses and lobules of closely packed, uniform-appearing basaloid cells with scant cytoplasm and spherical or oval dark nuclei. Peripheral margination by columnar cells is usually prominent. In larger tumor nodules, there may be areas of central degeneration and necrosis.

If a sufficiently wide local excision is not performed, there is a tendency for local recurrence, estimated to be about 20%. If a basal-squamous cell type tumor is diagnosed, appropriate therapy for invasive epidermoid cancer of the vulva should be undertaken.

**D. Malignant Melanoma:** About 5% of vulvar cancers are malignant melanomas. Since only 0.1% of all nevi in women are on vulvar skin, the disproportionate frequency of occurrence of melanoma in this area may be due to the fact that nearly all vulvar nevi are of the junctional variety. Malignant melanoma most commonly arises in the region of the labia minor and clitoris, and there is a tendency for superficial spread toward the urethra and vagina. A nonpigmented melanoma may closely resemble squamous cell carcinoma on clinical examination. A darkly pigmented, raised lesion at the mucocutaneous junction is a characteristic finding; however, the degree of melanin pigmentation is variable, and amelanotic lesions do occur. The lesion spreads primarily through lymphatic channels and tends to metastasize early in the course of the disease; local or remote cutaneous satellite lesions may be found. All small pigmented lesions of the vulva are suspect and should be removed by excision biopsy with a 0.5- to 1-cm margin of normal skin. In the case of large tumors, the diagnosis should be confirmed by a generous biopsy.

**E. Unusual Vulvar Malignancies:** Sarcomas of the vulva constitute a variety of malignant neoplasms that account for less than 2% of vulvar cancers. The most common is leiomyosarcoma, followed in frequency of occurrence by the fibrous histiocytoma group and an array of other sarcomas. Clinically, the tumor may be a subcutaneous nodule or may be exophytic and fleshy. Prognosis depends on histologic type, extent of local invasion, and treatment. In general, radical vulvectomy and regional lymphadenectomy are indicated, with the exception of tumors such as dermatofibrosarcoma protuberans, which is a locally aggressive tumor that tends to recur locally but does not metastasize.

Adenocarcinoma of the vulva is exceptionally rare unless it arises from Bartholin's gland or the urethra. Primary cancer of the breast from ectopic breast tissue has been reported. Rarely, a malignant tumor will arise from a vulvar sweat gland.

Metastatic cancers of the vulva have received scant attention in the medical literature. They usually originate from a genital tract tumor, and 18% arise from the kidney or urethra. Advanced cervical cancer is the most common primary tumor. Other primary tumors have been reported, including malignant melanoma, choriocarcinoma, and adenocarcinoma of the rectum or breast. Cloacogenic carcinoma is primarily an anorectal neoplasm occurring twice as often in women than in men; it may arise in anal ducts and present as a submucosal mass.

Metastatic epidermoid cancer tends to form nests of cells within the dermis. Adenocarcinoma, regardless of the primary site, invades the surface squamous epithelium. Because these tumors are a manifestation of advanced disease, the prognosis is uniformly grave.

## Clinical Findings

The patient with vulvar cancer characteristically has had infrequent medical examinations. About 10% are diabetic, and 30–50% are obese or hypertensive or demonstrate other evidence of cardiovascular disease. The incidence of complicating medical illness exceeds that expected in the age group under consideration.

Invasive epidermoid cancer is a disease mainly of the seventh and eighth decades of life, though about 15% of patients are age 40 or younger. During the past decade, the diagnosis of carcinoma in situ of the vulva in women in the third or fourth decade of life has increased remarkably, along with an apparent increased incidence of cervical neoplasia. About 20% of patients have a second primary cancer that was diagnosed prior to, at the time of, or subsequent to the diagnosis of vulvar cancer; 75% of these second primaries are in the cervix. Young patients in particular have a propensity for multicentric disease in the lower genital tract.

**A. Symptoms and Signs:** Pruritus vulvae or a vulvar mass is the presenting complaint in over 50% of patients with vulvar cancer. Other patients complain of bleeding or vulvar pain, whereas approximately 20% of patients have no complaints, and the tumor is found incidentally during routine pelvic examination. A significant number of patients, about 25%, have seen a physician and received various medical treatments without benefit of a biopsy of the tumor or have undergone incomplete therapy consisting of a simple excision biopsy of an invasive tumor. The importance of performing a biopsy of any vulvar lesion cannot be overemphasized.

### Differential Diagnosis

Differential diagnosis of vulvar disease and exclusion of cancer depend on an adequate biopsy. The tumor may be a diffuse white lesion, a discrete tumor, an ulcer, or diffuse papules, which may not be appreciated without thorough colposcopic examination of the skin of the vulva, perineum, and perianal area.

A white lesion of the vulva may be sampled in one or more areas, using a dermatologic punch biopsy to remove a full thickness of vulvar skin. The toluidine blue test may be of value in localizing areas of epithelial hyperactivity, although markedly hyperkeratotic lesions do not stain well and benign ulcers may give a false-positive stain. In the absence of epithelial dysplasia, a dystrophic lesion should be treated as recommended on p. 907; however, periodic examinations are necessary.

Ulcerative lesions can be due to a sexually transmitted disease (syphilis or granuloma inguinale), pyogenic infections, a benign tumor (granular cell myoblastoma), or viral infection (herpes simplex).

Tumors of the vulva must be diagnosed by biopsy or excision. Isolated enlargement of a groin lymph node may require fine-needle aspiration to establish a histologic diagnosis. The staging of vulvar cancer is based on surgical findings (Table 46–1). The primary treatment for all invasive vulvar cancers is complete surgical removal of all tumor whenever possible.

**Table 46–1.** International Federation of Gynecology and Obstetrics (FIGO) staging of invasive cancer.

| | | | |
|---|---|---|---|
| **Stage 0** | | | |
| Cis | | | Carcinoma in situ, intraepithelial carcinoma |
| **Stage I** | | | |
| T1 | N0 | M0 | Tumor confined to the vulva and/or perineum—2 cm or less in greatest dimension (no nodal metastasis) |
| **Stage II** | | | |
| T2 | N0 | M0 | Tumor confined to the vulva and/or perineum—no more than 2 cm in greatest dimension (no nodal metastasis) |
| **Stage III** | | | |
| T3 | N0 | M0 | Tumor of any size with |
| T3 | N1 | M0 | (1) Adjacent spread to the lower urethra and/or the vagina, or the anus, and/or |
| T1 | N1 | M0 | (2) Unilateral regional lymph |
| T2 | N1 | M0 | node metastasis |
| **Stage IVA** | | | |
| T1 | N2 | M0 | Tumor invades any of the following: Upper urethra, bladder mucosa, rectal mucosa, pelvic bone, and/or bilateral regional node metastasis |
| T2 | N2 | M0 | |
| T3 | N2 | M0 | |
| T4 | Any N | M0 | |
| **Stage IVb** | Any T | Any N | Any distant metastasis including |
| | M1 | | pelvic lymph nodes |

### Treatment

Invasive cancers of the vulva progressively increase in size, encroach upon adjacent structures such as the vagina, urethra, and anus, and metastasize to the inguinal lymph nodes, which may become very large and ulcerate through the overlying skin. Exophytic tumors can reach an exceptionally large size and become secondarily infected. The enlarged inguinal lymph nodes may impinge on the lymphatic and venous drainage from the leg, resulting in chronic lymphedema and thrombophlebitis. Invasion of the base of the bladder or urethra or the rectovaginal septum can cause a fistula. Patients eventually die from hemorrhage or inanition due to locally advanced and metastatic disease.

Local or remote persistence or recurrence of invasive cancer may be the result of undetected disease outside the treatment field or development of a new tumor. Most recurrences tend to occur within 2 years after surgery. Local recurrences may be amenable to secondary excision or radiation therapy. Therefore, the primary treatment of cancer of the vulva is wide excision of the tumor and extirpation of potential routes of dissemination.

Prior to surgery the number of preoperative studies ordered depends on the extent of disease and the general condition of the patient. A complete history with particular reference to medical diseases and a thorough physical examination that includes cytologic study of the cervix should be performed. A large tumor may interfere with adequate pelvic examination. Bleeding may be caused by a lesion higher in the genital tract rather than the obvious vulvar tumor. In that case, the pelvic examination may be performed under anesthesia and endometrial biopsy or D&C considered.

Chest x-ray, complete blood count, and urinalysis are performed on all patients. Older patients require an electrocardiogram (ECG) and a biochemical profile. Other studies such as proctoscopy, pyelography, barium enema, and CT scans are ordered on an individual basis. Enlarged lymph nodes do not require biopsy; they will be excised by lymphadenectomy or thoroughly sampled at the time of operation. Mechanical bowel cleansing is recommended for most patients, particularly if the perineal skin is involved. An antibiotic bowel preparation is prescribed if extensive perianal dissection, skin grafting, or intestinal surgery (such as abdominoperineal resection) is anticipated.

Large tumors are infected with aerobic and anaerobic organisms, and prophylactic antibiotic therapy beginning 2 hours before and for 24 hours after surgery may be desirable. Although an attempt must be made to isolate a large tumor during the operation, it may be difficult to accomplish vulvectomy without contaminating the operative wound. For this reason, groin dissection should be performed before vulvectomy. At least 2 units of packed red cells should be available for transfusion. Less than 50% of patients require a transfusion during or after the operation.

Whether the tumor is an epidermoid carcinoma, malignant melanoma, sarcoma, or Bartholin's gland tumor amenable to operative removal, the basic operation is radical vulvectomy and regional lymphadenectomy. The extent of the operative procedure may be modified in the aged or medically compromised patient. One might exclude the lymphadenectomy and confine the surgical procedure to removal of the primary tumor by vulvectomy. If the tumor extends anteriorly into the bladder, the involved organ must be removed by anterior exenteration with urinary diversion. If the cancer involves the rectum, abdominoperineal resection with a sigmoid colostomy is indicated. Cancer of a Bartholin's gland has a propensity for local recurrence. For that reason, in addition to vulvectomy, the tumor bed should be widely excised, including removal of fat from the ischiorectal fossa and partial excision of the adjacent levator ani muscle and vaginal mucosa.

Regional lymphadenectomy involves bilateral deep and superficial inguinal lymphadenectomy. The highest deep inguinal lymph nodes beneath the inguinal ligament (Cloquet's node) should be submitted for separate examination. If metastatic disease is found, whole-pelvis irradiation has been used to control potential pelvic nodal disease. With a relatively small lesion in the midportion of the labia on one side, one may consider ipsilateral deep and superficial inguinal lymphadenectomy; if all lymph nodes are negative, one may then choose not to perform a contralateral lymphadenectomy. Contralateral inguinal lymph node metastases are seldom found if none is found in the ipsilateral inguinal lymph nodes. Lymphadenectomy may be performed through a transverse lower abdominal incision (butterfly incision) that removes the lymph node-bearing tissues and vulvar structures in continuity or through separate vulvectomy and bilateral vertical groin incisions.

Therapy may also be modified in young women who exhibit a small primary lesion on the posterior vulva. In selected cases, the anterior vulva and clitoris can be preserved. Potential complications from a superficial and deep inguinal lymphadenectomy may be avoided by thorough sampling of the superficial inguinal lymph nodes. In general, lymphatic spread occurs in a sequential manner from the superficial to the deep inguinal lymph nodes. Therefore, if the superficial nodes harbor no metastatic disease, there is reasonable assurance that the deeper nodes are not involved. A similar approach has been recommended for the management of superficially invasive vulvar carcinoma.

Few patients survive who have metastatic disease in the deep pelvic lymph nodes. For that reason, extraperitoneal pelvic lymphadenectomy should not be performed. Bilateral pelvic lymphadenectomy may be a planned part of the operative procedure if a pelvic exenteration is performed or the primary tumor is a deeply seated Bartholin's gland cancer. Primary pelvic lymphadenectomy is no longer recommended for treatment of midline or clitoral tumors.

Locally advanced vulvar cancer in this older population of patients is a difficult therapeutic problem. The mortality and morbidity rates from ultraradical surgery have led to consideration of combined-modality treatment consisting of preoperative irradiation followed by less extensive surgery. This approach has also been used for treatment of recurrent disease. The irradiation field encompasses the primary vulvar disease in addition to the regional lymph nodes consisting of the groin and deep pelvic lymph nodes. Subsequent surgery is tailored to the extent of residual disease. Irradiation alone, without supplemental surgery, is rarely successful.

Chemotherapeutic agents such as cisplatin and 5-FU have been combined with radiation therapy in the treatment of locally advanced squamous cell carcinomas of the vulva. These chemotherapeutic agents are used as radiation sensitizers in large necrotic tumor beds in which radiation alone has minimal effect. Following chemotherapy combined with radiation, many advanced vulvar lesions can be surgically removed with less radical surgery and sparing of either the rectum or bladder.

There is controversy concerning the extent of surgery required for treatment of malignant melanoma of the vulva. For some years, standard treatment consisted of vulvectomy with superficial and deep inguinal and pelvic lymphadenectomy. Identification of metastases to the inguinal lymph nodes almost uniformly resulted in a fatal outcome. For that reason, some authors have suggested that vulvectomy alone should be performed at the initial operation.

Locally invasive but nonmetastasizing sarcomas such as dermatofibrosarcoma protuberans can be removed by wide local resection. Most other sarcomas are treated by radical vulvectomy and regional lymphadenectomy. The primary determinant of cure appears to be adequate wide removal of the primary lesion.

## Operative Morbidity & Mortality

About 80–90% of patients are candidates for operation despite the advanced age and complicating medical illness in the average patient. In the last decade the operative mortality rate for radical vulvectomy and bilateral inguinal lymphadenectomy is 1–2%. Frequently this procedure is performed in the ninth decade of life with few complications.

The most frequently encountered complication is wound breakdown, which occurs in well over 50% of patients undergoing radical vulvectomy and bilateral inguinal dissection. This complication is related to the amount of skin removed during the procedure, particularly at the groin areas. Separate groin incisions and careful handling of skin flaps have reduced the incidence of wound breakdown. Vigorous wound care with debridement almost always results in adequate healing.

Lymphedema of the lower extremities is another major complication that occurs in approximately 65% of patients who have had inguinal node dissections. Although lymphedema can occur in varying degrees, this long-term complication can be reduced by use of support hose during the first postoperative year. Collateral lymph drainage pathways develop in most cases; however, this complication can be permanent.

Lymphocyst formation in the groin area is a less common complication of inguinal node dissection, but it usually resolves spontaneously. The incidence of lymphocysts can be reduced by the use of suction catheters placed under the skin flaps at the time of surgery and remain in place postoperatively for 5–7 days.

Development of cystocele or rectocele is sometimes reported. Both conditions are caused by loss of tissue supporting the lower end of the vagina and introitus. These conditions can be surgically corrected, depending on how symptomatic the patient is.

## Follow-up

After the immediate postoperative period, patients should be examined every 3 months for 2 years and every 6 months thereafter to detect recurrent disease or a second primary cancer. Malignant melanomas and sarcomas may recur locally or metastasize to the liver or lungs.

## Prognosis

The principal prognostic factors in cancer of the vulva are the size and location of the lesion, the histologic type, and the presence or absence of regional lymph node metastases. As the tumor increases in size, the incidence of metastasis increases.

Approximately a 5-year survival rate of 75% should be expected after complete surgical treatment of invasive epidermoid cancer. Several authors have reported no deaths from cancer among patients who were found to have negative lymph nodes. With tumors less than 2 cm in diameter, the incidence of nodal metastases is 10–15%. Unfortunately, approximately 25% of patients who have nodal metastases do not have suspicious nodal enlargement on physical examination. In general, about 30% of patients undergoing surgery will be found to have positive lymph nodes. With nodal metastases, the approximate 5-year cure rates are as follows: 1 node, 94%; 2 nodes, 80%; 3 nodes or more, less than 15%. Patients who have 3 or more positive lymph nodes in the groin usually demonstrate palpably suspicious nodes preoperatively. These patients have a high incidence of metastases to the pelvic lymph nodes; however, pelvic lymphadenectomy apparently does not improve survival rates. Involvement of contiguous organs such as the bladder or rectum increases the incidence of nodal metastases and worsens the prognosis accordingly.

The cure rate for adequately treated cancer of Bartholin's gland has not been established. There is a propensity for unresectable local recurrences under the pubic ramus despite a thorough primary operation.

Wide local excision of basal cell carcinoma should be curative. Some authors have reported an approximately 20% recurrence rate after local excision that may represent cases of incomplete excision.

Results of treatment of malignant melanoma are related to the level of penetration of the tumor into the dermis of the vulvar skin or the lamina propria of the vaginal mucosa and to the presence or absence of nodal metastases. The 5-year survival rate ranges from 14 to 50%, but patients who have metastases to groin lymph nodes have a survival rate below 14%. Amelanotic cutaneous melanomas are particularly virulent tumors. The survival rate for patients with superficial spreading melanomas is much better than for those with the nodular variety, which tend to have a smaller diameter and exhibit aggressive vertical invasion, increased incidence of nodal metastases, treatment failures, and distant recurrences. The most common site of recurrence is at the site of resection or the groin lymph nodes (if not previously resected).

Sarcomas of the vulva tend to recur locally, particularly if the initial resection is not extensive, and metastasize to the liver and lungs.

The outcome of metastatic vulvar tumors depends on the primary tumor but, in general, is very poor.

## PREINVASIVE DISEASE OF THE VAGINA

### General Considerations

Vaginal intraepithelial neoplasia (VAIN) can occur as an isolated lesion, but multifocal disease is more common. Many patients may have similar intraepithelial neoplastic lesions involving the cervix or vulva. At least one-half to two-thirds of patients with VAIN have been treated for similar disease in either the cervix or the vulva. In addition, VAIN can reappear several years later necessitating long-term follow-up in these patients. Several investigators have recognized a "field response" involving the squamous epithelium of the lower genital tract including the cervix, vagina, and vulva to be affected simultaneously by the same carcinogenic agent.

The upper third of the vagina is vulnerable to the development of dysplasia and carcinoma in situ whether or not hysterectomy has been performed previously for intraepithelial neoplasia. Each of these entities has a potential for progression to invasive cancer. For this reason, women who have had a hysterectomy should continue to have periodic cytologic study of the vaginal apex. A similar lesion may develop after prior irradiation for a pelvic malignancy; some authors report a 20% incidence of cervical or vaginal dysplasia. These tumors are usually asymptomatic and detected by routine vaginal cytologic studies. New invasive tumors in an irradiated field usually develop 15–30 years after therapeutic irradiation.

Condylomatous lesions of the lower genital tract often demonstrate associated dysplasias. For this reason a biopsy should be made of condylomatous growth of the vagina prior to treatment.

### Pathology

As with other intraepithelial neoplasias occurring in the lower genital tract, VAIN is characterized by a loss of epithelial cell maturation. This is associated with nuclear hyperchromosis and pleomorphism with cellular crowding. The thickness of the epithelial abnormality designates the various lesions as VAIN I, II, or III. VAIN III is a synonymous term for carcinoma in situ of the vagina.

### Diagnosis

Almost all lesions of VAIN are asymptomatic. An abnormal Pap smear is usually the first sign of disease. The diagnosis is ultimately made by colposcopic examination of the vagina with a directed biopsy. Colposcopic examination of the vagina can be difficult to perform, particularly if a hysterectomy

has already been done. Similar techniques used for colposcopic examination of the cervix are used for examination of the vagina. Application of 3% acetic acid to the vagina will give a lesion under the colposcope appear like white epithelium, mosaicism, or punctation. Occasionally, iodine stains (Schiller's stain) can be used to identify lesions; however, this technique is not widely accepted as colposcopic-directed biopsies. Since the disease process tends to be multifocal, a thorough examination of the vagina from the introitus to the apex must be conducted.

### Treatment

The primary treatment modality for VAIN is surgical resection. If the lesion is focal, it can be removed in its entirety with local resection or partial colpectomy. When carcinoma in situ of the cervix extends to the upper vagina, the upper third of the vagina can be removed at the time of hysterectomy. When other treatment modalities have failed, a total vaginectomy can be performed with a split-thickness skin graft vaginal reconstruction.

Other treatment options include vaporization with $CO_2$ laser or intervaginal applicational fluorouracil cream. Isolated large lesions, if thoroughly examined by biopsy to exclude invasive disease, can be vaporized with the $CO_2$ laser. However, lesions are commonly multifocal at the time of diagnosis, or new lesions develop at a later date in apparently normal adjacent vaginal mucosa. Topical applications of fluorouracil cream have proved successful in such cases. The medication is caustic, and significant reaction around the vaginal introitus may cause urinary retention. Various regimens of administration have been recommended; however, 2 g of cream high in the vagina nightly for 5 days appears to be effective. Most patients require no more than two 5-day courses of treatment with a hiatus of several days. Immunosuppressed patients may require repeated short courses of treatment at perhaps 3-month intervals.

Carcinoma in situ or dysplasia after irradiation for cancer of the cervix usually occurs in the upper vagina. Care should be taken to exclude coexisting recurrent or persistent invasive disease of the cervix. Because the tissues have been compromised by a therapeutic dose of radiation, surgical excision—even an extensive biopsy—could precipitate development of a vesicovaginal or rectovaginal fistula.

In patients with persistent disease who are not candidates for total vaginectomy, intracavitary radium may be a satisfactory treatment choice. Colpostats or a specially designed (Bloedorn) vaginal applicator may be used to deliver 6000–7000 cGy surface dose to the vagina in approximately 72 hours. Irradiation of the entire length of the vagina causes stenosis and loss of vaginal function.

### Follow-up

Intraepithelial neoplasia of the vagina tends to be

multifocal with involvement of the cervix and vulva in many cases. These lesions can be difficult to eradicate with only one treatment modality or treatment session. This group of patients must be monitored closely every 3 to 4 months with colposcopic examinations of not only the vagina but also the entire lower genital tract.

## CANCER OF THE VAGINA

### Essentials of Diagnosis

- Asymptomatic: abnormal vaginal cytology.
- Early: painless bleeding from ulcerated tumor.
- Late: bleeding, pain, weight loss, swelling.

### General Considerations

Primary cancers of the vagina represent about 1–2% of gynecologic cancers. About 85% are epidermoid cancers, and the remainder, in decreasing order of frequency, are adenocarcinomas, sarcomas, and melanomas. A tumor should not be considered to be a primary vaginal cancer unless the cervix is uninvolved or only minimally involved by a tumor obviously arising in the vagina. By convention, any malignancy involving both cervix and vagina that is histologically compatible with the origin in either organ is classified as cervical cancer. Tumors involving the vulva should be classified as vulvar cancers. Secondary carcinoma of the vagina is seen more frequently than primary vaginal cancers. Extension of cervical cancer to the vagina is probably the most common malignancy involving the vagina. Primary adenocarcinoma of the vagina should not be diagnosed unless adenocarcinoma of the endometrium, ovary, urethra, bladder, and rectum has been excluded. Malignant trophoblastic disease can also metastasize to the vagina.

### Pathology

Invasive epidermoid cancer of the vagina occurs in postmenopausal women, usually in the sixth or seventh decade. The tumors may be ulcerative or exophytic, usually involve the posterior wall of the upper third of the vagina, and are often grade II or III tumors. Direct invasion of the bladder or rectum may occur. The incidence of lymph node metastases is directly related to the size of the tumor. The route of nodal metastases depends on the location of the tumor in the vagina. Tumors in the lower third metastasize like cancer of the vulva, primarily to the inguinal lymph nodes (Fig 46–8). Cancers of the upper vagina, which is the most common site, metastasize in a manner similar to cancer of the cervix. The lymphatic drainage of the vagina consists of a fine capillary meshwork in the mucosa and submucosa with multiple anastomoses. As a consequence, lesions in the middle third of the vagina may metastasize to the in-

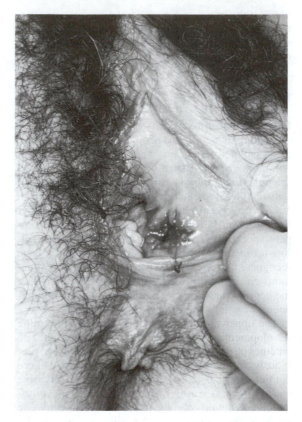

**Figure 46–8.** An ulcerated epidermoid cancer of the lower third of the vagina.

guinal lymph nodes or directly to the deep pelvic lymph nodes.

Melanomas and sarcomas of the vagina metastasize like epidermoid cancer, although liver and pulmonary metastases are more common. Nevi rarely occur in the vagina; therefore, any pigmented lesion of the vagina should be excised or biopsied. The anterior surface and lower half of the vagina are the most common sites. Grossly, the tumors are usually exophytic and described as polypoid or pedunculated with secondary necrosis.

Sarcomas of the vagina occur in children under 5 years of age and in women in the fifth to sixth decades. Embryonal rhabdomyosarcomas replace the vaginal mucosa of young girls and consist of polypoid, edematous, translucent masses that may protrude from the vaginal introitus. Leiomyosarcomas, reticulum cell sarcomas, and unclassified sarcomas occur in older women. The upper anterior vaginal wall is the most common site of origin. The appearance of these tumors depends on the size and the extent of disease at the time of diagnosis.

Clear cell adenocarcinomas arise in conjunction with vaginal adenosis, which in recent years has been detected most frequently in young women with a history of exposure to diethylstilbestrol (DES) in utero (Fig 46–9). The Registry of Clear Cell Adenocarcinoma of the Genital Tract in Young Females was established in 1971 to study the clinicopathologic and epidemiologic aspects of these tumors in girls born in 1940 or later, the years during which DES was used during pregnancy. The risk of developing clear cell adenocarcinoma by age 24 has been calculated to be 0.14–1.4 per 1000 exposed female fetuses. Adenosis vaginae and adenocarcinoma do occur in sexually mature and postmenopausal women.

Metastatic adenocarcinoma to the vagina may arise from the urethra, Bartholin's gland, the rectum or bladder, the endometrial cavity, the endocervix, or an ovary; or it may be metastatic from a distant site. Hypernephroma of the kidney characteristically metastasizes to the anterior wall of the vagina in the lower third. These tumors would not be primary vaginal cancers.

## Clinical Findings

The mean age of women with invasive cancer of the vagina is about 55 years; carcinoma in situ patients are about 10 years younger. There is no racial predisposition. Intraepithelial cancer is usually asymptomatic, discovered by routine vaginal cytologic examination, and confirmed by biopsy after delineation of the location and extent of the tumor by colposcopy.

Bleeding (or a bloody discharge) is the most common symptom associated with invasive vaginal cancer of any histologic type. About 50% of patients with invasive cancer vaginal cancer report for examination within 6 months after symptoms are noted. Advanced tumors cause a vaginal discharge and vulvar pruritus; impinge upon the rectum or bladder; extend to the pelvic wall and cause pain or leg edema; or metastasize to the lungs or inguinal lymph nodes.

A diagnosis of primary cancer of the vagina cannot be established unless metastasis from another source is eliminated; therefore, a complete history and physical examination are performed, including a thorough pelvic examination, cervical cytologic examination, endometrial biopsy when indicated, complete inspection of the vagina, including colposcopy, and biopsy of the vaginal tumor. Careful bimanual examination with palpation of the entire length of the vagina can detect small submucosal nodules that have not been visualized during the examination.

The staging system for cancer of the vagina is clinical and not surgical (Table 46–2).

## Differential Diagnosis

Benign tumors of the vagina are uncommon, are usually cystic, arise from the mesonephric (wolffian) or paramesonephric ducts, and are usually an incidental finding on examination of the anterolateral wall of the vagina (Gartner's duct cyst).

An ulcerative lesion may occur at the site of direct trauma, following an inflammatory reaction due to prolonged retention of a pessary or other foreign body, or, occasionally, following a chemical burn. Granulomatous venereal diseases seldom affect the vagina but may be diagnosed with appropriate laboratory studies and a biopsy.

Endometriosis that penetrates the cul-de-sac of Douglas into the upper vagina cannot be differentiated from cancer except by biopsy.

Cancer of the urethra, bladder, rectum, or Bartholin's gland may penetrate or extend into the vagina. Cloacogenic carcinoma is a rare tumor of the anorectal region originating from a persistent remnant of the cloacal membrane of the embryo. The tumor accounts for 2–3% of anorectal carcinomas and occurs more than twice as often in women. Although these metastatic tumors often penetrate into the vagina as fungating or ulcerating lesions, they may present as a submucosal mass.

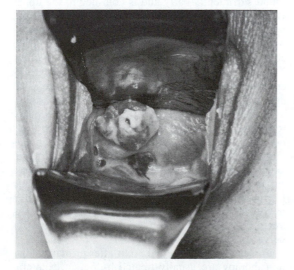

**Figure 46–9.** A clear cell adenocarcinoma of the vagina in a 19-year-old patient. The lesion is on the posterior wall of the upper third of the vagina.

**Table 46–2.** FIGO staging of carcinoma of the vagina.

**Preinvasive carcinoma**

| | |
|---|---|
| Stage 0 | Carcinoma in situ, intraepithelial carcinoma. |

**Invasive carcinoma**

| | |
|---|---|
| Stage I | The carcinoma is limited to the vaginal mucosa. |
| Stage II | The carcinoma has involved the subvaginal tissue but has not extended to the pelvic wall. |
| Stage III | The carcinoma has extended to the pelvic wall. |
| Stage IV | The carcinoma has extended beyond the true pelvis or has involved the mucosa of the bladder or rectum. A bullous edema as such does not permit allotment of a case to stage IV. |
| Stage IVA | Spread of the growth to adjacent organs. |
| Stage IVB | Spread to distant organs. |

FIGO, Federation of Gynecology and Obstetrics.

In decreasing order of frequency of occurrence, malignant tumors of the following organs or tissues of the genital tract may extend onto or metastasize to the vagina: cervix, endometrium, trophoblast, and ovary. Metastatic spread from a distant site is uncommon but does occur.

Biopsy establishes a histologic diagnosis. An epidermoid cancer is usually primary unless it is an extension of a tumor from the cervix, vulva, or a Bartholin's gland duct. Adenocarcinoma may arise from several sources; however, the diagnosis is apparent in young girls with associated adenosis of the cervix and upper vagina, a clear cell histologic pattern, and a history of DES exposure in utero. However, active benign squamous metaplasia in the adenomatous epithelium of the cervix and vagina may exhibit colposcopic characteristics that could be confused with dysplastic change. Primary adenocarcinoma in a postmenopausal patient may not be associated with adenosis and usually arises on the anterior wall of the lower third of the vagina in close proximity to the urethra.

## Treatment

The treatment of patients with primary invasive vaginal cancer may be surgical or radiologic. The treatment field must encompass the entire vaginal tumor and primary routes of dissemination. Pretreatment evaluation consists of a complete blood count, urinalysis, chest x-ray, ECG, biochemical profile, and intravenous urogram. A posterior vaginal wall lesion necessitates proctoscopy, and an anterior wall lesion requires cystoscopy. The inguinal lymph node area should be carefully palpated, although a negative examination does not mean that metastases are not present. CT scans are ordered on an individual basis. It must be established that the tumor is primary in the vagina and that distant metastases have not occurred. Most patients are postmenopausal and have a higher incidence of associated medical illness to be evaluated and treated.

Treatment of primary invasive cancer of the vagina depends on the location of the tumor within the vagina and the stage of the disease. Therapy is complicated by the anatomic proximity to the vagina of the rectum, bladder, and urethra. Most primary invasive epidermoid cancers of the vagina are treated by irradiation. Small stage I or II tumors involving the upper portion of the vagina can be treated by radical abdominal hysterectomy, partial vaginectomy, and pelvic lymphadenectomy. In young women, ovarian function can be preserved. If the vagina would be significantly shortened, length can be maintained by insertion of a split-thickness skin graft over a vaginal mold at the time of operation. Irradiation consists of whole-pelvis external therapy supplemented by intracavitary radium. If the cervix is absent, there is a greater incidence of complications involving the rectum, bladder, or bowel because of intestinal adhesions to the vaginal cuff. Stage I or II tumors in the middle or lower third of the vagina may be amenable to surgical excision; however, irradiation is usually the treatment of choice.

Surgical therapy is not applicable to stage III or IV lesions unless the tumor is confined to the midline and has invaded anteriorly into the bladder or posteriorly into the rectum, in which case an exenteration operation may be considered. However, most affected patients are treated by irradiation, which consists of whole-pelvis external irradiation followed by intracavitary or interstitial radium, or additional external therapy through a treatment field that has been reduced in size and localized to the affected parametrium. A colostomy may be performed if the tumor has penetrated the rectovaginal septum.

In some cases carcinoma at the introitus may be treated like cancer of the vulva, utilizing radical vulvectomy and bilateral superficial and deep inguinal lymphadenectomy. A very small and early lesion may be treated by total vaginectomy. However, the close proximity of the bladder and the rectum often precludes conservative surgery. Irradiation is essentially the same as that used for cancers of the upper vagina. When the lower third of the vagina is involved, the inguinal nodes must be treated with either irradiation or inguinal lymphadenectomy.

The principles of treatment of primary adenocarcinoma of the vagina are the same as those for epidermoid cancer. However, preferred therapy for clear cell carcinoma of the vagina and cervix in young women has not been established. Approximately 60% of tumors occur in the upper half of the vagina, and the remainder occur in the cervix. The incidence of nodal metastases is approximately 18% in stage I and 30% or more in stage II disease. If the disease is found sufficiently early and is confined to the upper vagina and cervix, radical abdominal hysterectomy, upper vaginectomy, and pelvic lymphadenectomy with ovarian preservation can be performed. More advanced lesions are treated with irradiation.

Sarcoma botryoides, a variety of rhabdomyosarcoma found in patients usually less than 5 years of age, has responded well to preoperative chemotherapy, allowing less radical surgery than previously recommended. In adult patients, chemotherapy has been less successful in the treatment of sarcomas. Radiation therapy has demonstrated some benefit, but no cures have been reported. Consequently, extensive surgery, usually a form of pelvic exenteration, is the treatment of choice. Many of these tumors occur in a previously irradiated field. Melanoma of the vagina is treated surgically, usually by anterior or posterior pelvic exenteration.

Epidermoid cancers that recur after primary radiation therapy are usually treated by pelvic exenteration. Chemotherapy for recurrent disease has been relatively ineffective, but multidrug regimens incorporating cisplatin may prove to be more useful.

## Prognosis

The size and stage of the disease at the time of diagnosis are the most important prognostic indicators in epidermoid cancers. The 5-year cure rate is 70–75% in patients with stage I and II disease. In stage III disease, the cure rate is 30–40%. In stage IV disease, there are few survivors.

Melanomas—even small ones—are very malignant, and few respond to therapy. The tumor recurs locally and metastasizes to the liver and lungs. Chemotherapy and immunotherapy have been used as adjunctive treatment.

Too few sarcomas of the vagina have been reported to generate survival data; these tumors have a propensity for local recurrence and distant metastases, and the prognosis is usually poor.

# REFERENCES

## GENERAL

Stening M: *Cancer and Related Lesions of the Vulva.* ADIS Press, 1980.

Van Nagell JR, Barber HRK: *Modern Concepts of Gynecologic Oncology.* PSG, 1982.

Way S: *Malignant Disease of the Vulva.* Churchill Livingstone, 1982.

## PREINVASIVE DISEASE OF THE VULVA & VAGINA

Benedet JL, Wilson PS, Matisic JP: Epidermal thickness measurements in vaginal intraepithelial neoplasia: A basis for optimal $CO_2$ laser vaporization. J Reprod Med 1992;37(9):899.

Davis GD: Colposcopic examination of the vagina. Obstet Gynecol Clin North Am 1993;20(1):217.

Hatch K: Colposcopy of vaginal and vulvar human papilloma virus and adjacent sites. Obstet Gynecol Clin North Am 1993;20(1):203.

Jones RW, Park JS, McLean MR et al: Human papilloma virus in women with VIN III. J Reprod Med 1990;35:1124.

Petrilli ES et al: Vaginal intraepithelial neoplasias: biologic aspects and treatment with topical 5-fluorouracil and the carbon dioxide laser. Am J Obstet Gynecol 1980;138:321.

Rettenmaier MA, Berman ML, DiSaia PJ: Skinning vulvectomy for the treatment of multifocal vulvar intraepithelial neoplasia. Obstet Gynecol 1987;69:247.

Schneider A, de Villiers E-M, Schndeider V: Multifocal squamous neoplasia of the female genital tract: Significance of human papillomavirus infection of the vagina after hysterectomy. Obstet Gynecol 1987;70:294.

Sillman FH, Sedlis A, Boyce JG: A review of lower genital intraepithelial neoplasia and the use of topical 5-fluorouracil. Obstet Gynecol Surv 1985;40:190.

Twiggs LB et al: A clinical, histopathologic and molecular biologic investigation of vulvar intraepithelial neoplasia. Int J Gynecol Pathol 1988;7:48.

Wright VC, Davies E: Laser surgery for vulvar intraepithelial neoplasia: Principles and results. Am J Obstet Gynecol 1987;156:374.

## EXTRAMAMMARY PAGET'S DISEASE.

Bergen S, DiSaia PJ, Liao SY, Berman ML: Conservative management of extramammary Paget's disease of the vulva. Gynecol Oncol 1989;33(2):151.

Creasman WT, Gallager HS, Rutledge F: Paget's disease of the vulva. Gynecol Oncol 1975;3:133.

Curtin JP, Rubin SC, Jones WB et al: Paget's disease of the vulva. Gynecol Oncol 1990;39:374.

Degefu S, O'Quinn AG, Dhurandhar HN: Paget's disease of the vulva and urogenital malignancies: A case report and review of the literature. Gynecology 1986;25:347.

Feuer GA. Shevchuk M. Calanog A: Vulvar Paget's disease: the need to exclude an invasive lesion. Gynecol Oncol 1990;38:81

Gunn RA, Gallager HS: Vulvar Paget's disease: A topographic study. Cancer 1980;46:590.

James LP: Apocrine adenocarcinoma of the vulva with associated Paget's disease. Acta Cytol 1984;28:178.

## CANCER OF THE VULVA

Andreasson B, Nyboe J: Predictive factors with reference to low risk of metastases in squamous cell carcinoma in the vulvar region. Gynecol Oncol 1985;21:196.

Berek JS, Heaps JM, Fu YS et al: Concurrent cisplatin and 5-fluorouracil chemotherapy and radiation therapy for advanced stage squamous cell carcinoma of the vulva. Gynecol Oncol 1991;42:197

Boice CR et al: Microinvasive squamous carcinoma of the vulva: Present status and reassessment. Gynecol Oncol 1984;18:71.

Bradgate MG, Rollason TP, McConkey CC, Powell J: Malignant melanoma of the vulva: A clinicopathological study of 50 women. Br J Obstet Gynecol 12990;97(2):124.

Copeland LJ et al: Bartholin gland carcinoma. Obstet Gynecol 1986;67:794.

Crosby JH, Bryan AB, Gallup DG et al: Fine-needle aspiration of inguinal lymph nodes in gynecologic practice. Obstet Gynecol 1989;73:281.

Crowther ME, Lowe DG, Shepherd JH: Verrucous carcinoma of the female genital tract: A review. Obstet Gynecol Surv 1988;43:263.

DiSaia PJ, Rutledge FN, Smith JP: Sarcoma of the vulva. Obstet Gynecol 1971;38:180.

Hacker NF et al: Individualization of treatment for stage I squamous cell vulvar carcinoma. Obstet Gynecol 1984;63:155.

Hacker NF et al: Management of regional lymph nodes and their prognostic influence in vulvar cancer. Obstet Gynecol 1983;61:408.

Hacker NF et al: Preoperative radiation therapy for locally advanced vulvar cancer. Cancer 1984;54:2056.

zur Hausen H: Papillomaviruses in human cancer. Cancer 1987;10:1692.

Homesley HD, Bundy BN, Sedlis A et al: Assessment of current International Federation of Gynecology and Obstetrics staging of vulvar carcinoma relative to prognostic factors for survival (a Gynecologic Oncology Group study). Am J Obstet Gynecol 1991;164(4): 997.

Homesley HD et al: Radiation therapy versus pelvic node resection for carcinoma of the vulva with positive groin nodes. Obstet Gynecol 1986;68:733.

Johnson TL et al: Prognostic features of vulvar melanoma: A clinicopathologic analysis. Int J Gynecol Pathol 1986;5:110.

Levin W: The use of concomitant chemotherapy and radiotherapy prior to surgery in advanced stage carcinoma of the vulva. Gynecol Oncol 1986;25:20.

Lin JY, DuBeshter B, Angel C, Dvoretsky PM.: Morbidity and recurrence with modifications of radical vulvectomy and groin dissection. Gynecol Oncol 1992; 47(1):80.

Microinvasive cancer of the vulva: Report of the ISSVD Task Force. J Reprod Med 1984;29:454.

Rotmensch J, Rubin SJ, Sutton HG et al: Preoperative radiotherapy followed by radical vulvectomy with inguinal lymphadenectomy for advanced vulvar carcinomas. Gynecol Oncol 1990;36(2):181.

Sedlis A et al: Positive groin lymph nodes in superficial squamous cell vulvar cancer. Am J Obstet Gynecol 1987;156:1159.

## CANCER OF THE VAGINA

Andersen ES: Primary carcinoma of the vagina: A study of 29 cases. Gynecol Oncol 1989;33:317.

Borazjani G, Prem KA, Okagaki T et al: Primary malignant melanoma of the vagina: A clinicopathological analysis of 10 cases. Gynecol Oncol 1990;37:264.

Chu AM, Beechinor R: Survival and recurrence patterns in the radiation treatment of carcinoma of the vagina. Gynecol Oncol 1984;19:298.

Copeland LJ, et al: Sarcoma botryoides of the female genital tract. Gynecol Oncol 1985;66:262.

Davis KP, Stanhope CR, Garton GR et al: Invasive vaginal carcinoma: Analysis of early-stage disease. Gynecol Oncol 1991;42:131.

Friedman M et al: Modern treatment of vaginal embryonal rhabdomyosarcoma. Obstet Gynecol Surv 1986; 41:614.

Gallup DG et al: Invasive squamous cell carcinoma of the vagina: A 14-year study. Obstet Gynecol 1987;69: 782.

Herbst A, Anderson D: Clear cell adenocarcinoma of the vagina and cervix secondary to intrauterine exposure to diethylstilbestrol. Semin Surg Oncol 1990;6(6): 343.

Herbst AL et al: Clear cell adenocarcinoma of the genital tract in young females: Registry report. N Engl J Med 1972;287:1259.

Herbst AL et al: Risk factors of the development of diethylstilbestrol-associated clear cell adenocarcinoma. Am J Obstet Gynecol 1986;154:814.

Jefferies JA et al: Structural anomalies of the cervix and vagina in women enrolled in the diethylstilbestrol adenosis (DESAD) Project. Am J Obstet Gynecol 1984; 148:59.

Kucera H, Vavra N: Radiation management of primary carcinoma of the vagina: Clinical and histopathological variables with survival. Gynecol Oncol 1991; 40:12.

Kucera H et al: Radiotherapy of primary carcinoma of the vagina: Management and results of different therapy schemes. Gynecol Oncol 1985;21:87.

Mahesh Kumar AP et al: Combined therapy to prevent complete pelvic exenteration for rhabdomyosarcoma of the vagina or uterus. Cancer 1976;37:118.

Melnick S et al: Rates and risks of diethylstilbestrol-related clear-cell adenocarcinoma of the vagina and cervix. N Engl J Med 1987;316:514.

Peters WA et al: Primary sarcoma of the adult vagina: A clinico-pathologic study. Obstet Gynecol 1985;65: 699.

Peters WA, Kumar NB, Morley GW: Carcinoma of the vagina: Factors influencing treatment outcome. Cancer 1985;55:892.

Reddy S et al: Radiation therapy in primary carcinoma of the vagina. Gynecol Oncol 1987;26:19.

Rubin SC, Young J, Mikuta JJ: Squamous carcinoma of the vagina: Treatment, complications, and long-term follow-up. Gynecol Oncol 1985;20:346.

Thigpen JT et al: A phase II trial of cisplatin in advanced recurrent cancer of the vagina: A GOG study. Gynecol Oncol 1986;23:101.

# Premalignant & Malignant Disorders of the Uterine Cervix

# 47

*Annekathryn Goodman, MD, & Edward C. Hill, MD*

## DYSPLASIA & CARCINOMA IN SITU OF THE CERVIX
### (Cervical Intraepithelial Neoplasia)

### Essentials of Diagnosis

- The cervix often appears grossly normal.
- Dysplastic or carcinoma in situ cells are noted in cytologic smear preparations (Papanicolaou [Pap] smears).
- Colposcopic examination reveals coarse punctate or mosaic patterns of surface capillaries, an atypical transformation zone, and thickened "white epithelium."
- Iodine-nonstaining (Schiller-positive) area of squamous epithelium is typical.
- Biopsy diagnosis of dysplasia or carcinoma in situ.

### General Considerations

Dysplasia or cervical intraepithelial neoplasia (CIN) means disordered growth and development of the epithelial lining of the cervix. The various degrees of CIN represent a continuum in the neoplastic process. Mild dysplasia or CIN I is defined as disordered growth of the lower one third of the epithelial lining. Abnormal maturation of two-thirds of the lining is called moderate dysplasia or CIN II. Severe dysplasia, CIN III, and carcinoma in situ (CIS) are equivalent terms for full-thickness dysmaturity. CIN may be suspected because of an abnormal Pap smear, but the diagnosis is established by cervical biopsy. Spontaneous regression, especially of CIN I, occurs in a significant number of patients; therefore, the process is reversible. In others, CIN appears to remain static for years. A certain percentage of all degrees of dysplasia will progress to an invasive cancer if followed for up to 20 years. Because it is not presently possible to predict which lesions will progress, it is recommended that all dysplasias be treated when diagnosed.

### Etiology

The field theory of the origin of squamous cell carcinoma of the cervix maintains that cancer begins in areas that have been previously altered to make them potentially neoplastic. Most cervical cancers make their initial appearance in zones of atypical or dysplastic epithelium and develop very slowly. Human papillomaviruses (HPV) are the prime etiologic suspects, and analysis of almost all CIN lesions shows the presence of a subtype of HPV. The epidemiologic factors in dysplasia are similar to those of cancer of the cervix and include smegma, repeated infections, smoking, oral contraceptives, and immunosupresion (see Cancer of the Cervix).

Prevalence figures for cervical dysplasia vary from 1.2–3.8% in nonpregnant patients. Pregnancy may produce changes in the cervical epithelium that mimic those of cervical dysplasia. Some of these variations may be related to folic acid deficiency. Morphologically, these changes cannot be distinguished from those of true neoplasia. Seventy-five percent of the pregnancy changes are involuted within 6 months postpartum with a return of the cytologic picture to normal. The incidence of true neoplastic dysplasia in pregnant women is not known. Nonetheless, dysplasia occurs in females age 15 and older, with a peak incidence in the age group from 25 to 35 years.

### Pathology

On cytologic examination, the dysplastic cell is characterized by anaplasia, an increased nuclear/cytoplasmic ratio (ie, the nucleus is larger), hyperchromatism with changes in the nuclear chromatin, multinucleation, and abnormalities in differentiation.

Histologically, involvement of varying degrees of thickness of the stratified squamous epithelium is typical of dysplasia. The cells are anaplastic and hyperchromatic, and show a loss of polarity in the deeper layers as well as abnormal mitotic figures in increased numbers. Benign epithelial alterations, particularly those of an inflammatory nature, the cytopathic effects of HPV and technical artifacts may be mistaken for CIN and CIN II. Retrospective studies have shown that about 50% of CIN I and 25% of CIN I lesions have been reclassified as flat condylomata.

The columnar epithelium of the mucus-secreting endocervical glands can also undergo neoplastic transformation. Adenocarcinoma in situ (ACIS), a

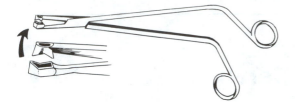

**Figure 47–1.** Tischler cervical biopsy forceps.

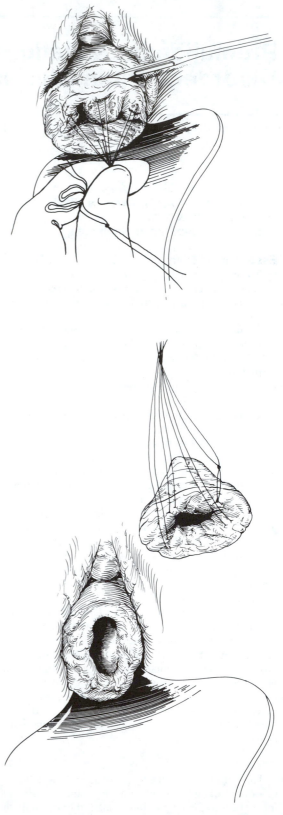

controversial diagnosis, is described as a lesion that retains the general characteristics of endocervical epithelium. This lesion shows an increase in architectural complexity with nuclear stratification, nuclear enlargement, and abnormal mitotic figures. Three criteria must be used to distinguish ACIS from an invasive adenocarcinoma: (1) its presence is limited to 3–5-mm depth; (2) there must be a combination of normal and neoplastic glands; (3) a stromal response such as edema or an inflammatory cell infiltrate must be absent. The diagnosis of ACIS can be made only by cone biopsy.

## Clinical Findings

**A. Symptoms and Signs:** There are usually no symptoms or signs of dysplasia, and the diagnosis is most often based on cytologic findings obtained in the course of a routine cervical Pap smear evaluation. Because dysplasia probably is a transitional phase in the pathogenesis of many cervical cancers, early detection is extremely important. All postpubertal women should have a pelvic and cytologic examination at least once a year. All abnormal Pap smears need to be evaluated by colposcopy with directed biopsies to confirm the diagnosis histologically, to determine the extent of the lesion, and to rule out an invasive cancer.

**B. Special Examinations:** In addition to gross inspection of the cervix, the diagnostic procedures include the Schiller test, colposcopic examination, directed biopsy, endocervical curettage, and cone biopsy of the cervix (Figs 47–1 to 47–4).

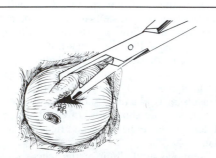

**Figure 47–2.** Multiple punch biopsy of the cervix with Tischler forceps.

**Figure 47–3.** Conization of the cervix.

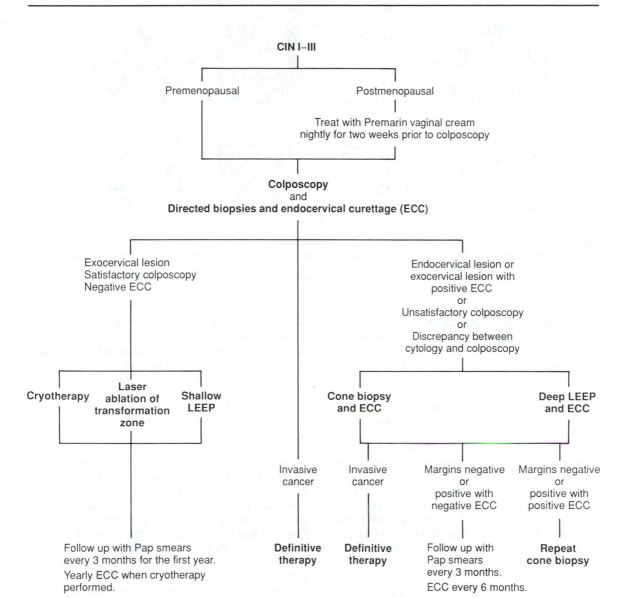

**Figure 47–4.** Plan for management of the abnormal cytologic smear in which there is no visible lesion **(A)** and a visible lesion **(B)**.

**1. Schiller test**–The Schiller test is based on the principle that normal squamous epithelium of the cervix contains glycogen, which combines with iodine to produce a deep mahogany-brown color. Nonstaining, therefore, indicates abnormal squamous (or columnar) epithelium, scarring, cyst formation, etc, and constitutes a positive Schiller test. The test is not specific for cancer but merely reveals non-glycogen-containing epithelium. Immature metaplastic epithelium frequently is nonstaining.

Schiller's solution is an aqueous iodine preparation. Lugol's solution is commonly used for the Schiller test, because it is readily available. Although the stronger Lugol's solution stains the glycogen-rich epithelium more quickly, it is a satisfactory substitute for Schiller's solution.

(Figures 47–4 through 47–7 are reproduced, with permission, from Johannisson E, Kolstat P, Soderberg G: Cytologic, vascular, and histologic patterns of dysplasia, carcinoma in situ and early invasive carcinoma of the cervix. Acta Radiol Suppl [Stockh] 1966;258.)

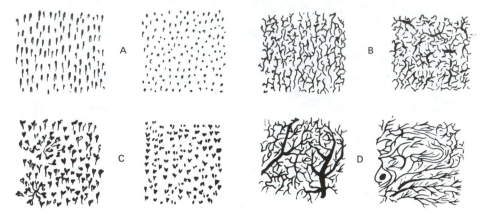

**Figure 47–5.** Schematic drawing of different types of terminal vessels as observed in the normal squamous epithelium: hairpin capillaries **(A)**, network capillaries **(B)**, both found in normal states; double capillaries **(C)**, seen in *Trichomonas* inflammation; and branching vessels **(D)**, seen in the transformation zone.

**2. Colposcopic examination**–(See also Chapter 30.) Colposcopy requires an instrument that allows inspection of the cervix under low-power magnification (6–40 ×) and an intense light source. It is especially useful in the evaluation of patients with an abnormal cytologic examination. Abnormalities in the appearance of the epithelium and its capillary blood supply often are not visible to the naked eye but can be identified by colposcopy, particularly after the application of 3% aqueous acetic acid solution. CIN produces recognizable abnormalities on the portio vaginalis of the cervix in the majority of patients.

Normal colposcopic findings are those of (1) original squamous epithelium, (2) transformation zone (metaplastic squamous epithelium), and (3) columnar epithelium. Abnormal findings indicative of dysplasia and CIS are those of (1) "white epithelium" and (2) mosaicism or coarse punctate pattern of the sur-face capillaries. Early stromal invasion should be suspected when bizarre capillaries with so-called corkscrew, comma-shaped, or spaghetti-like configurations are found (Figs 47–5 to 47–8). A colposcopically directed punch biopsy of such areas should be done. Except in pregnancy, evaluation of the endocervical canal by endocervical curettage should be performed in every case. In 20% of patients with abnormal Pap smears, the endocervical curettage is positive for dysplasia.

Colposcopically directed punch biopsy (the Younge-Kevorkian square jaw alligator punch forceps serve well) is most revealing in the diagnosis of CIN. The colposcopic evaluation is considered "adequate" or "satisfactory" if the complete transformation zone and the full extent of the lesion are visualized. If the squamocolumnar junction of the cervix is visible by colposcopy, the false-negative rate for colposcopically directed punch biopsy is less than 1%. Unfortunately, the transformation zone extends into

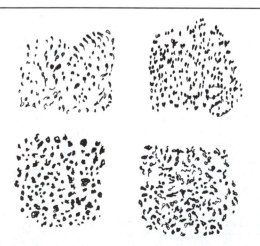

**Figure 47–6.** Punctuation terminal vessels.

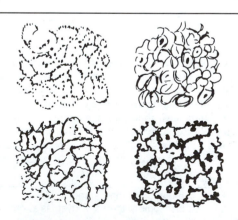

**Figure 47–7.** Mosaic terminal vessels.

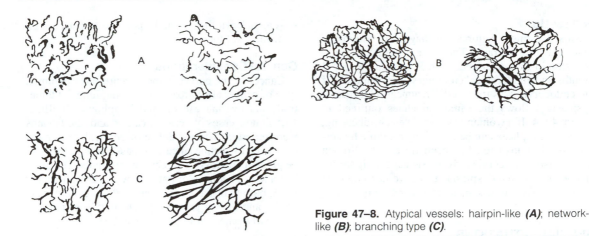

**Figure 47–8.** Atypical vessels: hairpin-like **(A)**; network-like **(B)**; branching type **(C)**.

the endocervical canal beyond the field of vision in 12–15% of premenopausal women and in a significantly higher percentage of postmenopausal women.

**3. Diagnostic cone biopsy**–Following expert colposcopic evaluation, diagnostic cone biopsy of the cervix (Fig 47–3) is indicated (1) if the lesion extends into the cervical canal beyond the view afforded by the colposcope (unsatisfactory colposcopic examination); (2) if there is a significant discrepancy between the histologic diagnosis of the directed biopsy specimen and the cytologic examination; or (3) if microinvasive carcinoma is diagnosed or suspected on the basis of a colposcopically directed punch biopsy.

## Treatment

CIN I regresses in at least 30% of patients and may be followed closely with repeat evaluations every 3 months if the patient appears reliable for follow-up or does not have any risk factors for rapid progression (such as immunosuppression; see Special Situations). However, most CIN lesions, regardless of the degree of severity, are treated immediately after diagnosis. Treatment for cervical dysplasia is essentially destructive and involves freezing, vaporization, or excision depending on the location of the lesion. If the lesion is confined to the exocervix, treatment with cryotherapy, laser ablation, or a superficial excision by the loop electrosurgical excision procedure (LEEP) is appropriate. If the lesion extends into the endocervical canal, the endocervical curettage contains dysplastic epithelium, or the colposcopic examination is otherwise unsatisfactory, the endocervical canal must be included in the treatment by a deep LEEP or cone biopsy (Fig 47–4).

**A. Cryotherapy:** In cryotherapy, an office procedure, nitrous oxide is used as the refrigerant and anesthesia is not required. The cryoprobe is positioned on the exocervix and an ice ball must extend at least 5 mm onto colposcopically normal cervix. If the lesion is 1.5 times greater than the surface area of the tip, 2 freeze cycles of 3 minutes each should be performed.

Side effects include mild uterine cramping, facial flushing, and a watery discharge for up to 3 weeks. Complications include cervical stenosis with possible increase in dysmenorrhea, and rarely pyometria. Follow-up colposcopic examinations can be unsatisfactory because of the inability to visualize the squamocolumnar junction. It is important to evaluate the endocervical canal with curettage at least once a year.

**B. Carbon Dioxide Laser:** Carbon dioxide ($CO_2$) laser can be used either to ablate the transformation zone or as a tool for cone biopsies. The procedure requires either local or general anesthesia. Laser destroys tissue with a very narrow zone of injury around the treated tissue. For exocervical lesions, the complete transformation zone is vaporized to a depth of 7 mm. Dysplastic lesions can extend into glands which can reach a maximum depth of 7 mm. Laser is considered more effective than cryotherapy for completely destroying these lesions. Bleeding that requires reexamination can occur in 1% of patients. Laser is less likely to cause cervical stenosis and follow up colposcopy is rarely unsatisfactory.

**C. Loop Electrosurgical Excision Procedure (LEEP):** LEEP uses a small fine wire loop attached to an electrosurgical generator. Various sizes of wire loop are available. LEEP is performed under local anesthesia using lidocaine and a vasoconstrictor such as 1:100,000 epinephrine. An insulated speculum to prevent conduction of electricity, a grounding pad, and a vacuum to remove the plume are necessary. The anesthetic is injected into the cervix to the planned depth of the excision. With this powerful technique, it is very easy to remove more cervical tissue than is necessary. Complications include cervical stenosis, cervical amputation, entering the cul-de-sac if the excision is taken too deeply, bleeding, and infection.

**D. Cone Biopsy:** Cervical cone biopsy may be performed under local or general anesthesia. Either a scalpel ("cold knife") or a $CO_2$ laser can be used. Complications include bleeding, infection, cervical stenosis, and cervical incompetence.

## Follow-Up

Most treatment failures are diagnosed within the first year after therapy. Therefore, careful examination should be performed, with Pap smears every 3 months and endocervical curettages every 6 months if the endocervix was involved. Treatment of recurrent dysplasia follows the same guidelines outlined in Figure 47–4. If a woman has completed childbearing, recurrent dysplasia can be treated by a simple hysterectomy after invasion has been ruled out. Women with a history of cervical dysplasia have a higher incidence of vaginal dysplasia. These women continue to need yearly Pap smears after hysterectomy.

## SPECIAL SITUATIONS

**A. In Utero Diethylstilbestrol (DES) Exposure:** Women with DES exposure have an increased incidence of cervical dysplasia of two to four times that of the general population. Some authorities recommend yearly or biennial colposcopic examinations regardless of the Pap smear findings.

**B. Pregnancy:** Abnormal Pap smears in pregnancy should be evaluated immediately by colposcopy to rule out an invasive lesion. Although the gravid cervix is more vascular, directed exocervical biopsies can be performed safely. Endocervical curettages are not performed in pregnancy because of the potential risk of abortion and infection. After the diagnosis of dysplasia has been established, the patient can be carefully followed with serial colposcopic examinations and treated postpartum. If an invasive lesion cannot be ruled out, a cone biopsy must be performed. Complications of a cone biopsy in pregnancy include abortion, hemorrhage, infection, and incompetent cervix.

**C. Immunosuppresion:** Women who are immunosuppressed, such as those on immunosuppressive agents after organ transplant or for autoimmune diseases, have an increased incidence of lower genital tract dysplasia. Women who are seropositive for the human immunodeficiency virus (HIV) are at increased risk for dysplasia. Some authorities recommend yearly routine colposcopy for these women because of concerns of an increased risk of false-negative Pap smears secondary to obscuring inflammation. In 1993, the Centers for Disease Control added invasive cervical cancer to the list of acquired immunodeficiency syndrome (AIDS) defining events.

## CANCER OF THE CERVIX

### Essentials of Diagnosis

- Abnormal uterine bleeding and vaginal discharge.
- Cervical lesion possibly visible on inspection as a tumor or ulceration; cancer within the cervical canal possibly occult.
- Vaginal cytology, usually positive (must be confirmed by biopsy).

### General Considerations

Cancer of the cervix is the seventh most common type of cancer after breast, colorectal, lung, endometrial, and ovarian cancer, and lymphoma. In 1992, 13,500 new cases of cervical cancer and 4500 deaths were reported. The incidence of cervical cancer has continued to decline since 1947, and partial credit can be given to aggressive screening programs. The average age at diagnosis of patients with cervical cancer is 45, but the disease can occur in the second decade of life and during pregnancy. Over 95% of patients with early cancer of the cervix can be cured.

### Etiology & Epidemiology

The cause of cervical cancer is not known, but certain predisposing factors are recognized.

Sexual activity seems to be positively correlated with the disease, and coitus at an early age, especially within 1 year of menarche. The number of sexual partners is also a highly significant risk factor. Cancer of the cervix is 4 times as frequent in prostitutes as in other women and is unusual in celibate women.

Cervical cancer occurs more frequently in North African women than in European and American Jewish women. It appears to be an independent risk factor in women of lower socioeconomic backgrounds.

HPV types 16 and 18 are strongly associated with malignant cervical transformation. Viral DNA sequences have been found in dysplastic and malignant cells of the cervix. Other associated risk factors are tobacco use, oral contraceptive use, a history of herpes simplex infection, an immunocompromised host, and a high-risk male sexual partner (male who has had multiple sexual partners, a history of sexually transmitted diseases, especially HPV, a previous sexual partner with cervical dysplasia or cancer, or a personal history of penile cancer).

### Pathogenesis & Natural History

Incipient cancer of the cervix is a slowly developing process. Most cervical cancers probably begin as a dysplastic change (see previous section) with gradual progression over a period of several years to a preinvasive form: CIS. At least 90% of squamous cell carcinomas of the cervix develop in the intraepithelial layers, almost always at the squamocolumnar junction of the cervix either on the portio vaginalis of the cervix or slightly higher in the endocervical canal (the transformation zone). In most instances, the preinvasive form of the disease remains static for another 7–10 years. During this time, however, it may extend over the surface to involve larger areas of squamous (and columnar) epithelium. Eventually the dysplasia breaks free of its restraints and invades the subjacent cervical stroma.

Early stromal invasion (stage IA) to a depth of 1–3 mm* below the basement membrane is a localized process, provided there is no pathologic evidence of confluence or vascular space involvement. Penetration of the stroma beyond this point carries an increased risk of lymphatic or hematogenous metastasis. The tumor also spreads by direct extension to the parametrium. When the lymphatics are involved, tumor cells are carried to the regional pelvic lymph nodes (parametrial, hypogastric, obturator, external iliac, and sacral) (Fig 47–9). The more pleomorphic or extensive the local disease, the greater the likelihood of lymph node involvement. Squamous cell carcinoma clinically confined to the cervix involves the regional pelvic lymph nodes in 15–20% of cases. When the cancer involves the parametrium (stage IIB), tumor cells can be found in the pelvic lymph nodes in 30–40% and in the para-aortic nodes in about 10% of cases. The more advanced the local disease, the greater the likelihood of distant metastases. The para-aortic nodes are involved in about 45% of patients with stage III disease.

The liver is the most common site of blood-borne metastasis, but the tumor may involve the lungs, brain, bones, adrenal glands, spleen, or pancreas.

Death can occur from uremia, pulmonary embolism, or hemorrhage from direct extension of tumor into blood vessels. Life-threatening sepsis from complications of pyelonephritis or vesicovaginal and rectovaginal fistulas is possible. Large bowel obstruction from direct extension of tumor into the rectosigmoid can be the terminal event. Pain from perineural extension is a significant management problem of advanced disease.

## Pathology

About 70–80% of cervical carcinomas are squamous cell; the remainder are composed of various types of adenocarcinomas, adenosquamous carcinomas, and undifferentiated carcinomas.

**A. Squamous Cell (Epidermoid) Carcinomas:** Cervical squamous cell carcinomas have been classified according to the predominant cell type: large cell nonkeratinizing, large cell keratinizing, and small cell carcinomas. The large cell nonkeratinizing variety is reputed to carry the best prognosis (68.3%), whereas the small cell nonkeratinizing tumor has the lowest 5-year survival rate (20%). However, other researchers have not found a significant difference in prognosis among those with the different types of cervical squamous tumors.

**Verrucous carcinoma–**Verrucous carcinoma, which has been associated with HPV 6, is a rare subtype of well-differentiated squamous carcinoma. It is

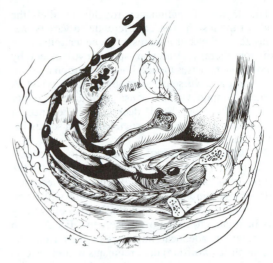

**Figure 47–9.** Lymphatic spread of carcinoma of the cervix.

a slow-growing, locally invasive neoplasm. Histologically, this tumor is composed of well-differentiated squamous cells with frond-like papillae and little apparent stromal invasion, but it is potentially lethal. Accelerated growth and metastases may occur after radiation and wide resection is considered the treatment of choice.

The most widely used classification system is based on the degree of differentiation, which may be expressed more specifically as follows:

**Well-differentiated (grade I)–**Squamous cells demonstrate well-defined intercellular bridges and cytoplasmic keratohyalin in the well-differentiated variety. Epithelial pearls are a common feature of this type of tumor, and mitotic figures are not too numerous—fewer than 2 mitoses per high-power field—with minimal variation in the size and shape of tumor cells.

**Moderately differentiated (grade II)–**This is an intermediate group. Varieties of all 3 patterns may be found in the same tumor, rendering accuracy of tumor grading on the basis of degree of differentiation somewhat difficult. There are infrequent epithelial pearls, moderate keratinization, occasional intercellular bridges, 2–4 mitoses per high-power field, and moderate variation in size and shape of tumor cells.

**Poor differentiated (grade III)–**Poorly differentiated cancers present nests and cords of small, deeply stained cells barely resembling mature squamous epithelium. These have scant cytoplasm surrounding hyperchromatic nuclei and show little tendency to differentiate. There are no epithelial pearls, slight keratinization, no intercellular bridges, more than 4 mitoses per high-power field, often marked variation in size and shape of tumor cells, occasional small, elongated, closely packed tumor cells, and numerous giant cells.

---

*Currently, FIGO staging for early stromal invasion (stage IA) accepts penetration to a depth of less than 5 mm, but the GOG (Gynecology Oncology Group) accepts penetration only to the depths of less than 3 mm.

The degree of malignancy roughly parallels the grade of the lesion. The undifferentiated variety metastasizes earlier but also responds better initially to radiation therapy. Vascular space involvement by tumor cells increases the likelihood of lymph node involvement and worsens the prognosis for survival. A marked lymphocytic response surrounding tumor cells, on the other hand, decreases the chance of lymph node spread and is associated with a somewhat better prognosis.

**B. Adenocarcinoma:** Adenocarcinoma of the cervix is derived from the glandular elements of the cervix. It is composed of tall, columnar secretory cells arranged in an adenomatous pattern with scant supporting stroma. The so-called clear cell variety may be related to in utero exposure to DES. A much less common adenocarcinoma is derived from the mesonephric (wolffian) duct remnants within the cervix. In these, the cells are small, cuboid, and irregular and the glandular pattern less well defined. Adenoma malignum or minimal deviation adenocarcinoma is an extremely well-differentiated adenocarcinoma that may be difficult to recognize as a malignant process. It has been associated with Peutz-Jeghers syndrome. Another uncommon variant of adenocarcinoma is adenoid cystic carcinoma. This lesion is considered more aggressive than most cervical adenocarcinomas and occurs in women in their sixth and seventh decades. It should not be confused with adenoid basal carcinomas which have an indolent growth pattern.

Adenocarcinoma is graded as well differentiated, moderately well differentiated, and poorly differentiated. When the initial growth of adenocarcinoma of the cervix is within the endocervical canal and the exocervix appears normal, this lesion may not be diagnosed until it is advanced and ulcerative.

**C. Mixed Epithelial Carcinoma:** Adenosquamous carcinomas contain an admixture of malignant squamous and glandular cells. Glassy cell carcinoma is a poorly differentiated form of adenosquamous carcinoma and is considered to have an extremely aggressive course. It accounts for about 1–2% of cervical cancers. Another poor prognosis variant is the mucoepidermoid carcinomas, which contain mainly malignant squamous cells with interspersed mucin-secreting cells. Synchronous adenocarcinomas and squamous cell carcinomas that invade each other are called **collision tumors.**

**D. Neuroendocrine Carcinomas:** Carcinoid tumors, arising from the argyrophil cells of the endocervical epithelium, are malignant but have not been associated with the carcinoid syndrome. Small cell carcinoma can be well differentiated or poorly differentiated. The poorly differentiated form of tumor resembles the oat cell tumor of the lung and has a worse prognosis than the well-differentiated form. These tumors need to be distinguished from small cell type of squamous tumors by immunohistochemical staining for argyrophilic granules.

**E. Other Malignant Tumors:** Direct extension of metastatic tumors to the cervix include those originating from the endometrium, rectum, and bladder. Lymphatic or vascular metastases occur less often but are associated with ovarian and endometrial carcinomas. Sarcomas, lymphomas, choriocarcinomas, and melanomas are encountered rarely in the cervix. Pure cervical sarcomas are rare tumors arising from those elements of the paramesonephric duct that differentiate into various mesodermal tissue—connective tissue, cartilage, smooth muscle, skeletal muscle, and others. The following types are recognized: (1) leiomyosarcoma, (2) mixed mesodermal tumors (including carcinosarcoma and sarcoma botryoides), (3) stromal cell sarcoma, (4) lymphosarcoma, and (5) angiosarcoma. These tumors may spread by direct extension or by lymphatic or hematogenous routes. Metastases appear in the lungs, brain, liver, kidney, and bone. Surgical excision is the best treatment. Leiomyosarcomas that arise in cervical myomas have the best prognosis, with 5-year survival rates of more than 50%. The remaining types of sarcomas have dismal prognoses. Most patients are postmenopausal, and the majority succumb within 2 years.

## Clinical Staging

It is important to estimate the extent of the disease not only to aid in making the prognosis but also to plan treatment. Clinical staging also affords a means of comparing methods of therapy.

The International Classification adopted by the International Federation of Gynecology and Obstetrics (FIGO) is the most widely used staging system (Table 47–1).

## Clinical Findings

**A. Symptoms and Signs:** Intermenstrual bleeding is the most common symptom of invasive cancer and may take the form of a blood-stained leukorrheal discharge, scant spotting, or frank bleeding. Leukorrhea, usually sanguineous or purulent, odorous, and nonpruritic, usually is present. A history of postcoital bleeding may be elicited on specific questioning.

Pelvic pain, often unilateral and radiating to the hip or thigh, is a manifestation of advanced disease, as is the involuntary loss of urine or feces through the vagina, a sign of fistula formation. Weakness, weight loss, and anemia are characteristic of the late stages of the disease, although acute blood loss and anemia may occur in an ulcerating stage I lesion.

In stage IA tumors, there are no symptoms (preclinical carcinoma) and only a remote chance of metastases. However, as the local disease progresses, physical signs appear. Infiltrative cancer produces enlargement, irregularity, and a firm consistency of the cervix and eventually of the adjacent parametria.

**Table 47–1.** International classification of cancer of the cervix (FIGO).

**Preinvasive carcinoma**

| | |
|---|---|
| Stage 0 | Carcinoma in situ, intraepithelial carcinoma. |

**Invasive carcinoma**

| | |
|---|---|
| Stage I | Strictly confined to the cervix. |
| IA | Preclinical carcinomas of the cervix (those diagnosed only by microscopy). |
| IA1 | Minimal microscopically evident stromal invasion. |
| IA2 | Lesions detected microscopically that can be measured. The upper limit of the measurement should not show a depth of invasion of > 5 mm from the base of the epithelium, either surface or glandular, and the horizontal spread must not exceed 7 mm. |
| IB | Lesions of greater dimensions than stage IA2 lesions, whether seen clinically or not. |
| Stage II | Carcinoma extends beyond the cervix but has not extended onto the pelvic wall. The carcinoma involves the vagina, but not the lower third. |
| IIA | No obvious parametrial involvement. |
| IIB | Obvious parametrial involvement. |
| Stage III | Carcinoma has extended onto the pelvic wall. On rectal examination, there is no cancer-free space between the tumor and the pelvic wall. The tumor involves the lower third of the vagina. All cases with hydronephrosis or nonfunctioning kidney. |
| IIIA | No extension onto the pelvic wall, but involvement of lower third of vagina. |
| IIIB | Extension onto the pelvic wall and/or hydronephrosis or nonfunctioning kidney due to tumor. |
| Stage IV | Carcinoma extended beyond the true pelvis or clinically involving the mucosa of the bladder or rectum. |
| IVA | Spread of growth to adjacent organs (that is, rectum or bladder with positive biopsy from these organs). |
| IVB | Spread of growth to distant organs. |

An exophytic growth generally appears as a friable, bleeding, cauliflower-like lesion of the portio vaginalis. Ulceration may be the primary manifestation of invasive carcinoma; in the early stages the change often is superficial, so that it may resemble cervical ectopy or chronic cervicitis. With further progression of the disease, the ulcer becomes deeper and necrotic, with indurated edges and a friable, bleeding surface. The adjacent vaginal fornices may become involved next. Eventually, extensive parametrial involvement by the infiltrative process may produce a nodular thickening of the uterosacral and cardinal ligaments with resultant loss of mobility and fixation of the cervix.

**B. X-Ray Findings:** Magnetic resonance imaging (MRI), computed tomography (CT) scan, or pelvic lymphangiography may demonstrate involvement of the pelvic or periaortic lymph nodes. Chest x-rays are indicated. A significant finding on intravenous urography in advanced cervical cancer is terminal ureteral obstruction. This produces hydroureter,

hydronephrosis, and, if complete obstruction occurs, MRI may be helpful in defining the extent of the more advanced lesions.

**C. Laboratory Findings:**

**1. Cytologic (Pap smear) studies**–Preclinical lesions usually are initially diagnosed by cytologic examination or colposcopy (see following text). Suspect or positive Pap smear calls for further investigation (see section on dysplasia); however, about 6% of cytologic smears are falsely negative.

Because of the presence of inflammatory cells and the failure of cells to shed in large numbers, false-negative smears are more common in invasive than in intraepithelial neoplasms. Moreover, in an area of invasive cancer, deficient blood supply or infection causes cytolysis. Clinical signs and symptoms suggestive of cancer call for continued investigation even if cytologic examination is negative.

Cytologic study and biopsy of suspect areas have greatly facilitated the early diagnosis and cure of cancer of the cervix.

**D. Special Examination:**

**1. Biopsy**–Because of the failure of malignant cells to desquamate and because of the obscuring effect of inflammatory cells, it is not uncommon for an invasive carcinoma of the cervix to exist despite a negative cytologic smear. Any suspicious lesion of the cervix should be sampled by adequate biopsy, regardless of cytologic examination result. Biopsy of any Schiller-positive areas or of any ulcerative, granular, nodular, or papillary lesion provide the diagnosis in most cases. Colposcopically directed biopsies with endocervical curettage or conization of the cervix may be required when repeated, confirmed reports of suspicious or probable exfoliated carcinoma cells are made by the pathologist and a visible or palpable lesion of the cervix is not evident.

**2. Colposcopy**–Early invasive carcinoma in a field of CIN should be suspected when the surface capillaries are markedly irregular, appearing as commas, corkscrews, and spaghetti-shaped capillaries. Directed biopsy of these areas often show microscopic evidence of early stromal invasion. Frank invasion frequently produces ulceration, and this is seen colposcopically as a markedly irregular surface with a waxy, yellowish surface and numerous bizarre, atypical blood vessels. Bleeding may occur also after slight irritation. Once carcinomatous invasion begins, ulceration and spotting occur. By the time sanguineous vaginal discharge or abnormal bleeding occurs, penetration of the malignant tumor into the substance of the cervix is certain.

Colposcopically directed biopsies have been useful in pinpointing the most severe epithelial change in a given cervix, and use of the colposcope, combined with light curettage of the endocervix (ECC), may abolish the need for cone biopsy in certain circumstances.

**3. Conization**–When the biopsy reveals CIS and invasion cannot be ruled out or when there are no suspicious areas on the portio vaginalis, conization of the cervix should be performed to determine the presence or absence of invasion. If a cervical biopsy shows microinvasive cancer (less than 3 mm of invasion), a cone biopsy is necessary to rule out deeper invasion before definitive therapy can be planned. This is usually performed in conjunction with a D&C, which is performed after conization to avoid denuding the cervix of malignant surface epithelium. The specimen should be properly marked for the pathologist, eg, with a pin or small suture, so that the area of involvement can be specifically localized in relation to the circumference and the upper and lower margins of the cervix.

Conization for a lesion grossly suggestive of invasive cancer only delays the initiation of appropriate radiation therapy and predisposes the patient to serious pelvic infections in the event that radical surgery is chosen as definitive therapy. The diagnosis of such a lesion can almost always be confirmed by simple cervical biopsy. An effective instrument for this purpose is the Tischler cervical biopsy forceps (Fig 47–1).

**4. Staging**–Cervical cancer is staged by clinical examination, evaluation of the bladder, ureters, and rectum. If the lesion is clearly confined to the cervix by office examination, only chest x-ray and evaluation of the ureters by intravenous pyelogram or CT scan with intravenous contrast is necessary to assign the stage. If it is not possible to evaluate the parametria in the office, cystoscopy and proctoscopy examinations with the patient under anesthesia are necessary. Although CT scan, MRI, or periaortic or scalene lymph node biopsies to evaluate lymphatic spread may be important in treatment planning, this information does not change the stage of disease.

## Differential Diagnosis

A variety of lesions of the cervix may be confused with cancer. Entities that must sometimes be ruled out include cervical ectopy, acute or chronic cervicitis, condyloma acuminatum, cervical tuberculosis, ulceration secondary to sexually transmitted disease (syphilis, granuloma inguinale, lymphogranuloma venereum, chancroid), abortion of a cervical pregnancy, metastatic choriocarcinoma, and rare lesions such as those of actinomycosis or schistosomiasis. Histopathologic examination is usually definitive.

## Complications

The complications of cervical cancer, for the most part, are those related to tumor size or invasion, necrosis of the tumor, infection, and metastatic disease (Figs 47–9, 47–10). There are also problems pertaining to treatment of the disease (eg, radical surgery or radiation therapy). (See Treatment, below.)

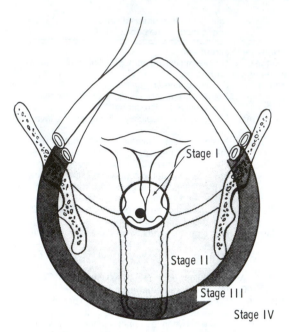

**Figure 47–10.** Staging of metastases of cervical cancer (corresponding to the International Federation of Gynecology and Obstetrics [FIGO] Classification; see Table 47–1.)

## Prevention

The causes of cervical cancer are unknown. Nevertheless, chastity is associated with almost total freedom from cervical cancers that are associated with HPV infections. Theoretically, carcinoma of the cervix (and penis), particularly before a person reaches middle age, may be considered to be a carcinogen-induced neoplasm involving intercourse.

Prevention of morbidity and death from cervical cancer largely involves early recognition and treatment. Risk factors must be recognized, ie, early sexual experience and promiscuity or a history of cervical dysplasia. Universal cytologic screening of all postpubertal women must be continued on a regular annual basis. Particular attention should be paid to women in the lower socioeconomic groups and those who are sexually active. Women with cervical dysplasia should be treated and followed up closely. (See Fig 47–4). Since inflammation and vaginitis may obscure a dysplastic or invasive lesion on Pap smear, these conditions should be treated and the Pap smear repeated.

Sexual abstinence is an effective but impractical prophylactic measure. Education of young women and men about risk factors and information about the association of smoking with the development of cervical cancers (as well as others) is crucial.

## Treatment

**A. General Measures:** Vaginal, urinary, and

pelvic infections should be eradicated before surgery or irradiation is initiated. Anemia must be corrected and nutrition improved. The debilitated patient should be kept in the hospital for supportive therapy during x-ray and radium treatment; if exposures are poorly tolerated, discharged patients should be readmitted.

Pain may be controlled with analgesics such as aspirin with codeine. Give diphenoxylate with atropine (Lomotil) as necessary for diarrhea. For urinary frequency and dysuria, give a bladder sedative mixture.

Plain warm water douches are permitted when necessary during x-ray therapy and after radium treatments for comfort and hygiene.

### B. Surgical Measures:

**1. Microinvasive carcinoma**–When thorough pathologic examination of a conization specimen reveals questionable invasion or early stromal penetration to a depth of no more than 3 mm and no confluence of tumor or vascular space involvement, simple or extended hysterectomy (without lymph node or extensive ureteral or bladder dissection) should be curative. Conization may be considered therapeutic in very carefully selected patients who strongly desire preservation of reproductive function. Such relatively conservative therapy is improper if the margins of the specimen are not adequate, if the tumor penetrates to a depth of more than 3 mm, if its lateral spread is greater than 4 mm, or if tumor cells are found in vascular (lymphatic or capillary-like) spaces.

**2. Invasive carcinoma**–There are 2 effective methods for the treatment of invasive carcinoma: radiation therapy and radical surgery. Radiation therapy (discussed separately below) is more widely used throughout the world because it is applicable to all primary cervical cancers, whereas radical hysterectomy is definitive only in stage I to stage IIA lesions. The overall 5-year cure rates for surgery and for radiation therapy in operable patients are approximately equal. The rate of severe complications for both surgery and radiation is 1%. Irradiation may be used either as a curative or a palliative measure.

There are specific circumstances in which the surgical approach to carcinoma of the cervix may be indicated or preferred. Radical hysterectomy may be considered in the young woman in whom preservation of the ovaries is important. Carcinoma of the cervix metastatic to the ovaries is rare in stage I–IIA patients. Moreover, because much of the ovarian blood supply is directly from the aorta, the ovaries may be detached and displaced into the abdomen during surgery without compromising the radical nature of the operation. Surgery is also more appropriate in sexually active women with early stage disease since radiation causes vaginal stenosis and atrophy. Radical surgery may be better for patients who are poor candidates for radiation therapy (eg, those with chronic salpingitis, extensive bowel adhesions from endome-triosis or previous peritonitis, diverticulitis, or ulcerative colitis); for those who cannot tolerate radiation therapy; and for those whose tumor demonstrates a poor response to radiation.

Finally, surgery is the only effective method of treating cancers that persist or recur centrally following adequate radiation therapy. In such instances, pelvic exenteration is often necessary to make certain that all the cancer has been removed.

The surgical treatment for invasive cancer of the cervix consists of one of the following: (1) extended hysterectomy with pelvic lymph node dissection (abdominal or vaginal); (2) radical hysterectomy with pelvic lymph node dissection; (3) extrafascial hysterectomy after radiation therapy for stage Ib barrel-shaped carcinomas; or (4)pelvic exenteration––anterior, posterior, or total.

**a. Extended hysterectomy**–Extended hysterectomy involves removal of the uterus, tubes, and ovaries together with most of the parametrial tissues and the upper vagina. Surgery involves dissection of the ureters from the paracervical structures so that the ligaments supporting the uterus and upper vagina can be removed. When the operation is done vaginally, a deep Schuchardt (paravaginal) incision is required for exposure. Extended hysterectomy is required for exposure. Extended hysterectomy is performed primarily for the removal of minimally invasive lesions (stage IA1) in which the chances of lymph node involvement are extremely small.

**b. Radical hysterectomy and node dissection**–Radical hysterectomy (Meigs or Okabayashi) with pelvic lymph node dissection is the customary surgical procedure for invasive cancer limited to the cervix (stages I and II). This operation requires careful preoperative evaluation and preparation of the patient. The operation is technically difficult and should be performed only by those experienced in radical pelvic surgery. The so-called Wertheim operation, initiated by Clark but popularized and expanded by Meigs and modified by Okabayashi and others, involves en bloc dissection with careful removal of all of the recognizable pelvic lymph nodes together with wide removal of the uterus, tubes and ovaries, supporting ligaments, and upper vagina. Obviously, the operation involves extensive dissection of the ureters and the bladder. The 5-year arrest rate of cervical cancer by this operation is as good as with radiation therapy in selected cases.

Obesity, advanced age, and serious medical problems, which are likely to complicate surgery or convalescence, greatly reduce the number of candidates for elective cancer surgery. Radical hysterectomy and pelvic lymphadenectomy are often used as the definitive method of treatment of cancer of the cervix if (1) the patient is pregnant; (2) large uterine or adnexal tumors are present; (3) the patient has chronic salpingitis; (4) the small or large bowel adheres to the uterus; (5) the patient is under 35 years of age and desires ovarian conservation; or (6) the patient refuses or abandons radiation but is a good surgical risk.

In a small proportion of patients with cancer of the cervix treated initially with radium and x-ray, recurrence or persistence of the cancer will be noted within the cervix or vaginal vault. A radical hysterectomy and lymph node resection (or pelvic exenteration) may be indicated for patients in this group because of the ineffectiveness and serious hazards of repeated irradiation.

**c. Extrafascial hysterectomy after radiation for barrel-shaped lesions–**Stage Ib cervical lesions that measure more than 3–5 cm have been described as bulky or barrel-shaped. These tumors may not be adequately treated by either surgery or radiation alone. Because of their size, there may not be adequate surgical margins. Radiation may not completely encompass such large tumors with resulting persistent central disease. Pelvic recurrence has been reduced from 19–2% by the combination of radiation therapy followed by extrafascial hysterectomy. However, the rate of severe complications when both treatment modalities are used increases to over 5%.

**d. Pelvic exenteration–**This operation was popularized by Brunschwig as a method of salvaging patients with central recurrences following radiation therapy (or radical hysterectomy) for cancer of the cervix. Pelvic exenteration is one of the most formidable of all gynecologic operations and requires removal of the bladder or rectum, the vagina, and perhaps even the vulva, along with radical hysterectomy and pelvic lymph node dissection. Urinary diversion necessitates the creation of a reservoir from an isolated loop of intestine (eg, ileum or transverse colon), one end of which is brought through the anterior abdominal wall. A sigmoid colostomy serves for the passage of feces. The vagina can be reconstructed using bilateral gracilis myocutaneous flaps. In the appropriate settings, a continent urostomy or low rectal reanastomosis or both can be performed.

Because of the high surgical morbidity and mortality rates, stringent criteria are necessary to justify these procedures. Pelvic exenteration should be reserved primarily for problems that cannot be effectively managed in any other manner. In essence, this means (1) a biopsy-proved persistence or recurrence of cervical cancer following an adequate course of radiation therapy or radical surgery in which the recurrent or persistent tumor occupies the central portion of the pelvis (without metastases) and is completely removable; and (2) a patient who is able to cope with the urinary and fecal stomas in the abdomen created by the operation. Both psychologic and physical preparation of the patient for this operation and its aftermath are of vital importance. This means making the patient's physical condition as favorable as possible by restoring good nutrition and normal blood volume, preparation of the bowel with low-residue diet and antibiotics, correction of anemia, and control of diabetes. The extent of the procedure is determined by the direction of tumor growth in the pelvis.

Because of the extreme difficulties encountered in making an accurate assessment, even at the time of surgical exploration, total exenteration rather than partial (anterior or posterior) exenteration has been advocated as being the definitive procedure in a critical clinical situation.

**4. Complications of radical surgery–**The operative mortality rate in radical hysterectomy with pelvic lymph node dissection has been reduced to less than 1%. The most common complication is fistula formation; ureterovaginal fistula is the most common type (1–2%), followed by vesicovaginal and rectovaginal fistulas. Modifications in technique to preserve the blood supply to the distal ureter and bladder and the use of prolonged catheter drainage of the urinary bladder (6–8 weeks) have reduced the incidence of urinary tract fistulas from 10% to less than 3%.

Other complications are urinary tract infections, bladder atony, lymphocysts in the retroperitoneal space, wound sepsis, dehiscence, thromboembolic disease, ileus, postoperative hemorrhage, and intestinal obstruction.

The surgical mortality rate from pelvic exenteration has been reduced from about 25% to about 2.5%. Bowel obstruction is a common complication. Electrolyte disturbances, leakage of urine from the urinary diversion, ureteral stricture, pyelonephritis, hemorrhage, sepsis, thromboembolism, enteric fistulas, stomal retraction, and other complications may also occur.

**C. Radiation Therapy:** See Chapter 51.

**D. Chemotherapy:** The use of chemotherapeutic agents in the treatment of cervical carcinoma has been discouraging. This is partly because most patients who may be candidates for this type of treatment have far-advanced cancer that has already failed to respond to radical surgery or radiation therapy. As a result of the neoplastic process or because of prior therapy, there is often diminished vascularity of the pelvic tissues causing impaired pelvic vascular perfusion. Furthermore, there may be ureteral obstruction causing decreased renal function or compromised bone marrow from radiation therapy. Both severely limit effective chemotherapy.

Doxorubicin, bleomycin, and cisplatin are the most active chemotherapeutic agents against squamous cell cancers of the cervix. Initial reports from Japanese investigators described complete remission rates in 65% of patients who had received a combination of bleomycin and mitomycin, but these results have not been reproduced in the USA, where complete remission rates have ranged from nil to 15%. Combinations of agents with methotrexate have not added to the number of responders, and this drug is very toxic in patients with poor renal function.

To date, the best results appear to be achieved with the use of cisplatin alone in doses of 50 mg/m$^2$ every

3 weeks with response rates of 20%. Most responses are short-lived and are accompanied by considerable toxicity. Bleomycin given by infusion over a period of 4 days is less toxic and is associated with a longer duration of response than when given in twice-weekly injections, but pulmonary toxicity (respiratory failure) is a problem when more than 2 cycles are administered. Complete remissions ranging from 8 to 21 months have been reported in several patients receiving cisplatin, vincristine, bleomycin, and mitomycin. However, a randomized trial comparing this regimen with single-agent cisplatin showed no difference in response. Ifosfamide and dibromodulcitol have shown response rates of 29% in early trials of advanced squamous cell carcinoma of the cervix. These drugs are being studied in combination with platinum agents.

Although there is a theoretic advantage to the direct intra-arterial administration of chemotherapeutic agents in advanced pelvic disease, this route has not been particularly helpful in clinical practice and has been accompanied by considerable morbidity.

Chemotherapy as a radiation sensitizer or enhancer has been evaluated for locally advanced disease. Hydoxyurea has been shown to enhance the action of radiation in both nonrandomized and randomized trials. Radiation with concurrent hydroxyurea or with cisplatin and 5-fluorouracil in advanced local disease is being studied.

## Management of Carcinoma of the Cervix During Pregnancy

Abnormal cytologic examination in pregnancy calls for immediate colposcopic evaluation and any other diagnostic modalities necessary to exclude invasive cancer.

Invasive carcinoma of the cervix in pregnancy is found more frequently in areas where routine prenatal cytologic examination is done; the incidence may be as high as 1 in 350 pregnancies depending on the population sampled. As is the case with nonpregnant patients also, the principal symptom is bleeding, but the diagnosis is frequently missed because the bleeding is assumed to be related to the pregnancy rather than to cancer. The possibility of cancer must be kept in mind. Cervical biopsy will lead to the correct diagnosis.

Radiation therapy may be used in treating invasive cancers of the cervix discovered during pregnancy. In the first trimester, irradiation may be carried out with the expectation of spontaneous abortion. The dosage is 6000 cGy of x-radiation to the pelvis through each of 4 ports. Concurrently, 2 courses of intra- and paracervical radium are given.

In the second trimester, interruption of the pregnancy by hysterotomy prior to radiation therapy is preferred, although some physicians advocate proceeding with treatment and ignoring the pregnancy, again awaiting spontaneous evacuation of the uterus. Another method is to place intra- and contracervical radium and then, 7–10 days later, perform an abdominal (classic) hysterotomy. Two weeks after surgery, 6000 cGy of x-radiation is begun, and a further course of intra- and contracervical radiation is administered during the last week of external therapy.

In the third trimester, the decision must be made whether to allow the pregnancy to proceed to viability (28–32 weeks' gestation) before performing a cesarean section and then instituting radiation therapy. In 7–10 days, 6000 cGy of external x-radiation is given, followed by 2 courses of intra- and paracervical radium 1 week apart, the first during the last 7–10 days of x-ray therapy.

Radical surgery may be chosen in all 3 trimesters for stage I and IIA lesions because it simultaneously eliminates the pregnancy and the cancer.

## Palliative Care of Cervical Cancer

About 50% of patients cannot be cured of cervical cancer and thus are candidates for management of persistent or recurrent disease. The majority of these women would not benefit from pelvic exenteration operations. Eventually, they develop symptoms related principally to the site and extent of the malignant disease. Ulceration of the cervix and adjacent vagina produces a foul-smelling discharge. Tissue necrosis and slough may initiate life-threatening hemorrhage. If the bladder or rectum is involved in the tissue breakdown, fistulas result in incontinence of urine and feces. Pain due to involvement of the lumbosacral plexus, soft tissues of the pelvis, or bone is frequently encountered in advanced disease. Ureteral compression leading to hydronephrosis and, if bilateral, to renal failure and uremia is a common terminal event.

The expert management of the patient with incurable cancer is an integral part of cancer therapy. The comfort and well-being of the patient can be considerably enhanced even though cure cannot be effected.

A foul, purulent discharge may be ameliorated by astringent douches (potassium permanganate, 1:4000) and antimicrobial vaginal creams (eg, sulfathiazole, sulfacetamide, and benzoylsulfanilamide cream [Sultrin Cream]) and nitrofurazone suppositories. Necrotic ulcers may be treated with enzymatic debridement (fibrinolysin and desoxyribonuclease, combined [bovine] ointment [Elase]), or the necrotic tissue may be removed by coating the normal vaginal mucosa with petrolatum and packing the ulcer with small cotton balls wrung out in acetone and left in place for several minutes. Occasionally, ulcerated areas heal with the administration of high-dose estrogen therapy (DES, 100 mg daily), although this may cause some nausea.

Hemorrhage from the vagina often can be controlled by packing the area with gauze impregnated with a hemostatic agent. Exposed, bleeding vessels should be ligated. Embolization of the pelvic blood vessels by an interventional radiologist often controls intractable bleeding and may abolish the need for a major operative procedure. Rarely, it may be necessary to bilaterally ligate the hypogastric arteries to control an exsanguinating vaginal hemorrhage.

Pain relief may be afforded by the liberal use of nonsteroidal antiinflammatory agents and codeine or oxycodone.

Severe pain requires the use of more potent, addicting drugs such as morphine, hydromorphone, and levorphanol (Levo-Dromoran). Present management of severe pain combines the use of a long-acting narcotic such as MS Contin or a transdermal fentanyl patch with a nonsteroidal antiinflammatory agent and an anxiolytic agent such as chlorpromazine or an antidepressant such as amitriptyline. For patients with significant pain who are no longer responding to oral medications, a subcutaneous or intravenous morphine drip can be started.

Radiation therapy may be of great value in the relief of pain due to bony metastases or in the treatment of lesions that recur following primary surgical treatment of cervical cancer. In general, if initial therapy has been accomplished by adequate radiation therapy, re-treatment is contraindicated since it does little good and carries the potential of massive radiation necrosis.

In patients with lower back or extremity pain, placement of a peridural catheter can be made, which is connected to a subcutaneous pump with a reservoir well for continuous morphine instillation. This method gives pain relief without the sedating effects of oral and parenteral narcotics. In the setting of unilateral lower abdominal or extremity pain that is unresponsive to other intervention, percutaneous cordotomy can be tried. However, the patient may commonly experience rebound pain on the contralateral side after hemicordotomy.

The general management of incurable cancer demands that the physician maintain a sympathetic and understanding relationship with the patient. Her nutritional status and general body functions must be maintained. Anxiety, fear, and depression should be dealt with by means of friendly counseling, reassurance, and the discreet use of psychic energizing drugs. The cancer patient should be encouraged to continue her normal activities as long as she can and should be given every possible support in the effort. The hospice concept of patient care, which originated in the United Kingdom, has gained wide acceptance in the USA.

## Prognosis

The factors to be considered in the assessment of prognosis in cervical cancer are the following: (1) age of the patient, (2) patient's general physical condition, (3) socioeconomic status, (4) gross features of the cancer, (5) cytologic features of the cancer, (6) histologic characteristics of the cancer, (7) skill of the therapist, and (8) clinical staging (extent of disease, lymph node metastases).

The age of the patient is important because the more aggressive, anaplastic tumors are more frequently encountered in young women with cervical cancer. Older persons are more likely to harbor well-differentiated, slow-growing malignant tumors. However, this clinical impression may not significantly influence the ultimate prognosis.

The patient's general physical condition influences survival figures in several ways. Death from intercurrent disease is more common in patients who have serious chronic illnesses, such as diabetes, heart disease, and kidney disease. Obesity imposes a handicap, making adequate therapy more difficult. Coincidental pelvic infection also worsens the prognosis.

Patients who are economically deprived have more advanced disease when first diagnosed and generally do not respond as well to therapy.

Exophytic or papillary tumors—those with a cauliflower-like appearance—are usually seen at an earlier clinical stage than endophytic, ulcerative, or nodular lesions, and everting cancers often are more responsive to radiation therapy.

Although more sensitive to radiation, the small cell carcinoma carries a poorer prognosis than the large cell, keratinizing variety. The large cell nonkeratinizing tumor is intermediate in radiation sensitivity.

Tumors that demonstrate a rapid reduction in the numbers of so-called resting cells and mitotic cells with an increase in differentiating and degenerating cells on serial biopsy during radiation therapy may have a better prognosis.

The experience and skill of the therapist are of obvious importance. Stage for stage, a higher cure rate of cancer of the cervix is reported from larger treatment centers than from smaller community hospitals. Experience and dedicated interest in the care and treatment of cancer are significant factors in the outcome, whether treatment is by radical surgery or by radiation therapy. Precision and individualization of therapy are often necessary and may make the difference between success and failure.

Involvement of the regional lymph nodes has a profound influence on the prognosis. The external iliac nodes are the most frequently involved, followed by the obturator, common iliac, and hypogastric nodes. Small cancers less than 1 cm in diameter rarely show regional node involvement. Well-differentiated lesions appear to metastasize to the lymph nodes less frequently than poorly differentiated ones.

The more extensive the tumor, the higher the incidence of regional lymph node metastases: stage I, 15%; stage II, 30%; and stage III, 60%. The cure rate for stage I lesions when the nodes are involved is about 40% of what can be achieved if the nodes are free of cancer. Evidence shows that this is true of both radiation treatment and radical surgery.

Although clinical staging admittedly is not precise, it is the best guide we have to the ultimate prognosis. The results of treatment stage by stage for cancer of the cervix are reported by 125 institutions from 26 countries in the *Annual Report* of the International Federation of Gynecology and Obstetrics in Stockholm. The results are equated in terms of 5-year cure rates, or those patients who are living and show no evidence of cervical cancer 5 years after the beginning of therapy. The following representative results were achieved in all 4 stages for squamous cell carcinomas in cancer treatment centers using radiation therapy alone as the method of treatment: stage I, 69.4%; stage II, 59.5%; stage III, 38.2%; and stage IV, 12.5%. For those cancers in stages I and II that were treated by surgery alone, the 5-year survival rates were 92.2% and 75.2% respectively. Five-year survival rates for patients with stages I and II tumors treated with surgery followed by radiation were 78.8% and 67.1%, respectively.

When cancer of the cervix is untreated or fails to respond to treatment, death occurs in 95% of patients within 2 years after the onset of symptoms.

Recurrences following radiation therapy are not often centrally located and thus amenable to exenteration procedures. Only about 25% of recurrences are localized to the central portion of the pelvis. The most common site of recurrence is the pelvic side wall. The signs and symptoms of recurrent malignant disease are (1) positive cytologic examination 2 months or more following therapy; (2) palpable tumor in the pelvis or abdomen; (3) ulceration of the cervix or vagina; (4) pain in the pelvis, back, groin, and lower extremity; (5) unilateral lower extremity edema; (6) vaginal bleeding or discharge; (7) supraclavicular lymphadenopathy; and (8) ascites.

# REFERENCES

## CERVICAL INTRAEPITHELIAL NEOPLASIA

Anderson MC, Harley RB: Cervical crypt involvement by intraepithelial neoplasia. Obstet Gynecol 1980;55: 546.

Baggish MS: A comparison between laser excisional conization and laser vaporization for the treatment of cervical intraepithelial neoplasia. Am J Obstet Gynecol 1986;155:39.

Benedet JL, Miller DM, Nickerson KG: Results of conservative management of cervical intraepithelial neoplasia. Obstet Gynecol 1992;79:105.

Benedet JL, Nickerson KG, Anderson GH: Cryotherapy in the treatment of cervical intraepithelial neoplasia. Obstet Gynecol 1981;58:725.

Brown MS, Phillips GL: Management of the mildly abnormal pap smear: A conservative approach. Gynecol Oncol 1985;22:149.

Buller RE, Jones HW 3rd: Pregnancy following cervical conization. Am J Obstet Gynecol 1982;142:506.

Centers for Disease Control and Prevention: 1993 Revised classification system for HIV infection and expanded surveillance case definition for AIDS among adolescents and adults. MMWR 1992;41(RR-17):4.

Evans AS, Monaghan JM, Beattie AB: Carbon dioxide laser treatment of cervical warty atypias. Gynecol Oncol 1984;17:296.

Gunasekers PC, Phipps JH, Lewis BV: Large loop excision of the transformation zone compared to $CO_2$ laser in the treatment of CIN: A superior mode of treatment. Br J Obstet Gynecol 1990;97:995.

Hatch KD et al: Cryosurgery of cervical intraepithelial neoplasia. Obstet Gynecol 1981;57:692.

Holdt DG et al: Diagnostic significance and sequelae of cone biopsy. Am J Obstet Gynecol 1982;143:312.

Jones HW III: Cone biopsy in the management of cervical intraepithelial neoplasia. Clin Obstet 1983;26:968.

Kohan S et al: Colposcopic screening of women with atypical Papanicolaou smears. J Reprod Med 1985;30: 383.

Koss LG: Human papillomaviruses and genital cancer. The Female Patient 1992;17:25.

Maiman M, et al: Colposcopic evaluation of human immunodeficiency virus-seropositive women. Obstet Gynecol 1991;78:84.

Ostor AG et al: Adenocarcinoma in situ of the cervix. Int J Gynaecol Pathol 1984;3:179.

Robboy SJ et al: Role of hormones including diethylstilbestrol (DES) in the pathogenesis of cervical and vaginal intraepithelial neoplasia. Gynecol Oncol 1981; 12(2-Part 2):S98.

Townsend DE, Richart RM: Cryotherapy and carbon dioxide laser management of cervical intraepithelial neoplasia: A controlled comparison. Obstet Gynecol 1983;61:75.

Wright TC et al: Treatment of cervical intraepithelial neoplasia using the loop electrosurgical excision procedure. Obstet Gynecol 1992;79:173.

Wright VC, Davies E, Riopelle MA: Laser surgery for cervical intraepithelial neoplasia: Principles and results. Am J Obstet Gynecol 1983;145:181.

## CANCER OF THE CERVIX

Allen HH, Nisker JA, Anderson RJ: Primary surgical treatment in 195 cases of stage IB carcinomas of the cervix. Am J Obstet Gynecol 1982;143:581.

Arneson AN, Kao MS: Long-term observation of cervical cancer. Am J Obstet Gynecol 1987;156:614.

Baker L et al: Combination chemotherapy for patients with disseminated carcinoma of the uterine cervix. Proc ASCO 1985;4:120.

Bandy LC et al: Computed tomography in evaluation of extrapelvic lymphadenectomy in carcinoma of the cervix. Obstet Gynecol 1985;65:73.

Bonomi P et al: A phase II evaluation of cisplatin and

5-fluorouracil in patients with advanced squamous cell carcinoma of the cervix: A Gynecologic Oncology Group Study. Gynecol Oncol 1989;34:357.

Brenner DE: Carcinoma of the cervix: A review. Am J Med Sci 1982;284:31.

Coppleson LW, Brown B: Prevention of carcinoma of cervix. Am J Obstet Gynecol 1976;125:53.

Greer BE et al: Stage Ia2 squamous cell carcinoma of the cervix: Difficult diagnosis and therapeutic dilemma. Am J Obstet Gynecol 1990;162:1406.

Hacker NF et al: Carcinoma of the cervix associated with pregnancy. Obstet Gynecol 1982;59:735.

Herbst AL et al: Analysis of 346 cases of clear cell adenocarcinoma of the vagina and cervix, with emphasis on recurrence and survival. Gynecol Oncol 1979;7:111.

Hopkins MP, Morley GW: Squamous cell cancer of the cervix: Prognostic factors related to survival. Int J Gynecol Cancer 1991;1:173.

Hreshchyshyn MM et al: Hydroxyurea or placebo combined with radiation to treat stage IIIb or IV cervical cancer confined to the pelvis. Int J Radiat Oncol Biol Phys 1979;5:317.

Hricak H et al: Gynecologic masses: Value of magnetic resonance imaging. Am J Obstet Gynecol 1985;153: 31.

Jones MW, Silverberg SG: Cervical adenocarcinoma in young women: Possible relationship to microglandular hyperplasia and use of oral contraceptives. Obstet Gynecol 1989;73:984.

Katz HJ, Daires JNP: Death from cervix uteri carcinoma: The changing pattern. Gynecol Oncol 1980;9:86.

Kolstad P: Follow-up study of 232 patients with stage Ia1 and 411 patients with stage Ia2 squamous cell carcinoma of the cervix (microinvasive carcinoma). Gynecol Oncol 1989;33:265.

Kuhnle H et al: Phase II study of carboplatin: Ifosfamide in untreated advanced cervical cancer. Cancer Chemother Pharmacol 1990;26(Suppl):S33.

Lawhead RA et al: Pelvic exenteration for recurrent or persistent gynecologic malignancies: A 10 year review of the Memorial Sloan-Kettering Cancer Center experience (1972–1981). Gynecol Oncol 1989;33:279.

Lee YN et al: Radical hysterectomy with pelvic lymph node dissection for treatment of cervical cancer: A clinical review of 954 cases. Gynecol Oncol 1989;32:135.

Maruyama Y, van Nagell JR, Yoneda J: Dose-response and failure pattern for bulky or barrel-shaped stage IB cervical cancer treated by combined photon irradiation and extrafascial hysterectomy. Cancer 1989;63:70.

Nisker JA, Shubat M: Stage IB cervical carcinoma and pregnancy: Report of 49 cases. Am J Obstet Gynecol 1983;145:203.

O'Quinn AG, Fetcher GH, Wharton JT: Guidelines for conservative hysterectomy after irradiation. Gynecol Oncol 1980;9:68.

Penalver MA et al: Continent urinary diversion in gynecologic oncology. Gynecol Oncol 1989;34:274.

Pettersson F (editor): Annual report on the results of treatment in gynecological cancer, vol 21. International Federation of Gynecology and Obstetrics, 1991.

Pisco JM, Martins JM, Correia MG: Internal iliac artery embolization to control hemorrhage from pelvic neoplasms. Radiology 1989;172:337.

Rutledge FN, Mitchell MF, Munsell M: Youth as a prognostic factor in carcinoma of the cervix: A matched analysis. Gynecol Oncol 1992;44:123.

Sheets EE et al: Surgically treated early-stage neuroendocrine small-cell cervical carcinoma. Obstet Gynecol 1988;71:10.

Sorbe B, Frankendal B: Bleomycin-adriamycin-cisplatin combination chemotherapy in the treatment of primary advanced and recurrent cervical carcinoma. Obstet Gynecol 1984;63:167.

Sutton GP et al: Ovarian metastases in stage IB carcinoma of the cervix: A Gynecologic Oncology Group study. Am J Obstet Gynecol 1992;166:50.

Twycross RG: The management of pain in cancer: A guide to drugs and dosages. Oncology 1988;2:35.

Webb MJ, Symmonds RE: Site of recurrence of cervical cancer after radical hysterectomy. Am J Obstet Gynecol 1980;138:813.

# Premalignant & Malignant Disorders of the Uterine Corpus

*Annekathryn Goodman, MD*

## ENDOMETRIAL HYPERPLASIA & CARCINOMA

### Essentials of Diagnosis

- Bleeding: hypermenorrhea, intermenstrual or postmenopausal.
- Hyperestrogenism: conditions with possible alterations in estrogen metabolism, ie, ovarian granulosa cell tumor, polycystic ovarian syndrome, obesity, late menopause, and exogenous estrogens, and tamoxifen use.
- Susceptible persons: classic–obese, white, diabetic, hypertensive, anovulatory; other–thin, genetic predisposition, no hyperestrogenic state, unusual histologic subtypes.
- Diagnosis: endometrial sampling, ultrasonography.

### General Considerations

In the USA, white women have a lifetime risk of endometrial carcinoma of 2.4% compared with 1.3% for black women. The peak incidence of onset is in the sixth and seventh decades, but 2–5% occur before age 40 years, and the disease has been reported in women aged 20–30. Endometrial carcinoma is now the most common pelvic genital cancer in women. A doubling of the incidence of endometrial cancer in the 1970s correlated with unopposed estrogen use in hormone replacement and sequential oral contraceptives over the previous 10 years. The declining incidence in the 1980s paralleled progesterone use in hormone replacement regimens and low-dose estrogen combination birth control pills. The incidence of endometrial cancer has now remained stable over the past 10 years. The onset of endometrial bleeding facilitates detection in the earlier stages of disease. Consequently, the overall prognosis is considerably better than for the other major gynecologic cancers.

Ovarian cancer and cervical cancer are decidedly more lethal than endometrial carcinoma. In the USA,

there were 33,000 new cases of endometrial cancer in 1991, but only 5500 deaths. In contrast, of the 21,000 new cases of ovarian cancer, 12,500 women died. For cervical cancer, 13,500 new cases and 4500 deaths were reported.

Estrogens have been implicated as a causative factor in endometrial carcinoma, because there is a high incidence of this disease in patients with presumed alterations in estrogen metabolism and in those who take exogenous estrogens. Classically, it affects the affluent obese, nulliparous, infertile, hypertensive, and diabetic white woman, but it can occur in the absence of all these factors. Unlike cervical cancer, it is not related to sexual history. Fortunately for the victim, there is a warning; abnormal bleeding usually occurs early in the course of the disease and alerts the patient or physician to an endometrial abnormality. In the elderly patient with an obliterated endocervical canal, severe cramps from hematometra or pyometra may be the presenting symptom. In the asymptomatic patient, a fortuitous diagnosis may occur from an abnormal Papanicolaou (Pap) smear, but cytologic discovery of endometrial cancer is not consistent and should not be relied on for early diagnosis. A total hysterectomy with bilateral salpingo-oophorectomy is usually the first step in treatment. Further postoperative therapy depends on the particular histologic characteristics and the extent of the tumor.

### Etiology

Although the exact cause of endometrial cancer remains unknown, the argument that estrogens are somehow implicated is becoming increasingly more difficult to refute. It has been known for many years that the administration of estrogen to laboratory animals can produce endometrial hyperplasia and carcinoma. Furthermore, certain constitutional states such as diabetes mellitus, hypertension, polycystic ovary syndrome, and obesity, perhaps having in common elevated endogenous estrogen levels, are associated with a higher incidence of endometrial carcinoma. Patients receiving exogenous estrogen replacement therapy for Turner's syndrome or gonadal agenesis and patients with endogenous elevations from granulosa cell tumors of the ovary are also more susceptible to endometrial carcinoma. Recently tamoxifen, which has weak estrogenic effects on the endometrium, has been associated with both endometrial hyperplasia and carcinoma.

More than a dozen case-control studies indicate an association between estrogen administration and endometrial carcinoma. These studies report a 2- to 10-fold increase in the incidence of endometrial carcinoma in women receiving exogenous estrogens. The risk of cancer is related to both the dose and the duration of exposure and diminishes with cessation of estrogen use. The risk seems to be neutralized by the addition of cyclic progestin for 10 days each month. Basic research also reveals increased conversion of androstenedione to estrone in women with recognized risk factors for endometrial cancer (advanced age, obesity, and polycystic ovary syndrome). This collective body of information has raised serious questions about the carcinogenic effects of unopposed estrogens on the endometrium. Women on replacement estrogens or women suspected of having elevated levels of endogenous estrogen require close clinical follow-up. Progestin should be added to the treatment program to counteract the effect of estrogen on the endometrium. Periodic endometrial biopsies to rule out endometrial hyperplasia or pelvic ultrasonography to evaluate the thickness of the endometrial stripe should be obtained.

Evidence is accumulating that there is a genetic factor in the development of endometrial cancer. Those women with a personal history of ovarian, colon, or breast cancer as well as those with a family history of endometrial cancer may be at higher risk. Certain oncogenes such as Ha-, K-, and N-*ras*, c-*myc*, and Her-2/neu have been found in endometrial cancers.

## Surgical Staging
## (Table 48–1)

Prior to 1988, a clinical staging system classified cancers of the endometrium. Presently the stage of an endometrial carcinoma is based on abdominal exploration, pelvic washings, total hysterectomy with salpingo-oophorectomy, and selective pelvic and periaortic lymph node biopsies. Grade of the tumor is included in the staging description. Grade 1 tumors have less than 5% of a nonsquamous solid growth pattern. Grade 2 tumors contain 6–50% of a nonsquamous solid growth pattern. Tumors with more than 50% of a solid pattern are classified as grade 3. Notable nuclear atypia that is not congruent with architectural grade, raises the grade of a tumor by 1 point.

Surgical stage I tumors account for 75% of all endometrial carcinomas, which explains the relatively good overall prognosis. Eleven percent of cancers are surgical stage II, and the remaining 11% and 3% are surgical stage III and IV, respectively.

**Table 48–1.** FIGO surgical staging of carcinoma of the corpus uteri (1988)[1].

| |
| --- |
| Stage I |
|   Stage Ia G123 Tumor limited to endometrium |
|   Stage Ib G123 Invasion to less than one-half the myometrium |
|   Stage Ic G123 Invasion to more than one-half the myometrium |
| Stage II |
|   Stage IIa G123 Endocervical glandular involvement only |
|   Stage IIb G123 Cervical stromal invasion |
| Stage III |
|   Stage IIIa G123 Tumor invades serosa and/or adnexa, and/or positive peritoneal cytology |
|   Stage IIIb G123 Vaginal metastases |
|   Stage IIIc G123 Metastases to pelvic and/or para-aortic lymph nodes |
| Stage IV |
|   Stage IVa G123 Tumor invades bladder and/or bowel mucosa |
|   Stage IVb Distant metastases including intra-abdominal and/or inguinal lymph nodes |

[1]From International Federation of Gynecology and Obstetrics: Annual Report on the results of treatment in gynecologic cancer. Int J Gynecol Obstet 36[Suppl]: 1991.

## Classification

**A. Endometrial Hyperplasia:** The glandular hyperplasias of the endometrium are benign conditions that may produce symptoms clinically indistinguishable from early endometrial carcinoma. Because of their association with hyperestrogenic states, some of the hyperplasias, even though reversible, are considered premalignant lesions. Since endometrial hyperplasia and endometrial carcinoma present clinically as abnormal bleeding, thorough fractional curettage is always necessary when hyperplasia is present to rule out coexisting carcinoma. Hyperplasia can be classified as simple or complex and with or without atypia.

**1. Hyperplasia without atypia**–Microscopically, this type of hyperplasia has crowding of glands in the stroma. There is no nuclear atypia. In simple hyperplasia (previously called "cystic hyperplasia"), the glands are cystically dilated and give a "Swiss cheese" appearance histologically. Frequently this type of hyperplasia is asymptomatic and is an incidental finding at hysterectomy. When followed without treatment over a 15-year period, 1% progressed to a cancer whereas 80% spontaneously regressed.

Complex hyperplasia without atypia (previously designated "adenomatous hyperplasia") describes a complex, crowded appearance to the glands with very little intervening stroma. There can be epithelial stratification and mitotic activity. Left untreated over for 13 years, complex hyperplasia regresses in 83% of cases and progresses to cancer in 3% of cases. In general, the hyperplasias without atypia are not considered premalignant. Eighty-five percent of women have reversal of the lesions with progestin therapy.

**2. Hyperplasia with atypia**–Atypical hyperplasia may be simple or complex. It is characterized histologically by endometrial glands lined by enlarged cells with increased nuclear to cytoplasmic ratios. The nuclei may be irregular with coarse chromatin clumping and prominent nucleoli. These hyperplasias are generally considered premalignant. Progression to carcinoma occurs in 8% and 29% of simple atypical and complex atypical hyperplasias, respectively. Fifty to 94% of lesions regress with progestin therapy but have a higher rate of relapse when therapy is stopped compared with that of lesions without atypia. In peri- and postmenopausal patients with atypical hyperplasias who relapse after progestin therapy or who cannot tolerate its side effects, vaginal or abdominal hysterectomy is recommended.

**3. Carcinoma In Situ**—The term carcinoma in situ has been used to denote an entity at the extreme end of the continuum from hyperplasia to carcinoma. It is distinguished from carcinoma by the presence of intervening stoma between abnormal glands. There is no evidence of invasion, but sometimes this is impossible to identify in regions of crowded glands. Many authorities do not feel this is a uniform and replicable diagnosis.

**B. Endometrial Carcinoma:** This cancer is characterized by obvious hyperplasia and anaplasia of the glandular elements, with invasion of underlying stroma, myometrium, or vascular spaces. As previously noted, it has been postulated that it may represent the end process of a spectrum beginning with hyperplasia, passing through atypical hyperplasia, and ending with frank cancer. Despite the attractiveness of this theory, only about 25% of patients with endometrial carcinoma have a history of hyperplasia. What really happens is not known, but it is likely that endometrial cancer, although it may follow atypical hyperplasia, can develop independently of it.

In recent years, careful reevaluation of the pathologic findings and spread pattern of endometrial cancer has clarified our understanding of this disease. Important prognostic factors include histologic grade and cell type, depth of myometrial invasion, presence of lymph vascular space involvement, lymph node metastases, and positive peritoneal cytology. There is some evidence that tumor aneuploidy and an increased proportion of cells in S phase as determined by DNA flow cytometry is predictive of a poorer outcome.

Endometrial cancers of any grade are almost never associated with lymph node metastases if there has been no myometrial invasion. After myometrial invasion occurs, the incidence of pelvic and aortic lymph node metastases is directly proportional to the depth of invasion and the degree of differentiation. Patients with poorly differentiated deeply invasive cancers have about a 35% incidence of involved pelvic nodes and a 10–20% incidence of aortic node metastases. Since patients with lymph node metastases are at very

high risk for recurrence, these pathologic features have serious implications for treatment planning.

Endometrial cancer can spread by four possible routes: direct extension, lymphatic metastases, peritoneal implants after transtubal spread, and hematogenous spread. It is believed that the tumor remains confined to the body of the uterus for a relatively long time, but eventually it invades the myometrium and cervix. It may then spread to the parametria, the pelvic wall and aortic nodes, the serosa of the uterus, the ovaries, and ultimately the peritoneal surfaces. Undifferentiated lesions (grade 3) may spread to the pelvic and aortic nodes while still confined to the superficial myometrium. In serous and clear cell subtypes (see text that follows), the spread pattern is similar to that of ovarian cancer, and upper abdominal peritoneal relapses are common. Hematogenous metastases to the lungs are uncommon with primary tumors limited to the uterus but do occur with recurrent or disseminated disease. In contrast to the former belief that endometrial carcinoma spreads primarily to the aortic lymph nodes through infundibulopelvic and broad ligament lymphatics, recent studies indicate a dual pathway of spread to the pelvic and aortic lymph nodes (Fig 48–1). The aortic nodes are rarely involved when the

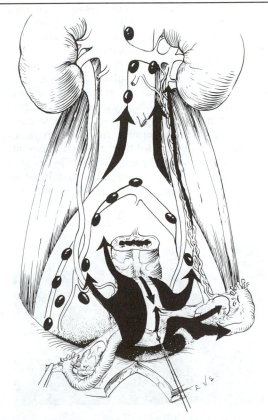

**Figure 48–1.** Dual lymphatic spread pattern of endometrial carcinoma.

pelvic nodes are free of metastases, but the pelvic nodes are sometimes involved when the aortic nodes are not.

Vaginal metastases occur by submucosal lymphatic or vascular metastases in approximately 3–8% of patients with clinical stage I disease. The concept that these metastases occur by spillage of tumor through the cervix at the time of surgery lacks convincing support. However, vaginal metastases are more common with higher histologic grade and with lower uterine segment or cervical involvement.

Malignant cells identified in the peritoneal washings obtained at the time of hysterectomy are usually associated with the finding of other risk factors such as deep myometrial invasion of lymph node metastases. When these cells are present in the absence of other risk factors, they convey a prognosis in proportion to their number and degree of differentiation. Vascular and lymphatic invasion in the hysterectomy specimen is also associated with a poorer outcome.

Pathologists recognize 3 major histologic types of endometrial carcinoma: adenocarcinoma, adenocarcinoma with squamous differentiation, and adenosquamous carcinoma. All 3 types have identical presenting symptoms and signs, patterns of spread, and general clinical behavior. For this reason, they can be considered collectively for purposes of clinical workup, differential diagnosis, and treatment. Papillary serous and clear cell carcinomas of the endometrium are other unusual histologic subtypes that appear to carry a poor prognosis even when apparently confined to the superficial myometrium.

**a. Adenocarcinoma**–The most common type of endometrial carcinoma is adenocarcinoma, composed of malignant glands that range from very well differentiated (grade 1)—barely distinguishable from atypical complex hyperplasia—to anaplastic carcinoma (grade 3). To determine stage and prognosis, the tumor is usually graded by the most undifferentiated area visible under the microscope (Fig 48–2). In the USA, adenocarcinoma comprises 70–80% of endometrial carcinomas, but this figure is higher in other countries.

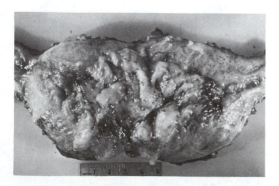

**Figure 48–2.** Adenocarcinoma of the endometrium. Note the sharp demarcation of the tumor at the isthmus.

**b. Adenocarcinoma with squamous differentiation**–This entity is composed of malignant glands and benign squamous metaplasia. It makes up approximately 5% of endometrial carcinomas. Although these cancers have a reputation for running a more benign course, this is probably due to the very well-differentiated pattern they usually display. Grade for grade, adenocarcinomas with squamous differentiation are probably no better or worse than other histologic types.

**c. Adenosquamous carcinoma**–Adenosquamous carcinoma of the endometrium is composed of malignant glands and malignant squamous epithelium and makes up approximately 10–20% of endometrial cancers in the USA. The reason for its high incidence in this country is unknown; however, there seems to be some variability in incidence from institution to institution, and the difference may be explained in the basis of pathologic interpretation. The tumor is often poorly differentiated (grade 3), which makes pathologic interpretation difficult. Because of the poor differentiation, prognosis is worse than that of endometrial carcinoma as a whole, since the overall statistics of endometrial carcinoma are heavily weighted in favor of better-differentiated lesions.

**d. Serous carcinoma**–Histologically, this cancer is identical with the complex papillary architecture seen in serous carcinomas of the ovary. Women with serous carcinoma are more likely to be older and less likely to have hyperestrogenic states. These tumors account for 50% of all relapses in stage I tumors. Serous tumors spread early and involve peritoneal surfaces of the pelvis and abdomen. The tumors also have a propensity for myometrial and lymphatic invasion. The prognosis is unfavorable, and patients with serous tumors should be treated in a manner similar to that of patients with ovarian tumors.

**e. Clear cell carcinoma**–This subtype is not associated with clear cell carcinomas of the cervix and vagina that are seen in young women with diethylstilbestrol exposure. Its microscopic appearance is significant for clear cells or hobnail cells. Solid, papillary, tubular, and cystic patterns are possible. Clear cell carcinoma is commonly high grade and aggressive with deep invasion and is seen at advanced stage. It occurs in older women (average age 67 years), and like the serous subtype is not associated with a hyperestrogenic state.

**f. Miscellaneous subtypes**–Mucinous carcinomas make up 9% of endometrial adenocarcinomas; they contain PAS-positive, diastase-resistant intracytoplasmic mucin. Secretory carcinoma, present in 1–2% of cases, exhibits subnuclear or supranuclear vacuoles resembling early secretory endometrium. These rare cancers behave in a manner similar to that of typical endometrial carcinomas. Pure squamous cell carcinomas are extremely rare and are associated with cervical stenosis, pyometra, and chronic inflammation.

## Clinical Findings

**A. Symptoms and Signs:** Abnormal bleeding occurs in about 80% of patients and is the most important warning sign of endometrial carcinoma. An abnormal vaginal discharge especially after menopause is present in some patients. During the premenopausal years, the bleeding is usually described as excessive flow at the time of menstruation. However, bleeding may occur as intermenstrual spotting or premenstrual and postmenstrual bleeding. In the postmenopausal woman, intermittent spotting, described as lighter than a normal menstrual period, is more common. As a presenting symptom, hemorrhage is rare. About 20% of patients with postmenopausal bleeding have underlying cancer; 12–15% have endometrial carcinoma; and the remainder have uterine sarcoma or cervical, vaginal, tubal, or ovarian carcinoma. Endometrial carcinoma as a cause of postmenopausal bleeding increases with age, so that after the age of 80, cancer is responsible in fully 50–60% of cases.

About 10% of patients complain of lower abdominal cramps and pain secondary to uterine contractions caused by entrapped detritus and blood behind a stenotic cervical os (hematometra). If the uterine contents become infected, an abscess develops and sepsis may supervene.

Physical examination is usually unremarkable but may reveal medical problems associated with advanced age. Speculum examination may confirm the presence of bleeding, but since it may be minimal and intermittent, blood may not be present. Atrophic vaginitis is frequently identified in these elderly women, but postmenopausal bleeding should never be ascribed to atrophy without a histologic sampling of the endometrium to rule out endometrial carcinoma. Bimanual and rectovaginal examination of the uterus in the early stages of the disease will be normal unless hematometra or pyometra is present. If the cancer is extensive at the time of presentation, the uterus may be enlarged and soft and may be confused with benign conditions such as leiomyoma. With very advanced cases, the uterus may be fixed and immobile from parametrial adnexal and intraperitoneal spread.

Vaginal metastases are rarely identified in early disease but are not uncommon in advanced cases or with recurrence following treatment. Ovarian metastases may cause marked enlargement of these organs.

When feasible, endocervical curettage with a small Kevorkian curet followed by endometrial biopsy may obviate the need, risk, and expense of fractional curettage.

**B. Laboratory Findings:** Routine laboratory findings are normal in most patients with endometrial carcinoma. If bleeding has been prolonged or profuse, anemia may be present.

Cytologic study of specimens taken from the endocervix and posterior vaginal fornix reveals adenocarcinoma in about 60% of symptomatic patients.

More important, endometrial carcinoma will be missed in 40% of symptomatic patients by routine cytologic examination. Accuracy has been greatly increased by aspiration cytologic study or biopsy (discussed under Special Examinations). The Pap smear is nevertheless an integral part of the examination of all patients, because it identifies a small but definite percentage of patients with asymptomatic disease. Furthermore, the presence of benign endometrial cells in the cervical or vaginal smear of a menopausal or postmenopausal woman is associated with occult endometrial carcinoma in 2–6% of cases. Thus, any postmenopausal woman who shows endometrial cells on a routine cervical Pap smear requires evaluation for endometrial cancer.

Routine blood counts, urinalysis, endocervical and vaginal pool cytology, chest x-ray, intravenous urography, stool guaiac, and sigmoidoscopy have proved to be useful ancillary diagnostic tests in patients with endometrial carcinoma. Liver function tests, blood urea nitrogen, serum creatinine, and a 2-hour postprandial blood glucose test (because of the known relationship to diabetes) and considered routine. Serum Ca-125, a well-established tumor marker for epithelial ovarian cancer, can also be useful for endometrial cancer. About 20% of patients with clinical stage I (preoperatively, the tumor appears to be confined to the uterus) have an elevated Ca-125. Eighty percent of surgically upstaged patients have an elevated preoperative value.

**C. X-Ray Findings:** Chest x-ray may reveal metastases in patients with advanced disease but is rarely positive in the early stages. Intravenous urography establishes the presence of a normal genitourinary system and rules out deviation or compression of the ureters by enlarged pelvic nodes or other unsuspected extrauterine spread. Barium enema is usually not necessary in a patient with a negative stool guaiac test and normal sigmoidoscopic examination but should always be performed in the patient with gross or occult gastrointestinal bleeding or symptoms.

Hysterosalpingography and hysteroscopy have been widely used in some foreign countries and in many institutions within the USA for the evaluation of endometrial carcinoma. Although investigators consistently report no adverse effects from these procedures, the possibility of transtubal spread of cancer is nevertheless real. Recent studies indicate that patients with stage I disease and positive intraperitoneal cytologic specimens obtained at hysterectomy are at very high risk for recurrence. For this reason, these procedures should not be used to evaluate this disease.

Magnetic resonance imaging (MRI) appears to improve the accuracy of clinical staging and is particularly helpful in identifying myometrial invasion and lower uterine segment or cervical involvement.

**D. Special Examinations:**

**1. Fractional curettage**–Dilatation and fractional curettage is the definitive procedure for diagnosis of endometrial carcinoma. It should be performed with the patient under anesthesia to afford an opportunity for thorough and more accurate pelvic examination. It is carried out by careful and complete curettage of the endocervical canal followed by dilatation of the canal and circumferential curettage of the endometrial cavity. When obvious cancer is present with the first passes of the curet, the procedure should be terminated as long as sufficient tissue for analysis has been obtained from the endocervix and endometrium. Perforation of the uterus followed by intraperitoneal contamination with malignant cells, blood, and bacteria is a common complication in patients with endometrial carcinoma and can usually be avoided by gentle surgical technique and limitation of the procedure to the extent necessary for accurate diagnosis and staging. D&C is never considered curative in these circumstances and should not be performed with the same vigor as therapeutic curettage.

**2. Endometrial biopsy–**This procedure is attractive because it can be performed in an outpatient setting, resulting in a substantial savings in cost. It can usually be done without anesthesia, although paracervical block is effective when necessary. Currently, some form of negative pressure attached to an aspiration curet is the most popular method, but gentle curettage with a Kevorkian nonaspirating curet is also successful.

All types of endometrial biopsy are notoriously inaccurate for diagnosing polyps and will miss a significant number of cases of endometrial hyperplasia as well. Therefore, it must be emphasized that when these tests cannot be completed for technical reasons or when the tissue obtained is insufficient for diagnosis or for accurate grading and staging of the lesion, complete fractional curettage must be performed.

**a. Aspiration biopsy–**This procedure is performed with a variety of aspirating or nonaspirating curets designed for easy entry into the endometrial cavity. The Novak curet is a good example (Fig 48–3). While slight negative pressure is maintained on the syringe, the endometrial cavity is sampled, preferably in all 4 quadrants. Overall, the procedure is 80–90% accurate for the diagnosis of endometrial carcinoma when the tissue sample is adequate and when it can be successfully accomplished. It does, however, have a wide range of accuracy (between 67% and 97%), and negative findings in the symptomatic (bleeding) patient should never be considered definitive. The pipelle, a thin plastic cannula, is another office instrument that can adequately sample the endometrium. Because of its small diameter, it usually causes less cramping than other curets.

**b. Aspiration curettage–**The Vabra aspirator is another form of endometrial biopsy technique using a 3- or 4-mm suction curet with approximately 300–600 mm of negative pressure (Fig 48–4). To date, aspiration curettage is the most accurate outpatient

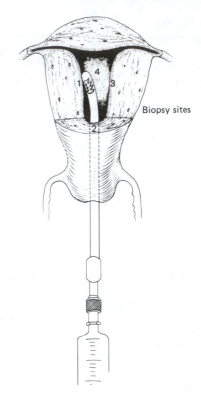

**Figure 48–3.** Technique of endometrial biopsy with Novak curet.

method for evaluating endometrial cancer, with an overall accuracy rate of 95–98%. However, the range of accuracy may be as low as 80%, and various technical problems preclude completion of the procedure in about 10% of cases. In another 6–7%, the sample is considered insufficient for histologic interpretation. Consequently, negative findings in a symptomatic patient cannot be considered definitive.

**3. Pelvic ultrasonography–**Ultrasonography can be helpful in deciding whether high-risk patients (such as those with a hyperestrogenic state, breast cancer patients on Tamoxifen, and women with strong family histories of endometrial cancer) who do not have symptoms should undergo endometrial sampling. In postmenopausal women, 5 mm is the cutoff for a normal unilateral endometrial stripe. Color flow imaging may increase specificity.

**4. Estrogen and progesterone receptor assays–**Estrogen and progesterone receptor assays should be obtained from the neoplastic tissue. This information helps in planning adjuvant or subsequent hormone therapy.

### Differential Diagnosis

Clinically, the differential diagnosis of endometrial carcinoma generally includes all the various causes of abnormal uterine bleeding. In the premeno-

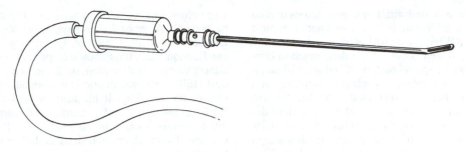

**Figure 48–4.** Vabra aspirator.

pausal or menopausal patient, complications of early pregnancy such as threatened or incomplete abortion must be high on the list; a pregnancy test usually clarifies the issue. Other causes of bleeding in this group are leiomyoma, endometrial hyperplasia and polyps, cervical polyps, and various genital or metastatic cancers. Cervical, endometrial, tubal, and ovarian neoplasms all can cause abnormal uterine bleeding. Although rare, metastatic cancers from the bowel, bladder, and breast have also been reported to cause abnormal uterine bleeding.

In the postmenopausal age group, the emphasis will be shifted to atrophic vaginitis, exogenous estrogens, endometrial hyperplasia and polyps, and various genital neoplasms. The older the patient, the more likely that her bleeding will prove to be due to endometrial cancer. In any event, the diagnosis will be evident following adequate evaluation of the endocervical and endometrial cavities. In the patient with a normal pelvic examination and recurrent postmenopausal bleeding following a recent negative D&C, tubal and ovarian cancer must be strongly considered. Patients with 2 unexplained episodes of postmenopausal uterine bleeding should undergo total hysterectomy and bilateral salpingo-oophorectomy.

Pathologically, the differential diagnosis of endometrial carcinoma is usually not difficult except in the well-differentiated forms, where the distinction from atypical hyperplasia can be perplexing. Whenever doubt or disagreement exists, consultation with a pathologist skilled in the diagnosis of gynecologic neoplasms usually resolves the problem.

## Complications

If the patient has ignored her symptoms of bleeding over a long period of time and allowed the cancer to extensively invade the myometrium, she may present with severe anemia secondary to chronic blood loss or acute hemorrhage. If bleeding is significant and continuous, high-dose bolus radiation therapy is usually effective in slowing the hemorrhage.

The presence of a hematometra can be confirmed by sounding the uterus under anesthesia, followed by dilatation of the cervix to allow adequate drainage. When a pyometra is present, the patient may present with peritonitis or generalized sepsis, with all the consequent complications.

Perforation of the uterus at the time of dilatation and fractional curettage or endometrial biopsy is not an uncommon problem. If the perforating instrument is large, loops of small bowel may be inadvertently retrieved through the cervical canal. A large perforation warrants laparoscopy or laparotomy to evaluate and repair the damage. If significant contamination of the peritoneal cavity with blood or necrotic tumor has occurred, the patient should be treated with broad-spectrum antibiotics to prevent peritonitis. Perforation in the patient with endometrial cancer should be viewed as a serious complication, since spill of tumor into the peritoneal cavity may drastically alter her prognosis.

## Prevention

The constitutional and other risk factors for endometrial carcinoma are well known. Obese, diabetic, hypertensive, nulliparous women with a history of infertility or repeated D&C for abnormal bleeding certainly require close surveillance. Women with late menopause or previous pelvic radiation therapy and those taking estrogens should be under closer observation than women in the general population. Very little can be done for the constitutional risk factors other than general health measures to control diabetes and hypertension and maintain ideal body weight.

Estrogens should be administered cyclically, 21–25 days each month, using the lowest dose that controls symptoms. Progesterone, 10 mg, should be added for the last 10–14 days of the cycle to neutralize the risk of endometrial carcinoma. Alternatively, estrogen and progesterone can be administered continuously; 2.5 mg of progesterone is given daily. It is not known whether continuous progesterone is as protective of endometrial hyperplasia and cancer as the cyclic method. Some authors recommend lifetime estrogen replacement to prevent the serious degenerative problems of osteoporosis.

## Treatment

The treatment of cancer anywhere in the body depends on its natural history and pattern of spread. The clinician is confronted with familiar questions in each case: What is it? Where is it now or where is it most likely to be? What are its pathways of dissemination or invasion? Recent studies have done much to clarify the lymphatic spread pattern of endometrial carcinoma; nodal metastases, vaginal recurrence, and survival have been demonstrated to be directly proportionate to the depth of myometrial invasion, degree of an aplasia, and the presence of cervical involvement. Any one of these features implies a high risk of treatment failure and recurrence. It follows that any rational treatment plan for endometrial carcinoma must take these risk factors into consideration.

Surgery and radiation therapy are the only methods of treatment that have consistently shown a high degree of success in treating this disease. It has been repeatedly demonstrated that radiation therapy can cure endometrial carcinoma in some patients, but when irradiation is used alone the survival rates have been clearly inferior to those achieved with surgery alone. Radiation therapy averages about a 20% lower cure rate than surgery in stage I disease. Surgery is therefore the treatment of choice whenever feasible, but some form of adjuvant therapy is necessary in patients at high risk for metastasis. Because chemotherapy is not reliable for this purpose, radiation therapy is the clear choice for adjuvant treatment. Even though preoperative or postoperative radiation therapy in combination with surgery for stage I disease has not significantly improved 5-year survival rates over rates achieved by surgery alone, considerable evidence supports the use of adjuvant radiation therapy in this disease.

It is well known that radiation therapy alone can cure endometrial carcinoma in some patients, and when used preoperatively it completely eradicates the primary tumor in over 50% of stage I cases. Furthermore, adjuvant radiation therapy has reduced the incidence of vaginal vault recurrence following surgery for stage I patients from an average of 3–8% to 1–3%. Also, regional radiation therapy has eliminated microscopic nodal metastases in other tumor systems, and some patients with surgically proved nodal metastases from endometrial carcinoma are now alive more than 5 years following adjuvant radiation therapy to pelvic and aortic nodes. Accordingly, in the presence of extrauterine extension, lower uterine segment or cervical involvement, poor histologic differentiation, papillary serous or clear cell histology, or myometrial penetration greater than one-third the full thickness, adjuvant radiation therapy is recommended. In the absence of these findings, it is difficult to justify the risk and morbidity of any additional treatment beyond simple total abdominal hysterectomy and bilateral salpingo-oophorectomy.

**A. Emergency Measures:** Infrequently, the patient with endometrial adenocarcinoma may present in a critical state. When bleeding has been ignored for long periods of time, profound anemia may exist; or when blood loss is acute and massive, the patient may be in shock. After vital signs have been stabilized and adequate blood is in reserve, emergency dilatation and fractional curettage should be performed with the utmost caution and gentleness. If the uterus is obviously full of necrotic tumor, instrumentation only increases the bleeding. If bleeding persists following D&C, high-dosage bolus radiation therapy to the whole pelvis should be administered. Rarely, in the face of very advanced lesions, embolization of the hypogastric arteries via percutaneous selective angiography may be required to control hemorrhage before treatment can be initiated. Hysterectomy should always be considered if it can be accomplished safely without jeopardizing curative therapy.

Elderly patients may present with severe lower abdominal pain and cramping secondary to hematometra or pyometra; these complications result from endometrial carcinoma in over 50% of cases. When adequate blood levels of broad-spectrum antibiotics are established, the cervix should be dilated and the endometrial cavity adequately drained. In this setting, vigorous D&C is contraindicated because of the high risk of uterine perforation. If the cervix is well dilated, an indwelling drain is usually not necessary; but if sepsis is not controlled within 24–48 hours, the patient should be reexamined to ascertain cervical patency. Once the infection has completely subsided and the patient has been afebrile for 7–10 days, gentle fractional curettage should be performed if the diagnosis was not confirmed at the initial procedure.

**B. Radiation Therapy:** Radiation therapy is used as primary therapy in patients considered medically unstable for laparotomy. Adjuvant preoperative radiation is no longer used unless the patient presents with gross cervical involvement. In this situation, after preoperative whole pelvic radiation and an intracavitary implant, an extrafascial hysterectomy is performed. Contraindications to preoperative radiation therapy include the presence of a pelvic mass, a pelvic kidney, pyometra, history of a pelvic abscess, prior pelvic radiation, and previous multiple laparotomies. See Chapter 51.

**C. Surgical Treatment:** Because bleeding is usually an early sign of endometrial carcinoma, most patients present with early disease and can be adequately and completely treated by simple hysterectomy. In this situation, the results are the same whether hysterectomy is accomplished vaginally or abdominally, but the abdominal approach is superior for removal of the ovaries and for assessment of the peritoneal cavity and retroperitoneal nodes. It also permits the surgeon to obtain peritoneal washings for cytologic identification of occult spread. For these reasons, the abdominal approach is preferred except in patients with very early disease and a small uterus, in whom the risk of occult cervical involvement or deep myometrial invasion is minimal and who also have other compelling reasons for vaginal surgery.

For grade 2 and 3 tumors, selective pelvic and peri-aortic nodes should be biopsied. For grade 1 tumors, the uterus should be opened in the operating room to assess depth of myometrial penetration. Although gross inspection is inaccurate, lymph node biopsies should be obtained in cases of an obviously large and deeply invading tumor. As stated previously, if risk factors are identified during the surgical staging procedure or on the operative specimen, postoperative adjuvant radiation therapy should be administered.

Radical hysterectomy has been recommended by some, particularly for stage II tumors, but the results have been no better than with simple hysterectomy combined with radiation therapy. Furthermore, most patients are elderly or have concurrent diabetes, hypertension, or other medical problems that preclude radical surgery. Radical hysterectomy can be effective treatment, however, for patients with recurrence following treatment with radiation therapy alone or for those who have previously received therapeutic doses of pelvic radiation therapy for other pelvic cancers. The high risk of bowel or urinary tract injury in this setting must be understood and accepted by both patient and physician.

As with patients presenting with gross cervical involvement, those with vaginal and parametrial involvement should receive initial pelvic radiation. Exploratory laparotomy should then be considered in patients whose disease seems resectable. Hormonal therapy or chemotherapy is most appropriate for patients with clinical evidence of extrapelvic metastases. Palliative radiation to bone or brain metastases is beneficial for symptomatic relief. Pelvic radiation can be helpful for local tumor control and alleviation of bleeding.

**D. Hormone Therapy:** Progesterone has been the time-honored agent for the treatment of recurrent endometrial carcinoma not amenable to irradiation or surgery. This type of therapy is not associated with side effects and can be administered orally or parenterally. Oral megestrol (Megace), parenteral medroxyprogesterone acetate suspension (Depo-Provera), and parenteral hydroxyprogesterone caproate (Delalutin) appear to have similar effectiveness. The frequently quoted response rate of 35% has been challenged by reports that indicate a lower overall response to progesterone therapy. The average duration of response is 20 months, and patients who respond survive more than 4 times longer than nonresponders. About 30% of responders survive 5 years; virtually all nonresponders die before this time. Patients who are young and have localized recurrence respond better than older patients and those with disseminated disease; those with well-differentiated tumors respond better than those with poorly differentiated ones; and patients with late recurrences respond better than those with early ones (indicating a more indolent, well-differentiated form of the disease). Because some patients do not achieve remission until after 10–12 weeks of therapy, the minimum duration of treatment should be over 3 months. Overall, about 13% of patients with recurrent disease appear to achieve long-term remissions with progesterone therapy.

The response to progesterone can be accurately predicted by levels of estrogen and progesterone receptors in the tumor. Levels of these receptors are inversely proportional to the grade of the tumor; poorly differentiated (grade 3) lesions have low levels of estrogen and progesterone receptors and usually do not respond to progesterone therapy.

Although progesterones have a somewhat encouraging record in the treatment of recurrent endometrial adenocarcinoma, they are disappointing as prophylactic agents. They have not improved survival or decreased recurrence when used following definitive treatment of early stage disease.

Tamoxifen has been used as another hormonal agent in advanced or recurrent endometrial cancer. It may be as effective as progesterone. As with progesterone, the patients who respond generally have well-differentiated tumors and long disease-free intervals. One report suggests a significantly better response to chemotherapy combined with both progesterone and tamoxifen than to chemotherapy alone.

**E. Antitumor Chemotherapy:** Doxorubicin (Adriamycin) and cisplatin are the two most active agents in the treatment of advanced or recurrent endometrial cancer. Response rates of 30% with a complete response rate of 5–10% have been reported. The alkylating agents cyclophosphamide and ifosfamide have also been used in this setting. No mature data are available on the use of adjuvant chemotherapy in patients with poor prognostic risk factors.

**F. General and Supportive Measures:** When the patient presents without acute symptoms of hemorrhage or sepsis, the workup, although it should be efficient and thorough, can be less urgent. Patients with endometrial carcinoma are often elderly and medically feeble. They may be weak, anemic, diabetic, or hypertensive, and specific attention to these problems is necessary before the cancer can be treated.

## Prognosis

Contemporary studies of the clinical, surgical, and pathologic findings in patients with endometrial carcinoma have identified subsets of patients at greater risk for recurrence. The prognosis is proportionately worse with increasing age, higher pathologic grade and clinical stage, and greater depth of myometrial invasion. Malignant cells in the peritoneal fluid or washings and adnexal metastases are ominous findings.

The 1991 report of the International Federation of Gynecology and Obstetrics (FIGO) on actuarial survival rates for surgical stages I–IV pooled data from 7646 cases at 147 institutions. Five-year survival rates are 85.3%, 70.2%, 49.2%, and 18.7% for stages I through IV, respectively.

These figures underline the increasing risk for treatment failure and recurrence with increasing bulk and extension of tumor. Consequently, identification of the known risk factors by thorough preoperative and intraoperative evaluation and careful examination of the histopathologic material is vital for treatment planning.

When no risk factors are identified, conservative surgery (simple total abdominal hysterectomy and bilateral salpingo-oophorectomy) should result in corrected survivals greater than 95% at 5 years. The presence of risk factors mandates an aggressive approach using adjuvant radiation therapy and, in some instances, chemotherapy as well. It is hoped that properly controlled prospective randomized studies will determine the success of such treatment.

## SARCOMA OF THE UTERUS (Leiomyosarcoma, Endometrial Sarcomas)

### Essentials of Diagnosis

- Bleeding: intermenstrual, hypermenorrhea, postmenopausal, preadolescent.
- Mass: rapid enlargement of the uterus or of a leiomyoma.
- Pain: discomfort in the pelvis from pressure on surrounding organs.
- Malignant tissue: obtained by biopsy, D&C, or hysterectomy, confirming uterine sarcoma.

### General Considerations

The uterine sarcomas, which are sometimes composed of a great variety of mesodermally derived elements, such as bone, cartilage, fat, and striated muscle, are the subject of great histogenetic speculation and innumerable pathologic classification systems. Consequently, they are surrounded by more confusion and controversy than most gynecologic tumors. In fact, for a group of cancers that make up only 2–3% of all malignant tumors of the corpus, they have received an inordinate amount of attention, and they occupy a disproportionate volume of controversial literature.

No common etiologic agent has been identified with uterine sarcomas, but in some reports prior pelvic radiation therapy has been associated with the mixed forms of uterine sarcoma in an unexpectedly high number of cases.

Sarcomas can occur at any age but are most prevalent after age 40. They are well known as a source of hematogenous metastases, but with the exception of leiomyosarcomas, lymphatic permeation and contiguous spread are probably the most common methods of extension. Endometrial sarcomas can usually be diagnosed by endometrial biopsy or dilatation and fractional curettage, but the sarcomas derived from the myometrium (leiomyosarcoma) frequently require hysterectomy to obtain adequate tissue for analysis.

There is no universal agreement on the histologic features that determine outcome, but most authorities agree that the number of mitotic figures per high-power field, vascular and lymphatic invasion, serosal extension, and in some cases degree of anaplasia are all helpful. Lack of discriminating histologic features and analytic sophistication often cause arbitrary assignment of a specific tumor to an improper category. This is regrettable, since treatment is largely predicated on correct histologic diagnosis. Historically, surgery has been the favored treatment for uterine sarcomas, but some evidence shows that a combination of radiation therapy and surgery is more beneficial for patients with endometrially derived uterine sarcomas. Chemotherapy has proved to be effective in treating some recurrences.

### Histogenesis, Classification, & Staging

From a clinical standpoint, the uterine sarcomas can be separated into 4 categories: leiomyosarcomas (LMS), endometrial stromal sarcomas (ESS), malignant mixed mesodermal tumors (MMMT), and adenosarcomas. A brief review of the histogenesis of these tumors will help the reader to understand the conflicting literature on this subject.

LMS is thought to arise from the myometrial smooth muscle cell or a similar cell lining blood vessels within the myometrium. A less plausible explanation proposes an origin from the endometrial stromal cell, but almost no data support this contention.

The ESS and MMMT arise from undifferentiated endometrial stromal cells, which retain the potential to differentiate into malignant cell lines that histologically appear native (homologous) or foreign (heterologous) to the human uterus. Because the undifferentiated stromal cells of the endometrium arise from specialized mesenchymal cells of the müllerian apparatus in the genital ridge and ultimately from the mesoderm during embryogenesis, endometrial sarcomas have been variously termed "mesodermal," "müllerian," or "mesenchymal" sarcomas. The prognoses of patients with homologous and heterologous tumors is similar stage for stage, and this terminology has limited clinical usefulness. ESS has been categorized in the older literature as a "pure" and homologous endometrial sarcoma because it is composed of a single cell line. MMMTs, previously designated as "mixed" because of containing 2 or more cell lines, arise from an undifferentiated malignant stem cell. MMMTs contain both a carcinomatous element and a sarcomatous element and have also been called "carcinosarcomas." The origin of this confusing terminology is better understood by study of Figure 48–5, which graphically represents the histogenesis of uterine sarcomas. Table 48–2 combines the prevailing histogenetic terminology for endometrial sarcomas and depicts the various possibilities in each category.

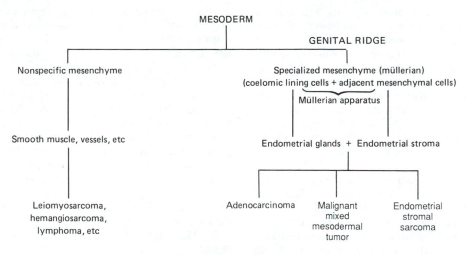

**Figure 48–5.** Histogenesis of uterine sarcomas.

Pure heterologous sarcomas such as rhabdomyosarcoma, chondrosarcoma, osteosarcoma, and liposarcoma are extremely rare. Finally, the other uterine sarcomas (hemangiosarcoma, fibrosarcoma, reticulum cell sarcoma, lymphosarcoma, and others) are exceedingly rare, and, being indistinguishable from identical sarcomas elsewhere in the body, are not considered specialized tumors of the uterus.

No staging system is designated for uterine sarcomas, but most authors use the FIGO system for endometrial carcinoma (Table 48–1).

## Major Types of Sarcomas of Uterus

**A. Leiomyosarcoma:** LMS make up 35–40% of all uterine sarcomas and 1–2% of all uterine cancers. It usually occurs between ages 25 and 75, with a mean incidence at about age 50. Younger patients with this disease seem to have a more favorable outcome than postmenopausal women. Like the benign leiomyomas, which are much more common in blacks, LMS are 1.5 times more common among black women than among white women. Leiomyomas are commonly identified in the uterus containing

leiomyosarcoma, but the incidence of malignant transformation of leiomyoma is only 0.1–0.5%. Only about 5–10% of LMS are reported to originate in a leiomyoma.

Abnormal uterine bleeding is the most common symptom of LMS, occurring in about 60% of patients; 50% describe some type of abdominal pain or discomfort; 30% complain of gastrointestinal or genitourinary symptoms; and only about 10% are aware of an abdominal mass. Occasionally a pedunculated tumor prolapses through the cervix, where it is accessible for biopsy. The deeply situated intramural position of most tumors impedes diagnosis by D&C, which is accurate in only 25% of cases. The Pap smear may be abnormal; more frequently, however, the true nature of the disease becomes evident after the fact, when pathologic analysis of a hysterectomy specimen reveals cancer.

LMS spread by contiguous growth, invading the myometrium, cervix, and surrounding supporting tissues. Lymphatic dissemination is common in the late stages. Pelvic recurrence and peritoneal dissemination following resection are also common. In the more malignant types, hematogenous metastasis to the lungs, liver, kidney, brain, and bones probably occurs early but is clinically evident only in the lungs until the advanced stages.

The clinical behavior of the tumor can usually be predicted by the number of mitotic figures identified on microscopic examination. Low-grade LMS are those with less than 5 mitoses per 10 high-power fields, with pushing rather than infiltrating margins. The outcome is favorable following simple hysterectomy. LMS with 5–10 mitoses per 10 high-power fields are considered to be of intermediate grade, but the outcome is unpredictable—usually favorable if the tumors are completely removed, but with poten-

**Table 48–2.** Classification of Uterine Sarcomas.

Leiomyosarcoma (tumors of the uterine smooth muscle)
Endometrial stromal sarcoma (pure homologous endometrial
   sarcoma)
   High grade
   Low grade (endolymphatic stromal myosis)
Malignant mixed mesodermal tumor (mixed epithelial/stromal
   tumors)
   Homologous carcinosarcoma
   Heterologous carcinosarcoma
Adenosarcoma (mixed epithelial/stromal tumors)
   Homologous
   Heterologous

tial to recur or metastasize. Tumors with mitosis counts greater than 10 per 10 high-power fields are highly malignant and usually lethal; less than 20% of these patients are alive at 5 years. Some authors emphasize that the mitosis count should not be the only criterion to evaluate the aggressiveness of LMS. An invasive pattern, particularly into the blood and lymphatic vessels and the surrounding smooth muscle, is important. By contrast, cellular characteristics such as atypia, anaplasia, and giant cells are not accurate prognosticators of aggressive behavior. Clinically, the most reliable prognostic feature of LMS stage; that is, when the tumor has extended beyond the uterus, the outcome is uniformly fatal. However, most patients with LMS present at stage I.

Other unusual smooth muscle tumors of the uterus such as benign metastasizing leiomyoma and intravenous leiomyomatosis should be considered low-grade LMS. Although they are histologically benign, they are notorious for local recurrence and can cause death by compression of contiguous or distant vital structures. Intravenous leiomyomatosis has been known to grow up the vena cava into the right atrium, impeding venous return and precipitating congestive heart failure. Because of their slow growth, they can frequently be controlled by repeated local excision. The metastatic lung lesions of benign metastasizing leiomyoma have disappeared following resection of the primary lesion in some cases, perhaps indicating hormone dependency.

### B. Endometrial Sarcomas:

### 1. Endometrial stromal sarcomas (ESS)–
ESS make up 8% of all sarcomas. They occur predominantly in postmenopausal women. Patients with these tumors most commonly present with bleeding or lower abdominal discomfort and pain. The diagnosis can be made accurately by D&C in approximately 75% of cases. Although no etiologic relationship to hormones has been established, a small number of metastatic lesions has responded to progesterone therapy.

ESS can be divided into two distinct subtypes; low-grade and high-grade. The indolent low-grade ESS—also called endolymphatic stromal myosis—have fewer than 10 mitoses per 10 high-power fields, with infiltrating margins and myometrial invasion. A benign form, the stromal nodule, has been described; it contains pushing rather than infiltrating margins and fewer than 15 mitoses per 10 high-power fields, with no vascular or myometrial invasion. The diagnosis of stromal nodule should be reserved for lesions with low mitotic counts, certainly fewer than 5 per 10 high-power fields.

The mean age at onset for endolymphatic stromal myosis is 5–10 years earlier than for high-grade sarcomas. This tumor infiltrates surrounding structures and is characterized by indolent growth and a propensity to vascular invasion. Patients frequently present with yellowish worm-like extensions into the peri-uterine vascular spaces. Under such circumstances, it may be confused grossly with intravenous leiomyomatosis, as previously described. It tends to recur late, sometimes after 5–10 years and can often be controlled by repeated local excisions.

The high-grade ESS display infiltrating margins and vascular and myometrial invasion and contain more than 10 mitoses per 10 high-power fields. These tumors are highly malignant and are associated with a poor prognosis, particularly when they extend beyond the uterus at the time of diagnosis. They spread by contiguous growth and lymphatic metastasis. After they move out to the serosal surface of the uterus, they spread to the adnexa and throughout the abdomen. Distant hematogenous metastases to the lungs and liver are usually a late event.

### 2. Malignant mixed mesodermal tumors (MMMT)–
MMMTs account for 50% of all uterine sarcomas and 3–6% of all uterine tumors. They characteristically occur in postmenopausal women, with the exception of embryonal rhabdomyosarcoma of the cervix or vagina (sarcoma botryoides), which occurs also in infants and children. Radiation therapy may be a predisposing cause. Many published series are available containing a significant number of patients with a history of pelvic radiation for benign or malignant conditions (Fig 48–6).

As with the other types, the presenting symptom of MMMT is usually bleeding. Abdominal discomfort and pain or a neoplastic mass prolapsed into the vagina also occur. Since the tumors are endometrial in origin, about 75% can be diagnosed accurately by D&C. In contrast to the other 2 major types—LMS and ESS—mitotic counts are not helpful in predicting the outcome of patients with these tumors. Histologically, they are usually highly anaplastic, with many bizarre nuclei and mitotic figures. They usually contain malignant glands and heterotopic elements such as bone, striated muscle, cartilage, or fat, and are then termed "carcinosarcoma." Like the high-grade ESS, MMMTs spread by contiguous infiltration of the surrounding tissues and by early lymphatic dissemination. Hematogenous metastases are common.

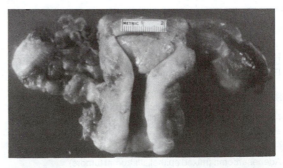

**Figure 48–6.** Mixed sarcoma of the uterine fundus. Prior full pelvic radiation therapy had little effect on the tumor.

The metastatic deposits are usually composed of malignant glands, but sarcomatous elements have been identified in some cases. The prognosis depends chiefly on the extent of the tumor at the time of primary surgery; there are virtually no long-term survivors among those whose tumor has extended beyond the confines of the uterus at the time of diagnosis.

**C. Adenosarcomas:** Adenosarcoma is a distinctive mixed müllerian tumor that accounts for 1–2% of uterine sarcomas. It arises from the endometrium and is composed of a combination of benign-appearing glands and a stromal sarcoma or fibrosarcoma. Adenosarcomas usually occur in the postmenopausal age group but have been reported in adolescents and women of reproduction age. Bleeding is the most common symptom. Recurrence occurs in 25% of patients and is usually late. The primary treatment is removal of uterus, tubes, and ovaries. Postoperative radiation therapy is recommended for those tumors with deep myometrial invasion.

**D. Other Uterine Sarcomas:** Embryonal rhabdomyosarcoma of the cervix (sarcoma botryoides), which occurs in infants and children was previously lethal. However, combination therapy using surgery, radiation, and chemotherapy has considerably improved the outlook for these patients.

Fibrosarcoma, hemangiosarcoma, reticulum cell sarcoma, hemangiopericytoma, and other esoteric and bizarre uterine sarcomas are rare. In general, these sarcomas behave like the other intermediate-grade uterine sarcomas, but treatment must be individualized according to age, histologic type, and the patient's state of health.

## Clinical Findings

**A. Symptoms and Signs:** Abnormal uterine bleeding is the most common manifestation of uterine sarcoma. Other recurring complaints include pelvic discomfort or pain, constipation, urinary frequency and urgency, and the presence of a mass low in the abdomen. Uterine sarcoma should be suspected in any nonpregnant woman with a rapidly enlarging uterus. Severe uterine cramps may exist if the tumor has prolapsed into the endometrial cavity or through the cervix. Pelvic examination may reveal the characteristic grape-like structures of sarcoma botryoides protruding from the cervix or the presence of velvety fronds of ESS in the cervical canal. A necrotic fungating mass at the vaginal apex should suggest an infarcted myoma, LMS, or MMMT. The uterus is usually enlarged and often soft and globular. If the cancer has involved the cervix, cul-de-sac, or cardinal ligaments, fixation or asymmetry of the parametria may be found. In advanced cases, inguinal or supraclavicular node metastases may be evident. Patients with advanced uterine sarcomas may present with a large omental mass or ascites secondary to abdominal carcinomatosis.

**B. Laboratory Findings:** Standard laboratory evaluation of patients with uterine sarcoma should include a complete blood count and urinalysis, liver function studies (especially serum alkaline phosphatase, prothrombin time, serum lactic dehydrogenase), blood urea nitrogen, and serum creatinine. CA-125 may be elevated. Estrogen and progesterone receptor analysis may indicate which patients are likely to respond to hormone therapy. Cytologic study of tissue recovered from the endometrial cavity or endocervical canal is often positive in endometrial sarcomas but not in the more deeply situated LMS. Office endometrial biopsy or punch biopsy of a prolapsed vaginal mass is helpful only if positive.

**C. X-Ray Findings:** The chest x-ray may contain metastatic coin lesions characteristic of uterine sarcomas. Because uterine sarcomas commonly metastasize to the lung, a chest computed tomography (CT) scan should be considered when the routine films are negative, particularly before any radical extirpative surgery in the pelvis is performed. An intravenous urogram is indispensable in the workup of any patient with a pelvic mass. It may reveal ureteral deviation, compression, obstruction, or anomaly, and will demonstrate clearly the number and location of the kidneys and ureters. The combination of the chest x-ray and the intravenous urogram (scout film) may be used as a survey of the axial skeleton, ribs, and pelvic bones, which are most frequently involved by metastases.

CT scan of the abdomen and pelvis is not warranted routinely but may delineate enlarged retroperitoneal nodes in advanced cases. MRI should provide an accurate preoperative assessment of uterine size and degree of involvement.

**D. Special Examinations:** Pelvic ultrasonography, although usually not indicated in the evaluation of palpable pelvic masses, may occasionally confirm the presence of a pelvic mass or help to differentiate an adnexal from a uterine mass in the obese patient. Sigmoidoscopy should always be performed in older women, or in young women if gastrointestinal bleeding or masses suspected of being malignant are present. Cystoscopy is indicated in locally advanced disease or in the presence of gross or microscopic hematuria.

## Differential Diagnosis

The clinical diagnosis of uterine sarcoma is frequently overlooked. Diagnostic accuracy can be increased if the physician keeps these tumors in mind while investigating any pelvic mass. The tumor frequently does not present the classic picture of abnormal bleeding accompanied by a symmetrically enlarged soft globular uterus. It can masquerade as any condition causing uterine enlargement or a pelvic mass; of these, pregnancy, leiomyoma, adenomyosis, and adherent ovarian neoplasms or pelvic inflammatory disease are most likely to cause misinterpretation. When cytologic studies, endometrial biopsy, or dilatation and fractional curettage fails to provide the diagnosis—a situation not uncommon with LMS—laparotomy is necessary. At laparotomy, thorough evaluation is critical to the future management of the patient with uterine sarcoma and must include inspection (where possible) and palpation of all abdominal viscera, peritoneal and mesenteric surfaces, liver, both diaphragms, and retroperitoneal structures, especially the pelvic and aortic lymph nodes. Cytologic examination of peritoneal exudate is indispensable for treatment planning; if no free fluid is present, samples may be obtained by instilling 50–100 mL of normal saline into the abdominal cavity. If a sarcoma is identified on frozen section of the hysterectomy specimen, suspicious lymph nodes should be removed. This information, gathered at the time of the initial exploration and carefully documented in the operative records, is critical for identification and staging of the neoplasm and for predicting outcome.

The pathologic diagnosis of uterine sarcoma is often extremely difficult and may require consultation with a gynecologic pathologist familiar with these tumors. As each cancer becomes more anaplastic, the parent cell or tissue becomes more difficult to identify histologically. Since proper treatment is predicated on accurate histologic diagnosis, every effort should be expended to identify the cell of origin.

## Complications

Severe anemia from chronic blood loss or acute hemorrhage may be present. The severity and extent of other complications due to uterine sarcomas are directly related to the size and virulence of the primary tumor. A pedunculated mass may protrude into the uterine cavity or prolapse through the cervix, causing bleeding or uterine cramps as the uterus attempts to expel the tumor. Infarction with subsequent infection and sepsis may ensue. Rupture of the uterus and kidney due to rapidly growing uterine sarcomas has been reported. Obstructed labor and postpartum uterine inversion secondary to endometrial sarcomas have also been noted. Extensive pulmonary metastases can produce hemoptysis and respiratory failure. Ascites is common in advanced disease with peritoneal metastases.

A wide variety of complications has been reported secondary to pressure or compression of a neighboring viscus or resulting from extension or metastases to other vital structures. Urethral elongation due to stretching of the bladder over a rapidly growing mass can simultaneously produce obstruction and loss of sphincter control, with subsequent overflow incontinence. Colon compression may result in ribbon stools and, eventually, complete bowel obstruction. Ureteral obstruction is common, especially with recurrent pelvic sarcomas. Urinary diversion or colostomy may be required prior to treatment if life-threatening viscus obstruction is present in an untreated patient, but urinary diversion should not be performed unless

there is some hope for cure or meaningful palliation, since it precludes a painless death from uremia.

## Prevention

Indiscriminate use of radiation therapy for benign conditions in the pelvis should be avoided, since several clinical studies have suggested an etiologic role of pelvic radiation in the development of MMMT.

## Treatment

**A. Emergency Measures:** Hemorrhage from uterine sarcomas can be exsanguinating and requires prompt attention. When there has been acute hemorrhage, blood volume should be replaced with whole blood; patients with severe or profound anemia secondary to chronic intermittent bleeding should have blood volume replaced with packed red blood cells over a somewhat prolonged time course. Rapid replacement with whole blood in these patients can precipitate congestive heart failure.

Emergency D&C should be used only to obtain tissue for analysis. Vigorous curettage is likely to aggravate or provoke bleeding. High-dose bolus radiation is a more reliable and safe method of controlling bleeding. A dose of 400–500 cGy administered daily to the whole pelvis over 2–3 days usually controls acute hemorrhage; this does not appreciably interfere with future management. If these measures are not successful, emergency embolization or ligation of the hypogastric arteries sometimes controls hemorrhage when hysterectomy is not indicated nor technically feasible.

**B. Surgical Measures:** Extirpative surgery provides the best chance for long-term palliation or cure for patients with uterine sarcomas. Surgery is the cornerstone of the treatment plan and should be the central focus of attack against these cancers.

Low-grade uterine sarcomas (some LMS, endolymphatic stromal myosis, intravenous leiomyomatosis) have a propensity for isolated local spread and central pelvic recurrence; therefore, such patients should be considered for radical hysterectomy and bilateral salpingo-oophorectomy. The benefits of this type of therapy have not been conclusively shown, but theoretically the problem of local recurrence should be improved by more radical excision of the primary tumor. Lymph node metastases in these low-grade tumors are negligible; consequently, pelvic lymphadenectomy can be reserved for patients with enlarged or suspicious nodes. Pelvic recurrences of low-grade uterine sarcomas have been successfully treated by repeated excisions of all resectable tumor. Patients have been known to survive for many years following this type of conservative treatment. Partial or complete pelvic exenteration may occasionally be useful for recurrence of indolent tumors.

The high-grade uterine sarcomas (some LMS, ESS, all MMMT) display early lymphatic, local, and hematogenous metastases even when apparently confined to the uterus. For this reason, radical surgery has been abandoned in favor of simple total abdominal hysterectomy and bilateral salpingo-oophorectomy preceded or followed by adjunctive radiation therapy. The addition of radiation therapy for LMS, although still controversial, is being discarded by many centers because it has not improved survival and because it substantially interferes with subsequent chemotherapy.

At the time of surgical exploration, a thorough examination and evaluation of the abdominal contents must be performed and documented. Cytologic specimens and omental tissue should be obtained, and suspicious papillations, excrescences, and adhesions should be excised for pathologic analysis. The more information obtained at the primary exploration, the less difficult will be the design of an appropriate postoperative treatment plan.

When uterine sarcomas recur in the lung and the metastatic survey is negative, unilateral isolated metastases should be excised after a chest CT scan has ruled out other lesions not apparent on the routine chest x-ray. Considering all sources, resection of isolated sarcoma metastases to the lung carries about a 25% 5-year cure rate.

**C. Chemotherapy:** Adjuvant doxorubicin has been shown to reduce the distant recurrence rate for LMS. Although the data are not statistically significant, some authorities recommend the use of doxorubicin-based chemotherapy in high-grade LMS.

Because of the high hormone receptor content in ESS, adjuvant progestin or tamoxifen therapy has been recommended. For receptor-negative tumors, doxorubicin-based chemotherapy is used.

Doxorubicin, cisplatin, and ifosfamide display significant activity against MMMTs. Cyclophosphamide and vincristine have also shown activity. Some data suggest that combination chemotherapy is more effective than single-agent therapy. In advanced or metastatic disease, adjuvant combination chemotherapy is recommended.

**D. Radiation Therapy:** When used as the only modality of treatment for uterine sarcomas, radiation has produced dismal results—very few survivors are reported in the literature following treatment with radiation therapy alone for any of the uterine sarcomas. Radiation therapy does seem to improve survival and reduce local recurrences when used in combination with surgery for the treatment of some endometrial sarcomas. Collected data indicate that adjuvant radiation therapy improves the 2-year survival rate in patients with ESS by approximately 20% and may also improve survival for those with MMMT, although less convincingly. Although an occasional 5-year survivor with LMS has been reported following radiation therapy alone, analysis of large numbers of patients from different institutions does not support its use for these tumors. Nevertheless, in advanced forms of LMS, radiation may prove useful for palliation and control of pelvic symptoms such as massive bleeding or pain.

**Prognosis**

In determining the prognosis for patients with uterine sarcomas, a constellation of factors must be examined simultaneously. Such considerations as the patient's age, state of health, and ability to withstand major surgery or radiation therapy (or both) must be evaluated. The most important clinical characteristic—and probably the overriding prognostic feature affecting the prognosis of these patients—is the stage of the disease at the time of diagnosis. In the high-grade sarcomas (LMS and mixed endometrial sarcoma), the presence of tumor outside the uterus at the time of diagnosis is a clear prognostic omen: fewer than 10% of patients survive 2 years. Even when the disease is apparently limited to the uterus, the prognosis is poor: 10–50% survive 5 years. In the intermediate-grade LMS and high-grade ESS, the outcome is improved, with up to 80–90% of patients surviving 5 years if the disease is clinically limited to the uterus at the time of surgery. Low-grade ESS and low-grade LMS have a generally favorable outcome: 80–100% of patients survive 5 years following complete excision of the uterus. Low-grade stromal tumors have been known to recur locally after 10–20 years; this confuses the survival statistics. Undoubtedly, these patients must be followed closely for life.

# REFERENCES

## ENDOMETRIAL HYPERPLASIA & CARCINOMA

Abeler V, Kjorstad KE: Clear cell carcinoma of the endometrium: A histopathological and clinical study of 97 cases. Gynecol Oncol 1991;40:207.

ACOG: Estrogen replacement therapy and endometrial cancer. Committee opinion: No. 126. American College of Obstetricians and Gynecologists, August 1993.

Belloni C et al: Magnetic resonance imaging in endometrial carcinoma staging. Gynecol Oncol 1990;37:172.

Bloss JD et al: Use of vaginal hysterectomy for the management of stage I endometrial cancer in the medically compromised patient. Gynecol Oncol 1991;40:74.

Boring CC et al: Cancer statistics, 1992. Ca 1992;42:19.

Borst MP et al: Oncogene alterations in endometrial carcinoma. Gynecol Oncol 1990;38:364.

Bourne TH et al: Detection of endometrial cancer by transvaginal ultrasonography with color flow imaging and blood flow analysis: A preliminary report. Gynecol Oncol 1991;40:253.

Britton LC et al: DNA ploidy in endometrial carcinoma: Major objective prognostic factor. Mayo Clin Proc 1990;65:543.

Burke TW et al: Treatment failure in endometrial carcinoma. Obstet Gynecol 1990;75:96.

Chen SS: Extrauterine spread in endometrial carcinoma clinically confined to the uterus. Gynecol Oncol 1985; 21:23.

Cherkis RC et al: Significance of normal endometrial cells detected by cervical cytology. Obstet Gynecol 1988;71:242.

Fox H, Buckley CH: The endometrial hyperplasia and their relationship to endometrial neoplasia. Histopathology 1982;2:493.

Gal D et al: Long-term effect of megestrol acetate in the treatment of endometrial hyperplasia. Am J Obstet Gynecol 1983;146:316.

Gallion, HH, van Nagell JR, Powell DF: Stage I serous papillary carcinoma of the endometrium. Cancer 1989; 63:2224.

Goff BA, Rice LW: Assessment of depth of myometrial invasion in endometrial adenocarcinoma. Gynecol Oncol 1990;38:46.

Granberg S et al: Endometrial thickness as measured by endovaginal ultrasonography for identifying endometrial abnormality. Am J Obstet Gynecol 1991;164:47.

Hendrickson RL: Endometrial epithelial metaplasias: Proliferations frequently misdiagnosed as adenocarcinomas. Am J Pathol 1980;4:525.

Holst J, Koskela O, Von Schaultz B: Endometrial findings following curettage in 2018 women according to age and indications. Ann Chir Gynaecol 1983;72:274.

Kurman RJ, Kaminski PF, Norris JH: The behavior of endometrial hyperplasia: A long-term study of "untreated" hyperplasia in 170 patients. Cancer 1985; 56:403.

Kurman RJ, Norris HJ: Evaluation of criteria for distinguishing atypical endometrial hyperplasia from well-differentiated carcinoma. Cancer 1982;49:2547.

Lehoczky O et al: Stage I endometrial adenocarcinoma: Treatment of nonoperable patients with intracavitary radiation alone. Gynecol Oncol 1991;43:211.

Morrow CP et al: Relationship between surgical-pathological risk factors and outcome in clinical stage I and II carcinoma of the endometrium: A gynecologic oncology group study. Gynecol Oncol 1991;40:55.

Morrow CP, Disaia, PJ, Townsend DE: The role of postoperative irradiation in the management of stage I adenocarcinoma of the endometrium. Am J Roentgenol 1976;127:325.

Patsner B et al: Predictive value of preoperative serum Ca125 levels in clinically localized and advanced endometrial carcinoma. Am J Obstet Gynecol 1988;158: 399.

Pettersson F: Annual report on the results of treatment in gynecological cancer. Int J Gynecol Obstet 1991;36 (Suppl):132.

Potish RA et al: Role of whole abdominal radiation therapy in the management of endometrial cancer: Prognostic importance of factors indicating peritoneal metastases. Gynecol Oncol 1985;21:80.

Quinn MA, Campbell JJ: Tamoxifen therapy in advanced/recurrent endometrial carcinoma. Gynecol Oncol 1989;32:1.

Rubin GL et al: Estrogen replacement therapy and the risk of endometrial cancer: Remaining controversies. Am J Obstet Gynecol 1990;162:148.

Salazar OM et al: The management of clinical stage I endometrial carcinoma. Cancer 1978;41:1016.

Scully RE: Definition of endometrial carcinoma precursors. Clin Obstet Gynecol 1982;25:39.

Seouid MAF, Johnson J, Weed JC: Gynecologic tumors in tamoxifen-treated women with breast cancer. Obstet Gynecol 1993;82:165.

Stringer CA, Gershenson DM, Burke TW: Adjuvant chemotherapy with cisplatin, doxorubicin, and cyclophosphamide (PAC) for early stage high-risk endometrial cancer: A preliminary analysis. Gynecol Oncol 1990;38:305.

Szpak CA et al: Prognostic value of cytologic examination of peritoneal washings in patients with endometrial carcinoma. Acta Cytol (Baltimore) 1981;225: 640.

Thigpen T et al: A randomized trial of medroxyprogesterone acetate (MPA) 200 mg versus 1000 mg daily in advanced or recurrent endometrial carcinoma: A gynecologic oncology group study. Proc ASCO 1991; 10:185.

Zaino RJ, Kurman RJ: Squamous differentiation in carcinoma of the endometrium: A critical appraisal of adenoacanthoma and adenosquamous carcinoma. Semin Diagn Pathol 1988;5:154.

## SARCOMA OF THE UTERUS

Antman KH et al: Response to ifosfamide and mesna:124 previously treated patients with metastatic or unresectable sarcoma. J Clin Oncol 1989;7:126.

Baker VV, Walton LA Jr, Currie JL: Steroid receptors in endolymphatic stromal myosis. Obstet Gynecol 1984; 63(Suppl 3):72S.

Berchuk A et al: Treatment of endometrial stromal tumors. Gynecol Oncol 1990;36:60.

Burns B, Curry RH, Bell ME: Morphologic features of prognostic significance in uterine smooth muscle tumors: A review of eighty-four cases. Am J Obstet Gynecol 1979;135:109.

Clement PB, Scully RE: Müllerian adenosarcoma of the uterus: A clinicopathologic analysis of 100 cases with a review of the literature. Hum Pathol 1990;21:363.

Echt G et al: Treatment of uterine sarcomas. Cancer 1990;66:35.

Evans HL: Endometrial stromal sarcoma and poorly differentiated endometrial sarcoma. Cancer 1982;50: 2170.

Fekete PS, Veillios F: The clinical and histologic spectrum of endometrial stromal neoplasms: A report of 41 cases. Int J Gynecol Pathol 1984;3:198.

Kahanpää KV et al: Sarcomas of the uterus: A clinicopathologic study of 119 patients. Obstet Gynecol 1986;67:417.

Leibsohn S et al: Leiomyosarcoma in a series of hysterectomies performed for presumed uterine leiomyomas. Am J Obstet Gynecol 1990;162:968.

Omura GA et al: A randomized clinical trial of adjuvant adriamycin in uterine sarcomas: A Gynecologic Oncology Group Study. J Clin Oncol 1985;3:1240.

Perez CA et al: Effects of irradiation on mixed müllerian tumors of the uterus. Cancer 1979;43:1274.

Peters WA et al: Cisplatin and adriamycin combination

chemotherapy for uterine stromal sarcomas and mixed mesodermal tumors. Gynecol Oncol 1989;34:323.

Silverberg SG et al: Carcinosarcoma (malignant mixed mesodermal tumor) of the uterus: A gynecology oncology group pathologic study of 203 cases. Int J Gynecol Pathol 1990;9:1.

Sorbe B: Radiotherapy and/or chemotherapy as adjuvant treatment of uterine sarcomas. Gynecol Oncol 1984; 20:281.

Spanos WJ Jr, Peters LJ, Oswald MJ: Patterns of recurrence in malignant mixed müllerian tumor of the uterus. Cancer 1986;57:155.

Sutton GP et al: Phase II trial of ifosfamide and mesna in mixed mesodermal tumors of the uterus: A gynecologic oncology group study. Am J Obstet Gynecol 1989 161:309.

Thigpen JT et al: Phase II trial of cisplatin as first line chemotherapy in patients with advanced or recurrent uterine sarcomas: A gynecologic oncology group study. J Clin Oncol 1991;9:1962.

Van Dinh T, Woodruff JD: Leiomyosarcoma of the uterus. Am J Obstet Gynecol 1982;144:817.

# Premalignant and Malignant Disorders of the Ovaries and Oviducts

*Vicki V. Baker, MD*

## General Introduction

Ovarian cancer is the fifth leading cause of cancer-related deaths in the USA. Although only 15–20% of all cancers of the female genital tract arise from the ovary or fallopian tube, these neoplasms account for more cancer-related deaths than all of the other primary pelvic cancers. About 23,000 cases were diagnosed in 1993, and 14,000 women died as a result of this disease. Approximately 1 in 70 newborn girls will develop ovarian cancer during her lifetime. In general, ovarian cancer is a disease of the postmenopausal woman and the prepubescent girl, although it is documented to occur in females of all ages.

## ETIOLOGY OF OVARIAN CANCER

The cause of ovarian cancer is unknown, although a number of risk factors have been identified. It has been proposed that repeated ovulation is causally related to the development of this disease. Ovulation is accompanied by disruption of the germinal epithelium and the activation of cellular repair mechanisms. Repeated ovulation may provide ample opportunity for somatic gene deletions and mutations to occur, which in turn can contribute to tumor initiation and progression. Supporting this theory are the observations that chronic anovulation, multiparity, and a history of breast feeding are protective. Pregnancy decreases the risk of ovarian cancer by 30–60%. Oral contraceptive use also decreases the risk by 30–60%, depending on the duration of use.

The role of diet as an etiologic factor in ovarian cancer has not been established, but several investigators have suggested that increased fat consumption is associated with an increased risk of ovarian cancer. Exposure to talc has also been proposed as a risk factor in women who place talcum powder on the external genitalia. The presence of talc granulomas in the ovaries of patients who have never been previously operated on has been well documented and can be explained by the continuity of the introitus and perito-

neal cavity via the endocervical canal, the endometrial cavity, and the fallopian tubes (Fig 49–1). The ability of foreign materials, including talc and asbestos, to act as carcinogenic substances is established in several models, but their role in ovarian carcinogenesis remains speculative.

Genetic factors also appear to play an important role in the development and progression of ovarian cancer. Patients with Turner's syndrome (45,XO) are at increased risk of dysgerminoma and gonadoblastoma. The presence of a Y chromosome, as found in Turner's syndrome with mosaicism (45,XO/46,XY) and Klinefelter's syndrome (XXY), further increases this risk. Other genetic disorders associated with an increased incidence of nonepithelial ovarian neoplasms include the familial occurrence of teratomas and the increased incidence of sex cord tumors in patients with Peutz-Jeghers syndrome. The molecular biologic explanation for these well-recognized associations is unknown.

Although most cases of epithelial ovarian cancer are sporadic and exhibit no heritable tendencies, approximately 7% occur in women with a suggestive family history. The most common pedigrees are sister/sister and mother/daughter patterns. Three heritable syndromes have been described: (1) site-specific ovarian cancer, (2) familial cases of breast and ovarian cancer, (3) the cancer family syndrome, characterized by the occurrence of colon cancer and adenocarcinoma of the ovary, breast, or uterus or a combination.

Persons affected by one of the heritable ovarian cancer syndromes are typically diagnosed in the fifth decade of life with poorly differentiated, bilateral ovarian neoplasms. Molecular biologic studies suggest the presence of one or more tumor suppressor genes on chromosome 17, which may play a role in the etiology of this disease. Chromosome 17 is the location of the p53 tumor suppressor gene, the HER-2/neu gene and the gene that encodes the epidermal growth factor receptor. In addition, the long arm of chromosome 17 appears to be the location of 2 putative tumor suppressor genes, the BRCA1 gene and the

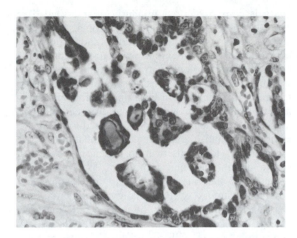

**Figure 49–1.** Papillary lesion with incorporated talc granules.

**Table 49–1.** Major histopathologic categories of ovarian cancer.

**Epithelial**
Serous, mucinous, endometrioid, clear cell, transitional cell, undifferentiated

**Germ Cell**
Dysgerminoma, endodermal sinus tumor, immature teratoma, embryonal carcinoma, choriocarcinoma, gonadoblastoma, mixed germ cell

**Sex Cord and Stromal**
Granulosa cell tumor, fibroma, thecoma, Sertoli-Leydig

**Neoplasms Metastatic to the Ovary**
Breast, colon, stomach, endometrium, lymphoma

prohibitin gene, both of which may play a role in the initiation and progression of familial ovarian cancer.

Additional evidence for a genetic basis for ovarian cancer comes from the observation that women diagnosed with breast and colon cancer are at increased risk of developing ovarian cancer.

## HISTOPATHOLOGY OF OVARIAN CANCER

Ovarian cancer may be divided into 3 major categories, based on the cell type of origin (Table 49–1). The ovary may also be the site of metastatic disease by primary cancer from another organ site. Unlike carcinomas of the cervix and endometrium, precursor lesions of ovarian carcinoma have not been defined.

## 1. EPITHELIAL NEOPLASMS

Epithelial neoplasms are derived from the ovarian surface mesothelial cells and include 6 cell types: **serous, mucinous, endometrioid, clear cell, transitional cell,** and **undifferentiated.** Epithelial tumors account for over 60% of all ovarian neoplasms and more than 90% of malignant ovarian tumors.

Ovarian **serous cystadenocarcinoma** is the most common malignant tumor of the ovary, accounting for 35–50% of all epithelial tumors. Grossly, these neoplasms are bilateral in 40–60% of cases, and 85% are associated with extraovarian spread at the time of diagnosis. Over 50% of serous tumors exceed 15 cm in diameter, and cut section reveals solid areas, areas of hemorrhage, necrosis, cyst wall invasion, and adhesions to adjacent structures. Unilocular or multilocular cysts often contain course papillae that project into the cystic lumen (Fig 49–2).

Histologically, serous carcinomas of the ovary exhibit mild to moderate nuclear atypia and occasional mitotic figures of the stratified squamous epithelium,

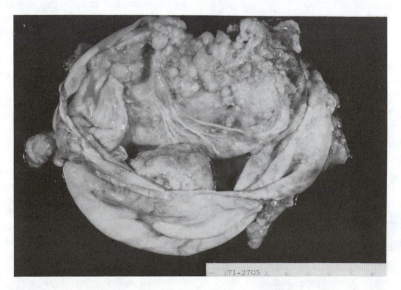

|71-2705|

**Figure 49–2.** Internal papillae characteristic of the papillary serous "cystadenocarcinoma."

which often forms budding tufts. Psammoma bodies, which are irregular calcifications, are characteristic of serous tumors. The grade of differentiation of these neoplasms is based on the degree of preservation of the papillary architecture. Most serous carcinomas are poorly differentiated with trabecular and solid growth patterns.

Serous ovarian neoplasms of low malignant potential exhibit histologic features suggestive of both carcinoma and benignity. Although marked cellular pleomorphism and mitotic figures are often present, there is no stromal invasion. Psammoma bodies are often present. As will be discussed in a later section, the prognosis and therapy of serous carcinoma of low malignant potential are different from invasive serous carcinoma, and an accurate diagnosis is essential.

**Mucinous neoplasms** of the ovary account for 10–20% of all epithelial ovarian tumors and are the second most common type of epithelial ovarian cancer. In contrast to serous tumors, mucinous tumors are bilateral in less than 10% of cases.

Mucinous tumors are notable for the large size that they may attain; neoplasms over 150 pounds have been reported. However, the average size of these lesions is 16–17 cm. Cut sections of these tumors typically reveal multilocular cysts filled with viscous mucin (Fig 49–3). The lining of these tumors is composed of atypical cells with numerous mitotic figures.

Histologically, mucinous adenocarcinoma of the

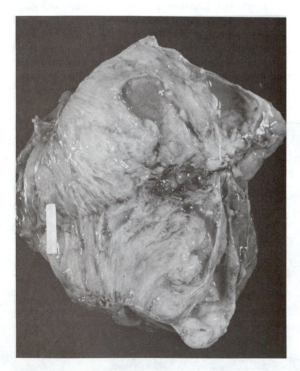

**Figure 49–3.** Mucinous cystadenocarcinoma, note the obvious mucinous component and the solid, more malignant areas.

ovary is composed predominantly of intestinal-like cells that invade the surrounding stroma. The cells have large hyperchromatic nuclei and prominent nucleoli. Invasive mucinous ovarian carcinoma exhibits marked histologic variability from area to area within the tumor, and extensive sampling is required. It is recommended that at least one section per centimeter of tumor be examined. The differentiation of mucinous cystadenocarcinoma is related to the preservation of gland-like architecture of the tumor.

Analogous to serous ovarian neoplasms, both invasive carcinomas and tumors of low malignant potential of the mucinous variety are recognized. Mucinous tumors of low malignant potential are characterized histologically by several cell types, including endocervical-like columnar cells, intestinal-like columnar cells with eosinophilic neoplasm, goblet cells, and basal endocrine cells. Although cellular atypia may be mild to moderate and a moderate number of mitotic figures may be present, cellular stratification does not exceed 2–3 layers and stromal invasion is absent.

**Pseudomyxoma peritonei** is an unusual condition that may occur in association with mucinous neoplasms of the ovary resulting from the progressive accumulation of mucin in the abdominal cavity following its slow leakage from a neoplasm. It most commonly occurs in association with lesions of low malignant potential, although it is also reported to occur in association with cystadenocarcinoma of the ovary and appendix as well as mucocele of the appendix. Although rare and histologically benign in appearance, pseudomyxoma peritonei has a protracted and potentially morbid course secondary to repeated bowel obstruction with a mortality rate that approaches 50%.

An **endometrioid neoplasm** of the ovary exhibits an adenomatoid pattern that resembles endometrial adenocarcinoma (Fig 49–4). It is bilateral in 30–50% of cases. Rarely, this neoplasm arises in foci of endometriosis (less than 10% of cases). The degree of differentiation is based on the extent to which the glandular architecture is retained. As many as 30% of patients with endometrioid carcinoma of the ovary also have a synchronous endometrial carcinoma of the uterus that is a second primary rather than a metastatic focus of disease.

**Clear cell carcinoma** of the ovary, also referred to as **mesonephroid carcinoma** of the ovary, accounts for approximately 5% of epithelial ovarian cancers. It rarely attains the size of serous and mucinous neoplasms of the ovary. Clear cell carcinomas of the ovary are biologically aggressive and may be associated with hypercalcemia and hyperpyrexia. On cut section, both cystic and solid areas are present. The external surface is smooth but has a bosselated contour. Histologically, 2 cell types may be present: the clear cell and the "hobnail cell" (Fig 49–5). Occasionally, clear cell carcinomas may be difficult to dif-

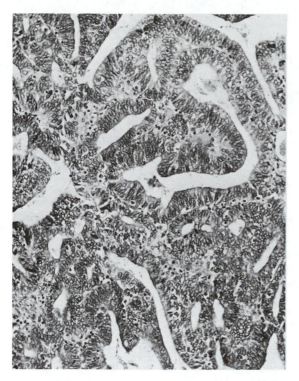

**Figure 49–4.** Endometrioid carcinoma as seen with high-power field. Note the tall epithelium—not a tubal type or the mucoid variety.

ferentiate from mucinous neoplasms. The periodic acid-Schiff reaction can be used to differentiate the 2 since it is only weakly positive in clear cell neoplasms but strikingly positive in mucinous tumors.

**Transitional cell carcinoma** of the ovary is a newly described entity composed of cells that resem-

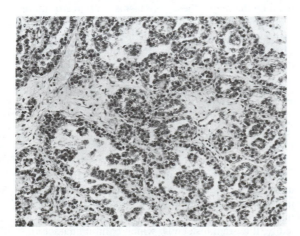

**Figure 49–5.** Adenomatous pattern with papillary infolding and "hobnail epithelium." In many areas, clear cells can be seen with transitions to the hobnail type.

ble low-grade transitional cell carcinoma of the urinary bladder. Patients typically present with advanced stage disease and exhibit a poorer prognosis when compared with that of other histologic types of epithelial ovarian cancer.

**Undifferentiated carcinoma** of the ovary accounts for less than 10% of epithelial neoplasms. This neoplasm is characterized by the absence of any distinguishing microscopic features that permit its placement in one of the other histologic categories.

## 2. GERM CELL NEOPLASMS

Germ cell neoplasms arise from the germ cell elements of the ovary and include dysgerminoma, endodermal sinus tumor, embryonal cell carcinoma, choriocarcinoma, teratoma, polyembryona, and mixed germ cell tumors. Unlike the epithelial neoplasms, which tend to occur during the sixth decade of life, this group of tumors tends to occur during the second and third decades and as a group is associated with a better prognosis. Many of these neoplasms produce biologic markers, which can be monitored to assess response to therapy (Table 49–2).

**Dysgerminoma** of the ovary is the female counterpart of the seminoma in the male. It occurs primarily in young females and accounts for about 50% of germ cell tumors. Grossly, the tumor is rather rubbery in consistency, smooth, rounded, and thinly encapsulated with a brown or grayish-brown color. This neoplasm is unilateral in 85–90% of cases. It is a solid neoplasm, which may contain areas of softening due to degeneration.

Histologically, dysgerminoma mimics the pattern seen in the primitive gonad, ie, with nests of germ cells that appear as large, rounded cells with central nuclei that contain 1 or 2 prominent nucleoli surrounded by undifferentiated stroma (Fig 49–6). Lymphocytes may invade the stroma and occasionally giant cells are identified. A lymphocytic infiltrate is considered a favorable prognostic indicator.

**Endodermal sinus tumor** of the ovary, previously called a **yolk sac tumor,** is the second most common germ cell neoplasm, occurring in approximately 20% of cases. It is bilateral in less than 5% of cases. It holds the distinction of being the most rapidly grow-

**Table 49–2.** Tumor markers that may be elevated in the presence of germ cell neoplasms.

| Neoplasm | AFP | HCG |
|---|---|---|
| Dysgerminoma | – | +/– |
| Endodermal sinus tumor | + | – |
| Immature teratoma | +/– | – |
| Mixed germ cell tumor | +/– | +/– |
| Choriocarcinoma | – | + |
| Embryonal carcinoma | – | + |

AFP, alpha-fetoprotein; HCG, human chorionic gonadotropin.

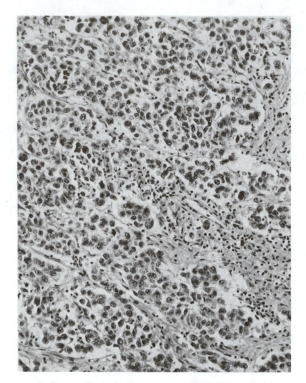

**Figure 49–6.** Classic histologic picture of germinoma. Note nests of germ cells of various sizes separated by fibrous trabeculae.

ing neoplasm that occurs at any site. These lesions are friable, focally necrotic, and hemorrhagic. Patients commonly present with an acute abdomen.

Microscopically, endodermal sinus tumor is composed of primitive epithelial cells that form architectural patterns that recapitulate the primitive gut and the primitive liver. The pathognomonic finding is the Schiller-Duval body, which is a single papilla lined by tumor cells with a central blood vessel. This neoplasm commonly contains cells that produce alpha-fetoprotein (AFP).

**Immature teratomas** of the ovary are the malignant counterpart of the mature cystic teratoma or dermoid and also account for about 20% of germ cell neoplasms. This malignancy is bilateral in less than 5% of cases, although the contralateral ovary commonly contains a dermoid cyst. The serum AFP is usually elevated in patients with an immature teratoma.

Microscopic examination reveals a disordered collection of tissues derived from the 3 germ layers with at least some of the components having an immature, embryonic appearance. The immature elements are commonly neuroectodermal and consist of small round malignant cells that may be associated with glia formation. Hyaline bodies stain positive for AFP. Immature teratomas are graded from 1 to 3 based on

the amount of immature neural tissue that they contain. Tumor grade is correlated with prognosis and also guides recommendations regarding the need for chemotherapy. Metastatic implants may be composed entirely of mature neuroectodermal tissue. In this circumstance, the stage of the tumor is not increased nor is the prognosis diminished.

Mature teratomas or dermoids are common ovarian neoplasms, occurring primarily in women ages 20–30 years. They represent the most common neoplasm diagnosed during pregnancy. Rarely, the squamous component undergoes malignant transformation (less than 2%) in women over the age of 40.

**Embryonal carcinoma** of the ovary is a very rare germ cell tumor in pure form, although foci may occasionally be found admixed with other germ cell neoplasms. Histologically, this neoplasm consists of solid sheets of large polygonal cells with pale, eosinophilic cytoplasms that appear to merge together as a syncytium because the cell membranes are poorly defined. Serum human chorionic gonadotropin hCG and AFP values are usually elevated.

**Choriocarcinoma** of the ovary is another rare germ cell tumor that is unrelated to pregnancy. Unlike gestational choriocarcinoma, primary ovarian choriocarcinoma is associated with somewhat lower elevations of hCG. The endocrine activity of this neoplasm may cause precocious puberty, uterine bleeding, or amenorrhea. Microscopically, this neoplasm is composed of cytotrophoblasts, intermediate trophoblasts, and syncytiotrophoblasts.

**Gonadoblastoma** of the ovary is a rare neoplasm composed of nests of germ cells and sex cord derivatives that are surrounded by connective tissue stroma (Fig 49–7). These tumors are more common in the right ovary than in the left and usually occur during the second decade of life.

**Mixed germ cell tumors** of the ovary account for approximately 10% of germ cell neoplasms. As implied by the name, these neoplasms contain 2 or more germ cell elements. A dysgerminoma and endodermal sinus tumor occur together most frequently. These neoplasms must be meticulously evaluated by the pathologist to identify all elements correctly, since different components may require treatment with different chemotherapeutic regimens.

## SEX-CORD AND STROMAL CELL NEOPLASMS

**Granulosa cell tumors** are associated with hyperestrogenism and may cause precocious puberty in young girls and adenomatous hyperplasia and vaginal bleeding in postmenopausal women. Microscopically, the granulosa cells, which exhibit characteristic grooved or coffee bean nuclei, may exhibit microfollicular, macrofollicular, trabecular, insular, or solid growth patterns. Call-Exner bodies are asso-

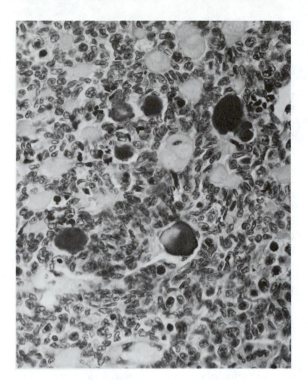

**Figure 49–7.** Gonadoblastoma with folliculoid pattern, focal calcifications, and concretions.

ciated with the microfollicular growth pattern and represent multiple small cavities that contain eosinophilic fluid. Theca cells are present in varying amounts.

Like the granulosa cell tumors, an ovarian thecoma is often associated with hyperestrogenism. This benign ovarian tumor consists of lipid-laden stromal cells, which gives the tumor a yellow color on cut section. An ovarian fibroma is another benign tumor that is noteworthy because of its association with Meigs' syndrome. Meigs' syndrome refers to the occurrence of an ovarian fibroma, ascites, and pleural effusion, which collectively mimic the presentation of ovarian cancer.

The **Sertoli-Leydig cell tumor** is usually virilizing and occurs most commonly during the third decade of life. It is rarely bilateral. Microscopically, both Sertoli and Leydig cells are present. A variety of architectural patterns have been described.

## NEOPLASMS METASTATIC TO THE OVARY

Cancer metastatic to the ovary accounts for as many as 25% of all ovarian malignancies. Clinically, these tumors often mimic primary ovarian cancer and usually present as bilateral adnexal masses, although

a unilateral mass occurs in as many as 25% of patients. These masses are usually smooth and bosselated, solid, and mobile (see Fig 49–14). The most common primary cancers that metastasize to the ovary are those of the breast, stomach, colon, and endometrium.

Microscopically, cancer metastatic to the ovary can present a variety of potentially confusing patterns. For example, when the primary lesion is a breast carcinoma, the histologic appearance of the ovary may vary from one that accurately reflects the primary pathology to a pattern of diffuse invasion of the stroma by undifferentiated cells. Gastrointestinal carcinoma metastatic to the ovary often simulates a primary mucin-secreting adenocarcinoma of the ovary with the presence of characteristic signet ring cells (Fig 49–8). Large locules lined by tall columnar mucin-secreting epithelial cells are separated by fibrous trabeculae. The epithelium may be well, moderately, or poorly differentiated.

Krukenberg tumors by definition represent carcinomas of the stomach metastatic to the ovary. However, common usage of the eponym reflects any gastrointestinal carcinoma metastatic to the ovary.

## DIAGNOSIS OF OVARIAN CANCER

Ovarian cancer typically develops as an insidious disease, with few warning signs or symptoms. Most neoplastic ovarian tumors produce few symptoms until the disease is widely disseminated throughout the abdominal cavity. A history of nonspecific gastrointestinal complaints, including nausea, dyspepsia, and altered bowel habits, is particularly common.

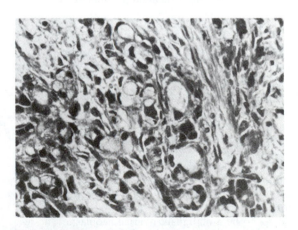

**Figure 49–8.** Metastatic ovarian cancer. Note the "signet cells," characteristic of the mucocellular nature of the tumor.

Early satiety and abdominal distention as a result of ascites are generally signs of advanced disease. A change in bowel habits, such as constipation and decreased stool caliber, is occasionally noted. Large tumors may cause a sensation of pelvic weight or pressure. Rarely, an ovarian tumor may become incarcerated in the cul-de-sac and cause severe pain, urinary retention, rectal discomfort, and bowel obstruction.

Menstrual abnormalities may be noted in as many as 15% of reproductive age patients with an ovarian neoplasm. Abnormal vaginal bleeding may occur in patients with ovarian cancer in the presence of a synchronous endometrial carcinoma or as a consequence of metastatic disease to the lower genital tract. Rarely, excess androgens or estrogens may be present in women with ovarian neoplasms, presumably because of stimulation of normal theca, granulosa, or hilar cells that surround the neoplasm. Ovarian stromal hyperplasia or hyperthecosis may also be associated with excess androgen production, which alters the normal menstrual cycle. Granulosa theca cell tumors are classically estrogen-producing tumors that present with abnormal vaginal bleeding.

The prognosis of ovarian cancer is significantly improved when the disease is detected while still confined to the ovary. Unfortunately, routine pelvic examination is a notoriously poor screening method with limited sensitivity and specificity. Ten percent of masses less than 10 cm in size are missed on routine examination, and the size of a mass is correctly predicted within 2 cm in only 68% of patients. Current strategies for screening revolve around the detection of tumor-associated antigens, such as CA-125, and ultrasound examinations of the adnexae. However, the limited prevalence of ovarian cancer in conjunction with the sensitivity and specificity of currently available tests such as ultrasound and CA-125 do not support the implementation of routine ovarian cancer screening in the general population.

## EVALUATION OF THE PATIENT WITH A SUSPECTED OVARIAN NEOPLASM

Patients found to have a pelvic mass must be evaluated in a timely and cost effective manner that is tailored to a realistic list of possible diagnoses. The differential diagnosis of a pelvic mass is influenced by the age of the patient, the characteristics of the mass on pelvic examination, and the radiographic appearance of the mass. In general, the prepubescent child and the postmenopausal woman are at greatest risk for developing a pelvic mass that subsequently proves to be a malignant ovarian neoplasm. The reproductive age woman is more likely to have a functional ovarian cyst or endometrioma.

## Physical Examination

Although the natural focus of the physical examination of the patient with a suspected adnexal neoplasm is the pelvis, it is important to perform a comprehensive examination. Particular attention should be paid to the lymph-node-bearing areas, particularly the supraclavicular and inguinal areas. Metastatic disease to the skin rarely occurs in the presence of ovarian cancer. **Sister Mary Joseph's nodule** is the term that refers to a metastatic implant in the umbilicus.

Examination of the abdomen often provides important information. Abdominal distention is one of the more common findings. The presence of flank fullness and shifting dullness implies the presence of ascites or a large pelvic-abdominal mass. Together with these signs, a tympanitic percussion note over the lateral abdomen is consistent with a large mass, which displaces the bowel to the periphery. In contrast, a central tympanitic percussion note is suggestive of ascites. Recent eversion of the umbilicus in a patient with abdominal distention may result from an increase in intra-abdominal pressure secondary to ascites.

A careful and thorough pelvic examination provides many helpful clues concerning the etiology of a pelvic mass and should never be replaced by a cursory examination or radiographic evaluation. The characteristics of the mass that should be noted on pelvic examination are listed in Table 49–3.

Unilateral, cystic masses in reproductive age women are benign in up to 95%. These masses, particularly when less than 6–8 cm in size, are observed through a menstrual cycle since many represent functional cysts and spontaneously resolve. An enlarging mass or one that is associated with pain merits prompt intervention. A cystic, somewhat immobile adnexal mass may represent a hydrosalpinx or tuboovarian abscess. Fixed, bilateral masses and firm masses with nodularity are suggestive of, but not diagnostic of, an ovarian malignancy. Because no features seen on physical examination consistently distinguish malignant from benign neoplasms, further characterization can be achieved with select radiographic examinations.

## Radiographic Evaluation

Ultrasonography is the most common radiographic

**Table 49–3.** Characteristics of a pelvic mass that should be noted on physical examination.

| Benign | Malignant |
| --- | --- |
| Mobility | Fixed |
| Consistency | Solid or firm |
| Bilateral or unilateral | Bilateral |
| Cul de sac | Nodular |
| Mobile | |
| Cystic | |
| Unilateral | |
| Smooth | |

test to evaluate adnexal masses. Transabdominal examinations require a full bladder as an acoustic window for optimal visualization of the adnexae. In contradistinction, a transvaginal examination does not have this requirement but may not be as useful for the assessment of large adnexal masses. The ultrasonographic characteristics that help differentiate benign from malignant masses are listed in Table 49–4. The correlation between the ultrasonic appearance of an adnexal mass and the pathologic findings is imprecise. Color flow Doppler studies that evaluate the vascular patterns of adnexal masses show promise as a means to improve the sensitivity and specificity of the radiographic prediction of benign and malignant lesions. Angiogenesis accompanying malignancy results in vascular abnormalities and increased blood flow compared with the vascular architecture and patterns of blood flow in nonmalignant lesions.

Characterization of adnexal masses by computerized tomography (CT) or magnetic resonance imaging (MRI) may provide clinically useful information in select instances. CT scanning provides information about the retroperitoneal structures in addition to the pelvic organs. Compared with ultrasonography, CT is a more accurate and sensitive way to differentiate benign from malignant lesions, although the specificity is comparable. The role of MRI in the evaluation of adnexal pathology has not been extensively evaluated. It is one of the most expensive and least available radiographic studies. However, it may be of particular benefit in the evaluation of pregnant patients because it avoids radiation exposure of the fetus.

When a patient has a suspected ovarian malignancy based on her clinical presentation, physical examination, and the ultrasonographic appearance of the mass, a radiograph of the chest is done to exclude metastatic parenchymal disease and to detect a pleural effusion.

If the patient notes a change in bowel habits or if guaiac-positive stools are detected, a barium enema should be obtained. Patients who appear to have advanced ovarian cancer, evidenced by a nodular pelvic mass with or without ascites may actually have colon cancer. Because of the genetic links among ovarian cancer, colon cancer, and breast cancer, a patient with a suspected ovarian malignancy should also undergo a screening mammogram study.

**Table 49–4.** Radiographic characteristics that help to differentiate benign and malignant adnexal masses.

| Benign | Malignant |
| --- | --- |
| Simple cyst, < 10 cm in size | Solid or cystic and solid |
| Septations < 3 mm in thickness | Multiple septations > 3 mm in size |
| Unilateral | Bilateral |
| Calcification, especially teeth | Ascites |
| Gravity-dependent layering of cyst contents | |

## Laboratory Evaluation

When an ovarian malignancy is included in the list of diagnostic possibilities, a limited number of laboratory tests are indicated. A complete blood count (CBC) and serum electrolytes tests should be obtained in all patients. Coagulation tests are not indicated in the absence of a suggestive history of bleeding after minor trauma or increased bruisability. Similarly, routine liver function tests are rarely helpful.

A serum hCG level should be measured in any female in whom pregnancy is a possibility. In addition, a serum AFP and lactate dehydrogenase (LDH) should be measured in young girls and adolescents who present with adnexal masses because the younger the patient, the greater the likelihood of a malignant germ cell tumor. The serum CA-125 level should also be determined whenever an ovarian malignancy is included in the differential diagnosis. An elevated CA-125 in the postmenopausal patient is particularly suggestive of the presence of an ovarian malignancy, although it is not specific for this diagnosis. Cancers of the colon, breast, pancreas, stomach, uterus, and fallopian tube are also associated with an elevated CA-125 value. Benign conditions commonly diagnosed in younger women, including pregnancy, endometriosis, leiomyomata, and adenomyosis, limit the usefulness of this test in premenopausal women. A normal CA-125 level does *not* exclude the diagnosis of cancer and does not represent a reason to delay surgery.

Paracentesis is not advocated as a routine procedure for the patient with ascites and a pelvic mass and in whom renal, cardiac, and hepatic failure has been excluded. False-negative results may occur in as many as 40% of patients with widespread intra-abdominal disease. The presence or absence of a malignant effusion does not diminish the need for surgery. Furthermore, insertion of a trocar may rupture an encapsulated neoplasm, spilling tumor cells into the peritoneal cavity, or it may result in implantation of neoplastic cells along the insertion site.

In contrast to the role of paracentesis, diagnostic thoracentesis to remove an aliquot of a pleural effusion for cytology is recommended prior to surgical intervention. In the presence of a malignant pleural effusion, the patient has stage IV disease. Many surgeons would not perform ultraradical surgical resections in patients with stage IV disease because of the very poor prognosis.

# SURGICAL TREATMENT OF EPITHELIAL OVARIAN CANCER

Surgery is the cornerstone of therapy for ovarian cancer, regardless of cell type or stage of disease. Whenever ovarian cancer is considered a likely diagnosis, a gynecologic oncologist should be consulted and actively involved in the evaluation and subsequent management of the patient. A gynecologic oncologist is trained to address both the surgical and the medical needs of these patients.

Ultrasonically directed cyst aspiration and laparoscopic cyst decompression are not generally recommended. Simple cyst aspiration is associated with a high recurrence rate, and the cytology of the cyst fluid is unreliable to establish or confidently exclude a diagnosis of cancer. In addition, the laparoscopic resection of a mass that is suggestive of malignancy is not advocated because of concerns related to the intra-abdominal spillage of neoplastic cells and the adequacy of surgical staging. Simply because a procedure can be accomplished using the laparoscope does not mean that it is in the patient's best interest to do so.

Intraoperatively, several features have been described that assist in the differentiation of malignant from benign adnexal masses (Table 49–5). However, gross examination of a mass is never a substitute for histologic examination. Whenever the pathology of a pelvic or adnexal mass is in question, a frozen section pathologic study should be requested. In the hands of experienced pathologists, false-positive and false-negative diagnoses occur in less than 2% of cases. Whenever the pathologic diagnosis is uncertain, it is best to remove the involved adnexa and perform the biopsies required for staging. The contralateral adnexa and uterus should not be removed if future fertility is an issue or if the patient's desires concerning future fertility are not known.

When patients are found to have ovarian cancer, regardless of cell type, it is of paramount importance that complete surgical staging be accomplished. The full extent of disease must be carefully documented.

At the time of diagnosis, over 70% of patients with epithelial ovarian cancer have metastases beyond the pelvis. The most common locations of metastases secondary to advanced stage ovarian cancer are the peritoneum (85%), omentum (70%), liver (35%), pleura (33%), lung (25%), and bone (15%). Approximately 80% of metastases involve the pelvic and para-aortic lymph nodes, and 50% involve the mediastinal or supraclavicular lymph nodes.

The information gained from accurate surgical staging guides discussion concerning prognosis and also influences treatment decisions. Surgical staging requires documentation of the primary neoplasm and determination of the extent of disease by inspection, biopsy of peritoneal and intra-abdominal lesions, and biopsy of the retroperitoneal lymph nodes. The procedures included in surgical staging of ovarian cancer are listed in Table 49–6. Any fluid in the peritoneal cavity should be aspirated. In the absence of free fluid, peritoneal washings should be obtained and submitted for cytologic study. It is recommended that 100 mL of saline be lavaged into the right paracolic gutter, the left paracolic gutter, the pelvic cul-de-sac, and the right subdiaphragmatic surface, and collected and submitted to the laboratory. Complete surgical staging of ovarian cancer requires biopsy of pelvic and para-aortic lymph nodes. It is emphasized that palpation of the retroperitoneal node-bearing areas is inaccurate and is not a substitute for biopsy and histologic examination. The current staging of ovarian cancer approved by the International Federation of Gynecology and Obstetrics (FIGO) is provided in Table 49–7.

In general, the contralateral adnexa should be removed even when it is grossly normal. It is often the site of occult metastatic disease, and there is a significant risk of subsequent cancer. Exceptions to this generalization are made for young women with an apparent stage I epithelial ovarian neoplasm. When future fertility is an issue and the patient fully understands the potential for recurrent disease, a more conservative approach may be followed when certain conditions are satisfied. Obviously, the conservative management of invasive ovarian cancer requires a

**Table 49–5.** Intraoperative differentiation of benign and malignant masses.

| Benign | Malignant |
|---|---|
| Simple cyst | Adhesions |
| Unilateral | Rupture |
| No adhesions | Ascites |
| Smooth surfaces | Solid areas |
| Intact capsule | Areas of hemorrhage or necrosis |
| | Papillary excrescences |
| | Multiloculated mass |
| | Bilateral |

**Table 49–6.** Procedures in the surgical staging of ovarian cancer.

Sample of ascites or peritoneal washings from the paracolic gutters and pelvic and subdiaphragmatic surface for cytology
Complete abdominal exploration
Intact removal of tumor
Hysterectomy
Infracolic omentectomy
Biopsies of abdominal peritoneal implants; if absent, random biopsies from the paracolic gutter peritoneum, pelvic peritoneum, and right subdiaphragmatic peritoneal surface
Pelvic and para-aortic lymph node biopsies
Cytoreductive surgery to remove all visible disease

**Table 49–7.** International Federation of Gynecologic and Obstetrics (FIGO) staging of ovarian neoplasms.

**Stage I. Growth limited to the ovaries**
Ia—one ovary involved
Ib—both ovaries involved
Ic—Ia or b and ovarian surface tumor, ruptured capsule, malignant ascites, or peritoneal cytology positive for malignant cells

**Stage II. Extension of the neoplasm from the ovary to the pelvis**
IIa—extension to the uterus or fallopian tube
IIb—extension to other pelvic tissues
IIc—IIa or b and ovarian surface tumor, ruptured capsule, malignant ascites, or peritoneal cytology positive for malignant cells

**Stage III. Disease extension to the abdominal cavity**
IIIa—abdominal peritoneal surfaces with microscopic metastases
IIIb—tumor metastases < 2 cm in size
IIIc—tumor metastases > 2 cm in size or metastatic disease in the pelvic, para-aortic or inguinal lymph nodes

**Stage IV. Distant metastic disease**
Malignant pleural effusion
Pulmonary parenchymal metastases
Liver or splenic parenchymal metastases (not surface implants)
Metastases to the supraclavicular lymph nodes or skin

thorough staging procedure. The histology and grade of the neoplasm, as well as the findings at the time of surgery, guide these decisions. Well-differentiated stage I lesions are associated with a much better 5-year survival rate than are moderately and poorly differentiated lesions. Mucinous and endometrioid neoplasms are associated with a better prognosis than those of serous and clear cell carcinomas of the ovary. The presence of adhesions, capsular rupture, ascites, or excrescences on the capsular surface constitute arguments against the performance of a conservative operation. When the decision to preserve or remove the contralateral adnexa is unclear, it is advisable to await the results of the permanent pathology before performing a bilateral adnexectomy.

A hysterectomy is generally performed because the uterus is a common site for metastatic disease. There is also a risk of synchronous endometrial cancer in patients with endometrioid carcinoma of the ovary. In addition, removal of the uterus facilitates subsequent follow-up examinations and obviates potential problems secondary to uterine bleeding.

An infracolic omentectomy is recommended, even in the absence of gross tumor involvement, because it is a common site of microscopic metastatic disease. In addition, removal of the omentum facilitates the distribution of intraperitoneal agents, may decrease the rate of accumulation of ascites postoperatively, and provides palliation to those patients with omental metastases.

Aggressive cytoreductive surgery should always be attempted. The rationale for removing as much of the gross tumor as possible includes removal of a

pharmacologic sanctuary provided by bulky tumors and a reduction in tumor burden, both of which may decrease the number of cycles of chemotherapy required. Theoretically, cytoreductive surgery also shifts the cell cycle kinetics of the neoplasm toward increased proliferation, which increases chemosensitivity. In addition, cytoreductive surgery is accompanied by improvement in host immune function.

Peritoneal implants should always be sampled to confirm the clinical impression of metastatic disease. Potential "look-alikes" include endometriosis, tuberculous peritonitis, and talc or suture granulomas. Nodular, roughened, or otherwise suspicious areas should be biopsied.

The role of second-look laparotomy in the management of patients with epithelial ovarian cancer has changed during the past decade. In the past, this procedure was performed routinely after completion of chemotherapy to evaluate the response to therapy and to guide subsequent treatment decisions. However, it has not been demonstrated that the decisions based on the information learned from the second-look operation significantly contributes to prolonged or improved patient survival. In addition, failure to diagnose persistent disease following platinum-based combination chemotherapy (eg, a negative second look) is no guarantee of long-term cure because 40–60% of these patients exhibit recurrent disease when followed up for over 2 years.

The indications for and realistic benefits of surgery in the patient with recurrent or persistent ovarian cancer are poorly defined and require individualization and considerable surgical judgment. Surgical therapy of recurrent ovarian cancer appears to be most beneficial for the patient who has an isolated mass in the absence of ascites several months after completion of first-line chemotherapy. The role of secondary debulking for persistent disease soon after the completion of first-line chemotherapy is more controversial.

# SURGICAL TREATMENT OF GERM CELL NEOPLASMS

In contrast to epithelial ovarian neoplasms, most germ cell neoplasms are early stage at the time of diagnosis. This observation, in conjunction with the low incidence of bilaterality and the young age of most patients, for whom future fertility is an issue, influence the surgical management of this group of neoplasms. For young women with a germ cell neoplasm of the ovary, removal of the involved adnexa with preservation of the normal-appearing contralateral adnexa and uterus is generally advocated. In view of the low incidence of bilaterality, biopsy or bivalving the contralateral ovary is not recommended because of the risk of peritubal and periovarian adhesions. Complete surgical staging of germ cell neoplasms is the same as for epithelial ovarian neoplasms and should be performed in all cases.

Certain characteristics unique to germ cell neoplasms make an impact on their surgical management. Dysgerminoma of the ovary has a propensity to metastasize to the pelvic and para-aortic lymph nodes in the absence of other evidence of metastatic disease; biopsies of these structures is particularly important. Endodermal sinus tumor of the ovary is the most rapidly growing neoplasm known to occur at any site. When a young woman presents with a rapidly enlarging mass and abdominal pain, this diagnosis must be considered and surgery undertaken as soon as possible. Immature teratoma of the ovary may present with numerous peritoneal implants consistent with metastatic disease. It is important to adequately sample these lesions to determine whether or not they contain malignant elements.

## CHEMOTHERAPY OF EPITHELIAL OVARIAN CANCER

Following surgery, cisplatin-based combination chemotherapy is administered. One common regimen includes cisplatin, 50–100 mg/m$^2$, and cyclophosphamide, 750–1000 mg/m$^2$, given every 3 weeks for 6–8 cycles. The potential toxicities of this regimen include alopecia, nephrotoxicity, ototoxicity, and myelosuppression.

Carboplatin is an analog of cisplatin, which demonstrates comparable activity against epithelial ovarian cancer. Unlike cisplatin, carboplatin can be administered on an outpatient basis, does not require pre- and posttreatment hydration, and is associated with minimal nephrotoxicity and neurotoxicity. Myelosuppression, including neutropenia and thrombocytopenia, is the dose-limiting toxicity of this regimen.

Assessment of response to combination chemotherapy is based on physical examination, changes in size of palpable or radiographically measurable lesions, and changes in the CA-125 level. Although the preoperative CA-125 level does not correlate with tumor burden, changes in response to chemotherapy appear to be of some prognostic benefit.

Unfortunately, most patients with epithelial ovarian cancer fail platinum-based combination chemotherapy. Salvage therapy for ovarian cancer is rarely curative, although significant prolongation of survival may be achieved in some instances. The response to retreatment with cisplatin is influenced by the time interval between completion of the initial regimen and subsequent disease recurrence—the greater the interval, the greater the likelihood of a beneficial response.

Other commercially available drugs that may be used to treat recurrent or persistent disease include hexamethylmelamine, VP16, and ifosfamide. Taxol (paclipaxel), a natural product extracted from the bark of the yew tree, and its synthetic derivative, Placitere, are new drugs in the armamentarium for treatment of epithelial ovarian cancer. These drugs stabilize the microtubules of dividing cells, resulting in mitotic arrest.

### Chemotherapy of Germ Cell Neoplasms

Significant advances have been made in the treatment of germ cell neoplasms of the ovary. Once associated with 5-year survival rates of less than 20–30%, these neoplasms are now considered curable in a majority of cases following the introduction and refinement of combination chemotherapy.

Dysgerminoma is the most radiation-sensitive neoplasm identified. Historically, it has been treated with whole abdominal radiation therapy with excellent results. More recently, chemotherapy with cisplatin-containing regimens has been administered with excellent results. A significant advantage of chemotherapy is the potential to preserve future reproductive potential compared with radiation therapy.

The other germ cell neoplasms are rare, and the optimal chemotherapy and duration of therapy have not been established. Regimens including vinblastine-bleomycin-cisplatin, vincristine-actinomycin D-cyclophosphamide, and bleomycin-etoposide-cisplatin have been used with encouraging results. Response to chemotherapy is based on physical examination and the decrease in serum tumor markers, if initially elevated.

### Complications of Chemotherapy

Combination chemotherapy invariably makes an impact on the patient's day-to-day activities and may be associated with a variety of potentially life-threatening side effects. The most common toxicities of some of the more commonly used drugs in the treatment of ovarian cancer are listed in Table 49–8.

Nausea, vomiting, and alopecia are side effects anticipated and feared by many patients. The development of new, more effective, antiemetics permit the improved control of nausea and a reduction in the number of emesis episodes. Unfortunately, suggested strategies to prevent alopecia, such as scalp tourniquets and local hypothermia, are generally ineffective. Patients should be counseled that all chemotherapy regimens do not invariably result in hair loss.

Myelosuppression is another common side effect of chemotherapy. CBCs with differential and platelet counts are typically monitored between cycles of therapy. Most regimens cause granulocytopenia and thrombocytopenia between days 10 and 18. Synthetic erythropoietin and colony-stimulating factor can be

**Table 49–8.** Chemotherapy-associated toxicities.

| Agent | Toxicity |
|-------|----------|
| Cisplatin | Nephrotoxicity, neurotoxicity, ototoxicity |
| Carboplatin | Thrombocytopenia, neutropenia |
| Cytoxan | Hemorrhagic cystitis, pulmonary fibrosis |
| Taxol | Myelosuppression |
| Hexalyn | Peripheral neuropathy |
| VP16 | Myelosuppression |
| Bleomycin | Pulmonary fibrosis |
| Doxorubicin | Cardiac toxicity |
| Vincristine | Neuropathy |
| Ifosfamide | Hemorrhagic cystitis, central neurotoxicity |

administered to lessen the severity and duration of anemia and granulocytopenia. In the future, agents to decrease chemotherapy-induced thrombocytopenia will be commercially available.

## RADIATION THERAPY

Currently, radiation therapy plays a very limited role in the treatment of patients with epithelial ovarian cancer. It is difficult to treat the entire abdominal cavity to therapeutic doses without causing life-threatening side effects because of damage to the small bowel, liver, and kidneys. Radioisotopes such as intraperitoneal $P^{32}$ may be of benefit in patients with stage Ic disease and those with microscopically positive second-look operations.

With respect to germ cell neoplasms, radiation therapy has been used successfully in the treatment of patients with dysgerminoma.

## PROGNOSIS

The prognosis for patients with ovarian cancer is primarily related to the stage of disease . The 5-year survival rate for patients with stage I epithelial ovarian cancer is approximately 80%. The 5-year survival rate for those with stage II disease is 40–50%. Stage III ovarian cancer is associated with a 5-year survival rate of approximately 30%. The survival rate for a patient with stage IV disease is less than 10%. Within each stage of disease, other factors are related to response to chemotherapy, disease-free survival, and overall survival. In general, patients with well-differentiated, diploid neoplasms with an S-phase fraction of less than 8–10% do better than patients who have poorly differentiated, aneuploid, rapidly proliferating (eg, high S-phase fraction) neoplasms.

In general, germ cell tumors are associated with better 5-year survival rates than epithelial ovarian neoplasms. Patients with dysgerminoma have a 5-year survival rate of 85%. Immature teratomas are associated with 5-year survival rates of 70–80%. An endodermal sinus tumor is associated with a 5-year survival rate of 60–70%. Embryonal carcinoma,

choriocarcinoma, and polyembryona are very rare lesions, and it is difficult to assess 5-year survival estimates.

Epithelial ovarian neoplasms of low malignant potential are characterized by 5- and 10-year survival rates of 90% and 80%, respectively, reflecting their protracted and indolent biologic behavior.

## DIAGNOSIS AND MANAGEMENT OF CANCER METASTATIC TO THE OVARY

Typically, patients with cancer metastatic to the ovary present as if they have primary ovarian cancer. Several clinical scenarios may be encountered. Primary colon cancer or gastric carcinoma may present as a pelvic mass, ascites, and a change in bowel habits or early satiety. Recurrent metastatic breast cancer may present as an asymptomatic pelvic mass.

The role of surgery in patients with cancer metastatic to the ovary must be individualized. When the diagnosis is unclear, exploratory laparotomy to establish the diagnosis is appropriate in most cases. However, the role of tumor-reductive surgery in patients with known metastatic disease is less clear. No long-term survivors of gastric cancer metastatic to the ovary are known, regardless of treatment. Survival following surgery and combination chemotherapy for breast and colon cancer metastatic to the ovary is poor, ranging from 4–12 months.

## MALIGNANT NEOPLASMS OF THE FALLOPIAN TUBE

### Etiology

Primary carcinoma of the fallopian tube is the least common cancer arising in the female genital tract, accounting for approximately 0.5% of all such cancers. Fewer than 3000 cases have been described in the literature to date.

### Clinical Presentation

The patient with carcinoma of the fallopian tube is usually in the sixth decade of life. The signs and symptoms are often similar to those noted in patients with ovarian cancer. In fact, it is difficult to differentiate tubal from ovarian carcinomas preoperatively.

Rarely, patients with carcinoma of the fallopian tube present with the symptom complex referred to as **hydrops tubae profluens** or **Latzko's sign,** which is a watery vaginal discharge and a palpable adnexal mass.

Positive vaginal cytology in the absence of endometrial or cervical neoplasia suggests the possibility of a tubal cancer but this is rarely diagnostic.

## Histopathology

At least 95% of all primary carcinomas of the fallopian tube are papillary carcinomas. Bilaterality is found in 40–50% of cases, and this is believed to represent synchronous neoplasms rather than metastatic disease from one tube to the other. Grossly, the affected tube is fusiform or sausage-shaped. On initial inspection, these neoplasms resemble pyosalpinx or tubo-ovarian inflammatory disease. However, there is usually little associated serosal reaction with adhesion formation, as is noted with an inflammatory process.

Classically, the neoplastic fallopian tube contains solid or necrotic cancer tissue and a dark-brown or serosanguinous fluid. The fimbriated end of the fallopian tube is patent in as many as 50% of cases, and often tumor extrudes from the ostium to adhere to adjacent structures. Histologically, papillary carcinomas may exhibit papillary, papillary-alveolar, and alveolar growth patterns. There is no prognostic significance attached to these differences.

## Treatment

The surgical therapy of fallopian tube carcinoma is the same as that recommended for epithelial ovarian cancer. In addition, the same type of surgical staging should be performed if for no other reason than it is often not clear at the time of surgery whether the primary cancer is of ovarian or fallopian tube origin. The staging system for ovarian cancer is often applied to neoplasms of the fallopian tube, although this is by custom rather than FIGO recommendations.

Chemotherapy for fallopian tube cancer has evolved along the same lines as that for epithelial ovarian cancer. Platinum-based combination chemotherapy is recommended, but the paucity of reported cases and relatively small series make it difficult to provide strong recommendations.

## Prognosis

The prognosis for patients with fallopian tube carcinoma is based on the stage of disease. The overall 5-year survival rate is roughly 35–40%.

## REFERENCES

Andolff E, Jorgensen C: Simple adnexal cysts diagnosed by ultrasound in postmenopausal women. JCU 1988;16: 301.

Bourne T, Campbell S, Steer C et al: Transvaginal colour flow imaging: A possible new screening technique for ovarian cancer. Br Med J 1989;299:1367.

Buy JN et al: Epithelial tumors of the ovary: CT findings and correlation with US. Radiology 1990;78:811.

Finkler NJ, Benacerraf B, Lavin PT et al: Comparison of serum CA125, clinical impression and ultrasound in the preoperative evaluation of ovarian masses. Obstet Gynecol 1988;72:659.

Gershenson DM: Update on malignant ovarian germ cell tumors. Cancer 1993;71(4 Suppl):1581.

Guidozzi F, Sonnendecker EW: Evaluation of preoperative investigations in patients admitted for ovarian primary cytoreductive surgery. Gynecol Oncol 1991;40:244.

Hasson HM: Laparoscopic management of ovarian cysts. J Reprod Med 1990;35:863.

Hoskins WJ: Surgical staging and cytoreductive surgery of epithelial ovarian cancer. Cancer 1993;71:(4 Suppl):1534.

Jacobs I, Oram D, Fairbanks J et al: A risk of malignancy incorporating CA125, ultrasound, and menopausal status for the accurate preoperative diagnosis of ovarian cancer. Br J Obstet Gynecol 1990;97:922.

Luxman D, Bergman A, Sagi J, David MP: The postmenopausal adnexal mass: Correlation between ultrasonic and pathologic findings. Obstet Gynecol 1991;77:726.

McGuire WP: Primary treatment of epithelial ovarian malignancies. Cancer 1993;71(4 Suppl):1541.

# Gestational Trophoblastic Diseases 50

*April Gale O'Quinn, MD, & David E. Barnard, MD*

## Essentials of Diagnosis

- Uterine bleeding in first trimester.
- Absence of fetal heart tones and fetal structures.
- Rapid enlargement of the uterus; uterine size greater than anticipated by dates.
- β-hCG titers greater than expected for gestational age.
- Expulsion of vesicles.
- Hyperemesis.
- Theca lutein cysts.
- Onset of preeclampsia in the first trimester.

## General Considerations

Gestational trophoblastic neoplasms include the tumor spectrum of hydatidiform mole, invasive mole (chlorioadenoma destruens), and choriocarcinoma. They arise from fetal tissue within the maternal host and are composed of both syncytiotrophoblastic and cytotrophoblastic cells. In addition to being the first and only disseminated solid tumors that have proved to be highly curable by chemotherapy, they elaborate a unique and characteristic tumor marker, human chorionic gonadotropin (hCG).

Hydatidiform mole is the most common gestational trophoblastic neoplasm. Its incidence varies worldwide from 1 in 125 deliveries in Mexico and Taiwan to 1 in 1500 deliveries in the USA. The incidence is higher in women under 20 and over 40 years of age, in patients of low economic status, and in those whose diets are deficient in protein and folic acid. Recent reports also indicate an increased incidence in patients with carotene deficiency. Molar pregnancy occurs in fewer than 5% of subsequent gestations in women with a history of mole.

Hydatidiform mole should be suspected in any woman with bleeding in the first half of pregnancy, passage of vesicles, hyperemesis gravidarum, or preeclampsia-eclampsia with onset before 24 weeks. Absent fetal heart tones and a uterus too large for the estimated duration of gestation on physical examination support the diagnosis. Ultrasonography and serial β-hCG determinations are necessary to establish a firm diagnosis of hydatidiform mole.

Invasive mole is reported in 10–15% of patients who have had primary molar pregnancy. Although considered a "benign" neoplasm, invasive mole is locally invasive and may produce distant metastases.

Choriocarcinoma is rare, reported in 2–5% of all cases of gestational trophoblastic neoplasia. The incidence in the USA is 1 in 40,000 pregnancies, but it is higher in the Orient. In about half of all cases of choriocarcinoma, the antecedent gestational event is hydatidiform mole. One-fourth follow term pregnancy, and the remainder occur following abortion.

A generalization worth repeating is that any woman presenting with bleeding or a tumor in any organ who has a recent history of molar pregnancy, abortion, or term pregnancy should have at least one β-hCG assay to be sure that metastatic gestational trophoblastic neoplasia is not the cause. This is important, for the cure rate of properly treated metastatic gestational trophoblastic neoplasia is approximately 90%.

## Etiology & Pathogenesis

Gestational trophoblastic tumors arise in fetal rather than maternal tissue. Cytogenetic studies have demonstrated that true moles are usually (perhaps always) euploiod and sex chromatin-positive 46,XX; transitional moles are usually trisomic; and partial moles are triploid. In 1977, Kajii reported that all chromosomes in true moles are paternal in origin. The development of an ovum under the influence of a sperm nucleus requires the absence or inactivation of the ovum nucleus and the presence of a diploid sperm or the duplication of its chromosomes. This provides important insight into the pathogenesis of gestational trophoblastic neoplasms, because this process results in a homozygous conceptus with a propensity for altered growth.

To date, hydatidiform mole has been considered to be derived from extraembryonic trophoblasts. Histologic similarities between molar vesicles and chorionic villi support the view that one is derived from the other. However, detailed morphologic study of a hysterectomy specimen containing an intact molar pregnancy presents a new concept regarding genesis of hydatidiform mole as a transformation of the embryonic inner cell mass at a stage just prior to the laying down of endoderm. At this stage in embryogenesis, the inner cell mass has the capability of developing into trophoblasts, ectoderm, and endoderm. If normal development is interrupted, such that the inner cell mass loses its capacity to differentiate into embryonic ectoderm and endoderm, a divergent development pathway is created. This pathway may then result in formation of trophoblasts (from the inner cell mass) that develop into cytotrophoblasts and syncytiotrophoblasts with sufficient differentiation to produce extraembryonic mesoderm, giving rise to molar vesicles with loose primitive mesoderm, in their villous core. In contrast, choriocarcinoma is less well differentiated and, lacking this capability, is composed of only cytotrophoblasts and syncytiotrophoblasts.

Thus, the ultimate cause of gestational trophoblastic disease may be genetic. Nonetheless, there are interesting clinical correlates, some of which are mentioned earlier. Additionally, evidence indicates that the distribution of ABO blood groups in women with gestational trophoblastic neoplasms and their sexual partners differs from that of the general population. The most remarkable findings are that group A women impregnated by group O men have an almost 10 times greater risk of developing choriocarcinoma than group A women with group A partners and that women with group AB have a relatively poor prognosis. A study of the ABO blood groups of children resulting from pregnancies prior or subsequent to choriocarcinoma revealed fewer instances than expected in which the child was ABO-incompatible with its mother. The leukocytes of these children frequently showed antigenic differences from the mothers' cells. Although these antigens are regarded as strong transplantation antigens, they seem notably weaker than the ABO factors—evidence that choriocarcinoma is able to grow and to kill in spite of the immune response it evokes.

## Pathology

Three distinct forms of gestational trophoblastic neoplasia are recognized: hydatidiform mole, invasive mole (chorioadenoma destruens), and choriocarcinoma.

**A. Hydatidiform Mole:** Hydatidiform mole is an abnormal pregnancy characterized grossly by multiple grapelike vesicles filling and distending the uterus, usually in the absence of an intact fetus (Fig 50–1). Most hydatidiform moles are recognizable on gross examination, but some are small and may seem to be ordinary abortuses.

Microscopically, moles may be identified by 3 classic findings: edema of the villous stroma, avascular villi, and nests of proliferating syncytiotrophoblastic or cytotrophoblastic elements surrounding villi (Fig 50–2). The likelihood of malignant sequelae is increased in patients whose trophoblastic cells

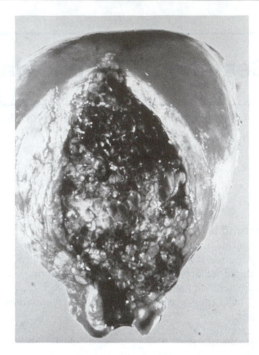

**Figure 50–1.** Hysterectomy specimen with anterior wall incised, displaying typical miliary, clear, "grapelike" vesicles filling the uterine cavity. Hysterectomy was performed for primary treatment for molar gestation.

show increased proliferation and anaplasia. Although histologic study of the trophoblast provides some basis for predicting a benign or malignant course for the mole, the correlation is not absolute, and it is essential to obtain accurate, sensitive gonadotropin assays in all patients who have had hydatidiform moles.

**B. Invasive Mole (Chorioadenoma Destruens):** Invasive mole is a hydatidiform mole that invades the myometrium or adjacent structures. It may totally penetrate the myometrium and be associated

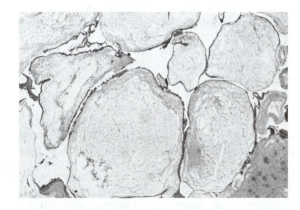

**Figure 50–2.** Photomicrograph of hydatidiform mole characterized by well-developed but avascular villi with stromal edema and minimal trophoblastic proliferation.

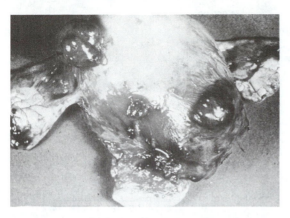

**Figure 50–3.** Hysterectomy specimen showing invasive mole penetrating the myometrium and serosal surface of the uterus that resulted in life-threatening intraperitoneal hemorrhage.

with uterine rupture and hemoperitoneum (Fig 50–3). The microscopic findings are the same as in hydatidiform mole (Fig 50–4). Since adequate myometrium is rarely obtained at curettage, the diagnosis is made by histologic study less frequently now than formerly, because fewer hysterectomies are performed in patients with trophoblastic disease. Metastatic lesions may contain invasive mole, but most will be choriocarcinoma regardless of the morphologic features of the uterine tumor.

**C. Choriocarcinoma:** Choriocarcinoma is a pure epithelial tumor composed of syncytiotrophoblastic and cytotrophoblastic cells. It may accompany or follow any type of pregnancy. Histologic examination discloses no villi but sheets or foci of trophoblasts on a background of hemorrhage and necrosis. A histopathologic diagnosis of choriocarcinoma in any site is an indication for prompt treatment after

confirmation by gonadotropin excretion measurements. Assessment of trophoblastic tissue following or accompanying pregnancy may be difficult because of the histologic similarity of the trophoblastic pattern in very early human pregnancy and in choriocarcinoma. The entire specimen must be processed for histologic study when curettage is done, because specimens may reveal only small, isolated areas of choriocarcinoma. Careful search usually discloses the villous pattern in the tissue of early normal pregnancy.

Choriocarcinoma may also arise from ectopic pregnancy. In confusing situations, β-hCG testing may clarify the diagnosis and document the need for therapy.

## Clinical Findings

**A. Symptoms and Signs:** Abnormal uterine bleeding, usually during the first trimester, is the most common symptoms, occurring in over 90% of patients with molar pregnancies. Three-fourths of patients with bleeding have this symptom before the end of the third month of pregnancy. Only one-third of patients have profuse vaginal bleeding. In over 80% of cases, the first evidence of hydatidiform mole is the passage of vesicular tissue.

Nausea and vomiting, frequently excessive but at times difficult to distinguish from similar complaints normally occurring in pregnancy, have been reported to occur in 14–32% of patients with hydatidiform mole. Ten percent of patients with molar pregnancies have nausea and vomiting severe enough to require hospitalization.

Disproportionate uterine size is the most common sign of molar gestation. About half of patients have excessive uterine size for gestational date, but in one-third the uterus is smaller than expected.

Multiple theca lutein cysts causing enlargement of one or both ovaries occur in 15–30% of women with molar pregnancies. In about half the cases, both ovaries are enlarged and may be a source of pain. Involution of the cysts proceeds over several weeks, usually paralleling the decline of hCG level. Operation is indicated only if rupture and hemorrhage occur or if the enlarged ovaries become infected. Patients with associated theca lutein cysts appear to have a greater likelihood of developing malignant sequelae of gestational trophoblastic neoplasia.

Preeclampsia in the first trimester or early second trimester—an unusual finding in normal pregnancy—has been said to be pathognomonic of hydatidiform mole, although it occurs in only 10–12% of those patients.

Hyperthyroidism from production of thyrotropin by molar tissue occurs in up to 10% of patients with hydatidiform mole. The manifestations disappear following evacuation of the mole. An occasional patient may require brief antithyroid therapy.

**B. Laboratory Findings:** A most important

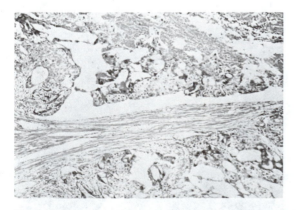

**Figure 50–4.** Photomicrograph of invasive mole. The pattern of hydatidiform mole is maintained with avascular villi and stromal edema, but they are deep within the uterine wall, interspersed among smooth-muscle bundles.

characteristic of gestational trophoblastic neoplasms is their capacity to produce hCG. This hormone may be detected in serum or urine in virtually all patients with hydatidiform mole or malignant trophoblastic disease. Careful monitoring of β-hCG levels is necessary for diagnosis, treatment, and follow-up in all cases of trophoblastic disease.

The amount of hCG found in the serum or excreted in the urine correlates closely with the number of viable tumor cells present. Studies indicate that one tumor cell produces from about $5 \times 10^{-5}$ to $5 \times 10^{-4}$ IU of hCG in 24 hours. Thus, a patient excreting $10^6$ IU of hCG in 24 hours has about $10^{11}$ viable tumor cells. At the point at which hCG is lost in the background of normal pituitary LH levels, there may remain $10^{5-6}$ viable tumor cells.

The usefulness of a gonadotropin assay depends on the level of the patient's β-hCG titer and the sensitivity of the test. A more sensitive bioassay or radioimmunoassay that will measure down to the basal pituitary range must be used.

Because hCG and LH have identical alpha chains, most tests do not differentiate between the 2 hormones. This is true of all biologic assays, immunoassays utilizing agglutination of particles, and radioimmunoassays utilizing agglutination of intact molecules of hCG. Therefore, a "normal" hCG titer is in the range of 20–30 IU (the pituitary level of LH). However, the beta chains of hCG and LH are not the same. A specific beta subunit assay for hCG is available that allows precise hCG determinations to a level approaching zero. With functioning gonads, a woman excretes less than 4 IU of hCG in 24 hours. It is in these lower ranges of gonadotropin excretion that specific assay for the beta subunit of hCG has been most useful.

The rate and constancy of the decline in hCG titer are important also. Using the serum β-hCG radioimmunoassay, a normal post molar pregnancy hCG regression curve based on weekly determinations in patients undergoing spontaneous remission has been constructed (Fig 50–5). This provides a reference with which random or serial values can be compared. In most instances, the β-hCG values exhibit a progressive decline to normal within 14 weeks following evacuation of a molar pregnancy. If metastases are detected or if the hCG titer rises or plateaus, it must be concluded that viable tumor persists.

**C. X-Ray Findings:** Because of its universal availability, transabdominal amniocentesis combined with amniography may be used to confirm the presence of hydatidiform mole. The uterus should be at or beyond 14 weeks in size, so that it is palpable above the symphysis pubica, allowing the bladder to be safely avoided when a needle is inserted into the uterine cavity. If amniotic fluid can be withdrawn after the needle is introduced, a diagnosis of pregnancy is presumed; radiopaque dye should not be injected in such cases, since there is a small risk that the hyper-

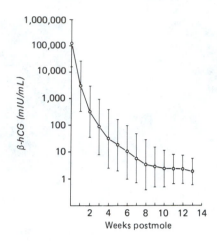

**Figure 50–5.** Normal post-molar pregnancy regression curve of serum gb-hCG measured by radioimmunoassay. Vertical bars indicate 95% confidence limits. (Reproduced, with permission of the American College of Obstetricians and Gynecologists, from Schlaerth JB et al: Prognostic characteristics of serum human chorionic gonadotropin titer regression following molar pregnancy. Obstet Gynecol 1981;58:478.)

osmolar contrast medium may induce premature labor. When little or no amniotic fluid is obtained on aspiration of the uterine cavity, radiopaque dye should be injected. The diagnosis of hydatidiform mole can be made by x-ray demonstration of the characteristic honeycomb pattern produced by the dispersion of dye around the vesicles (Fig 50–6).

**D. Special Examinations:** The simplicity, safety, and reliability of ultrasonography make it the diagnostic method of choice for patients with suspected molar pregnancy. In a molar pregnancy, the characteristic ultrasound pattern includes multiple echoes formed by the interface between the molar villi and the surrounding tissue without the presence

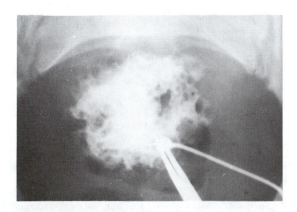

**Figure 50–6.** Amniogram of uterus with classic radiologic "honeycomb" appearance of unevacuated hydatidiform mole after intrauterine injection of radiopaque dye.

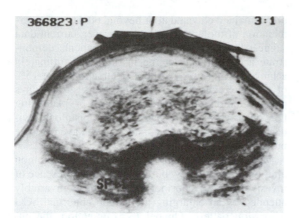

**Figure 50–7.** A gray-scale ultrasonogram depicting the typical intrauterine multiple-echo pattern of hydatidiform mole.

of a normal gestational sac or fetus (Fig 50–7). This study should be done in any patient who experiences bleeding in the first half of pregnancy and has a uterus greater than 12 weeks' gestational size. Even when the uterus is smaller or when an equivocal amniogram is present, ultrasonography may be very specific in differentiating between a normal pregnancy and hydatidiform mole.

### Differential Diagnosis

Gestational trophoblastic disease must be distinguished from normal pregnancy. Ultrasonography is useful, and quantitative hCG levels afford another means of differentiation. In general, β-hCG assays with values greater than 100,000 mIU/mL are usual with molar pregnancies, in contrast to normal pregnancy values below 60,000 mIU/mL.

### Complications

The maternal/fetal barrier contains leaks large enough to permit passage of cellular and tissue elements. Trophoblastic deportations to the lungs are frequent and have totally unpredictable manifestations, including spontaneous regression. A dramatic life-threatening complication of molar pregnancy in patients with uterine enlargement beyond 16 weeks' gestational size is a syndrome of acute pulmonary insufficiency characterized by sudden onset of dyspnea, often with cyanosis. Symptoms usually begin within 4–6 hours after evacuation. Historically, the syndrome has been attributed to massive deportation of trophoblasts to the pulmonary vasculature, but the most likely cause may be pulmonary edema secondary to cardiac dysfunction and excessive fluid administration. Nevertheless, massive fatal pulmonary embolization by gross deportation of villous tissue masses may occur, as documented by postmortem examination.

### Treatment

#### A. Hydatidiform Mole:

**1. Evacuation**–When the diagnosis has been confirmed, molar pregnancy should be terminated.

Suction curettage is the method of choice. It is safe, rapid, and effective in nearly all cases. Intravenous oxytocin should be started after a moderate amount of tissue has been removed. Suction curettage should be followed by gentle sharp curettage, and tissue from the decidua basalis should be submitted for pathologic study. Suction curettage can be safely accomplished even when the uterus is as large as in a 28-week pregnancy. Blood loss usually is moderate, but precautions should be taken for massive transfusion. When a large hydatidiform mole (>12 weeks in size) is evacuated by suction curettage, a laparotomy setup should be readily available, since hysterotomy, hysterectomy, or bilateral hypogastric artery ligation may be necessary if perforation or hemorrhage occurs.

Before the use of suction curettage, hysterectomy was frequently used for patients with uteri beyond 12–14 weeks in size. Hysterectomy remains an option for good surgical candidates not desirous of future pregnancy and for older women (who are more likely to develop malignant sequelae). If theca lutein cysts are encountered at hysterectomy, the ovaries should remain intact, because regression to normal size will occur as the hCG titer diminishes. Hysterectomy does not eliminate the need for careful follow-up and β-hCG testing, although the likelihood of metastatic disease following hysterectomy for gestational trophoblastic disease is low (3.5%).

Hysterotomy is no longer a method of choice in typical cases. The higher incidence of malignant disease following hysterotomy is probably attributable to greater uterine enlargement in patients selected for this therapy. Current recommendations restrict hysterotomy to cases complicated by hemorrhage.

Prostaglandin induction, oxytocin induction, and intra-amniotic instillation of prostaglandin or hypertonic solutions (saline, glucose, urea, etc) are no longer acceptable methods for evacuation of a molar pregnancy.

**2. Prophylactic chemotherapy**–Prophylactic dactinomycin therapy may be appropriate for patients with large uteri or in whom poor follow-up is anticipated. Caution is needed, since several deaths due to toxicity have been reported.

**3. Surveillance following molar pregnancy**–Regardless of method of termination, close follow-up with serial β-hCG titers is essential for every patient because of the incidence of malignant disease. The incidence is commonly thought to be 15% (10% for invasive mole and 5% for choriocarcinoma), although several recent reports indicate a 20–30% incidence. Three-fourths of patients with malignant nonmetastatic trophoblastic disease and half of patients with malignant metastatic disease develop these tumors as sequelae to hydatidiform mole. In the remainder, disease arises following term pregnancy, abortion, or ectopic pregnancy.

Several clinical features of hydatidiform mole are recognized as having a high association with malignant trophoblastic neoplasia. In general, at diagnosis, the larger the uterus, the higher the hCG titer; and the shorter the gestation, the greater the risk for malignant gestational trophoblastic disease. The combination of theca lutein cysts and uterine size excessive for gestational age is associated with an extremely high risk (57%) of malignant sequelae.

Effective contraceptive measures should be implemented and maintained throughout the period of surveillance in these patients. Oral contraceptives are the most widely used method.

Following evacuation of hydatidiform mole, the patient should have serial β-hCG determinations at weekly intervals until serum hCG declines to nondetectable levels (β-hCG radioimmunoassay) on 3 successive assays. If titer remission occurs spontaneously within 14 weeks and without a titer plateau, the β-hCG titer than should be repeated monthly for at least 1 year before the patient is released from close medical supervision. Thereafter, the patient may enter into a regular gynecologic care program.

Gynecologic examination should be done 1 week after evacuation, at which time blood may be taken for the first postevacuation hCG titer. Estimates of uterine size and adnexal masses (theca lutein cysts) and a careful search of the vulva, vagina, urethra, and cervix should be made for evidence of genital tract metastases. Unless symptoms develop, the examination should be repeated at 4-week intervals throughout the observation period.

Chest x-ray should be obtained prior to evacuation, and if pulmonary metastases are noted, at 4-week intervals thereafter until spontaneous remission is confirmed, then at 3-month intervals during the remainder of the surveillance period.

A patient who has entered into spontaneous remission with negative titers, examinations, and chest x-rays for 1 year and who is desirous of becoming pregnant may terminate contraceptive practices. Successful pregnancy is usual, and complications are similar to those of patients in the general population.

Therapy for progressive gestational trophoblastic neoplasia after delivery of a hydatidiform mole is usually instituted because of an abnormal hCG regression curve. While the hCG titer usually returns to normal within 1–2 weeks after evacuation of a hydatidiform mole, it should be normal by 8 weeks. The most critical period of observation is the first 4–6 weeks postevacuation. Few patients whose hCG titers are normal during this interval will require treatment. Approximately 70% of patients achieve a normal hCG level within 60 days postevacuation.

In the past, therapy was recommended if the hCG titer remained elevated at or beyond 60 days after termination of molar pregnancy. However, current data suggest that an additional 15% of patients demonstrate a continuous decline in titers and ultimately achieve normal titers without treatment. About 15% of patients who have elevated titers at 60 days postevacuation demonstrate a rising or plateauing titer. Nearly half these patients have histologic evidence of choriocarcinoma, and the rest have invasive mole.

Delayed postevacuation bleeding is uncommon after molar pregnancy, but it signifies the presence of invasive mole or choriocarcinoma and is invariably attended by an enlarging uterus and abnormal hCG regression pattern. On pelvic examination, the enlarged uterus may have the characteristics of an intrauterine pregnancy. Curettage is effective in stopping the bleeding, although little intracavitary tissue will be present in most of these cases.

In summary, the indications for initiating chemotherapy during the postmolar surveillance period are (1) β-hCG levels rising for 2 successive weeks or constant for 3 successive weeks; (2) β-hCG levels elevated at 15 weeks' postevacuation; (3) rising β-hCG titer after reaching normal levels; and (4) postevacuation hemorrhage. Too, treatment should be instituted whenever there is a tissue diagnosis of choriocarcinoma. However, histologic confirmation is unnecessary, because the development of metastasis is a sufficient justification for chemotherapy.

**B. Malignant Gestational Trophoblastic Neoplasia:** Once the diagnosis of malignant trophoblastic disease has been established, obtain an accurate history and perform a physical examination, including pelvic examination. Most patients have an enlarged uterus, and ovarian enlargement due to theca lutein cysts is common. Sites of metastasis must be sought, especially in the lower genital tract. Obtain a chest x-ray and scans of the liver and brain. CT scan is now the diagnostic procedure of choice for brain, lung, liver, and renal metastases. In brain metastasis, evaluation of the ratio of serum hCG to the concentration of hCG in cerebrospinal fluid may be helpful. Carefully consider the baseline hematologic counts as well as hepatic and renal function, which may be critical in the risk and monitoring of drug toxicity.

After sites of metastases or of abnormal function have been identified, the patient's desires for preservation of reproductive function are known, and the disease has been categorized as nonmetastatic or metastatic, specific therapy should be started.

**1. Nonmetastatic gestational trophoblastic disease**—Trophoblastic disease confined to the uterus is the most common malignant lesion seen in gestational trophoblastic neoplasia. The diagnosis is usually made during follow-up after evacuation of molar pregnancy. If there is no evidence of spread outside the uterus, histologic examination may be important, for nonmetastatic choriocarcinoma is a more serious condition than nonmetastatic hydatidiform mole. Therapy for patients with nonmetastatic malignant trophoblastic disease includes (1) single-agent chemotherapy; (2) combined chemotherapy and hysterectomy, with surgery done on the third day of drug therapy if the patient does not wish to preserve reproductive function and her disease is known to be confined to the uterus; and (3) intra-arterial infusion of chemotherapeutic agents in selected cases.

Single-agent chemotherapy using methotrexate or dactinomycin has demonstrated clear-cut superiority over other protocols (Table 50–1). The therapeutic efficacy of the 2 drugs is apparently equivalent, but dactinomycin is favored by some because it is less toxic. However, its hematologic toxicity is less predictable. Methotrexate is contraindicated in the presence of hepatocellular disease or when renal function is impaired. Each treatment cycle should be repeated as soon as normal tissues (bone marrow and gastrointestinal mucosa) have recovered, with a minimum 7-day window between the last day of one course and the first day of the next one.

---

**Table 50–1.** Single-agent chemotherapy.

A. Methotrexate, 0.4 mg/kg/d IV or IM, +
   or
   Dactinomycin, 10–12 µg/kg/d IV
   1. Give either one in 5-day course.
   2. Repeat cycle with minimum interval of 7–10 days as toxicity allows.
   3. Oral contraceptive agents, if not contraindicated.
B. Continue repeated chemotherapy cycles until–
   1. One course after a negative β-hCG titer.
   2. Remission, defined as 3 consecutive normal weekly β-hCG titers.
   Switch to alternative drug if–
      a. Titer rises (10-fold or more).
      b. Titer plateaus at an elevated level.
      c. New metastasis appears.
C. Laboratory values: Obtain daily during treatment cycle, weekly, or as indicated between treatment cycles. Take β-hCG titers weekly until remission induction. Do not begin or continue a course of chemotherapy if–
   1. White blood count <3000/µL.
   2. Granulocytes <1500/µL.
   3. Platelets <100,000/µL.
   4. BUN, AST (SGOT), ALT (SGPT), bilirubin significantly elevated.
D. Other toxicity mandating postponement of chemotherapy:
   1. Severe stomatitis or gastrointestinal ulceration.
   2. Febrile course (usually present only with leukopenia).
E. Follow-up program:
   1. β-hCG titer weekly until 3 consecutive normal titers; monthly β-hCG titers for 12 months thereafter; then β-hCG titers every 2 months for 12 additional months or every 6 months indefinitely.
   2. Physical examination including pelvic examination and chest x-ray monthly until remission is induced; at 3-month intervals for 1 year thereafter; then at 6-month intervals indefinitely.
   3. Continue contraception for minimum of 1 year after remission induction.

---

During treatment, weekly quantitative β-hCG titers and complete blood counts should be obtained. Before each course of therapy, liver and renal function assessments should be done. At least one course of drug therapy should be given after the first normal β-hCG determination. The number of treatment cycles necessary to induce remission is proportionate to the magnitude of the β-hCG concentration at the start of therapy. An average of 3 or 4 courses of single-agent therapy is required. After remission has been induced and treatment is completed, β-hCG assays should be obtained monthly for 12 months.

Methotrexate with leucovorin calcium* rescue also has been used to treat nonmetastatic trophoblastic disease (Table 50–2). This regimen requires hospitalization or daily outpatient visits. Blood counts are obtained on each day of methotrexate administration, and therapy is deferred if white blood cell and platelet counts are low.

Excellent results have been achieved with alternating sequential courses of dactinomycin and methotrexate (Table 50–3). This regimen avoids the cumulative toxicity of methotrexate and may retard the development of resistance.

**2. Metastatic gestational trophoblastic disease**–Therapy in metastatic disease depends on multiple factors that characterize patients as good-prognosis patients (Table 50–4). Therapy is based on this initial categorization as well as on factors governing selection of techniques (Table 50–5).

**a. Good-prognosis patients**–Patients can be expected to respond satisfactorily to single-agent chemotherapy if (1) metastases are confined to the lungs or pelvis and (2) serum β-hCG levels are below 40,000 mIU/mL at the onset of treatment and (3) therapy is started within 4 months of apparent onset of disease.

The most common site of metastasis is the lung. When a patient develops pulmonary metastases and elevation of hCG titer, choriocarcinoma is a more likely cause than metastatic mole. Invasive mole may also metastasize to the lungs, and hydatidiform mole has occasionally been reported to metastasize to the

---

**Table 50–2.** Methotrexate-leucovorin calcium rescue chemotherapy for nonmetastatic trophoblastic neoplasia.[1]

| Therapy | Time | Interval |
|---|---|---|
| Complete blood count; platelet count; AST (SGOT) | 8 AM | Days 1, 3, 5, 7 |
| Methotrexate, 1 mg/kg IM | 4 PM | Days 1, 3, 5, 7 |
| Leucovorin calcium, 0.1 mg/kg IM | 4 PM | Days 2, 4, 6, 8 |

[1]Modified from Goldstein DP et al: Methotrexate with citrovorum factor rescue for gestational trophoblastic neoplasms. Obstet Gynecol 1978;51:93.

---

*Formerly called citrovorum factor or folinic acid.

**Table 50–3.** Alternating sequential chemotherapy.[1]

Methotrexate, 15–30 mg/d IV daily for 5 days
Dactinomycin, 0.5 mg/kg IV daily for 5 days

The drugs are given sequentially and alternatively as soon as the oral and hematologic toxicity from the preceding drug has subsided.

[1]Modified from Smith JP: Chemotherapy in gynecologic cancer. Clin Obstet Gynecol 1975;18:109.

chest. Probably any form of metastasis (even benign deportation) should suggest metastatic trophoblastic disease.

In these patients, single-agent chemotherapy is almost uniformly successful. The complete remission rate in this group of patients has been 100%. Methotrexate is considered the drug of choice. Ideally, the 5-day treatment cycle is given every other week, because tumor regrowth becomes significant after treatment gaps of 2 weeks or longer. Once negative titers have been achieved, an additional course is administered. If resistance to methotrexate occurs, manifested either by rising or plateauing titers or by the development of new metastases—or if negative titers are not achieved by the fifth course of methotrexate—the patient should be given dactinomycin.

The advantage of single-agent chemotherapy is that it is less toxic and its toxicity is less apt to be irreversible than is the case with multiple-agent chemotherapy.

There is a tendency to approach the treatment of these patients too lightly, probably because of the "good-prognosis" (low-risk) designation. But failure of drug therapy does occur in about 10% of cases, and meticulous care by physicians familiar with these problems is necessary for good results.

**b. Poor-prognosis patients–**"Poor-prognosis" patients are those with (1) serum β-hCG titers greater than 40,00 mIU/mL or (2) disease diagnosed more than 4 months after molar pregnancy or (3) brain or liver metastases or (4) prior unsuccessful chemother-

**Table 50–4.** Categorization of gestational trophoblastic neoplasia.

**A. Nonmetastatic disease:** No evidence of disease outside uterus.
**B. Metastatic disease:** Any disease outside uterus.
  **1. Good-prognosis metastatic disease–**
    a. Short duration (< 4 months).
    b. Serum β-hCG (< 40,000 mIU/mL.
    c. No metastasis to brain or liver.
    d. No significant prior chemotherapy.
  **2. Poor-prognosis metastatic disease–**
    a. Long duration (> 4 months).
    b. Serum β-hCG > 40,000 mIU/mL.
    c. Metastasis to brain or liver.
    d. Unsuccessful prior chemotherapy.
    e. Gestational trophoblastic neoplasia following term pregnancy.

**Table 50–5.** Selection of therapy in metastatic trophoblastic disease.

**A. Good Prognosis:**
  1. Single-agent methotrexate or dactinomycin chemotherapy.
  2. Alternating sequential single-agent chemotherapy.
  3. Methotrexate with leucovorin calcium rescue chemotherapy.
  4. Delayed hysterectomy if residual resistant disease in uterus.
  5. Combination chemotherapy.
  6. Arterial infusion chemotherapy.
**B. Poor Prognosis:**
  1. Combination chemotherapy (MAC) [see Table 50–6]).
  2. Whole-brain irradiation to 3000 rads or whole-liver irradiation to 2000 rads (or both) given over 10–14 days concomitantly with chemotherapy.
  3. Delayed hysterectomy if residual resistant disease in uterus, and surgical "debulking" resection of isolated accessible resistant metastasis in pelvis, lung, brain.
  4. Other multiple-agent chemotherapeutic regimens (MBP [see Table 50–7], EMA-OC [see Table 50–8), or VBP [see Table 50–9]).
  5. Arterial infusion chemotherapy.
  6. Single-agent chemotherapy.

apy or (5) onset following term gestation. These patients present a serious challenge. Many have been previously treated with chemotherapy and have become resistant to that treatment while accumulating considerable toxicity and depleting bone marrow reserves. Prior unsuccessful chemotherapy is one of the worst prognostic factors.

Generally, these patients require prolonged hospitalization and many courses of chemotherapy. They often need specialized care and other life-support measures, including hyperalimentation, antibiotics, and transfusions to correct the effects of marrow depression.

Central nervous system involvement, particularly brain metastasis with focal neurologic signs suggestive of intracranial hemorrhage, is common in choriocarcinoma. Since patients with brain or liver metastases are at great risk of sudden death from hemorrhage from these lesions, it has been standard practice in the treatment of these patients to include immediate institution of whole-brain or whole-liver irradiation concomitantly with combination chemotherapy. It is uncertain whether radiation therapy exerts its beneficial effect by destroying tumor in combination with drug therapy or by preventing fatal hemorrhage and thus keeping the patient alive until remission with chemotherapy can be achieved.

Cerebral metastasis should be treated over a 2-week period with radiation given in a dosage of 300 rads daily, 5 days a week, to a total organ dose of 3000 rads. Whole-liver irradiation is usually accomplished over 10 days to attain a 2000-rad whole-organ dose given at a rate of 200 rads daily, 5 days a week.

The standard treatment regimen is with triple-agent MAC (methotrexate, dactinomycin, and chlor-

**Table 50–6.** Combination (MAC) chemotherapy.

A. Methotrexate, 10–15 mg/d IV or IM
   **and**
   Dactinomycin, 10–12 µg/kg/d I/V
   **and**
   Chlorambucil, 8–10 mg/d by mouth, or cyclophosphamide, 3–5 mg/kg/d IV.
   1. Given in 5-day courses.
   2. Repeat cycles with minimum interval of 10–14 days,
      as toxicity allows.
   3. Oral contraceptive agents, if not contraindicated.
B. Continue repetitive chemotherapy cycles until–
   1. Three courses after negative β-hCG titers.
   2. Remission, defined as 3 consecutive normal weekly β-
      hCG titers.
   Switch to alternative combination drug regimens if–
      a. Titer rises.
      b. Titer plateaus after 2 courses of MAC.
      c. Increasing metastatic disease is evident.
C. Laboratory values: Same as outlined in Table 50–1.
D. Complications:
   1. Severe stomatitis or gastrointestinal ulceration.
   2. Sever bone marrow suppression is major morbidity.
E. Follow-up program: Same as outlined in Table 50–1 except continue contraception for minimum of 2 years after
   remission induction.
F. Whole-brain irradiation to 3000 rads or whole-liver irradiation to 2000 rads (or both) given over 10–14 days concomitantly with chemotherapy.

**Table 50–7.** Modified Bagshawe protocol (MBP) for poor-prognosis trophoblastic disease.[1]

| Day | Hour | Drug | Dose |
|---|---|---|---|
| 1 | 6 AM | Hydroxyurea | 500 mg orally |
|  | 12 NOON | Hydroxyurea | 500 mg orally |
|  | 6 PM | Hydroxyurea | 500 mg orally |
|  | 7 PM | Dactinomycin | 200 µg IV |
|  | 12 MIDNIGHT | Hydroxyurea | 500 mg orally |
| 2 | 7 AM | Vincristine | 1 mg/m² IV |
|  | 7 PM | Methotrexate | 100 mg/m² IV |
|  |  | Methotrexate | 200 mg/m² In-fused over 12 hours |
|  |  | Dactinomycin | 200 µG IV |
| 3 | 7 PM | Dactinomycin | 200 µG IV |
|  |  | Cyclophosphamide | 500 mg/m² IV |
|  |  | Leucovorin calcium | 14 mg IM |
| 4 | 1 AM | Leucovorin calcium | 14 mg IM |
|  | 7 AM | Leucovorin calcium | 14 mg IM |
|  | 1 PM | Leucovorin calcium | 14 mg IM |
|  | 7 PM | Leucovorin calcium | 14 mg IM |
|  |  | Dactinomycin | 500 mg IV |
| 5 | 1 AM | Leucovorin calcium | 14 mg IM |
|  | 7 PM | Dactinomycin | 500 µG IV |
| 6 |  | No treatment |  |
| 7 |  | No treatment |  |
| 8 | 7 PM | Cyclophosphamide | 500 mg/m² IV |
|  |  | Doxorubicin | 30 mg/m² IV |

Wait 7–14 days for recovery and repeat cycles as toxicity allows.

[1]As currently used at the Southeastern Regional Center for Trophoblastic Disease.

ambucil or cyclophosphamide) chemotherapy (Table 50–6). These drugs are employed in 5-day intermittent courses with windows of 10–14 days between the last day of one course and the first day of the next one, depending on toxicity. The same tests must be employed to detect toxicity as are used when single-agent chemotherapy is given, but monitoring must be even more careful because of the possibility of combined toxicity.

Treatment of malignant trophoblastic disease must be continued with repeated courses of combination chemotherapy until β-hCG titers return to nondetectable levels. Complete remission is documented only after 3 consecutive weekly normal β-hCG titers have been achieved. It is recommended that all high-risk patients receive at least 3 courses of triple-agent chemotherapy after β-hCG titers have returned to normal. After remission is achieved, follow-up is the same as for hydatidiform mole and nonmetastatic or good-prognosis disease.

If the β-hCG titer rises or plateaus after 2 courses of MAC chemotherapy or if the patient fails to achieve a normal titer after 4 or 5 courses of MAC, an alternative method of therapy should be used. If toxicity is too severe, a less intensive regimen should be considered.

Three regimens are effective in management of MAC treatment failures: (1) the modified Bagshawe multidrug protocol (Table 50–7), (2) the alternating EMA-OC protocol of Bagshawe (Table 50–8), and (3) Einhorn's regimen of vinblastine, bleomycin, and

cisplatin (Table 50–9). These multiple-agent combinations appear to be effective adjuncts to MAC in resistant cases. Other drug protocols occasionally employed in resistant cases are methotrexate infusion and regimens containing etoposide.

In resistant cases, adjunctive measures along with chemotherapy may include hysterectomy, resection of metastatic tumors, or irradiation of unresectable lesions.

## Prognosis

The prognosis for hydatidiform mole following evacuation is uniformly excellent, though surveillance is needed as outlined in the text. The prognosis for malignant nonmetastatic disease with appropriate therapy is also quite good, since almost all patients are cured. Over 90% of patients have been able to preserve reproductive function, but first-line therapy failed in 6.5% of patients with nonmetastatic disease.

**Table 50–8.** Alternating EMA-OC chemotherapy for poor-prognosis trophoblastic disease.[1]

| Drug | Dose | Interval |
|---|---|---|
| Etoposide | 100 mg/m² IV | Days 1 and 2 |
| Methotrexate | 300 mg/m² IV | Day 1 |
| Dactinomycin | 0.5 mg IV | Days 1 and 2 |
| Leucovorin calcium | 15 mg orally, 3 times a day | Days 2 and 3 |
| Alternate weekly with: | | |
| Vincristine | 2 mg IV | Day 1 |
| Cyclophosphamide | 600 mg/m² IV | Day 1 |

Disregard bone marrow toxicity. Antibiotic prophylaxis with trimethoprim if WBC ≤1500. Treatment limiting mucosal toxicity is seldom encountered.

[1]As currently used by KD Bagshawe, Charing Cross Hospital, London.

**Table 50–9.** VBP Chemotherapy for poor-prognosis trophoblastic disease.[1]

| Drug | Dose | Interval |
|---|---|---|
| Vinblastine | 0.2 mg/kg IV | Days 1 and 2 |
| Bleomycin | 30 units IV | Weekly × 12 |
| Cisplatin | 20 mg/m² IV infusion | Days 1, 2, 3, 4, 5 |

Repeat cycle every 3 weeks for 3–4 cycles.

[1]Modified from Einhorn LH, Donohue JH: CIS-diamminedichloroplatinum, vinblastine and bleomycin: Combination chemotherapy in disseminated testicular cancer. Ann Intern Med 1977;87:293.

In one large reported series, no death from toxicity occurred, and only one patient died of the disease.

Prognostic factors in malignant metastatic disease are set forth in the discussion of treatment. In poor-prognosis metastatic disease, the best results are with chemotherapy plus concurrent radiation therapy, with 87% of patients or more achieving remission. This has been accomplished not only with newer chemotherapeutic regimens but also with an aggressive multimodal approach. Deaths from toxicity have decreased considerably. Recurrence, when it happens, is usually in the first several months after termination of therapy but may be as late as 3 years.

# REFERENCES

Bagshawe KD: Treatment of high risk choriocarcinoma. Repro Med 1984;29:813.

Balasubramaniam UN, Salem FA, Savage EW: Genesis of molar pregnancy: Neoplastic transformation of the inner cell mass with a case presentation. Gynecol Oncol 1982;14:62.

Berkowitz RS, Goldstein DP, Bernstein MR: Ten-year experience with methotrexate and folinic acid as primary treatment for gestational trophoblastic disease. Gynecol Oncol 1986;23:111.

Curry SL et al: A prospective randomized comparison of methotrexate, dactinomycin, and chlorambucil versus methotrexate, dactinomycin, cyclophosphamide, doxorubicin, melphalan, hydroxyurea, and vincristine in "poor prognosis" metastatic gestational trophoblastic disease: A Gynecologic Oncology Group Study. Obstet Gynecol 1989;73:357.

Dorreen MS: The gestational trophoblastic diseases: A review of their presentation and management. Clin Oncol 1993;5:46.

Fasoli M et al: Management of gestational trophoblastic disease: Results of a cooperative study. Obstet Gyne 1982; 60:205.

Jones WB: Management of low-risk metastatic gestational trophoblastic disease. J Reprod Med 1981;26:213.

Kajii T, Ohama K: Androgenetic origin of hydatidiform male. Nature 1977;268:633.

Kennedy RL, Darne J: The role of hCG in regulation of the thyroid gland in normal and abnormal pregnancy. Obstet Gynecol 1991;78:298.

Kohorn EI: Single-agent chemotherapy for nonmetastatic gestational trophoblastic neoplasia: Perspectives for the 21st century after three decades of use. J Reprod Med 1991;36:49.

Kurman RJ: Pathology of the trophoblast. Monogr Pathol 1991;33:195.

Lewis JL Jr: Diagnosis and management of gestational trophoblastic disease. Cancer 1993;71:1639.

Lurain JR: Gestational trophoblastic tumors. Semin Surg Oncol 1990;6:347.

Morrow CP et al: Clinical and laboratory correlates of molar pregnancy and trophoblastic disease. Am J Obstet Gynecol 1977;128:424.

Pattillo RA: Genetic origin, immunobiology, and gonadotropin expression in trophoblast and nontrophoblast neoplasms. Adv Exp Med Biol 1984;176:53.

Twiggs LB, Morrow CP, Schlaerth JB: Acute pulmonary complications of molar pregnancy. Am J Obstet Gynecol 1979;135:189.

Yordan EL, Jr et al: Radiation therapy in the management of gestational choriocarcinoma metastatic to the central nervous system. Obstet Gyne 1987;69:627.

# Radiation Therapy for Gynecologic Cancers

# 51

*Harrison G. Ball, MD, & David E. Barnard, MD*

Two discoveries in the late 1800s made the therapeutic use of radiation possible. While studying the penetrating power of cathode ray emission, Wilhelm Roentgen discovered x-rays by chance on November 8, 1895. The Curies isolated radium from uranium ore in 1898. The medical potential of these findings was quickly exploited. In the USA, Robert Abbe of New York City introduced radium for medical therapy, and Howard Kelly of Baltimore pioneered its application in cancer of the cervix. Evolution throughout this century has made radiation therapy a major modality in the treatment on many cancers, particularly those of the female reproductive tract.

## Definitions

**Radiation oncology** may be defined as the therapeutic manipulation of **ionizing radiation** (high-energy radiation capable of separating one or more orbital electrons from their affiliated atoms or molecules). This radiation may be electromagnetic or particulate, but in both types, the interactions of ionizing radiation transfer energy to the electrons or nuclei of cellular components. With **electromagnetic radiation,** the photons produced interact with water in the cell resulting in the formation of free radicals that then lead to cellular damage.

The most familiar forms of electromagnetic radiation, x-rays and gamma rays, are generated from different sources but possess the same physical characteristics (both lack mass and charge). When accelerated electrons strike the atoms of a positioned target, x-rays result from the energy liberated, whereas the decay of radioactive isotopes results in gamma rays.

**Particulate radiation** includes electrons and nuclear forms such as protons, neutrons, and pions (pimesons). These types of radiation also interact with atomic nuclei.

X-rays and gamma rays may be considered as discrete units of radiant energy called **photons.** The energy of each unit is proportional to the frequency of the wave associated with the photon. Radiation with a shorter wavelength has greater frequency and consequently carries greater energy per photon to allow deeper tissue penetration. It is the amount of energy imparted to the individual photons rather than the total invested energy that distinguishes ionizing from nonionizing radiation. Ionizing radiation possesses more energy per photon packet. The amount of energy per packet is in turn dependent on the creation process of the radiation.

The transfer of radiant energy in the form of photons to another material occurs either through the photoelectric effect, the Compton effect, or pair production. In the **photoelectric effect,** absorption is influenced by atomic number; the tissues bearing elements of higher atomic number (eg, calcium in bone) will absorb proportionately greater and possibly detrimental levels of radiation. In the photoelectric effect, electrons are ejected from matter when a photon strikes it. The **Compton effect** involves the interaction of incident photons with the outer shell electrons of bombarded atoms with resulting change in the wavelength of x-ray or gamma radiation due to production of a recoil electron and a scattered photon of reduced energy (Fig 51–1). The atomic number of the tissue elements does not determine the amount of absorbed radiation. **Pair production** refers to the complex interaction of an incident photon with the nucleus of a target atom. A positron electron pair results from this interaction.

In the lower range of energy transfer, the photoelectric effect predominates, while in the transfer of higher levels of energy, the Compton effect and pair production become more prevalent.

## Dosage Theory

Radiant energy is thought to produce biologic change by damaging the DNA molecule of target tissues and thus hampering further effective replication. This is brought about initially by the production of the hydroxyl radical, which is formed by the collision of radiant energy and water. Damage caused by the hydroxyl radical is irreversible only in the presence of molecular oxygen.

A common misconception is that therapeutic radiation severely affects malignant cells while sparing normal tissues. In actuality, the critical difference in the effect of radiation on various tissues is the relative

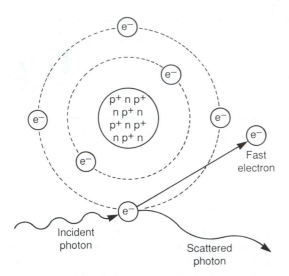

**Figure 51–1.** Absorption of an x-ray photon by the Compton process. The photon interacts with a loosely bound planetary electron of an atom of the absorbing material. Part of the photon energy is given to the electron as kinetic energy. The photon, deflected from its original direction, proceeds with reduced energy. $e^-$ = electron; $p^+$ = proton; n = neutron. (Reproduced, with permission, from Hall EJ: *Radiobiology for the Radiologist,* 4th ed. JB Lippincott, 1994:7.)

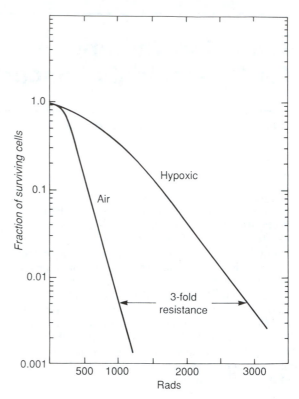

**Figure 51–2.** Typical radiation survival curve for mammalian cells. These cells have been irradiated and then plated out in culture, and the number of survivors has been determined by measuring the colonies (clones) of cells that survive. The curve is characterized by an initial shoulder followed by a log-linear region. Cells irradiated in air are considerably more sensitive than those irradiated in nitrogen (hypoxic), and the difference between the levels of killing is frequently about threefold. It is believed that most clinically demonstrable tumors have areas of hypoxia that lead to radioresistance. (Reproduced, with permission, from Morrow CP, Curtin JP, Townsend DE [editors]: *Synopsis of Gynecologic Oncology,* 4th ed. Churchill Livingstone, 1993:449.)

ability of the tissues to recover from radiation damage.

After exposure to radiation, the survival of tissues follows a predictable curve that essentially constitutes the number of viable clone cells (Fig 51–2). The shoulder occurring at the beginning of the curve represents the cell's enzymatic ability to reverse damage due to radiant energy. As radiation is increased, the cell becomes incapable of self-repair and a logarithmic pattern of cell destruction occurs. An important consequence is that for every increase in dosage that occurs beyond the shoulder, a constant fraction of cells is eliminated (**log-kill hypothesis**).

The implications of these observations provide some of the rationale for dividing (fractionating) the total dose of radiation therapy administered in the clinical setting. It is helpful to consider the so-called "4 R's" of radiobiology (Withers, 1975) to understand the effects of fractionated doses at the cellular level.

**A. Repair of Sublethal Injury:** When a specified radiation dose is divided into 2 doses given at separate times, the number of cells surviving is higher than that seen when the same total dose is given at one time. Fractionation allows the administration of amounts of radiation that would not be tolerated if the specified dose were given in only one treatment.

**B. Repopulation:** The reactivating of stem cells that occurs when radiation is stopped is necessary for further tissue growth; those tissues with increased numbers of progenitor cells have a greater ability to regenerate.

**C. Reoxygenation (Oxygen Effect):** Hypoxic cells are known to be relatively resistant to radiation. Experimental and clinical evidence has confirmed that molecular oxygen must be present before radiation damage can occur. Cells located farther than 100 mm from capillary flow are at risk for hypoxia. If these hypoxic cells are malignant, they may not be killed by radiation therapy. For this reason, it is important to correct anemia in patients undergoing radiation treatment so that tissue oxygen perfusion will be enhanced and tissues will become more radiosensitive. As tumor regresses with radiation treatment, previously anoxic areas may be brought into contact with capillary flow and, therefore, increased oxygenation. However, malignant cells in these sites may then be exposed to now sublethal amounts of radiation. This is due to the fact that cells undergoing reoxygenation only "begin" their treatment after surrounding tissues have received significant radiation doses. Therefore, the reoxygenated tumor will be able to receive only a portion of the optimum tumoricidal dose.

**D. Radiation-Induced Synchrony:** Malignant cells are most sensitive to radiation while in the mitotic phase of the cell cycle. If a segment of the malignant cell population can be destroyed in this phase of the cell cycle, the remaining malignant cells may be synchronized for selective destruction at a later time.

Clinical experience has shown that prolonged interruption of radiation therapy has a deleterious effect on cure, since malignant cells have a greater chance to regenerate.

It is important to remember that the larger the volume of body area irradiated, the more severely that normal tissues will be affected. For example, a total dose of 3000 cGy is tolerated quite well when given in standard pelvic radiation fields, but the same dose is lethal when administered as whole body irradiation. Total dose, fractionation design, dose per fraction, total treatment time, and field size are important in gauging the biologic effect of a course of radiation.

## Dosimetry

Dosimetry is the measurement of the amount of radiation absorbed by the tissue of interest and is expressed in rads or, more recently, the gray unit (Gy) which equals 100 rads (1 cGy = 1 rad). External pelvic irradiation is expressed in these terms, whereas internal irradiation is also described in milligram hours. This latter unit is obtained by multiplying the number of milligrams of radioactive substance (usually radium or cesium) used in the internal applicators by the number of hours the applicators have been in place.

The exact conversion factor between milligram hours and gray is difficult to determine, but computer-directed dosimetry permits the calculation of isodose curves (points of equal dose surrounding a radioactive source) that permit critical considerations in avoiding overdose to the bladder and rectum. The radiation tolerance of the bladder and rectum is close to the dosage levels required for curative radiation therapy of common pelvic cancers.

## TREATMENT METHODS

### External Irradiation (Teletherapy)

Early radiation therapists used electric x-ray sources that were basically modifications of Roentgen's experimental apparatus. Electrons were accelerated across a vacuum tube to strike a tungsten target with the subsequent liberation of photons. These ortho-voltage (140–400 keV) units were limited in their power to penetrate tissue effectively because of their relatively low energy output. Consequently, pronounced fibrotic skin changes and high absorbed bone radiation levels limited their usefulness in some patients.

As the energy of the projectile electrons was increased, significant clinical benefit accrued. As units generating higher levels of energy were developed, the penetrating power of the x-rays produced was enhanced, and less scattering of radiation was seen at the margins of the treatment area. The surface skin dose was also diminished (particularly important in the treatment of obese patients), and less toxic bone radiation was achieved (Fig 51–3).

Cobalt 60 teletherapy units are in the supervoltage range (500 keV–1 MeV) and use the radiant energy released by the nuclear decay of cobalt 60. Megavoltage (> 1 MeV) radiation sources, such as linear accelerators, allow even more precise delineation of the area requiring radiation therapy.

### Local Irradiation (Brachytherapy)

Brachytherapy is radiation therapy in which the source of therapeutic ionizing radiation is placed close to the treatment area. The appliances most commonly used in gynecologic cancer patients are intracavitary devices (tandem and colpostats containing radioactive materials) and interstitial implants.

The chief advantage of local irradiation is that a relatively high dose of radiation can be applied to a limited anatomic region. The **inverse square law** has critical implications in clinical applications. The principle of the inverse square law states that the intensity of radiation is inversely proportional to the square of the distance from the source. An important implication is that the rapid falloff of radiant energy supplied by a central source precludes the achievement of cancerocidal doses at the margins of the pelvis. External therapy therefore must be used as well to provide adequate radiation to eliminate tumor at the periphery of large lesions and at the pelvic side walls, where metastatic disease may be present.

An additional therapeutic possibility is the use of spacers in the vagina that increase the distance between vaginal epithelium and the source of radiation. The surface dose (and thus radiation damage) is diminished, but the effective radiation dose applied to the parametrial tissue is essentially unchanged (Fig 51–4).

Radium and cesium are the main elements used in intracavitary therapy, with the latter having the advantage of a long half-life and no gaseous by-products. Iridium is used most often for interstitial needle implants.

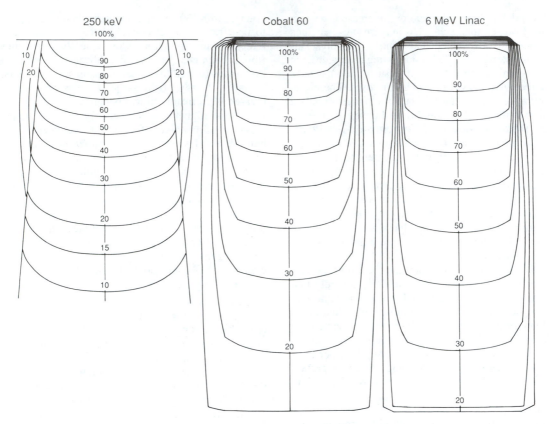

**Figure 51–3.** Typical isodose curves for orthovoltage (250 keV), cobalt 60, and a 6-MeV linear accelerator. The most important difference between the megavoltage (cobalt 60 and Linac) beams in comparison with the 250-keV unit is the movement of the 100% isodose line several millimeters beneath the surface. This results in elimination of the severe skin reactions characteristic of earlier radiation sources. In addition, it can be seen that the higher energy leads to deeper penetration as the energy of the beam increases. The lateral spreading of the beam (penumbra or shadow) is less with cobalt 60 than with the 250-keV unit and is further reduced in the accelerator beam. The reduction of the penumbra with the accelerator beam is due to its possessing a source with smaller physical dimensions. (Reproduced, with permission, from Morrow CP, Curtin JP, Townsend DE [editors]: *Synopsis of Gynecologic Oncology,* 4th ed. Churchill Livingstone, 1993:443.)

## TREATMENT OF GYNECOLOGIC CANCER

### Cervical Cancer

Treatment of cervical cancer is considered a prime example of the successful combination of internal and external radiation therapy. The relative accessibility of the central lesion, a metastatic pattern of cervical squamous cell carcinoma that can be predicted with reasonable accuracy, and the radiation tolerance of the cervix and surrounding tissues often permit curative radiation therapy.

Radiation therapy with curative intent uses both external-beam and intracavitary radiation. Palliative radiation for advanced cervix cancer may utilize either modality for control of bleeding, management of disease in the pelvis, and relief of pain.

The goal of external irradiation is to sterilize metastatic disease to pelvic lymph nodes and the parametria and to decrease the size of the cervix to allow optimal placement of intracavitary radioactive sources.

The size of the portal used to treat a patient with carcinoma of the cervix must be carefully designed to encompass those structures at risk for regional spread of the cancer. To spare normal structures within the pelvis, particularly bowel and bladder, a 4-field technique with both anterior-posterior and lateral portals can be used. The superior border of the anterior-posterior field is usually the L4–L5 interspace but may need to extend more cephalad if the common iliac lymph nodes are to be included in the treatment field. The inferior border is the obturator foramen, but if the vagina is involved by the cancer, the field may be extended to the introitus. Laterally the field should extend 1–2 cm lateral to the bony pelvis. The lateral field includes the pubic symphysis anteriorly and the sacral hollow posteriorly. For patients with stage IB

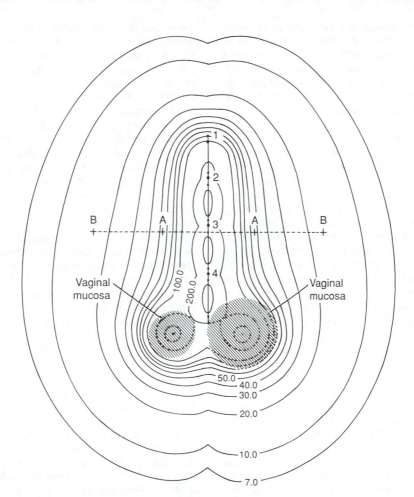

**Figure 51–4.** Isodose curve for a typical cesium insertion in cancer of the cervix. The numbers indicate the dose in cGy/h at various sites around the colpostat (colpostat centers indicated by the cross). The location of points A and B are as indicated. On the left side of the figure, a colpostat without plastic spacer (dotted lines in the outside circle) is shown, whereas on the right side the volume of the spacer has been increased by adding a large plastic cap. It can be seen that the larger spacer pushes the mucosa away from the radioactive source without significantly affecting the dose at points A or B. This improves the therapeutic ratio by significantly reducing the dose to the vaginal mucosa. (Reproduced, with permission, from Morrow CP, Curtin JP, Townsend DE [editors]: *Synopsis of Gynecologic Oncology,* 4th ed. Churchill Livingstone, 1993:442.)

cervical cancer a typical field would approximate 15 × 15 cm, whereas stage IIA to IVA cancer would require larger field sizes. Patients with known or suspected metastatic disease to periaortic lymph nodes may be considered for extended field irradiation. External irradiation is administered using a Cobalt 60 machine or a linear accelerator.

Various techniques are used to maximize the effect of therapy while decreasing the chances of damage to surrounding organs. With the aid of computerized dosimetry, radiation can be increased to compensate for asymmetric parametrial disease. In large lesions, the size of the field can be progressively restricted to concentrate on a defined tumor burden.

In the USA, most intracavitary therapy is delivered via the Fletcher-Suit afterloading applicator. This method permits optimal placement of the tandem and colpostats within the cervical canal and vagina in the operating room. Since the radioactive sources are placed in the devices later, this minimizes exposure to radiation in personnel involved in intracavitary placement. It is crucial that the devices be placed so as to maximize the dose to the target region and at the same time minimize the possibility of radiation damage to the bladder and rectum.

Calculation of the radiation dose given to the different areas of the pelvis has traditionally centered around the concept of point A and point B (Fig 51–4). Point A is 2 cm lateral to the endocervical canal and 2 cm superior to the lateral vaginal fornix; point B is 5 cm lateral to the endocervical canal and in the same plane as point A. Point A represents the point at which the uterine artery crosses the ureter, and point B represents the lymph nodes on the pelvic sidewall. The optimal dose from intracavitary radiation to point A is 6000–8000 cGy, depending on the anatomic limits of the central lesion.

## Endometrial Cancer

Adenocarcinoma of the endometrium tends to present with disease confined to the uterus. Although a variety of combinations of surgery and radiation therapy have been employed in treatment, there has been a trend in the United States toward surgical staging followed by individualized postoperative irradiation. Total abdominal hysterectomy with bilateral salpingo-oophorectomy and aspiration of peritoneal fluid for cytologic evaluation is performed for all patients. Patients chosen on the basis of poor prognostic factors undergo pelvic and periaortic lymph node biopsies.

After the pathologist examines the uterus, tubes, ovaries, and lymph nodes, a decision to use postoperative radiation therapy is based on the presence or absence of poor prognostic factors. Patients with deep myometrial invasion (greater than one-third) or with metastatic disease to fallopian tubes, ovaries, or pelvic lymph nodes receive 4500–5000 cGy of whole pelvis irradiation. If there is involvement of the cervix, additional treatment is given to the vaginal apex utilizing a vaginal cylinder delivering an additional 2500–3000 cGy to the vaginal mucosa. Metastatic disease to periaortic lymph nodes can be managed with extended-field radiation. Patients with stage III disease may be considered for whole abdominal radiation of 2500–3000 cGy with a pelvic boost of 4500–5000 cGy.

Patients with gross involvement of the cervix are ideally treated with preoperative whole pelvic and intracavitary radiation followed by extrafascial hysterectomy.

Endometrial cancer can be managed with radiation therapy alone for the high-risk patient with medical problems who is not a candidate for abdominal surgery. Patients with well-differentiated adenocarcinoma may be managed with tandem and ovoids or intrauterine Simon capsules. Patients with moderately or poorly differentiated cancers or those with involvement of the cervix are at risk for parametrial and pelvic lymph node spread and should receive whole pelvic irradiation prior to brachytherapy.

## Ovarian Cancer

Since the introduction of combination chemotherapy, the use of radiation therapy in the treatment of epithelial ovarian cancer has become increasingly uncommon in the USA. Irradiation is used as adjuvant therapy in patients with early-stage epithelial ovarian cancer, as definitive therapy for minimal residual advanced ovarian cancer, and in the management of re-current and persistent ovarian cancer. As with chemotherapy, the patients most likely to benefit from irradiation are those who have minimal residual disease.

Patients who have been adequately staged and have stage IA well-differentiated and moderately differentiated adenocarcinoma have not been shown to benefit from adjuvant therapy. All other patients with stage I disease and those with stage II disease currently receive adjuvant therapy. In these patients, a randomized trial has shown no difference in survival between those receiving intraperitoneal colloidal chromic phosphate ($^{32}$P) and single-agent melphalan. If $^{32}$P is considered for therapy, it is imperative that adequate staging has been performed including sampling of pelvic and periaortic nodes, since $^{32}$P has limited penetration and the dosage to pelvic and periaortic nodes is considered subtherapeutic. $^{32}$P has the advantages of convenience of a single treatment, minimal toxicity, and low cost. The Gynecologic Oncology Group recently has completed a trial of intraperitoneal $^{32}$P versus 3 courses of cisplatin plus cyclophosphamide in select patients with stage I and II disease, but the results are not yet available.

The use of whole abdominal irradiation in patients with stage III epithelial ovarian cancer has not been compared prospectively in a randomized trial with platinum-based combination chemotherapy. Since the tolerance of the kidneys, liver, and bone marrow limits the dose of radiation that can be delivered to the whole abdomen, the size of residual disease in the upper abdomen should be microscopic and not greater than 2 cm in the pelvis. Current treatment regimens use 2000–3000 cGy to the abdomen with appropriate shielding of the kidneys and liver and 4500–5500 cGy to the pelvis. The treatment can be delivered by either the moving-strip or the open-field technique; randomized studies have shown no differences in patient survival or in complications between the 2 methods.

Patients who complete chemotherapy for stage III ovarian cancer and are then found to have a negative second-look laparotomy remain at high risk for recurrence. As many as 50% of these patients eventually have recurrence. A number of investigators have reported improved survival in this group of patients following the administration of intraperitoneal $^{32}$P.

Whole abdominal irradiation has been used for recurrent and persistent disease, but the results generally have not been encouraging. Radiation therapy may play an important role in palliation for patients with advanced disease not responsive to chemotherapy. For example, recurrence in the pelvis impinging on the rectum may lead to large bowel obstruction. The judicious use of external-beam irradiation may control disease in the pelvis and prevent the need for a diverting colostomy.

## Vaginal Cancer

Because of the proximity of the bladder and rectum

to the vagina, most vaginal cancers are not amenable to resection. Occasional early superficial lesions may be treated with local excision followed by interstitial iridium 192 needle implants or a vaginal cylinder. Most patients with squamous cell carcinoma of the vagina are best managed with whole pelvic radiation therapy followed by a vaginal cylinder and interstitial needle irradiation. Patients with lesions involving the lower third of the vagina should have the inguinal and femoral lymph nodes included in the external-beam treatment field.

## Vulvar Cancer

The role of radiation therapy in the management of squamous cell carcinoma of the vulva has undergone a major change in the past decade. Although surgery remains the major modality in the treatment of patients with cancer of the vulva, the results of a randomized Gynecologic Oncology Group study has resulted in patients with more than one groin node containing cancer to be considered for treatment with groin and whole pelvic radiation therapy.

Patients with more advanced lesions may benefit from combinations of surgery and vulvar irradiation. This may include interstitial needle implants, external-beam irradiation, and concurrent chemoradiation with or without subsequent surgery.

## Complications of Radiation Therapy

The most serious complication of radiation therapy is failure to eradicate cancer. With this overriding goal in mind, radiation therapy regimens are formulated to maximize the chances for cure while incurring the smallest amount of damage to normal tissues. In gynecologic cancers, the most serious complications are those involving the gastrointestinal or genitourinary systems.

Complications of radiation therapy are classified as early or delayed. Early problems that occur especially with whole pelvis teletherapy include enteritis, proctosigmoiditis, cystitis, vulvitis, and, occasionally, depression of bone marrow elements. Bowel side effects usually take the form of painful cramping and diarrhea that require dietary adjustments and the judicious use of antidiarrheal agents. These problems usually respond to appropriate medication, but occasionally radiation therapy must be interrupted or curtailed because of fulminant acute reactions.

Delayed radiation injury may be manifested by chronic proctosigmoiditis, hemorrhagic cystitis, small and large bowel strictures, and the formation of rectovaginal and vesicovaginal fistulas. Pelvic fibrosis and loss of ovarian function may seriously cripple sexual activity in younger patients.

## New Directions in Radiation therapy

The evolution of combined-modality therapy and technologic advances are likely to benefit future patients with gynecologic malignancies. The role of radiation sensitizers and concurrent chemoradiation in the treatment of cancers of the cervix, vulva, and vagina continues to be explored. Prospective randomized trials of radiation therapy by the Gynecologic Oncology Group, the Radiation Therapy Oncology Group, and the Southwest Oncology Group will answer many important questions in the management of patients with gynecologic cancers. These include the need for extrafascial hysterectomy following radiation therapy for bulky (> 4 cm) cancer of the cervix and radiation sensitizers in locally advanced and periaortic node positive cancer of the cervix. In epithelial ovarian cancer, recent studies include adjuvant $^{32}$P versus combination platinum-based chemotherapy for early cancer and $^{32}$P versus no further treatment following negative second-look laparotomy in stage III disease. The benefit of whole pelvic irradiation for stage I endometrial cancer with intermediate-risk factors and whole abdominal irradiation for advanced endometrial cancer currently are being addressed. Finally, the role of irradiation in locally advanced cancer of the vulva will be evaluated in more detail.

In addition to radiation sensitizers, other treatment methods including hyperbaric oxygen administration, fast neutrons, hyperthermia, negative pions, and altered fractionation schemes are being evaluated for effectiveness against the tumor-protective effects of hypoxia, which is a common problem with gynecologic cancers. With the current emphasis on cost containment in medical care, continuing studies of high dose rate brachytherapy is likely to shorten the time course of intracavitary treatment. As newer computer technologies are wedded to imaging techniques, further advances in anatomic contouring for planning and treatment are certain. These advances ARE hoped to translate into better local control rates as well as improved survival with a wider margin of safety.

## REFERENCES

Delclos L et al: Can the Fletcher gamma ray colpostat system be extrapolated to other systems? Cancer 1978;41:970.

Dembo AJ: Epithelial ovarian cancer: The role of radiotherapy. Int J Radiat Oncol Biol Phys 1992;22:835.

DiSaia PJ, Creasman WT: *Clinical Gynecologic Oncology.* 4th ed. Mosby-Year Book, 1993.

Dusenbery KE, Carson LF, Potish RA: Perioperative morbidity and mortality of gynecologic brachytherapy. Cancer 1991;67:2786.

Eifel PJ et al: Twice-daily, split-course abdominopelvic radiation therapy after chemotherapy and positive second-look laparotomy for epithelial ovarian carcinoma. Int J Radiat Oncol Biol Phys 1991;21:1013.

Fanning J et al: Prognostic significance of the extent of cervical involvement by endometrial cancer. Gynecol Oncol 1991;40:46.

Fletcher GH: *Textbook of Radiotherapy.* 3rd ed. Lea & Febiger, 1980.

Fyles AW et al: Analysis of complications in patients treated with abdomino-pelvic radiation therapy for ovarian carcinoma. Int J Radiat Oncol Biol Phys 1992;22:847.

Greven KM et al: Analysis of complications in patients with endometrial carcinoma receiving adjuvant irradiation. Int J Radiat Oncol Biol Phys 1991;21:919.

Hall EJ: *Radiobiology for the Radiologist.* 4th ed. JB Lippincott, 1994.

Hoffman M et al: Interstitial radiotherapy for the treatment of advanced or recurrent vulvar and distal vaginal malignancy. Am J Obstet Gynecol 1990;162:1278.

Homesley HD et al: Radiation therapy versus pelvic node resection for carcinoma of the vulva with positive groin nodes. Obstet Gynecol 1986;68:733.

Hoskins WJ, Perez CA, Young RC (editors): *Principles and Practice of Gynecologic Oncology,* JB Lippincott, 1992.

Kim RY: Radiotherapeutic management in carcinoma of the uterine cervix: Current status. Int J Gynecol Cancer 1993;3:337.

Lanciano RM et al: Influence of age, prior abdominal surgery, fraction size, and dose on complications after radiation therapy for squamous cell cancer of the uterine cervix: A pattern of care study. Cancer 1992;69:2124.

Lindner H, Willich H, Atzinger A: Primary adjuvant whole abdominal irradiation in ovarian carcinoma. Int J Radiat Oncol Biol Phys 1990;19:1203.

Morrow CP, Curtin JP, Townsend DE (editors): *Synopsis of Gynecologic Oncology,* 4th ed. Churchill Livingstone, 1993.

Mychalczak BR, Fuks Z: The current role of radiotherapy in the management of ovarian cancer. Hematol Oncol Clin North Am 1992;6:895.

Perez CA, Brady LA (editors): *Principles and Practice of Radiation Oncology,* 2nd ed. JB Lippincott, 1992.

Perez CA et al: Radiation therapy in management of carcinoma of the vulva with emphasis on conservation therapy. Cancer 1993;71:3707.

Peters WA et al: Intraperitoneal P-32 is not an effective consolidation therapy after a negative second-look laparotomy for epithelial carcinoma of the ovary. Gynecol Oncol 1992;47:146.

Rubin SC et al: Management of endometrial adenocarcinoma with cervical involvement. Gynecol Oncol 1992;45:294.

Soper JT, Berchuck A, Clarke-Pearson DL: Adjuvant intraperitoneal chromic phosphate therapy for women with apparent early ovarian carcinoma who have not undergone comprehensive surgical staging. Cancer 1991;68:725.

Soper JT et al: Adjuvant therapy with intraperitoneal chromic phosphate ($^{32}$P) in women with early ovarian carcinoma after comprehensive surgical staging. Obstet Gynecol 1992;79:993.

Spanos WJ Jr et al: Complications in the use of intra-abdominal $^{32}$P for ovarian carcinoma. Gynecol Oncol 1992;45:243.

Speert H: *Obstetrics and Gynecology in America: A History.* The American College of Obstetricians and Gynecologists, 1980.

Stehman FB, Bundy BN: Carcinoma of the cervix treated with chemotherapy and radiation therapy: Cooperative studies in the Gynecologic Oncology Group. Cancer 1993;71:1697.

Stitt JA: High-dose-rate intracavitary brachytherapy for gynecologic malignancies. Oncology 1992;6:59.

Stock RG et al: The importance of brachytherapy technique in the management of primary carcinoma of the vagina. Int J Radiat Oncol Biol Phys 1992;24:747.

Vergote IB et al: Randomized trial comparing cisplatin with radioactive phosphorus or whole-abdomen irradiation as adjuvant treatment of ovarian cancer. Cancer 1992;69:741.

Vermorken JB: The role of chemotherapy in squamous cell carcinoma of the uterine cervix: A review. Int J Gynecol Cancer 1993;3:129.

Walton LA, Yadusky A, Rubinstein L: Intraperitoneal radioactive phosphate in early ovarian carcinoma: An analysis of complications. Int J Radiat Oncol Biol Phys 1991;20:939.

Withers HR: The four "R's" of radiotherapy. In: *Advances in Radiation Biology, Lett JT, Adler H (eds.), vol 5.* Academic Press, 1975.

Young RC et al: Adjuvant therapy in stage I and stage II epithelial ovarian cancer: Results of two prospective randomized trials. N Engl J Med 1990;322:1021.

# Chemotherapy for Gynecologic Cancers

# 52

*April Gale O'Quinn, MD, & Simie Degefu, MD*

## General Considerations

Effective chemotherapy for gynecologic cancers exploits characteristic differences between tumor cells and normal cells to selectively kill malignant cells without producing serious, irreversible harm to vital organs and tissues. Knowledge of the scientific basis of cancer chemotherapy is derived from research in molecular biology and cell kinetics and is indispensable to the development of better drugs, establishment of a more rational basis for the design of protocols, and the optimal use of presently available antineoplastic drugs.

Long-lasting remissions and occasional cures for several types of cancer have been achieved with antitumor drugs. For example, up to 90% of patients with metastatic choriocarcinoma achieve a normal life expectancy, and almost 100% of those without metastases are cured now that the effect of drugs may be monitored by the level of β-hCG (human chorionic gonadotropin), which provides a reliable index of tumor growth. For most tumors, however, no such specific and sensitive assay or tumor marker exists. Now that multiple-drug regimens are being used for primary chemotherapy of carcinoma of the ovary, objective response rates of 60–80% are achieved. The objective response rate of 20–40% achieved by chemotherapy in patients with primary carcinoma of the breast and endometrium warrants the use of chemotherapy as an integral part of an initial treatment program.

In spite of extensive experience, the use of cytotoxic agents for carcinomas of the cervix, vagina, and vulva is still on a clinical trial basis, since these tumors usually grow more slowly, and cytotoxic drug treatment has been palliative but not curative; these types of cancer are better controlled by surgery and radiation therapy, and chemotherapy should be considered only when these standard methods have proved ineffective.

Among the uncommon gynecologic cancers that may require chemotherapy are germ cell tumors of the ovary and primary ovarian, uterine, vaginal, or vulvar sarcomas. Because these tumors are rare, little is known about their sensitivity to antitumor drugs.

## The Normal Cell Cycle

Figure 52–1 represents the cell cycle in a clockwise progression. The phases and their durations are depicted, and the phases during which some specific chemotherapeutic agents exert their effects are included for reference.

## Cell Kinetics

Knowledge of tumor cells has been derived from clinical and laboratory methods of tumor growth measurement, including direct measurement of cell cycle parameters, clinical measurement of doubling times, and use of biologic markers such as hormone production or polyamines and other abnormal proteins. A knowledge of the terminology of cell kinetics is helpful in understanding the dynamics of tumor cells, in which some cells divide more slowly than others, some cells enter or leave a nondividing state, and some are lost from the tumor population entirely.

The **mitotic index (MI)** is the fraction of cells in mitosis in a steady-state condition. The MI may be calculated by giving a drug such as a *Vinca* alkaloid that halts further cellular progression through mitosis and then counting the number of cells in mitosis. Another method uses tritiated thymidine, which is incorporated only into the DNA of cells in the S phase; the tritiated thymidine emits β rays that can then expose the silver in a photographic emulsion during cell mitosis to produce **percent-labeled mitosis (PLM)** curves. Radioactive tagging of DNA during synthesis provides the **labeling index (LI)**, which is the percentage of cells in the S phase at a particular time.

**Growth fraction (GF)** is the overall proportion of proliferating tumor cells in a given tumor. The $G_1$–$G_0$ equilibrium is an important aspect of the growth fraction, because only the clonogenic, or stem, cells are considered. The growth fraction is important because most antitumor drugs inhibit only proliferating cells. Therefore, a major difference between tumor and normal cell populations may be the relative percentage of each in the growth fraction. The selective effect of antitumor drugs on tumor cells may be explained by the characteristic higher growth fraction of tumor cells. Toxicity results from the effects of antitumor drugs

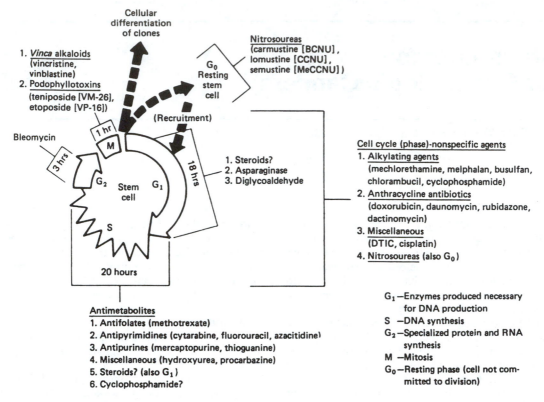

**Figure 52–1.** Model of the cell cycle, with progression proceeding clockwise. Phases and their durations are depicted, along with points in the cell cycle at which some chemotherapeutic agents exert their effects.

on normal cells in the mitotic cycle or growth fraction; consequently, the toxicity of most antitumor drugs occurs in those normal cell populations with rapid turnover, eg, the hematopoietic and gastrointestinal systems. Alopecia is a common manifestation of such toxicity.

**Cell cycle time** denotes the amount of time needed by a proliferating cell to progress through the cell cycle and produce a new daughter cell. Cell cycle times vary widely according to histologic type (18–217 hours in solid tumors) but are relatively constant for a specific tumor type.

**Doubling time** is the time required for the tumor cell population to double. Human tumors often have doubling times greater than those of comparable normal tissues and, in advanced stages of disease, may exhibit a range of doubling times, but 30–60 days is typical. In the model ascites system, cell doubling time remains constant at nearly 100% throughout almost the entire life cycle of the tumor, whereas in solid tumor systems, a gradual slowing of the tumor doubling time and reduction of the proliferation rate of cells occur with tumor enlargement as a result of decreased accessibility to nutrients.

Cell loss may be a major determinant of the tumor growth rate. Cells are lost from a tumor mass in vari-

ous ways, including death, migration, or metastases. Cell loss is frequently high in advanced tumors.

## Stem Cell Theory

The stem cell theory states that only certain relatively undifferentiated cells, or stem cells, of a particular tissue type are able to divide and reproduce the entire tissue. Examples include rapidly proliferating tissues such as bone marrow, the lining of the gastrointestinal tract, and the basal cell layer of the skin. In other words, most cells making up a particular tissue have matured or have become highly differentiated after clonal division from the reproducing cell or a specific stem cell.

Not all cells of a particular stem cell population are committed to division at a given time. A significant proportion of stem cells are in the $G_0$ or resting phase, as is the case in normal bone marrow, in which at any one time from 15 to 50% of stem cells are in $G_0$. Numerous stimuli may recruit this reserve (resting) population of stem cells into the cell cycle. The equilibrium between the number of cells in division and those at rest, and the requirement for controls on such growth, are important. Some of the controls are understood, whereas others are unknown.

The stem cell theory also describes neoplastic

growth. Tumors are thought to originate from a single stem cell, and in many tumor systems, it is possible to prove that all cells have a common ancestor. Most solid tumors are believed to contain only a relatively small stem cell population contributing to the bulk of the tumor mass. Theoretically, therapy should attempt to eradicate the stem cell population, since most of the tumor cell mass may be incapable of self-replication. Total eradication of the entire stem cell pool is a difficult task in most solid tumors, however, but advances in drug therapy for a growing number of tumors have demonstrated the possibility of cure.

Malignant tumors are thought to be composed of cells that have somehow escaped normal growth restrictions and controls. The principles of cell kinetics are invoked to describe and predict tumor growth and to assess the impact of therapy on that growth.

## Cell-Kill Hypothesis

The fundamental kinetic consideration in cancer chemotherapy is the cell-kill hypothesis, which states that the effects of cancer chemotherapy on tumor cell populations demonstrate first-order kinetics; ie, the proportion of tumor cells killed is a constant percentage of the total number of cells present. In other words, chemotherapy kills a constant proportion of cells, not a constant number of cells. The number of cells killed by a particular agent or combination of drugs is proportional to one variable: the dose used. The relative sensitivity of cells is not considered, and the growth rate is assumed to be constant.

Since chemotherapy follows an exponential (log-kill) model, treatment may be said to have a specific exponential, or log-kill, potential. For example, a log kill of 2 reduces a theoretical human tumor burden of $10^9$ cells to $10^7$ cells. Although this represents a reduction of 99%, at least 10 million ($10^7$) viable cells remain. A log kill of 3 achieves a reduction of 99.9%, but 1 million ($10^6$) cells remain. Theoretically, therefore, such fractional reductions by antineoplastic agents can never reduce a tumor cell population to zero. This traditional cell-kill model is based mainly on exponentially growing tumors in laboratory models, eg, L-1210 murine leukemia (Skipper and Schabel, 1982).

Although the cell-kill hypothesis probably explains some aspects of drug selectivity, other mechanisms are involved. The more responsive tumors are those with large growth fractions. Normal tissue can withstand greater cell loss due to chemotherapy than can tumors, although the proportion killed in both systems may be identical.

Norton and Simon have proposed an alternative to the constant first-order log-kill hypothesis of Skipper; it states that clinical tumor regression as a result of chemotherapy is best explained by the relative growth fraction in the tumor at the time of treatment. Thus, very small and very large tumors are less responsive than those of intermediate size, which have the biggest growth fraction. Therefore, log kills occur only at times of maximal tumor growth fraction. Although this hypothesis has not been directly confirmed clinically, it explains some clinical observations of responses to chemotherapy in large and small human tumors.

## Gompertzian Model of Tumor Growth

Gompertz, a German insurance actuary, depicted the relationship of an individual's age to the expected time of death by means of an asymmetric sigmoid curve. This mathematical model approximates tumor proliferation in experimental systems wherein tumors initially grow rapidly and a high percentage of stem cells replicate. As the tumor increases in size, a plateau effect develops, and the apparent doubling time is much longer than at the beginning.

Figure 52–2 demonstrates several current chemotherapeutic principles plotted against a Gompertzian tumor growth curve and the large tumor cell burden required to produce clinical expression of symptoms. The minimum palpable subcutaneous lesion is about 60 mg and contains $6 \times 10^7$ cells. In superficial tumors, 1 cm$^3$ or 1 g of tumor is not an uncommon size at the time of diagnosis and contains about $10^9$ cells, whereas most patients with visceral tumors of 10–100 g are estimated to have $10^{10}$–$10^{11}$ tumor cells at the time of diagnosis. Since death occurs with a tumor burden of $10^{12}$ cells, which is only 1–2 orders of magnitude less than the total number of cells in the human adult, a significant proportion of the life cycle of a clinically recognizable tumor has already transpired when it is finally detected. The importance of early diagnosis of malignant disease therefore becomes even more essential.

The outcome of the 2 chemotherapeutic treatment regimens A and B; the influence of the fractional kill achieved by drug therapy; and the effect of volume of tumor at the onset of therapy are illustrated in Figure 52–2. Chemotherapy treatment A in a patient with a visceral solid tumor composed of $10^{11}$ cells achieves a good response when the tumor cell population is reduced by the characteristic percentage of first-order kill, regardless of the actual number of tumor cells present. Thus, an agent with a one-log cell kill reduces the cell concentration by 90% from a palpable 10 g mass to a nonpalpable 1-g mass and induces an apparently tumor-free state; yet a residual tumor burden remains that may contain more than 1 billion cells. After a brief delay, the remaining 10% of tumor cells resume their former rate of proliferation. After tumor cell repopulation has occurred, treatment again results in reduction of tumor volume, but resistance develops that results in death of the host at a predictable time.

Although normal tissues do not develop resistance to antitumor drugs, the larger the initial tumor volume and the smaller the fractional kill, the more likely is the development of resistance in tumor cells. The ef-

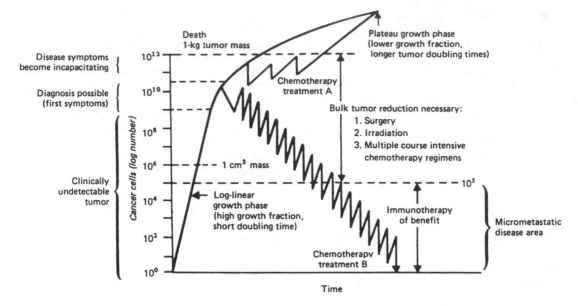

**Figure 52–2.** Gompertzian tumor growth curve. The model depicts the relationship between tumor growth and diagnosis, appearance of symptoms, and various treatment regimens.

fect of successive drug doses in sensitive tumors depends on the number of existing cells when treatment is begun, the fractional kill, the number of cells surviving the preceding treatment, and the tumor cell production between treatment cycles. Obviously, cell destruction must exceed cell production for chemotherapy to be successful.

Nonlethal damage to cells can occur due to chemotherapy and is well known after radiation therapy. A key principle of theory, therefore, is to schedule chemotherapy, radiation therapy, or both at appropriate intervals to allow normal cells to recover from nonlethal damage but to preclude the recovery of tumor cells, which is slower. It is important that the interval between treatments be reduced to the bare minimum required for restoration and recovery of normal tissues.

In chemotherapy treatment B, repeated doses of a chemotherapeutic agent are used to destroy a large tumor cell population. Such consecutive log-kill reductions cannot be consistently achieved because the cell-kill potential of a drug is limited in comparison with the size of the tumor cell population in most clinical situations; however, in Figure 52–2, a reduction of $10^{10}$ (10 billion) cell population by 90% as a result of a single course of drug therapy produces complete clinical remission. Repeated treatment at shorter intervals may result in enhanced destruction of tumor cells as long as toxic effects remain tolerable and resistant cell lines are not selected out by the drug. A drug becomes curative once the tumor cell kill exceeds the order of magnitude of repopulation

and (statistically) less than one tumor cell remains. Additional courses of drug therapy are required to eradicate the last surviving cell of the so-called exponential iceberg if each course kills the same fraction of cells and not the same number.

On the other hand, fewer cycles of chemotherapy may produce a tumor-free host if subclinical tumor containing only $10^4$ cells is present at diagnosis. Unfortunately, the usual inability to detect tumors so early in clinical situations makes this model less realistic.

Alternatively, the tumor population may be reduced by surgery or radiation so that subsequent adjuvant chemotherapy has a rational basis. Initial therapy for many solid tumors involves surgery or irradiation to reduce tumor bulk. Adjuvant chemotherapy, immunotherapy, or both are added as appropriate to eradicate micrometastatic or subclinical tumor masses. The same general principle guides therapy of hematologic cancer, in which intensive induction chemotherapy is used to achieve reduction of tumor bulk and induce remission; less intensive consolidation and remission maintenance doses of chemotherapy are then used to control subclinical tumor burdens.

## Effects of Chemotherapy on the Cell Cycle

Knowledge of the site of action of antitumor drugs within the mitotic cell cycle may help to explain the mechanism of their effectiveness and may suggest ways to enhance their carcinostatic properties. Chemotherapy and radiation therapy are thought to alter the proliferation kinetics of both tumor and normal cells. Initially, individual sensitive cells are killed or incapacitated, thereby leaving a more resistant residual population. This large reduction in tumor cell mass stimulates recruitment of quiescent cells from $G_0$ into $G_1$. This shift favors an increased growth fraction in the tumor, so that the LI and the MI are increased and tumor doubling times are decreased (ie, the tumor mass doubles in less time than before). The effect is a shift to the left along the Gompertzian curve.

Some drugs may not kill cells but can halt or slow the progression of a cell through a particular phase of the cell cycle. Because cells accumulate in a particular phase, this process has been termed **cell cycle synchronization.** Generally, these effects occur at lower doses than those necessary for cell killing. Blockage may be either temporary or permanent and does not occur predictably in all cell populations treated.

The effects of various classes of anticancer agents on tumors depend on the basic events occurring in the 4 main phases of the mitotic cell cycle and the pharmacologic mechanisms of drug action, and these cytotoxic effects influence the design of rational drug regimens. Two basic classes of antineoplastic drugs are recognized: cell cycle (phase)-specific agents and cell cycle (phase)-nonspecific agents.

**A. Cell Cycle (Phase)-Specific Drugs:** Cell cycle (phase)-specific drugs are much more effective in tumors in which a large proportion of cells are actively dividing, as occurs when the cell mass is low. The major cytotoxic activities of anticancer drugs in this class are manifested during a particular phase of the cell cycle, and these drugs are technically *phase-specific* rather than *cycle-specific* agents. These drugs have been termed schedule-dependent agents because they produce a greater cell kill if the drug is given in multiple, repeated fractions rather than as a large single dose.

In pharmacologic terms, these cell cycle (phase)-specific agents are most often described as antimetabolites, because each drug causes some type of unique biochemical blockade of a particular reaction that occurs in a single phase of the cell cycle.

Most cell cycle (phase)-specific agents, such as methotrexate and fluorouracil, exert their most significant activities in the S phase. Corticosteroids and asparaginase appear to be most active in $G_1$, bleomycin appears to be most active in $G_2$, and the *Vinca* and podophyllin alkaloids have marked activity in the M and $G_2$ phases.

**B. Cell Cycle (Phase)-Nonspecific Agents:** In contrast, the cell cycle (phase)-nonspecific agents are effective in large tumors in which the growth fraction, LI, and MI are low. Drugs in this group are dose-dependent, since a single bolus injection generally kills the same number of cells as do repeated doses totaling the same amount; ie, the degree of cell kill is directly proportionate to the absolute dose given.

In pharmacologic terms, the alkylating agents are the prototypes of this class, which also includes the nitrosoureas, the anthracyclines, and others.

The cell cycle (phase)-nonspecific drugs do not require a large growth fraction to exert maximal effects. The effectiveness of their cytotoxic activities generally depends on cellular attempts either to divide or to repair drug-induced damage. The attempt to perform these activities triggers expression of the damage already sustained, and the cell dies. This mechanism of cell death is important, since cancer cells in $G_0$ (resting phase) are not generally susceptible to cytotoxic agents, with the possible exception of the cell cycle (phase)-nonspecific mustard-type alkylators and the nitrosoureas.

A few cell cycle (phase)-nonspecific agents, such as some alkylators and the nitrosoureas, appear to have uncharacteristically nonselective actions on normal as well as on tumor stem cell populations.

### Selectivity of Anticancer Drugs

There is a common belief that cancer chemotherapy is generally nonselective and kills normal as well as cancerous tissues. However, most anticancer drugs are more active against tumor than normal tissues. The cell-kill hypothesis probably explains some drug selectivity, but other mechanisms are involved as well. The selectivity of cytotoxic agents appears to correlate inversely with cell cycle specificity, since cell cycle (phase)-nonspecific agents such as the nitrosoureas and mechlorethamine (an alkylator) tend to be more toxic in normal bone marrow than in tumor cells. The selectivity of most antitumor drugs must still be based largely on differences in the cell kinetics of normal and neoplastic cell lines. Normal systems can withstand greater cellular losses due to chemotherapy than can tumors, even though the proportion of cells killed in both might be identical. Recovery from damage produced by a tumor-inhibiting drug may be more protracted in tumor cells than in normal host cells. Increased antitumor selectivity can be provided by the judicious use of a second dose of drug following return of normal tissue function but before recovery of tumor cell function. This approach to selective recovery from chemotherapeutic damage may provide enormous benefit by enhancing the antitumor activity of presently available drugs.

The hormonal agents are probably the best examples of truly selective anticancer agents because of their action on specific target tissues. Prostatic tumors and tumors rich in acid phosphatase can selectively activate the hormone diethylstilbestrol within the cells.

Most agents are equally effective at key enzymatic sites in either normal or neoplastic cells, but some anticancer drugs kill cancer cells by taking advantage of unique biochemical differences in the cancer cells; eg, the enzyme asparaginase takes advantage of a relative deficiency of aspartic acid synthetase in some leukemic cells to cause cell death. Cancer cells demonstrate a selective uptake of high concentrations of methotrexate, and this selectivity can be experimentally enhanced by vincristine or asparaginase and inhibited by aminoglycosides and cephalosporins.

Sensitivity to drugs based on the type of tissue is recognized in some anticancer agents; eg, the antimetabolite fluorouracil is more active in neoplasms arising from endodermal tissues such as the gastrointestinal tract and the breast. Dacarbazine has some selective action for melanoma cells, and bleomycin is active against epithelial tumors such as squamous cell cancers of the lung and cervix. When a tumor is derived from an organ characterized by a distinct biochemical feature (eg, the thyroid gland's ability to accumulate iodine, the sensitivity of the adrenal cortex to mitotane, or the selective destruction of the pancreatic islet cells by streptozocin), chemotherapy can be devised that attacks that tumor preferentially.

Although individual differences between the cells of a particular tumor and normal cells have been discovered, no single biochemical feature has been detected that pertains exclusively to one or the other. Studies suggest numerous possibilities for exploiting small quantitative differences between tumor and normal tissue. These include selective uptake of drugs into tumors, enhanced anabolism in tumors of ápro-drugs" requiring activation, diminished catabolism of drugs by tumors, diminished repair of tumor cell damage, and reduced availability of a protecting metabolite in tumor tissue.

## Poor Host Defenses

The normal individual's immunologic defenses against an invading tumor cell population are unreliable and still poorly understood; they operate only if the tumor mass is relatively small, and they become less effective as the person ages. As tumor growth progresses, the body's diminishing immunocompetence compounds the difficulties of therapy. A complicating factor is the immunosuppressant properties of most antitumor drugs. Treatment schedules to minimize immunosuppression while permitting adequate therapeutic effectiveness should be more intensive but actually must be practiced sparingly because of the lack of antitumor selectivity. Current studies are attempting to enhance immunologic host defenses by immunostimulation with reagents such as bacillus Calmette-Guaaerin (BCG) or *Corynebacterium parvum* and by restoration of immunocompetence with agents such as levamisole, thymosin, or interferon, as well as with combinations of 2 or more kinds of immunotherapy.

## Protected Tumor Sanctuaries

Antitumor drugs frequently fail to reach all sites of tumor cells, and so-called "sanctuaries" may exist that permit the establishment and unimpeded prolif-

eration of a tumor once it has been successfully eradicated from the remainder of the body. Sanctuaries may develop because of the metastatic spread of tumors to distant sites, and the problem may be accentuated by a lack of knowledge regarding the mechanism of drug access to such secondary neoplasms and their susceptibility to various drugs.

The central nervous system is impervious to many drugs and often represents such a protected site. Attempts to reach sequestered cells have included intrathecal administration of drugs or use of more highly lipid-soluble drugs capable of rapidly penetrating the blood-brain barrier. The success of peripheral chemotherapy in the leukemias is due in part to the ease with which high levels of drug can be achieved in tumor cells; on the other hand, leukemic cells that have penetrated the central nervous system are no longer affected by most drugs, and disease progresses.

A more common problem, however, is the diminished blood supply in many solid tumors that blocks delivery of antitumor drugs to the tumor core, which, although necrotic, may still contain active cells sensitive to antitumor drugs. It should be remembered that high doses of radiation (as used in the primary treatment of many gynecologic cancers) produce vascular damage leading to the formation of ischemic sanctuaries for cells that might otherwise be sensitive to drug treatment.

Many antitumor drugs are also carcinogenic, a danger recognized only recently, when patients receiving antitumor therapy began to live longer and the development of secondary tumors occurred.

## Principles of Clinical Chemotherapy

The chief aim of therapy is to achieve maximum cell kill with minimum toxicity. To this end, the dose and schedule of drugs critically influence the therapeutic index. The steep dose-response curve for most drugs indicates that the highest tolerable dose producing an acceptable degree of reversible toxicity should be used in the treatment of sensitive tumors, in which a 2-fold increase in dose may produce a 10-fold increase in the fractional kill.

Therapy must also consider the length of time a therapeutic concentration of drug is maintained. The maximal effectiveness of some oncolytic drugs depends mainly on peak tissue concentration, whereas that of others depends on the duration of exposure.

In general, a therapeutic concentration of the cell cycle (phase)-specific drugs is best maintained by 5-day courses of treatment (about 2 average cell generation times). Such prolonged exposure permits a higher fraction of proliferating cells to pass through vulnerable phases of the cell cycle, since proliferating cells do not progress through the cell cycle in a synchronized fashion. In contrast, the cell cycle (phase)-nonspecific drugs are best administered as an intravenous bolus of the highest tolerable dose, and the dose repeated when normal target tissues have recovered.

High-dose, intermittent therapy has been the most successful schedule against tumors with a large growth fraction. Slow-growing tumors have a large component of permanently nondividing cells and a small growth fraction. Theoretically, drugs active against cells in $G_0$ and given on a continuous basis should produce the best results in these tumors.

Chronic therapy is feasible only if toxicity is negligible. Some myelosuppression is acceptable, since recovery occurs between treatment cycles. Immunosuppression is a side effect of most cytotoxic drugs and is more pronounced when drugs are given continuously.

Antitumor drugs have been combined concurrently or sequentially in an effort to increase their effectiveness. It is logical to suppose that drugs with different dose-limiting toxicities and different modes of action may increase the fractional cell kill without a parallel rise in damage to normal tissues and immunocompetent cells. Since tumors are composed of numerous cell clones that vary in their sensitivity to drugs, the use of multiple agents should lessen the chance of development of resistance and repopulation of the tumor by a resistant cell clone. Sequential, concomitant, or complementary blockade of metabolic pathways should avoid the problem of drug resistance secondary either to the utilization of alternative pathways or the emergence of a protective random mutation.

As a rule, drugs selected for multidrug therapy must be effective as single agents if improved results are to be expected. Unfortunately, the toxicities of most antitumor drugs are similar, and selecting drugs that have no overlapping side effects is usually not possible. Nevertheless, combination chemotherapy has proved superior to single-agent therapy in leukemia, lymphoma, and some rapidly proliferating solid tumors. Because the risk of serious toxicity does not seem to be justified by the small chance of substantial tumor control, drug combinations have not been used extensively in slow-growing solid tumors.

In summary, successful drug therapy requires the administration of an effective agent using the best possible dose and schedule. The tumor must have a high growth fraction and must be accessible to drugs so that they can exert their antitumor effects (ie, cells must not be in tumor "sanctuaries"). The tumor volume must be small or the fractional cell kill large to avoid the emergence of a resistant cell clone or the development of tolerance in previously sensitive cell clones. Normal tissue must recover from drug injury faster than tumor can regenerate to pretreatment levels.

# CANCER CHEMOTHERAPEUTIC AGENTS

Cancer chemotherapeutic agents are commonly classified on the basis of their mechanism of action into 6 general categories: alkylating agents, antimetabolites, plant alkaloids, miscellaneous agents, hormonal agents, and immunotherapeutic agents.

This section presents a broad overview of the mechanism of action and general toxicities of the 4 major groups of cytotoxic cancer chemotherapy drugs.

## Alkylating Agents

**A. Classic Alkylating Agents:** The alkylating agents evolved from products developed for chemical warfare. The parent chemical, dichloroethyl sulfide (sulfur mustard), was first synthesized during the mid-19th century and used during World War I because of its blistering properties on skin and mucous membranes. These agents also produced atrophy of lymphoid and myeloid tissues, a finding that led workers to explore their use in treating lymphomas and leukemias.

The 3 chemical subgroups of classic alkylating agents in use today are (1) the bis(chloroethyl)amines, which include chlorambucil, cyclophosphamide, ifosfamide, mechlorethamine, melphalan, and uracil mustard; (2) the ethylenimines, which include triethylenethiophosphoramide (Thiotepa); and (3) the alkylsulfonates, which include busulfan and improsulfan hydrochloride (Yoshi 864).

Inability of DNA to replicate and the actual breaking of DNA strands caused by depurination occur at the cellular level. In addition to these cytotoxic and mutagenic effects, alkylating agents also inhibit cellular glycolysis, respiration, and synthesis of various enzymes, protein, and nucleic acids. The major effect of the alkylators appears to be cross-linking of DNA strands. Synthesis of most other cellular constituents (eg, RNA and protein) continues, which causes an imbalance in cell growth, and the cell eventually dies.

Most alkylating agents are cell cycle (phase)-nonspecific drugs that are active against both resting and dividing cells; they may therefore be used effectively in tumors with a small growth fraction. **Cyclophosphamide** is unique in that it appears to inhibit DNA synthesis in certain tumors and may therefore have some cell cycle (phase) specificity in the S phase not possessed by the other alkylating agents.

The major toxicities associated with the classic alkylating agents are related to their cytotoxic effects, although each drug has its own unique side effects. Normal tissues most affected are those with a rapid growth rate, eg, the hematopoietic system, the gastrointestinal tract, and gonadal tissue. Nausea and vomiting occur with use of most of these agents, particularly with the intravenous route, and may result from a direct effect on the chemoreceptor trigger zone in the medulla. If extravasation of mechlorethamine occurs during administration or if skin or mucous membranes are exposed to this agent, tissue necrosis develops, and sloughing will occur later, producing a slow-healing ulcer. The myelosuppression associated with classic alkylating agents is mainly a leukopenia, with the lowest cell counts occurring in 10–14 days and recovery occurring in 21–28 days. Busulfan and chlorambucil have slightly more prolonged myelosuppressive effects. Bone marrow depression causes the most serious complications of therapy associated with the alkylating agents; patients are at increased risk for bleeding episodes due to thrombocytopenia and infection due to leukopenia. Anemia from depressed levels of erythrocyte production occurs less frequently.

**B. Nitrosoureas:** The nitrosoureas include carmustine (BCNU), lomustine (CCNU), semustine (methyl CCNU), estramustine, streptozocin, and chlorozotocin. Although nitrosoureas probably act mainly as alkylating agents, they may also cause the inhibition of several key enzymatic steps necessary for the formation of DNA. The cytotoxic activity of these drugs is thought to be mediated through the action of metabolites that can alkylate DNA. Like other alkylating agents, the nitrosoureas are cell cycle (phase)-nonspecific. The nitrosoureas are lipid-soluble and cross the blood-brain barrier. These agents may undergo some enterohepatic circulation, but they are rapidly metabolized. The largest fraction of these drugs is excreted in the urine as metabolites, with only a small fraction excreted in the active form. Streptozocin is a naturally occurring nitrosourea that is particularly useful in the treatment of insulinomas because of its marked specificity for pancreatic B and exocrine cells.

The major adverse reaction associated with the nitrosoureas is a notable delayed and dose-dependent depression of the hematopoietic system occurring with commonly used dosage levels. In contrast to the classic alkylating agents, maximal depression of the white cell count occurs in 3–5 weeks with use of the nitrosoureas; it may persist for several weeks or longer. Severe nausea and vomiting may limit the dosage that can be given. Pain at the injection site is associated with the use of carmustine.

**C. Antitumor Antibiotics:** The antitumor antibiotics are products of microbial fermentation and include the anthracyclines and the chromomycins. Although most antitumor antibiotics exert some antimicrobial properties, the cytotoxic effects of these agents generally preclude their use as such.

**1. Anthracyclines–**The anthracyclines include daunorubicin, doxorubicin, and rubidazone. These drugs effectively interfere with nucleic acid synthesis and block DNA-directed RNA and DNA transcription. The anthracyclines are probably effective in all phases of the cell cycle and are therefore cell cycle (phase)-nonspecific.

Disposition kinetics of the anthracyclines are complex. Their half-life is relatively long, ranging from 15 hours to several days for doxorubicin. These drugs are extensively metabolized in the liver, and some of the metabolites retain antitumor activity. Biliary excretion appears to be the major means of elimination, but a small portion of drug is excreted in the urine.

Many of the adverse effects of the anthracyclines are similar to those of the alkylating agents. Acute toxicity is manifested as bone marrow depression that may be severe enough to require limiting of dosage; the nadir usually occurs in 10–14 days, with recovery by 21 days in most patients. The anthracyclines also produce tissue necrosis and sloughing if extravasation occurs during intravenous injection. A unique cardiomyopathy has been observed when high cumulative doses of the anthracyclines have been administered.

**2. Chromomycins–**Another group of antitumor antibiotics is the chromomycins, which include chromomycin $A_3$, mithramycin (plicamycin), and dactinomycin. All act similarly to block DNA-directed RNA synthesis by intercalating and anchoring in DNA, as do the anthracyclines. Bone marrow depression due to chromomycins is a significant but usually not dose-limiting toxicity characterized by thrombocytopenia with some leukopenia.

**Chromomycin $A_3$** (Toyomycin) is rapidly cleared from plasma, is excreted via the urinary and biliary tracts, and causes nausea and vomiting, renal toxicity, and severe local reactions at the injection site.

**Mithramycin** crosses the blood-brain barrier and is well distributed in the cerebrospinal fluid. It is excreted mainly in the urine. Gastrointestinal effects include nausea and vomiting, anorexia, and diarrhea. Liver and kidney toxicity is common. A toxicity unique to this agent is a hemorrhagic syndrome heralded by facial flushing. Mithramycin has been used to lower serum calcium levels in patients with hypercalcemia.

**Dactinomycin** is rapidly cleared from serum and is excreted mainly in the bile with minimal biotransformation. Gastrointestinal effects include mucositis characterized by oral ulceration. Nausea and vomiting may be severe enough to limit the dosage. Other toxicities include bone marrow depression and alopecia.

**3. Other antitumor antibiotics–**Other antitumor antibiotics include mitomycin, piperazinedione, and bleomycin. Mitomycin probably functions as an alkylating agent by causing cross-linking of DNA. **Mitomycin** is rapidly cleared from the vascular compartment and is found in most body tissues except the brain; it is excreted via the kidneys and in bile. Delayed bone marrow depression may occur, with the nadir occurring 3–5 weeks after administration. Myelosuppression may be more severe with repeated doses and is the major dose-limiting toxicity. Renal toxicity may be observed, whereas gastrointestinal effects and alopecia occur less frequently.

**Piperazinedione** appears to function as an alkylating agent by inhibiting the incorporation of several DNA nucleotides into DNA synthesis. Although cell progression through $G_2$ is delayed, piperazinedione is probably not cell cycle (phase)-specific. Myelosuppression is the major dose-limiting toxic effect and is manifested as granulocytopenia followed by thrombocytopenia, with the nadir and recovery from myelosuppression varying by patient. The level of activity against neoplasms resistant to alternative alkylating agents and antimetabolites has not been high enough to warrant expanded clinical trials.

**Bleomycins** are antineoplastic antibiotics produced by fermentation of *Streptomyces verticillus*. More than a dozen fractions have been isolated, but the major constituent of commercially available preparations is bleomycin $A_2$. Inasmuch as the exact composition of the drug may vary, the drug is rated in units of activity. The exact mechanism of action is unknown, but bleomycin may exert cytostatic effects by binding to DNA to cause splitting of DNA strands and inhibition of replication, thereby inhibiting DNA synthesis and, to a lesser extent, RNA and protein synthesis. Bleomycin is cell cycle (phase)-specific for mitosis and $G_2$. This cycle specificity has been useful experimentally to achieve cell cycle synchronization in combination chemotherapy. Bleomycin appears to exert much less myelosuppressive activity than most other antineoplastic drugs and is therefore useful in patients who already have depressed bone marrow counts. Cutaneous reactions are dose-related and include hyperpigmentation, edema, erythema, and thickening of the nail beds. They are the most common side effects, because the drug is concentrated in the skin. The most serious toxicity is pneumonitis related to the total dose received; the disease is characterized by dyspnea, rales, and infiltrates that progress to fibrosis. A high incidence of hypersensitivity reactions ranging from fever and chills to anaphylaxis is also associated with bleomycin.

**D. Miscellaneous Alkylator-like Agents:** Other drugs that probably act as alkylating agents include cisplatin, dacarbazine, hexamethylmelamine, galactitol (DAG; investigational in the USA), and pipobroman.

**Cisplatin** was the first inorganic compound to be used to treat human cancers. Cross-linking of DNA may be somewhat different from that of other alkylators, in that the interatomic distance is much smaller than with the traditional alkylating agents; this characteristic may account for some of the toxicity associated with cisplatin. Cisplatin is cell cycle (phase)-nonspecific and is excreted mainly unchanged in the urine. Adverse reactions include anaphylaxis, nausea and vomiting, nephrotoxicity, ototoxicity, and myelosuppression that is usually mild.

**Dacarbazine** was originally thought to be an antimetabolite but is now recognized as an alkylating agent that is activated in the liver and excreted in the urine. It has somewhat less bone marrow toxicity than standard alkylating agents but typically causes severe nausea and vomiting similar to that due to cisplatin.

**Hexamethylmelamine** does not act as an alkylating agent in vitro, although it is structurally similar to triethylenemelamine, which is an alkylator. Although the precise mechanism is unknown, it is possible that hexamethylmelamine is activated to an alkylating agent in vivo. Hexamethylmelamine is rapidly metabolized in the liver and excreted in the urine. Gastrointestinal, neurologic, and hematologic toxicities occur.

**Galactitol** and **pipobroman** are thought to act as alkylating agents; major associated toxicities are myelosuppression and nausea and vomiting.

## Antimetabolites

The antimetabolites exert their major activity during the S phase and therefore are most effective against tumors that have a high growth fraction. The antimetabolites are structural analogs of naturally occurring metabolites and interfere with normal synthesis of nucleic acids by substituting different compounds for the normal purines or pyrimidines in metabolic pathways. The antimetabolites are subdivided into the folate antagonists, the purine antagonists, and the pyrimidine antagonists.

**A. Folate Antagonists:** Methotrexate is a 4-amino-4-deoxy-N-methyl analog of folic acid and is the classic antimetabolite prototype. Methotrexate is a cell cycle (phase)-specific agent that exerts its cytotoxic effect in the S phase by binding to dihydrofolate reductase and thereby blocking the reduction of folic acid. Thymidine and purine synthesis are halted, thus arresting DNA, RNA, and protein synthesis. For maximal effect, intracellular levels of methotrexate must be sufficiently high to bind almost all of the dihydrofolate reductase, of which only small quantities are required to maintain adequate levels of the reduced folate pool. Resistance is thought to develop as a consequence either of increased levels of dihydrofolate reductase or of decreased cell uptake.

Methotrexate enters the cell through an active carrier-mediated cell membrane transport system that it shares with leucovorin calcium (folinic acid, citrovorum factor) and its metabolite, 5-methyltetrahydrofolate. When this transport system is functional in tumor cells, adequate intracellular levels of methotrexate are easily achieved. Because some tumors lack or have reduced transport capabilities, high levels of methotrexate are required to facilitate transport by a passive method instead. To limit toxicity, treatment requiring high doses of methotrexate is followed by "rescue" of normal cells with leucovorin calcium.

Another antifolate is **ethane sulfonic acid compound,** or **Baker's antifol (triazinate)**. It is actively transported into the cell by a different transport carrier than is methotrexate, but the target enzyme is the same. Thus, these 2 antifolates may have different tumor specificity even though their general mechanism of action is the same.

Both compounds produce bone marrow depression, with the lowest cell counts occurring in 7–14 days. Stomatitis and gastrointestinal distress are frequent. Skin rashes are common side effects of ethane sulfonic acid compound but occur in fewer patients treated with methotrexate. Central nervous system abnormalities may also occur with either agent.

**B. Purine Antagonists:** Mercaptopurine and thioguanine are analogs of the natural purines hypoxanthine and guanine. The purine antagonists have specific antitumor effects on the S phase.

**Mercaptopurine** acts as a false metabolite because of its close chemical similarity to hypoxanthine. It competes for the enzymes responsible for the conversion of inosinic acid to adenine and xanthine ribotides and thus interferes with normal DNA and RNA synthesis. Simultaneous administration of allopurinol may block the metabolism of mercaptopurine and azathioprine by xanthine oxidase and require reduction of the dose to one-fourth or one-third the normal amount. This drug interaction does not occur with thioguanine, because its detoxification occurs by methylation.

**Thioguanine** also acts as a false metabolite; its substitution for the corresponding guanine nucleotide blocks purine synthesis.

The indications for use and efficacy of thioguanine and mercaptopurine are the same. Their toxicities are identical, and the 2 drugs are mutually cross-resistant.

**Azathioprine** is an imidazolyl derivative and mercaptopurine. It is used as an immunosuppressant but has cytotoxic properties similar to those of mercaptopurine and thioguanine because it is extensively metabolized to mercaptopurine.

The major dose-limiting toxicity of the purine antagonists is myelosuppression consisting mainly of leukopenia, with lesser effects on platelets and red blood cells. Gastrointestinal distress is common, and hepatotoxicity may occur with use of any of the purine antagonists.

**C. Pyrimidine Antagonists: Fluorouracil** (5-fluorouracil, 5-FU) is the classic antimetabolite. It is cell cycle (phase)-specific and inhibits the enzyme thymidylate synthetase to block DNA synthesis. It is catabolized in the liver by dihydrouracil dehydrogenase.

Two other closely related fluoropyrimidines, ftorafur and floxuridine (FUDR, 5-fluorodeoxyuridine), have recently been used in clinical trials.

Ftorafur is hydrolyzed to 5-FU in the liver and stomach and therefore may act as a depot form of 5-FU.

Fluorouracil and ftorafur cause myelosuppression that reaches a nadir in 1–14 days, but ftorafur appears to cause less myelosuppression, which may be due to its slower release of 5-FU. Both agents commonly produce gastrointestinal toxicities, including occasional glossitis and stomatitis. Neurotoxicities may also occur because these drugs cross the blood-brain barrier.

The cytidine and deoxycytidine analogs include **cytarabine, cyclocytidine** (ancitabine), and **azacitidine.** The active form of these nucleoside analogs stops DNA synthesis by competitively inhibiting DNA polymerase and production of deoxycytidine.

Cytarabine is metabolized by cytidine deaminase in the liver, granulocytes, and gastrointestinal tract. Small amounts of cytarabine cross the blood-brain barrier. Because cyclocytidine is not inactivated by cytidine deaminase, it slowly releases the more active cytarabine, which prolongs plasma levels; cyclocytidine can therefore be regarded as a depot form of cytarabine that has a biphasic half-life occurring at 3–15 minutes and at 2 hours.

Cytarabine and cyclocytidine are active only in the S phase. Although azacitidine is most active during the S phase, it appears to exert activity in all phases of the cell cycle by inhibiting DNA, RNA, and protein synthesis. Although it has some cross-resistance with the other cytidine analogs, this is not complete. These facts suggest that azacitidine has an additional mechanism of action not found in cytarabine and cyclocytidine.

The toxicities of cytarabine, cyclocytidine, and azacitidine are similar to those of other pyrimidine antagonists and include myelosuppression and gastrointestinal abnormalities, which may be severe. Cytarabine produces a flu-like syndrome, and cyclocytidine commonly produces unusual jaw pain and hypotension.

## Plant Alkaloids

**A. *Vinca* Alkaloids:** Although the periwinkle plant has a long history in folklore medicine, clinical research to evaluate its possible therapeutic effects was not begun until 1945; by 1958, several active alkaloids had been isolated, but to date, only vinblastine and vincristine have had extensive clinical use. Although they are quite similar chemically and structurally, vincristine and vinblastine have markedly different clinical activities and toxicities. The precise mechanism of action of these compounds is not clearly understood, but they appear to cause arrest of metaphase by crystallization of the microtubular spindle proteins. *Vinca* alkaloids may also inhibit nucleic acid and protein synthesis, but these effects become apparent only after high concentrations are reached. There appears to be no cross-resistance between the *Vinca* alkaloids and radiation therapy, alkylating agents, or each other. The differences in their therapeutic spectrum, toxicity, and potency may be related to each drug's ability to enter different types of cells.

The dose-limiting toxicity of vinblastine and vindesine is bone marrow depression, manifested chiefly by leukopenia 4–10 days after administration, with recovery occurring within 10–21 days. Vincristine does not usually cause leukopenia and can be given with relative safety to leukopenic patients.

Neurotoxicity is a major dose-limiting effect of vincristine and vindesine but occurs infrequently with vinblastine. Vincristine neurotoxicity consists of peripheral neuropathy with loss of deep tendon reflexes, numbness, and eventually severe weakness.

Cranial nerve palsies, vocal cord paralysis, and autonomic nervous system dysfunction, manifested as urinary retention, tachycardia, or gastrointestinal symptoms of constipation or paralytic ileus, may occur. All of the *Vinca* alkaloids cause severe local necrosis if extravasation occurs, and vindesine may produce pain and phlebitis even without evidence of infiltration.

**Maytansine,** an ansa macrolide, has a mechanism of action similar to that of the *Vinca* alkaloids. It is found in the wood and bark of several varieties of the mandrake plant. The drug exerts a stathmokinetic effect by blocking cell cycle progression in late $G_2$ and the M phase. Toxicities have consisted of mild gastrointestinal complaints with fewer neurologic and hepatic effects. Myelosuppression has not been a problem.

**B. Podophyllotoxins:** The 2 podophyllotoxins presently used are semisynthetic compounds derived from the root of the mayapple plant. The mechanism of action of **etoposide** (VP-16) and **teniposide** (VM-26) is similar to that of *Vinca* alkaloids in that they cause a mitotic spindle toxicity resulting in arrest of metaphase. Podophyllotoxins prevent cells from entering mitosis, thereby causing an increase in the MI; at high concentrations, the drugs cause lysis of cells entering mitosis. They also suppress DNA synthesis and, to a lesser degree, RNA and protein synthesis. Thus, both the *Vinca* alkaloids and podophyllotoxins are cell cycle (phase)-specific and exert their major activity in the M phase; they also demonstrate some activity in the $G_2$ and S phases.

Etoposide and teniposide are extensively protein-bound and are mainly eliminated by biliary excretion, with some enterohepatic recirculation. Both drugs may cause severe hypotension if infused too rapidly. Other adverse effects include nausea and vomiting, diarrhea, alopecia, and phlebitis at the injection site. The podophyllotoxins produce mild bone marrow depression and leukopenia, with the nadir occurring from 3 to 14 days following therapy.

## Miscellaneous Agents

**Hydroxyurea** is cell cycle (phase)-specific for the S phase. In addition to holding cells in $G_1$, the drug exerts a lethal effect on cells in the S phase by inhibiting ribonucleotide reductase and DNA synthesis without interfering with RNA or protein synthesis. Hydroxyurea may exercise some activity as an antimetabolite in that incorporation of thymidine into DNA appears to be inhibited. The major adverse reactions are bone marrow depression, gastrointestinal disturbances, and, rarely, dermatologic reactions and renal impairment.

**Procarbazine** appears to be cell cycle (phase)-specific for the S phase; it apparently interferes with DNA synthesis, but its exact mechanism of action is unclear. Oxidative breakdown products, hydrogen peroxide, formaldehyde, azoprocarbazine, and free hydroxyl radicals may be responsible for the characteristic chromosomal breakage observed after use of procarbazine. Procarbazine may demonstrate dangerous interactions with a number of other drugs. Adverse reactions include myelosuppression, a flu-like syndrome, and dermatologic and various central nervous system reactions.

Most normal cells possess the ability to synthesize the amino acid asparagine. Some tumor cells, such as those in acute lymphoblastic leukemia, do not possess this ability and require exogenous asparagine. **Asparaginase** converts asparagine to nonfunctional aspartic acid and thereby deprives the tumor cell of this crucial amino acid to block protein synthesis. Side effects include protein depletion and pancreatic and hepatic damage. Allergic reactions are frequent, since asparaginase is a biologic product obtained from bacteria.

## REFERENCES

Blum RH, Frei E III, Holland JF: Principles of dose, schedule, and combination chemotherapy. Chap XII-8, pp 730–751. In: *Cancer Medicine,* 2nd ed. Holland JF, Frei E III (eds.). Lea & Febiger, 1982.

Chabner BA, Myers CE: Clinical pharmacology of cancer chemotherapy. Chap 9, pp 156–197. In: *Cancer: Principles and Practice of Oncology.* DeVita VT Jr, Hellman S, Rosenberg SA (eds.). Lippincott, 1982.

DeVita VT Jr: Principles of chemotherapy. Chap 8, pp 132–155. In: *Cancer: Principles and Practice of Oncology.* DeVita VT Jr, Hellman S, Rosenberg SA (eds.). Lippincott, 1982.

Norton L, Simon R: Tumor size, sensitivity to therapy and design of treatment schedules. Cancer Treat Rep 1977; 61:1307.

Pardee AB: Cell biology and biochemistry of cancer. Chap 3, pp 59–72, in: Cancer: Principles and Practice of Oncology. DeVita VT Jr, Hellman S, Rosenberg SA (eds.). Lippincott, 1982.

Skipper HE: Combination therapy: Some concepts and results. Cancer Chemother Rep 1974;4 (Part 2):137.

Skipper HE, Schabel FM Jr: Quantitative and cytokinetic studies in experimental tumor systems. Chap XII-3, pp 663–684. In: *Cancer Medicine,* 2nd ed. Holland JR, Freid E III (eds.). Lea & Febiger, 1982.

Tattersall MHN: Pharmacology and selection of cytotoxic drugs. Chap 9, pp 121–138. In: *Gynecologic Oncology: Fundamental Principles and Clinical Practice.* Coppleson M (ed.). Churchill Livingstone, 1981.

# 53 Infertility

*Mary C. Martin, MD*

## Definitions & Statistics

Although infertility involves the loss of fundamental reproductive choices and the denial of expectations, it defies categorization as a single disease entity. There are few symptoms and few definitive tests, and there is an unrelenting confrontation with time as an enemy rather than an ally in the healing process. Furthermore, a sense of progress is seldom felt, since the goal—a successful delivery—is absolute. Strategies for treating infertility should encompass management of the frustration and the sense of personal loss that accompany the process of investigation and treatment.

Eighty percent of couples experiencing unprotected intercourse will achieve pregnancy within 1 year; an additional 10% will achieve pregnancy in the second year. **Infertility** is usually defined as the failure to conceive after 1 year of intercourse without contraception. **Sterility** implies an intrinsic inability to achieve pregnancy, whereas infertility implies a decrease in the ability to conceive; infertility is synonymous with **subfertility. Primary infertility** applies to those who have never conceived, whereas **secondary infertility** designates those who have conceived at some time in the past. **Fecundity** is the capacity to participate in the production of a child. To express the chances of pregnancy occurring in any interval of time, the term **fecundability** is used and is usually expressed as the likelihood of pregnancy per month of exposure. In young healthy couples having frequent intercourse, the chances of pregnancy are estimated to be only 25–30% per month.

It is estimated that 1 in 6 couples in the USA will experience difficulty in conceiving during 1 year and that 1–2% of couples are involuntarily sterile. An apparent increase in the prevalence of infertility is suggested by analysis of trends in medical visits, which reveals an exponential increase in the number of visits for infertility in the last decade. The reasons for the increase in attention given to infertility are multiple. Couples in some cases have voluntarily delayed childbearing in favor of establishing careers and may experience an age-related decline in fertility; in some cases the choice of prior contraception may have contributed to infertility, as with the use of some intrauterine devices (IUDs); having an increased number of sexual partners leads to a greater potential for exposure to sexually transmitted diseases, which may contribute to infertility; and couples are less willing to simply accept childlessness and are increasingly aware of the available services and options for resolving infertility.

Both partners in a relationship contribute to potential fertility, and both may be subfertile. A primary diagnosis of a male factor (see section on Evaluation of Male Factors) is made in about 30% of infertile couples, and the man may be contributory in another 20–30%. An abnormality in the woman is responsible for the remaining 40–50% of cases.

Fecundability is influenced by the ages of the partners, especially that of the female. The age-related decline in fertility reflects the influence of the "biological clock," which modulates the chances of success of any infertility therapy. The decline in fecundability occurs for most women in the fourth decade, as evidenced by a modest decline in population fertility statistics; the decline becomes more pronounced in the age range of 35–40 years, with a sharp decline evident in most women in their 40s.

A conscientious evaluation of the factors contributing to fertility usually indicates a probable cause in 85–90% of couples. Appropriate therapy will achieve pregnancy in about 50–60% of couples, excluding application of advanced reproductive technologies such as in vitro fertilization (IVF). Pregnancy will occur without treatment in about 15–20% of couples diagnosed as infertile. For the others, guidance toward other options for resolution of their infertility can still be provided during the course of assessment and treatment.

## PSYCHOLOGIC ASPECTS OF INFERTILITY

Along with the increasing level of sophistication in evaluation and treatment of infertility has come a growing awareness of the psychologic consequences of this problem. When an anticipated conception fails to occur in a timely fashion, and a couple begin to approach the thought of infertility as a diagnosis that may pertain to them, their reactions can be intense and overwhelming. Self-images are threatened, sexuality can be affected, and feelings of adequacy may be destroyed; feelings of loss of control, anger, guilt, shame, and resentment can alter behavior and become contributing factors as relationships are threatened. As an individual or couple actually confront infertility, they may progress through stages, including denial, anger, grief, and resolution. A recognition of these stages may assist the practitioner in providing appropriate support and counseling. Particularly when denial gives way to anger, the practitioner may be the recipient of the frustration, rage, or resentment expressed by couples in response to the results of tests or the failure of a proposed therapy. Insight into these profound reactions may assist partners in maintaining and strengthening their relationship, reaffirming the desirability of their mates, and preventing depression from becoming despair.

The advent of new therapies, while expanding the options for some, may open old wounds for others. Couples who had resolved their infertility may feel obligated to explore all options when they hear of yet another treatment or technique. Infertility, even when secondary, remains a chronic reality, and honest advice about probabilities for success should be offered at frequent intervals to assist couples in maintaining an appropriate perspective.

When confronted with monthly testing and monthly reminders of failure, couples can become obsessed with reproductive events and cycles, and time becomes marked by temperature curves, urine kits, and calendars of menstrual cycles. In some cases, the greatest service that the infertility specialist can provide is a thoughtfully determined time frame for completion of tests and evaluation. Even when ambiguity remains, it is usually helpful to make a best assessment of the causes of infertility and progress to a time-limited period of therapy. Since average fecundabilities will predict that most therapies, if correcting a true cause of infertility, will be successful within 6–9 cycles, it is appropriate to avoid endless chronic treatment and to chart appropriate steps toward completion of treatment. This "time contract" will be influenced by the age of the couple, by the diagnosis, by the affordability of various treatment options, and by the acceptability of alternatives such as adoption. In some cases, when a couple have been involved in testing and treatment for an extended interval, it is wise to suggest that they obtain a second opinion or to have the case reviewed by colleagues so that all possibilities will have been considered and presented.

The feelings of grief experienced by many infertile couples may be exacerbated by well-meaning but hurtful advice from friends, relatives, and even strangers. Often, support groups for infertile couples can be a surprising source of comfort and strength. Informal support and referral for professional counseling are provided by Resolve, a national organization.

## DIAGNOSIS OF INFERTILITY

The goals of the infertility evaluation are to determine the probable cause of infertility; to provide accurate information regarding prognosis; to provide counseling and support and education throughout the process of evaluation; and to provide guidance regarding options for treatment. It is hoped that, in the process of their infertility evaluation and treatment, a couple may achieve their goal of a desired child; it is also hoped that they may benefit from a strengthened relationship, gain information about the causes of their difficulty, and achieve the certainty that all that could reasonably be done was done in an expeditious and conscientious manner.

The organization of the infertility evaluation is based on a consideration of the various individual factors required for successful reproduction. These factors are discussed in terms of whether they are male or female (ovulatory, pelvic, and cervical); a detailed list of male and female factors is contained in Table 53–1. The efficiency in completing the evaluation is determined in large part at the initial assessment visit, when the expenses, invasiveness, risks, and probabilities of significant findings of various procedures and tests are discussed. Reassessment will occur at intervals determined by the completion of various evaluations or the discovery of a contributing factor.

### The Initial Assessment

The initial visit should be the opportunity to begin to accomplish several of the stated goals of the infertility evaluation. Participation of both partners is ideal and can assist the practitioner in assessing the dynamics of the relationship. Some determination of the couple's level of understanding of the problem and of their individual acceptance of the concept of infertility can be made.

The initial clinical assessment, while focusing on the history and physical status of the female partner, should also include the historical factors of importance that pertain to the male partner and to the couple. Important historical information beyond that obtained in a general medical history is outlined in Table 53–2 for the female and in Table 53–3 for the male.

General information regarding reproduction and the timing of events may assist in correcting any misunderstandings about coital frequency, and some myths regarding infertility may be dispelled. The timing of various investigative studies, which should be conducted within the framework of the work and life

**Table 53–1.** Causes of infertility.

**Male Factor**
Endocrine disorders
Hypothalamic dysfunction (Kallmann's syndrome)
Pituitary failure (tumor, radiation, surgery)
Hyperprolactinemia (drug, tumor)
Exogenous androgens
Thyroid disorders
Adrenal hyperplasia
Anatomic disorders
Congenital absence of vas deferens
Obstruction of vas deferens
Congenital abnormalities of ejaculatory system
Abnormal spermatogenesis
Chromosomal abnormalities
Mumps orchitis
Cryptorchidism
Chemical or radiation exposure
Varicocele
Abnormal motility
Absent cilia (Kartagener's syndrome)
Varicocele
Antibody formation
Sexual dysfunction
Retrograde ejaculation
Impotence
Decreased libido
**Ovulatory Factor**
Central defects
Chronic hyperandrogenemic anovulation
Hyperprolactinemia (drug, tumor, empty sella)
Hypothalamic insufficiency
Pituitary insufficiency (trauma, tumor, congenital)
Peripheral defects
Gonadal dysgenesis
Premature ovarian failure
Ovarian tumor
Ovarian resistance
Metabolic disease
Thyroid disease
Liver disease
Renal disease
Obesity
Androgen excess, adrenal or neoplastic
**Pelvic Factor**
Infection
Appendicitis
Pelvic inflammatory disease
Uterine adhesions (Asherman's syndrome)
Endometriosis
Structural abnormalities
DES exposure
Failure of normal fusion of the reproductive tract
Myoma
**Cervical Factor**
Congenital
DES exposure
Müllerian duct abnormality
Acquired
Surgical treatment
Infection

**Table 53–2.** Medical history for female factor infertility.

In utero DES exposure
History of pubertal development
Present menstrual cycle characteristics (length, duration, molimina)
Contraceptive history
Prior pregnancies, outcomes
Previous surgeries, especially pelvic
Prior infection
History of abnormal Pap smear, treatment
Drugs and medications
General health (diet, weight stability, exercise patterns, review of systems)

A realistic schedule of tests should be planned, and then an estimate of costs determined, with a discussion of their potential financial obligation and the variability of insurance policies. After the anticipated time investment and expenses have been discussed, a planned consultation for evaluation of test results should be offered, so that a discussion of diagnoses and appropriate therapies can then be held. When a team approach to the infertility evaluation is utilized, the members of the team and their roles should be identified and the strategies for providing emotional support and counseling discussed. In many cases, the couple will be attempting to absorb significant amounts of information, some of which may be highly technical, at a time of heightened emotion. It is therefore helpful to offer literature or a written summary of the discussion and to plan a subsequent review of the information; this written summary and plan can form the basis for the chart note, which assists in maintaining a consistent approach.

Frequently, the initial history will have indicated a probable diagnosis or a contributing cause of infertility, but it is important to complete a basic evaluation of all of the major factors so that a secondary diagnosis is not ignored.

## Evaluation of Male Factors

The initial evaluation of the male should include a general health history and a specific assessment of factors contributing to infertility, as listed in Table 53–3.

**A. Semen Analysis:** A normal semen analysis will usually exclude a significant male factor. Optimum parameters are usually observed after 2–3 days of abstinence, and the specimen should be received in

**Table 53–3.** Medical history for male factor infertility.

In utero DES exposure
Congenital abnormalities
Prior paternity
Frequency of intercourse
Exposure to toxins
Previous surgery
Previous infections, treatment
Drugs and medications
General health (diet, exercise, review of systems)

situation of the couple, can be discussed. In most cases, an initial basic investigation can be completed in 6–8 weeks. The aggressiveness of the approach taken should be agreed on and is determined by the age of the couple, any historical factors suggesting a cause of infertility, the affordability of various tests, and the availability of each partner for testing.

**Table 53–4.** Normal semen parameters.

| Liquification | 30 minutes |
|---|---|
| Count | 20–250 million/mL |
| Motility | > 50% |
| Volume | 2–5 mL |
| Morphology | > 50% normal |
|    Strict criteria | > 14% normal |
| pH | 7.2–7.8 |

the laboratory within 30–60 minutes of production. Normal values are given in Table 53–4. If fundamental parameters of count and motility are normal, the assessment morphology of the sperm becomes more critical. Specialized expertise in determining sperm morphology and applying strict criteria should be used before considering the semen normal.

If the semen analysis reveals abnormal or borderline parameters, the history should be reviewed for any proximate cause of an abnormality, keeping in mind that the cycle of spermiogenesis takes about 74 days. The semen parameters in normal fertile males may vary significantly over time, and the first response to any abnormal result should be to wait an interval of several days to weeks and repeat the test. Although low counts, decreased motility, and increased numbers of abnormal forms are more frequently associated with infertility, unfavorable semen parameters may still be found in 20% of males undergoing vasectomy after having completed their families. Abnormal parameters warrant further investigation and possible referral to a urologist with a special interest and expertise in infertility.

**B. Mucus Studies:** The functional sperm must interact normally with the egg and surrounding cells in the uterine tube. The normal migration of sperm is affected by attrition and filtering, so that of the normal ejaculate deposited in the vagina, it is estimated that less than 1000 sperm will be found in the environment of the oocyte. The initial interaction of sperm and female genital tract can be determined by postcoital examination of the cervical mucus (Sims-Huhner test).

When mucus is obtained from the cervical canal in the preovulatory phase, it normally exhibits a response to the high estrogen environment. The mucus is thin, watery, and acellular; it dries in a crystalline pattern (ferning), and acts as a facilitative reservoir for the sperm. When mucus is collected several hours after intercourse at the appropriate time in the cycle and examined under a coverslip under high power, the number of sperm seen and the extent and quality of motility can be assessed. A satisfactory test results in large numbers of forwardly progressive sperm seen in thin, acellular mucus and indicates a healthy sperm-mucus interaction. The absence of sperm suggests an investigation of coital technique or a reevaluation of the semen analysis. Intermediate results, eg, the presence of either one or a few sperm, are not interpretable in terms of assigning a contributing cause

of infertility if the semen analysis is normal and the mucus is favorable. Findings of few to rare sperm have been observed in cycles of conception and in many fertile couples serving as controls for studies of sperm-mucus interaction. Furthermore, when laparoscopic findings were correlated with postcoital assessment, numbers of sperm were identified in the peritoneal fluid of women from whom zero to rare sperm could be seen in the postcoital test performed at the same time.

In cases of sufficient numbers of sperm seen with poor motility, an assessment of the quality of the mucus and timing of the test is critical to interpretation. When the mucus and timing appear favorable, but the sperm appear immobile, tests for autoantibodies, in the male or serum antibodies in the female are appropriate. When the mucus is unfavorable in appearance or amount, the timing of the test should be investigated. Evaluation of a contributing female factor may also be necessary. Immediate feedback regarding the timing of the test can be obtained during an office visit by use of vaginal ultrasound to determine the presence or absence of a dominant follicle.

**C. Other Tests:** When the initial evaluation of both partners does not reveal a probable cause of infertility or when repeated semen analyses are abnormal, the male factor should be investigated further. More detailed assessment of sperm function may include antibody studies, a sperm penetration assay (hamster egg penetration assay), or more sophisticated assessment of the sperm parameters previously described. Such assessments are designed to investigate more subtle abnormalities or abnormalities of function not revealed by the determination of sperm number and motility. Although helpful in some cases, the predictability of these assays for ultimate fertility is still uncertain and varies with the particular laboratory where the test is performed; no universal methodology has yet been accepted, and consequently the interpretation of these tests requires close communication with the laboratory selected.

Antibody studies can determine the presence of autoantibodies. Use of immunobead tests can determine the class of antibody present and the antigenic site (head, tail or midpiece). These factors will influence the prognosis for in vivo fertility and guide subsequent recommendations. Autoimmunity is more likely in men with a history of trauma, infection, or previous surgery.

A sperm penetration assay tests the ability of the sperm to penetrate the zona-free hamster egg, with the test semen specimen compared to a known fertile donor similarly exposed to hamster eggs. The assay has a high degree of predictability for the normal male with a positive test. In cases of unfavorable sperm parameters, the correlation of assay results with ultimate fertility, or ability to fertilize human eggs in vitro, is less clear. The negative assay, usually expressed as less than 10% penetration, may correlate with IVF and will sometimes confirm a suspected male factor; it is somewhat less likely to predict behavior in IVF conditions.

The hemizona assay provides an alternate or additional assessment of sperm functional capacity. Human zonae are exposed to sperm and the ability of the sperm to penetrate and/or to bind to zonae is determined and compared with a simultaneous test done using a fertile donor specimen.

In some cases, more detailed analysis of the sperm morphology, of the type of flagellar movement, or of the capacity for sperm to undergo the acrosome reaction can be assessed in special centers. Subtle abnormalities in these parameters may explain a previously undiagnosed cause of infertility.

The ultimate test of sperm function may occur with IVF, and this may be the ultimate recourse for both diagnosis and attempted therapy for cases of poor sperm parameters or unexplained infertility. Failure to achieve fertilization in a cycle of IVF when an adequate number of apparently healthy mature fertilizable eggs are exposed to sperm may lead to an acceptance of the diagnosis of male factor infertility; the diagnosis is strengthened if a negative sperm penetration assay is obtained, and it is further substantiated if donor sperm are able to penetrate eggs when partner sperm has failed to do so.

## Evaluation of Female Factors

**A. Ovulatory Factors:** An ovulatory dysfunction is responsible for approximately 20–25% of infertility cases. The problem should be investigated first by review of historical factors, including the onset of menarche, present cycle length (intermenstrual interval) and presence or absence of molimina. Signs and symptoms of systemic disease, particularly of hyperthyroidism or hypothyroidism, and physical signs of endocrine disease, eg, hirsutism, galactorrhea, and obesity, should be noted. The degree and intensity of exercise, a history of weight loss, and complaints of hot flushes all are clinical clues to possible endocrine or ovulatory dysfunction.

The investigation of the normalcy of ovulation is aided by the ability to assess multiple parameters, but the number of tests performed and the extent of investigation is usually determined by the initial history and physical examination. If regular menses, with molimina and mild dysmenorrhea, occur at intervals of 28–32 days, and particularly if the patient notes reliable mittelschmerz, then the initial evaluation can focus on confirming ovulation with a serum progesterone assay performed in the third week of the cycle. The value accepted as confirming ovulation must be determined in each endocrine laboratory. Using very specific assay reagents, the follicular-phase progesterone will be less than 1 ng/mL, and values greater than 5 ng/mL are consistent with ovulation having occurred. In the case of oligomenorrhea, amenorrhea, or short or very irregular menstrual cycles, evaluation

of the hypothalamic-pituitary-ovarian axis is warranted, beginning with determination of the serum concentrations of luteinizing hormone (LH), follicle-stimulating hormone (FSH), and prolactin.

In some women with delayed childbearing who are seeking evaluation in their fifth decade, an evaluation of the level of FSH and estradiol in the early follicular phase may provide helpful guidance in terms of the likelihood of achieving success, as mild elevations in either FSH or estradiol may precede overt ovulatory dysfunction but still indicate a poor prognosis for successful pregnancy. The specific cause of oligo-ovulation or anovulation is determined by the history, physical examination, and appropriate laboratory studies.

**1. Follicular phase—**If menstrual cycles are normal by history, but no cause for infertility is determined after completing the initial testing, a more detailed assessment of the normalcy of the cycle is indicated. The follicular phase can be examined with the assistance of vaginal ultrasound monitoring, so that the development of a normal dominant follicle of adequate size can be detected. The dominant follicle usually is selected early in the follicular phase and can be detected by ultrasound around or before the 10th day of the cycle, with subsequent linear growth of about 1–2 mm per day, ultimately achieving a preovulatory size of 18–26 mm prior to rupture. The occurrence of ovulation can be suggested by the disappearance of, or change in, the preovulatory follicle as it becomes the corpus luteum. This change can be predicted by using either serum testing or home monitoring with commercially available urinary LH kits to detect the LH surge, which predicts the occurrence of ovulation within 24 hours. The LH surge effects the final maturation of the egg within the follicle, induces the preovulatory changes in the follicle that lead to rupture and extrusion of the egg in the cumulus mass, and initiates the luteinization of the granulosa cells.

**2. Luteal phase—**The luteal phase is characterized by the production of progesterone, and the clinical assessment of the luteal phase relies on determination of the adequacy of progesterone effects. Indirect evidence of progesterone production can be determined by assessing the following biologic effects of progesterone.

**a. Basal body temperature—** The basal body temperature (BBT) is the temperature obtained in the resting state, usually just before arising in the morning. It is most easily obtained by use of a basal body thermometer. Progesterone has a central thermogenic effect; when it is produced in sufficient concentrations, it causes the basal body temperature to become elevated. Usually, the rise represents a change of 0.5–0.8° F, or about 0.3° C, during the luteal phase. Some women exhibit a greater sensitivity to the thermogenic effect than others. When a biphasic monthly temperature pattern is recorded, it is confirmatory evidence of luteinization, but the absence of a biphasic pattern may be seen in ovulatory cycles. In some cases, use of an electric blanket or of a heated waterbed may reduce the observed fluctuations. The BBT is not useful for predicting ovulation, and no statement of the adequacy of ovulation can be made based on the BBT chart. The pattern of temperature rise, whether abrupt or gradual, also has no significance in fertility assessment. For some couples, the daily ritual of taking morning temperatures can be a symbol of frustration; since the information to be gained from BBT charts is usually more readily available by other means, the assignment of maintaining daily temperature charts can be individualized and, in any case, need not be continued indefinitely.

**b. Secretory endometrium–**The true adequacy of ovulation and of progesterone production is determined only by the establishment of a successful pregnancy, but the use of an endometrial biopsy near the end of the luteal phase can provide reassurance of an adequate maturational effect on the endometrial lining. An endometrial biopsy can be timed either from the LH surge or by noting the onset of the next menstrual period, and the cycle day should be within 1–2 days of the cycle day determined by the examination of the morphology of glands and stroma by a trained pathologist. Unfortunately, the diagnosis of a true inadequate luteal phase requires repetitive testing, as an occasional out-of-phase biopsy can be a random cycle-to-cycle occurrence.

**c. Premenstrual molimina–**Premenstrual molimina are largely due to the cyclic hormonal influences of estrogen followed by progesterone with estrogen. The particular constellation of symptoms that affect each woman is usually fairly constant, so that headaches, bloating, cramping, and emotional lability may be experienced differently, but often repetitively, by different women. When questioned, over 95% of ovulatory women can identify molimina associated with the premenstrual interval.

**d. Mucus changes–** Within 48 hours of ovulation, the cervical mucus changes under the influence of progesterone to become thick, tacky, and cellular, with loss of the crystalline fern pattern on drying.

As stated above, the only absolute documentation of release of a fertilizable egg is the establishment of pregnancy. The production of progesterone, whether determined by clinical signs or by assay of serum concentration, is usually accepted as evidence of the luteinization of the follicle that normally follows the LH surge. The value of serum progesterone adequate to prepare and maintain the secretory endometrium is difficult to determine by measurement. If serum concentrations are measured at the midluteal phase in several cycles, consistently low values (eg, < 10 ng/mL or as determined by the individual laboratory standards used) should be confirmed by assessment of the endometrial biopsy to diagnose a possible inadequate luteal phase.

The subject of the inadequate luteal phase remains an area of controversy. There is disagreement on how to make the diagnosis, when the diagnosis is significant, and how best to treat the problem if diagnosed. Since progesterone concentration fluctuates, serum measurements are usually helpful only if reassuringly elevated. Endometrial biopsies can be misinterpreted, or inappropriately timed, and out-of-phase biopsies have been obtained in normal fertile women as well as in women during the cycle of successful conception. A repetitive pattern of endometrial biopsies out of phase with the postovulatory day as determined by the LH surge is of significance in patients with habitual abortion, but the contribution to infertility is less clear. In 3–4% of women, endometrial biopsies suggest a true luteal phase defect, and these women should be offered treatment. Women with repetitive short cycles, galactorrhea, persistent low levels of progesterone, or repetitive out-of-phase endometrial biopsies should also have a serum prolactin determined. Elevated prolactin secretion has been shown to be associated with luteal phase defects.

**B. The Pelvic Factor:**

**1. History and pelvic examination–**The pelvic factor includes abnormalities of the uterus, fallopian tubes, ovaries, and adjacent pelvic structures. Factors in the history that are suggestive of a pelvic factor include any history of pelvic infection, such as salpingitis, appendicitis, use of intrauterine devices, endometritis, and septic abortion. Endometriosis is included as a pelvic factor in infertility and may be suggested by worsening dysmenorrhea, dyspareunia, or previous surgical reports. Any history of ectopic pregnancy, adnexal surgery, leiomyomas, or exposure to diethylstilbestrol (DES) in utero should be noted as possibly contributory to diagnosis of a pelvic factor. A transvaginal office ultrasound examination can be an efficient means of supplementing information gained from the standard bimanual examination. Hydrosalpinges, leiomyoma, and ovarian cysts and tumors can be often be observed, and the appropriate focused evaluations initiated sooner.

**2. Hysterosalpingogram–**After the pelvic examination, the evaluation of the pelvic factor usually begins with the hysterosalpingogram. Radiographic liquid dye is instilled into the uterine cavity using either a pediatric Foley catheter, to occlude the cervical canal, or a suction catheter. After 3–5 mL of dye is insufflated, an image is obtained, and additional dye is added to fill the uterine tubes. The procedure is witnessed by the practitioner under image intensification—or key films are obtained by a radiologist skilled in the procedure—in order to determine and demonstrate the uterine contour, the patency of the tubes, and the ability of the dye to freely spill into the pelvis. Abnormal findings include congenital malformations of the uterus, submucous leiomyomas, intrauterine synechiae (Asherman's syndrome) intrauterine polyps, salpingitis isthmica nodosa, and proximal or distal tubal occlusion. The hysterosalpingogram can be obtained in an outpatient setting, with minimal analgesia consisting of premedication with an antiprostaglandin synthetase medication. The test is usually scheduled for the interval after menstrual bleeding and prior to ovulation. Either water-based dye or oil-based dye may be selected; the advantages and disadvantages of each are summarized in Table 53–5. Several studies have suggested a fertility-enhancing effect of the procedure that is more pronounced with the oil-based dye.

If tubal patency is verified on the hysterosalpingogram and no infertility factor is identified, it is sometimes appropriate to allow an interval of several months without further therapy in order to capitalize on the benefit of the procedure. In studies of high-risk populations, an exacerbation of apparent preexisting salpingitis has been observed in 1–3% of women. For women with a history suggestive of salpingitis, a sedimentation rate may be obtained prior to the procedure—to decrease the likelihood of testing in the face of active disease—and a short interval of broad-spectrum antibiotics is frequently advocated when tubal occlusion is demonstrated. A lack of correlation between the interpretation of the hysterosalpingogram and subsequent findings at laparoscopy has been reported in up to 35% of cases. A hysterosalpingogram is contraindicated in the presence of an adnexal mass or an allergy to iodine or radiocontrast dye. Dye embolization is rare and is usually preceded by dye intravasation, which can be seen during the procedure. If dye intravasation occurs, infusion of dye should be terminated.

Some studies investigating the use of ultrasonography instead of fluoroscopy to monitor the passage of injected fluid suggest that in some cases a diagnosis of tubal patency may be established without exposure to diagnostic radiation.

**3. Laparoscopy–**The information regarding the pelvic factor obtained with a hysterosalpingogram is complemented by a laparoscopy with dye insufflation. When hysteroscopy is also done, supplementary information about the uterine contour can be obtained at the same time as the laparoscopy. Tubal abnormalities such as agglutinated fimbria or filmy adhesions, which restrict motion of the tubes, or peritubal cysts, may suggest tubal disease that would not necessarily

**Table 53–5.** Comparison of oil-based versus water-based dye used in the hysterosalpingogram.

| Fertility enhancement | Oil: higher pregnancy rates |
|---|---|
| Patient discomfort | Water: less cramping |
| Image quality | Water: rugae seen<br>Oil: better image |
| Embolization | Minimal risk with either dye |
| Granuloma | Greater risk for retained oil |

be detected on hysterosalpingogram. The diagnosis of endometriosis is usually based on laparoscopic findings. Endometriosis may be suggested by the history but can be diagnosed only by laparoscopy or laparotomy. The association between endometriosis and infertility is strong, although the understanding of the mechanism by which the disease contributes to infertility is as yet poor. In some cases, significant anatomic distortion can result from the irritative foci of endometriosis leading to dense adhesions, but in other cases extensive disease may be present without significant compromise of pelvic structures, and the disease is an unpredictable finding at laparoscopy.

The timing of the laparoscopy is one of the key aspects of the discussion of the pace at which the couple and the practitioner feel the investigation should proceed. In a young couple with a negative history, it is usually offered after all other tests are completed and discussed; in an older couple, or if the history suggests a pelvic factor, it is often indicated as one of the primary evaluations. In some patients with long-standing infertility, laparoscopy might be offered in conjunction with stimulation of the ovaries and ovum retrieval in order to combine the diagnostic potential with an attempt to achieve pregnancy. This may be done either by IVF, to confirm the ability of the eggs and sperm to interact, or by placing sperm and egg in the normal uterine tube to attempt normal transport to the uterus (see Chapter 56).

Documentation of the laparoscopic procedure, by either video or still photography, can be a valuable aid for the couple and may assist in determining subsequent therapy, particularly if referral to a consultant is indicated. With thoughtful preparation and discussion prior to the procedure, it is frequently possible to accomplish treatment of pathologic findings with either laser laparoscopy or operative pelviscopy. Particularly if significant endometriosis is encountered, it may be possible to eliminate much of the disease at the time of diagnosis. If uterine abnormalities are encountered during hysteroscopy, they can be required through the hysteroscope in some cases. The skill and training of the surgeon will determine the extent of intervention that can be offered, and this should be considered in discussion with the couple.

Laparoscopy is usually done in an outpatient surgery center with the patient under general anesthesia, although in some settings it is offered under local anesthesia with good results. The expense of the procedure, as well as the fact that it is the most invasive of the diagnostic strategies, are factors that may influence a couple's decision whether or not to progress to this step.

**C. The Cervical Factor:** A cervical factor may be indicated by a history of abnormal Pap smears, postcoital bleeding, cryotherapy, conization, or DES exposure in utero. The major evaluation of the cervical factor is by physical examination and properly timed postcoital test. In some cases of apparently normal cervical mucus that repeatedly fails to yield reassuring numbers of sperm, a cross-check of donor sperm and donor mucus can be performed to determine the possible contribution of the cervical mucus as opposed to that of the sperm. The value of routine cervical cultures is controversial, and the role of infectious agents, such as *Chlamydia* and *Ureaplasma*, is not universally accepted, particularly when the organisms are identified in cervical or vaginal cultures.

## Combined Factors & Unexplained Infertility

After completion of the basic evaluation, it is frequently necessary to repeat some of the initial tests in order to confirm abnormalities or validly time some assessments. This can be frustrating for the couple and the investigator and requires careful communication regarding anticipation of progress. After all test results are available and interpretable, an opportunity exists for review and discussion of the factors contributing to infertility. A review of what has been found to be normal as well as any probable cause of subfertility should be presented. This will then permit a discussion of treatment options available (see text that follows), with an attempt to convey prognosis for success with each approach. Because infertility statistics are the result of population studies and are seldom derived from controlled comparisons, it is very difficult to give unbiased recommendations.

Often, certain treatments will have been popularized in the mass media without substantiation of benefit, and the practitioner may be pressured to participate in unproved therapies. The individual circumstances, including attitudes toward surgery, financial status, previous experiences, and reports from friends, may determine the choice of therapy. The costs of each possible option, in terms of time and energy, required visits, side effects, loss of intimacy, and expense, should be presented. In some cases seeking a second opinion might be suggested, so that the couple may feel comfortable with the therapeutic choices they have made and ready for whatever degree of commitment is required.

In about 20% of couples, combinations of factors will have been found to be suboptimal, and multiple therapies need to be arranged, either sequentially or simultaneously. Perhaps the most disheartening situation confronting a couple may be when the initial evaluation has been completed and no diagnosis made. When this occurs, a review of more subtle causes of infertility is appropriate, and additional testing should be described and offered. For the couple with unexplained infertility, the options for testing may seem endless, and a discussion regarding the statistics that apply to unexplained infertility may lead them to choose to delay additional intervention, since up to 60% may ultimately achieve pregnancy. If age and length of time of infertility limit this option, empiric therapy and advanced reproductive technologies should be discussed.

## THERAPY FOR INFERTILITY

### Male Factor Infertility

Most causes of male factor infertility require therapy in consultation with a urologist. When no remedy is presently available, such as with azoospermia associated with elevated serum concentration of FSH, congenital anomalies, or chromosomal anomalies, donor insemination may be offered. Patients with azoospermia due to hypothalamic insufficiency or pituitary insufficiency may be given hormone replacement therapy; response is variable. In azoospermia due to congenital absence of the vas, successful aspiration of sperm from the epididymis, with IVF, offers potential paternity. For azoospermia secondary to vasectomy, microsurgical vasovasostomy is frequently successful in restoring patency; ultimate successful outcome is dependent on the quality of the sperm, which is in turn influenced by the length of time since occlusion and the presence or absence of sperm auto antibodies. In experienced centers, 75–90% patency rates, with 33–70% pregnancy rates, have been reported.

For infertile men with normal findings on physical examination and normal hormonal profiles, and in whom no clear etiology for infertility exists, a number of therapies with no clear substantiation of benefit have been suggested. Particularly where borderline sperm counts and motilities are reported, the benefit in improving the semen parameters may not reflect any real increase in prognosis for pregnancy. Use of clomiphene citrate is the most common therapy recommended, but the literature fails to substantiate improved pregnancy rates. Use of thyroid hormone cannot be justified in the euthyroid individual. Administration of gonadotropins, gonadotropin hormone-releasing hormone (GnRH), and androgen-rebound therapies have been proposed but have not been shown to be efficacious. Hypothermia has been advocated in idiopathic subfertile males, particularly where scrotal temperatures are demonstrated to be higher than normal. Trials have to date included only a small number of males. Where occupation or environment contribute to consistently elevated scrotal temperatures, modification of these circumstances should be advised. In cases where excessive exercise may be contributing to decreased testosterone, a change in exercise regimen—such as swimming instead of running—may improve parameters, but, again, there are no data correlating pregnancy rates with such measures.

In some men with high titers of autoantibodies to sperm, the immune response can be suppressed with steroid therapy, but the risk of complication and low probability of improvement in fertility lead to recommendation for a trial of IVF.

The role of varicocelectomy in the treatment of male infertility continues to be controversial. A varicocele can be demonstrated in 15% of men, but the incidence of infertility in males is much less. A varicocele has been diagnosed in up to one-third of men in infertility clinics. Abnormal sperm counts, motility, and morphology are often found in association with a varicocele, and two-thirds of patients demonstrate improved parameters after surgical correction. However, the efficacy of the procedure in terms of pregnancy rates is less well substantiated; postoperative pregnancy rates of 25–50% have been reported, but some controlled studies showed no difference between treated and untreated groups when life table analysis was performed. When no other cause for infertility has been identified, ligation of a documented varicocele is offered as empiric treatment.

When semen parameters are normal but results from postcoital examinations are repeatedly poor, treatment with intrauterine insemination of washed concentrated sperm has been effective in overcoming an apparent barrier to fertility. However, the use of artificial insemination when postcoital testing is normal or when sperm parameters are abnormal is associated with very little supporting data. In cases where oligospermia has been treated by artificial insemination with the male partner's sperm, success rates in the range of 12–16% are expected. It is tempting to offer this therapy to couples when the alternative is no treatment, and most couples find the therapy logically appealing acceptable, since it places the "best" sperm into the uterus at the proper time, removing any uncertainty regarding adequacy of technique or timing. However, for oligospermic individuals, the procedure offers little hope for success and should be discouraged. For the treatment of unexplained infertility, the success rates for artificial insemination by the male partner appear not to be different from treatment-independent pregnancy rates. In some series, the strategy of deliberate hyperstimulation of the ovary combined with IVF has been associated with pregnancy rates of 25–40% if 3–5 cycles are completed. Placement of the sperm directly into the uterine tube during laparoscopy timed to occur near ovulation and direct intraperitoneal insemination by culdocentesis are investigational therapies. A higher risk of infectious complications is associated with these therapies.

The ultimate therapy for male factor infertility as shown by unfavorable sperm parameters, a negative sperm penetration assay, or both, is IVF or gamete or zygote intrafallopian transfer (GIFT or ZIFT; see Chapter 56). When male infertility is not amenable to therapy, donor insemination offers an opportunity for pregnancy. The use of a donor raises medical, emotional, ethical, and legal issues for the potential parents and the practitioner. The husband may experience grief, confusion regarding the concepts of fertility versus masculinity, concern over acceptance of the child, and guilt. Decisions about what to tell the child are often difficult to face. Because of the potential for infection with use of fresh sperm, and the concern for risk of AIDS in particular, it is the recommendation of the American Fertility Society to rely on frozen semen. The freezing process results in semen with slightly lower fecundability and consequently a longer interval to pregnancy for most couples. Most pregnancies will result within 6–9 cycles; if this method is not successful, a reappraisal of female fertility factors is in order.

### Female Factor Infertility

**A. The Ovulatory Factor:** The treatment of specific ovulatory disorders is determined by the diagnosis. In offering treatment to induce ovulation, the premise that normal fertility should result from the correction of the anovulation implies that pregnancy should occur within the first 6 cycles for the majority of patients and within 1 year for up to 80%. If repetitive ovulatory cycles are established without achieving pregnancy, a reevaluation of other factors, or other treatment, should be offered.

If an elevated FSH is detected, ovarian failure or resistance is present and fertility cannot be restored; no biopsy information is necessary or helpful. The options that may then be considered include adoption, surrogate pregnancy, embryo donation, or egg donation. Success rates for embryo and egg donation are in the range of 40% pregnancies achieved per transfer with fresh embryos, and they are lower if cryopreservation has been used. The ethical, psychologic, and legal issues are similar to those involved in donor sperm options.

Induction of ovulation can be accomplished in 90–95% of patients with chronic anovulation and normal FSH and prolactin. Usually, a progression of therapy will be planned, with the use of clomiphene citrate as the first approach. Success with clomiphene may require adjustment of dosage and of timing and combination with other supplementary medications, such as corticosteroids, estrogen, or midcycle human chorionic gonadotropin (hCG). The amount of monitoring required depends on the response. Until a normal follicle with apparent ovulation has been consistently achieved, ultrasound and hormonal testing may be required for interpretation of response. After a regimen has been shown to achieve ovulation, 3–6 cycles with timed intercourse should be attempted. Clomiphene will be successful in inducing ovulation in about 70% of women with ovaries that are producing estrogen but not ovulating regularly. In more than 50% of the stimulated cycles, more than 1 follicle can be shown to be stimulated and will progress to dominance, correlating with an incidence of twins of 8%. Side effects with clomiphene are common, including hot flushes, emotional lability or depression, bloating, and visual changes; most are mild and all disappear with discontinuation of the drug. The clomiphene acts as an antiestrogen to provoke a response from the pituitary and is usually taken for 5 days in the early follicular phase. Adjustment of the dose or time of administration may be required from cycle to cycle. If ovulation occurs but no pregnancy results (60% of cases), reevaluation of the regimen and possible progression to more aggressive therapy may be considered.

Patients in whom there is no response to clomiphene, or those in whom there is ovulatory response to clomiphene but no pregnancy, patients with pituitary insufficiency, those with hypothalamic insufficiency, and patients with unexplained infertility usually respond to stimulation with human menopausal gonadotropins (hMG). Usually hCG is required as an ovulatory trigger, and monitoring is required to determine the intensity of the ovarian response. A combination of frequent ultrasonic scanning and estrogen determinations will indicate the number of follicles stimulated and their degree of maturity, so that hCG can be appropriately administered or withheld. With perseverance and appropriate adjustment of therapy, 85–90% of patients can be stimulated to ovulate with hMG treatment, but even with careful monitoring there is a 20% risk of multiple births. The cost of treatment is high owing to the expense of the drug and requisite monitoring. Used judiciously, the major complication of hyperstimulation from hMG will occur in 1–3% of cycles. The expense, risk, and side effects of these therapies will determine their feasibility.

When modification of lifestyle or body habitus does not successfully restore ovulation in the patient diagnosed with hypothalamic insufficiency, pulsatile GnRH is successful in restoring normal ovulation in nearly 100% of correctly diagnosed patients. Normal fertility is then restored during cycles of treatment, and most pregnancies occur within 3–6 cycles.

Elevated prolactin levels can cause abnormalities of ovulation, including inadequate luteal phase or amenorrhea. An elevated prolactin should lead to a verification of normal thyroid-stimulating hormone (TSH) secretion, because primary hypothyroidism can cause increased prolactin. Prolactin elevations are attributable to many different medications and drugs, and the history should be reviewed. The elevated prolactin can often be treated with bromocriptine, leading to normalization of the endocrinology of the cycle. The woman can be advised to discontinue the drug once pregnancy is verified, but she can be reassured by a growing body of information confirming the safety of the medication when it is taken during early pregnancy.

There is no consensus regarding the best treatment strategy for patients with a diagnosis of inadequate luteal phase. Some specialists interpret the luteal phase defect as an abnormality derived from an abnormal follicular development and recommend clomiphene augmentation of the early follicular phase. Since this usually results in the recruitment of an additional follicle, it may also contribute additional progesterone during the luteal phase. Other treatments that may be attempted are progesterone supplementation of the luteal phase or hCG injections. The progesterone can be administered as injections, as specially formulated suppositories, or as a micronized oral preparation. The various treatment methods have been advocated in the literature and supported by data, but because diagnosis is difficult to establish with certainty, the spontaneous cure rate will be high.

**B. The Pelvic Factor:** Endometriosis and the effects of salpingitis are 2 of the most common problems confronting infertile couples. When definitive treatment cannot be accomplished during diagnosis at laparoscopy, referral to experienced surgical specialists is advised, as the best opportunity for pregnancy will usually occur following the primary conservative procedure. The treatment of these problems is discussed elsewhere in this text (see Chapters 37 and 39).

The role of fibroids in infertility is unclear, and most surgeons reserve myomectomy for treatment of recurrent abortion, to relieve symptoms of discomfort or excessive blood loss, or when a submucosal fibroid has been demonstrated. The fibroids considered to be of significance will usually distort the endometrial cavity and may be diagnosed by hysterosalpingogram, ultrasonography, hysteroscopy, or magnetic resonance imaging.

When to abandon conservative surgical therapy in favor of IVF is a matter of assessing multiple factors that will influence the probabilities. The nature and extent of pelvic adhesions, the presence of hydrosalpinges, the age of the patient, and associated fertility factors will influence the degree of enthusiasm for recommendation of surgical treatment. The success rates associated with the various approaches need to be carefully explained to the couple. For example, cumulative success rates for populations of patients are usually quoted for surgical treatment (eg, 30% will conceive within 2 years), whereas pregnancy per cycle rates are usually quoted for IVF (eg, 15–20% pregnancies per transfer).

**C. The Cervical Factor:** The absence of adequate nurturing mucus at midcycle can be treated either by attempts to improve the mucus or by bypassing the mucus with intrauterine insemination. To improve the amount of mucus, estrogen can be administered during the mid- to late follicular phase of the cycle. The potential for interfering with the normal follicular dynamics exists, and if low doses of estrogen are ineffective, an attempt to increase endogenous follicular estrogen using hMG may result in improved cervical mucus. In most cases, this will be a direct result of the recruitment of additional follicles and must be carefully monitored for the intensity of the response in order to reduce the risk of multiple gestation and prevent hyperstimulation syndrome. When the cervical mucus appears to be affected by cervicitis and inflammatory changes, empiric treatment of patient and partner with doxycycline is advocated by some authors. When the cervix is altered by congenital malformation or by past surgical treatment that has rendered endocervical glands absent or nonfunctional, intrauterine insemination with washed sperm can be anticipated to result in pregnancy in 20–30% of patients who complete at least 3 cycles of treatment. Cervical factor patients who do not respond to these therapies can be offered IVF or GIFT or ZIFT (see Chapter 56).

## Unexplained Infertility

Because no diagnosis is achieved, there is no specific treatment that can be offered with confidence to couples with unexplained fertility. The cumulative pregnancy rate may be close to 60% over 3–5 years, but the chances of pregnancy in an individual couple decrease with the duration of infertility. There may be pressure to attempt some form of treatment, and this group of patients is vulnerable to exploitation. They are most likely to seek multiple providers and to be influenced by the popular literature or by the anecdotal experiences of friends and acquaintances. Most therapies (eg, artificial insemination with sperm from the partner or administration of clomiphene, Pergonal, or bromocriptine) have not been shown to be more effective than no treatment. In evaluating results of these therapies, it is important to note that few controlled studies are available. There is at present some enthusiasm for offering IVF or GIFT to these couples for both diagnosis and treatment, because populations of patients with unexplained infertility appear in most series to have a success rate equivalent or just below that of patients with tubal disease. Prior to entering an IVF cycle, most programs will offer these patients 3–6 cycles of Pergonal stimulation combined with timed inseminations, in the hope that pregnancy will result without the actual retrieval of the oocytes.

The success rates for these maneuvers are under investigation but have been reported to result in monthly fecundability of 10–15%. The treatment requires considerable time, expense, and expertise to accomplish but is less demanding than an IVF treatment program.

The use of an unproved remedy may be justified if some rationale exists for its use in a particular couple or if a study is undertaken to determine its efficacy; however, the couple must clearly understand the lack of proved benefit. For many, the hardest course to contemplate is no therapy at all. A time limit with expectation of resolution of infertility should be presented, and in some cases guidance toward acceptance of childless living, adoption, use of surrogate pregnancy, or donor insemination should be offered before extensive time and resources are expended on procedures or regimens that offer little potential.

## REFERENCES

Daniluk JC: Infertility: Intrapersonal and interpersonal impact. Fertil Steril 1988;49:982.

Glass, Robert H: Infertility. In: *Reproductive Endocrinology*, 2nd ed. Yen SSC, Jaffe RB (eds.). WB Saunders, 1986.

Griffiths CS, Grimes DA: The validity of the postcoital test. Am J Obstet Gynecol 1990;162:615.

Lobo RA: Unexplained infertility. J Reprod Med 1993; 38(4):241.

Meldrum DR: Female reproductive aging: Ovarian and uterine factors. Fertil Steril 1993;59:1.

Nulsen JC, Walsh J, Dumez S, Metzer DA: A randomized and longitudinal study of human menopausal gonadotropin with intrauterine insemination in the treatment of infertility. Obstet Gynecol 1993;82(5):780.

Obstet Gynecol Clin North Am 1987;14:entire volume.

Rasmussen F, Lindequist S, Larsen C, Justesen PL: Therapeutic effect of hysterosalpingography: Oil versus water soluble contrast media—a randomized prospective study. Radiology 1991;179:75.

Smarr SC, Wing R, Hammond MG: Effect of therapy on infertile couples with antisperm antibodies. Am J Obstet Gynecol 1988;158:969.

Wentz AC, Kossoy L, Parker RA: The impact of luteal phase inadequacy in an infertile population. Am J Obstet Gynecol 1990;162:937.

# Amenorrhea

# 54

*Ian H. Thorneycroft, MD, PhD*

## DEFINITION & INCIDENCE

**Primary amenorrhea** is the absence of menses by age 16. **Secondary amenorrhea** is the absence of menses for 6 months in a woman in whom normal menstruation has been established or for 3 normal intervals in a woman with oligomenorrhea. **Oligomenorrhea** is menses occurring at an interval exceeding 35 days.

About 97.5% of females begin normal menstruation cycles by age 16 in the USA; thus, the incidence of primary amenorrhea is 2.5%. The incidence of secondary amenorrhea is quite variable—from 3% in the general population to 100% under conditions of extreme physical or emotional stress (eg, in prisoners awaiting execution). In assessing possible causes of amenorrhea, the clinician must keep in mind the rate in the general population. For example, the incidence of amenorrhea following discontinuation of oral contraceptives is not strikingly higher than the 3% incidence in the general population.

Amenorrhea is important for several reasons: (1) Since amenorrheic women do not ovulate, they cannot conceive. (2) Amenorrhea with no estrogen production may lead to osteoporosis and genital atrophy. (3) Amenorrhea with some estrogen production can result in increased endometrial hyperplasia, which can increase the possibility of endometrial carcinoma from unopposed estrogen secretion. (4) Primary amenorrhea in a girl who has not already developed secondary sexual characteristics may give rise to major social and psychosexual problems.

## ETIOLOGY & PATHOGENESIS

A major cause of amenorrhea is pregnancy, which must be ruled out in every patient presenting with amenorrhea. Amenorrhea caused by aberrations of the normal menstrual cycle is discussed in Chapter 6. Other causes of amenorrhea not discussed in this chapter are developmental anomalies of the reproductive organs (Chapter 31) and masculinization at puberty (Chapter 55).

In this chapter, we will discuss amenorrhea associated with both 46,XX and 46,XX karyotypes, anatomic defects, hypothalamic defects, pituitary disorders, ovarian failure, ovarian dysfunction, and systemic disorders.

## Amenorrhea in Women With 46,XY Karyotype

The details of embryonic sexual differentiation are discussed in Chapter 3. Briefly, the sexually undifferentiated male fetal testis secretes müllerian inhibiting factor (MIF) and testosterone. MIF promotes regression of all müllerian structures: the uterine tubes, the uterus, and the upper two-thirds of the vagina. Testosterone and its active metabolite dihydrotestosterone (DHT) are responsible for embryonic differentiation of the male internal and external genitalia.

**A. Testicular Feminization:** In testicular feminization, all müllerian-derived structures are absent. The external genital anlagen and mesonephric ducts cannot respond to androgens, because androgen receptors are either absent or defective. Affected individuals are therefore phenotypic females lacking a uterus and a complete vagina. They produce some estrogen, develop breasts, and are reared as girls and therefore present with primary amenorrhea.

**B. Pure Gonadal Dysgenesis:** If the primitive germ cells do not migrate to the genital ridge, a testis will not develop, and a streak gonad will be present. Affected individuals have normal female internal and external genitalia, since neither MIF nor androgens are secreted by the streaks. Because these individuals produce no estrogen, they will not develop breasts. They are reared as girls and present clinically with either delayed puberty or primary amenorrhea.

**C. Anorchia:** If the fetal testes regress before 7 weeks' gestation, neither MIF nor testosterone is secreted, and affected individuals will present with a clinical picture identical to that of pure gonadal dysgenesis. Individuals whose testes regress between 7 and 13 weeks' gestation present with ambiguous genitalia.

**D. Testicular Steroid Enzyme Defects:** A testis with defective enzymes 1–4 will produce MIF but not testosterone (Fig 54–1). Affected individuals have

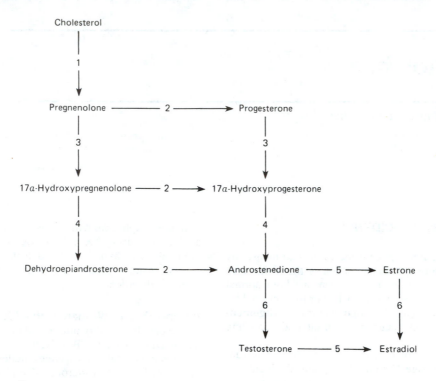

Cholesterol

1

Pregnenolone ——— 2 ———→ Progesterone

3               3

17α-Hydroxypregnenolone ——— 2 ———→ 17α-Hydroxyprogesterone

4               4

Dehydroepiandrosterone ——— 2 ———→ Androstenedione ——— 5 ——→ Estrone

6               6

Testosterone ——— 5 ——→ Estradiol

**Key to enzymes**
1 = Cholesterol 20- and 22-desmolase and 20-hydroxylase
2 = 3β-Hydroxysteroid dehydrogenase
3 = 17α-Hydroxylase
4 = 17- and 20-Desmolase
5 = Aromatase
6 = 17-Hydroxysteroid dehydrogenase

**Figure 54–1.** Steroidogenesis in the ovary and testis.

female external genitalia and no müllerian structures. They will be reared as girls and present clinically with either delayed puberty or primary amenorrhea.

A defect in enzyme 6 (17-hydroxysteroid dehydrogenase) results in ambiguous genitalia and virilization at puberty.

## Anatomic Abnormalities Associated with Amenorrhea (see Chapter 31).

**A. Müllerian Dysgenesis:** Müllerian dysgenesis is characterized by congenital absence of the uterus and the upper two-thirds of the vagina. Affected individuals have a 46,XX karyotype.

**B. Vaginal Agenesis:** Vaginal agenesis is characterized by failure of the vagina to develop.

**C. Transverse Vaginal Septum:** This anomaly results from failure of fusion of the müllerian and urogenital sinus-derived portions of the vagina.

**D. Imperforate Hymen:** If the hymen is complete, menstrual efflux cannot occur.

**E. Asherman's Syndrome:** In Asherman's syndrome, amenorrhea is due to intrauterine synechiae. The usual cause is a complicated D&C (eg, infected products of conception, vigorous elimination

of the endometrium), but the syndrome can occur after myomectomy, cesarean section, and tuberculous endometritis.

## Hypothalamic Defects

Under normal physiologic circumstances, the arcuate nucleus releases pulses of luteinizing hormone-releasing hormone (LHRH) into the hypophyseal portal system approximately every hour. Discharge of LHRH releases luteinizing hormone (LH) and follicle stimulating hormone (FSH) from the pituitary; LH and FSH in turn stimulate ovarian follicular growth and ovulation. Anovulation and amenorrhea will occur as a result of interference with LHRH transport, LHRH pulse discharge, or congenital absence of LHRH (Kallmann's syndrome). Any of these situations will lead to hypogonadotropic hypogonadism.

**A. Defects of LHRH Transport:** Interference with the transport of LHRH from the hypothalamus to the pituitary may occur with pituitary stalk compression or destruction of the arcuate nucleus. Pituitary stalk section from trauma, craniopharyngioma, germinoma, glioma, Hand-Schüller-Christian disease, midline teratomas, endodermal sinus tumor, tuberculosis, sarcoidosis, and irradiation will all either destroy parts of the hypothalamus or prevent transport of hypothalamic hormones to the pituitary.

**B. Defects of LHRH Pulse Production:** The metabolic consequence of any significant reduction in the normal LHRH pulse frequency or amplitude is that little or no LH or FSH can be released, with the result that no ovarian follicles develop, virtually no estradiol is secreted, and the patient is amenorrheic. This is the biochemical status in normal prepubertal girls and those with constitutional delayed puberty, in anorexia nervosa, in amenorrhea associated with severe stress, extreme weight loss, or prolonged vigorous athletic exertion, and in hyperprolactinemia. Amenorrhea on this basis may also be an idiopathic phenomenon.

Less severe reductions in LHRH pulse amplitude and frequency result in diminished LH and FSH secretion with some follicular stimulation. The stimulation is insufficient to result in full follicular development and ovulation, but estradiol is secreted. Amenorrhea on this basis may occur with stress or hyperprolactinemia, as a result of vigorous athletic activity, or in the early stages of eating disorders, or it may be idiopathic.

**C. Kallmann's Syndrome:** These patients have a congenital absence of LHRH and, consequently, do not release LH or FSH from the pituitary. Ovulation does not occur. Anosmia is an associated phenomenon.

## Pituitary Defects

Pituitary causes of amenorrhea are rare; most are secondary to hypothalamic dysfunction.

**A. Congenital Pituitary Dysfunction:** Congenital absence of the entire pituitary is a rare and lethal condition. Isolated defects of LH or FSH production do occur (rarely), resulting in anovulation and amenorrhea.

**B. Acquired Pituitary Dysfunction:** Sheehan's syndrome, characterized by postpartum amenorrhea, results from postpartum pituitary necrosis secondary to severe hemorrhage and hypotension and is a rare cause of amenorrhea. Surgical ablation and irradiation of the pituitary as management of pituitary tumors also cause amenorrhea.

Iron deposition in the pituitary may result in destruction of the cells that produce LH and FSH. This occurs only in patients with markedly elevated serum iron levels (ie, hemosiderosis) usually resulting from extensive red cell destruction. Thalassemia major is an example of a disease that causes hemosiderosis.

High prolactin levels resulting from pituitary hyperplasia or pituitary adenomas are associated with amenorrhea. The mechanism is not clear. Elevated prolactin levels probably trigger an increase in hypothalamic dopamine in an effort to decrease pituitary prolactin secretion. Elevated hypothalamic levels of dopamine decrease LHRH secretion.

## Ovarian Failure

Primary ovarian failure is characterized by elevated gonadotropins and low estradiol (**hypergonadotropic hypogonadism**). Secondary failure is almost always due to hypothalamic dysfunction and is characterized by normal or low gonadotropins and low estradiol (**hypogonadotropic hypogonadism**).

Causes of primary ovarian failure are listed in Table 54–1. The more important ones are discussed briefly later (also see Rebar, 1982).

**A. Steroid Enzyme Defects:** Genetic females with defects in enzymes 1–4 have primary amenorrhea and absence of breast development, since the ovaries cannot synthesize estradiol (see Fig 54–1). The internal genitalia are normal, the karyotype is 46,XX (female), and MIF production does not occur.

**B. Ovarian Resistance (Savage's) Syndrome:** Patients with this syndrome have elevated LH and FSH levels, and the ovaries contain primordial germ cells. A defect in the cell receptor mechanism is the presumed cause.

**C. Ovarian Dysgenesis:** If the primitive oogonia do not migrate to the genital ridge, the ovaries fail to develop. Streak gonads, which do not secrete hormones, develop instead, and the result is primary amenorrhea (pure gonadal dysgenesis; **Swyer's syndrome**).

In patient's with **Turner's syndrome** (45,XO) or mosaicism (45,XO/XX), the oogonia migrate normally to the ovary but undergo rapid atresia, so that by puberty no oogonia remain. These patients usually have primary amenorrhea, but some—particularly those with the mosaic abnormality—may menstruate briefly, and a few have conceived (see Chapter 5).

**D. Premature Ovarian Failure:** Menopause occurs when the ovaries fail secondary to depletion of ova. If this occurs before age 35, it is considered premature.

**Table 54–1.** Causes of primary gonadal failure (hypergonadotropic hypogonadism).

---

Idiopathic premature ovarian failure
Steroidogenic enzyme defects (primary amenorrhea)
    Cholesterol side-chain cleavage
    3β-ol-dehydrogenase
    17-hydroxylase
    17-desmolase
    17-ketoreductase
Testicular regression syndrome
True hermaphroditism
Gonadal dysgenesis
    Pure gonadal dysgenesis (Swyer syndrome) (46,XX and 46,XY)
    Turner's syndrome (45,XO)
    Turner variants
Mixed gonadal dysgenesis
Ovarian resistance syndrome (Savage syndrome)
Autoimmune oophoritis
Postinfection (eg, mumps)
Postoophorectomy (also wedge resections and bivalving)
Postirradiation
Postchemotherapy

## Ovarian Dysfunction

Patients presenting with primary or secondary amenorrhea may have polycystic ovaries (**Stein-Leventhal syndrome**; see Chapter 37). The ovaries in such cases are characterized by multiple small antral follicles, a thick capsule, and well-developed stromal tissue. Patients have elevated androgens and associated hirsutism and are usually obese. The exact pathophysiologic mechanism is unknown but is believed to include a "vicious cycle" feature. Insulin resistance plays a role in the development of polycystic ovaries (PCOD). Elevated insulin levels are believed to stimulate IGF-I receptors in the CA interna resulting in elevated androgen production. The event initiating anovulation is probably an increase in androgen secretion from the ovary or from the adrenal gland. The androgens are converted to estrogens in adipose tissue. The level of sex steroid-binding globulin (SSBG) is lower than normal, giving rise to higher than normal free estrogen levels. The pituitary responds to this hyperestrogenic state by yielding an elevated LH:FSH ratio. The altered ratio leads to aberrant follicular development, anovulation, and continued ovarian androgen production. The increased androgens are converted to estrogens and aggravate an already hyperestrogenic state.

## Obesity as a Cause of Amenorrhea

Obesity as such may be associated with amenor-rhea by the mechanism outlined in the preceding paragraph.

## DIAGNOSIS

The diagnostic workup for amenorrhea is diagrammed and summarized in Figures 54–2 to 54–4. It is important at the outset to determine which organ is dysfunctional and then to identify the exact cause. Once this has been done, specific therapy can be planned.

Any patient with amenorrhea who has a uterus should be tested for pregnancy and for serum levels of thyroid-stimulating hormone (TSH) and prolactin. A cone view of the sella turcica is also necessary. Galactorrhea should be identified or ruled out by physical examination.

### Diagnosis of Primary Amenorrhea

The diagnostic scheme for primary amenorrhea is outlined in Figure 54–2. Pelvic examination should be done to establish the presence of a vagina and uterus and no vaginal septum or imperforate hymen that might account for the failure of appearance of menses. Because pelvic examination of an adolescent girl may be difficult, pelvic ultrasound or examination under anesthesia may be required to establish the presence of a uterus.

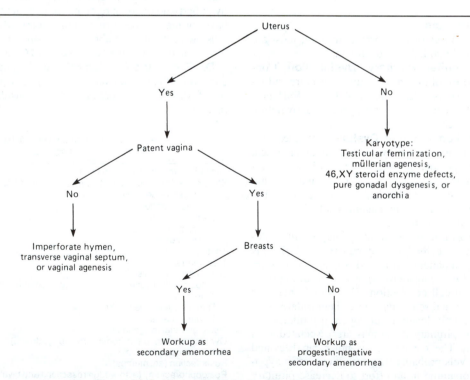

**Figure 54–2.** Workup for patients with primary amenorrhea.

If no uterus is present, serum testosterone levels should be measured and karyotyping done to differentiate between müllerian agenesis and testicular feminization.

## Diagnosis of Amenorrhea Associated With Galactorrhea-Hyperprolactinemia

The diagnostic workup of patients with galactorrhea or hyperprolactinemia is outlined in Figure 54–3. The differential diagnosis of galactorrhea-amenorrhea is summarized in Table 54–2.

An elevated serum TSH signifies hypothyroidism, which should be treated. Serum prolactin must be measured again after thyroid function has become normal. If prolactin remains elevated or is initially higher than 50–200 ng/mL, the patient should be further studied as outlined below.

If the prolactin level is under 50–100 ng/mL and the cone view of the sella turcica is normal, a pituitary macroadenoma (>10mm) is a very unlikely diagnosis. If the prolactin level exceeds 50–100 ng/mL, the cone view of the sella is abnormal, or the patient has restricted visual fields, then computed tomography (CT)or magnetic resonance imaging (MRI) scan of the sella is required to rule out pituitary macroadenoma.

A meticulous history must be taken to ascertain whether the hyperprolactinemia is due to ingestion of drugs. Prolactin secretion is inhibited by dopamine and stimulated by serotonin and thyrotropin-releasing hormone (TRH). Any drug that blocks the synthesis or binding of dopamine will increase the prolactin level. Prolactin is increased by serotonin agonists and decreased by serotonin antagonists. Pituitary macroadenoma should be ruled out if prolactin levels are higher than 50–100 ng/mL, even if the patient is taking drugs that lead to raised prolactin levels.

## Diagnosis of Amenorrhea Not Associated With Galactorrhea-Hyperprolactinemia

These patients are studied according to the scheme outlined in Figure 54–4.

The first step is the progestin challenge, which indirectly determines whether the ovary is producing estrogen. If the endometrium has been primed with estrogen, exogenous progestin will produce menses. Give either medroxyprogesterone acetate, 10 mg orally daily for 5 days, or progesterone, 100–200 mg intramuscularly as a single dose. If vaginal bleeding follows, the ovaries are secreting estrogen. If it does not, it can be concluded that there is no estrogen or that the patient has Asherman's syndrome.

From a practical standpoint, if a patient has not had a dilation and curettage (D&C), it is virtually impossible for her to have Asherman's syndrome, so that the diagnostic steps summarized in the following paragraphs can be disregarded.

Asherman's syndrome can be ruled out by administration of conjugated estrogen, 2.5 mg orally daily for 25 days, plus medroxyprogesterone acetate, 10 mg orally on days 16 through 25. Patients with Asherman's syndrome do not bleed following this regimen.

Asherman's syndrome can also be diagnosed by

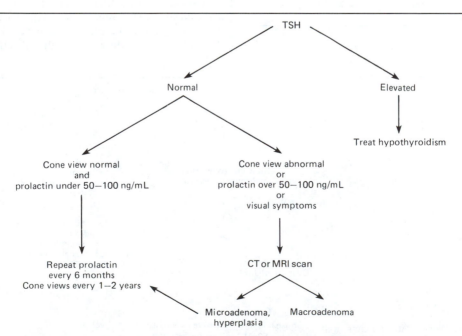

**Figure 54–3.** Workup for patients with amenorrhea-galactorrhea-hyperprolactinemia.

**Table 54–2.** Differential diagnosis of galactorrhea-hyperprolactinemia.

Pituitary tumors secreting prolactin
  Macroadenomas (>10 mm)
  Microadenomas (<10 mm)
Hypothyroidism
Idiopathic hyperprolactinemia
Drug-induced hyperprolactinemia
  Dopamine antagonists
    Phenothiazines
    Thioxanthenes
    Butyrophenone
    Diphenylbutylpiperidine
    Dibenzoxazepine
    Dihydroindolone
    Procainamide derivatives
  Catecholamine-depleting agents
  False transmitters (α-methyldopa)
Interruption of normal hypothalamic-pituitary relationship
Pituitary stalk section
Peripheral neural stimulation
  Chest wall stimulation
    Thoracotomy
    Mastectomy
    Thoracoplasty
    Burns
    Herpes zoster
    Bronchogenic tumors
    Bronchiectasis
    Chronic bronchitis
  Nipple stimulation
    Stimulation of nipples
    Chronic nipple irritation
  Spinal cord lesion
    Tabes dorsalis
    Syringomyelia
  Central nervous system disease
    Encephalitis
    Craniopharyngioma
    Pineal tumors
    Hypothalamic tumors
    Pseudotumor cerebri

weekly serum progesterone tests. Any value in the ovulatory range (>3 ng/mL) not associated with menses is indicative of Asherman's syndrome. Hysterosalpingography or hysteroscopy can also lead to a diagnosis of Asherman's syndrome.

In a patient who does not have Asherman's syndrome and does not respond to the progestin challenge, ovarian dysfunction may be of hypothalamic or ovarian origin. The distinction is based on the FSH level. Primary ovarian dysfunction resulting in low estradiol secretion is associated with high serum FSH. Values vary in different laboratories, but in general an FSH level higher than 40 mIU/mL indicates primary ovarian failure. A patient whose FSH level is less than 40 mIU/mL has hypothalamic-pituitary dysfunction and secondary ovarian failure.

## Diagnosis of Amenorrhea Due to Primary Gonadal Failure

The causes of primary gonadal failure are set forth in Table 54–1.

Karyotyping is indicated for all women who present with premature menopause, particularly if their amenorrhea is primary. Patients with primary amenorrhea may have a steroid enzyme defect. Autoimmune oophoritis is a reversible cause of ovarian failure that must be investigated (see Rebar, 1982).

## Diagnosis of Amenorrhea Associated With Hypothalamic-Pituitary Dysfunction

The differential diagnosis of this disorder is presented in Table 54–3. The category includes amenorrhea associated with athletic activity and weight loss and with stress. Differentiation of hypothalamic from pituitary dysfunction can be achieved by giving LHRH but is generally not a worthwhile effort, since

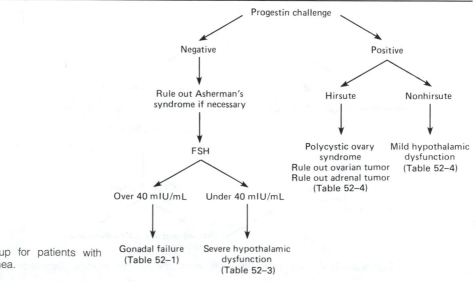

**Figure 54–4.** Workup for patients with secondary amenorrhea.

**Table 54–3.** Differential diagnosis of hypoestrogenic amenorrhea (hypogonadotropic hypogonadism).

**Hypothalamic dysfunction**
  Kallmann's syndrome
  Tumors of hypothalamus (craniopharyngioma)
  Constitutional delay of puberty
  Severe hypothalamic dysfunction
  Anorexia nervosa
  Severe weight loss
  Severe stress
  Exercise
**Pituitary disorder**
  Sheehans' syndrome
  Panhypopituitarism
  Isolated gonadotropin deficiency
  Hemosiderosis (primarily from thalassemia major)

**Table 54–4.** Differential diagnosis of eugonadotropic eugonadism (progestin-challenge positive).

**Mild hypothalamic dysfunction**
  Emotional stress
  Psychologic disorder
  Weight loss
  Obesity
  Exercise-induced
  Idiopathic
**Hirsutism-virilism**
  Polycystic ovary syndrome (Stein-Leventhal syndrome)
  Ovarian tumor
  Adrenal tumor
  Cushing's syndrome
  Congenital and maturity-onset adrenal hyperplasia
**Systemic disease**
  Hypothyroidism
  Hyperthyroidism
  Addison's disease
  Cushing's syndrome
  Chronic renal failure
  Many others

pituitary causes are rare and can often be diagnosed on the basis of the history. Moreover, in Kallmann's syndrome, a single bolus dose of LHRH may not elicit a normal response. Up to 40 doses of LHRH have been required to prime the pituitary so that it will respond normally.

CT or MRI scan is indicted to rule out hypothalamic or pituitary tumor, particularly if the cone view is abnormal or the amenorrhea is of long standing or is primary.

If there is a significant history consistent with Sheehan's syndrome, pituitary function testing is indicated in order to determine the functional capacity of the gland—particularly the integrity of the pituitary-adrenal axis.

In girls with primary amenorrhea, observing the pattern of LH and FSH release after administration of LHRH will help to determine whether the patient is undergoing late pubertal changes.

Patients who bleed in response to the progestin challenge (ie, whose ovaries are secreting estrogen) fit into one of 4 categories: (1) virilized, with or without ambiguous genitalia; (2) hirsute, with polycystic ovaries, hyperthecosis, or mild maturity-onset adrenal hyperplasia; (3) nonhirsute, with hypothalamic dysfunction; or (4) amenorrheic secondary to systemic disease. The differential diagnosis is set forth in Table 54–4. The LH:FSH ratio is a helpful clue to etiologic diagnosis. If the ratio exceeds 3:1 or if the LH level is persistently above 26–30 mIU/mL, a diagnosis of polycystic ovaries is a strong possibility. A vaginal ultrasound may be helpful in making the diagnosis of PCOD. However, 25% of normal patients have polycystic ovaries. Ultrasound cannot therefore be the sole criterion for diagnosis.

Virilism and hirsutism are discussed in Chapter 55.

## TREATMENT

### 1.  OVULATION INDUCTION

**Ovulation Induction in Patients With Amenorrhea-Galactorrhea With Pituitary Macroadenoma**

Transsphenoidal or frontal removal of the pituitary adenoma or the entire gland is required. About half of such patients will menstruate normally after this treatment. Bromocriptine may be required to induce ovulation. Many patients have been treated successfully with high doses of bromocriptine alone (up to 10 mg/d).

**Ovulation Induction in Patients With Amenorrhea-Galactorrhea Without Macroadenoma (Including Patients With Microadenomas)**

These patients ovulate readily in response to bromocriptine therapy. The usual dose is 2.5 mg orally twice daily, but it is generally titrated until serum prolactin is normal—often possible with as little as 1.25 mg daily. Once ovulation has been documented by basal body temperature monitoring, bromocriptine can be discontinued and then resumed after menses or it can be continued until pregnancy occurs. Continuous therapy avoids the nausea associated with intermittent therapy.

Patients taking drugs that raise the prolactin level should discontinue them if possible, but continued use of such drugs is not a contraindication to bromocriptine therapy.

## Ovulation Induction in Patients
## With Hypothyroidism

Amenorrheic patients with hypothyroidism frequently respond to thyroid replacement therapy.

## Ovulation Induction in Patients
## With Primary Ovarian Failure

According to Rebar and associates, patients with primary ovarian failure can be made to ovulate only under very rare circumstances. Patients with reversible ovarian failure include those with autoimmune oophoritis, who can be successfully treated with corticosteroids. Otherwise, almost all patients with primary ovarian failure fall into the category of idiopathic premature ovarian failure and cannot be made to ovulate. In vitro fertilization (IVF) with donor oocytes is the only way they can have children.

Any patient with a Y chromosome should undergo oophorectomy to prevent tumor development.

## Ovulation Induction in Patients
## With Hypoestrogenic Hypothalamic
## Amenorrhea (Progestin-Challenge Negative)

In these patients with low estrogen levels, the pituitary does not release high quantities of LH and FSH (as would be expected with an intact, normally functioning negative feedback mechanism). Therefore, even though clomiphene citrate (an antiestrogen) is not likely to stimulate gonadotropin release, many reproductive endocrinologists treat such patients successfully with a single course of clomiphene citrate, 150 or 250 mg daily for 5 days, on the chance that ovulation will occur.

Human menopausal gonadotropin (hMG) is usually the drug of choice. Patients showing some ovarian stimulation by clomiphene can be treated with a combination of clomiphene and hMG—the advantage being a reduction in the amount of hMG required and thus a substantial cost savings. Ovulation induction with hMG must be carefully monitored with serial ultrasound and estradiol determinations to avoid hyperstimulation. Hyperstimulation is the stimulation of too many follicles, with associated ovarian enlargement and ascites.

Because these patients are deficient in LHRH or have an abnormal LHRH pulse frequency and amplitude, ovulation can also be induced by administration of pulsatile LHRH subcutaneously or intravenously.

If a specific and potentially reversible cause of amenorrhea can be identified (eg, marked weight loss), it should be corrected.

## Ovulation Induction in Patients Who Bleed
## in Response to Progestin Challenge

Virtually all of these patients respond to clomiphene citrate. The starting dose is 50 mg orally daily for 5 days. This can be increased to a maximum of 250 mg orally daily in 50-mg increments until ovulation is induced. Ovulation occurs 5–10 days after the last dose. Patients with elevated androgens who do not respond to clomiphene citrate respond to combined treatment with corticosteroids and clomiphene.

If clomiphene therapy with or without corticosteroids is not effective, hMG or Metrodin can be given as outlined above for severe hypothalamic amenorrhea. Care must be taken in using hMG in these patients, as they are likely to become hyperstimulated.

Surgical wedge resection of the ovary in patients with polycystic ovary disease will frequently lead to ovulation. Unfortunately, wedge resection may cause postoperative pelvic adhesions, resulting in mechanical infertility. There is no place for a wedge resection today. The placement of multiple holes in the ovary with either cautery or the $CO_2$ laser appears to give similar results to wedge resection. Adhesions have also been noted with this technique.

Again—if a specific reversible cause of amenorrhea can be identified as outlined in Table 54–4, it should be corrected before drug therapy is attempted.

## 2. MANAGEMENT OF PATIENTS NOT WISHING OVULATION INDUCTION

Patients who are hypoestrogenic must be treated with a combination of estrogen and progesterone to maintain bone density and prevent genital atrophy. The dose of estrogen varies with the age of the patient. Oral contraceptives are good replacement therapy for women under age 35 and for women over 35 who do not smoke. Combinations of 0.625–1.25 mg of conjugated estrogens orally daily on days 1 through 25 of the cycle with 5–10 mg of medroxyprogesterone acetate on days 16 through 25 are suitable for women of all ages. Calcium intake should be adjusted to 1–1.5 g of elemental calcium daily.

Patients who respond to the progestin challenge require occasional progestin administration to prevent the development of endometrial hyperplasia and carcinoma. Again, if the patient is under 35, or for those over 35 who do not smoke, oral contraceptives are good therapy. Oral contraceptives also help with management of hirsutism. Alternatively, medroxyprogesterone acetate, 10 mg orally daily for 10–13 days every month or every other month, is sufficient to induce withdrawal bleeding and to prevent the development of endometrial hyperplasia.

Patients with hyperprolactinemia without macroadenoma need periodic prolactin measurements and radiographic cone views of the sellaturcica to rule out the development of macroadenoma, as outlined in Figure 54–3.

## COMPLICATIONS

The complications of amenorrhea are those of the disease entities listed in Tables 54–1 to 54–4. Hypoestrogenic patients can develop severe osteoporosis and fractures, the most hazardous to life being femoral neck fracture (see Chapter 57). The complications associated with amenorrhea in patients who respond to progestin challenge are endometrial hyperplasia and carcinoma (see Chapter 48) resulting from unopposed estrogen stimulation.

## PROGNOSIS

The prognosis for amenorrhea is good. It is not usually a life-threatening clinical event, since with proper workup, tumors can be recognized and treated. Many patients with hypothalamic amenorrhea will spontaneously recover normal menstrual cycles.

Virtually all amenorrheic women who do not have premature ovarian failure can be made to ovulate with bromocriptine, clomiphene citrate, corticosteroids, hMG, or LHRH.

## REFERENCES

Rebar RW, Erickson GF, Yen SSC: Idiopathic premature ovarian failure: Clinical and endocrine characteristics. Fertil Steril 1982;37:35.

Wilson JD, Foster DW (editors): Chapters 9 and 11 in: *Williams Textbook of Endocrinology*, 7th ed. Saunders, 1985.

Yen SSC, Jaffe RB (editors): *Reproductive Endocrinology: Physiology, Pathophysiology, and Clinical Management*. Saunders, 1986.

# Hirsutism

D. Ellene Andrew, MD, Carol L. Gagliardi, MD, & Adelina M. Emmi, MD

## Definition

Hirsutism is defined as excessive growth of androgen-dependent sexual hair, most often manifested as increased hair on the upper lip, chin, ears, cheeks, lower abdomen, back, chest, and proximal limbs. The interpretation of what constitutes excessive growth is subjective and may range from an occasional hair on the upper lip to a full male-pattern beard. The psychologic implications of hirsutism must not be underestimated. In Western society, excessive facial or body hair in women is unacceptable. Women who do not conform to a prevailing feminine ideal of physical appearance because of hirsutism may feel unattractive and suffer from low self-esteem, and they may find social interaction difficult. Hirsutism is more than a cosmetic problem, however, because it usually represents a hormonal imbalance resulting from a subtle excess of androgens that may be of ovarian origin, adrenal origin, or both.

## Etiology (Table 55–1)

Excessive growth of sexual hair is almost always due to excessive production of androgens, although (rarely) increased sensitivity of the hair follicle to androgens may be responsible. Potential sources of increased androgens include the ovaries, adrenals, and exogenous hormones and other medications.

### A. Ovarian Disorders Causing Hirsutism:

**1. Nonneoplastic disorders**–The most common cause of hirsutism is **polycystic ovary disease.** Polycystic ovary disease is typically associated with menstrual irregularities, infertility, obesity, and hirsutism. The pathophysiology of this disease is not fully understood; proposed causes include ovarian lesions, a disturbance of the hypothalamic-pituitary axis that causes ovarian dysfunction, and adrenal androgen excess. Regardless of the underlying defect, associated anovulation may result in increased androgen levels and lead to the complaint of hirsutism in 70% of patients. The histologic changes seen in polycystic ovary disease include a thickened ovarian capsule and numerous follicular cysts surrounded by a hyperplastic theca interna with luteinization.

Other nonneoplastic endocrine disorders of the ovary associated with increased androgen levels leading to hirsutism include stromal hyperplasia, stromal hyperthecosis, and hilar cell hyperplasia. **Stromal hyperplasia,** a relatively common phenomenon with a peak incidence between 50 and 70 years of age, is usually associated with equal enlargement of both ovaries. **Stromal hyperthecosis** is stromal proliferation with foci of luteinization and is usually bilateral. It may be caused by deficiency of a necessary enzyme in the biosynthetic pathway and is more apt than is simple stromal hyperplasia to be associated with virilism, obesity, hypertension, and disturbances of glucose metabolism. A few patients with stromal hyperthecosis have a more complicated syndrome that includes acanthosis nigricans and insulin resistance.

**Theca lutein cysts** (hyperreactio luteinalis) is a nonneoplastic disorder that can cause bilateral ovarian enlargement, hirsutism, and, infrequently, virilization. These cysts occur almost exclusively in normal pregnancy as well as pregnancy complicated by gestational trophoblastic disease. Ovarian biopsy reveals cysts lined mostly with luteinized theca cells, but luteinized granulosa cells may also be present.

**2. Neoplastic disorders**–Androgen-secreting ovarian neoplasms usually present with rapidly developing hirsutism, amenorrhea, and virilization, including breast atrophy, voice changes, clitoromegaly, and temporal balding. The most common androgen secreted by these tumors is testosterone, with the serum testosterone level being greater than 200 ng/dL. Most hormone-secreting neoplasms are palpable on pelvic examination and are unilateral.

**Sertoli-Leydig cell tumors** and **hilar (Leydig) cell tumors** are ovarian neoplasms typically associated with hirsutism and virilization. Sertoli-Leydig cell tumors constitute less than 0.5% of all ovarian tumors and occur mainly in young, menstruating females. Hilar cell tumors are rarer than Sertoli-Leydig cell tumors and are usually encountered in older women. Other ovarian neoplasms that may be associated with hirsutism are the gynandroblastomas, some germ cell tumors, and gonadoblastomas. The last occur mainly in patients with gonadal dysgenesis,

**Table 55–1.** Differential diagnosis of causes of hirsutism.

**Ovarian disorders**
  Polycystic ovary disease
  Stromal hyperplasia
  Stromal hyperthecosis
  Theca lutein cysts
  Luteoma of pregnancy
  Sertoli-Leydig cell tumor (arrhenoblastoma)
  Hilar cell (Leydig cell) tumor
  Gynandroblastoma
  Germ cell tumor
  Gonadoblastoma
  Ovarian tumor with functional stroma
**Adrenal disorders**
  Cushing's syndrome
  Cushing's disease
  Adult-onset congenital adrenal hyperplasia
  Hyperfunction of the adrenal gland
**Drugs**
  Testosterone
  Danazol (Danocrine)
  Anabolic steroids
  Synthetic progestins
**Other disorders**
  Idiopathic hirsutism

who usually have a Y chromosome in the karyotype although they are phenotypically normal women.

**Ovarian tumors with functional stroma** constitute another important category of androgenic ovarian tumors. In these tumors, the neoplastic cells do not secrete steroid hormones directly but stimulate steroid hormone secretion by the ovarian stroma. These tumors may be benign or malignant and metastatic or primary.

During pregnancy, elevated androgen levels that lead to severe hirsutism and virilization may be due to any of the neoplasms mentioned above or may be due to luteoma of pregnancy. Luteoma of pregnancy is a benign human chorionic gonadotropin (hCG)-dependent ovarian tumor that may develop during pregnancy. High levels of testosterone and androstenedione are present, and virilization may occur in the mother (25%) as well as in female fetuses (65%). In most patients, spontaneous regression of the neoplasm and return of androgen levels to normal occur in the postpartum period.

**B. Adrenal Disorders Causing Hirsutism:** Adrenal sources of excess androgens that lead to hirsutism include neoplasms, enzyme deficiencies within the biosynthetic pathways of the adrenal gland, and inappropriate stimulation of the adrenal gland. The main androgen produced by adrenal neoplasms is dehydroepiandrosterone sulfate (DHEAS), with serum levels usually greater than 7000 ng/mL. Rarely, adrenal neoplasms may secrete testosterone; when this occurs, testosterone values are usually higher than 200 ng/dL.

Since androgens are formed as intermediates in the synthesis of cortisol, disorders that lead to increased synthesis of cortisol, such as Cushing's syndrome, may increase androgen levels. **Cushing's syndrome**

may occur as a result of 3 different abnormalities: (1) adrenal tumor, (2) ectopic production of adrenocorticotropic hormone (ACTH) by a nonpituitary tumor, or (3) excess production of ACTH by the pituitary (**Cushing's disease**). The clinical picture is the same regardless of the underlying cause, and hirsutism may occur with any of the abnormalities.

Adrenal disorders that cause excessive androgen production include the various forms of **congenital adrenal hyperplasia,** all of which are inherited as autosomal recessive traits. The most common form of congenital adrenal hyperplasia is characterized by a deficiency of 21-hydroxylase enzyme. Endocrine studies show increased serum levels of 17-hydroxyprogesterone with elevated urinary excretion of 17-ketosteroids and pregnanetriol. A deficiency of 11β-hydroxylase is characterized by increased testosterone and deoxycortisol levels, whereas deficiency of 3β-ol-dehydrogenase can lead to increased DHEA (dehydroepiandrosterone), DHEAS (DHEA sulfate), and 17-hydroxypregnenolone levels. Congenital adrenal hyperplasia is usually diagnosed in females during the neonatal period because of androgen-induced ambiguous genitalia; however, a mild enzyme deficiency may go unrecognized until puberty or later when hirsutism, amenorrhea, and virilization may occur. Such disease is termed acquired, late-onset, or adult-onset congenital adrenal hyperplasia.

The adrenal gland may be the source of excess androgen production in the absence of congenital adrenal hyperplasia or tumors. The cause of this adrenal hyperactivity is not clear, but mild enzyme deficiencies, stress, hyperfunctioning of the entire adrenal, and even hyperprolactinemia have been postulated as probable causes. Several investigators have reported increased DHEAS levels with hyperprolactinemia; however, the mechanism by which this occurs is unknown at present.

**C. Drugs Causing Hirsutism:** Exogenous sources of androgens should also be considered as possible causes of hirsutism. Methyltestosterone, danazol, and anabolic steroids such as oxandrolone may lead to excessive hair growth. The 19-nortestosterones in low-dose oral contraceptives rarely cause hirsutism or acne.

**D. Idiopathic Hirsutism:** Hirsutism that occurs without adrenal or ovarian dysfunction and in the absence of any exogenous source of steroid hormones is termed **idiopathic hirsutism.** When normal levels of testosterone, unbound testosterone, DHEAS, dihydrotestosterone, and androstenedione are present, increased peripheral androgen metabolism may be responsible for excessive hair growth. Many patients with idiopathic hirsutism have an elevated level of serum androstanediol glucuronide, which is thought to reflect increased peripheral androgen metabolism in the skin and hair follicle.

In summary, hirsutism may suggest the presence of ovarian neoplasm or significant adrenal disease such as Cushing's syndrome, adrenal neoplasm, or congenital adrenal hyperplasia. Rarely, other endocrinologic disturbances such as hypothyroidism or acromegaly may be associated with excessive hair growth. Infertility may also accompany androgen excess and subsequent hirsutism either through anovulation or as a result of inadequate levels of progesterone in the luteal phase; this deficiency may lead to a shortened luteal phase, an endometrium incapable of supporting implantation of an embryo, or both.

## Physiology of Androgens

Androgens are steroids that stimulate the development of male secondary sex characteristics and consequently promote the growth of sexual hair. The major androgens are dihydrotestosterone, testosterone, DHEA, DHEAS, and androstenedione. In the nonpregnant woman, androgens are produced by both the ovaries and the adrenals as well as by peripheral conversion. In order to comprehend the role played by elevated levels of androgens in the development of hirsutism, one must understand the sources of androgens, their metabolic pathways and sites of action, and their interrelationship with other steroid hormones such as progestins, corticosteroids, and estrogens.

**A. Ovarian Production of Androgens:** Androgens are produced by the normal ovary as precursors in the synthesis of estrogen. In response to luteinizing hormone (LH), the theca cells of the preantral (secondary) ovarian follicle produce androstenedione and testosterone, whereas in response to follicle-stimulating hormone (FSH), the granulosa cells aromatize these androgens to the estrogens estrone and estradiol. This relationship between gonadotropins and follicular cells correlates well with the observed increase in androgens in anovulatory cycles. Many anovulatory women have increased levels of LH in their blood, as manifested by an increased LH:FSH ratio. Elevated levels of LH result in increased production of testosterone and androstenedione by the theca cells, whereas relatively lower levels of FSH result in a decreased conversion of these androgens to estrogens. Anovulation may lead to elevated levels of testosterone and androstenedione that may be manifested as hirsutism, dysfunctional uterine bleeding, or infertility.

**B. Adrenal Production of Androgens:** Androgens are produced by the adrenal cortex mainly as intermediates in the formation of cortisol. Consequently, when corticosteroid production is increased, as in Cushing's syndrome, the production of androgens in the zona reticularis and zona fasciculata of the adrenal cortex may increase and lead to hirsutism.

Elevated levels of androgens, including DHEA, DHEAS, androstenedione, and androstanediol, may occur in congenital adrenal hyperplasia. Certain enzyme defects, eg, deficiency of 21-hydroxylase, 11β-hydroxylase, or 3β-ol-dehydrogenase, result in impaired synthesis of cortisol. As a consequence, the pituitary increases ACTH secretion in an effort to normalize cortisol levels. Higher levels of ACTH stimulate adrenal production of certain intermediates in the biosynthetic pathway of cortisol. Because of enzyme defects, however, these intermediates cannot be used for cortisol production but are instead shunted into biosynthetic pathways for androgen production. When these enzymatic defects are manifested in the neonatal period, ambiguous genitalia are seen in female infants. When the enzymatic defects in cortisol metabolism occur later in life, as in adult-onset congenital adrenal hyperplasia, hirsutism may result.

**1. Testosterone–**Testosterone, by virtue of its plasma concentration and its potency, is one of the major androgens. It is the second most potent androgen after dihydrotestosterone, and circulating levels are 20–80 ng/dL in adult women. The ovary and the adrenal contribute equally to testosterone production, with each supplying about 25% of the total circulating level. The other 50% of circulating testosterone is derived from peripheral conversion of androstenedione, although the ovarian contribution to testosterone levels may increase during the periovulatory portion of the menstrual cycle. Peripheral levels of testosterone display a slight diurnal variation that parallels that of cortisol. In normal women, 99% of testosterone is protein-bound, with 80% bound to sex hormone-binding globulin (SHBG), about 19% loosely bound to albumin, and 1% free and unbound. In hirsute women, increased androgen levels may decrease production of SHBG by the liver, and the free, biologically active fraction of testosterone may increase to 2–3%. Therefore, normal total serum levels of testosterone in a hirsute woman can reflect a decreased level of SHBG with an increase in the free testosterone fraction.

**2. Dihydrotestosterone–**Circulating levels of dihydrotestosterone, the most potent androgen, are only one-tenth those of testosterone (2–8 ng/dL). Although it is secreted by both the ovary and the adrenal gland, most dihydrotestosterone is produced by peripheral conversion of testosterone by 5α-reductase. In tissues sensitive to dihydrotestosterone (eg, the hair follicle), dihydrotestosterone enters the cell and binds to cytosol receptors. The dihydrotestosterone receptor complex then enters the cell nucleus, where it binds to DNA, leading to increased hair growth and initiating the conversion of vellus to terminal hair.

**3. Androstenedione–**Androstenedione, one of the 17-ketosteroids, is not very potent, exerting only 20% of the effect of testosterone. Synthesis and secretion occur mostly in the ovaries and adrenals in equal amounts, with the remaining 10% being produced peripherally. Androstenedione levels display a diurnal variation paralleling that of cortisol and may simultaneously increase by as much as 50% when cortisol levels rise. Moreover, periovulatory increases in androstenedione levels can also be observed. In contrast to testosterone, androstenedione is bound mainly to albumin and secondarily to SHBG.

**4. DHEA and DHEAS**–DHEA and DHEAS, both weak androgens exerting approximately 3% of the effect of testosterone, are the other major precursors of 17-ketosteroids. DHEA is primarily produced by the adrenal (60–70%), with ovarian production and hydrolysis of DHEAS accounting for the remainder. DHEA has a large diurnal variation similar to that of cortisol. Conversely, DHEAS is derived almost entirely from the adrenal, has only slight diurnal variation, and circulates in high concentrations. DHEAS level may provide a good clinical assessment of adrenal function.

## Physiology of Hair Growth

The hair follicle and its sebaceous gland, which together make up the pilosebaceous unit, are sensitive to the effects of sex hormones, especially androgens. Testosterone and dihydrotestosterone can initiate growth and increase both the diameter and pigmentation of hair. Conversely, estrogens can retard the growth rate and result in finer hair with less pigmentation.

The growth and development of the hair follicle may also be influenced by genetic factors. Although males and females are born with equal numbers of hair follicles, racial and ethnic differences are noted in the concentration of hair follicles; Whites have a greater number of hair follicles than blacks, who in turn have a greater number than Asians. Different ethnic groups within each race may also exhibit differences in hair follicle concentrations; eg, whites of Mediterranean ancestry have a greater concentration of hair follicles than those of Nordic ancestry.

Hair growth is cyclic. The three phases of the cycle are (1) anagen (growth), (2) catagen (rapid involution), (3) telogen (inactivity). The length of each hair is determined by the relative durations of anagen and telogen and varies with different locations on the body, although each hair follicle has its own growth cycle independent of adjacent hair follicles. Scalp hair has a long anagen, from 2 to 6 years, with a short telogen. Conversely, short hair, such as eyelashes or eyebrows, has a long telogen and a short anagen.

The hair follicle begins to develop within the first 2 months of gestation, and by birth, a child possesses all of the hair follicles he or she will ever have. Hair first appears as vellus hair, which is fine, short, and lightly pigmented. During puberty, adrenal and ovarian androgen levels rise, converting vellus hair to terminal hair, which is coarse, long, and more heavily pigmented. Although conversion of vellus hair to terminal hair is essentially irreversible, removal of the androgenic stimulus will slow hair growth and thereby stop the conversion of vellus to terminal hair.

The skin and hair follicles are androgen-responsive and thus have the capacity to metabolize androgens. DHEA, androstenedione, or testosterone enters the target cell and is reduced to dihydrotestosterone by 5α-reductase. Dihydrotestosterone is then bound to a cytoplasmic receptor protein that transports the androgen into the cell nucleus, where it is bound to chromatin and initiates transcription of stored genetic information. In the hair follicle, this promotes hair growth. In hirsute women, metabolic conversion of androgens to dihydrotestosterone appears to be accelerated. This results in irreversible conversion of vellus hair to terminal hair in areas of androgen-sensitive skin.

## Diagnosis & Clinical Findings

The diagnosis of hirsutism begins with a careful medical history, menstrual history, and physical examination. Care should be taken to distinguish hypertrichosis from hirsutism and to rule out any history of drug ingestion that might cause excessive hair growth. The menstrual history is particularly important; if the patient presents with a long history of irregular menses with slow onset of hirsutism beginning at puberty or in the early 20s, polycystic ovary disease is suggested. However, an androgen-producing tumor should be strongly suspected when a woman with a normal menstrual history presents with sudden onset of irregular menses followed by amenorrhea, hirsutism, and virilization. The patient's age at the onset of hirsutism is also important. Genetic anomalies such as mosaic cells containing Y chromosomes or incomplete androgen insensitivity syndrome may produce signs of androgen stimulation (eg, hirsutism) at puberty, as is also noted in cases of late-onset congenital adrenal hyperplasia. Hirsutism presenting in childhood may be due to congenital adrenal hyperplasia or androgen-producing tumors. Hirsutism or virilization during pregnancy raises the suspicion of a luteoma of pregnancy or bilateral theca-lutein cysts.

**A. Symptoms and Signs:** During physical examination of the hirsute female, particular attention is paid to body habitus, hair pattern, and pelvic examination. The physical stigmas of Cushing's syndrome, including centripetal obesity, wasting of the extremities, fat deposition in supraclavicular areas as well as in the neck and face, facial plethora, and wide cutaneous striae are usually apparent if this syndrome is present. When acromegaly is present, overgrowth of the viscera and soft body tissues, as well as that of the bones of the hands, feet, and face, can be seen on physical examination. If hypothyroidism is present, thickening of the skin of the lips, fingers, lower leg, or lower eyelid may be present, along with complaints of lethargy, cold intolerance, constipation, and voice changes.

**B. Laboratory Findings:** Investigators disagree about which androgens should be measured in the evaluation of hirsutism. Laboratory evaluation should seek to identify life-threatening conditions associated with hyperandrogenism, such as Cushing's syndrome, congenital adrenal hyperplasia, and ovarian or adrenal tumors. Serum testosterone, DHEAS, and 17-hydroxyprogesterone can be obtained for screening purposes. The presence of hirsutism in a patient with a normal testosterone level already indicates increased androgen effects. The determination of the serum free testosterone level is expensive and does not add any useful clinical information. Further testing is dictated based on history and physical examination. If a woman is oligo-ovulatory or anovulatory, determination of FSH, LH, and prolactin levels is helpful. Elevated levels of LH, particularly when the LH:FSH ratio is 3 or higher, suggest polycystic ovary disease. A mildly elevated prolactin may be seen in patients with polycystic ovarian disease, or prolactin may be elevated suggesting a prolactinoma as the source of menstrual dysfunction and as a possible contributing factor in hirsutism as a result of increased adrenal stimulation.

**1. Testosterone levels**–A serum testosterone level of less than 200 ng/dL will rule out almost all of the testosterone-secreting neoplasms. A total testosterone level higher than 200 ng/dL should be considered evidence of ovarian tumor until proven otherwise; few adrenal tumors produce testosterone. Pelvic examination generally reveals a palpable ovarian mass; however, if the examination is limited by the patient's body habitus, pelvic ultrasonography may help delineate an ovarian mass. A history of rapidly developing hirsutism, palpable ovarian tumor, and testosterone levels higher than 200 ng/ dL necessitate laparotomy. However, if the testosterone level is higher than 200 ng/dL and no ovarian mass is identified, computed tomography (CT) scan or magnetic resonance imaging (MRI) of the adrenal glands should be performed before laparotomy to rule out the rare testosterone-producing adrenal tumor. CT scan and MRI of the adrenal glands have proven to be sensitive diagnostic techniques that have generally replaced selective venous sampling and selective angiography. Selective bilateral venous catheterization of adrenal and ovarian veins has limited clinical usefulness, since it is technically difficult and hazardous to perform, and its diagnostic sensitivity is poor.

**2. DHEAS levels**–A normal or slightly elevated DHEAS level will exclude a significant adrenal pathology. Adrenal tumors usually produce markedly elevated serum DHEAS levels or increased 17-ketosteroids in 24-hour urine collections. The serum DHEAS level is reliable and convenient and has replaced the 24-hour urine collection for measurement of 17-ketosteroids in most laboratories. If the DHEAS level is elevated or if Cushing's syndrome is suspected, then either a 24-hour urinary free cortisol level should be obtained or an overnight dexamethasone suppression test should be performed.

**3. Hypercortisolism (Cushing's syndrome)**–An overnight dexamethasone suppression test may be used as a simple outpatient screening test. It is easily performed on an outpatient basis and has a low incidence of false-negative results. A baseline morning plasma cortisol level is drawn and then dexamethasone, 1 mg orally, is given at 11:00 PM, a plasma cortisol level is obtained at 8:00 AM the next morning. In normal patients, cortisol levels are suppressed to 5 ng/dL, whereas in patients with Cushing's syndrome cortisol levels fall but do not go below 5 ng/dL. This test has a false-negative rate of less than 2% and a false-positive rate of 1%. The false-positive rate is much higher in obese patients, chronically ill patients, and patients taking phenytoin.

The most accurate screening test for documentation of hypercortisolism is measurement of urinary free cortisol over a 24-hour period. Values greater than 100 ng/d are considered abnormal and further evaluation is warranted. Values greater than 250 ng/d are virtually diagnostic of Cushing's syndrome. The 24-hour urinary free cortisol determination is an excellent screening test because it has a low incidence of false-positive and false-negative results and clearly distinguishes between patients with Cushing's syndrome and normal subjects.

If screening tests give equivocal results, the low-dose dexamethasone suppression test can be performed for verification of the diagnosis of Cushing's syndrome. Two baseline 24-hour urine collections for measurement of 17-hydroxycorticosteroids (17-OHCS) are obtained. Low-dose dexamethasone, 0.5 mg orally every 6 hours, is then given to 2 consecutive days. During the second day, urine is collected for 24 hours. In normal women, 17-OHCS levels are suppressed to less than 3 mg/d or to values 50% less than baseline. Failure to suppress is diagnostic of Cushing's syndrome.

**a. Differentiation of Cushing's disease and Cushing's syndrome**–After Cushing's syndrome is diagnosed, further testing differentiates the underlying disorder. ACTH-dependent hypercortisolism may be secondary to excess production of ACTH by the pituitary gland (Cushing's disease) or ectopic production of ACTH by a nonpituitary tumor. ACTH-independent hypercortisolism results from an adrenal tumor. Increasingly, as reliable ACTH radioimmunoassays become more widely available, an ACTH-directed approach will be used. Since this method is not readily available, the high-dose dexamethasone suppression test is most frequently used for differential diagnosis.

In the **ACTH-directed approach,** baseline ACTH levels are measured. Levels are normal or elevated in Cushing's disease and ectopic ACTH production. Levels are low or undetectable with primary adrenal disease. Differentiation of Cushing's disease from ectopic ACTH production requires administration of corticotropin-releasing hormone. Increased ACTH secretion in response to corticotropin-releasing hormone is diagnostic of Cushing's disease.

The **high-dose dexamethasone suppression test**

has recently been reevaluated. It requires 6 days of urine collection. On days 1 and 2, no dexamethasone is administered. The patient then receives 0.5 mg of dexamethasone every 6 hours on days 3 and 4 (low dose). The dose of dexamethasone is then increased to 2 mg every 6 hours on days 5 and 6. Urine volume and creatinine are measured to confirm collection completeness. The diagnosis of Cushing's disease can be made with 100% specificity when both urinary free cortisol and 17-OHCS are measured and suppression of urinary free cortisol by 90% and 17-OHCS by 64% are noted.

**b. Further studies**–To confirm the diagnosis of Cushing's disease and to localize the lesion, bilateral inferior petrosal sinus sampling is usually necessary. A petrosal sinus to peripheral venous ACTH ratio greater than 2:1 is diagnostic of Cushing's disease. More available are CT scan or MRI of the sella turcica, which may be used to attempt localization of an ACTH-secreting tumor. Primary adrenal disease is most often confirmed with adrenal CT scan. CT scan or MRI of the lung is indicated with ectopic ACTH secretion since this is the most common site of ectopic ACTH production.

**4. Congenital adrenal hyperplasia**–Late-onset congenital adrenal hyperplasia is present in 1–5% of women who complain of hirsutism. The most common form of this disease is due to deficiency of the 21-hydroxylase enzyme. This results in increased levels of circulating 17-hydroxyprogesterone. Suspicion of adult-onset congenital adrenal hyperplasia increases with severe hirsutism, typically beginning at puberty, a strong family history of hirsutism, short stature, and evidence of defeminization on examination (eg, flattening of the breasts). The 2 laboratory tests used to diagnose congenital adrenal hyperplasia are basal morning 17-hydroxyprogesterone and the ACTH stimulation test.

**a. Basal 17-hydroxyprogesterone**–17-hydroxyprogesterone is the single most accurate diagnostic test for congenital adrenal hyperplasia due to 21-hydroxylase deficiency. It is a cost-effective screen for women with hirsutism and other clinical findings suggestive of congenital adrenal hyperplasia. 17-Hydroxyprogesterone should be measured first thing in the morning and only during the follicular phase of the menstrual cycle. Normal levels are less than 200 ng/dL. Levels ranging between 200 and 1000 ng/dL warrant further evaluation. Levels greater than 1000 ng/dL are virtually diagnostic of 21-hydroxylase deficiency. In patients with a mild enzyme deficiency or a partial block at the 21-hydroxylation step in the biosynthesis of cortisol, basal 17-hydroxyprogesterone levels may not be elevated and ACTH stimulation may be required for diagnosis.

**b. ACTH stimulation test**–The ACTH-induced increase in 17-hydroxyprogesterone is a sensitive diagnostic test for congenital adrenal hyperplasia. 17-Hydroxyprogesterone is measured 30 minutes after an intravenous injection of 250 μg of synthetic ACTH. Values rarely exceed 400 ng/dL in normal women. When values are elevated the nomogram by Marie New can be used to differentiate patients with nonclassic and classic disease. Patients with classic disease will have the highest values after stimulation.

**5. Androstanediol glucuronide levels**–The measurement of serum androstanediol glucuronide has been proposed as a good marker of peripheral androgen production and activity in hirsutism. Serum androstanediol glucuronide may be elevated in idiopathic hirsutism as a result of altered metabolism or increased utilization of androgen in the skin and hair follicle. Although this test is useful for research, its clinical applicability remains limited. Because of high costs and limited usefulness, the test for androstanediol glucuronide levels is not currently recommended in the routine evaluation of hirsutism.

## Differential Diagnosis

Hirsutism should be differentiated from both virilization and hypertrichosis, since the cause and treatment of these disorders may be different. **Virilization** is characterized by more extensive androgen-induced changes than hirsutism alone; these changes include acne, increased oiliness of the skin, temporal balding, clitoromegaly, deepening of the voice, development of the male muscular pattern and body habitus (in extreme cases), and atrophy of the breasts.

**Hypertrichosis** is also characterized by excessive growth of hair, but the term denotes increased growth of nonsexual hair, eg, hair on the forehead, lower leg, or forearm. The hair is usually fine-textured and is not caused by androgen excess or abnormal androgen metabolism; heredity, certain drugs, physical irritation (trauma to the skin), or even starvation may be responsible. Drug ingestion is the most common cause, however. Phenytoin, diazoxide, and minoxidil are known to cause a generalized increase in hair growth. Penicillamine and streptomycin have been associated with increased hair growth in infants and children. In addition, inadvertent ingestion of the fungicide hexachlorobenzene has also caused hypertrichosis. Diseases such as porphyria, hypothyroidism, dermatomyositis, acromegaly, Hurler's syndrome, trisomy E, and Cornelia de Lange's syndrome may be associated with hypertrichosis.

## Treatment

The selection of therapy for hirsutism (Table 55–2) depends on the physical and laboratory findings as well as on the patient's desire for childbearing. After evaluation has ruled out neoplasm or a serious disease process, a mildly hirsute woman with normal menstrual cycles may require only reassurance. A moderately or severely hirsute woman with menstrual irregularities requires treatment. For women not desiring childbearing in the near future, medical therapy consisting of adrenal or ovarian suppression or the block-

**Table 55–2.** Treatment of hirsutism.

| Medical | Cosmetic |
|---|---|
| Oral contraceptives | Waxing |
| Progestins | Depilatories |
| Spironolactone | Electrolysis |
| Corticosteroids | Shaving |
| GnRH analogs | Surgical depilation |
| Cyproterone acetate* | |

*Not available in the USA.

ing of peripheral androgen effects is advised. If, on the other hand, infertility is a major concern, ovulation induction with the appropriate drug (eg, clomiphene, bromocriptine, hMG, or gonatropin-releasing hormones [GnRH]) is started after appropriate evaluation.

In the minority of hirsute patients in whom a specific cause can be identified, therapy should be directed toward the underlying disorder. Ovarian and adrenal tumors should be surgically excised. Patients with congenital or acquired adrenal hyperplasia should receive hydrocortisone to decrease ACTH levels and thereby decrease formation of the androgenic precursors of cortisol. Women with Cushing's disease may be treated with transsphenoidal pituitary microsurgery or, if that fails, with bilateral adrenalectomy or pituitary irradiation. When Cushing's syndrome is caused by an adrenal tumor, simple adrenalectomy is sufficient. Acromegaly can be treated by transsphenoidal hypophysectomy.

In most hirsute, hyperandrogenic women, no specific cause can be identified. Androgen excess may derive from the ovary, adrenal, or both, with ovarian origin being the most common. Androgen levels obtained during the preliminary evaluation may assist in determining the source of the hyperandrogenism, and therapy can be directed accordingly.

The medical treatment of hirsutism is not completely successful, and the response rate has been reported to be between 23% and 95%, depending on the drug and the dosage used. The drugs most commonly used to treat hirsutism include oral contraceptives, spironolactone, GnRH analogs, medroxyprogesterone acetate, and corticosteroids (eg dexamethasone).

All drug therapy should seek to change at least one of the 5 major aspects of androgen metabolism: (1) production of androgens can be decreased; (2) the metabolic clearance rate of androgens can be increased; (3) androgen receptors can be competitively inhibited; (4) enzymes involved in the peripheral production of testosterone or conversion of testosterone to dihydrotestosterone can be competitively inhibited or blocked; and (5) the amount of SHBG can be increased.

**A. Combination Oral Contraceptives:** Oral contraceptives have been extensively used to treat hirsutism. Their effect is exerted through a wide range of actions. The combination pill contains both estrogen and progestins and prevents ovulation by inhibiting gonadotropin secretion. Inhibition of LH secretion is mainly accomplished by the addition of the progestational component. When adequate suppression of LH is achieved, ovarian steroidogenesis is suppressed, leading to decreased testosterone production by the ovary. Testosterone levels can be decreased with the use of any combination birth control pill, including the low-dose pill (0.03 mg of estrogen). A decline in plasma testosterone can be seen as soon as 1 week after treatment has been started; levels may decrease to normal by 3 months. Hair growth is reportedly decreased in 50–60% of patients taking combination birth control pills. Use of a low-dose pill (less than or equal to 35 ng of estrogen) allows for suppression of testosterone production while minimizing estrogen-related side effects.

The estrogen component decreases the androgenic effects of plasma testosterone by elevating SHBG levels. Since only the unbound form of testosterone is available to initiate a biologic response, increasing the bound fraction of testosterone by increasing SHBG levels leads to a decrease in testosterone-mediated effects.

Most progestins used in the combination pill are derivatives of testosterone. Known as 19-nortestosterones, their major hormonal effect is progestational; however, androgenic properties are not totally eliminated. Thus, side effects can include acne, oily skin, and hirsutism. Recently, a new generation of oral contraceptives containing newly available progestins has been released. Studies suggest that these new progestins, desogestrel, gestodene, and norgestimate, have fewer androgenic side effects. If confirmed, they may represent first-line oral contraceptive therapy for patients with mild to moderate hirsutism.

Several studies have shown decreased levels of DHEAS in both hirsute and normal women taking oral contraceptives. Since DHEAS is mainly of adrenal origin, combination birth control pills may exert a significant suppressive effect on the production of adrenal androgens. Although the mechanism of action is presently unclear, this effect is probably due (at least in part) to suppression of ACTH release. The ability of combination birth control pills to lower the serum levels of DHEAS has several therapeutic implications. First, although DHEAS is low in biologic potency, it can serve as a precursor for peripheral conversion to more biologically potent androgens, and elevated levels of DHEAS can therefore be clinically manifested as hirsutism. Second, the ability of combination birth control pills to suppress both adrenal and ovarian androgen production, resulting in a significant reduction of androstenedione, DHEAS, and testosterone, may make these pills an even more attractive therapeutic option.

**B. Spironolactone:** Spironolactone, an aldosterone antagonist traditionally used as a diuretic in the treatment of hypertension, is now also used to treat hirsutism. It possesses antiandrogenic properties and exerts its peripheral antiandrogenic effects in the hair follicle by competing for androgenic receptors and displacing dihydrotestosterone at both nuclear and cytosol receptors. It also lowers testosterone levels by inhibiting the cytochrome P-450 mono-oxygenases that are required for biosynthesis of androgens in gonadal and adrenal steroid-producing cells. Serum levels of SHBG, DHEAS, and DHEA are unaltered by treatment with spironolactone. The dosage used for treatment of hirsutism has varied between 50 and 200 mg/d. Serum androgen levels will drop within a few days of treatment, and a clinical response can usually be seen within 2–5 months. Side effects are mild; transient diuresis and polydipsia have been noted in the first few days of treatment, and some disturbance of the menstrual cycle has been found, but no long-term problems have been encountered. Because spironolactone is a potent antiandrogen, all women using spironolactone should practice adequate contraception.

**C. Dexamethasone:** Dexamethasone is used mainly to treat hirsutism in patients with hyperandrogenism of adrenal origin. Chronic low-dose dexamethasone, 0.5–1 mg orally at night, will provide adequate adrenal androgen suppression. Diminution of hair growth is reported in 16–70% of patients. Therapy must be closely monitored by determination of morning cortisol levels to prevent oversuppression of the pituitary-adrenal axis. Aside from the obvious medical implications of long-term adrenal suppression, frequent side effects of dexamethasone therapy are fluid retention and weight gain.

**D. Gonadotropin-releasing Hormone (GnRH) Agonists:** GnRH analogs inhibit the secretion of gonadotropins from the pituitary gland, thereby inhibiting the secretion of androgens and estrogens from the ovary. Although GnRH agonists acutely stimulate ovarian production of androgens and estrogens, continued therapy causes a sustained decrease in ovarian steroid production compared with pretreatment levels. This suppression continues for the duration of GnRH agonist therapy. Significant decreases in serum levels of estradiol, testosterone, and androstenedione occur during treatment, although androgens of adrenal origin (such as DHEAS) are usually not affected.

GnRH analogs are particularly useful in moderate to severe hirsutism due to ovarian hyperthecosis and hyperandrogenism secondary to insulin resistance (HAIR-AN syndrome). A potential risk of osteoporosis exists with long-term use of GnRH analogs since estradiol levels, as well as androgen levels, are decreased during continued therapy. However, concomitant use of estrogen and progesterone replacement therapy may counteract the adverse effects of hypoestrogenism.

**E. Medroxyprogesterone Acetate:** Hirsute women who cannot or will not take the combination birth control pill may benefit from progestins alone.

Medroxyprogesterone acetate in either the regular form (eg, Provera, 30–40 mg/d orally) or depot form (Depo-Provera, 150–400 mg intramuscularly every 3 months) is an effective treatment for hirsutism; however, the depot form may cause long-term ovarian suppression and should not be used in women desiring pregnancy in the near future. The mechanism of action of these progestins is 2-fold. First, LH production is decreased, leading to decreased production of testosterone. Second, metabolic clearance of testosterone is increased. Medroxyprogesterone acetate induces hepatic testosterone A ring 5α-reductase activity, leading to increased removal of testosterone from the blood. Decreased production and increased clearance result in decreased testosterone levels that produce the clinically desired effect.

**F. Cyproterone Acetate:** This potent progestational agent is widely used in Europe to treat hirsutism. Antiandrogenic effects result from competitive displacement of dihydrotestosterone from its receptor and reduction of 5α-reductase activity in the skin. Progestational activity results in gonadotropin suppression with subsequent suppression of ovarian testosterone secretion. Administered orally each day or by intramuscular injection monthly, cyproterone acetate is combined with oral or topical estrogen to counter hypoestrogenic effects of gonadotropin suppression. Although highly effective, it is not available in the USA.

**G. Other Agents: Flutamide** is a potent, highly specific, nonsteroidal antiandrogen with no intrinsic hormonal or antigonadotropin activity. Although the exact mechanism of action is unknown, it competitively inhibits target tissue androgen receptor sites. Recent studies suggest that 250 mg 1–3 times daily is a highly effective treatment for moderate to severe hirsutism. No side effects occur at low doses. Higher doses may cause menstrual irregularity, amenorrhea, or dry skin. Because of possible teratogenic effects, contraception must be used with this therapy.

**Cimetidine**, an $H_2$ receptor antagonist, has weak antiandrogenic properties. Recent studies show minimal or no beneficial effect on hirsutism.

**Ketoconazole** is a synthetic imidazole derivative, which blocks adrenal and gonadal steroidogenesis; it has been advocated by some as a treatment for hirsutism. However, serious side effects result in poor compliance and preclude long-term use. Its use should be avoided since safer therapeutic regimens exist.

**H. Surgical Treatment:**

**1. Bilateral Oophorectomy:** Failure to respond to an adequate trial of medical management often reflects noncompliance. However, older women despite good compliance may fail medical management due to ovarian hyperthecosis. For these women, bilateral oophorectomy may be justified as definitive therapy.

**2. Wedge Resection of the Ovary:** Although

wedge resection of the ovary has been successfully used to induce ovulation, it is not recommended for the treatment of hirsutism. As a surgical procedure, it exposes patients to the risks of both anesthesia and possible formation of adhesions. More importantly, this procedure results in only a transient decrease in androgen levels and has successfully reduced the rate of hair growth in only 16% of patients. Wedge resection should not be used as a treatment for hirsutism.

## Complications & Prognosis

The treatment for hirsutism can be frustrating for both patient and physician because of the physiologic properties of hair itself. The growth cycle of hair is long, varying between 6 and 24 months, and the conversion of vellus hair to terminal hair is essentially irreversible. Also, once hair growth has been stimulated by excessive androgen levels, maintenance of that same growth rate requires much less androgen. Patients must be advised that a response to therapy may not be seen for 6–12 months and that although it is possible to prevent further conversion of vellus hair to terminal hair, little change will be seen in the total number of terminal hairs. Some patients may note a lighter hair color and a decrease in the diameter of the hair shaft with therapy. Cosmetic treatment of excess hair consists of shaving, plucking, bleaching, waxing, or use of depilatories; however, shaving and plucking may cause infection and scarring and are not recommended. Permanent hair removal may be accomplished only by electrolysis (electrocoagulation of the hair root, or papilla), which is costly and uncomfortable, or by depilation. Unless there is excessive hirsutism, electrolysis should be delayed until after 6–12 months of medical therapy have been completed.

Patients who exhibit progressive hirsutism while receiving hormonal therapy or patients whose circulating androgen levels fail to decrease as expected should undergo further evaluation. If androgen levels are not suppressed with appropriate therapy, the possibility of a slowly developing neoplasm should be considered. Levels of testosterone and DHEAS should be monitored and the adrenal glands and ovaries reevaluated.

When adequate suppression of DHEAS and testosterone has been maintained for 6–12 months but a satisfactory reduction in new hair growth has not occurred, several options are available. The dose of the current medication can be increased; a new medication can be substituted; or a new medication can be added. It is frequently impossible to increase the dose of the initial medication, since the incidence of side effects may increase as the drug dosage increases. Likewise, it is not always easy to switch medications, since choice of the initial drug may have been guided by specific therapeutic considerations (eg, hirsute women who desire contraception may be treated with combination birth control pills, whereas hirsutism associated with hypertension may be treated with spironolactone). Some authors have recommended adding a second medication to the treatment regimen for hirsutism unresponsive to therapy. Although there is little experience with combination drug treatment for hirsutism, drugs that act at different sites may offer the best results; eg, combination birth control pills that act chiefly through decreased production of ovarian steroids may be combined with spironolactone, which acts mainly at the peripheral androgen receptors.

Treatment for hirsutism must be individualized and based on the results of a thorough history, physical examination, and laboratory studies. After therapy has begun, the patient's progress can be monitored on the basis of both clinical appearance and laboratory values. The patient should be educated about her disorder in order to prevent unrealistic expectations of therapy and to become aware of any side effects that might appear during therapy. Adjunctive therapy is almost always necessary with any medical treatment for hirsutism. Depilatories and electrolysis are frequently needed to remove the terminal hair already present; these methods, when combined with medical therapy, offer the best cosmetic result.

## REFERENCES

Adashi EY: Potential utility of gonadotropin-releasing hormone agonists in the management of ovarian hyperandrogenism. Fertil Steril 1990;52:765.

Andreyko JL, Monroe SE, Jaffe RB: Treatment of hirsutism with a gonadotrophin-releasing hormone agonist (Nafarelin). J Clin Endocrinol Metab 1986;63:854.

Barnes RB: Adrenal dysfunction and hirsutism. Clin Obstet Gynecol 1991;34:827.

Barth JH et al: Spironolactone is an effective and well tolerated systemic antiandrogen therapy for hirsute women. J Clin Endocrinol Metab 1989;68:966.

Carmina E, Lobo RA: Peripheral androgen blockade versus glandular androgen suppression in the treatment of hirsutism. Obstet Gynecol 1991;78:845.

Chang RJ et al: Steroid secretion in polycystic ovarian disease after ovarian suppression by a long-acting gonadotropin-releasing hormone agonist. J Clin Endocrinol Metab 1983;56:897.

Chetkowski RJ et al: The incidence of late-onset congenital adrenal hyperplasia due to 21-hydroxylase deficiency among hirsute women. J Clin Endocrinol Metab 1984;58:595.

Cusan L et al: Treatment of hirsutism with the pure antiandrogen flutamide. J Am Acad Dermatol 1990;23:462.

Falsetti L, Galbignani E: Long-term treatment with the combination ethinylestradiol and cyproterone acetate in polycystic ovary syndrome. Contraception 1990;42:611.

Fern M, Rose DP, Fern EB: Effect of oral contraceptives on plasma androgenic steroids and their precursors. Obstet Gynecol 1978;51:541.

Flack MR et al: Urine free cortisol in the high-dose dexamethasone suppression test for the differential diagnosis of the Cushing syndrome. Ann Intern Med 1992;116: 221.

Golditch IM, Price VH: Treatment of hirsutism with cimetidine. Obstet Gynecol 1990;75:911.

Hage JJ, Bouman FG: Surgical depilation for the treatment of pseudofolliculitis or local hirsutism of the face: Experience in the first 40 patients. Plastic Reconstr Surg 1991;88:446.

Hauner H et al: Fat distribution, endocrine and metabolic profile in obese women with and without hirsutism. Metabolism 1988;37:281.

Jasonni VM et al: treatment of hirsutism by an association of cyproterone acetate and transdermal 17β-estradiol. Fertil Steril 1991;55:742.

Kessell B, Liu J: Clinical and laboratory evaluation of hirsutism. Clin Obstet Gynecol 1991;34:805.

Kuttenn F et al: Late-onset adrenal hyperplasia in hirsutism. N Engl J Med 1985;313:224.

Lissak A et al: Treatment of hirsutism with cimetidine: A prospective randomized controlled trial. Fertil Steril 1989;51:247.

Lobo RA, Goebelsmann U: Adult manifestation of congenital adrenal hyperplasia due to incomplete 21-hydroxylase deficiency mimicking polycystic ovarian disease. Am J Obstet Gynecol 1980;138:720.

Marcondes JA et al: Monthly cyproterone acetate in the treatment of hirsute women: Clinical and laboratory effects. Fertil Steril 1990;53:40.

Marcondes JA et al: Treatment of hirsutism in women with flutamide. Fertil Steril 1992;57:543.

Mongioi A et al: Effect of gonadotrophin-releasing hormone analogue administration on serum gonadotrophin and steroid levels in patients with polycystic ovarian disease. Acta Endocrinol 1986;111:228.

Motta T et al: Flutamide in the treatment of hirsutism. Int J Gynecol Obstet 1991;35:155.

New MI et al: Genotyping steroid 21-hydroxylase deficiency: Hormonal reference data. J Clin Endocrinol Metab 1983;57:320.

O'Brien RC et al: Comparison of sequential cyproterone acetate/estrogen versus spironolactone/oral contraceptive in the treatment of hirsutism. J Clin Endocrinol Metab 1991;72:1008.

Pang SY et al: Hirsutism, polycystic ovarian disease, and ovarian 17-ketosteroid reductase deficiency. N Engl J Med 1987;316:1295.

Pittaway DE: Evaluation and treatment of unresponsive hirsutism. Sex Med Today 1985;9:14.

Pittaway DE, Maxson WS, Wentz AC: Spironolactone in combination drug therapy for unresponsive hirsutism. Fertil Steril 1985;43:878.

Porcile A, Gallardo E: Long-term treatment of hirsutism: Desogestrel compared with cyproterone acetate in oral contraceptives. Fertil Steril 1991;55:877.

Rebar RW: Practical evaluation of hormonal status. Chap 24, pp 830–886. In: *Reproductive Endocrinology: Physiology, Pathology and Clinical Management,* 3rd ed. Yen SSC, Jaffe RB (editors). WB Saunders, 1991.

Rittmaster RS, Givner ML: Effect of daily and alternate day low dose prednisone on serum cortisol and adrenal androgens in hirsute women. J Clin Endocrinol Metab 1988;67:400.

Rittmaster RS, thompson DL: Effect of leuprolide and dexamethasone on hair growth and hormone levels in hirsute women: The relative importance of the ovary and the adrenal in the pathogenesis of hirsutism. J Clin Endocrinol Metab 1990;79:1096.

Ruutiainen K et al: Androgen parameters in hirsute women: Correlations with body mass index and age. Fertil Steril 1988;50:255.

Ruutiainen K et al: Influence of body mass index and age on the grade of hair growth in hirsute women or reproductive ages. Fertil Steril 1988;50:260.

Sciarra F, Concolino TG, DiSilverio FD: Antiandrogens: Clinical applications. J Steroid Biochem Molec Biol 1990;37:349.

Shaw JC: Spironolactone in dermatologic therapy. J Am Acad Dermatol 1991;24:236.

Speroff L, DeCherney A: Evaluation of a new generation of oral contraceptives. Obstet Gynecol 1992;81:1034.

Speroff L, Glass RH, Kase NG: Hirsutism. Chap 7, pp 233–263. In: *Blaustein's Pathology of the Female Genital Tract,* 3rd ed. Kurman RJ (editor). Springer-Verlag, 1987.

Venturoli S et al: Ketoconazole therapy for women with acne and/or hirsutism. J Clin Endocrinol Metab 1990; 71:335.

Vermeulen A, Rubens R: Effects of cyproterone acetate plus ethinylestradiol low dose on plasma androgens and lipids in mildly hirsute or acneic young women. Contraception 1988;38:419.

Wagner RF: Physical methods for the management of hirsutism. Cutis 1990;45:319.

Wajchenberg BL et al: The source(s) of estrogen production in hirsute women with polycystic ovarian disease as determined by simultaneous adrenal and ovarian venous catheterization. Fertil Steril 1988;49:56.

Wiebe RH, Morris CV: Effect of an oral contraceptive on adrenal and ovarian androgenic steroids. Obstet Gynecol 1984;63:12.

Yen SSC: Chronic anovulation caused by peripheral endocrine disorders. Chap 17, pp 576–630. In: *Reproductive Endocrinology: Physiology, Pathology and Clinical Management,* 3rd ed. Yen SSC, Jaffe RB (editors). WB Saunders, 1991.

Young RH, Scully RE: Sex cord-stromal, steroid cell, and other ovarian tumors with endocrine, paracrine, and paraneoplastic manifestations. Chap 19, pp 607–658. In: *Blaustein's Pathology of the Female Genital Tract,* 3rd ed. Kurman RJ (editor). Springer-Verlag, 1987.

# 56

# In Vitro Fertilization & Related Techniques

*Alan H. DeCherney, MD, Alan S. Penzias, MD, & Ian H. Thorneycroft, MD, PhD*

## IN VITRO FERTILIZATION

In vitro fertilization and embryo transfer (IVF-ET) involves removing eggs from the ovary, fertilizing them in the laboratory, and replacing them into the patient's uterus. The first live birth resulting from this technique occurred in June 1978. Since then, thousands of children have been born throughout the world after IVF-ET was used to help women who otherwise could not conceive.

IVF-ET techniques, as outlined here, are not experimental; they are part of the armamentarium of every fully equipped infertility service. As the success rate of IVF-ET improves with new developments, many conventional infertility therapies may become second-line treatments, and in vitro fertilization will become the primary therapy. Such is the case today for severe tubal disease, when pregnancy following tuboplasty is much less likely than pregnancy following in vitro fertilization.

Table 56–1 was drawn from the United States In Vitro Fertilization and Embryo Transfer registry for 1990. The table depicts the percentage of patients entering an IVF program who progress to oocyte retrieval and embryo transfer along with cycle outcome. This table shows that not all patients who begin an IVF cycle reach the egg retrieval stage. Some patients may respond poorly to stimulatory medications or ovulate prior to oocyte aspiration. An additional group of patients may undergo oocyte retrieval but not have an embryo transfer. These cases generally reflect couples with a severe male factor in whom oocyte fertilization fails to occur.

Approximately 20% of patients who undergo egg retrieval will become pregnant with sonographic documentation of an intrauterine pregnancy (clinical pregnancy); 80% of these patients will carry to term. Many "biochemical pregnancies" occur, but these should not be included in pregnancy statistics. (A biochemical pregnancy is one in which serum levels of human chorionic gonadotropin (hCG) rise and then fall before sonographic detection of pregnancy is possible.) Eggs are almost always obtained by aspiration, and under ordinary circumstances, approximately 85% of eggs will fertilize and cleave. The clinical pregnancy rate of approximately 20% per embryo transfer per IVF cycle, is close to the 20–25% pregnancy rate per cycle observed in spontaneous conceptions in the general population.

The success rate in IVF has been improved by replacing more than one embryo, but doing so increases the likelihood of multiple gestation. The ethical questions and medical problems associated with multiple gestation as IVF-ET becomes more successful are discussed at the end of this chapter.

## Indications

IVF-ET bypasses the mechanical transport functions of the female reproductive tract. It was first developed for patients with severe tubal disease, and it clearly offers the only hope of conception to patients who have had a bilateral salpingectomy or whose tubes are so badly damaged that they cannot function. Subsequently, in vitro fertilization has been applied to a variety of other infertility problems such as antisperm antibodies, endometriosis, oligospermia, and unexplained infertility. When the probability of conception by IVF-ET exceeds that of conception by conventional therapy, IVF-ET appears to be the procedure of choice.

Although IVF is successful in treating a large number of infertility problems, its success hinges upon entry of sperm into the egg. It was initially hoped that routine IVF-ET could be used to compensate for severe oligospermia (< 5 million sperm per mL). However, early results were highly variable. Recent advances in this area are now being applied in clinical practice. Newly developed microsurgical techniques now permit placement of sperm under the protective egg shell (zona pellucida) or even directly into the cytoplasm of the oocyte.

## Technique

**A. Superovulation:** All IVF-ET programs use superovulation to stimulate several eggs and to better time egg aspiration. The type of ovulation induction

**Table 56–1.** Success of IVF-ET at various stages.

| | |
|---|---|
| % of patients starting IVF | 100% |
| % undergoing oocyte retrieval | 82% |
| % having an embryo transfer (ET) | 69% |
| % Clinical pregnancies/ET | 20% |
| % Ectopic pregnancies/ET | 1% |
| % Deliveries/ET | 16% |
| % Multiple Deliveries/ET | 4% |

therapy varies from group to group and is constantly changing. The following methods are currently used:

(1) Clomiphene citrate alone.

(2) Human menopausal gonadotropins (hMG) and/or human follicle-stimulating hormone (hFSH) alone.

(3) A combination of clomiphene citrate and hMG/hFSH.

(4) Gonadotropin-releasing hormone agonist (GnRH-a) in combination with hMG and/or hFSH.

Superovulation is carefully monitored with ultrasound scanning and serum estradiol and luteinizing hormone (LH) determinations. Ultrasound scanning monitors the numbers and growth of ovarian follicles. At least 2 or 3 follicles should be developing before proceeding with egg aspiration. Otherwise, the cycle is abandoned and an alternative stimulation regimen is selected during a subsequent cycle. Serum estradiol levels are complementary to ultrasonography in evaluating the maturation and growth of the developing follicles. There is evidence that the pattern of serum estradiol may predict the cycles most likely to result in pregnancy. A declining estradiol level prior to hCG administration is associated with a lower pregnancy rate. hCG is given to mature the oocytes when ultrasonography has determined the presence of an adequate number of preovulatory follicles (17–20 mm). Ovulation ordinarily begins 36 hours after hCG injection. Serum LH measurement is extremely important, since spontaneous LH peaks, which result in ovulation prior to egg aspiration, can occur. Detection of a premature LH peak permits either immediate egg aspiration or abandonment of the cycle. The introduction of GnRH-a to superovulation regimens has drastically reduced the likelihood of a premature LH surge; therefore, it is used in the majority of IVF patients in the USA.

**B. Aspiration of Eggs:** Aspiration of the preovulatory follicles is performed approximately 34 hours after the hCG injection or 24 hours after the beginning of the natural LH surge.

Egg aspiration is performed using 1 of 2 methods. Laparoscopy was the first method to be used and is only rarely used today. The second method uses ultrasonography to direct transvaginal aspiration. In transvaginal aspiration, a needle is passed through the posterior vaginal fornix using a vaginal ultrasound probe and directed into the ovary.

The advantage of ultrasound aspiration is that it can be performed on an outpatient basis with the patient awake.

**C. Fertilization With Capacitated Sperm:** Freshly ejaculated sperm cannot fertilize an egg; the sperm must be capacitated. Fortunately, capacitation is a very simple process in humans and involves only a short incubation period in a culture medium.

Due to the nature of the superovulatory process, eggs will be in different stages of maturation. Therefore, once the eggs have been identified, they are classified by the embryologist as either mature (preovulatory) or immature. Mature eggs have an expanded cumulus oophorus, whereas immature eggs have a very compact cumulus. Mature eggs have undergone the first meiotic division; immature eggs have not. Mature eggs are usually fertilized 5 hours after aspiration. Immature eggs are incubated in the laboratory for up to 36 hours prior to fertilization. If sperm and eggs are mixed too early, fertilization and cleavage will not take place. Between 10,000 and 50,000 motile sperm are placed with each egg.

**D. Culture of Fertilized Eggs in the Laboratory:** All eggs are incubated in an atmosphere of 5% carbon dioxide. Some physicians advocate an oxygen content of 5%; others use atmospheric oxygen (20%). Various culture media are used and are often supplemented with either the patient's serum or bovine serum albumin. At various intervals after the attempted fertilization, the eggs are examined in order to identify pronuclei, which confirm fertilization, as well as blastomeres, which confirm cleavage.

Fertilization and culture of the eggs are probably the most crucial stages of IVF-ET. All media must be carefully prepared. As a means of quality control, mouse pronuclear or 2-cell embryos or human sperm are incubated in all media made for IVF-ET and in all Petri dishes and test tubes used. Nontoxicity is established if virtually all embryos develop to the blastocyst stage or if sperm maintain complete motility for 24 hours. If nontoxicity cannot be established, new media are prepared or that particular batch of plastic ware is discarded.

**E. Replacement of Fertilized Egg into the Uterus:** After 48–72 hours of laboratory culture, the fertilized eggs are replaced into the patient's uterus, usually at the 2-cell to 8-cell stage. The embryos are aspirated into a small catheter, the catheter is passed transcervically into the uterus, and the eggs are injected into the uterine cavity.

## Multiple Gestation

As IVF-ET becomes more successful, the probability of multiple gestation, particularly of triplets and quadruplets, increases.

IVF-ET clinics with the highest success rates transfer only 3–4 embryos, even though they may have cultured a larger number of fertilized embryos from a particular IVF-ET cycle. The remaining embryos can be (1) donated to another woman; or (2) frozen for later use in the same woman.

## Donation of Embryos in IVF-ET

Embryos have been donated from one woman to another with resultant live births. Women who receive donated embryos may be among those who are not candidates for IVF-ET because of ovarian failure or absence, or gonadal dysgenesis. In these women the endometrium must be primed with estrogen and progesterone prior to transfer of the donated embryo, and progesterone supplementation must be maintained for at least 10 weeks.

## Frozen Embryos

Human births have followed the transfer of frozen-thawed embryos. Each frozen embryo is thought to have approximately half the potential for implantation as a fresh embryo. The endometrium of the hyperstimulated cycle is thought by many not to be the most hospitable environment to an implanting embryo, and the success of frozen-thawed embryo transfer is likely related to placement into an unstimulated endometrium. Finally, there is no difference in the rate of birth defects in children born from frozen-thawed embryos when compared with the general population.

## Scientific Study of Human Embryos

Scientific study of human embryos is a very controversial subject and is generally restricted to abnormally fertilized embryos that are not compatible with life. Karyotyping of apparently normal embryos in some European centers has revealed interesting findings (eg, haploid and aneuploid embryos have appeared morphologically normal at the 8-cell stage).

No one advocates the discarding of healthy-appearing embryos.

## Complications

Few risks are associated with IVF-ET. Congenital anomalies occur no more frequently than in normally conceived embryos. Ectopic pregnancies, however, do occur, and these carry a significant maternal risk.

## TECHNIQUES RELATED TO IVF-ET

### Ovum Donation

Ovum donation can occur under 1 of 2 circumstances. One is the infertile patient who produces a large number of oocytes during her own IVF or GIFT cycle and elects to donate some of them to another woman who is otherwise incapable of producing eggs. The other circumstance involves the recruitment of a woman who undergoes superovulation and oocyte retrieval purely for the purpose of donating her oocytes. Although the genetics of the resulting pregnancy is derived from the husband and the donor, the infertile woman incapable of producing her own eggs goes through the pregnancy. This technique has resulted in live births, with remarkable success.

## EMBRYO BIOPSY

Certain genetically heritable diseases can be identified using a variety of molecular biologic techniques. These techniques include but are not limited to the polymerase chain reaction (PCR) and fluorescent in situ hybridization (FISH). Recent advances in embryo manipulation have made possible the removal of 1 or 2 cells from a developing 8-cell human embryo without harm to the embryo. In patients at risk of passing along a heritable genetic disease, application of PCR and FISH have made possible the identification of the normal embryos (which have no risk of passing on the lethal heritable disease). These normal embryos without risk are then transferred back to the patient. Several live births have been reported following application of these techniques. The number of centers performing these techniques are few but growing.

## GIFT
### (Gamete Intra-Fallopian Tube Transfer)

GIFT is similar to IVF-ET. Superovulation is induced as in IVF-ET; an hCG injection is given; and the follicles are aspirated via laparoscopy. Prior to laparoscopy, semen is collected and capacitated. The eggs are identified in the laboratory. Sperm are then mixed with the eggs and drawn up into a catheter. The sperm and eggs can also be separated by an air bubble in the catheter. The eggs and sperm are then transferred to the uterine tubes, permitting natural fertilization and cleavage. A 20–30% pregnancy rate per cycle has been reported for this technique.

Obviously, GIFT is applicable only in patients who have normal tube function. It has been argued that the requirement of normal tubal function renders the direct comparison of IVF-ET and GIFT results impossible. Among proponents of each technique, there is vigorous ongoing debate as to the advantages of GIFT over IVF-ET .

In unexplained infertility, IVF-ET will identify etiologic fertilization problems between egg and sperm; GIFT will not. Additionally, GIFT exposes patients to the risks of general anesthesia and laparoscopy. An alternative technique has been described whereby eggs are obtained transvaginally and the egg and sperm are then transferred into the uterine tubes by catheterizing them transcervically under ultrasound guidance.

# REFERENCES

## IN VITRO FERTILIZATION

Beral V et al: Outcome of pregnancies resulting from assisted conception. Br Med Bull 1990;46:753.

Bonnicksen A: Some consumer aspects of in vitro fertilization and embryo transfer. Birth 1988;15:148.

Dandekar PV, Quigley MM: Laboratory setup for human in vitro fertilization. Fertil Steril 1984;42:1.

Diamond MP, DeCherney AH: In-vitro fertilization (IVF) and gamete intrafallopian transfer (GIFT). Obstet Gynecol Clin North Am 1987;14:1087.

Edwards RG: Test-tube babies, 1981. Nature 1981;293:253.

Edwards RG, Steptoe PC, Purdy JM: Establishing full-term human pregnancies using cleaving embryos grown in vitro. Br J Obstet Gynaecol 1980;87:737.

Garrisi GJ et al: Analysis of factors contributing to success in a program of micromanipulation-assisted fertilization. Fertil Steril 1993;59:366.

Gordon JW et al: Fertilization of human oocytes by sperm from infertile males after zona pellucida drilling. Fertil Steril 1988;50:68.

Handyside AH et al: Birth of a normal girl after in vitro fertilization and preimplantation diagnostic testing for cystic fibrosis. N Engl J Med 1992;327:905.

Hertig AT et al: Thirty-four fertilized human ova good, bad and indifferent recovered from 210 women of known fertility. Pediatrics 1959;23:202.

Laufer N, Simon A: Treatment of male infertility by gamete micromanipulation. Hum Reprod 1992;7(Suppl 1):73.

Leridon H: *Human Fertility, the Basic Components* (Translated by JF Helzner). University of Chicago Press, 1977.

Marrs RP (editor): Human in-vitro fertilization. Clin Obstet Gynecol 1986;29:117.

Navot D et al: An insight into early reproductive processes through the in vivo model of ovum donation. J Clin Endocrinol Metab 1991;72:408.

Plachot M, Crozet N: Fertilization abnormalities in human in-vitro fertilization. Hum Reprod 1992;7 (Suppl 1):89.

Plachot M: Viability of preimplantation embryos. Baillieres Clin Obstet Gynaecol 1992;6:327.

Salat Baroux J et al: The management of multiple pregnancies after induction for superovulation. Hum Reprod 1988;3:399.

Seoud MA et al: Outcome of twin, triplet, and quadruplet in vitro fertilization pregnancies: The Norfolk experience. Fertil Steril 1992;57:825.

Shamma FN et al: Corpus luteum function in in vitro fertilization cycles. Fertil Steril 1992;57:1107.

Steptoe PC, Edwards RG: Birth after the reimplantation of a human embryo. (Letter.) Lancet 1978;2:366.

Toth TL et al: Embryo transfer to the uterus or the fallopian tube after in vitro fertilization yields similar results. Fertil Steril 1992;57:1110.

Trounson AO: Cryopreservation. Br Med Bull 1990;46:695.

Veeck LL et al: Significantly enhanced pregnancy rates per cycle through cryopreservation and thaw of pronuclear stage oocytes. Fertil Steril 1993;59:1202.

## OVUM DONATION

Sauer MV, Paulson RJ, Lobo RA: Reversing the natural decline in human fertility. An extended clinical trial of oocyte donation to women of advanced reproductive age. JAMA 1992;268:1275.

## GIFT

Asch RH et al: Pregnancy after translaparoscopic gamete intrafallopian transfer. (Letter.) Lancet 1984;2:1034.

Craft I et al: Analysis of 1071 gift procedures: The case for a flexible approach to treatment. Lancet 1988;1:1094.

Penzias AS et al: Successful use of gamete intrafallopian transfer (GIFT) does not reverse the decline in fertility in women over 40 years of age. Obstet Gynecol 1991;77:37.

Penzias AS et al: Gamete intrafallopian transfer (GIFT): Assessment of the optimal number of oocytes to transfer. Fertil Steril 1991;55:311.

# Menopause & Postmenopause

*Kristen E. Smith, MD, & Howard L. Judd, MD*

## General Considerations

According to the 1980 census of the USA, of the 128 million women in this country, 35 million were 50 years of age or older. Most of these women had or shortly would have their last menstrual period, thus becoming postmenopausal. Since a woman at age 50 can expect to live another 29 years, a large minority of the female population are without ovarian function and live about one-third of their lives after this function ceases. Consequently, physicians caring for women must understand the hormonal and metabolic changes associated with the menopause, or "change of life," and the potential benefits and risks of hormone replacement therapy.

According to the Comité des Nomenclatures de la Fédération Internationale de Gynécologie et d'Obstétrique, the **climacteric** is the phase of the aging process during which a woman passes from the reproductive to the nonreproductive stage. The signals that this period of life has been reached are referred to as "climacteric symptoms" or, if more serious, as "climacteric complaints" (not as "menopause symptomatology" or "menopausal complaints"). **Premenopause** refers to the part of the climacteric before the menopause occurs, the time during which the menstrual cycle is likely to be irregular and when other climacteric symptoms or complaints may be experienced. The **menopause** is the final menstruation, which occurs during the climacteric. **Postmenopause** refers to the phase of life that comes after the menopause. It is uncertain whether this term should refer to the remainder of a woman's life or just to the period in which climacteric symptoms occur.

## Etiology & Pathogenesis

**A. Menopause:** There are 2 types of menopause, classified according to cause.

**1. Physiologic menopause**—In the human embryo, oogenesis begins in the ovary around the third week of gestation. Primordial germ cells appear in the yolk sac, migrate to the germinal ridge, and undergo cellular divisions. It has been estimated that the fetal ovaries contain approximately 7 million oogonia at 20 weeks' gestation. After 7 months' gestation, no new oocytes are formed. At birth, there are approximately 2 million oocytes, and by puberty this number has been reduced to 300,000. Continued reduction of oocyte number occurs during the reproductive years through ovulation and atresia. Nearly all oocytes vanish by atresia, with only 400–500 actually being ovulated. Very little is known about oocyte atresia. Animal studies have shown that estrogens prevent whereas androgens enhance the atretic process.

Menopause apparently occurs in the human female because of 2 processes. First, oocytes responsive to gonadotropins disappear from the ovary, and, second, the few remaining oocytes do not respond to gonadotropins. Isolated oocytes can be found in postmenopausal ovaries on very careful histologic inspection. Some of them show a limited degree of development, but most reveal no sign of development in the presence of excess endogenous gonadotropins.

Because of logistic problems, it has been difficult to determine the average age at physiologic menopause currently or in the past. There may have been an increase in the age at menopause in the USA and Western Europe, but this is not clear. At this time, the average age at menopause in the USA is 50–51 years. There does not appear to be any consistent relationship between age at menarche and age at menopause. Marriage, childbearing, height, weight, and prolonged use of oral contraceptives do not appear to influence the age of menopause. Smoking, however, is associated with early menopause.

Spontaneous cessation of menses before age 40 is called **premature menopause** or **premature ovarian cessation.** It appears that 0.9% of women in the USA may experience this early cessation of function. Cessation of menstruation and the development of climacteric symptoms and complaints can occur as early as a few years after menarche. The reasons for premature ovarian failure are unknown.

Disease processes, especially severe infections or tumors of the reproductive tract, can occasionally damage the ovarian follicular structures so severely as to precipitate the menopause. The menopause can also be hastened by excessive exposure to ionizing radiation; chemotherapeutic drugs, particularly alkylating agents; and surgical procedures that impair ovarian blood supply.

**2. Artificial menopause–** The permanent cessation of ovarian function brought about by surgical removal of the ovaries or by radiation therapy is called an artificial menopause. Irradiation to ablate ovarian function is rarely used today. Artificial menopause is employed as a treatment for endometriosis and estrogen-sensitive neoplasms of the breast and endometrium. More frequently, artificial menopause is a side effect of treatment of intra-abdominal disease; eg, ovaries are removed in premenopausal women because the gonads have been damaged by infection or neoplasia. When laparotomy affords the opportunity, elective bilateral oophorectomy is also employed to prevent ovarian cancer. For premenopausal women, this practice is still highly controversial. For postmenopausal women, it is now generally accepted as good medical practice.

**B. Premenopausal State:** The decades of mature reproductive life are characterized by generally regular menses and a slow, steady decrease in cycle length. Mean cycle length at age 15 is 35 days, at age 25 it is 30 days, and at age 35 it is 28 days. This decrease is due to shortening of the follicular phase of the cycle, with the luteal phase length remaining constant. After age 45, altered function of the aging ovary is detectable in regularly menstruating women (Fig 57–1). The mean cycle length is significantly shorter than in younger women and is attributable, in all cases, to a shortened follicular phase. The luteal phase is of similar length, and progesterone levels are not different from those observed in younger women. Estradiol levels are lower during portions of the cycle, including active follicular maturation, the midcycle peak, and the luteal phase. Concentrations of follicle-stimulating hormone (FSH) are strikingly elevated during the early follicular phase and fall as estradiol increases during follicular maturation. FSH levels at the midcycle peak and late in the luteal phase are also consistently higher than those found in younger women and decrease during the midluteal phase. Luteinizing hormone (LH) concentrations are indistinguishable from those observed in younger women. The mechanism responsible for this early rise of FSH is probably related to inhibin. **Inhibin** is a polypeptide hormone that is synthesized and secreted by granulosa cells. It causes negative feedback on FSH release by the pituitary. As the oocyte number decreases, inhibin levels fall resulting in a rise of FSH.

The transition from regular cycle intervals to the permanent amenorrhea of menopause is characterized by a phase of marked menstrual irregularity. The duration of this transition varies greatly among women. Those experiencing the menopause at an early age have a relatively short duration of cycle variability before amenorrhea ensues. Those experiencing it at a later age usually have a phase of menstrual irregular-

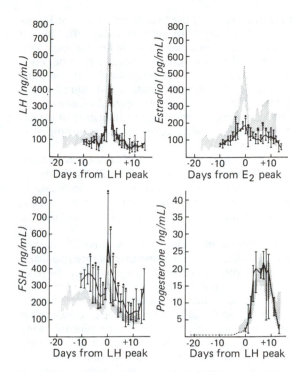

**Figure 57–1.** Mean and range of LH, FSH, estradiol ($E_2$), and progesterone levels in women over age 45 with regular menstrual cycles. Shaded area represents the mean ± 2 SEM in cycles found in young women. (Reproduced, with permission, from Sherman BM, Korenman SG: Hormonal characteristics of the human menstrual cycle throughout reproductive life. J Clin Invest 1975;55:699.)

ity characterized by unusually long and short intermenstrual intervals and an overall increase of mean cycle length and variance.

The hormonal characteristics of this transitional phase are of special interest and importance. The irregular episodes of vaginal bleeding in premenopausal women represent the irregular maturation of ovarian follicles with or without hormonal evidence of ovulation. The potential for hormone secretion by these remaining follicles is diminished and variable. Menses are sometimes preceded by maturation of a follicle with limited secretion of both estradiol and progesterone. Vaginal bleeding also happens after a rise and fall of estradiol without a measurable increase in progesterone, such as is seen during anovulatory menses. It is not known whether ovulation actually occurs during any of these cycles. Nevertheless, the potential for conception during this time is minimal.

From these findings, it is clear that the transitional phase of menstrual irregularity is not one of marked estrogen deficiency. During the menopausal transition, high levels of FSH appear to stimulate residual follicles to secrete bursts of estradiol. Occasionally, estradiol levels will rise to concentrations 2 or 3 times higher than is normally seen, probably reflecting the recruitment of more than 1 follicle for ovulation. This may be followed by corpus luteum formation, often with limited secretion of progesterone. Because the episodes of follicular maturation and vaginal bleeding are widely spaced, premenopausal women may be exposed to persistent estrogen stimulation of the endometrium in the absence of regular cyclic progesterone secretion.

### C. Changes in Hormone Metabolism Associated With the Menopause: (Fig 57–2)

Following the menopause, there are major changes in androgen, estrogen, progesterone, and gonadotropin secretion, much of which occurs because of cessation of ovarian follicular activity.

**1. Androgens**–During reproductive life, the primary ovarian androgen is androstenedione, the major secretory product of developing follicles. In postmenopausal women, there is a reduction of circulating androstenedione to approximately 50% of the concentration found in young women, reflecting the absence of follicular activity. In the year following the last menstrual period, the levels of this hormone are steady. In older women, there is a circadian variation of androstenedione, with peak concentration between 8:00 AM and noon, and the nadir occurring between 3:00 PM and 4:00 AM. This rhythm reflects adrenal activity. The clearance rate of androstenedione is similar in pre- and postmenopausal women; therefore, the level of circulating hormone reflects

production. Thus, the average production rate of androstenedione is approximately 1.5 mg/24 h in older women, a rate that is 50% of the rate found in premenopausal women. The source of most of this circulating androstenedione appears to be the adrenal glands, but continued secretion by the postmenopausal ovary accounts for approximately 20%.

For testosterone, the level found is postmenopausal women is minimally lower than that found in premenopausal women before ovariectomy and is distinctly higher than the level observed in ovariectomized young women. There is also a prominent nyctohemeral variation of this androgen, with the highest levels occurring at 8:00 AM and the nadir at 4:00 PM. There is no difference in the clearance rate of testosterone before and after the menopause. Thus, the production rate in older women is approximately 150 μg/24 h, a rate that is only one-third lower than the rate seen in young women.

The source of circulating testosterone is more complex than that of androstenedione. After the menopause, ovariectomy is associated with a nearly 60% decrease in testosterone. There is no change in the metabolic clearance rate of the androgen with ovariectomy; therefore, the fall in the circulating level reflects alterations of its production rate. About 15% of circulating androstenedione is converted to testosterone. The small simultaneous fall of androstenedione after ovariectomy can only account for a small portion of the total decrease of testosterone. The remainder presumably represents direct ovarian secretion and is larger than the amount secreted directly by the premenopausal ovary. Large increments in testosterone have been found in the ovarian compared with the peripheral veins of postmenopausal women. These increments are greater than those observed in premenopausal women, supporting the hypothesis that the postmenopausal ovary secretes more testosterone directly than the premenopausal ovary. Hilar cells and luteinized stromal cells (hyperthecosis) are present in most postmenopausal ovaries and have been shown to produce testosterone in premenopausal women. Presumably, these cells could do the same in postmenopausal subjects.

A proposed mechanism for increased ovarian testosterone production by postmenopausal ovaries is the stimulation of gonadal cells still capable of androgen production by excess endogenous gonadotropins, which in turn are increased because of reduced estrogen production by the ovaries. This increased ovarian testosterone secretion, coupled with a reduction of estrogen production, may in part explain the development of symptoms of defeminization, hirsutism, and even virilism occasionally seen in older women.

Levels of the adrenal androgens dehydroepiandrosterone (DHEA) and dehydroepiandrosterone sulfate (DHEAS) are reduced by 60% and 80%, respectively, with age. Whether these reductions are related to the menopause or to aging has not been deter-

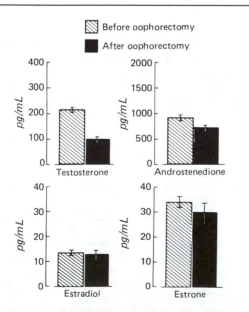

**Figure 57–2.** Serum androgen and estrogen levels in 16 postmenopausal women with endometrial cancer before and after oophorectomy. (Reproduced, with permission, from Judd HL: Hormonal dynamics associated with the menopause. Clin Obstet Gynecol 1976;1:775.)

mined. Again, a marked circadian variation of DHEA has been observed. Whether a similar rhythm is present for DHEAS is not known. As with younger subjects, the primary source of these 2 androgens is thought to be the adrenal glands, with the ovary contributing less than 15%. Thus, the marked decreases of DHEA and DHEAS reflect altered adrenal androgen secretion, and this phenomenon has been called the "adrenopause." The mechanism responsible for it is not known.

**2. Estrogens**–After a woman has passed the menopause, there is good clinical evidence of reduced endogenous estrogen production in most subjects. When circulating levels have been assessed, the greatest decrease is in estradiol. Its concentration is distinctly lower than that found in young women during any phase of their menstrual cycle and is similar to the level seen in premenopausal women following ovariectomy. A decrease of this estrogen occurs up to 1 year following the last menstrual period. There does not appear to be a nyctohemeral variation of the circulating concentration of estradiol following the menopause. The metabolic clearance rate of estradiol is reduced by 30%. The average production rate is 12 μg/24 h.

The source of the small amount of estradiol found in older women has been established. Direct ovarian secretion contributes minimally. The adrenal glands are the major source. Investigators who have examined the concentrations of estradiol in adrenal veins have reported minimal increments, arguing against direct adrenal secretion being a major contributor. Although both estrone and testosterone are converted in peripheral tissues to estradiol, it is conversion from estrone that accounts for most estradiol in older women.

After the menopause, the circulating level of estrone decreases—not as much as that of estradiol—and overlaps with values seen in premenopausal women during the early follicular phase in menstrual cycles. There is a nyctohemeral variation of circulating estrone, with the peak in the morning and the nadir in late afternoon or early evening. This variation is not as prominent as that observed for the androgens. In postmenopausal women, there is a 20% reduction of estrone clearance, and the average production rate is approximately 55 μg/24 h.

The adrenal gland is the major source of estrone. Direct adrenal or ovarian secretion is minimal. Most estrone results from the peripheral aromatization of androstenedione. The average percent conversion is double that found in ovulatory women and can account for the total daily production of this estrogen. Aromatization of androstenedione has been shown to occur in fat, muscle, liver, bone marrow, brain, fibroblasts, and hair roots. Other tissues may also contribute but have not been evaluated. To what extent each cell type contributes to total conversion has not been determined, but fat cells and muscle may be responsi-

ble for only 30–40%. This conversion has been shown to correlate with body size, with heavy women having higher conversion rates and circulating estrogen levels than slender women.

**3. Progesterone**–In young women, the major source of progesterone is the ovarian corpus luteum following ovulation. During the follicular phase of the cycle, progesterone levels are low. With ovulation, the levels rise greatly, reflecting the secretory activity of the corpus luteum. In postmenopausal women, the levels of progesterone are only 30% of the concentrations seen in young women during the follicular phase. Since postmenopausal ovaries do not contain functional follicles, ovulation does not occur and progesterone levels remain low. The source of the small amount of progesterone present in older women is felt to be due to adrenal secretion, since dexamethasone suppresses its level adrenocorticotrophic hormone (ACTH) stimulates its concentration, and human chorionic gonadotropin (hcg) administration has no effect.

**4. Gonadotropins**–With the menopause, both LH and FSH levels rise substantially, with FSH usually higher than LH. This is thought to reflect the slower clearance of FSH from the circulation. The reason for the marked increase in circulating gonadotropins is the absence of the negative feed back of ovarian steroids and inhibin on gonadotropin release. As in young women, the levels of both gonadotropins are not steady but show random oscillations. These oscillations are thought to represent pulsatile secretion by the pituitary. In older women, these pulsatile bursts occur every 1–2 hours, a frequency similar to that seen during the follicular phase of premenopausal subjects. Although the frequency is similar, the amplitude is much greater. This increased amplitude is secondary to increased release by the hypothalamic hormone gonadotropin-releasing hormone (GnRH) and enhanced responsiveness of the pituitary to GnRH due to low estrogen levels. Studies with rhesus monkeys suggest that the site governing pulsatile LH release is in the arcuate nucleus of the hypothalamus. The large pulses of gonadotropin in the peripheral circulation are believed to maintain the high levels of the hormones found in postmenopausal women.

### Clinical Findings

#### A. Symptoms and Signs:

**1. Reduced endogenous estrogens**–

**a. Reproductive tract**–Alteration of menstrual function is the first clinical symptom of the climacteric, although a gradual reduction of fertility starts by age 25 and is prominent after age 40. Some premenopausal women also complain of hot flushes. Changes in menstrual function may conform to one or more of the following patterns:

(1) Abrupt cessation of menstruation is fairly rare, because the decline of ovarian function usually proceeds slowly.

(2) The most common pattern is a gradual decrease in both amount and duration of menstrual flow, tapering to spotting only and eventually to cessation. Irregularity of the cycle appears sooner or later, with skips and delays of menses occurring.

(3) A minority of patients have more frequent or heavier vaginal bleeding. Bleeding between periods may also occur. As mentioned earlier, the occurrence of this type of bleeding usually reflects continued follicular estrogen production with or without ovulation. However, it may also reflect organic disease, eg, atypical endometrial hyperplasia or endometrial carcinoma.

The diagnosis of permanent cessation of menses is of necessity retrospective. Amenorrhea lasting 6 months to 1 year is commonly accepted as establishing the diagnosis. Only rarely will vaginal bleeding reflecting ovarian follicular activity recur after 1 year of amenorrhea. In older women, when uterine bleeding does happen after prolonged amenorrhea, it is more suggestive of organic disease. As menstrual function declines, associated symptoms such as mastodynia, abdominal bloating, edema, headache, and cyclic emotional disturbances also subside, reflecting the decrease in ovarian hormone secretion.

Because estrogen functions as the major growth factor of the female reproductive tract, there are substantial changes in the appearance of all the reproductive organs. Most postmenopausal women experience varying degrees of atrophic changes of the vaginal epithelium. The vaginal rugae progressively flatten. As the epithelium thins, the capillary bed shines through as a diffuse or patchy reddening. Rupture of surface capillaries produces irregularly scattered petechiae, and a brownish discharge may be noted. Minimal trauma with douching or coitus may result in slight vaginal bleeding. Early in the process, local bacterial invasion is likely to initiate vaginal pruritus and leukorrhea. Further atrophy of the vaginal epithelium renders its capillary bed increasingly sparse, so that the hyperemic appearance gives way to a smooth, shiny, pale epithelial surface.

There are also atrophic changes of the cervix. It usually decreases in size, and there is a reduction of secretion of cervical mucus. This may contribute to excessive vaginal dryness, which may cause dyspareunia.

Atrophy of the uterus also is seen, with shrinkage of both the endometrium and myometrium. This shrinkage is actually beneficial to women who enter the climacteric with small to moderate-sized uterine myomas. Reduction in size and elimination of symptoms frequently prevent the necessity for surgical treatment. The same applies to adenomyosis and endometriosis, both of which usually become asymptomatic. With cessation of follicular activity, hormonal stimulation of the endometrium comes to an end. This tissue usually is atrophic and inactive, not only inside the uterus but also at ectopic sites. Hence, palpable and symptomatic areas of endometriosis generally become progressively smaller and less troublesome.

The oviducts and ovaries also decrease in size postmenopausally. Although this produces no symptoms, the smallness of the ovaries makes them difficult to palpate during pelvic examination. A palpable ovary in a postmenopausal woman must be viewed with suspicion, and the presence of an ovarian neoplasm must be considered.

The supporting structures of the reproductive organs suffer loss of tone as estrogen levels decline. Postmenopausal estrogen deficiency may lead to symptomatic progressive pelvic relaxation.

**b. Urinary tract**–Estrogen plays an important role in maintaining the epithelium of the bladder and urethra. Marked estrogen deficiency may produce atrophic changes in these organs similar to those that occur in the vaginal epithelium. This may give rise to atrophic cystitis, characterized by urinary urgency, incontinence, and frequency without pyuria or dysuria. Loss of urethral tone, with pouting of the meatus and thinning of the epithelium, favors the formation of a urethral caruncle with resultant dysuria, meatal tenderness, and occasionally hematuria.

**c. Mammary glands**–Regression of breast size during and after menopause is psychologically distressing to some women. To those who have been bothered by cyclic symptoms of breast pain and cystic formation, the disappearance of these symptoms postmenopausally is a great relief.

**d. Hot flushes**–The most common and characteristic symptom of the climacteric is an episodic disturbance consisting of sudden flushing and perspiration, referred to as a **hot flash** or **flush.** It has been observed in about 75% of women who go through the physiologic menopause or have a bilateral ovariectomy. Of those having flushes, 82% experience the disturbance for more than 1 year and 25–50% complain of the symptom for more than 5 years. Most women indicate that hot flushes begin with a sensation of pressure in the head, much like a headache. This increases in intensity until the physiologic flush occurs. Palpitations may also be experienced. The actual flush is characterized as a feeling of heat or burning in the face, neck, and chest, followed immediately by an outbreak of sweating that affects the entire body but is particularly prominent over the head, neck, upper chest, and back. Less common symptoms include weakness, fatigue, faintness, and vertigo. The duration of the whole episode varies from momentary to as long as 10 minutes; the average length is 4 minutes. The frequency varies from 1–2 an hour to 1–2 a week. In women with severe flushes, the mean frequency is 54 minutes.

Investigators have now characterized the physiologic changes associated with hot flushes and have shown that the symptoms result from true alterations in cutaneous vasodilation, perspiration, reductions of

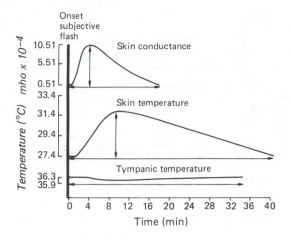

**Figure 57–3.** Skin conductance and temperature and core temperature changes associated with climacteric hot flashes. (Reproduced, with permission, from Tataryn IV et al: Postmenopausal hot flashes: A disorder of thermoregulation. Maturitas 1980;2:101.)

core temperature, and elevations of pulse rate (Fig 57–3). Fluctuations on baseline electrocardiographic recordings probably reflect changes in skin conductance. Changes in heart rhythm and blood pressure have not been observed.

The patient's awareness of symptoms does not correspond exactly with physiologic changes. Women become conscious of symptoms approximately 1 minute after the onset of measurable cutaneous vasodilatation, and discomfort persists for an average of 4 minutes, whereas physical changes persist for several minutes longer.

The exact mechanism responsible for hot flushes is not known, but physiologic and behavioral data indicate that symptoms result from a defect in central thermoregulatory function. Several observations support this conclusion: (1) The 2 major physiologic changes associated with hot flushes—perspiration and cutaneous vasodilatation—are the result of different peripheral sympathetic functions. Excitation of sweat glands results from sympathetic cholinergic fibers, and cutaneous vasodilatation is under the control of tonic alpha-adrenergic fibers. It seems unlikely that any peripheral event could cause both cholinergic excitation of sweat glands and alpha-adrenergic blockade of cutaneous vessels, and it is well recognized that these are the 2 basic functions triggered by central thermoregulatory mechanisms that lower the central temperature. (2) During a hot flush, the central temperature decreases because of cutaneous vasodilatation and perspiration. If hot flushes were the result of some peripheral event, the body's regulatory mechanisms would be expected to prevent such a decrease. (3) There is also a change in behavior associated with hot flushes. Women feel warm and have a

conscious desire to cool themselves by throwing off the bedcovers, standing by open windows or doors, fanning themselves, etc. This behavior is observed even in the presence of a steady or decreasing central temperature.

Most investigators believe the core temperature of the body is regulated around a central set point temperature that is controlled by central thermoregulatory centers, particularly those in the rostral hypothalamus. This central set point temperature is analogous to a thermostat setting. Hot flushes appear to be triggered by a sudden lowering of the central hypothalamic "thermostat." As a consequence, heat loss mechanisms, both physiologic and behavioral, are activated so that the core temperature will be brought in line with the new set point; this results in a fall of central temperature.

Because hot flushes occur after the spontaneous cessation of ovarian function or following ovariectomy, it has been presumed that the underlying mechanism is endocrinologic, related either to reduction of ovarian estrogen secretion or to enhancement of pituitary gonadotropin secretion. Low estrogen levels alone do not appear to trigger hot flushes; prepubertal children and patients with gonadal dysgenesis have low estrogen levels but not flushing. Patients with gonadal dysgenesis do experience symptoms if they are given estrogens that are later withdrawn. Thus, it appears that estrogen must be present and then withdrawn in order for hot flushes to be experienced.

Hot flushes appear to be related to gonadotropins. A close temporal association between the occurrence of flushes and the pulsatile release of LH has been demonstrated. The observation that flushes occur after hypophysectomy suggests that the mechanism is not due directly to LH release (Fig 57–4). The appearance of hot flushes in women with defects in GnRH release or synthesis, Kallman's syndrome, also suggests GnRH itself is not involved in the flushing mechanisms. The absence of hot flushes in women with hypothalamic amenorrhea and hypoestrogenemia is intriguing. These women have been shown to have defects in neurotransmitter or neurochemical input to their GnRH neurons. In particular, excessive endogenous opioid and dopamine input to GnRH neurons may account for chronic suppression of GnRH release leading to hypothalamic amenorrhea. The absence of hot flushes in these women suggests that altered afferent input of neurotransmitters or neurochemicals to the GnRH neuron that is secondary to hypogonadism leads to hot flushes. Two likely candidates are norepinephrine and endogenous opioids.

Hot flushes are a greater annoyance than most physicians have recognized. Patients frequently complain of "night sweats" and insomnia. A close temporal relationship has been shown between the occurrence of hot flushes and waking episodes. Women with frequent flushes may experience flushes and awakening episodes hourly; this may cause a profound sleep dis-

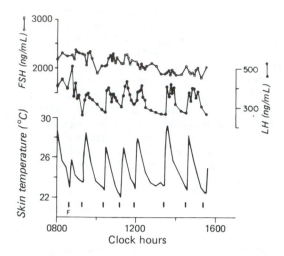

**Figure 57–4.** Skin temperature and LH and FSH levels in a woman with hot flashes. Note close temporal relationship between the rises in skin temperature and the occurrence of pulsatile LH release. (Reproduced, with permission, from Tataryn IV et al: LH, FSH, and skin temperature during the menopausal hot flash. J Clin Endocrinol Metab 1979;49:152.)

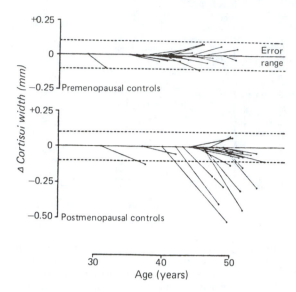

**Figure 57–5.** Changes in metacarpal cortical width, as determined by sequential measurements in pre- and postmenopausal women, age range 30–50. Note bone loss in postmenopausal women. (Reproduced, with permission, from Nordin BEC et al: Postmenopausal osteopenia and osteoporosis. Front Horm Res 1975;3:131.)

turbance that may in turn cause cognitive (memory) and affective (anxiety) disorders in some women.

Estrogens are the principal medications used to relieve hot flushes. All good studies show beneficial effects. Estrogens block both the perceived symptoms and the physiologic changes. Their use also relieves some aspects of the sleeping disorder. Estrogen administration has been shown to enhance hypothalamic opioid activity in postmenopausal women. This increase of hypothalamic opiates may be involved in the relief of hot flushes with estrogen administration.

Progestins also block hot flushes and represent a reasonable form of substitutional therapy in women who can't take estrogens. Clonidine, an alpha-adrenergic antagonist, is more effective than a placebo but is associated with side effects. Vitamins E and K, mineral supplements, and belladonna alkaloids used in combination with mild sedatives, tranquilizers, or antidepressants have all been tried, but their benefits have not been critically evaluated.

**e. Osteoporosis**–Osteoporosis is 1 of the 2 most important health hazards influenced by the climacteric. It is a disorder characterized by a reduction in the quantity of bone without changes in chemical composition. This loss occurs primarily in trabecular bone and is therefore most noticeable in the vertebra and distal radius. Although gradual bone loss occurs in all humans with aging, this loss is accelerated in women after cessation of ovarian function. Postmenopausal osteoporosis is responsible for fractures in 1 of every 2 postmenopausal women and is sometimes called type I osteoporosis (Fig 57-5). It is most severe in women who have sustained early ovariectomy or who have gonadal dysgenesis. Type II osteoporosis is age-related, is seen in both men and women, and affects both cortical and trabecular bone. The arguments for categorizing osteoporosis this way are reasonable, but are not supported by all experts. Symptomatic osteoporosis occurs most often in whites followed by Asians and then African-Americans, although 20% of African-American women also develop osteoporosis. Smoking and slender body size are also risk factors.

Bone loss produces minimal symptoms, but lead to reduced skeletal strength. Thus, osteoporotic bones are more susceptible to fractures. The most common site of fracture is in the vertebral body but, fractures also occur in the humerus, upper femur, distal forearm, and ribs. The 1990 figures from the National Osteoporosis Foundation show that osteoporosis is responsible for 1.5 million fractures per year and that more than 20 million women are affected. Forty percent of all women will have one or more spinal fractures by the age of 80 (Fig 57-6). More than 275,000 hip fractures occur annually in the USA at a cost of more than $10 billion per year. The incidence of hip fractures in women is 2–3 times that in men. The mortality rate associated with hip fractures is between 5% and 20% within 12 months following the injury. Fifteen to 25% of survivors are permanently disabled.

The proposed pathophysiology of osteoporosis is that monocytes contain collagen receptors that allow them to adhere to the bone. With adherence, the

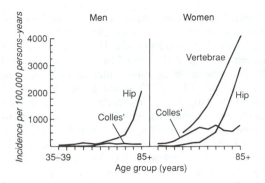

**Figure 57–6.** Incidences of the 3 common osteoporotic fractures (Colles', hip, and vertebral) in men and women, plotted as a function of age at time of fracture in the community population of Rochester, Minnesota. (Reproduced, with permission, from Riggs BL, Melton LJ III: Involutional osteoporosis. N Engl J Med 1986;314:1677.)

monocyte releases interleukin-1 (IL-1). This is the most potent known stimulator of osteoclast activity. Parathyroid hormone (PTH) is also involved in the genesis of osteoporosis. PTH stimulates bone resorption and absence of this hormone inhibits development of osteoporosis in animal and human studies. PTH receptors have been demonstrated on rat osteoblasts and PTH-stimulates release of insulin-like growth factor 1 (IGF-1) in vitro. IGF-1 has several actions on bone: it stimulates differentiation of osteoclast precursors into mature osteoclasts; it is produced by osteoblasts and stimulates osteoblast proliferation; and it increases local density of trabecular bone. To date, it does not appear that PTH is elevated in most women with osteoporosis or that the sensitivity of bone to PTH is enhanced. It is interesting that the amino-terminus of PTH (1-34) has been shown to inhibit bone resorption in experimental settings. Worth mentioning is that growth hormone receptors

have been demonstrated on osteoblasts, but their role in osteoporosis has not been determined.

Ovarian estrogen production and hormone replacement after the menopause are protective against osteoporosis. It is likely that estrogens have direct effects on bone, since estrogen receptors exist in osteoblasts, osteoclasts, macrophages, and T cells. IL-1 activity in bone has been shown to increase immediately after the menopause or oophorectomy, but remains increased in osteoporotic women, whereas IL-1 levels return to the premenopausal range after 2 or 3 years in those who do not develop the disease. Estrogen inhibits release of IL-1 by monocytes and may also have a direct effect on osteoclasts, although more study needs to be done in this area. Estrogen also seems to enhance bone formation by a direct local action on osteoblasts. A possible mediator for this action is transforming growth factor B.

Although much has been done to study urinary and serum factors as predictors of osteoporosis, the most predictive test remains bone densitometry. Several different types of densitometry are available (Table 57–1). Single-energy absorptiometry can be used to measure appendicular bone mineral density (BMD). In order to measure axial bone, however, dual-energy absorptiometry is required for an accurate assessment. The variability of soft tissue density around the spine and pelvis decreases the accuracy of single-photon testing. Radionuclides were initially used, but recently used of x-ray tubes has improved the precision of testing. Results are given in grams or g/cm². In most studies, decreased by 1 SD in mass was associated with an increase of 50–100% in fracture risk. The assessment of specific bones for fracture has increased the predictive value. A decrease of hip density of 1 SD increases the risk of future hip fracture by 250–300%.

Assessment of risk factors has not been nearly as predictive of fracture risk as density measurement. Assessment of serum osteocalcin, a marker of bone

**Table 57–1.** Selected Techniques for the Measurement of Bone Mass.

| Technique | Site | Precision | Accuracy | Examination Time (Minutes) | Radiation Dose Internal Organs (μSv) | Skin (mrem) | Approximate Cost |
|---|---|---|---|---|---|---|---|
| Radiographic absorptiometry (RA) | Hand | 1–2% | 4% | 3–5 | 1 | 100 | $ 75–150 |
| Single-photon absorptiometry (SPA) | Wrist, heel | 1–3% | 5% | 15 | 1 | 10–20 | $ 75–150 |
| Dual-photon absorptiometry (DPA) | Spine, hip, total body | 2–4% | 4–10% | 20–40 | 1 | 5 | $150–200 |
| Dual-energy x-ray absorptiometry (DXA) | Spine, hip, total body | 0.5–2% | 3–9% | 3–7 | 1 | 1–3 | $150–200 |
| Quantitative computed tomography (QCT) | Spine | 2–5% | 5–20% | 10–15 | 60 | 150–250 | $150–250 |

At least 1 of the 5 specific methods of bone mass measurement should be available to any clinician.

formation, or of urinary pyridinium cross-links, a marker of bone resorption, has not been shown to be predictive of fracture risk.

Current recommendations for testing are that some dual-energy techniques be performed to measure density of the hip and spine in any woman who is estrogen-deficient and has no climacteric symptoms. Testing should also be done on any patients who display osteopenia on x-ray or who are receiving long-term glucocorticoids.

Estrogen remains the mainstay of prevention of postmenopausal osteoporosis. It decreases the risk of hip fractures by 50% and reduces the risk of other fractures. Current recommendations are that all postmenopausal women, including those with established osteoporosis and the elderly, be treated with estrogen unless contraindications exist or the therapy is not tolerated. Daily dosages of 0.625 mg of conjugated estrogens, 1.25 mg piperazine estrone sulfate, 1 mg micronized estradiol, and 0.05 mg of transdermal estradiol all have been approved for the prevention of osteoporosis. For best results, early commencement of therapy after the menopause and long-term use are recommended.

Alternatives exist for those patients who cannot take estrogen. Second-line therapy consists of calcitonin or etidronate. Calcitonin is peptide hormone that inhibits osteoclast activity and therefore inhibits bone resorption. Salmon calcitonin is the most potent form and is available intranasally or as a subcutaneous injection. Calcitonin, 50–100 IU, is given subcutaneously daily or every other day. The intranasal calcitonin dose is 100–400 IU daily. Discontinuous regimens have been studied with withdrawal periods of up to 1 year may be taken without adverse effects after at least 1 year of therapy. This approach may decrease the cost of therapy. Besides expense, other disadvantages of calcitonin are that serum calcium levels must be followed, resistance may occur, and actual improvement in fracture rate has not been demonstrated.

Etidronate is a biphosphonate that inhibits osteoclastic activity. The dosage of etidronate is 400 mg daily by mouth and is usually given in 2-week cycles followed by a 10-week cycle of calcium supplementation to allow resumption of osteoblastic function. Some investigators recommend phosphate supplementation as the potassium and sodium salt, 1 g 3 times daily with meals for 3 days before beginning etidronate therapy to activate the osteoclasts.

High-dose progestins may have a similar effect on bone as estrogens, but are unlikely to be a practical alternative. Fluoride has been used in Europe and the USA and was associated with a marked increase intrabecular bone but did not improve fracture rates and in some studies, fracture rates were increased. This may be due to a lack of increase in cortical bone. Fluoride is not available for the treatment of osteoporosis in the USA.

Finally, all postmenopausal women should receive calcium supplementation to achieve a total daily dose of calcium of 1000–1500 mg/d. Therefore, additional supplementation to diet should be at least 400–600 mg. One chewable calcium tablet taken with each meal will provide this. Vitamin D supplements of 400–800 U daily are recommended. Postmenopausal women should be encouraged to exercise regularly to improve grace and agility, which will decrease their risk of falls. Diet should be modified to decrease salt, animal protein, alcohol, and caffeine, all of which may increase the risk of osteoporotic fractures.

**f. Cardiovascular system–**The incidence of death from cardiovascular disease increases with age in all populations and both sexes (Table 57–2). Substantially more heart disease is seen in younger men, with the onset of cardiovascular problems occurring an average of 10 years later in women. Before the age of menopause, very few women die of a heart attack. After the menopause, a woman's risk increases progressively until age 70 when it becomes equal to men. Heart disease affects nearly 3 million women in the USA. Deaths due to heart disease are more than 478,000 per year, which is greater than the deaths in men. The rate in women has nearly doubled since 1984.

Two types of studies have attempted to determine whether cessation of ovarian function is associated with increased incidence of heart disease. The first has examined the relationship between the menopause and carefully defined cardiovascular disease in an entire population. For example, the Framingham study, in which nearly 3000 women are examined biennially, revealed that following the menopause, there is indeed an increased incidence of heart disease that is not just age-related. In this study, the impact of the menopause was abrupt, and further (age-related) increases in incidence occurred only slowly, if at all. In the Nurses' Health Study cohort, of 121,700 women after controlling for age and cigarette smoking, women who had a natural menopause had no appreciable increase in risk compared with that of premenopausal women. However, women who underwent a bilateral oophorectomy and no estrogen replacement had an increased risk (RR 2.2) compared with that seen in premenopausal women.

**Table 57–2.** Deaths Due to Cardiovascular Disease in the US, 1988.

| Ages (in years) | Men | Women |
|---|---|---|
| 40–59 | 17,440 | 6,837 |
| 50–59 | 42,816 | 18,803 |
| 60–69 | 100,911 | 56,981 |
| 70–79 | 147,451 | 124,394 |
| 80–89 | 118,016 | 185,201 |
| 90–> | 33,165 | 101,580 |
| Total | 461,799 | 493,796 |

(Vital Statistics, 1988.)

In the second type of investigation, case-control studies have been performed comparing the degree of coronary heart disease or the incidence of myocardial infarction in women who had undergone early ovariectomy with age-matched premenopausal controls. Most of these studies revealed an increased risk of cardiovascular disease after ovarian excision. All these reports have been criticized because of patient selection bias, particularly the controls.

The evidence that supports a protective role of estrogen replacement on coronary artery disease is impressive (Table 57–3). Numerous case-control and large cohort studies have been published with most

showing a beneficial impact of estrogens. A recent meta-analysis found that estrogen use provided a 50% decrease in risk of mortality from heart disease. Although the magnitude of change and the consistency of results appear compelling, it must be recognized that all these studies are observational, and the choice of controls has been questioned. In particular, women who take estrogens are more health-conscious and must see a doctor regularly to receive their medication, whereas women who don't take estrogens may or may not receive regular medical checkups. Thus, some or all of the apparent benefits of estrogens on heart disease may be due to these other considera-

**Table 57–3.** Postmenopausal Hormone Use and Coronary Heart Disease

| Reference (Year) | Unopposed Estrogen | | | Estrogen and Progestin |
|---|---|---|---|---|
| | Ever Use Relative Risk | Duration of Use | | Ever Use Relative Risk |
| | | Years of Use | Relative Risk | |
| Case-control | | | | |
| Rosenberg (238) (1976) | 1.0* | | | |
| Talbott (83) (1977) | 0.3*† | | | |
| Jick (70) (1978) | 4.2*† | | | |
| Pfeffer (237) (1978) | 0.9 | | | |
| Rosenberg (113) (1980) | 1.0* | ≥5 | 0.6* | |
| Adam (77) (1981) | 0.6† | >4 | 1.0† | |
| Bain (229) (1981) | 0.8 | | | |
| Ross (81) (1981) | 0.5†‡ | | | |
| Szklo (241) (1984) | 0.6 | | | |
| La Vecchia (233) (1987) | 3.0* | | | |
| Beard (230) (1989) | 0.6 | | | |
| Croft (231) (1989) | 0.8 | | | |
| Thompson (114) (1989) | 1.1§ | | | 1.2§ |
| Cross-sectional | | | | |
| Gruchow (96) (1988) | 0.6‡‖ | | | |
| | 0.4‡¶ | | | |
| Sullivan (240) (1988) | 0.6‡ | | | |
| McFarland (235) (1989) | 0.5‡ | | | |
| Uncontrolled cohort | | | | |
| Byrd (61) (1977) | 0.4†‡ | | | |
| MacMahon (234) (1978) | 0.3 | ≥15 | 0.8 | |
| Hunt (63) (1990) | 0.4‡ | | | |
| Cohort | | | | |
| Hammond (117) (1979) | 0.3†‡ | | | |
| Lafferty (204) (1985) | 0.2† | | | |
| Wilson (73) (1985) | 1.9‡ | | | |
| Bush (78) (1987) | 0.4‡ | | | |
| Petitti (80) (1987) | 1.3 | | | |
| Criqui (79) (1988) | 1.0* | | | |
| Avila (228) (1990) | 0.7* | ≥1 | 0.3* | |
| Persson (101) (1990) | 0.8‡ | | | 0.5‡ |
| Sullivan (82) (1990) | 0.2*‡ | | | |
| Henderson (76) (1991) | 0.7†‡ | ≥15 | 0.5‡ | |
| Stampfer (85) (1991) | 0.6*‡ | | | |
| Wolf (84) (1991) | 0.7‡ | | | |
| Randomized, controlled trial | | | | |
| Nachtigall (64) (1979) | | | | 0.3† |

*Current estrogen use.
†The relative risk or $P$ value or both are estimated from data provided in the published study.
‡$P \leq 0.05$.
§End points include both stroke and myocardial infarction.
‖Moderate versus low coronary occlusion score.
¶Severe versus low coronary occlusion score.
(Reproduced, with permission, from Grady D et al: Hormone therapy to prevent disease and prolong life in postmenopausal women. Ann Intern Med 1992;117:1016.)

tions. It is essential that a long-term randomized drug trial be conducted to prove this benefit or not. Studies of this nature are currently underway.

Estrogen probably protects against coronary artery disease by more than one mechanism. Evidence for both an indirect effect on circulating lipids and a direct action on the vascular system now exists. For years, the greatest emphasis of research has been to study the impact of estrogens on lipoproteins. Orally administered estrogens influence hepatic lipid metabolism and raise HDL cholesterol and triglycerides and lower LDL cholesterol. The impact of nonorally administered estrogens is of lesser magnitude and takes longer to become apparent. Efforts to link these lipid changes with the benefits of estrogens on heart disease have been sparse. The Lipid Research Clinic study suggests that approximately 50% of the benefit of estrogen on heart disease is elicited through the action of estrogens on lipoproteins, whereas the remainder is through other mechanisms.

Numerous studies have shown that estrogen and progesterone receptors are present in the heart and aorta. Thus, the subcellular components necessary for hormonal action exist in these tissues. Studies in castrated cynomolgus monkeys given atherogenic diets have shown estradiol administered by subcutaneous pellets prevents coronary atherogenesis in the absence of any measurable change in circulating lipoproteins.

Endothelial cells of the arteries produce factors in response to estrogen. The most potent of these is believed to be nitric oxide (NO). NO exerts several effects on the arterial wall. It increases intracellular cyclic guanosine monophosphate in the arterial smooth muscle, which results in vasodilatation. It also inhibits platelet and macrophage adherence to the arterial endothelium. Both are important first steps to atheromatous plaque formation. Estrogen appears to increase NO production. Basal release of NO is greater in intact female rabbits than in either male rabbits or castrated females. Acetylcholine is known to stimulate vasodilatation of the coronary arteries of humans and monkeys. This effect is dependent on an intact vascular endothelium. Because superoxide radicals inhibit both NO and this acetylcholine-induced vasodilatation, NO is felt to be the endothelial factor responsible for this acetylcholine-induced vasodilatation. It has been theorized that estrogens may increase muscarinic receptors on endothelial cells leading to acetylcholine-induced, endothelial-dependent vasodilatation. Although these mechanisms are only partially understood, they emphasize the importance of studying the direct effects of estrogen on the vascular system.

Studies have suggested that the protective effect of estrogens on the heart is greatest in women with known risk factors for heart disease. These include obesity, smoking, hypertension, etc. Thus, physicians

are beginning to concentrate hormone replacement in women at risk for this disease.

**g. Skin and hair–** With aging, noticeable changes of the skin occur. There is generalized thinning and an accompanying loss of elasticity, resulting in wrinkling. These changes are particularly prominent in the areas exposed to light, ie, the face, neck, and hands. "Purse-string" wrinkling around the mouth and "crow's feet" around the eyes are characteristic. Skin changes on the dorsum of the hands are particularly noticeable. In this area, the skin may be so thin as to become almost transparent, with details of the underlying veins easily visible.

Histologically, the epidermis is thinned, and the basal layers become inactive with age. Dehydration is typical. Reduction in the number of blood vessels to the skin is also seen. Degeneration of elastic and collagenous fibers in the dermis also appears to be part of the process of aging.

These skin changes are of cosmetic importance and have been related to the onset of the climacteric by women. It is commonly stated that women undergoing estrogen replacement look younger, and the cosmetic industry has been placing estrogens in skin creams for years for precisely this purpose.

The possibility that estrogens may have effects on skin was suggested by the recent demonstration of estrogen receptors in skin. The number of receptors is highest in facial skin, followed by skin of the breasts and thighs. This gives credence to the hypothesis that estrogens affect the skin.

Skin circulation has been found to be decreased in women after oophorectomy. Radiolabeled thymidine incorporation (an index of new DNA metabolism) has been reported to decrease during the several months following ovariectomy. In animals, estrogens have been shown to increase the mitotic rate (a reflection of growth) of skin in some studies. Estrogens may alter the vascularization of skin. They also change the collagen content of the dermis, as reflected by mucopolysaccharide incorporation, hydroxyproline turnover, and alterations of the ground substance. In addition, dermal synthesis of hyaluronic acid and dermal water content are enhanced.

Skin collagen content and thickness have been studied in postmenopausal women. Decreases of both have been observed at a rate of 1–2% per year. The losses correlated with the number of years since the menopause, but not with chronologic age. Estrogen replacement has been shown to prevent or restore both parameters to premenopausal values. The greatest recovery is observed in women who began with low values. This data was interpreted to indicate that estrogen can prevent loss in women with high skin collagen levels, whereas it can restore content as well as prevent further loss in women with low collagen levels. Although these results are promising, it must be realized that randomized studies have not been performed, and the skin areas studied are the forearm and abdomen.

After the menopause, most women note some change in patterns of body hair. Usually, there is a variable loss of pubic and axillary hair. Often, there is loss of lanugo hair on the upper lip, chin, and cheeks, together with increase growth of course terminal hairs; a slight mustache may become noticeable. Hair on the body and extremities may either increase or decrease. Slight balding is seen occasionally. All of these changes may be due in part to reduced levels of estrogen in the face of fairly well maintained levels of testosterone.

**h. Psychologic changes**–Early cross-sectional surveys of community or large general medical practice-based populations attempted to measure the temporal association of depression and irritability to the cessation of the menses. Some reports indicated an increased incidence of minor symptoms such as irritability, dysphoria, and nervousness early in the menopausal transition.

Reports from community-based cohort studies have refined knowledge in the area of mood, mentation, and menopause. The initial longitudinal report of the USA cohort found an increase in overall non-specific symptom reporting at the menopause. Depression for more than 2 interviews was noted in 26%. Perceived health, rather than menopause or coincident life stresses, was most related to depression in this study. These findings are consistent with the concept of variability in a woman's response to the menopause; individual characteristics and self-perceptions appear to be important determinants of each woman's experience of the climacteric.

Hypotheses as to the etiology of the affective complaints at the menopause also include a primary biologic cause (eg, an alteration in brain amines). Studies using the opioid antagonist naloxone have demonstrated that estrogen deficiency is associated with low levels of endogenous opioid activity and that estrogen supplementation increases opioid activity. These findings suggest that central neurotransmitters may contribute to the etiology of affective/cognitive complaints. Sociologic factors postulated to cause psychologic symptoms, such as negative cultural values attached to aging, may also promote a negative climacteric experience.

Double-masked studies have found improvements in self-reported irritability, mild anxiety, and dysphoria in women treated with estrogen alone or combined with progestin. Improvement of the Beck depression score in women without hot flashes indicate that estrogens likely have direct effects on brain function.

The determinants of sexual behavior are complex and interrelated. Sexual function is believed to be regulated by 3 general components: the individual's motivation (also called desire or libido), endocrine competence, and social-cultural beliefs. Decreased libido is reported with increasing age. However, the relative contributions to this observation of a primary decrease in desire, anatomic limitations to sexual function, or beliefs that sexual behavior is inappropriate in older age are unknown.

The hypoestrogenemic state leads to atrophy of the internal genitalia. Although dyspareunia is the most obvious symptom of vaginal atrophy, suboptimal sexual functions can occur without frank dyspareunia. Diminished genital sensation, (and, therefore, decreased sensory output in the sexual arousal phase), lessened glandular secretions, less vasocongestion, and decreased vaginal expansion may not be perceived as discrete symptoms by the postmenopausal female but may influence her perception that she is less responsive.

Genital atrophy, one cause of postmenopausal sexual dysfunction, responds to estrogen therapy. The specific impact of estrogen on libido has been difficult to determine. Improved anatomy may also have a positive psychologic impact and may indirectly encourage sexual motivation.

**2. Excess endogenous estrogens**–Not all women experiencing the climacteric have symptoms of estrogen deprivation. Some have no symptoms, whereas other actually experience symptoms and signs of estrogen excess, usually uterine bleeding but in some cases mastodynia, abdominal bloating, edema, growth of uterine myomas, and exacerbation of endometriosis as well. The problems of postmenopausal uterine bleeding are of particular concern, because this bleeding may reflect the presence of endometrial hyperplasia or adenocarcinoma.

Based on a variety of evidence, it has been suggested that continuous estrogen stimulation of the endometrium, unopposed by progesterone, can lead to a progression of changes from benign proliferation to cystic or simple hyperplasia, adenomatous hyperplasia, and varying degrees of anaplasia, including invasive adenocarcinoma. When postmenopausal patients with hyperplasia or adenocarcinoma are studied, many have higher than usual levels of circulatory estrogens.

As mentioned earlier, the principal source of estrogens in older women is the peripheral aromatization of circulating androgens. Thus, there are 3 mechanisms that could conceivably result in increased endogenous estrogen production: (1) increased production of precursor androgens, (2) enhanced aromatization of precursor androgens, and (3) increased production of estrogens directly. The occurrence of each has been reported and has been associated with signs of estrogen excess.

Of particular importance is enhanced aromatization of androgens. A variety of conditions are associated with this including obesity, liver disease, and hyperthyroidism. The association of obesity with endometrial cancer has been known for years.

Comparisons have been made between postmenopausal women with and without endometrial cancer. When these comparisons have been conducted using control subjects matched to the cancer patients by age, there have been no differences in androgen and estrogen levels or in the conversion rate of androstenedione to estrone between the 2 groups. However, body size has always shown positive correlations with endogenous estrogen levels and with conversion rates of androstenedione to estrone, and it is well recognized that obese women are at greater risk of developing endometrial hyperplasia and adenocarcinoma than slender women. The high concentrations of endogenous estrogens found in obese subjects presumably play a role in the increased incidence of this tumor in obese older women.

**3. Miscellaneous postmenopausal symptoms**–Many other symptoms have been attributed to the endocrine changes of the postmenopausal state, but a direct cause-and-effect relationship has not been established for them. Some of these so-called climacteric symptoms are so common that they deserve brief mention.

Symptoms possibly related to specific autonomic nervous system instability—but equally attributable to anxiety or other emotional disturbances—are paresthesias (pricking, itching, formication), dizziness, tinnitus, fainting, scotomas, and dyspnea. Symptoms clearly not of endocrine origin are weakness, fatigue, nausea, vomiting, flatulence, anorexia, constipation, diarrhea, arthralgia, and myalgia.

Many women believe erroneously that the endocrine changes accompanying menopause will produce a steady weight gain. Women and men do tend to gain weight at this time of life, but the cause is a combination of decreased exercise and possibly increased caloric intake. There may be some redistribution of body weight occasioned by the deposition of fat over the hips and abdomen. Perhaps this is partly an endocrine effect, but more likely it is the result of decreased physical activity, reduced muscle tone, and other effects of aging.

Many of the previously mentioned symptoms occasionally respond promptly to administration of estrogen. This should not mislead physicians into assuming a specific endocrine action for what is actually a placebo effect.

**B. Laboratory Findings:**

**1. Vaginal cytologic smears**–In certain laboratory animals, the degree of maturation of exfoliated vaginal epithelial cells, as revealed by stained vaginal smears, is an accurate index of estrogenic activity. When this method is applied to women, several staining techniques are available. Among the various methods of assessing the smears, the following are most commonly used: (1) The **maturation index** consists of a differential count of 3 types of squamous cells—parabasal cells, intermediate cells, and superficial cells, in that order—expressed as percentages, eg, 10/85/5. (2) The **cornification count** is the percentage of precornified and cornified cells among total squamous cells counted. This is actually a simplified maturation index, because this percentage is essentially the same as that of the superficial cells.

The assessment of exfoliated vaginal epithelial cells is influenced not only by the level of estrogenic activity but also by other hormones (particularly progesterone and testosterone), local vaginal inflammation, local medication ("hygiene"), vaginal bleeding, the presence of genital cancer, the location of the vaginal area sampled, and variations in end organ (epithelial) responses to estrogenic influence. Thus, women with identical levels of circulating estrogens may have quite different cytograms. Moreover, even with extraneous factors eliminated, the vaginal smear does not indicate absolute levels of estrogenic function; rather, it reflects the net balance of the influence on vaginal epithelium of endogenous and exogenous estrogens, androgens, and progestogens. This is well demonstrated in women taking oral contraceptives. Despite the intake of relatively large doses of estrogen, the cornification counts are usually lower because of the concomitant effect of the progestin.

The great variation in cytologic findings leads to the following conclusions regarding the use of smears in the clinical management of postmenopausal women: (1) The smear is only a rough measure of estrogenic status, and it may sometimes be grossly misleading. (2) The vaginal cytogram cannot predict whether or not an individual woman is experiencing climacteric signs and symptoms, ie, it cannot be used as a "femininity index." (3) The smear cannot be used as the sole guide to steroid supplementation therapy; clinical signs and symptoms are more dependable for this purpose. (4) The smear can be helpful in determining the dosage of estrogen needed to reverse vaginal atrophy.

**2. Hormone production**–For the past 2 decades techniques of radioisotopic protein binding or radioimmunoassay have been available for the determination of hormone levels in blood and other body fluids (Table 57–4).

**Table 57–4.** Serum concentrations (mean ± SE) of steroids in premenopausal and postmenopausal women.

| Steroid | Premenopausal (ng/mL) | Postmenopausal (ng/mL) |
|---|---|---|
| Progesterone | $0.47 \pm 0.03$ | $0.17 \pm 0.02$ |
| Dehydroepiandrosterone | $4.2 \pm 0.5$ | $1.8 \pm 0.2$ |
| Dehydroepiandrosterone sulfate | $1600 \pm 350$ | $300 \pm 70$ |
| Androstenedione | $1.5 \pm 0.1$ | $0.6 \pm 0.01$ |
| Testosterone | $0.32 \pm 0.02$ | $0.25 \pm 0.03$ |
| Estrone | $0.08 \pm 0.01$ | $0.029 \pm 0.002$ |
| Estradiol | $0.05 \pm 0.005$ | $0.013 \pm 0.001$ |

**a. Androgens**–In premenopausal women, plasma androstenedione is approximately 1.5ng/mL. Plasma testosterone is about 0.3 ng/mL. Mean DHEA and DHEAS levels are approximately 4 ng/mL and 1600 ng/mL, respectively, in samples drawn at 8:00 AM.

In postmenopausal women, the mean plasma androstenedione concentration is reduced by at least 50%, to approximately 0.6 ng/mL. Plasma testosterone levels are only slightly reduced (about 0.25 ng/mL). Plasma DHEA and DHEAS levels are decreased to mean levels of 1.8 ng/mL and 300 ng/mL in women in their 60s and 70s.

**b. Estrogens**–During normal menstrual life, the mean plasma estradiol fluctuates from 50 to 350 pg/mL and estrone from 30 to 110 pg/mL. These fluctuations reflect the development and involution of the follicle and corpus luteum. In postmenopausal women, cyclic fluctuations disappear. The mean estradiol level is approximately 12 pg/mL, with a range of 5–25 pg/mL. The mean estrone level is approximately 30 pg/mL, with a range of 20–70 pg/mL. Estradiol levels in normal young women do not overlap those observed in postmenopausal subjects. The measurement of estradiol levels below 20 pg/mL can be helpful in establishing the diagnosis of the menopause, since the fall of this estrogen is the last hormonal change associated with loss of ovarian function. There is substantial overlap of estrone levels in younger and older women. Measurement of this estrogen is not helpful in determining the ovarian status of a patient.

**c. Progesterone**–In young cycling women, the mean progesterone level is approximately 0.4 ng/mL during the follicular phase of the cycle, with a range of 0.2–0.7 ng/mL. During the luteal phase, progesterone levels rise and fall, reflecting corpus luteum function; the mean level is approximately 11 ng/mL with a range of 3–21 ng/mL. In postmenopausal women, the mean progesterone level is 0.17 ng/mL. To date, no clinical use has been established for the measurement of progesterone in postmenopausal women.

**d. Pituitary gonadotropins**–One of the striking hormonal changes associated with the menopause is the increase in secretion of pituitary gonadotropins. During reproductive life, the levels of both FSH and LH range from 4 to 30 mU/mL except during the preovulatory surge, when they may exceed 50 mU/mL and 100 mU/mL, respectively. After the menopause, both rise to levels above 100 mU/mL, with FSH rising earlier and to greater levels than LH.

When contradictory or uncertain clinical findings make the diagnosis of the postmenopausal state questionable, measurement of plasma FSH, LH, and estradiol levels may be helpful. This situation occurs frequently in women following hysterectomy without ovariectomy. The findings of plasma estradiol below 20 pg/mL and elevated FSH and LH levels are consistent with cessation of ovarian function. In practical terms, it is not necessary to measure LH.

**e. Thyroid function**–There are changes of thyroid function with aging. Thyroxine ($T_4$) and free $T_4$ concentrations are similar in young and older women, but triiodothyronine ($T_3$) levels fall by approximately 25–40% during aging. This decrease of $T_3$ does not seem to reflect hypothyroidism, since the thyroid-stimulating hormone (TSH) concentration, a sensitive indicator of primary hypothyroidism, is not elevated. In addition, there is an age-related decrease in the responsiveness of TSH to thyrotropin-releasing hormone (TRH) rather than the increase seen in patients with hypothyroidism. $T_4$-binding globulin levels rise slightly and $T_4$-binding prealbumin falls, but the latter is a minor carrier of $T_4$. All these changes in thyroid function appear to be related to aging, not the climacteric, since they also occur in men.

There is an increased incidence of hypothyroidism (Hashimoto's thyroiditis) in older people, and this should be remembered in caring for the elderly.

**3. Endometrial histology**–As long as menses and occasional ovulation persist, all phases of endometrial growth may be found on histologic examination. After ovulation ceases, no further secretory changes are seen. After menopause, endometrial biopsy may reveal anything from a very scanty, atrophic endometrium to one that is moderately proliferative. Spontaneous postmenopausal bleeding may occur in the presence of any of these patterns. Endometrial tissue revealing glandular hyperplasia (with or without uterine bleeding) is an indication of enhanced estrogenic stimulation from either endogenous estrogen production (eg, increased conversion of androgen), or from exogenous intake of estrogen.

**C. Ultrasonography:** Increasingly, physicians are using vaginal ultrasonography to evaluate the pelvis in postmenopausal women. Besides the evaluation of pelvic masses, 2 other indications for pelvic ultrasound examination have been proposed. The first is evaluation of the endometrium or "endometrial stripe" to determine whether a woman has endometrial hyperplasia or cancer. This has been controversial with investigators reporting the demarcation between normal and abnormal endometrium being in the range of 4–10 mm. Others have recommended setting the criteria at a low thickness to exclude most people with a potential endometrial lesion. If the criteria are set low, such as at 4mm, then published results indicate that the rare patient (1 in 128) will have endometrial hyperplasia or cancer with a stripe greater than 4 mm. Conversely, approximately 20% will have normal endometrium with a stripe greater than 4 mm.

## Differential Diagnosis

Signs and symptoms similar to those of the climacteric can be caused by a variety of other diseases. In general, the total clinical picture is helpful in establishing the proper diagnosis. The absence of evidence of other disease will point to cessation of ovarian function, whereas the presence of prominent features of other conditions, in the absence of other climacteric symptoms, will suggest a nonclimacteric origin.

**A. Amenorrhea:** By definition, the primary symptom of the menopause is the absence of menstruation. Amenorrhea can occur for many reasons, of which physiologic menopause is only one. Cessation of ovarian function is by far the most common reason for amenorrhea to occur in women in their 40s or early 50s. Persistent amenorrhea in younger women may be due to premature cessation of ovarian function but must be differentiated from other causes. Obvious features of specific disease often suggest the proper diagnosis (eg, extreme weight loss in anorexia nervosa, galactorrhea in hyperprolactinemia, hirsutism and obesity in polycystic ovarian disease). Although the reproductive tract commonly shows evidence of lowered estrogenic activity in these and other diseases associated with amenorrhea, true vasomotor symptoms are rare. Rarely it is necessary to measure estrogen or gonadotropins in women with a uterus to establish cessation of ovarian function.

**B. Vasomotor Flushes:** Several diseases can produce sensations of flushing that may be misinterpreted as hot flushes. Notable are hyperthyroidism, pheochromocytoma, carcinoid syndrome, diabetes mellitus, tuberculosis, and other chronic infections. None of these disorders produces the specific symptoms associated with the climacteric (ie, short duration and specific body distribution). Moreover, the absence of other signs or symptoms of the climacteric suggest further search for the cause of the flushes.

**C. Abnormal Vaginal Bleeding:** Prior to the menopause, irregular vaginal bleeding is expected and does not necessitate a diagnostic workup in most cases. However, organic disease can occur at this time, and some patients require evaluation. If a woman is in her 40s or 50s and experiences an increase in cycle length and a decrease in the quantity of bleeding, menopausal involution can be presumed and endometrial sampling is not necessary. However, if the periods become more frequent and heavier or spotting between periods occurs, assessment of the endometrium should be done. The usual procedure is outpatient endometrial biopsy or inpatient D&C. The disadvantage of the former is that it may not be as accurate as D&C, and the drawbacks of the latter are greater expense and risk. If normal endometrium is found, no further investigation is required. If hyperplastic or cancerous endometrium is obtained, treatment should be instituted.

It is most unusual for a woman to experience vaginal bleeding because of ovarian activity by 6 months after the menopause. Thus, postmenopausal bleeding is much more ominous and necessitates evaluation each time it occurs. The only exception to this rule is the uterine bleeding associated with estrogen replacement therapy. Other guidelines are recommended for this type of bleeding (see Treatment).

Organic disease is commonly associated with postmenopausal bleeding. Endometrial polyps may be found. If so, D&C may be therapeutic. Endometrial hyperplasia may be discovered, frequently in obese women. This can be treated by the periodic administration of progestin or by hysterectomy. If hyperplasia develops in a woman taking estrogens, the addition of progestins should be considered. If hyperplasia develops unrelated to hormone replacement, surgery should be considered if the patient is a good surgical risk or is not reliable in taking progestins. The finding of endometrial cancer necessitates appropriate therapy depending on the stage and grade of the tumor.

**D. Vulvovaginitis:** Many specific vulvar and vaginal diseases (eg, trichomoniasis and candidiasis) may mimic the atrophic vulvovaginitis of estrogen deficiency. Their special clinical characteristics usually suggest more specific diagnostic testing. When pruritus and thinning of the vaginal epithelium or the vulvar skin are the only manifestations, therapeutic testing with local applications of estrogen may help to establish the diagnosis of vulvovaginitis. When any whitening, thickening, or cracking of vulvar tissues is present, biopsy to rule out carcinoma is mandatory. (This can easily be accomplished under local anesthesia by using the dermatologist's skin punch.) Biopsy to rule out carcinoma is also necessary for a suspicious-looking localized vaginal or cervical lesion.

**E. Osteoporosis:** Occasionally, the pain of vertebral compression may mimic that of gastric ulcer, renal colic, pyelonephritis, pancreatitis, spondylolisthesis, acute back strain, or herniated intervertebral disk.

## Prevention

Nothing can prevent the physiologic menopause (ie, ovarian function cannot be prolonged indefinitely), and nothing can be done to postpone its onset or slow its progress. However, artificial menopause can often be prevented. When ionizing radiation is used for the treatment of intra-abdominal disease, incidental ablation of ovarian function often cannot be avoided. In such cases, if an operation will serve equally well, it should be used in preference to radiation therapy in order to preserve the ovaries.

Elective removal of the ovaries to prevent ovarian cancer is frequently performed at laparotomy in premenopausal women, with deliberate acceptance of artificial menopause. This form of therapy, however, remains controversial, and we discourage its use.

## Treatment

As long as ovarian function is sufficient to maintain some uterine bleeding, no treatment is usually required. Occasionally, women complain of hot flushes while menstrual function is still present, and treatment with estrogen will relieve these symptoms. As the menstrual pattern alters and symptoms commence, patients begin to seek help.

**A. Counseling:** Every woman with climacteric symptoms deserves an adequate explanation of the physiologic event she is experiencing, in order to dispel her fears and minimize symptoms such as anxiety, depression, and sleep disturbance. Reassurance should emphasize what the climacteric is not—that contrary to anything the patient may have heard, she need not expect sudden aging or personal disasters of any sort. Specific reassurance about continued sexual activity is important.

**B. Estrogen Replacement:**

**1. Complications**–Before discussing the management of estrogen replacement, it is necessary to review the complications and contraindications of this type of therapy. These play an important role in the ultimate decision regarding treatment for all patients.

**a. Endometrial cancer**–The role of estrogen therapy in the development of endometrial cancer has been one of the most highly charged issues related to the climacteric. Current concerns are based on several lines of investigation. Although none has been conclusive, the scope of investigative efforts and the consistent incrimination of estrogen lead to the conclusion that estrogen stimulation of the endometrium, unopposed by progesterone, causes endometrial proliferation, hyperplasia, and, finally, neoplasia.

The reports of estrogen replacement and endometrial carcinoma have received the greatest attention; in most studies, a strong association has been found, with 2- to 8-fold overall risk ratios. High dosage and prolonged treatment increased the risk. Disease is local in most cases, although invasive tumors have been reported. Concerns have been raised about these studies, particularly regarding the selection of controls. In most studies, controls had not undergone sampling of the endometrium to rule out asymptomatic endometrial cancer. Studies using controls who have undergone endometrial sampling have shown no greater incidence of estrogen use in women with cancer than in women without cancer. Based on autopsy studies, approximately 50% of the endometrial cancers found at postmortem examination were not apparent in the women while they were alive. Thus, debates persist, and prudent physicians should discuss the risks with their patients and employ preventative measures.

**b. Breast cancer**–Early age at menarche and older age at menopause are known risk factors for breast cancer, and early oophorectomy is known to give protection against this disease. Ovarian activity is thus shown to be an important determinant of risk, and estrogen may play a role in the development of breast cancer. Studies in rodents support that view. More than 30 epidemiologic studies have been published since 1974 to determine the possible link between postmenopausal estrogen use and breast cancer. In general, the later studies have had better design, quality, and analytic strategies. The number of subjects in the later studies has also increased. However, statistically significant differences in one study are not confirmed in the next report. At least 6 meta-analyses of this topic also have been conducted. Again, these results have not always agreed.

Despite this inconsistency in studies, some trends have been observed. (1) The overall risk of breast cancer with estrogen use has uniformly not been shown to be increased. (2) Long-term use has been associated with mild increased risk (risk ratio 1.2–1.5) in some of the meta-analyses. (3) Increased estrogen dosage does not appear to increase risk. (4) The addition of a progestin does not appear to decrease risk. (5) Finally, risk does not vary in strata of family history of breast cancer or with benign breast disease.

Although these findings are somewhat reassuring, it must be remembered that all women are at risk for breast cancer. Thus, instructions for breast self-examination, a careful breast assessment, and routine screening mammography should be a part of the medical care of all older women.

**c. Hypertension**– Hypertension may develop during or may be exacerbated by use of oral contraceptives and usually disappears when the medications are discontinued. Hypertension has not been shown to be a risk of hormone replacement in women who are either normotensive or hypertensive at the beginning of replacement.

**d. Thromboembolic disease**–Use of oral contraceptives increases the risk of overt venous thromboembolic disease and subclinical disease extensive enough to be detected by laboratory procedures such as $_{125}$I fibrinogen uptake and plasma fibrinogen chromatography. In uncontrolled studies, thrombophlebitis has been reported following estrogen replacement therapy, but this has not been found in controlled experiments.

The effects of estrogen on the clotting mechanism may contribute to or be responsible for a generalized hypercoagulable state. Estrogen increases vascular endothelial proliferation; decreased venous blood flow; and enhances coagulability of blood, involving changes in the platelet, coagulation, and fibrinolytic systems. Reports have found decreased platelet counts. Evaluation of clotting factors has shown increases in factors VII, IX, X, and X complex; these factors are hepatic in origin. Estrogen replacement therapy can also cause decreases in anticoagulant factors such as antithrombin III and antithrombin Xa. Antithrombin III is of particular interest; it is also hepatic in origin and inactivates thrombin, activated factor X, and other enzymes involved with the generation of thrombin. Ingestion of conjugated estrogens, 1.25 mg/d, have been reported to have no effect on this anticlotting factor. Studies have reported increases of plasminogen and $\alpha_1$-antitrypsin with 1.25 mg of conjugated equine estrogens. The same has not been observed with nonoral estrogen administration.

**e. Lipid metabolism**–An increased incidence of gallbladder disease has been reported following estrogen replacement therapy. Estrogens cause increased amounts of cholesterol to collect in bile. Two primary bile salts, cholate and chenodeoxycholate, are produced by liver cells. In women taking estrogen, decreased levels of chenodeoxycholate and increased levels of cholate are found in bile. Chenodeoxycholate inhibits activity of the enzyme $\beta$-hydroxy-$\beta$-methylglutaryl-CoA reductase, which regulates cholesterol synthesis, and a decrease in chenodeoxycholate may therefore cause increased activity of $\beta$-hydroxy-$\beta$-methylglutaryl-CoA reductase, leading to increased synthesis of cholesterol. Bile normally has a 75–90% saturation in cholesterol, and even small increases of this substance can initiate cholesterol precipitation and stone formation. Three-fourths of gallstones are composed predominantly of cholesterol.

Estrogen replacement also makes an impact on circulating lipids. Most lipids are bound to proteins in the blood, and the concentrations of the various types of lipoproteins are associated with varying risks of heart disease. Lower levels of high-density lipoprotein cholesterol (HDL) and higher concentrations of total cholesterol, low-density (LDL) and very low-density lipoprotein cholesterol, and triglycerides are associated with increased risk of atherosclerosis and coronary artery disease. Estrogen replacement decreases LDL cholesterol and increases HDL cholesterol and triglycerides. Use of conjugated estrogens, 0.625 mg/d or less, causes approximately a 10% increase in HDL cholesterol. Much attention has been focused on the impact of estrogens on lipoproteins to explain its apparent beneficial effect on heart disease.

In patients with familial defects of lipoprotein metabolism, estrogen replacement therapy has been associated with massive elevations of plasma triglycerides, leading to pancreatitis and other complications. However, this is a very unusual complication of estrogen replacement.

**f. Miscellaneous**–Other side effects of estrogen therapy include uterine bleeding, generalized edema, mastodynia and breast enlargement, abdominal bloating, signs and symptoms resembling those of premenstrual tension, headaches (particularly of a "menstrual migraine" type), and excessive cervical mucus. These side effects may be dose-related or idiosyncratic and are managed by lowering the dosage, by use of another agent, or by discontinuation of the medication.

**2. Contraindications to estrogen replacement therapy**–Undiagnosed vaginal bleeding, acute liver disease, chronic impaired liver function, acute vascular thrombosis (with or without emboli), neuro-

ophthalmologic vascular disease, and endometrial or breast carcinoma are contraindications to estrogen replacement. Estrogen therapy may stimulate growth of malignant cells remaining after treatment of breast or endometrial carcinoma and may thus hasten the recurrence of cancer. Therefore, it is prudent to avoid estrogen therapy until arrest is likely. Recently, it has been suggested that women with early (stage 1) and well-differentiated (grade 1) endometrial cancer can be administered estrogens following primary treatment of the cancer. Care must be exercised in following this recommendation until properly studied. Patients who have had estrogen receptor-positive malignant tumors of the breast probably should not receive estrogen supplements. Recently, this concept has also been questioned. Again, until properly studied, physicians should avoid administering estrogens to such patients. A history of treated carcinoma of the cervix or ovary is not a contraindication to estrogen therapy. Estrogens may have undesirable effects on some patients with preexisting seizures, hypertension, fibrocystic disease of the breast, uterine leiomyoma, collagen disease, familial hyperlipidemia, diabetes mellitus, migraine headaches, chronic thrombophlebitis, and gallbladder disease. At the low dosages recommended for replacement therapy, increased growth of uterine myomas, endometriosis, or chronic cystic mastitis is rarely a concern.

**3. Management guidelines for estrogen replacement therapy**–Only general guidelines can be offered, because risks and benefits must be evaluated for each patient. Current indications for estrogen therapy are relief of menopausal symptoms including hot flushes and vaginal atrophy and prevention of osteoporosis. Caution should be exercised in providing therapy for other reasons until more definitive studies have been performed. If symptoms of hot flushes and vaginal atrophy are severe, therapy should be recommended; minimal or no symptoms may not require hormones. Prevention of osteoporosis depends on the bone density of a woman as measured by the newer techniques. The relative potency of the various estrogenic preparations has been only partially worked out.

In women with menopausal symptoms, a standard dosage of estrogen, such as 0.625 mg of conjugated equine estrogens, should be given daily (Table 57–5). Higher doses may be necessary to relieve hot flashes. Progressive reduction of dosage should be attempted as soon as feasible. Either systemic estrogen or vaginal creams can be used for vaginal symptoms. Treatment is usually required until sexual activity has ceased.

Prevention of osteoporosis, several guidelines are important. The lowest effective dosage has been established for several of the preparations. The 0.625 mg dosage of conjugated equine estrogens, the 1.25 mg dosage of piperazine estrone sulfate, and the 0.05 mg dosage of transdermal estradiol all have been

**Table 57–5.** Preparations of estrogens and progestins available in the USA for hormone replacement.

| Agent | How Supplied | Special Features |
|---|---|---|
| **Oral estrogens** | | |
| Conjugated equine estrogens | 0.3 mg, 0.625 mg,* 0.9 mg, 1.25 mg, 2.5 mg | Well studied, well tolerated, long use. |
| Micronized estradiol | 1 mg* scored tablet, 2 mg scored | Well tolerated. |
| Piperazine estrone (estropipate) | 0.625 mg, 1.25 mg,* 2.5 mg, 5.0 mg | The 1.25-mg dosage prevents bone loss from spine and hip. |
| Ethinyl estradiol | 0.02 mg, 0.05 mg, 0.5 mg | Not approved for prevention of osteoporosis. |
| Quinestrol | 100 μg | Not approved for prevention of osteoporosis. |
| Chlorotrianisene | 12 to 25 mg capsules | Not approved for prevention of osteoporosis. |
| Diethylstilbestrol | 1 mg, 5 mg enseals (enteric release), 1 mg, 5 mg tablets | Not approved for treatment of estrogen deficiency. |
| **Systemic estrogens** | | |
| Transdermal estradiol | 0.05 mg,* 0.1 mg patch | Well tolerated, 10% skin rash. |
| Injectable estrogens | | |
| Estradiol valerate | 20 mg/10 mL, 40 mg/10 mL, 4 mg/10 mL with 90 mg testosterone enanthanate | Certainty of administration; peak blood levels<br>Not approved for prevention of osteoporosis. |
| Polyestradiol phosphate | 40 mg ampules | Approved for use in prostate cancer only: not approved for treatment of estrogen deficiency. |
| **Vaginal estrogens** | | |
| Conjugated equine estrogens | 0.625 mg/g creme | Not approved for prevention of osteoporosis. |
| Micronized estradiol | 0.1 mg/g creme | Not approved for prevention of osteoporosis. |
| Piperazine estrone sulfate | 1.5 mg/g creme | Not approved for prevention of osteoporosis. |
| **Oral progestins** | | |
| Medroxyprogesterone acetate | 2.5 mg, 5 mg, 10 mg tablets | Well tolerated. |
| Megestrol acetate | 20 mg, 40 mg scored tablets | Well tolerated; dosage probably too large for routine use in hormone replacement. |
| Norethindrone | 0.35 μg | Available only as minipill. |
| Norethindrone acetate | 5 mg scored tablets | Dosage probably too large for routine use in hormone replacement. |
| **Injectable progestins** | | |
| Depoprovera | 100 mg/mL, 400 mg/mL | Approved for inoperable cancer and contraception. |

*Indicates lowest dosage of estrogen approved by FDA for prevention of osteoporosis.

shown to prevent bone loss from both the spine and the hip. The 0.5 mg dosage of micronized estradiol has been shown to prevent bone loss from the spine, but the FDA has approved only the 1- and 2-mg dosages. Early commencement of prophylaxis following cessation of ovarian function will maintain the highest bone density. Delay in administration will stop bone loss when estrogen is begun, but will not return bone density to that which was present at the time of the menopause. Long-term prophylaxis is essential to prevent fractures. At least 5 years appears necessary to reduce the occurrence of fracture and increase bone density in older women. Treatment for 1 or 2 years will have little impact on the occurrence of fractures.

All preparations—synthetic, naturally occurring, and nonsteroidal estrogens—probably yield equally good results, but only a few have been studied. We usually restrict the use of specific preparations to those that have been approved by the FDA for the prevention of osteoporosis. Many US physicians are now using continuous instead of interrupted estrogen administration.

**a. Progestin-estrogen therapy–**The most serious concern about estrogen replacement is the occurrence of endometrial hyperplasia or cancer. Progestins oppose the action of estrogen on the endometrium. Progestins reduce the number of estrogen receptors in glandular and stromal cells of the endometrium. These agents also block estrogen-induced synthesis of DNA, and they induce the intracellular enzymes, estradiol dehydrogenase and estrogen sulfotransferase. The former reduces estradiol to the much less potent estrone, while the later converts estrogen to estrogen sulfates for rapid elimination from endometrial cells. In addition, full secretory transformation occurs if the progestin is given at a large enough dosage for a sufficient length of time.

Progestins have been shown to reduce the occurrence of endometrial cancer. Three recently published epidemiologic studies have shown significant reduction of the occurrence of endometrial cancer with estrogen plus progestin compared with estrogen alone. One study indicated use of the progestin for greater than 10 days a month reduced the occurrence more than a shorter interval. In treating women with hormones, a more practical concern is the prevention of endometrial hyperplasia. Initially, British investigators showed that high-dose estrogens (1.25 mg or greater of conjugated equine estrogens) resulted in 32% hyperplasia, whereas low doses (0.625 mg or less) stimulated 16% hyperplasias in women followed for 15 months. In women given estrogen plus progestins, the occurrence of hyperplasia was 6% and 3%, respectively. In comparison to length of therapy, 7 days of progestin reduced the occurrence of hyperplasia to 4%, 10 days reduced it to 2%, and 12 days eliminated hyperplasia. Direct comparisons in drug trials have also shown reductions of hyperplasia in women given estrogens and progestins compared with those given estrogen alone. It should be pointed out that the majority of endometrial lesions observed in women in these trials were either cystic or simple hyperplasias, which could be reversed by giving a progestin or discontinuing the estrogen.

It is recommended to administer a progestin such as medroxyprogesterone acetate at a dosage of 10 mg, for 12–14 days each month (see Table 57–5). If this is accomplished, 80–90% of women will experience some vaginal bleeding monthly toward the end of or after the progestin is administered. An alternative is to prescribe a lower dosage, 2.5 mg, continuously. The combined, continuous administration of estrogen plus progestin promotes endometrial atrophy and results in amenorrhea in 70–90% of women who use continuous therapy for more than 1 year. The remainder will bleed occasionally, with the bleeding usually being less frequent, shorter, and lighter than with sequential therapy.

Administration of progestins can be associated with other uncomfortable side effects including fatigue, depression, breast tenderness, bloating, menstrual cramps, and headaches. It may not be possible to use the amounts of progestins recommended above. If lesser dosages or duration of progestins are necessary, endometrial sampling to diagnose the development of hyperplasia should be performed.

## Special Treatment Problems

**A. Alternatives to Estrogen Therapy:** Estrogen replacement is contraindicated in some patients, and others may want to avoid the risks of this type of therapy. Alternative medications are available for control of some of the symptoms and complaints associated with the climacteric.

For hot flushes, depo-medroxyprogesterone acetate, 150 mg/mo intramuscularly, oral administration

of the same agent, 10–40 mg/d, or megestrol acetate 20–80 mg/d, have all been shown to be more effective than placebo but less efficacious than estrogen in reducing hot flashes. Clonidine and methyldopa have also been shown to reduce flushes, but cause their own side effects and usually have not been satisfactory medications.

For prevention of osteoporosis, calcium supplements have been shown to significantly reduce the loss of calcium from bone, particularly several years after menopause. Elemental calcium, 1000–1500 mg, should be given. Cyclic administration of the biphosphonate, etidronate, has also been effective in preventing bone loss, but is not FDA approved. Calcitonin also prevents bone loss, but requires frequent injections. Vitamin D with calcium may also be effective but needs more study. For vaginal atrophy, no good substitution therapy has been devised.

**B. Uterine Bleeding:** If patients are given sequential estrogen and progestins, the majority will experience some uterine bleeding. This bleeding can occur during the treatment-free interval (scheduled bleeding) or while the medications are being administered (unscheduled bleeding). Hyperplastic endometrium can develop with this type of therapy. If the bleeding is heavy or prolonged, a biopsy should be performed. If endometrial hyperplasia is present, the medications can be discontinued, or a progestin can be given each day of estrogen administration. Whichever approach is adopted, a repeat biopsy should be performed to make certain that the hyperplastic endometrium has resolved. The cost-effectiveness ratio for periodic biopsy in women who do not bleed or bleed only during the medication-free interval is poor and indicates that such biopsy is probably not necessary.

In women taking estrogen only, the incidence of endometrial hyperplasia can be as high as 25% after only 12 months of therapy. Hyperplasia occurs in women who do not experience vaginal bleeding, bleed only during the medication-free interval, or bleed during drug administration. Thus, a pretreatment biopsy and yearly endometrial biopsies are necessary in all women receiving estrogens alone to determine the presence of hyperplasia. Again, estrogen withdrawal or combined estrogen-progesterone therapy may be employed to treat the hyperplasia. It is presumed, but not established, that the incidence of endometrial cancer will be reduced if the programs discussed above are instituted.

## Prognosis

The prognosis for the postmenopausal woman who does not develop clinically manifest estrogen deficiency includes only the ordinary hazards of disease and aging. For the woman who does develop signs of estrogen deficiency, steroid therapy can correct physical symptoms and signs, ameliorate associated emotional disturbances, and prevent the development of major metabolic estrogen deficiency disorders. Correction of minor distressing symptoms and signs can improve the general well-being of the postmenopausal woman and help her to pursue a vigorous life.

On the other hand, steroid therapy for the postmenopausal woman who does not need it serves no purpose and can cause unpleasant side effects and impose unnecessary risks to her health.

## REFERENCES

Abraham GE, Maroulis GB: Effect of exogenous estrogen on serum pregnenolone, cortisol, and androgens in postmenopausal women, Obstet Gyne 1975;45:271.

Adams MR et al: Inhibition of coronary artery atherosclerosis by 17-beta estradiol in ovariectomized monkeys: Lack of an effect of added progesterone. Arteriosclerosis 1990;10:1051.

Antunes CM et al: Endometrial cancer and estrogen use. N Engl J Med 1979;300;9.

Barrett-Connor E, Bush TL: Estrogen replacement and coronary heart disease. Cardiovasc Clin 1989;19:159.

Barrett-Connor E, Miller V: Estrogens, lipids, and heart disease. Clin Geriatr Med 1993;9:57.

Bergkvist L et al: The risk of breast cancer after estrogen and estrogen-progestin replacement. N Engl J Med 1989; 321:293.

Bolognia J: Aging skin, epidermal and dermal changes. Prog Clin Biol Res 1989;320:121.

Boston Collaborative Drug Surveillance Program, Boston University Medical Center: Surgically confirmed gallbladder disease, venous thromboembolism, and breast tumors in relation to postmenopausal estrogen therapy. N Engl J Med 1974;290:15.

Brincat M et al: Long-term effects of the menopause and sex hormones on skin thickness. Br J Obstet Gynecol 1985; 92:256.

Brincat M et al: Skin collagen changes in postmenopausal women receiving different regimens of estrogen therapy. Obstet Gynecol 1987;70:123.

Brincat M et al: A study of the decrease of skin collagen content, skin thickness, and bone mass in the postmenopausal woman. Obstet Gyneol 1987;70:840.

Buckler HM et al: Gonadotropin, steroid, and inhibin levels in women with incipient ovarian failure during anovulatory and ovulatory rebound cycles. J Clin Endocrinol Metab 1991;72:116.

Campbell S, Whitehead M: Estrogen therapy and the postmenopausal syndrome. Clin Obstet Gynecol 1977;4:31.

Chetkowski RJ et al: Biologic effects of transdermal estradiol. N Engl J Med 1986;314:1615.

Creasman WT: Estrogen replacement therapy: is previously treated cancer a contraindication? Obstet Gynecol 1991; 77:308.

Cummings SR et al: Bone density at various sites for prediction of hip fractures. Lancet 1993;341:962.

Dawson-Hughes B: Calcium supplementation and bone loss: A review of controlled clinical trials (1-3). Am J Clin Nutr 1991;54:274S.

Delmas PD: Biochemical markers of bone turnover: Methodology and clinical use in osteoporosis. Am J Med 1991;91:59S.

Erickson GE: Normal ovarian function. Clin Obstet Gynecol 1978;21:31.

Ettinger B et al: Low-dosage micronized 17β-estradiol prevents bone loss in postmenopausal women. Am J Obstet Gynecol 1992;166:479.

Ewertz M: Influence of noncontraceptive exogenous and endogenous sex hormones on breast cancer risk in Denmark. Int J Cancer 1988;42:832.

Falkeborn M et al: The risk of acute myocardial infarction after estrogen and estrogen-progesterone replacement. Br J Obstet Gynaecol 1992;99:821.

Field CS et al: Preventive effects of transdermal 17β- estradiol on osteoporotic changes after surgical menopause: A two-year placebo-controlled trial. Am J Obstet Gynecol 1993;168:114.

Furchgott RF, Vanhoutte PM: Endothelium-derived relaxing and contracting factors. FASEB J 1989;3:2007.

Gambone J et al: Further delineation of hypothalamic dysfunction responsible for menopausal hot flashes. J Clin Endocrinol Metab 1985;59:1097.

Gibbons WE et al: Biochemical and biological effects of sequential estrogen/progestin therapy on the endometrium of postmenopausal women. Am J Obstet Gynecol 1986; 154:456.

Hammond MG, Hatley L, Talbert LM: A double blind study to evaluate the effect of methyldopa on menopausal vasomotor flushes. J Clin Endocrinol Metab 1984;58:1158.

Hasselquist MB et al: Isolation and characterization of the estrogen receptor in human skin. J Clin Endocrinol Metab 1980;50:76.

Hayashi T et al: Basal release of nitric oxide from aortic rings is greater in female rabbits than in male rabbits: Implications for atherosclerosis. Proc Natl Acad Sci USA 1992;89:11259.

Henderson BE et al: Re-evaluating the role of progestogen therapy after the menopause. Fertil Steril 1988;49 (Suppl):9S.

Horwitz RI et al: Necropsy diagnosis of endometrial cancer and detection-bias in case/control studies. Lancet 1981; 2:66.

Jensen J et al: Long-term effects of percutaneous estrogens and oral progesterone on serum lipoproteins in postmenopausal women. Am J Obstet Gynecol 1987;156:66.

Johnston CC Jr, Slemenda CW, Melton LJ III: Clinical use of bone densitometry. N Engl J Med 1991;324:1105.

Judd HL: Hormonal dynamics associated with the menopause. Clin Obstet Gynecol 1976;19:775.

Judd HL et al: Endocrine function of the postmenopausal ovary: Concentrations of androgens and estrogens in ovarian and peripheral vein blood. J Clin Endocrinol Metab 1974;39:1020.

Judd HL et al: Estrogen replacement therapy: Indications and complications. Ann Intern Med 1983;98:195.

Judd HL et al: Origin of serum estradiol in postmenopausal women. Obstet Gynecol 1982;59:680.

Judd HL et al: Serum androgens and estrogens in postmenopausal women with and without endometrial cancer. Am J Obstet Gynecol 1980;136:859.

Laufer LR et al: Effect of clonidine on hot flashes in postmenopausal women. Obstet Gynecol 1982;60:583.

Lindsay R et al: Bone response to termination of estrogen treatment. Lancet 1978;1:1325.

Lindsay R et al: Prevention and treatment of osteoporosis. Lancet 1993;341:801.

Meldrum DR et al: Elevations in skin temperature of the finger as an objective index of postmenopausal hot flashes: Standardization of the technique. Am J Obstet Gynecol 1979;135:713.

Nabulsi AA et al: Association of hormone-replacement therapy with various cardiovascular risk factors in postmenopausal women. N Engl J Med 1993;328:1069.

Phillips SM, Sherwin BB: Effects of estrogen on memory function in surgically menopausal women. Psychoneuroendocrinology 1992;17(5):485.

Reid IR et al: Effect of calcium supplementation on bone loss in postmenopausal women. N Engl J Med 1993;328:460.

Rickard DJ, Gowen M, MacDonald BR: Proliferative responses to estradiol IL-1 alpha and TGF beta by cells expressing alkaline phosphatase in human osteoblast-like cell cultures. Calcif Tissue Int 1993;52:227.

Rigg LA et al: Absorption of estrogens from vaginal creams. N Engl J Med 1978;298:195.

Roberts WC, Giraldo AA: Bilateral oophorectomy in menstruating women and accelerated coronary atherosclerosis: An unproved connection. Am J Med 1979;67:363.

Rubin SM, Cummings SR: Results of bone densitometry affect women's decisions about taking measures to prevent fractures. Ann Intern Med 1992;116:990.

Shahrad P, Marks R: A pharmacologic effect of estrogen on human epidermis. Br J Dermatol 1977;97:383.

Sherman BM, Korenman SG: Hormonal characteristics of the human menstrual cycle throughout reproductive life. J Clin Invest 1975;55:669.

Sitteri PK, MacDonald PC: Role of extraglandular estrogen in human endocrinology. Chap 28, pp 615–629. In: **Handbook of Physiology: Endocrinology.** 7. Vol 2 (1). Green RO, Astwood E (editors). Williams & Wilkins, 1973.

Storm T et al: Effect of intermittent cyclical etidronate therapy on bone mass and fracture rate in women with postmenopausal osteoporosis. N Engl J Med 1990;322:1265.

Stumpf WE et al: Estrogen target cells in the skin. Experientia 1974;30:196.

Tataryn IV et al: LH, FSH, and skin temperature during the menopausal hot flash. J Clin Endocrinol Metab 1979;49:152.

Tsai KS, Ebeling PR, Riggs BL: Bone responsiveness to parathyroid hormone in normal and osteoporotic postmenopausal women. J Clin Endocrinol Metabl 1989;69:1024.

Vermeulen A: The hormonal activity of the postmenopausal ovary. J Clin Endocrinol Metab 1976;42:247.

Vollman RF: *The Menstrual Cycle.* WB Saunders, vol. 7, 1977:193.

Weiss NS et al: Decreased risk of fractures of the hip and lower forearm with postmenopausal use of estrogen. N Engl J Med 1980;302:551.

Whitehead MI et al: Effects of estrogens and progestins on the biochemistry and morphology of the postmenopausal endometrium. N Engl J Med 1981;305:1599.

Williams JK, Adams MR, Klopfenstein HS: Estrogen modulates responses of atherosclerotic coronary arteries. Circulation 1990;81:1680.

Williams JK et al: Short-term administration of estrogen and vascular responses of atherosclerotic coronary arteries. J Am Coll Cardiol 1992;20:452.

# Microsurgery in Gynecology

# 58

*Victor Gomel, MD, & Timothy C. Rowe, MD*

The past 3 decades have been witness to profound social changes, and prominent among these changes have been altered contraceptive practices and sexual behavior. In the late 1960s and through the 1970s, the introduction of oral contraception led to increased sexual activity without the use of barrier contraception. Inevitably, sexually transmitted diseases became more prevalent. North American demographic data have shown a significant rise in the incidence of pelvic inflammatory disease (PID) in young women during the early 1980s. The resulting pelvic adhesions and damage to the uterine tubes have been shown to cause involuntary infertility in about 20% of women after 1 episode of acute salpingitis and in more than 50% of women after 3 or more episodes. Tubal damage as a result of PID may also increase the risk of ectopic pregnancy.

Although there is early evidence that the incidence of gonorrhea in the population has been reduced, the incidence of other infections is not known. An estimated 20% of infertility is due directly to tubal damage resulting from PID, with this percentage showing little sign of decreasing.

Conventional techniques for surgical management of tubal infertility have produced disappointing results (Table 58-1). These results led to the introduction of microsurgical techniques for fertility surgery. Swolin (1975) was the first to use magnification in performing salpingostomy. Microsurgical techniques were subsequently expanded and applied to the treatment of other conditions and reconstruction of other parts of the fallopian tube (Gomel, 1977).

## APPROACH TO THE INFERTILE COUPLE

Even when tubal or peritoneal factors are the suspected cause of infertility, other fertility parameters must also be assessed. Semen analysis, appropriate assessment of ovulation, and, when necessary, other hormonal and immunologic parameters, must be performed.

In the assessment of tubal factors, hysterosalpingographic examination is the first step. A properly performed hysterosalpingogram is most valuable in evaluation of the uterine cavity and of intratubal architecture. An aqueous contrast medium (diatrizoate meglumine 60% [Hypaque 60%]) is preferred because the better penetrating ability of the aqueous medium permits delineation of the tubal mucosa and the subtle radiologic signs of intratubal disease. Hysterosalpingography also permits assessment of the length and internal patency and architecture of the proximal segments in the presence of midtubal obstruction or in women seeking sterilization reversal. In the event of cornual obstruction or sterilization procedures causing damage to the oviducts near the cornu, hysterosalpingography permits assessment of the intramural segments. With terminal tubal occlusion, the presence of rugal markings implies a favorable prognosis for future pregnancies; conversely, intratubal adhesions are an unfavorable prognostic sign.

Laparoscopy and hysterosalpingography are complementary procedures in the evaluation of tubal or peritoneal factors. It is recommended that laparoscopy follow hysterosalpingography, since information about the uterine tubes and their patency is especially important in cases that will prove amenable to laparoscopic surgery. In view of the possible therapeutic effect of hysterosalpingography, laparoscopy should be delayed for some months when the oviducts are found to be patent. Laparoscopy will permit assessment of the nature and extent of pelvic and periadnexal adhesions. The judicious decision to perform laparoscopic inferility surgery will frequently avoid the need for laparotomy. Indeed, laparoscopic surgery is recommended as the primary approach to peritubal and fimbrial disease.

If hysterosalpingography demonstrates the presence of intrauterine lesions (synechiae, submucous fibroids, polyps), hysteroscopy is performed in conjunction with laparoscopy. Hysteroscopy also allows direct visualization and assessment of the internal tubal ostia and the proximal 1–2 mm of the intramural segments.

If cornual obstruction of the tubes is shown at hysterosalpingography (in the absence of previous surgical occlusion), a number of options for subsequent assessment are available. It is possible that a tube is patent despite the failure of dye to pass, which may be due to cornual spasm, to the presence of a mucous plug or synechiae obstructing the intramural or isthmic portion of the tube, or simply to poor technique. The use of tubal cannulation under either radiologic or hysteroscopic control usually permits the differentiation of apparent from true obstructions; the value of cannulation in overcoming true pathologic occlusion remains to be established by controlled randomized study. Given the minimal risk of morbidity, however, it is reasonable to attempt tubal cannulation in women whose initial test of tubal patency indicates occlusion. If patency cannot be established, the choices for therapy are microsurgery and in vitro fertilization (IVF).

The choice of therapy between surgery and IVF depends on both technical and nontechnical factors; discussion of this issue is beyond the scope of this chapter.

# BASIC PRINCIPLES OF MICROSURGERY

Microsurgery is more than the use of an operating microscope—it is a *concept* of surgery requiring the surgeon to be as atraumatic as possible, by means of gentle tissue handling, careful dissection, meticulous hemostasis, the use of delicate instruments and fine sutures, avoidance of tissue drying, and accurate approximation of tissues.

The basic tenet of all abdominal surgery is to minimize tissue injury and avoid introducing foreign material into the peritoneal cavity. This is especially important in microsurgery. Peritoneal trauma, regardless of its nature (mechanical, thermal, desiccative, chemical, bacterial), induces an inflammatory reaction. The inflammatory exudate contains fibrinogen, which is converted into fibrin. Fibrin deposition and fibroblastic proliferation over this matrix are the basis for adhesion formation. Tissue handling must be gentle, with elevation, retraction, or grasping done by means of rounded Teflon rods or simply with the gloved fingers. To prevent desiccation, exposed peritoneal surfaces are kept moistened with irrigating solution. The addition of heparin to the irrigating solution (5000 U of heparin per liter of Ringer's lactate [Ringer's irrigation USP]) minimizes clot formation during the procedure and prevents collection of fibrin in the peritoneal cavity. Precise reperitonealization of denuded serosal surfaces is achieved without tension. Total excision of diseased tissues and accurate approximation of tissue planes enhance reestablishment of function.

The use of magnification enhances the surgeon's ability to prevent tissue trauma and to recognize pathologic changes and serosal disturbances. Magnification also allows precise hemostasis with pinpoint electrocoagulation, minimizing destruction of adjacent tissues.

## INSTRUMENTATION

Very few instruments are needed in gynecologic microsurgery, the basic requirements being a microneedleholder, platform microforceps (plain and toothed), and microscissors (Fig 58–1). The needle driver and forceps have rounded rather than pointed tips, and the needleholder has a concave-convex jaw configuration for firm grasping of the needle. Iristype scissors are usually used for tubal transection. Teflon-coated rods of different configuration and with rounded tips are used for retraction and elevation of tissues and adhesions.

Electromicrosurgery requires the use of a fine microelectrode. An insulated microelectrode with 100-micron shaft and conical pointed tip is used for both cutting (ie, division of adhesions) and coagulation of bleeders. A microbipolar jeweler's forceps may also be used for electrodesiccation.

The ValleyLab electrosurgical unit can be used in many commonly performed surgical and gynecologic procedures. It delivers steady current at low levels that allow use of a microelectrode for microsurgical procedures. The handle is equipped with a rocker switch that permits fingertip control of both cutting and coagulation modes. Although some physicans

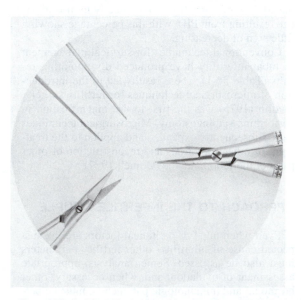

**Figure 58–1.** Magnified view of the tips of 3 essential microsurgical instruments. Clockwise from right: needle holder, scissors, forceps.

use a $CO_2$ laser routinely for division of adhesions and tubal transection, there is no evidence that the $CO_2$ laser is superior to either electromicrosurgery or mechanical surgery with fine sharp instruments.

Synthetic 8-0 sutures are best for gynecologic microsurgery; we employ absorbable sutures except where specific reason exists to use nonabsorbable ones. It is essential that these sutures be armed with fine tapercut type needles; otherwise the benefit of using fine sutures will be negated by needle trauma. A suture commonly employed is 8-0 polyglactin on a 130-micron, 4 mm or 5 mm long tapercut needle.

## MAGNIFICATION

The use of an operating microscope allows high magnification, clear vision with coaxial illumination, and an unchanging visual field. An objective lens with a focal length of 275 or 300 mm is recommended because it leaves an adequate working distance between the lens and the pelvic organs. The magnification, focus, and attitude of the microscope may be altered during the procedure by hand or foot controls, depending on the type of microscope.

The use of magnifying loupes is reserved for the division of adhesions at their distal extremities (ie, the pelvic sidewall, cul-de-sac) and for excision and repair of lesions located deep in the pelvis (eg, endometriotic lesions).

## MICROSURGICAL TECHNIQUE

### PROCEDURAL SETUP

Proper attention to details in setting up for infertility microsurgery facilitates the procedure itself and reduces unnecessary irritations and delays. Steps prior to induction of anesthesia are as follows: (1) The surgeon ensures that all necessary instruments are available and in working order. (2) The microscope is checked and adjusted for the surgeon's needs. (3) Any ancillary equipment (electrosurgical unit, television camera and monitor, etc) is checked to be sure it is in working order.

Once the patient is anesthetized, a Foley catheter is inserted into the bladder. A pediatric Foley catheter is inserted into the uterine cavity for intraoperative chromopertubation. A sterile extension tubing is connected at one end to the catheter and at the other to a syringe filled with dilute dye solution. This permits the syringe to be brought into the sterile field. The vagina is packed to elevate the uterine fundus under the abdominal incision.

Physicians and nurses assisting at surgery wash their gloves thoroughly before the instruments are handled and the patient is draped. This reduces the introduction of starch into the peritoneal cavity.

A minilaparotomy incision is usually adequate for tubal reconstructive procedures. We have used this type of access, and the following measures, since 1986. The site of the incision is infiltrated with 0.25% bupivacaine (Marcaine) or 0.5% lidocaine (Xylocaine) solution before and after the operation. In addition, once the incision has been closed a regional nerve block is established. Because of these measures, and minimal bowel manipulation, the patients require only small amounts of systemic analgesics administered postoperatively. Patients are admitted to hospital on the day of surgery and discharged usually within 24 hours of admission.

Good hemostasis of the abdominal wound is important to keep blood from dripping into the peritoneal cavity during the procedure. The gloves are rinsed once again before the peritoneal cavity is entered. Once access to the peritoneal cavity is gained and the pelvic organs are examined, the operation goes forward:

(1) A wound protector is inserted and a modified Dennis-Brown retractor is put in place.

(2) Bowel is displaced into the upper peritoneal cavity and retained with a Kerlex pad soaked in heparinized lactated Ringer's solution. Manipulation of bowel is kept to an absolute minimum.

(3) The table is placed in a slight Trendelenburg position (10–15 degrees); if desired, it may also be tilted toward the surgeon.

(4) The uterus and adnexa are elevated by packing the pouch of Douglas loosely with Kerlex pads washed in the irrigating solution.

(5) The microscope is then brought over the operative field. (The microscope need not be draped; it is cleansed before the procedure and sterile neoprene caps are applied to the controls.)

## MICROSURGICAL PROCEDURES

### SALPINGO-OVARIOLYSIS

If the tubes are patent, the primary approach to periadnexal disease is laparoscopic salpingo-ovariolysis, generally performed during the initial diagnostic laparoscopy. Laparotomy for this purpose is performed rarely and is usually part of a reconstructive tubal operation.

Periadnexal adhesions usually encapsulate parts or all of the tube and ovary and extend to the lateral pelvic wall, the posterior aspect of the broad ligaments, and the uterus. The adhesions are exposed at their distal margins with Teflon rods and are divided electrosurgically one layer at a time without damaging the adjacent pelvic peritoneum. The use of an elongating adaptor attached to the handle of the electrosurgical unit facilitates divisions deep in the pelvis. Division of the adhesions is effected electrosurgically over a Teflon rod using a microelectrode. For transection, either pure cutting or blended current is used. Pure coagulating current is usually employed for electrodesiccation of individual vessels. Magnification with loupes and proper illumination enhance accuracy.

Once the adhesions are freed from their distal attachments, the adnexa are elevated by packing the pouch of Douglas loosely with Kerlex pads soaked in irrigating solution. The microscope is brought over the operating field. The adhesions are then divided in a similar manner at the level of the tubal serosa or ovarian surface and are thus excised. Care must be taken not to damage the tubal serosa or ovarian surface. Inadvertently created defects in the peritoneum may be closed without tension using 6-0 to 8-0 polyglactin suture.

## FIMBRIOPLASTY

Fimbrioplasty involves reconstruction of existing fimbriae in a partially or totally occluded oviduct. The specific procedure necessary to reconstruct the fimbriae depends on whether they are agglutinated or intimately covered by serosa and whether the principal lesion is prefimbrial phimosis (stenosis at the level of the abdominal tubal ostium). In the latter case, the fimbriae may have a relatively normal external appearance.

Agglutinated fimbriae may be separated by gentle dilatation with closed mosquito forceps introduced through the phimotic opening. In some cases, electrosurgical dissection may also be necessary.

If agglutination of the fimbria is associated with a serosal layer that covers or constricts the terminal end of the tube, it is necessary first to incise or excise the serosal layer.

Prefimbrial phimosis is best treated by electrosurgical incision on the antimesosalpingeal edge of the tube, commencing at the fimbriated end and extending over the phimotic area and for a short distance into the ampulla. The edges of the incised area are everted with 2 interrupted 8-0 polyglactin sutures to maintain the enlarged stoma.

## SALPINGOSTOMY
## (Salpingoneostomy)

As with fimbrioplasty and salpingo-ovariolysis, the primary approach to the management of distal tubal occlusion has evolved to become a laparoscopic approach. However, under some circumstances (for example, distal tubal occlusion in a patient with contralateral cornual occlusion) a microsurgical approach to salpingostomy is indicated.

Salpingostomy is the surgical creation of a new ostium in a tube whose fimbrial end is totally occluded, forming a hydrosalpinx or sactosalpinx. Depending on its location on the tube, salpingostomy may be terminal, ampullary, or isthmic.

**Terminal salpingostomy** is preferable, since the tube is conserved in its entirety and the tubo-ovarian relationship is maintained. However, localized lesions such as intratubal adhesions may oblige the surgeon to excise a portion of the distal oviduct and to resort to **ampullary salpingostomy.** Similarly, reversal of a prior fimbriectomy (Kroener sterilization) also requires ampullary salpingostomy. In view of the extremely poor chance for a successful outcome, salpingostomy should not be undertaken unless at least 60% of the ampulla has been preserved.

Before undertaking a terminal salpingostomy, it is necessary to assess the tube and ovary and the tubo-ovarian ligament. It is essential for the tube (especially the fimbrial end) to be free. If the tube is adherent to the ovary or other structure, it is dissected free using sharp or blunt dissection or electrosurgery as necessary.

Once the normal anatomic relationships are restored, the tube is distended by transcervical chromopertubation. The occluded terminal end of the distended tube is examined through the microscope. It usually exhibits relatively avascular lines extending radially from a central punctum. This central point is entered first, and the incision is continued toward the ovary over an avascular line using the microelectrode and blend current. This step fashions a fimbria ovarica. After the initial incision is made, additional incisions are made along the circumference of the tube over avascular areas by everting the mucosa and working from within the tube. In this manner, it is possible to avoid cutting through the vascular mucosal folds, which will be shaped as neofimbriae. Salpingostomy is usually associated with minimal bleeding. Bleeding points are coagulated individually with the microelectrode, using coagulating current. Once a satisfactory stoma has been fashioned, the mucosal edges are everted slightly and without tension and secured with interrupted 8-0 sutures (Fig 58–2).

Depending on circumstances, it may be necessary to modify this technique.

## TUBOCORNUAL ANASTOMOSIS FOR PATHOLOGIC CORNUAL OCCLUSION OF THE TUBES

The traditional surgical approach to cornual occlusion associated with a variety of conditions (eg, infec-

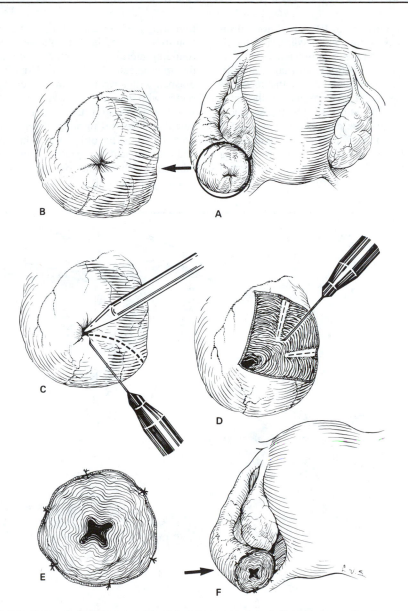

**Figure 58–2.** Salpingostomy. **A:** Salpingo-ovariolysis has been completed. **B:** Under magnification, the occluded terminal end of the tube exhibits a central dimple with avascular lines extending radially. **C:** The central point has been entered, and the initial incision will be continued toward the ovary over an avascular line. **D:** The mucosa is everted. Working from within the tube, additional incisions will be made along the circumference of the tube over avascular areas: **E:** Once a satisfactory stoma has been fashioned, the mucosal edges are everted slightly and secured with interrupted sutures. **F:** The completed salpingostomy.

tion, salpingitis isthmica nodosa, and endometriosis) has been tubouterine implantation. Microsurgical techniques and instrumentation have permitted anastomosis to be performed instead, after removal of the affected tubal segment.

Selective salpingography and tubal cannulation are useful techniques in differentiating between true occlusion occurring as a result of a disease process and obstructions due to cornual spasm, mucus plug, or in-

tratubal synechiae. However, the value of these techniques in the management of cornual occlusion associated with disease processes such as salpingitis isthmica nodosa remains to be determined. In such cases, microsurgical reconstruction remains the treatment of choice.

Initially, the cornual region of the uterus is injected superficially in a circular manner 1 cm proximal to the uterotubal junction with a dilute solution of vasopressin (10 U of vasopressin in 100 mL of normal saline). This approach minimizes bleeding and facilitates the procedure. The tube is incised adjacent to the uterus (at the uterotubal junction), with care not to divide the arcade of artery and vein at the mesosalpingeal margin (Fig 58–3A). The patency of the intramural portion of the tube is assessed by transcervical chromopertubation, and the cut surface is examined under the highest magnification for pathologic changes. It may be necessary to excise varying lengths of the intramural tube until patent and normal oviduct is reached. With the uterus distended, the in-

tramural tube is excised 1 or 2 mm at a time. The portion to be excised is first dissected free from the surrounding uterine musculature electrosurgically using the microelectrode (Fig 58–3B). The tube is then grasped with a strong toothed microforceps and transected with the use of a curved blade (Gomel Cornual Blade) (Fig 58–3C). Excision is continued until the patent and normal intramural segment is reached. A normal tube is free of fibrosis; it has normal muscular architecture, and the mucosal folds are intact and exhibit a pristine vascular pattern.

The approach described prevents creation of a

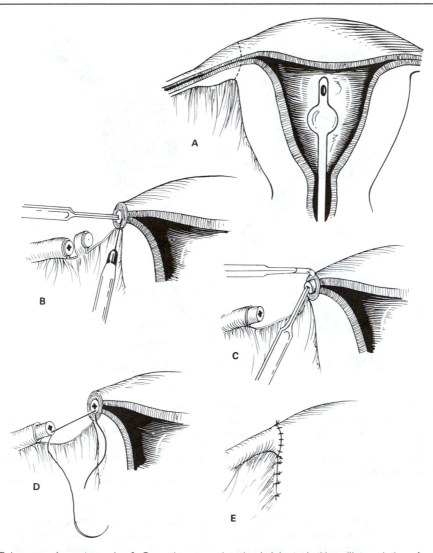

**Figure 58–3.** Tubocornual anastomosis. **A:** Once the cornual region is injected with a dilute solution of vasopressin and oxytocin, the tube is incised at the uterotubal junction. **B:** Serial incisions are placed on the isthmus, until normal patent tube is reached. The occluded portion of the intramural tube is dissected from the surrounding uterine musculature electrosurgically. **C:** The intramural portion already dissected from the surrounding uterine musculature is grasped and excised with a curved blade. **D:** The muscularis of the 2 segments is approximated with interrupted sutures, the first of which is placed at the 6 o'clock position. **E:** The seromuscularis of the cornu is approximated to the tubal serosa, and the mesosalpinx is joined to the uterus.

large defect in the cornu. Depending on the extent of excision of the intramural segment, tubocornual anastomosis may be juxtamural, intramural, or juxtauterine.

The occluded and abnormal segment of isthmus is then excised. Serial incisions are placed with iris scissors on this segment of tube, starting at the uterotubal junction, until normal isthmus is reached (Fig 58–3B). The patency of the distal segment of tube is confirmed by injecting irrigating solution through the fimbriated end (descending hydrotubation). The small transected segments of affected isthmus are excised from the mesosalpinx, remaining close to the tube in order to spare the tubal vessels. Hemostasis is achieved by desiccating only the more significant bleeders; overzealous electrocauterization must be resisted to avoid devitalization of the anastomosis site.

End-to-end anastomosis between the apparently healthy intramural and isthmic segments is then performed. The muscularis and epithelium are approximated with interrupted 8-0 polyglactin sutures placed at cardinal points in such a way that the knots remain external. Except in the case of juxtamural anastomosis, it is necessary to place all the sutures before they are tied. With anastomosis deeper in the cornu, tying the first suture would make placement of the subsequent sutures difficult or impossible.

The first muscular suture is placed at the 6 o'clock position (Fig 58–3D); it is not tied and is identified with a small Weck clip. The other sutures are placed using a single strand. This approach facilitates suture placement and prevents entanglement of sutures. The isthmus is held close to the intramural segment, and the 6 o'clock suture is tied. Sutures must be tied without undue tension. It may be necessary to approximate the isthmic mesosalpinx to the uterus with a single 7-0 suture before tying the muscular sutures. Once the 6 o'clock suture has been tied, further muscular sutures are tied individually after the loop between successive sutures has been divided. After apposition of the epithelium and muscularis, the seromuscularis of the cornu is approximated to the tubal serosa with 8-0 polyglactin sutures. The mesosalpinx is then joined to the uterus in a similar fashion (Fig 58–3E).

Tubocornual anastomosis may also be performed for the purpose of sterilization reversal. Such cases commonly require juxtamural anastomosis, since the intramural segment of the tube is usually intact.

## TUBOTUBAL ANASTOMOSIS

Tubotubal anastomosis is performed most frequently for reversal of a prior sterilization procedure. Tubal occlusions associated with disease processes are rare at sites other than the cornu; they may be due to endometriosis or follicular salpingitis but are more frequently associated with tubal pregnancy which has arrested or has been treated conservatively.

The occluded segment—or, in the previously sterilized group, the occluded ends—is resected (Fig 58–4). Transection of the tube is effected with iris scissors, and the occluded stump is excised from the mesosalpinx electrosurgically. In this process, it is mandatory to stay close to the tube to avoid broaching the mesosalpingeal vessels. Patency of the proximal and distal tubal segments is confirmed (respectively) by transcervical chromopertubation and descending hydropertubation, and the cut surfaces are examined under high magnification to ascertain normalcy.

End-to-end anastomosis of the tubal segments is performed in 2 layers using 8-0 suture material as described for tubocornual anastomosis. The first layer apposes the epithelium and muscularis, and the first suture is placed at the mesosalpingeal edge of the tube (6 o'clock position), and tied. These sutures incorporate the muscularis and submucosa, avoiding the mucosa. However, there is no evidence that inclusion of the epithelium adversely affects outcome. These sutures are placed so that the knots lie externally. Depending on the luminal caliber of the tubal segments, 3 or more additional sutures are placed to complete the approximation of the epithelial and muscular layers. The anastomosis is completed by apposition of the serosa and mesosalpinx using the same caliber of suture.

## PREOPERATIVE MANAGEMENT

In the normal, healthy patient, preoperative management differs little from what is required for any major gynecologic procedure (see Chapter 43). With placement of an intrauterine catheter for tubal reconstructive procedures, prophylactic antibiotics are employed, usually in the form of cefazolin sodium or cefoxitin sodium, in 2 intravenous doses—one administered 30 minutes before the procedure and one 6 hours after the first dose. Operation is deferred if there is any suggestion of recent pelvic infection. Systemic corticosteroids are of no proven value. However, as described in the following text, intraperitoneal corticosteroids may be used at the completion of surgery to reduce postoperative adhesion formation.

## POSTOPERATIVE MANAGEMENT

At the time of abdominal closure, 150–200 mL of lactated Ringer's solution containing 1000 mg of hydrocortisone sodium succinate may be left in the pelvis. Prostheses, stents, and postoperative hydrotubation are not required.

Postoperative morbidity is rare, and patients are usually discharged from the hospital on the first postoperative day. Depending on the procedure, hystero-

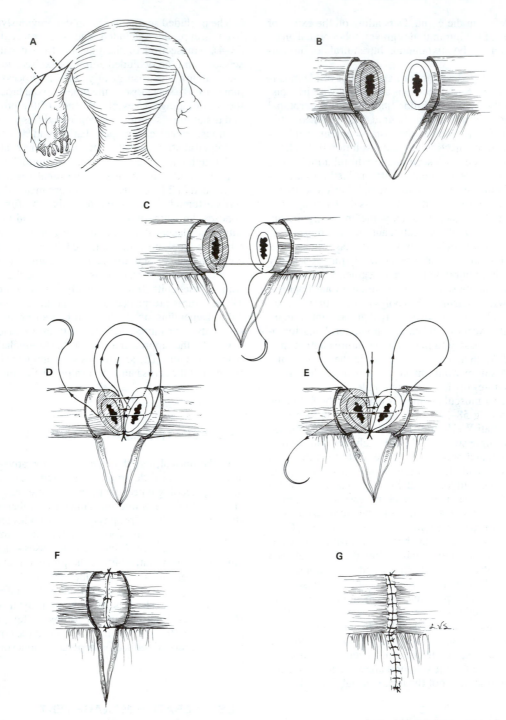

**Figure 58–4.** Tubotubal anastomosis. **A** and **B:** The occluded segment is excised and hemostasis obtained. **C:** The first muscular suture is placed at the 6 o'clock position. **D** and **E:** Subsequent sutures may be placed using a single strand; they are tied individually after the division of the loop between successive sutures. **F:** The muscularis has been approximated. **G:** Approximation of the serosa and mesosalpinx complete the anastomosis.

**Table 58–1.** Results obtained by conventional fertility surgery.

| Operation | Number of Patients | Viable Pregnancy (%) | Ectopic Pregnancy (%) |
|---|---|---|---|
| Salpingo-ovariolysis | 347 | 41.0 | 4.0 |
| Salpingostomy | 621 | 13.2 | 3.8 |
| Tubouterine implantation | 429 | 26.3 | Not stated |
| Tubotubal anastomosis (sterilization reversal) | 83 | 27.7 | Not Stated |

Reproduced, with permission, from Gomel V: *Microsurgery in Female Infertility.* Little, Brown, 1983.

salpingography is performed 3–6 months postoperatively to assess the outcome.

Early second-look laparoscopy (1–6 weeks after microsurgery) is recommended by some authors. There is no proven value to this approach. We reserve early second-look laparoscopy, generally, for women in the late reproductive age group subjected to salpingostomy and for those who had extensive pelvic adhesions preoperatively. If a patient fails to achieve pregnancy within 12–18 months following salpingostomy, a second-look laparoscopy may be considered to reassess the pelvis and to consider other therapies.

## COURSE & PROGNOSIS

The results in any given series of patients undergoing reconstructive tubal surgery are affected by numerous factors: (1) the nature and extent of pelvic adhesions, (2) the severity and extent of the disease process affecting the oviduct, (3) the extent of tubal damage caused by a previous disease process or intervention (eg, salpingitis, tubal pregnancy, sterilization procedure), (4) the length of the reconstructed oviduct, (5) the presence of additional pelvic disease, (6) the status of other fertility factors, (7) the surgical technique and perioperative care, (8) the preoperative selection process, (9) the method of classification of cases, and (10) reporting methods. Whereas the first 6 factors are associated with the extent of disease or damage resulting from prior pelvic inflammatory processes or intervention, the last 4 are related to the surgeon.

Obviously, surgical skill and good perioperative care favor a good outcome. Similarly, proper selection of cases for the specific procedure undertaken will affect the results. If difficult procedures are not attempted, the series will undoubtedly produce better results. The same applies to the classification of cases and reporting methods. If cases are not classified on the basis of the adnexa with the least pathology (most favorable) and if patients lost to follow-up are simply eliminated from the series, artificially more favorable results can be reported.

The results of major series of reconstructive infertility operations by conventional techniques are summarized in Table 58–1. The results obtained by the senior author on series of cases performed up to the end of December 1980 are summarized in Table 58–2. The reported results of salpingostomy by microsurgery by various authors are summarized in Table 58–3 and those on reversal of sterilization by microsurgery in Table 58–4.

Microsurgical techniques appear to offer significantly better results than those obtained by conventional techniques. The use of microsurgical instruments and microelectrosurgery appear to provide the best balance of optimal outcome and reasonable cost. Although some surgeons advocate the use of lasers as a preferred instrument for fertility surgery, to date no data indicate that the use of lasers in these procedures offers any advantage over the techniques described here.

## CONSERVATIVE SURGICAL MANAGEMENT OF ECTOPIC PREGNANCY

The availability of quantitative plasma $\beta$-hCG (human chorionic gonadotropin) and progesterone assays and ultrasonography (especially endovaginal)

**Table 58–2.** Results of reconstructive microsurgery.

| Operation | Number of Patients | Viable Pregnancy (%) | Ectopic Pregnancy (%) |
|---|---|---|---|
| Salpingostomy | 89 | 31.5 | 9 |
| Tubocornual anastomosis | 48 | 56.2 | 6.2 |
| Tubotubal anastomosis (sterilization reversal) | 118 | 78.8 | 1.7 |

**Table 58–3.** Results of salpingostomy by microsurgery.

| Author | Year | Number of Patients | Intrauterine Pregnancy (%) | Ectopic Pregnancy (%) |
|---|---|---|---|---|
| DeCherney et al | 1981 | 54 | 25.9 | 7.4 |
| Larsson | 1982 | 54 | 31.5 | 0 |
| Frantzen et al | 1982 | 85 | 14.1 | 3.5 |
| Verhoeven et al | 1983 | 143 | 19.6 | 2.1 |
| Boer-Meisel et al | 1986 | 108 | 22 | 18 |
| Kitchin et al | 1986 | 81 | 23 | 12 |
| Kosasa et al | 1988 | 93 | 40 | 14 |

has made early diagnosis of ectopic pregnancy easier and has limited the importance of laparoscopy for that purpose. Laparoscopy permits confirmation of the diagnosis and also usually allows surgical treatment of tubal gestation. Conservative surgical management is usually reserved for patients who wish to maintain their fertility potential. Although conservative management is more commonly elected when tubal gestation is intact, it is frequently possible to treat a ruptured tubal pregnancy conservatively if sufficient tube can be salvaged. Wherever possible, the options of conservative and definitive treatment (ie, preserving or not preserving potential for spontaneous conception) should be discussed with the patient before surgery is undertaken. A woman with a history of ectopic pregnancy is at greater risk thereafter of having another ectopic pregnancy, and some may not want to accept this risk.

Conservative surgical management of ectopic pregnancy must be followed by serial determinations of β-hCG in plasma to ensure complete removal of the trophoblast.

## LAPAROSCOPIC SURGERY

There are numerous prerequisites for the use of laparoscopic surgery in conservative management of tubal pregnancy, one being appropriate training of the surgeon. The use of a multiple puncture technique is recommended because this approach separates the visual and operative axis. This separation facilitates the procedure and permits more precise technique, which lowers the incidence of complications. Once the diagnosis is confirmed by laparoscopy, it is necessary to examine the site of the gestation and the condition of the tube in which it is contained. Before surgical treatment is undertaken, it is also mandatory to assess the ipsilateral ovary and the contralateral adnexa.

Laparoscopic management is generally reserved for tubal gestations that have not ruptured; however, in the hands of an experienced surgeon, most ruptures will also be amenable to this type of treatment.

Laparoscopic conservative surgical procedures for the treatment of tubal pregnancy include segmental ablation and segmental excision of the tube and linear salpingotomy. When necessary, a salpingectomy or adnexectomy can also be carried out by laparoscopy. The description that follows is confined to conservative procedures.

With the exception of segmental ablation, which can be performed with a single ancillary portal, 2 ancillary portals are required for these procedures. We usually place one of these ancillary portals suprapubically in the midline and the other at McBurney's point or its equivalent on the left side.

### Ablation

An unruptured isthmic or proximal ampullary pregnancy 1.5 cm or less in diameter may be ablated under laparoscopic guidance. The segment containing the tubal pregnancy is grasped with a bipolar grasping forceps, and the affected section of tube is

**Table 58–4.** Results of tubotubal anastomosis for reversal of sterilization.

| Author | Year | Number of Patients | Intrauterine Pregnancy (%) | Ectopic Pregnancy (%) |
|---|---|---|---|---|
| Winston | 1980 | 105 | 60 | 2.9 |
| Bremond (collect) | 1982 | 140 | 45.7 | 3.6 |
| DeCherney et al | 1983 | 124 | 58[1] | 6.5 |
| Paterson | 1985 | 140 | 61.4 | 3.6 |
| Pei Xue et al | 1989 | 117 | 81[1] | 1.7 |

thoroughly electrodesiccated. The procedure is akin to tubal sterilization and results in destruction of a tubal segment. The principal drawback to this approach is the lack of specimen for histologic examination. Tubotubal anastomosis may be undertaken later if reconstruction of the tube becomes desirable.

## Linear Salpingotomy

Linear salpingotomy is the conservative procedure of choice for ampullary gestations. A grasping forceps is introduced suprapubically through an appropriate cannula. A third puncture is made at McBurney's point, through which the hooked scissors are introduced.

The mesosalpinx adjacent to the ectopic gestation is infiltrated with 2–3 mL of a dilute vasopressin solution, using a narrow-gauge long spinal needle. The use of vasopressin minimizes oozing during the procedure and facilitates clotting in small vessels. The tube is immobilized with grasping forceps. Using the hooked scissors or a needle electrode inserted through the second portal, a longitudinal incision is made on the antimesosalpingeal edge of the tubal segment containing the pregnancy. The cutting instrument is replaced by a second pair of grasping forceps. Gentle compression of the tube with the forceps helps in extrusion of the products of conception, which are then teased out of the tube. The second grasping forceps is replaced by a bipolar suction coagulator. The opening into the tube and the edges of the tubal incision are irrigated with warm, heparinized lactated Ringer's solution injected through the cannula. Bleeding points on the margins of the tubal incision may be coagulated using a bipolar microelectrode or probe.

The conceptus is then removed from the peritoneal cavity. Pelvic lavage completes the procedure.

## Segmental Excision

Excision of the segment of tube containing the ectopic pregnancy is usually indicated for gestations of isthmic location, or for ampullary gestations if this segment of tube is clearly devitalized or diseased. To perform a segmental excision, the tube is immobilized with a grasping forceps inserted suprapubically. A pair of bipolar grasping forceps are introduced through an appropriate cannula inserted at McBurney's point. The oviduct is desiccated just proximal and distal to the gestation site. Replacing these forceps with scissors, the desiccated areas are divided. The affected segment of the tube is grasped and elevated, and the adjacent exposed mesosalpinx is successively electrodesiccated and divided. The excised segment of tube is removed from the peritoneal cavity.

## Surgical Treatment by Laparotomy

If laparotomy is performed for conservative surgical treatment of a tubal pregnancy, a small abdominal incision is usually sufficient, especially if the diag-

nosis has been confirmed by laparoscopy and the contralateral adnexa carefully inspected. Exposure through a small incision may be enhanced by the use of a uterine cannula affixed to the cervix. With the cannula, the uterus is positioned so as to expose the tube under the incision.

Magnification is not mandatory—though low power loupes are useful—but the tenets of microsurgical technique must be observed during conservative treatment of tubal pregnancy in a woman who wishes to remain fertile. Other principles of conservative surgical management are (1) to excise all gestational tissue, (2) to obtain hemostasis, (3) to conserve as much healthy oviduct as possible, and (4) to conclude the procedure by suctioning all blood and by performing pelvic lavage.

The segment of tube containing the conceptus is el-

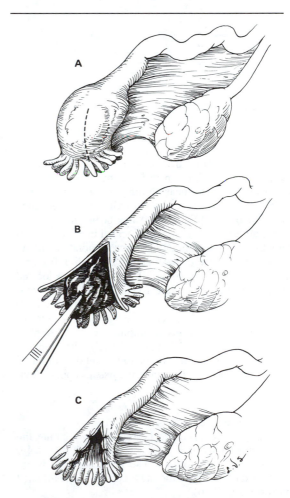

**Figure 58–5.** Conservative treatment of a distal ampullary pregnancy. **A:** An incision is placed on the antimesosalpingeal aspect of the distal ampulla. **B:** The conceptus is removed. **C:** Hemostasis of the edges is obtained either electrosurgically or with interrupted fine sutures.

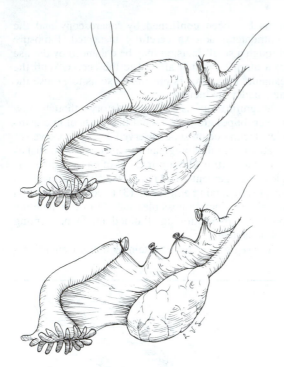

**Figure 58–6.** Segmental excision of a tubal pregnancy.

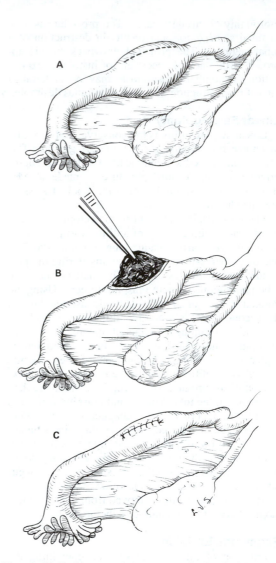

**Figure 58–7.** Linear salpingotomy. **A:** An incision is made electrosurgically on the antemesosalpingeal aspect of the affected portion. **B:** The conceptus is shelled out. **C:** The salpingotomy incision is closed with a fine suture.

evated on a Kerlex pad soaked in lactated Ringer's solution. Depending on the site, one may then proceed either with linear salpingotomy or segmental excision. Tubal abortion (milking the pregnancy through the fimbriated end) has been employed by some authors with gestations located in the distal ampulla, but this technique has been associated with an unacceptable rate of postoperative bleeding from retained trophoblastic tissue. With pregnancies located in the distal ampulla, linear salpingotomy is preferable even if the incision extends to the fimbrial extremity (Fig 58–5). Linear salpingotomy is used for pregnancies located in the ampulla or distal isthmus, while segmental excision is employed with pregnancies located in the proximal isthmus and in ruptured ampullary pregnancies where the tissues appear devitalized.

## Segmental Excision

Segmental excision is performed by ligating the tube on both sides of the conceptus with 3-0 or 4-0 Vicryl or Dexon sutures. The tubal segment is excised after ligation of the mesosalpinx of the affected portion (Fig 58–6).

## Linear Salpingotomy

A longitudinal incision is made on the antimesosalpingeal surface of the involved tubal segment, using a small scalpel blade or needle electrode

and blended current (Fig 58–7A). The tube is held between finger and thumb; gentle external pressure helps in extrusion of the products of conception through the salpingotomy incision. The conceptus is shelled out either with the back of a scalpel handle or by guiding the tissue through the incision with a pair of forceps (Fig 58–7B). The implantation site is then irrigated to ensure complete removal of the products of conception. Mild venous oozing from the margins of the tubal incision usually stops spontaneously. It may be necessary to electrocoagulate bleeders individually. Persistent bleeding from the implantation site after a period of compression is treated either by injection of 2–3 mL of a dilute vasopressin solution subserosally on the mesosalpingeal margin of the tube. The salpingotomy incision may be closed with 6-0 Vicryl or Dexon sutures, (Fig 58–7C), or may be left open to heal by secondary intention.

## REFERENCES

Boer-Meisel ME et al: Predicting the pregnancy outcome in patients treated for hydrosalpinx: A prospective study. Fertil Steril 1986;45:23.

Daniell JF: The role of lasers in infertility surgery. Fertil Steril 1984;42:815.

DeCherney AH, Kase N: A comparison of treatment for bilateral fimbrial occlusion. Fertil Steril 1981;35:162.

DeCherney AH, Mezer HC, Naftolin F: Analysis of failure of microsurgical anastomosis after midsegment, non-coagulation tubal ligation. Fertil Steril 1983;39:618.

Fayez JA, McComb JS, Harper MA: Comparison of tubal surgery with the CO2 laser and the unipolar microelectrode. Fertil Steril 1983;40:476.

Filmar S, Gomel V, McComb P: The effectiveness of CO2 laser and electromicrosurgery in adhesiolysis: A comparative study. Fertil Steril 1986;45:407.

Frantzen, C, Schloausser HW: Microsurgery and postinfectious tubal infertility. Fertil Steril 1982;38:397.

Gomel V: Laparoscopic tubal surgery in inferility. Obstet Gynecol 1975;46:47.

Gomel V: *Microsurgery in Female Infertility.* Little, Brown, Boston, 1983.

Gomel V: Microsurgical reversal of female sterilization: A reappraisal. Fertil Steril 1980;33:587.

Gomel V: An odyssey through the oviduct. Fertil Steril 1983;39:144.

Gomel V: Operative laparoscopy: Time for acceptance. Fertil Steril 1989;52:1.

Gomel V: Salpingo-ovariolysis by laparoscopy in infertility. Fertil Steril 1983;40:607.

Gomel V: Salpingostomy by laparoscopy. J Reprod Med 1977;18:265.

Gomel V: Salpingostomy by microsurgery. Fertil Steril 1978;29:380.

Gomel V: Tubal reanastomosis by microsurgery. Fertil Steril 1977;28:59.

Gomel V, Swolin K: Salpingostomy: Microsurgical technique and results. Clin Obstet Gynecol 1980;23:1243.

Gomel V, Taylor PJ: In vitro fertilization versus reconstructive tubal surgery. JARGE 1992;4:306.

Gomel V et al: *Laparoscopy and Hysteroscopy in Gynecologic Practice.* Year Book, 1986.

Kitchin JD, Nunley WC, Bateman BG: Surgical management of distal tubal occlusion. Am J Obstet Gynecol 1986;155:524.

Kosasa TS, Hale RW: Treatment of hydrosalpinx using a single incision eversion procedure. Int J Fertil 1988;33:319.

Larsson B: Late results of salpingostomy combined with salpingolysis and ovariolysis by electromicrosurgery in 54 women. Fertil Steril 1982;37:156.

McComb P, Gomel V: Cornual occlusion and its microsurgical reconstruction. Clin Obstet Gynecol 1980;23:1229.

Paterson PJ: Factors influencing the success of microsurgical tuboplasty for sterilization reversal. Clin Reprod Fertil 1985;3:57.

Pei Xue, Fa Y-Y: Microsurgical reversal of female sterilization. J Reprod Med 1989;34:451.

Royal Commission on New Reproductive Technologies: Proceed With Care. Final Report of the Royal Commission on New Reproductive Technologies, Ministry of Government Services Canada 1993, p 211.

Svensson L, Manardh PA, Westrauom L: Infertility after acute salpingitis with special reference to *Chlamydia trachomatis.* Fertil Steril 1983;40:322.

Swolin K: Electromicrosurgery and salpingostomy: Long-term results. Am J Obstet Gynecol 1975;121:418.

Tulandi T: Salpingo-ovariolysis: A comparison between laser surgery and electrosurgery. Fertil Steril 1986;45:489.

Tulandi T, Vilos GA: A comparison between laser surgery and electrosurgery for bilateral hydrosalpinx: A 2-year follow-up. Fertil Steril 1985;44:846.

Verhoeven HC et al: Surgical treatment for distal tubal occlusion. J Reprod Med 1983;28:293.

Winston RMJ: Microsurgical tubocornual anastomosis for reversal of sterilization. Lancet 1977;1:284.

Winston RML: Microsurgery of the fallopian tube: From fantasy to reality. Fertil Steril 1980;34:521.

*Ramada S. Smith, MD, Wesley Lee, MD, & David B. Cotton, MD*

Critical care medicine has increasingly become an area of interest to the obstetrician-gynecologist. Pregnancy complications such as shock, thromboembolism, adult respiratory distress syndrome, and coagulation disorders can lead to significant morbidity. Furthermore, the approach to these patients can be influenced by a variety of physiologic changes that are unique to pregnancy. This chapter provides a basic approach to some of the commom clinical problems that often require complex multidisciplinary care and a knowledge of invasive hemodynamic monitoring.

## PULMONARY ARTERY CATHETERIZATION

The flow-directed pulmonary artery catheter has been a major addition to the clinician's armamentarium because of its applicability to a wide range of cardiorespiratory disorders. The catheter allows simultaneous measurement of central venous pressure (CVP), pulmonary artery pressure (PAP), pulmonary capillary wedge pressure (PCWP), cardiac output, and mixed venous oxygen saturation. The pulmonary artery catheter is a 7F triple-lumen polyvinylchloride catheter with a balloon and thermodilution cardiac output sensor at the tip. Oximetric catheters also have 2 optical fibers that permit continuous measurement of mixed venous oxygen saturation by reflection spectrophotometry.

### Insertion Technique

A 16-gauge catheter is used to gain access to the internal jugular or subclavian vein (Fig 59–1). Pertinent anatomic landmarks for the internal jugular vein approach are shown in Figure 59–2. A guide wire is then introduced into the vein through the catheter, and the 16-gauge catheter sheath is removed. A pulmonary artery catheter is inserted over the guide wire, and the guide wire is removed. The central venous and pulmonary artery ports are connected to a pressure transducer, so that the characteristic waveforms of the various heart chambers can be identified as the catheter is advanced (Fig 59–3). When the catheter is in the superior vena cava, the balloon is inflated with

1–1.5 mL of air, and the catheter is advanced forward into the main pulmonary artery. Table 59–1 shows the average distance in centimeters the catheter must be advanced from various insertion sites. From the main pulmonary artery, the flow of blood moves the catheter into a branch of the pulmonary artery, where it wedges and records the PCWP.

Criteria for verification of the true PCWP include (1) x-ray confirmation of catheter placement, (2) characteristic left atrial waveform configuration, (3) mean PCWP lower than mean PAP, (4) respiratory variation demonstrated by fluctuation of the PCWP waveform baseline with inspiration and expiration, and (5) blood samples showing higher oxygen tension and lower $CO_2$ tension than in arterial blood.

After deflation of the balloon, the pulmonary artery waveform should again be visualized. Fiberoptic catheters allow verification of PCWP by showing a sudden increase in mixed venous saturation to 95% or greater.

### Indications for Invasive Monitoring

According to the American College of Obstetricians and Gynecologists, invasive hemodynamic monitoring may provide useful information for critical conditions during pregnancy such as:

- Shock (septic, hemorrhagic, cardiogenic).
- Pulmonary edema (eg, severe pregnancy-induced hypertension [PHI], congestive heart failure [CHF], unexplained or refractory.
- Severe PIH with persistent oliguria unresponsive to fluid challenge.
- Adult respiratory distress syndrome.
- Severe cardiac disease.

### Hemodynamic Parameters Available With Pulmonary Artery Catheterization

During the diastolic period of the cardiac cycle, the left ventricle, left atrium, and pulmonary vascular bed essentially become a common chamber (Fig 59–4). In a normal cardiovascular system, the left ventricular end-diastolic pressure (LVEDP), left atrial pressure, and PCWP are essentially interchangeable. A dispar-

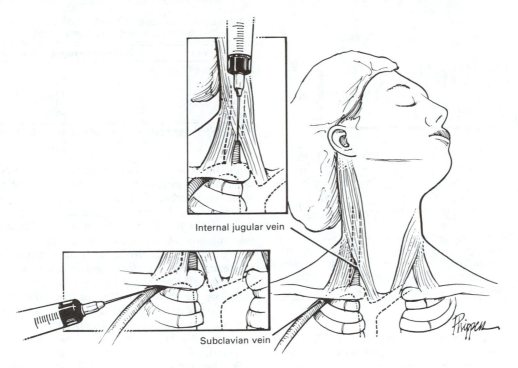

**Figure 59–1.** Comparison of right internal jugular vein and subclavian vein vascular access sites for right heart catheterization.

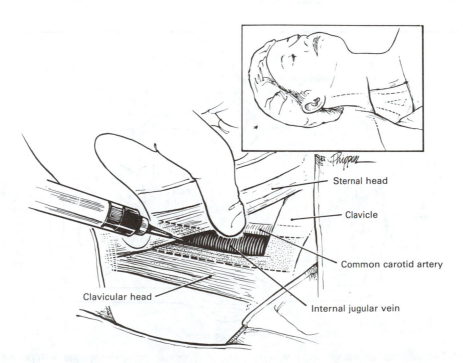

**Figure 59–2.** Important anatomic landmarks associated with the internal jugular vein approach for right heart catheterization.

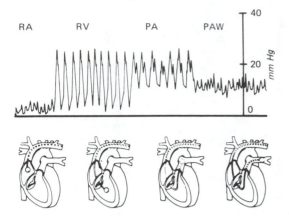

**Figure 59–3.** Changes in waveforms observed during placement of a pulmonary artery catheter. (Reproduced, with permission, from Rosenthal MH: Intrapartum intensive care management of the cardiac patient. Clin Obstet Gynecol 1981;24:796.)

**Table 59–1.** Distance to right atrium from various sites of insertion in pulmonary artery catheterization.

| Vein | Distance to Right Atrium[1] (cm) |
|---|---|
| Internal jugular | 15 |
| Subclavian | 15 |
| Right antecubital | 40 |
| Left antecubital | 50 |
| Femoral | 30 |

[1]Distance from right atrium to pulmonary artery is 8–15 cm.

ity may develop between PCWP and LVEDP when LVEDP is greater than 15 mm Hg; however, for clinical purposes, the PCWP provides a fairly accurate index of LVEDP, especially if the "a" wave (caused by retrograde transmission of the left atrial contraction) can be identified in the wedge tracing. The relationships described earlier can be substantially altered by mitral or aortic valvular disease.

**A. Cardiac Output:** The thermal sensing device in the tip of a pulmonary artery catheter allows for rapid determination of cardiac output by the thermodilution method. Five milliliters of 5% dextrose in water is injected through the central venous port at a constant distance from the thermistor tip. The use of this solution at room temperature can minimize sources of potential error associated with inaccurate temperature measurements and catheter warming. The change in pulmonary artery temperature is detected by the thermistor. The cardiac output is inversely proportionate to the fall in temperature and is computed by planimetric or computer methods. The average of 3 values within 10% of each other is typically utilized to calculate cardiac output.

**B. Systemic Vascular Resistance:** Systemic vascular resistance (SVR) represents the total resistance to forward flow of blood through the body's vascular tree. SVR is calculated as follows:

$$SVR = \frac{[(MAP - CVP)] \times 80}{CO}$$

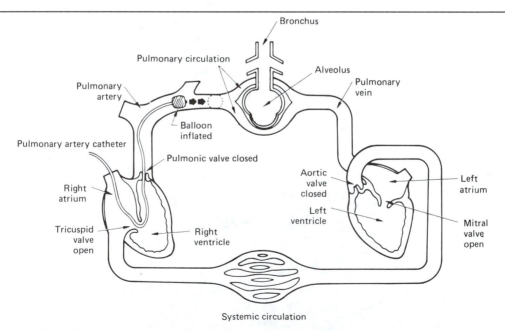

**Figure 59–4.** Pulmonary capillary wedge pressure in diastole (ventricles relaxed). (Reproduced, with permission, from Understanding Hemodynamic Measurements Made With the Swan-Ganz Catheter. American Edward Laboratories, 1982.)

(MAP = mean arterial pressure; CVP = central venous pressure; CO = cardiac output.)

During pregnancy, this parameter is usually in the range of $800–1200$ dyne $\cdot$ s $\cdot$ cm$^{-5}$. Depending on the clinical condition, a reduction or increase in SVR may be desirable in the presence of normal blood pressure, eg, septic shock, in which a very low SVR may be seen despite normal or low blood pressure. In order to maintain vital organ perfusion, vasopressor therapy may be indicated to increase SVR.

**C. Pulmonary Capillary Wedge Pressure:** The PCWP provides important information on 2 basic parameters of cardiopulmonary function: (1) pulmonary venous pressure, which is a major determinant of pulmonary congestion; and (2) the left atrial and left ventricular filling pressures, from which ventricular function curves can be constructed.

Pulmonary capillary wedge pressure can be reliably assessed by CVP monitoring only in the absence of significant myocardial dysfunction. The measurement of PCWP has certain advantages over measurement of CVP alone. A disparity between right and left ventricular function may exist in conditions such as myocardial infarction, valvular disease, sepsis, and severe pregnancy-induced hypertension. Under these circumstances, the management of fluid therapy based on CVP alone could have adverse results. Additionally, cardiac output and mixed venous oxygen tension cannot be determined with a simple CVP catheter.

**D. Ventricular Function Curves:** Myocardial performance is best interpreted in terms of left ventricular function curves (ie, the Frank-Starling relationship). The cardiac output and PCWP are used to construct the ventricular function curve by plotting the ventricular stroke work index against the mean atrial pressure or ventricular end-diastolic pressure (usually the PCWP). The left ventricular stroke work index is calculated by the following formula:

$$\text{LVSWI} = \text{SVI} \times (\text{MAP} - \text{PCWP}) \times 0.0136$$

(LVSWI = left ventricular stroke work index [g-m/m$^2$]; SVI = stroke volume index [mL/beat/m$^2$]; MAP = mean arterial pressure [mm Hg]; PCWP = pulmonary capillary wedge pressure [mm Hg].

Ventricular function curves provide a useful index of cardiovascular status to guide inotropic and vasoactive drug therapy. Evaluation of myocardial contractility by ventricular function curves allows one to obtain optimal filling pressures and stroke volume index in critically ill patients. The effects of therapy (eg, diuretics, antihypertensive agents, or volume expanders) can be evaluated on the basis of performance. Under normal conditions, a small rise in filling pressure is accompanied by a rapid rise in stroke work. Unfavorable conditions such as hypoxia or myocardial depression produce a shift in the curve to the right and downward such that lower stroke work indices are seen at higher filling pressures.

**E. Mixed Venous Oxygen Saturation:** The mixed venous oxygen saturation (SvO$_2$) reflects the body's capacity to provide adequate tissue oxygenation. This parameter is affected by cardiac output, hemoglobin concentration, arterial oxygen saturation, and tissue oxygen consumption. A mixed venous oxygen saturation of $60–80\%$ usually indicates normal oxygen delivery and demand with adequate tissue perfusion. An SvO$_2$ greater than $80\%$ reflects increased oxygen delivery and decreased oxygen utilization. This situation may be seen in patients with hypothermia or sepsis who are receiving supplemental oxygen. A high SvO$_2$ may also provide confirmatory evidence that the pulmonary artery catheter is in the wedge position. Finally, a low SvO$_2$ ($< 60\%$) indicates increased oxygen demands with decreased oxygen delivery due to anemia, low cardiac output state, or decreased arterial oxygen saturation.

Measurement of SvO$_2$ allows for continuous monitoring of cardiorespiratory reserve by providing an index of tissue oxygen delivery and utilization. Changes in SvO$_2$ will be apparent with infusion of vasoactive drugs, volume loading, or afterload reduction. While many intensive care units rely on direct measurement of cardiac output alone, this parameter does not always accurately reflect tissue oxygenation. For instance, normal cardiac output might not be adequate to meet increased oxygen requirements in malignant hyperthermia or thyroid storm.

**F. Maternal Oxygen Consumption:** Mixed venous oxygen saturation results can be used with arterial blood gas analysis to provide useful information about the metabolic status of the critically ill obstetric patient. Resting maternal oxygen consumption progressively increases during pregnancy. Occasionally, one needs to pay particular attention to the metabolic status of critically ill women or adult respiratory distress syndrome (ARDS). Factors such as tachycardia of fever that are associated with increased oxygen consumption should be minimized under these circumstances.

The Fick relationship:

$$\text{CO} = \frac{\text{VO}_2}{\text{AVO}_2 \text{ diff.}} \times 100$$

provides a method for calculating oxygen consumption (VO$_2$), if the CO and systemic arteriovenous oxygen (AVO$_2$) concentration difference is known. The (AVO$_2$) difference can be calculated by subtracting the oxygen content between arterial blood and desaturated mixed venous blood through the pulmonary artery catheter. For example, a patient with a cardiac output mL and an (AVO$_2$) difference of 5 mL would have an oxygen consumption (VO$_2$) of 300 mL.

$$6000 \text{ mL min}^{-1} \times 5 \text{ mL per 100 mL blood}$$
$$Vo_2 \text{ 100} = 300 \text{ mL min}^{-1}$$

An understanding of these relationships will allow the clinician to understand better how to use physiologic variables for interpreting the hemodynamic and pulmonary condition of critically ill patients.

**G. Colloid Osmotic Pressure:** The plasma colloid oncotic pressure (COP) is another measurement that can be useful in critical care (Table 59–2). Plasma COP is the pressure exerted by certain plasma proteins that hold fluid in the intravascular space. Albumin accounts for 75% of the oncotic pressure of plasma, with the rest coming from globulin and fibrinogen. The clinical importance of COP was first recognized by Guyton in 1959. He demonstrated in dogs that iatrogenic reduction in plasma proteins resulted in pulmonary edema with only minimal increases in left atrial pressure. Subsequent studies in humans identified cases of pulmonary edema in which normal or slightly elevated PCWP was present. From these studies, the important concept of a COP-PCWP gradient evolved. It appears that when the COP-PCWP gradient is less than 4 mm Hg, the likelihood of pulmonary edema is increased, although not all patients with a decreased gradient will develop pulmonary edema. The determination of COP and its relationship to the PCWP can play a crucial role in the detection of patients likely to develop pulmonary edema in the face of normal left-sided filling pressures.

Since the advent in the late 1960s of membrane transducer systems, clinical application of COP measurement has become a reality. Studies of pregnant women have demonstrated that patients with certain conditions in which the risk of pulmonary edema is markedly increased tend to have lowered COP, eg, hypovolemic shock, severe pregnancy-induced hypertension, prolonged tocolytic therapy, and frank pulmonary edema.

### Complications

The most common complication associated with pulmonary artery catheter placement is dysrhythmia. More serious complications also include pulmonary infarction, thromboembolism, balloon rupture with air embolism, pulmonary artery or valve rupture, catheter knotting, infection, and pulmonary hemorrhage. Table 59–3 summarizes the complication rates for pulmonary artery catheterization.

**Table 59–2.** Serum colloid oncotic pressure during pregnancy.

| | Normotensive (mm Hg) | Hypertensive (mm Hg) |
|---|---|---|
| Antepartum (term) | 22.4 ± 0.5 | 17.9 ± 0.7 |
| Postpartum (first 24 hours) | 15.4 ± 2.1 | 13.7 ± 0.5 |

**Table 59–3.** Complications of pulmonary-artery catheterization.[1]

| Complication | Incidence (%) |
|---|---|
| Premature ventricular contractions | 15–27 |
| Arterial puncture | 8 |
| Superficial cellulitis | 3 |
| Thromboembolism | ? |
| Pneumothorax | 1–2 |
| Balloon rupture | < 1 |
| Pulmonary infarction/ischemia | 1–7 |
| Pulmonary artery rupture | < 1 |
| Catheter knotting | < 1 |
| Catheter-related sepsis | 1 |

[1]Reproduced, with permission, from Hankins GDV, Cunningham FG: Severe preeclampsia and eclampsia: Controversies in management. Williams Obstetrics 1991;18(suppl):11. Appleton & Lange.

**A. Dysrhythmia:** Premature ventricular contractions may transiently occur as the catheter tip enters the right ventricle. However, they usually resolve following advancement of the catheter into the pulmonary artery. If the dysrhythmia is refractory to lidocaine, 50–100 mg given intravenously, the catheter should be withdrawn from the cardiac chambers.

**B. Pulmonary Infarction:** Pulmonary infarction may occur when the catheter migrates distally and wedges spontaneously for a prolonged period. This complication, as well as thromboembolism, may be avoided by monitoring the PCWP at brief intervals and by using a continuous heparinized flow system.

**C. Balloon Rupture:** Balloon rupture can be avoided by limiting the number of balloon inflations and by inflating only to the smallest necessary volume. Inflation of the balloon beyond 2 mL of air is unnecessary and may be harmful. To avoid rupture of a pulmonary artery branch, inflation of the balloon should be stopped immediately when the wedge tracing is seen.

**D. Catheter Knotting:** Catheter knotting is usually the result of advancing the catheter 10–15 cm farther than is necessary to reach the right ventricle or pulmonary artery. Withdrawing the catheter while the balloon is still inflated may cause tricuspid rupture or chordae tendineae tears.

**E. Infection and Phlebitis:** Infection and phlebitis can be minimized by using aseptic technique. The risk of associated sepsis is related to excessive catheter manipulation and the duration of catheterization.

## NONINVASIVE MONITORING FOR CRITICALLY ILL PATIENTS

Pulse oximetry is a simple tool that can be used with invasive monitoring for patients with cardiovascular or respiratory compromise. The correlation between pulse oximetry and direct blood oxygen saturation is excellent when oxygen saturation is greater than 60%. Factors adversely affecting the accuracy of pulse oximetry may include movement, peripheral vasoconstriction, hypotension, anemia, hypothermia, intravascular dye, and possibly nail polish.

# OBSTETRIC DISORDERS REQUIRING CRITICAL CARE

## OBSTETRIC SHOCK

Shock may be defined as an imbalance between oxygen supply and demand. The basic underlying defect is a significant reduction in the supply of oxygenated blood to various tissues due to inadequate perfusion. In obstetrics, this reduction often results from hemorrhage, sepsis, or pump failure. The physiologic compensation common to all shock states involves tachycardia and peripheral vasoconstriction to maximize cerebral and cardiac perfusion by way of the sympathetic nervous system. Failure of these compensatory mechanisms will lead to a predominance of anaerobic metabolism and lactic acidosis, which can be potentially devastating to the patient and fetus. Cardiogenic shock may be seen in pregnant women with cardiac dysrhythmias, congenital heart disease, peripartum cardiomyopathy, and congestive heart failure. The following discussion will focus on 2 of the more common shock syndromes complicating pregnancy— those related to hemorrhage and sepsis.

## 1. HYPOVOLEMIC SHOCK

### Essentials of Diagnosis
- Recent history of acute blood loss or excessive diuresis.
- Hypotension, tachycardia, tachypnea, oliguria with progression to altered mental status.
- Precipitous drop in hematocrit.

### General Considerations
Hypovolemic shock is a leading cause of maternal morality in the USA and is most commonly associated with obstetric hemorrhage. Bleeding severe enough to cause hemorrhagic shock may result from a wide variety of conditions, including ruptured ectopic pregnancy; abruptio placentae; placenta accreta; rupture, atony, or inversion of the uterus; surgical procedures; obstetric lacerations; or retained products of conception.

### Pathophysiology
During normal pregnancy, the blood volume expands by approximately 1500 mL. This hypervolemia results from hormonal alterations and may be considered protective against peripartum bleeding. During acute hemorrhage, the body responds to volume loss by hemodynamic, volume-altering, and hormonal mechanisms.

Hemodynamic adjustments result from activation of the sympathetic nervous system. These changes include vasoconstriction of arteriolar resistance vessels, constriction of venous capacitance vessels, and redistribution of blood flow away from peripheral organs to preserve adequate cerebral and cardiac blood flow.

Volume adjustments occur from extravascular fluid shifts into the intravascular compartment. The rate of plasma refill depends on the magnitude of volume depletion.

The secretion of epinephrine by the adrenal medulla will have inotropic and chronotropic effects on the heart. Additionally, epinephrine will contribute to peripheral vasoconstriction. Over a more prolonged period, water and salt will be conserved by the combined actions of antidiuretic hormone and aldosterone.

These homeostatic mechanisms serve to maintain adequate tissue perfusion until approximately 20–25% of the circulating blood volume is lost. Inadequate tissue perfusion and oxygenation will then lead to anaerobic metabolism and lactic acidosis. Observations on blood flow regulation during pregnancy suggest that uterine arteries have limited capacity to autoregulate fetoplacental perfusion. Thus, uteroplacental blood flow is critically dependent upon systemic maternal cardiac output.

### Clinical Findings
The clinical manifestations of hemorrhagic shock depend on the quantity and rate of volume depletion. Orthostatic signs and symptoms may be masked by the hypervolemia of pregnancy, especially if a source of bleeding is not evident. Obvious hypotension and tachycardia in the presence of external bleeding should alert the clinician to the possibility of shock. A careful physical examination will identify decreased tissue perfusion in several different organ systems, including the heart, brain, kidneys, lungs, and skin. Altered mental status, dizziness, diaphoresis, and cold, clammy extremities are common findings in significant hemorrhagic shock. Oliguria (< 30 mL/h), CVP of less than 5 cm $H_2O$, and PCWP of less than 5 mm Hg are all consistent with significant volume depletion. The identification of intra-abdominal bleeding may require culdocentesis or peritoneal lavage. Fetal heart monitoring may reveal bradycardia or late decelerations.

### Differential Diagnosis
Hypovolemic shock should be differentiated from

other shock syndromes resulting from sepsis or heart failure. Usually, there is a history of profound bleeding. Since shock may affect several organ systems, it is essential that its underlying cause be identified. Patients with septic shock will tend to be febrile, with associated abnormal white blood cell counts and clinical evidence of infection. Cardiogenic shock may be associated with clinical and radiographic evidence of pulmonary congestion or a previous history of heart disease.

## Complications

Electrolyte imbalance, acidosis, acute tubular necrosis, pulmonary edema, and adult respiratory distress, syndrome are common complications associated with hemorrhagic shock.

## Treatment

The treatment of hemorrhagic shock should be directed toward replacing blood volume and optimizing cardiac performance. If possible, the source of bleeding should be controlled. Uterine atony that is unresponsive to massage and oxytocin may benefit from methylergonovine (0.2 mg intramuscularly), or 15-methyl prostaglandin $F_{2\alpha}$ (0.25 mg intramuscularly). Persistent bleeding may require hypogastric artery ligation or even cesarean hysterectomy (see Fig 28–1 and Chapter 22). Decisions regarding blood and fluid replacement should be guided by central pressures and urine output. Military antishock trousers (MAST suit) will mobilize blood pooled in the lower body and return it to the central circulation, improving systemic cardiac output and organ perfusion. Supplemental oxygen will minimize tissue hypoxia and fetal acidosis.

Initial rapid volume replacement with crystalloid solution given through a large-bore intravenous site is a temporizing measure until blood replacement is possible. Typically, 1–2 L of lactated Ringer's solution can be administered as rapidly as possible. Compared with normal saline, the electrolyte composition of lactated Ringer's solution more closely approximates plasma, and the metabolism of lactate to bicarbonate provides some buffering capacity for acidosis. There is concern that lactated Ringer's solution may worsen any associated lactate metabolic acidemia. However, experience with casualties in Vietnam has shown no clinical difference in either arterial lactate levels or acid-base status in blood-transfused patients resuscitated with lactated Ringer's solution or normal saline.

Guidelines for perioperative transfusion of red blood cells have been recommended by the National Institutes of Health. Initial treatment of hemorrhagic shock should involve volume replacement by crystalloid or colloid solutions that do not carry risks for disease transmission or transfusion reaction. The use of perioperative red blood cell transfusion should not rely solely upon the dogma of "transfusing to a hematocrit above 30%" as a single criterion since there is poor evidence supporting its usefulness. The decision whether or not to transfuse red cells should also take into account other factors such as a patient age, hemodynamic status, anticipated bleeding, and medical or obstetrical complications.

The risk of posttransfusion hepatitis should be dramatically decreased by testing blood products with a new hepatitis C assay that has recently become commercially available. The test is a qualitative, enzyme-linked imunosorbant assay (ELISA) for the detection of antibody to hepatits C Virus (anti-HCV) in human serum or plasma. The ELISA test has a specificity of 99.84% in a low prevelance population. A supplemental assay, the recombinant immunoblot assay (RIBA), can be performed on blood that has a repeat reactive anti-HCV.

Fluid balance from intravenous (IV) infusions or urine output should be meticulously recorded with daily weights. Oliguria refractory to volume loading may be improved by the addition of IV dopamine in low doses (2–5 μg/kg/min) to improve renal perfusion. A diuretic such as bumetanide (Bumex$^R$) 0.5–1 mg IV, not to exceed 10 mg/day, should be considered for patients with prolonged oliguria despite normal elevated pulmonary capillary wedge pressures.

Blood tests should include complete blood count, serum electrolytes creatinine, arterial blood gas analysis, and coagulation profile. Urinalysis is also important. A baseline chest radiograph and electrocardiogram are desirable. Typed and cross-matched transfusion products should be available from the blood bank. One to 2 ampules of sodium bicarbonate (50–100 mEq) can be administered intravenously to correct acidosis (pH < 7.20. Frequent serial hematocrits may provide an index of acute blood loss. A baseline hematologic profile (PT, PTT, fibrinogen, platelets) is necessary to evaluate the possibility of coagulopathy.

## Prognosis

Maternal and fetal survial rates are directly related to the magnitude of volume depletion and length of time the patient remains in shock. If the hemorrhage is controlled and intravascular volume is restored within a reasonable interval, the prognosis is generally good in the absence of associated complications. The return of fetal blood flow, however, may lag behind correction of maternal flow.

## 2. SEPTIC SHOCK

### Essentials of Diagnosis

- History of recent hospitalization or surgery.
- Pelvic or abdominal infection with positive confirmatory cultures.

- Temperature instability, confusion, hypotension, oliguria, cardiopulmonary failure.

## General Considerations

Septic shock is a life-threatening disorder secondary to bacteremia that is characterized by inadequate tissue perfusion. It has been estimated that approximately 10% of women with obstetric infections also have bacteremia. Although gram-negative bacteria are usually responsible for most of these infections, septic shock may also result from infection with other bacteria, fungi, protozoa, or viruses. Commonly associated obstetric conditions include antepartum pyelonephritis, septic abortion, chorioamnionitis, and postpartum endometritis.

## Pathophysiology

Sepsis may lead to a systemic inflammatory response that can be triggered not only by infections but also by noninfectious disorders, such as trauma and pancreatitis. However, there is strong evidence to support the concept that endotoxin is responsible for the pathogenesis of gram-negative septic shock. The precise cause of circulatory insufficiency associated with gram-negative sepsis remains unclear. *Escherichia coli* has been implicated in 25–50% of cases of septic hypotension, but a variety of other organisms may be causative, including *Klebsiella, Enterobacter, Serratia, Proteus, Pseudomonas, Streptococcus, Peptostreptococcus, Clostridium, and Bacterioides*. The gram-negative endotoxin theory does not explain gram-positive shock, although an understanding of the proposed mechanisms will serve to exemplify the multisystemic effects of this disorder.

Endotoxin is a complex lipopolysaccharide present in the cell walls of gram-negative bacteria. The active component of endotoxin, lipid A, is responsible for initiating activation of the coagulation, fibrinolysis, complement, prostaglandin, and kinin systems. Activation of the coagulation and fibrinolysis systems may lead to consumptive coagulopathy. Complement activation leads to the release of mediators by leukocytes that are responsible for damage to vascular endothelium, platelet aggregation, intensification of the coagulation cascade, and degranulation of mast cells with histamine release. Histamine will cause increased capillary permeability, decreased plasma volume, vasodilatation, and hypotension. Release of bradykinin and β-endorphins also contributes to systemic hypotension. Early stages of septic shock involve low systemic vascular resistance and high cardiac output with a relative decrease in intravascular volume. Late or cold shock subsequently involves an endogenous myocardial depressant factor that has not been isolated. This factor is associated with decreased cardiac output and continued low systemic vascular resistance in the absence of pressor agents. Animal studies suggest that tumor necrosis factor (TNF) may lead to depressed myocardial function during septic

shock. TFN is a 17 kd polypeptide produced by monocytes, macrophages, and other cells exposed to endotoxin or microorganisms.

## Clinical Findings

**A. Symptoms and Signs:** The earliest symptom resulting from septic shock may be altered mental status, which is usually associated with temperature instability from the effect of endotoxin on hypothalamic temperature regulation. Vascular instability may be reflected by sinusoidal fluctuations in arterial blood pressure. The reduction in afterload results in systemic hypotension and will manifest itself clinically as warm shock. As this condition progresses, activation of the sympathetic nervous system with release of catecholamines will lead to intense vasoconstriction, which serves to shunt blood from the peripheral tissues to the heart and brain (cold shock). The compensatory vasoconstriction results in increased cardiac work. Lactic acidosis, poor coronary perfusion, and the influence of myocardial depressant factor may also contribute to poor cardiac performance. A significant number of pregnant women with septic shock exhibit depressed myocardial performance when analyzed by left ventricular function curves (Fig 59–5).

The clinical manifestations of septic shock depend on the target organs affected (Table 59–4). The most common cause of death in patients with this condition is respiratory insufficiency secondary to adult respiratory distress syndrome.

**B. Laboratory Findings:** Complete blood cell count, serum electrolytes, urinalysis, baseline arterial blood gases, chest radiograph, and a coagulation profile are laboratory studies important in the management of these patients. Hematologic findings may include significant anemia, thrombocytopenia, and leukocytosis. Serum electrolytes are often abnormal because of acidosis, fluid shifts, or decreased renal perfusion. Urinalysis permits evaluation of renal involvement. In addition to urine cultures, aerobic and anaerobic blood cultures may be helpful to confirm the diagnosis and guide antibiotic therapy.

Arterial blood gas measurements and a chest radiograph will facilitate clinical assessment of the ventilatory and oxygenation status. Early stages of septic shock will be associated with respiratory alkalosis, which later progresses to metabolic acidosis.

A baseline electrocadiogram (ECG) should be performed to rule out myocardial infarction or cardiac dysrhythmia. Abdominal radiographic studies may be useful to rule out other intrapelvic or intra-abdominal sources of obstetric sepsis (eg, bowel perforation, uterine perforation, tubo-ovarian abscess). Significant disseminated intravascular coagulation will be identified by abnormal PT, PTT, or fibrinogen levels.

## Differential Diagnosis

The differential diagnosis should include other

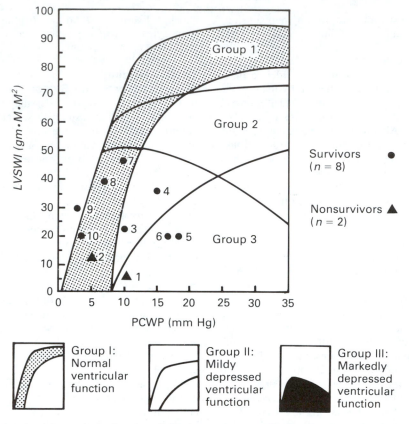

**Figure 59–5.** Presenting left ventricular function of 10 pregnant women with septic hypotension. LVSWI = left ventricular stroke work index; PCWP = pulmonary capillary wedge pressure. (Reproduced, with permission, from Lee W et al: Septic shock during pregnancy. Am J Obstet Gynecol 1988;159:410.

hypovolemic and cardiogenic shock syndromes. Additional causes of acute cardiopulmonary compromise include amniotic fluid embolism, pulmonary thromboembolism, cardiac tamponade, aortic dissection, and diabetic ketoacidosis. The history, physical examination, and laboratory studies will usually be sufficient to distinguish between these diagnoses.

**Table 59–4.** Effects on target organs in septic shock.[1]

| Organ System | Clinical and Laboratory Findings |
| --- | --- |
| Brain | Confusion, obtundation |
| Hypothalamus | Hypothermia, hyperthermia |
| Cardiovascular | Myocardial depression, arrhythmias, tachycardia, hypotension |
| Pulmonary | Tachypnea, arteriovenous shunting, hypoxemia |
| Gastrointestinal | Vomiting, diarrhea |
| Hepatic | Increased AST (SGOT) and bilirubin |
| Kidneys | Oliguria, renal failure |
| Hematologic | Hemoconcentration, thrombocytopenia, leukocytosis, coagulopathy |

[1]Adapted and reproduced, with permission, from ACOG: *Septic Shock.* Technical Bulletin No. 75. American College of Obstetricians and Gynecologists. March, 1984.

## Complications

Numerous complications may occur with septic shock, depending on the target organs involved. Aside from adult respiratory distress syndrome, some of the more serious complications include congestive heart failure and cardiac dysrhythmias. Systemic hypotension and ischemic end-organ damage can lead to hepatic failure or renal insufficiency. Inability to maintain cardiopulmonary support will lead to death.

## Treatment

Successful management of obstetric septic shock depends on early identification and aggressive treatment focused on stabilization of the patient, removal of underlying causes of sepsis, broad-spectrum antibiotic coverage, and treatment of associated complications. Febrile patients with mild hypotension who respond rapidly to volume infusion alone do not require invasive monitoring. In other cases, the pulmonary artery catheter should be used to guide specific therapeutic maneuvers for optimizing myocardial performance and maintaining systemic cardiac output and blood pressure. A hemodynamic approach for stabilizing pregnant women with septic shock should include: (1) volume repletion and hemostasis; (2) inotropic therapy with dopamine on the basis of left ventricular function curves; and (3) addition of peripheral vasoconstrictors (phenylephrine first, then norepinephrine) to maintain afterload (Fig 59–6).

**A. General Measures:** Septic shock during pregnancy should be treated with a broadspectrum antibiotic regimen such as ampicillin (2 g IV every 6 hours), gentamicin (2 mg/kg IV [loading dose], followed by 1.5 mg/kg IV every 8 hours [maintenance dose]), and clindamycin (900 mg IV every 8 hours). This regimen provides preliminary broadspectrum coverage against organisms such as *coli, Enterococcus*, and anaerobic bacteria until culture results are available. Aminoglycoside maintenance doses should be titrated in relation to serum peak and trough levels. There must be a careful search for infected or necrotic foci that can result in persistent bacteremia, eg, in women whose septic conditions are related to retained products of conception. Supportive care should also include control of fever with antipyretics, hypothermic cooling blankets, or both. In the antepartum patient, correction of maternal acidosis, hypoxemia, and systemic hypotension will usually improve any associated fetal heart decelerations.

**B. Cardiovascular Support:** Aggressive treatment of obstetric septic shock must rapidly and effectively reverse organ hypoperfusion, improve oxygen delivery, and correct acidosis. Priority should be given to cardiopulmonary support with the additional understanding that other major organ systems can also be severely affected.

A sequential hemodynamic approach for stabilizing obstetric septic shock with volume repletion, inotropic therapy, and peripheral vasoconstrictors is recommended. Volume therapy initially begins with 1–2 L of lactated Ringer's solution infused over approximately 15 minutes. However, it is important that volume infusion not be withheld in a hypotensive patient pending placement of a pulmonary artery catheter. The total amount of crystalloid administered should be guided by the presence or absence of maternal hypoxemia secondary to pulmonary edema and left ventricular filling pressures, as estimated by PCWP.

In general, myocardial performance will be optimized according to the Starling mechanism at a

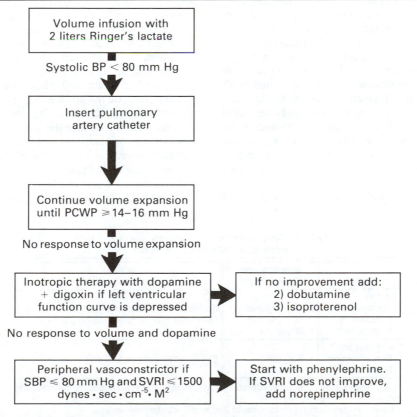

**Figure 59–6.** Hemodynamic algorithm for treatment of obstetric septic shock. (Reproduced, with permission, from Lee W et al: Septic shock during pregnancy. Am J Obstet Gynecol 1988;159:410.)

PCWP of 14–16 mm Hg. Such preload optimization is mandatory prior to the initiation of inotropic therapy. Blood component therapy can also be an important adjunctive measure if the patient has experienced significant hemorrhage and has developed an associated coagulopathy.

If the shock state persists despite volume replacement and adequate hemostasis, efforts should be directed toward improving myocardial performance and vascular tone. Inotropic agents such as dopamine, dobutamine, or isoproterenol are excellent choices for improving myocardial contractility in an obstetric patient with a failing heart (Table 59–5). We recommend dopamine as the first-line drug of choice for treating septic hypotension when inotropic therapy is indicated. This substance is a chemical precursor of norepinephrine that has alpha-adrenergic, beta-adrenergic, and dopaminergic receptor stimulating actions. The dopamine infusion is initiated at 2–5 µg/kg/min and titrated against its effect on improving cardiac output and blood pressure in patients with obstetric septic shock. At low doses (0.5–5.0 µg/kg/min), this sympathomimetic amine acts primarily on the dopaminergic receptors, leading to vasodilation and improved perfusion of the renal and mesenteric vascular beds. Higher dopamine doses (5.0–15.0 µg/kg/min) are associated with predominant effects on the β receptors of the heart. The beta-adrenergic effects are responsible for improved myocardial contractility, stroke volume, and cardiac output. Much higher dopamine dosages (15–20 µg/kg/min) will elicit an alpha-adrenergic effect, similiar to a norepinephrine infusion, and result in generalized vasoconstriction. Vasoconstrictive action associated with high doses of infused dopamine can actually be detrimental to organ perfusion and will rarely be useful under these clinical circumstances. Although myocardial performance after dopamine therapy is best evaluated by ventricular function curves, it is reasonable to maintain a systemic cardiac index above 3 L/min/M$^2$

If satisfactory ventricular function is not achieved with dopamine, a second inotropic agent such as dobutamine (2–20 µg/kg) should be added to the dopamine regimen. Dobutamine is a direct myocardial β$_1$ stimulant that increases cardiac output with only minimal tachycardia. Isoproterenol should be considered a third-line agent, which can be titrated at 1–20 µg/min. This drug acts primarily on beta adrenergic receptors to increase contractility and heart rate. However, potential side effects may include ventricular ectopy, excessive tachycardia, and undesired vasodilatation. Digoxin is commonly added to the previously described regimen to improve the force and velocity of myocardial contraction. This agent is given in a loading dose of 0.5 mg IV, followed by 0.25 mg every 4 hours for a total dose of 1.0 mg. Intravenous digoxin should be given under continuous ECG monitoring with special attention to serum potassium levels. The usual maintenance dosage during pregnancy is 0.25–0.37 mg/dL depending on plasma drug levels.

A peripheral vasoconstrictor may be initiated if there is a reduced systemic vascular resistance index (less than 1500 dyne $\cdot$ m $\cdot$ s $\cdot$ cm$^{-5}$) accompanied by a systolic blood pressure of less than 80 mm Hg despite inotropic therapy. It should be emphasized that maintenance of afterload appears to be a major hemodynamic determinant associated with maternal survival. Because of its pure alpha-adrenergic activity (which increases systemic vascular resistance), phenylephrine (1–5 µg/kg/min) is the initial drug of choice. Norepinephrine is only indicated for septic shock patients with decreased afterload who do not respond to volume loading, inotropic therapy, and phenylephrine. This drug is a mixed adrenergic agonist with a primary effect on the alpha receptors leading to generalized vasoconstriction and increased systemic vascular resistance. Although the therapy of septic shock should focus primarily on stabilization of maternal factors, vasopressor agents should be administered cautiously during pregnancy since they have been reported to decrease uterine blood flow in animals with experimentally induced spinal hypotension.

**Table 59–5.** Sympathomimetic and vasopressor drugs useful for therapy of obstetric septic shock.

| Agent | Maintenance Dose Range[1] | Therapeutic Goals |
|---|---|---|
| Inotropic<br>  Dopamine<br>  Dobutamine<br>  Isoproterenol | 2–10 µg/kg/min<br>2–10 µg/kg/min<br>1–20 µg/min | Cardiac index ≥3 L/min/M$^2$ SBP ≥80 mm Hg<br>Optimize left ventricular function curves |
| Vasopressors<br>  Phenylephrine<br>  Norepinephrine | 1–5 µg/kg/min<br>1–4 µg/min | SVRI ≥ 1500 dyne$\cdot$se$\cdot$cm$^{-5}\cdot$M$^2$ |

[1]Drug dosages that are administered by (µg/kg/min) can be prepared by the following method:
1.5 mg × body weight (kg) = total mg in 250 mL 5% dextrose in water
10 mL/h = 1 µg/kg/min
20 mL/h = 2 µg/kg/min

Some investigators have advocated large doses of corticosteroids for the acute management of septic shock, but human clinical trials have failed to demonstrate any conclusive benefit.

Finally, anti-endotoxin therapy has been recently investigated for the treatment of septic shock. In animals, antibodies against the lipid A (the biologically toxic) portion of the endotoxin molecule have been successful against gram-negative infection. Multicenter trials of endotoxin antibodies have suggested a possible improvement in mortality rate and organ failure in some subgroups of nonpregnant septic patients.

## Prognosis

Despite all medical and surgical therapeutic options, the overall maternal mortality rate in septic shock is approximately 50%. The prognosis is worsened by the presence of adult respiratory distress syndrome or preexisting medical problems.

## AMNIOTIC FLUID EMBOLISM

### Essentials of Diagnosis

- Sudden, unexplained peripartum respiratory distress, cardiovascular collapse, and coagulopathy.
- Bleeding secondary to coagulopathy or uterine atony (common).
- Chest pain or bronchospasm (unusual).
- Amniotic fluid debris in right side of the heart on autopsy.

### General Considerations

Amniotic fluid embolism is a rare but potentially devastating complication of pregnancy that often results in poor obstetric outcome. Between 1968 and 1973, the incidence was 1:47,300–1:63,500 live births in the USA.

### Pathophysiology

The basic mechanism of disease is related to the effects of amniotic fluid on the respiratory, cardiovascular, and coagulation systems. One of the more popular theories hypothesizes that the following 3 primary acute events occur: (1) pulmonary vascular obstruction, leading to sudden decreases in left ventricular filling pressures and cardiac output; (2) pulmonary hypertension with acute cor pulmonale; and (3) ventilation-perfusion inequality of lung tissue, leading to arterial hypoxemia and its metabolic consequences. In a histologic study of 220 maternal deaths, Attwood and Park (1961) demonstrated trophoblastic material in the lungs in 43.6% of cases, although fewer than 1% had evidence of amniotic fluid embolus.

Only a small volume of amniotic fluid (1–2 mL) is transferred to the maternal circulation during normal labor. Thus, enhanced communication between the amniotic fluid sac and the maternal venous system is necessary for amniotic fluid embolism to occur. Sites of entry may include endocervical veins lacerated during normal labor, a disrupted placental implantation site, and traumatized uterine veins. Once amniotic debris enters the venous system, it travels rapidly to the cardiopulmonary circulation, leading to shock and arterial hypoxemia. Some experimental evidence suggests that pulmonary hypertension may result from the release of prostaglandins or biogenic amines (eg, serotonin). The effects of systemic hypotension and hypoxemia may lead to cardiopulmonary collapse, renal insufficiency, hepatic failure, seizures, and coma.

The etiology of coagulopathy associated with amniotic fluid embolism is incompletely understood. Amniotic fluid may have a thromboplastin-like effect that causes platelet aggregation, release of platelet factor III, and intravascular coagulation.

Hankins and colleagues (1993) have recently reported marked pulmonary and systemic hypertension resulting from amniotic infusion into animals. The addition of meconium led to greater hemodynamic responses that were associated with transient left ventricular dysfunction and increased extravascular lung fluid.

Limited hemodynamic observations with pulmonary artery catheterization suggest that in humans with amniotic fluid embolism, left ventricular dysfunction is the only significant hemodynamic alteration that is consistently documented (Clark, 1985). The response to amniotic fluid embolus in humans may be biphasic, initially resulting in intense vasospasm, severe pulmonary hypertension, and hypoxia. The transient period of right heart failure with hypoxia is later followed by a secondary phase of left heart failure, as reflected by elevated pulmonary artery pressure with subsequent return of right heart function. This biphasic theory may account for the extremely high maternal mortality rate within the first hour (25–34%) and explains why pulmonary hypertension can be difficult to document in patients with this disorder.

### Clinical Findings

**A. Symptoms and Signs:** In his classic review of 272 patients with amniotic fluid embolus, Morgan (1979) characterized the main presenting clinical features: 51% presented with respiratory distress and cyanosis, 27% with hypotension, and only 10% with seizures. Approximately 100 women (37%) subsequently exhibited an associated bleeding diathesis, and nearly one-fourth of the 272 women developed pulmonary edema. Typically, the patient was multiparous (88%), and the disorder was diagnosed during labor (90%). Tumultuous labor or tetanic uterine contractions were found in only 28% of patients. Importantly, the use of uterine stimulants was associated with amniotic fluid embolus in only 22% of cases.

There did not appear to be an association between intrauterine death and amniotic fluid embolism. Bronchospasm and chest pain were unusual features of this syndrome.

**B. Laboratory Findings:** Arterial blood oxygen tension typically indicates severe maternal hypoxemia. This hypoxemia may result from ventilation-perfusion inequality with atelectasis and associated pulmonary edema. The diagnosis of significant coagulopathy is manifested by the presence of microangiopathic hemolysis, hypofibrinogenemia, prolonged clotting times, prolonged bleeding time, and elevated fibrin split products. The chest radiograph is nonspecific, although pulmonary edema is often noted. The ECG typically reveals unexplained tachycardia, nonspecific ST and T wave changes, and a right ventricular strain pattern. Lung scans occasionally identify perfusion defects resulting from amniotic fluid embolism even though chest radiographic findings are normal.

### Differential Diagnosis

Many conditions may mimic the effects of amniotic fluid embolism on the respiratory, cardiovascular, and coagulation systems. Pulmonary thromboembolism can result in severe hypoxemia with pulmonary edema. In contrast to amniotic fluid embolism, chest pain is a relatively common finding. Congestive heart failure due to fluid overload or preexisting heart disease may mimic the cardiorespiratory compromise observed during amniotic fluid embolism. Hypotension may result from several disorders, including septic chorioamnionitis or postpartum hemorrhage. Pulmonary aspiration (Mendelson's syndrome) is associated with tachycardia, shock, respiratory distress, and production of a frothy pink sputum. Although similar findings are also observed in patients with amniotic fluid embolism, pulmonary aspiration with resultant chemical pneumonitis is more frequently associated with bronchospasm and wheezing. Severe placental abruption has also been associated with disorders of maternal coagulation. Convulsions resulting from eclampsia or preexisting neurologic disease may confuse the clinical presentation of patients with amniotic fluid embolism.

### Treatment

Amniotic fluid embolism remains one of the most devastating and unpreventable conditions complicating pregnancy. Therapeutic measures are supportive and should be directed toward minimizing hypoxemia with supplemental oxygen, maintaining blood pressure, and managing associated coagulopathies. Patients with poor oxygenation often require intubation and positive end-expiratory pressure. Adequate oxygenation will minimize related cerebral and myocardial ischemia and acidosis-induced pulmonary artery vasospasm. Pulmonary artery catheterization should be considered in the absence of coagulopathy

to guide inotropic therapy with dopamine. If invasive hemodynamic monitoring is not available, rapid digitalization should be considered. Finally, the development of consumptive coagulopathy may require replacement of depleted hemostatic components in the case of significant uncontrollable bleeding or abnormal clotting parameters.

### Prognosis

Maternal mortality rates are high. In the 272 cases reviewed by Morgan (1979), only 39 women (14%) survived. Although no specific data regarding fetal outcome were reported in this series, correspondingly high perinatal morbidity and mortality rates would be expected.

## PULMONARY THROMBOEMBOLISM

### Essentials of Diagnosis

- Unexplained chest pain and dyspnea (most frequent presenting symptoms).
- History of pulmonary embolism, deep venous thrombosis, prolonged immobilization, or recent surgery.
- Occurrence of symptoms during postpartum period.
- Physical examination: usually nonspecific, depending on extent of cardiopulmonary involvement; may include wheezing, pleural friction rub, and pulmonary rales.
- Laboratory evaluation: decreased arterial blood oxygen tension less than 90 mm Hg in the sitting position.
- Diagnostic studies: pulmonary radionuclide ventilation-perfusion scanning, angiography.

### General Considerations

Pulmonary thromboembolism is a rare complication of pregnancy (0.09%) but is a significant cause of maternal death. From 1974 to 1978, pulmonary thromboembolism accounted for 11% of all maternal deaths in the USA. The diagnosis is more commonly made (75% of cases) postpartum. Interestingly, the incidence of superficial thrombophlebitis (1.2%) far exceeds that of deep venous thrombosis (0.2%) in patients with pulmonary thromboembolism. Predisposing factors commonly include advanced maternal age, obesity, traumatic delivery, abdominal delivery, thrombophlebitis, and endometritis.

### Pathophysiology

More than 100 years ago, Virchow postulated that the basic mechanism of thrombus formation is related to a combination of vessel injury, vascular stasis, and alterations in blood coagulability. Venous thrombi consist of fibrin deposits and red blood cells with varying amounts of platelet and white blood cell components. In most cases, lower extremity and pelvic thrombi are responsible for the pathologic sequelae.

Ordinarily, the vascular endothelium does not react with either platelets or the blood coagulation system unless it is disrupted by vessel injury. Such injury exposes subendothelial cells to blood elements responsible for activation of the extrinsic coagulation cascade. Disruption of the vascular endothelium may occur during traumatic vaginal delivery or cesarean section.

Pregnancy is also associated with venous stasis, especially in the lower extremities, because the enlarging uterus reduces blood return to the inferior vena cava by direct mechanical effects. Hormonal factors may contribute to venodilatation and stasis during pregnancy. Stasis prevents the hepatic clearance of activated coagulation factors and minimizes mixing of these factors with their serum inhibitors. In this manner, venous stasis becomes another predisposing factor for the formation of thrombi. Stasis secondary to prolonged bed rest for medical complications will predispose a pregnant women to increased venous stasis and formation of vascular thrombi. The period of greatest risk for thrombosis and embolism appears to be the immediate postpartum, especially after cesarean delivery. Postpartum deep venous thrombis has been reported to be 3–5 times more common than antepartum deep venous thrombosis and 3–16 times more common after cesarean versus vaginal delivery.

The maternal circulation becomes hypercoagulable from alterations in the coagulation and fibrinolytic systems. Serum concentrations of most coagulation proteins, such as fibrinogen and factors II, VII, VIII, IX, and X, increase during pregnancy. These changes are also associated with decreased fibrinolytic activity, which is responsible for the conversion of plasminogen to the active proteolytic enzyme plasmin.

A vitamin-K dependent protein, protein C produces a hypocoagulant action by releasing tissue plasminogen activator from the endothelial cells to facilitate fibrinolysis. A deficiency of protein C can increase maternal risk for thrombosis. Protein S, a protein C cofactor, also produces a hypocoagulant action. Finally, individuals with congenital or acquired antithrombin III (AT III) deficiency are also at increased risk for developing thrombosis. Thrombosis occurs in almost 70% of women with congenital AT III deficiency.

Once a venous thrombus is formed, it may dislodge from its peripheral vascular origin and enter the central maternal circulation. Propagation of the original venous clot or recurrent pulmonary emboli are possible. Deep venous thromboses limited to the calf rarely embolize, but approximately 20% extend to the proximal lower extremity.

### Clinical Findings

**A. Symptoms and Signs:** The subsequent cardiopulmonary effects of pulmonary embolus will depend on the location and size of thrombi in the lung. A patient with a large embolus affecting the central pulmonary circulation may present with acute syncope, respiratory embarrassment, and shock. Smaller emboli may not have significant clinical sequelae.

A collaborative study by the National Heart and Lung Institute (Bell et al, 1977) has provided a summary of clinical findings in 167 nonpregnant patients with angiographically established massive and submassive pulmonary emboli. This investigation, the largest of its kind, demonstrated that no single symptom or combination of symptoms is specific for this diagnosis. Classic triads (hemoptysis, chest pain, and dyspnea; or dyspnea, chest pain, and apprehension) were seldom identified. As seen in Table 59–6, chest pain and dyspnea were the most common symptoms in patients with angiographically documented pulmonary emboli (over 80%). Physical findings were nonspecific, except for tachypnea (rate > 16/min), which was noted in approximately 90% of the patients. Other findings may include pulmonary rales, wheezing, and pleural friction rub.

**B. Laboratory Findings:** There are no specific routine laboratory findings associated with the diagnosis of pulmonary embolus, although arterial blood gas measurements will often reveal significant hypoxemia. In the upright position, almost all healthy young pregnant women will have an arterial blood oxygen tension greater than 90 mm Hg. The ECG may reveal unexplained tachycardia associated with cor pulmonale (right axis deviation, S wave in lead I, Q wave plus T wave inversion in lead III). A chest roentgenogram may be normal or may show infiltrates, atelectasis, or effusions. Thirty percent of pa-

**Table 59–6.** Symptoms and signs in 327 patients with pulmonary embolus confirmed by angiography.[1]

| Symptom or Sign | Frequency (%) |
|---|---|
| Chest pain | 88 |
| Pleuritic | 74 |
| Nonpleuritic | 14 |
| Dyspnea | 84 |
| Apprehension | 59 |
| Cough | 53 |
| Hemoptysis | 30 |
| Sweating | 27 |
| Syncope | 13 |
| Respiration more than 16/min | 92 |
| Pulmonary rales | 58 |
| Pulse more than 100/min | 44 |
| Fever (> 37.8°C [99.7°F]) | 43 |
| Phlebitis | 32 |
| Heart gallop | 34 |
| Diaphoresis | 36 |
| Edema | 24 |
| Heart murmur | 23 |
| Cyanosis | 19 |

[1]Adapted and reproduced, with permission, from Bell WR, Simon TL, DeMets DL: The clinical features of submassive and massive pulmonary emboli. *Am J Med* 1977;62:355.

tients with a pulmonary embolus (PE) will have a normal chest x-ray.

It is generally accepted that a normal radionuclide perfusion study can effectively rule out pulmonary embolus. Perfusion studies are occasionally equivocal, and ventilation scanning may be required to clarify the diagnosis. Ventilation scanning will improve the specificity of the perfusion study, since this will rule out airway disorders that may be responsible for reduced pulmonary perfusion. Since radioactive technetium (ventilation scan) can cross the placenta, first-trimester exposure should be avoided if possible. The reliability of diagnosis of PE using both ventilation and perfusion scans, with or without noninvasive testing for deep vein thrombosis (DVT), is approximately 90%.

Pulmonary embolism will usually show abnormal perfusion and normal ventilation scans. If ventilation-perfusion studies are also equivocal, pulmonary angiography should be considered. Subsequent exposure of the fetus to the relatively low levels of ionizing radiation from angiography can be minimized with appropriate pelvic shielding and selective angiography on the basis of prior radionuclide scanning.

Noninvasive Doppler should be considered as an initial diagnostic test for suspected deep venous thrombosis involving the lower extremities. Real-time ultrasonographic imaging including duplex Doppler has become a valuable addition to continuous-wave Doppler. Imaging is most useful for the distal iliac, femoral, and popliteal veins. Doppler is also useful for the proximal iliac veins. Collateral venous channels however, are responsible for missing at least 50% of small calf thrombi. In one study of nonpregnant patients, the combination of continuous-wave Doppler and imaging resulted in 98% detection of calf or proximal DVT, with 95% specificity compared with venography. Impedence plethysmorgraphy is another noninvasive technique that has a diagnostic sensitivity of 95% and specificity of 98% in nonpregnant patients with proximal vein thrombi. Compression of the inferior vena cava by the gravid second or third trimester uterus may yield false-positive results.

If the above noninvasive tests are inconclusive, it may be helpful to confirm the extent of the original thrombotic event by venography with pelvic shielding. The soleal calf sinuses and the valves involving the popliteal and femoral veins are the sources of most deep venous thrombi. Venography is associated with induced phlebitis in approximately 3–5% of procedures performed. Radiofibrinogen methods to detect thrombus formation will result in placental transfer of radioactive iodine and are contraindicated in pregnant or nursing women.

### Differential Diagnosis

Any condition potentially related to cardiopulmo-nary compromise during pregnancy should be included in the differential diagnosis. This includes amniotic fluid and air emboli, spontaneous pneumothorax, septic shock, and preexisting heart disease.

### Treatment

**A. Preventive Treatment:** Once predisposing risk factors to pulmonary embolus are identified, it is important to minimize the possibility of further complications. In patients at higher risk for deep venous thrombosis, prophylactic measures should be directed toward preventing venous stasis leading to clot formation. Mechanical maneuvers such as raising the lower extremities 15 degrees above the horizontal, keeping the legs straight rather than bent at the knees when sitting, or performing calf flexion exercises may be useful, as may external pneumatic compression. One method used to prevent perioperative thrombophlebitis includes minidose heparin prophylaxis, 5000 U subcutaneously 2 hours before surgery and every 12 hours until routine ambulation is achieved. Mini-dose heparin prophylaxis significantly decreases not only the incidence of deep venous thrombosis but also the incidence of fatal pulmonary emboli. Prophylaxis is indicated for women with a previous history of deep venous thrombosis during pregnancy, thrombophlebitis, atrial fibrillation, or pulmonary embolism. Women with severe varicosities or morbid obesity who are awaiting surgery may also benefit from this regimen. Prophylaxis should be discontinued at the onset of surgery. Subcutaneous mini-dose heparin may be reinstituted approximately 6 hours after delivery. Postpartum or postoperative ambulation is important in minimizing thromboembolic complications during this high-risk period.

**B. Treatment of Documented Pulmonary Embolism:** Once pulmonary embolism is documented, therapeutic intervention should be directed to correction of arterial hypoxemia and any associated hypotension. Other measures should prevent clot propagation or recurrent emboli. Supplemental oxygen should be given to achieve an arterial oxygen tension of at least 70 mm Hg. A loading dose of 5,000–10,000 U of heparin should be given IV by continuous infusion, followed by a maintenance dose of approximately 1000 U/h. Alternatively, the loading dose may be followed by intermittent IV heparin in a dosage of 5000–7500 units every 4–6 hours. The partial thromboplastin time (PTT) should be maintained at 1.5–2 times control values. There are some laboratories that advocate the use of the activated clotting time (ACT) instead of following PTT values. The ACT is an accelerated version of the Lee-White clotting time. With the addition of celite from diatomaceous earth, the test can be interpreted in a few minutes as opposed to waiting 10 minutes or longer. Other investigators recommend the use of heparin levels for monitoring anticoagulation therapy. Heparin levels may be measured on the third or fourth day and should be about 0.2 μ/mL, not to exceed 0.4 μ/mL. Leg elevation, bed rest, and local heat will be beneficial to patients who have associated deep venous thrombosis. IV morphine may be helpful in alleviating anxiety and ameliorating chest pain. IV aminophylline should be considered in the presence of bronchospasm.

Selected patients with recent pulmonary thromboboembolism, ileofemoral DVT, or heart valve prosthesis should probably continue full anticoagulation with high-dose heparin during labor or surgical procedures. Under these circumstances, the risk for potential bleeding complications from anticoagulant needs to be balanced against the risk of thromboembolism. Although there is a higher incidence of wound hematomas associated with peripartum anticoagulation, there is no clear evidence that this regimen is associated with excessive postpartum hemorrhage after normal vaginal delivery. During labor and delivery, continuous heparin should be titrated to a prothrombin clotting time of 1.5–2 times control values.

Postpartum patients receiving heparin may be switched over to warfarin once oral intake is tolerated. Heparin should be continued for the first 5–7 days of warfarin therapy. By the time heparin is discontinued, the prothrombin time (PT) should be 1.5–2 times the control value. Alternatively, it may be desirable to continue moderate doses of subcutaneous heparin (10,000 U twice daily), especially in nursing mothers. Postpartum anticoagulation should be continued for at least 3 months if the patient developed pulmonary embolus in the third trimester.

**C. Complications of Treatment:** The major complication of anticoagulant therapy is maternal or fetal hemorrhage. Heparin does not cross the placenta due to its large molecular weight, but it has been associated with maternal thrombocytopenia and osteoporosis. Warfarin is known to cross the placental barrier, and its use in the first trimester has been associated with embryopathy (nasal hypoplasia and stippled epiphyses). Fetal nervous system abnormalities (eg, hydrocephalus) have also been noted with the use of warfarin during pregnancy.

A small percentage of patients will experience recurrent pulmonary emboli despite full anticoagulation. These patients may be candidates for vena caval ligation by a transabdominal approach under general or regional anesthesia. If the pelvis is suspected as the source of embolus, the right ovarian vein should also be ligated. It has been estimated that approximately 95% of patients with pulmonary embolism massive enough to cause hypotension eventually die. In this context, pulmonary artery embolectomy may be life-saving.

Placement of a vena caval umbrella via the internal jugular vein is an option for unstable patients with recurrent emboli who would not be prime surgical candidates. Although abdominal radiography is required for this procedure, placement of the umbrella filter does not require general anesthesia. This strategy will prevent larger emboli from reaching the pulmonary circulation.

There is evidence that thrombolytic agents such as streptokinase, tissue plasminogen activator and urokinase may effectively dissolve massive thrombotic emboli of recent origin. These drugs are associated with significant hemorrhagic complications in nearly one-half of treated patients. Obstetric experience with thrombolytic agents is limited to a few case reports, and firm recommendations regarding use of these agents cannot be offered at this time. Therefore, selected use of thrombolytic agents should only be considered as a last resort for life-threatening thrombotic complications during pregnancy.

### Prognosis

Pulmonary embolus, with a mortality rate of 15% (Wessler, 1976), will develop in approximately one-fourth of untreated patients with antenatal deep venous thrombosis. In a review of pregnancies complicated by deep venous thrombosis treated with anticoagulant therapy, the incidence of pulmonary embolus was 4.5% of patients, with a maternal mortality rate of less than 1% (Villasanta, 1965).

## DISSEMINATED INTRAVASCULAR COAGULATION (DIC)

### Essentials of Diagnosis

- History of recent bleeding diathesis, especially concurrent with placental abruption, amniotic fluid embolism, fetal demise, sepsis, preeclampsia-eclampsia, or saline abortion.
- Clinical evidence of multiple bleeding points associated with purpura and petechiae on physical examination.
- Laboratory findings classically include thrombocytopenia, hypofibrinogenemia, and elevated PT.

### General Considerations

Disseminated intravascular coagulation (DIC) is a pathologic condition associated with inappropriate activation of coagulation and fibrinolytic systems. It should be considered a secondary phenomenon resulting from an underlying disease state. DeLee (1901) described a syphilitic patient who developed "temporary hemophilia" in association with placental abruption and fetal death. The most common obstetric conditions associated with DIC are intrauterine fetal death, amniotic fluid embolism, preeclampsia-eclampsia, and placental abruption. Saline-induced abortion is also a common cause.

INTRINSIC PATHWAY (PTT)

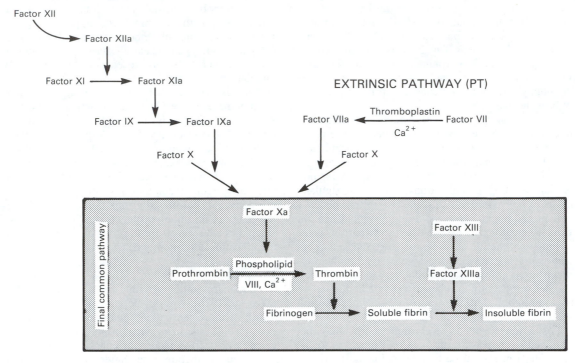

**Figure 59–7.** Coagulation cascade mechanism.

## Pathophysiology

The most widely accepted theory of blood coagulation has been popularized by Ratnoff and Bennett (1973) and entails a "cascade theory" (Fig 59–7). Basically, the coagulation system is divided into intrinsic and extrinsic systems. The intrinsic system contains all the intravascular components required to activate thrombin by sequential activation of factors XII, XI, IX, X, V, and II (prothrombin). The extrinsic system is initially activated by tissue thromboplastin, leading to sequential activation of factors VII, X, V, and prothrombin. Both the intrinsic and extrinsic pathways converge to activate factor X, which subsequently reacts with activated factor V in the presence of calcium and phospholipid to convert prothrombin to thrombin.

Thrombin is a proteolytic enzyme responsible for splitting fibrinogen chains into fibrinopeptides, leading to the formation of fibrin monomer. This central enzyme is capable of activating factor XIII to stabilize the newly formed fibrin clot and will enhance the activity of factors V and VIII.

Activation of the coagulation system also stimulates the conversion of plasminogen to plasmin as a protective mechanism against intravascular thrombosis. Plasmin is an enzyme that inactivates factors V and VIII and is capable of lysing fibrin and fibrinogen to form degradation products. Thus, the normal physiologic hemostatic mechanism represents a delicate and complex balance between the coagulation and fibrinolytic systems.

Pregnancy is considered to represent a hypercoagulable state. With the exception of factors XI and XIII, there is an overall increase in the activity of coagulation factors. Fibrinogen rises as early as 12 weeks' gestation and reaches a peak level of 400–650 mg/dL in late pregnancy. The fibrinolytic system is depressed during pregnancy and labor but returns to normal levels within 1 hour of placental delivery. The early puerperium is accompanied by a secondary rise in fibrinogen, factors VIII, IX, X, and antithrombin III; a return to nonpregnant levels occurs by 3–4 weeks postpartum.

DIC occurs as a secondary event in a wide variety of illnesses associated with excess production of circulating thrombin. The pathophysiologic factors responsible for inappropriate activation of the clotting mechanism include endothelial cell injury, liberation of thromboplastin from injured tissue, and release of phospholipid from red cell or platelet injury. All these mechanisms may contribute to development of a bleeding diathesis resulting from increased thrombin activity. Additionally, widespread DIC will cause increased platelet aggregation, consumption of coagulation factors, secondary activation of the fibrinolytic system, and deposition of fibrin into multiple organ sites, which can result in ischemic tissue damage. The associated thrombocytopenia and presence of fibrin split products will impair satisfactory hemostasis.

Specific obstetric conditions associated with DIC include the following:

**A. Placental Abruption:** DIC may occur in placental abruption involving liberation of tissuethromboplastin or possible intrauterine consumption of fibrinogen and coagulation factors during the formation of retroplacental clot. This leads to activation of the extrinsic coagulation mechanism. Placental abruption severe enough to cause fetal death has been associated with significant coagulopathy in approximately one-third of cases (Pritchard and Brekken, 1967) and is the most common obstetric cause of DIC.

**B. Retained Dead Fetus Syndrome:** Another cause of DIC is retained dead fetus syndrome involving liberation of tissue thromboplastin from nonviable tissue. Jimenez and Pritchard (1968) studied approximately 100 patients who had retained a dead fetus for more than 1 week. For 5 weeks after detection of fetal death, all patients had fibrinogen concentrations of at least 150 mg/dL. After 5 weeks, approximately one-third had fibrinogen levels below 150 mg/dL.

**C. Amniotic Fluid Embolism:** This involves not only the release of tissue thromboplastin but also the intrinsic procoagulant properties of amniotic fluid itself. It is likely that the associated hypotension, hypoxemia, and tissue acidosis will encourage the activation of coagulation factors.

**D. Preeclampsia-Eclampsia:** This condition is associated with chronic coagulation abnormalities that may lead to thrombocytopenia and elevation of fibrin degradation products. Pritchard and associates (1976) have postulated that the coagulation abnormalities reflect platelet adherence to exposed collagen at the sites of damaged endothelium. Maternal fibrinogen levels in normal pregnancies were not significantly different from those in the preeclamptic-eclamptic state unless some degree of placental abruption was also present.

**E. Saline or Septic Abortion:** Saline-induced abortion has been associated with subclinical DIC. Severe cases of DIC have occurred in 1:400–1:1000 cases. Disease may be related to the release of tissue thromboplastin from the placenta. Septic abortion may also cause release of tissue thromboplastin or release of bacterial endotoxin (phospholipids).

## Clinical Findings

**A. Symptoms and Signs:** Acute clinical manifestations of DIC are variable and include generalized bleeding, localized hemorrhage, purpura, petechiae, and thromboembolic phenomena. Widespread fibrin deposits may affect any organ system, including the lungs, kidneys, brain, and liver. Chronic DIC (eg, fetal demise) is associated with slower production of thrombin and may be associated with minimal or absent clinical signs and symptoms.

**B. Laboratory Findings:** Although histologic diagnosis of fibrin deposits is the only definitive manner by which DIC may be confirmed, there are a host of indirect tests suitable for the clinical evaluation of coagulopathy. Platelets, PT, PTT, TT, fibrinogen, fibrin split products, clotting time, clot retraction, peripheral blood smear, and bleeding time should be performed in all patients with suspected bleeding abnormalities.

**1. Platelets**–Platelets are decreased (< 100,000/μL) in more than 90% of cases. In the absence of other causes, spontaneous purpura usually does not occur when platelet counts are greater than 30,000/μL.

**2. Prothrombin time (PT)**–PT measures the time required for clotting by the extrinsic pathway and is prolonged in more than 90% of patients with DIC. This measurement evaluates the extrinsic and final common pathways of the coagulation cascade.

**3. Partial thromboplastin time (PTT)**–PTT is frequently normal in DIC and is not as helpful for establishing the diagnosis. This test measures the function of the intrinsic and final common pathways of the coagulation cascade.

**4. Thrombin time (TT)**–TT is elevated in 80% of patients with DIC. It is affected only by the amount of circulating fibrinogen or the presence of thrombin inhibitors such as fibrin degradation products and heparin. This test specifically measures the time necessary for conversion of fibrinogen to fibrin.

**5. Fibrinogen**–Fibrinogen is often decreased, with approximately 70% of patients with DIC having a serum level less than 150 mg/dL. The normal physiologic increase of serum fibrinogen levels during pregnancy may mask a pathologic decrease in this parameter.

**6. Fibrin split products**–Fibrin split products are best measured by the tanned red cell hemagglutination inhibition immunoassay. Values greater than 40 μg/mL are suggestive of DIC. The half-life of low-molecular-weight (5–15 hours) and high-molecular-weight (24–72 hours) fragments indicates that their presence does not necessarily imply continuing fibrinolysis. More recently, monoclonal antibodies to the D-dimer have been used. The D-dimer is a cross-linked fragment from the fibrin molecule. It is a more specific test for the presence of active fibrinolysis as compared with fibrin split products, which is more of a screening test. Fibrin degradation products from a significant consumptive coagulopathy are always abnormally high.

**7. Clotting time and clot retraction**–Observation of clotting time and ability of the clot to retract can be performed by using 2 mL of blood in a 5-mL glass test tube. These are relatively simple bedside tests that can provide qualitative evidence of hypofibrinogenemia. When the clot forms, it is usually soft but not reduced in volume (adding celite will hasten this reaction). Over the next half hour, the clot should retract, with the volume of serum exceeding that of the formed clot. If this phenomenon does not occur, low serum fibrinogen levels can be suspected.

**8. Peripheral blood smear**—A peripheral blood smear reveals schistocytes in approximately 40% of patients with DIC.

**9. Bleeding time**—The time required for hemostasis after skin puncture will become progressively prolonged as the platelet count falls below 100,000/μL. Spontaneous continuous bleeding from puncture sites may develop if the platelet count falls below 30,000/μL.

### Differential Diagnosis

Most acute episodes of generalized bleeding in obstetric patients will be related to pregnancy, but other rare causes of congenital or acquired coagulopathies need to be considered. These include idiopathic thrombocytopenic purpura, hemophilia, and von Willebrand's disease. Placental abruption is often associated with uterine tenderness, fetal bradycardia, and uterine bleeding. DIC associated with fetal demise usually does not become apparent until at least 5 weeks after the absence of heart tones has been documented. Amniotic fluid embolus is typically associated with acute onset of respiratory distress and shock. Preeclampsia is characterized by hypertension and proteinuria, which may lead to eclamptic seizures.

### Complications

In addition to the potential complications of uncontrolled hemorrhage previously discussed, widespread fibrin deposition may affect any major organ system. This may include the liver (hepatic failure), kidneys (tubular necrosis), and lungs (hypoxemia).

### Treatment

Although individual measures will be dictated by the specific obstetric condition, the primary, most important treatment of pregnancy-related DIC is correction of the underlying cause. In most cases, prompt termination of the pregnancy is required. Moderate or low-grade DIC may not be associated with clinical evidence of excessive bleeding and often will require close observation but no further therapy.

Supportive therapy should be directed to the correction of shock, acidosis, and tissue ischemia. Cardiopulmonary support, including inotropic therapy, blood replacement, and assisted ventilation, should be implemented with the patient in close proximity to a delivery suite. Fetal monitoring, careful recording of maternal fluid balance, and serial evaluation of coagulation parameters are extremely important. If sepsis is suspected, antibiotics should be employed. Central monitoring with a pulmonary artery catheter is relatively contraindicated due to potential bleeding complications. Vaginal delivery, without episiotomy if possible, is preferable to cesarean section. Failure of improvement in the coagulopathy within several hours after delivery suggests sepsis, liver disease, re-

tained products of conception, or a congenital coagulation defect.

Blood component therapy should be initiated on the basis of transfusion guidelines reported by the National Institutes of Health. Criteria for red cell transfusions were previously discussed earlier (see Hypovolemic Shock). Fresh-frozen plasma has only limited and specific indications, which include massive hemorrhage, isolated factor deficiencies, reversal of warfarin, antithrombin II deficiency, immunodeficiencies, and thrombocytopenic purpura. Although most cases of severe obstetric hemorrhage will lead to laboratory evidence of coagulation abnormalities, transfusion of fresh-frozen plasma may not always benefit these patients; the amount transfused is usually insufficient for replacing coagulation factors lost by dilution or clot formation. Even with massive obstetric hemorrhage, most procoagulant levels are above 30% of normal values, which is sufficient for maintaining clinical hemostasis in most patients. Specific replacement of fibrinogen should be accomplished by cryoprecipitate. Each unit of cryoprecipitate carries approximately 250 mg of fibrinogen. Platelets should only be administered in the face of active bleeding with a platelet count < 50 μL or prophylactically with platelet count 20–30 μL or less or following massive tranfusion (< 2 blood vol). Platelets should be tranfused on the basis of 1 U/10 kg body weight to raise the cell count above 50,000/μL. Obstetricians should remember that Rh immune globulin should be given to Rh-negative recipients of platelets from Rh-positive donors.

Although heparin therapy is indicated when there is evidence of large-vessel thrombosis or a thromboembolic event, this drug is generally ineffective for treatment of DIC. Heparin acts as an anticoagulant by activating antithrombin III but has little effect on activated coagulation factors. There is one instance, however, where heparin has been demonstrated to benefit pregnancy-related DIC. In the case of the retained dead fetus with an intact vascular system, heparin may be administered to interrupt the coagulation process and thrombocytopenia for several days until safe delivery may be implemented.

### Prognosis

Most cases of obstetric DIC will improve with delivery of the fetus or evacuation of the uterus. The maternal and fetal prognosis will be more closely related to the associated obstetric condition than to the coagulopathy.

## ARDS

### Essentials of Diagnosis

- History of gastric aspiration, seizure, sepsis, blood transfusion, coagulopathy, or amniotic fluid embolism.

- Progressive respiratory distress with decreased lung compliance.
- Severe hypoxemia refractory to oxygen therapy.
- Diffuse infiltrates on chest roentgenogram.
- Normal PCWP, with absence of radiographic evidence of congestive heart failure.

## General Considerations

ARDS is a serious disorder of pulmonary function that has many causes, including gastric aspiration, amniotic fluid embolism, sepsis, coagulopathy, massive blood transfusion, and shock. It can be easily confused with cardiogenic pulmonary edema secondary to alterations in preload, myocardial contractility, or afterload. A basic understanding of the differences between cardiogenic and noncardiogenic pulmonary edema is essential before rational therapeutic intervention may be implemented.

## Pathophysiology

The basic underlying pathologic change responsible for ARDS is lung injury resulting in enhanced permeability of the alveolar epithelium and capillary endothelium. Factors determining the net flux of lung fluid between the capillary lumen and interstitial space are quantitatively related by the Starling equation:

$$\text{Net fluid flux} = k[(Pcap - Pis) - (\pi cap - \pi is)]$$

(k = filtration coefficient, Pcap = pulmonary capillary hydrostatic pressure, Pis = interstitial space hydrostatic pressure, gpcap = pulmonary capillary serum colloid osmotic pressure, gpis = interstitial space fluid colloid osmotic pressure.)

Normally, fluid flows from the capillary system to the interstitial space and is returned to the systemic circulation by the pulmonary lymphatic system. An increase in left atrial pressure is observed when the left ventricle is unable to pump all the returning blood into the left atrium. Accordingly, the pulmonary capillary hydrostatic pressure increases, facilitating net movement of lung fluid into the interstitial space. When capillary fluid efflux into the interstitial space exceeds lymphatic resorption, the clinical presentation of pulmonary edema will occur. Although colloid osmotic pressure in the interstitial space and serum also plays a role in pulmonary edema, the most common factor is increased capillary hydrostatic pressure secondary to increased preload (fluid overload), afterload (severe hypertension), and decreased myocardial contractility (postpartum cardiomyopathy).

Capillary membrane permeability is not important in the development of cardiogenic pulmonary edema but is very significant in the genesis of noncardiogenic pulmonary edema (ARDS). Such injury due to hypoxic ischemia, vasoactive substances, chemical irritation, or microthrombi facilitates further efflux of capillary fluid and plasma proteins into the interstit-

ium. Additionally; the loss of cell membrane integrity will allow loss of the protective transmural protein osmotic pressure difference, which normally protects against the development of ARDS. Thus, the development of either cardiogenic pulmonary edema or ARDS results in a final common pathway leading to increased interstitial and intraalveolar fluid.

The most common obstetric cause of ARDS includes infection and aspiration. Aspiration of acidic gastric contents (**Mendelson's syndrome**), causes alveolar damage by chemical irritation. Endotoxin from gram-negative septic shock, vasoactive substances released by amniotic fluid emboli, and microthrombi secondary to DIC can also lead to injury, with subsequent increases in lung fluid. The potential effects of endotoxin include acute hemolysis, thrombocytopenia, toxic hepatitis, renal injury, and release of endogenous pyrogen affecting the hypothalamic thermoregulatory center. Maternal physiologic changes can contribute to the severity of ARDS. Mabie and colleagues (1992), have suggested that decreased extrathoracic compliance, decreased functional residual capacity, higher oxygen deficit, limited cardiac output increases, and anemia may adversely affect the clinical presentation and course of ARDS during pregnancy.

## Clinical Findings

**A. Symptoms and Signs:** Classic signs of respiratory distress are tachypnea, intercostal retractions, and even cyanosis, depending on the degree of hypoxemia. Fetal tachycardia or late decelerations may reflect maternal hypoxemia and uteroplacental insufficiency. Pulmonary rales in noncardiogenic pulmonary edema will be indistinguishable from those of cardiogenic pulmonary edema, but physical findings consistent with the cardiogenic disorder (ventricular gallop, jugular venous distention, and peripheral edema) are not typical features of ARDS. Unfortunately, the physiologic changes of pregnancy may mask the significance of these physical findings during the more subtle stages of respiratory distress.

**B. Laboratory Findings:** Arterial blood gas determinations will reveal a progressive moderate to severe hypoxemia despite oxygen therapy. Depending on the obstetric cause of ARDS, other laboratory findings will be variable or nonspecific. The initial chest roentgenogram will often be normal, even in the presence of clinically significant respiratory distress. Within the next 24–48 hours, patchy or diffuse infiltrates will progress to prominent alveolar infiltrates (Fig 59–8). Unlike in cardiogenic pulmonary edema, the heart will most likely be of normal size in a patient with ARDS. PCWP measured by right heart catheterization is the procedure most helpful in differentiating ARDS and pulmonary edema. The PCWP is elevated (< 20 mm Hg) in cardiogenic pulmonary edema but is often normal in ARDS.

Measurement of endobronchial fluid COP has also

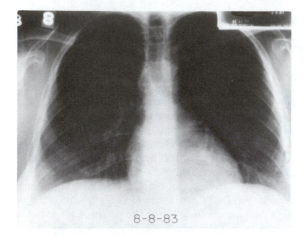

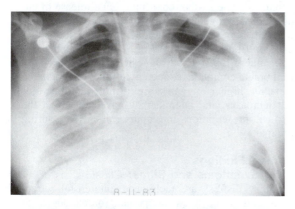

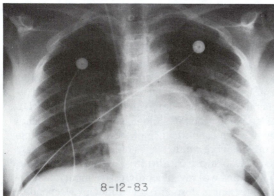

**Figure 59–8.** Sequence of chest radiographs from a 21-year-old woman during her first pregnancy with antepartum pyelonephritis and ARDS. **A:** Normal chest film. **B:** Bilateral patchy pulmonary densities have developed consistent with the diagnosis of ARDS. Much of the apparent increase in heart size is related to shallow inspiration and supine technique. **C:** ARDS has improved dramatically with only minimal residual pulmonary densities.

been utilized to differentiate capillary permeability-induced pulmonary edema from hydrostatic or cardiogenic pulmonary edema. In pulmonary edema secondary to capillary permeability, the COP of endobronchial fluid obtained from endotracheal tube suctioning is usually greater than 75% of the simultaneously obtained plasma COP. In cardiogenic pulmonary edema, the COP of the endobronchial fluid is usually less than 60% that of plasma.

Histopathologically, idiopathic pulmonary fibrosis and ARDS are remarkably similar. Both show evidence of acute alveolar injury, which is characterized by interstitial inflammation, hemorrhage, and edema. This is followed by a hypercellular phase, loss of alveolar structure, and pulmonary fibrosis.

### Differential Diagnosis

ARDS should be differentiated from infectious pneumonitis and cardiogenic causes of pulmonary edema. Cardiogenic pulmonary edema will usually respond more rapidly to diuretic therapy than will ARDS, in which abnormalities in capillary membrane permeability are not quickly resolved by such intervention.

### Treatment

Therapy should be directed toward the prevention of hypoxemia, correcting acid-base abnormalities, removal of inciting factors, and hemodynamic support appropriate for the specific cause (eg, amniotic fluid embolus, DIC). Cardiogenic pulmonary edema is usually treated with a combination of diuretics, inotropic therapy, and afterload reduction. If a hemodynamic profile is not immediately available by pulmonary artery catheter, the clinician may elect to begin oxygen and furosemide (20 mg IV) for the presumptive diagnosis of cardiogenic pulmonary edema. By contrast, it should be apparent that the basic therapy for ARDS is supportive. Supplemental oxygen by mask or nasal prongs represents initial therapy. If the work of breathing is excessive or arterial oxygenation cannot be maintained, oxygen given by endotracheal intubation and mechanical ventilation is recommended. Positive end-expiratory pressure (PEEP) has been shown to be advantageous for the treatment of ARDS, presumably because it improves functional residual capacity and alveolar ventilation. The pulmonary artery catheter will be helpful in guiding fluid management and optimizing cardiac performance. Additionally, mixed venous oxygen saturation from the distal port of the pulmonary artery catheter will provide an index of oxygen utilization.

Reasonable therapeutic goals for cardiorespiratory support include a mechanical venilator tidal volume of 10–20 mL/kg, with PEEP 5–35 cm $H_2O$, PCWP 8–12 mm Hg, arterial blood oxygen tension greater than 60 mm Hg, and mixed venous oxygen tension greater than 30 mm Hg. If the mixed venous tension is low, transfusion of red blood cells or inotropic therapy may improve oxygen transport and delivery.

Since the presence of capillary membrane abnormalities in ARDS is associated with rapid equilibration of proteinaceous material between the capillaries and interstitial spaces, IV colloid replacement should be discouraged in lieu of crystalloid resuscitation. Prospective controlled studies have not demonstrated the benefit of steroid therapy for ARDS. Once therapy for cardiopulmonary support has been implemented, a thorough search for predisposing factors to ARDS must be identified for specific intervention.

Potential future therapies for ARDS include surfactant replacement, oxygen-free radical scavengers, arachidonic acid metabolite inhibitors, anti-protease agents, anti-endotoxin antibodies, anti-tumor necrosis factor antibodies and other immunologic therapies for sepsis.

The timing of delivery in these patients is unclear in the literature. Theoretically, absence of the gravid uterus should improve ventilatory efforts, but there have been too few cases to uniformly recommend elective delivery. Cesarean section should be reserved for standard obstetrical indications.

### Prognosis

Collected series from some centers suggest a mortality rate as high as 50–60% for patients with ARDS. However, the diagnostic criteria for ARDS have not been uniformly applied, and some cases have been confused with cardiogenic pulmonary edema. The Memphis series had a 56% survival rate with the majority of survivors having an infectious etiology for ARDS. Many of these affected patients developed pulmonary complications that include barotrauma and pneumothorax. Fortunately, survivors of ARDS usually do not demonstrate permanent long-term pulmonary dysfunction.

## CARDIOPULMONARY RESUSCITATION DURING PREGNANCY

Many of the critical conditions discussed in this chapter can lead to cardiopulmonary arrest, which can be difficult to effectively implement secondary to the gravid uterus. The left lateral decubitus position will help facilitate cardiopulmonary resuscitation under these circumstances. However, this position will also make chest compressions very difficult. Some have found the use of a specially designed wedge to be helpful for uterine displacement away from the great vessels. Defibrillation has been successfully used during pregnancy without disturbance of the fetal cardiac conduction system. Finally, the decision to perform a perimortem cesarean section should be made rapidly within 4–5 minutes of cardiac arrest. This extreme measure can maximize maternal survival by relieving aortocaval compression and increasing blood flow return back to the heart.

## REFERENCES

### INVASIVE HEMODYNAMIC MONITORING

Clark SL, Horenstein JM, Phelan JP, et al: Experience with the pulmonary artery catheter in obstetrics and gynecology. Am J Obstet Gynecol 1985;152:374.

Cotton DB, Gonik B, Dorman K, et al: Cardiovascular alterations in severe pregnancy-induced hypertension: Relationship of central venous pressure to pulmonary capillary wedge pressure. Am J Obstet Gynecol 1985; 151:762.

Cotton DB, Benedetti TJ: Use of the Swan-Ganz catheter in obstetrics and gynecology. Obstet Gynecol 1980; 56:641.

Invasive Hemodynamic Monitoring in Obstetrics and Gynecology. Technical Bulletin No. 175. American College of Obstetrics and Gynecology, 1992; No. 175.

Kandel G, Aberman A: Mixed venous oxygen saturation: Its role in the assessment of the critically ill patient. Arch Intern Med 1983;143:1400.

### HYPOVOLEMIC SHOCK

Bottoms S: *Hemorrhagic Shock*. Technical Bulletin No. 82. American College of Obstetricians and Gynecologists, Washington, DC. December, 1984.

Clark, SL. Shock in pregnant patient. Semin Perinatol 1990;14:52.

Office of Medical Applications of Research, National Institutes of Health: Perioperative red cell transfusion. JAMA 1988;260:2700.

Pearse CS, Magrina JF. Finley BE: Use of MAST suit in obstetrics and gynecology. Obstet Gynecol Surv 1984; 39:416.

### SEPTIC SHOCK

American College of Obstetricians and Gynecologists: Septic Shock. Technical Bulletin No. 75. American College of Obstetricians and Gynecologists, Washington, DC. March, 1984.

Duff WP, Ledger W: Management of septic shock in the pelvic surgery patient. Infect Surgery (Feb) 1985;101.

Epstein FH, Pathogenic mechanisms of septic shock. N Engl J Med 1993;328:1471.

Lee W et al: Septic shock during pregnancy. Am J Obstet Gynecol 1988;159:410.

Sprung CL et al: The effects of high-dose corticosteroids in patients with septic shock: A prospective, controlled study. N Engl J Med 1985;311:1137.

## AMNIOTIC FLUID EMBOLISM

Attwood HD, Park WW: Embolism to the lungs by trophoblast. J Obstet Gynecol Br Commonw 1961;68: 611.

Clark SL, Montz FJ, Phelan JP: Hemodynamic alterations associated with amniotic fluid embolism: A reappraisal. Am J Obstet Gynecol 1985;151:617.

Hankins GDV, Snyder RR, Clark SL, et al: Acute hemodynamic and respiratory effects of amniotic fluid embolism in the pregnant goat model. Am J Obstet Gynecol 1993;168:1113.

Morgan M: Amniotic fluid embolism. Anaesthesia 1979;34:20.

## PULMONARY THROMBOEMBOLISM

Awe RJ et al: Arterial oxygenation and alveolar-arterial gradients in term pregnancy. Obstet Gynecol 1978;53: 182.

Bell WR, Simon TL, DeMets DL: The clinical features of submassive and massive pulmonary emboli. Am J Med 1977;62:355.

Hall JFG, Pauli RM, Wilson KM: Maternal and fetal sequelae of anticoagulation during pregnancy. Am J Med 1980;68:122.

Kaunitz AM et al: Causes of maternal mortality in the United States. Obstet Gynecol 1985;65:605.

## DISSEMINATED INTRAVASCULAR COAGULATION

DeLee JB: A case of fatal hemorrhagic diathesis with premature detachment of the placenta. Am J Ob 1901; 44:45.

Jimenez JM, Pritchard JA: Pathogenesis and treatment of coagulation defects resulting from fetal death. Obstet Gynecol 1968;32:449.

Naumann RO, Weinstein L: Disseminated intravascular coagulation: The clinician's dilemma. Obstet Gynecol Surv 1985;40:487.

Office of Medical Applications of Research, National Institutes of Health: Fresh frozen plasma: Indications and risks. JAMA 1985;253:551.

Office of Medical Applications of Research, National Institutes of Health: Platelet transfusion therapy. JAMA 1987;257:1777.

Pritchard JA, Brekken AL: Clinical and laboratory studies on severe abruptio placentae. Am J Obstet Gynecol 1967;97:681.

Pritchard JA, Cunningham FG, Mason RA: Coagulation changes in eclampsia: Their frequency and pathogenesis. Am J Obstet Gynecol 1976;124:855.

Ratnoff OD, Bennett B: The genetics of hereditary disorders of blood coagulation. Science 1973;179:1291.

Rutherford SE, Phelan JP. Deep venous thrombosis and pulmonary embolism in pregnancy. Critical Care Obstet 1991;18:345.

Wehrmacher WH, Messmore HL. Thromboembolic disease during pregnancy: Problems with anticoagulant therapy. Compr Ther 1990;16:31.

## ADULT RESPIRATORY DISTRESS SYNDROME

Andersen HF, Lynch JP, Johnson TR Jr: Adult respiratory distress syndrome in obstetrics and gynecology. Obstet Gynecol 1980;55:291.

Bone RC et al: Early methylprednisolone treatment for septic syndrome and the adult respiratory distress syndrome. N Engl J Med 1987;317:653.

Cunningham FG et al: Respiratory insufficiency associated with pyelonephritis during pregnancy. Obstet Gynecol 1984;63:121.

Mabie WC, Barton JR, Sibai BM. Adult respiratory distress syndrome in pregnancy. Am J Obstet Gynecol 1992;167:950.

Martin JN et al: Categorization of clinical conditions associated with adult respiratory distress syndrome (ARDS) in the pregnant patient. Proceedings of the Eighth Annual Meeting of the Society of Perinatal Obstetricians, Feb 3-6, 1988. Abstract No. 112.

Petty TL: *Acute respiratory distress syndrome: Disease of the month.* Year Book, 1990.

Rinaldo JE, Rogers RM: Adult respiratory distress syndrome: Changing concepts of lung injury and repair. N Engl J Med 1982;306:900.

## CARDIOPULMONARY ARREST

Katz BL, Dotters DJ, Droegemueller W; Perimortem cesarean delivery. Obstet Gynecol 1986;60:571.

Lee RV, Rodgers BD, White LM: Cardiopulmonary resuscitation of pregnant women. Am J Med 1986; 81:311.

Emergency Cardiac Care Committee and Subcommittee, Am Heart Assoc. Guidelines for Cardiopulmonary Resuscitation & Emergency Cardiac Care IV: Special resuscitation situations. JAMA 1992;268:2243.

# Psychological Aspects of Obstetrics & Gynecology

# 60

*Miriam B. Rosenthal, MD*

## PSYCHOLOGIC ASPECTS OF OBSTETRICS

Pregnancy has always been a time of psychologic adjustment for many women. In recent decades, there have been many additional changes in women's lifestyles and attitudes that have an effect on the psychologic aspects of pregnancy. Family structure is changing. Many women now work outside the home, are single or divorced, or are having first babies in the teenage years or after age 35. Sexual values and practices have changed and more changes will occur as AIDS continues. Women have more knowledge about their bodies, and most want to participate in important decisions regarding fertility, pregnancy, delivery, and infant care. Many men want a greater part in sharing their partner's pregnancy. Finally, the legal climate has greatly affected medical practice. These alterations significantly influence the practice of obstetrics and gynecology. Indeed, the clinician is faced with new challenges and stresses in caring for women from diverse ethnic, economic, and social backgrounds in a sensitive, caring, and highly skilled way.

Good obstetric and gynecologic care requires the consideration of each woman as an individual. To establish an effective working alliance with women who seek treatment, the clinician must not only be knowledgeable in medicine but also be a good observer and an able communicator. With a biopsychosocial approach, the clinician sees a "person" and not a "disease." The collaboration of physicians with nurses, social workers, and psychiatrists or psychologists is useful.

This chapter presents an overview of the important normal and abnormal psychologic aspects of pregnancy, and the puerperium, gynecologic practice and describes some of the syndromes that have prominent psychologic features. However, clinicians should bear in mind that all major physiologic or pathologic conditions have psychosocial overtones.

## Motivations for Pregnancy

Procreation is a compelling goal for many women, but not for all. Motivations for pregnancy are varied and complex, and only some of them are conscious. The desire for a pregnancy is not always the same as the wish for a child. For example, a pregnancy may be wanted to confirm one's sexual identity or to give proof of one's reproductive integrity and capability. Desire for a pregnancy may also be a response to loss or feelings of loneliness. A woman may identify with a fantasied child as someone to love who will love her in return. She may wish to preserve a relationship with a partner, or she may be responding to family or cultural pressures to have a baby. In adolescents, peer pressure, rebellion against family, and feelings of depression are frequent motivations for pregnancy. In women in their 30s, the biologic clock is ticking away, leaving them only limited time in which to conceive. Many of these feelings also exist in men. In some cultures, children represent immortality for the parents, and it is natural for many people, as they grow older, to hope that some part of them will live on in future generations.

## Pregnancy as a Developmental Transition

Pregnancy like menarche and menopause, is a major developmental step in the lives of women. It is often the fulfillment of deep and powerful wishes and can be a chance for creativity, self-realization, and an opportunity for new growth. While pregnancy may bring a sense of joy and well-being, it is also a stressful experience. Conflicts may arise, such as the relationship with one's parents and siblings, responsibilities of motherhood, demands of a career and obligations as wife and mother. How a woman responds to pregnancy is related to her early childhood experiences, coping mechanisms, personality style, life situation, emotional supports, and physical problems.

The father-to-be is also presented with many conflicts. Men may have unusual symptoms during their partner's pregnancy and will visit physicians more often with complaints reflecting their own anxieties and concerns about their new role. They may envy their partner's new condition and may wish for the attention they used to receive that may now be directed toward the baby.

Women and their partners often welcome the chance to discuss their feelings with an empathetic professional or with others in a group setting at prenatal classes.

## Normal Psychologic Processes During Pregnancy and the Puerperium

The basic developmental and psychologic tasks of pregnancy vary with the stage of pregnancy. During the first trimester, the woman's main task is to incorporate the fetus—part of the woman and part of her partner—as an integral part of her body and self. In the second trimester, with recognition of fetal movement, it is necessary to perceive the fetus as a separate entity and to begin to visualize the fetus as a baby with needs of its own. In the third trimester and postpartum, the patient comes to see herself as a mother and begins to establish a nurturing relationship with the infant. To mother an infant adequately, a woman must herself have had the experience of being nurtured as an infant. She may have to resolve some lingering conflicts with her own parents. Her relationship with her partner may also change for better or worse.

**A. First Trimester:** The diagnosis of a wanted pregnancy is usually accompanied by a sense of excitement and anxiety. Even the most wanted pregnancy can cause ambivalence on the part of both parents because of the recognized major life transition. An unplanned pregnancy is not necessarily unwanted and may be readily accepted. However, the woman and her partner need time to process their feelings and thoughts. If a termination is being considered, counseling should begin as soon as possible and without ambivalence on the part of the professional staff. Such counseling should allow the woman, and her partner if possible, to understand the implications of each of their possible choices and to weigh the risks, benefits, and alternatives before making a decision.

The first trimester, with its attendant fatigue, breast tenderness, nausea, and urinary frequency, is often accompanied by an increased preoccupation with self and with the growth of the fetus. There may be a sense of fulfillment and well-being, but emotions may be labile. Sexual interest may decline, while a desire for affection may increase. Apprehension concerning miscarriage, the baby's health, and role changes is common. Even the most educated individuals may harbor superstitious beliefs in the cause and effect of unrelated events.

Ultrasound has led to earlier maternal and paternal bonding. It has also allowed earlier prenatal knowledge of the baby's sex. This information can have either positive or negative effects. If parents are displeased with the fetal sex, counseling during the pregnancy can often help them adapt.

**B. Second Trimester:** During the second trimester, there is an increased sense of well-being and the resumption of outside interests. Fetal movement, at approximately 16–18 weeks, often results in a greater sense of reality about the pregnancy. The fetus is perceived as a separate entity, and the parents fantasize about how the baby will look. The mother may experience increased feelings of dependency; sexual desire varies greatly, and changes in body image may be distressing.

**C. Third Trimester:** During the latter part of pregnancy, fear or anxiety about labor and delivery may increase. Concerns arise about pain, injury, and the baby's health; about being a responsive mother; and about how relationships may be changed. Sleep is often disturbed, and somatic preoccupations may increase.

Childbirth education, in a setting where the woman, and her partner are free to ask questions, regardless of how inconsequential she may think they are, is invaluable. Questions to the mother-to-be should be open-ended, not "Yes" or "No" questions. For example, "What worries or concerns are you having?" is far more likely to evoke a meaningful response than "Are you having any worries?"

Some difficulties arise when a woman considers herself a "failure" if she does not fulfill her own expectations concerning the numerous birth options and delivery methods, eg giving birth without anesthesia or surgical interventions. Prospective discussion of these issues may be helpful in preventing such problems. Another potential problem may arise around informed consent. There is an increasingly high parental expectation that with modern technology in obstetrics nothing can go wrong; however, the inherent nature of informed consent involves telling women the potential for what could go wrong. Thus, without adequate preparation and information exchange, communication may break down. Good communication usually does not require much time. In fact, many physicians who spend considerable time do so because they have not listened or communicated well while trying to correct the problem. Patience in listening is an invaluable aid to lessening patient anxiety and fear and improving the chance of successful communication.

**D. Labor and Delivery:** Labor and delivery are unique experiences for each woman. The professional support team's goals are to enhance the health and safety of mother and infant, to free the mother from excessive pain or complications without complete loss of fulfillment, and to establish a strong and loving relationship among mother, infant, and family.

Emphasis today is on active mastery of the birth experience with as much patient participation as possible. However, women vary tremendously in their ability to meet this goal. Fear and unfamiliarity can increase tension and pain. Some of the fear can be reduced by childbirth education classes, relaxation techniques, knowledge of both usual and unusual obstetric procedures, and familiarity with hospital facilities and delivery rooms. The presence during the labor of the partner, a close female friend, or a family member offers invaluable support to the mother. She should not be left alone under any circumstance. Pain is related not only to biologic factors, length of labor, and complications, but also to fear, past experiences with pain, personality, style of expression, and cultural factors. The reassuring presence of a labor companion and childbirth preparation classes can help the mother handle the pain of labor and delivery.

The patient's attitude during pregnancy may *not* be a good predictor of her psychologic status in labor. Giving up the unity, the oneness with the child, is reported by some women as a stressor. Fears exist about death, bodily injury, loss of adequacy or control, and especially about exposing bodily functions. While women should be encouraged to take an active part in both labor and delivery, some women don't want to.

The number of home births in the USA remains low. The major concern is that there may be complications that can be handled only in a hospital. One-third of infants requiring immediate intensive care from home deliveries have been products of normal pregnancies. While the safety of mother and infant must be the first concern, hospitals should strive to provide a more homelike and less institutional atmosphere for the birthing experience.

Electronic fetal monitoring during labor is now commonly employed. Some patients find this practice intrusive, while others find it reassuring. Women who have experienced prior fetal loss are more accepting of its presence and find it reduces their anxiety. However, highly technical equipment does not eliminate the possibility of complications, nor is it a replacement for human skill. More studies are needed to relate psychologic factors to obstetric progress and complications. Women who freely express their concerns may do better than passive patients who suppress them. Communication between physician and patient remains crucial.

**E. Puerperium:** "Mothering" is a learned skill, but the attachment of mother and infant begins long before birth. The term **bonding** refers to a sensitive period after birth, where interactions between mother and infant lock them together. The attachment direction is from mother to infant, making her a more effective parent. Early visual and physical contact between mother and baby facilitates the attachment. Attachment behaviors include fondling, kissing, cuddling, and gazing—practices that maintain contact between mother and infant. Factors that may interfere with early bonding include lack of instinctual response, psychologic problems, inadequate preparation, physical illness in mother or baby, and hospital practices that separate mother and infant. To facilitate

early bonding, sedation and separation should be minimal. Separation may have physical, biologic, and emotional consequences. However, a mother should not believe she will be a failure because something has interfered with her earliest contact with her infant. There is evidence that later bonding is also successful.

Bonding is especially important for women and infants who may have attachment problems. Some of these high-risk individuals are mothers who are very young, ill, or ambivalent about pregnancy, or who have suffered child abuse, have relational difficulties with their partner, or have a psychiatric disorder. Intervention includes recognition of the problem and referral to an appropriately trained mental health professional.

The father's presence in the labor and delivery room has contributed to earlier father-infant bonding, but fathers must be prepared for attending the delivery and must have a role in it (eg, coaching the mother's efforts). Whether the father will be present when complications occur or when operative delivery is required should be discussed in advance.

**F. Transition to Motherhood:** As noted earlier, although mothering has instinctual roots, it is largely a learned behavior. A mother's early experiences with a loving caregiver in her own infancy strengthen her capacity for mothering. Mothers of new and young infants in our culture are often isolated from family and friends, which makes the early days even more difficult. During this stressful time, the new mother needs supportive individuals in her environment. It is helpful if the professional staff knows of unusual home circumstances. Indeed, an evaluation of this environment should be part of discharge planning. Will this new mother be alone or with numerous relatives? Are there religious or cultural practices that will interfere with sexuality, reproduction, nursing, or motherhood? Will this woman be returning to work? If so, when? Finally, if she was known to the staff during the pregnancy, have her personality and coping ability undergone abrupt changes?

Breastfeeding may have advantages, but women who bottle-feed their babies must not be made to feel guilty or inadequate.

It is helpful for a woman to review her labor and delivery with her physician if she feels she has performed inadequately—whatever the setting and procedures may have been. Such communication may be encouraged by asking the woman, "How do you feel about your labor and delivery?"

## Sources of Stress in Pregnancy and the Puerperium

Endocrine, somatic, and psychologic changes contribute to making pregnancy and the puerperium times of stress. The confirmation of pregnancy may be thrilling for some but devastating for others. Indeed, a degree of ambivalence is probably the usual response.

Women with preexisting health problems may be concerned about the availability of resources to withstand additional physiologic demands. Most healthy women have some physical distress from the discomforts of abdominal enlargement, nausea, heartburn, or urinary frequency. Most women also experience psychologic distress from worries about body image, genetic problems, and role changes as well as the effect of the pregnancy on her partner, career, education plans, finances, or her ability to be a mother. A worry often not voiced, especially by a primigravida, is "Will I live through this experience?"

Interpersonal relationships with husband (or partner), mother, coworkers, and friends change during and after the pregnancy. Partner satisfactions often decline during pregnancy. Women who are sexually responsive are more likely to experience pregnancy with pleasure; however, pregnancy is a public statement of a woman's sexual activity, which may be a source of pride or embarrassment.

While anxiety, emotional lability, and worries are normal during this time, the ability to cope depends on each woman's life experiences, personality style, social supports, and the care and technical expertise of the obstetric staff.

**A. Denial of Pregnancy:** Good prenatal care improves pregnancy outcome. Early recognition of pregnancy by a woman and her family leads her to seek prenatal health care, take extra care of herself, eat well, and get sufficient rest. Denial of pregnancy may interfere with the patient obtaining proper care. The women most prone to denial of pregnancy may fit into one of the following categories: psychotic, borderline personality, or women from extremely rigid backgrounds. The denial is usually an unconscious process in which the individual keeps the unpleasant reality of an unwanted pregnancy out of her awareness. She is often joined in this negativity by family and, on rare occasions, by physicians. She may go through an entire pregnancy forgetting missed periods, and unaware of breast changes, abdominal enlargement, or fetal movements. She may present in the emergency room in labor or deliver the infant at home. With the birth, a psychotic reaction may occur. The neonates are at high risk for injury or death. Obviously, these women need extra support in the postnatal period and, if identified during the course of pregnancy, may benefit from psychologic assistance.

**B. Sexuality:** There are many variations in sexual functioning during pregnancy and the puerperium. In general, woman note a decrease of sexual interest during the first trimester, which is related to fatigue, nausea, and a feeling of turning inward. Women without a history of miscarriage, genital bleeding, or dyspareunia need not fear that intercourse will harm the fetus. In the second trimester there is often an increased interest and desire for sexual experience. Many women have an increased wish to be held or to masturbate. Some become orgasmic for the first time, possibly because of increased pelvic vasocongestion.

In the third trimester, sexual interest and performance are even more variable. The woman may feel awkward and have increased fears of harming the fetus. If there are no obstetric complications or physical discomfort, intercourse is not contraindicated; there is no evidence that intercourse precipitates premature labor, although orgasm does cause uterine contractions. Some men lose their sexual interest during their partner's pregnancy, or they fear harming the fetus. Noncoital techniques can be satisfying to the couple. Couples should be told that oral-genital sex must not include air blown into the vagina as this practice may cause an air embolism, which is potentially fatal to mother and fetus.

Sexual desire postpartum may not return for many weeks or months. This may be due to new interest in the baby, fatigue, depression, hormonal status, or concerns about body image. Breast feeding may alter sexual feelings in the new mother or her partner. Fathers may feel excluded. The obstetrician can be helpful to a couple by discussing sexuality changes with them.

**C. Vomiting in Pregnancy:** Vomiting in pregnancy may be of 4 varieties: the usual causes as in the nonpregnant state (eg, influenza, viral disorders, drug reactions); hormonal changes in the first trimester, which affect approximately 50% of pregnant women and are not associated with any particular psychologic syndrome (see Chapter 9), preeclampsia, liver disease, or other obstetric complication; or hyperemesis gravidarum (pernicious vomiting of pregnancy). The latter is a severe form of nausea occurring at any time during pregnancy. The woman may become severely dehydrated, lose weight, and have metabolic disturbances and electrolyte imbalances. The incidence in the USA is 1 in 1000 pregnancies.

Biologic, psychologic, and social etiologies have been suggested for hyperemesis gravidarum. Biologic causes, still unconfirmed, relate to endocrine, metabolic, or immune function disorders. There is some support for an association with multiple birth and past pregnancy loss. Psychologically, this condition is considered to be a somatization disorder in which dysphoric feelings or psychic conflicts are expressed via physical symptoms, which are much more acceptable in our culture. There is often a past history of early life experienced colored by abdominal pain and nausea. The condition is not related to any one psychiatric diagnosis, although more severe psychiatric illness may be present. Social stress may contribute to its severity.

Treatment may require rehydration, antiemetics, or antihistamines; hospitalization may be necessary. A good response has been noted with hypnosis and relaxation techniques. Identification of stress in the individual's life and help with stress reduction is often useful.

**D. Sleep in Pregnancy and the Puerperium:** Sleep disturbances during pregnancy and the puerperium are common. There is often increased sleepiness in the early prepartum period associated with high levels of estrogen and progesterone. In the postpartum period, a demanding infant together with decreased ovarian hormone levels may lead to sleep deficiency. During pregnancy and the puerperium sleep latency, the frequency of awakening and stage 0 sleep are increased; REM sleep is decreased. Hormonal fluctuations are related to sleep pattern changes. Medication should be used cautiously.

## ADOLESCENT PREGNANCY: PSYCHOLOGIC ISSUES

Approximately 1 million adolescents 15–19 years old (one-tenth of all women in this age range in the USA) become pregnant each year, and 500,000 give birth. This high teenage pregnancy rate is due to many factors, including a subculture in which there is glorification of sexual activity without education of young people regarding its consequences. Other motivations for pregnancy in adolescence may be related to peer pressure, rebellion, keeping a relationship, and desiring more emotional intimacy. Adolescent girls rarely enjoy their early sexual experiences as boys do, and a large number of teenage mothers have been sexually abused. First intercourse often takes place within a relationship the girl wants to keep, and contraception is rarely used. Psychologic traits related to contraceptive use in adolescents are high self-esteem, an orientation toward the future, feelings of control over life, and acceptance of the sexual self.

Three psychologic subsets of adolescent mothers have been described. The **problem prone** use alcohol, drugs, or both, are truant from school, and get poor grades in school. They act on impulse and are often part of a peer counterculture who reject conventional society. The **adequate copers** are competent and open to alternative lifestyles but characteristically go through life transitions at an earlier age than their peers. The **depressed** idealize pregnancy as a way of dealing with their feelings of loss, sadness, and emptiness. It is useful to distinguish from among these 3 groups and to offer assistance in response to their various needs.

Adolescents often strain the patience of healthcare personnel because they may be difficult to talk with, have values very different from those of the staff, arrive late for prenatal care, or be noncompliant. If the physician understands more about preadult development and sexuality, adolescent care can be extremely gratifying. Counseling adolescents requires an ability to educate and communicate with them while offering privacy and confidentiality.

## PSYCHIATRIC DISORDERS OF PREGNANCY AND THE PUERPERIUM

Pregnancy and the puerperium are emotionally stressful periods for many women. Mood swings are commonly manifested by emotional lability, weepiness, irritability, and feeling blue or high. Prenatal assessment for psychological difficulties should include the following:

(1) Prior personal or family history of psychiatric illness

(2) Psychiatric disorder

(3) Psychologic problems that accompanied maturational periods, eg, puberty

(4) History of early maternal deprivation or mother's death

(5) Difficulty separating from parents

(6) Conflicts about mothering

(7) Marital or family difficulties, including separation

(8) Past difficulty with pregnancy, delivery, or postpartum depression

(9) Recent death of family member or close friend

(10) Familial or congenital disorders

(11) History of infertility

(12) History of repeat abortion

(13) History of pseudocyesis or hyperemesis

(14) Prior fetal death, miscarriage, or congenital abnormality extreme age range

(15) History of sexual, physical, or emotional abuse current or past

(16) History of premenstrual syndrome

Psychiatric disorders during pregnancy and in the puerperium have been described throughout history. There may be disagreement as to whether these disorders are the same or different from those occurring at other times. However, no one denies that they occur frequently postpartum in the first 2–4 weeks and that the most frequent disorder is major depression.

### Depressive Disorders

The term depression refers to a mood, symptom, or group of syndromes. The mood—feeling "blue"—is part of human experience related to sadness, frustration, discouragement, and of feeling "down." Many women experience such moods, in greater or lesser degrees, in the weeks following delivery. The **symptom** can be part of another physical or psychologic illness such as alcoholism, schizophrenia, or viral illness. The **syndrome**, known as a major depression or affective disorder, is characterized by a specific set of symptoms associated with a change in mood. This lasts for a period of at least 2 weeks and is severe enough to interfere with activities of daily life. The severity can vary considerably from a very mild transient period of feeling blue, such as in the postpartum period, (blues) to major clinical depression with vegetative signs and symptoms but normal reality testing, to severe psychotic depressions with hallucinations, delusions, and a possibility of suicide or infanticide. In the first 2 weeks to few months postpartum, most new mothers report feeling tired, weepy, moody, anxious about caring for a new baby, trapped, afraid, angry at the baby's father and at the baby, and guilty at having hostile thoughts. This has been called the "new mother syndrome." Treatment consists of support from family, healthcare providers, and other mothers. Generally the depressive reactions may be divided into 2 types.

**A. Postpartum Blues:** This condition (also called postnatal blues, 3-day blues, or baby blues) is a transitory mood disturbance following delivery (usually from days 3 to 10) and usually occurs at the height of hormonal changes. It is frequent, occurring in about 50–70% of women. It is characterized by crying, irritability, anxiety, forgetfulness, sadness, or elation. It is unrelated to the health of mother or baby, obstetric complications, hospitalization, social class, or breast or formula feeding, although any of these factors can affect the patient's mood. It occurs cross-culturally but is less noticeable in cultures where emotions are expressed freely and when relatives and friends surround the new mother offering care and support. It may last a few days to 2–3 weeks.

**B. Major Depression:** This condition is a non-psychotic depressive syndrome during pregnancy but most commonly occurs in the weeks and months after delivery. The incidence of moderate depression is 10–15%. Its symptoms include change in mood, sleep patterns, eating, mental concentration, or libido and may involve somatic preoccupations, phobias, and fear of harming self or infant.

Discussion of her feelings may offer relief. To facilitate such discussion, a woman with symptoms of moderate depression should be asked about her symptoms. To elicit suicidal, or homicidal ideas, the physician might ask "Have you felt so overwhelmed or trapped that you might hurt yourself or your baby?" There seem to be few predictive factors, but there is a higher occurrence in women with past psychiatric disorders, family history of such disorders, life event and partner problems, and possibly the premenstrual syndrome. Depressions during pregnancy may differ from those occurring postpartum, but this is unclear.

Postpartum depressions have a high rate of recurrence in subsequent pregnancies. Mental health consultation is advisable. Treatment may include providing the mother with environmental support, psychotherapy (with the partner included when possible), and antidepressant medication (carefully weighed against adverse effects in a pregnant or lactating woman and her fetus or infant). Suicidal or homicidal patients should be assessed immediately and should not be left alone. Hospitalization may be necessary.

**Postpartum Psychoses**

Postpartum psychoses occur in 1–2 of 1000 births. These are severe mental illnesses, usually requiring admission to mental hospitals because of delusions and the concern that the woman may harm herself or the infant. They are most frequently **depressive illnesses** (70–80%) but must be differentiated from **schizophrenia** or **organic brain syndromes**. There is often a family history of mental illness, past psychiatric history, marital and family problems, recent stressful life situations, and a lack of social supports, although none of these risk factors may be present. No single obstetric complication imposes a higher risk for these disorders. These individuals appear to be biologically vulnerable to mental disorder. The discovery of neurotransmitter disorders in these conditions has led to the development of medications that are useful in therapy. Risk of recurrence in subsequent pregnancies may be as high as 20–30%.

Symptoms develop most commonly from a few days to 4–6 weeks postpartum, although a careful history often reveals that the illness began in the third trimester of pregnancy. The woman may become restless, unable to sleep, irritable, have pressured speech, or become very withdrawn. Drug dependency, endocrinopathies such as thyroid disease, and other neurologic disorders must be ruled out.

Most postpartum psychoses are similar to those noted in nonpregnant women, although atypical disorders may not fit traditional classifications. Women at high risk for psychotic states are those with a past psychiatric history of psychosis. Other symptomatologies to be followed closely after delivery are confusion, sleep disorders, increased emotional lability, unusual behavior, and obsessional or delusional thinking. Infant injury or infanticide by the mother is rare but does occur in serious cases. Treatment of affective disorders is with antidepressant drugs or lithium and care in a psychiatric environment. Because antidepressant drugs are secreted in breast milk, breast feeding must be discontinued.

**Schizophrenia** is a psychiatric disorder at least 6 months' duration characterized in its acute phase by symptoms of delusions, hallucinations, incoherent speech, catatonia, or flat affect. Generally, the level of the individual's function declines, with withdrawal and social isolation. The onset is usually during adolescence or young adulthood. Genetic as well as environmental and psychologic factors are involved. Schizophrenic women may have exacerbations during pregnancy and the puerperium and should be carefully monitored. Delusions in pregnancy often relate to bodily changes and fetal movements. The disease is considered to have an organic basis with biochemical abnormalities, and drug treatment is usually with neuroleptic antipsychotics such as phenothiazones, butyrophenones, and thioxanthenes. A psychiatric referral is indicated. Suicidal risk should be assessed.

**Organic brain disease** (delirium, organic brain syndrome) is often confused with acute psychosis. Toxic states, drugs, metabolic disorders, infection, and hemorrhage can cause neurodysfunction. There may be impairment of orientation, memory, intellectual functions, and judgment as well as emotional lability. The individual is usually conscious and symptoms fluctuate. A neuropsychiatric consultation is indicated. It is best to avoid sedative drugs until an evaluation and diagnosis are made and treatment of the underlying disorder is begun.

In-hospital management includes keeping the surroundings familiar, the room lighted, and the woman oriented by using her name. The clinician must be alert to changes in mood, behavior, and thinking.

Psychoses require specialized psychiatric care, but a patient who becomes acutely disturbed or confused requires emergency management until the psychiatric consultation can be achieved. Such patients can be roughly divided into 5 categories according to the following features (Schatzberg):

(1) Acute psychoses with disordered thought, hallucinations, and fear possibly due to psychotic illness or drug reaction

(2) Delirium due to an underlying medical problem with fluctuating disorientation to time, place, and person

(3) Severe anxiety with somatic symptoms

(4) Anger and belligerence with or without alcohol or drug abuse

(5) Depression with suicidal ideas

A medical and drug history should be obtained from relatives or friends. Accuracy is essential, eg, insulin shock in a diabetic may be confused with "psychogenic seizures." If possible, a blood sample should be drawn for toxic screening. The patient is calmed, and a relative or friend may remain with her unless she becomes violent. In such instances, security personnel should be alerted and the patient transferred to a psychiatric facility as quickly as possible. Haloperidol may be given orally or parenterally to facilitate immediate management.

### Anxiety Disorders in Pregnancy

Anxiety during pregnancy and the puerperium is normal; its total absence is as pathologic as is its excess. When anxiety increases enough to be considered a disorder, there are 2 major classifications: phobic disorders and anxiety state disorders. **Phobic disorders** include persistent and irrational fear of a specific object, activity, or situation that may lead to avoidance. In pregnancy, women with these disorders have irrational fears, eg, nonsubstantiated worries about food that might harm the fetus. Treatment ranges from simple reassurance to behavior modification.

**Anxiety states** are divided into 4 categories. **Panic disorders** include recurrent attacks of anxiety with sudden onset of intense fear and apprehension. There may be physical symptoms such as dyspnea, chest pains, palpitations, choking, and dizziness. Attacks may last minutes to hours with anxiety between attacks. They are thought to have a biochemical basis, but there is often a precipitating event. Their occurrence in pregnancy is not uncommon. Panic disorders may be part of the syndrome of depression. Treatment, if necessary, is with antianxiety drugs, eg, alprazolam.

**Generalized anxiety disorders** last a month or more with signs of motor tension, vigilance, scanning, autonomic hyperactivity, and apprehension. Other conditions causing anxiety must be ruled out.

Patients with **obsessive compulsive** disorder have ideas or thoughts that make them do or over-do certain things. In pregnancy, these may relate to harming the fetus or the infant after birth. This may interfere with function and compliance. Diagnosis and therapy by a mental health professional is usually necessary.

**Posttraumatic stress disorders** develop after a known traumatic event. The individual may recurrently experience thoughts or dreams, and the symptomatology may include sleep disturbance, hyperalertness, guilt, and memory impairment. The posttraumatic event may be a stressful labor and delivery, fetal loss, infertility, or the death of a close relative or friend.

When counseling a woman with any of the above disorders, the clinician needs answers to 3 questions: (1) Is there a medical condition causing the disorder, eg, as endocrine problem? (2) Is there a basic psychiatric disorder such as depression or schizophrenia present? (3) Is this patient abusing alcohol or other drugs?

Consultation with a mental health professional is recommended.

### Substance Abuse and Alcohol Abuse

Substance abuse can cause major problems in pregnancy and the puerperium; the problems may be mild or may be severe enough to lead to fetal abnormalities, morbidity, and death of infant and mother. Therefore, inquiry concerning drug use should be made during prenatal visits and documented in the records.

### Management of Psychiatric Illness in Pregnancy and Lactation

Psychotropic drugs should be avoided if at all possible during pregnancy and lactation. However, there are many instances when this is not possible because there are psychiatric illnesses that do require medication. Nonpharmacologic methods such as psychotherapy, cognitive behavioral therapies, family and marital treatment, and even psychiatric hospitalization may be indicated before medications are used. A major problem is that there are not good data on the effects of these drugs on the fetus.

An antipsychotic drug of choice might be haldoperidol in lowest possible divided dosages and avoided in the first trimester. It would be used for the treatment of psychosis. Antidepressant drugs have not been proven safe in pregnancy and lactation, and there is very little data on the newer serotonin re-uptake inhibitors or the monoamine oxidase inhibitors. Nortriptilene and desipramine are often used because they have less anticholinergic side effects and because serum levels can be obtained in mother and neonate, when the depressive disorder is of significant enough magnitude to require medication. Lithium and carbamazine should be avoided because of their teratogenic effects. If they must be used, then patients should be warned of their possible harm, and those patients should be carefully monitored.

## GRIEF & GRIEVING: PERINATAL LOSS

Despite modern medical technology, there is still significant pregnancy loss due to spontaneous abortion, stillbirth, or neonatal death. Relinquishment of a baby for adoption may have the same psychologic effects as loss due to death. While the fetus is in utero it becomes perceived by the mother as part of herself. Death of a fetus or baby is often felt to be a loss of part of the mother's self. Grief is the process of adapting to such a loss by detaching little by little through anger, pain, and sadness. The mother and father may feel an emptiness. Thoughtless comments, eg, "You can always have another," "You didn't know the baby anyway," or "Plan another pregnancy right away" may serve only to increase the couple's emotional pain.

Parents grieve for the lost fetus or infant in their own way and in their own time. One difficulty in grieving for a lost pregnancy is the lack of identification that is useful in detaching from a known person. Parents should be encouraged to make their own decisions concerning seeing or holding the baby, disposition of the remains (burial or cremation), religious observances, and naming the baby. They should not be discouraged from seeing a malformed infant; they often recall the positive aspects. Photos may be obtained if desired. Autopsies often give parents more information about the normal as well as the abnormal features. Mothers, perhaps more than fathers, suffer from guilt and helplessness. Participation in decision making can help them achieve more control in dealing with their loss.

Physicians may also feel helpless and sad. They must talk with patients, give them as much information as possible and assure them (if possible) that nothing the mother did caused the fetal or infant demise. Often, the anger that is part of the grieving process is displaced to hospital staff, especially physicians. It is helpful to individualize each set of parents, meet with them, encourage their own form of grieving, and encourage them to wait at least 6 months before starting another pregnancy. If severe grief persists beyond several months, psychiatric consultation should be obtained.

## PSEUDOCYESIS

Pseudocyesis is a syndrome in which a nonpregnant woman believes she is pregnant and develops signs and symptoms suggestive of pregnancy. Pseudocyesis is a conversion reaction in which a psychic conflict is expressed in physical terms. It is an example of how a false belief may affect physiologic processes. It has been known since ancient times, and many cases have been described in women aged 7–79 years. The most common symptoms include menstrual abnormalities (oligomenorrhea, amenorrhea), abdominal enlargement, and breast changes. There may be nausea and vomiting. On examination, the uterus is not enlarged; the abdomen is firm to palpation and often tympanic to percussion. "Fetal movement" has been reported; it is usually intestinal activity or unconscious contractions of abdominal muscles. A supposed fetal heart rate may be maternal tachycardia. Galactorrhea may be present because of increased prolactin levels from other causes (ie, pituitary adenomas), long-term breast stimulation, or use of drugs such as phenothiazines. There are usually neuroendocrine abnormalities, eg, hypothalamic amenorrhea. Duration varies from 9 months to several years. Diagnosis of true pregnancy can be obtained with pregnancy tests and ultrasonography. However, test results may not convince a woman with this syndrome that she is not pregnant.

The clinical variants of pseudocyesis include "true" pseudocyesis, which should be distinguished from psychosis in women in whom the false belief in pregnancy is a delusion; factitious illness in which the woman knows she is not pregnant but simulates pregnancy for some secondary gain, eg, keeping a straying partner; organic diseases such as a pelvic tumor; and iatrogenic pseudopregnancy administration of hCG with positive pregnancy tests in infertile women.

Management consists of a careful history, physical examination, and laboratory tests to rule out pregnancy and organic disease. Psychologic assessment and treatment are also indicated.

# PSYCHOLOGIC ASPECTS OF GYNECOLOGY

Gynecologic practice in all cultures has always been affected by folklore, taboos, and religious and civil sanctions to control and regulate sexual activity and reproduction. Recent changes in gynecologic practice have been greatly influenced by significant alterations in women's perceptions of what gynecologic care should be and by the growing numbers of younger women physicians specializing in gynecology.

The gynecologist is a primary care physician for women, often from childhood across the life cycle—from menarche through adolescence, young adulthood, pregnancy, menopause, and old age. To perform this function well, gynecologists need to know about the psychosexual as well as the physical development of women. They need to be prepared to be a pelvic surgeon, a reproductive endocrinologist, a sex counselor, and an educator. Gynecologists need to be sensitive to their own attitudes, values, prejudices, and personality, and they must understand how these characteristics will influence their practice and their patients' decision to trust and work collaboratively with them.

## THE DOCTOR-PATIENT RELATIONSHIP IN GYNECOLOGY

In the past, doctors and patients generally related to each other in accordance with a model in which a compliant, conforming patient viewed the doctor as omnipotent. Today, many women reject this model and demand a more active part in making decisions relating to their health care. Health and disease-related information is much more widely available. Thus, patients are much better informed than in the past and have access to specific material relating to the concern that brings them to the physician. They often want their partners or family involved. An appropriate doctor-patient relationship is an essential part of the therapeutic process and can lead to a healthy compliance with medical and surgical regimens. To accomplish this relationship, it is essential to have some understanding of the personality style of the woman and her response to stress, as well as knowledge of oneself.

There are still many women who do not want to participate in decisions about health care and who view their physicians as all-good and protective. They believe they will be protected and that nothing will go wrong. While these beliefs may be flattering to the physician, unrealistic expectations often lead to anger and disappointment on the part of the patient. The collaborative model of doctor-patient interaction, when possible, is most effective. The patient interview is the place to begin this collaboration and to assess the woman's personality.

### The Patient Interview

Gathering historical data and subsequent decision making based on that information is essential for the practice of all clinical medicine. Failure to obtain an essential bit of information can be disastrous. The clinician must use both direct and indirect methods in history taking plus active listening, noting not only the words but also the effect and the nonverbal cues accompanying them such as facial expressions, body posture, gestures, voice quality, or tears. Physicians need to learn why these complaints are being brought to his or her attention now. Open-ended questions, followed by specific ones, allow information to flow. For example, in talking to a woman with pelvic pain, it is better to ask the open-ended question, "What is the pain like?" rather than the closed-ended, "Does the pain hurt badly?"

An insight into the patient's basic life situation and knowing something about her work and social situations is important. Again, open-ended questions such as, "How are things at home?" can better assist in eliciting this information. Psychologic symptoms such as problems with sleep, eating, fatigue, libido, and anxiety all have a part in the current physical disorder.

### Personality Style

Some of the following personality styles are seen in practice, and an understanding of how each type views illness can assist with planning a patient's care.

1. The dependent, overdemanding personality has insatiable needs. This patient becomes increasingly dependent on the physician, calls frequently and creates realistic anger. The physician needs to set limits, but with some concessions, telling the patient she can call at specific times. Interviews can be limited in frequency and duration. The dependent patient can make the physician angry by venting hostility in an indirect way. Illness is seen as a threat of abandonment. Assuring her of continued care that has definite limits is helpful.

2. The orderly, obsessive, controlled, anxious personality has needs for control and uses the defense mechanisms of isolation and intellectualization. This patient needs much information and participation in decisions regarding care. Illness is seen as a punishment for letting things get out of control.

3. The histrionic, dramatic, vivid, anxious personality is often seductive and flirtatious. This patient needs a physician with a caring, but firm professional manner. Illness is seen as punishment or an attack on her femininity. This patient needs support but not overly detailed explanations.

4. The long-suffering personality needs somatic symptoms to function. Illness may be considered as justly deserved and a punishment for worthlessness. The patient may need the physician to acknowledge her courage and not give too much reassurance.

5. The paranoid personality is suspicious, blaming, and hypersensitive and is threatened by intimacy. A respectful distance is necessary to help this individual. Illness is viewed as an annihilating assault coming from outside the self. Honest and simple explanations, including the assurance that no one is trying to hurt the patient, are needed.

6. The schizoid personality is remote, unsociable, uninvolved. Illness is viewed as a force that threatens to invade her privacy. A respect for privacy and distance is helpful.

### Acute Gynecologic Emergency

Whenever emergency or urgent medical or surgical care is needed, the relationship with the patient changes at once to one that requires almost total submission of a passive patient to the swift intervention of the physician. This role may be one the physician likes best. However, just as a patient may have to be weaned from a drug by tapering the dosage to nil over time, so each patient whose personal decision-making function has been taken over by a doctor acting in an emergency must be permitted to gradually resume responsibility for her emotional and physical welfare as soon as possible after the crisis has passed. Prolongation of the dominant role by the physician may easily lead to continued dependency after its justification has ceased. The patient recovering from surgery or regaining health after a serious illness must not be suddenly abandoned to her own devices as long as she needs her doctor's help and support, but every effort should be made to hasten her return to full health without dependency on her doctor.

## PSYCHOLOGIC ASPECTS OF SPECIFIC GYNECOLOGIC PROBLEMS

### Chronic Pelvic Pain

Pain is one of the commonest symptoms that women present to their gynecologists. It is also one of the most frustrating. Many patients coming to a gynecologist's office bring complaints of pain excluding dysmenorrhea. Ten to 60% have no pathology when examined at laparoscopy. Thus, in a large number of these women, no pelvic disease can be found. These women are often labeled as having psychiatric problems, and the pain is seen as a result of emotional conflicts when for many this may not be the case. There are at least 4 reasons why women may complain of pain in the apparent absence of organic pelvic disease. (1) Disease processes are present but cannot yet be detected; endometriosis is an example. (2) Pain may be associated with vascular disorders where no disease process can be observed (migraine variant). (3) Pain may be due to nongynecologic causes such as gastrointestinal, genitourinary, or skeletal system problems. (4) Complaints may be psychogenic.

The perception of pain can be influenced by several psychologic variables, including the individual's expectations of pain from past experiences, the anxiety that accompanies pain, childhood experiences with pain and punishment, the ability of the individual to control pain with cognitive and behavioral means, experiences with physical and sexual abuse, previous painful illnesses, the patient's current psychic state, and the patient's cultural expression of pain.

Chronic pain is pain of at least 6 months' duration. In persons who have had pain for 6 months or longer, it is not possible to distinguish organic from psychogenic pain. Chronic pain may cause emotional problems, and psychologic disorders may be related etiologically to pain. However, a reasonable approach is to determine what organic factors are present and what psychiatric disorders are present and to treat each type, following the person over time. Patients with chronic pelvic pain are found to be more depressed, to suffer more from substance abuse, and to have more sexual dysfunctions, somatization disorders, and histories of childhood and adult sexual abuse.

The most common psychiatric disorder related to pain is depression that is being expressed in physical terms. Somatization disorders are psychiatric ones in which recurrent somatic complaints occur over many months and years, and no physical causes are found. Psychologic problems are present. The disorders are more common in women and occur in 0.2–2% of patients. No one type of personality style is more prone to chronic pain than another.

The management of chronic pain requires careful history taking, physical examination, laboratory studies, laparoscopy, and psychologic assessment. Unnecessary surgery should be avoided, and psychologic treatments along with suitable medications are helpful. Biofeedback with pelvic vaginal blood flow as one physiologic variable has been used, as has relaxation training, hypnosis, and psychotherapy. Amitriptyline and some other antidepressants have been used with good results. Advances in this field will come from research that integrates the biologic, psychologic, and cultural approaches, not from the labeling of the unknown as psychologic.

### Eating Disorders

Eating disorders have been markedly increasing in recent years and are seen frequently in gynecologic practice. There is a cultural bias toward thinness for beauty as well as for health. The diagnostic criteria for the major entities of obesity, anorexia nervosa, and bulimia are still imprecise, and the relationship among these 3 disorders is unclear. However, 2 general principles in understanding these patients are (1) most physical and laboratory abnormalities seem to be the result, not the cause, of the disorders; and (2) anorexia, bulimia, and obesity are heterogeneous conditions with biologic, psychologic, and social dimensions. For each patient being evaluated, particular attention should be paid to history of the eating problem, weight and eating history, physical examination, and family dynamics, including affective mental disturbances in the family, personality style, substance abuse, and cultural background. Patients with anorexia nervosa or bulimia should have a psychologic assessment. Eating disorders may also reappear during pregnancy and interfere with appropriate nutrition.

**A. Obesity:** Obesity is the excessive accumulation of fat; it is usually defined as a 20% increase over standard weight and a 20% increase in skin-fold thickness. It affects approximately 25% of the adult population, is more common in women, increases with age, and is more prevalent in the USA in lower socioeconomic classes. There is no correlation with psychologic disturbance except for overeating behaviors, diet complications, and body image problems. Many treatment modalities are popular; nutritional–behavioral methods and self-help groups are useful for moderate obesity.

**B. Anorexia Nervosa:** Anorexia nervosa is a disorder characterized by refusal to maintain body weight to within 85% for age and height, by markedly decreasing food intake, by a preoccupation with a fear of becoming fat, by a distorted body image, and usually by amenorrhea for at least 3 consecutive menstrual cycles. People with this condition consider themselves obese, although they appear thin. There is often self-induced vomiting, excessive exercising, and use of laxatives and diuretics. The weight loss may be very marked, but the patient often comes to the attention of the gynecologist because of the amenorrhea. Associated physiologic signs may include hypothermia, bradycardia, hypotension, edema, lanugo, and other metabolic changes.

The onset of anorexia nervosa is usually from early adolescence to early adult life. Ninety-five percent of patients are female, and its occurrence is rare in heterosexual males. Its prevalence is 0.13–1% in females 12–18 years old. The course may be episodic or chronic: 40% of patients recover, 30% significantly improve, 20% remain ill, and death occurs in more than 5%. Family patterns show the disorder more common in sisters and mothers of affected individuals. Other family members may have a history of major depression or bipolar affective disorder. The onset may or may not occur with a stressful life event. These patients often were model children and are perfectionists.

Management consists of referral to specialists trained in the treatment of this disorder, usually as a team with behavioral medicine specialists and nutritionists. Hospital treatment is indicated for severe cases. As this time there is no specific treatment shown to be effective. Outcome studies still are not clear, but good prognosis is related to earlier age of onset and poor prognosis to premorbid obesity, bulimia, vomiting, and laxative abuse. These complex disorders require considerably more research.

**C. Bulimia:** Bulimia is an eating disorder characterized by recurrent bouts of rapid consumption of large amounts of food in a short time alternating with little or no food intake. There is accompanying depression, a lack of control over the eating, low self-esteem, and often social isolation. Other features include self-induced vomiting, use of laxatives and diuretics, dieting, fasting, and vigorous exercise all designed to keep weight down. There is preoccupation with food, weight, and body shape. The diagnosis is made when there are at least 2 large binge-eating episodes per week for at least 3 months. The food eaten is usually high in calories, easily ingested, and eaten secretly. The binge may be followed by abdominal pain, distention, and vomiting. The individual may be obese, thin, or of normal weight. Stress or eating itself may precipitate binges, which usually occur in the late afternoon or evening after school or work.

Many bulimics are depressed, and an association with affective disorders is suggested. There is also frequent association with alcohol or drug abuse (especially sedatives, amphetamines, and cocaine). A variety of personality types, including those with borderline personality disorders, develop this condition. Some physical complications include lethargy, impaired concentration, abdominal pain, dehydration, electrolyte disturbances (ie, hypokalemia, metabolic alkalosis, hypochloremia, and rarely metabolic acidosis) related to fasting or acute diarrhea. Other complications are gastric rupture, salivary gland swelling (usually the parotid), and dental problems with decalcification of teeth.

The neuroendocrine abnormalities include blunted thyroid-stimulating hormone (TSH) response to thyroid-releasing hormone (TRH) administration, increase in growth hormone following TRH or glucose administration, and elevated basal serum prolactin. Menstrual dysfunction may be due to disturbed gonadotropin production.

The cause is unknown, but etiologic theories relate to onset being associated with traumatic events, especially separation or loss, history of being overweight, association with anorexia nervosa, and cultural context in a society where food is abundant and thinness is very desirable. The onset is usually in adolescence and young adulthood. In a mild form bulimia is fairly common among women in college (4.5% women, 0.4% men reported in one study of college freshmen). Severe bulimia occurs in approximately 1% of the population. The course is chronic and intermittent over many years. The differential diagnosis must include schizophrenia, certain neurologic diseases such as central nervous system tumors, and epileptic equivalent seizures.

Management and treatment begin with a very careful history of eating patterns and psychologic function. This may be difficult to obtain since the patients are secretive. Behaviors to inquire about include binge eating and use of diuretics, laxatives, diet pills, and enemas. The next step is careful physical examination including a neurologic workup, noting the state of hydration, teeth, salivary glands, and cardiac function. Minimal laboratory work should include plasma glucose, complete blood count, liver function tests, thyroid function, and, if indicated, skull films with visual fields or CT scan. Hospitalization may be necessary. Psychologic approaches are usually behavioral or cognitive behavioral, group therapy, and patient education (especially about nutrition). Drug treatment consists of anticonvulsants or antidepressants. As with anorexia, the course, outcome, and response to therapy require considerable more research before the data may be considered conclusive.

## Sleep Disorders

A national survey indicates that one-third of the US population has some degree of sleep disturbance. Complaints are frequently presented to gynecologists in the context of other disorders and may be minor or be part of a more serious physical or psychiatric disorder. Considerable diagnostic and treatment options are available.

Recent advances in the study of sleep have related sleep physiology and the stages of the sleep cycle. Stage 0 is wakefulness with closed eyes, high muscle tone, and some eye movement. Stages 1–4 are non-REM sleep in humans and are characterized by specific encephalographic changes. REM or "desynchronized" sleep is characterized by extreme hypotonia, rapid eye movements, blood pressure and heart rate variability, muscle twitches, and nocturnal penile tumescence. There is high dream recall if one wakens during REM sleep. Sleep cycles vary with age, sex, and numerous other influences. In an ordinary 8-hour period of sleep, an adult age 25 years will go through 4–6 cycles, with the average cycle taking 90 minutes and REM periods 15 minutes.

Sleep and arousal problems have been classified into 4 groups. (1) The insomnias are disorders of initiating and maintaining sleep. They are a heterogenous group associated with organic and psychiatric conditions. A history of the sleep-wakefulness pattern helps with diagnosis. A disturbance in falling asleep may be due to anxiety or worry. Staying asleep or early-morning awakening is often seen in depressive illness. Myoclonus or central apnea can disturb sleep. (2) Disorders of excessive somnolence can be due to narcolepsy, obstructive airway syndrome, depression, substance abuse, or other conditions. (3) Disorders of the sleep-wake schedule are those in which there is a misalignment between the individual's usual sleep-wake cycle and the internal circadian rhythms, eg, jet lag. (4) Parasomnias are a group of clinical conditions that happen during sleep, sleep stages, and partial arousals. Examples include somnambulism (sleep walking) and asthma (which may get worse during sleep). They are manifestations of atypical central nervous system activation during sleep with discharge into skeletal muscle or into channels of autonomic activity.

Treatment of sleep problems requires an accurate diagnosis. Insomnias that do not respond to treatment with relaxation, sleep hygiene methods, and benzodiazepines should be referred to a sleep laboratory for diagnosis and treatment. Sleep hygiene suggestions generally include (1) curtail excess sleep; (2) maintain regular awakening times; (3) exercise regularly; (4) avoid loud noises during sleep; (5) keep sleeping room temperature comfortable; (6) avoid hunger; (7) limit caffeine and do not smoke; (8) avoid alcohol; (9) try to stop worrying; (10) keep busy after a sleepless night; (11) be flexible, but limit daytime naps. Hypnotic drugs are among the most widely used drugs in the USA. The 3 most commonly used groups are the barbiturates, the benzodiazepines, and nonbarbiturates, nonbenzodiazepines (eg, chloral hydrate, methaqualone). It is essential to be familiar with their pharmacology, action, potential for addiction or use for suicide, and teratogenicity before prescribing these drugs.

## Premenstrual Syndrome

Premenstrual syndrome is a psychoneuroendocrine disorder related to menses with biologic, psychologic, and social parameters. A complete discussion of premenstrual syndrome can be found in Chapter 32.

# PSYCHOLOGIC ASPECTS OF GYNECOLOGIC SURGERY

## Hysterectomy

In most cases of gynecologic surgery, there are clear-cut indications for the procedures and psychologically adaptable patients. When this situation does not exist, 3 principal participants must communicate well: the patient, her family, and the physician. Stress often impairs communication for the patient undergoing surgery. There are several sources of fear: death and injury, physiologic stress, separation from family, and the forced dependency of being a "patient." It is not abnormal to have a recurrence of childhood fears, especially related to punishment and abandonment, and feelings of aggression. The person who is the best surgical risk is intellectually intact, copes well with stress, has some anxiety, understands the risks of surgery, expects a reasonable outcome, is motivated to be healthy, and is not depressed.

The reproductive tract, uterus, ovaries, and vagina have special meanings to women including, but extending beyond, how she views her anatomy, physiology, and the psychologic symbolism derived from developmental experiences. Menstruation is an important confirmation of feminine identity for many, and body image is influenced by sensations from inner pelvic organs as well as from the vagina and labia. However, many women, even those with considerable education, are not comfortable with or knowledgeable about their bodies and inner organs.

A woman's adaptation to hysterectomy is related to her age, stage of development, personality, style of coping, pathophysiology of disease affecting the uterus, whether she has children or wants them, the relationships in her life, past experiences with close relatives or friends who had this operation, and the communication she establishes with health caretakers, especially her physician.

Premenopausal women interviewed prior to undergoing hysterectomy have worries about loss of childbearing ability, loss of menstruation, changes in sexual function and in their partner's sexual interest in them, loss of strength, aging, and pain. Some feel they are being punished. Others feel positively about not having further pregnancies, and having enhanced sexual pleasure and physical attractiveness. Preoperatively, it is helpful to inquire about attitudes toward femininity, prior losses, attitudes and expectations about surgery, baseline sexual functioning, and past history of anxiety or depression. Those with positive attitudes about femininity, ability to adapt to loss, and some anxiety do best. The patients with no anxiety, indifference, or very high degrees of anxiety are of concern.

Patients at high risk for psychologic difficulties after hysterectomy are those who repeatedly request surgery for less-than-clear reasons, those with chronic pelvic pain without any apparent pelvic disease, those who are depressed or who have past psychiatric history, those who have conflicts over sexuality and childbearing, those who have inappropriate levels of preoperative anxiety, and those with premonitions of death during surgery. Patients with somatization disorders should be identified prior to surgery.

Postoperatively, the surgeon needs to be alert for delirium, a form of encephalopathy, with clouding of consciousness and disorientation, perceptual abnormalities, and agitation or withdrawal. Other postoperative syndromes include delirium, tremors, ie, withdrawal from alcohol (or drugs), postoperative depression or psychosis, or excessive pain. Interestingly, patients may recall comments made in the operating room during anesthesia if it is light, and care should be taken about conversation while believing the patient is unconscious.

**A. Management:** Patients who are well prepared for surgery, compared with nonprepared patients, show less postoperative pain, use fewer pain medications, and have shorter hospital stays. A team effort is helpful with office staff providing as much information as is necessary. Preparation means more than reassurance that "everything will be all right." Sharing with the patient the indications for the contemplated surgery and the risks and side effects is helpful. However, it has been shown that patients who are very anxious do not hear the information well. An assessment of the patient's social supports and personality style can be very useful in assessing whether she is able to assimilate the information. Her husband, partner, or family should be included to enhance her support.

Postoperatively, patients require orientation to the hospital, an explanation of procedures, and adequate medication for pain. Early identification of patients who might need further psychologic assessment and treatment is imperative for success. There is no indication that women with a history of depression have more depressive episodes after surgery than other women. Sexual activity after hysterectomy may feel different, but can be as pleasurable as before.

### Gynecologic Oncology

The improved prognosis for many cancers makes the quality of life an increasingly important issue in the management of malignant disorders. The physician who cares for patients with gynecologic cancer needs not only to be familiar with the most current technical material, but also must be able to respond to the patient with empathy and understanding at all stages of the illness. For some patients, gynecologic cancers often have symbolic meanings related to sexuality and reproduction and are therefore extremely emotionally laden.

With the diagnosis there is often a grief response characterized by shock, disbelief, anger, and fears of death, pain, losing a body part, and abandonment. This can occur even when the malignancy is treatable. The treatment plan discussion should cover expected functional losses, side effects of treatment, and effects on sexual functioning. Psychiatric disorders that may occur in the course of malignant disease (eg, organic brain syndromes, depressive syndromes, and anxiety syndromes) need recognition and treatment.

### SEXUAL PROBLEMS IN GYNECOLOGIC PRACTICE

The most available resource for women with sexual difficulties is their gynecologist or family physician. Thus, a minimal sexual history is part of every gynecologic history. The gynecologist should be familiar with the sexual response cycle, with taking a sexual history, with the ability to make diagnoses of the commonest sexual disorders, with the effects on sexuality of organic problems and drugs, and with the kind of sexual therapies that are available. Most sexual problems are managed by education, corrections of organic problems, and reassurance. More intense psychologic problems should be managed by gynecologists with added training in sexual therapy. Certain common dimensions of sexual identity warrant discussion for those providing primary sexual counseling. Sexuality and reproduction are central to one's identity as a male or female whether or not one wants children. The sexual identity of any adult can be described along 3 major dimensions: gender identity, sexual orientation, and sexual intention.

**Gender identity** is the earliest aspect of sexual identity to form. Core gender identity is the sense one has of being male or female. It develops in the second year of life and is the result of: (1) biologic factors originating in fetal life and with the organization of the fetal brain; (2) sex assignment at birth by parents and medical staff; (3) parental attitudes; (4) conditioning and imprinting; and (5) development of body ego and body image, which comes in part from sensations from the genitals and body parts. Masculinity and femininity are those behaviors that a person, parents, society, or the culture define as male or female. These may change from time to time. While many children show some evidence of gender confusion, 90% develop a core gender identity consistent with their biologic sex. **Gender role** is the sum of what one does that indicates to others the degree of maleness or femaleness. Gender identity continues to be influenced by identification with important adults as the child grows to adulthood.

**Sexual orientation** refers to the sex of the person in fantasy or reality that causes sexual arousal. Heterosexual individuals are sexually aroused by persons of the opposite sex, homosexual individuals by persons of the same sex, and bisexual individuals by persons of both sexes. There is increasing evidence of biologic contributions to sexual orientation. Further research is needed.

**Sexual intention** refers to what a person wants to do with his or her sexual partner, eg, kissing, caressing, intercourse, etc. There are dimensions: fantasy and actual behavior. The usual intention is giving and receiving pleasure. Some examples of abnormal sexual intention related to aggression are sadism, exhibitionism, rape, and pedophilia.

The ability to function sexually in adulthood begins at birth with the earliest parent-infant bonds. The loving care a person receives in infancy and childhood prepares him or her for intimate relationships in adult life.

## Phases of the Sexual Response Cycle*

Stages in the sexual response cycle are described below. A broader description can be found in the classic work of Masters and Johnson, *Human Sexual Response*.

**A. Excitement Phase:** Early sexual arousal in the male, whether initiated by tactile, visual, or psychic stimuli, results in engorgement and erection of the penis, with an increase in penile size and in the angle of protrusion from the body. In the woman, arousal in the excitement phase, also initiated by tactile, visual, or psychic stimuli, involves vaginal lubrication. This lubrication, previously thought to be of uterine or cervical origin, has been demonstrated by Masters and Johnson to be a "sweating reaction" of the vagina; it is probably a true transudation that continues throughout sexual excitement. Coalescence of droplets provides a lubricating film; later in the response cycle, Bartholin's glands make a small contribution. The glans clitoridis swells, often to almost double its size, as a result of engorgement, but the degree of enlargement is apparently unrelated either to the woman's capacity for sexual response or to her ability to achieve orgasm. The shaft of the clitoris also increases in diameter. Engorgement of the glans clitoridis and shaft occur most rapidly with direct manual stimulation of the glans clitoridis and the mons veneris, by means of fantasy, or by stroking the breasts.

Breast changes in the sexually aroused woman consist of nipple erection and, later in the excitement phase, an increase in total size of the breasts. The labia majora, which in a resting state meet in the midline of the vagina, gape slightly and may be displaced toward the clitoris. In nulliparous women, the outer labia may also thin out and flatten against the surrounding tissue. In multiparous women, they may extend and be engorged to an exaggerated degree. The labia minora also swell. The vagina, which is in a collapsed state normally, now begins to expand in the inner two-thirds of the vaginal canal, alternating with a tendency to relax. As excitement increases, progressive distention of the vagina occurs. The vaginal walls also "tent" in response to upward and backward posterior movement of the cervix and uterus, so that the inner portion of the vagina swells dramatically. Engorgement changes the color of the vaginal wall to dark purple and causes the vaginal rugae to become smooth.

In both men and women, erotic tension causes increased muscle tone accompanied by tachycardia and blood pressure elevation. A "sex flush" begins over the upper abdomen and later spreads over the breasts as a morbilliform rash; this occurs in about 75% of women and 25% of men before orgasm. In the late

---

*This section contributed by Ralph Benson.

phase, the man experiences shortening of the spermatic cords and retraction of the testes. The scrotum thickens and is flattened against the body.

**B. The Plateau Phase:** The distinction between the excitement and the plateau phases is imprecise. Ordinarily, the penis is completely erect in the first phase. In the plateau phase, there is usually a slight increase in the diameter of the coronal ridge and, in some men, a deepening of color of the glans to reddish-purple. Progressive excitement may increase testicular size by about 50%; at this point, the man is very close to orgasm and approaches an inevitable stage. In the late plateau phase, respiratory rate, muscle tone, pulse rate, and blood pressure changes intensify, and muscle tension increases in the buttocks and anal sphincter. A few drops of fluid may appear in the male urethra from the bulbourethral (Cowper's) gland. Although this is not semen, it can contain large numbers of active sperm, which means that impregnation is possible before ejaculation.

In the woman, the "orgasmic platform" consists of engorgement and swelling of the tissues of the outer third of the vagina, which reduces its interior diameter by 30–50%, forming a grip on the penis and indicating that she is rapidly approaching orgasm. Elevation and ballooning of the inner two-thirds of the vagina increase, as does the size of the uterus (especially in multiparous women). The clitoris, now erect, rises from its position over the pubic bone, and retracts into its hood, shorter by about 50%. In this position the clitoris continues to respond, either to manual stimulation or to penile thrusts. Engorgement of the labia continues until they take on a deep wine color, indicating that climax is imminent.

**C. Orgasmic Phase:** In the woman, a series of rhythmic muscular contractions of the orgasmic platform signals the onset of climax. These contractions vary in number from 3 to 5 per minute to as many as 8–12 per minute in some women. They are intense at first but subside quickly. A series of uterine contractions quickly follows, beginning in the superior portion and moving downward toward the cervix. Occasionally, rhythmic contractions in the anal sphincter occur. In the man, the rhythmic contractions stimulate a discharge in the perineal floor, particularly in the bulbocavernosus muscle. Just before orgasm, increasing tension in the seminal vesicles causes the semen to empty into the bulbous urethra. Simultaneously, the prostate begins to contract, expelling fluid and distending the bulbous portion of the urethra as semen and prostatic fluid mingle. A series of rhythmic contractions at the bulb now eject the semen with great pressure. A series of minor contractions persists in the urethra for several seconds, continuing even after complete expulsion of the semen.

Changes in pulse rate, blood pressure, and respiratory rate reach a peak and quickly dissipate, but for both the man and the woman the height of orgasm is marked by generalized muscle tension. The facial muscles tighten, and the muscles of the neck, extremities, abdomen, and buttocks are strongly contracted. There may be grasping movements by both partners, followed by clutching and even carpopedal spasm. A fleeting period occurs in which each individual withdraws physiologically but not physically, concentrating almost solely on genital sensation, unaware perhaps of cries and uncontrollable behavior.

**D. Resolution Phase:** Muscle tension is released and engorgement subsides in the genitals and skin. The sex flush slowly fades. In the woman the nipples appear slightly prominent, but only because the swelling around them is subsiding. As the sex fades, slight perspiration appears. In some women, perspiration appears uniformly, and in men it occurs over the soles and palms as well; but in either case it is unrelated to the degree of muscular effort before or during orgasm.

In the woman, the clitoris promptly returns to its unstimulated state but will not reach normal size for 5–10 minutes. Relaxation of the orgasmic platform then occurs, and the diameter of the outer third of the vagina increases. Vaginal ballooning diminishes, the uterus shrinks, and the cervix descends into its normal position. The slight enlargement of the cervical canal is maintained. Total resolution time varies; as much as 30 minutes may elapse before the woman is in a truly unstimulated state.

In men, loss of erection occurs in 2 stages: in the first, most of the erectile volume is lost; the second is a refractory stage during which he is unable to be aroused again, and the remainder of the shrinkage occurs. In young men, the refractory period may be very short, but it lengthens with age. In most men it will last for several minutes; in others it may last for hours or even days. Women are capable of multiple orgasms.

## Sexual History Taking

A sexual history should be part of every gynecologic examination, although the amount of detail may vary.

Sexual dysfunctions are very common, and patients usually appreciate suitable inquiry. Physicians need a knowledge base to respond to concerns, although their own anxiety may get in the way of adequate questioning. Time is usually not a major deterrent if one is skilled enough. The sexual history belongs in the review of systems. Language should begin with biologic terms and then move to simpler terms. General questions precede more specific ones. The physician should maintain a positive, empathetic, and professional manner with a patient and ask questions in a logical sequence. The sexual history can cover (1) Areas of the sexual response cycle: sexual desire, sexual arousal (erection in males, lubrication in females), orgasm, and satisfaction. (2) Concerns about gender identity and sexual orientation. (3) Classification of problems: onset, course, best and worst functioning, frequency of sexual behaviors, and relationship of sexual behaviors to other life circumstances, ie, relationships, losses, financial problems, illness, medication, surgery, family difficulties, infertility, and contraception.

Sexual history taking should include the following information:

1. Identifying data
   a. Patient: age, sex, number of pregnancies, marriages
   b. Parents, family
   c. Partner
   d. Children
2. Childhood sexuality
   a. Family and religious attitudes toward sex
   b. Sexual learning
   c. Childhood sexual activity
   d. Childhood sexual abuse or incest
3. Adolescence
   a. Preparation for menses
   b. Menarche
   c. Masturbation
   d. Partner petting
   e. Intercourse
   f. Gender issues
4. Adolescence and adulthood
   a. Sexual fantasies
   b. Sexual orientation (heterosexual, homosexual)
   c. Partner choice
   d. Sexual activity
   e. Sexual deviations
   f. Sexual orientation
   g. Sexual function and dysfunction
   h. Contraception
5. Life changes in past year
   a. Losses
   b. Moves
   c. Pregnancy
   d. Other

## Female Sexual Dysfunctions

Considerable advances in the knowledge of female sexuality have occurred in the past decade. The major contributions of gynecologist William Masters and his colleague Virginia Johnson to the physiology and psychology of sexuality are well recognized. Women had been so inhibited by their culture that some had lived through courtship, marriage, childbearing, and menopause without ever experiencing their bodies in sexual arousal or orgasm. Most women today want to participate actively in their sexual lives and do so. This is a major change in sexual functioning. The following discussion applies to both heterosexual and lesbian women.

The most common female sexual dysfunctions are inhibited sexual desire, orgasmic dysfunction, and

**Table 60–1.** Classification of female sexual dysfunctions.

| Component | Symptom | Term |
|---|---|---|
| Desire | Decreased interest in sex | Inhibited sexual desire (ISD) |
| Excitement or arousal | Decreased lubrication | Excitement-phase dysfunction |
| Orgasm | No orgasm | Orgasmic dysfunction |
| Satisfaction | Decreased satisfaction | — |
| Other | Pain with intercourse | Dyspareunia |
|  | Spasm of circumvaginal musculature | Vaginismus |
|  | Fear of sex; fear of penetration | Sexual phobias Sexual panic |

All: Primary or secondary; situational or absolute.

dyspareunia (Table 60–1). Inhibited sexual desire may be lifelong (primary) or occur after a period of normal functioning (secondary). Its presence does not necessarily imply a lack of ability to respond physiologically. Many women with primary inhibited sexual desire come from very sexually repressive backgrounds, have been sexually traumatized in childhood or adolescence, or have a poor partner relationship. They may avoid relationships in order to avoid sex. Treatment consists of behavioral and psychologic methods.

Secondary inhibited sexual desire often develops after problems with a partner, physical or emotional traumas, physical illnesses, drug or alcohol abuse, surgery, or psychologic depression. A careful history will usually reveal recent life changes, losses, and medical or drug problems. Other contributions to difficulties in sexual desire come from concern about pregnancy, partners with very different sexual appetites, and changes in body image.

Sexual phobias occur in many women who then develop patterns of avoidance and are thought to have low desire. The thought of sex arouses panic and anxiety. There may be avoidance of any mention of sex and social isolation. Treatment consists of education, support, psychotherapy, and behavioral desensitization. In severe cases, antianxiety medications such as imipramine have been used with success.

**A. Orgasmic Problems:** Orgasm is a genital reflex with sensory input from the brain and periphery (clitoris, nipples, and other body parts) that enter the spinal cord in the pudendal nerve at the sacral level. The efferent outflow is from T-11 to L-2 and involves the contraction of the perivaginal musculature. The reflex centers are close to those for bowel and bladder control, so that injuries to the lower cord may affect all 3 functions.

Orgasmic problems are very common. About 8–10% of adult women in the USA have never been orgasmic; another 10% may achieve orgasm with fantasy alone. Most women fall somewhere in between the 2 extremes, demonstrating a variety of responses. Women with primary orgasmic problems have never experienced orgasm in any situation, even after prolonged and effective sexual stimulation. Those with secondary orgasmic problems have had periods of normal functioning. In both primary and secondary cases, the women may lubricate easily, enjoy lovemaking, and feel satisfaction. Somehow, they get "stuck" in the plateau phase of the sexual response cycle. Some women are not sure if they have reached orgasm; others regularly "fake" orgasm in order to please their partner. A number of women are orgasmic with clitoral stimulation but not during intercourse; this is a normal variant. For others, the presence of the penis, a strong erotic stimulus, is necessary for orgasm.

In the female with adequate sensory stimulation, orgasm will bring about rhythmic contractions of pelvic musculature around the vagina at 8/min, plus pleasurable feelings. The uterus may also contract.

Because of the connection between brain and spinal cord centers for orgasm, learned inhibition can happen as with other reflexes. Orgasm is under voluntary control so that there may be neural connections between the orgasm center and voluntary motor conscious perception areas of the brain.

The woman with primary orgasmic dysfunction is likely to have some very basic fears about sexuality and relationships. She may fear losing control, urinating, getting pregnant, or giving herself pleasure. She may experience performance anxiety and may or may not be sexually inhibited in general. Not having a trusted partner is sometimes a factor.

There are innumerable orgasmic variations. Theories that labeled vaginal orgasms mature and clitoral orgasms immature have been laid to rest. The goal of any treatment is to help the individual achieve her first orgasm, if she has never had one, or to reestablish orgasmic achievement if it has ceased. Although every woman is physiologically capable of having an orgasm, the orgasm mania of our current climate sometimes makes its achievement more difficult for some women. Pressure may also come from partners who insist that a women's lack of orgasm is due to her partner's failure.

Treatment is aimed at enhancing sensory stimulation and extinguishing the woman's involuntary overcontrol. The therapist's first task is to make certain that the woman understands sufficient clitoral stimulation and is able to communicate her needs to her partner. She needs to know that it is all right to be sexual. Sometimes these educational techniques are enough to overcome the problem. Barbach's book, *For Yourself*, has been very helpful to many women.

A woman with primary orgasmic dysfunction needs to learn what it feels like to have an orgasm. She may have to disregard her obsessive thoughts and distractions and focus on the erotic thoughts and premonitory feelings that directly precede orgasm. The use of fantasy can be very helpful. Women with very religious backgrounds may find the idea of erotic fantasy, ie, thinking of other partners and being overcome by a loving partner, more guilt-provoking than sex itself. Self-stimulation is often recommended as a means of learning what feels good and helps the woman become sexually aroused. The longstanding prohibition against masturbation in her value system may be difficult to overcome. She may prefer to masturbate in privacy, rather than with a partner. Some women have marked success with a vibrator, at first alone and then, possibly, with the partner. In addition to mastering the physical aspects of achieving orgasm, women need to understand and discuss their fears. Many patients find it helpful to join a women's discussion group. Besides discussing educational issues, members are assigned specific sexual tasks to do at home alone. Tasks are performed in privacy and responses are later shared with the group members. They may also be able to share fantasies and give one another support.

Transferring orgasmic achievement to a partner situation is the final step in most treatment situations. Heterosexual women are encouraged to heighten arousal before penetration. They learn the clitoris may be stimulated by indirect friction of the hood being pulled back and forth over this organ, eg, during penile thrusting. Each woman needs to learn the most effective means of increasing her own pleasure, eg, active thrusting and use of pelvic and thigh musculature, avoidance of distracting thoughts, and free use of erotic and exciting fantasies. When there is a beloved, trusted partner, the prognosis is good.

**B. Dyspareunia:** Pain during sexual intercourse can be especially distressing. Even when the actual pain is gone, memory of the pain may persist and interfere with pleasure. Some women with no background of trauma or major inhibitions may assume that sex will be painful because they associate menstruation and childbirth with pain. A careful history and physical examination are essential. Table 60–2 lists the physical reasons for dyspareunia. It is also important to look for psychologic contributions. Management consists of treating the specific problem.

**Vaginismus** is the painful reflex spasm of the perivaginal and thigh adductor muscles that occurs in anticipation of any vaginal penetration. It occurs most often in young, inexperienced women from strict homes. Some patients may have been subjected to rape or incest as children or adults. Severe pain secondary to trauma or medical procedures in the vaginal area may sometimes cause the problem. Insufficient lubrication from lack of arousal or sexual phobias may also cause pain with intercourse and vaginismus.

Vaginismus must be diagnosed by history and physical examination. Gynecologists often institute a program of gradual vaginal dilation, using dilators,

**Table 60–2.** Some physical reasons for dyspareunia.

**Vaginal opening**
  Hymen—rare
  Tender episiotomy scar
  Aging—with decreased elasticity
  Labia—Bartholin gland abscess
  Other lesions
**Clitoris**
  Irritations
  Infections
**Vagina**
  Infections
  Sensitivity reactions
  Atrophic reactions
  Decreased lubrication
**Uterus, uterine tubes, ovaries**
  Endometriosis
  Pelvic inflammatory disease
  Ectopic pregnancy
**Numerous others**

the woman's finger, or the partner's finger; not all women will respond to this prescription. Some may have more serious problems that require psychotherapy. It is not unusual for a woman who has overcome her difficulty to find that her partner has developed erectile problems. This finding supports the belief that sexual problems are rarely limited to one partner.

## Male Sexual Dysfunction

The term *impotence* used to refer to most male performance problems. Today, the word has an imprecise meaning since there has been a great increase in knowledge about sexual dysfunctions and classification based on the physiology of the sexual response cycle (Table 60–3). The term impotence usually refers to erectile problems or the inability to sustain an erection for the time necessary for a desired sexual act. Erectile problems are common and increase with age.

Male sexual dysfunctions have been classified on the basis of an understanding of the sexual response cycle. The classification includes (1) problems of desire—diminished or excessive; (2) problems with arousal, ie, erectile difficulties (or impotence); (3)

**Table 60–3.** Classification of male sexual dysfunctions.

| Component | Symptom | Term |
|---|---|---|
| Desire | Decreased interest in sex | Inhibited sexual desire (ISD) |
| Arousal or excitement | Difficulty with erection | "Impotence," erectile difficulty |
| Orgasm | No ejaculation No emission | Premature ejaculation, inhibited orgasm, retrograde ejaculation |
| Satisfaction | Decreased satisfaction | — |

All: primary or secondary, situational or absolute.

problems with orgasm, premature ejaculation, inhibited orgasm, or retrograde ejaculation. These conditions may be caused by psychogenic, organic, or mixed psychogenic and organic reasons. Performance anxiety leads to "spectatoring" in which a person becomes preoccupied in watching his or her own sexual responses. They may be primary—present all of one's life—or secondary—having developed after a period of normal functioning. The history should focus on the stages of life of the man, the quality of his sexual desire, the role of his partner, and significance of early and past life experiences. Organic contributions are more common than was previously thought and are related to illness, surgery, medication, drugs, alcohol, vascular disorders, and neuropathies.

Psychologic causes in addition to performance anxiety include fears of women and intimacy, relationship problems, and depression or other mental illnesses. The purely psychogenic dysfunctions show more variability in erectile responses and are associated with normal nocturnal tumescence studies. Often, evaluation by a urologist knowledgeable about sexual function is indicated.

Treatment is based on etiology. Organic causes need treatment if possible. The psychogenic forms of dysfunction are best managed by behavioral treatment approaches. Partners are seen together and their relationship helped with improved communication as well as special techniques for specific problems.

Drugs that cause sexual dysfunction commonly include antihypertensives, cimetidine, antipsychotic drugs, tricyclic antidepressants, and central nervous system depressants—sedatives, anxiolytics, cannabis, alcohol, and heroin.

## Sexual Activity with Aging

Sexual changes occur in men and women as they grow older. Perimenopausal and postmenopausal women may have less sexual desire, with fewer sexual fantasies and a slower and lessened lubrication response to arousal with more vaginal dryness and discomfort with intercourse. Their breasts may have less nipple erection and enlargement. Sex flush diminishes, and the clitoris and labia enlarge to a lesser degree. The vaginal walls are thinner and less able to expand. Orgasm may be less intense, with weaker muscle contractions, and uterine contractions may be uncomfortable. Atrophic skin changes and altered peripheral nerve endings may diminish sensory perceptions.

Men show decreased sexual activity with aging. By age 60 men are having about one erection a week. Sexual desire may diminish and erections take longer, require more stimulation, and are less firm. Ejaculation takes longer, with the feeling of ejaculatory inevitability less pronounced. There is less ejaculate, and the refractory period is longer. The sex flush is diminished.

Despite these normal changes with aging, the capacity for sexual activity and enjoyment persists. Many couples, freed from the worries of pregnancy, feel more able than ever to have the pleasure of an active sex life. An overly tight vagina after surgical procedures may make it difficult for a man with a less firm erection. Noncoital sexual activity may be a very satisfying form of intimacy and pleasure for some couples. The gynecologist can help the aging couple through educating them about normal changes, using estrogen and progesterone replacement when indicated, and accepting sexual activity as a suitable activity for older people.

## The Referral Process

Referral to mental health professionals may be indicated for any psychologic processes the gynecologist sees as beyond his or her ability, training, or willingness to treat. The gynecologist may prefer to work closely with a psychiatrist, psychologist, social worker, or psychiatric nurse. There should be comfort in the feeling that counseling would be helpful, not that the patient is bothersome and therefore should be labeled or stigmatized by such referrals. Consultation-liaison psychiatrists have expertise in the psychologic aspects of medical and surgical problems as well as in the use of psychopharmacologic drugs. Most hospital staffs include social workers and psychiatric nurses who specialize in psychosocial issues. Marriage counselors offer much to those with relationship problems. As with obstetrics, the biopsychosocial approach is extremely useful.

# REFERENCES

## PSYCHOLOGIC ASPECTS OF OBSTETRICS

Anderson BL, Sexual functioning complications in women with gynecologic cancer. Cancer 1987;60: 2123.

Asch A, Rubin L: Postpartum reactions: Some unrecognized variations. Am J Psychiatry 1974;131:870.

Astrachan JM: The psychological management of the family whose child is born dead. In: *Gynecology and Obstetrics*. Sciavia JJ (ed.). Harper & Row, 1983.

Blume SB, Russell M: Alcohol and substance abuse in the practice of obstetrics and gynecology. in: *Psychological Aspects of Women's Health Care*. Stewart D, Stotland N (eds.). American Psychiatric Press, Inc, 1993.

Campbell J, Winokur G: Postpartum affective disorders: Selected biological aspects. Pages 20–35 in: *Recent Advances in Postpartum Psychiatric Disorders*. Inwood D (ed.). American Psychiatric Press, 1985.

Cohen L: The use of psychotropic drugs during pregnancy and the puerperium. Currents in Affective Illness 1992;11(9):5.

Dagg P: The psychological sequelae of therapeutic abortion—denied and completed. Am J Psychiatry 1991; 148:578.

Edlund MJ, Craig TJ: Antipsychotic drug use and birth defects: An epidemiologic reassessment. Compr Psychiatry 1984;25:32.

Fairburn CG, Stein A, Jones R: Eating habits and eating disorders during pregnancy. Psychosom Med 1992; 54:665.

Gyves MT: The psychosocial impact of high risk pregnancy. Adv Psychosom Med 1985;12:71.

Jacobson J, et al: Prospective multicenter study of pregnancy outcome after lithium exposure during first trimester. Lancet 1992;339:530.

Kellner K, Donnelly WH, Gould S: Parental behavior after perinatal death: Lack of predictive demographic and obstetric variables. Obstet Gynecol 1982;63:809.

Kennell J, Trause M: Helping parents cope with neonatal death. Contemp Obstet Gynecol 1978;12:53.

Lancaster J, Hamburg S (eds.): *School-Age Pregnancy and Parenthood: Biosocial Dimensions*. Aldine DeGruyter, 1986.

Leon IG: *When a Baby Dies*. Yale University Press, 1990.

Nadelson CC: "Normal" and special aspects of pregnancy: A psychological approach. In: *The Woman Patient: Medical and Psychological Interfaces*. Nadelson CC, Notman MT (eds.). Vol. 1, pages 73–85 in: *Sexual and Reproductive Aspects of Women's Health Care*. Plenum Press, 1978.

Nurnberg HG, Prudic J: Guidelines for treatment of psychosis in pregnancy. Hosp Commun Psych 1984;35: 67.

O'Hara MW, et al: Prospective study of postpartum blues: Biologic and psychosocial factors. Arch Gen Psychiatry 1991;48:801.

Pasnau R (editor): *Diagnosis and Treatment of Anxiety Disorders*. American Psychiatric Press, 1984.

Pasnau R: Psychiatry and obstetrics-gynecology: Report of a five year experience in psychiatry liaison. In: *Consultation Liaison Psychiatry*. Pasnau R (ed.). Grune & Stratton, 1975.

Raphael B: *The Anatomy of Bereavement*. Basic Books, 1983.

Reamy K, White S: Sexuality in pregnancy and puerperium: A review. Obstet Gyn Surv 1985;40:1.

Robinson G, Stewart D, Flak E: The rational use of psychotropic drugs in pregnancy and postpartum. Can J Psychiatry 1986;31:183.

Rosenthal M: Adolescent pregnancy. In: *Psychological Aspects of Women's Health Care. Stewart D, Stotland N (editors). American Psychiatric Press, Inc, 1993.*

Schatzberg A, Cole J: *Manual of Clinical Psychopharmacology*. American Psychiatric Press, 1986.

Seiden A: The sense of mastery in the childbirth experience. In: Sexual and Reproduction Aspects of Women's Health Care. Vol. 1 in: *The Woman Patient*. Plenum Press, 1978.

Starkman MN: Psychological responses to the use of the fetal monitor during labor. Psychosom Med 1976;38: 269.

Stewart DE, et al: Anorexia nervosa, bulimia, and pregnancy. Am J Obstet Gynecol 1987;157:1194.

Stirtzinger R, Robinson GE: The psychologic effects of spontaneous abortion. Can Med Assoc J 1989;140: 799.

Wilson AL, et al: The death of a newborn twin: An analysis of parental bereavement. Pediatrics 1982;70:587.

Wise TN: Assessing emotional problems in medical practice. Primary Care 1979;6:233.

Youngs DD, Starkman MN: Psychological and physiological aspects of electronic fetal monitoring. Primary Care 1976;3:691.

## PSYCHOLOGIC ASPECTS OF GYNECOLOGY

Bachmann GA: Psychosexual aspects of hysterectomy. Health Issues 1990;1:41.

Barbach L: For Yourself: *The Fulfillment of Female Sexuality*. Doubleday, New York, 1975.

Barbach L: *For Each Other— Sharing Sexual Intimacy*. Anchor Books/Doubleday, 1983.

Bird B: *Talking with Patients*, 2nd ed. Lippincott, 1973.

Budoff PW: *No More Menstrual Cramps and Other Good News*. Penguin Books, 1980.

Cooper A, Bishop M: Hysterectomy, hormones and behavior: A prospective study. Lancet 1981;1:126.

Dalton K: *The Premenstrual Syndrome and Progesterone Study*. Heinemann Medical Books, 1977.

Dalton K: Progesterone, fluid, and electrolytes in premenstrual syndrome. Br Med J 1980;281:61.

Dickstein L: Spouse abuse and other domestic violence. Psychiatr Clin North Am 1988;11:611.

Hamilton JA et al: An update on premenstrual depressions: Evaluation and treatment. In: *The Psychiatric Implications of Menstruation*. Gold J.(ed.). American Psychiatric Press, 1985.

Kaplan H: *The New Sex Therapy*. Bruner/Mazel, 1974.

Kaplan H: *The New Sex Therapy*. Vol 2. *Disorders of Sexual Desire*. Bruner/Mazel, 1979.

Kennedy S, Garfinkel P: *Anorexia Nervosa*. American Psychiatric Association Annual Review. Hales R, Frances A (eds.) American Psychiatric Press, 1985.

Kolodny RD: Sexual dysfunction in diabetic females. Diabetes 1971;20:557.

Martin R, Roberts W, Clayton P: Psychiatric status after hysterectomy. JAMA 1980;244:350.

Masters W, Johnson V: *Human Sexual Inadequacy*. Little, Brown, 1970.

Notman M, Nadelson C: *The Woman Patient*. Vol. 1. *Sexual and Reproductive Aspects of Women's Health Care*. Plenum Press, 1978.

Pasnae RO: Psychiatric consultation for obstetric and gynecologic patients. Psychiatr Digest 1979;40:25.

Pearce, S, Beard RW: Chronic pelvic pain. In: *Psychology and Gynecological Problems*. Broome A, Wallace L (eds.). Tavistock Publications, 1984.

Reich J, Tupin J, Abramowitz S: Psychiatric diagnosis of chronic pain patients. Am J Psychiatry 1983;140: 1495.

Reid RL, Yen SSC: Premenstrual syndrome. Am J Obstet Gynecol 1981;139:85.

Renaer M, Guzinski G: Pain in gynecologic practice. Pain 1978;5:305.

Steege J, Stout A: Chronic gynecologic pain in Psychological Aspects of Women's Health Care. American Psychiatric Press, Inc., 1993:249.

Stewart DE, et al: Psychosocial aspects of chronic clinically unconfirmed vulvovaginitis. Obstet Gynecol 1990;76:852.

Stoller R: *Presentations of Gender*. Yale Univ Press, 1985.

Stunkard AJ: The current status of treatment for obesity in adults. In: *Eating and Its Disorders*. Stunkard AJ, Stellar E (eds.). Raven Press, 1984.

Walker EW, et al: Relationship of chronic pelvic pain to psychiatric diagnosis and childhood sexual abuse. Am J Psychiatry 1988;145:75.

Wise, TN: Assessing emotional problems in medical practice. Primary Care 1979;6:233.

Youngs D, Wise T: Preparing a patient for hysterectomy surgery: Consent, information, and emotional support. Clin Obstet Gynecol 1976;19:431.

# Domestic Violence and Sexual Assault

# 61

*Vivian Halfin, MD, & Deborah Lehmann, MD*

For many victims of domestic violence and sexual assault, the first contact with the health care system is with the obstetrician-gynecologist or primary care doctor. Therefore, it is critical that these physicians be knowledgeable in the identification, evaluation, and treatment of such patients.

## DOMESTIC VIOLENCE

While the home is often thought of as a safe haven, it is the site of the most common manifestations of violence in our society today. Domestic violence is the abuse of a family or household member. It is a behavior pattern that is manifested in physical, sexual, and emotional forms. The abuser utilizes the behavior in order to establish and maintain power and control over the victim, who is most often a woman. Because abuse is accompanied by shame and guilt, the victim often does not report the abuse.

As a result of significant underreporting, it is difficult to compile exact data on the incidence of domestic violence. The FBI and the department of Justice estimate the following in the United States:

- A woman is beaten every 18 seconds.
- Over 20% of women who use emergency rooms are battered women.
- Almost half the injuries sustained by women who present to emergency rooms are the result of battering, but fewer than 5% are recognized as such.
- Thirty percent of all women who are murdered are murdered by their husbands, boyfriends or ex-partners.

Overall, it is thought that domestic violence occurs in half the homes in the United States at least once a year.

Some of the factors associated with domestic violence for both the victim and the perpetrator include increased life stresses, having been abused, or having witnessed marital violence during childhood. The abuser often feels inadequate and may be worried about finances. The victim typically has low self-esteem and feels dependent and helpless. Excessive use of alcohol or other substances may occur in the home. Unemployment, economic strains, and crowding also contribute to the likelihood of abuse. Nevertheless, domestic violence cuts across all ethnic, religious, and socioeconomic backgrounds, and women from virtually any group can be potential victims.

It is not uncommon to find that both women and children in the same household are the victims of domestic violence. Children may suffer abuse in a variety of forms: physical, sexual, verbal, emotional, as well as physical neglect. Sexual abuse of children is characterized by the sexual exploitation of the child by virtue of age or a caretaking relationship and/or the use of threat or force. While a stranger may be the abuser, it is estimated that 85% of child abuse occurs with a person whom the child knows. All too often, that person may be a parent, grandparent, or other close relative. The prevalence of sexual abuse of children is thought to be in the range of 12–20%.

### Clinical Evaluation and Presentation

Survivors of domestic violence or sexual abuse may present to health care professionals in a variety of clinical settings. Such patients commonly report chronic pelvic pain to their gynecologists. Others may complain of sexual dysfunctions such as decreased interest or arousal, dyspareunia, or anorgasmia. Incest victims have a very high rate of sexual dysfunction and may avoid sex or seek it out compulsively. Some women may present for a routine gynecologic appointment but become anxious and tearful before or during the pelvic examination. Still others may voice multiple physical complaints or pains. A history of sexual abuse has been found in significantly more women with chronic pelvic pain as compared with other gynecologic conditions.

Some women with persistent multiple bodily complaints may have a somatoform disorder. This condition is characterized by physical symptoms suggesting a physical condition for which there are no demonstrable organic findings or physiologic mechanisms. In the face of a negative workup, there may be evidence or presumption that the symptoms are linked to psychologic factors or conflicts. Women who meet the criteria for somatoform disorder often have a history of abuse.

In a mental health setting, victims of domestic violence or sexual assault may note feeling depressed or suicidal. They may have anxiety or sleep disorders that they may self-medicate with alcohol or other substances. Most commonly, these women have post-traumatic stress disorder (PTSD), which occurs in individuals who have experienced a psychologically distressing event that is outside the range of usual human experience. Such events include natural disasters (hurricanes, tornadoes) and acts of violence (war, terrorism, physical/sexual assault) that threaten one's life or that of one's loved ones, or one's home or community. Witnessing such stressful events can also precipitate the disorder.

Symptoms of PTSD include reexperiencing the traumatic event through intrusive memories, dreams, flashbacks, or exposure to events symbolic of the trauma. Thus, a benign gynecologic history or examination may reopen a past experience of abuse that may have been repressed. Patients with PTSD also exhibit a "psychic numbing," ie, they are detached from other people and have difficulty feeling emotions, especially those associated with intimacy or sexuality. They avoid thoughts, feelings and situations that are linked to the trauma. At the same time, they may show symptoms of increased arousal such as hypervigilance, sleep or concentration disturbance, an exaggerated startle response, and physiologic reactivity when exposed to something symbolic of the trauma.

Other clinical syndromes that occur with increased frequency in victims of abuse are eating disorders and personality disorders. In the latter, character traits are inflexible and maladaptive and cause functional impairment or subjective distress. Patients with multiple personality disorder (MPD), a dissociation, ie, the removal of some aspect of sensation or knowledge from consciousness, is used to escape mentally from danger. MPD patients have a disturbance in the normally integrated functions of identity, memory, and consciousness, and they have two or more distinct personalities existing within them.

## Domestic Violence in Pregnancy

The problem of domestic violence in pregnancy merits special mention because it is a threat to both the mother and her developing fetus. Estimates of prevalence of domestic violence in pregnancy are in the range of 8–15%. There is some controversy as to whether pregnancy results in an increase or decrease in abuse. For some men, ambivalence about the pregnancy, growing financial pressures, increased dependency by the woman, and her decreased sexual availability may contribute to a heightened risk of violence. At the same time, some women report that the only time their partner doesn't hurt them is when they are pregnant.

Battering, which often goes unreported in the pregnant patient, is thought to be associated with adverse pregnancy outcome. Abdominal trauma, which can cause abruptio placentae, may result in fetal demise, premature labor, and a low-birth-weight infant. Other consequences of physical abuse to the gravid female include damage to maternal or fetal organs, premature rupture of membranes, and infection. The psychological sequelae of violence include increased anxiety, behavioral risks (smoking and substance abuse), and inadequate nutrition. The pregnant victim may present in a clinical setting, yet she may not report the abuse, fearing reprisal from her partner. An increased sense of isolation, as well as the shame and guilt associated with potential discovery of the abuse, can result in the victim obtaining little, if any prenatal care, thereby further increasing the risk of poor pregnancy outcome.

## Diagnosis and Treatment

The critical factor in making a diagnosis of domestic violence or abuse is taking a thorough and pointed history. The obstetrician-gynecologist or primary care physician can screen each patient by asking about the patient's relationship as part of the routine social history. Possible questions include the following:

- How are you and your partner getting along?
- What happens when you disagree about something? (ie, How do you resolve conflict?)
- Have you been physically hurt by anybody in the last year?
- Have you ever been pressured or forced into a sexual situation against your will?

An inquiry of this kind can uncover past or ongoing traumatic experiences. It is most productive to ask these questions of the patient privately, without the partner present. When the answers to any of the screening questions are positive, the physician can then obtain more detailed data about the nature of the abuse, its frequency and severity. While some standard medical intake forms include such questions, and other abuse screening questionnaires have been developed, it is noteworthy that there is a significantly higher yield of positive responses when the questions are asked face-to-face by a health care provider.

Once identified, the victim of domestic violence or abuse must be examined and her injuries treated. Further treatment planning should, whenever possible, include the patient as an active participant. Assessment of the patient's comfort with returning home may indicate that she needs a setting that will insure greater safety, such as with family or friends, or in a shelter. Self-help and advocacy programs, often based at shelters, work toward empowering the victim. This goal encompasses strengthening her coping skills, having her involve the legal system, and ultimately enabling the victim to leave the abusive situation permanently.

Given the high rate of psychiatric symptomatology in this population, psychiatric screening can be useful. Patients who are experiencing posttraumatic stress disorder can benefit from psychotherapy and possibly medication as well. Those with depression, substance abuse, anxiety, personality, or dissociative disorders will also require ongoing treatment. Psychiatrists or other mental health professionals can serve to coordinate a variety of treatment modalities for the victims: individual, couples, and family therapy detoxification and substance abuse treatment, and advocacy groups. Local organizations run battered women's shelters and support groups, and they educate the public about this problem of epidemic proportions. Such organizations often staff regional 24-hour-a-day domestic violence hotlines that provide information and shelter referral. These phone numbers can be posted in clinic waiting rooms in recognition of the problem and as a resource for those who do not openly acknowledge their distressing home environment.

Despite the best efforts of physicians and other health care professionals, some women may initially be unable to extirpate themselves from victimization. For such women, an encounter with a health care system that they experience as nonblaming, accessible, and supportive will hopefully maximize the chances of their making a positive life change at some future point.

## SEXUAL ASSAULT

Sexual assault (*rape*) is a violent crime directed predominantly against women. It is becoming increasingly prevalent in industrialized societies. In the USA, as many women will be sexually assaulted during their lifetimes as will develop breast cancer. Thus, rape is one of the most common threats to a woman's well-being. Physicians responsible for the care of women bear a responsibility for treatment and prevention of rape, just as they do for other less common gynecologic problems. To understand the ramifications of rape, it is essential to understand the wide variation in the specifics of assault, the general characteristics of rapists, and the physical and emotional consequences to the victims.

In the USA, rape is classified as a violent crime. The legal definition of rape varies widely from state to state. Legal statutes may categorize sexual assault as forcible, statutory, attempted, carnal knowledge of a juvenile, or a crime against nature. Legal codes may categorize rape according to the anatomic site of assault (eg, oral, anal, or vaginal) and according to the degree of penetration (eg, none, slight, or full). The psychologic effect of rape on the victim cannot be predicted according to the degree of penetration or the anatomic site of assault. Distinctions in the site and extent of sexual assault do, however, carry medical importance, since the risk of injury, impregnation, or acquisition of sexually transmitted disease will vary according to the specifics of the assault. Therefore, an accurate detailed history of the assault is essential for proper diagnosis, documentation, and treatment.

For the physician attempting to care for the victim-patient, rape would be defined as physical assault involving the genitalia of either the victim or the assailant. The effects of such an assault are both physical and emotional.

### Incidence

Rape is the most underreported violent crime in the USA. Current estimates are that no more than 20% of all sexual assaults are reported to the authorities. Despite such extensive underreporting, rape is still one of the most rapidly growing of all violent crimes. The most recent trend index of the FBI Unified Crime Report records 106,593 reported forcible rapes in the United States in 1991, with an extrapolated total of 532,695 rapes. This constitutes a 3.9% increase over 1990 and a 21.6% increase over the 87,671 forcible rapes reported in 1985. It is estimated that 83 of every 100,000 females in this country were reported rape victims in 1991. By using crude population statistics, the risk is roughly 1 in 10 that a woman will be sexually assaulted in her lifetime.

Rape is more prevalent in urban areas. Approximately 50% of all sexual assaults occur in the victim's own home. The rapist usually gains access by breaking and entering or by obtaining entrance under false pretense (eg, requesting to use the telephone or impersonating a building inspector or repairman). More than 80% of sexual assaults occur within the victim's own neighborhood, and more than 50% of rapists reside in the same neighborhood. In fact, approximately 20% of victims are able to identify the rapist by name, and another 20% of victims have seen the rapist before the assault.

The widespread societal assumption that the victim of rape is somehow the culpable party is antiquated and erroneous. Records show that over 50% of homicide victims are related to or acquainted with their murderers, and yet it is not commonly assumed that the victim in some way acquiesced to the murder. Similarly, the fact that rapists may be known to their victims should not form a basis for assumption that the victim is actually culpable for the assault.

### General Characteristics of Rapists

Rapists most often choose as victims individuals who seem vulnerable (eg, women who live nearby; are small in size or elderly; or are unaccompanied, intoxicated, or disabled). For some rapists, the victim need only be female to become a target.

Approximately 45% of rapists are under 25 years

of age, with 30% between ages 18 and 24. Most are repeat offenders and average more than 10 rapes before being apprehended. Careful retrospective evaluation reveals emotional and sociopathic disturbances. Motivation for the assault seems not to be sexual gratification but rather degradation, terrorization, and humiliation of the victim. The incidence of nonejaculation in rape episodes is much greater than that in the general male population. Most rapists who are unable to ejaculate during a sexual assault have no difficulty ejaculating during consensual sexual intercourse. This finding reinforces the theory that the purpose of sexual assault is debasement of the victim rather than an impulsive or aggressive extension of normal sexual activity on the part of the rapist.

## General Characteristics of Rape Episodes

A thorough understanding of the victim's short- and long-term responses to sexual assault requires an awareness of the 3 basic types of rape episodes: the power rape, the anger rape, and the sadistic rape. Examination of these 3 variations makes it even more apparent that rape is not an extension of ordinary sexual drives encouraged by the behavior or appearance of the victim.

**Power Rape:** Power rape is the type most commonly reported and accounts for slightly more than 50% of episodes. The rapist is generally an immature male, often under age 18. The assault is premeditated, and the rapist usually acknowledges precrime rape fantasies. For this type of rapist, the motivation is to demonstrate power through sexual assault rather than through overt injury of the victim, although injury may occur from coercion. In many cases, the victim is kidnapped, held for a period of time ranging from hours to days, and repeatedly assaulted. Power rape is also more likely to involve multiple assailants. Psychiatrists have characterized these rapists as insecure and immature, fearful of sexual inadequacy, and needful of forcing submission in order to derive a sense of power and self-worth. The power rapist is likely to ask his victim whether or not she "enjoyed it" or to attempt to win her approval in some fashion. In fact, the event does not fulfill the power rapist's expectations, and he will usually repeat the crime in an effort to ameliorate his feelings of inadequacy and powerlessness.

**Anger Rape:** The second most common type of rape is anger rape, which accounts for approximately 40% of all reported rapes. These rapists are characterized as impulsive and episodic, generally subjecting their victims to greater physical abuse than do power rapists. The psychologic objective is humiliation and degradation of the victim, motivated by anger and a need to obtain revenge. Anger rapes are not as carefully premeditated and seem to be triggered by a stressful situation in which the rapist feels he has been wronged. He acts out his anger on the victim, who is perceived as a convenient object on whom to

vent his rage. He typically threatens to return and repeat the assault or to kill the victim if she reports the rape.

**Sadistic Rape:** Sadistic rape accounts for approximately 5% of reported rapes and is characterized by extensive violent injury to the victim that may result in death. Of note is the fact that victims murdered by the rapist or those who die as a result of injuries sustained during the rape are entered into the crime statistics as homicides rather than rape victims. In 1991, approximately 2% of all female homicides were combined with sexual assault; thus, the actual percentage of sadistic rapes is greater than reports would indicate. These assaults are premeditated and frequently involve ritualized torture or mutilation of the victim, especially of the genital region. They seem primarily designed to degrade, injure, and even destroy the victim. Sadistic rapists often have a history of wife and child abuse, and they are more likely to be diagnosed as psychotic than are other rapists.

## Response of the Victim

Understanding the characteristics of sexual assault as well as prevailing societal attitudes is germinal to understanding the rape victim's immediate and long-term response to the assault. Victims often exhibit or express feelings of continued fear of repeated violation, as well as feelings of isolation and disorientation. Because of prevailing societal attitudes that the victim is ultimately to blame for the incident, there are often feelings of deep anguish and guilt.

The victim's primary response during the assault is one of survival, and most victims will relate that they were afraid their assailant might kill them. This explains the usually limited resistance that the victim offers, as well as her feeling of culpability after the episode, when she berates herself for "not fighting him off." The victim's assumption of guilt is greater when less physical force has been used to coerce submission to intercourse and is, therefore, more prevalent in victims of the more common power rape. Thus, because of "assumed guilt," victims of power rape are frequently reluctant to report the assault to the authorities or to inform their families. Victims of anger rape are also frequently reluctant to report the assault, usually out of fear that the assailant will somehow obtain revenge. After any form of sexual assault, almost all victims experience a posttraumatic stress disorder that may be of long duration.

## Physical Examination & Evaluation

A victim who has survived sexual assault must deal with her feelings of helplessness and, usually, worthlessness. For this reason, it is most important that medical personnel approach such patients in a nonjudgmental fashion, with an attitude of respect and concern for their well-being. Indeed, many rape victims relate that they found their exposure to the emergency room and its personnel only marginally less traumatic than the sexual assault.

The majority of rape victims who come to emergency rooms do not openly admit to having been sexually assaulted. Instead, they may complain of having been mugged or may voice concerns about AIDS or other sexually transmitted diseases. Others may present with psychiatric symptoms including depression, anxiety, or a suicide attempt. Unless the primary care physician, obstetrician-gynecologist, and/or psychiatrist obtains a sexual history, assault victims will remain unidentified as such and, therefore, inadequately treated.

The patient who presents for examination and treatment reporting that she has been raped abandons one of her most powerful defense mechanisms, denial. Other coping mechanisms are substituted, and patients generally appear withdrawn, detached, and overly calm when first seen. This behavior represents the patient's need to reestablish control over herself and her environment while simultaneously abandoning the defense mechanism of denial and allowing the renewed invasion of privacy represented by the questioning and examination.

Aside from emotional trauma and varying ranges of physical trauma, several specific medical problems must be addressed. This requires a structured, skillful physical examination. Carefully organized evaluations and examinations also allow law enforcement agencies to pursue and prosecute rapists successfully.

The physician must accurately obtain and record the details of the assault, preferably from the patient. The physician must also obtain a detailed gynecologic history in order to evaluate fully the risks of impregnation and acquisition of sexually transmitted disease. The patient's activities in the interval between the assault and the examination—whether the patient has eaten, drunk, bathed, douched, voided, or defecated—might affect findings on physical examination; such activities must be recorded.

The physical examination should document the location, nature, and extent of external trauma (ecchymoses, abrasions, lacerations, bite marks, rope burns). If possible, these lesions should be photographed. The patient should then be examined and specimens collected. Relevant areas of the patient's body should be examined with an ultraviolet, or Wood's, light, because dried seminal fluid will fluoresce. Saline-moistened filter paper should be used to blot each examined area, and the filter paper specimens from each area should be packaged separately. Scrapings should be taken from underneath the victim's fingernails. The pubic hair should be combed for foreign material; the comb and specimens thus obtained are packaged together. Pubic hair cuttings should also be obtained. Each specimen is placed in a sealed envelope or container and carefully labeled with the source, patient's name, and date. All collected specimens are placed in a larger sealed container and processed in a "chain of evidence" fashion. The person who collects the specimens verifies their completeness by signature on the sealed "master container." The individual to whom they are transferred must verify by signature that all specimens were received in an untampered state. Thus, each individual who has "custody" of the specimens during processing must verify that they were transmitted without alteration until log-in with the responsible law enforcement agency. The name of the law enforcement agent who receives the specimens should be noted in the medical record.

Meticulous inspection of the perineum and vulva for ecchymoses, abrasions, and lacerations should be performed and a careful diagram made. The walls of the vagina and vaginal fornices must be carefully inspected for trauma. The patient should never be coerced into or restrained for an examination. When indicated, it may be preferable to perform the examination in the operating room with the patient under anesthesia.

The speculum must be moistened only with saline. Nonabsorbent cotton swabs should be used to sample fluid from the vaginal pool and should then be placed in sterile glass tubes. Air-dried, nonfixed smears of this same fluid should be placed on glass slides. Two milliliters of normal saline are injected into the vaginal vault, respirated, and examined for the presence of sperm, which usually remain motile in the vagina for 4–6 hours. A Papanicolaou smear taken from the cervix will provide a permanent record of the presence of sperm. In addition, culture of material from the endocervical canal should be performed for gonorrhea.

If oral or anal penetration occurred, the same procedures (omitting the use of a speculum) should be repeated on the mouth and rectum. A sample of the patient's saliva should be obtained to determine the secretory status of the patient. Blood should be drawn for blood type and VDRL tests. If it is known that the assailant is in a high-risk group for hepatitis B or AIDS, serologic testing for those diseases can be done. Alternatively, a tube of serum may be frozen and saved for future testing. If the possibility exists that the patient was already pregnant at the time of the assault, levels of $\beta$-hCG should be determined.

Proper processing and labeling of collected specimens is crucial. If sexual assault is viewed as a common, serious injury of women, then attention should be directed not only toward diagnosis and treatment but also toward prevention and eradication. Our contribution to the efforts of law enforcement agencies and the judicial system to prevent and eradicate sexual assault is the collection of accurate information that can be used as reliable evidence. For this reason, the examination must be concise and thorough.

### Diagnosis & Treatment

When one is completing the medical record, it is crucial to be descriptive and to detail a diagnosis that can stand legal scrutiny. The legal definition of rape may require integration of information not available to the physician. Therefore, it is recommended that "rape" or "alleged rape" not be given as a diagnosis. If one is filling out a standard emergency room sheet, it is recommended that the diagnosis be stated as "deferred" or as "findings on physical examination consistent with the history obtained."

Treatment of physical injuries sustained at the time of assault should be initiated immediately; prophylactic medical treatment may be indicated for prevention of pregnancy or sexually transmitted infections.

Medical care for victims of sexual assault is directed not only to the treatment of obvious physical trauma but also to the prevention of sexually transmitted disease and pregnancy. The potential for acquiring sexually transmitted infections is increased when sexual contact during the episode is extensive, the assailant is nonwhite, or there are multiple assailants. Treatment is usually given only for gonorrhea and syphilis, but other sexually transmitted infections are also commonly encountered, and prophylactic treatment for these should also be considered (eg, infection due to *Trichomonas vaginalis, Candida albicans,* and *Gardnerella vaginalis*). Other possible infections are those due to herpesvirus, papillomavirus, hepatitis virus, cytomegalovirus, and human immunodeficiency virus (HIV).

Numerous treatment protocols exist for prophylaxis, and they usually include penicillin or tetracycline (Table 61–1). In patients who have sustained

**Table 61–1.** Incidence and treatment of sexually transmitted infection associated with sexual assault.

|  | Incidence | Treatment |
|---|---|---|
| *Neisseria gonorrhoeae* | 2.4–12% | Penicillin, 4.8 million units, plus probenecid, 1 g |
|  |  | Amoxicillin 3.0 g, plus probenecid, 1 g |
|  |  | Doxycycline, 300 mg orally; repeat in 1 hour |
|  |  | Doxycycline, 100 mg orally twice a day for 7 days |
| *Treponema pallidum* (incubating) | < 4% | Penicillin |
| Herpesvirus | < 3% | (?) None |
| *Trichomonas vaginalis* | > 6% | Metronidazole |
| *Candida albicans* | > 6% | Topical imidazoles |
| *Gardnerella vaginalis* | > 6% | Metronidazole |
| *Chlamydia trachomatis* | > 4% | Doxycycline 100 mg orally twice a day for 7 days |
| Hepatitis B virus | Unknown | None |
| Cytomegalovirus | Unknown | None |
| HIV | Unknown | None |

contaminated extragenital injury, tetanus toxoid should be administered. It is also important to schedule a follow-up appointment at 7–14 days after the assault so that the patient may be examined for evidence of new infections.

Prevention of pregnancy as a result of rape is crucial. If there is any possibility that the patient is already pregnant, β-hCG levels should be determined immediately before any medication is prescribed. Hormonal pregnancy prophylaxis may be used within 72 hours of the assault. Hormonal methods of pregnancy prevention are 95–98% effective and, if ineffective, are associated with a small risk of fetal damage. Prevention of pregnancy should be discussed with the patient in the event that she would be unwilling to abort a pregnancy resulting from the assault or to risk potential damage to a retained fetus.

There are several regimens for postcoital contraception. A combination of ethinyl estradiol, 50 µg, plus norgestrel, 0.5 µg (Ovral), 2 tablets orally at the time of examination followed by 2 additional tablets in 12 hours, is an effective postcoital contraceptive. It has a failure rate of 0.9% and a nausea rate of 50%. This regimen is preferred because it has the highest efficacy and a comparatively low rate of side effects.

## Prognosis

The prognosis for complete recovery is improved if persons responsible for the victim's care have a well-developed understanding of the emotional, as well as physical, consequences of sexual assault. Competent management requires health personnel to remain nonjudgmental in their approach, to have a thorough understanding of the different types of rape, and to be able to collect an accurate history from the patient. Knowing how to approach the problem on several levels helps the physician to perform a thorough physical examination, ensuring collection of all appropriate specimens. The meticulous labeling of materials and their transfer to the legal authorities are of crucial legal importance. As most patients suffer significant emotional trauma as a consequence of sexual assault, the physician must be prepared to provide access to counseling. It is preferable that follow-up psychologic counseling be provided by individuals who have extensive experience in the management of crisis-response to rape.

The reintegration of the ego following sexual assault is a slow process, fluctuating in its rate of progress and usually taking at least several months. Many patients never fully recover emotionally. In addition, the woman's family and friends experience their own emotional responses to the assault episode. The victim's responses and those of her community frequently result in permanent alterations in her personal relationships.

In addition to viewing the aftermath of rape as a manifestation of posttraumatic stress disorder, one can conceptualize the sequelae in terms of the phases of crisis resolution. In this context, the emotional recovery process following sexual assault is similar to the processes involved in recovery from other life crises and can be divided into 2 phases: acute and long-term. The acute phase extends from the moment that the woman realizes she is being assaulted until such time as she begins to reorganize and reintegrate her emotions and behavior. The long-term phase usually begins 2–3 weeks after the assault, typically with alteration in the victim's life-style and emotional equilibrium. This phase may persist for an extended period of time. All follow-up studies of rape victims have identified emotional sequelae to the assault extending for varying periods of time, often for several years.

The acute-phase reaction is characterized by fear, shock and disbelief, or denial. The wide range of emotions experienced in this phase is usually demonstrated in 1 of 2 ways: the patient may become agitated and appear visibly upset, or, more commonly, she may become withdrawn and appear surprisingly calm and controlled. Somatic symptoms are prevalent during the acute phase and include sleep disturbances, gastrointestinal upset (with nausea predominating), headaches, and musculoskeletal pain from tension. Symptoms of vaginal irritation occur in more than 50% of victims, and rectal pain and bleeding are frequent in patients subjected to anal penetration.

Victims also experience psychiatric symptoms during the acute phase. They may be distracted, disorganized, fearful, or easily startled, or they may experience nightmares. They are generally emotionally labile, and their feelings may fluctuate rapidly from fear and guilt to anger and desire for revenge.

The long-term phase of recovery is also characterized by somatic and psychiatric symptoms as well as by overt and frequently permanent alterations in behavior and life-style. Victims will often change their phone numbers, change jobs, move to another location within the city, or move to another city altogether. There is frequently an increase in personal contact with family members. Repeated nightmares are common, as is the development of phobias related to the specific or general circumstances of the assault. Victims may be unable to tolerate being indoors (especially in the bedroom), or, conversely, they may be unable to tolerate being outdoors, especially if unaccompanied. Solitude may lead to panic. An overwhelming fear of crowds and strangers, especially men, may develop.

More than half of rape victims experience substantial difficulty in reestablishing sexual and emotional relationships with spouses or boyfriends. The negative effect of sexual assault is even more pronounced in women who have never been sexually active. Victims with preexisting psychiatric problems or partially resolved personal conflicts can be expected to reactivate previously existent maladaptive behavior patterns. Thus, neurotic and psychotic behavior disorders, suicidal behavior, and substance abuse may become more prevalent following sexual assault. Because of this emergence or exacerbation of psychiatric symptoms, it is important to offer psychiatric follow-up to all rape victims.

## REFERENCES

American Psychiatric Association: *Diagnostic and Statistical Manual of Mental Disorders*. 3rd Rev (DSM-III-R). American Psychiatric Association, 1987.

Bolen JD: The impact of sexual abuse on women's health. Psychiatr Ann 1993;8:446.

Burgess AW, Holmstrom LL: Rape trauma syndrome. Am J Psychiatry 1974:131:981.

Dickstein LJ: Spouse abuse and other domestic violence. Psychiatr Clin North Am 1988;11:611.

Dickstein LJ, Nadelson CC (editors): *Family Violence Emerging Issues of a National Crisis*. American Psychiatric Press, Inc, 1989.

Federal Bureau of Investigation: *Uniform Crime Reports for the United States*. US Department of Justice, 1991.

Gise LH, Paddison P: Rape, sexual abuse and its victims. Psychiatr Clin North Am 1988;11:629.

Groth AN, Birnbaum HJ: *Men Who Rape: The Psychology of the Offender*. Plenum Press, 1979.

Groth AN, Burgess AW: Sexual dysfunction during rape. N Engl J Med 1977;297:764.

Herman JL: *Trauma and Recovery*. Basic Books, 1992.

Hicks DJ: Rape: Sexual assault. Am J Obstet Gynecol 1980; 137:931.

Hochbaum SR: The evaluation and treatment of the sexually assaulted patient. Emerg Clin North AM 1987;5: 601.

Jenny C: Sexual assault and sexually transmitted diseases. In: *Sexually Transmitted Diseases*. Holmes KK et al (editors). McGraw-Hill, 1990.

Kanin EJ et al: Personal sexual history and punitive judgments for rape. Psychol Rep 1987;61:439.

Martin PY, DiNitto DM: The rape exam: Beyond the hospital emergency room. Women & Health 1987;12:5.

McFarlane J et al: Assessing for abuse during pregnancy: Severity and frequency of injuries and associated entry into prenatal care. JAMA 1992;267:3176.

Nadelson CC et al: A follow-up study of rape victims. Am J Psychiatry 1982;139:1266.

Newberger EH et al: Abuse of pregnant women and adverse birth outcome: Current knowledge and implications for practice. JAMA 1992;267:2370.

Renshaw DC: Treatment of sexual exploitation: Rape and incest. Psychiatr Clin North Am 1989;2:257.

Rose DS: Sexual assault, domestic violence, and incest. In: *Psychological Aspects of Women's Health Care: The Interface Between Psychiatry and Obstetrics and Gynecol-*

*ogy*. Stewart DE, Stotland NL (editors). American Psychiatric Press 1993.

Scott RL et al: Attitudes of rapists and other violent offenders toward women. J Soc Psychol 1987;127:375.

Sonnenberg SM: Victims of violence and posttraumatic stress disorder. Psychiatr Clin North Am 1988;11:581.

Walker E et al: Relationship of chronic pelvic pain to psychiatric diagnoses and childhood sexual abuse. Am J Psychiatry 1988;145:75.

Yuzpe AA, Smith RP, Rademaker AW: A multicenter clinical investigation employing ethinyl estradiol combined with dl-norgestrel as postcoital contraceptive agent. Fertil Steril 1982;37:508.

# The Breast

# 62

*Kathleen F. Harney, MD, & Leonard F. Smith, MD*

## ANATOMY OF THE FEMALE BREAST

The breasts (mammae) are secondary reproductive glands of ectodermal modified sweat gland origin. Each breast lies on the superior midsurface of the chest wall. In women, the breasts are the organs of lactation; in men, the breasts are normally functionless and undeveloped.

### HISTOLOGY

The adult female breast contains glandular and ductal tissue, a stroma of fibrous tissue that binds the individual lobes together, and fatty tissue within and between the lobes.

Each breast consists of 12–20 conical lobes. The base of each lobe is close to the ribs; the apex, which contains the major excretory duct of the lobe, is situated close to the areola and nipple. Each lobe consists of a group of lobules, and the many lactiferous ducts in each lobule unite to form a major duct that drains a lobe as it converges toward the areola. Each of the major ducts widens to form an ampulla as it reaches the areola and then narrows for its individual opening on the nipple. The lobules are held in place by a mesh work of fatty areolar tissue. The fatty tissue increases toward the periphery of the lobule and gives the breast its bulk and its hemispheric shape.

About 80–85% of the normal breast is fat. The breast tissues are joined to the overlying skin and subcutaneous tissue by fibrous strands.

In the nonpregnant, nonlactating breast, the alveoli are small and tightly packed. During pregnancy, the alveoli enlarge and their lining cells increase in number. During lactation, the alveolar cells secrete milk proteins and lipids.

The deep surface of the breast lies on the fascia that covers the chest muscles. The fascial stroma, derived from the superficial fascia of the chest wall, is condensed into multiple fascial bands that run from the breast into the subcutaneous tissues and the corium of the skin overlying the breast. These fascial bands—Cooper's ligaments—support the breast in its upright position on the chest wall. These bands may be distorted by a tumor, resulting in skin dimpling.

### HISTOLOGIC CHANGES IN THE FEMALE BREAST DURING THE LIFE SPAN

During puberty, in response to multiglandular stimulation, the female breast begins to enlarge and eventually assumes its conical or spherical shape. Growth is due to increase in acinar tissue, ductal size and branching, and deposits of fat (the main factor in breast enlargement). Also during puberty, the nipple and areola enlarge. Smooth muscle fibers surround the base of the nipple, and the nipple becomes more sensitive to touch.

Once menses are established, the breast undergoes a periodic **premenstrual phase** during which the acinar cells increase in number and size, the ductal lumens widen, and breast size and turgor increase slightly. Many women have breast tenderness during this phase of the cycle. Menstrual bleeding is followed by a **postmenstrual phase**, characterized by decrease in size and turgor, reduction in the number and size of the breast acini, and decrease in diameter of the lactiferous ducts. Individual response of the breast to cyclic hormonal influences is variable. This is true not only of breast size and turgor but also of the degree of hypertrophic and regressive histologic changes that may occur.

During pregnancy, in response to progesterone—the corpus luteum hormone secreted by the ovary—breast size and turgidity increase markedly. These changes are accompanied by deepening nipple and areolar pigmentation, nipple enlargement, areolar widening, and an increase in the number and size of the lubricating glands in the areola. The breast ductal system branches markedly, and the individual ducts widen. The acini increase in number and size. In late pregnancy, the fatty tissues of the breasts are almost completely replaced by cellular breast parenchyma. After delivery, the breasts, now fully mature, start to secrete milk. With cessation of nursing or administration of estrogens to inhibit lactation, the gland rapidly returns to its prepregnancy state, with marked diminution of cellular elements and an increase in fat deposits.

Between the fifth and sixth decades of life, when menses cease, the breast undergoes a gradual process of involution. There is a decrease in the number and size of acinar and ductal elements, so that the breast tissue regresses to an almost infantile state. Adipose tissue may or may not atrophy, with disappearance of the parenchymal elements.

## GROSS ANATOMY
### (Fig 62–1)

The adult female breast usually forms an almost hemispheric protrusion on each side of the chest wall, usually extending from just below the level of the second rib inferiorly to the sixth or seventh rib. The gland is usually situated between the lateral sternal border and the anterior axillary fold. The superior surface of the breast emerges gradually from the chest wall, whereas the lateral and inferior borders are quite well defined. The major portion of the breast, lying atop the pectoralis major muscle, projects ventrally; smaller portions extend laterally and inferiorly to lie atop the serratus anterior and external oblique muscles and as far caudad as the rectus abdominis. A triangular tongue-shaped tail of breast tissue (the axillary tail of Spence) extends superiorly and laterally toward the axilla, perforates the deep axillary fascia, and enters the axilla, where it terminates

in close apposition to the axillary lymph vessels and nodes and the axillary blood vessels and nerves.

### The Nipple & Areola

The areola is a circular pigmented zone 2–6 cm in diameter at the tip of the breast. Its color varies from pale pink to deep brown depending on age, parity, and skin pigmentation. The skin of the areola contains multiple small elevated nodules beneath which lie the sebaceous glands (glands of Montgomery). The glands are responsible for lubrication of the nipple and help prevent nipple and areolar cracks and fissures. During the third trimester of pregnancy, the sebaceous glands hypertrophy markedly.

A circular smooth muscle band surrounds the base of the nipple. Longitudinal smooth muscle fibers branch out from the ring of circular smooth muscle to encircle the lactiferous ducts as they converge toward the nipple. The many small punctate openings situated at the top of the nipple are the terminals of the major lactiferous ducts. The ampullae of the lactiferous ducts lie just deep to the nipple and the areola.

### Blood Vessels, Lymphatics, & Nerves
**A. Arteries: (Fig 62–2)** The breast has a multiple arterial supply. Perforating branches from the internal thoracic artery that appear in interspaces 2, 3, and 4 supply blood to the medial quadrants of the breast. These arteries perforate the intercostal muscles and the anterior intercostal membrane to supply both the breast and the pectoralis major and minor muscles. During pregnancy and in advanced breast disease, the intercostal perforators generally enlarge. The breast is also supplied medially by small branches from the anterior intercostal arteries. It is nourished laterally by the pectoral branch of the thoracoacromial branch of the axillary artery and by the external mammary branch of the lateral thoracic artery, which also is a branch of the second segment of the axillary artery. The external mammary artery passes along the lateral free border of the pectoralis major muscle to reach the lateral half of the breast, the artery usually lying medial to the long thoracic nerve.

The medial and lateral arteries, as they reach the breast, tend to arborize mainly in the supra-areolar area; consequently, the arterial supply to the upper half of the breast is almost twice that of the lower half.

**B. Veins:** Venous return from the breast closely follows the routes of arterial supply. Blood returns to the superior vena cava via the axillary and internal thoracic veins. It also returns via the vertebral venous plexuses, which are fed by the intercostal and azygos veins. There is some minor flow into the portal system via the azygos system. There is a rich subareolar anastomotic plexus of superficial breast veins. In thin-skinned, fair individuals, these veins are normally visible. They almost always become visible

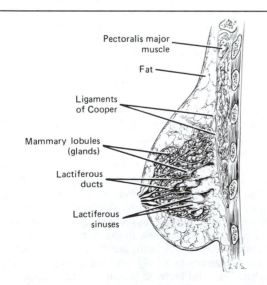

Pectoralis major muscle

Fat

Ligaments of Cooper

Mammary lobules (glands)

Lactiferous ducts

Lactiferous sinuses

**Figure 62–1.** Sagittal section of mammary gland.

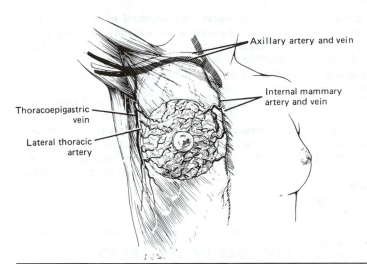

**Figure 62–2.** Arteries and veins of the breast.

during pregnancy. Their presence makes for marked vascularity of sub- and para-areolar incisions. Venous flow in the superior quadrants is greater than in the inferior quadrants of the breast.

**C. Lymphatics: (Fig 62–3)** Study of the lymphatic drainage from the breast is of great importance for its implications in breast cancer. Modern surgical concepts of management of breast cancer are based to a large extent on an understanding of the pattern of lymphatic drainage from the breast.

Lymphatic drainage from the breast may be divided into 2 main categories: superficial (including cutaneous) drainage and deep parenchymatous drainage.

**1. Superficial drainage**–A large lymphatic plexus lies in the subcutaneous tissues of the breast just beneath the areola and nipple. This plexus drains the areola and nipple areas and the cutaneous and subcutaneous tissues adjacent to the areola. It also drains the deep central parenchymatous region of the breast; the lymph rising from these areas pools in the superficial plexus.

**2. Deep parenchymatous drainage**–The deep parenchymatous lymph channels drain most of the breast as well as some lymph from the skin and subcutaneous tissues of the areolar and nipple areas. Small periductal and periacinal lymph channels collect parenchymal lymph and deliver it to the larger interlobar lymphatics. Lymph from the cutaneous and areolar areas may drain either directly into the subareolar plexus or deeply into the parenchymatous lymph channels and is secondarily delivered to the subareolar plexus for efferent transport.

From both the retroareolar and the deep interlobar lymphatics, most breast lymph usually passes to the ipsilateral axillary group of lymph nodes. There are no predetermined pathways by which breast lymph reaches the highest axillary node or nodes. Lymph flowing in either the superior or inferior mammary trunk may bypass the inferior or central group of axillary nodes and flow directly to the highest group of axillary nodes. However, most breast lymph usually goes first to the anterior axillary or subpectoral group of nodes that lie just beneath the lateral border of the pectoralis major muscle, close to the course of the lateral thoracic artery. From these nodes, lymph usually passes to nodes lying close to the lateral portion of the axillary vein. The lymph then passes superiorly, via the axillary chain of lymph vessels and nodes. The

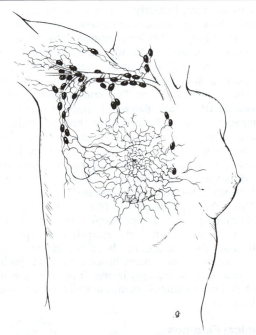

**Figure 62–3.** Lymphatics of the breast and axilla.

lymph eventually reaches the highest nodes of the axilla. Although this is the so-called normal pattern of lateral and superior breast lymphatic drainage, other paths of drainage are fairly common, particularly when the lateral and superiorly directed channels are obstructed by tumor masses. When plugging occurs, the following pathways are available for lymphatic flow from the breast:

a. From the breast directly to the highest axillary node, completely bypassing all other axillary nodal tissue. This may occur with superior quadrant breast tumors.

b. From the breast directly to the subscapular group of axillary nodes, subsequently progressing ventrally and superiorly through channels lying close to the axillary vein.

c. From the breast directly to the most inferior group of supraclavicular cervical nodes. Supraclavicular nodes are more commonly involved via direct extension from the apical axillary nodes.

d. From the breast across the sternal midline to the lymphatics of the contralateral breast.

e. From the breast directly to the contralateral axilla.

f. From the breast to the internal mammary group of nodes when the primary breast tumor is in the medial quadrant.

g. Rarely, from the breast to lymphatics that run to lymphatics closely related to the sheaths of the superior segments of the rectus abdominis and external oblique muscles and thence inferiorly toward the upper abdominal wall, the diaphragm, and the intra-abdominal viscera (especially the liver).

**D. Nerves Encountered During Axillary Dissection:** The lateral and anterior cutaneous branches of T4–6 supply the cutaneous tissues covering the breasts. Two major nerves and 2 smaller groups of nerves lie close to the breast area and thus assume importance in breast surgery:

(1) The **thoracodorsal nerve**, a branch of the posterior cord of the brachial plexus (C5–7), runs inferiorly along with the subscapular artery lying close to the posterior axillary wall and the ventral surface of the subscapular muscle. The nerve innervates the superior half of the latissimus dorsimuscle and is usually surrounded by a large venous plexus that drains into the subscapular veins.

(2) The **long thoracic nerve** (nerve of Bell) arises from the anterior primary divisions of C5–7 at the level of the lower half of the anterior scalene muscle. In the neck, the nerve descends dorsal to the trunks of the brachial plexus on the inferior segment of the middle scalene muscle. Further descent places it dorsal to the clavicle and the axillary vessels. On the lateral thoracic wall, it descends on the external surface of the serratus anterior muscle along the anterior axillary line. The long thoracic nerve supplies filaments to each of the digitations of the serratus anterior muscle. Injury to this nerve results in a "winged" scapula.

(3) The **intercostal brachial nerves** are 3 relatively minor cutaneous nerves that supply the skin of the medial surface of the upper arm. They cross transversely from the lateral chest wall to the upper inner surface of the arm, passing across the base of the axilla.

(4) The **medial and lateral pectoral nerves** that supply the 2 pectoral muscles pass from the axilla to the lateral chest wall, reaching it by piercing the costocoracoid membrane. The medial pectoral nerve arises from the medial cord of the brachial plexus; the lateral pectoral nerve arises from the lateral cord of the plexus.

# DISEASES OF THE BREAST

## FIBROCYSTIC CHANGE

### Essentials of Diagnosis

- Painful, often multiple, usually bilateral masses in the breast.
- Rapid fluctuation in the size of the masses is common.
- Frequently, pain occurs or increases and size increases during premenstrual phase of cycle.
- Most common age is 30–50. Rare in postmenopausal women.

### General Considerations

This disorder, formerly known as mammary dysplasia, fibrocystic disease, or chronic cystic mastitis, is the most frequent benign condition of the breast. It is common in women 30–50 years of age but rare in postmenopausal women; this suggests that it is related to ovarian activity. Estrogen hormone is considered a causative factor. The term **mammary dysplasia,** or **fibrocystic disease**, is imprecise and encompasses a wide variety of pathologic entities. These lesions are always associated with benign changes in the breast epithelium, some of which are found so commonly in normal breasts that they are probably variants of normal breast histology but have unfortunately been termed a "disease."

The microscopic findings of fibrocystic change include cysts (gross and microscopic), papillomatosis, adenosis, fibrosis, and ductal epithelial hyperplasia. Although this condition has been considered to increase the risk of subsequent breast cancer, it is probable that only the variants in which proliferation of epithelial components is demonstrated represent true risk factors.

### Clinical Findings

Fibrocystic change may produce an asymptomatic

lump in the breast that is discovered by palpation, but pain or tenderness often calls attention to the mass. There may be discharge from the nipple. In many cases, discomfort occurs or is increased during the premenstrual phase of the cycle, at which time the cysts tend to enlarge. Some women seem to have more severe pain that is constant and not related to the menstrual cycle (**mastodynia**). Fluctuation in size and rapid appearance or disappearance of a breast tumor are common in cystic changes. Multiple or bilateral masses are common, and many patients will give a history of transient lump in the breast or cyclic breast pain. Pain, fluctuation in size, and multiplicity of lesions are the features most helpful in differentiation from carcinoma. However, if a dominant mass is present, it should be evaluated by biopsy.

### Differential Diagnosis

Pain, fluctuation in size, and multiplicity of lesions help to differentiate these lesions from carcinoma and fibroadenoma. Final diagnosis often depends on biopsy. Mammography may be helpful, but the breast tissue in these young women is usually too radiodense to permit a worthwhile study. Aspiration and/or sonography may be useful in differentiating a cystic from a solid mass.

### Treatment

Because the condition of fibrocystic change is frequently indistinguishable from carcinoma on the basis of clinical findings, it is advisable to perform biopsy examination of suspicious lesions, which is usually done under local anesthesia. Surgery should be conservative, since the primary object is to exclude cancer. Simple mastectomy or extensive removal of breast tissue is rarely, if ever, indicated for fibrocystic change.

When the diagnosis of fibrocystic change has been established by previous biopsy or is practically certain, because the history is classic, aspiration of a discrete mass suggestive of a cyst is indicated. The patient is reexamined at intervals thereafter. If no fluid is obtained, or if fluid is bloody, if a mass persists after aspiration, or if anytime during follow-up a persistent lump is noted, biopsy should be performed (Fig 62–4).

Breast pain associated with generalized fibrocystic change is best treated by avoiding trauma and by wearing a bra with good support.

The role of caffeine consumption in the development and treatment of fibrocystic change is controversial. Many patients report relief of symptoms after giving up coffee, tea, and chocolate.

### Prognosis

Exacerbations of pain, tenderness, and cyst formation may occur at any time until the menopause, when symptoms subside. The patient should be advised to examine her own breasts each month just after menstruation and to inform her physician if a mass appears. The risk of breast cancer in women with fibrocystic change showing proliferative or atypical changes in the epithelium is higher than that of women in general. Follow-up examinations at regular intervals should therefore be arranged.

### FIBROADENOMA OF THE BREAST

This common benign neoplasm occurs most frequently in young women, usually within 20 years after puberty. It is somewhat more frequent and tends to occur at an earlier age in black than in white women. Multiple tumors in one or both breasts are found in 10–15% of patients.

The typical fibroadenoma is a round, firm, discrete, relatively movable, nontender mass 1–5 cm in diameter. The tumor is usually discovered accidentally. Clinical diagnosis in young patients is generally not difficult. In women over 30, cystic disease of the

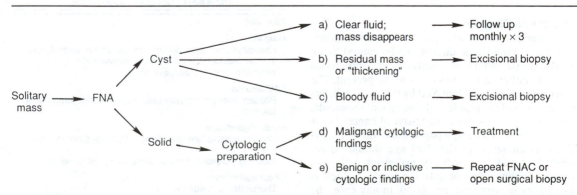

**Figure 62–4.** Algorithm for the use of fine needle aspiration (FNA) and fine needle aspiration cytology (FNAC for office triage of breast lumps. (Reproduced, with permission, from Hindle WH: *Breast Disease for Gynecologists.* Appleton & Lange, 1990.

breast and carcinoma of the breast must be considered. Cysts can be identified by aspiration. Fibroadenoma does not normally occur after the menopause, but postmenopausal women may occasionally develop fibroadenoma after administration of estrogenic hormone.

Treatment is excision under local anesthesia, or careful clinical observation.

**Cystosarcoma phyllodes** is a type of fibroadenoma with cellular stroma that tends to grow rapidly. This tumor may reach a large size and if inadequately excised will recur locally. The lesion is rarely malignant. Treatment is by local excision of the mass with a margin of surrounding breast tissue. The treatment of malignant cystosarcoma phyllodes is more controversial. In general, complete removal of the tumor and a rim of normal tissue should avoid recurrence. Since these tumors tend to be large, simple mastectomy is often necessary to achieve complete control.

## NIPPLE DISCHARGE

### General Considerations

The most common causes of nipple discharge in the nonlactating breast are carcinoma, intraductal papilloma, and fibrocystic change with ectasia of the ducts. The important characteristics of the discharge and some other factors to be evaluated by history and physical examination are as follows:

(1) Nature of discharge (serous, bloody, or other).

(2) Association with a mass or not.

(3) Unilateral or bilateral.

(4) Single duct or multiple duct discharge.

(5) Discharge is spontaneous (persistent or intermittent) or must be expressed.

(6) Discharge produced by pressure at a single site or by general pressure on the breast.

(7) Relation to menses.

(8) Premenopausal or postmenopausal.

(9) Patient taking contraceptive pills, or estrogen for postmenopausal symptoms.

### Differential Diagnosis

Unilateral, spontaneous serous or serosanguineous discharge from a single duct is usually caused by an intraductal papilloma or, rarely, by an intraductal cancer. In either case, a mass may not be present. The involved duct may be identified by pressure at different sites around the nipple at the margin of the areola. Bloody discharge is more suggestive of cancer but is usually caused by a benign papilloma in the duct. Cytologic examination of the discharge should be accomplished and may identify malignant cells, but negative findings do not rule out cancer, which is more likely in women over age 50. In any case, the involved duct, and a mass if present, should be excised.

In premenopausal women, spontaneous multiple duct discharge, unilateral or bilateral, most marked just before menstruation, is often due to fibrocystic change. Discharge may be green or brownish. Papillomatosis and ductal ectasia are also diagnostic possibilities. Biopsy may be necessary to establish the diagnosis of a diffuse nonmalignant process. If a mass is present, it should be removed.

Milky discharge (galactorrhea) from multiple ducts in the nonlactating breast may occur in certain syndromes (Chiari-Frommel syndrome, Argonz-Del Castillo[Forbes-Albright] syndrome), presumably as a result of increased secretion of pituitary prolactin. An endocrine workup may be indicated. Drugs of the chlorpromazine type and contraceptive pills may also cause milky discharge that ceases on discontinuance of the medication. Other medical illnesses may rarely cause galactorrhea (Table 62–1).

Oral contraceptive agents may cause clear, serous, or milky discharge from a single duct, but multiple duct discharge is more common. The discharge is more evident just before menstruation and disappears on stopping the medication. If it does not and is from a single duct, exploration should be considered.

Purulent discharge may originate in a subareolar abscess and require excision of the abscess and related lactiferous sinus.

When localization is not possible and no mass is palpable, the patient should be reexamined every week for 1 month. When unilateral discharge persists, even without definite localization or tumor, exploration must be considered. The alternative is careful follow-up at intervals of 1–3 months. Mammography should be done. Cytologic examination of nipple discharge for exfoliated cancer cells may be helpful in diagnosis.

Chronic unilateral nipple discharge, especially if bloody, is an indication for resection of the involved ducts.

**Table 62–1.** Causes of galactorrhea.

| |
|---|
| *Idiopathic* |
| *Drug induced* |
|    Phenothiazines, butyrophenones, reserpine, methyldopa, imipramine, amphetamine, metaclopramide, sulpride, pimozide, oral contraceptive agents. |
| *CNS lesions* |
|    Pituitary adenoma, empty sella, hypothalamic tumor, head trauma. |
| *Medical conditions* |
|    Chronic renal failure, sarcoidosis, Schuller-Christian disease. |
|    Cushing's disease, hepatic cirrhosis, hypothyroidism. |
| *Chest wall lesions* |
|    Thoracotomy, herpes zoster |

Reproduced, with permission, from Hindle WH: *Breast Disease for Gynecologists*. Appleton & Lange, 1990.

# FAT NECROSIS

Fat necrosis is a rare lesion of the breast but is of clinical importance because it produces a mass, often accompanied by skin or nipple retraction, that is indistinguishable from carcinoma. Trauma is presumed to be the cause, although only about half of patients give a history of injury to the breast. Ecchymosis is occasionally seen near the tumor. Tenderness may or may not be present. If untreated, the mass associated with fat necrosis gradually disappears. Should the mass not resolve in several weeks, a biopsy should be considered. The entire mass should be excised, primarily to rule out carcinoma. Fat necrosis is common after segmental resection and radiation therapy.

# BREAST ABSCESS

During nursing, an area of redness, tenderness, and induration not infrequently develops in the breast. In the early stages, the infection can often be reversed while continuing nursing with that breast and administering an antibiotic. If the lesion progresses to form a localized mass with local and systemic signs of infection, an abscess is present and should be drained, and nursing should be discontinued.

A subareolar abscess may develop (rarely) in young or middle-aged women who are not lactating. These infections tend to recur after incision and drainage unless the area is explored in a quiescent interval with excision of the involved lactiferous duct or ducts at the base of the nipple. Except for the subareolar type of abscess, infection in the breast is very rare unless the patient is lactating. Therefore, findings suggestive of abscess in the nonlactating breast require incision and biopsy of an indurated tissue.

## Malformation of the Breast

Many women consult their physicians for abnormalities in either the size or the symmetry of their breasts. It is not infrequent for there to be some difference in size between the two breasts, which, if extreme, may be corrected by plastic surgery. However, the breast tissue in these individuals is otherwise normal.

Similarly, woman may complain of overly large breasts (macromastia). Studies have failed to show any endocrinologic or pathologic abnormalities, and these patients may also be considered candidates for plastic surgery (breast reduction).

Less common malformations of the breast include amastia (complete absence of one or both breasts) or the presence of accessory breast tissue along the embryologic milk line (occurring in 1–2% of Caucasians).

# PUERPERAL MASTITIS

See Chapter 29.

# CARCINOMA OF THE FEMALE BREAST

## Essentials of Diagnosis

- Early findings: Single, nontender, firm to hard mass with ill-defined margins; mammographic abnormalities and no palpable mass.
- Later findings: Skin or nipple retraction; axillary lymphadenopathy; breast enlargement, redness, edema, pain, fixation of mass to skin or chest wall.
- Late findings: Ulceration; supraclavicular lymphadenopathy; edema of arm; bone, lung, liver, brain, or other distant metastases.

## General Considerations

Cancer of the breast is the most common invasive cancer in women from the ages of 15 to 54. It is the second most common cause of death in the age group 55–74. The American Cancer Society predicted 182,000 new cases of cancer of the breast and 46,000 deaths for 1993. The probability of developing the disease increases throughout life. The mean and the median age of women with breast cancer is 60–61 years.

At the present rate of incidence, one of every 9 American women will develop breast cancer during her lifetime. Women whose mothers or sisters had breast cancer are more likely to develop the disease than controls. Risk is increased when breast cancer has occurred before menopause, was bilateral, or was present in 2 or more first-degree relatives. However, there is no history of breast cancer among female relatives in over 90% of patients with breast cancer. Nulliparous women and women whose first full-term pregnancy was after age 35 have a slightly higher incidence of breast cancer than multiparous women. Late menarche and artificial menopause are associated with a lower incidence of breast cancer, whereas early menarche (under age 12) and late natural menopause (after age 50) are associated with a slight increase in risk of developing breast cancer. Fibrocystic change of the breast, when accompanied by proliferative changes, papillomatosis, or atypical epithelial hyperplasia, is associated with an increased incidence of cancer. A woman who has had cancer in one breast is at increased risk of developing cancer in the other breast. Women with cancer of the uterine corpus have a breast cancer risk significantly higher than that of the general population, and women with breast cancer have a comparably increased risk of endometrial cancer. In the USA, breast cancer is more common in whites than in nonwhites. The incidence of the disease among nonwhites (mostly blacks), however, is increasing, especially in younger women. In general, rates reported from developing countries are low, whereas rates are high in developed countries, with the notable exception of Japan. Some of the variability may be due to underreporting in the developing countries, but a real difference probably exists.

Women who are at greater than normal risk of developing breast cancer should be identified by their physicians and followed carefully. Screening programs involving periodic physical examination and mammography of asymptomatic high-risk women increase the detection rate of breast cancer and may improve the survival rate. Unfortunately, most women who develop breast cancer do not have significant identifiable risk factors.

Growth potential of tumor and resistance of host vary over a wide range from patient to patient and may be altered during the course of the disease. The doubling time of breast cancer cells ranges from several weeks in a rapidly growing lesion to nearly a year in a slowly growing one. If one assumes that the rate of doubling is constant and that the neoplasm originates in one cell, a carcinoma with a doubling time of 100 days may not reach clinically detectable size (1 cm) for about 8 years. On the other hand, rapidly growing cancers have a much shorter preclinical course and a greater tendency to metastasize to regional nodes or more distant sites before a breast mass is discovered.

The relatively long preclinical growth phase and the tendency of breast cancers to metastasize have led many clinicians to believe that breast cancer is a systemic disease at the time of diagnosis. Although it may be true that breast cancer cells are released from the tumor prior to diagnosis, variations in the host-tumor relationship may prohibit the growth of disseminated disease in many patients. For this reason, a pessimistic attitude concerning the management of localized breast cancer is not warranted, and many patients can be cured with proper treatment.

**Table 62–2.** Clinical and histologic staging of breast carcinoma.

**Clinical Staging
(American Joint Committee)**

**Stage I**
  Tumor < 2 cm in diameter
  Nodes, if present, not felt to contain metastases
  Without distant metastases
**Stage II**
  Tumor < 5 cm in diameter
  Nodes, if palpable, not fixed
  Without distant metastases
**Stage III**
  Tumor > 5 cm or-
  Tumor any size with invasion of skin or attached to chest wall
  Nodes in supraclavicular area
  Without distant metastases
**Stage IV**
  With distant metastases

## Staging

The physical examination of the breast and additional preoperative studies are used to determine the clinical stage of a breast cancer. Clinical staging is based on the TNM system (of the International Union Against Cancer). This classification considers tumor size, clinical assessment of axillary nodes, and the presence or absence of metastases. The assessment of the clinical stage is important in planning therapy. Histologic (or pathologic) staging is determined following surgery and along with clinical staging helps determine prognosis (Table 62–2).

## Clinical Findings

The patient with breast cancer usually presents with a lump in the breast. Clinical evaluation should include assessment of the local lesion and a search for evidence of metastases in regional nodes or distant sites. After the diagnosis of breast cancer has been confirmed by biopsy, additional studies are often needed to complete the search for distant metastases or an occult primary lesion in the other breast. Then, before any decision is made about treatment, all the available clinical data are used to determine the extent or "stage" of the patient's disease.

**A. Symptoms:** When the history is taken, special note should be made of menarche, pregnancies, parity, artificial or natural menopause, date of last menstrual period, previous breast lesions, and a family history of breast cancer. Back or other bone pain may be the result of osseous metastases. Systemic complaints or weight loss should raise the question of metastases, which may involve any organ but most frequently the bones, liver, and lungs. The more advanced the cancer in terms of size of primary lesion, local invasion, and extent of regional node involvement, the higher is the incidence of metastatic spread to distant sites.

The presenting complaint in about 70% of patients with breast cancer is a lump (usually painless) in the breast. About 90% of breast masses are discovered by the patient herself. Less frequent symptoms are breast pain; nipple discharge; erosion, retraction, enlargement, or itching of the nipple; and redness, generalized hardness, enlargement, or shrinking of the breast. Rarely, an axillary mass, swelling of the arm, or bone pain (from metastases) may be the first symptom. Thirty-five to 50% of women involved in organized screening programs have cancers detected by mammography only.

**B. Signs:** The relative frequency of carcinoma in various anatomic sites in the breast is shown in Figure 62–5.

Inspection of the breast is the first step in physical examination and should be carried out with the patient sitting, arms at sides and then overhead. Abnormal variations in breast size and contour, minimal nipple retraction, and slight edema, redness, or retraction of the skin can be identified. Asymmetry of the

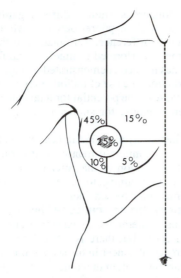

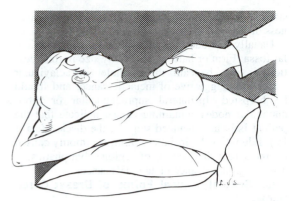

**Figure 62–7.** Palpation of breasts. Palpation is performed with the patient supine and the arm abducted.

**Figure 62–5.** Frequency of breast carcinoma at various anatomic sites.

breasts and retraction or dimpling of the skin can often be accentuated by having the patient raise her arms overhead or press her hands on her hips in order to contract the pectoralis muscles. Axillary and supraclavicular areas should be thoroughly palpated for enlarged nodes with the patient sitting (Fig 62–6). Palpation of the breast for masses or other changes should be performed with the patient both seated and supine with the arm abducted (Fig 62–7).

Breast cancer usually consists of a nontender, firm, or hard lump with poorly delineated margins (caused by local infiltration). Slight skin or nipple retraction

is an important sign. Minimal asymmetry of the breast may be noted. Very small (1–2 mm) erosions of the nipple epithelium may be the only manifestation of Paget's carcinoma. Watery, serous, or bloody discharge from the nipple is an occasional early sign but is more often associated with benign disease.

A lesion smaller than 1 cm in diameter may be difficult or impossible for the examiner to feel and yet may be discovered by the patient. She should always be asked to demonstrate the location of the mass; if the physician fails to confirm the patient's suspicions, the examination should be repeated in 1 month. During the premenstrual phase of the cycle, increased innocuous nodularity may suggest neoplasm or may obscure an underlying lesion. If there is any question regarding the nature of an abnormality under these circumstances, the patient should be asked to return after her period.

The following are characteristic of advanced carcinoma: edema, redness, nodularity, or ulceration of the skin; the presence of a large primary tumor; fixation to the chest wall; enlargement, shrinkage, or retraction of the breast; marked axillary lymphadenopathy; supraclavicular lymphadenopathy; edema of the ipsilateral arm; and distant metastases.

Metastases tend to involve regional lymph nodes, which may be clinically palpable. With regard to the axilla, one or 2 movable, nontender, not particularly firm lymph nodes 5 mm or less in diameter are frequently present and are generally of no significance. Firm or hard nodes larger than 5 mm in diameter usually contain metastases. Axillary nodes that are matted or fixed to skin or deep structures indicate advanced disease (at least stage III). Histologic studies show that microscopic metastases are present in about 30% of patients with clinically negative nodes. On the other hand, if the examiner thinks that the axillary nodes are involved, this will prove on histologic section to be correct in about 85% of cases. The incidence of positive axillary nodes increases with the

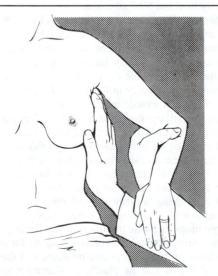

**Figure 62–6.** Palpation of axillary region for enlarged lymph nodes.

size of the primary tumor and with the local invasiveness of the neoplasm.

Usually no nodes are palpable in the supraclavicular fossa. Firm or hard nodes of any size in this location or just beneath the clavicle (infraclavicular nodes) are suggestive of metastic cancer and should be biopsied. Ipsilateral supraclavicular or infraclavicular nodes containing cancer indicate that the patient is in an advanced stage of the disease (stage IV). Edema of the ipsilateral arm, commonly caused by metastatic infiltration of regional lymphatics, is also a sign of advanced (stage IV) cancer.

**C. Special Clinical Forms of Breast Carcinoma:**

**1. Paget's carcinoma**–The basic lesion is usually an infiltrating intraductal carcinoma, usually well differentiated and multicentric in the nipple and breast ducts. The nipple epithelium is infiltrated, but gross nipple changes are often minimal, and a tumor mass may not be palpable. The first symptom is often itching or burning of the nipple, with a superficial erosion or ulceration. The diagnosis is established by biopsy of the erosion.

Paget's carcinoma is not common (about 1% of all breast cancers), but it is important because it appears innocuous. It is frequently diagnosed and treated as dermatitis or bacterial infection, leading to unfortunate delay in detection. When the lesion consists of nipple changes only, the incidence of axillary metastases is about 5%. When a breast tumor is also present, the incidence of axillary metastases rises, with an associated marked decrease in prospects for cure by surgical or other treatment.

**2. Inflammatory carcinoma**–This is the most malignant form of breast cancer and constitutes less than 3% of all cases. The clinical findings consist of a rapidly growing, sometimes painful mass that enlarges the breast. The overlying skin becomes erythematous, edematous, and warm. Often there is no distinct mass, since the tumor infiltrates the involved breast diffusely. The diagnosis should be made when the redness involves more than one-third of the skin over the breast and biopsy shows invasion of the subdermal lymphatics. The inflammatory changes, often mistaken for an infectious process, are caused by carcinomatous invasion of the dermal lymphatics, with resulting edema and hyperemia. If the physician suspects infection but the lesion does not respond rapidly (1–2 weeks) to antibiotics, a biopsy must be performed. Metastases tend to occur early and widely, and for this reason inflammatory carcinoma is rarely curable. Mastectomy is seldom, if ever, indicated. Radiation, hormone therapy, and anticancer chemotherapy are the measures most likely to be of value.

**3. Occurrence during pregnancy or lactation**–Cancer of the breast diagnosed in pregnancy has a ratio of occurrence from 1:3000 to 1:10,000. The association of pregnancy and breast cancer presents a therapeutic dilemma for the patient and the physician. Numerous studies differ regarding the prognosis; some show poorer outcome, while others demonstrate no difference. Termination of the pregnancy, formerly performed routinely in the first two trimesters, has not been demonstrated to improve outcome. In addition, the use of radiotherapy is contraindicated because of the potential for fetal damage. The use of chemotherapy, for similar reasons, is debatable.

In most instances, modified radical mastectomy in pregnancy is the minimal treatment of choice, with the possible exception of the latter part of the third trimester, wherein lumpectomy and radiotherapy in the puerperium may be considered.

**4. Bilateral breast cancer**–Clinically evident simultaneous bilateral breast cancer occurs in less than 1% of cases, but there is a 5–8% incidence of later occurrence of cancer in the second breast. Bilaterality occurs more often in women under age 50 and is more frequent when the tumor in the primary breast is lobular. The incidence of second breast cancers increases directly with the length of time the patient is alive after her first cancer, and is approximately 0.5% per year.

In patients with breast cancer, mammography should be performed before primary treatment and at regular intervals thereafter, to search for occult cancer in the opposite breast. Routine biopsy of the opposite breast is usually not warranted.

**D. Mammography:** Mammography is the only reliable means of detecting breast cancer before a mass can be palpated in the breast. Some breast cancers can be identified by mammography as long as 2 years before reaching a size detectable by palpation.

Although false-positive and false-negative results are occasionally obtained with mammography, the experienced radiologist can interpret mammograms correctly in about 90% of cases.

Other than for screening, indications for mammography are as follows: (1) to evaluate each breast when a diagnosis of potentially curable breast cancer has been made, and at yearly intervals thereafter; (2) to evaluate a questionable or ill-defined breast mass or other suspicious change in the breast; (3) to search for an occult breast cancer in a woman with metastatic disease in axillary nodes or elsewhere from an unknown primary; (4) to screen at regular intervals a selected group of women who are at high risk for developing breast cancer (see below), (5) to screen women prior to cosmetic operations or prior to biopsy; and (6) to follow women who have been treated with breast-conserving surgery and radiation.

Patients with a dominant or suspicious mass must undergo biopsy despite mammographic findings. The mammogram should be obtained prior to biopsy so that other suspicious areas can be noted and the contralateral breast can be checked. Mammography is never a substitute for biopsy, because it may not reveal clinical cancer in a very dense breast, as may be seen in young women with fibrocystic change, and often does not reveal medullary type cancer.

**E. Cytology:** Cytologic examination of nipple discharge or cyst fluid may be helpful on rare occasions. As a rule, mammography and breast biopsy are required when nipple discharge or cyst fluid is bloody or cytologically questionable.

**F. Biopsy:** The diagnosis of breast cancer depends ultimately upon examination of tissue removed by biopsy. Treatment should never be undertaken without an unequivocal histologic diagnosis of cancer. The safest course is biopsy examination of all suspicious masses found on physical examination and, in the absence of a mass, of suspicious lesions demonstrated by mammography. About 30% of lesions thought to be definitely cancer prove on biopsy to be benign, and about 15% of lesions believed to be benign are found to be malignant. These findings demonstrate the fallibility of clinical judgment and the necessity for biopsy.

The simplest method is needle biopsy, either by aspiration of tumor cells or, preferably, by obtaining a small core of tissue with a Vim–Silverman or other special needle. A negative needle biopsy should be followed by open biopsy, because false-negative needle biopsies may occur in 15–20% of cancers.

The preferred method is open biopsy under local anesthesia as a separate procedure prior to deciding upon definitive treatment. The patient need not be admitted to the hospital. Decisions on additional workup for metastatic disease and on definitive therapy can be made and discussed with the patient after the histologic diagnosis of cancer has been established. This approach has the advantage of avoiding unnecessary hospitalization and diagnostic procedures in many patients, since cancer is found in the minority of patients who require biopsy for diagnosis of a breast lump.

In general, the 2-step approach—that is, outpatient biopsy followed by definitive operation at a later date—allows patients to be given time to adjust to the diagnosis of cancer, to carefully consider alternative forms of therapy, and to seek a second opinion should they feel it important. Studies have shown no adverse effect from the short (1–2 weeks) delay of the 2-step procedure, and this is the current recommendation of the National Cancer Institute.

At the time of the initial biopsy of breast cancer, it is important for the physician to preserve a portion of the specimen for determination of estrogen receptors.

**G. Laboratory Findings:** A consistently elevated sedimentation rate may be the result of disseminated cancer. Liver or bone metastases may be associated with elevation of serum alkaline phosphatase. Hypercalcemia is an occasional important finding in advanced cancer of the breast. Carcinoembryonic antigen (CEA) may be used as a marker for recurrent breast cancer.

**H. X-Ray Findings:** Chest x-rays may show pulmonary metastases. CT scan of liver and brain is of value only when metastases are suspected in these areas.

**I. Radionuclide Scanning:** Bone scans utilizing technetium 99m-labeled phosphates or phosphonates are more sensitive than skeletal x-rays in detecting metastic breast cancer. Bone scanning has not proved to be of clinical value as a routine preoperative test in the absence of symptoms, physical findings, or abnormal alkaline phosphatase levels. the frequency of abnormal findings on bone scan parallels the status of the axillary lymph nodes on pathologic examination.

### Early Detection

**A. Screening Programs:** A number of mass screening programs consisting of physical and mammographic examination of the breasts of asymptomatic women have been conducted. They are identifying more than 6 cancers per 1000 women. About 80% of these women have negative axillary lymph nodes at the time of surgery, whereas, by contrast, only 45% of patients found in the course of usual medical practice have uninvolved axillary nodes. Detecting breast cancer before it has spread to the axillary nodes greatly increases the chance of survival, and about 85% of such women will survive at least 5 years.

Both physical examination and mammography are necessary for maximum yield in screening programs, since about 40% of early breast cancers can be discovered only by mammography, and another 40% can be detected only by palpation. Women 20–40 years of age should have a breast examination as part of routine medical care every 2–3 years. Women over age 40 should have yearly breast examinations.

The American College of Radiology and the American Cancer Society have revised their recommendations regarding use of mammography in asymptomatic women. A baseline mammogram should be performed on all women between ages 35 and 40 years. Women aged 40–49 years should have a mammogram every 1–2 years. Annual mammograms are indicated for women age 50 years or older. High-risk women—those whose mothers or sisters had bilateral or premenopausal breast cancer, those who have had cancer of one breast, and those with histologic abnormalities associated with subsequent cancer (eg, atypical epithelial hyperplasia, papillomatosis, lobular carcinoma in situ)—should have an annual mammogram and biannual examinations. In a recent large study of women under age 50, nearly half of all cancers were detected by mammography alone. Mammographic patterns are not a reliable predictor of the risk of developing breast cancer.

Automated breast ultrasonography is very useful in distinguishing cystic from solid lesions but should be used only as a supplement to physical examination and mammography in screening for breast cancer.

**B. Self-Examination:** All women over age 20

should be advised to examine their breasts monthly. Premenopausal women should perform the examination 7–8 days after the menstrual period, and high-risk patients may be asked to perform a second examination in midcycle. The breasts should be inspected initially while standing before a mirror with the hands at the sides, overhead, and pressed firmly on the hips to contract the pectoralis muscles. Masses, asymmetry of breasts, and slight dimpling of the skin may become apparent as a result of these maneuvers. Next, in a supine position, each breast should be carefully palpated with the fingers of the opposite hand. Physicians should instruct women in the technique of self-examination and advise them to report at once for medical evaluation if a mass or other abnormality is noted. Some women discover small breast lumps more readily when their skin is moist while bathing or showering.

## Differential Diagnosis

The lesions most often to be considered in the differential diagnosis of breast cancer include, in order of frequency, fibrocystic change, fibroadenoma, intraductal papilloma, and fat necrosis. The differential diagnosis of a breast lump should be established without delay by biopsy, by aspiration of a cyst, or by observing the patient until disappearance of the lump within a period of a few weeks.

## Pathologic Types

Numerous pathologic subtypes of breast cancer can be identified histologically (Table 62–3). These pathologic types are distinguished by the histologic appearance and growth pattern of the tumor. In general, breast cancer arises either from the epithelial lining of the large or intermediate-sized ducts (ductal) or from the epithelium of the terminal ducts of the lobules (lobular). The cancer may be invasive or in situ. Most breast cancers arise from the intermediate ducts and are invasive (invasive ductal, infiltrating ductal), and most histologic types are merely subtypes of in-

**Table 62–3.** Histologic types of breast cancer.

| Type | Percent Occurrence |
|---|---|
| Infiltrating ductal (not otherwise specified) | 70–80 |
|    Medullary | 5–8 |
|    Colloid (mucinous) | 2–4 |
|    Tubular | 1–2 |
|    Papillary | 1–2 |
| Invasive lobular | 6–8 |
| Noninvasive | 4–6 |
|    Intraductal | 2–3 |
|    Lobular in situ | 2–3 |
| Rare cancers | < 1 |
|    Juvenile (secretory) | — |
|    Adenoid cystic | — |
|    Epidermoid | — |
|    Sudiferous | — |

vasive ductal cancer with unusual growth patterns (colloid, medullary, scirrhous, etc). Ductal carcinoma that has not invaded the extraductal tissue is intraductal or in situ ductal. Lobular carcinoma may be either invasive or in situ.

The histologic subtypes have only a little bearing on prognosis when outcomes are compared after accurate staging. Various histologic parameters, such as invasion of blood vessels, tumor differentiation, invasion of breast lymphatics, and tumor necrosis have been examined, but they too seem to have little prognostic value.

The noninvasive cancers by definition lack the ability to spread. However, in patients whose biopsies show noninvasive intraductal cancer, associated invasive ductal cancers are present in 1–3% of cases. Lobular carcinoma in situ is considered by some to be a premalignant lesion that by itself is not a true cancer. It lacks the ability to spread but is associated with the subsequent development of invasive cancer in at least 30% of cases.

## Hormone Receptor Sites

The presence of absence of estrogen receptors in the cytoplasm of tumor cells is of paramount importance in managing patients with recurrent or metastatic disease. Up to 60% of patients with metastatic breast cancer will respond to hormonal manipulation if their tumors contain estrogen receptors. However, fewer than 10% of patients with metastatic, estrogen receptor-negative tumors can be successfully treated with hormonal manipulation.

Progesterone receptors may be an even more sensitive indicator than estrogen receptors of patients who may respond to hormonal manipulation. Up to 80% of patients with metastatic progesterone receptor-positive tumors seem to respond to hormonal manipulation. Receptors probably have no relationship to response to chemotherapy.

Some studies suggest that estrogen receptors are of prognostic significance. Patients whose primary tumors are receptor-positive have a more favorable course after mastectomy than those whose tumors are receptor-negative.

Receptor status is not only valuable for the management of metastatic disease but also may help in the selection of patients for adjuvant therapy. Some studies suggest that hormonal therapy (tamoxifen) for patients with receptor-positive tumors treated by mastectomy may improve survival rates.

It is advisable to obtain an estrogen-receptor assay for every breast cancer at the time of initial diagnosis. Receptor status may change after hormonal therapy, radiotherapy, or chemotherapy. The specimen requires special handling, and the laboratory should be prepared to process the specimen correctly.

## Curative Treatment

Treatment may be curative or palliative. Curative treatment is advised for clinical stage I and II disease (see Table 62–2). Treatment can only be palliative for patients in stage IV and for previously treated patients who develop distant metastases or unresectable local recurrence.

**A. Therapeutic Options: Radical mastectomy** involves en bloc removal of the breast, pectoral muscles, and axillary nodes and was the standard curative procedure for breast cancer from the turn of the century until about 10 years ago. Radical mastectomy removes the primary lesion and the axillary nodes with a wide margin of surrounding tissue, including the pectoral muscles. **Extended radical mastectomy** involves, in addition to standard radical mastectomy, removal of the internal mammary nodes. It has been recommended by a few surgeons for medially or centrally placed breast lesions and for tumors associated with positive axillary nodes, because of the known frequency of internal mammary node metastases under these circumstances. **Modified radical mastectomy** (total mastectomy plus axillary dissection) consists of en bloc removal of the breast with the underlying pectoralis major fascia (but not the muscle) and axillary lymph nodes. Some surgeons remove the pectoralis minor muscle. Others retract or transect the muscle to facilitate removal of the axillary lymph nodes. Modified radical mastectomy gives superior cosmetic and functional results compared with standard radical mastectomy. **Simple mastectomy** (total mastectomy) consists of removing the entire breast, leaving the axillary nodes intact. Limited procedures such as **segmental mastectomy** (lumpectomy, quadrant excision, partial mastectomy) are becoming more popular as definitive treatment for early breast cancer (eg, stage I). The proved efficacy of **irradiation** in sterilizing the primary lesion and the axillary and internal mammary nodes has made radiation therapy with segmental mastectomy a reasonable option for primary treatment of most breast cancers.

**B. Choice of Primary Therapy:** The extent of disease and its biologic aggressiveness are the principal determinants of the outcome of primary therapy. Clinical and pathologic staging help in assessing extent of disease (see Table 62–2), but each is to some extent imprecise. Since about two-thirds of patients eventually manifest distant disease regardless of the form of primary therapy, there is a tendency to think of breast carcinoma as being systemic in most patients at the time they first present for treatment.

There is a great deal of controversy regarding the optimal method of primary therapy of stage I, II, and III breast carcinoma, and opinions on this subject have changed considerably in the past decade. Legislation initiated in California and Massachusetts and now adopted in numerous states requires physicians to inform patients of alternative treatment methods in the management of breast cancer.

## Radical Mastectomy

For about three-quarters of a century, radical mastectomy was considered standard therapy for this disease. The procedure was designed to remove the primary lesion, the breast in which it arose, the underlying muscle, and, by dissection in continuity, the axillary lymph nodes that were thought to be the first site of spread beyond the breast. When radical mastectomy was introduced by Halsted, the average patient presented for treatment with advanced local disease (stage III), and a relatively extensive procedure was often necessary just to remove all gross cancer. This is no longer the case. Patients present now with much smaller, less locally advanced lesions. Most of the patients in Halsted's original series would now be considered incurable by surgery alone, since they had extensive involvement of the chest wall, skin, and supraclavicular regions.

Although radical mastectomy is extremely effective in controlling local disease, it has the disadvantage of being one of the most deforming of any of the available treatments for management of primary breast cancer. The surgeon and patient are both eager to find therapy that is less deforming but does not jeopardize the chance for cure.

## Less Radical Surgery & Radiation Therapy

A number of clinical trials have been performed in the past decade in which the magnitude of the surgical procedure undertaken for removal of cancer in the breast and adjacent lymph nodes has been varied, with and without the use of local radiotherapy to the chest wall and node-bearing areas.

Radical mastectomy, modified radical mastectomy, and simple mastectomy have been compared in numerous clinical trials. In general, radical mastectomy has a slightly lower local recurrence rate than modified radical or simple mastectomy. Simple mastectomy has the highest regional recurrence rate, since the lymph nodes are not removed, and as many as 30% of patients with clinically negative nodes will have metastatic breast cancer within these nodes. At least half of these patients subsequently develop regional recurrences. Despite these differences in local and regional effect, no significant differences in survival have been consistently demonstrated among these 3 types of treatment. The addition of radiotherapy to mastectomy will also reduce the incidence of local recurrence, but in general, radiotherapy does not improve overall survival rates. Even the removal of occult cancer in axillary lymph nodes generally is not reflected in improvement in over all survival rates, although regional failures will be much lower.

The most significant recent advance in the management of primary breast cancer has been the realization that less than total mastectomy combined with radiotherapy may be as effective as more radical operations alone for certain patients with small primary tumors. Studies are still relatively recent, however, and long-term follow-up is necessary for definite conclusions. Patients with large or stage III breast cancers may benefit from a combination of surgery, radiotherapy, and systemic chemotherapy.

Radiation therapy alone (without surgery) in the treatment of primary breast cancer fails to achieve local control in about 50% of cases. Small, nonrandomized studies have suggested that removal of the tumor by segmental mastectomy, or "lumpectomy," combined with postoperative irradiation is as effective as mastectomy in achieving local control without diminishing long-term survival.

The results of the Milan trial and a large randomized trial conducted by the National Surgical Adjuvant Breast Project (NSABP) in the USA showed that disease-free survival rates were similar for patients treated by partial mastectomy plus axillary dissection followed by radiation therapy and for those treated by modified radical mastectomy (total mastectomy plus axillary dissection). All patients whose axillary nodes contained tumor- received adjuvant chemotherapy.

In an earlier NSABP trial, patients were randomized to one of the following treatments: (1) radical mastectomy, (2) total mastectomy plus radiation therapy, and (3) total mastectomy followed by axillary dissection if clinically negative axillary nodes later became clinically positive. Among patients with clinically negative nodes, there were no differences in disease-free or overall survival rates with the 3 modes of treatment. Among those with clinically positive axillary nodes, there were no differences in outcome following radical mastectomy or total mastectomy plus radiation therapy.

The results of these and other trials have demonstrated that much less aggressive surgical treatment of the primary lesion than has previously been thought necessary gives equivalent results.

It is important to recognize that axillary dissection is valuable both in planning therapy and in staging of the cancer. Operation is extremely effective in preventing axillary recurrences. In addition, lymph nodes removed during the procedure can be pathologically assessed. This assessment is essential for the planning of adjuvant therapy, which is often recommended for patients with gross or occult involvement of axillary nodes.

## Current Recommendations

We believe that partial mastectomy plus axillary dissection and radiation therapy or total mastectomy plus axillary dissection (modified radical mastectomy) in the best initial treatment for most patients with potentially curable carcinoma of the breast. Radical mastectomy may rarely be required for some cases of advanced local disease if the tumor invades the muscle but otherwise is not advisable for the average patient. Similarly, extended radical mastectomy would rarely be appropriate. Treatment of the axillary nodes is not indicated for noninfiltrating cancers, be-

cause nodal metastases are present in only 1% of such patients.

Preoperatively, full discussion with the patient regarding the rationale for mastectomy and the manner of coping with the cosmetic and psychologic effects of the operation is essential. Patients often have questions about possible alternatives to standard or modified radical mastectomy—eg, local excision, simple mastectomy, and radiotherapy—and wish detailed explanations of the risks and benefits of the various procedures. Women with small tumors (ie, < 2 cm) and clinically negative axillary nodes should have the option of treatment by partial mastectomy (lumpectomy) plus axillary dissection and radiotherapy. Breast reconstruction should be discussed with the patient. Time spent preoperatively in educating the patient and her family is time well spent.

## Adjuvant Therapy

Chemotherapy is now used as adjunctive treatment of patients with curable breast cancer and positive axillary nodes, since there is a great likelihood that these patients harbor occult metastases. Overall, about 75% of such patients eventually succumb within 10 years, even though the initial therapy, either surgery or irradiation, eradicated all neoplasm evident at that time. The objective of adjuvant chemotherapy is to eliminate the occult metastases responsible for late recurrences while they are microscopic and theoretically most vulnerable to anticancer agents.

Numerous clinical trials with various adjuvant chemotherapeutic regimens have been completed. The most extensive clinical experience to date is with the CMF regimen (*c*yclophosphamide, *m*ethotrexate, and *f*luorouracil). The regimen should be repeated for 6 months in patients with axillary metastases. Follow-up studies at 8 years show that premenopausal women definitely benefit from receiving adjuvant chemotherapy, whereas postmenopausal women may not. The recurrence rate in premenopausal patients who received no adjuvant chemotherapy was more that $1\frac{1}{2}$ times that of those who received therapy. No therapeutic effect with CMF has been shown in postmenopausal women, perhaps because therapy was modified so often in response to side effects that the total amount of drugs administered was less than planned. Other trials with different agents support the value of adjuvant chemotherapy; in some cases, postmenopausal women appear to benefit. Combinations of drugs are clearly superior to single drugs.

Adjuvant chemotherapy can be offered confidently to premenopausal women with metastases in axillary lymph nodes, but the use of adjuvant chemotherapy in postmenopausal women and patients with negative findings in axillary lymph nodes is more controversial. It is difficult to determine which regimen is appropriate for which subgroup of women with breast cancer. Some studies show a beneficial effect in premenopausal but not postmenopausal women, while other studies utilizing different combinations of agents show a beneficial effect in postmenopausal but not premenopausal women. In addition, the estrogen receptor status of the tumor must be taken into consideration when chemotherapy is being planned. Some agents were shown to be effective in randomized studies, and others have been shown to be effective when compared with historical controls. In general, comparison with historical controls is less convincing proof of effect than are concurrent randomized prospective trials. For this reason, controversy persists regarding which agents are most beneficial for particular patients with breast cancer.

The addition of hormones may improve the results of adjuvant therapy. For example, tamoxifen has been shown to enhance the beneficial effects of melphalan and fluorouracil in women whose tumors are estrogen receptor-positive. Interestingly, in this study, improvement in disease-free survival rates was seen only in postmenopausal women. Tamoxifen has been used alone with some success as adjuvant treatment for postmenopausal women with estrogen receptor-positive tumors.

The length of time adjuvant therapy must be administered remains uncertain. Several studies suggest that shorter treatment periods may be as effective as longer ones. The Milan group has compared 6 versus 12 cycles of postoperative CMF and found 5-year disease-free survival rates to be comparable. One of the earliest adjuvant trials (Nissen-Meyer, 1982) used a 6-day perioperative regimen of intravenous cyclophosphamide alone, follow-up at 15 years shows a 15% improvement in disease-free survival rates for treated patients, suggesting that short-term therapy may be effective.

Patients with estrogen receptor-negative tumors, even without axillary lymph node involvement, may have a recurrence rate as high as 30% within the first 2 years after operation. For this reason, a number of clinical studies are investigating the value of adjuvant chemotherapy in women with estrogen receptor-negative tumors and no evidence of axillary lymph node involvement. Preliminary results suggest that these patients may benefit from adjuvant systemic chemotherapy; however, these studies are not yet conclusive.

An NIH consensus development conference in 1985 summarized the studies of adjuvant treatment of breast cancer. In 1988, a Clinical Alert from the National Cancer Institute was mailed to practicing physicians. The conclusions from these 2 publications may be summarized as follows:

1. Premenopausal women with positive lymph-nodes and either estrogen receptor-positive or estrogen receptor-negative tumors should be treated with adjuvant combination chemotherapy.

2. Premenopausal women with negative nodes whose tumors are estrogen receptor-positive may

benefit from tamoxifen. Premenopausal women with negative axillary nodes whose tumors are estrogen receptor-negative may benefit from combination chemotherapy.

3. Postmenopausal patients with positive lymph-nodes whose tumors are estrogen receptor-negative may benefit from adjuvant combination chemotherapy.

4. Postmenopausal women with negative axillary nodes whose tumors are estrogen receptor-positive may benefit from tamoxifen. Postmenopausal women with negative axillary lymph nodes whose tumors are estrogen receptor-negative may benefit from adjuvant chemotherapy.

The NIH concluded in the Clinical Alert that "adjuvant hormonal or adjuvant cytotoxic chemotherapy can have a meaningful impact on the natural history of node negative breast cancer patients." However, the short follow-up in the node-negative studies and the lack of an observed effect on survival has still not completely clarified the role of adjuvant therapy for these patients. (See Tables 62–4 and 62–5.)

Important questions remaining to be answered are the timing and duration of adjuvant chemotherapy, which chemotherapeutic agents should be applied for which subgroups of patients, how best to coordinate adjuvant chemotherapy with postoperative radiation therapy, the use of hormonal therapy, and the use of combinations of hormonal and chemotherapy.

## Follow-Up Care

After primary therapy, patients with breast cancer should be followed for life for at least 2 reasons: to detect recurrences and to observe the opposite breast for a second primary carcinoma. Local and distant metastases occur most frequently within the first 3 years. During this period, the patient is examined every 3–4 months. Thereafter, examination is done every 6 months until 5 years postoperatively and then every 6–12 months. Special attention is given to the remaining breast, because of the increased risk of developing a second primary tumor. The patient should examine her own breast monthly, and a mammogram should be obtained annually. In some cases, metastases are dormant for long periods and may appear up to 10–15 years or longer after removal of the primary tumor. Because there has been no definitive evidence

**Table 62–4.** Summary of NIH Consensus Conference and Clinical Alert on adjuvant chemotherapy for premenopausal women.

| Nodal Involvement | Estrogen Receptors | Adjuvant Systemic Therapy |
|---|---|---|
| Yes | Positive | Combination chemotherapy |
| Yes | Negative | Combination chemotherapy |
| No | Positive | Probably tamoxifen |
| No | Negative | Probably combination chemotherapy |

**Table 62–5.** Summary of NIH Consensus Conference and Clinical Alert on adjuvant chemotherapy for postmenopausal women.

| Nodal Involvement | Estrogen Receptors | Adjuvant Systemic Therapy |
|---|---|---|
| Yes | Positive | Tamoxifen |
| Yes | Negative | Probably combination chemotherapy |
| No | Positive | Probably tamoxifen |
| No | Negative | Probably combination chemotherapy |

of deleterious effects of estrogen replacement therapy in postmenopausal women with previous breast cancer, until further studies are done, such patients should be counseled regarding the theoretic adverse effects of the estrogen replacement versus the proven beneficial effects (DiSaia, 1993).

**A. Local Recurrence:** The incidence of local recurrence correlates with tumor size, the presence and number of involved axillary nodes, the histologic type of tumor, and the presence of skin edema or skin and fascia fixation with the primary tumor. About 15% of patients develop local recurrence after total mastectomy and axillary dissection. When the axillary nodes are not involved, the local recurrence rate is 5%, but the rate is 25% when they are involved. A similar difference in local recurrence rate was noted between small and large tumors. Factors that affect the rate of local recurrence in patients who have had partial mastectomies are not yet determined. However, early studies show that such things as multifocal cancer, in situ tumors, positive resection margins, chemotherapy, and timing of radiotherapy are likely to be important.

Chest wall recurrences usually appear within the first 2 years but may occur as late as 15 or more years after mastectomy. Suspect nodules should be biopsied. Local excision or localized radiotherapy may be feasible if an isolated nodule is present. If lesions are multiple or accompanied by evidence of regional involvement in the internal mammary or supraclavicular nodes, the disease is best managed by radiation treatment of the whole chest wall including the parasternal, supraclavicular, and axillary areas.

Local recurrence may signal the presence of widespread disease and is an indication for bone and liver scans, posteroanterior and lateral chest x-rays, and other examinations as needed to search for evidence of metastases. When there is no evidence of metastases beyond the chest wall and regional nodes, radical irradiation for cure of complete local excision should be attempted. Most patients with locally recurrent tumor will develop distant metastases within 2 years. For this reason, many physicians use systemic therapy for treatment of patients with local recurrence. Although this seems reasonable, it should be pointed out that patients with local recurrence may be cured with local resection or radiation. Systemic chemotherapy or hormonal treatment should be used for patients who develop disseminated disease or those in whom local recurrence occurs following adequate local therapy.

**B. Edema of the Arm:** Significant edema of the arm occurs in 10–30% of patients after radical mastectomy and in about 5% after modified radical mastectomy. Edema of the arm is less frequent after modified radical mastectomy than after radical mastectomy and occurs more commonly if radiotherapy has been given or if there was postoperative infection. Early trials suggest that partial mastectomy with radiation to the axillary lymph nodes is followed by chronic edema of the arm in 10–20% of patients. To avoid this complication, many authorities advocate axillary lymph node sampling rather than complete axillary dissection. Judicious use of radiotherapy, with treatment fields carefully planned to spare the axilla as much as possible, can greatly diminish the incidence of edema. Since axillary dissection is a more accurate staging operation than axillary sampling, we recommend axillary dissection, with removal of at least level I and II lymph nodes, in combination with partial mastectomy.

Late or secondary edema of the arm may develop years after radical mastectomy, as a result of axillary recurrence or of infection in the hand or arm, with obliteration of lymphatic channels. There is usually no obvious cause of late arm swelling.

**C. Breast Reconstruction:** Breast reconstruction, with the implantation of a prosthesis, is usually feasible after standard or modified radical mastectomy. Reconstruction should be discussed with patients prior to mastectomy, because it offers an important psychologic focal point for recovery. Reconstruction is not an obstacle to the diagnosis of recurrent cancer.

**Prognosis**

The stage of breast cancer is the single most reliable indicator of prognosis. Patients with disease localized to the breast and no evidence of regional spread after microscopic examination of the lymph nodes have by far the most favorable prognosis. Estrogen and progesterone receptors appear to be an important prognostic variable, because patients with hormone receptor-negative tumors and no evidence of metastases to the axillary lymph nodes have a much higher recurrence rate than do patients with hormone receptor-positive tumors and no regional metastases. The histologic subtype of breast cancer (eg, medullary, lobular, comedo) seems to have little, if any, significance in prognosis once these tumors are truly invasive. Flow cytometry to analyze DNA ploidy may aid in prognosis.

As mentioned above, several different treatment regimens achieve approximately the same results when given to the appropriate patient. Localized disease can be controlled with local therapy—either surgery alone or limited surgery in combination with radiation therapy. However, the criteria for selection of patients to be treated with conservative resection and radiation therapy require further clarification.

Most patients who develop breast cancer will ultimately die of breast cancer. The mortality rate of breast cancer patients exceeds that of age-matched normal controls for nearly 20 years. Thereafter, the mortality rates are equal, although deaths that occur among the breast cancer patients are often directly the result of tumor. Five-year statistics do not accurately reflect the final outcome of therapy.

When cancer is localized to the breast, with no evidence of regional spread after pathologic examination, the clinical cure rate with most accepted methods of therapy is 75–90%. Exceptions to this may be related to the hormonal receptor content of the tumor, tumor size, host resistance, or associated illness. Patients with small estrogen and progesterone receptor-positive tumors and no evidence of axillary spread probably have a 5-year survival rate of nearly 90%. When the axillary lymph nodes are involved with tumor, the survival rate drops to 40–50% at 5 years and probably less than 25% at 10 years. In general, breast cancer appears to be somewhat more malignant in younger than older women, and this may be related to the fact that fewer younger women have estrogen receptor-positive tumors.

## TREATMENT OF ADVANCED BREAST CANCER

This section covers palliative therapy of disseminated disease incurable by surgery (stage IV).

### Radiotherapy

Palliative radiotherapy may be advised for locally advanced cancers with distant metastases in order to control ulceration, pain, and other manifestations in the breast and regional nodes. Radical irradiation of the breast and chest wall and the axillary, internal mammary, and supraclavicular nodes should be undertaken in an attempt to cure locally advanced and inoperable lesions when there is no evidence of distant metastases. A small number of patients in this group are cured in spite of extensive breast and regional node involvement. Adjuvant chemotherapy should be considered for such patients.

Palliative irradiation is also of value in the treatment of certain bone or soft tissue metastases to control pain or avoid fracture. Radiotherapy is especially useful in the treatment of the isolated bony metastasis and chest wall recurrences.

### Hormone Therapy

Disseminated disease may respond to prolonged endocrine therapy such as administration of hormones; or administration of drugs that block hormone receptor sites (eg, antiestrogens) or drugs that block the synthesis of hormones (eg, amino-glutethimide). Hormonal manipulation is usually more successful in postmenopausal women. If treatment is based on the presence of estrogen receptor protein in the primary tumor or metastases, however, the rate of response is nearly equal in premenopausal and postmenopausal women. A favorable response to hormonal manipulation occurs in about one-third of patients with metastatic breast cancer. Of those whose tumors contain estrogen receptors, the response is about 60% and perhaps as high as 80% for patients whose tumors contain progesterone receptors as well. Because only 5–10% of women whose tumors do not contain estrogen receptors respond, they should not receive hormonal therapy except in unusual circumstances.

Since the quality of life during a remission induced by endocrine manipulation is usually superior to a remission following cytotoxic chemotherapy, it is usually best to try endocrine manipulation first in cases where the estrogen receptor status of the tumor is unknown. However, if the estrogen receptor status is unknown but the disease is progressing rapidly or involves visceral organs, endocrine therapy is rarely successful, and introducing it may waste valuable time.

In general, only one type of systemic therapy should be given at a time, unless it is necessary to irradiate a destructive lesion of weight-bearing bone while the patient is on another regimen. The regimen should be changed only if the disease is clearly progressing but not if it appears to be stable. This is especially important for patients with destructive bone metastases, since minor changes in the status of these lesions are difficult to determine radiographically. A plan of therapy that would simultaneously minimize toxicity and maximize benefits is often best achieved by hormonal manipulation.

The choice of endocrine therapy depends on the menopausal status of the patient. Women with 1 year of their last menstrual period are considered to be premenopausal, while women whose menstruation ceased more than a year ago are postmenopausal. The initial choice of therapy is referred to as primary hormonal manipulation; subsequent endocrine treatment is called secondary or tertiary hormonal manipulation.

### Treatment of Advanced Breast Cancer Hormone Therapy

**A. The Premenopausal Patient:**

**1. Primary hormonal therapy**–In the past, bilateral oophorectomy had been the standard method of hormone manipulation employed in premenopausal women with advanced breast cancer. However, it has subsequently become clear that the antiestrogen tamoxifen is equally effective and has none of the attendant risks of surgical ablation of the ovaries. Tamoxifen, therefore, is now recommended as the treatment of choice for hormonal therapy in the premenopausal woman with advanced breast cancer.

**2. Secondary or tertiary hormonal therapy–** A favorable response to initial hormonal therapy with tamoxifen is predictive of future responses to hormonal maneuver.

Other hormonal agents have been found effective in premenopausal patients. GnRH analogies that result in down regulation of the pituitary with eventual suppression of FSH and LH, and subsequent decrease in estrogen production by the ovary, have equivalent response rates to tamoxifen in some situations.

The use of aminoglutethimide, an antiadrenal agent, which works by blocking the conversion of testosterone to estradiol and androstenedione to estrogen both in the adrenal cortex and in peripheral tissue including breast cancers themselves, has been shown to be effective.

Progestins, megestrol acetate, and medroxyprogesterone acetate have also yielded good tumor response. Finally, new antitumorigenic agents such as somatostatin analogues (probably mediated through growth hormone) are being investigated.

**B. The Postmenopausal Patient:**

**1. Primary hormonal therapy–**Tamoxifen, 10 mg twice daily, is now the initial therapy of choice for postmenopausal women with metastatic breast cancer amenable to endocrine manipulation.

## Chemotherapy

Cytotoxic drugs should be considered for the treatment of metastatic breast cancer (1) if visceral metastases are present (especially brain or lymphangitic pulmonary), (2) if hormonal treatment is unsuccessful or the disease has progressed after an initial response to hormonal manipulation, or (3) if the tumor is estrogen receptor-negative. The most useful single chemotherapeutic agent to date is doxorubicin (Adriamycin), with a response rate of 40–50%. The remissions tend to be brief, and, in general, experience with single-agent chemotherapy in patients with disseminated disease has not been encouraging.

Combination chemotherapy using multiple agents has proved to be more effective, with objectively observed favorable responses achieved in 60–80% of patients with stage IV disease. Various combinations of drugs have been used, and clinical trials are continuing in an effort to improve results and to reduce undesirable side effects. Doxorubicin and cyclophosphamide produced an objective response in 87% of 46 patients who had an adequate trial of therapy. Other chemotherapeutic regimens have consisted of various combinations of drugs, including cyclphosphamide, vincristine, methotrexate, and fluorouracil, with response rates ranging up to 60–70%. Prior adjuvant chemotherapy does not seem to alter response rates in patients who relapse. Few new drugs or combinations of drugs have been sufficiently effective in breast cancer to warrant wide acceptance.

## REFERENCES

### GENERAL

Aamdal S et al: Estrogen receptors and long-term prognosis in breast cancer. Cancer 1984;53:2525.

American Cancer Society: *Cancer Facts and Figures: 1993*. American Cancer Society, 1993.

DiSaia PJ: Hormone-replacement therapy in patients with breast cancer. A reappraisal. Cancer 1993;71 (suppl):1490.

Glauber JG, Kiang DT: The changing role of hormonal therapy in advanced breast cancer. Semin Oncol 1992; 19:308.

Haagensen CD: *Diseases of the Breast*, 3rd ed. Saunders, 1985.

Harris JR et al. (editors): *Breast Diseases*, 2nd ed. Lippincott, 1985.

Hindle WH: *Breast Disease for Gynecologists*. Appleton & Lange, 1990.

Marchant DJ: Breast Cancer: challenge and responsibility. Cancer 1993;71(suppl):1518.

Zeigler LD, Buzdar AU: Recent advances in the treatment of breast cancer. AM J Med Sci 1991;301:337.

### FIBROCYSTIC CHANGE

Dupont WD, Page DL: Risk factor for breast cancer in women with proliferative breast disease. N Engl J Med 1985;312:146.

Hutter RVP: Goodbye to "fibrocystic disease." (Editorial.) N Engl J Med 1985;312:179.

### CYSTOSARCOMA OF THE BREAST

Briggs RM, Walters M, Rosenthal D: Cystosarcoma phyllodes in adolescent female patients. Am J Surg 1983;146:712.

Pietruszka M, Barnes L: Cystosarcoma phyllodes: A clinicopathologic analysis of 42 cases. Cancer 1978; 41:1974.

# The Borderland of Law & Medicine

# 63

Stewart E. Niles, Jr., JD

Professional liability claims against obstetrician-gynecologists have increased dramatically in the past decade. Most of these lawsuits are initiated when there have been undesired or unavoidable results from medical intervention. Such results are then used to obscure assessment of compliance to requisite standards. When there have been catastrophic results, even minor criticism of compliance can potentiate adverse judgments. Thus, the most reliable defense against such lawsuits is appreciation of and conformance to principles of laws that establish prevailing standards. Medical professional liability claims are supported by numerous legal theories; the most commonly applied is that of tort, although claims may be premised upon other contract law theories.

## ELEMENTS OF TORT

A **tort** is an act that causes harm to another person or his or her property for which the injured party is seeking monetary damages. All personal injury claims, eg, automobile accidents, slip and fall, and medical professional liability, are types of torts. Tort law is divided into 4 categories: intentional, negligence, strict liability, and concomitant torts. In medical malpractice suits, most claims are based on intentional or negligence torts.

### Intentional Torts

Intentional torts include battery, assault, and false imprisonment. Intent to put harmful action into motion is common to each type; however, intent to cause harm is not required. Assault and battery are similar but not quite the same. **Battery** is harmful or offensive bodily contact with another. *Assault* is the intention to create the apprehension of harmful or offensive bodily contact, although no contact occurs.

In medical malpractice claims, battery is the significant intentional tort. Most common is surgery performed on an anatomic structure for which patient consent was not obtained, for example, if bilateral oophorectomy is performed when consent was obtained only for one side. Another example is if an obstetrician–gynecologist obtains permission to perform a

cesarean section, and during the procedure also performs a bilateral tubal ligation. Unless there were extraordinary mitigating factors, the physician has exceeded the scope of the obtained consent and has committed battery.

Although some medical professional liability actions are based on intentional torts, particularly battery, the incidence is quite low. The importance of intentional tort claims must not be overlooked, however, because most insurance policies exclude coverage for intentional acts. Thus, some insurance protection may not cover a claim for battery.

Consent, either actual or implied, is the available defense against an intentional tort claim. Thus, if the patient has consented to harmful bodily contact, eg, surgery or digital physical examination, an intentional tort claim may be defeated. However, it is the burden of the physician to prove consent. Consent will be discussed in a later section of this chapter.

### Negligence Torts

Negligence torts represent the overwhelming majority of medical professional liability actions. In essence, the patient must demonstrate that in violating a standard of care, the physician caused the patient damage. The patient must prove 4 elements in a negligence action: duty, breach of duty, causation, and damages.

**Duty** is the physician's responsibility to act in accordance with a standard of care to prevent or avoid patient injury. It is the duty of the physician to use reasonable care or diligence, along with his or her best judgment, in the application of skill. In medical malpractice claims, duty is best perceived as a test to determine whether the physician acted as would other average reasonable physicians practicing in the same field of medical specialty and confronted with the same or similar circumstances.

**Breach of duty** concerns violation or deviation from a standard of care. In general, it is the patient's burden to prove by a preponderance of evidence that it is more likely than not that the physician breached a duty owed to the patient.

Standards of care are imposed on physicians by statutes, regulations, hospital bylaws, and medical specialty protocols. Expert testimony is generally required to establish whether or not a physician's conduct conformed to a particular standard of care. For example, the American College of Obstetricians and Gynecologists (ACOG) has protocol standards for management of fetal distress to which the physician, when confronted with such circumstances, may be compelled to conform. To meet the burden of proof, the patient would engage an expert to testify that the defendant physician deviated from the prevailing standard of care by specifically deviating from the ACOG protocol.

Expert testimony, however, is not the sole means of establishing the requisite standard of care. In some instances, the burden of proof is shifted to the physician. One exception to the general rule is the doctrine of *res ipsa loquitur*, which translates as "the thing speaks for itself." If the event causing damage would not have occurred in the ordinary course of patient management, with the physician exercising proper care, then *res ipsa loquitur* may be applied to shift the burden of proof to the physician. The patient actuates this result by demonstrating that the physician had exclusive control over the injury-producing circumstances, that the injury ordinarily does not happen unless the physician is negligent, and that the patient is free from fault. The classic example would be a sponge left in the peritoneal cavity following surgery.

The modern tendency is for a physician's conduct or judgment to be judged by national standards. Custom and practice in the physician's local community is no longer conclusive; instead, physicians, particularly specialists, are now held to national standards. This approach recognizes the availability of information, training, and continuing medical education on a national level.

If a specialist such as an obstetrician–gynecologist deviates from the standard of care practiced by others in the same field of medicine, a negligent act or negligent exercise of judgment occurs to make the physician liable for damages. Breach of duty is more encompassing than surgical error. Failing to remain current in the state of knowledge, failing to refer the patient to a specialist or subspecialist, or failing to exercise appropriate judgment at a critical time constitute a few of the many negligent acts for which the obstetrician–gynecologist may be liable.

The third element that patients must prove is **proximate cause**. This is an essential element that links the physician's negligent act to the damages. Multiple causes for plaintiff's damages makes proof of causation difficult. The physical injuries claimed in the medical professional liability law suit might be as attributable to the original disease or disorder as to the physician's alleged negligence.

Discussions of legal causation in tort claims have challenged and delighted legal scholars for centuries. From a physician's vantage, the issue is whether it was foreseeable that the physician's action would have caused or contributed to the resultant injury or loss or whether these results were a recognized risk of the original medical condition. The primary question at issue is whether the consequences are an unavoidable result of the treatment or of negligence in its administration. If the damages in question were an unforeseeable idiosyncrasy of the patient or a recognized result of the disease or condition, proof of causation is not established.

Damages must be actual. This element is simplest for plaintiffs, to prove; however, the extent, duration, and profoundness of the injuries are seldom as severe as claimed by plaintiffs.

## DOCUMENTATION

The wise physician recognizes that proper documentation of information contemporaneous with decisions is not only good medical practice but also good legal "medicine" to protect against meritless or unjustified claims. Regardless of the plaintiff's theory of recovery, the physician's defense is materially jeopardized by improper documentation, whether it is illegible, incomplete, inaccurate, imprecise, or critical of others. In circumstances wherein judgment or skill can be defended, improper documentation can become the primary focus of a plaintiff's claim.

The office or hospital chart contains a contemporaneous record of the patient's history, physical examination, progress notes, laboratory data, views of consultants, nursing assessment, and related data. Therapeutic or surgical plans are outlined in the chart and shared with other healthcare providers. Records from any other sources are also included in charts. In medical-liability claims, the test often becomes whether the office or hospital chart represents a complete and accurate record of all relevant information necessary to support the decisions and actions of the physician. If the chart contains sufficient data to support the diagnosis or physician action, defense of meritless claims is advanced. On the other hand, the absence of critical data can hurt a physician's claim to appropriate action even to the extent that the defense may not succeed in proving a meritless claim.

Since the chart is a contemporaneous chronicle of the information it purports to present, its evidentiary value cannot be underestimated by either side. Records can be enlarged into graphics for the judge or jury. Enlarged graphics of legible, well-maintained records supporting a defendant's testimony, are compelling, persuasive evidence. Conversely, illegible, incomplete records can endorse a plaintiff's theory that the physician hastily reviewed or failed to consider all information or that the physician's sloppy practices validate the plaintiff's complaints.

Documentation is the physician's greatest ally or

enemy in the courtroom. It is inexcusable for physicians to allow records under their dominion to become key to a plaintiff's success. Records poorly maintained by others cannot be altered, but if reviewed and considered, the relevant information should be incorporated into the physician's notes to portray the precise information analyzed and relied upon.

## ABANDONMENT OR LACK OF DILIGENCE

Throughout the duration of the physician–patient relationship, the physician is obliged to give the patient medical services as may be required. Abandonment or lack of diligence constituting actionable medical malpractices results from breach of this duty. To succeed in this type of claim, the plaintiff must prove that the physician's abandonment or lack of diligence in attending the patient was the proximate cause of the injury for which damages are sought. Thus, merely showing physician neglect, without proving the cause of damages, is insufficient to sustain the claim.

The issue of **lack of diligence** in attending a patient can arise only during the physician–patient relationship. Diligence concerns physician liability based on omissions in the course of applying proper treatment. The patient's complaint often involves a physician's failure to give the patient the attention necessary or proper to make the correct diagnosis of the ailment or to apply appropriate treatment.

Cases of **abandonment**, or termination of the relationship between the physician and patient, must have been brought about by a unilateral act of the physician. There can be no abandonment if the relationship was terminated by mutual consent, by the dismissal of the physician by the patient, or if the physician's services are no longer required. Physicians have the right to withdraw from a case but may do so only after giving the patient reasonable notice so as to enable the patient to secure other medical attention. Such withdrawal does not constitute abandonment.

While physicians have the right to withdraw with proper notice, they are under a duty to continue attendance until the patient is no longer in need or the patient has had reasonable opportunity to procure the attendance of another physician. Instances of abandonment are as follows: unqualified refusal to attend, leaving a patient during or immediately after an operation, failure to attend a patient despite a promise to do so, refusal to treat a patient at a particular time and place, premature discharge of a patient, or failure to give the patient proper instruction at discharge.

The frequency of evaluation or examination of the patient must be determined with reasonable care. If prolonged intervals of time elapse, the physician may be negligent. The surrounding circumstances ultimately determine whether the interval was appropriate. A theory of recovery based on unreasonable frequency of evaluation is less likely to render the physician liable than is a specific request for the physician's services that went unheeded. The failure of due diligence in attending the patient is often coupled with other complaints, and this accusation can have an impact on the jury's determination of liability.

Consider, for instance, the case of a macrosomic fetus delivered by cesarean section after 36 hours of labor and attempted vaginal delivery, with the infant subsequently having brain damage secondary to hypoxia. Among other complaints, the plaintiff could assert that antepartum evaluations were so infrequent that the attending physician failed to determine that the fetus was macrosomic, that fetopelvic disproportion required immediate cesarean section, and that other antepartum decisions were inappropriate. The physician's response to each of these allegations is significantly stronger if the patient's antepartum status has been evaluated frequently, adequately, and in a timely manner. Secondary considerations would include the physician's response to the patient's request for specific action.

Allegations of lack of due diligence or abandonment can be defended by proving physician availability by telephone, temporary absence from practice after providing reasonable alternatives, or the intervening illness of the physician or a family member. The requisites for each defense are different. For example, a physician may not be negligent if telephone contact is maintained with the patient; the physician's physical presence is not absolutely necessary. However, this factor is usually troublesome, because after catastrophic results it is always difficult to prove that the physician's absence was justified.

If the physician temporarily leaves or interrupts practice, arrangements for reasonable alternatives must be made. A competent substitute must be secured, and patients must be informed of the substitution. In no event may the physician be absent while a patient is in a critical condition that cannot be managed by another. Similarly, if a physician temporarily interrupts the treatment of a patient because of illness (of his or her own or of a family member), failure to attend will be excused if the patient is notified and afforded an opportunity to secure another physician, or if a competent substitute is provided.

Liability cannot be avoided for neglecting a patient because the physician has taken on more patients than can be managed. It is not an excuse to fail to attend a patient because the physician is busy with another patient.

The physician-patient relationship continues until ended by mutual consent, the patient dismisses the physician, the medical necessity that gave rise to the relationship ends, or the physician withdraws after reasonable notice and gives reasonable opportunity to secure alternative medical care.

## CONSENT

A rogue who slashes a victim's abdomen is subject to criminal penalties. The physician who incises the patient's abdomen is authorized by consent of the patient or the patient's duly authorized representative. However, the physician's superior knowledge of the patient's need for surgery or invasive treatment neither authorize, nor justifies the surgery or invasive treatment—the patient's consent is required. The wise physician recognizes and appreciates the role of guiding the patient in alternative treatment decisions and consequences thereof. Yet, the ultimate decision must rest with the patient.

**Capacity** to consent varies from state to state. Certainly, any competent adult may consent to medical treatment. A majority of states have enacted the Uniform Consent Law, which establishes a ranking of persons who are empowered to consent to medical treatment for an incapacitated or incompetent person. Usually, a parent may consent to medical treatment for a minor child. A spouse may consent for an incapacitated spouse. In certain instances, other family members, guardians, or persons standing *in loco parentis* may consent. In the foregoing instances, consent may be provided for necessary treatment or surgery but not for elective procedures. For example, a husband may not consent to a tubal ligation of his wife as a secondary procedure to cesarean section or other abdominal procedure.

An adult retains the right to refuse medical treatment or surgery. Regardless of the strength of the physician's belief that treatment or surgery would benefit the patient, the adult, competent patient has an inviolate right to refuse treatment. For example, if prior to surgery, for reasons of religious conviction a patient absolutely refuses blood transfusion, unexpected bleeding during the course of a hysterectomy will not justify blood transfusion.

If the refusal is absolute, ie, refusal for surgery or chemotherapy, the physician should document the diagnosis, the treatment alternatives, the informed discussions with the patient, and the patient's refusal. The patient, and a family member if available, should sign an acknowledgment in the office chart or hospital record confirming the informed discussion and refusal. If confronted with such absolute refusal for surgery or treatment, the obstetrician–gynecologist is presented with less complicated issues from a liability standpoint than from relative refusal.

If the refusal is relative, ie, consent to surgery but no blood transfusion, again the physician should document the diagnosis, the alternative treatment, and the informed discussion, and should obtain signed acknowledgment from the patient. If the patient has

confronted the risk of irreversible impairment or death arising from refusal to authorize blood transfusion, and if during surgery such blood transfusion is required to avoid irreversible impairment or death, the physician who has appropriately documented the record is legally comfortable with the patient's decision—although the patient's decision may be contrary to the philosophy, experience, and training of the physician. Ethical issues of patient management must be decided prior to surgery or institution of risky treatment, because decisions made during crises seldom allow for complete balance of competing interests.

Consent may be **actual** or **implied**. The foregoing discussion addressed actual consent, which is usually documented in writing, but expression of actual consent may be proved by other means. Consent may be implied from the circumstances though neither actually written nor expressed. Emergencies best exemplify implied consent. An emergency situation exists upon a finding of 3 factors: (1) the medical treatment or surgical procedure is immediately necessary to avoid unreasonable risk of irreversible impairment or death; (2) the person who should authorize consent, or such person's representative, is incapacitated or unavailable; and (3) any delay in treatment could jeopardize life, limb, or bodily function of the person threatened. Most states recognize implied consent in consideration of these circumstances. On the other hand, the emergency can be neither created nor abetted by the physician in order to attain a goal established by the physician but previously rejected by the patient.

In a true emergency situation, good-faith medical treatment by the physician will be protected or would constitute a substantial defense in mitigation of claim for damage. Similar analysis is presented when the risk of harm arising from the patient's refusal to treatment or surgery was not foreseeable. If such a rare circumstance is truly presented, society generally supports the physician's decision to intervene in favor of avoiding irreversible impairment or death. However, physician intervention contrary to patient desire or objection is unreasonable if the physician could have foreseen the risk.

## INFORMED CONSENT

From the physician's perspective, the doctrine of informed consent poses the most disconcerting theory available to plaintiffs. Recovery is not sought for physician negligence or fault. The patient sustains a less-than-desirable result and seeks to impose liability upon the physician for failure to disclose a risk of the procedure or its consequences, for which the patient now claims consent would have been withheld. From the physician's vantage, the result at law is imposition of liability in the absence of fault.

Heritage for this theory is quite simple. The physician-patient relationship places a unique obligation upon the physician. Since the physician is afforded great power to prescribe drugs, perform surgery, and affect the well-being of the patient, the physician is placed in a position of great trust. Not unlike the fiduciary, the trustee, the guardian, or the executor, the physician accepts an obligation to protect the best interests of the patient. The patient may rely upon such trust and will always claim to have done so during the course of litigation premised upon lack of informed consent.

The physician has superior knowledge of medicine and the patient's condition. Training, experience, and thorough knowledge of prevailing circumstances often tempt the physician to substitute judgment on behalf of the patient. The recognized risks of therapy or surgery may be perceived by the physician with a sense of "routineness." Yet, the patient is the master, and the physician is the servant obligated not to exceed the patient's decisions as evidenced by proper consent. No longer may the physician dictate the course of medical management and merely obtain blanket authorization from the patient.

To avoid lawsuits claiming damages for lack of informed consent, the physician must impart to the patient information that is complete and understandable. It is the physician's duty to reveal all the facts that are necessary to form an intelligent consent to the proposed treatment. Unfortunately, the extent of disclosure necessary to inform adequately has eluded specific, uniform formulation. Various articulations have been adopted by state courts or legislatures. The most consistent theme is that the law, not the medical profession, will establish the standard measuring performance of the physician's duty. The difference is profound. Initially, courts relied upon expert testimony to describe the scope of the physician's duty to inform. The standard reflected the medical community's philosophy. Although some jurisdictions retain this approach, a majority of states have rejected it. Of concern was the necessity to establish an appropriate standard that was not limited by self-interest of the medical community. To safeguard the patient's right to achieve his or her own determination of treatment, the law must set the standard for adequate disclosure. The duty is whether the physician disclosed sufficient risks for the patient's informational needs. The courts have noted that all risks potentially affecting the decision must be unmasked. For a meaningful decision by the patient, the physician must divulge all information relevant to the procedure or treatment. Compliance with a full disclosure requirement often conflicts with the physician's philosophy and is virtually impossible to ensure; however, a few basic suggestions provide guidance.

Do not overlook the opportunity to document informed discussion of risks and benefits of proposed medical treatment. Office notes or progress notes reinforce such discussions. Complete notes prove the scope and nature of the discussions. Instead of ignoring information shared with the patient, the patient's questions and the facts supporting the patient's decision should be noted. Broad statements are sufficient. For example, "Risks and benefits of anesthesia discussed. Patient wants epidural." Although brief, the note demonstrates the patient's decision-making process and ultimate decision.

Allow the patient to sign the note. Since some patients are suspicious about the notes charted, the chart or record is "demystified" when the patient is asked to review the note and to co-sign. When a co-signed note in controversy is enlarged for trial, claimed lack of consent is dealt a serious blow.

The attending physician should obtain written consent from the patient. A nurse, resident, or substitute physician presenting written consent forms to a patient cannot meet the requirements of full disclosure with opportunity to respond to all questions raised by the patient. The attending obstetrician-gynecologist must present the consent form, completely inform, answer all questions, and obtain the patient's signature. This is the only method to avoid a claim of misrepresentation of material fact or failure to adequately disclose benefits and risks.

The degree of disclosure of risks varies throughout the USA. Nevertheless, emphasis is placed on completeness of disclosure. If a risk poses at least a 1% possibility of occurrence, it must be disclosed and discussed. Since medical or surgical management of a condition will probably carry the same risks in most patients, the most common risks can be routinely listed, and risks peculiar to the patient can be added.

Alternative treatment must be made known to the patient. Since the patient has the ultimate right to decide, the obstetrician-gynecologist cannot unilaterally decide the elements of treatment. The patient must participate in the decision-making process.

A claim based on lack of consent is the easiest to avoid. Documentation of the decision-making process, coupled with complete disclosure of risks, reduces the obstetrician-gynecologist's greatest risk—litigation.

## PRESCRIPTION DRUG CONSIDERATIONS

A physician is required to use reasonable skill and care in the prescription and administration of drugs. All drugs are "unavoidably unsafe," ie, all drugs have recognized side effects. The mere occurrence of side effects does not permit an inference of negligence, but the physician has a duty to warn the patients of recognized risks and to advise on the benefits versus the risks.

After review of the manufacturer's accompanying literature, *Physician's Desk Reference*, and other source material, the physician must determine whether the drug can be safely prescribed for a particular patient. Do the benefits outweigh the risk of adverse reaction? The physician becomes the "learned intermediary" who assists the patient in deciding whether to accept the recognized risks to obtain the potential benefits. As "learned intermediary," the physician advises; however, the patient retains the ultimate right to determine the course of treatment. Frequently, the physician seeks to substitute personal judgment in lieu of the patient's right to decide. Such substituted judgment exceeds the bounds of the physician–patient relationship and creates circumstances vulnerable to substantial litigation exposure. The physician must advise, and the patient must make an informed decision.

Deviation from the manufacturer's instructions for the prescription and administration of a particular drug is extremely difficult to defend and should be avoided. If a drug is used for unapproved purposes or in excess or at variance from the manufacturer's recommendations, the greatest care must be taken to obtain patient consent, to document the justification and consent, and to maintain close observation. Even so, a lawsuit may not be avoided and may, in fact, be invited.

The physician must inquire into the patient's susceptibility to the recognized risks. Adequate testing for hypersensitivity may be required. The patient's medical history of prior reactions to particular drugs should be explored.

Regarding all contraceptives or contraceptive devices, the issue of informed consent is extremely vital. The patient must be informed of all risks associated with every method of contraception to allow the patient to make an informed decision. The incidence of pregnancy occurring with each method of contraception must be addressed as a risk. The physician must advise whether certain methods of contraception are contraindicated for the patient.

Risks subsequently discovered in medical literature or manufacturer's publications must be revealed to the patient. Information vital to the patient must be transmitted before and during drug administration.

## THE PHYSICIAN AS EXPERT WITNESS

The techniques of testifying, whether in the courtroom or in deposition, are similar. (A few notable exceptions will be discussed in the following section.) There is no substitute for preparation. Regardless of the nature of the testimony, a thoroughly prepared medical witness is a formidable foe to counsel opposing the witness's finding and opinions.

A good medical witness knows in advance the nature and scope of the subject matter of the testimony. Identify the side—plaintiff or defendant—calling for expert witness testimony. Review the issues relating to the testimony. Review all available medical records and medical literature on the subject matter. Unless the obstetrician–gynecologist is employed as a witness for the plaintiff, contact counsel for the defendant to discuss the legal issues. Understand the relationship between the medical and legal issues. Complete preparation reduces the risk that the testimony will be rejected or that the witness will be embarrassed. A completely prepared medical expert witness is less likely to encounter unforeseen difficulty in the interrogation process.

Patience, discipline, control, and professional demeanor must be maintained at all times. The technique to attain these goals is quite simple. First, listen to the attorney's question. Second, formulate a response to the question as posed. Third, reformulate the response in as few words as possible. Fourth, deliver the response in as few words as possible. This method has universal application. Dispersed throughout this technique are several "do's" and "don'ts."

*Do not* interrupt the interrogating attorney. Interruption can only lead to miscommunication. By interrupting, the witness is assuming an element not yet revealed and potentially different from what the attorney is seeking. The witness should answer the attorney's question as posed.

*Do not* anticipate questions. By attempting to lead counsel into or away from areas of inquiry, the interrogator is provided valuable information about the witness's sensitivities to the facts, issues, or opinions under consideration.

*Do* maintain a professional demeanor at all times. Discourtesy undermines the witness's credibility. Contentious or argumentative statements educate opposing counsel. Emotional outbursts discredit the witness and provide opportunity to divert the witness's attention, weaken the testimony, or diminish the witness's believability.

*Do* listen to the questions. The form of the question is important. Generally, opposing counsel may ask leading questions—ie, the question may suggest an answer. However, it is never proper for counsel to suggest incorrect information. If so, the question is no longer leading, it is misleading. Never categorically affirm or deny a question that contains incorrect or misleading information. Identify the misleading information and request opposing counsel to restate the question to incorporate the corrected information. Further, if the question poses a multitude of questions, request the question to be broken into its component parts. For example, if asked, "Did the fetus have one loop of cord wrapped around its neck and was the fetus hypoxic because of shoulder dystocia?" the witness should request that the question be divided into its component parts.

*Do* know the difference between possibility and probability. The issues in the case must be proved to a reasonable medical probability. In essence, is it more likely than not that a particular fact or conclusion is true. Speculation or possibility is insufficient to establish medical probability. Accordingly, any question that seeks possibility should be countered with the response equivalent to "I can only formulate opinions based on probability, not on sheer speculation or possibility." If further pressed, a continuing response might be, "Admittedly, almost anything is possible, but in this case the [fact in question] is not a reasonable medical probability."

*Do* compel the interrogating attorney to declare whether his or her question is hypothetical or whether it is based on the case under review. Hypothetical questions are allowed. A primary purpose is to allow the interrogating attorney to ask a question based upon facts that will be proved after the witness has testified. Ultimately, the party posing the hypothetical question must prove the probability of the underlying facts; otherwise, the hypothetical question is subject to objection. When confronted with a hypothetical question, it is appropriate to include a statement that advises, "My answer is hypothetical and has nothing to do with this case" or "If your question is hypothetical, I can only provide a hypothetical answer that is unrelated to these facts." Also, it is particularly important for the witness to avoid assumptions when responding to hypothetical questions. It is even more important for the witness to answer the question "as posed." If insufficient information has been provided to formulate a response to the hypothetical question, it is appropriate for the witness to respond, "I don't know" or "I can't answer." Each hypothetical question must contain sufficient information or assumptions upon which an opinion may be formulated to that particular hypothetical question. The witness diminishes the testimony if the opposing attorney is allowed to link several hypothetical questions together, to force the witness to make certain assumptions about the combination, and to express an opinion based thereon. Whatever the witness's response, it is subject to mischaracterization and confusion.

*Do* require counsel to define vague and indefinite terms such as "normal," "customary," or "average." Often, counsel will be confronted with the dilemma of defining such terms. If counsel is unable to do so, it is likely that the response to the question would have been misconstrued at a later date. If adequate definition is provided, the witness can specifically respond within the limits, qualifiers, or standards interjected into the question.

*Do* admit lack of knowledge or opinion where appropriate. "I can't answer the question as posed" or "I don't know" are commonly used by good, well-prepared witnesses. Testimony must be premised upon facts, not speculation.

*Do* review all documentary materials prior to commenting thereon. Rather than rely upon memory, the witness should review reference to office notes, hospital charts, or other documentary information after a relevant question is asked but before the response is supplied. Conflicts in testimony or deviation from readily available facts will thus be avoided. The witness is entitled to review the witness's records prepared contemporaneously with the circumstances under review or business records customarily relied upon by the witness in the course of ordinary affairs. At time of deposition, it is to the witness's advantage to review each relevant document when review would assist in refreshing the witness's recollection or would positively corroborate the witness's testimony. At trial, although this technique is generally available, all relevant record entries may be memorized in order to demonstrate total command of the facts and circumstances.

*Do not* interpret the meaning of a document prepared by another person. If asked, "What did the nurse mean at 0200 hours when she wrote 'tachycardia and decelerations noted on fetal monitor strip'?" the witness may respond, "That is what the entry says" or "Please ask the nurse the meaning of her notes." Although the witness can define the terms used, the witness should not interpret the statements in the context of the facts in litigation. In doing so, the witness will be viewed as adopting the statements. On the other hand, most rules allow for exception. In medical professional liability cases, if the information is favorable to the defendant or if the information is a necessary part of the defense and the nurse is unavailable, the defense witness may interpret the information. The adequately prepared witness will have reviewed this exception with the counsel for the defendant prior to opposing counsel's interrogation. If the information is sufficiently important for the exception to apply, it was foreseeable during testimony preparation.

*Do not* defer to another physician or author as an authoritative expert. Written medical documentation may be recognized as accepted medical information. However, if the witness defers to a medical writing as authoritative, counsel will next seek the witness to accept a statement or proposition from the writing as authoritative and inviolate. Since the statement or proposition does not take into consideration the prevailing circumstances in the case under review, the statement or proposition is never in proper context. Further, if the statement or proposition were inviolate, exception would never be allowed, and the prevailing circumstances would never be a significant factor. The witness may acknowledge that the medical writing is accepted; the degree to which it is accepted; its application in the instant circumstances; the extent to which it should be considered by the witness; or the impact, or lack thereof, of the statement or proposition, thereof. Otherwise, the medical writing will supersede and override the witness's testimony.

Similarly, the witness should not defer to another physician. The following represents typical dialogue. *Question*: "Since Dr Jones is an expert in neonatology, would you defer to his opinions in the area of neonatology?" *Answer*: "Dr Jones is a well-respected neonatologist, and I would enjoy reviewing his opinions on the subject." *Question*: "But, doctor, if Dr Jones was of the opinion that [fact in dispute], wouldn't you agree and defer to his opinion?" *Answer*: "I would consider his opinions, but I would want to know the facts and opinions he relied upon and the medical writings he took into account." The witness has sidestepped the issue and retained an independent role.

*Do not* respond until objections are completed. Often, the objection describes information or an issue that the witness should take into account before responding. Further, all parties have the right to protect the record. Interrupting the objection places the witness in the same position as interrupting the question—the witness may assume information that is incorrect.

*Do* depersonalize the plaintiff. Do not refer to the plaintiff as the minister's daughter, the deceased, the newborn infant, or the good-natured elderly person you affectionately refer to as "grandmother." The patient should be referred to as "the patient."

*Do* use medical language in depositions. The art of medicine employs precise vocabulary. Precision may be lost if medical terms are avoided. If the interrogating counsel requires definition, the opportunity is afforded to request same. On the other hand, at the time of trial, it is necessary to use medical terms only in combination with a readily understood definition. The witness will lose rapport with the judge or jury if the demeanor is bombastic or incomprehensible.

*Do not* allow the interrogating attorney to intimidate. During deposition, the witness should look directly at the interrogating attorney at all times. At trial, the witness should look at the trier of fact, a judge or jury, in order to develop and maintain rapport. The witness should not allow the attorney to "invade the witness's space." For example, counsel should not be allowed to look over the witness's shoulder, stand beside the witness, review records simultaneously with the witness, or tolerate circumstances that allow the counsel to come "face to face" with the witness. Counsel will attempt to use this tactic to obtain additional information, to break the witness's train of thought, or to force the witness to step out of character of professional demeanor.

*Do* admit deposition or trial preparation with your attorney or the attorney who has employed you to testify. Judges and juries expect such discussions. Denial of pretestimony meetings is an untruth that will discredit the testimony. There should be no hesitancy in admitting the amount and basis of the witness fee.

## THE PHYSICIAN AS DEFENDANT

In preparing to testify as a defendant in a professional medical liability case, the foregoing guidelines are valid, with some exceptions to accommodate the best strategy available. Preparation begins with receipt of notice of claim or suit papers. While notifying his or her insurance carrier or medical professional liability attorney, the defendant should make every effort to obtain all medical records. These medical records will provide the basis for a narrative medical summary to be used by the defense team in preparation for litigation. The medical summary should not be prepared until requested by counsel, in order to reduce the possibility that the statement could be obtained by opposing parties.

Within an extremely short period after receipt of notice of claim and the medical records, a meeting should be scheduled with defense counsel. Adequate time should be allowed. The meeting should be conducted at the defense counsel's office, where counsel is best prepared to use resources on the defendant's behalf. The conference should be conducted prior to filing responsive pleadings.

The initial conference should achieve several goals. All issues should be identified and the component elements of each issue discussed. All witnesses must be identified. Witnesses potentially unfavorable or unavailable should be discussed. If all medical records have been reviewed and a narrative summary completed, the favorable or challenging aspects of the case can be considered to prevent surprise issues or witnesses.

The need for expert witnesses, the medical specialty required, and the litigation personality of potential expert witnesses should be thoroughly discussed.

Joint strategy with codefendants should be developed. In medical professional liability cases, seldom is a defendant benefitted by adopting an adversarial position to another defendant. In those rare circumstances, claims against codefendants or other persons should be considered.

The discovery stage of litigation allows the parties to develop facts, documents, and testimony to be used at the time of trial. The type, timing, and strategy of informal and formal discovery should be outlined. Agreement should be obtained as to whether aggressive or passive strategy will be used in whole or in part.

In addition to all medical records, the physician should provide an up-to-date curriculum vitae and extracts from relevant medical literature. A well-conceived and well-organized initial conference will save considerable time in preparing the defense team for the challenge, will remove mystery from the litigation, and should alleviate the physician's natural anxieties.

Preparing for deposition necessitates additional work. The physician should meet with defense counsel as often as is necessary to prepare completely. Deposition preparation should not be rushed. Each of the plaintiff's areas of inquiry must be analyzed and response prepared. On the day of the deposition, meet with the defense attorney prior to the deposition for an adequate period of time to update and finalize strategy.

Throughout the deposition, trial demeanor should be maintained. Plaintiff's counsel must conclude that the defendant physician will be a worthy opponent. In final trial preparation, schedule adequate time for trial appearance and preparation. All depositions, pleadings, documents, or summaries thereof must be reviewed. Discuss the strategy and tactics on each of the critical points in the case with defendant counsel.

Trial tactics and testimony must be individualized to the case under consideration. Generalities may serve as a basis for a broadly structured approach; however, each element of the trial must be precisely conceived and executed. One observation, however, is germane to all medical professional liability trials—it is important to maintain patient, controlled, and authoritative demeanor at all times, even though it may appear that the judge, the jury, or the opposing counsel are not present. In numerous instances, an unintended action when the defendant believed observation or monitoring was not possible has damaged the psychology or strategy developed after long and arduous work.

As an expert witness or as a defendant, the physician should derived comfort from one overriding consideration. As the investigating or attending physician, he or she is in the best position to know the facts and circumstances. The truthfulness of the testimony transcends all procedures, methodologies, or strategies. Truthful testimony disarms opposing counsel and remains the fundamental basis for successful litigation.

## MEDICAL LIABILITY LIMITATION STATUTES

In light of the liability crisis and increasing malpractice premiums, several states have enacted statutes limiting damages in medical professional liability claims. In Indiana, the total amount recoverable for injury or death of a patient may not exceed $500,000. This applies to all "qualified health-care providers."

Kansas provides that punitive damages may not exceed the lesser of $3 million or 25% of the defendant's highest gross income during 5 years before the wrongful act. Half the punitive damages collected revert to a health-care stabilization fund and half are awarded to the plaintiff.

If the hospital or health-care facility is insured for not less than $100,000, Maryland provides an immunity for the excess over the insurance limits.

Under Missouri statutes, recovery in medical professional liability actions is limited to $350,000 for noneconomic damages from any one defendant. Puni-

tive damages can be awarded only if there was willful, wanton, or malicious misconduct. Damages are divided into (1) past economic damages, (2) past noneconomic damages, (3) future medical damages, (4) future economic damages other than medical, and (5) future noneconomic damages. Future damages are expressed at present value. Past damages are available in lump sum. Any party may request that future damages be paid, in whole or in part, in periodic payments if the total future damages exceeds $100,000.

Nevada limitation statutes provide that damages awarded against a health-care professional must be reduced by the amount of any prior payment made by or on behalf of the provider to the claimant as reasonable expenses in medical care, other essential goods and services, or reasonable living expenses.

Louisiana's statute, similar to Indiana's, provides that a total amount recoverable for any injury or death of patient may not exceed $500,000, plus future medical expenses. This limitation applies to all "qualified health-care providers." Each qualified health-care provider is liable for $100,000, with the patient compensation fund being liable for any remainder up to $500,000. This $500,000 limit does not include future medical expenses that are covered by the patient compensation fund.

In Ohio, damages against a physician or hospital not involving death may not exceed $200,000. South Dakota provides that, for medical professional liability claims, total damages are limited to $1 million. New Mexico's statute succinctly provides that damages are limited to $500,000 excluding punitive damages and past medical care.

Under Utah's statute, the plaintiff may recover noneconomic losses to compensate for pain, suffering, and inconvenience up to $250,000. This limitation does not affect awards for punitive damages. Future damages that equal or exceed $100,000, less attorneys' fees and costs, may be paid by periodic rather than lump-sum payment. Lost future earnings may be paid over the creditor's work life expectancy.

Similar statutes in Virginia and Texas have been declared unconstitutional by several district courts and the state supreme court, respectively. In other states, the courts have invalidated statutes of limitation. Some states, such as Alaska and Oregon, have statutory limits of $500,000 on noneconomic damagees on all tort cases.

## PEER REVIEW

In 1988, the United States Supreme Court refused to extend antitrust immunity to members of peer review committees. In a case of first impression, the Court held that a physician whose hospital privileges were wrongfully denied could seek redress pursuant to the treble-damage provision of antitrust laws. To succeed, the physician must prove that members of the peer review process were competitors of the accused physician and were motivated by economic self-interest.

Viewed in its most expansive light, peer review was dealt a chilling blow. Potential peer review is subjective by the very nature of the case-by-case analysis. Issues of medical judgment are usually evaluated by physicians of the same practice or specialty as the accused physician. Thus, competitors have been traditionally relied upon. While it may be difficult to prove to a jury a physician's incompetence or lack of compliance with requisite standards, it is considerably easier to demonstrate economic interest by competitors.

Yet, Congress enacted the Health Care Quality Act of 1986 to promote peer review and the reporting of deviation from the standard of care. Within these provisions, limited immunity is provided. Members of the peer review process are immune from civil liability if found to be acting in "good faith," which is absent if motivated by economic self-interest.

Considering the balance of these principles, it would be wise for hospital-based peer review committees to redefine the review process. First, all competitors of the accused physician must be excused from deliberating or participating in any aspect of the proceedings. Second, noncompeting experts in the practice or specialty of the accused physician should be retained to evaluate matters of patient care, competence, judgment, or skill. Third, peer review should be pursued aggressively, but all rights and privileges of the accused physician must be meticulously observed.

Once the pitfalls of peer review have been identified and avoided, the practitioner should not refuse to assist in legitimate, objective review to strengthen the medical profession.

## REFERENCES

American College of Obstetricians & Gynecologists, Department of Professional Liability: *Litigation Assistant. A Guide for the Defendant Physician.* ACOG, 1986.

Harney M: *Medical Malpractice,* 2nd ed. Michie Co., 1987.

King, JH Jr: *The Law of Medical Malpractice in a Nutshell.* West, 1986.

Lawyers Co-Op Editorial Staff: *Medical Malpractice: ALR 2nd, 3rd, & 4th eds, Cases & Annotations.* Lawyers Co-Op, 1987.

Pegalis S, Wachsman H: *American Law of Medical Malpractice.* 3 vols. Lawyers Co-Op, 1986.

Robertson WO: *Medical Malpractice: A Preventive Approach.* Univ of Washington Press, 1985.

Schwartz SS, Tucker ND: *Handling Birth Trauma Cases.* Wiley, 1985.

# Subject Index

NOTE: Page numbers in bold face type indicate a major discussion. A *t* following a page number indicates tabular material and an *i* following a page number indicates an illustration. Drugs are listed under their generic names. When a drug trade name is listed, the reader is referred to the generic name.

unicollis, 78, 79*i*
Bicuspid aortic valve, in pregnancy, 442
Bifid clitoris, 90, 640
Bifidus factor, in breast milk, 263
Biischial diameter (intertuberous diameter), 30, 205
   assessment of in initial prenatal visit, 193
   contraction of, 205
Bilateral renal agenesis, 68
Bilirubin levels, for phototherapy or exchange transfusion,
   604*t*
Billings method of contraception, 673
Bill's rotation, 553
Bimanual pelvic examination, 620–621
Bimanual uterine compression, in postpartum hemorrhage,
   577
Biologic tests, for pregnancy, 188
Biophysical profile, **292–293**
   accuracy of, 294*t*
Bipartite placenta, 52
Biphosphonate, for osteoporosis prevention, 1048
Birth. *See also* Delivery
   live, 183–184
Birth anoxia, in breech delivery, 419
Birth control. *See* Contraception
Birth control pills (oral contraceptives), **674–678**
   for amenorrhea, 1014
   in breast milk, 266*t*, 271
   for dysmenorrhea, 664
   ectopic pregnancy and, 315
   for endometriosis, 805
   failure rate of, 142*t*
   for hirsutism, 1022
   nipple discharge caused by, 1120
   for premenstrual syndrome, 663
Birth injury, in breech delivery, 419
Birth rate, 184
Birthing chairs/tables, 217
Bishop method, for pelvic scoring for elective induction of
   labor, 224
Bite wounds, genital, sexual abuse and, 649
Bivalents, formation of in meiosis, 98
Bladder (urinary)
   in acute abdomen, 848
   anatomy of, **31–32**
   arteries supplying, 32
   care of, during puerperium, 256
   damage to
      during gynecologic surgery, 868
      during hysterectomy, 903
   emptying, during labor, 216
   exstrophy of, 645
   fascia/ligaments/muscle of, 32
   formation of, 78
      in female, 80–83, 82*i*
      in male, 80, 81*i*
   irritability of, in pregnancy, 186
   lymphatics draining, 32, 37*t*
   in midforceps delivery, 550
   mucous membrane of, 32
   nerves supplying, 32
   palpation of, 833
   postmenopausal estrogen deficiency affecting, 1034
   postoperative drainage of, 880
   during pregnancy, 148
   preparation of for gynecologic surgery, 863
   during puerperium, 242
   relationships of, 31–32
   trigone of, development of, 76, 80

unstable, **840–842**
   veins draining, 32
Bladder retraining, for unstable bladder, 842
Blastema, metanephric, 67, 68*i*
Blastocyst, 155
Blastomycosis, female genital tract involvement and, 706
Bleeding. *See also* Hemorrhage
   in cesarean section, control of, 564
   and history taking in gynecologic exam, 614
   after laparoscopy, 891
   uterine/vaginal
      abnormal, **665–669**
         cervical polyps causing, 727
         evaluation of, **665–666**, 886*t*
         in gestational trophoblastic disease, 969
         gynecologic diseases and disorders causing, **667**
         hysteroscopy for, 886*t*
         menopause and, 1034
         nongynecologic diseases and disorders causing, **667**
         principles of management of, 666
      contact, 665
      dysfunctional, **667–668**
      in ectopic pregnancy, 316
      intermenstrual, 665
         in cervical cancer, 928
         cervical polyps causing, 727
         in von Willebrand's disease, 858
      postcoital, 665
         cervical polyps causing, 717
      postmenopausal, **668–669**
         differential diagnosis of, 1044
         estrogen replacement therapy and, 1048
         excess endogenous estrogens and, 1041
      premature labor and, 331
      in premenarcheal child, **654–655**
      third-trimester, 280–281, **398–409**. *See also specific cause*
         initial evaluation of, 398–400
      uterine leiomyoma causing, 733
   withdrawal, after discontinuation of estrogen therapy, 134
Bleeding disorders, during pregnancy, **454**
Bleeding time, in disseminated intravascular coagulation, 1082
Bleomycin, 993
   for cervical cancer, 932–933
   for gestational trophoblastic disease, 976*t*
   toxicities associated with, 965*t*
Blood clotting
   disorders of
      postpartum hemorrhage and, 575
      during pregnancy, **454**
   during pregnancy, 149–150
      preeclampsia and, 383
   during puerperium, 243–244
Blood count, complete
   in acute abdomen, 848
   in ovarian cancer, 961
   in spontaneous abortion, 308
Blood flow, changes in during pregnancy, 150
Blood gases
   cord, 173*t*, 304*t*
      in premature labor, 336
   in respiratory distress syndrome, 601–602
Blood group incompatibilities, **339–342**. *See also* Rh
      isoimmunization
Blood mole, 307
Blood pressure
   increased. *See* Hypertension
   maternal
      changes in during pregnancy, 150, 429*t*

Cardiac rhythms, during pregnancy, 150
Cardiac surgery, during pregnancy, **502–503**
   for mitral stenosis, 434
Cardiac tamponade, during pregnancy, 436
Cardinal ligaments (ligaments of Mackenrodt), 41, 42
Cardiogenic shock, characteristics of, 872*t*
Cardiomyopathy
   postpartum, 254, 437–438, 591
   in pregnancy, **437–438**
      hypertrophic, 438
Cardiopulmonary resuscitation, during pregnancy, **1085**
Cardiovascular drugs, use of in pregnancy, 446, 447*t*
Cardiovascular system. *See also specific organ or structure*
   maternal
      labor affecting, 151
      during pregnancy, **150–151**, **428**, 429*t*, 430*t*
         disorders of, **428–448**. *See also specific disorder*
            preeclampsia and, 382–383
         during puerperium, 243–245
      menopausal changes in, 1038–1040
      in newborn
         assessment of, 233
         risk assessment and, 284
      perioperative risks and, **856–857**
      postoperative complications and, **871–875**
      in septic shock, 1072*t*
         support of, 1073–1075
Carmustine, 992
Carneous mole, 307
Carneous (red) degeneration, of uterine leiomyoma, 733
Carpal tunnel syndrome, in pregnancy, 474–475
Carpenter's syndrome, large-for-gestational age infant/pregnancy and, 353
Carriers, genetic
   counseling and, 104–106
   identification of, 94–95
Carrying angle, estrogen affecting, 134
Caruncula myrtiformes, 20, 242
Carus, curve of, 205
Cascara sagrada, in breast milk, 266*t*
Catecholamines, in preeclampsia, 384
Catheter knotting, in pulmonary artery catheterization, 1068
Caudal block
   for obstetric analgesia and anesthesia, 529
   for premature labor, 534
Cauterization, for cervicitis, 722–723
Cautery, laparoscopic sterilization with, 890
Cavernous hemangiomas, vulvovaginal, in premenarcheal
      child, 650, 702
CBC. *See* Complete blood count
CCNU. *See* Lomustine
   methyl. *See* Semustine
Cefadroxil, 791
Cefazolin, 791
   for cesarean section prophylaxis, 588, 799
Cefixime, for gonorrhea, 755, 756
Cefonicid, 792
Cefoperazone, 792
Ceforanide, 792
Cefotaxime
   for gonorrhea, 756
   for pelvic abscess, 773
   for salpingitis, 771
   for tubo-ovarian abscess, 776
Cefotetan, 792
   for gonorrhea, 755
   for salpingitis, 771
Cefoxitin, 792

   for gonorrhea, 755
   for pelvic abscess, 773
   for salpingitis, 771
Ceftazidime, 792
Ceftizoxime, 792
   for gonorrhea, 755, 756
   for salpingitis, 771
Ceftriaxone, 792
   for chancroid, 763
   for gonorrhea, 755, 756
   for salpingitis, 771
Cell cycle
   chemotherapy affecting, 988–989
   normal, 985, 986*i*
Cell cycle (phase)-nonspecific drugs, for cancer chemotherapy, 989
Cell cycle (phase)-specific drugs, for cancer chemotherapy, 989
Cell cycle synchronization, cancer chemotherapy and, 989
Cell cycle time, 986
Cell division, **97–99**
Cell-kill hypothesis, in cancer chemotherapy, 987
Cell kinetics, tumor cell dynamics and, 985–986
Cellular immunity, defects in, endometriosis and, 801, 804
Cellulitis, fungal, **706**
Central nervous system
   drugs affecting, in breast milk, 265–266*t*
   in fetus, **176–177**
   in newborn, **176–177**
      assessment of, 234–235
      disorders of, **606–607**
   in preeclampsia, 381–382
Central venous monitoring, for gynecologic surgery, 857
Centromere, 98
Cephalexin, 791
Cephalhematoma, vacuum extraction and, 558
Cephalic version, external, **420–421**
Cephalopelvic disproportion
   cesarean section delivery and, 561–562
   forceps delivery and, 545
   midforceps delivery and, 551
Cephalosporins, **791–793**
   adverse effects of, **792–793**
   in breast milk, 265*t*
   first-generation, **791**
   for salpingitis, 771
   second-generation, **792**
   third-generation, **792**
   for urinary tract infection, 835*t*
Cephalothin, 791
Cephapirin, 791
Cephradine, 791
   for *Gardnerella vaginalis* vaginitis, 697
Ceptometrics, in cystocele and urethrocele, 810
Cerclage
   for incompetent cervix, 310, 311*i*, 312, 313*i*
   in multiple pregnancy, 362
Cerebral blood flow, preeclampsia and, 381–382
Cerebral embolism, and cerebrovascular disease in pregnancy, 468
Cerebral neoplasms, in pregnancy, **469–470**
Cerebral thrombosis, oral contraceptive use and, 675–676
Cerebrovascular disorders, in pregnancy, **468–469**
Cervical cap, for contraception, **672**
Cervical cultures, in cervicitis, 721
Cervical dystocia
   cesarean section and, 563
   chronic cervicitis and, 721

Imidazoles, 798
Imipenem, 793
Imipramine
  fetal exposure to, risk/benefit assessment of, 328*t*
  for unstable bladder, 842*t*
Immature fetus, 165
Immature infant, definition of, 183
Immature teratoma, of ovary, 958
  surgical management of, 964
  tumor markers for, 957*t*
Immune thrombocytopenic purpura, in pregnancy, 454
Immunization
  for newborn, 239
  postpartum, 257–258
  during pregnancy, 200
Immunoglobulins, 169. *See also specific type under Ig*
  in breast milk, 263
Immunologic system
  abnormalities of
    endometriosis and, 801, 804
    gynecologic surgery and, 861–862
    recurrent abortion and, 313
  fetal, 167–169
Immunologic pregnancy tests, 188, 189*t*
  for home use, 189
Immunosuppression, cervical dysplasia and, 926
Immunosuppressive agents
  in breast milk, 266*t*
  use of during pregnancy, small-for-gestational age in-
    fant/pregnancy and, 348
Impedance plethysmography, in thromboembolization in preg-
    nancy, 455
Imperforate anus, 91
Imperforate hymen, 19, 85, 619, 641
  amenorrhea and, 1008
  assessment of, 637
Impetigo
  herpetiformis, in pregnancy, **477**
  vulvar, **706**
Impotence, 1104
Improsulfan, 991
In vitro fertilization and embryo transfer, **1026–1028**
  complications of, 1028
  embryo biopsy and, **1028**
  embryo donation for, 1028
  frozen embryos and, 1028
  gamete intra-fallopian tube transfer (GIFT) and, **1028**
  indications for, 1026
  for male factor infertility, 1004
  multiple gestation and, 1027–1028
  ovum donation and, 1028
  for pelvic factor infertility, 1005
  technique for, 1026–1027
  techniques related to, **1028**
Inborn errors of metabolism
  and drug-induced hemolytic anemia, 450
  prenatal detection of, 286*t*
Incisions, abdominal, 9, 11*i*
  arterial vasculature and, 11–12
  for cesarean section, 564
Incompetent cervix
  cerclage closure of, 310, 311*i*, 312, 313*i*
  habitual abortion and, 312
  as high-risk factor in pregnancy, 278
  laceration causing, 716
Incomplete abortion, 308–309
  definition of, 307
Incontinence, urinary, **835–844**

bypass, **843**
cystocele associated with, 809–810
detrusor instability and, 840–842
overflow, **843**
psychogenic, **843–844**
stress, 832, **836–840**
  cystocele associated with, 809–810, 837
  unstable bladder and, 840–842
urge, 832
  motor, **840–842**
  sensory, **842–843**
Inderal. *See* Propranolol
Indifferent (sexless) stage of development, 71
  of external genitalia, 86–89, 89*i*
  of genital ducts, 74
  of gonads, 71–72
    adult derivatives and vestigial remains of, 64*t*
Indomethacin
  in breast milk, 266*t*
  for patent ductus arteriosus, 603
Induced abortion, **682–686**
  definition of, 307
  evaluation of patients requesting, 683
  follow-up after, 686
  legal aspects of, 683
  methods of, 683–686
  sequelae of, 686
Induction of labor, **223–225**
  in diabetic pregnancy, 377, 378
  premature separation of placenta and, 402
Inertia, uterine
  cesarean section and, 562
  forceps delivery and, 545
Inevitable abortion, 308
  definition of, 307
Infant. *See also under Neonatal and Perinatal and* Newborn
  average-for-gestational age, 230*i*
  definition of, 183
  of diabetic mother, **377**
    congenital anomalies in, 369, 370*t*
  of excessive size, 183–184
  gynecologic examination in, 635–636
  immature, 183
  large-for-gestational age. *See* Large-for-gestational age in-
    fant/pregnancy
  low-birth-weight, 183
  macrosomic. *See* Macrosomia
  mature, 183
  oversized, 183
  postmature, 183, 281
  premature. *See* Premature infant
  reproductive system in, 633
  at risk, **594–612**
    adolescent pregnancy and, 659
    central nervous system disorders in, **606–607**
    developmental disorders in, **608–610**
    fluid balance in, 599
    gastrointestinal disorders in, **605–606**
    heart disease in, **602–603**
    hematologic disorders in, **604–605**
    history of, 277
    hyperbilirubinemia in, **603–604**
    infections in, **607–608**
    multiple pregnancy and, 365
    nutritional considerations and, 599–600
    renal failure in, **606**
    respiratory distress syndrome in, **600–602**
    resuscitation of, **594–599**

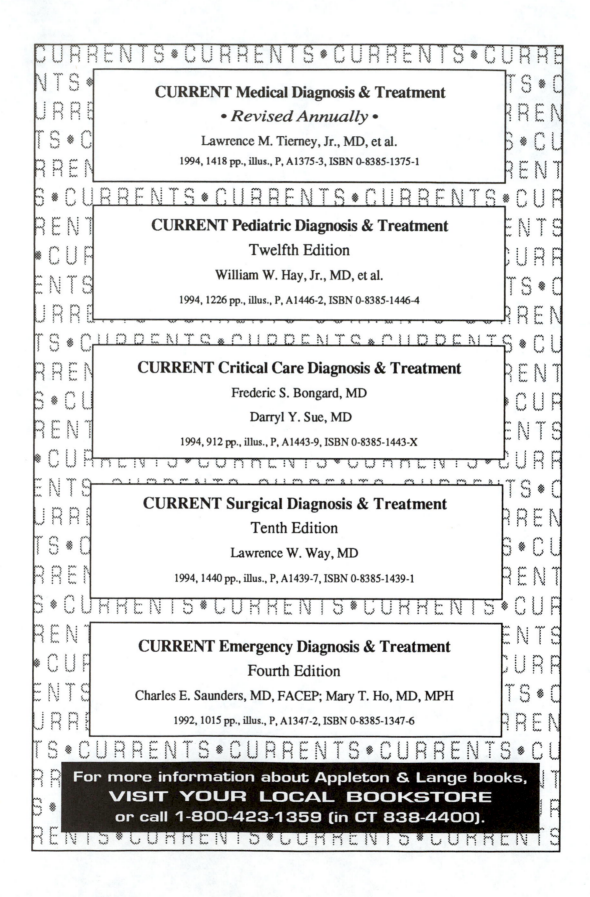

**CURRENT Medical Diagnosis & Treatment**

• *Revised Annually* •

Lawrence M. Tierney, Jr., MD, et al.

1994, 1418 pp., illus., P, A1375-3, ISBN 0-8385-1375-1

**CURRENT Pediatric Diagnosis & Treatment**

Twelfth Edition

William W. Hay, Jr., MD, et al.

1994, 1226 pp., illus., P, A1446-2, ISBN 0-8385-1446-4

**CURRENT Critical Care Diagnosis & Treatment**

Frederic S. Bongard, MD

Darryl Y. Sue, MD

1994, 912 pp., illus., P, A1443-9, ISBN 0-8385-1443-X

**CURRENT Surgical Diagnosis & Treatment**

Tenth Edition

Lawrence W. Way, MD

1994, 1440 pp., illus., P, A1439-7, ISBN 0-8385-1439-1

**CURRENT Emergency Diagnosis & Treatment**

Fourth Edition

Charles E. Saunders, MD, FACEP; Mary T. Ho, MD, MPH

1992, 1015 pp., illus., P, A1347-2, ISBN 0-8385-1347-6